MEDICAL CARE
OF
CANCER PATIENTS

MEDICAL CARE
OF
CANCER PATIENTS

Sai-Ching Jim Yeung, MD, PhD
Deputy Section Chief of Emergency Care
Associate Medical Director of Emergency Center (Ad Interim)
Associate Professor
Department of General Internal Medicine,
Ambulatory Treatment and Emergency Care
Department of Endocrine Neoplasia & Hormonal Disorders
The University of Texas
M. D. Anderson Cancer Center
Houston, Texas

Carmen P. Escalante, MD
Professor and Chair
Department of General Internal Medicine,
Ambulatory Treatment and Emergency Care
The University of Texas
M. D. Anderson Cancer Center
Houston, Texas

Robert F. Gagel, MD
Professor and Division Head
Division of Internal Medicine
The University of Texas
M. D. Anderson Cancer Center
Houston, Texas

2009

PEOPLE'S MEDICAL PUBLISHING HOUSE—USA
SHELTON, CONNECTICUT

People's Medical Publishing House—USA
2 Enterprise Drive, Suite 509
Shelton, CT 06484
Tel: 203-402-0646
Fax:203-402-0854
E-mail: info@pmph-usa.com

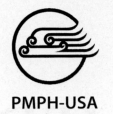

PMPH-USA

09 10 11 12 13 14 / PMPH / 9 8 7 6 5 4 3 2

ISBN 978-1-60795-008-0
Printed in China by People`s Medical Publishing House
Typesetter (1st Printing) : Charlesworth
Typesetter (2nd Printing) : diacriTech

Sales and Distribution

Canada
McGraw-Hill Ryerson Education
Customer Care
300 Water St.
Whitby, Ontario   L1N 9B6
Tel: 1-800-565-5758
Fax: 1-800-463-5885

Foreign Rights
John Scott & Company
International Publishers' Agency
P.O. Box 878
Kimberton, PA 19442
Tel: 610-827-1640
Fax: 610-827-1671
E-mail: jsco@voicenet.com

Japan
United Publishers Services Limited
1-32-5 Higashi-Shinagawa
Shinagawa-Ku, Tokyo 140-0002
Tel: 03 5479 7251
Fax: 03 5479 7307
Email: kakimoto@ups.co.jp

UK, Europe, Middle East, Africa
McGraw-Hill Education
Shoppenhangers Road, Maidenhead
Berkshire, England SL6 2QL
Tel: 44-0-1628-502500
Fax: 44-0-1628-635895
www.mcgraw-hill.co.uk

**Singapore, Thailand, Philippines,
Indonesia, Vietnam, Pacific Rim, Korea**
McGraw-Hill Education
60 Tuas Basin Link, Singapore 638775
Tel: 65-6863-1580
Fax: 65-6862-3354

Australia, New Zealand
Elsevier Australia, Tower 1, 475 Victoria Ave.
Chatswood NSW 2067, Australia
Tel: 0-9422-8553
Fax: 0-9422-8562
www.elsevier.com.au

Customer Service New Zealand
Phone (Free Phone): +64 (0) 800 449 312
Fax (Free Phone): +64 (0) 800 449 318
Email: cservice@mcgraw-hill.co.nz

Brazil
Tecmedd Importadora E Distribuidora De
Livros Ltda.
Avenida Maurílio Biagi, 2850
City Ribeirão, Ribeirão Preto – SP – Brasil
CEP: 14021-000
Tel: 0800 992236
Fax: (16) 3993-9000
E-mail: tecmedd@tecmedd.com.br

**India, Bangladesh, Pakistan, Sri Lanka,
Malaysia**
CBS Publishers
4819/X1 Prahlad Street 24, Ansari Road
Darya, New Delhi-11002, India
Tel: 91-11-23266861/67
Fax: 91-11-23266818
Email: cbspubs@vsnl.com

People's Republic of China
PMPH, Bldg 3, 3rd District, Fangqunyuan,
Fangzhuang, Beijing 100078, P..R. China,
Tel: 8610-676533423
Fax: 8610-67691034
www.pmph.com

SECTION EDITORS

W. Michael Alberts, MD, MBA
Vice President Medical Affairs
Chief Medical Officer
H. Lee Moffitt Cancer Center & Research Institute
Tampa, Florida

Frank C. Arnett, MD
Professor of Internal Medicine and Pathology and
Laboratory Medicine
Elizabeth Bidgood Chair in Rheumatology
Department of Internal Medicine
The University of Texas Medical School at Houston
Houston, Texas

Diane C. Bodurka, MD
Associate Professor
Department of Gynecologic Oncology
The University of Texas
  M. D. Anderson Cancer Center
Houston, Texas

Robert Bresalier, MD
Professor
Department of GI Medicine and Nutrition
The University of Texas
  M. D. Anderson Cancer Center
Houston, Texas

Charles Cleeland, PhD
Chair and Professor
Symptom Research CAO
The University of Texas
  M. D. Anderson Cancer Center
Houston, Texas

Kevin W. Finkel, MD
Professor
Division Director
Division of Renal Diseases and Hypertension
Department of Internal Medicine
The University of Texas Medical School at Houston
Houston, Texas

Ellen F. Manzullo, MD
Professor
Department of General Internal Medicine,
  Ambulatory Treatment and Emergency Care
The University of Texas
  M. D. Anderson Cancer Center
Houston, Texas

Issam I. Raad, MD
Chair and Professor
Department of Infectious Diseases,
Infection Control & Employee Health
The University of Texas
  M. D. Anderson Cancer Center
Houston, Texas

Ronald P. Rapini, MD
Chair and Professor
Department of Dermatology
The University of Texas
  M. D. Anderson Cancer Center
Houston, Texas

David Schiff, MD
Professor
Division of Neuro-Oncology
University of Virginia
Charlottesville, Virginia

Steven I. Sherman, MD
Chair and Professor
Department of General Internal Medicine,
  Ambulatory Treatment and Emergency Care
The University of Texas
  M. D. Anderson Cancer Center
Houston, Texas

Edward Yeh, MD
Chair and Professor
Department of Cardiology
The University of Texas
  M. D. Anderson Cancer Center
Houston, Texas

PREFACE

The last decade has seen a remarkable improvement in clinical outcomes for most patients with cancer. The development of targeted therapies, the direct result of the sweeping discoveries of the past two decades related to the causation of cancer, has revolutionized treatment of cancer. The sweeping events of the past two decades have resulted in the mapping and sequencing of the human genome, the identification of molecular causation for many types of cancer, and the use of this information to develop targeted therapy has initiated a change, not only in the outcomes associated with cancer, but also the modes and approaches of therapy.

These changes have induced several profound changes in the medical needs of cancer patients. The first is that a larger percentage of cancer patients are living for longer periods of time. Unlike previous generations of patients treated for cancer in which survival was often poor, these "survivors" live longer and are in many cases undergoing chronic therapy for cancer. The important point is that they are surviving. Along with survivorship go many of the co-morbidities associated with cancer or short- and long-term side-effects of therapy. For example, survival in patients with myeloma was very poor as short a time ago as five years. Advances over the past two to three years using combinations of proteasome inhibitors and thalidomide derivatives have created a significant population of myeloma patients who are well controlled while they are on chronic therapy. Along with the beneficial effects of these medications, however, are a constellation of side effects that include fatigue, thromboembolism, peripheral neuropathy, and bone and cardiac abnormalities.

The goal of this textbook is to focus on existing and newly emerging internal medicine problems associated with cancer or its treatments. These problems include not only those associated with older chemotherapeutic agents, but also newer classes of drugs such as monoclonal antibodies and signaling pathway-specific small molecules. This textbook will also address emerging management issues for comorbid conditions in cancer patients.

This text is a focused attempt to systematically categorize and describe the complex and rapidly evolving field of internal medicine in cancer survivors. Although the pace of new therapies for cancer treatment is moving so rapidly that any textbook is likely to be out of date at the time of publication, we believe that the contents will provide you with a different perspective and a framework to organize rapidly accumulating new information.

"To cure the curable and make life livable for the incurable!" 'Tis our motto.

CONTENTS

SECTION V: Endocrinologic and Metabolic Disorders

SECTION VI: Disorders of the Digestive Tract and Nutrition

SECTION VII: Disorders of the Respiratory Tract

SECTION VIII: Neurologic and Psychiatric Disorders

CONTRIBUTORS

Eddie K. Abdalla, MD
Assistant Professor
Department of Surgical Oncology
The University of Texas
  M. D. Anderson Cancer Center
Houston, Texas
Hepatobiliary and Pancreatic Disorders

Javier A. Adachi, MD
Assistant Professor
Department of Infectious Diseases,
Infection Control and Employee Health
The University of Texas
  M. D. Anderson Cancer Center
Houston, Texas
Parasitic Disease Issues in Cancer Patients

Asra Ali, MD
Associate Professor
Department of Dermatology
The University of Texas
  M. D. Anderson Cancer Center
Houston, Texas
Alopecia

Firas Alkassab, MD
Division of Rheumatology
The University of Texas Medical School at Houston
Houston, Texas
Rheumatologic Issues in Cancer Patients

Ricardo H. Alvarez, MD
Medical Oncology Fellow
Division of Cancer Medicine
Department of Medical Oncology
The University of Texas
  M. D. Anderson Cancer Center
Houston, Texas
Fever

Karen O. Anderson, PhD, MPH
Associate Professor
Symptom Research CAO
The University of Texas
  M. D. Anderson Cancer Center
Houston, Texas
Sleep Disorders in the Cancer Patient

Donald Armstrong, MD
Member Emeritus
Infectious Disease Service
Memorial Sloan-Kettering Cancer Center
New York, New York
Mycobacterial Infections in Patients with Cancer

Frank C. Arnett, MD
Professor of Internal Medicine and Pathology
and Laboratory Medicine
Elizabeth Bidgood Chair in Rheumatology
Department of Internal Medicine
The University of Texas Medical School at Houston
Houston, Texas
Rheumatologic Paraneoplastic Syndromes
Rheumatologic Issues in Cancer Patients

Donald M. Arnold, MD, MSc, FRCP(C)
Assistant Professor
Division of Hematology
Department of Medicine
McMaster University, New Investigator,
Canadian Institutes for Health Research
Hamilton, Ontario, Canada
Hematological Complications in Patients with Malignancy

Lodovico Balducci, MD
Professor
Division of Geriatric Oncology
Department of Oncology
University of South Florida
College of Medicine
Tampa, Florida
Geriatric Considerations in the Care of Cancer Patients

Shehzad Basaria, MD
Department of Medicine
Division of Endocrinology and Metabolism
Johns Hopkins University School of Medicine
Bayview Medical Center
Baltimore, MD
Hypogonadism and Hormone Replacement in Men with Cancers

Lora D. Baum, PhD
Assistant Professor of Clinical Psychiatric Medicine
Cancer Center
University of Virginia Health System
Charlottesville, Virginia
Psychiatric Issues in Oncology

Isabelle Bedrosian, MD
Assistant Professor
Department of Surgical Oncology
The University of Texas
  M. D. Anderson Cancer Center
Houston, Texas
Long-Term Consequences of Cancer Surgery

Claudia Beghe, MD
Associate Professor
Division of Geriatrics
Department of Medicine
University of South Florida
College of Medicine
Tampa, Florida
Geriatric Considerations in the Care of Cancer Patients

Kathleen Young Bellamy, MSW, LISW
Patient Care Resource Manager
Division of Head and Neck Oncology
Department of Patient Care Resource Management
Arthur Janes Cancer Hospital
Columbus, Ohio
Psychosocial Issues

Leslie J. Blackhall, MD, MTS
Associate Professor of Medicine
Division of Geriatric, General Medicine
  and Palliative Care
Department of Medicine
University of Virginia
School of Medicine
Charlottesville, Virginia
Neuropathic Pain

Diane C. Bodurka, MD
Associate Professor
Department of Gynecologic Oncology
The University of Texas
  M. D. Anderson Cancer Center
Houston, Texas
Obstetric and Gynecologic Issues
Reproductive Issues
Sexual Function Issues

Michael Boeckh, MD
Associate Professor of Medicine
Division of Allergy and Infectious
  Disease Center
University of Washington
Seattle, Washington
Viral Infections

H. Leon Bradlow, PhD
Senior Scientist
Alice and David Jurist Institute for Research
Hackensack University Medical Center
Hackensack, New Jersey
Obesity and Cancer

Daniel J. Brotman, MD
Director
Hospitalist Program
Associate Professor of Medicine
Johns Hopkins Hospital
Baltimore, Maryland
Prevention of Postoperative Venous Thromboembolism
  and Perioperative Management of Anticoagulation in
  the Cancer Patient

Naifa L. Busaidy, MD
Assistant Professor
Department of Endocrine Neoplasia and Hormonal Disorders
The University of Texas
  M. D. Anderson Cancer Center
Houston, Texas
Diabetes and the Cancer Patient

Maria E. Cabanillas, MD
Assistant Professor
Department of General Internal Medicine,
  Ambulatory Treatment and Emergency Care
The University of Texas
  M. D. Anderson Cancer Center
Houston, Texas
Fever

Jeffrey P. Callen, MD
Professor of Medicine (Dermatology)
Division of Dermatology
Department of Medicine
University of Louisville
School of Medicine
Louisville, Kentucky
Paraneoplastic Dermatoses

Barrie R. Cassileth, PhD, MS
Chief, Integrative Medicine Service
Laurance S. Rockefeller Chair in
  Internal Medicine
Memorial Sloan-Kettering Cancer Center
New York, New York
Integrative Medicine: Complementary and Alternative Therapies

Spero Cataland, MD
Clinical Assistant Professor
Division of Hematology
Ohio State University
Columbus, Ohio
Hematologic Issues

Robert Cavaliere, MD
Assistant Professor of Neurology
Division of Neuro-Oncology
Department of Neurology
The Ohio State University
Columbus, Ohio
Direct Complications of Cancer
Direct Neurologic Complications of Cancer

Mark S. Chambers, DMD, MS
Deputy Chief, Section of Oncologic
  Dentistry and Prosthodontics
Associate Professor
Head and Neck Surgery
Radiation Oncology
University of Texas
  M. D. Anderson Cancer Center
Houston, Texas
Oral and Orofacial Considerations in Oncology

J. Christopher Champion, MD
Assistant Professor
Department of Cardiology
The University of Texas
  M. D. Anderson Cancer Center
Houston, Texas
Congestive Heart Failure

Wassim Chemaitilly, MD
Children's Hospital of Pittsburgh
University of Pittsburgh
Pittsburgh, Pennsylvania
Disturbances of Growth and Pubertal
  Development in Childhood Cancer Survivors

Roy F. Chemaly, MD, MPH
Assistant Professor
Department of Infectious Diseases
The University of Texas
  M. D. Anderson Cancer Center
Houston, Texas
Viral Infections

Gregory A. Clines, MD, PhD
Assistant Professor of Internal Medicine
Department of Medicine
Division of Endocrinology & Metabolism
University of Virginia
Charlottesville, Virginia
Hypercalcemia of Malignancy

Gene L. Colice, MD
Professor of Medicine
Division of Pulmonary/Critical Care
Department of Medicine
The George Washington University
School of Medicine
Washington, District of Columbia
Noninfectious Pulmonary Problems in the Patient with Cancer

Sarah E. Cooper, BS
Division of Internal Medicine
The University of Texas
  M. D. Anderson Cancer Center
Mechanisms of Complications of Malignancy

Daniel R. Couriel, MD
Associate Professor
Department of Stem Cell Transplantation
  and Cellular Therapy
The University of Texas
  M. D. Anderson Cancer Center
Houston, Texas
Graft-versus-Host Skin Disease

Denise M. Damek, MD
Associate Professor of Neurology and Neurosurgery
Department of Neurology
University of Colorado at Denver
  Health Sciences Center
Aurora, Colorado
Neurologic Complications of Chemotherapy

Alexander A. Dekovich, MD
Associate Professor
Department of GI Medicine and Nutrition
The University of Texas
  M. D. Anderson Cancer Center
Houston, Texas
Gastroesophageal Issues

Gary E. Deng, MD, PhD
Assistant Professor
Integrative Medicine
Memorial Sloan-Kettering Cancer Center
New York, New York
Integrative Medicine: Complementary and Alternative Therapies

Adrian Dobs, MD, MHS
Professor
Division of Endocrinology & Metabolism
Johns Hopkins University
Baltimore, MD
Hypogonadism and Hormone Replacement in Men with Cancers

Herbert L. DuPont, MD
Professor and Vice-Chairman
Division of Infectious Diseases
Department of Medicine
Baylor College of Medicine
Houston, Texas
Parasitic Disease Issues in Cancer Patients

Carmen P. Escalante, MD
Professor and Chair
Department of General Internal Medicine,
  Ambulatory Treatment and Emergency Care
The University of Texas
  M. D. Anderson Cancer Center
Houston, Texas
Cancer-Related Fatigue
Survivorship—A Reversal of Fortune

Michael S. Ewer, MD, JD
Professor
Department of Cardiology
The University of Texas
  M. D. Anderson Cancer Center
Houston, Texas
The Pericardium in the Cancer Patient

Steven M. Ewer, MD
Cardiovascular Research Fellow
Division of Cardiology
Department of Internal Medicine
Washington University
St. Louis, Missouri
The Pericardium in the Cancer Patient

Kevin W. Finkel, MD
Professor
Division Director
Division of Renal Diseases and Hypertension
Department of Internal Medicine
The University of Texas Medical School at Houston
Houston, Texas
Renal Failure and Renal Tubular Defects

Anne L. Flamm, JD
Clinical Ethicist
Department of Clinical Ethics
The University of Texas
  M. D. Anderson Cancer Center
Houston, Texas
Ethical and Legal Issues in the Care of a Cancer Patient

John R. Foringer, MD
Assistant Professor
Division of Renal Diseases & Hypertension
Department of Internal Medicine
The University of Texas Medical School at Houston
Houston, Texas
Renal Failure and Renal Tubular Defects
Urologic Disorders

Graeme A. M. Fraser, MD, MSc, FRCPC
Clinical Scholar
Department of Medicine
McMaster University
Hamilton, Ontario, Canada
Hematologic Complications in Patients with Malignancy

Michael Frumovitz, MD, MPH
Assistant Professor
Department of Gynecologic Oncology
The University of Texas
  M. D. Anderson Cancer Center
Houston, Texas
Obstetric and Gynecologic Issues

Robert F. Gagel, MD
Professor
Division Head
Division of Internal Medicine
The University of Texas
  M. D. Anderson Cancer Center
Houston, Texas
Endocrine Paraneoplastic Syndromes
Pituitary and Adrenal Complications in Cancer Patients
Endocrine Neoplastic Syndromes
Introduction to the Care of the Cancer Patient
Mechanisms of Complications of Malignancy
Survivorship—A Reversal of Fortune

Adam S. Garden, MD
Professor
Radiation Oncology
Associate Clinical Medical Director for Head and Neck Cancer
The University of Texas
  M. D. Anderson Cancer Center
Houston, Texas
Oral and Orofacial Considerations in Oncology

Jane M. Geraci, MD, MPH
Staff Physician
Department of Internal Medicine
Providence St. Peter Hospital
Olympia, Washington
Diabetes and the Cancer Patient

Daniel N. Ginn, MPH
Medical Student
Georgia Campus
Philadelphia College of Osteopathic Medicine
Suwanee, Georgia
Pneumonia in Cancer Patients

Gregory W. Gladish, MD
Associate Professor
Department of Diagnostic Radiology
The University of Texas
  M. D. Anderson Cancer Center
Houston, Texas
Imaging

Dominick I. Golio, MD
Assistant Clinical Professor
Ophthalmology
Downstate Medical Center
State University of New York
Brooklyn, New York
Orbital Cellulitis

Dan S. Gombos, MD, FACS
Associate Professor
Department of Ophthalmology
The University of Texas
  M. D. Anderson Cancer Center
Houston, Texas
Orbital Cellulitis
Endogenous Endophthalmitis
Metastatic Disease to the Eye and Orbit

John N. Greene, MD, FACP
Professor
Division of Infectious Diseases
Department of Interdisciplinary Oncology
University of South Florida
College of Medicine
Tampa, Florida
Pneumonia in Cancer Patients

Theresa A. Guise, MD
University of Virginia
Fountaine Research Facility
Charlottesville, Virginia
Hypercalcemia of Malignancy

Ying Guo, MD
Associate Professor
Department of Palliative Care and
  Rehabilitation Medicine
The University of Texas
  M. D. Anderson Cancer Center
Houston, Texas
Cancer Rehabilitation

Sanjay Gupta, MD
Associate Professor
Department of Diagnostic Radiology
The University of Texas
  M. D. Anderson Cancer Center
Houston, Texas
Imaging

Melissa Hamilton, RD
Clinical Dietician
Department of Clinical Nutrition
The University of Texas
  M. D. Anderson Cancer Center
Houston, Texas
Diabetes and the Cancer Patient

Beverly C. Handy, MD, MS
Assistant Professor
Division of Pathology and Laboratory
  Medicine
Department of Laboratory Medicine
The University of Texas
  M. D. Anderson Cancer Center
Houston, Texas
Laboratory Investigation

Hend Hanna, MD, MPH
Assistant Professor
Department of Infectious Diseases,
  Infection Control & Employee Health
The University of Texas
  M. D. Anderson Cancer Center
Houston, Texas
Bacterial Infectious Disease Issues: Catheter-Related Infections

Mimi I. Hu, MD
Assistant Professor
Department of Endocrine Neoplasia & Hormonal
Disorders
The University of Texas
  M. D. Anderson Cancer Center
Houston, Texas
Endocrine Paraneoplastic Syndromes

Auris Huen, PharmD
Clinical Pharmacist
Department of Infectious Diseases,
Infection Control and Employee Health
The University of Texas
  M. D. Anderson Cancer Center
Houston, Texas
Systemic Sequelae of Bioimmunotherapy

Jessica P. Hwang, MD, MPH
Assistant Professor
Department of General Internal Medicine,
  Ambulatory Treatment and Emergency Care
The University of Texas
  M. D. Anderson Cancer Center
Houston, Texas
Mechanisms of Complications of Malignancy

Sharon R. Hymes, MD
Professor
Department of Dermatology
The University of Texas
  M. D. Anderson Cancer Center
Houston, Texas
Graft-versus-Host Skin Disease
Radiation Dermatitis

Amir K. Jaffer, MD
Director, IMPACT Center
Department of General Internal Medicine
The Cleveland Clinic Foundation
Solon, Ohio
Prevention of Postoperative Venous Thromboembolism and
  Perioperative Management of Anticoagulation in the
  Cancer Patient

Diana I. Jalal, MD
Assistant Professor
Division of Renal Disease and Hypertension
Department of Internal Medicine
The University of Texas Medical School at Houston
Houston, Texas
Urinary Tract Infections

Carolyn Jonas-Accardi, PhD
Emory University School of Medicine
Atlanta, Georgia
Cancer and Depression: Phenomenology and Pathophysiology

Kimberly Keene, MD
Assistant Professor
Department of Radiation Oncology
Office of the Chairman
Wallace Tumor Institute
University of Alabama
Birmingham AL
Neurologic Toxicity of Radiotherapy

Merrill S. Kies, MD
Professor
Department of Thoracic/Head & Neck Medical Oncology
The University of Texas
  M. D. Anderson Cancer Center
Houston, Texas
Oral and Orofacial Considerations in Oncology

Angela W. Kim, MD
Assistant Professor
Department of Ophthalmology
The University of Texas
  M. D. Anderson Cancer Center
Houston, Texas
Ocular Side Effects Associated with Chemotherapy
Vascular Events, Optic Neuropathies, Paraneoplastic
  Syndromes, and Visual Loss
Metastatic Disease to the Eye and Orbit

Dimitrios P. Kontoyiannis, MD, ScD, FACP
Professor
Department of Infectious Diseases,
  Infection Control & Employee Health
The University of Texas
  M. D. Anderson Cancer Center
Houston, Texas
Fungal Infections in Immunocompromised Hosts with Cancer

Benedict Konzen, MD
Assistant Professor
Department of Physical Medicine
  and Rehabilitation
The University of Texas
  M. D. Anderson Cancer Center
Houston, Texas
Cancer Rehabilitation

Bruce P. Krieger, MD, FCCP
Professor
Department of Pulmonary Medicine
Mount Sinai Medical Center
Miami Beach, Florida
Cancer-Related Issues in Mechanical Ventilation

Ashok J. Kumar, MD
Professor
Department of Diagnostic Radiology
The University of Texas
  M. D. Anderson Cancer Center
Houston, Texas
Imaging

Joy Kunishige, MD
Department of Dermatology
The University of Texas
  M. D. Anderson Cancer Center
Houston, Texas
Cutaneous Reactions to Medications

Laura A. Lambert, MD
Assistant Professor
Department of Surgical Oncology
The University of Texas
  M. D. Anderson Cancer Center
Houston, Texas
Long-Term Consequences of Cancer Surgery

Colleen G. Lance, MD
Assistant Professor
Department of General Internal Medicine,
  Ambulatory Treatment and Emergency Care
The University of Texas
  M. D. Anderson Cancer Center
Houston, Texas
Sleep Disorders in the Cancer Patient

James Larner, MD
Professor and Chair
Department of Radiation Oncology
University of Virginia
Charlottesville, Virginia
Neurologic Toxicity of Radiotherapy

Agnes Y. Y. Lee, MD, MSc, FRCP(C)
Associate Professor
Division of Hematology
Department of Medicine
McMaster University
Hamilton, Ontario, Canada
Hematologic Complications in Patients with Malignancy

Christine Lee, MD
Department of Medicine
Division of Endocrinology and Metabolism
Johns Hopkins University School of Medicine
Bayview Medical Center
Baltimore, MD
Hypogonadism and Hormone Replacement in Men with Cancers

Jeffrey H. Lee, MD
Associate Professor
Department of GI Medicine and Nutrition
The University of Texas
  M. D. Anderson Cancer Center
Houston, Texas
Interventional Gastroenterology

James C. Lemon, DDS
Professor
Department of Head and Neck Surgery
The University of Texas
  M. D. Anderson Cancer Center
Houston, Texas
Oral and Orofacial Considerations in Oncology

Daniel J. Lenihan, MD
Professor, Department of Cardiology
The University of Texas
  M. D. Anderson Cancer Center
Houston, Texas
Vascular Disease

Russell E. Lewis, PharmD
Assistant Professor
University of Houston
College of Pharmacy
Houston, Texas
Fungal Infections in Immunocompromised Hosts with Cancer

Robert H. Lustig, MD
Professor
Division of Endocrinology
Director of the Weight Assessment for
  Teen and Child Health (WATCH) Program
University of California at San Francisco
San Francisco, California
Obesity and Cancer

Megan C. MacNeil, MD
Division of Rheumatology
The University of Texas Medical School at Houston
Houston, Texas
Rheumatologic Paraneoplastic Syndromes

Dennis G. Maki, MD
Ovid O. Meyer Professor of Medicine
Head of the Section of Infectious Diseases
University of Wisconsin Medical School
Madison, Wisconsin
Bacterial Infectious Disease Issues: Catheter-Related Infections

Sean Malone, MD, FACP
Clinical Assistant Professor
Department of Internal Medicine
Wake Forest University
Baptist Medical Center
Winston-Salem, North Carolina
Perioperative Nutritional Issues
Preoperative Considerations in the Cancer Patient
  Undergoing Surgery

Jack W. Martin, DDS, MS
Section Chief of Oncologic Dentistry and Prosthodontics
Professor
Department of Head and Neck Surgery
The University of Texas
  M. D. Anderson Cancer Center
Houston, Texas
Oral and Orofacial Considerations in Oncology

Gabrielle Marzani-Nissen, MD
Assistant Professor
Department of Psychiatry and Neurobehavioral Sciences
University of Virginia
Charlottesville, Virginia
Psychiatric Issues in Oncology

Aurelio Matamoros, Jr., MD
Professor
Department of Diagnostic Radiology
The University of Texas
  M. D. Anderson Cancer Center
Houston, Texas
Imaging

Gaurav Mathur, MD
Medical Director
VITAS Innovative Hospice Care
Mt. Laurel, New Jersey,
Cancer Pain

Karen F. Mauck, MD, MSc
Assistant Professor
General Internal Medicine
Mayo Clinic
Rochester, Minnesota
Surgery in the Patient with Endocrine Disease

Steven R. Mays, MD
Associate Professor, Dermatology
Division of Internal Medicine
Department of Dermatology
The University of Texas
  M. D. Anderson Cancer Center
Houston, Texas
Cutaneous Reactions to Medications

Glenn A. McDonald, MD
Assistant Professor
Division of Renal Diseases and Hypertension
Department of Medicine
The University of Texas Medical School at Houston
  Houston, Texas
Urologic Disorders

Sanjay Mehta, MD
Department of Dermatology
The University of Texas
  M. D. Anderson Cancer Center
Houston, Texas
Alopecia

Andrew H. Miller, MD
William P. Timmie Professor of Psychiatry
  and Behavioral Sciences
Director of Psychiatric Oncology
Winship Cancer Institute
Emory University School of Medicine
Atlanta, Georgia
Cancer and Depression: Phenomenology and Pathophysiology

John T. Mullen, MD
Instructor
Surgery
Harvard Medical School
Boston, Massachusetts
Hepatobiliary and Pancreatic Disorders

Major Michael Murphy, MC, USA, MD
Department of Dermatology
The University of Texas Medical School at Houston
Houston, Texas
Skin Neoplasms Related to Internal Malignancy

William A. Murphy, Jr., MD
Professor and John S. Dunn, Sr.
  Distinguished Chair in Diagnostic Imaging
Department of Diagnostic Radiology
The University of Texas
  M. D. Anderson Cancer Center
Houston, Texas
Imaging

Bhamidipati V.R. Murthy, MD
Assistant Professor
Division of Renal Diseases and Hypertension
Department of Internal Medicine
The University of Texas Medical School at Houston
Houston, Texas
Urinary Tract Infections

Yakir Muszkat, MD
Division of Gastroenterology
Henry Ford Health Science Center
West Bloomfield, Michigan
Nutritional Issues in Cancer Patients

Tri H. Nguyen, M.D
Director of Mohs Micrographic
  and Dermatologic Surgery
Associate Professor
Department of Dermatology
The University of Texas
  M. D. Anderson Cancer Center
Houston, Texas
Skin Neoplasms Related to Internal Malignancy

Herbert B. Newton, MD
Professor of Neurology, Pediatrics
  and Oncology
Division of Neuro-Oncology
Ohio State University Medical Center
Columbus, Ohio
Perioperative Neurologic Issues

John T. Patlan, MD
Assistant Professor
Department of General Internal Medicine,
  Ambulatory Treatment & Emergency Care
The University of Texas
  M. D. Anderson Cancer Center
Houston, Texas
Nausea

Rebecca D. Pentz, PhD
Winship Cancer Institute
Emory University
Atlanta, Georgia
Ethical and Legal Issues in the Care of a Cancer Patient

Raphael E. Pollock, MD, PhD
Professor and Division Head
Division of Surgery
Department of Surgical Oncology
The University of Texas
  M. D. Anderson Cancer Center
Houston, Texas
Long-Term Consequences of Cancer Surgery

Russell K. Portenoy, MD
Chairman
Pain Medicine & Palliative Care
Beth Israel Medical Center
New York, New York
Cancer Pain

Issam I. Raad, MD
Chair and Professor
Department of Infectious Diseases,
  Infection Control & Employee Health
The University of Texas
  M. D. Anderson Cancer Center
Houston, Texas
Bacterial Infectious Disease Issues: Catheter-Related Infections

Atiar M. Rahman, MD, PhD
Associate Professor
Department of Cardiology
The University of Texas
  M. D. Anderson Cancer Center
Houston, Texas
Ischemic Heart Disease in Cancer Patients
Vascular Disease

Charles L. Raison, MD
Professor of Psychiatry
Emory University School of Medicine
Atlanta, Georgia
Cancer and Depression: Phenomenology and Pathophysiology

Kenneth V. I. Rolston, MD
Professor
Department of Infectious Diseases
The University of Texas
  M. D. Anderson Cancer Center
Houston, Texas
Risk Assessment and the Management of Neutropenia and Fever

William A. Ross, MD, MBA
Associate Professor
Department of GI Medicine and Nutrition
The University of Texas
  M. D. Anderson Cancer Center
Houston, Texas
Graft-versus-Host Disease and the Immunologic Complications
 of Cancer Interventional Gastroenterology

Margaret B. Row, MD, MBA
Associate Vice President
Global Clinical Programs
Associate Professor
Department of General Internal Medicine,
  Ambulatory Treatment & Emergency Care
The University of Texas
  M. D. Anderson Cancer Center
Houston, Texas
Emergency Care: Special Considerations in Cancer Patients

Jeffrey Rubins, MD
Minneapolis VA Medical Centers
Pulmonary Section
Minneapolis, Minnesota
Noninfectious Pulmonary Problems in the Patient with Cancer

Mark Rumbak, MD, FCCP
H. Lee Moffitt Cancer Center
James A. Haley Veterans Administration
Tampa, Florida
Cancer-Related Issues in Mechanical Ventilation

Amar Safdar, MD
Associate Professor
Department of Infectious Diseases,
  Infection Control & Employee Health
The University of Texas
  M. D. Anderson Cancer Center
Houston, Texas
Mycobacterial Infections in Patients with Cancer

David Schiff, MD
Professor
Division of Neuro-Oncology
University of Virginia
Charlottesville, Virginia
Direct Neurologic Complications of Cancer

Kathleen M. Schmeler, MD
Assistant Professor
Department of Gynecologic Oncology
The University of Texas
  M. D. Anderson Cancer Center
Houston, Texas
Reproductive Issues
Sexual Function Issues

Christoph Schmidt-Hieber, MD
Post-Doctoral Fellow
Institute of Physiology
University of Freiburg
Freiburg, Germany
Pneumonia in Cancer Patients

Pamela N. Schultz, PhD, RN
Department of Endocrine Neoplasia
& Hormonal Disorders
The University of Texas
  M. D. Anderson Cancer Center
Houston, Texas
Life After Cancer

Valerie Seabaugh, MD
Assistant Professor
Anesthesiology
School of Medicine
Loma Linda University
Loma Linda, California
*Perioperative Cardiopulmonary Complications
  and Consideration in the Cancer Patient*

Shirin Shafazand, MD, MS
Assistant Professor of Medicine
Assistant Director, Transplant Clinic
University of Miami
Miami, Florida
Noninfectious Pulmonary Problems in the Patient with Cancer

Pankaj Shah, MD
Division of Endocrinology Metabolism Diabetes and Nutrition
Mayo Clinic
Rochester, Minnesota
Diabetes and the Cancer Patient

Steven I. Sherman, MD
Chair and Professor
Department of Endocrine Neoplasia
& Hormonal Disorders
The University of Texas
  M. D. Anderson Cancer Center
Houston, Texas
Thyroid Disorders in Cancer Patients

Ki Y. Shin, MD
Assistant Professor
Department of Rehabilitation Medicine
The University of Texas
  M. D. Anderson Cancer Center
Houston, Texas
Cancer Rehabilitation

Michael J. Simoff, MD
Assistant Professor of Medicine
Department of Internal Medicine
Wayne State University
Detroit, Michigan
*Bronchoscopy and Lung Cancer:
  Diagnostic and Therapeutic Modalities*

Charles Sklar, MD
Director
Long-term Follow-Up Program
Memorial Sloan-Kettering Cancer Center
New York, New York
*Disturbances of Growth and Pubertal
  Development in Childhood Cancer Survivors*

Brian M. Slomovitz, MD
Assistant Professor
Division of Gynecologic Oncology
Department of Obstetrics & Gynecology
Weill Cornell Medical College
New York, New York
Obstetric and Gynecologic Issues

Martin L. Smith, STD
Associate Professor
Department of Critical Care
The University of Texas
  M. D. Anderson Cancer Center
Houston, Texas
Ethical and Legal Issues in the Care of a Cancer Patient

Pamela T. Soliman, MD
Assistant Professor
Department of Gynecologic Oncology
The University of Texas
  M. D. Anderson Cancer Center
Houston, Texas
Reproductive Issues
Sexual Function Issues

David J. Stewart, MD
Professor
Department of Thoracic/Head & Neck Medicine Oncology
The University of Texas
  M. D. Anderson Cancer Center
Houston, Texas
Collateral Damage Associated with Chemotherapy

John R. Stroehlein, MD
Chair (Ad interim) and Professor
Department of GI Medicine and Nutrition
The University of Texas
  M. D. Anderson Cancer Center
Houston, Texas
Disorders of the Digestive Tract and Nutrition: Intestinal Issues

Eric A. Strom, MD
Professor
Department of Radiation Oncology
The University of Texas
  M. D. Anderson Cancer Center
Houston, Texas
Radiation Dermatitis

Joseph Swafford, MD, FACC
Deputy Division Head
Division of Internal Medicine
Professor
Department of Cardiology
The University of Texas
  M. D. Anderson Cancer Center
Houston, Texas
Cardiac Manifestations of Malignancy

Bruce H. Thiers, MD
Professor and Chair
Department of Dermatology
Medical University of South Carolina
Charleston, South Carolina
Paraneoplastic Dermatoses

Diane S. Thompson, MD
Department of Psychiatry
Winship Cancer Institute
Emory University School of Medicine
Atlanta, Georgia
Cancer and Depression: Phenomenology and Pathophysiology

Harrys A. Torres, MD
Medical Oncology Fellow
Division of Cancer Medicine
Department of Medical Oncology
The University of Texas
  M. D. Anderson Cancer Center
Houston, Texas
Viral Infections

Anne S. Tsao, MD
Assistant Professor
Department of Thoracic/Head and Neck
  Medical Oncology
The University of Texas
  M. D. Anderson Cancer Center
Houston, Texas
Collateral Damage Associated with Chemotherapy

Saroj Vadhan-Raj, MD
Professor
Department of Bioimmunotherapy
The University of Texas
  M. D. Anderson Cancer Center
Houston, Texas
Systemic Sequelae of Bioimmunotherapy

Rena Vassilopoulou-Sellin, MD
Medical Director
Life After Cancer Care program
Clinical Professor
Department of Endocrine Neoplasia & Hormonal Disorders
The University of Texas
  M. D. Anderson Cancer Center
Houston, Texas
Life After Cancer

Steven Vernino, MD, PhD
Associate Professor
Department of Neurology
The University of Texas
  Southwestern Medical Center
Dallas, Texas
Paraneoplastic Neurologic Disorders

T. J. Walsh, MD
Immunocompromised Host Section
Pediatric Oncology Branch
National Cancer Institute
Bethesda, Maryland
Fungal Infections in Immunocompromised Hosts with Cancer

Xin Shelley Wang, MD, MPH
Associate Professor
Symptom Research CAO
The University of Texas
  M. D. Anderson Cancer Center
Houston, Texas
Cancer-Related Fatigue

Randal S. Weber, MD
Chairman
Department of Head and Neck Surgery
Hubert L. and Olive Stringer Distinguished
  Professor in Cancer Research
The University of Texas
  M. D. Anderson Cancer Center
Houston, Texas
Oral and Orofacial Considerations in Oncology

Harrison G. Weed, MD, MS, FACP
Professor
Department of Internal Medicine
Ohio State University
College of Medicine
Columbus, Ohio
Perioperative Neurologic Issues
Perioperative Nutritional Issues
Preoperative Considerations in the Cancer
  Patient Undergoing Surgery
Psychosocial Issues

Mary Ann Weiser, MD, PhD
Professor
Department of General Internal Medicine
  Ambulatory Treatment & Emergency Care
The University of Texas
  M. D. Anderson Cancer Center
Houston, Texas
Diabetes and the Cancer Patient

Gail A. Welsh, MD
Assistant Professor
General Internal Medicine
Mayo Clinic
Rochester, Minnesota
Surgery in the Patient with Endocrine Disease

Franklin C. Wong, MD, PhD, JD
Professor
Department of Nuclear Medicine
The University of Texas
  M. D. Anderson Cancer Center
Houston, Texas
Imaging

Rajesh Yadav, MD
Assistant Professor
Section of Physical Medicine and Rehabilitation
The University of Texas
  M. D. Anderson Cancer Center
Houston, Texas
Cancer Rehabilitation

Sai-Ching Jim Yeung, MD, PhD, FACP
Associate Medical Director of Emergency Center (Ad Interim)
Deputy Section Chief of Emergency Care
Associate Professor
Department of General Internal Medicine,
  Ambulatory Treatment and Emergency Care
Department of Endocrine Neoplasia & Hormonal Disorders
The University of Texas
  M. D. Anderson Cancer Center
Houston, Texas
Cancer Screening in Cancer Survivors
Endocrine Paraneoplastic Syndromes
Endocrine Neoplastic Syndromes
Emergency Care: Special Considerations in Cancer Patients
Pituitary and Adrenal Complications in Cancer Patients
Survivorship—A Reversal of Fortune

Rex C. Yung, MD, FCCP
Assistant Professor
Department of Pulmonary Medicine
Johns Hopkins University
East Baltimore Campus
Baltimore, Maryland
Upper Airway Problems

S. Wamique Yusuf, MD, FACC
Assistant Professor
Department of Cardiology
The University of Texas
  M. D. Anderson Cancer Center
Houston, Texas
Cardiac Manifestations of Malignancy
Treatment-Induced Arrhythmia, Pacemakers, and Automatic
  Implantable Cardioverter Defibrillators

Introduction to the Care of the Cancer Patient

Robert F. Gagel, MD

The beginnings of medical oncology in the middle of the twentith century pitted the enterprising and aggressive young internist, the newly minted "oncologist," against cancer, a terrifying disease. Other than those tumors that could be treated effectively with surgery or radiotherapy, there were few tools in the oncologist's armamentarium to treat malignancy. The advent and rise of cytotoxic chemotherapy during the first 25 years following the Second World War resulted in a number of therapeutic successes. These included the development of successful treatment protocols for testicular cancer, Hodgkin's lymphoma, and several other tumors. The next 20 to 25 years were characterized by the introduction of several new agents but, more importantly, by the combining of several chemotherapeutic agents and other forms of therapy. Notable among the successes were the impact of adjuvant chemotherapy in the management of breast cancer, the use of multiple chemotherapeutic agents in acute lymphoblastic leukemia, and the combined use of chemotherapy and surgery in sarcoma.

The past 10 to 15 years have been defined by molecular biology and genomics. The identification of oncogenes and tumor suppressor genes, and the insight gained from the deciphering of the genome and characterizations of signal transduction pathways important for regulation of cell growth have led to targeted therapies. Most newly developed therapeutic agents target specific signal transduction pathways. These therapies include small organic molecules, monoclonal antibodies, genetic treatments, vaccines, and other compounds. The first high-impact success of this period has been the development of imatinib, a specific tyrosine kinase inhibitor, as a highly effective oral therapy for chronic myelogenous leukemia and gastrointestinal stromal tumors. The success of these agents has led to a proliferation of activity by the biotechnology and pharmaceutical industries, leading to additional improvement in therapies for a number of malignancies and the prospect of more to come.

This recent frenetic activity occurs on a background of already improving outcomes for a wide range of malignancies. In a broad spectrum of malignancies, there has been a significant improvement in survival over the past 30 years (Figure 1). Even more remarkably, much of the improvement, particularly during the period covered in this table, occurred during a time when relatively few new therapeutic agents were approved for use. Although the reasons for this improvement are unclear, the application of combined chemotherapy and new surgical and radiotherapy approaches are the most likely explanations.

The current pace of therapeutic discovery superimposed on the steady improvement in outcomes observed over an extended period of time, creates on expectation that this trend will continue over the next several decades. The result may be that cancer is turned into a chronic disease akin to many others, such as diabetes mellitus, immunologic disease, kidney disease, or coronary artery disease. In each of these examples, affected individuals live with chronic disease that is controlled for years or decades, often dying from other causes.

The evolving paradigm of cancer as a chronic disease is filled with both hope and a growing sense among survivors that the long-term price, both financially and the loss of quality of life, of cancer cure or control is substantial. For many patients, this is a rollercoaster ride with terrifying periods when the cancer is diagnosed and treated, and extended periods of relief when the disease is arrested or its growth rate slowed. Unfortunately, for many, the control of the cancer is associated with a variety of medical problems caused by the malignancy, its therapy, or the stress associated with the treatment process.

The success of oncology has spawned a new discipline of internal medicine, separable from

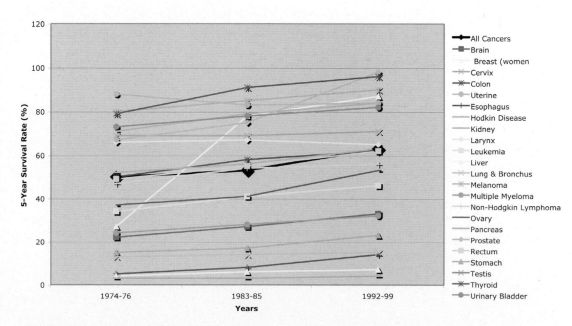

FIGURE 1 Trends in 5-year relative survival rates by year of diagnosis, 1974–1999. The figures shows survival rates during the 1974–1976, 1983–1985, and 1992–1999 periods for many different malignancies. The *thick black line* shows the improvement in 5-year survival for patients with cancer over this 25-year period. Adapted from Cancer facts and figures 2004. Atlanta (GA): American Cancer Society; 2004.

oncology, and focused on the management of the multitude of problems, acute and chronic, experienced by patients treated for cancer. Some of these problems are caused by the underlying malignancy; others result directly from the therapy; and still others evolve over years and decades caused by some combination of the natural aging process, other disease states, and long-term toxicity of the cancer treatment. Although most of these patients are joyous in their victory over a dreaded disease, they are uniformly disappointed that they have traded one problem for others they had not anticipated. I vividly recall a patient who approached me following a patient education lecture on bone loss following breast cancer who thrust a book of poetry into my hands. The book, *Reflections on Facing Cancer Fear & Loneliness*, by Lois Tschetter Hjelmstad, describes the cancer experience from a patient's perspective.[1] She opened the book she had authored to show me the following poem:

> The test show
> I have osteoporosis
> The doctor seems surprised
> I am dismayed.
> I feel betrayed again-
> Alienated from my body-
>
> I was counting on
> My bones to hold me up
> The rest of my life

This example illustrates the anxiety felt by many and, more importantly, the uncertainty about where patients should turn to obtain help for a variety of unanticipated problems — fatigue, sleep disorders, depression, and the more specific organ-related effects of cancer or its treatment. This confusion has only worsened in recent years as new treatment protocols have proliferated. Inevitably, each of the new therapies targets a pathway important not only for the growth of cancer but also compromises a variety of normal physiologic functions.

When patients are discharged from oncology care, they have a difficult time identifying physicians comfortable with management of disorders that occur in the context of the cancer patient. Their reintegration into the community is often challenging. Oncology patients who have been successfully treated feel, at times, like Sisyphus, the king of Corinth, who was condemned in Hades to roll a huge stone up a hill only to have it roll back down when it neared the top, necessitating that it be pushed back up again. Having defeated their malignancy, they are dismayed having to confront a new set of problems. The frustration experienced by these patients is palpable, and their increasing numbers have, in turn, spawned the development of patient advocacy programs focused on survivorship.

The good news is that the growth in this patient population has stimulated major cancer centers to develop broad-based expertise focused on these problems. There is an increasing emphasis, not only on the therapeutic benefit of a particular oncologic agent, but also its impact on quality of life. Physicians who are not oncologists routinely work alongside oncologic investigators to assess the broader impact of therapies and to develop management strategies. Specific examples include bone loss and fractures associated with aromatase inhibitors, hypertension and bleeding disorders associated with certain tyrosine kinase inhibitors, the cardiac effects of certain monoclonal antibodies, and many others.

The goal of this textbook is to begin to identify, organize, and catalog the broad spectrum of nononcologic problems experienced by oncology patients. We see this textbook as a companion to the standard internal medicine and oncology textbooks, whose content will inevitably overlap each of these subject areas. We also recognize that as the number and complexity of therapies for cancer have increased, oncology texts have systematically shortened the discussion of the long-term side effects of therapy and other medical problems associated with cancer. We seek to fill this void.

Please join us in this inaugural edition. If you are convinced of its value and place it on your bookshelf adjacent to standard internal medicine and oncology texts, pulling it down periodically to address specific medical problems, then we will have been successful.

REFERENCE

1. Tschetter Hjelmstad L. Reflections on facing cancer fear & loneliness. Mulberry Hill Press; 1992.

2

Mechanisms of Complications of Malignancy

Jessica P. Hwang, MD, MPH

Sarah E. Cooper, BS

Robert F. Gagel, MD

What differentiates internal medicine from most other subspecialties is its focus on deciphering complex symptoms to identify and treat the underlying disease processes. In no other disease state is the internist challenged as in the management of patients with cancer. Cancer is a protean disorder in which broad and confusing symptom complexes occur with some regularity. The challenge for the internist is to sort through these symptom complexes to identify those caused by the underlying malignancy or its therapy or associated with another disorder unrelated to the malignant process. The steady improvement in cancer outcomes over the past several decades heightens the need for sharpening this skill set. Two to three decades ago, most common malignancies evolved over a period of weeks, to months, to years, making palliative care and comfort measures most important. The steady improvement in outcomes for most malignancies has changed the evolution of cancer to years, to decades, to a lifetime. In other words, most cancer patients will live with their disease for prolonged periods of time and develop the broad spectrum of health problems seen in the noncancer population. This improvement in cancer outcomes has occurred so rapidly that most general internists and family practice physicians who manage the bulk of these patients long term have insufficient experience with the management of patients in this new paradigm. Under the new paradigm of cancer care, patients may continue therapy indefinitely. The prolongation of therapy for cancer, particularly in older individuals, in whom most cancer develops, leads to a situation in which the cancer patient is likely to develop a host of other medical problems. Those of us who work in cancer centers have struggled with the appropriate management of such patients. Should the oncologist, the person most knowledgeable about the malignancy, direct general internal medicine care for these patients? Although this is logical and makes sense, the sheer

volume of patients who live with cancer has made this impractical. In most large cancer centers, departments of internal medicine have developed to provide general and subspecialty internal medicine to patients.

This chapter is an introduction to a thought process and knowledge base that, it is hoped, will enable the reader to sort through the complaints of a patient with cancer and identify clinical complexes that are unique and separable from those seen in patients without cancer. In subsequent chapters, other authors expand on each of the subspecialty areas of internal medicine with the goal of identifying medical problems in cancer patients as separable from more general medical problems.

It is important for the clinician to reject the concept that symptoms in patients with cancer (eg, weakness, fatigue, weight loss) are indecipherable. Patients with specific types of cancers and treatments develop reproducible clinical syndromes that can be understood and, in many cases, treated. Patients with cancer are also subject to the broad variety of age-related diseases seen in the general population, many of which cause symptoms that can be confused with cancer-related disorders. This text is not meant to replace the excellent general internal medicine or oncology texts but rather to fill a gap that exists between the more active treatment role of the oncologist and the broad perspective of the general or subspecialty internist or family practitioner.

In this chapter, we introduce a conceptual framework for thinking about the interplay between cancer and the broad spectrum of disorders that fall under the rubric of internal medicine. The themes that are discussed are not new: they can be outlined under several straightforward headings (Table 1). What is new is the proliferation of information about these disorders and therapeutic options that makes it worthwhile for the clinician to better understand these

mechanisms and to differentiate them from the more common mechanisms of disease in patients without cancer.

We seek to provide examples that will highlight specific mechanisms and focus on what is known rather than what is not, anticipating that we should encourage clinicians to think analytically and positively about impacting the care of a particular patient. Most importantly, it is important to complement the efforts of the oncology community, which is appropriately focused on development and application of therapies to positively impact the outcomes in patients with cancer. There is value for the patient in this complementary approach.

How does the thought process of an internist in the oncology environment differ from that of the oncologist? The most important distinction is that the oncologist is focused primarily on the therapy and management of the malignancy, whereas the internist thinks more broadly about the spectrum of disorders that might explain the symptom complex in a particular patient. Most

Table 1 Mechanisms of Disease in Patients with Cancer

Local effects
   Compression
   Obstruction
   Infiltration
Systemic effects
   Hormonal
   Nutrition
   Immunologic
   Idiopathic
Treatment-related effects
   Cytotoxic chemotherapy
   Bystander effects caused by death of tumor cells
   Unintended effects of targeting specific signal transduction pathways
   Toxic effects of radiation therapy

oncologists are far more knowledgeable about the specific patterns of cancer behavior; on the other hand, nononcology internists who work in the cancer environment are focused on the broader spectrum of medical problems. Although these two thought processes intersect at many points, there are also substantial differences.

Fundamental Characteristics of Cancer

In the accompanying text in this series, *Cancer Medicine*, the senior editor, James Holland, defines the cardinal manifestations of cancer.[1] One of the primary concepts he develops is the failure of cancer cells to adhere to normal biologic principles of cellular physiology. This manifests in a number of different ways: cancer cells do not die at appropriate times, they do not conform to the normal spatial constraints of organs, and they have developed mechanisms to grow in tissues in which one would not normally expect to find them. Transformed cells also activate transcriptional pathways that are normally silenced, resulting in aberrant production of a broad spectrum of tumor products, some of which have biologic effects. These observations form the beginning of our discussion of how cancer interfaces with the broader discipline of internal medicine.

Mechanisms of Organ Dysfunction in Cancer

To grasp the spectrum of clinical presentations that may impact oncology care, it is important to describe the multiple ways in which malignant tumors can impact normal physiology. Table 1 provides an overview of major mechanisms. Of equal importance is to consider that the symptom complex may have nothing to do with cancer. Perhaps this characteristic—the ability to blend knowledge of oncology clinical syndromes with a broad, in-depth knowledge of internal medicine—defines the nononcology internal medicine specialist.

To outline the broad spectrum of potential causes for a particular problem, it may be helpful to describe a common problem in an oncology center: a patient with lung cancer who presents with a grand mal seizure and confusion that extends beyond the postictal period. This hypothetical patient is being treated with a tyrosine kinase inhibitor that targets several tyrosine kinase receptors (vascular endothelial growth factor, epidermal growth factor, and fibroblast growth factor receptors). In the evaluation of such a patient, a broad spectrum of causes needs to be considered. It is important to recognize that neurologic problems are one of the most common reasons that cancer patients are admitted to the hospital.[2,3] These include spinal cord compression, brain metastases, brachial and lumbosacral plexopathies, and leptomeningeal metastases. Although brain metastases are the most common neurologic complication in the general cancer population,[4] the incidence of these complications also depends on the primary cancer.

Given the frequency of brain and spinal metastasis in lung cancer, it would be appropriate to examine the patient for a mass effect or to consider the possibility of leptomeningeal metastasis of the lung cancer. It would also be important to consider other potential causes, which would include metabolic (hypo- or hyperglycemia, hyponatremia,[5] hypercalcemia, or severe hypothyroidism), a paraneoplastic syndrome, drug-induced (hemorrhagic effect at a site of tumor metastasis of a tyrosine kinase inhibitor that targets the vascular endothelial growth factor receptor), an infectious cause, or the broad spectrum of neurologic disorders (cerebrovascular, hemorrhagic, demyelinating) that might contribute to or cause the presenting complaint. In this particular case, the patient had no evidence of brain metastasis or hemorrhage but was found to have hyponatremia caused by excessive production of vasopressin by the malignancy. Correction of the hyponatremia quickly reversed the neurologic abnormalities. This example highlights the importance of a broad perspective. The sections that follow amplify the basic outline in Table 1.

Compression, Obstruction, and Infiltration

Airway Obstruction

One particularly important example is airway compression, obstruction, or infiltration. Common symptoms of airway involvement and obstruction include dyspnea, wheezing, stridor, and cough. Hemoptysis, recurrent respiratory infections, atelectasis, and hoarseness may also be associated with this complication. Obstruction of the airway can occur through several mechanisms, such as invasion through or compression of the airway by an adjacent tumor, direct invasion of the larynx, and bilateral vocal cord paralysis.[6,7] Invasion from a primary adjacent tumor, usually of the lung, is the most common cause of airway obstruction. This complication is also found frequently in esophageal, thyroid, and mediastinal malignancies.[6] Tumors involving the trachea or carina may be asymptomatic until the airway narrowing has become life threatening, whereas obstruction involving the bronchi is typically not immediately life threatening.[6] Airway obstruction can also be caused by tumor invasion through the bilateral vocal cords causing subsequent paralysis. Lung cancer is the most common cancer associated with bilateral vocal cord paralysis.[8] In this condition, the flaccid vocal cords are drawn inward during inspiration, obstructing the upper airway. A vocal cord lesion may precede, succeed, or be concurrent with the tracheal occlusion. Bilateral vocal cord paralysis can occur concurrently with malignant tracheal stenosis and a respiratory-digestive fistula.[9]

Hemoptysis with life-threatening bleeding into the airway is a particularly difficult management problem. This is particularly evident in pulmonary metastasis associated with renal cell carcinoma in which there is a tendency for even small tumors to bleed. In the past, little could be done in this clinical situation, but the rapid evolution of interventional bronchoscopy, using laser techniques to cauterize a hemorrhagic tumor, has positively impacted outcomes.[10] Similarly, these same techniques have made it possible to clear obstructing tracheal or bronchial lesions or to place a stent that bypasses the obstructive process.

In this situation, it is also important to recognize that obstruction can mimic other disorders of the respiratory system, including pneumonia, tuberculosis or fungal infection, lung abscess, asthma, or chronic obstructive pulmonary disease. Indeed, postobstructive pneumonia or abscess is a common occurrence,[11–13] further clouding the differential diagnosis.

Blood Vessel Obstruction

Obstruction can also affect other structures in the chest. A relatively well-documented complication associated with solid tumors is superior vena cava syndrome (SVCS). This syndrome often progresses slowly, although cases with acute onset have been reported. Dyspnea and swelling of the face, torso, and upper extremities are the most common symptoms. Patients may also experience chest pain, cough, dysphagia, venous distention, and, rarely, vocal cord paralysis. Headache and seizures, Horner's syndrome, changes in consciousness, and cyanosis have also been reported. If left untreated, obstruction of the superior vena cava may progress to tracheal obstruction, cerebral herniation, and even death.

The superior vena cava is particularly susceptible to occlusion owing to tumor compression, invasion, or thrombus formation because of its low pressure and thin vein wall. Its close proximity to several organs also makes it vulnerable to tumor-related complications.[34] Lung cancer is most commonly associated with SVCS,[14–16] causing 75 to 85% of cases, whereas lymphomas account for 10 to 15%.[14] Metastatic cancers, especially breast cancer, account for the rest of the cases of SVCS of neoplastic origin.[14,15] Three to 5% of lung cancer patients develop SVCS, with the small cell variant being the most common type.[15,16]

Neoplasms can also cause injury and stasis in other vessel walls, leading to deep venous thrombosis and pulmonary embolism.[15] Along with vessel wall stasis caused by the infiltration of cancer cells, activation of thrombotic mechanisms adds to the increased risk of clot formation.

Gastrointestinal Compression, Obstruction, or Infiltration

Assessing gastrointestinal symptoms is among the more challenging tasks facing a clinician in the context of cancer. Not only does a broad spectrum of therapeutic agents for cancer cause gastrointestinal symptoms that mimic intestinal obstruction such as abdominal distention and vomiting, but metabolic disorders may also cause ileus and other gastrointestinal symptoms. Indeed, there are no clinical signs or symptoms that differentiate malignant from benign causes, but establishing the correct etiology is important to determine treatment. Like airway obstruction, intestinal obstruction can be caused by either extrinsic pressure or tumor invasion, but, surprisingly, 26 to 38% of intestinal obstructions in patients with a cancer history are not due to recurrent or metastatic disease.[17] This is somewhat less true for ovarian cancer patients, who are more likely to have cancer as the cause of their obstruction than the general cancer population.[18] The cancers most commonly associated with obstruction are local abdominal cancers such as colorectal, ovarian, and gastric cancers.[4,17] Tumors from outside the abdomen associated with this complication include breast cancer, melanoma, and soft tissue sarcoma. Approximately a quarter to as many as half of patients with ovarian cancer will develop intestinal obstruction,[4,17] usually from extrinsic compression rather than intraluminal tumor invasion.[19] In addition to mechanical intestinal obstruction, motility problems may occur from the invasion of the tumor to the leaves of the mesenteries.[18] Gastric outlet obstruction, although uncommon, is frequently caused by malignancy. In one series, 61% of patients presenting with this disorder were found to have a causative malignancy.[20]

Signs and symptoms vary with the site of obstruction. Pain is the most common symptom, usually at the site of obstruction, whereas vomiting is generally common only with high small bowel obstruction. Abdominal distention is the most pronounced in patients with large bowel obstruction. Dehydration and electrolyte and acid-base imbalances are most likely to be a severe problem in patients with a low small bowel obstruction.[4]

As with other organ systems, it is important to consider noncancer causes of obstruction. Infection or abscess in immunosuppressed patients, adhesions from previous surgical procedures, and abscesses resulting from perforation, volvulus, or obstruction to normal blood flow in the intestine should be considered as well.

Hepatic or Biliary Infiltration or Obstruction

The liver is the second most common metastatic site for cancer, after regional lymph nodes. Forty to 50% of patients with solid tumors develop hepatic metastasis in the course of their disease.[21] Neoplasms that most commonly metastasize to the liver are those of the gastrointestinal tract, followed by tumors of the lung, breast, and skin.[21] Many other tumors, such as renal cell carcinoma, metastasize to the liver as well. A serious complication of these metastases is liver failure. In some cases, liver metastases occur and cause liver failure rapidly after the initial primary cancer diagnosis. Diffuse liver metastases can cause liver failure without producing identifiable lesions in the liver,[22] and, occasionally, there is selective interference with a particular aspect of hepatic function, such as gluconeogenesis (causing fasting hypoglycemia) or production of important clotting factors.

Biliary obstruction can occur intra- or extra-hepatically. Intrahepatic obstruction requires the compression or infiltration of both sides of the intrahepatic bile duct. Extrahepatic obstruction can be caused by tumor infiltration of the extrahepatic duct, a fragment from a necrotic tumor traveling to the bile duct, or hemorrhage caused by the tumor.[23] Primary cancers causing this complication include tumors of the bile duct, ampulla, duodenum, and pancreas.[24] Obstructive jaundice can also have a metastatic cause. Although this is extremely rare, gastric carcinoma is commonly the cause when metastatic biliary obstruction occurs,[25] although any metastatic cancer can cause this complication. Common signs and symptoms of biliary obstruction other than jaundice include nausea, pruritis, and nutritional deficiencies.[26] It is important to keep in mind that cholecystitis and obstructive biliary disease caused by stones occur with the same or greater frequency than is observed in the normal population. Therefore, the entire spectrum of hepatobiliary disease should be considered before concluding that the cause is related to malignancy.

Systemic Effects

Some of the most challenging manifestations of cancer are those caused by production and secretion of proteins and other substances by malignant neoplasms. For some, we understand the underlying pathophysiology; for others, we associate the clinical syndrome with cancer but cannot identify a specific mechanism.

Hormone Production by Malignant Tumors

Perhaps the best characterized of the paraneoplastic syndromes are those associated with hormonal production. These fall into two broad categories: those in which the malignant cell type normally produces the causative hormone and in which the symptoms are related to excessive or unregulated hormone secretion or the "ectopic" or unexpected production of a hormonal substance by a cell type that does not normally produce this product. Specific examples of the former are carcinoid tumors (serotonin and its metabolites) that cause flushing, diarrhea, and carcinoid heart disease or islet cell malignancies in which excessive insulin, gastrin, or glucagon causes clearly defined clinical syndromes. Examples of the latter include ectopic production of adrenocorticotropic hormone by lung carcinoma. In each of these examples and others, a clearly defined hormonal agent has been implicated in the causation of these clinical syndromes. This is an important point: in situations in which a specific hormone has been implicated, it has often been possible to develop therapeutic approaches that abrogate the effects of the hormone. The most recent example is the development of vasopressin receptor antagonists for treatment of the syndrome of inappropriate antidiuretic hormone secretion described at the beginning of this chapter.[27]

Disordered Production of Clotting Factors

Coagulation disorders occur commonly in patients with malignancy. Tumor cells have been shown to produce a variety of factors that either activate the clotting system or alter the normal balance between pro- and anticoagulation.[7] Many of the coagulation disorders associated with cancer can be traced to over functioning of the clotting system. Tumors may secrete substances that cause the abnormal activation of the clotting system.[28] Neoplastic cells have been shown to generate thrombin and procoagulants.[15] Tissue factor, a cofactor for factor VII/VIIa that helps activate procoagulation factor X,[29] has been seen in solid tumors and in the macrophages of patients with cancer. Elevated levels of the coagulation factors V, VIII, IX, and XI have been seen in patients with malignancy in which vesicles shed from tumor cells bind to factor V, accelerating the coagulation pathway.[29] Fibrinolysis is impaired in tumors with increased levels of plasminogen activator inhibitor 1.[29] In addition to producing proclotting factors, tumors may also decrease the levels of proteins that inhibit thrombosis, such as protein C, protein S, and antithrombin III.

Common complications caused by increased clotting activity include deep venous thrombosis, pulmonary embolism, and inferior vena cava obstruction. There is an increased risk of pulmonary embolus in patients with mucin-producing tumors, particularly those with pancreatic, lung, stomach, colon, kidney, and ovarian cancer.[14] Most symptomatic cerebrovascular infarctions are related to the tumor in cancer patients.[3] Whereas SVCS is usually caused by compression or invasion from a tumor, inferior vena cava obstruction is usually caused by thrombosis.[28]

Nutritional Effects in Cancer

A common complaint of patients with cancer is weight loss. More importantly, there is abundant evidence that anorexia and weight loss are highly correlated with performance status and clinical outcomes in most types of metastatic cancer. Several overlapping mechanisms contribute to weight loss. The first is iatrogenic: the nausea and vomiting induced by many therapeutic agents, including radiotherapy.[30] In most cases, these symptoms can be managed by use of pharmacologic agents that selectively antagonize 5-hydroxytryptamine 3 receptors or by short-term enteral or parenteral feeding methods. The second is more complicated and incompletely understood at present: the complex interplay between cytokines and other substances produced or induced by cancer cells and the hypothalamic neuroendocrine system that controls orexigenic and anorexigenic signaling pathways.[31] There has been progress toward understanding the normal physiologic pathways that regulate appetitite and satiety. These include leptin, melanocortin, orexin, neuropeptide Y, and endocannabinoid signaling pathways.[32–35] One hypothesis, partially supported by current information, is that cytokines (eg, interleukin [IL]-1β, IL-6, interferon [IFN]-γ, tumor necrosis factor –[TNF] α) produced by malignancies impact serotoninergic or dopaminergic pathways that, in turn, regulate the neuroendocrine pathways that control appetite and satiety.[36,37] In addition, tumors produce other factors, such as proteolysis-inducing factor and lipid-mobilizing factor, that cause protein and fat degradation, leading to a cachectic state.[37,38] The development of competitive inhibitors for several cytokines and their application in patients with cancer will make it possible to determine whether these hypotheses are correct. The third factor that almost certainly impacts eating behavior is the development of depression. Depression is a common occurrence in patients with cancer metastasis and has been shown to have an effect on the outcome of treatment.[39] Although patients with metastatic cancer may have good reason to be depressed, it seems likely that a cytokine cascade that depresses serotoninergic pathways is also involved in the development of depression in cancer patients.[40,41]

The important point for the general internist dealing with the cancer patient is to understand the complexity of weight loss in the cancer patient. In many cases, the diagnosis of cancer-related cachexia or weight loss may be complicated by other underlying treatable medical conditions. In the absence of specific diagnostic criteria or diagnostic markers for cancer-related weight loss, it is important to search for treatable causes, including anemia, liver or renal dysfunction, endocrine deficiency or excess, cardiomyopathy, malabsorption, or pulmonary failure.

It is also important to identify and correct nutritional deficiency syndromes, a point often overlooked. All patients with cancer should be given a daily oral multivitamin. In patients who are losing weight or otherwise not faring well, studies should be performed to determine whether vitamin deficiency is a factor. If there is suspicion of malabsorption, parenteral vitamin supplementation should be considered.

Immunologic Effects

The immune system is normally activated in response to invasion by a pathogen or to facilitate clearance of a protein recognized as foreign. Substances such as bacteria or other foreign antigens are recognized by macrophages, natural killer cells, or dendritic cells and then presented to T cells, which, in turn, activate B or antibody-producing cells or other components of the immune system. Once the offending antigen has been eliminated, the immune system returns to its basal state. In many types of cancer, there is chronic activation of the immune system by the aforementioned production or activation of cytokine pathways. Cytokines can be broadly classified as proinflammatory (IL-1α, IL-1β, IL-2, IL-12p35, IL12p40, IL-15, TNF-α, and IFN-γ) or anti-inflammatory (IL-4, IL-8, IL-10, and IL-5), with some uncategorized. Normally, there is a balance between these two classes of cytokines; during periods of infection or inflammation, there is activation, but under normal circumstances, this system is quiescent.[42]

In the cancer environment, production or activation of proinflammatory cytokine pathways continues unabated, leading to chronic stimulation not only of the immune system but also of the tumor cells by cytokines. For example, in chronic hepatitis B infection, there is often a failure of the immune system to clear the virus, leading to chronic activation of cytokine production.[43] This, in turn, leads to recruitment of activated immune cells to the liver, resulting in chronic stimulation of hepatocytes and resultant fibrosis, cirrhosis, and hepatocellular carcinoma. In varying ways, this same type of process can affect the progression of many other tumors.

Activation of the immune system can also be used to treat cancer. There is ample evidence that cytokine treatment of several hematologic malignancies is effective and in some cases has caused long-term remission of disease. Antigenic stimulation has also been used with success in melanoma. The challenge for the future will be to identify those features of the immune system that promote tumor regression without causing other detrimental bystander effects.

Other aspects of the immune system contribute to morbidity and mortality in the cancer patient. Therapies used to treat specific cancer types, including cytotoxic chemotherapy and corticosteroids, can have profound suppressive effects on cellular and humoral immunity, leading to an increased risk of infection. After death from cancer metastasis, infection is the leading cause of death in patients treated for cancer. There is the strongly held belief that better understanding of the immune system and the development of strategies to manipulate the immune system will improve outcomes of cancer therapy and prevent infections.

Idiopathic or Clinical Syndromes without an Identifiable Cause

A number of protean manifestations of cancer occur with some frequency. These clinical syndromes fall into three broad categories: neurologic, systemic or hematologic, and endocrine (Table 2). The pathophysiology is understood for some; for others, there is no identifiable explanation. These clinical syndromes are discussed in greater detail in several subspecialty sections in this book. Internists caring for oncology patients should have a working knowledge of these syndromes as they can be confused with their counterparts in patients without a malignancy.

In addition, each of these syndromes challenges the skills of the internist. One example, hypoglycemia, has a multiplicity of causes, which can include increased use of glucose, such as is seen in tumors that produce insulin or insulin-like growth factor 2, decreased production of glucose when there is hepatic infiltration by tumor, or combinations of the two, such as in cortisol or growth hormone deficiency.[44] The neurologic presentations of myopathy and neuropathy can also be challenging.

Treatment-Related Effects

Cytotoxic Chemotherapy

Cancer therapy has evolved from single-agent therapy to the current use of multiple agents that target different cellular processes. These combination chemotherapies are designed to deliver a lethal blow to the rapidly dividing cancer cell. In the evolution of chemotherapy use, at each stage, there has been the need to balance the efficacy of the therapeutic regimen with short- and long-term toxicity. The short-term effects of chemotherapy can include leukopenia, anemia, mucositis, nausea and vomiting, hepatic dysfunction, renal damage leading to decreased glomerular filtration, and cardiac and endocrine dysfunction. As one observes the progression of treatment paradigms for specific malignancies for the past several decades, a pattern emerges

Table 2 Categorization of Paraneoplastic Syndromes
Neurologic paraneoplastic syndromes
Autonomic and sensory neuropathy
Cord and brain lesions, including myelopathy, cerebellar degeneration, limbic encephalitis, encephalopathy
Muscle disorders, including myasthenia gravis, neuromyotonia, rippling muscle syndrome, stiff-man syndrome, and myoclonus
Gastrointestinal pseudo-obstruction
Systemic and dermatologic paraneoplastic syndromes
Hypogammaglobulinemia, acquired
Red cell aplasia
Alopecia
Pemphigus
Endocrine paraneoplastic syndromes
Hypercalcemia caused by parathyroid hormone–related protein
Carcinoid syndrome
Hyperpigmentation
Hyperthyroidism
Syndrome of inappropriate antidiuretic hormone
Hypoglycemia
Diabetes mellitus

Earlier treatment regimens applied to malignancies in which survival was poor tended to be more toxic while the oncology community searched for efficacious treatments. In tumor types in which successful combinations of chemotherapeutic agents were identified, there have been systematic efforts to identify therapies with as great or better efficacy but with lower toxicity. The example of breast cancer is illustrative. Earlier chemotherapeutic regimens used to treat breast cancer had greater side effects than those used after outcomes improved. There is a continuing trend to use less chemotherapy, particularly in early breast cancer, or to combine other treatment modalities with the use of aromatase inhibitors, whose effect on reducing the recurrence of breast cancer is related primarily to the lowering of plasma estrogen levels.

Toxicities tend to be of two types: those directly related to therapy and those whose effects are indirect. Perhaps the single best example of the former is the effect of anthracyclines (doxorubicin) on cardiac function. Anthracyclines remain an effective therapy for a broad spectrum of malignancies and remain front-line therapy in the treatment of a number of malignancies. Cardiac toxicity caused by anthracyclines is dose related and cumulative, occurring in approximately 30% of individuals who receive doses greater than 500 mg/m^2,[45] and cardiac mortality in this group of patients is significant. The introduction of liposomal forms of anthracycline has lowered but not eliminated short-term toxicity.[46] Over the longer term, anthracycline toxicity contributes to overall cardiac mortality. Indeed, as coronary artery disease has receded as the most important cause of middle-age death, cardiac muscle dysfunction or cardiomyopathy has assumed greater importance. Thus, patients who are cured of their underlying malignancy by anthracycline-based chemotherapy have a significant probability of developing later cardiac failure. Although active efforts are under way to ameliorate the effects of anthracycline toxicity on the heart or to replace this effective chemotherapeutic agent, progress has been slow.

The second type of effect from chemotherapy is one that is a secondary effect. One good example of this phenomenon is the induction of an early menopause in women with breast cancer treated with adjuvant chemotherapy. A significant percentage of these women develop an early menopause, with its attendant problems of bone loss, memory and cognitive dysfunction, and symptoms of hot flashes, vaginal dryness, and loss of libido. In recent years, these issues have been exacerbated by the further lowering of plasma estrogen levels by use of aromatase inhibitors, a class of agents that further lower breast cancer recurrence rates.[47] The efficacy of aromatase inhibitors has been so recently demonstrated that the long-term effects of decades of estrogen deficiency, particularly for young women, have not been clearly defined.

The general or subspecialty internist will have the greatest impact in the area of long-term effects. Most short-term effects of cancer therapy are managed skillfully by oncologists. Once a suitable period of observation (5–10 years) following treatment has passed, most patients will be returned to the care of a general physician. In-depth knowledge of potential long-term problems and their management is essential.

Unintended Effects of Targeting Specific Signal Transduction Pathways

Another new and rapidly evolving area of interest for the internist caring for cancer patients is the side effects of targeted therapy. These agents, many of which are small organic molecules or monoclonal antibodies that target specific signal transduction pathways, were developed with the intent of being cancer specific. As might be predicted, many of these pathways are also important in normal cells, leading to a variety of unexpected side effects. Examples of side effects are developing almost as rapidly as these agents are being introduced into clinical trials. Prominent among this group because of their success in the treatment of cancer are tyrosine kinase inhibitors that target the family of vascular endothelial growth factor receptors.[48] In addition to effects on vascular endothelial growth, inhibition of this class of receptors causes hypertension and through its effects on vascularity may cause tumor-related hemorrhage. In addition, this group of tyrosine kinase receptors shares considerable homology with receptors for epidermal growth factor, glial cell–derived neurotrophic factor, and fibroblast growth factor.[49] As a result, skin rashes (from targeting of the epidermal growth factor receptor) and nausea, vomiting, and diarrhea are common side effects. In the new paradigm of cancer treatment, patients whose tumors respond to these therapeutic agents are expected to remain on these agents for long periods of time, in some cases for life. Longevity of therapy has led to increasing concern regarding these side effects. For example, the recent observation that sunitinib, an agent with efficacy in renal cell carcinoma, causes cardiac dysfunction and failure in approximately 10% of patients treated with this agent is of concern, particularly if long-term therapy is envisioned.[50] The paradox presented by this rapidly evolving literature is that agents effective for treatment of malignancy as chronic (lifetime?) therapy may have to be discarded unless strategies are developed to deal effectively with these problems. As internists in cancer centers, we will have to be in the forefront of the effort to collate these side effects and develop effective preventive strategies.

Bystander Effects Caused by the Death of Tumor Cells

Tumor lysis syndrome is characterized by the release of neoplastic cellular contents into the circulation following an exuberant response to a cancer therapeutic agent.[51] This clinical syndrome occurs most often within the first 48 to 72 hours after initiation of therapy for a rapidly proliferating tumor that is responsive to therapy. It occurs most commonly with leukemia or lymphoma but may be seen with any solid tumor. The major manifestations result from a failure of the kidney, liver, and other buffering mechanisms to clear or inactivate the large volume of cellular material released following a therapeutic response. Manifestations include hyperkalemia, hyperuricemia, hyperphosphatemia, and hypocalcemia. Acute renal failure occurs with some frequency and is, most commonly, caused by precipitation of uric acid or calcium phosphate crystals. Subsequent life-threatening events include cardiac arrhythmias, metabolic acidosis, and fluid overload causing pulmonary edema and hypertension.

Detrimental Effects of Radiation Therapy

Radiation for treatment of malignancy is a well-established and effective form of therapy for multiple forms of cancer. Its use has been incorporated into the primary management of multiple forms of cancer, and it is routinely used to treat metastasis in the central and peripheral nervous systems, skeleton, and many other sites. Older techniques for delivering radiation therapy used higher doses of radiation and were less focused, thereby resulting in a large field of exposure. Newer techniques using computerized imaging (intensity-modulated radiation therapy [IMRT] and gamma knife) to more narrowly defined fields of radiation exposure and the increasing use of proton beam therapy have reduced but not completely eliminated some of these effects. As these newer techniques have been used only during the past decade and rarely outside major cancer centers, there is still a substantial group of patients who have received radiation therapy using older technologies. It is important that the practicing internist be aware of radiation effects and include appropriate screening techniques for these effects in long-term management approaches. In the following sections, we provide some illustrative examples to highlight the concerns.

Radiation to the Central Nervous System

Irradiation to the brain is used to treat a number of benign and malignant conditions, including primary malignancies of the brain, metastasis of many types of cancer, and benign processes, such as pituitary tumors. The long-term effects of cranial radiation may be dramatic, such as the development of a secondary primary malignancy, or subtle, as evidenced by gradual development of endocrine deficiency and associated loss of regulatory control over appetite and energy consumption. For example, more than half of patients who have received skull-based or neck radiation will develop some evidence of endocrine deficiency (growth hormone deficiency, hypothyroidism, hypogonadism, or adrenal insufficiency) over the course of a lifetime.[44] These effects are particularly evident in children treated for benign or malignant brain tumors in whom growth retardation, hypothalamic obesity, memory loss, fatigue, and other endocrine deficiency syndromes occur

with some regularity.[44] It is important to consider these possibilities, particularly those that are easily treated by hormonal replacement, in patients who develop ill- or vaguely defined symptoms in the years or decades following cranial irradiation.

Long-Term Effects of Breast Radiation

Over the past two decades, there has been a trend to combine less aggressive surgical resection with radiotherapy to the affected breast for treatment of localized breast carcinoma with comparable or better results than earlier and more aggressive surgical approaches. Unfortunately, application of this type of radiation has had unintended effects. In a number of studies, including a large analysis of the Surveillance, Epidemiology, and End Results (SEER) database, the incidence of lung cancer and cardiac dysfunction is increased in irradiated regions.[52–56] Although most of these analyses were conducted on cohorts that received radiation more than a decade ago using techniques that are currently outdated, they highlight the concerns. Fortunately, radiation techniques have improved, there is clear evidence of benefit in patients with localized breast cancer with one to three positive nodes, and it can be expected that the incidence of these complications will fall in future years.[57] The important point is that the internist, oncologist, or cardiologist who follows these patients should incorporate cardiac and cancer screening (breast and lung) into long-term management.

Effects of Abdominal Radiation

Radiation is applied to treat many malignancies that occur in the abdomen or adjacent structures. A broad spectrum of side effects is observed following abdominal radiation. The most serious is radiation-induced enteritis. Symptoms of this disorder include nausea, vomiting, pain, diarrhea, and rectal bleeding. Patients with severe enteritis may develop sepsis, a condition resulting from acute radiation impairment of normal cell division, micro- and macroulceration, and resultant passage of bacteria and/or endotoxin into the circulation. Radiation damage to blood vessels supplying the intestine may also contribute to this process. Cotreatment with several chemotherapeutic agents, including 5-fluorouracil, methotrexate, and doxorubicin, may increase the radiation-induced damage to normal tissues. In most patients, these acute effects will resolve within a period of 1 week, although complete recovery may take months or longer.

There are also long-term effects of radiation therapy to multiple structures within the abdomen. These may include hepatic or renal injury, ureteral strictures, narrowing of the aorta, impairment of uterine development in young patients, premature ovarian failure, and skeletal effects,

such as insufficiency fractures or failure of normal skeletal development.

Moreover, recent advances in the use of more focused radiation, such as IMRT and proton beam therapy, have already had an impact on the bystander effects of radiation. It is likely that this trend will continue, reducing the effects of abdominal radiation.

Conclusions

There are several inescapable trends in oncology. The first is that survival in cancer patients is improving, with more than 50% of patients treated for cancer now surviving long term. Moreover, this trend is likely to continue and accelerate in the coming years as newer pathway-specific agents enter routine therapy. In this new world of oncology, long-term management of patients treated for cancer will merge with the broad spectrum of other disease processes. This will necessitate the active collaboration of oncologists and a group of general and subspecialty internists or family physicians conversant in the management of cancer, the side effects of therapeutic agents, and the broader spectrum of disorders that affect the general population. Success in oncology therapy will almost certainly lead to a new and interesting discipline of internal and general medicine that will be defined as a discrete subspecialty. We look forward to the challenges that successful therapy of cancer will bring.

REFERENCES

1. Holland JF. The cardinal manifestations of cancer. In: Holland JF, editor. Cancer medicine. 6th ed. Toronto: BC Decker; 2003. p. XX–XX.
2. Gilbert MR GS. Incidence and nature of neurologic problems in patients with solid tumors. Am J Med 1986; 81:951–4.
3. Newton HB. Neurologic complications of systemic cancer. Am Fam Physician 1999;59:878–86.
4. Labovich TM. Selected complications in the patient with cancer: spinal cord compression, malignant bowel obstruction, malignant ascites, and gastrointestinal bleeding. Semin Oncol Nurs 1994;10:189–97.
5. Soria JC, Fizazi K, Merad M, Le Chevalier T. [Inappropriate antidiuretic hormone secretion disclosing a second primary lung cancer 5 years after complete remission of a small cell lung carcinoma]. Bull Cancer 1996;83:605–8.
6. Wood DE. Management of malignant tracheobronchial obstruction. Surg Clin North Am 2002;82:621–42.
7. Lore JM Jr. Complications in management of thyroid cancer. Semin Surg Oncol 1991;7:120–5.
8. Baumann MH, Heffner JE. Bilateral vocal cord paralysis with respiratory failure. A presenting manifestation of bronchogenic carcinoma. Arch Intern Med 1989;149:1453–4.
9. Wassermann K, Mathen F, Edmund Eckel H. Malignant laryngotracheal obstruction: a way to treat serial stenoses of the upper airways. Ann Thorac Surg 2000;70: 1197–201.
10. Bolliger CT, Sutedja TG, Strausz J, Freitag L. Therapeutic bronchoscopy with immediate effect: laser, electrocautery, argon plasma coagulation and stents. Eur Respir J 2006;27:1258–71.
11. Casey KR. Neoplastic mimics of pneumonia. Semin Respir Infect 1995;10:131–42.
12. Putinati S, Trevisani L, Gualandi M, et al. Pulmonary infections in lung cancer patients at diagnosis. Lung Cancer 1994;11:243–9.

13. Burke M, Fraser R. Obstructive pneumonitis: a pathologic and pathogenetic reappraisal. Radiology 1988;166: 699–704.

14. Shuey KM. Heart, lung, and endocrine complications of solid tumors. Semin Oncol Nurs 1994;10:177–88.

15. Aurora R, Milite F, Vander Els NJ. Respiratory emergencies. Semin Oncol 2000;27:256–69.

16. Stewart IE. Superior vena cava syndrome: an oncologic complication. Semin Oncol Nurs 1996;12:312–7.

17. Stellato TA, Shenk RR. Gastrointestinal emergencies in the oncology patient. Semin Oncol 1989;16:521–31.

18. Tunca JC, Buchler DA, Mack EA, et al. The management of ovarian-cancer-caused bowel obstruction. Gynecol Oncol 1981;12(2 Pt 1):186–92.

19. Randall TC, Rubin SC. Management of intestinal obstruction in the patient with ovarian cancer. Oncology (Huntingt) 2000;14:1159–63; discussion 67–8, 71–5.

20. Shone DN, Nikoomanesh P, Smith-Meek MM, Bender JS. Malignancy is the most common cause of gastric outlet obstruction in the era of H2 blockers. Am J Gastroenterol 1995;90:1769–70.

21. Bhattacharya R, Rao S, Kowdley KV. Liver involvement in patients with solid tumors of nonhepatic origin. Clin Liver Dis 2002;6:1033–43, x.

22. Martelli O, Coppola L, De Quarto AL, et al. Fulminant hepatic failure caused by diffuse intrasinusoidal metastatic liver disease: a case report. Tumori 2000;86:424–7.

23. Lau WY, Leung KL, Leung TW, et al. Obstructive jaundice secondary to hepatocellular carcinoma. Surg Oncol 1995;4:303–8.

24. Rubin RA, Lichtenstein GR, Morris JB. Acute esophageal obstruction: a unique presentation of a giant intramural esophageal leiomyoma. Am J Gastroenterol 1992;87: 1669–71.

25. Chu KM, Law S, Branicki FJ, Wong J. Extrahepatic biliary obstruction by metastatic gastric carcinoma. J Clin Gastroenterol 1998;27:63–6.

26. Moazzam N, Mir A, Potti A. Pancreatic metastasis and extrahepatic biliary obstruction in squamous cell lung carcinoma. Med Oncol 2002;19:273–6.

27. Ghali JK, Koren MJ, Taylor JR, et al. Efficacy and safety of oral conivaptan: a V1A/V2 vasopressin receptor antagonist, assessed in a randomized, placebo-controlled trial in patients with euvolemic or hypervolemic hyponatremia. J Clin Endocrinol Metab 2006;91:2145–52.

28. Nelson KA WD, Abdullah O, McDonnell F, et al. Common complications of advanced cancer. In: Seminars in oncology. Cleveland (OH): W.B. Saunders; 2000. p. 34–44.

29. Arkel YS. Thrombosis and cancer. Semin Oncol 2000;27: 362–74.

30. Munshi A, Pandey MB, Durga T, et al. Weight loss during radiotherapy for head and neck malignancies: what factors impact it? Nutr Cancer 2003;47:136–40.

31. Gordon JN, Green SR, Goggin PM. Cancer cachexia. QJM 2005;98:779–88.

32. Pagotto U, Marsicano G, Cota D, et al. The emerging role of the endocannabinoid system in endocrine regulation and energy balance. Endocr Rev 2006;27:73–100.

33. Hanusch-Enserer U, Roden M. News in gut-brain communication: a role of peptide YY (PYY) in human obesity and following bariatric surgery. Eur J Clin Invest 2005;35: 425–30.

34. Adan RA, van Dijk G. Melanocortin receptors as drug targets for disorders of energy balance. CNS Neurol Disord Drug Targets 2006;5:251–61.

35. Park AJ, Bloom SR. Neuroendocrine control of food intake. Curr Opin Gastroenterol 2005;21:228–33.

36. Morely JE, Thomas DR, Wilson MM. Cachexia: pathophysiology and clinical relevance. Am J Clin Nutr 2006;130: 735–43.

37. Argiles JM, Busquets S, Lopez-Soriano FJ. Cytokines as mediators and targets for cancer cachexia. Cancer Treat Res 2006;130:199–217.

38. Todorov PT, Field WN, Tisdale MJ. Role of proteolysis-inducing factor (PIF) in cachexia induced by a human melanoma (G361). Br J Cancer 1999;80:1734–7.

39. Onitilo AA, Nietert PJ, Egede LE. Effect of depression on all-cause mortality in adults with cancer and differential effects by cancer site. Gen Hosp Psychiatry 2006;28: 396–402.

40. Menzies H, Chochinov HM, Breitbart W. Cytokines, cancer and depression: connecting the dots. J Support Oncol 2005;3:55–7.

41. Illman J, Corringham R, Robinson D, et al. Are inflammatory cytokines the common link between cancer-associated cachexia and depression? J Support Oncol 2005;3:37–50.

42. Kim R, Emi M, Tanabe K, Arihiro K. Tumor-driven evolution of immunosuppressive networks during malignant progression. Cancer Res 2006;66:5527–36.

43. Budhu A, Wang XW. The role of cytokines in hepatocellular carcinoma. J Leukoc Biol 2006. [In press]

44. Yeung SC, Chiu AC, Vassilopoulou-Sellin R, Gagel RF. The endocrine effects of nonhormonal antineoplastic therapy. Endocr Rev 1998;19:144–72.

45. Yeh ET, Tong AT, Lenihan DJ, et al. Cardiovascular complications of cancer therapy: diagnosis, pathogenesis, and management. Circulation 2004;109:3122–31.

46. Ewer MS, Martin FJ, Henderson C, et al. Cardiac safety of liposomal anthracyclines. Semin Oncol 2004;31(6 Suppl 13):161–81.

47. Buzdar AU. Aromatase inhibitors: change the face of endocrine therapy for breast cancer. Breast Dis 2005–2006; 24:107–17.

48. Isobe T, Herbst RS, Onn A. Current management of advanced non-small cell lung cancer: targeted therapy. Semin Oncol 2005;32:315–28.

49. Sandler A, Herbst R. Combining targeted agents: blocking the epidermal growth factor and vascular endothelial growth factor pathways. Clin Cancer Res 2006;12: 4421s–5s.

50. Demetri GD. Phase 3, multicenter, randomized, double-blind, placebo-controlled trial of SU11248 in patients following failure of imatinib for metastatic GIST. J Clin Oncol 2005;24:138.

51. Rampello E, Fricia T, Malaguarnera M. The management of tumor lysis syndrome. Nat Clin Pract Oncol 2006;3: 438–47.

52. Katelyn AR, Marks LB, Prosnitz RG. Late effects of breast radiotherapy in young women. Breast Dis 2005;23: 53–65.

53. Darby SC, McGale P, Taylor CW, Peto R. Long-term mortality from heart disease and lung cancer after radiotherapy for early breast cancer: prospective cohort study of about 300,000 women in US SEER cancer registries. Lancet Oncol 2005;6:557–65.

54. Taylor CW, McGale P, Darby SC. Cardiac risks of breast-cancer radiotherapy: a contemporary view. Clin Oncol (R Coll Radiol) 2006;18:236–46.

55. Jarvenpaa R, Holli K, Pitkanen M, et al. Radiological pulmonary findings after breast cancer irradiation: a prospective study. Acta Oncol 2006;45:16–22.

56. Prochazka M, Hall P, Gagliardi G, et al. Ionizing radiation and tobacco use increases the risk of a subsequent lung carcinoma in women with breast cancer: case-only design. J Clin Oncol 2005;23:7467–74.

57. Whelan T, Levine M. More evidence that locoregional radiation therapy improves survival: what should we do? J Natl Cancer Inst 2005;97:82–4.

Long-Term Consequences of Cancer Surgery

Isabelle Bedrosian, MD

Laura A. Lambert, MD

Raphael E. Pollock, MD, PhD

Over the last several decades, significant improvements in outcomes have been achieved for many patients with cancer. Surgical treatment has been and remains a principal modality for cure. Technological improvements and advances in surgical management have allowed for more extensive operative interventions, and multidisciplinary approaches have expanded surgical options for previously nonoperative patients. The increase in long-term survivorship has led to an increased focus on the functional outcomes and quality of life of cancer survivors. In this chapter, we discuss the long-term management of some of the more commonly encountered consequences of cancer surgery.

Management of Lymphedema

Regional lymph node dissection is routinely employed in the management of invasive breast cancer or malignant melanoma following a positive sentinel node biopsy or in the setting of breast cancer with known axillary metastases or stage III melanoma. Aside from disease recurrence, lymphedema is the most dreaded sequela of these procedures, with reported rates of 6 to 70% after level II axillary dissection for breast cancer[1] and 6 to 20% following inguinal and pelvic lymph node dissection for melanoma.[2] Patients who are obese and patients who undergo adjuvant radiation therapy are at an additionally increased risk of developing lymphedema.[1,3] Although rarely life-threatening, lymphedema is a problem of significant clinical importance. In addition to causing pain, swelling, tightness, and heaviness of the affected extremity, it places the patient at risk of recurrent skin infections, and chronic lymphedema increases the risk of developing lymphangiosarcoma (Stewart-Treves syndrome) in the affected limb. Other studies have documented a significant degree of functional impairment, psychological morbidity,

and reduced quality of life in patients suffering from lymphedema.[4,5] Furthermore, the psychosocial impact of lymphedema has been reported by patients to be as distressing as their initial cancer diagnosis as it serves as a reminder of the cancer and can be an overt physical disfigurement.[6]

The diagnosis of postoperative lymphedema is usually first considered by the clinical finding of unilateral enlargement of the operated limb. Lymphedema can occur immediately postoperatively or weeks, months, or even years later.[7] Other symptoms of lymphedema include a sense of fullness in the affected limb; decreased flexibility in the hand, wrist, or ankle; and difficulty fitting into clothes or jewelry.[8] Although a variety of methods are available for the detection of lymphedema (circumferential measurements at various points, volumetric measures using water displacement, optoelectronic scanning), there are neither established guidelines for the use of many of these methods nor consensus within the literature regarding the degree of enlargement or impairment that defines lymphedema. Currently, a circumferential measurement of selected points along the limb is the most commonly used anthropometric assessment in the clinical setting. A recent prospective study of 90 breast cancer patients evaluated the sensitivity and specificity of several different criteria for circumferential measurements and volume assessment for the detection of lymphedema. Lymphedema was identified in 43% of patients, and the authors concluded that a change in the circumference of greater than 1 cm at specific sites along the length of the arm provided reliable detection of lymphedema, with 91% sensitivity and 46% specificity.[9] Regardless of the method used, limb volume changes compared over time and with the contralateral limb provide the most complete objective assessment for lymphedema diagnosis and treatment. Early diagnosis and treatment help improve both the prognosis and the clinical condition.

Unfortunately, there is no cure for lymphedema. Therapeutic efforts focus on minimizing the edema to reduce the risk of chronic and recurrent infections and to restore the functional and cosmetic nature of the limb. Options for the treatment of lymphedema include compression therapy with fitted compression garments, complex decongestive therapy (CDT) (manual lymphatic drainage, bandaging, proper skin care, compression garments, and remedial exercises), or pneumatic compression pumps (chambered pumps that deliver compression distally to proximally along the limb) (Table 1). Comparison of the relative success of these methods is difficult owing to substantial variation in the definitions of lymphedema, treatment interventions, and outcome measures. Since 1989, four randomized controlled trials (RCTs) and two cohort studies of the nonpharmacologic treatment of lymphedema in patients with breast cancer have shown a significant reduction in lymphedema with the use of standard compression therapy (11–86%).[10–15] Similar findings were seen in three RCTs and eight cohort studies with CDT (10–79% volume reduction).[12–22] Three small RCTs and two cohort studies have shown a 15 to 50% volume reduction with the use of the pneumatic compression pump.[10,11,15,18,23]

Prior to initiating any form of therapy, it is important to identify and treat other possible sources of limb swelling, such as infection, deep venous thrombosis, or recurrent or metastatic disease. Compression therapy, CDT, and pneumatic compression pumps all require a referral to a certified physical therapist. Patients with a

Table 1 Results of Treatment for Lymphedema

Treatment Modality	Percent Volume Reduction
Standard compression therapy	11–86
Complex decongestive therapy	10–79
Pneumatic compression pump	15–50

history of congestive heart failure may not be eligible for CDT or pneumatic compression pump therapy. Recommendations for the prevention of lymphedema include but are not limited to close surveillance for any swelling, avoiding venipuncture or blood pressure measurement on the at-risk limb, meticulous skin care, avoiding vigorous, repetitive movements and heavy lifting, avoiding tight jewelry or clothing, avoiding trauma, and wearing a well-fitted compression garment when flying.[24] Currently, these lifelong precautions apply to all patients until further studies better stratify an individual patient's risk of lymphedema.

Endocrine and Exocrine Function after Pancreatectomy

Surgical treatment for pancreatic malignancy frequently requires resection of either the pancreatic head and duodenum (pancreaticoduodenectomy or Whipple procedure) or distal pancreatectomy. These procedures commonly result in intestinal disturbances and may also lead to glucose intolerance and the development of anastomotic ulcers. Patients with tumors limited to the neck or body may be treated with a segmental resection, often termed central or median pancreatectomy. Such limited resection is well tolerated and rarely leads to the development of the complications discussed below.[25–27]

Exocrine Insufficiency

The incidence of pancreatic exocrine insufficiency has been reported to range from approximately 30% to as high as 100% following pancreatic resection.[28–31] This wide range is due to variations across studies in how this is defined, the type of pancreatic resection, and the duration of follow-up. Reports of pancreatic insufficiency may define this biochemically (serum para-aminobenzoic acid [PABA] levels, fecal elastase 1 assay) or clinically by the presence of diarrhea or symptoms requiring pancreatic enzyme supplementation. Studies that have measured pancreatic insufficiency by fecal stool content and fecal elastase assay have shown that biochemical alterations in pancreatic exocrine dysfunction can be found in nearly 100% of patients following pancreaticoduodenectomy.[28,29] However, clinical determinations of pancreatic insufficiency based on the presence of steatorrhea and/or the requirement for pancreatic enzyme replacement have identified one-third to two-thirds of patients who continue to show signs of exocrine insufficiency at 1 to 2 years of follow-up after pancreatic head resection.[28–30,32]

A number of factors lead to the development of exocrine dysfunction after pancreatectomy. These include the extent of resection, the presence of fibrosis in the remnant pancreas,

occlusion of the pancreatic duct, inactivation of pancreatic enzymes by gastric content, and the rate of gastric emptying. Notably, although the extent of resection is clearly important, there is no linear relationship between the volume of pancreatic parenchymal loss and the development of pancreatic insufficiency.[33]

The clinical manifestations of pancreatic exocrine insufficiency are primarily diarrhea, abdominal pain, malabsorption, and, ultimately, weight loss (or lack of weight gain postoperatively to a preillness state).[29,30] Some groups have suggested that preservation of the pylorus during pancreaticoduodenectomy is associated with improved long-term nutritional status.[31,34,35] However, recently reported results of a prospective randomized trial of 170 patients showed no statistical differences in weight loss up to 6 months postoperatively between patients who had preservation of the pylorus and those who had standard pancreaticoduodenectomy with distal gastric resection.[36] van Berge Henegouwen and colleagues suggested that differences in postoperative weight gain between patients undergoing pancreatic resection have more to do with positive margins of resection rather than the type of pancreaticoduodenectomy.[30] Patients with distal pancreatectomy appear to be at a substantially lower risk of development of pancreatic exocrine insufficiency.[27]

Management of pancreatic exocrine insufficiency is usually based on clinical symptoms and is aimed at reversing the malabsorption and associated weight loss. The hallmark signs and symptoms include steatorrhea and abdominal pain. Confirmation of the diagnosis can be achieved with a number of tests, including direct measurements of fecal fat, an enzyme-linked immunosorbent assay for assessment of fecal elastase 1 levels,[121] and serum PABA levels.[37,38] Patients with clinical symptoms of pancreatic insufficiency should be treated with pancreatic enzyme supplementation. Treatment with pancreatic enzymes is titrated to relief of gastrointestinal symptoms. Significant dosage may be necessary in some patients, and high-dose preparations are available. Dietary alterations, in particular restriction of dietary fat intake, are not required. Given the sensitivity of pancreatic enzymes to degradation within the acid environment of the stomach, pancreatic enzyme preparations are frequently enteric coated and release enzyme only at nearly neutral pH levels. Acid-reducing agents such as H_2 blockers may sometimes be necessary to enhance the activity of oral pancreatic enzyme preparations. Subsequently, patients should closely monitor the efficacy of combining pancreatic enzymes with H_2 blockers because this may lead to premature dissolution of the enzyme preparation within the stomach, with a possible reduction in the efficacy of pancreatic enzyme therapy.

There has also been interest in the clinical use of agents that may ameliorate the sequelae of pancreatic exocrine insufficiency by promoting the regeneration of the remnant pancreas. Although regeneration of the pancreas is seen in animal models of pancreatic resection, in humans, atrophy of the remnant pancreas is the more common occurrence.[28] One hormone believed to be important in the growth of the pancreas is gastrin. Jang and colleagues used proton pump inhibitors (PPIs) in patients with pancreatic resection to increase serum gastrin levels.[33] Patients treated with PPIs for 3 months postoperatively had less atrophy of the remnant pancreas, were able to maintain pancreatic enzyme levels, and demonstrated improved nutritional status compared with those who did not receive PPIs. However, although such data are encouraging, longer-term data from such a strategy are required. In addition, the possible role of gastrin as a growth factor in pancreatic cancer has been raised by some groups,[39,40] and the use of an antigastrin antibody has been investigated therapeutically in patients with advanced pancreatic carcinoma.[41] Therefore, the impact of long-term PPI treatment on the survival of patients with pancreatic cancer needs to be evaluated prior to generalized use of PPIs to stimulate pancreatic regeneration following resection for carcinoma.

Alterations in Glucose Metabolism

Pancreatic cancer has been associated with impaired glucose metabolism,[42] with an improvement in diabetic status noted following resection.[43] These observations have led some to propose that a diabetogenic factor may be produced by pancreatic adenocarcinoma.[43] For those patients who do not have diabetes at presentation, the risk of developing de novo glucose intolerance and frank diabetes following pancreatic resection is primarily related to the extent of surgery and the duration of follow-up. The relative concentration of islets is denser in the tail of the pancreas compared with the head or body of the gland.[44] This would suggest that patients undergoing distal pancreatectomy may be at greatest risk of the long-term development of diabetes.

Some authors have suggested that overt diabetes is unlikely to occur in patients undergoing pancreaticoduodenectomy despite the reduced capacity to secrete insulin and glucagon in the remnant pancreas.[45] However, most series with longer-term follow-up demonstrate that pancreatic head resection does, in fact, increase the likelihood of new-onset diabetes, although it is difficult to ascertain the exact incidence. At 1 year of follow-up, Anderson and colleagues reported that 2 of 47 patients (4%) not previously diabetic developed diabetes after pancreaticoduodenectomy.[46] A similarly low incidence was reported by Lemaire and colleagues, who followed a cohort of 19 patients after pancreaticoduodenectomy for a median of 3 years.[28] Of 17 patients with normal fasting blood glucose preoperatively, 3 showed impaired glucose tolerance at 42, 73, and 120 months postoperatively, although none had overt diabetes. The two remaining patients had non–insulin-dependent diabetes preoperatively, and both required insulin after pancreatic resection.

In contrast, van Berge Henegouwen and colleagues reported a 24% incidence of patients requiring oral hypoglycemics or insulin for management of endocrine insufficiency at 1 year after pancreaticoduodenectomy.[30] Furthermore, of patients who show early signs of abnormal glucose metabolism postoperatively, long-term follow-up studies suggest that further deterioration may occur over time. Ishikawa and colleagues followed 51 patients who were treated with pancreaticoduodenectomy and survived more than 7 years without recurrence of tumor.[47] At 3 months after surgery, 30 patients had a normal oral glucose tolerance test; none of these patients developed glucose intolerance or diabetes at 7 years. Of the 21 patients with abnormal glucose tolerance or diabetes at the 3-month analysis, 14 patients (67%) had further deterioration in pancreatic endocrine function at the longer-term follow-up. The incidence of diabetes in these latter studies appears to approach that seen in patients following distal pancreatectomy. From a group of 24 nondiabetic patients treated with distal pancreatectomy, Yamaguchi and colleagues found that nearly half had deterioration of glucose tolerance at 6 months of follow-up.[27]

The data clearly suggest that irrespective of the type of pancreatic resection, patients need to be monitored closely and consistently over time for development of alterations in glucose metabolism.

Postgastrectomy Syndromes

Postgastrectomy syndromes have been described in approximately 20% of patients. These syndromes encompass a number of specific conditions, including dumping, postvagotomy diarrhea, alkaline reflux gastritis, atonic gastric remnant, and Roux stasis syndrome, as well as more generalized consequences, such as malnutrition and anemia. They occur as a result of loss of gastric reservoir capacity, loss of the pyloric valve mechanism, and loss of vagal innervation important for both the reservoir and emptying functions of the stomach. The likelihood of occurrence of any one of these specific conditions depends on both the type of gastric resection (total, subtotal proximal, subtotal distal) and the method used to restore gastrointestinal continuity (Billroth I, Billroth II, or Roux-en-Y gastrojejunostomy).

Management of these syndromes depends on recognizing those that are amenable to medical treatment and those for which surgery is the preferred intervention (Table 2). The clinical manifestations of postgastrectomy syndromes are described below. In general, they can be categorized as disorders secondary to rapid gastric transit (dumping, postvagotomy diarrhea), disorders secondary to functional and mechanical obstruction (Roux stasis, atonic gastric remnant), and disorders secondary to reflux of intestinal content (bile reflux gastritis). For patients with postgastrectomy syndromes, a clinical history, upper endoscopy, barium radiography, and nuclear medicine gastric emptying studies are important elements for accurate diagnosis of the specific disorder.

Dumping

Dumping syndrome occurs in approximately 20 to 30% of patients[48,49] and is divided into early and late forms based on the interval between oral intake and the development of symptoms. Early dumping symptoms occur within 30 minutes of ingestion; patients experience gastrointestinal discomfort (abdominal pain, nausea, vomiting, and diarrhea) and vasomotor symptoms (diaphoresis, palpitations, hypotension, dizziness). These changes are mediated by gastrointestinal peptide hormones in response to rapid gastric emptying into the small intestine.[50] The sudden appearance of a large volume of hyperosmolar, high-carbohydrate load in particular tends to generate the symptoms of early dumping.

Late dumping occurs in approximately 2% of postgastrectomy patients and consists of vasomotor symptoms alone seen 2 to 4 hours after oral intake. The underlying pathophysiology is the presence of hyperosmolar food within the small intestine that triggers an exaggerated insulin response and subsequent hypoglycemia.

Management of dumping is aimed at altering the pattern of oral intake by reducing intake of concentrated carbohydrates, taking frequent, small meals, and avoiding concomitant intake of solids and liquids. In patients with late dumping, the development of symptoms can be alleviated by intake of carbohydrates to counter the hypoglycemia. In patients with severe symptoms that cannot be managed by behavioral alterations, 50 μg of octreotide taken 15 to 30 minutes before meals appears to counter the effects of gastrointestinal hormones and alleviate dumping symptoms in many patients.[51–53] In general, the symptoms of dumping improve during the course of the first year with conservative measures.

Postvagotomy Diarrhea

The pathophysiology of this disorder is likely a combination of decreased gastric relaxation secondary to vagal denervation and rapid gastrointestinal transit. Postvagotomy diarrhea is characterized primarily by watery diarrhea that occurs after eating and may be confused with dumping syndrome. However, unlike dumping syndrome, there is no clear and consistent association with the type or volume of oral intake. Postvagotomy diarrhea is also frequently episodic.

The highest incidence of postvagotomy diarrhea occurs immediately after gastric resection, and symptoms generally abate over time. Treatment is largely symptomatic with the use of antidiarrheal and antimotility agents. The use of cholestyramine, which binds bile acids, has also been described.[54] Dietary modifications of reducing fluid intake and avoidance of dairy products should also be attempted. In contrast to dumping syndrome, octreotide appears to be less effective in the treatment of postvagotomy diarrhea.[55] In addition to symptomatic treatment, it is important to rule out other causes of diarrhea, including infection and malabsorption syndromes.

Bile Reflux Gastritis

Bile reflux gastritis occurs as a result of loss of the normal pyloric function and consequent reflux of intestinal content into the gastric remnant. Whether delayed gastric emptying is also a primary component of the pathophysiology of this disorder[56] or the secondary effects of bile injury to the gastric pouch remains unclear.[57]

Table 2 Postgastrectomy Syndromes		
Syndrome	*Symptoms*	*Primary Management*
Dumping	Postprandial gastrointestinal distress and vasomotor symptoms	Dietary modification; octreotide in refractory cases
Postvagotomy diarrhea	Postprandial diarrhea	Dietary modification; antidiarrheal agents
Bile reflux gastritis	Epigastric pain, bilious emesis	Prokinetics/acid-reducing agents/cholestyramine
		Surgical revision may be required
Gastric atony	Epigastric pain, nausea, vomiting	Prokinetic agents
		Surgical revision may be required
Roux stasis	Epigastric pain, nausea, vomiting	Surgical revision

The incidence may be as high as 50% after some gastric operations.[49] Patients with bile reflux experience burning epigastric pain, nausea, and bilious vomiting. Eating exacerbates symptoms; therefore, many patients reduce their food intake with consequent weight loss.

Diagnosis is based on the clinical history and confirmation by endoscopic biopsy to distinguish bile reflux gastritis from bile staining of the gastric mucosa. Other etiologies, such as gastric outlet obstruction, gastroesophageal reflux, ulcer disease, and *Helicobacter pylori*, should be ruled out. Nuclear medicine scans may be a helpful adjunct but cannot be used as the primary diagnostic modality because transient reflux can also be seen in asymptomatic patients. Gastric emptying studies will usually demonstrate delay.

Single-agent treatments with bile-chelating agents, sucralfate, and prostaglandins have generally shown disappointing results.[58–61] Nonetheless, an initial trial of intensive therapy with a combination of prokinetic agents, cholestyramine, and acid-reducing agents is recommended. Patients whose symptoms persist should be referred for consideration of surgical treatment.

Gastric Atony

Gastric atony results from loss of vagal innervation that controls gastric contractility and emptying. Symptoms include postprandial epigastric pain, nausea, and vomiting. Gastric emptying scans will show marked delay. Endoscopy and contrast radiography are important components of the workup to rule out mechanical causes of obstruction. Upper gastrointestinal series will typically demonstrate a large, flaccid gastric reservoir. Treatment with prokinetic agents is generally unsuccessful, and many patients ultimately require surgical revision.[62]

Roux Stasis Syndrome

Roux stasis syndrome presents as a functional obstruction in patients who have had gastrointestinal continuity reestablished using a Roux-en-Y gastroenterostomy. The underlying pathophysiology is likely due to altered motility in the jejunal limb as a result of disruption of the intestinal pacemaker by resection of the jejunum to fashion the Roux-en-Y gastroenterostomy. Symptoms are similar to those of gastric atony and consist of abdominal pain, nausea, and vomiting after meals. Roux stasis has been described in approximately 30% of patients and appears to be related to the length of the Roux-Y limb.[63]

As with gastric atony, an important part of the differential that needs to be excluded is mechanical obstruction. Upper endoscopy and upper gastrointestinal series should be used to exclude this possibility. Nuclear medicine scans to document transit times through the Roux-Y limb are also helpful for making the diagnosis. The treatment is surgical revision.

Malnutrition and Anemia

Malnutrition and weight loss are not uncommon after gastrectomy. Although in some cases, these may be due to malabsorption, in many patients, there is inadequate caloric intake to avoid adverse symptoms. For such patients, emphasis on altering eating behaviors, in particular switching from three meals daily to frequent small meals, is essential. Additionally, some patients with no preoperative history of lactose intolerance have been known to develop intolerance of dairy products after gastrectomy. The increase in intestinal pH levels with a subsequent change in the bacterial flora can lead to anaerobic bacterial overgrowth and malabsorption.[64]

The most frequently noted etiology for anemia after total or distal gastrectomy is loss of the intrinsic factor and subsequent malabsorption of vitamin B_{12}. Parenteral vitamin B_{12} replacement is therefore necessary. In addition, iron deficiency anemia and deficiency in folic acid are also described, and these sources should be sought out and treated in patients with chronic anemia following gastrectomy.

Functional Complications of Esophageal Surgery

A number of functional consequences of esophageal surgery are recognized. These include dysphagia, vocal cord paralysis, regurgitation, delayed emptying of the neoesophagus, and dumping syndrome. Most of these complications may be seen irrespective of the surgical approach to resection (transhiatal, transthoracic) or the conduit used. Although many patients will continue to have some long-term functional complaints, studies suggest that quality of life for many returns to national norms.[65,66]

Dysphagia

Some degree of dysphagia has been reported by as many as 45% of patients after esophagectomy followed for over 5 years.[66] Dysphagia may be a symptom of underlying mechanical obstruction, commonly from anastomotic strictures. The severity of symptoms has been shown to correlate with the probability of stricture, those patients with severe symptoms all having evidence of mechanical obstruction.[67] Patients with complaints of dysphagia should be evaluated with endoscopy and cine-esophagrams.

Most strictures are seen within the first 3 months of surgery, and early postoperative dilatation may be required for as many as 30 to 50% of patients after esophagectomy.[68,69] Most strictures can be successfully managed by dilation.[68–70] Multiple sessions are frequently required. By 1 year after surgery, only about 5 to 10% of patients will continue to have symptomatic strictures that require continued dilatation.[69,70]

These patients may be candidates for surgical intervention. In addition, stricture dilatation in patients with colonic or jejunal interpositions carries a higher risk of perforation, and surgical revision should be considered earlier in these patients.

A neurogenic etiology should be considered in patients with dysphagia who do not have radiographic or endoscopic evidence of obstruction.[67] Injury to branches of the recurrent laryngeal nerve is the most likely cause.[67] These patients are managed supportively, in particular with greater emphasis on thorough chewing. Most symptoms resolve with time.

Vocal Cord Paralysis

The incidence of vocal cord paralysis has been reported to be 20 to 30% after esophagectomy[67,71] and is a result of injury to the recurrent laryngeal nerve. Paralysis may be either unilateral or bilateral. The primary symptom is that of hoarseness; however, additional difficulties with swallowing, breathing, and pulmonary complications may also be present. In the majority of patients with recurrent nerve injury, the hoarseness is transient, and many patients have resolution of symptoms within the first 4 to 6 months.[67,71] Patients with recurrent nerve injury have been reported to have a higher incidence of postoperative pulmonary complications,[71,72] and those with severe hoarseness are more likely to have problems with activity and quality of life.[72]

Patients with persistent hoarseness should be referred for laryngoscopy to confirm the clinical diagnosis. Patients with repeated pulmonary complications after esophagectomy should be similarly evaluated. Treatment is aimed at medialization of the vocal cord by intracordal injection with silicone or Gelfoam. The success rate in improving patient symptoms is 90%.[73]

Regurgitation

Many patients will experience occasional reflux after esophagectomy, with some reports showing approximately 60% of patients with intermittent symptoms.[66,74]

The factors that contribute to reflux are multiple, including loss of the natural antireflux mechanism, impaired motility of the neoesophagus, and delay in gastric emptying.[74] In addition to typical symptoms of burning, patients may also complain of chronic cough and recurrent pneumonia.[74] Lying supine frequently exacerbates symptoms. Treatment is supportive. Avoidance of large meals, particularly prior to sleep, can minimize the occurrence of regurgitation. Use of prokinetics in patients with motility disorders may also be of benefit. Regurgitation that necessitates that the patient sleep upright at night is uncommon.[69]

Delayed Conduit Emptying

Delayed conduit emptying may be the result of either poor motility of the neoesophagus or a delay in gastric emptying as a result of denervation of the gastric tube. Patients will frequently complain of early satiety. Contrast radiography can help elucidate the underlying etiology of delayed motility. Treatment is primarily pharmacologic, using promotility agents such as metoclopramide or erythromycin.[75,76] In addition, for patients who have delayed gastric emptying as a result of pyloric narrowing, upper endoscopy with balloon dilatation should be performed.

Dumping

Postvagotomy dumping syndrome is noted in approximately 25% of patients after esophagectomy.[74] As with dumping after gastrectomy, the management is alteration of dietary behavior, with emphasis on frequent, small meals, separating liquids and solid intake by about 30 minutes, and the use of antidiarrheal agents.

Pelvic Operations

The complex neuroanatomy of the pelvis, the close proximity of pelvic organs, and extended multivisceral resections for advanced disease place patients undergoing pelvic surgery for bladder, prostate, gynecologic, and rectal malignancy at risk of the development of urinary, sexual, and anorectal dysfunction after such operations. In addition, patients with stomas for fecal or urinary diversion can present with long-term complications of stenosis and prolapse and may also develop significant metabolic problems.

Sexual Dysfunction

Injury to the parasympathetic and sympathetic nerves in the pelvis plays a primary role in the development of sexual dysfunction following pelvic operations. Additional factors that may contribute include vascular injury, psychosocial factors, and, particularly in women, pelvic scarring. Data regarding postoperative sexual function are more readily available in men than women. In part, this reflects the availability of clearly defined end points of sexual function in men, namely potency and ejaculation.

Erectile dysfunction (ED) in men is defined as an inability to achieve and maintain erections sufficient for sexual intercourse. The incidence of ED after pelvic surgery is highly variable and depends on several factors, including the type of surgery and the patient's age.[77–83] The relationship with the type of surgery in large part reflects the ability to preserve the parasympathetic and sympathetic innervation of the pelvis during the procedure. Preservation of neurovascular bundles bilaterally correlates with an increased likelihood of recovering sexual function; data

from prostatectomy studies indicate that, depending on age, 50 to 90% of men with full erections preoperatively can be expected to recover potency after bilateral nerve preservation compared with only approximately 25 to 50% for those with unilateral nerve preservation.[77–79] Importantly, for men who were potent preoperatively, recovery of sexual function after pelvic surgery can take as long as 40 months.[77,84,85]

Given that the primary etiology of ED in men after pelvic surgery is nerve injury, specialized testing to evaluate for the causes of ED in this setting is not warranted. However, exclusion of metabolic and endocrine conditions that impact sexual activity, such as measurement of serum testosterone, lipid profile, and thyroid function, is appropriate, particularly for men with complaints of decreased libido.[86,87]

Treatment of ED was substantially advanced with the introduction of sildenafil. The initial reports of the efficacy of sildenafil in ED included patients with both organic and psychogenic disorders.[88] More recent reports, specifically on patients with ED after pelvic operations, have similarly confirmed the effectiveness of sildenafil in this cohort.[89,90] Overall, approximately 80% of patients with partial or total ED after pelvic operations can be expected to respond. Doses of 100 mg will often be required to achieve satisfactory results.[88–90] However, the success of recovery of sexual function with sildenafil is also dependent on the preservation of pelvic neuroanatomy.[90] The rates of response to sildenafil according to the status of the neurovascular bundles are 72%, 50%, and 15% for bilateral, unilateral, and non–nerve-preserving operations, respectively.[90]

The reported side effects of sildenafil include headache, flushing, and dyspepsia, although few men discontinued the medication secondary to these side effects.[88] Sildenafil should be used with caution in patients with cardiovascular disease and is contraindicated for those patients on nitrates.[91] For patients who do not respond to sildenafil or for whom sildenafil is contraindicated, alternative treatments include implantation of a penile prosthesis, vacuum constriction devices, and intracorporeal injection or transurethral delivery of alprostadil.

Data on sexual function in women after pelvic surgery are not as readily available. Physical factors are known to be altered after pelvic operations, particularly after gynecologic and rectal operations. These include a shortened vagina, pain, vaginal dryness, and bleeding.[92–94] In patients who have had proctectomy, leakage of stool during intercourse is also reported.[92–94] Reports on sexual function and activity are more varied. Data from women following proctectomy suggest that despite some complaints of physical changes, sexual arousal, sensitivity, and frequency were unchanged postoperatively.[92,94] However, in a

long-term follow-up of 105 women after radical pelvic surgery, Corney and colleagues found that 66% of patients had persistent sexual difficulties, including nearly half who reported a lack of desire.[93] They found that psychogenic causes, in addition to organic ones, had a significant impact on postoperative sexual function. The management of sexual dysfunction in female patients is primarily supportive counseling. The role of sildenafil for treatment of sexual dysfunction in women has been investigated, with studies showing mixed results.[95–97] These studies have not included women experiencing deterioration of sexual function following pelvic surgery.

Anorectal Function after Pelvic Surgery

Alterations in bowel habits are primarily seen in patients following resection of the rectum. Loss of the rectal reservoir and loss of rectal compliance contribute to an increase in stool frequency, urgency, incontinence to stool and/or flatus, and, in some instances, constipation.[98–101] The probability of these functional outcomes is usually inversely correlated with the level of the colorectal anastomosis.[98–101] As the residual rectum gains in compliance and capacitance, in many patients, these symptoms improve over the first 6 to 12 months, and in some series, functional outcomes have continued to improve 2 to 5 years after surgery.[100,102,103]

Treatment is directed at management of these symptoms. A rectal examination is important to confirm that rectal tone is normal and there is no impaction. Furthermore, for patients with severe symptoms that show no sign of abating over time, a barium enema or endoscopy to rule out stricture or secondary causes is important. Increasing stool bulk through the use of fiber is the mainstay of management. Intake of fiber supplements is gradually titrated upward to achieve a more formed bowel movement. Occasionally, antidiarrheal agents are necessary to control loose bowel movements, but these should be used cautiously to avoid alternating cycles of constipation and diarrhea.

In addition to pharmacologic treatments, patients should be encouraged to perform Kegel exercises daily to strengthen the muscles of the pelvic floor. Lastly, education and management of expectations are important components of care in these patients. Despite improvements in anorectal function that occur over many months postoperatively, most patients will ultimately stabilize at an average of two to three bowel movements daily,[102,104] and only 50 to 75% will be completely continent.[98,103,104]

Urologic Dysfunction

As with sexual function, preservation of the pelvic autonomic nerves is important for maintenance of normal bladder function postoperatively.[105–108] Depending on the type of nerve injury, patients may present with symptoms of urinary retention, such as urinary strain, overflow incontinence, and loss of sensation of bladder fullness. Alternatively, patients may complain of urgency and stress incontinence.

Although transient postoperative difficulties requiring intermittent catheterization are not uncommon after pelvic operations,[107,109] the persistence of voiding problems 6 to 8 weeks after surgery requires further evaluation. Such a workup should start with a postvoid residual as measured by catheterization or bladder ultrasonography, as well as a urinalysis and culture to rule out infection. Patients with postvoid bladder volumes exceeding 500 mL should be started on a regimen of clean intermittent catheterization. Further workup will require formal urodynamic studies to better define the etiology of urinary dysfunction and initiate appropriate pharmacologic treatment.

Metabolic Consequences of Urinary and Bowel Diversion

Urinary Diversion

For patients undergoing cystectomy, diversion of urine flow is generally through a segment of bowel, typically the distal ileum or a segment of colon. These urinary diversions may serve simply as a conduit to an external stoma or may be fashioned such that they form a continent urinary pouch. Among the most common complications of such urinary diversions is the development of acidosis, renal insufficiency, and renal calculi, occurring in 15 to 20% of patients (Table 3).[86,87,110]

The incidence of metabolic acidosis depends on the method of follow-up. Electrolyte analysis

---

Table 3 Metabolic Consequences of Urinary Diversion

Renal
  Metabolic acidosis
  Hypokalemia
  Renal insufficiency
  Renal calculi
Bone
  Demineralization
Nutritional
  Vitamin B_{12} deficiency
  Steatorrhea/malabsorption
Infection
  Urinary tract infection
  Pyelonephritis
Liver
  Hyperammonemia
Other
  Altered drug metabolism

---

of venous blood samples will demonstrate an incidence of approximately 15% of patients.[86,87,110] The incidence is much higher if patients are monitored by arterial blood gas measurements.[111] Whether these acid-base abnormalities impact bone metabolism is not clear.[110] However, alkalinizing agents, such as sodium or potassium bicarbonate, should be used in children with urinary diversion as chronic acidosis may lead to bone loss and orthopedic problems.[110] In addition, selective use of alkalinizing agents in patients with a base excess < −2.5 has been recommended.[112] In a series of 27 patients with urinary diversion, Stein and colleagues assessed the long-term impact of early alkalinization in individuals with a base excess < −2.5.[112] They found no abnormalities in bone mineral density in their cohort.

Development of stones, in both the kidney and the conduit, is also not uncommon in patients with urinary diversion and likely results from a combination of stasis and bacterial colonization of the conduit. Antibiotic treatment for colonization is not warranted, and such therapy is reserved for those patients with objective evidence of infection. The presence of bacteria has also been postulated to play a role in the risk of cancer developing at the ureteroenteric anastomosis. This risk was well documented when ureterosigmoid anastomoses were performed for urinary diversion,[113] and sigmoidoscopy every 2 years is warranted in these patients. More recently, isolated ileal or colonic conduits for urinary diversion have replaced ureterosigmoidoscopy. Long-term data on the cancer risk in these isolated bowel conduits have not been established.

Additional complications following urinary diversion that require monitoring include renal insufficiency, deficiency of vitamin B_{12} and malabsorption of bile salts as a result of resection of the terminal ileum for conduit formation, hyperammonemia, especially in patients with liver insufficiency, and drug intoxication with drugs that are excreted unchanged by the kidney and reabsorbed by the bowel conduit.

Bowel Diversion

Although reestablishment of intestinal continuity after gastrointestinal surgery is the primary objective, ostomy formation, either temporary or permanent, is occasionally required in the management of the cancer patient. Long-term complications of such ostomies include prolapse, stenosis, peristomal fistula, parastomal hernia, and retraction of the stoma.[114–116] In addition, patients with ileostomy are prone to dehydration and electrolyte abnormalities. Control of high ileostomy output (generally > 1 L/d) is important and can be accomplished through the use of fiber and antimotility agents. Alterations in uric acid levels are also seen in patients with ileostomy,

which predisposes patients toward the formation of uric acid stones.[117,118] Treatment of patients with aciduria has been suggested to prevent the formation of such stones.[119] An increased incidence of cholelithiasis has also been reported.[120]

REFERENCES

1. Harris SR, Hugi MR, Olivotto IA, Levine M. Clinical practice guidelines for the care and treatment of breast cancer: 11. Lymphedema. CMAJ 2001;164:191–9.
2. Hughes TM, Thomas JM. Combined inguinal and pelvic lymph node dissection for stage III melanoma. Br J Surg 1999;86:1493–8.
3. Schunemann H, Willich N. [Lymphedema after breast carcinoma. A study of 5868 cases]. Dtsch Med Wochenschr 1997;122:536–41.
4. Beaulac SM, McNair LA, Scott TE, et al. Lymphedema and quality of life in survivors of early-stage breast cancer. Arch Surg 2002;137:1253–7.
5. Velanovich V, Szymanski W. Quality of life of breast cancer patients with lymphedema. Am J Surg 1999;177:184–7; discussion 188.
6. Tobin MB, Lacey HJ, Meyer L, Mortimer PS. The psychological morbidity of breast cancer-related arm swelling. Psychological morbidity of lymphoedema. Cancer 1993; 72:3248–52.
7. Guedes Neto HJ. Arm edema after treatment for breast cancer. Lymphology 1997;30:35–6.
8. Armer JM, Radina ME, Porock D, Culbertson SD. Predicting breast cancer-related lymphedema using self-reported symptoms. Nurs Res 2003;52:370–9.
9. Bland KL, Perczyk R, Du W, et al. Can a practicing surgeon detect early lymphedema reliably? Am J Surg 2003; 186:509–13.
10. Bertelli G, Venturini M, Forno G, et al. Conservative treatment of postmastectomy lymphedema: a controlled, randomized trial. Ann Oncol 1991;2:575–8.
11. Bertelli G, Venturini M, Forno G, et al. An analysis of prognostic factors in response to conservative treatment of postmastectomy lymphedema. Surg Gynecol Obstet 1992;175:455–60.
12. Andersen L, Hojris I, Erlandsen M, Andersen J. Treatment of breast-cancer-related lymphedema with or without manual lymphatic drainage—a randomized study. Acta Oncol 2000;39:399–405.
13. Hornsby R. The use of compression to treat lymphoedema. Prof Nurse 1995;11:127–8.
14. Williams AF, Vadgama A, Franks PJ, Mortimer PS. A randomized controlled crossover study of manual lymphatic drainage therapy in women with breast cancer-related lymphoedema. Eur J Cancer Care (Engl) 2002;11: 254–61.
15. Szuba A, Achalu R, Rockson SG. Decongestive lymphatic therapy for patients with breast carcinoma-associated lymphedema. A randomized, prospective study of a role for adjunctive intermittent pneumatic compression. Cancer 2002;95:2260–7.
16. Boris M, Weindorf S, Lasinski B, Boris G. Lymphedema reduction by noninvasive complex lymphedema therapy. Oncology (Huntingt) 1994;8:95–106; discussion 109–10.
17. Boris M, Weindorf S, Lasinkski S. Persistence of lymphedema reduction after noninvasive complex lymphedema therapy. Oncology (Huntingt) 1997;11:99–109; discussion 110, 113–4.
18. Bunce IH, Mirolo BR, Hennessy JM, et al. Post-mastectomy lymphoedema treatment and measurement. Med J Aust 1994;161:125–8.
19. Daane S, Poltoratszy P, Rockwell WB. Postmastectomy lymphedema management: evolution of the complex decongestive therapy technique. Ann Plast Surg 1998;40: 128–34.
20. Ko DS, Lerner R, Klose G, Cosimi AB. Effective treatment of lymphedema of the extremities. Arch Surg 1998;133: 452–8.
21. Morgan RG, Casley-Smith JR, Mason MR. Complex physical therapy for the lymphoedematous arm. J Hand Surg [Br] 1992;17:437–41.
22. Foldi E, Foldi M, Clodius L. The lymphedema chaos: a lancet. Ann Plast Surg 1989;22:505–15.
23. Dini D, Del Mastro L, Gozza A, et al. The role of pneumatic compression in the treatment of postmastectomy lymphedema. A randomized phase III study. Ann Oncol 1998; 9:187–90.

24. Petrek JA, Pressman PI, Smith RA. Lymphedema: current issues in research and management. CA Cancer J Clin 2000;50:292–307; quiz 308–11.
25. Sperti C, Pasquali C, Ferronato A, Pedrazzoli S. Median pancreatectomy for tumors of the neck and body of the pancreas. J Am Coll Surg 2000;190:711–6.
26. Warshaw AL, Rattner DW, Fernandez-del Castillo C, Z'Graggen K. Middle segment pancreatectomy: a novel technique for conserving pancreatic tissue. Arch Surg 1998;133:327–31.
27. Yamaguchi K, Yokohata K, Ohkido M, et al. Which is less invasive—distal pancreatectomy or segmental resection? Int Surg 2000;85:297–302.
28. Lemaire E, O'Toole D, Sauvanet A, et al. Functional and morphological changes in the pancreatic remnant following pancreaticoduodenectomy with pancreaticogastric anastomosis. Br J Surg 2000;87:434–8.
29. Jang JY, Kim SW, Park SJ, Park YH. Comparison of the functional outcome after pylorus-preserving pancreatoduodenectomy: pancreatogastrostomy and pancreatojejunostomy. World J Surg 2002;26:366–71.
30. van Berge Henegouwen MI, Moojen TM, van Gulik TM, et al. Postoperative weight gain after standard Whipple's procedure versus pylorus-preserving pancreatoduodenectomy: the influence of tumour status. Br J Surg 1998; 85:922–6.
31. Crucitti F, Doglietto G, Bellantone R, et al. Digestive and nutritional consequences of pancreatic resections. The classical vs the pylorus-sparing procedure. Int J Pancreatol 1995;17:37–45.
32. Andersen HB, Baden H, Brahe NE, Burcharth F. Pancreaticoduodenectomy for periampullary adenocarcinoma. J Am Coll Surg 1994;179:545–52.
33. Jang JY, Kim SW, Han JK, et al. Randomized prospective trial of the effect of induced hypergastrinemia on the prevention of pancreatic atrophy after pancreatoduodenectomy in humans. Ann Surg 2003;237:522–9.
34. Kozuschek W, Reith HB, Waleczek H, et al. A comparison of long term results of the standard Whipple procedure and the pylorus preserving pancreatoduodenectomy. J Am Coll Surg 1994;178:443–53.
35. Zerbi A, Balzano G, Patuzzo R, et al. Comparison between pylorus-preserving and Whipple pancreatoduodenectomy. Br J Surg 1995;82:975–9.
36. Tran KT, Smeenk HG, van Eijck CH, et al. Pylorus preserving pancreaticoduodenectomy versus standard Whipple procedure: a prospective, randomized, multicenter analysis of 170 patients with pancreatic and periampullary tumors. Ann Surg 2004;240:738–45.
37. Delchier JC, Soule JC. BT-PABA test with plasma PABA measurements: evaluation of sensitivity and specificity. Gut 1983;24:318–25.
38. Hall RI, Rhodes M, Isabel-Martinez L, et al. Pancreatic exocrine function after a sutureless pancreatico-jejunostomy following pancreaticoduodenectomy. Br J Surg 1990;77: 83–5.
39. Goetze JP, Nielsen FC, Burcharth F, Rehfeld JF. Closing the gastrin loop in pancreatic carcinoma: coexpression of gastrin and its receptor in solid human pancreatic adenocarcinoma. Cancer 2000;88:2487–94.
40. Smith JP, Fantaskey AP, Liu G, Zagon IS. Identification of gastrin as a growth peptide in human pancreatic cancer. Am J Physiol 1995;268(1 Pt 2):R135–41.
41. Brett BT, Smith SC, Bouvier CV, et al. Phase II study of anti-gastrin-17 antibodies, raised to G17DT, in advanced pancreatic cancer. J Clin Oncol 2002;20:4225–31.
42. Permert J, Ihse I, Jorfeldt L, et al. Pancreatic cancer is associated with impaired glucose metabolism. Eur J Surg 1993;159:101–7.
43. Permert J, Ihse I, Jorfeldt L, et al. Improved glucose metabolism after subtotal pancreatectomy for pancreatic cancer. Br J Surg 1993;80:1047–50.
44. Wittingen J, Frey CF. Islet concentration in the head, body, tail and uncinate process of the pancreas. Ann Surg 1974;179:412–4.
45. Ahren B, Andren-Sandberg A. Capacity to secrete islet hormones after subtotal pancreatectomy for pancreatic cancer. Eur J Surg 1993;159:223–7.
46. Anderson TJ, Lamb J, Alexander F, et al. Comparative pathology of prevalent and incident cancers detected by breast screening. Edinburgh Breast Screening Project. Lancet 1986;1:519–23.
47. Ishikawa O, Ohigashi H, Eguchi H, et al. Long-term follow-up of glucose tolerance function after pancreaticoduodenectomy: comparison between pancreaticogastrostomy and pancreaticojejunostomy. Surgery 2004;136:617–23.
48. Svennevig JL, Vetvik K, Bernstein O, Sigstad H. Dumping following partial gastrectomy. Ann Chir Gynaecol 1977; 66:4–7.
49. Hotta T, Taniguchi K, Kobayashi Y, et al. Postoperative evaluation of pylorus-preserving procedures compared with conventional distal gastrectomy for early gastric cancer. Surg Today 2001;31:774–9.
50. Sirinek KR, O'Dorisio TM, Howe B, McFee AS. Neurotensin, vasoactive intestinal peptide, and Roux-en-Y gastrojejunostomy. Their role in the dumping syndrome. Arch Surg 1985;120:605–9.
51. Gray JL, Debas HT, Mulvihill SJ. Control of dumping symptoms by somatostatin analogue in patients after gastric surgery. Arch Surg 1991;126:1231–5; discussion 1235–6.
52. Geer RJ, Richards WO, O'Dorisio TM, et al. Efficacy of octreotide acetate in treatment of severe postgastrectomy dumping syndrome. Ann Surg 1990;212:678–87.
53. Tulassay Z, Tulassay T, Gupta R, Cierny G. Long acting somatostatin analogue in dumping syndrome. Br J Surg 1989;76:1294–5.
54. Allan JG, Russell RI. Cholestyramine in treatment of postvagotomy diarrhoea—double-blind controlled trial. Br Med J 1977;1:674–6.
55. Mackie CR, Jenkins SA, Hartley MN. Treatment of severe postvagotomy/postgastrectomy symptoms with the somatostatin analogue octreotide. Br J Surg 1991;78: 1338–43.
56. Mackie C, Hulks G, Cuschieri A. Enterogastric reflux and gastric clearance of refluxate in normal subjects and in patients with and without bile vomiting following peptic ulcer surgery. Ann Surg 1986;204:537–42.
57. Madura J. Primary bile reflux gastritis: which treatment is better, Roux-en-Y or biliary diversion? Presented at the 42nd Annual Meeting of the Midwest Surgical Association; 1999 August 15–18; Galena, IL.
58. Nicolai JJ, Speelman P, Tytgat GN, van der Stadt J. Comparison of the combination of cholestyramine/alginates with placebo in the treatment of postgastrectomy biliary reflux gastritis. Eur J Clin Pharmacol 1981;21:189–94.
59. Nicolai JJ, van de Stadt J, Tytgat GN. Double-blind crossover trial of prostaglandin E2 in postgastrectomy reflux gastritis. Dig Dis Sci 1986;31:1281–6.
60. Meshkinpour H, Elashoff J, Stewart H, Sturdevant RAL. Effect of cholestyramine on symptoms of reflux gastritis-randomized, double-blind, crossover study. Gastroenterology 1977;73:441–3.
61. Buch KL, Weinstein WM, Hill TA, et al. Sucralfate therapy in patients with symptoms of alkaline reflux gastritis. A randomized, double-blind study. Am J Med 1985; 79(2C):49–54.
62. Eckhauser FE, Conrad M, Knol JA, et al. Safety and long-term durability of completion gastrectomy in 81 patients with postsurgical gastroparesis syndrome. Am Surg 1998;64:711–6; discussion 716–7.
63. Gustavsson S, Ilstrup DM, Morrison P, Kelly KA. Roux-Y stasis syndrome after gastrectomy. Am J Surg 1988; 155:490–4.
64. Bradley EL, Isaacs J, Hersh T, et al. Nutritional consequences of total gastrectomy. Ann Surg 1975;182:415–29.
65. Collard JM, Otte JB, Reynaert M, Kestens PJ. Quality of life three years or more after esophagectomy for cancer. J Thorac Cardiovasc Surg 1992;104:391–4.
66. McLarty AJ, Deschamps C, Trastek VF, et al. Esophageal resection for cancer of the esophagus: long-term function and quality of life. Ann Thorac Surg 1997;63:1568–72.
67. Pierie JP, Goedegebuure S, Schuerman FA, Leguit P. Relation between functional dysphagia and vocal cord palsy after transhiatal oesophagectomy. Eur J Surg 2000;166: 207–9.
68. Pierie JP, de Graaf PW, Poen H, et al. Incidence and management of benign anastomotic stricture after cervical oesophagogastrostomy. Br J Surg 1993;80:471–4.
69. Orringer MB, Marshall B, Iannettoni MD. Transhiatal esophagectomy: clinical experience and refinements. Ann Surg 1999;230:392–400; discussion 400–393.
70. Finley FJ, Lamy A, Clifton J, et al. Gastrointestinal function following esophagectomy for malignancy. Am J Surg 1995;169:471–5.
71. Hulscher JB, van Sandick JW, Devriese PP, et al. Vocal cord paralysis after subtotal oesophagectomy. Br J Surg 1999; 86:1583–7.
72. Baba M, Natsugoe S, Shimada M, et al. Does hoarseness of voice from recurrent nerve paralysis after esophagectomy for carcinoma influence patient quality of life? J Am Coll Surg 1999;188:231–6.
73. Kraus DH, Ali MK, Ginsberg RJ, et al. Vocal cord medialization for unilateral paralysis associated with intrathoracic malignancies. J Thorac Cardiovasc Surg 1996;111:334–9; discussion 339–41.
74. Aly A, Jamieson GG. Reflux after oesophagectomy. Br J Surg 2004;91:137–41.
75. Hill AD, Walsh TN, Hamilton D, et al. Erythromycin improves emptying of the denervated stomach after oesophagectomy. Br J Surg 1993;80:879–81.
76. Collard JM, Romagnoli R, Otte JB, Kestens PJ. Erythromycin enhances early postoperative contractility of the denervated whole stomach as an esophageal substitute. Ann Surg 1999;229:337–43.
77. Rabbani F, Stapleton AM, Kattan MW, et al. Factors predicting recovery of erections after radical prostatectomy. J Urol 2000;164:1929–34.
78. Quinlan DM, Epstein JI, Carter BS, Walsh PC. Sexual function following radical prostatectomy: influence of preservation of neurovascular bundles. J Urol 1991;145: 998–1002.
79. Catalona WJ, Carvalhal GF, Mager DE, Smith DS. Potency, continence and complication rates in 1,870 consecutive radical retropubic prostatectomies. J Urol 1999;162: 433–8.
80. Cosimelli M, Mannella E, Giannarelli D, et al. Nerve-sparing surgery in 302 resectable rectosigmoid cancer patients: genitourinary morbidity and 10-year survival. Dis Colon Rectum 1994;37(2 Suppl):S42–6.
81. Danzi M, Ferulano GP, Abate S, Califano G. Male sexual function after abdominoperineal resection for rectal cancer. Dis Colon Rectum 1983;26:665–8.
82. Fazio VW, Fletcher J, Montague D. Prospective study of the effect of resection of the rectum on male sexual function. World J Surg 1980;4:149–52.
83. Banerjee AK. Sexual dysfunction after surgery for rectal cancer. Lancet 1999;353:1900–2.
84. Litwin MS, Flanders SC, Pasta DJ, et al. Sexual function and bother after radical prostatectomy or radiation for prostate cancer: multivariate quality-of-life analysis from CaPSURE. Cancer of the Prostate Strategic Urologic Research Endeavor. Urology 1999;54:503–8.
85. Balslev I, Harling H. Sexual dysfunction following operation for carcinoma of the rectum. Dis Colon Rectum 1983;26: 785–8.
86. Wagner JR, Russo P. Urologic complications of major pelvic surgery. Semin Surg Oncol 2000;18:216–28.
87. Russo V, Traversari C, Verrecchia A, et al. Expression of the MAGE gene family in primary and metastatic human breast cancer: implications for tumor antigen-specific immunotherapy. Int J Cancer 1995;64:216–21.
88. Goldstein I, Lue TF, Padma-Nathan H, et al. Oral sildenafil in the treatment of erectile dysfunction. Sildenafil Study Group. N Engl J Med 1998;338:1397–404.
89. Lindsey I, George B, Kettlewell M, Mortensen N. Randomized, double-blind, placebo-controlled trial of sildenafil (Viagra) for erectile dysfunction after rectal excision for cancer and inflammatory bowel disease. Dis Colon Rectum 2002;45:727–32.
90. Zippe CD, Jhaveri FM, Klein EA, et al. Role of Viagra after radical prostatectomy. Urology 2000;55:241–5.
91. Alboni P, Bettiol K, Fuca G, et al. Sexual activity with and without the use of sildenafil: risk of cardiovascular events in patients with heart disease. Ital Heart J 2004;5:343–9.
92. Bambrick M, Fazio VW, Hull TL, Pucel G. Sexual function following restorative proctocolectomy in women. Dis Colon Rectum 1996;39:610–4.
93. Corney RH, Crowther ME, Everett H, et al. Psychosexual dysfunction in women with gynaecological cancer following radical pelvic surgery. Br J Obstet Gynaecol 1993; 100:73–8.
94. Platell CF, Thompson PJ, Makin GB. Sexual health in women following pelvic surgery for rectal cancer. Br J Surg 2004;91:465–8.
95. Berman JR, Berman LA, Lin H, et al. Effect of sildenafil on subjective and physiologic parameters of the female sexual response in women with sexual arousal disorder. J Sex Marital Ther 2001;27:411–20.
96. Berman JR, Berman LA, Toler SM, et al. Safety and efficacy of sildenafil citrate for the treatment of female sexual arousal disorder: a double-blind, placebo controlled study. J Urol 2003;170(6 Pt 1):2333–8.
97. Basson R, McInnes R, Smith MD, et al. Efficacy and safety of sildenafil citrate in women with sexual dysfunction

associated with female sexual arousal disorder. J Womens Health Gend Based Med 2002;11:367–77.

98. Rasmussen OO, Petersen IK, Christiansen J. Anorectal function following low anterior resection. Colorectal Dis 2003;5:258–61.

99. Nesbakken A, Nygaard K, Lunde OC. Mesorectal excision for rectal cancer: functional outcome after low anterior resection and colorectal anastomosis without a reservoir. Colorectal Dis 2002;4:172–6.

100. Lee SJ, Park YS. Serial evaluation of anorectal function following low anterior resection of the rectum. Int J Colorectal Dis 1998;13:241–6.

101. Williamson ME, Lewis WG, Finan PJ, et al. Recovery of physiologic and clinical function after low anterior resection of the rectum for carcinoma: myth or reality? Dis Colon Rectum 1995;38:411–8.

102. Kim NK, Lim DJ, Yun SH, et al. Ultralow anterior resection and coloanal anastomosis for distal rectal cancer: functional and oncological results. Int J Colorectal Dis 2001;16:234–7.

103. Fichera A, Michelassi F. Long-term prospective assessment of functional results after proctectomy with coloanal anastomosis. J Gastrointest Surg 2001;5:153–7.

104. Paty PB, Enker WE, Cohen AM, et al. Long-term functional results of coloanal anastomosis for rectal cancer. Am J Surg 1994;167:90–4; discussion 94–5.

105. Havenga K, Maas CP, DeRuiter MC, et al. Avoiding long-term disturbance to bladder and sexual function in pelvic surgery, particularly with rectal cancer. Semin Surg Oncol 2000;18:235–43.

106. Maas CP, Moriya Y, Steup WH, et al. A prospective study on radical and nerve-preserving surgery for rectal cancer in the Netherlands. Eur J Surg Oncol 2000;26:751–7.

107. Junginger T, Kneist W, Heintz A. Influence of identification and preservation of pelvic autonomic nerves in rectal cancer surgery on bladder dysfunction after total mesorectal excision. Dis Colon Rectum 2003;46:621–8.

108. Sugihara K, Moriya Y, Akasu T, Fujita S. Pelvic autonomic nerve preservation for patients with rectal carcinoma. Oncologic and functional outcome. Cancer 1996;78:1871–80.

109. Leveckis J, Boucher NR, Parys BT, et al. Bladder and erectile dysfunction before and after rectal surgery for cancer. Br J Urol 1995;76:752–6.

110. Mundy AR. Metabolic complications of urinary diversion. Lancet 1999;353:1813–4.

111. Nurse DE, Mundy AR. Metabolic complications of cystoplasty. Br J Urol 1989;63:165–70.

112. Stein R, Fisch M, Andreas J, et al. Whole-body potassium and bone mineral density up to 30 years after urinary diversion. Br J Urol 1998;82:798–803.

113. Stewart M. Urinary diversion and bowel cancer. Ann R Coll Surg Engl 1986;68:98–102.

114. Duchesne JC, Wang YZ, Weintraub SL, et al. Stoma complications: a multivariate analysis. Am Surg 2002;68:961–6; discussion 966.

115. Park JJ, Del Pino A, Orsay CP, et al. Stoma complications: the Cook County Hospital experience. Dis Colon Rectum 1999;42:1575–80.

116. Carlsen E, Bergan A. Technical aspects and complications of end-ileostomies. World J Surg 1995;19:632–6.

117. Christie PM, Knight GS, Hill GL. Comparison of relative risks of urinary stone formation after surgery for ulcerative colitis: conventional ileostomy vs. J-pouch. A comparative study. Dis Colon Rectum 1996;39:50–4.

118. Kennedy HJ, Fletcher EW, Truelove SC. Urinary stones in subjects with a permanent ileostomy. Br J Surg 1982;69:661–4.

119. Arai K, Fukushima T, Sugita A, Shimada H. Urinary changes in patients following restorative proctocolectomy. Surg Today 1997;27:801–5.

120. Giunchi F, Balbi B, Giulianini G, Cacciaguerra G. Cholelithiasis and urolithiasis in ileostomy patients. Ital J Surg Sci 1989;19:37–40.

121. Loser C, Mollgaard A, Folsch UR. Faecal elastase 1: a novel, highly sensitive, and specific tubeless pancreatic function test. Gut. 1996 Oct;39(4):580–586.

Collateral Damage Associated with Chemotherapy

Anne S. Tsao, MD
David J. Stewart, MD

A major problem with chemotherapy is the occurrence of marked toxic effects that patients experience. Extensive research has been conducted to understand the pathogenesis of toxic effects so that they might be prevented; however, acute intratherapeutic effects of nausea, vomiting, diarrhea, and myelosuppression remain limiting factors in cancer treatment. Long-term sequelae of the chemotherapy can include infertility, carcinogenesis, and damage to the heart, kidney, lung, and nervous system. Standardized systemic symptoms are helpful for uniform management of patients on clinical trials and for initiation of appropriate dose adjustments. Several toxicity definition and grading systems are in use, largely in cooperative groups; one used frequently is the National Cancer Institute (NCI) Common Toxicity Criteria for Adverse Events (version 3) (<http://www.fda.gov/cder/cancer/toxicityframe.htm>), which grades each symptom on a scale of 0 to 4 by severity. A dose-limiting toxicity (DLT) is the clinical toxic response that determines the maximum tolerated dose.[1]

Additional factors to consider when evaluating toxicities of chemotherapy include determining whether they are acute or chronic and whether they are cumulative. The DLT of a single agent may differ depending on the method of administration (intravenous bolus or infusion over hours).[1] Treatment schedule, route of administration, other agents' used, and patient comorbidities can also affect a patient's tolerance to chemotherapy. In addition, such patient characteristics as age, renal and hepatic function, pharmacogenomic status, and previous amount of therapy are major contributors to patient tolerance of therapy.[1–3]

This chapter provides a general overview of both the systemic and nonsystemic toxic effects of cancer chemotherapies, along with a discussion of the various classes of chemotherapy and their mechanisms of action.

Systemic Toxic Effects

Myelosuppression

One of the most common DLTs of chemotherapy is hematopoietic toxicity causing myelosuppression.[1] The severity of any toxic effect is dependent on the drug type, dose and bioavailability, duration of exposure, and frequency of administration.[4] Because most cytotoxic chemotherapy agents target proliferating cells, most hematopoietic progenitor cells (mature granulocytes, erythrocytes, and thrombocytes) that are in the peripheral circulation are affected by the therapy. Pluripotent hematopoietic stem cells do not divide frequently, and in normal cases, stem cells will produce one daughter cell that differentiates and another daughter cell that becomes another stem cell.[5] Bone marrow stem cells may also be affected, especially by alkylating agents, which can result in an even longer period of myelosuppression.[1,4] High doses of chemotherapy will prolong the bone marrow recovery period, and studies have found that a decrease in granulocyte-macrophage colony-forming unit cells can be seen for up to 3 years after therapy.[4]

Different chemotherapy agents will affect a patient's bone marrow reserve differently. These agents target different phases of the cell cycle (Figure 1). For example, alkylating agents cause 1 to 4 weeks of myelosuppression, with recovery within 4 weeks, whereas antimetabolite agents will nadir granulocyte counts within 1 week, with recovery approximately 3 weeks later. Myelosuppression can also be delayed by agents such as mitomycin-C, nitrosoureas, and procarbazine, which depress granulocyte counts 3 to 4 weeks after treatment.[4]

Anemia is reported in up to 90% of patients receiving chemotherapy. Clinical symptoms include fatigue, lethargy, weakness, irritability, dyspnea, and reduced performance status.[6] The severity of chemotherapy-induced anemia depends on the dose of the agent, the duration of treatment, and the patient's bone marrow reserve.[6,7] Younger patients with more cellular bone marrow are likely to tolerate chemotherapy better than older patients. Patients with iron deficiency anemia or marked bone marrow infiltration by tumor will have more complicated cases of chemotherapy-induced anemia.[7] Chemotherapy may also complicate preexisting anemia; anemia owing to chronic disease is associated with erythroid hypoplasia of the bone marrow, and chemotherapy agents compound the problem by delaying the maturation of the erythroid lineage cells.[8] Treatment for anemia consists of red blood cell transfusions, administration of recombinant erythropoietin, and vitamin supplementation and should be initiated based on the clinical presentation.[9,10] In general, patients who are symptomatic and have hemoglobin levels below 10 g/dL should receive intervention.[11] Patients with a cardiac history of angina may require more aggressive therapy. Iron supplementation should be initiated if the ferritin level drops below 100 ng/mL.[7] Cisplatin may cause anemia through reduced erythropoietin production resulting from the agent's nephrotoxicity.

Thrombocytopenia occurs 8 to 14 days after chemotherapy and can occur concomitantly with neutropenia.[7] As a general rule, chemotherapy should be delayed if platelets are below 100,000/mm^3. Thrombocytopenia places patients at increased risk of bleeding, but spontaneous bleeding rarely occurs when the platelet level is above 20,000/μL.[7] Patients who are not bleeding should still receive platelet transfusions when their platelet counts drop below 10,000/mm^3. Other factors that complicate thrombocytopenia include hypersplenism, concomitant use of antiplatelet and anticoagulant medications, and sepsis. Thrombocytopenia has been reported as a DLT for gemcitabine, carboplatin, darcarbazine, 5-fluorouracil (5-FU), lomustine, mitomycin, and thiotepa. Cumulative effects from carmustine, fludarabine, lomustine, mitomycin-C, streptozocin, and thiotepa have also been reported,

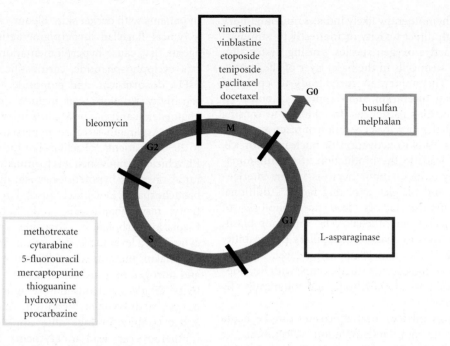

Table 1 Emetogenicity of Commonly Used Chemotherapy Agents

High
  Cisplatin
  HD cyclophosphamide
  HD carmustine
  Dacarbazine
  Dactinomycin

Moderate
  SD cyclophosphamide
  SD carmustine
  Doxorubicin
  Cytarabine
  Irinotecan
  Ifosfamide
  Melphalan
  Carboplatin
  Mitoxantrone

Low
  5-Fluorouracil
  Methotrexate
  Gemcitabine
  Etoposide
  Paclitaxel
  Docetaxel
  Topotecan

Minimal
  Bleomycin
  Capecitabine
  Vinca alkaloids

Adapted from Grunberg S.[15]
HD = high dose; SD = standard dose.

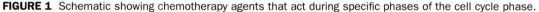

FIGURE 1 Schematic showing chemotherapy agents that act during specific phases of the cell cycle phase.

and agents that have cumulative bone marrow toxicity are also more likely to cause thrombocytopenia than are agents with relatively little cumulative effect.

Neutropenia is a common DLT chemotherapy. Neutrophils have life spans of 6 to 8 hours after their release from the bone marrow and are the initial responders to infection and development of a host reaction to infectious agents. Neutropenia occurs within 5 to 14 days after chemotherapy, with recovery of counts in 721 days.[7] Neutropenia is defined as an absolute neutrophil count (ANC) less than 1,500/mm^3 by some authors, whereas others define it as a count less than 1,000 or 500/mm^3. The risk of infection rises as the neutrophil count falls below 1,000/mm^3 and is inversely related to the neutrophil count during neutropenia. As a general guideline, chemotherapy should be withheld if the ANC drops below 1,000 to 1,500/mm^3. The NCI toxicity grading scale quantifies neutropenic toxic responses on a scale of 1 to 4. A grade 4 or life-threatening, toxic response is defined as an ANC less than 500/mm^3.

Patients with hematologic malignancies are at higher risk of neutropenic complications owing to the underlying disease.[12] Febrile neutropenia is considered a life-threatening oncologic emergency and requires immediate intervention with antibiotics and evaluation for sepsis.[12] Febrile neutropenia has been defined in several ways. For example, some authors have defined it as a temperature greater than 38.2°C (101°F) with a granulocyte count of less than 1,000/mm^3, whereas others have defined it as fever greater than 38.2°C for over 1 hour associated with a grade 4 ANC.[1] Neutropenia can be treated using human granulocyte colony-stimulating factor (CSFs).[12] The current American Society of

Clinical Oncology (ASCO) guidelines recommend primary prophylactic use of CSFs when the anticipated risk of febrile neutropenia exceeds 40% in patients who are at high risk of febrile neutropenia or infection. Patients who have had one episode of febrile neutropenia after chemotherapy are considered high risk and should receive CSF support during subsequent cycles of chemotherapy unless the chemotherapy dose is reduced. However, CSFs have not shown any benefit in disease-free or overall survival, and their use in febrile patients receiving chemotherapy is not recommended except in a high-risk situation.[13]

Gastrointestinal Symptoms

The gastrointestinal toxic effects of chemotherapy include nausea, vomiting, diarrhea, and mucositis. Chemotherapy-induced nausea and vomiting (CINV) may markedly affect a patient's quality of life during chemotherapy and can be a factor in determining a patient's ability to tolerate further treatment. The risk factors for CINV include a high level of chemotherapy emetogenicity (Table 1), young patient age, female gender, history of pregnancy-related or motion sickness, nausea, patient anxiety, history of CINV with previous chemotherapy, and low social functioning. Patients with a history of heavy alcohol use appear to have a reduced risk of CINV.[14–16]

Acute CINV (defined as CINV occurring within the first 24 hours after chemotherapy administration) arises when chemotherapy damages enterochromaffin cells in the gastrointestinal tract, resulting in the release of serotonin. The serotonin binds to 5-hydroxytryptamine$_3$ (5-HT$_3$) receptors in vagal afferent nerves and the chemoreceptor trigger zone, activating the vomiting

center in the medulla lateral reticular formation.[15] The release of dopamine and its interaction with dopamine receptors play a lesser role than the serotonin pathway. CINV may also be "delayed" or "anticipatory."[15] Delayed emesis is defined as emesis occurring after 24 hours and maintained for several hours (sometimes 120 hours or more) afterward and is thought to be mediated by substance P neurokinin-1(NK-1) receptor pathways.[15,17] NK-1 receptors line the intestinal tract and the nucleus tractus solitarius of the brain. Substance P, a tachykinin, binds to the NK-1 receptors at the nucleus tractus solitarius and induces vomiting.[16] Substance P is released in two phases, first from the direct cytotoxic effect of chemotherapy on the chemoreceptor zone and then from the damaged enterochromaffin cells in the gastrointestinal tract. CINV is also regulated by dopamine 2 receptors. Dopamine receptors are located in the chemoreceptor trigger zone, and blockade enables some control over emesis.

Anticipatory nausea is nausea that occurs prior to chemotherapy administration and is a conditioned response to chemotherapy. In this setting, antiemetic prophylaxis is less effective and behavioral modification is recommended.[15] Two additional minor categories of CINV are reported: breakthrough CINV and refractory

CINV.[16] Breakthrough CINV occurs in patients who are receiving preventive antiemetic therapy. Patients with refractory CINV develop adverse symptoms after initially responding to antiemetic therapy during the first few cycles of chemotherapy.

If effective antiemetics are not given, acute CINV can occur in up to 98% of patients receiving highly emetogenic agents, such as cisplatin. Delayed CINV has been reported in up to 61% of patients. The incidence is lower for less emetogenic agents.[15] Antiemetic regimens for acute CINV include 5-HT$_3$ receptor antagonists in combination with corticosteroids. Corticosteroids are thought to prevent emesis by prostaglandin antagonism, although the exact mechanism is unclear. Delayed CINV requires additional therapy with steroids, possibly 5-HT$_3$ antagonists, dopamine 2 receptor antagonists such as (metoclopramide), and NK-1 receptor antagonists. Control of acute CINV may decrease the incidence of delayed CINV.[15,16]

Diarrhea, if prolonged and severe, can lead to dehydration and malabsorption. Chemotherapy-induced diarrhea is graded by the number of additional bowel movements above a normal baseline. The pathophysiology of chemotherapy-induced diarrhea is not clear but is partly due to chemotherapy-induced damage to intestinal crypt cells, which divide rapidly, and a delay in regeneration of the intestinal villi and intestinal absorptive surface. Changes in absorptive capability lead to diarrhea by altering the osmotic gradient in the intestine. Inflammatory cytokines, which promote secretion of intestinal fluids and electrolytes from the crypt cells, are also secreted.[18] Chemotherapy itself will occasionally lead to the development of *Clostridium difficile*–induced diarrhea.

Agents that commonly cause diarrhea include 5-FU, irinotecan, methotrexate, docetaxel, and doxorubicin. Diarrhea is dose limiting in irinotecan and 5-FU combinations. Patients who develop chemotherapy-induced diarrhea should modify their diet to avoid greasy, spicy, or fried foods and any milk products. The BRAT diet (bananas, rice, applesauce, and toast) with clear liquids is recommended until the diarrhea lessens.[18] Maintaining fluid intake is critical to replace the volume lost and can require up to 3 to 4 L of fluid per day. Antidiarrheal agents such as loperamide, diphenoxylate or atropine, and, in severe cases, octreotide can be used.[18]

Mucositis can occur at any mucosal surface between the mouth and the rectum or vagina and is characterized by inflammation of the mucosa. The patients most likely to develop mucositis include those undergoing high-dose chemotherapy with hematopoietic stem cell transplantation or patients with head and neck cancer receiving concomitant radiotherapy. The agents most likely to cause mucositis are methotrexate, etoposide, 5-FU, and irinotecan.[19]

Chemotherapy likely induces mucosal injury through direct toxicity or indirectly by stimulating reactive oxygen species, causing destruction of the stem cells in the basal layer of the epithelium. This injury, in turn, leads to epithelial thinning, ulceration, and secondary colonization by infectious pathogens. In addition to causing epithelial injury, the generation of reactive oxygen species leads to activation of nuclear factor κB, which leads to the production of proinflammatory cytokines, tumor necrosis factor, interleukin-6, and platelet-activating factor. Additional transcription factors lead to apoptosis of submucosal endothelial cells and fibroblasts, which leads to changes in capillary permeability and the submucosal supportive layer. Mucosal injury with ulceration then occurs, with development of a pseudomembrane and colonization by bacteria.[20]

Stomatitis or oral mucositis can be acute (with mucosal inflammation, ulceration, or bleeding) or chronic (with xerostomia, taste alterations, trismus, or soft tissue and bone necrosis).[20] With chemotherapy-induced stomatitis, the injury occurs within 1 to 2 weeks of treatment. The risk factors for development of stomatitis include poor nutritional status, alterations in oral flora, poor salivary function, old age, male gender, and the presence of inflammation.[20,21] Symptoms will generally improve with the restoration of bone marrow products. Several agents are under investigation to prevent oral mucositis, among them amifostine, benzydamine, and *N*-acetylcysteine.[20] Taste alterations can occur, with more perception of bitterness, a metallic taste, or increased perception of sweetness. The agents that most commonly affect taste perception are cyclophosphamide, dacarbazine, doxorubicin, 5-FU, levamisole, methotrexate, nitrogen mustard, cisplatin, and vincristine. Esophagitis may have symptoms of dysphagia, odynophagia, and epigastric pain. Substernal symptoms indicate worsening esophagitis. Previous or concurrent radiation will worsen the effects of chemotherapy. Dactinomycin, doxorubicin, and gemcitabine may markedly potentiate radiation injury to the esophagus, whereas 5-FU, hydroxyurea, procarbazine, and vinblastine have a lesser potentiation effect.[22] Severe esophagitis may require placement of a feeding tube. Vaginitis is uncommon but can occur 3 to 5 days after therapy and resolve within 7 to 10 days. Superimposed *Candida* infections may complicate esophagitis and vaginitis.

Skin Changes

Chemotherapy can induce skin hyperpigmentation, hypersensitivity, acral erythema, pruritus, photosensitivity, alopecia, nail pigmentation or Beau's lines, and onycholysis. Hyperpigmentation can be seen in the skin, nails, and mucous membranes and tends to be more prominent in patients with darker skin. Bleomycin can cause a typical flagellate hyperpigmentation.[23] Other agents that cause hyperpigmentation are busulfan, cyclophosphamide, carmustine, irinotecan, 5-FU, doxorubicin, and etoposide. Skin hypersensitivity reactions can include urticaria and angioedema and can be accompanied by anaphylaxis. L-Asparaginase causes hypersensitivity in 10 to 20% of patients.[23] Paclitaxel or the Cremophor EL vehicle within which it is formulated can cause rapid onset of hypotension, rash, dyspnea, and bronchospasm. Docetaxel causes skin hypersensitivity, rash, anaphylaxis, and fluid retention. Cisplatin, carboplatin, etoposide, procarbazine, cytarabine, levamisole, topotecan, trimetrexate, melphalan, methotrexate, all-*trans* retinoic acid, and nitrogen mustard can also cause hypersensitivity. Single-agent busulfan, etoposide, procarbazine, hydroxyurea, bleomycin, methotrexate, and cytarabine or high-dose combination chemotherapy can lead to erythema multiforme. Skin desquamation, "hand-foot" syndrome, acral erythema, or erythrodysesthesia is typically associated with cytarabine, doxorubicin, 5-FU, paclitaxel, or docetaxel.[23] This reaction may increase with subsequent therapy, and the cause is unknown. Photosensitivity to ultraviolet light may be caused by 5-FU, dacarbazine, all-*trans* retinoic acid, vinblastine, and high-dose methotrexate.

Alopecia, or hair loss, is a common toxic effect and is often seen with trimetrexate, cyclophosphamide, doxorubicin, dactinomycin, daunorubicin, etoposide, idarubicin, ifosfamide, irinotecan, mechlorethamine, paclitaxel, topotecan, and vincristine. Milder hair loss is seen with bleomycin, carmustine, epirubicin, 5-FU, methotrexate, melphalan, mitomycin, mitoxantrone, teniposide, and vinorelbine. Hair is the most rapidly proliferating cell population in the body and is therefore susceptible to the effects of chemotherapy. Chemotherapy can also cause mitotic arrest and atrophy of the root bulb. Alopecia has been reported to be more severe when more highly lipophilic metabolites are used as these agents can penetrate the hair follicles more easily.[24] Chemotherapy also may decrease nail-bed growth in a similar manner and manifest as Beau's lines or onycholysis.

Cardiotoxic Effects

Cardiotoxicity may have immediate or delayed effects. Toxic effects can occur during or immediately after the chemotherapy infusion or within a few days or weeks. Acute toxicity can manifest as pericarditis, arrhythmias, electrocardiographic changes, and pump dysfunction and is likely to resolve once therapy is stopped. Chronic cardiotoxic effects occur months or years after therapy and can consist of nonreversible cardiomyopathy and congestive heart failure.[25,26]

Anthracyclines are the agents most often associated with acute and chronic cardiotoxic effects. Several risk factors are associated with a greater likelihood of cardiotoxic response: a higher cumulative dose, preexisting heart disease, older patient age, mediastinal irradiation, female gender, hypertension, high rate of administration, bolus administration, and combination chemotherapy (doxorubicin with trastuzumab or cyclophosphamide).[25,26] The exact mechanism of action is not proven, but the cardiotoxic effects of anthracyclines are suspected to result from the generation of free oxygen radicals and oxidative stress.[26] These free oxygen radicals are directly toxic to myocytes and lead to the loss of myocardial fibrils, mitochondrial changes, and apoptosis.[26–28] Unfortunately, anthracycline-induced cardiomyopathy is irreversible and carries a poor prognosis. Current recommendations for anthracycline use include limiting the cumulative dose (eg, to less than 550 mg/m² in the case of doxorubicin), prolonging the drug infusion time, and considering the use of liposomal formulations in high-risk patients. Dexrazoxane, an iron-chelating cardioprotectant, may sometimes be used during chemotherapy. However, this agent should be used only on selected patients as its effect on the antitumor efficacy of the anthracycline is unknown.[25]

High-dose cyclophosphamide has been associated with acute pericarditis, myocarditis, and congestive heart failure. Although rare, these side effects can be fatal.[26] The cardiotoxic effects are not cumulative, and the risk factors include concurrent doxorubicin use, a higher dose (> 1.5 g/m²/d), and previous irradiation.[26] The toxic effect can be reversed once the agent is stopped. Patients treated with ifosfamide have similar findings, but up to 17% of them may experience cardiotoxicity.[25]

5-FU is cardiotoxic in 8% of patients. The effects generally occur within the first 72 hours of infusion and include angina, acute ischemia, arrhythmia, myocardial infarction, and even cardiac arrest.[25] Risk factors include concurrent radiation, preexisting heart disease, and the continuous infusion route of administration. Patients who have experienced cardiotoxicity should cease therapy immediately and should not be rechallenged.[25,26]

Paclitaxel can cause asymptomatic bradycardia, hypotension during infusion, and myocardial infarction or other arrhythmias (including atrioventricular conduction blocks, left bundle branch blocks, ventricular tachycardia, and atrial fibrillation).[25] Approximately 30% of patients develop asymptomatic bradycardia. Symptoms can be exacerbated with concomitant cisplatin administration.[26]

Neurotoxic Effects

The neurotoxic effects of chemotherapy can occur in the central nervous system (CNS) or peripheral nervous system (PNS). Cerebellar toxicity causing ataxia may be caused by 5-FU and by high-dose cytarabine. Potentially serious metabolic encephalopathy may occur with ifosfamide (particularly at high doses or in the presence of hypoalbuminemia) and is also seen occasionally with high-dose paclitaxel, cisplatin, nitrosoureas, and (rarely) cytarabine.[29] The encephalopathy is usually reversible after the cessation of therapy. In rare situations, carboplatin can cause cortical blindness, and cisplatin can lead to headaches, strokes, and seizures.[29]

High-dose systemic methotrexate given intravenously can cause a transient leukoencephalopathy, and intrathecal methotrexate can cause aseptic meningitis, with onset 2 to 4 hours after methotrexate injection and a duration of up to 3 days. In some cases, transverse myelopathy can develop,[29] but the risk may be reduced by ensuring that the saline used as a diluent is preservative free. A combination of delayed neurotoxic effects and leukoencephalopathy has been seen in patients who received high-dose methotrexate with brain irradiation. This condition carries a poor prognosis and is characterized by progressive dementia, gait disturbances, aphasia, hemiparesis, and death. The etiology is unclear.[29]

PNS toxic effects most frequently consist of a pure sensory neuropathy (possibly owing to the lack of a blood-nerve barrier in the dorsal root ganglion), with motor neuropathies being seen less frequently and cranial neuropathies rarely. With the vinca alkaloids and taxanes, the neuropathy is often acute, with symptoms coming on soon after drug exposure and frequently accompanied by neuralgic pain. Conversely, with cisplatin, the peripheral neuropathy is often delayed in onset and may not first appear until several weeks after the completion of therapy. The more severe the neuropathic symptoms, the lower the probability that they will resolve, although very gradual improvement may occur in some patients, even in the face of severe symptoms. In some cases, the neuropathy can be disabling, either owing to neuropathic pain or to the patient's inability to feel his or her feet (making it very difficult to maintain balance and walk in the dark).[29,30] Motor neuropathy, with weakness and loss of ankle reflexes, can be seen in patients with severe neuropathy, particularly those who received vinca alkaloids. Patients at higher risk of chemotherapy-related peripheral neuropathy include diabetics, patients with preexisting peripheral neuropathy, patients with hepatic insufficiency, and those receiving large cumulative doses of neurotoxic agents (eg, cisplatin doses > 400 mg/m²).[29] The degree of neurotoxicity varies within families of drugs, with vincristine being the most neurotoxic of the currently used vinca alkaloids and vinorelbine being the least neurotoxic, paclitaxel being more neurotoxic than docetaxel, and oxaliplatin being more neurotoxic than cisplatin, which, in turn, is more neurotoxic than carboplatin.[31] Cytarabine is rarely associated with painful sensory neuropathy, brachial plexopathy, and lateral rectus muscle palsy.[29] Neuropathic pain can occur in the PNS as axons regenerate. As the axons repair damaged endings, the threshold for stimuli is lowered and patients have an increased perception of sensitivity and pain. Another mechanism that has been suggested is abnormal sensitivity of the afferent neurons to the sympathetic nervous system response and noradrenergic agonist receptor binding. Also, tumor necrosis factor α is reported to activate nociceptors.[30]

In addition to causing sensory and motor neuropathies, vincristine (and, to a lesser extent, other neurotoxic agents) may cause autonomic neuropathy, manifesting as constipation, bladder atony, impotence, orthostatic hypotension, and an altered cardiac rate. Ototoxic effects consisting of tinnitus and high-frequency hearing loss owing to the loss of hairs in the organ of Corti may be caused by cisplatin and, to a lesser extent, by carboplatin. This condition is permanent, cumulative, and dose related and is more likely to occur in pediatric patients, in older patients with preexisting hearing loss, and in patients receiving cranial irradiation. Nitrogen mustard, vincristine, and vinblastine also have been reported to be ototoxic.[31] Nitrogen mustard causes loss of the outer hair cells in the cochlea and leads to irreversible sensorineural hearing loss and tinnitus. Vincristine and vinblastine are suspected to affect the organ of Corti sensory cells, and vincristine also affects the spiral ganglion cells and fibers.[31]

Pulmonary Toxic Effects

Pulmonary toxic effects may be irreversible and serious. Presenting clinical symptoms can include a nonproductive cough and dyspnea. Symptoms of progression are heralded by basilar rales, hypoxia, and cyanosis. Eventually, pulmonary insufficiency may become irreversible and death can occur.[32] Generally, destruction of endothelial cells is followed by pneumocyte necrosis, with altered pulmonary parenchyma and connective tissue, and obliteration of alveoli, manifested as restrictive lung disease and decreased diffusion capacity. Toxicity can manifest as diffuse alveolar damage (DAD), nonspecific interstitial pneumonia (NSIP), bronchiolitis obliterans organizing pneumonia (BOOP), or pulmonary hemorrhage.[33]

DAD can result from bleomycin, busulfan, carmustine, cyclophosphamide, mitomycin, or melphalan exposure. The acute phase of DAD occurs 1 week after exposure and manifests as alveolar and interstitial edema. Type II pneumocytes then proliferate, and pulmonary fibrosis develops a few weeks later. This can progress to a honeycomb lung. A drop in diffusing capacity is seen in severe cases.[33] NSIP is characterized by inflammation and hyperplastic type II pneumocytes. NSIP can occur in isolated patches of the lung and is associated with methotrexate, carmustine, and chlorambucil.[33]

BOOP is characterized by the proliferation of immature fibroblastic plugs located in the respiratory bronchioles, alveolar ducts, and spaces. Radiographs show bilateral peripheral opacities that are distributed equally throughout the lungs.[33] BOOP is associated with bleomycin, cyclophosphamide, and methotrexate. Pulmonary hemorrhage is uncommon but can result from high-dose cyclophosphamide, mitomycin, and cytarabine.[33]

Bleomycin causes lung toxicity in 3 to 5% of the patients who receive it.[34] Bleomycin is inactivated by hydrolase enzyme, which is not present in lung tissue; hence, bleomycin can accumulate in the lung. Endothelial cell type I pneumocytes are damaged early on, resulting in type II pneumocyte migration into alveolar spaces and interstitial changes. Fibroblasts then proliferate, causing pulmonary fibrosis.[33]

Cytarabine is directly toxic to pneumocytes and endothelial cells. Both cytarabine and mitomycin-C can cause capillary leak syndrome. This leads to pulmonary edema and respiratory failure. Cyclophosphamide can lead to alveolar hemorrhage and fibrin deposition. Carmustine inhibits lung glutathione disulfide reductase and can cause pulmonary toxic effects 6 weeks to 3 years after therapy. Among all patients exposed to carmustine, 20 to 30% will experience pulmonary toxicity. This percentage can increase to 50% when a cumulative dose above 1,500 mg/m[2] is given.[35] Methotrexate can damage type I pneumocytes and stimulate the formation of hyaline membranes.

Hepatotoxic Effects

Hepatotoxic agents can act by damaging the parenchymal cells. Also, obstruction of hepatic blood flow leads to hepatocellular necrosis, cholestasis, hepatitis, and veno-oclusive disease. Hepatotoxic effects range from elevation of hepatic enzymes to cirrhosis.[36] High-dose methotrexate, high-dose cytarabine, 5-FU, gemcitabine, irinotecan, and trimetrexate can all lead to elevated hepatic enzymes.[37] Fluorodeoxyuridine given intra-arterially causes chemical hepatitis and stricture of intra- and extrahepatic bile ducts. Irreversible biliary sclerosis also can develop.[36] Most chemotherapy agents are not hepatotoxic, however. Dose modifications of certain chemotherapy agents are recommended in some patients with hepatic compromise (see the Appendix).

Genitourinary Toxic Effects

Hemorrhagic cystitis can result from cyclophosphamide or ifosfamide therapy and can manifest as microscopic hematuria or frank bleeding. It is caused by binding of the metabolite acrolein to the bladder mucosa, resulting in inflammation and ulceration.[38,39] Cyclophosphamide induces microscopic hematuria in 10% of patients. Mesna, a uroprotectant, contains sulfhydryl, which binds and inactivates acrolein. Chronic complications, such as long-term cystitis, bladder fibrosis, contraction, and bladder cancer, can occur.[40–42] Ifosfamide is also metabolized to acrolein and requires mesna administration. Gemcitabine can cause microscopic hematuria and proteinuria.

Chemotherapy can cause both acute and chronic nephrotoxic effects, ranging from direct renal cell damage to obstructive nephropathy caused by metabolite precipitate formation.[43] Renal tubules are highly vulnerable to chemotherapy-induced damage because of their generous blood supply and their resorption of drugs, which prolongs exposure time. Tumor lysis syndrome can also lead to urate nephropathy and renal failure. A list of chemotherapy agents that require dose modification with renal compromise is found in the Appendix.

Cisplatin damages both proximal and distal tubules, with acute focal tubular necrosis of the distal convoluted tubules and collecting ducts. Casts can also form, with dilatation of the convoluted tubules.[42,44] Acute damage often occurs 3 to 21 hours after cisplatin administration and may be irreversible. Patients can have permanent decreases of 20 to 30% in glomerular filtration rates.[44] The histologic changes seen in chronic renal damage include thickening of the tubular basement membrane, interstitial fibrosis, and degeneration of the renal tubule epithelium. Magnesium wasting caused by changes in renal tubular function is a common chronic problem.[44] When tubular damage occurs, urinary excretion of endothelin 1 and Tamm-Horsfall protein may occur.

Ifosfamide can also cause widespread damage throughout the nephron. Often glomerular, proximal, and distal tubule damage is seen, along with renal tubular acidosis. Risk factors include a high cumulative dose, young patient age, concurrent use with cisplatin, and preexisting renal abnormalities.[43] The exact pathogenesis is not certain but is suspected to be related to the metabolite chloroacetaldehyde. Other agents that can cause renal dysfunction are lomustine and carmustine, which cause delayed renal failure; mitomycin-C, which causes microangiopathic hemolytic anemia; and gemcitabine, which causes hemolytic-uremic syndrome (HUS).

Thrombotic thrombocytopenic purpura–hemolytic-uremic syndrome (TTP-HUS) has been associated with mitomycin-C and gemcitabine. To a lesser degree, cisplatin, 5-FU, cytarabine, and daunorubicin have also been reported to cause TTP-HUS.[45] This condition is characterized by thrombocytopenia, anemia, neurologic deficits, renal failure, and fever. Although rare, it is a serious complication of chemotherapy. Mitomycin-C is thought to cause a decrease in prostacyclin, which leads to direct damage to the renal endothelium and platelet aggregation.[45]

Rheumatologic Toxic Effects

Arthralgias and myalgias commonly occur after chemotherapy. In general, the symptoms begin 1 to 2 days after therapy and last for 3 to 5 days. Taxanes have been reported to induce moderate to severe arthralgia and myalgia.[46,47] The mechanism of action is unclear, and supportive analgesia is the recommended treatment. Treatment should begin with nonsteroidal or codeine-containing agents and can be advanced to short courses of glucocorticoids, if needed, in more severe cases.[47]

Agents and Mechanisms of Action

Antimetabolite Toxic Effects

Antimetabolites are weakly acidic molecules that inhibit cellular metabolism. These agents are all cell cycle phase specific and act as false substrates for deoxyribonucleic acid (DNA) or ribonucleic acid (RNA) synthesis.[48] Methotrexate is an antifolate with activity against leukemia, lymphoma, breast cancer, head and neck cancer, osteogenic sarcoma, colon cancer, bladder cancer, and choriocarcinoma. This agent inhibits de novo purine and pyrimidine biosynthesis and demonstrates the majority of its activity during the S phase of the cell cycle. Methotrexate is a highly specific inhibitor of dihydrofolate reductase that regulates the intracellular tetrahydrofolate pool. When methotrexate becomes polyglutamated, inhibition of thymidylate synthase also occurs.[49]

The primary route of elimination for methotrexate is renal.[49] The methotrexate half-life may be prolonged and toxicity increased in patients with third-space fluid collections (ascites or pleural effusions, which ideally should be drained prior to methotrexate administration) and in bladder cancer with ileal conduits. Intrathecal administration of methotrexate to treat meningeal cancer can also result in myelosuppression or mucositis because therapeutic blood levels may be reached. If high-dose methotrexate with leucovorin rescue is used, patients must receive aggressive intravenous hydration and the urine should be kept at a pH > 7 for 24 to 48 hours by intravenous sodium bicarbonate to ensure that the methotrexate does not precipitate in renal tubules. Blood levels should be monitored every 24 hours starting 24 hours after high-dose methotrexate administration. Leucovorin must be given 24 hours after infusion and continued until the methotrexate blood level is < 50 nM.[49]

The DLT of intravenous methotrexate is myelosuppression. Another common toxic effect is mucositis, which occurs 3 to 7 days after systemic administration.[49] Renal toxic effects result from intratubular precipitation of methotrexate. Pneumonitis and hepatotoxicity may be seen with chronic daily oral administration.[49] High-dose methotrexate may cause acute encephalopathy (starting within 6 days and resolving 48 to 72 hours later), with paresis, aphasia, behavioral abnormalities, and seizures.[29,50] Chronic encephalopathy may develop 2 to 3 months after high-dose therapy, with dementia and paralysis.[29]

Intrathecal methotrexate may cause acute chemical arachnoiditis, subacute arachnoiditis, and chronic encephalopathy. Acute chemical arachnoiditis occurs immediately after intrathecal therapy. Patients present with nuchal rigidity, vomiting, fever, and inflammatory cell infiltrate in the cerebrospinal fluid. Subacute arachnoiditis occurs in 10% of patients after the third or fourth course of intrathecal therapy and causes cranial nerve palsies, seizures, motor paralysis, or coma.[29,51] Chronic encephalopathy occurs months to years after intrathecal therapy and presents as dementia, limb spasticity, and, in advanced cases, coma.[29]

5-FU is most commonly used in colorectal, breast, head and neck, pancreatic, gastric, anal, and esophageal cancers and hepatocellular carcinoma. Within the cell, 5-FU is converted into active metabolites that are incorporated into DNA or RNA or that inhibit DNA synthesis. 5-FU is eliminated by metabolic conversion by dihydropyrimidine dehydrogenase (DPD). Patients who are DPD deficient because of an inborn error of metabolism experience greater myelosuppression, gastrointestinal toxicity, and neurotoxicity and should not be rechallenged with 5-FU.[49,52] 5-FU is not usually markedly neurotoxic unless administered in the setting of DPD deficiency.[29]

5-FU has a short plasma half-life of 7 to 20 minutes and is generally administered by bolus injection daily for ≥ 5 consecutive days or as a multiday continuous intravenous infusion.[49] The main DLT is myelosuppression, which occurs more often with a bolus administration route. Mucositis, diarrhea, and hand-foot syndrome occur more often with continuous drug infusion. 5-FU occasionally causes angina, coronary vasospasm, electrocardiographic changes, cerebellar ataxia, or encephalopathy with somnolence, confusion, seizures, and, rarely, coma.[49,53] Ocular toxic effects include blepharitis, tear duct stenosis, and acute and chronic conjunctivitis.[54] With hepatic artery infusion, cholestatic jaundice with biliary sclerosis can occur.

5-FU interacts with several drugs, which increase its toxicity.[49] When methotrexate is given before 5-FU, 5-FU metabolite formation increases, as does toxicity. When 5-FU is combined with allopurinol, acute or subacute cerebellar dysfunction, visual disturbances, or seizures can occur.[29] Leucovorin enhances 5-FU's effect by forming a ternary complex with thymidylate synthase and the 5-FU metabolite 5-fluorodeoxyuridine monophosphate.

Capecitabine (Xeloda) is a third-generation oral fluoropyrimidine that is absorbed intact by the gastrointestinal mucosa and is activated by three successive enzymatic steps in the intestine, liver, and tumor (by thymidine phosphorylase). Thymidine phosphorylase is expressed at higher levels in tumor than in normal tissue.[49] Capecitabine is used in breast cancer and in cancers in which 5-FU has clinical activity. Capecitabine is contraindicated in patients with CrCl < 30 m/min and requires dose reductions in patients with moderate renal impairment. The most common toxic effects include hand-foot syndrome and diarrhea.[49,55] Infrequently, mucositis, myelosuppression, alopecia, and hyperbilirubinemia can be seen.[56] Drug interactions can occur with warfarin and phenytoin.

Cytarabine (Ara-C) is an arabinose nucleoside isolated from the *Cryptotethya crypta* sponge. It is commonly used in leukemias, non-Hodgkin's lymphoma, and meningeal carcinomatosis. Intracellular activation to the triphosphate ara-CTP is required for therapeutic activity. Cytarabine inhibits DNA synthesis and repair. Cytarabine has a short plasma half-life (7–20 minutes) and is excreted in the urine as an inactive metabolite.[49] Intrathecal cytarabine rarely causes encephalopathy, seizures, aseptic meningitis, and myelopathy.[29] The pathophysiology of action of intrathecal cytarabine neurotoxicity is unknown, but the risk appears to be reduced by using preservative-free saline as a diluent. Standard-dose intravenous cytarabine can lead to myelosuppression (neutropenia and thrombocytopenia), nausea, vomiting, diarrhea, intrahepatic cholestasis, and, rarely, pancreatitis. In rare cases, "Ara-C syndrome" can occur, characterized by an allergic reaction presenting as fever, myalgia, bone pain, skin rash, and conjunctivitis. High-dose cytarabine can cause severe myelosuppression, mucositis, cerebral and cerebellar dysfunction, noncardiogenic pulmonary edema, pneumonia, conjunctivitis, and hand-foot syndrome.[49]

Gemcitabine is a fluorine-substituted analogue of deoxycytidine and requires intracellular activation by deoxycytidine kinase. This agent has activity in cancers of the pancreas, lung, ovary, bladder, breast, and colon. Gemcitabine inhibits DNA synthesis and repair and alters RNA processing and messenger RNA translation. Gemcitabine also targets ribonucleotide reductase. Gemcitabine is metabolized in the liver, plasma, and peripheral tissues; most of the drug is excreted in the urine within 24 hours of administration. Common toxic effects of gemcitabine include myelosuppression (neutropenia and thrombocytopenia), flu-like syndrome, mild nausea and vomiting, mild proteinuria or hematuria, and transient elevations in liver function test values. An infusion reaction, characterized by acute onset of dyspnea, flushing, facial swelling, headache, or hypotension, occurs in a small proportion of patients. In addition, HUS has been reported.[49,57]

Purine Analogues

6-Thiopurines are used to treat acute leukemia. They inhibit de novo purine synthesis in the cell after conversion by hypoxanthine-guanine phosphoribosyltransferase to ribonucleoside monophosphates. At high doses, most of the agents are eliminated renally. The main toxic effects include myelosuppression (neutropenia and thrombocytopenia), nausea and vomiting, diarrhea, mucositis, cholestatic jaundice, and altered cell-mediated immunity.[49] Drug interactions can occur with allopurinol, which inhibits xanthine oxidase, an enzyme that regulates the thiopurine 6-mercaptopurine. A 6-mercaptopurine dose reduction of 50 to 75% from the standard single-agent dose is needed when this agent is used in conjunction with allopurinol. No dose reductions are needed, however, when using the related agent 6-thioguanine.

The fluorinated antimetabolite fludarabine enters cells and undergoes phosphorylation by deoxycytidine kinase to the triphosphate metabolite fludarabine triphosphate (F-Ara-ATP), which competes with deoxyadenosine triphosphate for incorporation into DNA. This process leads to the inhibition of DNA synthesis and repair and RNA processing. Fludarabine is used primarily in the lymphoid malignancies chronic lymphocytic leukemia and non-Hodgkin's lymphoma. The main route of elimination is renal. The main toxic effects include myelosuppression (neutropenia and thrombocytopenia), nausea and vomiting, diarrhea, fatigue, mild elevation in liver function test values, and fever. In addition, immune system abnormalities can occur.[49] Fludarabine can suppress CD4[+] and CD8[+] T cells, leaving patients with an increased risk of opportunistic infections.[58,59] It may be more than a year after treatment before CD4 counts normalize, and patients should receive trimethoprim-sulfamethoxazole prophylaxis against *Pneumocystis* pneumonia. In rare situations, autoimmune hemolytic anemia and thrombocytopenia can occur.[60]

Cladribine is a purine nucleoside analogue primarily used in the treatment of hairy cell leukemia. This agent can also be used in indolent lymphoid malignancies, such as chronic lymphocytic leukemia, low-grade non-Hodgkin's lymphoma, and some T-cell leukemias. Cladribine enters cells, becomes metabolized to cladribine triphosphate, and accumulates until reaching lymphotoxic levels. This agent also inhibits ribonucleotide reductase and DNA synthesis and repair and can initiate apoptosis of quiescent lymphocytes. A single course of therapy can induce complete remission in 65 to 91% of patients with hairy cell leukemia.[49] Cladribine is eliminated renally, with 25% of the drug excreted unchanged. The most common toxic effects include myelosuppression (neutropenia and thrombocytopenia), nausea and vomiting, and fever.[61] Approximately 40 to 50% of patients with hairy cell leukemia receiving cladribine develop a fever,[49] which may be related to tumor cell apoptosis and release of cytokines or pyrogens.[62] Cladribine also induces marked immunosuppression, with both T and B cells being affected. Some patients require up to 1 year after cladribine therapy to recover their T-cell counts and up to 2 to 3 years for the B cells to normalize.[63]

Alkylating Agents

The alkylating agents consist of a wide spectrum of drugs, including cyclophosphamide, ifosfamide, nitrogen mustard, melphalan, chlorambucil, carmustine, procarbazine, dacarbazine, busulfan, and thiotepa. Alkylating agents attack negatively charged, electron-rich nucleophilic sites on DNA, most commonly the N7 of guanine, the N3 of cytosine, and the O6 of guanine. This action alters DNA structure and function and interferes with DNA base pairing, replication, and transcription. Alkylating agents can react with one or two strands of DNA to form a covalent "cross-link."[32] The main toxic effects of alkylating agents include myelosuppression (which is the DLT), nausea and vomiting, mucositis, diarrhea, oligospermia, amenorrhea, and infertility with prolonged use[32]; teratogenicity with fetal malformations in the first trimester of pregnancy; and carcinogenesis (which is more likely with melphalan than cyclophosphamide). Infrequently, pulmonary interstitial pneumonitis and fibrosis can be seen after treatment with busulfan, melphalan, chlorambucil, cyclophosphamide (particularly with prolonged daily, low-dose oral administration), mitomycin-C, and carmustine.[32] Melphalan, an amino acid analogue, is used in multiple myelomas, high-dose myeloablative therapy, and isolated limb perfusion for melanoma and sarcoma.[32]

Cyclophosphamide is activated by liver P-450 microsomal enzymes into cytotoxic metabolites that cross-link DNA and inhibit DNA synthesis and function at all phases of the cell cycle.[32] Although cyclophosphamide is metabolized extensively in the liver, it is eliminated in the urine. The toxic metabolite acrolein causes hemorrhagic cystitis in 5 to 10% of patients.[64,65] Cyclophosphamide doses must be reduced in patients with renal dysfunction. The major toxic effects associated with cyclophosphamide include myelosuppression (nadir at 1.5 to 2.5 weeks and recovery within 3 weeks for granulocytes), nausea and vomiting, syndrome of inappropriate secretion of antidiuretic hormone (SIADH) with hyponatremia, and hypersensitivity. High-doses may be cardiotoxic. Cyclophosphamide has marked immunosuppressive effects and is often used in the treatment of autoimmune diseases and as part of the preparative regimen for bone marrow transplantation.[32] Rare cases of neurotoxicity have occurred, causing vision changes, confusion, and dizziness.[29] An uncommon late sequela of cyclophosphamide use is bladder contracture or fibrosis with bladder cancer.[40,64] An increased risk of treatment-related acute myelogenous leukemia is also reported.[66]

Ifosfamide is an isomer of cyclophosphamide and has a similar mechanism of action. Ifosfamide is activated at a slower rate than cyclophosphamide but is more likely to cause hematuria and therefore must be administered with mesna and hydration to provide uroprotection.[32] Ifosfamide is metabolized to chloroacetaldehyde, which is thought to contribute to both its neurotoxicity and renal toxicity.[67] Ifosfamide can cause acute encephalopathy characterized by cerebellar and extrapyramidal symptoms, seizures, and sometimes coma. The clinical findings begin within 1 day of drug infusion and resolve within 3 to 4 days. The risk factors associated with encephalopathy include hypocalcemia, low serum albumin, high dose of the drug, rapid infusion, renal or hepatic impairment, and previous cisplatin exposure.[29] Marked drug interactions can occur, with precipitation of the anticoagulant effect of warfarin and an increased risk of neurotoxicity when given with phenobarbital.[29]

Carmustine, a nitrosourea, can cross the blood-brain barrier and enter the CNS,[32,68,69] where concentrations can reach more than 50% of plasma drug levels. Carmustine is mainly used to treat brain tumors either in an adjuvant setting or for advanced disease.[70] Carmustine spontaneously decomposes into chloromethylisocyanate, which is a known pulmonary toxin.[32,71] Higher cumulative doses of the drug are associated with greater pulmonary toxicity, and pulmonary function tests may be considered at baseline and periodically during treatment. An increased risk of pulmonary toxic effects is seen in patients with a baseline carbon monoxide diffusing capacity < 70%. Nitrosoureas often produces two granulocyte nadirs, with an early drop during the first 3 weeks of treatment, apparent recovery, and then a subsequent drop at 5 to 6 weeks after treatment.[32] Nausea and vomiting are also prominent with carmustine. Carmustine is formulated in ethanol at concentrations that are high enough to cause symptoms in some patients.

Hydrazine and triazine derivatives are agents that methylate the O6 position of the guanylic acid in DNA.[32] Procarbazine, a phenylhydrazine derivative, has clinical activity against brain tumors, Hodgkin's disease, and non-Hodgkin's lymphoma.[32] It was originally developed as a monoamine oxidase inhibitor and can potentiate other CNS agents (eg, barbiturates, opiates, antihistamines, and phenothiazines). Hypertensive reactions can occur when using procarbazine with other sympathomimetics, tricyclic antidepressants, or tyramine-rich foods (eg, wine, dark beer, bananas, yogurt, and ripe cheese). Alcohol use can precipitate a disulfiram (Antabuse) effect, with symptoms of sweating, flushing, and headache. Procarbazine also causes nausea, vomiting and myelosuppression. Procarbazine is activated by the P-450 system; the interaction leads to the formation of a metabolite that methylates DNA. Procarbazine is rapidly and completely absorbed after oral dosing, with peak plasma levels achieved within 1 hour.

Dacarbazine is a triazene derivative that is used in the treatment of melanoma and Hodgkin's disease.[32] After intravenous administration, dacarbazine is metabolized into a methyldiazonium that methylates DNA.[72,73] It is highly emetogenic and somewhat myelosuppressive. Temozolamide, another triazene analogue that decomposes into a methyldiazonium ion,[32] is administered orally and is much less emetogenic than dacarbazine. It is currently used in the treatment of CNS tumors and melanoma.

Anthracyclines

The anthracyclines include doxorubicin, daunorubicin, idarubicin, and epirubicin; they are related to the anthracenediones, such as mitoxantrone. Doxorubicin is used in cancers of the breast, lung, ovary, stomach, and bladder and in soft tissue sarcoma, hepatoma, Hodgkin's disease, and non-Hodgkin's lymphoma. Daunomycin is used in acute lymphoblastic leukemia and acute myelogenous leukemia. Mitoxantrone has activity in prostate cancer, lymphoma, leukemia, and breast cancer. Anthracyclines and anthracenediones form complexes with topoisomerase II and DNA strands, preventing rejoining of the DNA strands after topoisomerase II temporarily breaks it to enable DNA unwinding for replication. This leads to topoisomerase II–dependent DNA double-stranded breaks. In the presence of iron, these agents can also form free oxygen radicals and cause peroxidation of membrane lipids. These agents are primarily metabolized in the liver, with 40 to 50% excretion in the stool.[74] Dose reductions are required in patients with liver dysfunction.

The main toxic effects associated with anthracyclines are dose-limiting myelosuppression and mucositis, diarrhea, alopecia, skin radiation recall, severe local tissue damage if the drug extravasates into subcutaneous tissues, and red-orange discoloration of the urine for 1 to 2 days after therapy.[74] Cardiotoxicity may be experienced and can be severe. Acute pump failure within the first 2 to 3 days of treatment can occur, with arrhythmias or conduction problems, pericarditis, or myocarditis. Chronic cardiotoxic effects (eg, dilated cardiomyopathy) are associated with a high cumulative dose and are thought to arise from membrane lipid peroxidation related to the heart's decreased ability to detoxify oxygen free radicals.[28] Associated risk factors include age > 70 years, a history of hypertension or other cardiac disease, previous irradiation of the mediastinal region, and a high cumulative drug dose (eg, above 450 to 500 mg/m[2] for doxorubicin).[25,75] Giving the drug by prolonged administration reduces both the peak drug concentration and the risk of cardiomyopathy but increases the risk of both mucositis and extravasation. Epirubicin is somewhat less cardiotoxic than doxorubicin. Mitoxantrone, which is somewhat less likely to cause nausea and vomiting, alopecia, and cardiotoxic effects than anthracyclines, may cause bluish discoloration of the fingernails, sclera, and urine for 1 to 2 days.

Several drug interactions can occur between P-450 active drugs and the anthracyclines. Phenobarbital and phenytoin may enhance the metabolic clearance of doxorubicin. Cyclophosphamide, mitomycin-C, and trastuzumab can increase the risk of cardiotoxic effects.[25,28] Dexrazoxane, an iron chelator, can reduce the cardiotoxicity of doxorubicin but may also decrease its efficacy.[25]

Platinum Analogues

Commonly used platinum agents include cisplatin, carboplatin, and oxaliplatin. The platinums are among the most useful of all chemotherapy agents, with a very wide range of activity. Cisplatin has activity in breast, lung, head and neck, ovarian, bladder, testicular, esophageal, and gastric cancers.[76] The only common malignancies that are generally unresponsive to platinum are cancers of the colon and kidney. Cisplatin binds covalently to DNA, with preferential binding to the N7 of guanine and adenine, and forms intra- and interstrand DNA cross-links. DNA adduct formation leads to inhibition of DNA synthesis, transcription, and function and induction of apoptosis. The platinum compounds also form complexes with nuclear and cytoplasmic proteins, which contributes to their antitumor activity and toxicity.

Whereas cisplatin is excreted in the urine via glomerular filtration and tubular secretion, the major method by which cisplatin is detoxified is by rapid, irreversible binding to albumin. The active, toxic free drug has a plasma half-life of only about 30 minutes, whereas the half-life of protein-bound drug in the plasma is several days. The main DLT is nephrotoxicity, which affects 30 to 40% of patients.[76,77] Renal damage is cumulative and mainly involves the proximal and distal convoluted tubules. The risk of serious nephrotoxicity is decreased by ensuring adequate hydration during and after drug administration and by use of mannitol to induce diuresis. The risk increases with increasing doses and may be peak concentration related in that it may be more common in the case of rapid drug administration. Patients often have an asymptomatic, acute rise in serum creatinine in the first few days after cisplatin administration, followed by gradual improvement over the subsequent 2 to 3 weeks. Hypomagnesemia owing to renal wasting is very common and often requires magnesium replacement. In most patients, this condition gradually improves after discontinuation of therapy. Salt wasting, metabolic acidosis, hypocalcemia, hypokalemia, and SIADH caused by tubule damage occur occasionally.[76]

Neurotoxicity can also be dose limiting, with development of an irreversible sensory peripheral neuropathy.[76] Cumulative doses above 400 mg/m[2] will often cause paresthesias and numbness. Peripheral neuropathy may begin several weeks after the completion of therapy, very gradually worsen over time, and then very gradually improve. Cisplatin occasionally causes autonomic neuropathy. Rare cases of encephalopathy, stroke, and seizures have been reported.[29] Impairment of color vision can be detected by sensitive retinal test, but often the impairment is not clinically detectable.

Cisplatin is highly emetogenic. As in other emetogenic chemotherapies, acute nausea is due to damage to gastrointestinal enterochromaffin cells, which causes release of the neurotransmitter serotonin. As serotonin becomes elevated, it triggers nausea and vomiting by interacting with 5-HT$_3$ receptors in vagal nerve endings and in the chemoreceptor trigger zone. Typically, the nausea and vomiting begin 5 to 6 hours after therapy, although patients who become severely nauseated after one course of therapy may develop anticipatory nausea that occurs much earlier (potentially even while thinking about an upcoming appointment for treatment).

The acute nausea and vomiting generally last for 8 to 12 hours, and delayed nausea (thought to be due to the release of substance P) can last for 3 to 5 days. In addition, foods may taste metallic and the patient may experience a loss of appetite. Ototoxicity causing high-frequency hearing loss (4,000–8,000 Hz) or tinnitus by damaging the cochlear hair cells is very common. Although it is usually very mild, it is severe in some patients and irreversible.[77] The risk of ototoxic effects increases with an increase in the cisplatin dose per course, with an increase in the rate of drug administration (ie, with a high peak concentration) if cranial radiation is also given and with a preexisting hearing impairment. Ototoxic effects typically manifest within 24 hours of drug administration.

Myelosuppression is relatively uncommon with normal doses of cisplatin, and part of this agent's usefulness derives from the fact that full doses of it can be given with full doses of other myelosuppressive agents. Reduced erythropoietin production is a common consequence of cisplatin nephrotoxicity and causes anemia that is amenable to treatment by recombinant erythropoietin analogues. Anemia may also be caused by a direct effect of cisplatin on bone marrow. Rarely, hemolytic anemia arises.

In rare cases, side effects include arrhythmias, acute ischemic vascular events, Raynaud's syndrome, pulmonary fibrosis, glucose intolerance, and pancreatitis.[44,77] Although cisplatin is not generally regarded as a vesicant, intra-arterial administration may occasionally result in severe local tissue damage.

Several drug interactions do occur with cisplatin administration. Caution is particularly important when cisplatin is given with other nephrotoxic agents (eg, aminoglycosides and amphotericin B). Cisplatin reduces the renal clearance of etoposide, ifosfamide, methotrexate, and bleomycin, and systemic thiol-containing proteins (eg, amifostine and mesna) may inactivate cisplatin. In addition, cisplatin administered before paclitaxel will lower paclitaxel clearance rates, which may lead to increased myelosuppression. Cisplatin's toxicity is also increased if it is administered before topotecan instead of after it. The efficacy of the cisplatin-etoposide combination in small cell lung cancer is schedule dependent, with greater activity if cisplatin is given before etoposide.

Carboplatin is a second-generation compound; its mechanism of action is identical to that of cisplatin, and it has an identical spectrum of antitumor activity, although in some malignancies, it is felt to be somewhat less effective than cisplatin. Its spectrum of toxicity is substantially different from that of cisplatin; however, this is thought to be due to a reduced rate of conversion to the reactive aquated species that bind to DNA and proteins. The major toxic effect is induced by carboplatin myelosuppression, which is dose limiting, with other toxic effects being much less pronounced than with cisplatin.[76,78] Myelosuppression manifests mainly as thrombocytopenia, with a nadir at 17 to 21 days after therapy and recovery by day 28. Additional toxic effects include acute and delayed nausea and vomiting, alopecia, peripheral neuropathy, mild renal pathology, and, in some cases, an allergic reaction that arises after seven or eight courses of therapy.[76] The primary route of carboplatin excretion is renal; the rate of renal excretion is directly proportional to the glomerular filtration rate, permitting accurate prediction of drug pharmacology and toxicity (and adjustment of dose) based on renal function.

Oxaliplatin is a third-generation compound with the same mechanism of action as cisplatin and carboplatin. For reasons that are unclear, however, it has a markedly different spectrum of activity than cisplatin or carboplatin and is most effective against cancers of the colon, pancreas, and stomach. With oxaliplatin, neurotoxic effects are dose limiting and can present in two forms: acute (< 14 days) or persistent (> 14 days).[76] Acute neurotoxic effects include reversible paresthesias, hypersensitivity to cold, jaw and eye pain, ptosis, muscle cramping, and motor nerve hyperexcitability. Neurotoxicity can manifest a few minutes after drug infusion and resolve within a few days; it recurs after each cycle of treatment. The mechanism of action is suspected to involve axon conductance and neuronal excitability.[29] Neurotoxic effects can be triggered or enhanced by cold temperatures. Laryngopharyngeal dysesthesia, which may present with choking, difficulty breathing, or swallowing, is a dose-dependent effect and is seen in patients receiving more than 850 mg/m^2 oxaliplatin. This dysesthesia is reversible and may last 3 to 4 months. The persistent form of toxic effects occurs after a high cumulative dose of oxaliplatin and is similar to cisplatin-induced neuropathy.[29] This condition is reversible within 4 to 6 months after the cessation of therapy.[76] Oxaliplatin-induced myelosuppression is uncommon, but gastrointestinal toxic effects, such as nausea, vomiting, and diarrhea, may be seen.

Taxanes

Taxanes target the N-terminal of the β subunit of microtubules and prevent tubulin depolymerization, thereby stabilizing the mitotic spindle complex and preventing tumor cell proliferation.[79] Taxanes are administered intravenously and are primarily metabolized by the liver and excreted in the stool. The main DLT of paclitaxel is myelosuppression, specifically neutropenia.[79] Patients may also experience an acute hypersensitivity reaction to the Cremophor EL vehicle, with dyspnea, bronchospasm, skin flushing, urticaria, and hypotension; the reaction often occurs within the first 2 to 3 minutes of the initiation of infusion and almost always happens within the first 10 minutes.[80] Paclitaxel infusions require premedication with dexamethasone, diphenhydramine hydrochloride (Benadryl), and antihistamine agents. Additional toxic effects include a dose-dependent peripheral neuropathy (mainly sensory but motor or autonomic in some cases), bradycardia, ventricular arrhythmias, rarely mucositis, diarrhea, nausea and vomiting, alopecia, transient elevations of liver function test values, and onycholysis.[79] Paclitaxel has several drug interactions. Concomitant administration of cisplatin will lower paclitaxel clearance rates and increase myelosuppression. Cyclophosphamide can also increase symptoms of myelosuppression when administered before paclitaxel. Paclitaxel reduces the clearance of doxorubicin by 30 to 35%, and P-450 enzyme inducers (eg, phenytoin and phenobarbital) may accelerate the metabolism of paclitaxel and decrease drug levels.

Docetaxel is a semisynthetic derivative that stabilizes tubulin polymerization and has activity in breast, lung, head and neck, ovarian, bladder, testicular, and gastroesophageal cancers. The main toxic effect is myelosuppression, with dose-limiting neutropenia. Up to 25% of patients experience major or minor hypersensitivity reactions if they are not premedicated. Docetaxel can induce a fluid-retention syndrome, with edema, weight gain, pleural effusion, and ascites. The risk of fluid accumulation increases at cumulative doses > 400 mg/m^2. In 50% of patients, a rash develops on forearms and hands. Additional toxic effects include mild to moderate peripheral neuropathy, mucositis, general malaise, asthenia in up to 70% of patients, and alopecia.[79,81]

Topoisomerase I Inhibitors

Camptothecins act by binding topoisomerase I, a nuclear enzyme that temporarily breaks DNA and permits it to unwind for replication. Topoisomerase inhibitors permit the topoisomerase to break the DNA but do not permit it to subsequently rejoin the DNA strands, thereby giving rise to single-stranded DNA breaks for agents that inhibit topoisomerase I and double-stranded DNA breaks for agents that inhibit topoisomerase II. The camptothecin derivative irinotecan is active against colorectal, lung, cervical, ovarian, gastric, and esophageal cancers and lymphoma. This agent requires hepatic activation by a carboxylesterase enzyme to form the SN-38 metabolite.[74] The major toxic effects include a dose-limiting diarrhea (acute and delayed), nausea and vomiting, transient elevations in liver function test values, fatigue, and alopecia. In addition, myelosuppression can be dose limiting with an every 3-week schedule and is significantly more likely to arise after the third and fourth cycles of therapy. Less frequently, pneumonitis, arrhythmias, and paralytic ileus can occur.[82,83]

Topotecan is used in small cell lung and ovarian cancers. It can be administered intravenously or orally. Topotecan is eliminated by the kidney and requires a dose reduction in the setting of renal dysfunction. The major toxic effects are dose-limiting neutropenia and myelosuppression; flu-like symptoms with headache, fever, chills, malaise, mild nausea, and vomiting; transient elevation in liver function test values; diarrhea; generalized fatigue; and skin rash.[74,84]

Topoisomerase II Inhibitors

Topoisomerase II inhibitors include the anthracyclines, the anthracenediones, and etoposide; as noted, these inhibitors cause double-stranded DNA breaks by inhibiting the DNA-rejoining portion of the enzyme's activity. The anthracyclines have been described previously. Etoposide is an epipodophyllotoxin that is active in lung cancer, germ cell tumors, and non-Hodgkin's lymphoma; etoposide is also used in high-dose therapy with bone marrow or stem cell transplantation. Etoposide is metabolized in the liver by the cytochrome P-450 microsomal system by means of glucuronidation, with about 30 to 50% of the drug excreted in the urine.[74] Patients with renal dysfunction require dose reductions. The main toxic effects owing to etoposide include dose-limiting myelosuppression, nausea and vomiting, mucositis, alopecia, and, rarely, headache, seizures, and somnolence.[29] Patients are also at risk of a hypersensitivity reaction to the polysorbate 80 vehicles, which can manifest as chills, fever, bronchospasm, tachycardia, facial and tongue swelling, and hypotension. Hypersensitivity primarily occurs when the drug is administered rapidly intravenously, whereas it is rarely seen if the drug is given over an hour or more, and it is not seen with oral administration. Etoposide is also carcinogenic and associated with the t(11;23) translocation in acute myelogenous leukemia.[74]

Vinca Alkaloids

The vinca alkaloids include vincristine, vinblastine, vindesine, and vinorelbine. These agents bind to specific sites on tubulin, prevent tubulin dimer polymerization, and inhibit mitotic spindle apparatus formation. These effects result in mitotic arrest and tumor cell apoptosis. Vinca alkaloids are metabolized in the liver by the cytochrome P-450 system and are excreted in stool.[79] As a class, the vinca alkaloids are potent vesicants. Vincristine is used in pediatric and adult acute leukemias, Hodgkin's and non-Hodgkin's lymphoma, Wilms' tumor, Ewing's sarcoma, neuroblastoma, and rhabdomyosarcoma. The DLT is peripheral neuropathy. As with most other neurotoxic chemotherapy agents, peripheral neurotoxicity is dose dependent and primarily sensory, but it can also involve motor, autonomic, and cranial nerves. Additional toxic effects are paralytic ileus and intestinal obstruction, urinary retention, postural hypotension, and SIADH. Vinblastine is used in germ cell tumors, Hodgkin's lymphoma, and breast cancer. Myelosuppression is dose limiting, and mucositis, alopecia, peripheral neuropathy, and SIADH can also occur. Vindesine causes both myelosuppression and severe peripheral neuropathy. It is occasionally used in the treatment of non–small cell lung cancer.

Vinorelbine is a semisynthetic analogue of vinblastine and is active against non–small cell lung, breast, and head and neck cancers and against Hodgkin's lymphoma; it appears to be more effective than other vinca alkaloids. Vinorelbine is metabolized by the P-450 system, with excretion via the biliary tract and in stool.

Myelosuppression is dose limiting, with neutropenia being most prominent. In addition, nausea and vomiting, diarrhea, constipation, elevated liver function test values, alopecia, peripheral neuropathy, and SIADH can occur. Vinorelbine can cause severe phlebitis in the vein into which it is infused, but the risk of phlebitis is reduced by rapid administration and by postadministration flushing of the vein. Vinorelbine has several drug interactions and can reduce effective blood levels of phenytoin.[79]

Miscellaneous Agents

Bleomycin is extracted from the fungus *Streptomyces verticillus* and contains DNA-binding and iron-binding regions at opposite ends of the peptide. This agent requires activation by oxidized iron to form oxygen free radicals, which then cause single- and double-stranded DNA breaks and cell death. Up to 70% of bleomycin is excreted in the urine, and dose modification is required in the case of renal dysfunction.[85] The major concern when using bleomycin is its pulmonary toxicity. Patients may develop a reversible acute inflammatory reaction in the lungs, with pulmonary infiltrates evident on chest radiographs; rales may arise after exposure to even low cumulative doses, with a risk of much more serious chronic pulmonary pneumonitis and fibrosis occurring at higher cumulative doses. Approximately 3 to 5% of patients receiving a total of 400 to 450 units develop a subacute or chronic pneumonitis. The proportion increases to 10% in patients treated with higher doses. Presenting clinical symptoms include cough, bibasilar infiltrates, and pulmonary nodules. Additional predisposing factors include age > 70 years, underlying lung disease, previous pulmonary or mediastinal irradiation, and use of high-concentration oxygen.[33] Extreme caution is required to limit the fraction of inspired oxygen during surgery in patients previously treated with bleomycin. Additional toxic effects of bleomycin include hyperpigmentation of skin, thickening of nail beds, ulceration or desquamation in severe cases, vascular events (eg, Raynaud's syndrome, myocardial infarction, and stroke),[86] and hypersensitivity reactions in 25% of patients.[34,85] Cisplatin can decrease the renal clearance of bleomycin and may enhance its toxicity.

Chemotherapy-Induced Secondary Malignancies

Secondary malignancies induced by chemotherapy were first described in 1947 by Haddow.[87] Chemotherapy interacts with DNA and can cause irreversible genetic mutations that accumulate and progress to frank carcinogenesis. Most carcinogenic agents have long latency periods, and a multistep process involving initiators and promoters is required. Both the toxic agent and the host immune system and environment play a role in initiating a second malignancy. Combined exposure to chemotherapy and radiation will increase the risk of carcinogenesis (Table 2). Patients with preexisting germline mutations are especially at risk of second malignancies because of both their genetic makeup and the toxicity of the chemotherapy. Included in this category of patients are those who have microsatellite instability or impaired DNA repair mechanisms (eg, hereditary nonpolyposis colorectal cancer and retinoblastoma).[88]

Patients who have loss of heterozygosity in the *TP53* gene are more prone to therapy-related acute myelogenous leukemia after exposure to alkylating agents.[89] In addition, chemotherapy for certain disease types has an above-average risk of secondary malignancies. High-risk diseases (and the chemotherapy regimen or agent causing the secondary malignancy) include Hodgkin's disease (treated with the doxorubicin, bleomycin, vinblastine, and dacarbazine or the mechlorethamine hydrochloride, procarbazine, vincristine, and prednisone regimen), non-Hodgkin's lymphoma (cyclophosphamide, doxorubicin, vincristine, and prednisone), multiple myeloma (melphalan), acute lymphoblastic leukemia (etoposide), testicular cancer (bleomycin, etoposide, and cisplatin), ovarian cancer (cyclophosphamide, doxorubicin, and cisplatin), bone marrow transplantation (alkylator combination

Table 2 Carcinogenic Risk of Chemotherapy Agents

High
  Melphalan
  Nitrosoureas
  Etoposide
  Teniposide
  Mechlorethamine

Moderate
  Doxorubicin
  Thiotepa
  Cyclophosphamide
  Procarbazine
  Dacarbazine
  Cisplatin

Low
  Vinca alkyloids
  Methotrexate
  Cytarabine
  5-Fluorouracil
  L-Asparaginase
  Carboplatin

Unknown Bleomycin
  Taxanes
  Busulfan
  Gemcitabine
  Irinotecan
  Mitoxantrone

therapy), and breast cancer (high-dose cyclophosphamide-doxorubicin combinations).[90,91] The Surveillance, Epidemiology, and End Results (SEER) database review of 21,708 patients with breast cancer reported an 11.5-fold relative risk of developing a secondary leukemia at 4.2 years.[66] Further studies in 82,700 women with breast cancer reported a 10-fold increase in the relative risk of leukemia with chemotherapy alone and a 17.4-fold higher relative risk after chemotherapy and radiation.[92]

The exact carcinogenic mechanisms of action differ between the classes of chemotherapy drugs. Chemical carcinogens often require metabolic activation to an electrophilic intermediate, which reacts with DNA bases, particularly the negatively charged or nucleophilic N7 of guanine.[93] Cyclophosphamide and mitomycin-C also cause secondary tumors by means of this mechanism, whereas L-phenylalanine mustard and nitrogen mustard do not require metabolism to form alkylating species. Doxorubicin and mithramycin form reactive oxygen intermediates, which can cause DNA strand breaks and lead to carcinogenicity.

Therapy-Related Acute Myelogenous Leukemia

Therapy-related acute myelogenous leukemia accounts for 10 to 20% of all cases of this cancer.[88] There is no gender or ethnic predisposition, but older age at drug exposure appears to increase the risk.[91] Patients have developed therapy-related acute myelogenous leukemia in response to alkylating agents, topoisomerase II inhibitors, and combination regimens. Unfortunately, most therapy-related acute myelogenous leukemia carries a poor prognosis, with a median survival of 9 months. The exceptions to this general rule include patients with favorable cytogenetics (t(8;21), inv (16), and t(8;16)) who respond to therapy and patients with de novo disease who have the same translocations.[89]

There are two main groups of therapy-related leukemia. The first is acute myelogenous leukemia that results from exposure to topoisomerase II inhibitors and the second from exposure to alkylators.[94] Topoisomerase II inhibitor–related acute myelogenous leukemia occurs 2 to 3 years after treatment and typically has an M4 or M5 phenotype by the French-American-British (FAB) classification system. Alkylator therapy–related acute myelogenous leukemia occurs 5 to 7 years after treatment and is associated with myelodysplasia and loss of chromosomes 5 and 7.[94]

Etoposide, a topoisomerase II inhibitor, has been associated with secondary acute non-lymphocytic leukemia (ANLL), with a risk of 5.9% at 4 years in children.[95] At 6 years, the risk was reported as 3.8%.[96] Pui and colleagues noted that a schedule of twice-weekly or weekly etoposide or teniposide increased the risk of ANLL at 6 years to 12.3%.[96] Etoposide causes dose-dependent chromosomal damage that can be perpetuated in cells of the hematopoietic system. It is suspected that cytogenetic abnormalities are due to topoisomerase-induced abnormal sister chromatid exchanges.[97] In vitro studies of etoposide-treated cells have found frequent breaks in chromosomes 1, 11, and 17.[98] Translocations in the *MLL* gene at chromosome 11q23 have been reported.[99,100] Also associated with etoposide-induced ANLL is the lack of a preleukemic phase.[98] A meta-analysis conducted by the NCI Cancer Therapy Evaluation Program on 12 cooperative group trials (11 in the pediatric population) reported a cumulative dose-dependent increase in the risk of secondary leukemias at 6 years after treatment.[101] Patients with germ cell tumors treated with cisplatin, etoposide, and bleomycin have been reported to have a 1 to 4.7% cumulative risk of developing leukemia by 5.7 years after treatment.[98]

Alkylating agent–induced acute myelogenous leukemia has a peak incidence at 4 to 6 years after treatment and a range of onset of 1 to 20 years.[97] A cumulative dose-response effect is associated with an increased risk of myelodysplastic syndrome or acute myelogenous leukemia. Carcinogenesis is caused by direct alkylator therapy–induced stem cell damage. Alkylating agents form covalent bonds with the DNA bases and cause intra- and interstrand DNA cross-linking and breaks. Aberrant DNA coding then occurs, with the potential for malignant transformation.

Studies of multiple myeloma patients report a high incidence of ANLL attributed to previous alkylator-based therapy.[102,103] In an international collaborative group evaluation of cancer registries, alkylator-based chemotherapy had a relative risk of 12, was at greatest risk 4 to 5 years after treatment, and persisted for at least 8 years.[104] The conclusion of this study was that chlorambucil and melphalan were more leukemogenic than cyclophosphamide.[105] Several alkylating agents have been reported to cause therapy-related acute myelogenous leukemia. This list includes cyclophosphamide, ifosfamide, procarbazine, chlorambucil, melphalan, and busulfan.[88] Single-agent melphalan and busulfan reportedly confer the highest acute myelogenous leukemia risk, and combination therapies such as mechlorethamine, Oncovin (vincristine), procarbazine, and prednisone (MOPP) carry a higher risk than single agents.[97] Melphalan has been used in ovarian cancer and is associated with a marked increase in the risk of secondary acute leukemia in some reports, showing a 93- to 174.4-fold increase in risk.[102,105–108] The NCI and Connecticut Tumor Registry reported a relative risk of 4.1 for acute leukemia in 32,251 women treated for ovarian cancer.[109] In breast cancer patients, melphalan

carried a 5-fold higher risk of secondary leukemia.[110]

Anthracycline therapy does not appear to significantly increase the risk of leukemia. The University of Texas M.D. Anderson Cancer Center reported a 0.5% higher risk of secondary leukemia at 10 years in 1,474 patients treated with six cycles of 5-FU, doxorubicin, and cyclophosphamide.[111] Radiation increased the risk to 2.5% at 10 years. However, combination regimens for hematologic malignancies, such as Hodgkin's disease, have been reported to have a significantly greater risk of secondary leukemia. A case-control study conducted in the Netherlands reported that 1,939 patients with Hodgkin's disease had as much as a 40-fold increase in the risk of leukemia owing to treatment with (MOPP).[112–114]

Solid Tumors

Second primary solid tumors can arise from previous field defects in the aerodigestive tract or previously irradiated areas. In general, single-agent chemotherapy is infrequently associated with second primary solid tumor formation. However, the treatment of certain diseases is associated with higher rates of second primary solid tumors. Up to 20% of patients with Hodgkin's disease can develop second malignancies within 15 years of the primary therapy.[115–117] A German review of 1,500 Hodgkin's disease patients showed a 20-year cumulative risk of 19% for second primary solid tumors.[118] This statistic may be high as a significant proportion of the solid tumors arose from a previously irradiated field.

Cyclophosphamide is associated with bladder toxicity and the development of bladder cancer.[119,120] The risk appears to increase with the cumulative dose, with an overall 4.5-fold increase in risk.[120] The carcinogenic pathway is activated by the acrolein metabolite, which is toxic to bladder mucosa; bladder fibrosis and dysplasia can transform into a malignant phenotype.

Fertility and Mutagenicity

Cancer occurs in pregnant women at a rate of 1 per 1,000.[121,122] The most common malignancies encountered are breast cancer, melanoma, cervical cancer, lymphoma, and leukemia.[123,124] Chemotherapy agents have known teratogenicity, with the extent of the effect dependent on exposure time, dose, lipid solubility, molecular weight, and the stability of binding to plasma proteins.[122,125] As cytotoxic agents target rapidly dividing cells, the effects on a growing fetus are a major concern when considering the use of chemotherapy in pregnant patients. During pregnancy, the volume of distribution, protein binding, and renal clearance of drugs are typically increased. Other pharmacokinetic factors, such as drug

absorption, are also affected.[126] The timing of delivery is also a concern when pregnant patients undergo chemotherapy as thrombocytopenia can complicate labor.

First-trimester use of chemotherapy should be avoided if possible. Use of chemotherapy during this time will significantly increase the risk of major fetal malformations or spontaneous abortion.[122,125,127] If chemotherapy is necessary during the first trimester of pregnancy, doxorubicin and the vinca alkaloids have the lowest rates of teratogenic effects.[127] The gestational age of the fetus at the time of chemotherapy exposure is the most likely predictor of what type of malformation will occur.[122] The first 2 weeks of pregnancy are highly susceptible to fetal death and spontaneous abortion. This is when the zygote implants and develops amnion. During weeks 2 to 8 after conception, teratogenesis of major organs, such as the heart, neural tube, and limbs, can occur. Limb buds appear between the fourth and sixth weeks of gestation.[127] Even after embryonic organogenesis is completed, the hematopoietic system, CNS (visual), and genitalia remain vulnerable.[122] CNS congenital defects include neural tube defects and mental retardation. Cardiac abnormalities include truncus arteriosus, atrial septal defects, and ventricular septal defects. Amelia, meromelia, cleft lip, low-set malformed ears and deafness, microphthalmia, cataracts, and glaucoma can occur. Also, masculinization of female genitalia and enamel hypoplasia and staining may be seen.

Second- and third-trimester exposure to chemotherapy increases the risk of intrauterine growth retardation (IUGR) and low birth weight.[128] In addition, minor congenital anomalies and functional defects can occur. Some studies report that children exposed to chemotherapy in utero can have normal learning behavior and intact immune and hematologic systems.[129]

Fetal Effects owing to Specific Chemotherapies

Alkylating Agents

In 1968, a review of the literature on alkylating agents found that women treated during the first trimester of pregnancy had a 16% chance of giving birth to children with fetal malformation.[130] First-trimester treatment, but not second- or third-trimester exposure, with cyclophosphamide was associated with marked malformations.[126,131,132] Fetal malformations associated with cyclophosphamide include low-set ears, eye abnormalities, loss of toes, cleft palate, blepharophimosis, a flat nasal bridge, and microcephaly.[122,126] Although safe alkylator agent use in the second and third trimesters has been reported, the risks of fetal death and IUGR are increased, regardless of the timing of exposure.[122] The dacarbazine used in the ABVD regimen for Hodgkin's disease is associated with intrauterine growth retardation (IUGR) and minor malformations.[122] Busulfan in the second trimester can lead to malformations.[133]

Antimetabolites

Methotrexate given at doses greater than 10 mg per week is associated with fetal malformations, such as oxycephaly, low-set ears, skin folds, absence of toes, growth retardation, and rib abnormalities.[127,134] First-trimester exposure to methotrexate has been associated with fetal death.[122,122] 5-FU is very teratogenic and should be avoided in pregnancy, especially in the first trimester.[127] 5-FU in combination with other agents can lead to intrauterine fetal growth malformation and fetal death. Cytarabine exposure, even after the first trimester, leads to limb malformation, intrauterine fetal death (IUFD), fetal growth retardation, and neonatal death.[122] Cytarabine is highly teratogenic in animals and is recommended only in the second and third trimesters of pregnancy.[127] However, chromosome abnormalities have been reported with cytarabine exposure throughout all trimesters.[127] Cytarabine also causes low birth weight, perinatal seizures, cytopenias, and preterm labor.[127] 6-Mercaptopurine crosses the human placenta, but only a 1 to 2% fetal blood concentration is seen.[126] Mercaptopurine has been reported to cause IUGR and IUFD but has a lower degree of association with congenital abnormalities.[122] First-trimester use of 6-mercaptopurine has been associated with chromosomal, hematologic, and immunologic abnormalities in the fetus.[126] Second-trimester use of 6-mercaptopurine has also led to chromosomal changes.[126]

Anthracyclines

Anthracycline use during pregnancy has been associated with transient marrow hypoplasia, fetal limb malformations (after first-trimester exposure), IUGR, IUFD, and transient myelosuppression. Although cardiotoxicity is a concern in patients receiving anthracyclines, it is unclear whether fetal exposure leads to cardiotoxicity. Idarubicin, a more lipophilic agent, has been associated with IUFD and cardiomyopathy. In one study of a small number of cases, 23% of fetuses and neonates exposed to epirubicin-based combination chemotherapy died. Doxorubicin, with its higher protein binding, is recommended instead of epirubicin or idarubicin in pregnant women but only in the second or third trimester.[122,126]

Vinca Alkaloids

Vinca alkaloids are less teratogenic than the antimetabolite agents.[122,125,135] Fetal malformations can occur with first-trimester use, especially when vinca alkaloids are used in combination therapy. However, single-agent vinblastine has been used in all trimesters without evidence of teratogenicity.[127]

Taxanes

Taxanes have been reported to be lethal in animal models. Only a small number of case reports involving taxane exposure have been published, and although no malformations were seen, taxanes are not recommended in pregnancy because of the paucity of information.[122]

Platinum Agents

Platinum agents have been associated with fetal sensorineural hearing loss, cardiomegaly, CNS abnormalities, IUGR, and IUFD.[122] Cisplatin is preferred over carboplatin for use in pregnancy because carboplatin is more likely to cause thrombocytopenia and has the potential for higher placental transfer because it is less protein bound than cisplatin.[122] Published case reports suggest that use of cisplatin is safe in the second and third trimesters of pregnancy.[127]

Topoisomerase II Inhibitors

There is limited information about the use of etoposide in pregnancy. The agent has been associated with neonatal alopecia and ventriculomegaly.[136,137]

Male Fertility

In men, the seminiferous tubules are lined by spermatogenic and Sertoli's cells. Sertoli's cells regulate the release of spermatozoa from the germinal epithelium and maintain the blood-testis barrier.[138] Chemotherapy can be directly toxic to immature spermatozoa in the germinal epithelium or to Sertoli's and Leydig's cells. Cytotoxic agents can block maturation of spermatozoa and lead to incompetency.[138] Once the seminiferous tubules are damaged, testicular atrophy becomes clinically evident. Increased serum follicle-stimulating hormone is seen when spermatogenesis is impaired.

In animal models, Sertoli cell damage and abolition of sperm release from the germinal epithelium occur after doxorubicin, cisplatin, 5-FU, and methotrexate administration.[138,139] Doxorubicin has been shown to cause an absence of primary spermatocytes.[138,140] Cisplatin affects intermediate- and late-stage spermatids with Sertoli cell damage.[141] 5-FU leads to arrest in spermatid development.[139] Carmustine and procarbazine affect stem cells and early and intermediate spermatogonia.[141]

Alkylating agents are the chemotherapy agents most likely to cause male infertility.[138] Cyclophosphamide affects early and late spermatogonia and spermatocytes, resulting in decreased sperm counts.[138] Alkylator therapy has been shown to cause Leydig cell dysfunction in up to 30% of men.[142] In multiple-agent therapy, chromosome abnormalities in human sperm have been reported.[142]

In general, spermatogenesis can recover, even after high-dose chemotherapy is given. Standard or conventional doses of vinblastine, etoposide, bleomycin, and ifosfamide do not appear to impact long-term fertility.[143,144] However, cyclophosphamide at a cumulative dose higher than 7.5 g/m^2 can cause irreversible infertility.[145] Patients with testicular cancer who receive more than four cycles of chemotherapy also are at greater risk of infertility.[143] Fertility recovery depends on the amount of chemotherapy and its duration of administration. Treatment with multiple agents causes longer-lasting azoospermia than single-agent therapy and increases the risk of long-term infertility.

Female Fertility

During oogenesis, a primitive female germ cell gives rise to a mature ovum. Oocytes are coated by granulose cells and remain in prophase until they become a mature or graafian follicle prior to ovulation. Oocytes that are not ovulated become atresic and are resorbed.

Chemotherapy affects follicular growth and maturation. Ovarian fibrosis and follicle destruction may occur, followed by amenorrhea and elevation of serum follicle-stimulating hormone and luteinizing hormone.[146,147] Vaginal atrophy and endometrial hypoplasia then occur. Younger patients appear to recover from amenorrhea more quickly than older ones, although age and the amount of chemotherapy taken together will better predict the timing of ovarian function recovery.[47,148] Alkylating agents (particularly busulfan) are the most likely to cause ovarian dysfunction.[138]

In animal models, cyclophosphamide is directly toxic to ovarian follicles and decreases serum estradiol and progesterone.[149] Doxorubicin also causes apoptotic changes in oocytes, with bax protein up-regulation. In humans, busulfan at a dose of 0.5 to 14 mg daily for 3 months can cause permanent amenorrhea.[138,150] Antimetabolites such as methotrexate, conversely, do not appear to have ovarian toxicity.[151] Etoposide at doses up to 5 g causes oligo- or amenorrhea in 41% of women.[152] Despite the animal model data, doxorubicin is less toxic to ovaries than are alkylating agents.[138] Combination regimens have a higher risk of amenorrhea and ovarian failure.[47,138] Among women receiving 6 months of adjuvant chemotherapy (cyclophosphamide, methotrexate, and 5-FU) for breast cancer, those over 40 years old had a 70% ovarian failure rate and those younger than 40 years had a 40% failure rate.[47,153]

Effects on the Immune System: Autoimmunity

Postchemotherapy rheumatism is a disease characterized by noninflammatory musculoskeletal pain that is symmetric and associated with stiffness and mild swelling in both large and small upper and lower extremity joints.[154] This condition occurs in the absence of metastatic cancer or laboratory findings of rheumatologic disease. It has most often been reported in patients who received adjuvant chemotherapy for breast cancer (cyclophosphamide combined with methotrexate and 5-FU or doxorubicin and 5-FU). Many of the patients reported developed rheumatic complaints 2 to 6 months after completing chemotherapy.[155–157] Symptoms include myalgia, arthralgia, arthritis, periarticular swelling, and tenosynovitis. Postchemotherapy rheumatism has also been reported in patients with ovarian cancer who received cyclophosphamide-based therapy.[158] In addition, chemotherapy has been reported to worsen rheumatic complaints in patients with preexisting disease.[159] The biologic mechanism of postchemotherapy rheumatism is not known.[159]

Autoimmune vascular abnormalities have been associated with cytotoxic chemotherapy. It is well known that 5-FU induces a cardiotoxic effect, which can range from anginal symptoms to myocardial infarction and death. The exact mechanism of action is unknown but is suspected to involve either an autoimmune reaction to 5-FU or 5-FU-induced cell death that leads to an inflammatory response.[53] 5-FU may also induce acute coronary artery spasm while the drug is being administered. 5-FU has also been reported to induce Raynaud's syndrome, with digital ischemia and necrosis.[160] Raynaud's syndrome has also been reported in combination regimens using bleomycin, vinblastine, and cisplatin as measured by hand arteriography.[86]

Autoimmune reactions have been reported in patients receiving purine analogues, such as fludarabine and 2-chloro-2′-deoxyadenosine.[161] The proposed mechanism of action includes an allergic reaction to agents, cytokine release, or T-cell imbalance, leading to release of autoantibodies. The most common conditions that can result include hemolytic anemia, thrombocytopenia, bicytopenia (Evans's syndrome), and neutropenia.[161] In some instances, vasculitis, urticaria, pemphigus, interstitial pneumonia, and glomerulonephritis may also arise.

HUS is a serious condition characterized by renal failure, microangiopathic hemolytic anemia, and thrombocytopenia.[162] Mitomycin-C and gemcitabine have been associated with HUS.[163,164] Up to 10 to 15% of patients receiving mitomycin-C develop HUS,[164,165] and gemcitabine is reported to induce HUS in 0.015 to 0.25% of patients.[57,162,163] Chemotherapy-induced HUS carries a poor prognosis, with high mortality rates.[163]

Mitomycin-C-induced renal failure can develop 8 to 10 months after therapy and is associated with direct damage to renal endothelial cells.[164] Gemcitabine-induced HUS is associated with high cumulative doses of gemcitabine (2.5–40.3 g^2) and has a delayed presentation of 3.8 to 13.1 months.[163] Plasma exchange has been reported to benefit HUS therapy.

REFERENCES

1. Dale DC. Colony-stimulating factors for the management of neutropenia in cancer patients. Drugs 2002;62 Suppl 1:1–15.
2. Buratti S, Lavine JE. Drugs and the liver: advances in metabolism, toxicity, and therapeutics. Curr Opin Pediatr 2002;14:601–7.
3. Repetto L. Greater risks of chemotherapy toxicity in elderly patients with cancer. J Support Oncol 2003;1:18–24.
4. Aksentijevich I, Flinn I. Chemotherapy and bone marrow reserve: lessons learned from autologous stem cell transplantation. Cancer Biother Radiopharm 2002;17:399–403.
5. Kim SK, Demetri GD. Chemotherapy and neutropenia. Hematol Oncol Clin North Am 1996;10:377–95.
6. Vadhan-Raj S, et al. Assessment of hematologic effects and fatigue in cancer patients with chemotherapy-induced anemia given darbepoetin alfa every two weeks. J Support Oncol 2003;1:131–8.
7. Capo G, Waltzman R. Managing hematologic toxicities. J Support Oncol 2004;2:65–79.
8. Vose JM, Armitage JO. Clinical applications of hematopoietic growth factors. J Clin Oncol 1995;13:1023–35.
9. Smith RE Jr. Erythropoietic agents in the management of cancer patients. Part 1: anemia, quality of life, and possible effects on survival. J Support Oncol 2003;1:249–56, 258–9; discussion 257–8.
10. Smith RE Jr. Erythropoietic agents in the management of cancer patients. Part 2: studies on their role in neuroprotection and neurotherapy. J Support Oncol 2004;2:39–49.
11. Rizzo JD, Lichtin AE, Woolf SH, et al. Use of epoetin in patients with cancer: evidence-based clinical practice guidelines of the American Society of Clinical Oncology and the American Society of Hematology. J Clin Oncol 2002;20:4083–107.
12. Crawford J, Dale DC, Lyman GH. Chemotherapy-induced neutropenia: risks, consequences, and new directions for its management. Cancer 2004;100:228–37.
13. Ozer H, et al. 2000 update of recommendations for the use of hematopoietic colony-stimulating factors: evidence-based, clinical practice guidelines. American Society of Clinical Oncology Growth Factors Expert Panel. J Clin Oncol 2000;18:3558–85.
14. Osoba D, et al. Determinants of postchemotherapy nausea and vomiting in patients with cancer. Quality of Life and Symptom Control Committees of the National Cancer Institute of Canada Clinical Trials Group. J Clin Oncol 1997;15:116–23.
15. Grunberg S. Chemotherapy-induced nausea and vomiting: prevention, detection, and treatment—how are we doing? J Support Oncol 2004;2:1–23.
16. Navari RM. Pathogenesis-based treatment of chemotherapy-induced nausea and vomiting—two new agents. J Support Oncol 2003;1:89–103.
17. Stahl SM. The ups and downs of novel antiemetic drugs, part 1: substance P, 5-HT, and the neuropharmacology of vomiting. J Clin Psychiatry 2003;64:498–9.
18. Saltz LB. Understanding and managing chemotherapy-induced diarrhea. J Support Oncol 2003;1:35–46; discussion 38–41, 45–6.
19. Sonis ST. Oral mucositis in cancer therapy. J Support Oncol 2004;2:3–8.
20. Sonis ST. A biological approach to mucositis. J Support Oncol 2004;2:21–32; discussion 35–6.
21. Barasch A, Peterson DE. Risk factors for ulcerative oral mucositis in cancer patients: unanswered questions. Oral Oncol 2003;39:91–100.
22. Maule W. Gastrointestinal toxicity of chemotherapeutic agents. In: Perry M, editor. The chemotherapy source book. Baltimore: Williams & Wilkins; 1996. p. 697–707.
23. Remlinger KA. Cutaneous reactions to chemotherapy drugs: the art of consultation. Arch Dermatol 2003;139:77–81.
24. Feil VJ, Lamoureux CH. Alopecia activity of cyclophosphamide metabolites and related compounds in sheep. Cancer Res 1974;34:2596–8.
25. Chanan-Khan A, Srinivasan S, Czuczman MS. Prevention and management of cardiotoxicity from antineoplastic therapy. J Support Oncol 2004;2:251–6; discussion 259–61, 264–6.
26. Loerzel VW, Dow KH. Cardiac toxicity related to cancer treatment. Clin J Oncol Nurs 2003;7:557–62.
27. Singal PK, Deally CM, Weinberg LE. Subcellular effects of Adriamycin in the heart: a concise review. J Mol Cell Cardiol 1987;19:817–28.
28. Lefrak EA, Pitha J, Rosenheim S, Gottlieb JA. A clinicopathologic analysis of Adriamycin cardiotoxicity. Cancer 1973;32:302–14.
29. Verstappen CC, Heimans JJ, Hoekman K, Postma TJ. Neurotoxic complications of chemotherapy in patients with cancer: clinical signs and optimal management. Drugs 2003;63:1549–63.
30. Paice JA. Mechanisms and management of neuropathic pain in cancer. J Support Oncol 2003;1:107–20.
31. Schweitzer VG. Ototoxicity of chemotherapeutic agents. Otolaryngol Clin North Am 1993;26:759–89.
32. Colvin OM. Antitumor alkylating agents. In: DeVita VT, Hellman S, Rosenberg SA, editors. Cancer: principles & practice of oncology. Philadelphia: Lippincott Williams & Wilkins; 2001. p. 363–75.
33. Rossi SE, Erasmus JJ, McAdams HP, et al. Pulmonary drug toxicity: radiologic and pathologic manifestations. Radiographics 2000;20:1245–59.
34. Ginsberg SJ, Comis RL. The pulmonary toxicity of antineoplastic agents. Semin Oncol 1982;9:34–51.
35. Litam JP, et al. Early pulmonary toxicity after administration of high-dose BCNU. Cancer Treat Rep 1981;65:39–44.
36. King P, Perry M. Hepatotoxicity of chemotherapeutic agents. In: Perry M, editor. The chemotherapy source book. Baltimore: Williams & Wilkins; 1996. p. 709–26.
37. Moertel CG, Fleming TR, Macdonald JS, et al. Hepatic toxicity associated with fluorouracil plus levamisole adjuvant therapy. J Clin Oncol 1993;11:2386–90.
38. Furlanut M, Franceschi L. Pharmacology of ifosfamide. Oncology 2003;65:2–6.
39. Kurowski V, Wagner T. Urinary excretion of ifosfamide, 4-hydroxyifosfamide, 3- and 2-dechloroethylifosfamide, mesna, and dimesna in patients on fractionated intravenous ifosfamide and concomitant mesna therapy. Cancer Chemother Pharmacol 1997;39:431–9.
40. Cannon J, Linke CA, Cos LR. Cyclophosphamide-associated carcinoma of urothelium: modalities for prevention. Urology 1991;38:413–6.
41. Alexandre J, et al. [Bladder neoplasms and cyclophosphamide. Apropos of 3 cases amd review of the literature]. Bull Cancer 1996;83:945–50.
42. Choudhury D, Ahmed Z. Drug-induced nephrotoxicity. Med Clin North Am 1997;81:705–17.
43. Skinner R. Strategies to prevent nephrotoxicity of anticancer drugs. Curr Opin Oncol 1995;7:310–5.
44. Hartmann JT, Kollmannsberger C, Kanz L, Bokemeyer C. Platinum organ toxicity and possible prevention in patients with testicular cancer. Int J Cancer 1999;83:866–9.
45. Medina PJ, Sipols JM, George JN. Drug-associated thrombotic thrombocytopenic purpura-hemolytic uremic syndrome. Curr Opin Hematol 2001;8:286–93.
46. Jacobson SD, et al. Glutamine does not prevent paclitaxel-associated myalgias and arthralgias. J Support Oncol 2003;1:274–8.
47. Shapiro CL, Recht A. Side effects of adjuvant treatment of breast cancer. N Engl J Med 2001;344:1997–2008.
48. Calabresi P, Chabner B. Chemotherapy of neoplastic disease. In: Goodman A, Gilman TR, Nies A, Taylor P, editors. Goodman and Gilman's the pharmacological basis of therapeutics. New York: McGraw-Hill; 1990. p. 1811.
49. Chu E, Mota A, Fogarasi M. Antimetabolites. In: DeVita VT, Hellman S, Rosenberg, SA, editors. Cancer: principles & practice of oncology. Philadelphia: Lippincott Williams & Wilkins; 2001. p. 388–415.
50. Rubnitz JE, et al. Transient encephalopathy following high-dose methotrexate treatment in childhood acute lymphoblastic leukemia. Leukemia 1998;12:1176–81.
51. Brock S, Jennings HR. Fatal acute encephalomyelitis after a single dose of intrathecal methotrexate. Pharmacotherapy 2004;24:673–6.
52. Diasio RB, Lu Z. Dihydropyrimidine dehydrogenase activity and fluorouracil chemotherapy. J Clin Oncol 1994;12:2239–42.

53. Anand AJ. Fluorouracil cardiotoxicity. Ann Pharmacother 1994;28:374–8.

54. Eiseman AS, Flanagan JC, Brooks AB, et al. Ocular surface, ocular adnexal, and lacrimal complications associated with the use of systemic 5-fluorouracil. Ophthal Plast Reconstr Surg 2003;19:216–24.

55. Hoff PM, Royce M, Medgyesy D, et al. Oral fluoropyrimidines. Semin Oncol 1999;26:640–6.

56. Rothenberg ML. Current status of capecitabine in the treatment of colorectal cancer. Oncology (Huntingt) 2002; 16:16–22.

57. Fung MC, et al. A review of hemolytic uremic syndrome in patients treated with gemcitabine therapy. Cancer 1999;85:2023–32.

58. Gamberale R, et al. In vitro susceptibility of CD4+ and CD8+ T cell subsets to fludarabine. Biochem Pharmacol 2003; 66:2185–91.

59. Goodman ER, Fiedor PS, Fein S, et al. Fludarabine phosphate: a DNA synthesis inhibitor with potent immunosuppressive activity and minimal clinical toxicity. Am Surg 1996;62:435–42.

60. Di Raimondo F, et al. Autoimmune hemolytic anemia in chronic lymphocytic leukemia patients treated with fludarabine. Leuk Lymphoma 1993;11:63–8.

61. Bryson HM, Sorkin EM. Cladribine. A review of its pharmacodynamic and pharmacokinetic properties and therapeutic potential in haematological malignancies. Drugs 1993;46:872–94.

62. Van Den Neste E, et al. Infectious complications after 2-chlorodeoxyadenosine therapy. Eur J Haematol 1996; 56:235–40.

63. Robak T. Cladribine in the treatment of chronic lymphocytic leukemia. Leuk Lymphoma 2001;40:551–64.

64. Cox PJ. Cyclophosphamide cystitis and bladder cancer. A hypothesis. Eur J Cancer 1979;15:1071–2.

65. Cox PJ. Cyclophosphamide cystitis—identification of acrolein as the causative agent. Biochem Pharmacol 1979; 28:2045–9.

66. Curtis RE, Boice JD Jr, Moloney WC, et al. Leukemia following chemotherapy for breast cancer. Cancer Res 1990; 50:2741–6.

67. Pratt CB, et al. Central nervous system toxicity following the treatment of pediatric patients with ifosfamide/mesna. J Clin Oncol 1986;4:1253–61.

68. Kohn KW. Interstrand cross-linking of DNA by 1,3-bis(2-chloroethyl)-1-nitrosourea and other 1-(2-haloethyl)-1-nitrosoureas. Cancer Res 1977;37:1450–4.

69. Colvin M, Brundrett RB, Cowens W, et al. A chemical basis for the antitumor activity of chloroethylnitrosoureas. Biochem Pharmacol 1976;25:695–9.

70. Garfield J, Dayan AD, Weller RO. Postoperative intracavitary chemotherapy of malignant supratentorial astrocytomas using BCNU. Clin Oncol 1975;1:213–22.

71. Colvin M, Cowens JW, Brundrett RB, et al. Decomposition of BCNU (1,3-bis(2-chloroethyl)-1-nitrosourea) in aqueous solution. Biochem Biophys Res Commun 1974; 60:515–20.

72. Farina P, et al. Metabolism of the anticancer agent 1-(4-acetylphenyl)-3,3-dimethyltriazene. Biomed Mass Spectrom 1983;10:485–8.

73. Skibba JL, Beal DD, Ramirez G, Bryan GT. N-Demethylation the antineoplastic agent 4(5)-(3,3-dimethyl-1-triazeno)imidazole-5(4)-carboxamide by rats and man. Cancer Res 1970;30:147–50.

74. Stewart C, Ratain MJ. Topoisomerase interactive agents. In: DeVita VT, Hellman S, Rosenberg SA, editors. Cancer: principles & practice of oncology. Philadelphia: Lippincott Williams & Wilkins; 2001. p. 415–31.

75. Mackay B, Ewer MS, Carrasco CH, Benjamin RS. Assessment of anthracycline cardiomyopathy by endomyocardial biopsy. Ultrastruct Pathol 1994;18:203–11.

76. Johnson S, Stevenson J, O'Dwyer P. Cisplatin and its analogues. In: DeVita V, Hellman S, Rosenberg SA, editors. Cancer: principles & practice of oncology. Philadelphia: Lippincott Williams & Wilkins; 2001. p. 376–88.

77. Loehrer PJ, Einhorn LH. Drugs five years later. Cisplatin. Ann Intern Med 1984;100:704–13.

78. Evans BD, Raju KS, Calvert AH, et al. Phase II study of JM8, a new platinum analog, in advanced ovarian carcinoma. Cancer Treat Rep 1983;67:997–1000.

79. Rowinsky E, Tolcher A. Antimicrotubule agents. In: DeVita VT, Hellman S, Rosenberg SA, editors. Cancer: principles & practice of oncology. Philadelphia: Lippincott Williams & Wilkins; 2001. p. 431–52.

80. Shepherd GM. Hypersensitivity reactions to chemotherapeutic drugs. Clin Rev Allergy Immunol 2003;24:253–62.

81. Cortes JE, Pazdur R. Docetaxel. J Clin Oncol 1995;13: 2643–55.

82. Nikolic-Tomasevic Z, Jelic S, Popov I, Radosavljevic D. Colorectal cancer: dilemmas regarding patient selection and toxicity prediction. J Chemother 2000;12:244–51.

83. van Groeningen CJ, et al. Altered pharmacokinetics and metabolism of CPT-11 in liver dysfunction: a need for guidelines. Clin Cancer Res 2000;6:1342–6.

84. Creemers GJ, et al. Phase II and pharmacologic study of topotecan administered as a 21-day continuous infusion to patients with colorectal cancer. J Clin Oncol 1996; 14:2540–5.

85. Cheson B. Miscellaneous chemotherapeutic agents. In: DeVita VT, Hellman S, Rosenberg SA, editors. Cancer: principles & practice of oncology. Philadelphia: Lippincott Williams & Wilkins; 2001. p. 452–9.

86. Vogelzang NJ, Bosl GJ, Johnson K, Kennedy BJ. Raynaud's phenomenon: a common toxicity after combination chemotherapy for testicular cancer. Ann Intern Med 1981;95:288–92.

87. Haddow A. Mode of action of chemical carcinogens. Br Med Bull 1947;4:331–42.

88. Ng A, Taylor GM, Eden OB. Treatment-related leukaemia—a clinical and scientific challenge. Cancer Treat Rev 2000;26:377–91.

89. Ben-Yehuda D, et al. Microsatellite instability and p53 mutations in therapy-related leukemia suggest mutator phenotype. Blood 1996;88:4296–303.

90. Vega-Stromberg T. Chemotherapy-induced secondary malignancies. J Infus Nurs 2003;26:353–61.

91. Leone G, Voso MT, Sica S, et al. Therapy related leukemias: susceptibility, prevention and treatment. Leuk Lymphoma 2001;41:255–76.

92. Curtis RE, et al. Risk of leukemia after chemotherapy and radiation treatment for breast cancer. N Engl J Med 1992;326:1745–51.

93. Price C, Gaucher G, Koneru P, et al. Mechanism of action of alkylating agents. Ann N Y Acad Sci 1969;163:593–600.

94. Kollmannsberger C, Hartmann JT, Kanz L, Bokemeyer C. Therapy-related malignancies following treatment of germ cell cancer. Int J Cancer 1999;83:860–3.

95. Winick NJ, et al. Secondary acute myeloid leukemia in children with acute lymphoblastic leukemia treated with etoposide. J Clin Oncol 1993;11:209–17.

96. Pui CH, et al. Acute myeloid leukemia in children treated with epipodophyllotoxins for acute lymphoblastic leukemia. N Engl J Med 1991;325:1682–7.

97. Karp JE, Smith MA. The molecular pathogenesis of treatment-induced (secondary) leukemias: foundations for treatment and prevention. Semin Oncol 1997;24:103–13.

98. Kobayashi K, Ratain MJ. Pharmacodynamics and long-term toxicity of etoposide. Cancer Chemother Pharmacol 1994;34 Suppl:S64–8.

99. Felix CA. Secondary leukemias induced by topoisomerase-targeted drugs. Biochim Biophys Acta 1998;1400:233–55.

100. Smith MA, et al. Secondary leukemia or myelodysplastic syndrome after treatment with epipodophyllotoxins. J Clin Oncol 1999;17:569–77.

101. Smith MA, Rubinstein L, Ungerleider RS. Therapy-related acute myeloid leukemia following treatment with epipodophyllotoxins: estimating the risks. Med Pediatr Oncol 1994;23:86–98.

102. Rosner F, Grunwald H. Multiple myeloma terminating in acute leukemia. Report of 12 cases and review of the literature. Am J Med 1974;57:927–39.

103. Bergsagel DE, et al. The chemotherapy on plasma-cell myeloma and the incidence of acute leukemia. N Engl J Med 1979;301:743–8.

104. Kaldor JM, et al. Leukemia following chemotherapy for ovarian cancer. N Engl J Med 1990;322:1–6.

105. Greene MH, et al. Melphalan may be a more potent leukemogen than cyclophosphamide. Ann Intern Med 1986; 105:360–7.

106. Reimer RR, Hoover R, Fraumeni JF Jr, Young RC. Acute leukemia after alkylating-agent therapy of ovarian cancer. N Engl J Med 1977;297:177–81.

107. Rosner F, Grunwald H. Hodgkin's disease and acute leukemia. Report of eight cases and review of the literature. Am J Med 1975;58:339–53.

108. Einhorn N. Acute leukemia after chemotherapy (melphalan). Cancer 1978;41:444–7.

109. Travis LB, et al. Second malignant neoplasms among long-term survivors of ovarian cancer. Cancer Res 1996;56: 1564–70.

110. Fisher B, et al. Leukemia in breast cancer patients following adjuvant chemotherapy or postoperative radiation: the NSABP experience. J Clin Oncol 1985;3:1640–58.

111. Diamandidou E, et al. Treatment-related leukemia in breast cancer patients treated with fluorouracil-doxorubicin-cyclophosphamide combination adjuvant chemotherapy: The University of Texas M.D. Anderson Cancer Center experience. J Clin Oncol 1996;14:2722–30.

112. van Leeuwen FE, et al. Leukemia risk following Hodgkin's disease: relation to cumulative dose of alkylating agents, treatment with teniposide combinations, number of episodes of chemotherapy, and bone marrow damage. J Clin Oncol 1994;12:1063–73.

113. Brusamolino E, et al. The risk of acute leukemia in patients treated for Hodgkin's disease is significantly higher aft [see bined modality programs than after chemotherapy alone and is correlated with the extent of radiotherapy and type and duration of chemotherapy: a case-control study. Haematologica 1998;83:812–23.

114. Travis LB, et al. Risk of leukemia following treatment for non-Hodgkin's lymphoma. J Natl Cancer Inst 1994;86: 1450–7.

115. Hancock SL, Tucker MA, Hoppe RT. Breast cancer after treatment of Hodgkin's disease. J Natl Cancer Inst 1993; 85:25–31.

116. Sont JK, et al. Increased risk of second cancers in managing Hodgkin's disease: the 20-year Leiden experience. Ann Hematol 1992;65:213–8.

117. Henry-Amar M. [Second cancers after treatment of Hodgkin's disease: experience at the International Database on Hodgkin's disease (IDHD)]. Bull Cancer 1992;79: 389–91.

118. Slanina J, Heinemann F, Henne K, et al. [Second malignancies after the therapy of Hodgkin's disease: the Freiburg collective 1940 to 1991]. Strahlenther Onkol 1999;175: 154–61.

119. Siu LL, Moore MJ. Use of mesna to prevent ifosfamide-induced urotoxicity. Support Care Cancer 1998;6: 144–54.

120. Travis LB, et al. Bladder and kidney cancer following cyclophosphamide therapy for non-Hodgkin's lymphoma. J Natl Cancer Inst 1995;87:524–30.

121. Waalen J. Pregnancy poses tough questions for cancer treatment. J Natl Cancer Inst 1991;83:900–2.

122. Cardonick E, Iacobucci A. Use of chemotherapy during human pregnancy. Lancet Oncol 2004;5:283–91.

123. Donegan WL. Cancer and pregnancy. CA Cancer J Clin 1983;33:194–214.

124. Greenlund LJ, Letendre L, Tefferi A. Acute leukemia during pregnancy: a single institutional experience with 17 cases. Leuk Lymphoma 2001;41:571–7.

125. Doll DC, Ringenberg QS, Yarbro JW. Antineoplastic agents and pregnancy. Semin Oncol 1989;16:337–46.

126. Matalon ST, Ornoy A, Lishner M. Review of the potential effects of three commonly used antineoplastic and immunosuppressive drugs (cyclophosphamide, azathioprine, doxorubicin) on the embryo and placenta. Reprod Toxicol 2004;18:219–30.

127. Wiebe VJ, Sipila PE. Pharmacology of antineoplastic agents in pregnancy. Crit Rev Oncol Hematol 1994;16:75–112.

128. Zemlickis D, et al. Fetal outcome after in utero exposure to cancer chemotherapy. Arch Intern Med 1992;152:573–6.

129. Aviles A, Niz J. Long-term follow-up of children born to mothers with acute leukemia during pregnancy. Med Pediatr Oncol 1988;16:3–6.

130. Nicholson HO. Cytotoxic drugs in pregnancy. Review of reported cases. J Obstet Gynaecol Br Commonw 1968; 75:307–12.

131. Reichman BS, Green KB. Breast cancer in young women: effect of chemotherapy on ovarian function, fertility, and birth defects. J Natl Cancer Inst Monogr 1994;16:125–9.

132. Lergier JE, Jimenez E, Maldonado N, Veray F. Normal pregnancy in multiple myeloma treated with cyclophosphamide. Cancer 1974;34:1018–22.

133. Earll JM, May RL. Busulfan therapy of myelocytic leukemia during pregnancy. Am J Obstet Gynecol 1965;92:580–1.

134. Feldkamp M, Carey JC. Clinical teratology counseling and consultation case report: low dose methotrexate exposure in the early weeks of pregnancy. Teratology 1993;47: 533–9.

135. Williams SF, Schilsky RL. Antineoplastic drugs administered during pregnancy. Semin Oncol 2000;27:618–22.

136. Elit L, Bocking A, Kenyon C, Natale R. An endodermal sinus tumor diagnosed in pregnancy: case report and review of the literature. Gynecol Oncol 1999;72:123–7.

137. Henderson CE, et al. Platinum chemotherapy during pregnancy for serous cystadenocarcinoma of the ovary. Gynecol Oncol 1993;49:92–4.

138. Schilsky R. Infertility after cancer chemotherapy. In: Bruce A, Chabner DLL, editors. Cancer chemotherapy and biotherapy: principles and practice. Philadelphia: Lippincott Williams & Wilkins; 2001. p. 50–66.

139. Russell LD, Russell JA. Short-term morphological response of the rat testis to administration of five chemotherapeutic agents. Am J Anat 1991;192:142–68.

140. Lu CC, Meistrich ML. Cytotoxic effects of chemotherapeutic drugs on mouse testis cells. Cancer Res 1979;39:3575–82.

141. Meistrich ML, Finch M, da Cunha MF, et al. Damaging effects of fourteen chemotherapeutic drugs on mouse testis cells. Cancer Res 1982;42:122–31.

142. Genesca A, et al. Sperm chromosome studies in individuals treated for testicular cancer. Hum Reprod 1990;5:286–90.

143. DeSantis M, Albrecht W, Holtl W, Pont J. Impact of cytotoxic treatment on long-term fertility in patients with germ-cell cancer. Int J Cancer 1999;83:864–5.

144. Gulati SC, Van Poznak C. Pregnancy after bone marrow transplantation. J Clin Oncol 1998;16:1978–85.

145. Meistrich ML, Wilson G, Brown BW, et al. Impact of cyclophosphamide on long-term reduction in sperm count in men treated with combination chemotherapy for Ewing and soft tissue sarcomas. Cancer 1992;70:2703–12.

146. Sobrinho LG, Levine RA, DeConti RC. Amenorrhea in patients with Hodgkin's disease treated with antineoplastic agents. Am J Obstet Gynecol 1971;109:135–9.

147. Miller JJ III, Williams GF, Leissring JC. Multiple late complications of therapy with cyclophosphamide, including ovarian destruction. Am J Med 1971;50:530–5.

148. Dnistrian AM, et al. Endocrine consequences of CMF adjuvant therapy in premenopausal and postmenopausal breast cancer patients. Cancer 1983;51:803–7.

149. Jarrell J, et al. Ovarian toxicity of cyclophosphamide alone and in combination with ovarian irradiation in the rat. Cancer Res 1987;47:2340–3.

150. Galton DA, Till M, Wiltshaw E. Busulfan (1,4-dimethanesulfonyloxybutane, myleran); summary of clinical results. Ann N Y Acad Sci 1958;68:967–73.

151. Shamberger RC, Rosenberg SA, Seipp CA, Sherins RJ. Effects of high-dose methotrexate and vincristine on ovarian and testicular functions in patients undergoing postoperative adjuvant treatment of osteosarcoma. Cancer Treat Rep 1981;65:739–46.

152. Choo YC, Chan SY, Wong LC, Ma HK. Ovarian dysfunction in patients with gestational trophoblastic neoplasia treated with short intensive courses of etoposide (VP-16-213). Cancer 1985;55:2348–52.

153. Goodwin PJ, Ennis M, Pritchard KI, et al. Risk of menopause during the first year after breast cancer diagnosis. J Clin Oncol 1999;17:2365–70.

154. Andrykowski MA, et al. Rheumatoid symptoms following breast cancer treatment: a controlled comparison. J Pain Symptom Manage 1999;18:85–94.

155. Smith DE. Additional cases of postchemotherapy rheumatism. J Clin Oncol 1993;11:1625–6.

156. Loprinzi CL, Duffy J, Ingle JN. Postchemotherapy rheumatism. J Clin Oncol 1993;11:768–70.

157. Michl I, Zielinski CC. More postchemotherapy rheumatism. J Clin Oncol 1993;11:2051–2.

158. Raderer M, Scheithauer W. Postchemotherapy rheumatism following adjuvant therapy for ovarian cancer. Scand J Rheumatol 19994;23:291–2.

159. Abu-Shakra M, Buskila D, Ehrenfeld M, et al. Cancer and autoimmunity: autoimmune and rheumatic features in patients with malignancies. Ann Rheum Dis 2001;60:433–41.

160. Papamichael D, Amft N, Slevin ML, D'Cruz D. 5-Fluorouracil-induced Raynaud's phenomenon. Eur J Cancer 1998;34:1983.

161. Van Den Neste E, Delannoy A, Feremans W, et al. Second primary tumors and immune phenomena after fludarabine or 2-chloro-2{165}-deoxyadenosine treatment. Leuk Lymphoma 2001;40:541–50.

162. Walter RB, Joerger M, Pestalozzi BC. Gemcitabine-associated hemolytic-uremic syndrome. Am J Kidney Dis 2002;40:E16.

163. Muller S, Schutt P, Bojko P, et la. Hemolytic uremic syndrome following prolonged gemcitabine therapy: report of four cases from a single institution. Ann Hematol 2005;84(2):110–14.

164. Jain S, Seymour AE. Mitomycin C associated hemolytic uremic syndrome. Pathology 1987;19:58–61.

165. Lesesne JB, et al. Cancer-associated hemolytic-uremic syndrome: analysis of 85 cases from a national registry. J Clin Oncol 1989;7:781–9.

Appendix

Dose Reductions Required in Cases of Organ Dysfunction

Chemotherapy agents requiring dose reduction in patients with liver dysfunction

- Amsacrine
- Daunorubicin
- Doxorubicin
- Epirubicin
- Idarubicin
- Mitoxantrone
- Paclitaxel
- Docetaxel
- Vinblastine
- Vincristine
- Thiotepa
- Irinotecan

Chemotherapy agents requiring dose reduction in patients with renal dysfunction

- Methotrexate
- Capecitabine
- Fludarabine
- Cisplatin
- Carboplatin
- Oxaliplatin
- Bleomycin
- Cyclophosphamide
- Ifosfamide
- Etoposide
- Hydroxyurea
- Topotecan

Systemic Sequelae of Bioimmunotherapy

Auris Huen, PharmD
Saroj Vadhan-Raj, MD

In the last two decades, bioimmunotherapy has achieved great strides in establishing its role in medical treatment. Agents previously investigated for salvage or palliative purposes are considered part of standard treatment for untreated patients. Since the introduction of the first recombinant protein, human insulin, into the market, many biologic drugs have been approved by the Food and Drug Administration (FDA) for clinical use in the United States.

Bioimmunotherapy encompasses all therapy related to the modification of the immune system's response to infection or malignancy.[1] The roots of biotherapeutics trace back to before the nineteenth century, when manipulation of the immune response was used to treat cancer, but the inability to produce adequate quantities limited their broad clinical application. Advancements in production techniques in the 1970s to 1980s allowed for large quantities of purified product to be readily available for investigation. In the past two decades, many new biologic compounds have been identified with the use of powerful molecular biology tools.

Several classes of agents fall under the umbrella of bioimmunotherapy, including monoclonal antibodies (MoAbs), interferons, interleukins (ILs), cytokine antagonists, and growth factors. Although grouped together, agents in this category are vastly different in character and treatment indications. These agents generally differ from traditional chemotherapy in both side-effect profiles and dose-toxicity relationships.[2] This chapter will focuses on only the biologic agents that have been FDA approved or investigated for therapeutic applications in oncology or as supportive care agents. The goal is to provide an overview of their systemic effects.

Bioimmunotherapy Agents and Systemic Effects

Monoclonal Antibodies

The discovery of antibody-based therapy began in 1890 when transferable immunity was first described by von Behring and Kitasato in the animal model.[3] However, it was not until the discovery of hybridoma technology[4] by Kohler and Milstein in 1975 that the large-scale production of therapeutic monoclonal antibodies (MoAbs) became possible.

The MoAbs bind to specific antigens on the surface of the targeted cell and, once bound, incite an immune response to the antigen and consequently the cell bound to the antigen. Some antibodies may also directly induce apoptosis via other pathways.[5]

Early murine MoAb carried 100% murine protein sequences and incited severe hypersensitivity reactions owing to the development of human antimouse antibodies (HAMAs).[6,7] The HAMA response impairs targeting and accelerates MoAb clearance, subsequently decreasing its potency. Development of partly human (chimeric) and humanized (complementary determining region grafted) MoAb via recombinant deoxyribonucleic acid (DNA) technology significantly decreased this immunogenic response.[8] A chimeric molecule is still detectable in human circulation for 2 weeks compared with 2 days for a murine molecule.[6] Most therapeutic antibodies are chimeric (30–35% murine) or humanized (< 10% murine), but murine antibodies are also in use. Although occurring at a lower rate, human antichimeric antibody and human antihuman antibody have also been reported.[2]

MoAbs can be classified into three groups: unconjugated (naked), conjugated with immunotoxins, and radioimmunotherapy. Table 1 summarizes the currently approved MoAbs, their biologic targets, and FDA-approved indications.[9–24]

Unconjugated Antibodies

Unconjugated antibodies independently mediate cell death via recruitment of an immune response via antibody-dependent cell-mediated cytotoxicity (ADCC) and complement-dependent cytotoxicity. In ADCC, the Fc constant region of the antibody engages effector cells such as natural killer (NK) cells, monocytes, and macrophages. These effector cells function to illicit phagocytosis and cyctotoxicity. The Fc region additionally activates complement.[5] This mechanism requires high tumor expression of the antigen and tight antibody-antigen binding. Antibody-mediated calcium channel inhibition may also directly induce apoptosis independently of an immune response, such as with rituximab.[25] Examples of unconjugated MoAb include rituximab, alemtuzumab, trastuzumab, cetuximab, and bevacizumab, each specific to a spectrum of antigenic targets.

Unconjugated antibodies are used clinically for treatment of hematologic and solid tumor malignancies, as well as for management of infections. Single-agent response rates in hematologic malignancies range from 20 to 48%.[26–28] Given that the biologic targets of antibodies differ from those of traditional cytotoxic chemotherapy, MoAbs may also enhance the chemotherapy response without increasing toxicity and overlapping patterns of resistance.[29]

Adverse events of unconjugated MoAb predominantly involve hypersensitivity or infusion-related reactions. These symptoms can vary from rash, fevers, chills, and rigors to severe urticaria, hypotension, bronchospasm, dyspnea, and anaphylaxis. These reactions can occur in up to 77% of patients receiving MoAb infusion. Infusion reactions generally improve with subsequent doses and are managed successfully with supportive medications.[12] Other less common adverse effects reported with unconjugated MoAb include cardiotoxicity associated with trastuzumab; severe and prolonged immunosuppression and infections with alemtuzumab; hypertension, coagulopathy, and decreased wound healing with bevacizumab; and acneiform rash with cetuximab.

Cardiotoxicity is not uncommon among cancer agents.[30] The risk of development of cardiotoxicity with trastuzumab is 4% with monotherapy and 27% when used concurrently with anthracyclines and cyclophosphamide.[31] But unlike anthracycline-induced cardiotoxicity, the cardiac effects associated with trastuzumab are generally asymptomatic or mild and responsive to medical management. Cardiomyopathy with trastuzumab did not appear to be dose dependent, and some patients are able to continue with trastuzumab therapy with proper management

Table 1 Monoclonal Antibodies and Their Treatment Indications[9–24]

Drug	Target	Indication(s)
Unconjugated MoAb for oncology indication		
Alemtuzumab (Campath)	Anti-CD52 antibody	B-cell chronic lymphocytic leukemia in patients who have been treated with alkylating agents and who have failed fludarabine therapy
Bevacizumab (Avastin)	Anti-VEGF antibody	For use in combination with intravenous 5-fluorouracil-based chemotherapy as a first-line treatment for metastatic colorectal cancer
Cetuximab (Erbitux)	Anti-HER1 antibody	(1) In combination with radiation therapy, is indicated for the treatment of early stages of most types of head and neck cancer (2) Patients with head and neck cancer whose tumor has grown larger or has spread to other parts of the body after receiving treatment containing a platinum-based chemotherapy (3) EGFR-expressing metastatic colorectal carcinoma ± irinotecan-based chemotherapy
Rituximab (Rituxan)	Anti-CD20 antibody	(1) For relapsed or refractory low-grade or follicular, CD20-positive, B-cell NHL (2) For the first-line treatment of diffuse large B-cell, CD20-positive, NHL (a type of NHL) in combination with CHOP or other anthracycline-based chemotherapy regimens (3) For use in combination with methotrexate for reducing signs and symptoms in adult patients with moderately to severely active rheumatoid arthritis who have had an inadequate response to one or more TNF antagonist therapies
Trastuzumab (Herceptin)	Anti-HER2 antibody	For metastatic breast cancer in HER2-overexpressed tumors
Unconjugated MoAb for autoimmune diseases and other indications		
Adalimumab (Humira)	Anti-TNF antibody	(1) Reducing signs and symptoms, inducing major clinical response, inhibiting the progression of structural damage, and improving physical function in adult patients with moderately to severely active rheumatoid arthritis (2) Reducing signs and symptoms of active arthritis in patients with psoriatic arthritis
Basiliximab (Simulect)	Anti-IL-2 receptor antibody	Prophylaxis of acute organ rejection in patients receiving renal transplants
Daclizumab (Zenapax)	Anti-IL-2 receptor antibody	Prophylaxis of acute organ rejection in patients receiving renal transplants
Efalizumab (Raptiva)	Anti-CD11a antibody	For chronic moderate to severe plaque psoriasis in adults age 18 yr or older
Infliximab (Remicade)	Anti-TNF-α antibody	(1) Reducing signs and symptoms, achieving clinical remission and mucosal healing, and eliminating corticosteroid use in patients with moderately to severely active ulcerative colitis who have had an inadequate response to conventional therapy (2) Reducing signs and symptoms and inducing and maintaining clinical remission in patients with moderately to severely active Crohn's disease who have had an inadequate response to conventional therapy (3) Reducing the number of draining enterocutaneous and rectovaginal fistulae and maintaining fistula closure in patients with fistulizing Crohn's disease (4) Reducing signs and symptoms in patients with active ankylosing spondylitis (5) Reducing signs and symptoms of active arthritis in patients with psoriatic arthritis (6) In combination with methotrexate for reducing signs and symptoms, inhibiting the progression of structural damage, and improving physical function in patients with moderately to severely active rheumatoid arthritis
Muromonab CD3 (Orthoclone OKT3)	Anti-CD3 antibody	Treat rejection of transplanted organs, including the heart, kidneys, and liver
Omalizumab (Xolair)	Anti-IgE antibody	For moderate to severe persistent asthma in adults and adolescents
Unconjugated MoAb for infectious disease		
Palivizumab (Synagis)	Antibody directed at the epitope of the A antigenic site of the F protein of RSV	Prevention of serious lower respiratory tract disease caused by RSV in pediatric patients at high risk of RSV disease
Radioimmunotherapy		
Ibritumomab Tiuxetan (Zevalin)	Anti-CD20 antibody attached to ⁹⁰yttrium	Relapsed or refractory low-grade, follicular, or transformed B-cell NHL, including patients with rituximab (Rituxan) refractory follicular NHL
Tositumomab ¹³¹iodine (Bexxar)	Anti-CD20 antibody attached to ¹³¹iodine	Relapse or refractory low-grade follicular lymphoma or transformed NHL, including patients with rituximab refractory NHL
Immunoconjugate		
Gemtuzumab Ozogamicin (Mylotarg)	Anti-CD33 antibody attached to calicheamicin derivative	Relapsed acute myeloid leukemia in first relapse patients who are 60 yr of age or older and who are not considered candidates for cytotoxic chemotherapy

CHOP = cyclophosphamide, doxorubicin, Oncovin (vincristine), and prednisone; EGFR = epidermal growth factor receptor; IgE = immunoglobulin E; IL = interleukin; MoAb = monoclonal antibody; NHL = non-Hodgkin's lymphoma; RSV = respiratory syncytial virus; TNF = tumor necrosis factor; VEGF = vascular endothelial growth factor.

and monitoring.[32] The mechanism of trastuzumab-associated cardiotoxicity is still being investigated. It has been postulated that trastuzumab may have direct cardiotoxic effects on the heart mediated by the presence of HER2 receptors on cardiac tissue.[33]

Alemtuzumab targets the CD52 antigen expressed on B and T lymphocytes. Most treated patients will experience significant and prolonged lymphopenia by 2 to 4 weeks that may persist up to 1 year.[34,35] Concurrently, patients may also experience neutropenia between 2 and 12 weeks, with extreme cases lasting several months.[36] A combination of these factors leads to increased risk of infection and infection-related mortality. In addition to bacterial infections, atypical infections with *Pneumocystis jiroveci* (formerly *P. carinii*), viral reactivation, and invasive fungal infections are common.[37]

The use of bevacizumab to block angiogenesis by vascular endothelial growth factor (VEGF) is associated with cardiovascular adverse effects, coagulopathy, and decreased wound healing. Hypertension is a common adverse effect associated with bevacizumab. VEGF antagonism has been linked to inhibition of nitric oxide, leading to vasoconstriction. The reported incidence is 15 to 30%, with only 2% graded as severe.[10,38] Hemorrhage and thrombosis have been reported with bevacizumab. The risk of severe hemorrhage or thrombosis is low. VEGF inhibition has been proposed to decrease the ability of endothelial cells to respond to injury, thereby increasing the risk of bleeding. A prothrombotic state has been attributed to inhibition of nitric oxide–mediated platelet aggregation.[10,39,40] Wound complications and dehiscence have been associated with bevacizumab.[10]

Dermatologic toxicity has been reported in clinical trials with cetuximab. Up to 89% of treated patients reported dermatologic side effects, but only 11% were severe.[41] The most common presentation is a follicular rash, usually in an acneiform distribution. Although the precise mechanism of development of rash has not been elucidated, inhibition of the epidermal growth factor receptor pathway by cetuximab may interfere with development of hair follicles, leading to an inflammatory response.[42,43]

Unconjugated MoAbs are also indicated in the treatment of various autoimmune indications. Most of these agents are targeted at cytokines and are discussed in the cytokine antagonist section of this chapter.

Conjugated Antibodies

Therapeutic MoAbs may be used as delivery vehicles for toxins and cytotoxic therapy, theoretically targeting only specific diseased cells and sparing normal ones. Immunotoxins are conjugated antibodies with protein toxin bound to the MoAb.

Protein toxins disrupt protein synthesis and ultimately lead to cell death. This mechanism requires the antibody- (with toxin) antigen complex to undergo endocytosis once binding occurs at the cell surface, thereby delivering the toxin directly into the targeted cells.[5]

Gemtuzumab ozogamicin is a conjugated MoAb with activity in acute myeloid leukemia (AML) targeting CD33-positive cells. The antibody portion is attached to a derivative of the highly potent natural toxin calicheamicin via a carboxylic acid linker. An overall remission rate of 26% (defined as less than 5% bone marrow blasts, a normal white blood cell count without blasts, and transfusion independence) has been reported for elderly patients with relapsed AML (based on three multicenter phase II trials).[24] In addition to hypersensitivity reactions, gemtuzumab ozogamicin has also been associated with myelosuppression and hepatotoxicity. Venoocclusive disease (incidence up to 17% of treated patients) has been attributed to the calicheamicin derivative.[44]

Radioimmunotherapy

Historically, one of the drawbacks of radiotherapy had been the inability to target tumor cells while sparing normal tissue. Using the same principle as antibody-conjugated chemotherapy, radioimmunotherapies also use MoAb as a delivery mechanism to provide targeted therapy. MoAb conjugates are labeled with a β-emitting isotope, such as ^{90}yttrium and ^{131}iodine, and can deliver localized radiation therapy by binding to antigens on tumor cells. Additionally, radiation is emitted to surrounding tumor cells. This effect on neighboring cells is sometimes referred to as the "bystander effect."[5] Cytotoxicity occurs independently from receptor internalization and an immune-mediated response. For the treatment of relapsed non-Hodgkin's lymphoma, radioimmunoconjugates ^{90}yttrium ibritumomab tiuxetan and ^{131}iodine tositumomab ^{131}iodine have approximate overall response rates of 39 to 92%.[45] ^{90}Yttrium ibritumomab tiuxetan has demonstrated superior activity over the naked MoAb rituximab.[46] Both radioimmunotherapy agents are murine antibodies and target the CD20 antigen on B lymphocytes. The murine antibody was chosen in this class of agents to increase clearance and decrease prolonged radiation exposure. Adverse reactions are generally mild but primarily include prolonged myelosuppression, with nadirs occurring 5 to 8 weeks from therapy. Small fractions of patients receiving tositumomab ^{131}iodine may develop hypothyroidism despite thyroid protection during treatment.[45]

The MoAbs have been used successfully in the treatment of various diseases outside the oncology arena. Palivizumab is the first MoAb indicated for treatment of infection. It is directed

against the epitope of the A antigenic site on the F protein of respiratory syncytial virus (RSV), thereby inhibiting RSV replication. The agent is indicated for the prevention of RSV infections in high-risk pediatric patients.[21]

Research is ongoing uncovering new antigenic targets for which MoAbs may be used as part of a treatment modality. New routes of administration, such as intraperitoneal and intrathecal, are also currently being investigated, increasing the utility of these agents.[47,48]

Interferons

Over 40 years ago, Isaacs and Lindenmann described a protein that "interfered" with viral growth.[49] This substance, called interferon (IFN), has been investigated extensively for treatment of oncologic and nonmalignant diseases. Various mechanisms of action and biologic activity have been reported, but the details have only been partially elucidated.[50] IFNs impair viral replication by synthesis of a number of enzymes that interfere with cellular and viral processes. They also possess antitumor activity, which seems to be related to both modulation of the immune response to the tumor cells and direct antiproliferative effects.[49]

IFNs are divided into two major groups based on binding to either the type I or type II IFN receptor. The type I IFNs are IFN-α, IFN-β, IFN-ω, and IFN-tau. IFN-γ is the only type II IFN. On viral stimulation, almost all cells will produce type I IFNs, but the primary sites of production are leukocytes and fibroblasts. In contrast, type II IFNs are produced by T cells and NK cells following immunologic stimuli, such as with T cell–specific antigens and staphylococcal enterotoxin A.[49] IFNs are species specific and receptor dependent. Binding of IFNs to receptors outside the cell membrane leads to the phosphorylation of Janus-activated kinase (Jak) molecules intracellularly. Signal transducers and activators of transcription in the cytoplasm are activated by Jak, which translocates to the nucleus to activate transcription of IFN-stimulated genes.[49,50] Biologic activities of IFNs include inhibition of cell proliferation, enhanced phagocytic activity of macrophages, increased cytotoxic activity of NK cells, enhanced major histocompatibility complex (MHC) class I and II antigen presentation pathways, and antiangiogenic effects.[49–51]

The development of DNA technology for the sequencing and cloning of genes led to the ability to produce and purify large quantities of IFN for clinical application.[49] Table 2 lists the IFNs approved for treatment of various malignant and nonmalignant diseases.[52–60]

Interferon-α

The primary production sites for IFN-α are the leukocytes. This subgroup of IFNs possesses a multitude of modulatory activity in immune and

IFN	FDA Indication(s)
IFN-α2a, recombinant (Roferon-A)	AIDS-related Kaposi's sarcoma
	CML, chronic phase
	Hairy cell leukemia
	Chronic hepatitis C
Pegylated IFN-α2a (Pegasys)	Chronic hepatitis B and C
IFN-α2b, recombinant (Intron A)	AIDS-related Kaposi's sarcoma
	Condyloma acuminatum
	Follicular lymphoma
	Hairy cell leukemia
	Chronic hepatitis B and C
	Malignant melanoma
Pegylated IFN-α2b (Peg-Intron)	Chronic hepatitis C
IFN-αn3 (Alferon N)	Refractory or recurring condylomata acuminata
IFN alfacon-1 (Infergen)	Chronic hepatitis C
IFN-β1a (Avonex, Rebif)	Multiple sclerosis
IFN-β1b (Betaseron)	Multiple sclerosis
IFN-γ1b (Actimmune)	Chronic granulomatous disease Malignant osteopetrosis

Table 2 Types of Interferon and Treatment Indications[52–60]

AIDS = acquired immune deficiency syndrome; CML = chronic myeloid leukemia; FDA = US Food and Drug Administration; IFN = interferon.

tumor cells. In tumor cells, IFN-α has been observed to directly inhibit tumor proliferation, as well as up-regulation of tumor-specific antigens, MHC I, and adhesion molecules. Stimulatory effects are also reported in NK cells and macrophages. IFN-α can also lead to both stimulatory and inhibitory effects on T lymphocytes.[49] Currently, four forms of IFN-α are available in the United States. IFN-α2a and IFN-α2b are both recombinant proteins derived from *Escherichia coli*. The two agents differ by a single amino acid at position 23. IFN-αn3 is produced from pooled units of human leukocytes stimulated by the Sendai murine virus.[56] In contrast, IFN alfacon-1 is a recombinantly produced non-naturally occurring IFN. Its polypeptide sequence was derived by scanning sequences of several naturally occurring IFN-α subtypes.[57] Pegylated formulations of IFN-α combine the IFN molecule to a polyethylene glycol moiety. This slows the metabolism of the molecule and provides increased sustained exposure and increased efficacy.[61,62]

IFN-α has been used in both oncology and nononcologic diseases. IFNs exhibit antitumor activity in solid tumors and hematologic malignancies. IFN-α is indicated for the front-line treatment of chronic myeloid leukemia in the chronic phase. The median survival for patients with some evidence of cytogenetic response has been approximately 6 years, and over 90% of patients with a complete cytogenetic response are in remission at 10 years.[50] It has also been shown to prolong disease-free survival in chronic myeloid leukemia patients after allogeneic stem cell transplantation. Response rates of 40 to 50% as a single agent have been demonstrated in non-Hodgkin's lymphoma.[63] In addition, IFN-α

also has shown activity in multiple myeloma, melanoma, and renal cell carcinoma.[50]

Interferon-β

Many mechanisms of action of IFN-β have been proposed. IFN-β may exert antiproliferative effects through suppression of c-*myc* gene expression in tumor cells.[64] The two recombinant formulations IFN-β1a and IFN-β1b are currently available for the treatment of multiple sclerosis . IFN-β slows the frequency of neurologic disturbances and progression of physical debilitation in patients with multiple sclerosis.[62] The once-weekly injection of IFN-β1a may be preferred over IFN-β1b owing to decreased injection-site reactions and a lower incidence of neutralizing antibodies.

Interferon-γ

This IFN is also known as the immune IFN since it is derived from immune stimulation of T cells. It is an activator of T cells and macrophages in synergy with IL-2. It up-regulates both MHC classes I and II and possesses higher antiproliferative properties compared with IFN-α or IFN-β.[49,64] The recombinant protein is used in prevention of infection in patients with chronic granulomatous disease. In these patients, the risk of infection was decreased by 67% compared with placebo. IFN-γ has also been shown to delay time to progression in malignant osteopetrosis.[60]

Adverse Effects

IFNs have been associated with multiple systemic adverse effects. The incidence and severity of these effects are dependent on the dose, route,

and duration of therapy.[50] In general, short infusions and bolus administration are associated with decreased incidence of adverse effects compared with continuous infusion. IFN-mediated release of other cytokines, such as tumor necrosis factor (TNF)-α, IL-1, IL-2, and IL-6, may be responsible for the adverse effects observed with IFN.[65]

The most common acute toxicity associated with IFN is flu-like or constitutional symptoms (eg, fatigue, fever, chills, malaise, headache, rigors, anorexia). The cellular and inflammatory immune response incited by IFN and induced cytokines may result in these constitutional symptoms. Up to 96% of patients receiving systemic administration of IFN have reported this adverse effect.[54] Symptoms usually occur on initiation of therapy and subside within a few months with continued use.

Chronic side effects include fatigue, anorexia, weight loss, and alteration in mood. Fatigue may persist throughout therapy and may worsen over the length of treatment altering qualify of life. It may also contribute to the reasons for discontinuation of therapy.[49,65]

Depression is a serious and dose-limiting adverse effect associated with IFN therapy.[49] Suicide ideation and attempts have been attributed to IFN therapy.[66] The incidence tends to be greater among the type I IFN (IFN-α 6–26% and IFN-β 25–34%). The etiology is unclear but may stem from the direct and indirect effects of IFN on the hypothalamus and alterations in neurotransmitter levels.[65] Additionally, other neurologic and psychiatric disorders, such as mood instability (manic-depressive), psychosis, neuropathy, somnolence, and impairment of cognitive function, have been reported.[49] The incidence and severity of neurologic disorders are dose and duration dependent.

Thyroid dysfunction has also been associated with IFN therapy, manifesting as hypo- or hyperthyroidism.[67,68] The thyroid autoantibodies can develop in up to 40% of patients treated with IFN.[69] IFN's toxicity on the thyroid may be due to direct and indirect effects on the thyroid gland.[49] Direct mechanisms for IFN-induced thyroid disease include inhibition of thyroid-stimulating hormone–induced gene expression, decreased iodine organification, and decreased thyroxine release. Indirect effects relate to activation of secondary cytokines.[69] Hyperglycemia and hypertriglyceridemia have also been reported with IFN therapy.[50]

High-dose IFN therapy may result in the development of myelosuppression. Neutropenia (more common), thrombocytopenia, and anemia occurred in patients receiving IFN therapy. Other laboratory abnormalities include liver function test elevations, which are usually mild and reversible, and have been reported in up to 63% of patients receiving IFN-α.[62]

IFNs are a potent class of cytokines that modulate the immune response. These effects are harnessed for the treatment of various autoimmune, infectious, and oncologic conditions. Various challenges remain for this class of agents: better definition of the mechanism of action and the limitation of adverse effects associated with IFNs. Better understanding of these factors will further broaden the therapeutic application of these agents.

Interleukins

The ILs are a diverse group of cytokine proteins that are produced primarily from activated T lymphocytes and monocytes. These substances function primarily to enhance the immune response but have been reported to also stimulate cellular differentiation (as hematopoietic growth factors).[64] The ILs and their resultant signal proteins orchestrate the complex balance between cellular activation and immunomodulation. Interactions with ILs may be redundant, stimulatory, or inhibitory.[70,71] ILs display both inhibition of tumor growth, as seen in patients treated with IL-2 for renal cell carcinoma, and stimulation of tumor proliferation, demonstrated by IL-6 in multiple myeloma. Two ILs are approved by the FDA to date for clinical indications: IL-2 and IL-11. IL-11 is a platelet growth factor and is discussed under the section on growth factors.

Interleukin-2

In 1976, a T-cell growth factor was isolated in cultures of mitogen-stimulated human peripheral blood mononuclear cells. This protein, later termed IL-2, was also found to induce proliferation of B cells, NK cells, and lymphokine-activated killer cells. IL-2 was produced by activated T lymphocytes and by some T-cell leukemias.[72] There are two recombinant forms of IL-2: aldesleukin and teceleukin derived from *E. coli*. Only aldesleukin is FDA approved.[73] IL-2 binds to the specific cell surface receptor IL-2 receptor, expressed on both T and B lymphocytes. Recombinant IL-2 binds to IL-2 receptor, inducing tyrosine phosphorylation of multiple cellular proteins, resulting in the synthesis of a multitude of secondary cytokines, such as IL-1, TNF, and IFN-γ[72] IL-2 has also demonstrated activation of both humoral and cell-mediated immunity.[71]

Aldesleukin is indicated for the treatment of adults with metastatic renal cell carcinoma and melanoma.[73] In metastatic renal cell carcinoma in which treatment options are limited, high-dose intravenous IL-2 therapy demonstrated response rates ranging from 0 to 40%, with a median of 15% in all trials.[70] In patients with a complete response, IL-2 improved the quality and durability of tumor response. Lower subcutaneous doses of IL-2 and combination therapy with IFN-α and

5-fluorouracil have been evaluated in renal cell carcinoma. Continuous infusion IL-2 is used in combination with chemotherapy and IFN-α (biotherapy) in the treatment of metastatic melanoma. IL-2 has shown activity in non-Hodgkin's lymphoma and leukemia and in lymphoma following stem cell transplantation.[72]

Toxicities associated with IL-2 therapy are dose and schedule dependent.[74] Higher doses and continuous infusion of IL-2 correlate with more adverse effects, such as constitutional symptoms and capillary leak syndrome, compared with lower doses and bolus intermittent administration. Toxicities can be severe and life-threatening if not properly managed but usually resolve 2 to 3 days on discontinuation of IL-2 therapy.[72,75] In clinical trials for metastatic renal cell carcinoma and melanoma, the majority of patients were not able to receive all planned doses of IL-2 owing to toxicity.[73]

Capillary leak syndrome is a toxicity resulting from increased capillary permeability and decreased vascular resistance caused by secondary cytokines induced by IL-2.[72] Cytokines lead to generation of complement-activating products, endothelial cell antigens, and neutrophil activation. The result is fluid shifting to an extravascular space and consequently hypovolemia (oliguria, ischemia, confusion) and fluid retention (edema, weight gain, pulmonary congestion, pleural effusion, ascites).[71,72]

Cardiovascular adverse effects are a dose-limiting toxicity associated with IL-2 therapy, the majority of which manifests as hypotension (70% of patients with a 20 to 30 mm Hg decrease in systolic pressure). Tachycardia and other cardiac symptoms, such as arrhythmia, have been reported. Neurologic changes have also been reported in patients receiving IL-2 therapy. This toxicity can be dose limiting, with confusion and somnolence being the most common, at a reported incidence of 34 and 22%, respectively, in patients treated for renal cell carcinoma and melanoma.[71,72]

Constitutional symptoms are also common with IL-2 therapy, developing in more than 50% of patients.[73] Symptoms include chills, fever, and fatigue. Increased TNF-α serum levels stimulated by IL-2 have been implicated with the development of fever.[76] These symptoms appear to have an increased frequency in the high-dose regimens.[77] Other adverse effects associated with IL-2 therapy include gastrointestinal symptoms (nausea and vomiting), prerenal azotemia, hyperbilirubinemia, increased infection risk, and endocrine dysfunction (hypo- and hyperthyroidism).[72] Hypothyroidism is more common, with a reported incidence of 35% of patients receiving IL-2.[78] Proposed mechanisms include suppression of thyroid-stimulating hormone secretion and development of antithyroid antibodies.[79]

Although treatment with IL-2 is associated with significant toxicity and often requires close monitoring, with the prophylactic measures to prevent toxicity, the incidence of drug-related mortality is reported to be 2% (in single-agent studies).[73] Patient selection and determination of the optimal dose are the primary challenges with this treatment modality.

Denileukin Diftitox

Denileukin diftitox is a fusion protein consisting of a fragment of diphtheria toxin genetically fused to IL-2. Denileukin diftitox targets IL-2 receptors on the surface of malignant cells and some normal lymphocytes. Once bound, the fusion protein is internalized, cleaving the toxin moiety into the cytoplasm, leading to the death of these cells.[80] Denileukin diftitox was FDA approved in 1999 for the treatment of patients with persistent or recurrent cutaneous T-cell lymphoma (CTCL) whose malignant cells express the CD25 component of the IL-2 receptor.[81] Approximately 30% (21 of 71) of patients with CTCL demonstrated a reduction in tumor burden of 50% or greater.[82]

Significant adverse events included flu-like symptoms (91%), acute hypersensitivity-type reactions (69%), nausea and vomiting (64%), infections (48%), and vascular leak syndrome (27%), consistent with some of the IL-2-related toxicities.[82] CTCL patients are particularly susceptible to infections because of the compromised condition of their skin. It is unknown if increased infection may be related to denileukin diftitox therapy targeting some normal lymphocytes.

Growth Factors

Myelosuppression is a common dose-limiting factor of chemotherapy and increases the need for hospitalization, intravenous antibiotic administration, transfusion of blood products, dose reduction, and treatment delays. These factors may lead to significant negative effects on patient quality of life or even response to treatment. Recently, significant progress has been made in understanding the process of hematopoiesis by which mature cellular elements of blood are formed.[83] Hematopoietic growth factors are regulatory molecules that function by activating the mature blood cells and promoting the growth, survival, and differentiation of progenitor cells. Several growth factors are marketed for the minimization of chemotherapy-induced hematologic toxicity. The FDA-approved recombinant human hematopoietic growth factors are listed in Table 3.[84–90] Palifermin is the only growth factor not targeting hematopoiesis. The second-generation growth factors pegfilgrastim and darbepoetin alfa have long serum half-lives and have been approved by the FDA for use in the oncology setting.

Table 3 Hematopoietic Growth Factors and Their Indications		
Growth Factor	*Target*	*FDA-Approved Indication*
Filgrastim (G-CSF, Neupogen)	Committed granulocytes	Decrease the incidence of infection, febrile neutropenia, in patients with nonmyeloid malignancies receiving myelosuppressive anticancer drugs associated with a significant incidence of severe neutropenia with fever
Sargramostim (Leukine)	Committed and noncommitted cells	(1) Use following induction chemotherapy in older patients with acute myelogenous leukemia (2) Use in myeloid reconstitution after autologous and allogeneic BMT (3) Use in BMT failure or engraftment delay (4) Use in mobilization and following autologous BMT
Pegfilgrastim (pegylated G-CSF, Neulasta)	Committed granulocytes	To decrease the incidence of infection, as manifested by febrile neutropenia, in patients with nonmyeloid malignancies receiving myelosuppressive anticancer drugs associated with a clinically significant incidence of febrile neutropenia
Epoetin alfa (Procrit, Epogen)	Committed erythroid progenitor cells	(1) For the treatment of anemia in patients with nonmyeloid malignancies in whom anemia is due to the effect of concomitantly administered chemotherapy; to decrease the need for transfusions in patients who will be receiving concomitant chemotherapy for a minimum of 2 mo (2) For the treatment of anemia in chronic kidney disease patients not on dialysis; to elevate or maintain the red blood cell level and to decrease the need for transfusions (3) For the treatment of anemia related to therapy with zidovudine in HIV-infected patients (4) For the treatment of anemic patients (Hb >10 to ≤ 13 g/dL) scheduled to undergo elective, noncardiac, nonvascular surgery to reduce the need for allogeneic blood transfusions
Darbepoetin (Aranesp)	Committed erythroid progenitor cells	(1) For the treatment of anemia associated with chronic renal failure, including patients on dialysis and patients not on dialysis (2) For the treatment of anemia in patients with nonmyeloid malignancies in whom anemia is due to the effect of concomitantly administered chemotherapy
IL-11 (Oprelvekin, Neumega)	Committed megakaryocyte progenitor cells	For the prevention of severe thrombocytopenia and the reduction of the need for platelet transfusions following myelosuppressive chemotherapy in adult patients with nonmyeloid malignancies who are at high risk of severe thrombocytopenia
Palifermin (Kepivance)	Epidermal cells	To decrease the incidence and duration of severe oral mucositis in patients with hematologic malignancies receiving myelotoxic therapy requiring hematopoietic stem cell support

BMT = bone marrow transplantation; G-CSF = granulocyte colony-stimulating factor; Hb = hemoglobin; HIV = human immunodeficiency virus.

Anemia in cancer patients can be multifactorial, including nutritional deficiencies, hemolysis, blood loss, bone marrow involvement, anemia of chronic disease, a blunted endogenous erythropoietin (EPO) response, and cytotoxic treatment causing a damaging effect on bone marrow precursor cells, which is usually proportional to the intensity of the chemotherapy dose. Additionally, this anemia may be related to the renal toxicity of some chemotherapy agents, such as platinum agents.

EPO was the first hematopoietic growth factor to become commercially available in the United States. Several randomized and non-randomized trials have demonstrated that EPO can significantly reduce transfusion requirements and improve quality of life.[91,92] Approximately 60% of all cancer patients receiving chemotherapy will respond to EPO treatment. Darbepoetin has an efficacy similar to that of EPO for the management of chemotherapy-induced anemia.[93] Darbepoetin contains two additional *N*-glycosylation sites over EPO, giving it a longer half-life.[87] This allows for the drug to be given up to every 3 weeks compared with traditional weekly dosing with EPO.

Treatment with erythropoietic agents has been well tolerated in cancer patients. Rarely, hypertension associated with a dramatic rise in hemoglobin has been observed.[94] Occasionally, patients with underlying central nervous system disease may have increased seizure activity in the context of the aforementioned hypertension. The incidence of venous thrombosis has been reported to be somewhat higher with the use of these agents, with the incidence reported around 6% in patients receiving the active treatment compared with 4% with patients receiving the placebo in randomized trials for correction of anemia. However, the risk is significantly increased in the recent studies targeting higher hemoglobin values for reducing tumor hypoxia and for prevention of anemia. Two of these studies have also reported an adverse outcome on survival.[95,96] Although EPO has been widely used, with an excellent safety profile in the management of anemia in oncology and nephrology, these findings have raised concerns and caution against targeting higher hemoglobin levels.

Granulocyte colony-stimulating factor (G-CSF) is a myeloid lineage growth factor that stimulates the production and functions of mature neutrophils. G-CSF was first approved in 1991 for its ability to reduce the incidence of febrile neutropenia in cancer patients receiving myelosuppressive chemotherapy. This indication has been further expanded to include other areas of utility within the practice of oncology, including the mobilization of progenitor stem cells for use in blood and marrow transplantation and the stimulation of neutrophil recovery following high-dose chemotherapy with stem cell support. Additionally, G-CSF is indicated to increase neutrophil production in congenital neutropenic states and other endogenous myeloid disorders.[97]

Granulocyte-macrophage colony-stimulating factor (GM-CSF) stimulates the production of neutrophils, monocytes, and eosinophils and has been FDA approved since 1991 for use in patients with nonmyeloid malignancies undergoing autologous bone marrow transplantation. Since then, GM-CSF has received approval for other indications, such as the reduction of myelotoxicity for leukemia patients following induction chemotherapy. More recently, GM-CSF has been reportedly effective as an immune stimulant for management of infectious disease and in the oncology setting when used concurrently with other biologic agents.[98,99]

Myeloid growth factors are generally well tolerated. Mild to moderate bone pain, which usually manifests at the onset of therapy or at the time of neutrophil recovery, is the predominant side effect observed with the use of G-CSF. On occasion, the pain may be severe enough to require analgesics for control.[100] Other rare side effects include cutaneous vasculitis, activation of preexisting psoriasis, and Sweet's syndrome.[97] The most common side effects reported with the use of GM-CSF have included constitutional symptoms, such as fever, bone pain, myalgia, headaches, and chills. These side effects are more frequent when GM-CSF is administered at higher doses or by continuous intravenous infusion than with traditional subcutaneous dosing. In the transplant setting, no excessive toxicity has been reported with the use of GM-CSF compared with controls. Other rare side effects, such as first-dose phenomenon and capillary leak syndrome, are reported with *E. coli*–derived GM-CSF (not approved in the United States), and not with sargramostim (Leukine).[97]

Following standard-dose chemotherapy, severe thrombocytopenia requiring platelet transfusions is uncommon. However, it can be cumulative in patients treated with multiple chemotherapeutic regimens and represents a significant problem in patients receiving dose-intensive or myeloablative chemotherapy. Several hematopoietic cytokines with thrombopoietic activity have been evaluated in clinical trials, including IL-l, IL-3, IL-6, IL-11, thrombopoietin (TPO), megakaryocyte growth and development factor (MGDP) and granulocyte colony stimulating factor/IL-3 fusion molecule (PIXY 321). Most of these cytokines have shown modest thrombopoietic activity and mediate a number of biologic effects, including some untoward effects. At this time, IL-11 is the only thrombopoietic cytokine approved by the FDA for clinical use.[89]

IL-11 is a pleiotropic cytokine with hematopoietic, anti-inflammatory, and mucosa-protective activities. Based on its thombopoietic activity, IL-11 was FDA approved in 1997 for the prevention of severe thrombocytopenia and the reduction of platelet transfusion following myelosuppressive chemotherapy in patients with non-myeloid malignancies.[101] However, the systemic adverse effects have limited its wide clinical utility. The most common side effects experienced with IL-11 are injection-site reactions and mild to moderate fluid retention, which may be manifested by either peripheral edema or pulmonary edema with dyspnea. IL-11 administration has increased the size of preexisting pleural effusions in some patients.[97]

Additionally, reports of decreased hemoglobin values are thought to be related to the dilutional effect of fluid retention. In addition, palpitations, tachycardia, and atrial arrhythmias have also been reported with this agent, making it difficult to use in patients with a history of cardiac disease.[89]

Immunoglobulins

The immunoglobulins (Igs) are polyclonal antibodies collected from pooled human plasma. These antibodies are collected from 3,000 to 100,000 healthy blood donors, representing a diverse mixture of various antibodies present in normal serum.[102] These antibodies provide passive immunity directed against foreign pathogens and natural autoantibodies. These autoantibodies react against self-antigens, which are responsible for the immunomodulatory activity of Ig. Igs have been used for decades in the treatment of multiple diseases, ranging from antibody-mediated autoimmune states to infections. Controlled trials have demonstrated the efficacy of intravenous Ig in idiopathic thrombocytopenic purpura, dermatomyositis, Guillian-Barré syndrome, myasthenia gravis, graft-versus-host disease, Kawasaki disease, prevention of infection in leukemia patients, and others.[102,103] More recently, more specific forms of Ig are available with higher antibody titers specific to infectious pathogens, such as cytomegalovirus, hepatitis, or varicella zoster.

Adverse effects associated with Ig are generally mild and uncommon. Similar to administration of any allogeneic blood product, the most common adverse reaction is hypersensitivity or infusion-related reactions, which are infusion rate dependent. The symptoms may include fevers, chills, bronchospasms, skin rash or hives, and anaphylaxis. A rapid rate of antibody infusion may precipitate renal dysfunction in patients unable to tolerate the large protein load administered. Preparations of intravenous immunoglobulin (IVIG) stabilized with sucrose may be more prone to cause renal dysfunction owing to hyperosmolality.[62] Although often used interchangeably, various different commercial preparations of IVIG may have differences in adverse reaction profile owing to differences in the manufacturing process, Fc receptor function, and complement fixation.[104]

Cytokine Antagonists

Cytokines have varied cellular effects in the human body. Some of these effects are beneficial and are used to treat diseases. In some cases, cytokine activity is part of the pathogenesis of disease. Cytokines have also been identified as major mediators of systemic manifestations of several disease processes. Cytokine antagonists have been developed to block their effects and improve patient outcome. Several cytokine antagonists, such as TNF-α and IL-1 antagonists, have been evaluated for treatment of autoimmune states. IL-2 MoAbs have also been developed for use as immunosuppressants in the transplant setting.

TNF-α Antagonists

TNF is a proinflammatory cytokine produced by macrophages and T cells. Exposure to TNF at sites of inflammation leads to activation of proinflammatory cytokines and production of destructive enzymes, resulting in tissue damage.[105]

Currently, there are three TNF-α inhibitors (adalimumab, infliximab, etanercept) on the US market. These agents block the activity of TNF via different mechanisms and are indicated for the treatment of inflammatory conditions. Adalimumab (human antibody) and infliximab (chimeric mouse-human IgG1) are MoAbs directed at TNF-α and inhibit its binding to TNF receptors. A major clinical response has been observed in patients receiving these agents in combination with methotrexate chemotherapy compared with placebo and methotrexate in patients with rheumatoid arthritis. Infliximab has activity in multiple other diseases, such as Crohn's disease, ulcerative colitis, and ankylosing spondylitis.[18] Infliximab has also been investigated for the treatment of steroid-refractory graft-versus-host disease in bone marrow transplant recipients.[106] Adalimumab is indicated for psoriatic arthritis.[14]

Infliximab is associated with infusion-related adverse effects, observed in approximately 20% of patients.[18] The infusion reactions with infliximab may be related to development of antibodies against the drug. The incidence of antibody is lower in patients who receive a concurrent immunosuppressant (10–43%) versus those who did not (18–75%).[107] Treatment with infliximab is also associated with antibodies to double-stranded DNA and antinuclear antibodies.[107] The scheduled administration of infliximab is associated with a lower risk of immunogenicity compared with episodic treatment. Patients treated with adalimumab may also have infusion-related effects.[14,108]

Patients receiving these agents are at higher risk of infections associated with atypical organisms and opportunistic infections, such as cytomegalovirus, histoplasmosis, aspergillosis, and nocardiosis.[109,110] The microbial organisms responsible for these infections are generally intracellular pathogens or pathogens kept in check by cell-mediated immunity. This finding may be supported by experimental studies establishing the role of TNF in protective immunity.[111] Several cases of tuberculosis have been reported in patients receiving infliximab and adalimumab. The infections seem to be more reported with infliximab, presumably because of its potent TNF inhibitory activity. Therefore, it is recommended that patients are appropriately evaluated for latent infections prior to initiation of such treatment, and a high index of suspicion and appropriate surveillance cultures, with prompt empiric treatment, may be required to prevent morbidity and mortality.

More patients treated with anti-TNF-α antibodies developed malignancies compared with patients receiving placebo, although the direct causal relationship remains controversial. All TNF-α inhibitors were associated with an increased incidence of non-Hodgkin's and

Hodgkin's lymphoma in treated patients.[112] Up to a fourfold higher risk has been reported in patients receiving adalimumab. Other solid tumor malignancies have also been observed.[14]

Etanercept is a genetically engineered fusion protein with two identical chains of TNF receptor p75 monomer fused with the Fc domain of IgG1, binding to TNF and inhibiting its activity. Similar to infliximab, it is indicated for treatment of various autoimmune diseases, such as rheumatoid arthritis, ankylosing spondylitis, and plaque psoriasis. It is being investigated for treatment of graft-versus-host disease in stem cell transplant recipients and various hematologic malignancies.[113,114] Infections, injection-site reactions, flu-like symptoms, and headache have been reported in clinical trials with etanercept.[107] An increased incidence of lymphoma (three times the expected rate) has been observed in patients receiving etanercept for rheumatoid arthritis.[115]

IL-1 Antagonists

IL-1 is a proinflammatory cytokine produced in response to inflammation.[116] The activity of IL-1 includes stimulation of osteoclast activity, leading to increased inflammation and in synovial tissue possibly increasing bone and cartilage attrition in addition to other diverse activities, such as hematopoietic stimulation and augmentation of the T-cell response.[117]

Anakinra is a IL-1 antagonist indicated for the treatment of rheumatoid arthritis. It is a recombinant form of the human IL-1 receptor antagonist. In combination with methotrexate, anakinra improves response compared with methotrexate alone. Adverse reactions are generally mild but may include an increased risk of infections. The risk of infection with anakinra is lower compared with TNF inhibitors.[116] Neutropenia has also been associated with the use of this agent.[117]

IL-2 Antagonist

The stimulation of a T cell–mediated cellular immune response to allogeneic organ transplant is mediated by IL-2. Binding of IL-2 to high-affinity IL-2 receptors on activated T lymphocytes leads to activation of cell-mediated immunity associated with allograft rejection. MoAb targeting the IL-2 receptor blocks the activation pathway for T-cell activation and mutes its response to antigenic stimulation.[62] Basiliximab and daclizumab are both recombinant antibodies targeting the IL-2 receptor used to prevent acute organ rejection in the renal transplantation setting in combination with other immunosuppressants. Both agents are being investigated in oncology patients for the treatment of graft-versus-host disease following bone marrow transplantation.[118,119] Adverse effects attributable to the IL-2 receptor antagonists (compared with placebo)

were not found in these studies.[15,16] However, in other settings, such as ulcerative colitis, fever, and lethargy, upper respiratory infections with basiliximab and headache and skin rash with daclizumab have been reported.[107]

Thalidomide

Thalidomide, an immunomodulatory agent with multiple biologic activities, has been shown to have efficacy in the treatment of patients with refractory, relapsed myeloma. Although the precise mechanism of action responsible for this activity is unknown, the inhibitory effects of thalidomide on the various cytokines that stimulate angiogenesis (VEGF, basic fibroblast growth factor) and cytokines (IL-6, IL-1β, and IL-10 and TNF-α) secreted into the microenvironment of the marrow and modulating the growth and survival of myeloma cells may play an important role in its antitumor activity.[120] The clinical side effects of thalidomide include drowsiness or sedation, fatigue, constipation, dizziness, and peripheral neuropathy.[81] The efforts are directed at developing more potent analogues (lenalidomide) with fewer side effects.

Conclusions

Recent advances in biotechnology have accelerated the development of biologic agents, leading to novel therapeutic options and diagnostic tools. The number of biologic response modifiers will increase as understanding of cellular signaling processes improves. Manipulation of cell signaling and subsequent modulation of the immune system will continue to play an integral part in the management of immune-related diseases and malignancies. Research also continues with adoptive cellular therapy, a strategy intended to eliminate tumor either by a direct antitumor effect or by indirect effects on the immune system, although no form of cellular therapy has as yet been FDA approved.

Although the arsenal of biologic agents is growing, it is also important to understand the mechanisms responsible for the systemic effects of these agents to optimize their clinical utility and to develop more potent analogues with fewer side effects. Many of these side effects, although they may not be serious, nevertheless can have a significant impact on patients' quality of life. Furthermore, some systemic sequelae, such as opportunistic infections, can lead to life-threatening complications. Therefore, it is important to remain cognizant about the full spectrum of biologic effects and prevention or management of adverse events.

Significant advances are also being made in the area of supportive care for the prevention and attenuation of toxicity as the biology of the

underlying process is better understood and new tools are available to intervene and improve the tolerance of cytotoxic treatment. The targeting of various receptors, such as 5-hydroxytryptamine$_3$ and neurokinin-1, with novel antiemetics has significantly ameliorated nausea and vomiting. Recent progress in the understanding of biology of the bone disease has identified the role of RANK/RANKL pathways and other novel targets and opened up new possibilities for the treatment of malignant bone disease and the prevention of skeleton-related complications. The enhanced understanding of biologic effects and how to improve the therapeutic index by minimizing untoward systemic effects and enhancing clinical benefits will likely broaden the therapeutic applications of cytokines and other biologic response modifiers in the future.

REFERENCES

1. Oldhan R. Cancer biotherapy: general principles. In: Oldham R, editor. Principles of cancer biotherapy. Dordrecht (Netherlands): Kluwer Academic Press; 1998. p. 1–15.
2. Weinberg WC, Frazier-Jessen MR, Wu WJ, et al. Development and regulation of monoclonal antibody products: challenges and opportunities. Cancer Metastasis Rev 2005;24:569–84.
3. Forero A, Lobuglio AF. History of antibody therapy for non-Hodgkin's lymphoma. Semin Oncol 2003;30 (6 Suppl 17):1–5.
4. Kohler G, Milstein C. Continuous cultures of fused cells secreting antibody of predefined specificity. Nature 1975;256:495–7.
5. Scheinberg DA, Sgouros G, Junghans RP. Antibody-based immunotherapies for cancer. In: Chabner BA, Longo DL, editors. Cancer chemotherapy and biotherapy: principles and practice. Philadelphia: Lippincott Williams and Wilkins; 2001. p. 850–90.
6. Breedveld FC. Therapeutic monoclonal antibodies. Lancet 2000;355:735–40.
7. Weiner LM, Adams GP, Von Mehren M. Therapeutic monoclonal antibodies: general principles. In: Devita VT, Hellman S, Rosenberg SA, editors. Cancer: principles and practice of oncology. 6th ed. PhiladelphiaA: Lippincott Williams and Wilkins; 2001. p. 495–508.
8. Ross JS, Gray K, Gray GS, et al. Anticancer antibodies. Am J Clin Pathol 2003;119:472–85.
9. Campath [package insert]. Montville (NJ): Berlex. Revised 7/2005.
10. Avastin [package insert]. South San Francisco (CA): Genentech Biooncology. Revised 9/2005.
11. Erbitux [package insert]. Princeton (NJ): Bristol-Myers Squibb Company. 6/2004.
12. Rituxan [package insert]. South San Francisco (CA): Genentech Inc. 2/2006.
13. Herceptin [package insert]. South San Francisco (CA): Genentech Inc. 2/2005.
14. Humira [package insert]. Chicago: Abbott Laboratories. Revised 10/2005.
15. Simulect [package insert]. East Hanover (NJ): Novartis Pharmaceutical Corporation. Revised 11/2003.
16. Zenapax [package insert]. Nutley (NJ): Hoffman-La Roche Inc. Revised 9/2005.
17. Raptiva [package insert]. South San Francisco (CA): Genentech Inc. 6/2005.
18. Remicade [package insert]. Malvern (PA): Centocor Inc. Revised 3/2006.
19. Orthoclone OKT3 [package insert]. Raritan (NJ): Ortho Biothech. Revised 11/2004.
20. Xolair [package insert[. South San Francisco (CA): Genentech Inc. Revised 3/2005.
21. Synagis [package insert]. Gaithersburg (MD): MedImmune Inc. Revised 7/2004.
22. Zevalin [package insert]. Cambridge (MA): Biogen Idec Inc. 9/2005.
23. Bexxar [package insert]. Research Triangle Park (NC): Glaxo Smith Kline. 10/2005.

24. Mylotarg [package insert]. Philadelphia: Wyeth Pharmaceuticals Inc. Revised 1/2006.

25. Janas E, Priest R, Wilde JI, et al. Rituxan (anti-CD20 antibody)-induced translocation of CD20 into lipid rafts is crucial for calcium influx and apoptosis. Clin Exp Immunol 2005;139:439–46.

26. Lundin J, Osterborg A, Brittinger G, et al. CAMPATH-1H monoclonal antibody in therapy for previously treated low-grade non-Hodgkin's lymphomas: a phase II multi-center study. European Study Group of CAMPATH-1H Treatment in Low-Grade Non-Hodgkin's Lymphoma. J Clin Oncol 1998;16:3257–63.

27. McLaughlin P, Grillo-Lopez AJ, Link BK, et al. Rituximab chimeric anti-CD20 monoclonal antibody therapy for relapsed indolent lymphoma: half of patients respond to a four-dose treatment program. J Clin Oncol 1998;16:2825–33.

28. Berinstein NL, Grillo-Lopez AJ, White CA, et al. Association of serum rituximab (IDEC-C2B8) concentration and anti-tumor response in the treatment of recurrent low-grade or follicular non-Hodgkin's lymphoma. Ann Oncol 1998;9:995–1001.

29. Coiffier B, Lepage E, Briere J, et al. CHOP chemotherapy plus rituximab compared with CHOP alone in elderly patients with diffuse large-B-cell lymphoma. N Engl J Med 2002;346:235–42.

30. Yeh ET. Cardiotoxicity induced by chemotherapy and antibody therapy. Annu Rev Med 2006;57:485–98.

31. Seidman A, Hudis C, Pierri MK, et al. Cardiac dysfunction in the trastuzumab clinical trials experience. J Clin Oncol 2002;20:1215–21.

32. Keefe DL. Trastuzumab-associated cardiotoxicity. Cancer 2002;95:1592–600.

33. Fuchs I, Landt S, Buehler H, et al. HER2 expression in the myocardium as a cause for cardiotoxicity of trastuzumab. Proc Am Soc Clin Oncol 2000;19:102a.

34. Dearden CE, Matutes E, Cazin B, et al. High remission rate in T-cell prolymphocytic leukemia with CAMPATH-1H. Blood 2001;98:1721–6.

35. Rawstron AC, Kennedy B, Moreton P, et al. Early prediction of outcome and response to alemtuzumab therapy in chronic lymphocytic leukemia. Blood 2004;103:2027–31.

36. Gibbs SD, Westerman DA, McCormack C, et al. Severe and prolonged myeloid haematopoietic toxicity with myelodysplastic features following alemtuzumab therapy in patients with peripheral T-cell lymphoproliferative disorders. Br J Haematol 2005;130:87–91.

37. Thursky KA, Worth LJ, Seymour JF, et al. Spectrum of infection, risk and recommendations for prophylaxis and screening among patients with lymphoproliferative disorders treated with alemtuzumab. Br J Haematol 2006;132:3–12.

38. Sane DC, Anton L, Brosnihan KB. Angiogenic growth factors and hypertension. Angiogenesis 2004;7:193–201.

39. Ignoffo RJ. Overview of bevacizumab: a new cancer therapeutic strategy targeting vascular endothelial growth factor. Am J Health Syst Pharm 2004;61(21 Suppl 5): S21–6.

40. Motl S. Bevacizumab in combination chemotherapy for colorectal and other cancers. Am J Health Syst Pharm 2005;62:1021–32.

41. Rhee J, Oishi K, Garey J, Kim E. Management of rash and other toxicities in patients treated with epidermal growth factor receptor-targeted agents. Clin Colorectal Cancer 2005;5 Suppl 2:S101–6.

42. Kimyai-Asadi A, Jih MH. Follicular toxic effects of chimeric anti-epidermal growth factor receptor antibody cetuximab used to treat human solid tumors. Arch Dermatol 2002;138:129–31.

43. Monti M, Mancini LL, Ferrari B, et al. Complications of therapy and a diagnostic dilemma case. Case 2. Cutaneous toxicity induced by cetuximab. J Clin Oncol 2003;21: 4651–3.

44. Giles FJ, Kantarjian HM, Kornblau SM, et al. Mylotarg (gemtuzumab ozogamicin) therapy is associated with hepatic venoocclusive disease in patients who have not received stem cell transplantation. Cancer 2001;92:406–13.

45. Pohlman B, Sweetenham J, Macklis RM. Review of clinical radioimmunotherapy. Expert Rev Anticancer Ther 2006; 6:445–61.

46. Witzig TE, Gordon LI, Cabanillas F, et al. Randomized controlled trial of yttrium-90-labeled ibritumomab tiuxetan radioimmunotherapy versus rituximab immunotherapy for patients with relapsed or refractory low-grade, follicular, or transformed B-cell non-Hodgkin's lymphoma. J Clin Oncol 2002;20:2453–63.

47. Schulz H, Pels H, Schmidt-Wolf I, et al. Intraventricular treatment of relapsed central nervous system lymphoma with the anti-CD20 antibody rituximab. Haematologica 2004;89:753–54.

48. Ng T, Pagliuca A, Mufti GJ. Intraperitoneal rituximab: an effective measure to control recurrent abdominal ascites due to non-Hodgkin's lymphoma. Ann Hematol 2002;81: 405–6.

49. Isaacs A, Lindenmann J. Virus Interference. I. The interferon. Proc R Soc Lond B Biol Sci. 1957;147(927): 258–67.

50. Vestal DJ, Yi T, Borden EC. Pharmacology of interferons: induced proteins, cell activation and antitumor activity. In: Chabner BA, Longo DL, editors. Cancer chemotherapy and biotherapy: principles and practice. 3rd ed. Philadelphia: Lippincott Williams and Wilkins; 2001. p. 752–78.

51. Kirkwood JM. Interferons. In: Devita VT, Hellman S, Rosenberg SA, editors. Cancer: principles and practice of oncology. 6th ed. Philadelphia: Lippincott Williams and Wilkins; 2001. p. 461–71.

52. Roferon-A [package insert]. Nutley (NJ): Roche Pharmaceuticals. Revised 9/2003.

53. Pegasys [package insert]. Nutley (NJ): Roche Pharmaceuticals. Revised 1/2004.

54. Intron A [package insert]. Kenilworth (NJ): Schering Corp. Revised 3/2004.

55. Peg-Intron [package insert]. Kenilworth (NJ): Schering Corporation. Revised 2/2005.

56. Alferon N [package insert]. Hemispherx Biopharma Inc. 2004.

57. Infergen [package insert]. Brisbane (CA): InterMune Inc. Revised 2/2003.

58. Avonex [package insert]. Cambridge (MA): Biogen Idec Inc. 3/2005.

59. Betaseron [package insert]. Berlex Laboratories. Revised 2/2003.

60. Actimmune [package insert]. Brisbane (CA): InterMune Inc. Revised 5/2005.

61. Chung RT, Andersen J, Volberding P, et al. Peginterferon alfa-2a plus ribavirin versus interferon alfa-2a plus ribavirin for chronic hepatitis C in HIV-coinfected persons. N Engl J Med 2004;351:451–9.

62. McEvoy GK, editor. AHFS drug information 2005. Bethesda (MD): American Society of Health-System Pharmacists; 2005.

63. Steis RG, Foon KA, Longo DL. Current and future uses of recombinant interferon alpha in the treatment of low-grade non-Hodgkin's lymphoma. Cancer 1987;59 (3 Suppl):658–63.

64. Dorr RT, Von Hoff DD, editors. Cancer chemotherapy handbook. 2nd ed. East Norwalk (CT): Appletion and Lange; 1994.

65. Kirkwood JM, Bender C, Agarwala S, et al. Mechanisms and management of toxicities associated with high-dose interferon alfa-2b therapy. J Clin Oncol 2002;20: 3703–18.

66. Janssen HL, Brouwer JT, van der Mast RC, Schalm SW. Suicide associated with alfa-interferon therapy for chronic viral hepatitis. J Hepatol 1994;21:241–3.

67. Gisslinger H, Gilly B, Woloszczuk W, et al. Thyroid autoimmunity and hypothyroidism during long-term treatment with recombinant interferon-alpha. Clin Exp Immunol 1992;90:363–7.

68. Caraccio N, Dardano A, Manfredonia F, et al. Long-term follow-up of 106 multiple sclerosis patients undergoing interferon-beta 1a or 1b therapy: predictive factors of thyroid disease development and duration. J Clin Endocrinol Metab 2005;90:4133–7.

69. Mandac JC, Chaudhry S, Sherman KE, Tomer Y. The clinical and physiological spectrum of interferon-alpha induced thyroiditis: toward a new classification. Hepatology 2006; 43:661–72.

70. Schmidinger M, Hejna M, Zielinski CC. Aldesleukin in advanced renal cell carcinoma. Expert Rev Anticancer Ther 2004;4:957–80.

71. Bukowski RM, Tannenbaum CS, Finke JH. Clinical pharmacokinetics of interleukin 1, interleukin 2, interleukin 4, tumor necrosis factor, interleukin 12, and macrophage colony-stimulating factor. In: Chabner BA, Longo DL, editors. Cancer chemotherapy and biotherapy: principles and practice. Philadelphia: Lippincott Williams and Wilkins; 2001. p. 779–828.

72. Bruton JK, Koeller JM. Recombinant interleukin-2. Pharmacotherapy 1994;14:635–56.

73. Proleukin [package insert]. Emeryville (CA): Chiron Therapeutics. 9/2000.

74. Yang JC, Rosenberg SA. An ongoing prospective randomized comparison of interleukin-2 regimens for the treatment of metastatic renal cell cancer. Cancer J Sci Am 1997;3 Suppl 1:S79–84.

75. Schwartzentruber DJ. Guidelines for the safe administration of high-dose interleukin-2. J Immunother 2001;24: 287–93.

76. Mier JW, Vachino G, van der Meer JW, et al. Induction of circulating tumor necrosis factor (TNF alpha) as the mechanism for the febrile response to interleukin-2 (IL-2) in cancer patients. J Clin Immunol 1988;8:426–36.

77. Sundin DJ, Wolin MJ. Toxicity management in patients receiving low-dose aldesleukin therapy. Ann Pharmacother 1998;32:1344–52.

78. Weijl NI, Van der Harst D, Brand A, et al. Hypothyroidism during immunotherapy with interleukin-2 is associated with antithyroid antibodies and response to treatment. J Clin Oncol 1993;11:1376–83.

79. Krouse RS, Royal RE, Heywood G, et al. Thyroid dysfunction in 281 patients with metastatic melanoma or renal carcinoma treated with interleukin-2 alone. J Immunother Emphasis Tumor Immunol 1995;18:272–8.

80. Foss F. Clinical experience with denileukin diftitox (ONTAK). Semin Oncol 2006;33(1 Suppl 3):S11–6.

81. Micromedex® Healthcare Series: Thomson Micromedex, Greenwood Village, Colorado (edition expires [3/2006]).

82. Olsen E, Duvic M, Frankel A, et al. Pivotal phase III trial of two dose levels of denileukin diftitox for the treatment of cutaneous T-cell lymphoma. J Clin Oncol 2001;19: 376–88.

83. Demetri GD. Targeted approaches for the treatment of thrombocytopenia. Oncologist 2001;6 Suppl 5:15–23.

84. Neupogen [package insert]. Thousand Oaks (CA): Amgen Inc. Revised 12/2004.

85. Neulasta [package insert]. Thousand Oaks (CA): Amgen Inc. Revised 9/2005.

86. Leukine [package insert]. Seattle (WA) : Berlex Pharmaceutical Inc. Revised 5/2004.

87. Aranesp [package insert]. Thousand Oaks (CA): Amgen Inc. 3/2006.

88. Procrit [package insert]. Raritan (NJ): Ortho Biotech Products. Revised 11/2005.

89. Neumega [package insert]. Philadelphia: Wyeth Pharmaceuticals Inc. PA 2/2006.

90. Kepivance [package insert]. Thousand Oaks (CA): Amgen Inc. 12/2005.

91. Demetri GD, Kris M, Wade J, et al. Quality-of-life benefit in chemotherapy patients treated with epoetin alfa is independent of disease response or tumor type: results from a prospective community oncology study. Procrit Study Group. J Clin Oncol 1998;16:3412–25.

92. Glaspy J, Bukowski R, Steinberg D, et al. Impact of therapy with epoetin alfa on clinical outcomes in patients with nonmyeloid malignancies during cancer chemotherapy in community oncology practice. Procrit Study Group. J Clin Oncol 1997;15:1218–34.

93. Schwartzberg LS, Yee LK, Senecal FM, et al. A randomized comparison of every-2-week darbepoetin alfa and weekly epoetin alfa for the treatment of chemotherapy-induced anemia in patients with breast, lung, or gynecologic cancer. Oncologist 2004;9:696–707.

94. Smith KJ, Bleyer AJ, Little WC, Sane DC. The cardiovascular effects of erythropoietin. Cardiovasc Res 2003;59: 538–48.

95. Leyland-Jones B. Breast cancer trial with erythropoietin terminated unexpectedly. Lancet Oncol 2003;4:459–60.

96. Henke M, Laszig R, Rube C, et al. Erythropoietin to treat head and neck cancer patients with anaemia undergoing radiotherapy: randomised, double-blind, placebo-controlled trial. Lancet 2003;362:1255–60.

97. Demetri GD, Vadhan-Raj S. Hematopoietic growth factors. In: Pazdur R, Coia LR, Hoskins WJ, Wagman LD, editors. Cancer management: a multidisciplinary approach. 4th ed. Melville (NY): PRR; 2000. p. 747–62.

98. Ferrajoli A, O'Brien S, Faderl S, et al. Rituximab plus GM-CSF for patients with chronic lymphocytic leukemia. Presented at the American Society of Hematology; 2005 Dec; Atlanta, GA.

99. Bodey GP, Anaissie E, Gutterman J, Vadhan-Raj S. Role of granulocyte-macrophage colony-stimulating factor as adjuvant therapy for fungal infection in patients with cancer. Clin Infect Dis 1993;17:705–7.

100. Kubista E, Glaspy J, Holmes FA, et al. Bone pain associated with once-per-cycle pegfilgrastim is similar to daily

filgrastim in patients with breast cancer. Clin Breast Cancer 2003;3:391–8.

101. Tepler I, Elias L, Smith JW II, et al. A randomized placebo-controlled trial of recombinant human interleukin-11 in cancer patients with severe thrombocytopenia due to chemotherapy. Blood 1996;87:3607–14.

102. Ephrem A, Misra N, Hassan G, et al. Immunomodulation of autoimmune and inflammatory diseases with intravenous immunoglobulin. Clin Exp Med 2005;5:135–40.

103. Boughton BJ, Jackson N, Lim S, Smith N. Randomized trial of intravenous immunoglobulin prophylaxis for patients with chronic lymphocytic leukaemia and secondary hypogammaglobulinaemia. Clin Lab Haematol 1995;17:75–80.

104. Jolles S, Sewell WA, Misbah SA. Clinical uses of intravenous immunoglobulin. Clin Exp Immunol. 2005;142:1–11.

105. Vilcek J, Feldmann M. Historical review: Cytokines as therapeutics and targets of therapeutics. Trends Pharmacol Sci 2004;25:201–9.

106. Patriarca F, Sperotto A, Damiani D, et al. Infliximab treatment for steroid-refractory acute graft-versus-host disease. Haematologica 2004;89:1352–9.

107. Blonski W, Lichtenstein GR. Complications of biological therapy for inflammatory bowel diseases. Curr Opin Gastroenterol 2006;22:30–43.

108. Scheinfeld N. A comprehensive review and evaluation of the side effects of the tumor necrosis factor alpha blockers etanercept, infliximab and adalimumab. J Dermatolog Treat 2004;15:280–94.

109. Chang JT, Lichtenstein GR. Drug Insight: antagonists of tumor-necrosis factor-alpha in the treatment of inflammatory bowel disease. Nat Clin Pract Gastroenterol Hepatol 2006;3:220–8.

110. Hamilton CD. Infectious complications of treatment with biologic agents. Curr Opin Rheumatol 2004;16:393–8.

111. Havell EA. Evidence that tumor necrosis factor has an important role in antibacterial resistance. J Immunol 1989;143:2894–9.

112. Brown SL, Greene MH, Gershon SK, et al. Tumor necrosis factor antagonist therapy and lymphoma development: twenty-six cases reported to the Food and Drug Administration. Arthritis Rheum 2002;46:3151–8.

113. Uberti JP, Ayash L, Ratanatharathorn V, et al. Pilot trial on the use of etanercept and methylprednisolone as primary treatment for acute graft-versus-host disease. Biol Blood Marrow Transplant 2005;11:680–7.

114. Tsimberidou AM, Giles FJ. TNF-alpha targeted therapeutic approaches in patients with hematologic malignancies. Expert Rev Anticancer Ther 2002;2:277–86.

115. Enbrel [package insert]. Thousand Oaks (CA): Amgen Inc. 7/2005.

116. Dinarello CA. The many worlds of reducing interleukin-1. Arthritis Rheum 2005;52:1960–7.

117. Kineret [package insert]. Thousand Oaks (CA): Amgen Inc. 2/2006.

118. Funke VA, de Medeiros CR, Setubal DC, et al. Therapy for severe refractory acute graft-versus-host disease with basiliximab, a selective interleukin-2 receptor antagonist. Bone Marrow Transplant 2006;37:961–5.

119. Wolff D, Roessler V, Steiner B, et al. Treatment of steroid-resistant acute graft-versus-host disease with daclizumab and etanercept. Bone Marrow Transplant 2005;35:1003–10.

120. Anderson KC. Lenalidomide and thalidomide: mechanisms of action—similarities and differences. Semin Hematol 2005;42(4 Suppl 4):S3–8.

Ethical and Legal Issues in the Care of a Cancer Patient

Martin L. Smith, S.T.D.

Anne Lederman Flamm, J.D.

Rebecca D. Pentz, Ph.D.

The Shift from Paternalism to Partnership

Clinical decision making and the physician-patient relationship have undergone major revolutionary changes, starting in the last quarter of the twentieth century. Prior to the 1970s, the prevailing model for decision making was paternalism. This model was founded on physicians' commitment to patients' well-being and the ethical principles of beneficence and nonmaleficence and was dominated by physicians' expertise and authority. In this model, patients played a passive, almost child-like role of obediently and unquestioningly following doctors' orders. But paternalism has been replaced by an expectation of partnership between physicians and patients. The partnership model continues to affirm medical expertise but recognizes patients' expertise as well, that is, that patients are most knowledgeable about their own values, goals, and preferences, all of which should be incorporated into clinical decisions for a particular patient. A partnership model emphasizes mutuality and shared decisions between physicians and patients. The emergence and significance, as a standard of care, of engaging patients in an informed consent process are symbolic of the shift from paternalism to partnership.

Multiple forces and factors contributed to the changes noted above. The Civil Rights Movement in the United States during the 1950s and the 1960s, with its emphasis on individual freedom, rights, and liberties, provided a cultural basis and backdrop for similar emphases taking root in health care delivery. Revelations in the 1960s and 1970s of significant abuse and misuse of research subjects, in which the medical researchers failed to respect research participants as persons by ignoring their right to receive information about the research and to consent voluntarily to participate, produced public horror and shock. The US government responded by enacting federal regulations for protecting research subjects. Similar protections for clinical practice developed subsequently. Court cases also provided greater legal clarity regarding disclosure of information and patients' rights regarding consent or refusal of treatment. In *Canterbury v. Spence* (1972), the court affirmed that

> The patient's right of self-decision can be effectively exercised only if the patient possesses enough information to enable an intelligent choice. The patient should make his own determination on treatment.... Social policy does not accept the paternalistic view that the physician may remain silent because divulgence might prompt the patient to forego needed therapy. Rational, informed patients should not be expected to act uniformly, even under similar circumstances, in agreeing to or refusing treatment.[1]

The *Canterbury* court also attempted to set forth an objective standard for the disclosure of information to a patient: "what a prudent person in the patient's position would have decided if suitably informed of all perils bearing significance."[1] Applying informed consent standards to life-sustaining treatment, the New Jersey Supreme Court in *In re Quinlan* (1976) found the implied right to privacy under the US Constitution to be sufficiently broad to include a patient's right to refuse medical treatment.[2] Specifically, the court permitted Karen Quinlan's parents to authorize the discontinuation of a life-sustaining ventilator from their incompetent 21-year-old daughter, who had suffered a severe anoxic event 10 months before. In 1981, the Judicial Council of the American Medical Association (AMA), echoing *Canterbury v. Spence*, recognized informed consent and patients' participation in their own health care decisions, even if the physician disagrees, as "a basic social policy."[3]

The content of this chapter is framed by the ethical and legal changes to clinical decision making that were summarized above. Within this framework of the changed and changing physician-patient relationship—which we view as a positive development—we describe informed consent and the ethical and legal standards for decision making, the importance of assessing a patient's decisional capacity, the initiation of advance care planning and discussions about cardiopulmonary resuscitation (CPR), and the challenges arising when the physician-internist assumes the role of patient-confidant and coordinator of overall care.

Informed Consent: Process and Transparency

The shift from paternalism to partnership has not been without accompanying ambiguities. For example, how do physicians respect the autonomy and freedom of patients to make their own health care choices while at the same time not abandoning traditional duties of providing medical recommendations, advice, and counsel? Where is the line of demarcation between educating, advising, recommending, and persuading patients about particular courses of treatment judged by physicians to be best for their patients and the extremes of being coercive and manipulative or totally nondirective? In their discussion on the ethical and legal myths about informed consent, Meisel and Kuczewski noted that some physicians believe that respect for patient autonomy requires them to operate a medical cafeteria "in which they must set out all therapeutic options and let patients choose, each according to his or her own appetite."[4] These authors label medical practice in accordance with this myth as "a serious sin of omission" that abdicates a central part of the physician-patient partnership, namely, the physician's role as medical advisor, a professional with expert knowledge crucial for the patient's health. To actualize this role, physicians should see informed consent as a shared, collaborative, educative process that includes human interaction, conversation, questions, and answers. To avoid operating a medical cafeteria, Meisel and Kuczewksi suggested that physicians distinguish between particular treatment options (eg, chemotherapy, radiation) and the goals of those treatments (eg, cure, remission, palliation). In their view, treatments are often discussed in detail, but patients are not really sure what the treatments are ultimately meant to do. Further, as disease responds or progresses, treatments and the goals of treatment can change. They noted the relevance of the distinction between treatments and goals in the following way: "Patients are not experts at treatments; physicians are. However, patients' preferences are central to the choice of treatment goals. Thus, in selecting and revising treatment goals, physicians and patients need to form a partnership."[4] This partnership is particularly important as treatment goals shift from curative to palliative; if forged, the partnership supports communication during difficult end-of-life discussions.

Another ambiguity arising from the partnership model of the physician-patient relationship is how much information to disclose to patients so that they can make good and informed decisions. Ethics, law, and regulatory bodies (such as the Joint Commission for Accrediting Health Care Organizations) have clarified the general categories of information to be disclosed. These elements include the proposed treatment's (or diagnostic procedure's) nature, purpose, risks, and benefits; reasonable alternatives and their risks and benefits; and the likelihood of achieving treatment goals. Although helpful for structuring the kinds of information to be disclosed, this list of categories still does not identify how much information physicians need to disclose, and patients need to understand, to satisfy each element. State laws in the United States typically require physicians to meet either the "reasonable professional" or the "reasonable patient" standard. The former requires physicians to follow customary professional practice, that is, to disclose to patients the amount and kinds of information that a reasonable professional would customarily disclose. Beauchamp and Childress explained the rationale for this standard:

> Disclosure, like treatment, is a task that belongs to physicians because of their professional expertise and commitment to the patient's welfare. As a result, only expert testimony from members of this profession could count as evidence that a physician has violated a patient's right to information.[5]

The "reasonable patient" standard requires physicians to provide the amount and kind of information that a hypothetical reasonable patient would find material or pertinent to making a decision about a treatment or diagnostic procedure. This standard has gained increasing acceptance both in practice and in law because it is more compatible with the partnership model of the physician-patient relationship. Regarding this standard, Beauchamp and Childress provided a note of caution:

> Whatever its merits, the reasonable person standard encounters conceptual, moral, and practical difficulties. First, the concepts of "material information" and "reasonable person" have never been carefully defined. Second, questions arise about whether and how the reasonable person standard can be employed in practice. Its abstract and hypothetical character makes it difficult for physicians to use, because they have to project what a reasonable patient would need to know.[5]

Brody proposed "the transparency standard" as an alternative and as a "means to operationalize the best features of the conversation model in medical practice."[6] Contrasting his proposal with the reasonable professional and the reasonable patient standards, he stated:

> According to the transparency model, the key to reasonable disclosure is not adherence to existing standards of other practitioners, nor is it adherence to a list of risks that a hypothetical reasonable patient would want to know. Instead, disclosure is adequate when the physician's basic thinking has been rendered transparent to the patient.[6]

For example, if a physician determines which treatment to recommend based on the published literature on the risk and benefits of this treatment compared with alternative ones, the physician should explain those risks and benefits. If, on the other hand, the physician was convinced that the least risky treatment was unreasonably inconvenient for the patient (eg, it involved a lengthy hospital stay), the physician should explain that trade-off to the patient.

In summarizing this approach, Brody stated: "Essentially, the transparency standard requires the physician to engage in the typical patient-management thought process, only to *do it out loud in language understandable to the patient*."[6] To fulfill their partnership obligations, patients need to participate in medical decisions, to the extent that they wish, by asking questions prompted by the disclosure of the physician's reasoning. Such questions, of course, need to be answered by the physician to the patient's satisfaction. Given that patients sometimes do not even know which questions to ask, encouraging the presence of family members or anyone whom the patient views as a trusted advisor or advocate is important when crucial decisions must be made.

A transparency model of informed consent might also respond to the concerns raised by Cassell and colleagues regarding the potentially impaired thinking in sick patients.[7] The core of their concern is that sick patients, especially if they are hospitalized, may too easily or quickly consent to treatments and procedures, not because these are judged by patients to be in their best interests but because of the authoritative influence of their physicians. Cassell opined: "The biggest thief of autonomy is sickness."[8] The transparency model of informed consent, because it does not rely on authority but allows the patient to discern the thinking process underlying the physician's recommendation, may allow patients to determine if their physician's reasoning agrees with their own.

Informed consent as a conversational, educational, transparent process contrasts with an event-based model. According to Lidz and colleagues,

> The event model of informed consent treats medical decision making as a discrete act that takes place in a circumscribed period of time, usually shortly before the administration of treatment, and emphasizes the provision of information at that time…. The consent form, with its detailed recital of risks and benefits, can be seen as the central symbol of the event model.[9]

A view of informed consent as an event is the product of a reductionism, that is, a rich and multifaceted concept and process is reduced to a patient's signature on an informed consent form. Nothing could be farther from the truth. Although documenting consent via a printed form or a notation in the patient's medical record is important for a variety of practical and legal reasons, the patient's signature on a form is the least important element of informed consent. The human interaction, the respectful exchange of information, the dialogue that includes questions and satisfactory answers, and the establishment of mutual trust that occur before the event of signing all promote the core values and legally required elements of informed consent, as well as the physician-patient partnership. Moreover, these core values extend beyond the moment of a document's execution and continue throughout treatment so that a patient is free to withdraw consent or change treatment goals at any time during the treatment process. Informed consent neither starts nor ends with signing a document.

Assessing Decisional Capacity

The partnership model of the physician-patient relationship and the informed consent process presume that the patient has the cognitive skills to participate adequately in health care decision making. For various reasons (eg, sedating medication, cerebrovascular accident, head trauma), patients experience temporary or permanent loss or diminution of cognitive abilities. When doubts arise about a patient's cognition, the primary physician has the responsibility to assess the patient's decisional capacity. Seeking the assistance and input of mental health professionals (eg, a psychiatrist, a psychologist, or a social worker) can be helpful and appropriate. Whether or not assistance is sought, the patient should be assessed for specific cognitive skills or abilities to (1) express a choice, (2) understand relevant information, (3) appreciate the medical situation and its consequences, and (4) reason with relevant information.[10] This clinical assessment should be focused on the specific decision to be made and occur after a process of information disclosure about that specific decision. In other words, the question is not whether the patient has cognitive abilities to manage all spheres of his or her life but to make a specific medical decision after having received relevant and transparent information about the proposed therapeutic or diagnostic treatment and its goals. The assessment is not dependent on whether the patient is able to communicate orally. For example, a patient who is in an intensive care unit, intubated and supported by a ventilator, might still retain decisional capacity as long as the patient has some method of communicating his or her wishes.

Related to the four cognitive skills listed above, Grisso and Appelbaum recommended that the clinician performing the assessment (ie, the primary physician or the mental health professional) structure a set of questions around each skill being assessed.[10] For example, for the ability to express a choice, the patient could be asked: "Have you decided whether to go along with your doctor's suggestions for treatment? Can you tell me what your decision is?" For the ability to understand relevant information, the patient could be instructed as follows: "Tell me in your own words what your doctor told you about the nature of your condition, the recommended treatment (or diagnostic test, or research protocol), the possible benefits from the treatment or test or research, the possible risks or discomforts of the treatment or test or research, the possible risks and benefits of alternative treatments, and the possible risks and benefits of no treatment at all." Alternatively, for the second skill, the patient could be told and asked: "Your doctor gave you a percentage chance that [a named risk] might occur with treatment. In your own words, how likely do you think the occurrence of [the named risk] might be? Why is your doctor giving you all this information? What will happen if you decide not to go along with your doctor's recommendation?" For the ability to appreciate the situation and its consequences, the patient could be instructed as follows: "Tell me what you really believe is wrong with your health now." Then the patient could be asked: "Do you believe that you

need some kind of treatment? What is the treatment likely to do for you? Why do you think it will have that effect? What do you think will happen if you are not treated? Why do you think your doctor has recommended [a specific treatment] for you?" Finally, pertaining to the ability to reason with relevant information, the physician or other professional performing the assessment might inquire: "Tell me how you reached the decision to accept [or reject] the recommended treatment? What were the factors that were important to you in reaching the decision? How did you balance those factors?"

Standards for Decision Making

The gold standard for clinical decision making involves a patient who currently has decisional capacity and is able to engage presently in the process of informed consent. Most adult patients in the outpatient setting and many hospitalized patients meet this gold standard. Also, as some pediatricians and others have argued, some mature adolescents are able to meet this standard as well.[11–13]

But when a patient's decisional capacity is judged to be insufficient, the silver standard needs to be invoked and used, that is, turning to and using proxy or surrogate decision makers, when available. The ethical and legal expectations of the surrogate decision maker are to provide a substituted judgment, that is, voicing the values, preferences, and wishes of the patient and, based on those, making the decision that the patient would have made. In the words of Beauchamp and Childress:

> Accordingly, if the surrogate can reliably answer the question, 'What would *the patient* want in this circumstance?' substituted judgment is an appropriate standard. But if the surrogate can only answer the question, 'What do *you* want for the patient?' then this standard is inappropriate.[5]

Occasionally, patients express their wishes or preferences to their physicians, other health care professionals, or family and friends (see Advance Care Planning below). When this has occurred, and especially when a patient's wishes and statements have been documented in the patient's medical record, such indicators of a patient's directives can extend patient autonomy into the time period when the patient lacks decisional capacity. When the previously expressed wishes of the patient exist and have been well documented, the silver standard of substituted judgment is more confidently actualized.

When proxy or surrogate decision makers are unable to formulate a substituted judgment because of a lack of knowledge about the patient, a third or bronze standard for decision making should be used, the standard of best interests.

Strictly speaking, this standard is neither connected to nor an extension of patient autonomy and preferences. Rather, the best interest standard attempts objectively to weigh the benefits and burdens of the proposed treatment or diagnostic procedure, with the goal of maximizing benefit and minimizing risks and harms. This standard for decision making, which mirrors the paternalism of a former era, is useful not only when an available proxy or surrogate lacks specific knowledge about patient preferences but also for pediatric decision making for young patients[12] and when the medical team must make health care decisions for a patient because no patient surrogate has been found, designated, or identified.

Advance Care Planning

As noted above, a substituted judgment is only as good as the knowledge that the surrogate has about the patient's wishes, preferences, and values. Some patients will have had very specific and concrete discussions with family, friends, physicians, or other health care professionals about their wishes and treatment preferences related to particular clinical situations. But most adult patients have not engaged in such conversations or in what has been called "advance care planning."

Emanuel and colleagues described advance care planning as a multistage process by which individuals indicate their preferences for future medical care in the event of decisional incapacity.[14] This patient-centered process can be subdivided into three stages: (1) thinking about preferences and proxies, (2) communicating preferences to others, and (3) documenting preferences and designated proxies. The goals and benefits of advance care planning include extending patient self-determination and control into situations when decisional capacity has been lost; facilitating communication and minimizing future conflict; decreasing family anxiety, stress, and burden when significant decisions must be made for the patient; reducing overtreatment or undertreatment; saving health care resources and dollars because the treatments the patient would not have wanted are not initiated or continued; and providing legal protections for those with ultimate decision-making authority, especially when decisions lead to a patient's death.

Multiple barriers have been identified to explain why most patients seem to avoid thinking about their preferences and communicating them to others and why many physicians fail to initiate advance care planning discussions with their patients. An overarching cultural barrier is a general societal difficulty with thinking and talking about dying and death, whether one's own or someone else's. Metaphorically, death is "the elephant in the room"—present and obvious, especially in situations of serious illness, yet calling attention to it or conversation about it is to be avoided almost at all costs. A narrower but similar cultural barrier exists within US hospitals, ambulatory clinics, and other health care facilities, where the dying and death of patients (and talk of such) may be viewed as medical or patient failure. The military metaphors often associated with cancer (eg, the *war* or *battle* against cancer, the therapeutic *armamentarium* used to *counterattack* cancer, *defend* the body, and *defeat* disease) reinforce the expectation that patients and their physicians are to wage a courageous fight, subtly conveying that they have more control over illness than they actually do. Physicians sometimes fear that death talk or death preparation, especially early in an illness, can be interpreted as a sign that the battlefield is being surrendered prematurely. However, studies have shown that patients prefer a realistic approach, particularly if it is individualized to the patient's situation, and the physician projects confidence and competence during the discussion.[15,16]

Practical barriers to advance care planning, and the substantive conversations between patients and physicians they require, include time constraints and compensation concerns.[17] Advance care planning, by the very nature of its cognitive content and emotional evocations, can be time-intensive and psychologically difficult and draining. Physicians who experience constant pressures to see more patients in the course of a day to generate more revenue could easily relegate advance care planning to the bottom of a priority list of issues to be addressed during a 10- to 20-minute office visit.

Some studies report that patients and physicians have diverse views about who should initiate advance care planning.[18] Patients wait for physicians to initiate such discussions, and physicians wait for patients to initiate such discussions, resulting in mutual misunderstandings and silence. A physician's reluctance to initiate the discussion may be due to discomfort with talking about dying and death, fear of causing the patient distress, a desire to protect patients and maintain their hope, a belief that only older and seriously ill or terminal patients should be concerned about such issues, and a lack of training, skills, or knowledge about advance directives. Patients' reluctance to initiate advance care planning discussions may be due to fear of their own death, an overly optimistic view of medical prognosis, the absence of a trusting relationship with the physician, a perception that such issues and decisions should remain private, and cultural beliefs and practices that emphasize communal or familial decision making over the individualism, self-determination, and independence that characterize patient autonomy.

Overcoming this multitude of barriers is a significant challenge. But physicians committed to empowering patients to be partners in their own health care decisions are not without practical resources[19] and strategies. Back and colleagues addressed the common concern that frank conversation will destroy hope.[20] These authors recommended that physicians engage patients in a conversation that has a dual agenda of "hoping for the best while preparing for the worst." They asserted:

> Hoping for a cure and preparing for potential death need not be mutually exclusive. Both patients and physicians want to hope for the best. At the same time, some patients also want to discuss their concerns about dying, and others probably should prepare because they are likely to die sooner rather than later. Although it may seem contradictory, hoping for the best while *at the same time* preparing for the worst is a useful strategy for approaching patients with life-limiting illness. By acknowledging all the possible outcomes, patients and their physicians can expand their medical focus to include disease-modifying and symptomatic treatments and attend to underlying psychological, spiritual, and existential issues.[20]

Within this framework of a dual agenda, these authors offer five practical recommendations: (1) give equal time to hoping and preparing; (2) align patient and physician hopes, with a first step of directly inquiring from patients what they are hoping for; (3) encourage but do not impose the dual agenda of hoping and preparing; (4) support the evolution of hope and preparation over time; and (5) respect hopes and fears, responding to the patient's emotions.

Where, when, and with whom should physicians initiate discussions about advance care planning? We recommend ambulatory clinics as the preferred site because outpatients are often less stressed and anxious and are more likely to be able to focus on the issues, information, and recommendations associated with advance care planning. Further, if a physician incorporates advance care planning into routine clinical appointments with many or most patients, some of the patient's immediate worries and questions (such as "Why is my doctor bringing this up now? What does she know about my medical condition that I don't know?") may be quickly dispelled when the physician is able to say "I'm not singling you out and I'm not holding back medical information about you. I have these conversations with all my patients." Intending the process of advance care planning to occur over time during multiple outpatient visits allows the physician to introduce the topic, encourage the patient to think about preferences and discuss them with close family and friends, and provide the patient with take-home materials (eg, pamphlets, copies of advance directives, videotapes) aimed at reinforcing basic information. Using this kind of a strategy increases the likelihood that advance care planning will extend appointments only by a few minutes.

Not all physicians will routinely initiate advance care planning with patients. Nevertheless, there can be specific clinical indicators that signal a degree of urgency for physicians to initiate end-of-life discussions. Quill opined that the following situations are more urgent indicators for meaningful end-of-life discussions: patients facing imminent death, patients who talk about wanting to die, patients or families inquiring about a hospice, patients recently hospitalized for severe progressive illness, and patients suffering out of proportion to the prognosis.[21] In oncology, a relapsed patient or one found to have metastatic disease is a priority candidate for advance care planning. At a minimum, physicians need to be attentive to patients manifesting clinical "triggers" and to respond quickly by initiating advance care planning discussions with them.

Physicians should remember that they play a key but not an all-encompassing role in the advance care planning process. In addition to raising issues, helping patients understand their diagnoses and prognoses, and encouraging patients to reflect on their preferences and values, physicians can and should direct patients and their families to appropriate support persons and resources, such as social workers, chaplains, and midlevel practitioners (eg, physician assistants, advance practice nurses) who may be knowledgeable and skilled in this area.

The third stage for advance care planning is documenting preferences and designated proxies. One caution about this third stage is the tendency to reduce what should be a quality conversational and educational process to the signing of documents—similar to the tendency to reduce the informed consent process to the event of getting a patient's signature on an informed consent form. All states in the United States now have legislatively approved advance directive forms, which may provide instructions regarding medical treatment in the event of a terminal or irreversible condition (usually called a living will) or designate a surrogate or proxy decision maker when a person loses decisional capacity (a medical power of attorney or durable power of attorney for health care). Traditionally, a living will directs the limitation or cessation of treatment for specified medical conditions, but some states (eg, Texas) allow patients to request being kept alive in a terminal or irreversible condition using available life-sustaining treatment. In either case, physicians should be open and honest with patients about their willingness and ability to honor the advance directive. Most living will instructions are very general (eg, do not specify or distinguish which life-sustaining treatments a patient is declining) and apply narrowly in explicitly stated medical conditions (eg, terminal illness or irreversible conditions, such as a permanent vegetative state). Most commentators acknowledge that documents designating proxy decision makers are more flexible and more useful because instructional documents such as a living will could not practically list or anticipate all or most of the medical situations that could befall a patient. But the more flexible medical power of attorney is useful only if a patient designates a proxy decision maker who knows the patient well and his or her values and preferences or who has had substantive conversations with the patient about his or her wishes for various anticipated medical circumstances.

Since 1991, US federal law has required hospitals, health maintenance organizations, and hospices to inquire of patients, on admission, whether they have an advance directive.[22] A patient's response to this inquiry is to be recorded in the patient's medical record, and many health care organizations encourage patients to provide copies to be placed in their medical records. Federal law also states that access to care cannot be conditioned on whether a patient has completed an advance directive. Many patients will complete advance directive documents without the participation or knowledge of their primary care physician or oncologist. In an outpatient setting, routinely asking patients whether they have completed advance directives can be an excellent entry into a discussion about advance care planning.

Although the execution of legislatively approved forms is probably the most common manner for patients to document preferences and proxies, completion of these forms is not the only way to document patient wishes. When physicians engage patients in advance care planning, written summaries should be documented in the progress notes of a patient's medical record.

CPR and Do Not Resuscitate

Discussing patients' desires regarding CPR in the event of a cardiac or respiratory arrest can also be a part of advance care planning. Since the 1980s, discussions with patients about resuscitation status have become more commonplace. Most, if not all, hospitals have policies addressing CPR and "code status." Although most hospitals have chosen to designate decisions and corresponding medical orders to not provide CPR as do not resuscitate (DNR) orders, there is no uniform designation for such orders. For example, some hospitals and health care facilities have chosen instead to designate such orders as do not attempt resuscitation orders, as no CPR orders, or as allow natural death orders. Significantly, when patients

are in transit from one care setting to another (eg, via ground or air ambulance) or are able to be cared for in a private home, many states have passed legislation allowing emergency medical personnel to honor out-of-hospital DNR orders.[23]

Addressing resuscitation status in a proactive, timely way is crucial for many oncology patients, especially for those who have incurable or metastatic disease, comorbidities, or major organ failures. Within a context of "hoping for the best, preparing for the worst" (as discussed above), physicians should first help patients understand the realities of CPR and the resuscitative modalities that are entailed (ie, chest compressions, electric shock, intubation, pharmacologic agents). Further, physicians should include in such conversations empiric data that demonstrate relatively low rates of survival to discharge for all inpatient CPR attempts (approximately 17%)[24] and the even lower outcomes for inpatients who experience anticipated cardiac arrests as a result of their metastatic disease, comorbidities, or multiple organ failures.[25] Patients should also be informed that a DNR order does not mean that they will be abandoned by their physicians or health care teams (ie, a DNR order is not equivalent to a do not treat order) and that a DNR order is not incompatible with continuing other aggressive treatments. Discussions of treatments with a patient for whom a DNR order has been written should include the goals of particular treatments and the likelihood of achieving those goals. Continued chemotherapy, antibiotic administration, and blood transfusions may be appropriate when an acute condition is reversible, when a patient's quality of life can be enhanced, or when continued treatments or procedures can serve palliative purposes. A DNR order need not be rescinded during aggressive treatments, including surgery and anesthesia,[26-28] as long as the patient understands the risks involved and possible benefits of resuscitation during a specific procedure.

Discussions with patients about resuscitation status can be excellent opportunities to review and revise explicitly the goals of treatment. Initially, treatment goals may realistically include cure or remission. But over time, depending on whether a patient responds to treatment, the goals may need to incorporate palliation or eventually shift to comfort care only.

Confidant and Coordinator of Overall Care

Although emphasis on patient autonomy and individual choice has transformed the physician-patient relationship into one characterized by partnership rather than paternalism, physician-internists often retain the role, once held by the beloved "family doctor" or "general practitioner,"

as a patient's confidant and coordinator of overall care. These responsibilities can generate numerous ethical dilemmas in which internists must weigh their obligations to patients against compelling family and public interests. Managing patients' overall care also results in heightened obligations and challenges related to communication, information management, allocation of medical resources, and conflict resolution. This segment of the chapter identifies and analyzes specific conflicts arising in internists' roles as confidants and coordinators of overall care, reviews existing guidelines for managing these dilemmas, and proposes ethically justifiable responses.

Physician-Internist as Confidant

Since the implementation of the Health Insurance Portability and Accountability Act of 1996 (HIPAA),[29] physicians are more attuned than ever to the ethical obligation to maintain the confidentiality and privacy of patients' medical information. However, ethical dilemmas related to possessing sensitive information about patients' conditions and lives predate HIPAA by thousands of years. Ethical standards, as reflected in the ancient Hippocratic Oath and current professional guidelines, emphasize confidentiality as fundamental to the physician-patient relationship.[30] Physicians' duty of confidentiality is a corollary of the patients' right of individual autonomy, which encompasses the right to control the use of their own health care information. The legal relationship of physicians to patients is a fiduciary one; loyalty and the duty to act in patients' best interests obligate physicians to maintain the confidentiality of information entrusted to them by patients. An individual's right to privacy in personal matters is also constitutionally based.[31] Additionally, respect for confidentiality has practical advantages; patients will be more forthcoming with the information physicians need to provide effective medical care if they trust that the information will remain confidential.

Although the HIPAA clarifies the legal consequences of unauthorized disclosures, it also articulates circumstances that might justify disclosure of confidential information, for example, threats of violence to others or mandatory reporting of abuse. Other statutory requirements, societal norms, and ethical values can also guide internists when they feel some ethical compulsion to disclose patient information obtained in confidence by patients. In general, exceptions to the general rule of confidentiality require strong ethical justification. Yet the duty to maintain confidentiality can be outweighed, in some circumstances, by internists' competing duties of beneficence and nonmaleficence to patients themselves and broader obligations to patients' family members and the public. Existing legal and professional authorities' standards may offer guidance. We discuss these with several examples that occur with relative frequency.

Family Secrets

Internists frequently learn sensitive information about a patient that the patient wishes to maintain as a secret even from close family, such as the sexual activity of a teenager, a spouse's drug abuse problem, or a surprise finding of nonpaternity. The internist might anticipate benefit to the patient accruing from disclosure to family members yet fear potential harm as well. Exacerbated when an internist has more than one physician-patient relationship within a single family, these situations can pose grave ethical challenges and need to be evaluated on a case-by-case basis. Generally, if the physician judges disclosure to family members to be beneficial, persuading the patient to disclose is the best course of action.

HIV and Communicable Diseases and the Duty to Warn

Although human immunodeficiency virus/acquired immune deficiency syndrome (HIV/AIDS) is far from the first communicable disease to trouble physicians and public policy makers with whether to disclose the patient's condition to others, the epidemic nature of the disease and the absence of an effective cure generated controversy about how to balance the patient's privacy interest against the risks to others.[32,33] When a physician knows that a patient has a communicable disease, such as HIV/AIDS, and knows that the patient has not disclosed the condition to sexual partners or caregivers who will likely be exposed to the patient's bodily fluids, physicians' ethical and legal duties of confidentiality conflict with obligations to warn those who might be harmed by nondisclosure.

The duty to warn third parties to the physician-patient relationship derives in part from a 1976 court case decided by the Supreme Court of California. In *Tarasoff v. Regents of the University of California*,[34] the defendant-psychotherapist's patient, who had stated his intentions in therapy, killed the plaintiffs' daughter. In response to the plaintiffs' claim that the therapist should be liable for a duty to warn, the court ruled that a health care professional is required to take reasonable actions, breaching confidentiality as necessary, to warn an identifiable third party when the patient poses a serious and imminent threat to that party.

Statutory[35] and ethical[36] guidelines that attempt to define when a breach of confidentiality is justified by a duty to warn continue to recognize the factors emphasized by the *Tarasoff* court, specifically, the identifiability of the third party and the likelihood and magnitude of harm if the

third party is not warned. Additional factors include the preventability or treatability of the communicable disease. The case for disclosure diminishes when it is not possible to prevent, treat, or minimize the severity of the illness.

Individual autonomy is not an absolute right. If an individual's choice endangers innocent others or threatens the public health, restrictions may be ethically justified. Thus, whereas a patient might abdicate his or her duty to disclose information to their partners or intimates, physicians have an independent obligation to weigh their duty of confidentiality against the interests of others. At a minimum, physicians' disclosure of the HIV diagnosis or a communicable disease directly to patients should include counseling about implications for intimate partners. When counseling patients with communicable diseases, physicians should inform patients about the limitations of the physician's protection of privacy. For example, if a patient asks his physician not to tell his wife that he tested positive for HIV/AIDS, the physician could agree to maintain confidentiality while the patient was admitted to hospital but might inform the patient that the physician would not discharge him to his wife's care at home, where she might be exposed to his bodily fluids, as long as she remained unaware of his positive status.

Applicable laws may permit or mandate disclosure to sexual partners or other persons potentially exposed to a communicable disease, so physicians should be familiar with and obtain legal advice regarding legal parameters. However, legal guidance may not address all situations and will likely provide little practical advice regarding the methods of disclosure. Recommendations for breaking bad news to patients, which include ensuring privacy, empathic delivery, and adequate time for questions and emotional reactions, also apply to disclosure to partners. In cases in which disclosure is permitted but not mandated, physicians need to weigh the social and interpersonal implications of informing others, acknowledging the potential negative consequences of the information, societal stigma, employment and housing discrimination, and the impact on insurability.

Genetic Risks and the Results of Testing

Internists are increasingly likely to have patients who undergo genetic testing. Particularly if they were the referring physicians, internists may incur responsibility to participate in disclosure of results directly to patients. Positive results for an individual patient may imply an increased risk to that patient's relatives, potentially generating tension between an internist's obligations to respect the privacy of a patient's genetic information and a

duty to inform third parties about the heightened risk.

The availability of effective interventions that reduce the risk of developing a related disease or lessen the ensuing harm from a particular genetic susceptibility strengthens the ethical justification for breaching patient confidentiality. When a medical intervention, such as screening in hereditary breast, colon, or other cancers, or other means of prevention (eg, dietary restrictions for phenylketonuric patients), clearly reduces harm from a particular genetic disorder, the beneficial consequences more compellingly favor disclosure. In contrast, the impact of not informing relatives of their hereditary risks is less forceful when the genetic risks are indeterminate or when no effective medical intervention exists to prevent harm.

Existing case law recognizes that physicians' duties of beneficence can extend beyond an individual patient and has imposed obligations to disclose genetic information when the disclosure has the potential to prevent harm to third parties. However, courts have differed on whether the physician's duty to warn at-risk relatives is discharged by informing the patient of relatives' increased health risks. In *Pate v. Threlkel*, the Florida Supreme Court recognized that privacy limitations often prohibit physicians from disclosing the patient's medical condition to others, that patients can ordinarily be expected to pass on a warning, and that requiring a physician to seek out family members would place too heavy a burden on the physician.[37] Thus, the court said, "in any circumstances in which the physician has a duty to warn of a genetically transferable disease, that duty will be satisfied by warning the patient."[37]

A New Jersey court explicitly disagreed with *Pate v. Threlkel*, requiring instead that "reasonable steps be taken to assure that the information reaches those likely to be affected or is made available for their benefit."[38] Finally, in *Molloy v. Meier*, a Minnesota Supreme Court opinion held that "a physician's duty regarding genetic testing and diagnosis extends beyond the patient to biological parents who foreseeably may be harmed by a breach of that duty."[39] The facts of *Molloy v. Meier* involve primarily a failure to test for genetic traits and not specifically the failure to breach confidentiality to warn. However, *Molloy v. Meier* is significant because by allowing the lawsuit to continue, the court agreed that failure to warn in the context of genetic information can result in harm, in this case a conception that allegedly would not have occurred if the mother had been warned about fragile X syndrome.

The HIPAA also provides some guidance. Its stringent privacy rule requires that disclosure of protected information must be "necessary to prevent or lessen a serious and imminent threat to the health or safety of a person or the public; and [be] to a person or persons reasonably able to prevent or lessen the threat, including the target of the threat...."[35] Although this exception suggests that disclosure directly to the at-risk third party might be supportable, the internist would have to consider whether the specific threat met the substantive components of this exemption. Consider the case of a person with a genetic mutation predisposition to hereditary nonpolyposis colorectal cancer (HNPCC). Monitoring and early detection can prevent and lessen a serious threat to the person's health, with surveillance reducing the incidence of colorectal cancer by more than 50% and overall mortality by 65%.[40] Yet it is difficult to argue that the threat is imminent because the average age at onset of colorectal cancer in HNPCC families is 44 years. The HIPAA exception appears not to apply.

Several professional organizations recommend that the informed consent process prior to genetic testing include discussions of the patient's responsibility to warn at-risk relatives. The Council on Ethical and Judicial Affairs of the AMA asserts that, at the time of testing, physicians should discuss with patients "circumstances under which they would expect patients to notify biological relatives of the availability of information related to the risk of disease,"[41] with the responsibility for notification lying with the patient. Similarly, the American Society of Clinical Oncology concludes that "the cancer care provider's obligations (if any) to at-risk relatives are best fulfilled by communication of familial risk to the person undergoing testing."[42]

These guidelines notably do not recommend that physicians notify relatives directly in breach of patient confidentiality. The AMA's advice also acknowledges that some relatives may not want the genetic information, even though the patient's knowledge makes it available to them. Genetic counselors can contribute valuable expertise, insight, and guidance when physicians consider whether potential harm to third parties justifies a breach of patient confidentiality.

Risks to the Public

Internists encounter myriad situations in which they are aware that a patient's condition poses risks to the general public. In such circumstances, the *Tarasoff*-based duty to warn may be inapplicable because those at risk are not specifically identified. However, ethical and legal obligations to breach patient confidentiality may still be compelling.

Some examples involving breach of confidentiality for public safety have reached sufficient scope and threat so as to justify virtually national policies, such as state notification of tuberculosis patients. Other public health risks threatened by nondisclosure are more ambiguous yet likely are far more common. Internists must weigh when an elderly patient's vision problems or dementia results in an inability to drive a car safely. A patient who is a commercial truck driver, pilot, or physician may disclose to his internist that he regularly abuses alcohol or drugs.

Although each patient's situation deserves its own evaluation, existing law may provide guidance. Some state laws impose a legal duty to report dangerous conduct to an appropriate authority. For example, a physician may be legally obligated to report to the state department of transportation a truck driver's medical condition that poses a danger to the driver or others, although most states allow for physicians to report on a permissive basis.[43] Some states require physicians in specific circumstances to report to the state medical board their awareness of an impaired colleague.[44]

Ethical justification for disclosure of conditions that threaten the general public reflects the fact that an individual's right to self-determination, with its corollary right to control personal and medical information, does not encompass the right to harm others. Thus, when a patient's medical condition puts others at risk, the physician need not maintain confidentiality to respect autonomy. Autonomy is not a consequential benefit to be weighed against potential societal harms; rather, harm to others limits the autonomy of an individual member of a democratic society.

Legal reporting requirements, if they exist, may provide immunity against liability for the resulting breach of patient confidentiality, but they may not absolutely mitigate the negative consequences and ethical implications. If a physician elects disclosure, the physician should attempt to mitigate adverse consequences. Elderly patients may have been unaware of or in denial about their disabilities, and a physician's decision to disclose the risks they pose to others may threaten not only their independence but perhaps their self-image and psychological well-being. A better course would be to help the patient recognize disabilities and work with him or her toward alternative ways of meeting the goals of independence.

Limited disclosure to family caregivers or social supports, who may already have explicitly or implicitly authorized access to the patient's information, may constitute an alternative to legal or official mechanisms for protecting the public. The circumstances of the patient's communication may suggest other alternatives to disclosure. If the impaired patient disclosed the condition as a first step toward rehabilitation, the physician may be able to ascertain the patient's commitment to terms that sufficiently reduce the public threat. Some states have programs, authorized by licensing boards or unions, to permit impaired professionals to avoid disclosure as long as they participate in a treatment program. Specifically for physicians, the Federation of State Physician Health Programs offers programs in every state in the United States that address physician impairment.[45] Seeking the advice of mentors or legal and ethics consultants may also be helpful in hard cases. In all situations, however, physicians should avoid making explicit promises of confidentiality they cannot legally or ethically keep.

Coordinator of Overall Care

Increased specialization in health care contributes to the array of professionals who provide care for patients. Internists, as primary or central care providers, will encounter ethical challenges in their roles as frequent "gatekeepers"[46] to medical services and as mediators among consultants with divergent opinions. These roles illuminate the often competing interests internists must balance. Although patient best interest remains paramount, alliances with consultants, affiliations with institutions, and legitimate self-interest can create pressures running counter to this fundamental obligation.

As a backdrop to the specific ethical issues that arise, strong interpersonal and communication skills facilitate the fulfillment of the internist's obligations as coordinator. A physician's empathic manner[47] and effective style of communication support the provision of quality medical care.[48] Physicians' communication shortcomings have been shown to limit the collection of significant information from patients.[49] Studies done with oncology patients show that a substantial segment of the lay public does not understand the terms and medical jargon doctors used to describe diagnosis, prognosis, screening, and treatment procedures and that doctors overestimate patients' levels of understanding.[50] Such misunderstandings may affect patients' decision making, treatment preferences, and satisfaction with care.[51] Moreover, multiple studies have shown that poor physician-patient or physician-family communication and a perceived lack of caring correlate with increased exposure to litigation.[52,53]

Internists are no more or less likely than other physicians to have greater or fewer skills in communicating with and communicating caring to patients. However, the centrality of an internist's role as a coordinator of overall care increases the likelihood of the internist's responsibility for summarizing complex medical judgments and options, producing a single medical recommendation from multiple sources of information and possibly divergent opinions, and securing the patient's trust and affiliation amid numerous specialty consultants. These responsibilities heighten internists' need for empathy, competence, and expertise in communication.

Evidence that internal medicine trainees grow more cynical and less compassionate and that empathy as a trait is not easy to inculcate[54] suggests that cultivating communication skills and empathy is difficult. Moreover, the literature contains a litany of reasons why exhibiting these skills is so challenging in the modern medical setting, including inadequate[55] and potentially counterproductive[56] training, time and resource constraints,[57] and competitive pressures.[58]

Despite these obstacles, extensive resources exist to cultivate these characteristics and skills in medical professionals. The medical literature contains both empirically and experience-based guidance.[59–62] Commentaries written or contributed by patients poignantly offer insights and suggestions based on their positive and negative experiences.[63–66] Training courses that offer interactive techniques and role playing offer opportunities to practice and are a promising modality for increasing interpersonal skills.[67] The Internet is also a valuable resource for information about training opportunities to increase these skills.

Internist as Gatekeeper

Although the cost-saving strategies of managed care differ from the medical field's traditional fee-for-service practice, both systems raise ethical concerns related to physicians' financial interests. Physicians can just as easily overuse resources in the fee-for-service setting as underuse them in the context of managed care. Both inappropriate uses of health care resources pose a direct risk to patients. Moreover, individual physicians' primary duties to patients coexist with the profession's collective responsibility to advocate for the health and well-being of the public.[68] Adherence to the principle of justice, defined as the just distribution of health resources within the community, impels all physicians to practice responsible stewardship of resources they control.

Thus, whatever the organization of health care delivery, the principles for resource allocation remain consistent. The American College of Physicians (ACP) *Ethics Manual* posits two guiding principles: (1) all health-related resources should be used in a technically appropriate and efficient manner, avoiding unnecessary testing, interventions, and consultations, and (2) resource allocation decisions, such as rationing medical care among recipients, are most appropriately made at the level of policy, not at the bedside. In light of physicians' parallel obligations to patients and society, they are ethically bound to object to policies that undermine the fundamental ethical commitment of physicians to care appropriately for their patients.[68] The ACP has also published a more detailed statement of ethical principles, developed by a working group that included patients, clinicians, ethicists, and managed care leaders, to guide allocation of resources in current health care environment.[69]

Relationships with Consultants

The breadth and scope of medical knowledge necessitate internists' frequent use of specialized consultants, but consultants' participation magnifies the communication and interpersonal challenges already present in the physician-patient relationship. The ACP *Ethics Manual* encourages primary physicians to obtain competent consultation but recommends explicit clarification among professionals in advance of the consultation about its scope and durational authority for patient care.[68]

When disagreements arise, candid discussion between the internist and consultant about the medical bases for their divergent judgments not only creates reciprocal learning opportunities but also enhances the internist's ability, requisite for informed consent, to depict the patient's options accurately.[70] Patients ultimately need to elect the option that best meets their goals and risk orientation, but trust in a particular physician critically influences patients' choices.[71,72] Internists' medical recommendations are optimally informed by respectful discussion with consultants, thereby warranting patients' trust. Further, internists are often in the best position to understand the patient's entire medical and personal situation, key ingredients for formulating the best medical recommendations.

Ensuring adequate communication among the numerous diagnostic and treatment providers also poses potential ethical hazards. The relative insecurity of electronic communication methods such as transmission via facsimile, electronic mail, and cellular telephones has made the duty of confidentiality, now federally mandated by the HIPAA, harder to uphold. Simultaneously, concern about genetic discrimination and revelation of misuses of medical information have heightened the public's attention to the privacy of their information. Internists should clarify security mechanisms and policies within their organizations and should inform patients choosing to communicate by electronic means about security limitations. When communicating with consultants, brief electronic mail interchanges may not adequately capture the subtleties of the patient's condition; the internist must take care that the consultant's advice is based on adequate information.

Alternative Medicine

Coordinating overall care obligates internists to ascertain patients' use of complementary or alternative medical (CAM) therapies. The results of a US survey indicate that total visits to CAM providers (629 million) exceeded total visits to all primary care physicians (386 million) in 1997 and that total out-of-pocket expenditures for CAM therapies, including both products and

professional services, were estimated to be $27 billion, an amount comparable to projected out-of-pocket expenditures for all physician services.[73] Often these nontraditional interventions are complementary to and not exclusive of conventional medicine.[74]

Advising patients on CAM therapy represents a fundamental challenge. Although formal studies of some CAM therapies are under way, evidence for many types simply does not exist. Both their effectiveness and potential hazards, whether inherent in or in conjunction with conventional interventions, remain unknown. Many CAM practitioners are unregulated by any oversight body; thus, physicians and patients are ill-equipped to judge the quality of their services. Physicians interested in or willing to incorporate patients' use of CAM therapies into the care plan are disadvantaged in ensuring patient best interest. Finally, patients' refusals of or delays in conventional treatment owing to reliance on CAM therapies can complicate the provision of quality medical care and may even threaten the physician-patient relationship.

The routine balancing of risks and benefits in physician-patient decision making about CAM therapies versus conventional medical treatment must accommodate for the absence of evidence. Factors to consider include the severity and acuteness of the illness; curability with conventional treatment; degree of invasiveness, associated toxicities, and side effects of conventional treatment; quality of evidence of safety and efficacy of the desired CAM treatment; degree of understanding of the risks and benefits of CAM treatment; knowledge and voluntary acceptance of those risks by the patient; and persistence of the patient's intention to use CAM treatment.[75]

Physicians should clarify and attempt to incorporate the values and beliefs patients express by seeking CAM therapies, including patients' views of their own best interests. A helpful step-by-step strategy for advising and comanaging a patient who uses CAM therapy begins with an emphasis on patient safety, with continued monitoring, and includes clear documentation of clinical activity of both CAM and traditional medical interventions with ongoing conversations and advice related to the patient's treatment decisions.[76]

Terminating the Physician-Patient Relationship

Traditionally, physicians have been free to choose whom they will serve. Once the physician-patient relationship is established, however, physicians incur a legal and ethical duty to treat. Termination of the relationship can be justified, but improper termination constitutes abandonment, an act of negligence, and violates the fiduciary responsibility to act in the patient's best interest. The prospect of terminating the physician-patient relationship usually arises in the context of patients who exhibit extreme or repeated nonadherence to the physician's advice.

Recommendations for a proper termination process reflect a combination of ethical principles and legal guidance from common and statutory law.[77] Organizations may have internal policies or protocols as well. Generally, the physician must notify the patient in writing, preferably in a manner that establishes receipt, such as certified mail. The document should unequivocally state that the physician intends to discontinue providing medical care for the patient and may describe the reasons for, as well as previous efforts to avoid, termination. The letter should state that the physician will continue to treat the patient for a reasonable time period, the duration of which should reflect the patient's condition and how long it should reasonably take the patient to find another treating physician. The letter should also state clearly the date that termination becomes effective (eg, "March 30," not "10 days from receipt of this letter").

Liability concerns related to negligent referrals favor recommending or referring the patient to a local medical society or physician referral service rather than to a specific practitioner. The letter should also indicate agreement to transfer records to the new physician on receipt of the patient's signed authorization to do so. Finally, the letter should acknowledge that the physician will see the patient if a medical emergency arises within a stated period of time after termination.

Practical realities may prevent a provider from completely severing the relationship. Specialists may not have replacements available who can provide comparable care. Emergency centers cannot turn away patients if they need to be stabilized, even if the hospital notified the patient of termination. Physicians participating in managed care group plans may not be able to sever the patient's relationship with the entire group and thus may have to care for the patient as part of his or her group responsibility.

Moreover, the ethical and professional obligations of physicians to patients suggest that termination should be considered as a last resort. Physicians can inform patients directly at the outset of a relationship of patients' own obligations, such as arriving for scheduled appointments, paying for services, and participating in treatment, and can remind patients about these stipulations as problems arise. Written "care contracts" may be introduced to emphasize the need for the patient's participation in treatment and can state termination of the relationship as a consequence of nonadherence to a described treatment plan.

Reviewing some of the theories and empiric data that attempt to explain the reasons for patients' nonadherence suggests some considerations and approaches that might enable a physician to continue managing the patient.[78,79] A patient's decision not to adhere to medical recommendations may reflect the need to retain some measure of control, a serious denial of the reality of illness, or a more extreme personality disorder. These considerations might be worth exploring directly with the patient or, with the patient's permission, with family members, friends, or a therapist to inquire into the patient's motivations and characteristics. A formal assessment of decision-making capacity may determine whether compulsory treatment might be justified.

A patient's social circumstances should also be considered. Illiteracy, the inability to arrange for child care or transportation, or the inability to pay for treatment may be contributing to nonadherence. Problems deriving from the physician's own relationship with the patient may be a factor; for example, failures of communication and of trust or discordance between expectations may be yielding a dissatisfaction that leads to nonadherence.[80,81] Volitional disability, a patient's inability to prevent self-destructive nonadherence that might be compared to compulsive or addictive behavior, might also be the source of the problem.[82] Engaging patient advocates, social workers, behavioral therapists, addiction experts, or other allied health professionals may generate additional ideas for redressing the patient's nonadherence.[83,84]

Finally, physicians should consider whether the patient's nonadherence reflects the patient's individual rationality in the face of chronic illness.[85,86] A patient may not be willing to sacrifice a way of life that he or she singularly values, leaving the physician forced to accept the patient's life-threatening choices. When best efforts to understand and modify patients' nonadherent choices fail, terminating the physician-patient relationship may be necessary.

Conclusion

The goal of this chapter has been to create an ethical and legal framework that supports quality care of cancer patients in a variety of clinical settings. Significant elements of our framework include a partnership model for the physician-patient relationship; an informed consent process that emphasizes communication, education, and transparency; end-of-life care that helps patients retain hope while preparing for the reality of death when appropriate; and the physician's role of confidant and coordinator of patients' overall care.

Throughout the chapter, we have explicitly addressed a selected set of ethical and legal issues. In doing so, we hope that we have also created a framework for identifying, analyzing, and addressing other ethical and legal issues that time and space have prevented us from including.

REFERENCES

1. Canterbury v. Spence, 464 F.2d 772 (D.C. Cir. 1972), cert. Denied, 409 U.S. 1064 (1972).
2. In re Quinlan. 70 N.J. 10, 355 A.2d 647 (1976), cert. Denied, 429 U.S. 922 (1976).
3. American Medical Association, Judicial Council. Current opinions of the Judicial Council of the American Medical Association. Chicago, 1981.
4. Meisel A, Kuczewski M. Legal and ethical myths about informed consent. Arch Intern Med 1996;156:2521–6.
5. Beauchamp TL, Childress JF. Principles of biomedical ethics. 5th ed. New York: Oxford University Press; 2001.
6. Brody H. Transparency: informed consent in primary care. Hastings Cent Rep 1989;19(5):5–9.
7. Cassell EJ, Leon AC, Kaufman SG. Preliminary evidence of impaired thinking in sick patients. Ann Intern Med 2001;134:1120–3.
8. Cassell EJ. Consent or obedience? Power and authority in medicine. N Engl J Med 2005;352:328–30.
9. Lidz CW, Appelbaum PS, Meisel A. Two models of implementing informed consent. Arch Intern Med 1988;148:1385–9.
10. Grisso T, Appelbaum PS. Assessing competence to consent to treatment, a guide for physicians and other health professionals. New York: Oxford University Press; 1998.
11. Leikin SL. Minors' assent or dissent to medical treatment. J Pediatr 1983;102:169–76.
12. Weithorn LA, Campbell SB. The competency of children and adolescents to make informed treatment decisions. Child Dev 1982;53:1589–98.
13. Weir RF, Peters C. Affirming the decisions adolescents make about life and death. Hastings Cent Rep 1997;27:29–40.
14. Emanuel L, Danis M, Pearlman R, Singer P. Advance care planning as a process. J Am Geriatr Soc 1995;43:440–6.
15. Hagerty RG, Butow PN, Ellis PM. Communicating with realism and hope: incurable cancer patients' views on the disclosure of prognosis. J Clin Oncol 2005;23:1278–88.
16. Pentz RD, Lenzi R, Holmes F, Verschraegen C. Discussion of the do-not-resuscitate order: a pilot study of perceptions of patients with refractory cancer. Support Care Cancer 2002;10:573–8.
17. Morrison RS, Morrison EW, Glickman DF. Physician reluctance to discuss advance directives, an empiric investigation of potential barriers. Arch Intern Med 1994;154:2311–8.
18. Miles SH, Koepp R, Weber EP. Advance end-of-life treatment planning, a research review. Arch Intern Med 1996;156:1062–8.
19. Marquis DK. Advance care planning: a practical guide for physicians. Chicago: American Medical Association; 2001.
20. Back AL, Arnold RM, Quill TE. Hope for the best, and prepare for the worst. Ann Intern Med 2003;138:439–42.
21. Quill TE. Initiating end-of-life discussions with seriously ill patients, addressing the "elephant in the room." JAMA 2000;284:2502–7.
22. La Puma J, Orentlicher D, Moss RJ. Advance directives on admission, clinical implications and analysis of the Patient Self-Determination Act of 1990. JAMA 1991;266:402–5.
23. Sabatino CP. Survey of state EMS-DNR laws and protocols. J Law Med Ethics 1999;27:297–315.
24. Peberdy MA, Kaye W, Ornato JP, et al. Cardiopulmonary resuscitation of adults in the hospital: a report of 14,720 cardiac arrests from the National Registry of Cardiopulmonary Resuscitation. Resuscitation 2003;58:297–308.
25. Ewer MS, Kish SK, Martin CG, et al. Characteristics of cardiac arrest in cancer patients as a predictor of survival after cardiopulmonary resuscitation. Cancer 2001;92:1905–12.
26. Fine PG, Jackson SH. Do not resuscitate in the operating room: more than rights and wrongs. Am J Anesthesiol 1995;:46–51.
27. Walker RM. DNR in the OR, resuscitation as an operative risk. JAMA 1991;266:2407–12.
28. Cohen CB, Cohen PJ. Do-not-resuscitate orders in the operating room. N Engl J Med 1991;325:1879–82.

29. US Code of Federal Regulations, Title 45 Parts 160, 164.

30. American Medical Association Code of Ethics. IV, 5.05, and 10.01. Code of Medical Ethics, Current Opinions with Annotations (2004-2005 Edition). Chicago: AMA Press; 2004.

31. Whalen v. Roe, 429 U.S. 589, 599 (1977).

32. Carlson GA, Greeman M, McClellan TA. Management of HIV-positive psychiatric patients who fail to reduce high-risk behaviors. Hosp Community Psychiatry 1989; 40:511–4.

33. Mayo DJ. AIDS, quarantines, and noncompliant positives. In: AIDS: ethics & public policy. Belmont (CA): Wadsworth Publishing; 1988. p.113–23.

34. Tarasoff v. Regents of the University of California. 551 P.2d 334 (Cal. 1976).

35. Health Insurance Portability and Accountability Act. US Code of Federal Regulations, Title 45 §164.512(j).

36. American Medical Association Code of Ethics, E-2.23, HIV Testing, Updated June, 1994. Available at: www.ama-assn.org. Accessed August 21, 2007.

37. Pate v. Threlkel. 661 So.2d 278 (Fla. 1995), rehearing denied (Oct 10, 1995).

38. Safer v. Estate of Pack, 667 A.2d 1188 (NJ App, appeal denied, 683 A2d 1163 (N.J. 1996).

39. Molloy v. Meier, 679 N.W.2d 711 (Minn. 2004).

40. Jarvinen HJ, Aarnio M, Mustonen H, et al. Controlled 15-year trial on screening for colorectal cancer in families with hereditary nonpolyposis colorectal cancer. Gastroenterology 2000;118:829–34.

41. American Medical Association Code of Ethics, E-2.131, Disclosure of Familial Risk in Genetic Testing. Available at: www.ama-assn.org. Accessed August 21, 2007.

42. American Society of Clinical Oncology. Policy statement of the American Society of Clinical Oncology: update: genetic testing for cancer susceptibility. J Clin Oncol 2003;21:2397–406.

43. American Medical Association Code of Ethics, E-2.24, Impaired Drivers and Their Physicians. Available at www.ama-assn.org. Accessed August 21, 2007.

44. See, for example, New York State Public Health Laws 230–11(2007); Ohio Revised Code 4731.224(B)(2007).

45. Federation of State Physician Health Programs. Available at: www.fsphp.org. Accessed August 21, 2007.

46. Eisenberg JM. The internist as gatekeeper. Ann Intern Med 1985;102:537–43.

47. DiBlasi ZD, Harkness E, Earnst E, et al. Influence of context effects on health outcomes: a systematic review. Lancet 2001;357:757–62.

48. DiBlasi ZD, Kleijnen J. Context effects: powerful therapies or methodological bias? Eval Health Prof 2003;26:166–79.

49. Beckman HB, Frankel RM. The effect of physician behavior on the collection of data. Ann Intern Med 1984;101: 692–6.

50. Chapman K, Abraham C, Jenkins V, Fallowfield L, et al. Lay understanding of terms used in cancer consultations. Psychooncology 2003;12:557–66.

51. Weeks JC, Cook EF, O'Day SF, et al. Relationship between cancer patients' predictions of prognosis and their treatment related preference. JAMA 1998;279:1709–14.

52. Levinson W, Roter DL, Mullooly JP, Dull VT, Frankel RM, et al. Physician-patient communication: the relationship with malpractice claims among primary care physicians and surgeons. JAMA 1997;277:553–9.

53. Beckman HB, Markakis KM, Suchman AL, Frankel RM. The doctor-patient relationship and malpractice: lessons from plaintiff depositions. Arch Intern Med 1994;154: 1365–70.

54. Mangione S, Kane GC, Caruso JW, et al. Assessment of empathy in different years of internal medicine training. Med Teach 2002;24:370–3.

55. MacLeod RD. On reflection: doctors learning to care for people who are dying. Soc Sci Med 2001;52:1719–27.

56. Feudtner C, Christakis DA, Christakis NA. Do clinical clerks suffer ethical erosion? Students' perceptions of their ethical environment and personal development. Acad Med 1994;69:670–9.

57. Kash KM, Holland JC. Special problems of physicians and house staff in oncology. In: Holland JC, Rowland JH, editors. Handbook of psychooncology: psychological care of the patient with cancer. New York: Oxford University Press; 1989. p. 647–57.

58. Lu MC. Why it was hard for me to learn compassion as a third-year medical student. Camb Q Healthc Ethics 1995;4:454–8.

59. Baile WF, Buckman R, Lenzi R, et al. SPIKES—a six step protocol for delivering bad news: applications to the patient with cancer. Oncologist 2000;5:302–11.

60. Holland JC. The human side of cancer: living with hope, coping with uncertainty. New York: Harper Collins Publisher; 2000.

61. Larson EB, Yao X. Clinical empathy as emotional labor in the patient-physician relationship. JAMA 2005;293:1100–6.

62. Quill TE. Recognizing and adjusting to barriers in doctor-patient communication. Ann Intern Med 1989;111: 51–57.

63. Cleary PD. A hospitalization from hell: a patient's perspective on quality. Ann Intern Med 2003;138:33–9.

64. Verrees M; edited by Young RK. Touch me (a piece of my mind). JAMA 1996;276:1285–6.

65. Poulson J. Bitter pills to swallow. N Engl J Med 1998;338: 1844–6.

66. Yardley SJ, Davis CL. Receiving a diagnosis of lung cancer: patients' interpretations, perceptions and perspectives. Palliat Med 2001;15:379–86.

67. Baile WF, Kudelka AP, Beale EA, et al. Communication skills training in oncology: description and preliminary outcomes of workshops on breaking bad news and managing patient reactions to illness. Cancer 1999;86: 887–97.

68. American College of Physicians. Ethics Manual, 5th ed. Available at www.acponline.org/ethics/ethics_man.htm. Accessed August 21, 2007.

69. Povar GJ, Blumen H, Daniel J, et al. Ethics in practice: managed care and the changing health care environment: medicine as profession. Managed Care Ethics Working Group Statement. Ann Intern Med 2004;141:131–6.

70. Jones JW, McCullough LB, Richman BW. Management of disagreements between attending and consulting physicians. J Vasc Surg 2003;38:1137–8.

71. Kraetschmer N, Sharpe N, Urowitz S, Deber RB. How does trust affect patient preferences for participation in decision-making? Health Expect 2004;7:271–3.

72. Betting your life: when the author's doctors disagreed, she had to choose sides. The New Yorker 2001 Jan 29;38–42.

73. Eisenberg DM, Davis RB, Ettner SL, et al. Trends in alternative medicine use in the United States, 1990-1997: results of a follow-up national survey. JAMA 1998;280:1569–75.

74. Druss BG, Rosenheck RA. Association between use of unconventional therapies and conventional medical services. JAMA 1999;282:651–6.

75. Adams KE, Cohen MH, Eisenberg D, Jonsen AR. Ethical considerations of complementary and alternative medical therapies in conventional medical settings. Ann Intern Med 2002;137:660–4.

76. Eisenberg DM. Advising patients who seek alternative medical therapies. Ann Intern Med 1997;127:61–9.

77. Orentlicher D. Denying treatment to the noncompliant patient. JAMA 1991;265:1579–82.

78. Eraker SA, Kirscht JP, Becker MH. Understanding and improving patient compliance. Ann Intern Med 1984; 11:258–68.

79. Garrity TF. Medical compliance and the clinician-patient relationship: a review. Soc Sci Med 1981;15E:215–22.

80. Sledge WH, Feinstein AR. A clinimetric approach to the components of the patient-physician relationship. JAMA 1997;278:2043–8.

81. Groves JE. Taking care of the hateful patient. N Engl J Med 1978;298:883–7.

82. Ferrell RB, Price TR, Gert B, Bergen BJ. Volitional disability and physician attitudes toward noncompliance. J Med Philosophy 1984;9:333–51.

83. Faulk JS. Peer-to-peer transplant mentor program: the San Diego experience. Transplant Proc 1999;31 Suppl 4A: 75S.

84. Settle MA. Increased compliance through targeted behavioral interventions. Transplant Proc 1999;31 Suppl 4A: 45S.

85. Donovan JL, Blake DR. Patient non-compliance: deviance or reasoned decision-making? Soc Sci Med 1992;34:507–13.

86. Duffy B, Brent NJ, Pfaadt MJ, Rooney AL. What to do about Harry? Home Healthcare Nurse 1996;14:420–6.

Cancer-Related Fatigue

Carmen P. Escalante, MD
Xin Shelley Wang, MD, MPH

Cancer-related fatigue (CRF) is a significant problem that increases the stress and anxiety of both patients and caregivers. Because of successes over the last several years of being able to stabilize and even cure some patients, cancer has now been relegated to the status of a "chronic condition," similar to comorbidities such as hypertension, cardiac disease, congestive heart failure, and diabetes mellitus.

Fatigue is a common symptom of many serious illnesses, including cancer. Its presence adds little to the diagnosis,[1] and so far, it has no objective physiologic or behavioral markers. Often neglected and undertreated,[2,3] fatigue is commonly associated with other physical and psychological disorders and may decrease a patient's quality of life and functioning. Because more precise screening tools are available for some cancers, management of comorbidities has improved, and lives have been extended, we expect new cancer diagnoses to continue to increase. Most of these newly diagnosed cancer patients will receive treatment, and fatigue will continue to top the list of symptoms associated with cancer.

CRF must be addressed early in the patient's evaluation. The symptom must be acknowledged, and an attempt must be made to reverse the contributing conditions, given the fact that there is currently no gold standard regarding fatigue therapy. Multiple conditions that contribute to fatigue, such as pain, depression, anemia, and hypothyroidism, are treatable.

CRF may occur before, during, or after cancer treatment and as a result of any type of cancer treatment. Some patients experience fatigue before the cancer is diagnosed, and fatigue may seem to be one of the most severe symptoms, partly because of the type and extent of the malignancy at the initial diagnosis. Patients with a hematologic malignancy, for example, are more likely to exhibit significant anemia and have a high risk of infections because of low neutrophil counts. For these patients especially, collection of baseline data to establish the presence and intensity of CRF is often helpful in understanding the effect of cancer treatment.

Most patients experience fluctuations in fatigue during high-dose chemotherapy, with fatigue increasing as the patients' blood counts approach their nadir and improvement as the counts recover.[4] Patients who receive radiotherapy may experience a gradual deepening of fatigue as the treatment goes on.[5] Sometimes patients experience more fatigue during treatment than before it began but do not describe it as increasing.[6] They may hesitate to complain of growing fatigue because they believe it is an expected part of treatment, they do not wish to be a "complainer," or they may fear that the treatment will be modified or stopped as a result of the complaint. Many patients experience persistent fatigue between chemotherapy treatments. A relevant issue for patients cured of malignancy, CRF may continue for years following treatment and cure.[7,8]

Some cancer patients may need to maintain sufficient function either at work or at home after their diagnosis, and persistent fatigue may prevent them from doing so. Fatigue may affect both physical and cognitive functions. Many patients have trouble with short-term memory or concentration. Neurocognitive dysfunction may lead to loss of livelihood and increased dependence on caregivers for assistance in daily activities. Patients may feel increased anxiety and frustration from a loss of pleasurable activities, such as reading or solving puzzles. Increasing dependence on others and an assortment of associated negative emotions may cause patients to experience depression, which often compounds the fatigue.

Because of CRF's increased incidence, its complexity, and the profound effects it has on cancer patients, health care providers should be encouraged to evaluate and treat this symptom. The uncertainties of assessment and treatment can be cleared up only by a continuing focus on the symptom, with encouragement of further research to define its pathophysiologic mechanisms, development of targeted pharmaceutic agents, and well-designed clinical trials that will strengthen the armamentarium of treatment choices.

Here we examine the current state of knowledge of CRF, including frequently seen clinical manifestations and associated symptoms, proposed hypotheses related to pathophysiologic mechanisms, related etiologies, diagnostic tools available for measurement, and current treatments.

Clinical Manifestations

Several definitions of CRF are found in the literature. The National Comprehensive Cancer Network (NCCN) describes CRF as a persistent, subjective sense of tiredness related to cancer or cancer treatment that interferes with usual functioning.[9] Other words and phrases to describe fatigue include a lack of energy, weakness, tiredness, an increased effort in regard to a given task, increased sleepiness, and lassitude. It is important to have the patient describe the fatigue and how it affects her or him. Some patients may feel the effect only on physical stamina, whereas for others, cognitive aspects may be an issue as well.

Prevalence

The prevalence of CRF ranges from 60 to 90% of cancer patients, the variance depending on the CRF definition used and the presence of other factors in the population studied (cancer type, extent of disease, presence of comorbidities or treatment complications, cancer treatment received, medications, physical condition, and presence of other symptoms). Compared with other cancer-related symptoms, fatigue was the most severe symptom reported by a large outpatient sample who had various cancers and were receiving differing treatments in a comprehensive cancer center.[10] More than 30% of cancer patients reported severe fatigue, feeling weak, or not getting things done, whereas fewer than 30% reported other symptoms. Severe levels of fatigue are more common in cancer patients than in the general population. Half of the patients with hematologic malignancies described severe fatigue (defined as 7 or higher on a 0- to 10-point scale).[11] Approximately one-third of patients with solid tumors reported severe fatigue when asked, whereas only 17% of a community-dwelling sample reported this level of fatigue.[12] Newly diagnosed non–small cell lung cancer patients experienced significantly more fatigue than did patients with newly diagnosed breast or prostate cancer.[13]

Associations with Treatment

Surgery, chemotherapy, radiotherapy, biologic response modifiers, and hormonal treatment have been associated with fatigue, although more consistent data support the association of fatigue with chemotherapy, radiotherapy, and biologic response modifiers. The literature concerning the effects of surgery on fatigue is limited. Forsberg and colleagues asked patients with colon, rectal, or stomach cancer to complete surveys prior to surgery and 6 weeks postoperatively.[14] Similar fatigue levels were noted at each time point: 43% preoperatively and 49% postoperatively, with minimal variation in symptom patterns. Galloway and Graydon studied colon cancer patients postoperatively and noted the presence of fatigue before the patients' discharge.[15]

Haylock and Hart's first demonstration of the association between radiotherapy and fatigue was followed by numerous studies that examined fatigue incidence and symptom pattern during radiotherapy regimens.[16–30] These studies make known that fatigue commonly begins at the start of radiotherapy, usually increases, and then plateaus between the second and fourth week of treatment. On treatment completion, fatigue gradually decreases and usually resolves by 3 months post-treatment. The cause of fatigue owing to radiotherapy is unclear.

The association of fatigue and chemotherapy has been noted for about 20 years and has been studied in a variety of cancer types, although the association of fatigue and chemotherapy has been most thoroughly studied in breast cancer patients.[6,22,31–34] The symptom pattern of fatigue in patients undergoing chemotherapy is not consistent, probably because of the variation in disease and treatment characteristics (ie, chemotherapy regimen, stage and extent of disease, measurement method, and time). As the complexity of a chemotherapy regimen increases, fatigue levels increase apace. Greene and colleagues reported fatigue onset within 24 to 48 hours after treatment with pulsed therapy,[35] whereas Richardson and colleagues demonstrated that the least fatigue occurred directly before the next treatment course began.[34] Breast cancer patients receiving adjuvant chemotherapy have greater fatigue than matched controls without cancer.[6,35]

Patients on biologic response modifiers experience such intense and intolerable fatigue that this often limits their ability to continue treatment with these agents.[36–39] Extremely limited data about this treatment modality make symptom patterns difficult to describe. Similarly, the side effects of hormonal treatment have not been well assessed and are frequently underestimated.[40] Leonard reported lethargy and lack of energy related to hormonal treatment.[41]

Pathophysiology of CRF

The pathophysiology of CRF has not been elucidated; however, several mechanisms are proposed in the literature. According to the muscle metabolism hypothesis, cancer or cancer treatment results in a defect in adenosine triphosphate regeneration in skeletal muscle, decreasing the ability to perform mechanical work and producing the symptom of fatigue.[42,43]

The vagal afferent hypothesis suggests that cancer or cancer treatment causes release of neuroactive agents that activate vagal afferents, thereby decreasing somatic motor output and causing sustained changes in particular regions of the brain associated with fatigue.[44–46] The theory of serotonin dysregulation is based on an increase in brain serotonin (5-hydroxytryptamine [5-HT]) levels in localized regions of the brain and an up-regulation of certain 5-HT receptors, leading to decreases in somatomotor drive, modified hypothalamic-pituitary axis (HPA) function, and a sensation of decreased capacity to perform physical work.[47,48] The HPA dysfunction hypothesis proposes that cancer or its treatment either directly or indirectly causes change in the HPA function, leading to endocrine changes that either cause or contribute to fatigue.[49,50]

Many laboratory studies have identified cytokines as central mediators of "sickness behavior" owing to infections.[51] Sickness behavior includes decreased locomotor activity, decreased feeding, decreased exploration of the environment, less sexual activity and other social interactions, and increased sleep (specifically slow-wave sleep). CRF in humans may be similar to sickness behavior, with its characteristics of general malaise, lack of motivation to eat, and decreased interest in activities. Cytokines were linked recently to mental and physical functioning of cancer patients and were associated with pain, depression, sleep disturbances, and cachexia.[52–54]

Fatigue-Associated Symptoms

Rarely occurring alone, fatigue is frequently associated with a cluster of symptoms related to either cancer or cancer treatment.[55–58] The symptoms most often coupled with fatigue include pain, nausea, depression, sleep disturbances, and dyspnea.

Fatigue and depression were shown associated in several studies. Visser and Smets demonstrated, in a cohort of 308 adult outpatients treated with radiation therapy, that fatigue was not predictive of depression and vice versa.[59–63] Sleep disturbances have been less studied, yet fatigued cancer patients receiving treatment show severely disrupted sleep patterns.[63,64] Berger and Farr conducted a prospective repeated-measures study of 72 women free of unstable chronic illnesses during the first three chemotherapy cycles after surgery for stage I or II breast cancer.[64] The authors noted that women whose sleep is disrupted at chemotherapy cycle midpoints are at risk of CRF. The overall effects of less daytime activity, more daytime sleepiness, and night awakenings were associated with higher CRF levels. To manage fatigue, Visser and Smets suggested that CRF and night awakenings be assessed at the midpoint of chemotherapy cycles and that appropriate treatment interventions be developed to promote daytime activity and nighttime rest.[63]

Many cancer patients are anemic. Several large community-based studies demonstrated that treatment with erythropoietin alfa increased the patients' hemoglobin levels, decreased their red blood cell transfusion requirements, and showed an association between patient's quality of life and hemoglobin level.[33,65–68] Recently, treatment with darbepoetin alfa produced similar outcomes.[69,70]

CRF Assessment Tools

The first step of measuring fatigue is severity level currently and over time. The selection of fatigue assessment tool (with or without company of other measurements) depends on the specifics of the intervention or research. Specifically, it depends on the need for rapid screening versus a more comprehensive appraisal and consideration of psychometric qualities (standardization, reliability, validity).

Successful treatment and management of CRF depend on reliable and valid assessment tools. Patient self-report has become a standard method in clinical practice for assessing fatigue dimensions, including fatigue severity and interference with daily activities. A good assessment tool for measuring CRF is characterized by a small number of valid, simple items; patient-friendly scaling; understandable terms; standard administration and scoring methods; and demonstrated reliability and validity. Another characteristic should be easy translatability to other languages for comparisons in different populations.

Several CRF assessment tools offer variability in coverage, structure, standardization of administration and scoring, and high levels of reliability and validity. In Table 1, they are categorized as to whether they are unidimensional or multidimensional tools.

Evaluating the Patient with CRF

Whatever tool is chosen, it must be reproducible and practical. Patients with significant fatigue often feel overwhelmed, and when measurement requires much time, they may be unable to complete it. In clinical practice, a simple

Table 1 Selected Fatigue Assessment Tools

Tool	Total Items	Time Window
Unidimensional		
Cancer-Related Fatigue Distress Scale[110]	20	Past 7 d
Brief Fatigue Inventory[12]	9	Past 24 hs
Fatigue Symptom Inventory[111]	13	Past wk
Fatigue Severity Scale[94]	9	Past wk
Multidimensional		
Cancer Fatigue Scale[112]	15	Current state
Revised Piper Fatigue Scale[113]	22	Now
Schwartz Cancer Fatigue Scale[114]	28	Past 2–3 d
Multidimensional Fatigue Symptom Inventory[115]	83	Past 7 d
Multidimensional Fatigue Inventory[116]	20	Lately
Fatigue Assessment Instrument[117]	29	Past 2 wk

Table 2 Factors Contributing to Fatigue

Comorbidities
Adrenal insufficiency
Coronary artery disease
Connective tissue disease
Chronic obstructive pulmonary disease
Diabetes mellitus
Hepatic dysfunction
Neurologic dysfunction
Renal insufficiency
Thyroid dysfunction
Nutritional abnormalities
Weight changes
Variations in caloric intake
Electrolyte imbalances
Anemia (may be due to malignancy or treatment of malignancy or unrelated to either)
Other symptoms
Pain
Sleep disturbances
Emotional distress
Depression
Anxiety
Other psychiatric disorders
Dyspnea
Medications
Physical deconditioning
Direct effects of the malignancy
Cancer treatment–related effects
Chemotherapy
Radiation therapy
Surgery
Bone marrow transplantation
Biologic response modifiers
Hormonal treatment

one-question screening tool may be sufficient; for example, "What was your worst level of fatigue during the last 24 hours, on a scale of 1 to 10, with 10 being worst fatigue?" The NCCN Cancer-Related Fatigue Guideline screens are based on a patient's response to a single tool. If the patient has moderate to severe fatigue, completion of a more comprehensive fatigue assessment tool should be performed.[58]

The *International Classification of Diseases*, tenth revision (ICD-10), describes the CRF diagnostic criteria as follows[71–73]:

1. Six or more of 11 possible fatigue symptoms, with one being "significant fatigue," have been present every day or nearly every day during the same 2-week period in the past month.
2. The symptoms cause clinically significant distress or impairment in important aspects of functioning.
3. The symptoms are the result of cancer or cancer treatment.
4. The symptoms are not primarily due to a comorbid psychiatric disorder.

Use of consistent diagnostic criteria will improve consistency in condition- and treatment-related CRF epidemiologic estimates.

Patients with moderate to severe fatigue require a thorough medical evaluation, including a careful history that focuses on fatigue onset; duration, intensity, and changes over time; associated symptoms; and factors that may alleviate or worsen fatigue. The assessment should include the patient's current disease status, type and length of cancer treatment and its ability to cause fatigue, and the patient's response to treatment. For patients who are disease free, the evaluation should include the question of whether recurrence is a cause of fatigue, and for those with underlying malignancy, whether fatigue is related to disease progression. These questions often provoke extreme anxiety in the disease-free patient and family members, and reassurance that the fatigue is unrelated to the disease may reduce their fears. Other factors that may affect fatigue and should be considered include medications used (both prescribed and over-the-counter, including herbal and vitamin and mineral supplements), nutritional aspects (weight changes, variations in caloric intake, fluid and electrolyte imbalances); decreases in activity and physical deconditioning; and the presence of comorbidities (infection, hypothyroidism, or cardiac, pulmonary, renal, hepatic, neurologic, or endocrine dysfunction). Table 2 summarizes potential contributing factors to CRF.

CRF is an important outcome measure and should be considered when conducting trials of new pharmacologic agents to combat cancer. Decreases in CRF may be represented by a reduction in treatment toxicity, improved palliation for patients with progressive or advanced disease, or better functional and health status in cancer survivors. Fatigue may affect other aspects of care, such as morbidity and mortality, cost of care, and patient satisfaction with care. It may also serve as an indicator of quality of life.

Intervention in CRF

Given that the pathophysiologic mechanisms of CRF are still poorly understood, the root cause cannot be targeted. However, contributing and potentially reversible conditions are anemia, depression, and pain, all of which can be managed.

All patients should be provided with education concerning the side effects of specific tumors and cancer treatment regimens. This will often alleviate the anxiety and stress patients and caregivers feel if they assume that when fatigue is present, the malignancy is worsening or recurring. Patients and caregivers may also be able to make better lifestyle adjustments if they understand and expect certain symptoms. For example, patients on some chemotherapy regimens may expect decreasing blood counts beginning approximately on day 7, with a nadir usually between days 10 through 14; these will bring higher levels of fatigue, and patients should prioritize activities during this time period.

Treatment of CRF may be categorized into nonpharmacologic and pharmacologic treatments. Nonpharmacologic treatments include exercise, energy conservation, sleep enhancement, nutritional therapy, and cognitive and behavioral treatment strategies. Pharmacologic treatments include erythropoietin and darbepoetin; stimulants such as methylphenidate, pemoline, and modafinil; selective serotonin reuptake inhibitors; and corticosteroids.

Nonpharmacologic Treatments
Exercise

Graded aerobic exercise has been shown in randomized controlled trials to have a beneficial effect on fatigue,[74–80] and several trials demonstrated improvements in both fatigue and function.[74,76,80] The exercise types used in these trials included bed-cycle ergometer, home-based walking programs, and resistance exercise. Most studies included only patients with breast cancer.

Three studies showed reductions in fatigue and improvement in quality of life.[77–79]

Because patients with bone metastases, neutropenia, thrombocytopenia, and fever need to be cautious in pursuing an exercise program, the patient and health care provider should discuss the type of exercise, frequency, intensity, and duration. Exercise programs should be tailored to the patient's needs, considering her or his overall medical status, including significant comorbidities in addition to cancer, the status of physical conditioning, the extent of neoplastic disease, and the cancer treatment modality in which the patient is currently engaged. Age and gender may be less important but should be considered. Patients with significant comorbidities or deconditioning should have a medical evaluation before beginning an exercise program; they may benefit from being referred to a physical medicine and rehabilitation program.

Psychosocial Interventions

Randomized clinical trials of various psychosocial interventions have demonstrated significant improvements in fatigue levels.[81–87] The interventions included weekly support groups, individual psychotherapy, support groups providing education and stress management, coping strategy programs, tailored behavioral interventions, and professionally or self-administered stress management training. All resulted in decreased fatigue and improvement in various other symptoms. Recently, patients in a randomized clinical trial by Given and colleagues, in which a cognitive behavioral intervention was used, demonstrated significant improvement in both fatigue and pain after 10 weeks, and this was maintained at 20 weeks by patients who started the trial with moderate to severe symptoms.[86]

Restorative Therapy

Cimprich described the concept of attentional fatigue in cancer patients as decreased capacity to concentrate or focus attention during stressful or challenging situations.[88] Studies of attention-restoring interventions demonstrated improvement in concentration and problem-solving abilities, with earlier return to work by patients who used the intervention.[89,90] These studies also focused primarily on breast cancer patients.

Sleep Therapy

The sleep disturbances of cancer patients are often more of quality than quantity of sleep.[63] Research on this issue and its relationship to fatigue is limited. In two studies using actigraphy to measure sleep and activity, cancer patients were found to spend more time sleeping or resting than healthy individuals, and the sleep pattern of cancer patients was shown to be severely disrupted.[33,91] Berger and colleagues performed a prospective pilot study to test the feasibility of a sleep promotion plan, including aspects of sleep hygiene, relaxation therapy, stimulus control, and sleep restriction techniques, in 25 stage I and II breast cancer patients.[92] The intervention resulted in improved treatment adherence rates over time, and in most patients, sleep and wake patterns returned to normal values.

Patients with sleep disturbances may benefit from a consistent bedtime and wake-up regimen. They should avoid caffeine and stimulating activities such as an exercise regimen in the evening, avoid late or long afternoon naps, and limit bedtime to normal sleep time. Comforting activities before bed (warm bath, reading, tranquil music) and a favorable sleep environment (quiet, cool, dark, comfortable room) may be helpful.

Energy Conservation

Little research has been done on this issue, although patients commonly will prioritize activities if they have significant levels of fatigue. Barsevick and colleagues recently completed a randomized clinical trial that compared energy conservation and activity management (ECAM) by 200 patients with a control intervention including 196 patients focused on nutrition.[85] Patients in the ECAM group experienced a modest but significant improvement in fatigue, although the intervention was not associated with changes in overall functional performance.

Pharmacologic Treatments

Stimulants

No randomized controlled trials have been done to assess the use of stimulants in managing CRF, but some of the drugs have been studied in other conditions, such as fatigue related to human immunodeficiency virus (HIV) disease[93] and multiple sclerosis.[94,95]

Use of pemoline to treat fatigue related to multiple sclerosis produced inconsistent beneficial effects. It has not been used in patients with CRF, and its association with severe liver dysfunction in some patients resulted in its disfavor.[96]

Methylphenidate and modafinil have been used in most attempts to manage CRF. Methylphenidate is a central nervous system stimulant similar to amphetamine. It has a peak plasma concentration of 1 to 3 hours, a plasma half-life of 2 hours, and a duration of action of 3 to 6 hours.[97,98] Baseline doses generally are 5 mg in the morning and 5 mg at noon, with titration as necessary. The maximum recommended dosage is 1 mg/kg/d. The side effects of hypertension, tachycardia, nervousness, insomnia, and anorexia in children preclude its use in patient populations susceptible to these conditions. Three studies of methylphenidate, with fatigue as an end point, are summarized in Table 3. Sarhill and colleagues demonstrated a beneficial effect of methylphenidate in a small group of patients with advanced cancer.[99] The primary outcome variable was fatigue. Bruera and colleagues used a prospective open study of 31 patients with advanced cancer and fatigue.[100] Fatigue was the primary end point, although multiple symptoms were assessed. Patients took 5 mg methylphenidate by mouth every 2 hours as needed for 7 days (maximum 20 mg/d). They had significant improvement in fatigue using this treatment schedule without sleep disruption.

Modafinil is another central nervous system stimulant approved by the US Food and Drug Administration for treatment of narcolepsy. It has been studied in patients with fatigue induced by multiple sclerosis and has produced improvement in levels of fatigue at 200 mg per day.[101] The usual dose of modafinil is 100 to 200 mg in the morning, with another dose at noon or shortly thereafter. The maximum dosage used is 400 mg per day. No randomized clinical trials of the use of this agent have been done with cancer patients.

Antidepressants

In most patients, but particularly cancer patients, fatigue and depression are related, although if there is a shared pathophysiology, it is unknown. Because of the close association, questions have been raised whether treating patients with antidepressants will lower levels of fatigue. Morrow and Hickok conducted a double-blind, randomized, placebo-controlled study with 738 patients undergoing chemotherapy who received either 20 mg of paroxetine or placebo.[102] Patients who received paroxetine experienced significantly fewer depressive symptoms but no significant change in levels of fatigue. Other studies of particular classes of antidepressant and different modes of cancer therapy are necessary to determine whether fatigue can improve in these circumstances. Currently, antidepressants are reasonable medications to prescribe to patients with fatigue if patients are depressed. Patients with sleeping difficulties and depression may benefit from antidepressants such as nortriptyline and amitriptyline because of the drugs' sedative qualities. Bupropion may benefit patients with CRF because it has stimulant pharmacologic properties.

Steroids

Most trials concerning steroids and fatigue use end-point measures other than fatigue, such as strength, weakness, or activity level. There is no consensus that use of these end points demonstrates the benefits of steroids in fatigue management. In addition, the adverse side effects related to steroid administration must be taken into account.

Table 3 Pharmacologic Treatment of Cancer-Related Fatigue with Methylphenidate

Investigators	Type of Study	Number/Features of Patients	Fatigue Outcome
Sarhill et al[99]	Prospective open-label pilot	11/advanced cancer	Improved
Bruera et al[100]	Prospective open study	30/advanced cancer	Improved
Schwartz et al[118]	Prospective pilot/methylphenidate + aerobic exercise	12/melanoma patients on interferon	Improved

Moertel and colleagues studied 116 patients with advanced gastrointestinal cancer in a double-blind randomized trial, administering dexamethasone 0.75 mg/d, dexamethasone 1.5 mg 4 times a day, or placebo.[103] After 4 weeks of treatment, 34% of patients in the two dexamethasone groups showed improved "strength" compared with the placebo group. Bruera and colleagues, in a randomized, double-blind, placebo-controlled, crossover study including 40 patients with advanced cancer, used methylprednisolone 16 mg orally twice a day.[104] After 2 weeks of treatment, the activity levels of 61% of patients increased, but the changes became nonsignificant 2 weeks later. Della Cuna and colleagues, who enrolled 403 patients with advanced cancer in a blinded, randomized, parallel-group study, administered either intravenous methylprednisolone 125 mg/d or placebo.[105] Self-reported "weakness" scores did not improve.

In a similar study by Popiela and colleauges with 173 women with advanced cancer, an improvement in "weakness" was noted by the women in the steroid group after 2 weeks of treatment, but the improvement did not last past the first 2 weeks.[106]

Complementary Alternative Therapy

Although no well-designed trials have been done to test these therapies for CRF, there is much interest in herbal treatments, massage therapy, and acupuncture. Patients should be cautious in their use of herbal treatments because there may be profound drug interactions. Given that they are easily acquired at health food stores, patients may not think of them as medications, but patients should be asked about the use of herbal agents during their clinic visits.

Acupuncture, used to treat pain, nausea, and vomiting,[107] has not been well studied in patients with CRF. In a pilot study of 31 patients who had completed cytotoxic chemotherapy, Vickers and colleagues used acupuncture to determine whether this intervention might improve fatigue.[108] Randomized into two treatment arms, patients underwent acupuncture twice a week for 4 weeks or once a week for 6 weeks. The mean improvement following acupuncture, 31.1%, indicated that the question of whether this intervention is effective for CRF deserves further study.

Summary

CRF is the most common complaint of cancer patients and is frequently the most distressing symptom because it interferes with multiple aspects of daily life. Awareness and study of this symptom have grown tremendously in recent years, although much about the mechanism is still unknown.[109] In clinical evaluations of patients with CRF, health care professionals should focus attention on reversible causes for which therapies are readily available to ameliorate the symptom. Chemotherapy-induced anemia, for example, is easily treated with erythropoietin or darbepoetin, with significant improvement in or resolution of fatigue. CRF education should be made available to all patients and their family supporters. Such education often alleviates the stress and anxiety provoked by misinformation. Exercise interventions, which have been shown to lower fatigue levels, should be tailored to individual patients, taking into account such factors as comorbidities, extent of disease, and level of deconditioning. There is a great need for well-designed clinical trials to evaluate pharmacologic agents to treat fatigue in cancer populations. There is also a need for better understanding of the pathophysiologic mechanisms attributed to CRF so that interventions targeting these mechanisms may be designed and evaluated.

REFERENCES

1. Wessely S. Chronic fatigue: symptom and syndrome. Ann Intern Med 2001;134:838–43.
2. Curt GA. The impact of fatigue on patients with cancer: overview of FATIGUE 1 and 2. Oncologist 2000;5 Suppl 2:9–12.
3. Curt GA, Breitbart W, Cella D, et al. Impact of cancer-related fatigue on the lives of patients: new findings from the Fatigue Coalition. Oncologist 2000;5:353–60.
4. Knobel H, Loge JH, Nordoy T, et al. High level of fatigue in lymphoma patients treated with high dose therapy. J Pain Symptom Manage 2000;19:446–56.
5. Wang XS, Janjan NA, Guo H, et al. Fatigue during preoperative chemoradiation for resectable rectal cancer. Cancer 2001;92:1725–32.
6. Jacobsen PB, Hann DM, Azarello LM, et al. Fatigue in women receiving adjuvant chemotherapy for breast cancer: characteristics, course and correlates. J Pain Symptom Manage 1999;18:233–42.
7. Bower JE, Ganz PA, Desmond KA, et al. Fatigue in breast cancer survivors: occurrence, correlates, and impact on quality of life. J Clin Oncol 2000;18:743–53.
8. Servaes P, Verhagen S, Bleijenberg G. Determinants of chronic fatigue in disease-free breast cancer patients: a cross-sectional study. Ann Oncol 2002;13:589–98.
9. Mock V, Atkinson A, Barsevick A, et al. NCCN practice guidelines for cancer related fatigue. Oncology (Huntingt) 2000;14:151–61.
10. Cleeland CS, Mendoza TR, Wang SX, et al. Assessing symptom distress in cancer patients. The M D Anderson Symptom Inventory. Cancer 2000;89:1634–46.
11. Wang XS, Giralt SA, Mendoza TR, et al. Clinical factors associated with cancer-related fatigue in patients being treated for leukemia and non-Hodgkin's lymphoma. J Clin Oncol 2002;20:1319–28.
12. Mendoza TR, Wang XS, Cleeland CS, et al. The rapid assessment of fatigue severity in cancer patients: use of the Brief Fatigue Inventory. Cancer 1999;85:1186–96.
13. Stone P, Richards M, A'Hern R, Hardy J. A study to investigate the prevalence, severity and correlates of fatigue among patients with cancer in comparison with a control group of volunteers without cancer. Ann Oncol 2000;11:561–7.
14. Forsberg C, Bjorvell H, Cedermark B. Well-being and its relation to coping ability in patients with colo-rectal and gastric cancer before and after surgery. Scand J Caring Sci 1996;10:35–44.
15. Galloway SC, Graydon JE. Uncertainty, symptom distress, and information needs after surgery for cancer of the colon. Cancer Nurs 1996;19:112–7.
16. Haylock PJ, Hart LK. Fatigue in patients receiving localized radiation. Cancer Nurs 1979;2:461–7.
17. Kubricht DW. Therapeutic self-care demands expressed by outpatients receiving external radiation therapy. Cancer Nurs 1984;7:43–52.
18. King KB, Nail LM, Kreamer K, et al. Patients' descriptions of the experience of receiving radiation therapy. Oncol Nurs Forum 1985;12:55–61.
19. Kobashi-Schoot JA, Hanewald GJ, van Dam FS, Bruning PF. Assessment of malaise in cancer patients treated with radiotherapy. Cancer Nurs 1985;8:306–13.
20. Blesch KS, Paice JA, Wickham R, et al. Correlates of fatigue in people with breast or lung cancer. Oncol Nurs Forum 1991;18:81–7.
21. Greenberg DB, Sawicka J, Eisenthal S, Ross D. Fatigue syndrome due to localized radiation. J Pain Symptom Manage 1992;7:38–45.
22. Irvine D, Vincent L, Graydon JE, et al. The prevalence and correlates of fatigue in patients receiving treatment with chemotherapy and radiotherapy. A comparison with the fatigue experienced by healthy individuals. Cancer Nurs 1994;17:367–78.
23. Hickok JT, Morrow GR, McDonald S, Bellg AJ. Frequency and correlates of fatigue in lung cancer patients receiving radiation therapy: implications for management. J Pain Symptom Manage 1996;11:370–7.
24. Munro AJ, Potter S. A quantitative approach to the distress caused by symptoms in patients treated with radical radiotherapy. Br J Cancer 1996;74:640–7.
25. Mock V, Dow KH, Meores C, et al. Effects of exercise on fatigue, physical functioning, and emotional distress during radiation therapy for breast cancer. Oncol Nurs Forum 1997;24:991–1000.
26. Hann DM, Jacobsen P, Martin S, et al. Fatigue and quality of life following radiotherapy for breast cancer: a comparative study. J Clin Psychol Med Settings 1998;4:19–33.
27. Smets EM, Visser MR, Garssen B, et al. Understanding the level of fatigue in cancer patients undergoing radiotherapy. J Psychosom Res 1998;45:277–93.
28. Smets EM, Visser MR, Willems-Groot AF, et al. Fatigue and radiotherapy: (A) experience in patients undergoing treatment. Br J Cancer 1998;78:899–906.
29. Smets EM, Visser MR, Willems-Groot AF, et al. Fatigue and radiotherapy: (B) experience in patients 9 months following treatment. Br J Cancer 1998;78:907–12.
30. Miaskowski C, Lee KA. Pain, fatigue, and sleep disturbances in oncology outpatients receiving radiation therapy for bone metastasis: a pilot study. J Pain Symptom Manage 1999;17:320–32.
31. Jamar S. Fatigue in women receiving chemotherapy for ovarian cancer. In: Funk S, Tornquist E, Champagne M, et al, editors. Key aspects of comfort: management of pain, fatigue and nausea. New York: Springer; 1989. p. 224–8.
32. Pickard-Holley S. Fatigue in cancer patients. A descriptive study. Cancer Nurs 1991;14:13–9.
33. Berger AM. Patterns of fatigue and activity and rest during adjuvant breast cancer chemotherapy. Oncol Nurs Forum 1998;25:51–62.
34. Richardson A, Ream E, Wilson-Barnett J. Fatigue in patients receiving chemotherapy: patterns of change. Cancer Nurs 1998;21:17–30.
35. Greene D, Nail LM, Fieler VK, et al. A comparison of patient-reported side effects among three chemotherapy regimens for breast cancer. Cancer Pract 1994;2:57–62.

36. Davis C. Interferon induced fatigue. Oncol Nurs Forum 1985;11.

37. Rieger P. Interferon-induced fatigue: a study of fatigue measurement. Program proceedings: Sigma Theta Tau International. 1987.

38. Robinson KD, Posner JD. Patterns of self-care needs and interventions related to biologic response modifier therapy: fatigue as a model. Semin Oncol Nurs 1992;8:17–22.

39. Dean GE, Spears L, Ferrell BR, et al. Fatigue in patients with cancer receiving interferon alpha. Cancer Pract 1995;3:164–72.

40. Obe SD. Exploring the impact of treatment: communications, perceptions, reality! Eur J Cancer Care (Engl) 1996;5:3–4.

41. Leonard RCF. Impact of side effects associated with endocrine treatments for advanced breast cancer: clinicians' and patients' perception. Breast 1996;5:259–64.

42. Dimeo F, Stieglitz RD, Novelli-Fischer U, et al. Correlation between physical performance and fatigue in cancer patients. Ann Oncol 1997;8:1251–5.

43. Akechi T, Kugaya A, Okamura H, et al. Fatigue and its associated factors in ambulatory cancer patients: a preliminary study. J Pain Symptom Manage 1999;17:42–8.

44. Opp MR, Toth LA. Somnogenic and pyrogenic effects of interleukin-1beta and lipopolysaccharide in intact and vagotomized rats. Life Sci 1998;62:923–36.

45. Hansen MK, Krueger JM. Subdiaphragmatic vagotomy blocks the sleep- and fever-promoting effects of interleukin-1beta. Am J Physiol 1997;273:R1246–53.

46. Kapas L, Hansen MK, Chang HY, Krueger JM. Vagotomy attenuates but does not prevent the somnogenic and febrile effects of lipopolysaccharide in rats. Am J Physiol 1998;274:R406–11.

47. Newsholme EA, Blomstrand E. Tryptophan, 5-hydroxytryptamine and a possible explanation for central fatigue. Adv Exp Med Biol 1995;384:315–20.

48. Gandevia SC, Allen GM, McKenzie DK. Central fatigue. Critical issues, quantification and practical implications. Adv Exp Med Biol 1995;384:281–94.

49. Swain MG, Maric M. Defective corticotropin-releasing hormone mediated neuroendocrine and behavioral responses in cholestatic rats: implications for cholestatic liver disease-related sickness behaviors. Hepatology 1995;22:1560–4.

50. Bakheit AM, Behan PO, Dinan TG, et al. Possible upregulation of hypothalamic 5-hydroxytryptamine receptors in patients with postviral fatigue syndrome. BMJ 1992;304:1010–2.

51. Kelley KW, Bluthe RM, Dantzer R, et al. Cytokines and sickness behavior. Brain Behav Immun 2006. [In press]

52. Dunlop RJ, Campbell CW. Cytokines and advanced cancer. J Pain Symptom Manage 2000;20:214–32.

53. Cleeland CS, Bennett GJ, Dantzer R, et al. Are the symptoms of cancer and cancer treatment due to a shared biologic mechanism? A cytokine-immunologic model of cancer symptoms. Cancer 2003;97:2919–25.

54. Lee BN, Dantzer R, Langley KE, et al. A cytokine-based neuroimmunologic mechanism of cancer-related symptoms. Neuroimmunomodulation 2004;11:279–92.

55. Smets EM, Garssen B, Schuster-Uitterhoeve AL, de Haes JC. Fatigue in cancer patients. Br J Cancer 1993;68:220–4.

56. Winningham ML. Strategies for managing cancer-related fatigue syndrome: a rehabilitation approach. Cancer 2001;92:988–97.

57. Nail LM, Winningham ML. Fatigue and weakness in cancer patients: the symptoms experience. Semin Oncol Nurs 1995;11:272–8.

58. Mock V, Atkinson A, Barsevick AM, et al. Clinical practice guidelines in oncology for cancer-related fatigue. J Natl Compr Canc Netw 2003;1:308–31.

59. Richardson A. Fatigue in cancer patients: a review of the literature. Eur J Cancer Care (Engl) 1995;4:20–32.

60. Hopwood P, Stephens RJ. Depression in patients with lung cancer: prevalence and risk factors derived from quality-of-life data. J Clin Oncol 2000;18:893–903.

61. Newell S, Sanson-Fisher RW, Girgis A, Ackland S. The physical and psycho-social experiences of patients attending an outpatient medical oncology department: a cross-sectional study. Eur J Cancer Care (Engl) 1999;8:73–82.

62. Loge JH, Abrahamsen AF, Ekeberg, Kaasa S. Fatigue and psychiatric morbidity among Hodgkin's disease survivors. J Pain Symptom Manage 2000;19:91–9.

63. Visser MR, Smets EM. Fatigue, depression and quality of life in cancer patients: how are they related? Support Care Cancer 1998;6:101–8.

64. Berger AM, Farr L. The influence of daytime inactivity and nighttime restlessness on cancer-related fatigue. Oncol Nurs Forum 1999;26:1663–71.

65. Demetri GD, Kris M, Wade J, et al. Quality of life benefit in chemotherapy patients treated with epoetin alfa is independent of disease response or tumor type: results from a prospective community oncology study. J Clin Oncol 1998;16:3412–25.

66. Glaspy J, Bukowski R, Steinberg D, et al. Impact of therapy with epoetin alfa on clinical outcomes in patients with nonmyeloid malignancies during cancer chemotherapy in community oncology practice. Procrit Study Group. J Clin Oncol 1997;15:1218–34.

67. Gabrilove JL, Cleeland CS, Livingston RB, et al. Clinical evaluation of once-weekly dosing of epoetin alfa in chemotherapy patients: improvements in hemoglobin and quality of life are similar to three-times-weekly dosing. J Clin Oncol 2001;19:2875–82.

68. Crawford J, Cella D, Cleeland CS, et al. Relationship between changes in hemoglobin level and quality of life during chemotherapy in anemic cancer patients receiving epoetin alfa therapy. Cancer 2002;95:888–95.

69. Glaspy JA, Jadeja JS, Justice G, et al. Darbepoetin alfa given every 1 or 2 weeks alleviates anaemia associated with cancer chemotherapy. Br J Cancer 2002;87:268–76.

70. Vansteenkiste J, Pirker R, Massuti B, et al. Double-blind, placebo-controlled, randomized phase III trial of darbepoetin alfa in lung cancer patients receiving chemotherapy. J Natl Cancer Inst 2002;94:1211–20.

71. Portenoy RK, Itri LM. Cancer-related fatigue: guidelines for evaluation and management. Oncologist 1999;4:1–10.

72. Cella D, Davis K, Breitbart W, GC. Cancer-related fatigue: prevalence of proposed diagnostic criteria in a United States sample of cancer survivors. J Clin Oncol 2001;19:3385–91.

73. Sadler IJ, Jacobsen PB, Booth-Jones M, et al. Preliminary evaluation of a clinical syndrome approach to assessing cancer-related fatigue. J Pain Symptom Manage 2002;23:406–16.

74. Mock V, Dow KH, Meares CJ, et al. Effects of exercise on fatigue, physical functioning, and emotional distress during radiation therapy for breast cancer. Oncol Nurs Forum 1997;24:991–1000.

75. Dimeo FC, Stieglitz RD, Novelli-Fischer U, et al. Effects of physical activity on the fatigue and psychologic status of cancer patients during chemotherapy. Cancer 1999; 85:2273–7.

76. Mock V, Pickett M, Ropka ME, et al. Fatigue and quality of life outcomes of exercise during cancer treatment. Cancer Pract 2001;9:119–27.

77. Courneya KS, Mackey JR, Bell GJ, et al. Randomized controlled trial of exercise training in postmenopausal breast cancer survivors: cardiopulmonary and quality of life outcomes. J Clin Oncol 2003;21:1660–8.

78. Segal RJ, Reid RD, Courneya KS, et al. Resistance exercise in men receiving androgen deprivation therapy for prostate cancer. J Clin Oncol 2003;21:1653–9.

79. Courneya KS, Friedenreich CM. Physical exercise and quality of life following cancer diagnosis: a literature review. Ann Behav Med 1999;21:171–9.

80. Mock V, McCorkle R, Ropka ME, et al. Fatigue and physical functioning during breast cancer treatment. Presented at the Oncology Nursing Forum 27th Annual Congress; 2002; Washington, DC.

81. Fawzy FI, Cousins N, Fawzy NW, et al. A structured psychiatric intervention for cancer patients. I. Changes over time in methods of coping and affective disturbance. Arch Gen Psychiatry 1990;47:720–5.

82. Spiegel D, Bloom JR, Yalom I. Group support for patients with metastatic cancer. A randomized outcome study. Arch Gen Psychiatry 1981;38:527–33.

83. Fawzy NW. A psychoeducational nursing intervention to enhance coping and affective state in newly diagnosed malignant melanoma patients. Cancer Nurs 1995;18: 427–38.

84. Gaston-Johansson F, Fall-Dickson JM, Nanda J, et al. The effectiveness of the comprehensive coping strategy program on clinical outcomes in breast cancer autologous bone marrow transplantation. Cancer Nurs 2000;23: 277–85.

85. Barsevick AM, Sweeney C, Beck S, et al. A randomized clinical trial of energy conservation training versus attentional control during cancer treatment. Presented at the Oncology Nursing Forum 27th Annual Congress; 2002; Washington, DC.

86. Given B, Given CW, McCorkle R, et al. Pain and fatigue management: results of a nursing randomized clinical trial. Oncol Nurs Forum 2002;29:949–56.

87. Jacobsen PB, Meade CD, Stein KD, et al. Efficacy and costs of two forms of stress management training for cancer patients undergoing chemotherapy. J Clin Oncol 2002;20:2851–62.

88. Cimprich B. Attentional fatigue following breast cancer surgery. Res Nurs Health 1992;15:199–207.

89. Cimprich B, Ronis DL. An environmental intervention to restore attention in women with newly diagnosed breast cancer. Cancer Nurs 2003;26:284–92; quiz 293–84.

90. Cimprich B. Development of an intervention to restore attention in cancer patients. Cancer Nurs 1993;16:83–92.

91. Lee KA. Sleep and fatigue. Annu Rev Nurs Res 2001;19: 249–73.

92. Berger AM H, P, VonEssen S, Kuhn B, et al. Outcomes of a sleep intervention following adjuvant chemotherapy. Oncol Nurs Forum 2002;29:333.

93. Breitbart W, Rosenfeld B, Kaim M, Funesti-Esch J. A randomized, double-blind, placebo-controlled trial of psychostimulants for the treatment of fatigue in ambulatory patients with human immunodeficiency virus disease. Arch Intern Med 2001;161:411–20.

94. Krupp LB, LaRocca NG, Muir-Nash J, Steinberg AD. The fatigue severity scale. Application to patients with multiple sclerosis and systemic lupus erythematosus. Arch Neurol 1989;46:1121–3.

95. Weinshenker BG, Penman M, Bass B, et al. A double-blind, randomized, crossover trial of pemoline in fatigue associated with multiple sclerosis. Neurology 1992;42:1468–71.

96. Berkovitch M, Pope E, Phillips J, Koren G. Pemoline-associated fulminant liver failure: testing the evidence for causation. Clin Pharmacol Ther 1995;57:696–8.

97. Faraj BA, Israili ZH, Perel JM, et al. Metabolism and disposition of methylphenidate-14C: studies in man and animals. J Pharmacol Exp Ther 1974;191:535–47.

98. Wargin W, Patrick K, Kilts C, et al. Pharmacokinetics of methylphenidate in man, rat and monkey. J Pharmacol Exp Ther 1983;226:382–6.

99. Sarhill N, Walsh D, Nelson KA, et al. Methylphenidate for fatigue in advanced cancer: a prospective open-label pilot study. Am J Hosp Palliat Care 2001;18:187–92.

100. Bruera E, Driver L, Barnes EA, et al. Patient-controlled methylphenidate for the management of fatigue in patients with advanced cancer: a preliminary report. J Clin Oncol 2003;21:4439–43.

101. Rammohan KW, Rosenberg JH, Lynn DJ, et al. Efficacy and safety of modafinil (Provigil) for the treatment of fatigue in multiple sclerosis: a two centre phase 2 study. J Neurol Neurosurg Psychiatry 2002;72:179–83.

102. Morrow GR, Hickok JT. Effect of an SSRI antidepressant on fatigue and depression in seven hundred thirty-eight cancer patients treated with chemotherapy. Proc Am Soc Clin Oncol 2001.

103. Moertel CG, Schutt AJ, Reitemeier RJ, Hahn RG. Corticosteroid therapy of preterminal gastrointestinal cancer. Cancer 1974;33:1607–9.

104. Bruera E, Roca E, Cedaro L, et al. Action of oral methylprednisolone in terminal cancer patients: a prospective randomized double-blind study. Cancer Treat Rep 1985;69:751–4.

105. Della Cuna GR, Pellegrini A, Piazzi M. Effect of methylprednisolone sodium succinate on quality of life in preterminal cancer patients: a placebo-controlled, multicenter study. The Methylprednisolone Preterminal Cancer Study Group. Eur J Cancer Clin Oncol 1989;25:1817–21.

106. Popiela T, Lucchi R, Giongo F. Methylprednisolone as palliative therapy for female terminal cancer patients. The Methylprednisolone Female Preterminal Cancer Study Group. Eur J Cancer Clin Oncol 1989;25:1823–9.

107. Shen J, Glaspy J. Acupuncture: evidence and implications for cancer supportive care. Cancer Pract 2001;9:147–50.

108. Vickers AJ, Straus DJ, Fearon B, Cassileth BR. Acupuncture for postchemotherapy fatigue: a phase II study. J Clin Oncol 2004;22:1731–5.

109. Cleeland CS. Measuring and understanding fatigue. Oncology 1999;13:91–7.

110. Holley SK. Evaluating patient distress from cancer-related fatigue: an instrument development study. Oncol Nurs Forum 2000;27:1425–31.

111. Hann DM, Denniston MM, Baker F. Measurement of fatigue in cancer patients: further validation of the Fatigue Symptom Inventory. Qual Life Res 2000;9:847–54.

112. Okuyama T, Akechi T, Kugaya A, et al. Development and validation of the cancer fatigue scale: a brief, three-dimensional, self-rating scale for assessment of fatigue

in cancer patients. J Pain Symptom Manage 2000;19: 5–14.

113. Piper BF, Dibble SL, Dodd MJ, et al. The revised Piper Fatigue Scale: psychometric evaluation in women with breast cancer. Oncol Nurs Forum 1998;25:677–84.

114. Schwartz AL. The Schwartz Cancer Fatigue Scale: testing reliability and validity. Oncol Nurs Forum 1998;25:711–7.

115. Stein KD, Martin SC, Hann DM, Jacobsen PB. A multidimensional measure of fatigue for use with cancer patients. Cancer Pract 1998;6:143–52.

116. Smets EM, Garssen B, Bonke B, De Haes JC. The Multidimensional Fatigue Inventory (MFI) psychometric qualities of an instrument to assess fatigue. J Psychosom Res 1995;39:315–25.

117. Schwartz JE, Jandorf L, Krupp LB. The measurement of fatigue: a new instrument. J Psychosom Res 1993;37: 753–62.

118. Schwartz AL, Thompson JA, Masood N. Interferon-induced fatigue in patients with melanoma: a pilot study of exercise and methylphenidate. Oncol Nurs Forum Online 2002;29:E85–90.

8

Cancer Pain

Russell K. Portenoy, MD
Gaurav Mathur, MD

Approximately 30 to 50% of patients undergoing antineoplastic therapy and 75 to 90% of patients with advanced disease have chronic pain severe enough to warrant opioid therapy.[1-3] There are numerous obstacles to effective pain management, and inadequately treated pain is commonly encountered in practice. These obstacles relate to deficiencies in clinician knowledge and skills, health care systems that limit access to care, and the tendency to underreport pain on the part of patients. To improve patient outcomes, strategies are needed to address all of these obstacles. Clinician education based on well-accepted guidelines for treatment is central to this effort. Education must focus on both the assessment of pain and the many approaches that now exist to manage it.

Definitions

According to the International Association for the Study of Pain, pain is "an unpleasant sensory and emotional experience associated with actual or potential tissue damage, or described in terms of such damage."[4] To clarify the approach to pain assessment, it is useful to distinguish pain from both nociception and suffering.

Nociception is the activity produced in the afferent nervous system by potentially tissue-damaging stimuli. Nociception is clinically inferred whenever tissue damage is identified. Pain is the perception of nociception and can be sustained in the absence of ongoing tissue injury by any of a variety of factors. Neuropathic pain syndromes are presumably sustained through plastic changes in the nervous system; so-called psychogenic pains are attributed to psychological disturbances. Targeting only the nociceptive component without addressing these other factors can lead to a poor outcome, in which the focus of tissue damage is ameliorated but the pain continues.

Suffering has been described as a perceived threat to the integrity of the person, as a type of "total pain"[5] or overall impairment in the quality of life. Suffering may be driven by unrelieved symptoms (including pain), psychological or psychosocial disturbances, or spiritual distress.

Other factors, such as financial concerns, also may be prominent. Patients vary in psychosocial and spiritual strengths and weaknesses and consequently suffer in different ways when dealing with symptoms such as pain.

Models of Care

The assessment and management of pain must be positioned within a broader effort to preserve quality of life and address the nature of the suffering experienced by the patient and family. An understanding of the physical, psychosocial, and spiritual issues that may undermine quality of life or worsen suffering is fundamental to this process. The therapeutic approach that addresses these issues is known as palliative care. Palliative care is a therapeutic approach to the care of patients with any type of life-threatening illness and their families.[6] It is focused on maintaining quality of life throughout the course of the illness and must intensify as the end of life approaches. The goals of this model include symptom control; effective communication among patient, family, the treatment team, and others; management of psychological distress and comorbid psychiatric disorders; and support for efforts to address family stress, social isolation, and spiritual distress. Palliative care recognizes the need to provide practical support in the home and to manage caregiver distress and burden. If the disease progresses and the end of life is anticipated, palliative care strives to provide opportunities for a comfortable and dignified death and bereavement support for families.

Palliative care is now considered an approach that should be implemented at a generalist level by all physicians who care for patients with serious medical illnesses. It should also be available at a specialist level for those patients and families who have more complex needs. In the United States, specialist-level palliative care is now provided through a growing number of institution-based palliative care programs and through hospice programs. Physicians and nurses may now pursue subspecialty training and certification in palliative care. There is consensus about the elements that should be provided in institution-based programs.[6]

The United States established hospice as a government entitlement program in the early 1980s. Treatment by a hospice program is supported by a benefit available to eligible patients insured by Medicare or Medicaid; comparable benefits are available through most other insurances. When optimally delivered, hospice can provide specialist-level palliative care to patients with advanced illness. Eligibility is determined by patient election of the benefit and physician certification of a prognosis of 6 months or less should the disease run its expected course. It is a capitated health care system that provides most care at home but can also offer access to hospital beds if needed. By regulation, the care must include management by a hospice physician, nurse, social worker, and chaplain; access to medicines, supplies, and durable medical equipment related to the terminal illness at no cost to the patient; access to aides and other services as needed; and 13 months of bereavement support for the family after the death of the patient. This robust benefit now is provided through more than 3,300 hospice programs nationwide. About half of the more than 900,000 patients who are now served annually by these programs have cancer.

Despite the large population served, the hospice benefit is underused. The median length of stay in these programs is less than 20 days, reflecting the tendency to refer patients very late in the course of the illness. This tendency most likely results from a combination of factors, including the linkage of hospice with death and the misconception that the primary physician must relinquish care of a patient once admitted to the program.

Hospice programs vary in size and quality of the services provided. Many have little physician involvement and cope with the financial constraints of a capitated system by limiting the types of treatments that may be offered to patients. These factors also drive late referrals. The hospice industry in the United States now is attempting to address these limitations and is exploring a modern concept of hospice care, known as "open access." The future will likely bring expanded use of hospice services, with earlier referrals and better integration of hospice with ongoing oncologic care. This integration will also be supported by the continued development of institution-based palliative care programs, which lack the resources available to hospice but are well situated to assist with earlier treatment of the many concerns that may adversely affect quality of life during the course of the disease.

Evaluation of the Patient with Cancer Pain

Pain Characteristics

The pain complaint should be characterized in terms of clinically relevant descriptors. This information, combined with ancillary medical data, may allow the identification of the etiology for the pain, including its relationship to the underlying disease, and the development of inferences about pain pathophysiology.

Temporal Features

Acute pain usually has a well-defined onset and a readily identifiable cause (eg, surgical incision). If it is associated with other features, these usually are anxiety, overt pain behaviors (moaning or grimacing), and signs of sympathetic hyperactivity (including tachycardia, hypertension, and diaphoresis).

In contrast, chronic pain is characterized by an ill-defined onset and a prolonged, fluctuating course. Overt pain behaviors and sympathetic hyperactivity typically are absent, and vegetative signs, including lassitude, sleep disturbance, and anorexia, may be present. A clinical depression evolves in some patients.

Most patients with chronic cancer pain also experience periodic flares of pain, or "breakthrough pain."[7] An important subtype of breakthrough pain is "incident pain," which is precipitated by voluntary activity. A recent international study demonstrated an association between breakthrough pain and higher ratings on worst and average pain scales and higher pain interference with function.[8] The recognition of breakthrough pain as a significant problem has supported the use of so-called "rescue" doses—a short-acting opioid administered on an as-needed basis—during long-term opioid therapy.

Topographic Features

Focal pain is experienced at or near the causative lesion. Referred pains are experienced at a site distant from the lesion. Pain may be referred from any structure, including nerve, bone, muscle, soft tissue, and viscera.[9,10] Various subtypes can be distinguished. Pain may be referred along the course of an injured peripheral nerve (such as pain in the thigh or knee from a lumbar plexus lesion) or nerve root (radicular pain). Pain also may be referred to a site remote from the nociceptive lesion and outside the dermatome affected by the lesion (eg, shoulder pain from diaphragmatic irritation).

Knowledge of pain referral patterns is needed to guide the evaluation. For example, a patient with recurrent cervical cancer who reports progressive pain in the inguinal region may require evaluation of numerous structures to identify the underlying lesion, including the subjacent pelvic bones and hip joint, pelvic sidewall, paraspinal gutter at an upper lumbar spinal level, and intraspinal region at the upper lumbar level.

Intensity

Measurement of pain intensity may be accomplished using a numeric scale (0–10), a verbal rating scale (none, mild, moderate, severe), or a visual analogue scale. Pictorial scales are particularly useful for the very young and patients with mild to moderate cognitive impairment. The particular scale is less important than its consistent use to monitor and document the status of pain over time.

Pain measurement is best performed by providing a framework for the patient. A specific question about the experience of pain "on average during the past day" or "at its worst during the past week" will be most informative. Patients can usually provide a detailed response to such a question.

In assessing pain intensity, it is important to obtain information about factors that increase or decrease the pain. In some cases, this information highlights the need for additional evaluation or specific interventions.

Quality

The variation in pain phenomenology, including descriptors of quality (eg, aching, sharp, burning, stabbing), suggests the existence of multiple types of pain mechanisms. Research into pain mechanisms is proceeding rapidly, and there is reason to hope that the future may bring an opportunity to diagnose pain disorders according to the predominating mechanism and use this information to select a mechanism-based treatment. Unfortunately, clinicians presently are far from this level of sophistication.

Information about the quality of the pain, when combined with other elements in the pain assessment, may provide clues about the etiology of the pain and allow classification according to broad pathophysiologic categories (see below). Although these categories represent a gross simplification of complex mechanisms, they have clinical utility, potentially suggesting specific types of interventions.

Etiology and Inferred Pathophysiology

To the extent that credible conclusions can be drawn, an important goal of the pain evaluation is to determine etiology. In most patients with cancer, pain can be related to an underlying nociceptive lesion, usually direct invasion of pain-sensitive structures by the neoplasm.[11] The structures most often involved are bone and neural tissue, but pain also can occur when there is an obstruction of hollow viscus, distention of organ capsules, distortion or occlusion of blood vessels, and infiltration of soft tissues. The etiology of pain relates to an antineoplastic treatment in about one-quarter of patients, and fewer than 10% have pain unrelated to the neoplasm or its treatment.[11]

Identification of the etiology of the pain can provide an opportunity for a primary therapy, such as radiotherapy. A survey of patients referred to a pain service in a major cancer hospital noted that previously unsuspected lesions were identified in 63% of patients.[12] This outcome altered the known extent of disease in virtually all patients, changed the prognosis for some, and provided an opportunity for antineoplastic therapy in approximately 15%.

Information from the history, examination, and imaging studies also may identify a specific pain syndrome and allow inferences about underlying pathophysiology. Pathophysiology may be categorized as nociceptive, neuropathic, psychogenic, idiopathic, or mixed. Although these labels represent constructs that presumably reflect complex interactions among multiple processes, they are clinically relevant, in many cases suggesting the use of specific therapies.

Nociceptive pain indicates that an inference has been made that pain is sustained predominantly by ongoing tissue injury. Nociceptive pain can involve either somatic or visceral structures. Somatic pain is often described as aching, stabbing, throbbing, or pressure-like. Visceral pain is usually gnawing or crampy when arising from obstruction of a hollow viscus and aching or stabbing when arising from other visceral structures. Visceral pain is often referred to cutaneous sites or may be poorly localizable.

Pain is labeled neuropathic if the evaluation suggests that it is sustained by abnormal somatosensory processing in the peripheral or central nervous system. Neuropathic mechanisms are involved in approximately 40% of cancer pain syndromes and can be caused by disease or by treatment.[13] Dysesthesia, or abnormal uncomfortable sensations that may be described using words such as "burning," "shock-like," and "electrical," is suggestive of neuropathic mechanisms. On physical examination, the presence of allodynia (pain induced by nonpainful stimuli) and hyperalgesia (increased perception of painful stimuli) further suggests this diagnosis. Patients may or may not develop motor or autonomic dysfunction in the distribution of the involved nerve.

The term *psychogenic pain* refers to pain that is believed to be sustained predominantly by psychological factors. These pains may be more precisely characterized by applying the widely accepted taxonomy of somatoform disorders proposed by the American Psychiatric Association.[14] These pains share an assessment that reveals positive evidence for the psychopathology that is believed to be causally related to the pain. This is uncommon in the cancer population, notwithstanding the importance of psychological influences in the presentation of the pain complaint and the patient's adaptation. Given the complexity of these pains, the inability to identify a structural cause for the pain should not lead to the assumption that the pain is psychogenic. Similarly, the identification of a structural etiology should not be taken as the complete explanation if psychological factors are evident.

In the absence of a lesion capable of explaining the pain and positive evidence of a somatoform disorder, it is appropriate to label the pain idiopathic. In the cancer population, this label usually suggests the need to reassess etiology and pathophysiology at a later time.

Cancer Pain Syndromes

Efforts to improve the assessment of cancer pain have been greatly encouraged by the description of numerous pain syndromes, each of which is defined by a cluster of symptoms and signs.[11,13] Syndrome identification can help direct the diagnostic evaluation, clarify the prognosis, and target therapeutic interventions.

Acute pain syndromes are commonly caused by diagnostic or therapeutic interventions, including surgery (Table 1). Chronic pain syndromes may be directly related to the neoplasm or to antineoplastic therapy (Tables 2 and 3).

Chronic Pain Syndromes Related to Direct Tumor Invasion

The most common pain syndromes are nociceptive and result from metastatic injury to bone. Only a small proportion of bone metastases become painful, and the factors that result in pain are only beginning to be elucidated.[15] Multifocal bone pain is usually caused by widespread metastases. The spine is the most common site of bone metastasis, and back or neck pain is associated with varied discrete syndromes. For example, tumor invasion of the C1 or C2 vertebra can cause progressive neck or posterior occipital pain, which is exacerbated by flexion of the neck. Metastasis to the C7 or T1 vertebral bodies may cause pain that refers inferiorly to the interscapular region, and a lesion of the T12 or L1 vertebral bodies can refer pain to the ipsilateral sacroiliac joint or iliac crest. Without recognition of pain referral patterns, imaging can be directed to the wrong location.

Table 1 Acute Pain Syndromes in Cancer Patients

Acute pain associated with diagnostic procedures
  Lumbar puncture headache
  Bone marrow biopsy
  Lumbar puncture
  Venipuncture
  Paracentesis
  Thoracentesis
Acute pain associated with analgesic techniques
  Spinal opioid hyperalgesia syndrome
  Acute pain after radiopharmaceutical therapy of metastatic bone pain
Acute postoperative pain
Acute pain associated with other therapeutic procedures
  Pleurodesis
  Tumor embolization
  Nephrostomy insertion
  Pain associated with bone marrow transplantation
Acute pain associated with chemotherapy
  Pain from intravenous or intra-arterial infusion
  Intraperitoneal chemotherapy
  Headache owing to intrathecal chemotherapy
  Painful oropharyngeal mucositis
  Painful peripheral neuropathy
  Bone or muscle pain from colony-stimulating factors or chemotherapies
  5-Fluorouracil-induced angina
Acute pain associated with hormonal therapy
  Painful gynecomastia
  Luteinizing hormone–releasing factor tumor flare in prostate cancer
  Hormone-induced acute pain flare in breast cancer
Acute pain associated with immunotherapy
  Arthralgia and myalgia from interferon and interleukin
Acute pain associated with radiation therapy
  Painful oropharyngeal mucositis
  Acute radiation enteritis or proctitis
  Early-onset brachial plexopathy following radiation for breast cancer
Acute tumor-related pain
  Vertebral collapse and other pathologic fractures
  Acute obstruction of hollow viscus (eg, bowel, ureter, bladder outlet)
  Headache from intracranial hypertension
  Hemorrhage from tumor
Acute pain associated with infection
  Myalgia and arthralgia associated with sepsis
  Pain associated with superficial wounds or abscesses

Adapted from Portenoy RK. Pain syndromes in patients with cancer and HIV/AIDS. In: Portenoy RK, editor. Contemporary diagnosis and management of pain in oncologic and AIDS patients. Newton (PA): Handbooks on Healthcare; 1998.

Table 2 Chronic Pain Syndromes in Patients with Cancer: Tumor-Related Pain Syndromes

Nociceptive pain syndromes
Bone, joint, and soft tissue pain syndromes
  Multifocal or generalized pain (focal metastases or marrow expansion)
  Base of skull metastases
  Vertebral syndromes
  Pain syndromes of the bony pelvis and hip
  Tumor invasion of joint, soft tissue, or both
Paraneoplastic pain syndromes
  Hypertrophic osteoarthropathy
  Tumor-related gynecomastia
Neoplastic involvement of viscera
  Hepatic distention syndrome
  Rostral retroperitoneal syndrome
  Chronic intestinal obstruction and peritoneal carcinomatosis
  Malignant pelvic and perineal pain
  Chronic ureteral obstruction
Neuropathic pain syndromes
  Painful peripheral mononeuropathies
  Painful polyneuropathies
  Plexopathy
    Cervical
    Brachial
    Lumbosacral
    Sacral
  Radiculopathy
  Epidural spinal cord compression

Adapted from Portenoy RK, Lesage P. Management of cancer pain. Lancet 1999;353:1696–7.

Other nociceptive syndromes are caused by obstruction, infiltration, and compression of visceral structures. Patients with liver metastases may experience focal pain, which usually is sharp or pressure-like, in the right upper quadrant of the abdomen. Infrahepatic disease may refer pain to the right scapula. Diaphragmatic irritation may refer pain to the shoulder, and any lesion in the rostral retroperitoneum can produce pain that mimics the pain of pancreatic cancer, with referral to the midback. Chronic partial bowel obstruction is a common complication of many tumors, particularly ovarian and colorectal, and may produce frequent abdominal cramping or sharp and aching pains that may be worsened by eating, activity, and constipation.

Cancer-related neuropathic pain syndromes are usually caused by tumor infiltration or compression of peripheral nerves or nerve roots.[11,13] The resultant pain syndromes are highly variable and often challenging to treat. Painful mononeuropathies can occur after injury to any nerve that carries afferent fibers. A painful polyneuropathy may be paraneoplastic but more often has an etiology unrelated to the cancer, such as multiple vitamin deficiencies, metabolic derangements, or neurotoxic drugs. The paraneoplastic polyneuropathies include a dorsal root ganglionopathy

Table 3 Chronic Pain Syndromes in Patients with Cancer: Treatment-Related Pain Syndromes

Nociceptive pain syndromes
  Painful osteonecrosis
    Radiation- or corticosteroid-induced
      necrosis of femoral or humeral head
    Osteoradionecrosis of other bones
  Painful lymphedema
  Painful gynecomastia
  Chronic abdominal pain
    Due to intraperitoneal chemotherapy
    Due to radiation therapy
  Radiation-induced chronic pelvic pain

Neuropathic pain syndromes
  Postsurgical neuropathic pain syndromes
    Postmastectomy syndrome
    Post-thoracotomy syndrome
    Postradical neck dissection syndrome
    Postnephrectomy syndrome
    Stump pain and phantom pain
  Postradiotherapy pain syndrome
    Radiation fibrosis of cervical, brachial, or
      lumbosacral plexus
    Radiation-induced neoplasm
    Radiation myelopathy
  Postchemotherapy pain syndromes
    Polyneuropathies

Adapted from Portenoy RK, Lesage P. Management of cancer pain. Lancet 1999;353:1696–7.

and a painful sensorimotor neuropathy. Painful radiculopathy usually is caused by a metastatic tumor arising from the vertebral body. Other possible causes include leptomeningeal metastases, primary epidural metastases, and primary tumors that arise from the root.

Chronic Pain Syndromes Related to Cancer Therapy

Chronic nociceptive pain syndromes also may be related to cancer therapy. For example, radiation to bone and systemic corticosteroid therapy can cause focal painful osteonecrosis. Interruption of lymphatic channels by surgical manipulation or radiation can result in painful lymphedema.

Neuropathic pain following cancer treatment may be associated with mononeuropathy or polyneuropathy. Chemotherapy-induced polyneuropathy is common and may be a consequence of treatment with any number of agents, including vinca alkaloids, cisplatin, carboplatin, oxaliplatin, or paclitaxel. Most patients improve once chemotherapy is stopped, but some develop persistent pain.

Surgical incisions at any site can precipitate a neuropathic pain syndrome. The best described examples are associated with amputation at any site. Neuropathic pain at the site of the incision may be related to painful neuromas (stump pain in amputation) or to other processes in the peripheral nerve; injury also can initiate changes that are presumably central and result in a deafferentation pain syndrome (phantom limb when associated with amputation).

Radiation-induced fibrosis can injure peripheral nerves and cause neuropathic pain that may begin months to years following treatment. This pain is generally less prominent than nerve injury caused by neoplasm. Slowly progressive weakness, sensory disturbances, radiation changes of the skin, and lymphedema are often associated.

Overcoming Obstacles in Cancer Pain Treatment

Cancer pain is frequently undertreated, and the evaluation should attempt to identify the barriers that may compromise treatment efforts. Positive strategies may be needed to overcome these barriers and increase the likelihood of a favorable outcome.

Patient Education and Attitudes

Patients can hinder their own pain control. They may believe that pain is a "normal" part of cancer and that little can be (or should be) done to relieve it. A few believe that pain has redemptive power. Patients also may object to the use of an opioid for any of a variety of reasons: fear of becoming "addicted," fear of continually escalating the dose, or fear of side effects. Some of these concerns may arise from having witnessed destructive drug abuse in the family or having a personal history of abuse.

Most of these fears can be alleviated by careful listening and explanation by the clinician. A recent study demonstrated an improvement in cancer pain outcomes after a focused educational session with a trained nurse, which included self-assessment of pain, information about opioid use and side effects, and pointers on communication with the physician.[16] The clinician must explain that opioids can treat pain effectively and that side effects usually can be managed. Patients should be advised that physical dependence, the capacity to experience abstinence if the drug is stopped abruptly or an antagonist is administered, is a biologic phenomenon and poses no clinical problem as long as simple steps are followed to avoid abstinence. Patients also should be disabused of the concern that tolerance to analgesic effects commonly compromises long-term opioid efficacy. In the absence of worsening pain related to progressive disease, opioid doses typically remain stable.

Patients must be told specifically that physical dependence is not the same as addiction, a term that is commonly misused by both physicians and patients. Addiction is a biopsychosocial disorder with a strong hereditary component and behavioral manifestations characterized by compulsive drug use, loss of control over use, drug craving, and use despite harm.[17] Patients with no history of drug abuse or addiction must be reassured that addiction is a rare problem during treatment for pain; patients with a history of substance use disorder must be informed that pain usually can be managed concurrently with the addictive disease.

Biomedical Barriers

Patients may be unable to swallow, absorb, or metabolize the opioid because of comorbid disease. Mental status changes may prevent patients from expressing their symptoms or from understanding how and when to take pain medication. These barriers must be addressed by the clinician to ensure effective pain control. Alternative routes of opioid delivery are available if enteral intake is difficult (see below). Communication difficulties can be addressed, and caregivers, when properly educated about pain assessment and treatment, can be of invaluable assistance.

Physician Barriers

Concern about the risks associated with opioid use, including the risk of side effects and the risk of addiction, can lead a clinician to be unnecessarily wary and therefore undertreat pain.[18] Physicians, like patients, may stigmatize the use of opioids, despite the wide acceptance of their use for cancer pain treatment. Physicians treating cancer pain should be comfortable with opioid therapy and possess strategies to address side effects or problematic drug use. Physicians also must become familiar with the laws and regulations governing opioid use, including the elements of documentation that are required by those in the law enforcement and regulatory communities.

Other Barriers

Involved family members and caregivers can sometimes become unintentional barriers to effective pain control. Family members may fear the use of opioids in a loved one, especially in the context of cultural or community stigma. The physician should make every effort to include family members and educate them to alleviate such fears.

In the United States, a fragmented health care system continues to impose unnecessary burdens on patients, families, and health care providers. These difficulties can be particularly challenging for patients who are seriously ill. Home visits by professionals and home delivery of medicines can be invaluable services to the ailing cancer patient but are largely unavailable. A recent study found the use of morphine in home-care hospice patients to be safe and effective, even at very high doses.[19]

Other barriers are also important. For example, an increasing amount of literature suggests that access to optimal care may be compromised by minority status.[20] These barriers deserve further study.

Management of Chronic Cancer Pain

The evaluation of the patient with cancer pain should provide the information necessary to characterize the pain complaint, determine its etiology and presumed pathophysiology, understand its impact, and clarify relevant comorbidities. This understanding is the basis for therapeutic decision making.

Role of Primary Therapy

Primary treatments for the pain include antineoplastic therapies and interventions directed at other pathologies. Although the palliative role of chemotherapy is widely accepted,[21–23] the specifics have received limited study. Nonetheless, it is a common observation that patients who attain a partial or complete tumor response also experience symptom improvement. Two chemotherapies, mitoxantrone for prostate cancer and gemcitabine for pancreatic cancer, received regulatory approval largely on the basis of symptom palliation.

Radiation therapy has been reported to provide effective palliation of pain in up to 50% of patients treated for bone metastases,[24,25] and pain control is the reason for treatment in the majority of patients who receive this intervention. Analgesia also commonly results when radiation is used to treat other disorders, including epidural disease, tumor ulceration, cerebral metastases, superior vena cava obstruction, and bronchial obstruction. Patients with a limited prognosis (ie, months) may benefit from single doses or a shortened fractionation schedule, thereby decreasing treatment burden.[26]

Pharmacotherapy of Chronic Cancer Pain

Although primary therapies can be very helpful in selected patients, most patients require symptomatic analgesic therapy. Prospective trials indicate that 70 to 90% of patients can achieve adequate relief of cancer pain using a pharmacologic approach.[3,27,28] Effective pain management requires expertise in the use of nonsteroidal anti-inflammatory drugs (NSAIDs), opioid analgesics, and adjuvant analgesics. The term *adjuvant analgesic* is applied to a diverse group of drugs that have primary indications other than pain but can be effective analgesics in specific circumstances, such as the treatment of neuropathic pain.

A model approach to the selection of analgesic drugs for cancer pain, known as the "analgesic ladder," was developed in the 1980s by an expert panel for the World Health Organization (WHO).[3] Although the analgesic ladder approach has evolved since it was created and rigid adherence to its guidelines is no longer justified, key elements are still accepted. Most important, the approach reinforces the consensus view that persistent moderate to severe cancer pain should be treated with an opioid-based drug regimen. From this perspective, the analgesic ladder has been very useful as a tool to educate policy makers and others about the need for access to opioids.

According to the analgesic ladder approach, mild to moderate cancer pain is first treated with acetaminophen or an NSAID. This often is combined with an adjuvant drug to provide additional analgesia (ie, an adjuvant analgesic), treat a side effect of the analgesic, or help manage a coexisting symptom.

Patients who present with moderate to severe pain or who do not achieve adequate relief after a trial of an NSAID should be treated with a so-called "weak" opioid (see below). This is typically combined with an NSAID and may also be administered with an adjuvant drug. Those who present with severe pain or who do not achieve adequate relief following appropriate administration of drugs on the second rung of the ladder should receive a so-called "strong" opioid, which may be combined with an NSAID or an adjuvant drug as indicated.

Nonsteroidal Anti-inflammatory Drugs

The nonopioid analgesics include acetaminophen (also known as paracetamol), dipyrone, and the diverse NSAIDs. These drugs have a well-established role in the treatment of cancer pain.[29–31] Dipyrone is not available in the United States, and practice usually focuses on the use of the NSAIDs. These drugs may be the sole analgesics required by patients with generally mild pain and should be considered as adjunct therapy for opioid-based treatment of moderate or severe pain. NSAIDs appear to be especially useful in patients with nociceptive pain, particularly bone pain and pain related to grossly inflammatory lesions, and relatively less useful in patients with neuropathic pain.[32–34] In addition, NSAIDs have an opioid-sparing effect that may be helpful to prevent the occurrence of dose-related side effects.[33]

All NSAIDs have the potential for nephrotoxicity, with effects that range from peripheral edema to acute or chronic renal failure. Clinical effects and serum creatinine must be monitored periodically in the medically frail cancer patient who receives an NSAID for ongoing treatment of pain.

NSAIDs all increase the risk of gastrointestinal ulcers and bleeding. The selective cyclooxygenase (COX)-2 inhibitors appear to have a relatively reduced risk of these outcomes, and many clinicians recommend these drugs as first-line therapy for all patients at a relatively high risk of ulcer, including the elderly, those concurrently receiving a corticosteroid, and those with a history of peptic ulcer disease or NSAID-induced gastroduodenopathy, and medically frail patients who are less able to tolerate a gastrointestinal hemorrhage.

This approach is reasonable, notwithstanding recent data that have raised concerns about an increased risk of cardiovascular events in populations treated with the selective COX-2 inhibitors. Recently, rofecoxib was withdrawn from the US market by the manufacturer after a study revealed a doubling of cardiovascular risk after 18 months of use. Similar effects were suggested for high-dose celecoxib in a cancer prevention trial, valdecoxib in a trial of patient who underwent coronary bypass surgery, and naproxen in a dementia prevention trial. Other large studies of celecoxib have not shown this effect.[35]

At present, the extent to which cardiovascular toxicity may be an effect of specific drugs, a class effect of the COX-2 selective inhibitors, or possible with any NSAID is uncertain. Given the current evidence, it is appropriate to continue the preferential use of COX-2 selective inhibitors in populations with a relatively high risk of gastrointestinal toxicity. Many with cancer pain would be in this category.

Adjuvant Analgesics

The adjuvant analgesics comprise numerous drugs in diverse classes, most of which are commercially available for indications other than pain but may be analgesic in selected circumstances (Table 4).[36] Treatment with one of these drugs is generally considered if an optimally administered opioid regimen fails to provide a satisfactory balance between pain relief and side effects. These drugs are particularly useful in the treatment of neuropathic pain, bone pain, and pain related to bowel obstruction.

Corticosteroids are multipurpose adjuvant analgesics. In addition to their use in neuropathic pain, these drugs may improve anorexia, nausea, and fatigue and are often used in open-ended therapy when cancer is relatively advanced. They are empirically used to treat the pain associated with lymphedema, bowel obstruction, metastatic bone pain, headache associated with intracranial mass lesions, and superior vena cava syndrome. Dexamethasone and prednisone are typical choices, and long-term administration is common in advanced illness. Doses are typically modest, such as dexamethasone 1 to 4 mg or prednisone 5 to 10 mg daily. Higher doses are sometimes used when pain is severe and rapid control of pain cannot be obtained with an opioid.

Anticonvulsants, antidepressants, and sodium channel blockers have analgesic effects in neuropathic pain.[36] The safety and efficacy of

Table 4 Adjuvant Analgesics

Indication	Class	Examples
Neuropathic pain	Steroids	Dexamethasone
		Prednisone
	Antidepressants	
	Tricyclics	Amitryptiline
		Desipramine
		Nortriptyline
	SSRIs/SNRIs	Paroxetine
		Citalopram
		Venlafaxine
		Duloxetine
		Buproprion
	Anticonvulsants	Gabapentin
		Carbamazepine
		Valproate
		Clonazepam
		Lamotrigine
		Topiramate
		Oxcarbazepine
		Zonisamide
		Levetiracetam
		Tiagabine
	Sodium channel blockers	Mexilitine
		Tocainide
	α_2-Adrenergic agonists	Tizanidine
		Clonidine
	NMDA receptor antagonists	Ketamine
		Dextromethorphan
		Amantadine
		Memantine
	GABA agonists	Baclofen
	Topical agents	5% Lidocaine patch
		Local anesthetic creams
		Capsaicin
Bone pain	Bisphosphonates	Pamidronate
	Other osteoclast inhibitor	Calcitonin
	Radiopharmaceuticals	Strontium [89]
		Samarium [153]
Bowel obstruction	Steroid	Dexamethasone
	Anticholinergic drugs	Scopolamine
		Glycopyrrolate
	Somatostatin analogue	Octreotide

GABA = γ-aminobutyric acid; NMDA = N-methyl-D-aspartate; SNRI = serotonin-norepinephrine reuptake inhibitor; SSRI = selective serotonin reuptake inhibitor.

A trial with an oral sodium channel blocker, such as mexiletine, usually is considered after antidepressant and anticonvulsant drugs have been tried.[42] Intravenous or subcutaneous lidocaine may be useful in the treatment of severe, rapidly increasing neuropathic pain.

Other drugs are also used for neuropathic pain.[36] There is extensive experience with the γ-aminobutyric acid (GABA) agonist baclofen and limited experience with the α_2-adrenergic drugs tizanidine and clonidine. Recently, interest has focused on the use of the N-methyl-D-aspartate inhibitors. Dextromethorphan, memantine, amantadine, and ketamine are all considered among the agents that may be tried for neuropathic pain. Small studies have suggested benefit from ketamine in cancer patients with difficult neuropathic pain,[43,44] but this drug carries the risk of psychomimetic effects and must be used cautiously.

Topical agents represent another adjuvant analgesic strategy. A lidocaine patch (Lidoderm)[45,46] is now available and has been shown to be effective in postherpetic neuralgia. In a study in cancer patients with surgical neuropathic pain (eg, postmastectomy syndrome), topical capsaicin, a peptide that depletes substance P in small primary afferent neurons, was found to significantly decrease pain.[47]

Opioid-refractory malignant bone pain is another syndrome for which adjuvant analgesics often are considered. The preferred drugs include bisphosphonates, radiopharmaceuticals, and calcitonin. The bisphosphonates, including pamidronate, clodronate (not available in the United States), and zolendronate, are usually considered first. There has been increasing evidence that these drugs improve the overall morbidity associated with bone metastases.[48]

Adjuvant analgesics also are commonly employed in the setting of advanced bowel obstruction. Aggressive pharmacotherapy, particularly in those with advanced disease, may control symptoms and obviate the need for drainage procedures. Treatment usually involves the combination of anticholinergic drugs (eg, scopolamine or glycopyrrolate), octreotide, corticosteroids, and opioids.[49]

Opioid Analgesics

Expertise in the administration of opioid analgesics is the foundation of cancer pain management. The clinician should have knowledge of opioid pharmacology and a clear grasp of practical guidelines for dosing.

Opioid Selection

The distinction between so-called "weak" and "strong" opioids, which was originally incorporated into the WHO analgesic ladder approach, is

gabapentin are well established,[37–40] and this drug is typically tried first. Of the newer drugs, the evidence of analgesic efficacy is strongest for pregabalin, lamotrigine, topiramate, and levetiracetam. Pregabalin is now available in the United States, approved for the treatment of two types of neuropathic pain. Other anticonvulsants, including zonisamide, oxcarbazepine, tiagabine, and the older drug valproate, also may be tried for neuropathic pain. The benzodiazepine clonazepam also is commonly tried, particularly if anxiety is prominent.

Although there is substantial evidence for the analgesic efficacy of the tricyclic antidepressants, particularly amitriptyline,[41] the use of these drugs is often limited by the high likelihood of side effects. Newer antidepressants, such as duloxetine, venlafaxine, paroxetine, citalopram, and bupropion, are also analgesic and are better tolerated in the cancer population.

more operational than pharmacologic. The weak opioids are conventionally administered orally for moderate pain in those patients with limited previous opioid exposure. The strong opioids are conventionally used to treat severe pain and pain in those already receiving opioid therapy. In the United States, the former group includes codeine, hydrocodone (only with acetaminophen or ibuprofen), dihydrocodeine (only with aspirin), oxycodone (combined with aspirin, acetaminophen, or ibuprofen), propoxyphene, and, occasionally, meperidine. Tramadol, a unique centrally acting analgesic with a mechanism that is partly opioid, is also generally included in this group. Oxycodone is included only in terms of the formulation that combines this opioid with acetaminophen or an NSAID.

The designation of these medications as "weak" is inappropriate because none are characterized by a ceiling effect. Nonetheless, these drugs are used at doses that are potentially effective only in those patients with limited opioid exposure and often only with moderate pain. The opioids that are combined with acetaminophen or ibuprofen in a single tablet may be escalated until the dose of the coanalgesic reaches a level associated with toxicity. In the case of acetaminophen, this is usually a maximum of 4 g/d (and less in patients with known hepatic disease or a history of heavy alcohol consumption). Propoxyphene and meperidine usually are avoided because toxic metabolites may lead to neuroexcitatory effects, including seizures.

Opioids used conventionally for severe pain include morphine, fentanyl, oxycodone, (without acetaminophen or aspirin), hydromorphone, oxymorphone, levorphanol, and methadone. Historically, morphine was considered the preferred first-line drug, based on worldwide experience, ease of dosing, and the availability of numerous formulations. In recent years, however, recognition of large variation in the response to different opioids has reinforced the understanding that an alternative opioid may be preferable for individual patients. There is no one preferred opioid, and the decision to choose one over another is usually based on the available formulation, cost, and previous experience. Therapeutic failure with one drug may be followed by remarkable success with another.[50]

Morphine is metabolized to morphine-3-glucuronide (M3G) and morphine-6-glucuronide (M6G). Accumulation of these metabolites can result in side effects.[51–53] Liver dysfunction has only a small effect on morphine kinetics,[54] but renal insufficiency results in accumulation of M3G and M6G. For this reason, morphine should be administered cautiously to patients with renal insufficiency. An opioid with no known active metabolites, such as fentanyl, may be preferred.

The role of methadone is expanding in pain management. This drug is available as a racemic mixture of the L-isomer (an opioid compound) and the D-isomer (an N-methyl-D-aspartate receptor blocker). The D-isomer may yield independent analgesic effects and partially reverse opioid tolerance; these effects may be responsible for a greater than expected potency when methadone is administered. Methadone has reliable absorption and a low cost. Given its long half-life, consistent pain control usually is possible with dosing three to four times per day. The use of methadone presents challenges, however, because its half-life varies widely across patients and its potency in those with previous opioid exposure is difficult to predict accurately. To ensure safety, a switch to methadone from another drug should be accompanied by a large reduction in the equianalgesic dose and a prolonged observation period to judge the full effect. Recent reports also indicate a potential for Q–T prolongation from high doses of methadone, but the clinical significance of this effect is not clear.[55,56] Nonetheless, methadone should be used cautiously in patients at risk of arrhythmia or receiving other drugs that could prolong the Q–T interval.

Routes of Administration

Long-term administration of an opioid is best accomplished by the oral or transdermal route. Numerous oral formulations are available, including modified-release forms of morphine (with dosing intervals of 12 or 24 hours), oxycodone (12-hour dosing interval), and hydromorphone (24-hour interval). A modified-release oxymorphone is now available. The transdermal route is available for fentanyl and offers a 48- to 72-hour interval; this formulation is preferred by some patients and may be associated with less constipation.[57] A recent study supported the effectiveness of transdermal fentanyl even in both opioid-naive patients and patients converting from a "weak" opioid.[58]

Long-term parenteral dosing can be used for patients who are poor candidates for oral or transdermal formulations. Continuous intravenous infusion is most feasible for patients with an indwelling central venous port. This approach eliminates fluctuations in plasma concentration. Any opioid available in an injectable formulation may be administered in this manner. Ambulatory infusion via the subcutaneous route has been made possible with the development of small infusion pumps. Typically, a 25-gauge "butterfly" needle is inserted subcutaneously and can be left under the skin for as long as a week. High-concentration, low-volume infusions must be used to accommodate limited fluid volumes (eg, less than 5 mL/h).[59]

Opioids and other drugs may also be delivered into the epidural or intrathecal spaces.

Neuraxial infusion can provide opioid analgesia at doses far lower than those required systemically and can therefore provide equivalent or better analgesia with fewer side effects. The strongest indication for neuraxial analgesia is the presence of intolerable somnolence or confusion in patients who experience some degree of analgesia from systemic therapy. In a recent controlled trial, continuous intrathecal infusion of morphine via an implanted drug delivery system yielded better pain control, less fatigue, and improved survival than comprehensive medical management alone.[60] Other drugs can be combined with the opioid to further enhance analgesia. The preferred opioid drugs for chronic intraspinal infusion are morphine and hydromorphone, and the most common admixture drugs include bupivacaine, a local anesthetic, and clonidine, an α_2-agonist. A novel analgesic, ziconotide, was recently released in the United States for intrathecal therapy.

Many methods for neuraxial infusion are now in use.[61] They include a percutaneous epidural catheter, which is usually tunnelled to the anterior abdominal wall and connected to an ambulatory infusion pump; a totally implanted epidural catheter connected to a subcutaneous portal, which, in turn, is connected to an ambulatory pump; and an intrathecal catheter connected to a totally implanted continuous infusion device. Patients with life expectancies exceeding 3 months usually are considered for intrathecal infusion via an implanted pump.

The oral transmucosal form of fentanyl has been shown to be safe and efficacious when used to treat breakthrough pain in cancer patients receiving a fixed-dose opioid regimen for persistent pain.[7,62] Absorption through the oral cavity is theoretically possible with any opioid, particularly those that are, like fentanyl, highly lipophilic.[63] Although injectable formulations of any opioid therefore could be tried, practical considerations and the variable absorption of most drugs do not support wider use of this approach.

Rectal formulations of hydromorphone, and morphine are available in the United States and have potencies that are believed to approximate oral dosing. This route is generally used in opioid-naive patients who are transiently unable to take oral drugs.

Dosing

Following initiation of opioid therapy, dose adjustment usually is required. As the dose is titrated, most patients experience a favorable balance between analgesia and side effects, which generally persists unless there is progression in the pain-producing pathology. Recurrent pain necessitates another period of dose titration. In all cases, the dose of an opioid should be increased until acceptable analgesia is produced or unmanageable side effects supervene. The absolute dose of the opioid is immaterial as long as the balance between analgesia and side effects remains acceptable to the patient. Conventionally, the size of the increment at each dose escalation is between 30 and 100% of the total daily dose on the previous day. The lower end of this range is used if the pain is not severe or the patient is medically frail; the upper part of the range is appropriate for severe pain in the patient who is more robust.

For persistent or frequently recurring pain, the best outcome is achieved by administering an opioid according to a fixed, around-the-clock schedule. Long-acting opioids are preferred because of convenience and the likelihood that treatment adherence will be better than with frequent daily doses. Some clinicians prefer to start therapy with an "as-needed" regimen in the hope of facilitating dose finding. A recent study suggests, however, that dosing also can be initiated with a long-acting drug, without sacrificing effectiveness or increasing risk.[64]

Given the high prevalence of breakthrough pain, the coadministration of a short-acting drug along with a long-acting baseline regimen—a technique called "rescue" dosing—is common practice.[7] An oral rescue dose can be prescribed every 2 hours "as needed" at a dose equal to 5 to 15% of the total daily opioid consumption.

There is large variation in the response of an individual to each opioid. Some patients develop side effects rather than satisfactory analgesia, a scenario now termed "poor responsiveness." The development of poor responsiveness during an opioid trial should be considered specific to the drug, route, and clinical setting. The occurrence of poor responsiveness necessitates a change in the therapeutic strategy.

Among the approaches that may be used to manage the patient with a poor response to an opioid trial is a switch of the opioid, or so-called "opioid rotation." When patients are switched from one opioid to another, the dose of the new drug is calculated based on well-accepted equianalgesic doses (Table 5).[65] The calculated dose of the new drug is reduced to account for incomplete cross-tolerance and individual variation. A reduction in dose by 25 to 50% is typical practice. There are two exceptions, however: a safety factor has already been built into the conversion to transdermal fentanyl, and the dose of this formulation usually is not reduced. When converting to methadone, the dose should be reduced by 75 to 90% because of the possibility of a greater-than-expected potency from this drug.

Management of Side Effects

Effective side-effect management is a fundamental aspect of opioid therapy (Table 6).[66] Side-effect management may improve the quality of analgesia and the likelihood of treatment adherence. Patients who experience poor responsiveness during titration of an opioid may also become

Table 5 Opioid Analgesics Used for the Treatment of Persistent Cancer Pain

Drug	Dose (mg) Equianalgesic to Morphine 10 mg IM*		Half-Life	Duration	Comment
	PO	IM	(h)	(h)	
Morphine	20–30[†]	10	2–3	2–4	Standard for comparison
Morphine modified release	20–30	10	2–3	8–12	Various formulations are not bioequivalent
Oxycodone	20	—	2–3	3–4	
Oxycodone modified release	20	—	2–3	12	
Hydromorphone	7.5	1.5	2–3	2–4	Potency may be greater during prolonged use (ie, hydromorphone: morphine = 3:1 rather than 6.7:1)
Hydromorphone	7.5	1.5	2–3	24	
Methadone	20	10	12–190	4–12	Although 1:1 IM:IM potency ratio with morphine was found in a single-dose study, there is a change with chronic dosing and a large dose reduction (75–90%) is needed when switching to methadone
Oxymorphone	10	1	2–3	2–4	Available in injectable formulations
Levorphanol	4	2	12–15	4–6	
Fentanyl	—	—	7–12	—	Can be administered as a continuous IV or SQ infusion; based on clinical experience, 100 µg/h is roughly equianalgesic to morphine IV 4 mg/h
Fentanyl TTS	—	—	16–24	48–72	Based on clinical experience, 100 µg is roughly equianalgesic to morphine 4 mg/h IV. A ratio of oral morphine to transdermal fentanyl of 70:1 may also be used clinically.

Adapted from Derby S, Chin J, Portenoy RK. Systemic opioid therapy for chronic cancer pain: practical guidelines for converting drugs and routes of administration. CNS Drugs 1998;9:99–109.
IM = intramuscular; IV = intravenous; PO = oral; SQ = subcutaneous.
*Studies to determine equianalgesic doses of opioids have used morphine by the IM route. The IM and IV routes are considered to be equivalent, and IV is the most common route used in clinical practice.
†Although the PO to IM morphine ratio was 6:1 in a single-dose study, other observations indicate a ratio of 2 to 3:1 with repeated administration.

more responsive if the treatment-limiting toxicity can be addressed.

Constipation

The management of opioid-induced constipation begins with prevention. Nonessential constipating drugs should be eliminated and fluid and fiber intake increased. Fiber should not be increased in those with likely partial bowel obstruction or marked debility because of the potential for worsening obstruction. Laxative therapy should be administered prophylactically to patients who

are starting opioid therapy and have other risk factors for constipation, such as advanced age or limited mobility or fluid intake.

There are numerous types of laxatives, including bulk-forming agents, osmotic agents, lubricants, surfactants, contact cathartics, prokinetic drugs, agents for colonic lavage, and oral opioid antagonists.[67] The conventional first-line approach is a combination of a stool softener, such as docusate, and a cathartic agent, such as senna or bisacodyl. Most patients respond to this therapy. For patients who do not, lactulose (an

Table 6 Commonly Used Approaches in the Management of Opioid Side Effects

Side Effect	Treatment
Constipation	General approach
	Increase fluid intake and dietary fiber
	Encourage mobility and ambulation if appropriate
	Ensure comfort and convenience for defecation
	Rule out and treat impaction if present
	Pharmacologic approach
	Contact laxative plus stool softener (eg, senna plus docusate)
	Osmotic laxative (eg, Milk of Magnesia)
	Lavage agent (eg, oral propylethylene glycol)
	Prokinetic agent (eg, metoclopramide)
	Oral naloxone
Nausea	General approach
	Hydrate as appropriate
	Progressive alimentation
	Good mouth care
	Correct contributory factors
	Adjust medication
	Pharmacologic approach
	Vertigo→ antihistamine (eg, scopolamine, meclizine)
	Early satiety→ prokinetic (eg, metoclopramide)
	Dopamine antagonists (eg, prochlorperazine, chlorpromazine, haloperidol, metoclopramide)
Somnolence or cognitive impairment	General approach
	Reassurance
	Education
	Treatment of potential etiologies
	Pharmacologic approach
	If analgesia is satisfactory, reduce opioid dose by 25–50%
	If analgesia is satisfactory and the toxicity is somnolence, consider a trial of psychostimulant (eg, methylphenidate)

osmotic agent) or polyethylene glycol, a lavage agent, might be considered.[68] In refractory cases, a prokinetic drug, such as metoclopramide, can be added.

Oral opioid antagonist therapy can reverse opioid-induced constipation without causing systemic opioid withdrawal through local action on opioid receptors in the gut.[69,70] Oral naloxone can be administered at a starting dose of 0.8 mg daily; the dose is doubled every 2 to 3 days until favorable effects occur or side effects are experienced. Studies of other oral opioid antagonists, including alvimopan and methylnaltrexone,[71,72] have been favorable, and the advent of these drugs will expand the utility of this approach in the future.

Nausea and Vomiting

Opioid-induced nausea may affect as many as 10 to 30% of cancer patients.[73] Conventional antiemetic therapy can be administered on either an "as-needed" or fixed-schedule dosing regimen according to the persistence of symptoms.

Treatment of nausea is likely to be more effective if the drug is targeted toward the mechanism of nausea. Although the evidence in support of this approach is meager, it is often pursued on empiric grounds.[67] Nausea can be caused by a direct effect on the brainstem's chemoreceptor trigger zone, by gastroparesis and relaxation of the gastroesophageal sphincter, or by sensitization of the vestibular-labyrinthine system. Gastroparesis may be suspected if the patient complains of early satiety or postprandial nausea, and vestibular-related nausea is suspected if vertigo is present or nausea is worsened by movement.

Most patients with opioid-induced nausea respond promptly to drugs that are active at the chemoreceptor trigger zone. A dopamine agonist, such as prochlorperazine or haloperidol, is a reasonable initial therapy. Refractory nausea can be treated with a 5-hydroxytryptamine$_3$ antagonist, such as ondansetron, granisetron, or dolasetron. Although the antiemetic efficacy of corticosteroids is unexplained, these drugs are clearly beneficial for some patients. Others respond to the commercially available cannabinoid dronabinol.

Patients with postprandial nausea should be considered for a trial of a prokinetic drug, such as metoclopramide. A proton pump inhibitor often is added. Nausea that is associated with vertigo or movement may be alleviated by an anticholinergic (eg, scopolamine), an antihistamine (eg, meclizine or promethazine), or a benzodiazepine (eg, lorazepam).

Somnolence and Cognitive Impairment

Prospective studies indicate that sedation or mental clouding occurs in 20 to 60% of patients starting oral opioid therapy for cancer pain.[66] Significant impairment disappears in most patients with prolonged exposure to the drug. However, there is wide variation in response, and persistent alterations in cognition, perception, and mood can occur. Cognitive disturbances may be influenced by many factors, including the evolving medical condition and concurrent therapies.

If neuropsychological side effects are mild, reassurance and education may be sufficient. When toxicity is severe or persistent enough to compromise the benefits of therapy, other interventions are needed. Treatment of potential etiologies other than the opioid (eg, elimination of another nonessential drug or treatment of a metabolic disturbance) is the first step to consider. If pain is well controlled, it also is reasonable to try an opioid dose reduction of 25 to 50%.

A trial of specific therapy may be appropriate, but few have been well studied in clinical trials. Evidence suggests that psychostimulants may ameliorate somnolence, fatigue, cognitive impairment, pain, and depression. For example, methylphenidate has been shown to decrease sedation in cancer patients taking opioids.[74–76] Other psychostimulants that have been used empirically include dextroamphetamine and amphetamine. Modafinil, a newer psychostimulant, has fewer sympathomimetic effects than the older drugs and is now favored by some clinicians.[77]

The strongest indication for a psychostimulant trial is the presence of uncomfortable somnolence or cognitive impairment associated with significant analgesia. Patients who are dysphoric also might benefit from the antidepressant effects of these drugs.[78,79] The safety of these drugs in cognitively impaired patients who are restless or agitated has not been established.

Therapy with a psychostimulant usually is initiated with methylphenidate at a dose of 5 to 10 mg/d or modafinil 100 mg/d. Dextroamphetamine and amphetamine, each at doses of 5 to 10 mg/d, are alternatives. A repeat dose at midday often is required for the short-acting drugs. Dose escalation usually is needed. In some cases, favorable effects are attained but appear to wane over time.

Patients should be monitored for side effects

from psychostimulants, including anorexia, insomnia, anxiety, cognitive changes (eg, subtle paranoid thinking), and sympathomimetic effects, such as hypertension and tachycardia. Relative contraindications include preexisting anorexia, severe insomnia, psychiatric disorder characterized by anxiety or paranoid ideation, cardiac disease, or poorly controlled hypertension.

Other Approaches in the Management of Chronic Cancer Pain

Patients with pain that is poorly responsive to an opioid regimen also may be considered for any of a wide variety of alternative analgesic approaches, either pharmacologic or nonpharmacologic. If effective, these approaches reduce the need for the opioid regimen and sometimes eliminate it completely.

Interventional approaches include injection therapies, neural blockade, and the implantation of analgesic devices, usually providing spinal cord stimulation or neuraxial drug infusion. Neural blockade comprises a diverse group of procedures that transiently or permanently block sympathetic nerves, somatic nerves, or both.[61,80] Temporary nerve blocks may be diagnostic, prognostic, or therapeutic. Diagnostic blocks elucidate the afferent pathways involved in pain. Prognostic blocks are implemented prior to a proposed neurolytic procedure. The failure to achieve pain relief is a contraindication to a neurodestructive procedure. Therapeutic blocks include repeated use of a local anesthetic, continuous infusion of an epidural or perineural anesthetic, or administration of a neurolytic solution.

Neurolytic blockade is accomplished using a solution such as alcohol, phenol, or glycerol or through the use of intense heat or cold, to damage the peripheral nerve and partially denervate a particular area. The most widely accepted approach is celiac plexus blockade for the syndrome of rostral retroperitoneal pain, typically caused by pancreatic cancer. The favorable response to this block warrants its consideration whenever the typical pain syndrome occurs and the response to an opioid trial is not satisfactory.[81] Other neurolytic techniques are generally reserved for patients with far advanced cancer and the experience of severe regional pain that is poorly responsive to systemic therapies and occurs in an area that can be safely denervated without compromise of motor or autonomic function.

The role of neuraxial drug infusion for difficult-to-manage cancer pain may grow as a result of a controlled trial that demonstrated the benefits of this approach over conventional systemic opioid therapy in a population with cancer[60] and the recent availability of unique analgesic agents,

such as ziconotide. Neuraxial infusion should be considered in patients who are poorly responsive to a systemic opioid regimen as a result of treatment-limiting side effects.

Other analgesic strategies include the so-called rehabilitative treatments, psychological therapies, and complementary approaches. The potential for analgesia from rehabilitative approaches such as physical therapy, orthotics, and modalities such as heat and cold is insufficiently recognized. Although all of these techniques remain inadequately studied, clinical experience is favorable. Refractory movement–induced pain may be partially relieved by bracing the painful part, and a well-fitting prosthesis may reduce stump pain. Therapeutic exercise may lessen the pain associated with the complications of immobility, such as trigger points in muscle and joint ankylosis. The use of heat and cold, ultrasonography, and electrical stimulation for regional pain syndromes appears to benefit some patients.

Cognitive behavioral approaches have been applied successfully in the management of pain and related symptoms.[82–85] These approaches include specific techniques that may assist in pain control, such as relaxation training, distraction, hypnosis, and biofeedback. Several of these therapies can be taught by the nonspecialist. Other behavioral approaches designed specifically to improve functioning, which have achieved wide acceptance in the management of nonmalignant pain, are occasionally useful for patients whose functional impairment is disproportionate to the effects of the disease.

Complementary and alternative medicine approaches endorse a holistic strategy that may enhance a sense of personal control and lessen pain.[86,87] Some of these interventions, such as the mind-body therapies, nutritional support, acupuncture, and massage, have an emerging evidence base, are widely used, and should be considered mainstream. For example, one recent randomized controlled study demonstrated that auricular acupuncture significantly improved pain in cancer patients.[88] Others, such as homeopathy and naturopathy, have little scientific support. Clinicians should provide whatever data are available about complementary approaches and support informed decision making.

Cancer Pain at the End of Life: Special Considerations

As the illness progresses, some patients' pain or suffering cannot be controlled despite the optimal use of pharmacotherapy and other approaches. In such cases, treatment options include the use of a drug to induce somnolence, a technique known as "palliative sedation."[89] Sedation should

be considered a medical therapy with defined indications and practices and a strong ethical foundation.[90] Decisions about this intervention are grounded in the "principle of double effect," a well-accepted ethical tenet that describes the appropriateness of actions that may produce harm (such as hastened death), when the intention (to relieve suffering) is beneficent and the need to relieve suffering is the most important goal. Palliative sedation must be clearly distinguished from euthanasia, in which the intended goal is the death of the patient.

Palliative sedation should be implemented only after thorough discussion with the patient, if possible, the family or surrogate decision maker, and involved staff. Informed consent should be sought after clearly establishing the goals of care. Once sedation is activated, ongoing information should be provided to the family and staff, questions should be answered, and ethical and legal implications should be clarified. In some cases, plans should be made to lighten sedation when appropriate to allow interactions with the family.

Conclusion

Pain is a common and potentially devastating complication of cancer. Fortunately, relatively simple therapeutic approaches can provide effective relief in a large majority of patients. All clinicians who treat patients with cancer should develop competency in the assessment and management of pain, and pain management should be perceived as a clinical imperative in oncology practice.

REFERENCES

1. Kanner RM. The scope of the problem. In: Portenoy RK, Kanner RM, editors. Pain management: theory and practice. Philadelphia: FA Davis; 1996. p. 40.
2. Vainio A, Auvinen A. Prevalence of symptoms among patients with advanced cancer: an international collaborative study. J Pain Symptom Manage 1996;12:3–10.
3. World Health Organization. Cancer pain relief with a guide to opioid availability. 2nd ed. Geneva: World Health Organization; 1996.
4. Merskey H, Bogduk N, editors. Classification of chronic pain: descriptions of chronic pain syndromes and definitions of pain terms. 2nd ed. Seattle (WA): IASP Press; 1994.
5. Saunders C. A personal therapeutic journey. BMJ 1996;313:1599–601.
6. www.nationalconsensusproject.org.
7. Fine PG. Breakthrough pain. In: Bruera E, Portenoy R, editors. Cancer pain. New York: Cambridge University Press; 2003. p. 408–12.
8. Caraceni A, Martini C, Zecca E, et al. Breakthrough pain characteristics and syndromes in patients with cancer pain. An international survey. Palliat Med 2004;18:177–83.
9. Ness TJ, Gebhart GF. Visceral pain: a review of experimental studies. Pain 1990;41:167–234.
10. Torebjork HE, Ochoa JL, Schady W. Referred pain from intraneural stimulation of muscle fascicles in the median nerve. Pain 1984;18:145–6.
11. Cherny NI, Portenoy RK. Cancer pain: principles of assessment and syndromes. In: Wall PD, Melzack R, editors. Textbook of pain. 4th ed. Edinburgh: Churchill

Livingstone; 1999. p. 1017–64.
12. Gonzales GR, Elliott KJ, Portenoy RK, et al. The impact of a comprehensive evaluation in the management of cancer pain. Pain 1991;47:141–4.
13. Caraceni A, Portenoy RK. A working group of the IASP task force on cancer pain: an international survey of cancer pain characteristics and syndromes. Pain 1999;82: 263–74.
14. American Psychiatric Association. Diagnostic and statistical manual of mental disorders. 4th ed. Washington (DC): American Psychiatric Association; 1994.
15. Mantyh P, Schwei M, Honore P, et al. Neurochemical and cellular reorganization of the spinal cord in a murine model of bone cancer pain. J Neurosci 1999;19:10886–9.
16. Miaskowski C, Dodd M, West C, et al. Randomized clinical trial of the effectiveness of a self-care intervention to improve cancer pain management. J Clin Oncol 2004;22:1713–20.
17. Portenoy RK, Payne R, Passik S. Acute and chronic pain. In: Lowinson JH, Ruiz P, Millman RB, editors. Comprehensive textbook of substance abuse. 4th ed. Baltimore: Williams & Wilkins; 2005. p. 863–903.
18. Cleeland CS, Gonin R, Hatfield AK, et al. Pain and its treatment in outpatients with metastatic cancer. N Engl J Med 1994;330:592–6.
19. Bercovitch M, Adunsky A. Patterns of high-dose morphine use in a home-care hospice service: should we be afraid of it? Cancer 2004;101:1473–7.
20. Green CR, Anderson KO, Baker TA, et al. The unequal burden of pain: confronting racial and ethnic disparities in pain. Pain Med 2003;4:277–94.
21. Ellison NM. Palliative chemotherapy. In: Berger A, Weissman D, Portenoy RK, editors. Principles and practice of supportive oncology. Philadelphia: Lippincott-Raven; 2002. p. 667.
22. Hoy AM, Lucas CF. Radiotherapy, chemotherapy and hormone therapy: treatment for pain. In: Wall P, Melzack R, editors. Textbook of pain. 3rd ed. New York: Churchill Livingstone; 1994. p. 1279.
23. McIllmurry M. Palliative medicine and the treatment of cancer. In: Doyle D, Hanks GWC, Cherny NI, Calman K, editors. Oxford textbook of palliative medicine. 3rd ed. Oxford (UK): Oxford University Press; 2004. p. 229.
24. Hoskin PJ, Paice P, Easton D, et al. A prospective randomized trial of 4 Gy or 8 Gy single doses in the treatment of metastatic bone pain. Radiother Oncol 1992;23:74–8.
25. Pereira J. Management of bone pain. In: Portenoy RK, Bruera E, editors. Topics in palliative care. New York: Oxford University Press; 1998. p. 79.
26. Fine PG. Palliative radiation therapy in end-of-life care: evidence-based utilization. Am J Hosp Palliat Care 2002;19:166–70.
27. Zech DFJ, Grong S, Lynch J, et al. Validation of the World Health Organization guidelines for cancer pain relief: a 10-year prospective study. Pain 1995;63:5–76.
28. Schug SA, Zech D, Dorr U. Cancer pain management according to WHO analgesic guidelines. J Pain Symptom Manage 1990;5:27–32.
29. Eisenberg E, Berkey CS, Carr DB, et al. Efficacy and safety of nonsteroidal anti-inflammatory drugs for cancer pain: a meta-analysis. J Clin Oncol 1994;12:2756–65.
30. Mercadante S. The use of anti-inflammatory drugs in cancer pain. Cancer Treat Rev 2001;27:51–61.
31. Wallenstein DJ, Portenoy RK. Nonopioid and adjuvant analgesics. In: Berger AM, Portenoy RK, Weissman DE, editors. Principles and practice of palliative care and supportive oncology. Philadelphia: Lippincott-Raven; 2002. p. 84.
32. Mercadante S, Cassucio A, Agnello A, et al. Analgesic effects of nonsteroidal anti-inflammatory drugs in cancer pain due to somatic or visceral mechanisms. J Pain Symptom Manage 1999;17:351–6.
33. Mercadante S, Sapio M, Caligara M, et al. Opioid-sparing effect of diclofenac in cancer pain. J Pain Symptom Manage 1997;14:15–20.
34. Mercadante S, Fulfaro F, Casuccio A. A randomized controlled study on the use of anti-inflammatory drugs in patients with cancer pain on morphine therapy: effects of dose-escalation and a pharmacoeconomic analysis. Eur J Cancer 2002;38:1358–63.
35. Solomon DH, Schneeweiss S, Glynn RJ, et al. Relationship between selective cyclooxygenase-2 inhibitors and acute myocardial infarction in older adults. Circulation 2004;109:2068 73.
36. Lussier D, Portenoy RK. Adjuvant analgesics in pain management. In: Doyle D, Hanks GWC, Cherny NI, Calman K, editors. Oxford textbook of palliative medicine. 3rd ed. Oxford (UK): Oxford University Press; 2004. p. 349.
37. Backonja M, Beydoun A, Edwards KR, et al. Gabapentin for the symptomatic treatment of painful neuropathy in patients with diabetes mellitus: a randomized controlled trial. JAMA 1998;280:1831–6.
38. Rowbotham M, Harden N, Stacey B, et al. Gabapentin for the treatment of postherpetic neuralgia: a randomized controlled trial. JAMA 1998;280:1837–42.
39. Caraceni A, Zecca E, Bonezzi C, et al. Gabapentin for neuropathic cancer pain: a randomized controlled trial from the Gabapentin Cancer Pain Study Group. J Clin Oncol 2004;22:2909–17.
40. Bosnjak S, Jelic S, Susnjar S, et al. Gabapentin for relief of neuropathic pain related to anticancer treatment: a preliminary study. J Chemother 2002;14:214–9.
41. Kalso E, Tasmuth T, Neuronen PJ. Amitriptyline effectively relieves neuropathic pain following treatment of breast cancer. Pain 1995;64:293.
42. Sloan P, Basta M, Storey P, et al. Mexiletine as an adjuvant analgesic for the management of neuropathic cancer pain. Anesth Analg 1999;89:760–1.
43. Mercadante S, Arcuri E, Tirelli W, et al. Analgesic effect of intravenous ketamine in cancer patients on morphine therapy: a randomized, controlled, double-blind, crossover, double-dose study. J Pain Symptom Manage 2000;20:246–52.
44. Thogulava RK, Saxena A, Bhatnagar S, et al. Oral ketamine as an adjuvant to oral morphine for neuropathic pain in cancer patients. J Pain Symptom Manage 2002;23:60–5.
45. Galer BS, Rowbotham MC, Perander J, et al. Topical lidocaine patch relieves postherpetic neuralgia more effectively than a vehicle topical patch: results of an enriched enrollment study. Pain 1999;80:533–8.
46. Gammaitoni AR, Davis MW. Pharmacokinetics and tolerability of lidocaine patch 5% with extended dosing. Ann Pharmacother 2002;36:236–40.
47. Ellison N, Loprinzi CL, Kugler J, et al. Phase III placebo-controlled trial of capsaicin cream in the management of surgical neuropathic pain in cancer patients. J Clin Oncol 1997;15:2974–80.
48. Bloomfield DJ. Should bisphosphonates be part of the standard therapy of patients with multiple myeloma or bone metastases from other cancers? An evidence-based review. J Clin Oncol 1998;16:1218–25.
49. Ripamonti C. Management of bowel obstruction in advanced cancer patients. J Pain Symptom Manage 1994;9: 193–200.
50. Galer BS, Coyle N, Pasternak GW, et al. Individual variability in the response to different opioids: report of five cases. Pain 1992;49:87–91.
51. O'Honneur G, Gilton A, Sandouk P, et al. Plasma and cerebrospinal fluid concentration of morphine and morphine glucuronide after oral morphine. The influence of renal failure. Anesthesiology 1994;81:87–93.
52. Faura CC, Moore RA, Horga JF, et al. Morphine and morphine-6-glucuronide plasma concentrations and effect in cancer. J Pain Symptom Manage 1996;11: 95–102.
53. Tiseo PJ, Thaler HT, Lapin J, et al. Morphine 6-glucoronide concentrations and opioid-related side effects: a survey in cancer patients. Pain 1995;61:47–54.
54. Sawe J. High-dose morphine and methadone in cancer patients: clinical pharmacokinetic consideration of oral treatment. Clin Pharmacokinet 1986;11:87–106.
55. Cruciani RA, Homel P, Yap Y, et al. QTc measurements in patients on methadone. J Pain Symptom Manage 2006. [In press]
56. Krantz MJ, Lewkowiez I, Hays H, et al. Torsades de pointes associated with very-high-dose methadone. Ann Intern Med 2002;137:501–4.
57. Ahmedzai S, Brooks O. Transdermal fentanyl versus sustained-release oral morphine in cancer pain: preference, efficacy and quality of life. J Pain Symptom Manage 1997;13:254–61.
58. Mystakidou K, Parpa E, Tsilika E, et al. Pain management of cancer patients with transdermal fentanyl: a study of 1828 step I, II, & III transfers. J Pain 2004;5:119–32.
59. Coyle N, Adelhardt J. Cancer patients and subcutaneous infusions. Am J Nurs 1996;96:61.
60. Smith TJ, Staats PS, Stearns LJ, et al. Randomized clinical trial of an implantable drug delivery system compared with comprehensive medical management for refractory cancer pain: impact on pain, drug-related toxicity, and survival. J Clin Oncol 2002;19:4040–9.
61. Swarm RA, Karanikolas M, Cousins MJ. Anaesthetic techniques for pain control. In: Doyle D, Hanks G, Cherny NI, Calman K, editors. Oxford textbook of palliative medicine. 3rd ed. Oxford (UK): Oxford University Press; 2004. p. 378–95.
62. Christie JM, Simmonds M, Patt R, et al. A dose-titration, multicenter study of oral transmucosal fentanyl citrate (OTFC) for the treatment of breakthrough pain in cancer patients using transdermal fentanyl for persistent pain. J Clin Oncol 1998;16:3238–45.
63. Weinberg OS, Inturrisi CE, Reidenberg B, et al. Sublingual absorption of selected opioid analgesics. Clin Pharmacol Ther 1988;44:335–42.
64. Klepstad P, Kaasa S, Jystad A, et al. Immediate- or sustained-release morphine for dose finding during start of morphine to cancer patients: a randomized, double-blind trial. Pain 2003;101:193–8.
65. Indelicato RA, Portenoy RK. Opioid rotation in the management of refractory cancer pain. J Clin Oncol 2002;20: 348–52
66. Cherny N, Ripamonti C, Pereira J, et al. Strategies to manage the adverse effects of oral morphine: an evidence-based report. J Clin Oncol 2001;19:2542–54.
67. Sykes N. Constipation and diarrhoea. In: Doyle D, Hanks G, Cherny NI, Calman K, editors. Oxford textbook of palliative medicine. 3rd ed. Oxford (UK): Oxford University Press; 2004. p. 513–25.
68. Andorsky RI, Goldner F. Colonic lavage solution (polyethylene glycol electrolyte lavage solution) as a treatment for chronic constipation: a double-blind, placebo-controlled study. Am J Gastroenterol 1990;85:261–5.
69. Culpepper-Morgan JA, Inturrisi CE, Portenoy RK, et al. Treatment of opioid-induced constipation with oral naloxone: a pilot study. Clin Pharm 1992;52:90–5.
70. Sykes NP. An investigation of the ability of oral naloxone to correct opioid-related constipation in patients with advanced cancer. Palliat Med 1996;10:135–44.
71. Yuan CS, Foss JF, Osinki J, et al. The safety and efficacy of oral methylnaltrexone in preventing morphine-induced oral-cecal transit time. Clin Pharmacol Ther 1997;4: 467–75.
72. Liu SS, Hodgson PS, Carpenter RL, et al. ADL 8-2698, a trans-3,4-dimethyl-4-(3-hydroxyphenyl) piperidine, prevents gastrointestinal effects of intravenous morphine without affecting analgesia. Clin Pharmacol Ther 2001; 69:66–71.
73. Campora E, Malini L, Pace M, et al. The incidence of narcotic-induced emesis. J Pain Symptom Manage 1991;6: 428–30.
74. Bruera E, Brenneis C, Paterson AH, et al. Use of methylphenidate as an adjuvant to narcotic analgesics in patients with advanced cancer. J Pain Symptom Manage 1989;4: 3–6.
75. Bruera E, Chadwick S, Brenneis C, et al. Methylphenidate associated with narcotics for the treatment of cancer pain. Cancer Treat Rep 1987;71:67–70.
76. Bruera E, Miller MJ, Macmillian K, et al. Neuropsychological effects of methylphenidate in patients receiving a continuous infusion of narcotics for cancer pain. Pain 1992;48: 163–6.
77. Webster L, Andrews M, Stoddard G. Modafinil treatment of opioid-induced sedation. Pain Med 4:135–40.
78. Breitbart W, Mermelstein H. Pemoline. An alternative pyschostimulant for the management of depressive disorders in cancer patients. Psychosomatics 1992;33: 352–6.
79. Katon W, Raskind M. Treatment of depression in the medically ill elderly with methylphenidate. Am J Psychiatry 1980;137:963–5.
80. Patt RB, Cousins MJ. Techniques for neurolytic neural blockade. In: Cousins MJ, Bridenbaugh PO, editors. Neural blockade in clinical anesthesia and management of pain. Philadelphia: Lippincott-Raven; 1998. p. 1035.
81. Wong GY, Schroeder DR, Carns PE, et al. Effect of neurolytic celiac plexus block on pain relief, quality of life, and survival in patients with unresectable pancreatic cancer: a randomized controlled trial. JAMA 2004;291: 1092–9.
82. Breitbart W, Payne D, Passik S. Psychological and psychiatric

interventions in pain control. In: Doyle D, Hanks G, Cherny NI, Calman K, editors. Oxford textbook of palliative medicine. 3rd ed. Oxford (UK): Oxford University Press; 2004. p. 424–38.

83. Jacobsen PB, Hann DM. Cognitive-behavioral interventions. In: Holland JC, editor Psycho-oncology. New York: Oxford University Press; 1998. p. 717–30.

84. Meyer TJ, Mark MM. Effects of psychosocial interventions with adult cancer patients: a meta-analysis of randomized experiments. Health Psychol 1995;14:101–8.

85. Orne MT, Whitehouse WG. Nonpharmacologic approaches to pain relief: hypnosis, self-hypnosis, placebo effects. In: Aronoff GM, editor. Evaluation and treatment of chronic pain. 3rd ed. Baltimore: Williams & Wilkins; 1999. p. 579–87.

86. Pan CX, Morrison RS, Ness J, et al. Complementary and alternative medicine in the management of pain, dyspnea, nausea and vomiting near the end of life. A systematic review. J Pain Symptom Manage 2000;20:374–87.

87. Wu WH, Adewunni AA. Alternative medicine for chronic pain: a critical review. In: Aronoff GM, editor. Evaluation and treatment of chronic pain. 3rd ed. Baltimore: Williams & Wilkins; 1999. p. 627–32.

88. Alimi D, Rubino C, Pichard-Leandri E, et al. Analgesic effect of auricular acupuncture for cancer pain: a randomized, blinded, controlled trial. J Clin Oncol 2003;21:4120–6.

89. Chater S, Viola R, Paterson J, et al. Sedation for intractable distress in the dying: a survey of experts. Palliat Med 1998;12:255–69.

90. Cherny NI, Portenoy RK. Sedation in the management of refractory symptoms: guidelines for evaluation and treatment. J Palliat Care 1994;10:31–8.

Cancer and Depression: Phenomenology and Pathophysiology

Diane S. Thompson, MD

Charles L. Raison, MD

Carolyn Jonas-Accardi, PhD

Andrew H. Miller, MD

Receiving a diagnosis of cancer is a life-changing event that brings in its wake a host of psychological reactions, including fear, anger, denial, and intense uncertainty. This emotional turmoil is often compounded by the treatment for cancer, which can involve multiple bodily assaults, including surgery, radiation, and chemotherapy. Given these psychological and physiologic burdens, not surprisingly, a significant percentage of cancer patients develop an equally devastating emotional disorder: major depression. Although depression in the cancer patient can be readily managed, it is frequently not recognized (often being seen as a natural reaction to a difficult circumstance) and goes largely un- or undertreated. Complicating matters, many patients fail to present with the complaint of "depression" (and may actually deny it) and instead voice somatic concerns, including gastrointestinal distress, pain, or fatigue, coupled with worrisome social withdrawal (usually reported by family and friends) and a lack of interest in previously pleasurable pursuits. Of note, some cancer patients may be acutely aware of their depression but silently accept it as part of the cancer diagnosis, needlessly suffering while sparing the oncology staff the burden of their emotional distress.

Much attention has been paid to the psychosocial aspects of cancer and its treatment.[1] Nevertheless, more recently, advances have been made in understanding the biologic underpinnings of depression and other behavioral comorbidities in cancer patients.[2,3] Notable among these is an increasing appreciation of the role of neurobiologic, immunologic, and metabolic factors.

In an effort to support the recognition and treatment of depression in cancer patients, this chapter addresses relevant issues regarding the diagnosis of cancer-related depression. In addition, we explore potential biologic mechanisms that may provide clues as to when depressive symptoms may arise and how they can be treated. Finally, this chapter provides a scientific framework wherein mental health providers and oncologists can collaborate to uncover novel approaches to depression before, during, and after the treatment of cancer.

Clinical Manifestations

Although depressive symptoms may manifest differently depending on the type of cancer and its treatment, there are standardized psychiatric criteria that are used for making a diagnosis (Table 1). These criteria are based on the *Diagnostic and Statistical Manual of Mental Disorders, Fourth Edition (DSM-IV)*, published by the American Psychiatric Association.[4] To meet the criteria for major depressive disorder, at least five symptoms must be present for a period of not less than 2 weeks. Core symptoms that are required for every diagnosis include either depressed mood or anhedonia. As noted above, patients may be less likely to endorse "depressed" mood but may endorse symptoms of anhedonia (lack of enjoyment in activities that were previously found to be pleasurable). Other symptoms of depression include decreased concentration, low self-esteem, guilt, suicidal ideation, impaired sleep, altered appetite, fatigue, and psychomotor agitation or retardation.

Diagnosis

Diagnosing depression in patients with cancer has long been recognized to be problematic as a result of the symptom overlap between sickness and depression.[5] Indeed, nondepressed, sick individuals demonstrate many symptoms that are also experienced by medically healthy patients with major depression. Especially relevant in this regard are neurovegetative symptoms of depression that are often directly caused by pathophysiologic processes inherent to the illness itself or by concurrent treatment modalities, such as surgery, chemotherapy, or radiation. These symptoms include fatigue, weight loss, anorexia, loss of libido, sleep alterations, and psychomotor slowing. Thus, the clinical dilemma becomes when, if ever, neurovegetative symptoms should be counted toward a diagnosis of depression in cancer patients and who may have these symptoms simply because they are sick. How this question is answered significantly impacts the prevalence of depression in patients with cancer and affects when a clinician considers that treatment is appropriate.

Inclusive versus Exclusive Approach

Various strategies to resolve this issue have been proposed. In their simplest iteration, they take two forms: an inclusive approach that counts all depressive symptoms toward a diagnosis of depression, regardless of putative etiology, and an

Table 1 DSM-IV Diagnostic Criteria for Major Depression
5 or more symptoms for 2 wk or longer (must include depressed mood or decreased interest/enjoyment)
Depressed mood
Significant change in weight
Psychomotor agitation/retardation
Feelings of worthlessness or guilt
Suicidal ideation
Decreased interest/enjoyment in activities
Insomnia or hypersomnia
Fatigue/low energy
Poor concentration

DSM-IV = Diagnostic and Statistical Manual of Mental Disorders, Fourth Edition.

exclusive approach that removes neurovegetative symptoms when these symptoms could likely be caused by underlying illness.[6] Refinements of these simpler approaches include (1) replacing the removed neurovegetative symptoms with alternate emotional symptoms (thus keeping the total number of required diagnostic symptoms the same)[7] and (2) privileging the time course of symptoms in the evaluation of neurovegetative symptoms such that these symptoms are counted toward a diagnosis of depression only if their onset co-occurs with or follows the onset of depressed mood or anhedonia.[8] Studies support the validity of both symptom substitution and temporal approaches; however, other data suggest that these exclusive strategies underdiagnose depression in the medically ill when compared with inclusive approaches.[9]

Inclusive approaches increase the likelihood that all patients who have a depression will be identified but run the risk of misclassifying patients with a mild mood or hedonic disturbance as having a full major depression when, in fact, they are only mildly depressed and very sick.

A second diagnostic complication involves the question of how much depression is enough to merit recognition and treatment in patients with cancer. This question is embedded within the larger psychiatric issue of whether mood disorders are best understood as categorical entities with firm boundaries or as a spectrum of conditions that differ from "normalcy" only by matters of degree. Defining normalcy when one has just been diagnosed with cancer or informed of a tumor recurrence is a difficult proposition, given that grief, fear, and other symptoms that define depression are extremely common under these circumstances. Many solutions have been proposed for determining when normal sadness has progressed to a clinically relevant disorder, but the problem remains a vexing one with clear diagnostic and treatment implications. Much of the mood disturbance observed in studies of cancer patients falls under the rubric of "adjustment disorder," a diagnosis that is often interpreted as implying a mild and transient fluctuation in mood that requires little more than reassurance, support, and clinical patience.[4] However, studies increasingly indicate that even minor levels of depressive symptoms (regardless of putative etiology) significantly impair quality of life and physical functioning and may increase mortality in the context of medical illness.[10–15] Clearly, therapeutic errors of over- and undertreatment, can be committed; however, most data indicate that patients with cancer and depressive symptoms receive inadequate treatment.[16] We are increasingly aware that even mild cancer-related depressive syndromes respond to antidepressant treatment.[17,18] As data accumulate documenting the effectiveness of antidepressants in treating

many disease-related symptoms, there is growing support for treating even milder depressive presentations, especially in patients who are open to—or request—treatment and in patients with persistent symptoms.

A final diagnostic issue of great importance in the evaluation and treatment of dysphoric cancer patients involves distinguishing between mood disorders and delirium. Many patients with cancer will develop delirium as a result of chemotherapy or adjuvant pain medication or in the context of severe illness. Not infrequently, delirious patients demonstrate depressive affects and endorse profound dysphoria and/or anxiety. It is essential, therefore, for the clinician to carefully evaluate a patient's orientation to time, place, and situation in contexts in which delirium is likely. If a patient is disoriented, especially if the disorientation has a recent and acute onset, delirium should be suspected and addressed prior to embarking on further treatment for depression. This issue is important because delirium does not respond to antidepressant therapy but usually abates or resolves promptly with the initiation of antipsychotic therapy.[19,20] Thus, missing delirium incurs the risk of initiating an ineffectual treatment (ie, antidepressants or benzodiazepines) that will add to a patient's medication burden while depriving the patient of medications that resolve the dysphoria and anxiety that often accompany the condition.

Rating Scales

The widespread tendency to excuse depression as a natural reaction to cancer and the overlap between sickness and depressive symptoms both point to the importance of accurately assessing depression in the context of neoplastic illness. Standardized instruments are especially valuable in this regard, including the Zung Self-Rating Depression Scale (SDS),[21] the Beck Depression Inventory (BDI),[22] and the Center for Epidemiologic Studies Depression Scale (CESD)[23] (Table 2). Self-report questionnaires have the advantage of not requiring the presence of a trained psychiatric interviewer and can thus be completed by patients while waiting to see the physician. Having patients complete such scales prior to office visits often provides the clinician with additional key information that time pressures may have otherwise precluded. These

scales have been used and validated in oncology patients; however, each of the scales has strengths and weaknesses. For example, the BDI emphasizes mood and cognitive symptoms that are more specific to depression than are neurovegetative symptoms shared by major depression and physical illness.[22] Even if circumstances do not permit the administration of self-report questionnaires, recent data suggest that simply asking cancer patients the single question "Do you feel depressed most of the time?" effectively identifies most subjects with clinically relevant mood disorders.[24] At the very least, such a simplified approach identifies patients who require a more thorough evaluation.

Prevalence

The vast majority of studies indicate that the rates of both major depression and depressive symptoms are elevated in cancer patients compared with healthy controls. Reviews of the literature place median point prevalence rates between 15 and 29%,[24,25] which are significantly higher than prevalence rates for major depression in the general US population (Table 3).[26] Recent studies continue to report widely divergent rates of major depression in cancer patients, but findings from these studies are generally consistent with earlier work in terms of risk factors (see below) and depression prevalence. Moreover, even in studies with low rates of depression, prevalence is typically increased in cancer patients compared with rates in the general populations in the countries in which the studies were performed.[27–30]

Rather than being an impediment to managing depression in the context of cancer, we suggest that a great deal of useful clinical information can be gleaned from the factors that underlie the tremendous variations in depression prevalence

Table 3 Prevalence of Major Depression in Different Types of Cancer

Tumor Site	Prevalence of Major Depression (%)
Pancreas	50
Oropharynx	22–40
Colon	13–25
Breast	10–32
Gynecologic	23
Lymphoma	17
Gastric	11

Table 2 Representative Rating Scales for Assessing Depressive Symptom Severity

Scale	Relative Severity of Depressive Symptoms			
	Normal	Mild	Moderate	Severe
Zung Self-Rating Depression Scale	≤ 49	50–59	60–69	≥70
Beck Depression Inventory	0–9	10–16	17–29	30–63
Center for Epidemiologic Studies Depression Scale	≤15	16–20	21–25	26–60

reported in the world literature. We have already touched on one such reason: the lack of uniformity in how depression is defined in the context of medical illness. In this regard, depression is more common in cancer patients when it is diagnosed via inclusive methods. Indeed, several studies show that rates of depression approximately double in the same group of patients depending on whether an inclusive or exclusive diagnostic approach is employed.[24,31] This finding suggests that many cancer patients are significantly troubled by depression-related neurovegetative symptoms, such as fatigue and poor sleep or appetite, even while not endorsing sadness or loss of interest in life. This observation has clinical relevance for at least two reasons. First, the presence of neurovegetative and other sickness-related symptoms is a risk factor for the development of full depression in patients receiving cancer treatment. For example, sleep disturbance has been repeatedly found to predict both the future development of new depression and depressive relapse in remitted patients.[32] Second, increasing data demonstrate that antidepressants and related pharmacologic strategies effectively treat a number of sickness-related and neurovegetative symptoms, including sleep disturbance, decreased appetite, and pain (see below).[33]

A second debate that affects the prevalence of depression in cancer centers around how much depression is enough to qualify as a clinically relevant entity. Studies repeatedly show that the majority of cancer patients with mood disturbances meet the criteria for conditions other than major depression.[29,34–36] Consistent with this notion, a recent study found that although 23% of outpatients with cancer endorsed significant depressive symptoms, only a third of these patients met the criteria for major depression.[29] The most common mood-related *DSM* diagnosis in patients with cancer is adjustment disorder.[35] The essential components of an adjustment disorder with depressed mood include the following: (1) the presence of mood symptoms that do not meet the criteria for major depression, (2) the mood symptoms arise in response to an identifiable psychosocial stressor, and (3) the mood symptoms impair functioning.[4] These symptoms can persist indefinitely if the stressor is chronic. Given overwhelming data that stressors of all types profoundly increase the risk of depression[37,38] and given that many patients with cancer are, by definition, dealing with a severe and chronic stressor, the diagnosis of adjustment disorder seems impossible to credibly differentiate from a mild depression or dysthymic disorder. Increasing data consistently indicate that even mild depression profoundly interferes with both functioning and quality of life and has adverse health consequences.[10,39] These considerations raise the question of why a depressive syndrome that arises from the known stressor of cancer (ie, an adjustment disorder) should be treated differently from symptomatically similar syndromes that arise for other reasons, especially given ample data that depressive syndromes, even when not meeting the criteria for major depression, are amenable to therapeutic intervention. On the other hand, the fact that most patients with mood symptoms meet adjustment disorder criteria also suggests that at least some of these patients may have a syndrome that will resolve in a reasonable time period without specific pharmacologic intervention. In this regard, accurate assessment of each patient will require some clinical judgment, but, again, the fact that depression prevalence is greatly affected by where the lower limits are set has important and clinically meaningful treatment implications.

Risk Factors

In addition to diagnostic issues, prevalence rates of depression are affected by other factors, including premorbid patient characteristics, tumor characteristics, disease severity, the presence of pain, and the type of treatment administered (Table 4).[3,5,34] Several studies concur that patients with a history of psychiatric illness (including a history of depression) are at increased risk of developing depression in the context of cancer or its treatment.[28,40] Similarly, a family history of mood disorder has also been observed to be a risk factor for cancer-related depression.[41] Women appear to be more likely to develop mood disorders in the context of cancer, consistent with a worldwide body of literature suggesting that women are generally more prone to depression

Table 4 Risk Factors for Depression in Patients with Cancer
History of depression or anxiety disorder
Current subsyndromal depressive and/or anxiety symptoms
Lack of social support
Recent diagnosis or recurrence of illness

Type of cancer
  Pancreas > oropharynx > breast > colon >
  gynecologic > lymphoma > gastric >
  leukemia

Central nervous system tumor involvement
Severity of disease
Uncontrolled pain
Medications (see Table 5)
Medical conditions (eg, anemia, hypothyroidism, renal/liver failure, hypercalcemia)
Surgery type   Mastectomy > breast conservation

Depression criteria employed for diagnosis
  Inclusive > exclusive
  Symptomatic > categorical

than men.[42] It is increasingly recognized that patients' current mood and/or anxiety state strongly influence their emotional responses in the face of cancer's exigencies, both psychological and physiologic. So, for example, increased self-reported depression and anxiety at the time of cancer diagnosis (presumably caused or exacerbated by the psychological stress attendant on such a diagnosis) are associated with greater psychological distress 6 months later,[43] and numerous studies demonstrate that increased depressive and/or anxiety symptoms just prior to treatment predict the development of depression during interferon (IFN)-α2b therapy—a regimen known to activate inflammatory pathways and produce high rates of depression.[44] The clinical implications of these data are clear: patients recently diagnosed or about to undergo depressogenic treatments should be evaluated for past and current mood and anxiety symptoms, as well as for a family history of depression. Patients with positive histories in these domains will likely benefit from closer monitoring and in some cases (especially in the context of depressogenic treatments) may merit prophylactic antidepressant treatment or treatment at the earliest signs of mood disturbance.

Prevalence of depression also appears to vary with tumor type and location (see Table 3). Depression rates are generally reported to be highest for pancreatic, oropharyngeal, and breast carcinomas and lowest for lymphoma, leukemia, and gastric cancers.[5,45] Brain tumors are also associated with high rates of depression, especially when tumors are located in the frontal lobe, especially on the left side—a brain area implicated in the genesis and treatment of depression in general.[41,46] Delirium and seizures are also extremely common in these patients. Both of these conditions have high rates of associated mood disturbance and hence need to be evaluated and ruled out prior to ascribing mood or anxiety symptoms to a mood disorder diagnosis.[47] As with medical illnesses in general,[39] rates of depression in cancer patients increase as disease severity intensifies.[2,48,49] The presence of metastases and pain have also been shown to correlate with depression, whether measured by inclusive- or exclusive-type approaches.[49]

The type of treatment patients undergo also affects the likelihood of developing depression (Table 5). As discussed below, cytokines such as IFN-α or interleukin (IL)-2, which are used in the treatment of several malignancies, are notorious for inducing depressive symptoms.[50] For example, the rates of developing major depression approach 50% in patients receiving chronic, high-dose, IFN-α therapy.[51] Other chemotherapeutic agents frequently associated with depression include procarbazine, L-asparaginase, vinblastine, and vincristine.[52] All of these treatments, along with

Table 5 Antineoplastic Agents Associated with Depression in Patients with Cancer
Chemotherapeutic agents
Procarbazine
Vinblastine
Vincristine
L-Asparaginase
Hormonal therapies
Tamoxifen
Leuprolide
Flutamide
Bicalutamide
Glucocorticoids
Cytokine therapies
Interferon-α, interleukin-2

surgical interventions, are associated with significant metabolic stress and inflammation, which may, in turn, mediate their effects on mood and brain function (see below).

Hormonal treatments also pose a significant risk factor for the development of depression in cancer patients. Tamoxifen and other antiestrogen therapies for breast cancer are particularly relevant in this regard. By displacing estrogen from its receptor, tamoxifen obviates estrogen's neuroprotective functions. Tamoxifen also directly inhibits serotonin release in peripheral mast cells, an effect that may also occur in the brain.[53] Depression rates in both male and female cancer patients undergoing tamoxifen therapy are ≈15%.[54] Of note, antiestrogen therapies are typically initiated during a period when many patients consider themselves in a "survivorship phase." Hence, the risk of medication-induced depression may not be as anticipated as with the mood changes that occur during "active" treatment with other chemotherapeutic regimens. Like estrogen, testosterone also plays a role in mood regulation.[55] Indeed, testosterone has been used to treat depression in some medically ill patients, including patients with acquired immune deficiency syndrome (AIDS),[56] and appears to be especially effective in alleviating fatigue.[57] Therefore, it is not surprising that drugs that reduce the availability of testosterone (leuprolide) or antagonize the testosterone receptor (flutamide or bicalutamide) have been associated with depression.[58] Finally, glucocorticoid hormones are notorious for causing mood alterations, including both depression and mania (as well as psychosis).[47]

Aside from the acute effects of cancer treatment regimens on mood, recent data suggest that some chemotherapies may have long-term neuropsychiatric effects. In a large study of adults who had survived childhood leukemia, Hodgkin's disease, or non-Hodgkin's lymphoma, depressive symptoms were significantly more common in cancer survivors than in nonaffected siblings.[59]

The intensity of chemotherapeutic exposure in childhood predicted the prevalence of depressive symptoms in adulthood in these patients.[60] Cancer treatment may also be associated with long-term cognitive effects. For example, 128 adults with a history of breast cancer or lymphoma were assessed for neurocognitive impairment 5 years after either local therapy or systemic chemotherapy. Consistent with several other studies, cognitive impairment was significantly worse in the patients who received chemotherapy.[61]

Aside from depression and cognitive dysfunction, anxiety is another persisting problem for many cancer patients. There is little doubt that cancer survivors fear recurrence. Nevertheless, although most survivors may use this slightly elevated "somatic concern" to their advantage with good follow-up compliance and vigilant monitoring, some may experience excessive anxiety and intrusive cancer-related thoughts and memories. These symptoms may become severe enough to warrant a diagnosis of post-traumatic stress disorder (PTSD).[62] Interestingly, small volume of the hippocampus (a brain region involved in learning and memory) has been associated with recurrent and intrusive memories related to cancer diagnosis and treatment in breast cancer survivors.[63] Of note, both major depression and PTSD also have been associated with small hippocampal volume. Future studies are needed to determine if patients with small hippocampal volume at baseline (prior to cancer diagnosis and treatment) are more likely to experience post-treatment symptoms of PTSD versus the potential for cancer or cancer treatment to induce hippocampal atrophy and thereby lead to symptoms consist with PTSD.

Mechanisms

In exploring the mechanisms that underlie the development of significant depressive symptoms in patients with cancer, it is important to consider the possibility that manifest and treatable hematologic, infectious, endocrine, and metabolic alterations are relevant contributing factors. These factors must always be evaluated and treated before proceeding with other strategies that address nervous system pathways, including neurotransmitter function. Moreover, because mood disorders, regardless of etiology, may ultimately engage "downstream" brain processes involving serotonin, norepinephrine, and/or dopamine, amelioration of a depressive syndrome by antidepressants does not necessarily rule out the presence of "upstream" medical pathology that is treatable.

Recent advances in neurobiology and immunology have enriched our understanding of potential pathways that may play a role in the development of mood disorders in cancer patients. In this section, we consider how inflammation and oxidative stress represent two processes that have been associated with depression and are common to multiple aspects of having been and being treated for cancer.

Inflammation and Sickness Behavior

One explanation for the high rate of depression and other behavioral comorbidities in cancer patients is that depression in this context is an expression of "sickness behavior."

Sickness behavior is a constellation of signs and symptoms that accompany illness in general and inflammation or immune activation in particular. Caused by proinflammatory cytokines that are released in response to threats to bodily integrity (eg, infection, neoplasia, radiation treatment, and toxic chemotherapeutic regimens), sickness behavior includes behavioral symptoms of depressed mood, anhedonia, fatigue, psychomotor slowing, anorexia, social isolation, sleep disturbances, cognitive dysfunction, and increased sensitivity to pain (hyperalgesia).[64,65] The overlap of the symptoms of sickness behavior with the symptoms used to make a diagnosis of depression is considerable (Table 6) and has led many to consider that depression in many cancer patients is an outgrowth of the effects of cytokines and inflammation on the brain.

Relevant to understanding the pathophysiology and, ultimately, treatment of sickness behavior, an explosion of interest has focused on exploring how proinflammatory cytokines cause changes in the brain and behavior.[65] Cytokines are relatively large molecules that do not freely pass through the blood-brain barrier. Nevertheless, several pathways by which cytokine signals can reach the brain have been characterized, including (1) passage through leaky regions in the blood-brain barrier, (2) active transport, and (3) binding to relevant receptors on peripheral afferent nerve fibers, such as those derived from the vagus nerve. In addition, the complexity of the cytokine network within the brain, including the distribution of cytokine receptors and signaling pathways, is now being revealed. The contribution of specific cytokines to specific behaviors is also being explored.

At least five pathways have been elucidated by which proinflammatory cytokines may cause depression or sickness behavior (Table 7). First, proinflammatory cytokines have been shown to alter the metabolism of the monoamines, including norepinephrine, serotonin, and dopamine, all of which have been implicated in the pathophysiology of mood disorders.[66] Second, cytokines have been shown to have potent stimulatory effects on the hypothalamic-pituitary-adrenal (HPA) axis, in large part through activation of corticotropin-releasing hormone (CRH).[67,68] CRH has behavioral effects in animals that are similar to those

Table 6 Comparison of Symptoms in Sickness Behavior and Major Depression

Sickness behavior
  Anhedonia*
  Anorexia†
  Cognitive disturbance*
  Decreased libido*
  Fatigue*
  Psychomotor retardation†
  Sleep disturbance*
  Social isolation*
  Weight loss*
  Hyperalgesia*

Major depression
  Anhedonia*
  Anorexia
  Cognitive disturbance*
  Decreased libido*
  Fatigue*
  Psychomotor retardation
  Sleep disturbance*
  Social isolation*
  Weight loss*
  Increased pain complaints*
  Sad mood‡
  Suicidal ideation‡
  Worthlessness/guilt‡

*Common to both depression and sickness behavior.
†More common in sickness than depression.
‡More common in depression than sickness behavior.

Table 7 Cytokine Pathways to Sickness Behavior/Depression in Cancer Patients

Cytokine disruption of monoamine metabolism in the central nervous system
Cytokine induction of corticotropin-releasing factor
Cytokine disruption of glucocorticoid receptor–mediated feedback inhibition of inflammation and corticotropin-releasing factor
Cytokine induction of enzymes that metabolize tryptophan
Cytokine inhibition of pathways involved in thyroid hormone metabolism (euthyroid sick syndrome).

seen in patients suffering from depression or sickness behavior, including alterations in activity, appetite, and sleep.[69] Moreover, patients with depression have been found to exhibit increased CRH activity as manifested by elevated concentrations of CRH in cerebrospinal fluid, increased messenger ribonucleic acid in the paraventricular nucleus of the hypothalamus, a blunted adrenocorticotropic hormone (ACTH) response to CRH challenge (likely reflecting down-regulation of pituitary CRH receptors),[70,71] and down-regulation of receptors for CRH in the frontal cortex of victims of suicide (presumably secondary to hypersecretion of CRH). Third, in vivo and in vitro studies suggest that proinflammatory cytokines, including IL-1, may induce resistance of nervous, endocrine, and immune system tissues to circulating glucocorticoid hormones through direct inhibitory effects on the expression and/or function of glucocorticoid receptors.[72] Glucocorticoid resistance has been repeatedly demonstrated in medically healthy patients with depression (as reflected in nonsuppression on the dexamethasone suppression test),[73] as well as cancer patients with depression,[45,74] and may contribute to impaired feedback regulation of CRH and the release of proinflammatory cytokines. Fourth, cytokines, including IFN-α, have been shown to reduce serum concentrations of L-tryptophan (TRP), likely secondary to changes in dietary intake (owing to anorexia) and the induction of the enzyme indolamine 2,3-dioxygenase (IDO), which breaks down TRP into kynurenine.[75–77] TRP is the primary precursor of serotonin, and depletion of TRP has been associated with the precipitation of mood disturbances in vulnerable patients.[78] Finally, proinflammatory cytokines have been associated with euthyroid sick syndrome, which is characterized by normal thyroid-stimulating hormone (TSH) and thyroxine (T_4) levels and reduced triiodothyronine (T_3) levels in the early stages and by normal TSH and reduced T_3 and T_4 in the later stages.[79] Alterations in thyroid hormone availability are well known to influence mood regulation. The mechanism by which euthyroid sick syndrome occurs is believed to involve both direct effects of cytokines on thyroid gland function and inhibition of the metabolic enzymes (5′-deiodination) that convert peripheral T_4 to T_3 (the more biologically active form of thyroid hormone), especially in the liver.[79]

Early studies are beginning to provide support for the notion that inflammation and inflammatory cytokines may play a role in the development of depressive symptoms in cancer patients. In a study by Musselman and colleagues, depression was associated with significantly increased plasma concentrations of IL-6 in patients with a wide variety of cancers.[74] In addition, both IL-6 and IL-1 have been found to significantly correlate with fatigue in cancer patients undergoing treatment with radiation and/or chemotherapy.[80–82] Increased serum concentrations of IL-6 also have been found to correlate with increasing depressive symptom scores in patients undergoing abdominal surgery.[83] As discussed in detail below, treatment with cytokines such as IFN-α, which is a potent activator of the inflammatory cytokine network, including IL-6,[84] is associated with rates of depression that range from 30 to 50% depending on the dose.[44] Finally, it should be noted that there is a rich literature demonstrating increased inflammatory markers, including IL-6 and C-reactive protein, in depressed patients who are medically healthy,[85] suggesting that the immune system may play a more fundamental role in mood regulation, even in patients without medical illnesses.

Although the symptom overlap between sickness and depression complicates the task of identifying and treating patients with cancer, it also offers clues to mechanisms by which the physiology of illness may contribute to the pathophysiology of depression. Moreover, as often happens, expanding knowledge has provided support for dichotomous positions previously perceived as being exclusive, in this case, giving credence to both inclusive and exclusive ways of understanding depression in the context of sickness. Indeed, accumulating data lend support for an emerging paradigm in which immune system activation is seen to induce physical and behavioral symptoms common to both illness and depression and to induce changes in central nervous and stress system pathways that additionally predispose vulnerable individuals to the development of profound mood and hedonic alterations in the context of sickness.

Cytokine-Mediated Models

To aid in separating immune from psychosocial contributions to depression in the context of medical illnesses, including cancer, researchers have employed treatment with IFN-α as a model system to study cytokine-mediated behavioral disturbance. IFN-α is a cytokine released early in viral infection that has both antiviral and antiproliferative activities.[86] In addition to direct effects on the immune system, IFN-α also potently stimulates the production of proinflammatory cytokines, including IL-6 and, to a lesser extent, tumor necrosis factor (TNF)-α and IL-1α and IL-1β.[84,87] Because of its antiproliferative and antiviral activities, IFN-α is currently used for the treatment of several malignancies and viral infections.[88] Although frequently of benefit in each of these conditions, IFN-α has been repeatedly observed to cause a variety of neuropsychiatric side effects that closely resemble sickness behavior in animals and that meet symptom criteria for major depression in humans. Indeed, our group observed that nearly 50% of patients receiving high-dose IFN-α for malignant melanoma developed major depression over 3 months of treatment.[51] These results are especially striking given that depressive symptom scores were minimal in this population prior to treatment.

The possibility that antidepressant pretreatment might ameliorate neurobehavioral toxicity in patients receiving high doses of IFN-α for the treatment of malignant melanoma has been examined.[51] Forty patients with nonmetastatic disease were randomized in a double-blind manner to receive either the serotonin reuptake inhibitor (SRI) paroxetine or placebo. Antidepressant (or placebo) treatment was commenced 2 weeks prior to the initiation of IFN-α and continued for an additional 12 weeks of IFN-α therapy. At the end of the study period, only 11% of patients receiving paroxetine had developed symptoms sufficient to meet the diagnostic criteria for major depression compared with 45% of patients receiving placebo.[51] Moreover, the rates of discontinuation from IFN-α were significantly lower in paroxetine-treated patients, 5% versus 35% for patients receiving placebo.

A recent study in rodents suggested that the SRI fluoxetine prevents cytokine-induced decrements in the gustatory hedonic domain while having no impact on cytokine-induced anorexia.[89] Given that major depression is a syndrome consisting of both mood or hedonic and neurovegetative symptoms (such as anorexia),[4] these findings raise the possibility that serotoninergic antidepressants might be more effective in treating core depressive symptoms, such as hedonic drive, and less effective in resolving neurovegetative symptoms, such as anorexia. To examine this possibility, Capuron and colleagues evaluated whether paroxetine was equally effective in ameliorating all depressive symptoms in patients receiving INF-α for malignant melanoma or whether its ability to prevent major depression derived from a more limited spectrum of therapeutic efficacy.[90] A dimensional analysis revealed that symptoms more commonly seen in depression than in sickness, including depressed mood, loss of interest (anhedonia), suicidal thoughts, guilt, and anxiety, as well as subjective cognitive complaints, were prevented by SRI pretreatment, whereas neurovegetative symptoms, including fatigue, anorexia, and psychomotor retardation, were minimally responsive to the antidepressant. Additionally, neurovegetative and somatic complaints were noted to develop early during treatment (within the first 2 weeks) in the majority of patients, whereas depression-specific and cognitive symptoms developed later and tended to occur only in patients who met the *DSM-IV* criteria for major depression.

Similar patterns have been identified in the phenomenology and treatment response of behavioral disturbances in other cancer populations. In terms of phenomenology, a factor analysis in a large group of patients found that mood, anxiety, and cognitive symptoms clustered together, whereas fatigue, anorexia, and physical symptoms represented separate factors.[91] Consistent with SRI response patterns during IFN-α treatment, paroxetine was recently shown in a large, double-blind, placebo-controlled trial to ameliorate depression, but not fatigue, in cancer patients undergoing chemotherapy.[17] Taken together, these findings support the notion that behavioral changes during immune activation may represent an amalgam of at least two subsyndromes: a neurovegetative or somatic syndrome that develops in most sick individuals appears early in the course of inflammation and is minimally responsive to SRI treatment and a mood, anxiety, and cognition syndrome that occurs in a subset of patients (who are also most likely to meet the full criteria for major depression). This syndrome develops after more prolonged inflammatory exposure and responds to SRI treatment.

The finding that both IFN-α-induced and cancer-related depression can be meaningfully subdivided on the basis of phenomenology and treatment response into a more depression-specific syndrome of mood, anxiety, and cognitive symptoms and a more generalized sickness syndrome composed of neurovegetative and somatic symptoms strongly suggests that separate pathophysiologic mechanisms may underlie these syndromes, with the corollary that different symptoms may respond to different treatment strategies in depressed, medically ill patients (Figure 1).[90] Recent work aimed at delineating pathways by which immune activation produces behavioral disturbance is consistent with these ideas.

TRP Depletion and Serotonin   As mentioned above, inflammatory stimuli (including IFN-α exposure) lead to a depletion of TRP via an immune-mediated induction of the enzyme IDO, which metabolizes TRP to kynurenine and hence reduces the amount of TRP that is available for the synthesis of serotonin.[92,93] It has been argued that IDO induction serves several adaptive purposes, including diminishing TRP availability for bacterial pathogens (for which TRP is also an essential amino acid) and promoting maternal T-cell tolerance toward the fetus during pregnancy.[94] Despite these evolutionary benefits, however, IDO induction might also be expected to increase the risk of developing depressive symptoms during conditions of immune activation, given evidence that TRP depletion is capable of rapidly inducing depressive symptoms in nondepressed but vulnerable individuals.[60,95] Data from patients receiving high IFN-α suggest that this is true: several studies report that treatment results in decreases in serum TRP and increases in kynurenine,[92,93,96] consistent with activation of IDO.[97] Moreover, the amount of reduction in TRP during treatment has been correlated with depressive symptom severity scores.[93,96] Similarly, it has been observed that antidepressant-free patients who met the criteria

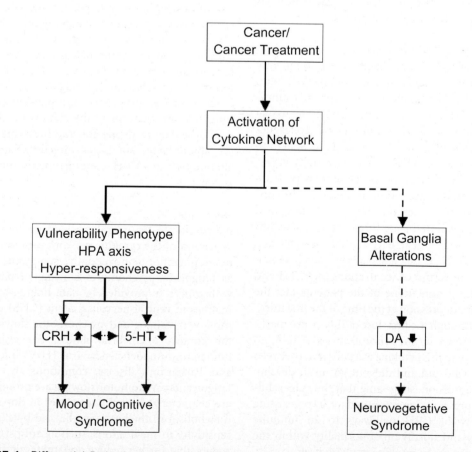

FIGURE 1 Differential Pathophysiological Mechanisms Underlying Interferon-Alpha-Induced Mood/Cognitive Syndrome and Neurovegetative Syndrome: A Model for Cytokine-Induced Neurobehavioral Alterations. *Solid arrow*: published data available. *Dashed arrow*: under investigation. (modified from Capuron, L., Miller, A.H. Cytokines and psychopathology: lessons from interferon alpha. *Biological Psychiatry*, 56(11):819–24, 2004).

for major depression during IFN-α therapy for malignant melanoma demonstrate significantly larger increases in kynurenine and the ratio of kynurenine to TRP and prolonged decreases in TRP during treatment when compared with patients who do not develop major depression.[92]

Interestingly, the relationship between major depression and TRP depletion resulted from a significant correlation between decreases in serum TRP concentrations and the development of mood, anxiety, and cognitive symptoms. No association was seen between TRP metabolism and neurovegetative symptoms or pain complaints. That alterations in TRP metabolism correlated with the same symptoms that responded to treatment with paroxetine but did not correlate with symptoms that were not responsive to the SRI[90] strongly suggests that serotoninergic mechanisms contribute significantly to the expression of mood, anxiety, and cognitive complaints in these patients, a finding strengthened by the fact that no such correlation was observed in patients pretreated with paroxetine, which might be expected, via the effects of this medication on the serotonin reuptake pump, to compensate for IDO-induced decrements in serotoninergic functioning. By the same logic, serotoninergic mechanisms did not appear to play a central role in the mediation of neurovegetative or pain symptoms.

Corticotropin-Releasing Hormone
Because CRH hyperactivity is a frequently reported abnormality in major depression,[73] and because the inflammatory system robustly stimulates the HPA axis in animals and humans via stimulation of CRH, Capuron and colleagues used treatment with IFN-α as a model system to examine whether HPA axis hyperactivity represents a risk factor for developing depression during immune activation in humans.[84] In antidepressant-free patients, those who developed major depression during IFN-α treatment exhibited increased CRH activity in response to the first dose of IFN-α (as assessed by postinjection increases in serum concentrations of ACTH and cortisol). Of note, none of the patients met the criteria for depression at the time of the first injection.[84] Although the first dose of IFN-α also markedly increased serum concentrations of IL-6, no differences in this cytokine were observed between patients who did and did not go on to develop major depression, suggesting that the vulnerability to depression was accounted for by preexisting sensitivity of CRH pathways to an immune stimulus and not by an abnormality within the proinflammatory cytokine network itself.

Interestingly, both CRH pathway and cytokine responses to IFN-α rapidly attenuated with repeated treatment, such that within a week of initiating therapy, no differences were observed

in postinjection ACTH or cortisol responses between patients who did and did not subsequently develop major depression.[84] This finding is quite different from the temporal pattern observed between IDO-induced TRP depletion and depression, in which changes in TRP levels and the development of depressive symptoms were contemporaneous.[92] However, it is intriguing that patients who demonstrated CRH hyperactivity in response to an initial dose of IFN-α were also more likely to later demonstrate increased TRP depletion, indicating a possible link between CRH and serotoninergic systems in the mediation of depressive symptoms in the context of immune activation. Moreover, as with IDO-induced TRP depletion, CRH hyperactivity predicted the subsequent development of major depression through an effect on mood, anxiety, and cognitive symptoms.[84] No correlation was observed between CRH hyperactivity and the later development of neurovegetative or somatic symptoms. Of note, previous studies have suggested that CRH hypersensitivity may result from early life stress or exposure to intense stressors in adulthood.[98] Family members of patients with depression have also exhibited evidence of CRH hypersensitivity.[99] Taken together, these findings suggest that patients with preexisting supersensitivity in CRH-mediated stress pathways may be at risk of developing mood, anxiety, and cognitive symptoms, not perhaps through ongoing abnormalities in stress system responses to immune stimulation but rather through as yet unidentified functional connections between CRH and serotoninergic metabolism (see Figure 1). On the other hand, neurovegetative and physical symptoms that are frequent in the context of illness, even when more depression-specific symptoms are absent, may not be as directly related to alterations in CRH and/or serotoninergic systems.

Dopamine
A first clue to the neural mechanisms by which activation of the cytokine network promotes the development of neurovegetative symptoms, such as fatigue or psychomotor slowing in patients with cancer, is provided by data linking abnormalities in central nervous system (CNS) dopamine with fatigue and psychomotor slowing in the context of medical illness. For example, human immunodeficiency virus (HIV) infection and Parkinson's disease, conditions in which fatigue and psychomotor slowing are prominent, are characterized by abnormalities in dopamine metabolism in the basal ganglia and by extreme sensitivity to medications, such as antipsychotic agents, that further reduce dopaminergic signaling via postsynaptic receptor blockade.[100,101] Consistent with this, even in medically healthy depressed patients, affective flattening and psychomotor retardation are associated with

evidence of altered dopaminergic functioning in the left caudate nucleus.[102] Finally, agents with dopaminergic activity have been repeatedly shown to effectively treat fatigue in a number of medical conditions.[103–105]

Chronic immune activation appears to inhibit dopamine signaling within frontostriatal circuits within the CNS. Rodents treated chronically with IFN-α demonstrate inhibition of dopaminergic neural activity and CNS dopamine metabolism, with concomitant decrements in motor activity.[106] In humans, high-dose IFN-α reliably slows reaction time on standardized neuropsychological tests and in extreme cases has been reported to produce frankly parkinsonian states that are responsive to treatment with levodopa.[50,107]

These findings support the possibility that psychomotor retardation and fatigue observed during states of immune activation may be related in part to cytokine-induced reductions in dopamine activity. Cytokine receptors are expressed in abundance in key areas of the basal ganglia–thalamocortical circuitry, including the striatum and cerebral cortex,[108] and therefore are uniquely poised to influence dopamine neuronal activity in these brain regions. Moreover, chronic infusion of bacterial endotoxin (a potent inducer of the inflammatory cytokine network) into rat brain leads to delayed and selective degeneration of dopaminergic neurons in the substantia nigra through microglial activation.[109] Finally, the targeting of basal ganglia and dopamine pathways during activation of the cytokine network is suggested by involvement of these pathways in infectious diseases associated with neuropsychiatric alterations, including HIV.[101]

Taken together, these data suggest that alterations in basal ganglia, notably in dopamine neurotransmission, may contribute to the development of core neurovegetative symptoms of IFN-α-induced depression, including psychomotor slowing (see Figure 1). Consistent with this, preliminary data from our group and others demonstrate altered glucose metabolism in the basal ganglia of IFN-α-treated patients.[110,111]

Implications

The concept of sickness behavior promotes an awareness that many symptoms of both physical and emotional distress in cancer patients may have a significant biologic component, arising out of the body's own attempt to fight disease and at the same time maintain homeostatic balance. This perspective discourages simple dichotomies between emotional and physical suffering in the context of cancer and points to the clinical utility of broadening therapeutic concerns beyond depression into the larger sickness syndrome, of which depression in the medically ill is a component. Such a perspective argues for an inclusive approach to identifying patients with clinically relevant behavioral disturbances, even when these disturbances do not meet the criteria for currently recognized *DSM-IV* mood disorders. Moreover, recognizing that inflammation provides a physiologic substrate that promotes mood disturbance implies that markers of inflammation may provide an additional diagnostic tool to identify individuals at risk of developing depressive disorders. Such inflammatory risk markers were recently identified for both diabetes and coronary artery disease—conditions that, like cancer, are associated with increased rates of depression. Relevant in this regard are the previously noted data that patients with cancer who develop depression have significantly higher levels of IL-6 than cancer patients without depression.[74] Other abnormalities that may hold promise as predictive markers for depressive disorders include IDO-mediated decreases in plasma TRP and alterations in the production of HPA axis hormones, such as ACTH and cortisol, as discussed above. Similarly, imaging studies of patients undergoing cytokine exposure may, in the future, cast light on neural circuits that mediate both the risk and expression of behavioral toxicity.

However, if the elucidation of sickness behavior promotes an inclusive approach to behavioral symptoms in patients with cancer, findings on depressive subsyndromes and the pathways that underlie these different symptom dimensions argue for the wisdom inherent in exclusive approaches that privilege more depression-specific symptoms and downplay the importance of neurovegetative symptoms. Specifically, studies in patients undergoing immune activation strongly suggest that sickness symptoms, including fatigue and other neurovegetative symptoms, are widespread and serve as a physiologic base from which a smaller number of vulnerable individuals progress to develop symptoms most classically associated with mood disturbances, including sadness, loss of pleasure, anxiety, hopelessness, helplessness, and suicidal ideation. A strong rationale for privileging these symptoms comes from studies over the last several years suggesting that these symptoms may be the primary mediators of the relationship between depression and poor health outcomes.[8,112]

Although the identification of vulnerability factors for depression-specific symptoms is in its infancy, data indicate that patients with sensitized CRH pathways—as a result of genetic endowment, previous stressor exposure, or both—are at increased risk of developing depression-specific symptoms and of meeting the full criteria for major depression when exposed to an immune challenge. Similarly, patients who respond to an immune challenge with heightened IDO activity and resultant decrements in TRP also appear to

be at increased risk of progressing from sickness to full depression when exposed to inflammatory activation.

Recent evidence suggests that both inclusive and exclusive approaches to depression in patients with cancer have important clinical implications and that, although apparently contradictory, both approaches should be held in mind for clinicians to optimally relieve suffering in the context of neoplasia. As discussed above, with the development of the concept of sickness behavior, a coherent rationale is provided for addressing a more inclusive range of emotional, neurovegetative, and physical symptoms than would be targeted under strict definitions of current *DSM-IV* mood disorders.

Although sickness behavior in general supports a broadening of the terrain that is appropriate for therapeutic intervention, recent evidence that cytokine and oxidative stress-induced depression is not a unitary phenomenon but rather represents an amalgam of at least two separable subsyndromes provides a rationale for privileging depression-specific symptoms that are core features of exclusive diagnostic approaches to depression in the medically ill.

Oxidative Stress

In addition to the effects of inflammation or cytokine pathology on behavior, another important potential mediator of behavioral pathology in cancer patients is oxidative stress. Considerable evidence implicates oxidative stress and depletion of the critical antioxidant glutathione (GSH) in neurodegenerative processes. GSH deficiency leaves the brain susceptible to oxidant-mediated injury that leads to neuronal cell dysfunction and death.[113,114] Significant loss of both systemic and brain GSH pools has been associated with a range of cognitive dysfunctions related to Parkinson's disease, Alzheimer's disease, and schizophrenia.[113-115] Furthermore, the extent of systemic GSH depletion was a highly significant and independent predictor of the severity of cognitive impairment in a recent prospective study of individuals with Alzheimer's disease.[116] It is not known whether perturbations in systemic GSH status contribute to chemotherapy-associated neurocognitive dysfunction; however, various chemotherapeutic agents have been shown to induce significant and acute declines in circulating GSH concentrations in cancer patients,[117,118] which may exacerbate hematologic toxicity, nephrotoxicity, and neurotoxicity.[119,120] Jonas and colleagues demonstrated that chemotherapy regimens administered during bone marrow transplantation progressively decreased and oxidized plasma GSH pools over a prolonged 14-day period posttreatment (Figure 2).[117] There are data suggesting a role for GSH deficiency in the development of neurotoxicity in patients receiving multiple

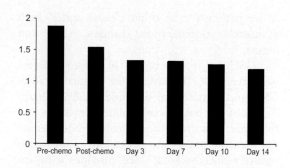

FIGURE 2 Mean (±SE) plasma GSH (umol/L) over time in patients receiving bone marrow transplantation. Pre-chemotherapy values were obtained at the time of admission and post-chemotherapy values were obtained on days 1, 3, 7, 10, and 14 after conditioning therapy. GSH concentrations decreased significantly over time reaching well below the normal reference range for healthy populations (P < 0.001; effect of time).

cycles of chemotherapy. In patients with advanced colorectal cancer, clinically evident neuropathy induced by oxaliplatin-based chemotherapy was markedly reduced with bimonthly GSH infusion by the eighth treatment cycle.[119]

GSH is an abundantly present antioxidant found in all cells and extracellular fluids in humans. GSH functions in detoxification, acts as a reservoir for cysteine, maintains other functional antioxidants, and is central to control of protein thiol-disulfide balance, ultimately regulating thiol-dependent cellular functions. Compromised GSH metabolism may contribute to oxidative stress, sensitivity to toxicants, and alterations in oxidative metabolism, all of which have been implicated in neurologic disorders.[121]

GSH depletion may represent a key mechanism in neuronal cell injury and dysfunction. The brain is particularly susceptible to oxidative stress owing to high rates of oxidative metabolism, the abundance of polyunsaturated fatty acids in cell membranes, and the comparatively low antioxidant activity relative to other tissues.[122] Oxidative stress and substantial GSH losses have been demonstrated in neurodegenerative disorders and have been linked with the progressive degeneration of dopaminergic neurons in preclinical stages of Parkinson's disease.[123] Evidence indicates that GSH deficiency may cause or worsen neuronal dysfunction through multiple mechanisms. In addition to increasing neuronal cell susceptibility to reactive oxygen species (eg, H_2O_2) and to neurotoxicants, GSH loss and oxidative stress result in neuronal dysfunction through the accumulation and aggregation of oxidized proteins and through the signaling of redox-sensitive cell death pathways.[114,124] Whether abnormalities in the systemic GSH redox state relate to defects in brain GSH metabolism, oxidative stress, and neuronal cell fate is not established. Nonetheless, blood GSH levels reflect oxidative stress found to be pathogenic in other disease states, such as macular degeneration, diabetes, AIDS, and cancer.[125–127]

GSH redox is a means to clinically assess oxidative stress. In humans, the balance between GSH and glutathione disulfide (GSSG), determined by the balance of oxidative reactions and the capacity of the reduced nicotinamide adenine dinucleotide phosphate–dependent reductase to reduce GSSG back to GSH, provides a means to clinically measure oxidative stress. Previous clinical studies show differences in plasma GSH redox in humans, which are related to states of oxidative stress, such as in aging, chemotherapy treatment, and critical illness.[118–120,128] Progressive oxidation of the plasma GSH pool may correlate with intracellular GSH depletion in various organ systems, as well as loss of redox potential in extracellular compartments particularly important to the CNS, as has been shown in cerebrospinal fluid during aging.[125] Because of continuous cycling of GSH pools between peripheral tissue or plasma and the brain (likely through substrate cycling via the blood-brain barrier) plasma measurements may indirectly reflect brain redox conditions of potential relevance to neurodegenerative changes.

Alterations in cytokines, such as TNF-α, IL-2, IL-6, and IFN-γ, are documented responses to chemotherapeutic regimens that may be important to treatment-induced toxicity in breast cancer patients. Oxidative stress is directly linked to proinflammatory cytokine activation. Given evidence (discussed above) that cytokine activation may contribute to neurobehavioral disturbances in the context of cancer and its treatment, the possibility arises that changes in oxidative state may be a mechanism by which inflammation alters neuronal and, ultimately, psychiatric functioning. Studies are currently under way to evaluate this intriguing hypothesis. If findings corroborate this idea, the road will be opened for nutritional intervention studies aimed at improving resilience to redox state perturbations during cancer chemotherapy. Indeed, diets rich in vegetables, plant-derived extracts, amino acid substrates, and micronutrients have been shown to protect against oxidative stress, and such dietary manipulations could be used to protect patients during chemotherapeutic treatments and prevent neuropsychiatric problems before they occur.

Although evidence has been provided that oxidative stress may contribute to the development of behavioral pathology in cancer patients, it should be noted that several studies have suggested that higher GSH concentrations in the mitochondria may act as a redox buffer and inhibit mitochondrial alterations associated with apoptosis secondary to chemotherapeutic agents, notably cisplatin.[129] Most recently, GSH synthesis has been identified as an essential component for the apoptotic inhibitor of cisplatin (Bcl-2). This activity cannot be explained by DNA adduct formation or damage repair and is likely to be regulated through mitochondrial or cellular homeostasis.[130] Thus, balancing levels of GSH to offer neuroprotective effects while maintaining the cytotoxic or apoptotic properties of chemotherapy agents represents a challenge for future translational studies.

Summary

Based on a rich literature, there is compelling evidence that depression is a common comorbidity in oncology patients. However, diagnosing depression in the cancer patient can present a challenge because both somatic and psychic complaints intertwine. Nevertheless, with the use of appropriate rating scales and a more "inclusive" approach to diagnosis, fewer depressed patients will go unrecognized and untreated. With new developments in the understanding of the potential pathophysiologic mechanisms involved in symptom expression, it is also becoming increasingly clear which patients are at risk and when. Moreover, therapeutic strategies targeting specific symptom dimensions have been identified and are available. Future studies investigating the multiple neurobiologic, immunologic, and genetic pathways involved in symptom development will help elaborate new treatment and prevention strategies and help patients better negotiate the short- and long-term neuropsychiatric challenges of cancer and its treatment.

REFERENCES

1. Spiegel D. Cancer and depression. Br J Psychiatry Suppl 1996;30:109–16.
2. Spiegel D, Giese-Davis J. Depression and cancer: mechanisms and disease progression. Biol Psychiatry 2003;54:269–82.
3. Raison CL, Miller AH. Depression in cancer: new developments regarding diagnosis and treatment. Biol Psychiatry 2003;54:283–94.
4. Diagnostic and statistical manual of mental disorders, — fourth edition. Washington (DC): American Psychiatric Association; 1994.
5. McDaniel JS, Musselman DL, Porter MR, et al. Depression in patients with cancer. Diagnosis, biology, and treatment. Arch Gen Psychiatry 1995;52:89–99.
6. Cohen-Cole SA, Brown FW, McDaniel JS. Diagnostic assessment of depression in the medically ill. In: Stoudemire A, Fogel B, editors. Psychiatric care of the medical patient. New York: Oxford University Press; 1993. p. 53–70.
7. Endicott J. Measurement of depression in patients with cancer. Cancer 1984;53(10 Suppl):2243–9.
8. von Ammon Cavanaugh S, Furlanetto LM, Creech SD, Powell LH. Medical illness, past depression, and present depression: a predictive triad for in-hospital mortality. Am J Psychiatry 2001;158:43–8.
9. Koenig HG, George LK, Peterson BL, Pieper CF. Depression in medically ill hospitalized older adults: prevalence, characteristics, and course of symptoms according to six diagnostic schemes. Am J Psychiatry 1997;154:1376–83.
10. Wells KB, Stewart A, Hays RD, et al. The functioning and well-being of depressed patients. Results from the Medical Outcomes Study. JAMA 1989;262:914–9.
11. Whooley MA, Browner WS. Association between depressive symptoms and mortality in older women. Study of Osteoporotic Fractures Research Group. Arch Intern Med 1998;158:2129–35.
12. Black SA, Markides KS. Depressive symptoms and mortality in older Mexican Americans. Ann Epidemiol 1999;9:45–52.
13. Bush DE, Ziegelstein RC, Tayback M, et al. Even minimal symptoms of depression increase mortality risk after acute myocardial infarction. Am J Cardiol 2001;88:337–41.
14. Barefoot JC, Schroll M. Symptoms of depression, acute myocardial infarction, and total mortality in a community sample. Circulation 1996;93:1976–80.
15. Everson SA, Goldberg DE, Kaplan GA, et al. Hopelessness and risk of mortality and incidence of myocardial infarction and cancer. Psychosom Med 1996;58:113–21.
16. Norton TR, Manne SL, Rubin S, et al. Prevalence and predictors of psychological distress among women with ovarian cancer. J Clin Oncol 2004;22:919–26.
17. Morrow GR, Hickok JT, Roscoe JA, et al. Differential effects of paroxetine on fatigue and depression: a randomized, double-blind trial from the University of Rochester Cancer Center Community Clinical Oncology Program. J Clin Oncol 2003;21:4635–41.
18. Fisch MJ, Loehrer PJ, Kristeller J, et al. Fluoxetine versus placebo in advanced cancer outpatients: a double-blinded trial of the Hoosier Oncology Group. J Clin Oncol 2003;21:1937–43.
19. Breitbart W, Marotta R, Platt MM, et al. A double-blind trial of haloperidol, chlorpromazine, and lorazepam in the treatment of delirium in hospitalized AIDS patients. Am J Psychiatry 1996;153:231–7.
20. Schwartz TL, Masand PS. The role of atypical antipsychotics in the treatment of delirium. Psychosomatics 2002;43:171–4.
21. Zung WW. A self-rating depression scale. Arch Gen Psychiatry 1965;12:63–70.
22. Beck AT. Psychometric properties of the Beck Depression Inventory: twenty-five years later. Clin Psychol Rev 1988;8:77–100.
23. Radloff LS. The CES-D scale: a self-report depression scale for research in the general population. Appl Psychol Measure 1977;1:385–401.
24. Chochinov HM. Depression in cancer patients. Lancet Oncol 2001;2:499–505.
25. Hotopf M, Chidgey J, Addington-Hall J, Ly KL. Depression in advanced disease: a systematic review part 1. Prevalence and case finding. Palliat Med 2002;16:81–97.
26. Kessler RC, Berglund P, Demler O, et al. The epidemiology of major depressive disorder: results from the National Comorbidity Survey Replication (NCS-R). JAMA 2003;289:3095–105.
27. Harter M, Reuter K, Aschenbrenner A, et al. Psychiatric disorders and associated factors in cancer: results of an interview study with patients in inpatient, rehabilitation and outpatient treatment. Eur J Cancer 2001;37:1385–93.
28. Pirl WF, Siegel GI, Goode MJ, Smith MR. Depression in men receiving androgen deprivation therapy for prostate cancer: a pilot study. Psychooncology 2002;11:518–23.
29. Sharpe M, Strong V, Allen K, et al. Major depression in outpatients attending a regional cancer centre: screening and unmet treatment needs. Br J Cancer 2004;90:314–20.
30. Smith EM, Gomm SA, Dickens CM. Assessing the independent contribution to quality of life from anxiety and depression in patients with advanced cancer. Palliat Med 2003;17:509–13.
31. Silverstone PH. Concise assessment for depression (CAD): a brief screening approach to depression in the medically ill. J Psychosom Res 1996;41:161–70.
32. Breslau N, Roth T, Rosenthal L, Andreski P. Sleep disturbance and psychiatric disorders: a longitudinal epidemiological study of young adults. Biol Psychiatry 1996;39:411–8.
33. Raison CL, Demetrashvili M, Capuron L, Miller AH. Neuropsychiatric side effects of interferon-alpha: recognition and management. CNS Drugs 2005;19:1–19.
34. Chochinov HM. Depression in cancer patients. Lancet Oncol 2001;2:499–505.
35. Akechi T, Nakano T, Okamura H, et al. Psychiatric disorders in cancer patients: descriptive analysis of 1721 psychiatric referrals at two Japanese cancer center hospitals. Jpn J Clin Oncol 2001;31:188–94.
36. Derogatis LR, Morrow GR, Fetting J, et al. The prevalence of psychiatric disorders among cancer patients. JAMA 1983;249:751–7.
37. Handwerker WP. Cultural diversity, stress, and depression: working women in the Americas. J Womens Health Gender Based Med 1999;8:1303–11.

38. Kendler KS, Karkowski LM, Prescott CA. Causal relationship between stressful life events and the onset of major depression. Am J Psychiatry 1999;156:837–41.

39. Evans DL, Staab JP, Petitto JM, et al. Depression in the medical setting: biopsychological interactions and treatment considerations. J Clin Psychiatry 1999;60 Suppl 4:40–55; discussion 6.

40. Burgess CC, Ramirez AJ, Richards MA, Potts HW. Does the method of detection of breast cancer affect subsequent psychiatric morbidity? Eur J Cancer 2002;38:1622–5.

41. Wellisch DK, Kaleita TA, Freeman D, et al. Predicting major depression in brain tumor patients. Psych Oncol 2002;11: 230–8.

42. Weissman MM, Bland RC, Canino GJ, et al. Cross-national epidemiology of major depression and bipolar disorder. JAMA 1996;276:293–9.

43. Akechi T, Okamura H, Nishiwaki Y, Uchitomi Y. Psychiatric disorders and associated and predictive factors in patients with unresectable nonsmall cell lung carcinoma: a longitudinal study. Cancer 2001;92:2609–22.

44. Raison CL, Demetrashvili M, Capuron L, Miller AH. Neuropsychiatric side effects of interferon-alpha: recognition and management. CNS Drugs;19:1–19.

45. Evans DL, McCartney CF, Nemeroff CB, et al. Depression in women treated for gynecological cancer: clinical and neuroendocrine assessment. Am J Psychiatry 1986;143: 447–52.

46. Krishnan KR, Delong M, Kraemer H, et al. Comorbidity of depression with other medical diseases in the elderly. Biol Psychiatry 2002;52:559–88.

47. Wise MG, Rundell JR, editors. The American Psychiatric Publishing textbook of consultation-liaison psychiatry: psychiatry in the medically ill. 2nd ed. Washington (DC): American Psychiatric Publishing; 2002.

48. Moffic HS, Paykel ES. Depression in medical in-patients. Br J Psychiatry 1975;126:346–53.

49. Ciaramella A, Poli P. Assessment of depression among cancer patients: the role of pain, cancer type and treatment. Psychooncology 2001;10:156–65.

50. Capuron L, Ravaud A, Dantzer R. Timing and specificity of the cognitive changes induced by interleukin-2 and interferon-alpha treatments in cancer patients. Psychosom Med 2001;63:376–86.

51. Musselman DL, Lawson DH, Gumnick JF, et al. Paroxetine for the prevention of depression induced by high-dose interferon alfa. N Engl J Med 2001;344:961–6.

52. Raison CL, Nemeroff C. Cancer and depression: prevalence, diagnosis and treatment. Home Health Care Consultant 2000;7:34–41.

53. Vliagoftis H, Dimitriadou V, Boucher W, et al. Estradiol augments while tamoxifen inhibits rat mast cell secretion. Int Arch Allergy Immunol 1992;98:398–409.

54. Cathcart CK, Jones SE, Pumroy CS, et al. Clinical recognition and management of depression in node negative breast cancer patients treated with tamoxifen. Breast Cancer Res Treat 1993;27:277–81.

55. Shores MM, Sloan KL, Matsumoto AM, et al. Increased incidence of diagnosed depressive illness in hypogonadal older men. Arch Gen Psychiatry 2004;61:162–7.

56. Rabkin JG, Wagner GJ, Rabkin R. A double-blind, placebo-controlled trial of testosterone therapy for HIV-positive men with hypogonadal symptoms. Arch Gen Psychiatry 2000;57:141–7; discussion 55–6.

57. Rabkin JG, Wagner GJ, McElhiney MC, et al. Testosterone versus fluoxetine for depression and fatigue in HIV/AIDS: a placebo-controlled trial. J Clin Psychopharmacol 2004; 24:379–85.

58. Almeida OP, Waterreus A, Spry N, et al. One year follow-up study of the association between chemical castration, sex hormones, beta-amyloid, memory and depression in men. Psychoneuroendocrinology 2004;29:1071–81.

59. Zebrack BJ, Zeltzer LK, Whitton J, et al. Psychological outcomes in long-term survivors of childhood leukemia, Hodgkin's disease, and non-Hodgkin's lymphoma: a report from the Childhood Cancer Survivor Study. Pediatrics 2002;110:42–52.

60. Moreno FA, Gelenberg AJ, Heninger GR, et al. Tryptophan depletion and depressive vulnerability. Biol Psychiatry 1999;46:498–505.

61. Ahles TA, Saykin AJ, Furstenberg CT, et al. Neuropsychologic impact of standard-dose systemic chemotherapy in long-term survivors of breast cancer and lymphoma. J Clin Oncol 2002;20:485–93.

62. Gurevich M, Devins GM, Rodin GM. Stress response syndromes and cancer: conceptual and assessment issues. Psychosomatics 2002;43:259–81.

63. Nakano T, Wenner M, Inagaki M, et al. Relationship between distressing cancer-related recollections and hippocampal volume in cancer survivors. Am J Psychiatry 2002;159: 2087–93.

64. Kent S, Bluthe RM, Kelley KW, Dantzer R. Sickness behavior as a new target for drug development. Trends Pharmacol Sci 1992;13:24–8.

65. Dantzer R. Cytokine-induced sickness behavior: where do we stand? Brain Behav Immun 2001;15:7–24.

66. Dunn AJ, Wang J, Ando T. Effects of cytokines on cerebral neurotransmission. Comparison with the effects of stress. Adv Exp Med Biol 1999;461:117–27.

67. Besedovsky H, del Rey A, Sorkin E, Dinarello CA. Immuno-regulatory feedback between interleukin-1 and glucocorticoid hormones. Science 1986;233:652–4.

68. Rivier C. Influence of immune signals on the hypothalamic-pituitary axis of the rodent. Front Neuroendocrinol 1995; 16:151–82.

69. Owens MJ, Nemeroff CB. Physiology and pharmacology of corticotropin-releasing factor. Pharmacol Rev 1991;43: 425–73.

70. Holsboer F, Barden N. Antidepressants and hypothalamic-pituitary-adrenocortical regulation. Endocr Rev 1996;17: 187–205.

71. Owens MJ, Nemeroff CB. The role of corticotropin-releasing factor in the pathophysiology of affective and anxiety disorders: laboratory and clinical studies. Ciba Found Symp 1993;172:296–308.

72. Pariante CM, Miller AH. Glucocorticoid receptors in major depression: relevance to pathophysiology and treatment. Biol Psychiatry 2001;49:391–404.

73. Holsboer F. The corticosteroid hypothesis of depression. Neuropsychopharmacology 2000;23:477–501.

74. Musselman DL, Miller AH, Porter MR, et al. Higher than normal plasma interleukin-6 concentrations in cancer patients with depression: preliminary findings. Am J Psychiatry 2001;158:1252–7.

75. Lestage J, Verrier D, Palin K, Dantzer R. The enzyme indoleamine 2,3-dioxygenase is induced in the mouse brain in response to peripheral administration of lipopolysaccharide and superantigen. Brain Behav Immun 2002;16: 596–601.

76. Capuron L, Hauser P, Hinze-Selch D, et al. Treatment of cytokine-induced depression. Brain Behav Immun 2002; 16:575–80.

77. Liebau C, Baltzer AW, Schmidt S, et al. Interleukin-12 and interleukin-18 induce indoleamine 2,3-dioxygenase (IDO) activity in human osteosarcoma cell lines independently from interferon-gamma. Anticancer Res 2002;22 Suppl 2A:931–6.

78. Moore P, Landolt HP, Seifritz E, et al. Clinical and physiological consequences of rapid tryptophan depletion. Neuropsychopharmacology 2000;23:601–22.

79. Papanicolaou DA. Euthyroid sick syndrome and the role of cytokines. Rev Endocrine Metab Disord 2000;1:43–8.

80. Greenberg DB, Gray JL, Mannix CM, et al. Treatment-related fatigue and serum interleukin-1 levels in patients during external beam irradiation for prostate cancer. J Pain Symptom Manage 1993;8:196–200.

81. Rigas JR, Hoopes PJ, Mayer LA, et al. Fatigue linked to plasma cytokines in patients with lung cancer undergoing combined modality therapy. Proc Am Soc Clin Oncol 1998;17:68a.

82. Bower JE, Ganz PA, Aziz N, Fahey JL. Fatigue and proinflammatory cytokine activity in breast cancer survivors. Psychosom Med 2002;64:604–11.

83. Kudoh A, Katagai H, Takazawa T. Plasma inflammatory cytokine response to surgical trauma in chronic depressed patients. Cytokine 2001;13:104–8.

84. Capuron L, Raison CL, Musselman DL, et al. Association of exaggerated HPA axis response to the initial injection of interferon-alpha with development of depression during interferon-alpha therapy. Am J Psychiatry 2003;160: 1342–5.

85. Raison CL, Miller AH. When not enough is too much: the role of insufficient glucocorticoid signaling in the pathophysiology of stress-related disorders. Am J Psychiatry 2003;160:1554–65.

86. Roitt I, Bostoff J, Male D. Immunology. 5th ed. New York: Mosby; 1998.

87. Taylor JL, Grossberg SE. The effects of interferon-alpha on the production and action of other cytokines. Semin Oncol 1998;25(1 Suppl 1):23–9.

88. Schaefer M, Engelbrecht MA, Gut O, et al. Interferon alpha (IFNa) and psychiatric syndromes: a review. Prog Neuropsychopharmacol Biol Psychiatry 2002;26:731–46.

89. Merali Z, Brennan K, Brau P, Anisman H. Dissociating anorexia and anhedonia elicited by interleukin-1beta: antidepressant and gender effects on responding for "free chow" and "earned" sucrose intake. Psychopharmacology 2003;165:413–8.

90. Capuron L, Gumnick JF, Musselman DL, et al. Neurobehavioral effects of interferon-alpha in cancer patients: phenomenology and paroxetine responsiveness of symptom dimensions. Neuropsychopharmacology 2002;26: 643–52.

91. Cleeland CS, Mendoza TR, Wang XS, et al. Assessing symptom distress in cancer patients: the M.D. Anderson Symptom Inventory. Cancer 2000;89:1634–46.

92. Capuron L, Neurauter G, Musselman DL, et al. Interferon-alpha-induced changes in tryptophan metabolism: relationship to depression and paroxetine treatment. Biol Psychiatry 2003;54:906–14.

93. Capuron L, Ravaud A, Neveu PJ, et al. Association between decreased serum tryptophan concentrations and depressive symptoms in cancer patients undergoing cytokine therapy. Mol Psychiatry 2002;7:468–73.

94. Mellor AL, Munn DH. Tryptophan catabolism and T-cell tolerance: immunosuppression by starvation? Immunol Today 1999;20:469–73.

95. Moreno FA, Heninger GR, McGahuey CA, Delgado PL. Tryptophan depletion and risk of depression relapse: a prospective study of tryptophan depletion as a potential predictor of depressive episodes. Biol Psychiatry 2000; 48:327–9.

96. Bonaccorso S, Marino V, Puzella A, et al. Increased depressive ratings in patients with hepatitis C receiving interferon-alpha-based immunotherapy are related to interferon-alpha-induced changes in the serotonergic system. J Clin Psychopharmacol 2002;22:86–90.

97. Widner B, Ledochowski M, Fuchs D. Interferon-gamma-induced tryptophan degradation: neuropsychiatric and immunological consequences. Curr Drug Metab 2000;1: 193–204.

98. Heim C, Newport DJ, Heit S, et al. Pituitary-adrenal and autonomic responses to stress in women after sexual and physical abuse in childhood. JAMA 2000;284:592–7.

99. Krieg JC, Lauer CJ, Schreiber W, et al. Neuroendocrine, polysomnographic and psychometric observations in healthy subjects at high familial risk for affective disorders: the current state of the 'Munich vulnerability study.' J Affect Disord 2001;62:33–7.

100. Cummings JL. Depression and Parkinson's disease: a review. Am J Psychiatry 1992;149:443–54.

101. Berger JR, Arendt G. HIV dementia: the role of the basal ganglia and dopaminergic systems. J Psychopharmacol 2000;14:214–21.

102. Martinot M, Bragulat V, Artiges E, et al. Decreased presynaptic dopamine function in the left caudate of depressed patients with affective flattening and psychomotor retardation. Am J Psychiatry 2001;158:314–6.

103. Sugawara Y, Akechi T, Shima Y, et al. Efficacy of methylphenidate for fatigue in advanced cancer patients: a preliminary study. Palliat Med 2002;16:261–3.

104. Sarhill N, Walsh D, Nelson KA, et al. Methylphenidate for fatigue in advanced cancer: a prospective open-label pilot study. Am J Hosp Palliat Care 2001;18:187–92.

105. Zifko UA, Rupp M, Schwarz S, et al. Modafinil in treatment of fatigue in multiple sclerosis. Results of an open-label study. J Neurol 2002;249:983–7.

106. Shuto H, Kataoka Y, Horikawa T, et al. Repeated interferonalpha administration inhibits dopaminergic neural activity in the mouse brain. Brain Res 1997;747:348–51.

107. Sunami M, Nishikawa T, Yorogi A, Shimoda M. Intravenous administration of levodopa ameliorated a refractory akathisia case induced by interferon-alpha. Clin Neuropharmacol 2000;23:59–61.

108. de Jonge P, Ormel J, Slaets JP, et al. Depressive symptoms in elderly patients predict poor adjustment after somatic events. Am J Geriatr Psychiatry 2004;12:57–64.

109. Gao HM, Jiang J, Wilson B, et al. Microglial activation-mediated delayed and progressive degeneration of rat nigral dopaminergic neurons: relevance to Parkinson's disease. J Neurochem 2002;81:1285–97.

110. Capuron L, Pagnoni G, Lawson D, et al. Altered fronto-pallidal activity during high-dose interferon-alpha treatment as determined by positron emission tomography. Soc Neurosci Abstr 2002;498:5.

111. Juengling FD, Ebert D, Gut O, et al. Prefrontal cortical hypometabolism during low-dose interferon alpha treatment. Psychopharmacology (Berl) 2000;152:383–9.

112. Evans DL, Ten Have TR, Douglas SD, et al. Association of depression with viral load, CD8 T lymphocytes, and natural killer cells in women with HIV infection. Am J Psychiatry 2002;159:1752–9.

113. Dringen R, Hirrlinger J. Glutathione pathways in the brain. Biol Chem 2003;384:505–16.

114. Bharath S, Hsu M, Kaur D, et al. Glutathione, iron and Parkinson's disease. Biochem Pharmacol 2002;64:1037–48.

115. Castagne V, Rougemont M, Cuenod M, Do KQ. Low brain glutathione and ascorbic acid associated with dopamine uptake inhibition during rat's development induce long-term cognitive deficit: relevance to schizophrenia. Neurobiol Dis 2004;15:93–105.

116. McCaddon A, Hudson P, Hill D, et al. Alzheimer's disease and total plasma aminothiols. Biol Psychiatry 2003;53:254–60.

117. Jonas CR, Puckett AB, Jones DP, et al. Plasma antioxidant status after high-dose chemotherapy: a randomized trial of parenteral nutrition in bone marrow transplantation patients. Am J Clin Nutr 2000;72:181–9.

118. Lauterburg BH, Nguyen T, Hartmann B, et al. Depletion of total cysteine, glutathione, and homocysteine in plasma by ifosfamide/mesna therapy. Cancer Chemother Pharmacol 1994;35:132–6.

119. Cascinu S, Catalano V, Cordella L, et al. Neuroprotective effect of reduced glutathione on oxaliplatin-based chemotherapy in advanced colorectal cancer: a randomized, double-blind, placebo-controlled trial. J Clin Oncol 2002;20:3478–83.

120. Bohm S, Oriana S, Spatti G, et al. Dose intensification of platinum compounds with glutathione protection as induction chemotherapy for advanced ovarian carcinoma. Oncology 1999;57:115–20.

121. Monks TJ, Ghersi-Egea JF, Philbert M, et al. Symposium overview: the role of glutathione in neuroprotection and neurotoxicity. Toxicol Sci 1999;51:161–77.

122. Pastore A, Federici G, Bertini E, Piemonte F. Analysis of glutathione: implication in redox and detoxification. Clin Chim Acta 2003;333:19–39.

123. Sofic E, Lange KW, Jellinger K, Riederer P. Reduced and oxidized glutathione in the substantia nigra of patients with Parkinson's disease. Neurosci Lett 1992;142:128–30.

124. Adams JD Jr, Chang ML, Klaidman L. Parkinson's disease—redox mechanisms. Curr Med Chem 2001;8:809–14.

125. Jones DP, Mody VC Jr, Carlson JL, et al. Redox analysis of human plasma allows separation of pro-oxidant events of aging from decline in antioxidant defenses. Free Radic Biol Med 2002;33:1290–300.

126. Samiec PS, Drews-Botsch C, Flagg EW, et al. Glutathione in human plasma: decline in association with aging, age-related macular degeneration, and diabetes. Free Radic Biol Med 1998;24:699–704.

127. Droge W. Cysteine and glutathione deficiency in AIDS patients: a rationale for the treatment with N-acetyl-cysteine. Pharmacology 1993;46:61–5.

128. Tsavaris N, Kosmas C, Vadiaka M, et al. Immune changes in patients with advanced breast cancer undergoing chemotherapy with taxanes. Br J Cancer 2002;87:21–7.

129. Nishimura T, Newkirk K, Sessions RB, et al. Association between expression of glutathione-associated enzymes and response to platinum-based chemotherapy in head and neck cancer. Chemicobiol Interact 1998;111–2:187–98.

130. Rudin CM, Yang Z, Schumaker LM, et al. Inhibition of glutathione synthesis reverses Bcl-2-mediated cisplatin resistance. Cancer Res 2003;63:312–8.

Sleep Disorders in the Cancer Patient

Colleen G. Lance, MD

Karen O. Anderson, PhD, MPH

Sleep disturbance is a frequent complaint among cancer patients, as clinicians caring for patients can attest. A sleep disturbance can be defined as any disruption that causes a person to have difficulty falling asleep or maintaining sleep, to feel not rested after a night's sleep, or to require a nap during the day.[1] Having a sleep disturbance affects all aspects of a patient's well-being, which, in turn, affects the patient's response to cancer treatment. The body of literature and amount of research invested into this common symptom are relatively limited. One reason might be the small amount of time clinicians spend on sleep disorders during medical school: on average, only 2 hours over the course of 4 years.[2] Also, sleep disturbance complaints are very subjective, which makes developing tools for quantitative measurement difficult.

Sleep disturbances within the cancer population, whether caused by the cancer itself, cancer-related adjustment disorders, or treatment interventions, are even more frequent than for the general population. Research among various cancer groups has found a prevalence of sleep disturbance ranging from as low as 24%[3] to as high as 95%.[4] One recent study found that 62% of those studied had moderate to severe sleep disturbance.[1] The importance of this symptom to cancer patients was brought to light by Derogatis and colleagues, who looked at psychotropic medications prescribed for almost 1,600 cancer patients.[5] Of all of the prescriptions written, 48% were for hypnotics.

Although most studies to date have been nonspecific questionnaire studies, they have helped bring quality of life issues to the forefront. For example, patients who received radiation treatment and who had lower Karnofsky Performance Status scores reported more sleep disturbances.[6] Also, a recent questionnaire study of metastatic breast cancer patients showed that 63% reported one or more kinds of sleep complaints.[7]

A few studies that focused on specific cancer populations used polysomnography to investigate sleep architecture. One such study examined the sleep architecture and psychological state of breast and lung cancer patients. Using insomniacs as a control group, investigators found that lung cancer patients had more disturbed sleep than insomniacs yet underreported their symptoms. The lung cancer patients had to stay in bed much longer to obtain the same quantity of sleep, had lengthy sleep disruptions through the night, and took longer daytime naps. The breast cancer group also reported more sleep difficulties than the controls, but an examination of the sleep architecture indicated that they actually had slept well.[8]

Diagnosing Sleep Disturbance

Prompt referral to a sleep medicine specialist should be made whenever a patient's sleep complaint is disrupting his or her daytime routine or cancer treatment. The following is what to expect from a sleep medicine consultation and may help the clinician in deciding when to refer a patient. Two helpful Web sites are <www.absm.org> for finding board-certified sleep physicians and <www.sleepfoundation.org> for sleep tools.

The Sleep History

The initial step in characterizing a patient's sleep disturbance is taking a sleep history. A cancer patient's sleep complaints are most often mixed with other complaints and may be far down on the patient's list of concerns. A sleep history asks the patient and, if possible, the patient's sleep partner a variety of descriptive questions about the nature of the patient's sleep experience (Table 1).

A sleep history may reveal that the sleep difficulties are being caused by treatable conditions. For example, certain medical ailments may have nocturnal presentations: patients may complain of shortness of breath or chest pain with cardiopulmonary conditions, heartburn or abdominal pain with gastrointestinal conditions, headaches with carbon dioxide retention, or jaw pain with temporomandibular joint disorder. Medications, such as bronchodilators and psychotropic, gastrointestinal, and pain medications, also may contribute to sleep difficulties. A detailed review of the patient's intake of medication, herbal supplements, nicotine, and caffeine may indicate the need to change a medication altogether or simply to change the time of day that it is given.

Social history provides useful information about normal daily routines and possible interruptions from the cancer or cancer treatment. A social history interview should include the patient and all household members as cancer treatment may be severely disruptive to the entire household and can require difficult adjustments from both the patient and the family. Particular attention should be given to the state of the

Table 1 Sleep History Sample Questions
What time do you go to bed?
Do you have difficulty falling asleep?*
Do you have racing thoughts while trying to fall asleep?*
How many times do you awaken during the night?*
What awakens you?
How long until you fall back to sleep?
What time do you awaken to start your day?
Do you wake up refreshed?
Do you snore at night?**
Are you sleepy during the day?
Do others tell you that you have pauses in breathing or gasping for air?†
Does your bed partner have to sleep in another room because of the way you sleep?†
Do you ever have sudden loss of strength in your arms or legs during the day?‡
If yes, are these episodes brought on by fright or laughter?
Do you take naps?‡
If yes, how often and for how long?
How do you feel after these naps?
Do you ever awaken feeling paralyzed?‡
Do you kick or twitch at night?§
How much caffeine or nicotine do you consume?§
Do you have a restless feeling in your legs while trying to sleep?§
If yes, how often?

*Insomnia.
†Sleep-disordered breathing.
‡Narcolepsy.
§Periodic limb movement and restless legs.

patient's relationships with his or her spouse, children, and coworkers.

The Sleep Physical

The physical examination of a patient with a sleep complaint begins the moment the physician enters the room. A disheveled appearance or altered affect may indicate a psychiatric disorder as a primary diagnosis. A large body habitus and central obesity may be indicators of sleep-disordered breathing or obesity hypoventilation.

The head and neck examination is of paramount importance. A neck circumference greater than 17 inches or thyromegaly may indicate increased adipose tissue around the airway. Craniofacial abnormalities associated with head and neck cancer or the treatment of such tumors may signify sleep-disordered breathing. Cardio-pulmonary examination may reveal medical conditions contributing to nocturnal sleep difficulties. Chest wall abnormalities such as kyphosis or pectus excavatum are associated with restrictive lung defects. Wheezing can signify nocturnal asthma attacks. Hypertension, cardiac thrust, or signs of pulmonary hypertension may be signs of sleep-disordered breathing, with signs of heart failure, such as hepatomegaly, ascites, and peripheral edema, in the most severe cases.

Neurologic examination may uncover reasons for disturbed sleep. Impaired mentation may suggest an underlying dementia that causes insomnia, hypersomnolence, or a circadian rhythm disorder. Use of sedatives and/or stimulants (prescription or illicit) may be apparent on initial examination. Prolonged alcohol abuse may be apparent, with hepatomegaly, ascites, spider telangiectasis, or jaundice. Peripheral neuropathy or joint abnormalities may cause nocturnal pain and sleep disturbance.

Diagnostic Tools

Given that neither patients nor clinicians may initiate a discussion of sleep problems, screening questionnaires can help identify patients who are experiencing sleep difficulties. A checklist of common cancer-related symptoms, such as the M.D. Anderson Symptom Inventory[9] or the Symptom Distress Scale,[10] can be used as an initial screening tool. These brief and easily administered scales include one sleep disturbance item that can be used to identify patients with potential sleep disorders. If the patient responds positively to a sleep disturbance item, then a more detailed sleep questionnaire can be used to further define the problem. For cancer populations that are particularly at risk of sleep disorders, it may be helpful to include a brief sleep questionnaire as part of the initial workup.

The 19-item Pittsburgh Sleep Quality Index (PSQI), developed to measure sleep quality and quantity, has been evaluated in healthy samples and samples of individuals with chronic diseases.[11] The scale yields a global sleep quality score and seven component scores: subjective sleep quality, sleep latency, duration, habitual sleep efficiency, sleep disturbances, use of sleeping medication, and daytime dysfunction. The PSQI has been evaluated in samples of patients with cancer.[12–15] This global sleep quality scale has demonstrated good internal reliability and construct validity in samples of breast cancer patients and patients with diverse cancer diagnoses.

The 12-item Medical Outcomes Study (MOS) Sleep Scale provides a concise assessment of several sleep dimensions and yields a sleep problems index and six scale scores: sleep disturbance, sleep adequacy, daytime somnolence, snoring, shortness of breath or headache, and quantity of sleep.[16] Evidence of the reliability and validity of the scale was provided in studies of individuals with chronic illness[17] and a nationally representative sample of adults.[16] In addition, the MOS Sleep Scale was sensitive to change in a sample of patients with neuropathic pain enrolled in a clinical drug trial.[16] This scale is brief and easy to administer, and a computer program is available for scoring. The scale has not been evaluated in samples of patients with cancer but appears to have potential utility owing to its brevity.

Other sleep questionnaires were designed to screen for obstructive sleep apnea (OSA), daytime somnolence, or other specific disorders.[18–21] These measures may be helpful if initial screening suggests a specific sleep disorder. The Epworth Sleepiness Scale was designed to differentiate persons with excessive daytime sleepiness from alert individuals by measuring their sleep propensity.[19] The scale asks individuals how likely they are to sleep in eight different situations.

The Sleep Diary

When a sleep problem is indicated by a screening questionnaire or medical history, a sleep log or diary is often used to obtain additional information. Sleep logs provide a daily account of all sleep activities, including sleep latency (the time from lights out until sleep onset), sleep duration, number of nighttime awakenings, perceived sleep quality, and daytime naps. Such sleep logs are relatively easy to complete and cost little. A sleep diary of at least 2 weeks' duration is one of the most important tools in evaluating a sleep disturbance. The diary tracks the bedtime, time to sleep onset, the number and timing of nocturnal awakenings, time of final awakening, naps, and the subject's feelings on arising. This is particularly helpful in diagnosing circadian rhythm disorders and in managing insomnia.

Actigraphy

Actigraphy is a tool used to assess activity level. It uses a device that can be worn on any limb for several days to several weeks and that transfers a mechanical or digital signal with movement of the limb. The information is downloaded at the end of the study period. Actigraphy is useful for clarifying the level of insomnia and diagnosing circadian rhythm disorders and is an accurate measure of the sleep-wake cycle, with only a few exceptions. Validation studies comparing actigraphy with minute-by-minute polysomnography scoring show an 80 to 90% agreement when differentiating the sleep state from the wakeful state.[22]

Polysomnography

The gold standard in sleep measurement is the attended nocturnal polysomnography (NPSG), in which a polygraphic recording of multiple physiologic variables is made during sleep. "Attended" means that a qualified technician remains with the subject throughout the study to monitor for technical adequacy and patient compliance. NPSG measures several biologic parameters simultaneously. These usually include electroencephalography, electro-oculography, electromyography, electrocardiography, body position, respiratory effort, airflow, and pulse oximetry. Other parameters may be added, such as esophageal pH to diagnose gastroesophageal reflux disease, esophageal pressure monitoring for the diagnosis of upper airway resistance syndrome, or end-tidal CO_2. The Multiple Sleep Latency Test is a series of nap opportunities and recording of electroencephalography, electro-oculography, and chin electromyography. Performed the day after NPSG, it is used to evaluate hypersomnias, such as narcolepsy and idiopathic hypersomnia. Indications for NPSG are found in Table 2.[23]

Specific Sleep Disorders in the Cancer Patient

Insomnias

Insomnia is characterized by difficulty initiating or maintaining sleep or by nonrestorative sleep that causes significant distress or impairment in daily functioning. Insomnia is considered acute if the sleep problem lasts for one to three nights per week, with no episode lasting longer than several weeks, or chronic if the sleep difficulties last for three or more nights per week for 1 month or longer.[24] Patients with insomnia may also complain of daytime fatigue, irritability, decreased memory and concentration, and general malaise. The variables associated with increased risk of insomnia are fatigue, younger age, leg restlessness, use of sedatives or hypnotics, depression, dreams, concerns, and recent surgery.

Epidemiologic surveys that use diagnostic criteria for insomnia estimate the prevalence in the general population as 9 to 12%.[25,26] Cancer

Table 2 Indications for Polysomnography	
Routine for Suspected	
Sleep-disordered breathing	
Titration of positive airway pressure	
Narcolepsy (with MSLT)	
Periodic limb movement disorder	
Not Routine for Suspected	**_Exceptions_**
Insomnia	Sleep maintenance insomnia
Restless legs syndrome	
Circadian rhythm disorder	
Parasomnias	Violent or atypical behavior
Seizures	
Snoring without daytime somnolence	Not responding to therapy
MSLT = Multiple Sleep Latency Test.	

- Coronary disease
- Reactive airway disease (Table 10-4)
- Movement disorders
  - Restless legs syndrome (RLS)
  - Periodic limb movement disorder (PLMD)
  - Nocturnal leg cramps
- Neurologic
  - Parkinson's disease
  - Dementia
  - Epilepsy
  - Tumor related
- Sleep-disordered breathing
  - Mild to moderate sleep apnea
  - Central sleep apnea (CSA)

patients appear to be at greater risk of insomnia than the general population. In a recent survey of over 900 cancer patients, 31% of the patients reported insomnia.[27] The most frequent patient-reported reasons for insomnia were pain, health concerns, concerns about family or friends, and the cancer itself.

The prevalence of insomnia among cancer patients has been evaluated in several descriptive studies. Savard and colleagues found that one-third of breast cancer patients with insomnia reported the onset of their sleep disturbance following their cancer diagnosis.[28] Thus, their insomnia appeared to be secondary to the cancer. In a larger heterogeneous sample of cancer patients, 48% indicated that their insomnia began around the time of cancer diagnosis.[27] Approximately 40% of the patients reported insomnia symptoms that began years prior to the cancer diagnosis. Another study of women with breast cancer found that 25% of the women reported difficulty falling asleep and 44% reported problems with nighttime awakenings.[7] Risk factors for sleep disturbance included pain, depression, and lower levels of social support. Another descriptive study of women with breast cancer found that 50% reported insomnia symptoms and 19% met diagnostic criteria for insomnia.[28]

The primary care physician or oncologist should screen patients for symptoms of insomnia during clinic visits. Patients with cancer may be reluctant to report poor sleep quality owing to a belief that insomnia is an expected reaction to having cancer or a reluctance to distract the physician from focusing on the cancer treatment. A telephone survey of breast and lung cancer patients experiencing sleep problems found that only 17% of the patients had discussed sleep with their physicians.[29] As noted previously, a brief symptom checklist completed prior to a clinic visit may help identify patients who are experiencing insomnia. When an initial screen indicates that insomnia is a problem, then a complete sleep history and physical examination, possibly by a sleep specialist, is needed to determine the etiology of the insomnia. Polysomnography is not recommended for routine screening or diagnosis of insomnia, unless a sleep-related breathing or movement disorder is suspected.[30] Below are listed the most common causes of insomnia in the cancer patient:

- Behavioral
  - Inadequate sleep hygiene
  - Psychophysiologic insomnia
- Environmental
  - Hospitalization
- Psychiatric
  - Psychosis
  - Mood disorders
  - Anxiety disorders
- Medications
  - Bronchodilators
  - Antihypertensives
  - Anticholinergics
  - Diuretics
  - Antidepressants (ie, selective serotonin reuptake inhibitors)
  - Decongestants
  - Chemotherapy (Table 10-3)
  - Hormone therapy: antiestrogens, antiandrogens
  - Substance abuse
- Medical conditions
  - Gastroesophageal reflux
  - Arrhythmias

Table 3 Biochemotherapy Agents Associated with Insomnia
Busulfan
Mechlorethamine
Cladribine
Pentostatin
Fludarabine
Procarbazine
Irinotecan
Rituximab

Pain also is a risk factor for insomnia in patients with cancer. Patients receiving active cancer treatment often experience pain, and more than 60% of patients with advanced disease report pain.[31,32] Descriptive studies of cancer patients with pain have found that over half of the patients experienced sleep disturbance that they attributed to pain.[32–35] Difficulty initiating sleep and nighttime awakenings were frequently reported. Optimal pain management is necessary to eliminate pain as a stimulus that can disrupt sleep. For patients with complicated pain syndromes, referral to a pain specialist may be indicated.

Certain behaviors may lead to insomnia. Inadequate sleep hygiene refers to insomnia resulting from behaviors that increase bedtime arousal or disrupt sleep patterns. Examples of such behaviors include working or exercising late at night, taking excessive daytime naps, and keeping irregular sleep hours. Using stimulants such as caffeine and nicotine or substances such as alcohol near bedtime also can disrupt sleep. Patients with cancer may develop maladaptive sleep hygiene behaviors if their cancer treatment interferes with their usual sleep schedule.

In descriptive studies of cancer patients, the prevalence of mood disorders ranges from 13% to as high as 50%.[36,37] Mood disorders alone, however, do not explain the high rate of sleep disorders among cancer patients. One survey study found that only 21% of cancer patients reported insomnia and demonstrated a concurrent psychiatric diagnosis.[38] Common patterns seen include early morning awakening in depressed patients and frequent arousals in those with anxiety disorders. Early referral to a psychiatrist in conjunction with a sleep specialist is warranted.

Nonpharmacologic Treatments of Insomnia

Behavioral and cognitive-behavioral treatments have been used successfully to treat insomnia in the general population. Two recent meta-analyses of research studies evaluating these treatments concluded that behavioral and cognitive-behavioral interventions were effective and typically produced significant improvements in sleep-onset latency, sleep quality ratings, the duration of nighttime awakenings, total sleep time, and the number of awakenings.[39,40] The amount of improvement demonstrated on most outcome variables was comparable to that seen in studies of hypnotic medications.[41] In addition, many studies have found that the improvements associated with behavioral and cognitive-behavioral interventions for insomnia were maintained up to 2 years after the initial treatment.[39,40]

Education on sleep hygiene is often included in behavioral and cognitive-behavioral treatments for insomnia. This education focuses on behaviors and environmental factors that affect sleep. Patients are taught to avoid alcohol and stimulants such as caffeine and nicotine close to bedtime. They also are advised to avoid heavy meals close to bedtime and to keep their bedroom a comfortable, dark, and quiet environment. Regular exercise is recommended, but not close to bedtime. Research evaluating sleep hygiene education alone has found that this intervention is modestly beneficial.

Cognitive-behavioral treatment usually requires the assistance of someone trained in these techniques, such as a psychologist. Techniques include

- Stimulus control
- Sleep restriction
- Relaxation techniques
  - Muscle relaxation
  - Biofeedback
  - Meditation
  - Imagery training
  - Hypnosis
  - Autogenic therapy
- Cognitive interventions

Only a few studies have evaluated behavioral and cognitive-behavioral interventions for insomnia in samples of cancer patients, but the results suggest that such interventions are effective for that population. In a small sample of patients with cancer, a cognitive-behavioral group intervention was associated with significant improvements in sleep efficiency, sleep quality, and nighttime awakenings.[42] A larger randomized controlled study of a stress reduction intervention for women with breast cancer found that women who reported frequent practice of mindfulness meditation improved more on a sleep quality measure than women who reported less practice.[43] A recent randomized controlled trial of cognitive-behavioral treatments for insomnia in cancer patients compared a multimodal package that included a relaxation technique with one that included an autogenic intervention.[44] Both treatment groups demonstrated significant improvements compared with a control group on measures of sleep latency, duration, efficiency, quality, use of sleep medication, and daytime dysfunction.

Pharmacologic Treatment of Insomnia

The first step in pharmacologic management of insomnia is to eliminate, if possible, any agents that may be causing insomnia. Common medications that cause insomnia include anticholinergics, antidepressants, bronchodilators, corticosteroids, central nervous system stimulants, weight loss medications, decongestants, and diuretics.

Insomnia may be treated with any of several available sedative-hypnotic agents, including benzodiazepines, nonbenzodiazepine hypnotics, and sedating antihistamines and antidepressants. Ideally, these agents should be prescribed at the lowest dose possible for the shortest time possible and combined with the nonpharmacologic treatments described previously. Sedating antihistamines and antidepressants usually have only a transitory effect on alleviating insomnia. Antihistamines have some undesirable side effects, including constipation, urinary retention, and dry mouth. Benzodiazepines cause muscle relaxation, which can be a problem for those with sleep-disordered breathing and can produce rebound insomnia when stopped. The newer nonbenzodiazepine hypnotics do not cause muscle relaxation or rebound insomnia, nor do they suppress rapid eye movement (REM) and slow-wave sleep. The newest class of drug is the melatonin agonist ramelteon, which has US Food and Drug Administration (FDA) approval for insomnia. This drug also does not suppress REM or slow-wave sleep as the benzodiazepines do. Figure 10-1 is for the treatment of insomnia; treatment options are not mutually exclusive.

Circadian Rhythm Disorders

We each have a 24-hour internal circadian "clock" that helps keep us synchronized with internal and external environments. This clock, the suprachiasmatic nucleus, is found in the anterior hypothalamus. It is entrained, or resynchronized, by external cues, the strongest being light.[45] When light stimulus is withdrawn from the suprachiasmatic nucleus, melatonin is released from the pineal gland, which, in turn, causes a decrease in body temperature and helps induce sleep. Abnormalities in this cycle are termed *circadian rhythm disorders*.

Delayed sleep phase syndrome is a disorder in which patients are unable to fall asleep until some time between 2:00 am and 6:00 am and then arise between 10:00 am and 1:00 pm; the clock is delayed. The prevalence of delayed sleep phase disorder in sleep clinics has been found to be as high as 16%.[46] The complaint is typically one of sleep initiation insomnia, and patients usually use sedative-hypnotics or alcohol to help initiate sleep; this is then followed by excessive daytime somnolence. Advanced sleep phase syndrome is a disorder in which the clock is advanced so that the patient falls asleep much earlier than expected and wakes between 2:00 and 5:00 am. Diagnosis is made by history, sleep diaries, and sometimes actigraphy.

Several studies have used actigraphy and diurnal cortisol levels to look at circadian rhythm disruption within the cancer population. On the whole, daytime inactivity was correlated with nighttime restlessness and excessive daytime fatigue. Breast cancer patients undergoing adjuvant chemotherapy were found to have levels of fatigue that followed a "roller-coaster" pattern throughout treatment and that was negatively correlated with nighttime restlessness.[47] This has also been found in patients receiving treatment for metastatic colorectal carcinoma and those undergoing radiation treatment for various cancers.[48] Advanced sleep phase syndrome was found in some groups undergoing cancer chemotherapy, whereas others remained normal.[49] There are also reports in the literature of children with central nervous system neoplasms having circadian rhythm disturbance.[50] These findings imply that, for cancer patients, daytime naps and inactivity cause disruption to the circadian rhythm and hence greater fatigue.

Accordingly, treatment of these disorders parallels the treatment of cancer-related fatigue. Patients are placed on a mild exercise regimen, if they are able, to keep them active during the daytime and thus help consolidate nocturnal sleep. Elimination of daytime naps also may help improve nocturnal sleep. The above recommendations are thought to increase a person's exposure to bright sunlight, which in itself promotes daytime alertness by activating certain centers in the brain that promote vigilance, as has been supported in animal research.[51]

Other treatment options include the use of melatonin in combination with bright-light therapy. Melatonin (5 mg) is taken at bedtime as a mild hypnotic; it must be combined with bright-light therapy because melatonin alone does not restore the circadian rhythm. Bright-light therapy attempts to promote alertness during the day and thus to adjust the patient's circadian rhythm toward appropriate nocturnal sleep. It also needs to be prescribed by a sleep medicine specialist since timing of the bright light is critical. A new pharmacologic agent, ramelteon, is a melatonin agonist that may prove to be helpful in the future; it does not yet have FDA approval in the use of circadian rhythm disorders.

Sleep-Disordered Breathing

The term *sleep-disordered breathing* refers to a spectrum of diseases that can be described as varying degrees of airway obstruction, in which increasing severity causes increased morbidity.

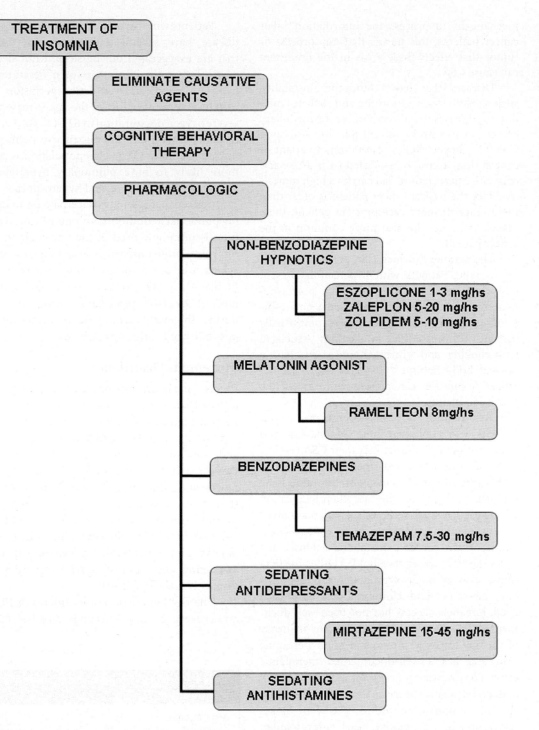

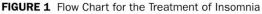

FIGURE 1 Flow Chart for the Treatment of Insomnia

These include primary snoring, upper airway resistance syndrome, obstructive sleep hypopnea syndrome, obstructive sleep apnea-hypopnea syndrome, obstructive sleep apnea (OSA) syndrome, and mixed sleep apnea syndrome. Apnea is defined as complete cessation of airflow for at least 10 seconds; the obstruction can occur anywhere from the nasal passages to the larynx.[52] A central apnea is one that has cessation of both airflow and ventilatory effort.

Obstructive Sleep Apnea Syndrome

The prevalence of OSA in the general population ranges from 2 to 9% among women and 4 to 24%

among men.[53,54] It is estimated that 80% of those with the disease have not yet been diagnosed,[53] which means that most cancer patients with OSA have not been diagnosed. Presentation of OSA includes both nocturnal and daytime symptomatology. The nighttime complaints include snoring, gasping for air, observed apneas, frequent arousals, nocturia, and palpitations; some patients with mild to moderate OSA complain of sleep maintenance insomnia. Daytime complaints include excessive daytime somnolence, decreased concentration, depression, impotence, dry mouth, morning headaches, and forgetfulness. Some patients with severe sleep-disordered

breathing may not have any complaints but are brought by family members for evaluation. Excessive daytime sleepiness can be evaluated with the Epworth Sleepiness Scale,[25] which can be used in the initial evaluation and in treatment follow-up.[55]

Although relatively few studies have described sleep-disordered breathing in those with head and neck cancer,[56] space-occupying lesions are known to impinge on the airway and cause OSA. Treatment of head and neck cancers has been associated with OSA after both radiation and resection. Radiation causes OSA through post-treatment inflammation and by scarring, although one theory postulates that scarring may actually reduce obstruction by tightening the soft tissue. One large study looked at the incidence of OSA in patients who were treated with radiation or surgical resection for head and neck cancer. Of 24 patients, 91.7% had significant OSA after treatment: 100% of the radiation group and 78.5% of the surgical resection group.[57] Mandibulectomy precipitates OSA by altering the anatomy of the skeletal structure, whereas flap procedures and rigid reconstruction of the lower jaw help prevent the development of OSA.[58] Laryngectomies have caused OSA at the reconstruction site in the postoperative setting, requiring prolonged treatment.[59] There are case reports of lymphoproliferative diseases leading to OSA, in which the apnea improves as patients receive chemotherapy.[60] The anatomy of the neck is also an important factor. A neck larger than 17 inches in a man or 16 inches in a woman is associated with OSA. More common in the head and neck cancer group is cervical kyphosis, which shortens the thyromental distance.

If sleep-disordered breathing is a diagnostic possibility in a cancer patient, then a full NPSG is indicated. Ideally, the test is performed for one full diagnostic night, and if sleep-disordered breathing is diagnosed, a second treatment night is added for titration of positive airway pressure. Alternatively, split-night polysomnography allows 2 to 4 hours for diagnosis and determination of disease severity, followed by titration of positive airway pressure.

Treatment of sleep-disordered breathing depends on its level of severity and usually requires the assistance of a sleep specialist. Control of body weight is key in an era of increasing obesity, even with cancer patients, for whom weight loss may be a distressing but inescapable subject. The avoidance of precipitating factors such as alcohol and sedating medications is also important, especially for the cancer patient, who may be tempted to increase the use of alcohol as a coping mechanism. Further, many pharmacologic agents used in this population adversely affect the upper airway. Benzodiazepines have a mixed reputation for patients with OSA: the older benzodiazepines have muscle-relaxant properties that may adversely affect the airway, whereas the newer nonbenzodiazepine hypnotics, such as zolpidem and zaleplon, do not have myorelaxant or respiratory depressant effects. Narcotics, on the other hand, have powerful respiratory depressant effects. It has been shown that a single dose of morphine 10 mg to a normal person can suppress the hypoxic and hypercapnic respiratory drives by 60% and increase arterial carbon dioxide partial pressure (Pco_2).[61] It may be difficult to avoid using these agents in a patient with cancer. Once the patient is adequately treated with positive airway pressure, however, these medications could be used with caution.

Continuous positive airway pressure (CPAP) given for OSA is delivered either by a nasal or an oral route to create a pneumatic splint for the airway.[62] If prescribed and used with close follow-up, CPAP can treat OSA with minimal side effects. It can be adjusted over time to suit a patient's changing needs and stopped at any time without untoward effect. Over the last decade, the equipment has improved exponentially. The units are small, quiet, portable, and adjustable to different altitudes. The masks are available in a number of types and styles, which is especially helpful for the head and neck cancer patient, whose anatomy may make using the older types of CPAP masks difficult. There are masks that deliver pressure either nasally or orally and heated humidifiers to help with nasal congestion. Some units can autotitrate so that the pressure will automatically adjust to the level needed by the patient. Patients who have difficulty adjusting to the amount of pressure needed to maintain an open airway can use either ramp CPAP, in which the pressure starts low and increases to therapeutic levels, or bilevel CPAP, in which the pressure at exhalation is lower than the pressure at inhalation.

For patients who have tumors causing the obstruction, CPAP is an effective means of treatment.[63] CPAP can be used by head and neck cancer patients who are awaiting surgery or who experience OSA as a result of their therapy. After resection of an obstructing tumor, polysomnography should be repeated to ensure that sleep-disordered breathing issues have been resolved.

Central Sleep Apnea

CSA is a condition in which there are repeated events of apnea with no ventilatory effort.[64] Diagnosis is also made with full NPSG. Patients with severe OSA may also have mixed apneic events with features of both CSA and OSA. The control of ventilation is a combination of metabolic and behavioral factors during wakefulness; during sleep, the control is predominantly metabolic. Ventilation is linked to input from chemoreceptors in the carotid body for hypoxemia, medullary chemoreceptors for hypercapnia, vagal intrapulmonary receptors, and brainstem

mechanisms to process the information.[65] For cancer patients, this means that any process or tumor that affects these areas in the brainstem can cause CSA.

Diseases that have autonomic instability, such as Shy-Drager syndrome and diabetes mellitus, or diseases that directly affect the medullary centers, such as stroke and encephalitis, also cause CSA.[66,67] Cheyne-Stokes respiration, a variant of central sleep apnea, is associated with stroke and congestive heart failure and carries a high mortality. Since the typical cancer patient is older than the average primary care practice patient, these disease processes are also more common in the cancer patient.

The manner in which CSA presents depends on its type. Patients with hypercapnia present with daytime somnolence, snoring, polycythemia, cor pulmonale, peripheral edema, and respiratory failure. Those with nonhypercapnia usually present with insomnia, awakenings associated with choking, and witnessed apneas and have a normal body habitus.[68] Patients with Cheyne-Stokes respiration can present with any of the above complaints.

Treatment of CSA also depends on its type. Patients with nonhypercapnic CSA have several treatment options. Sometimes their CSA resolves spontaneously, whereas at other times it improves with aggressive management of the underlying problem. If this is not the case, then medication can be tried. A small series of six patients showed improvement in hypersomnolence with acetazolamide, which causes a metabolic acidosis that shifts the Pco_2 lower threshold.[69] Other medications, such as medroxyprogesterone, theophylline, naloxone, and clomipramine, have been tried, but their success has not been well documented. Positive airway pressure is the mainstay of therapy for hypercapnic and nonhypercapnic CSA and has a well-documented therapeutic effect. For Cheyne-Stokes respiration, both CPAP and bilevel positive pressure ventilation have been shown to improve symptoms. If Cheyne-Stokes respiration in a congestive heart failure patient is treated, there is an 80% decrease in 2-year mortality.[70]

Asthma and Chronic Obstructive Pulmonary Disease

The circadian variation in airway caliber is exaggerated for those with asthma,[71] most of whom have their lowest peak flows between 10:00 pm and 8:00 am. The largest amount of REM sleep is obtained in the latter third of the rest period, and some data suggest that peak flows are lowest when subjects are awakened from REM sleep.[72] In addition to their cancer treatment, patients with asthma may also be receiving medication that decreases respiratory drive, worsens gastroesophageal reflux, or even causes bronchospasm.

Patients with chronic obstructive pulmonary disease have several pathophysiologic factors that are exaggerated during sleep. REM sleep is particularly vulnerable to oxygen desaturation, hypoventilation, and ventilation-perfusion mismatch. Hypoventilation is the main reason for severe oxygen desaturation in REM sleep. A subset of patients with chronic obstructive pulmonary disease also have OSA. This population is much more likely to have pulmonary hypertension, right-sided heart failure, and hypercapnea.[73]

Cancer therapy may exacerbate an underlying pulmonary condition. Amphotericin, an antifungal commonly used in the oncologic setting, can cause bronchospasm. Certain chemotherapy agents also are associated with bronchospasm (Table 4). When patients are receiving these medications, the physicians caring for them during the night should be prepared for the possibility of bronchoconstriction.

Movement Disorders

RLS is a persistent, uncomfortable feeling in the legs that is most noticeable when lying down to sleep at night. Patients with RLS describe a constant need to move the legs because of a "creeping and crawling" or "pins and needles" sensation that is aggravated by rest and relieved with limb movement. Although RLS typically presents with sleep-onset insomnia, it may also present with daytime somnolence since 80% of those with RLS also have PLMD, in which involuntary leg cramps or jerking movements during sleep cause frequent awakening and nonrestorative sleep. RLS is a diagnosis made by history.

The rhythmic jerking movements of PLMD occur every 20 to 40 seconds and last 0.5 to

Table 4 Oncologic Treatments Associated with Bronchospasm

Asparaginase
Mitomycin
Doxorubicin
Procarbazine
Epipodophyllotoxins
    Etoposide
    Tenoposide
Platinums
    Carboplatin
    Cisplatin
Interferons
Taxanes
    Docitaxel
    Paclitaxel
6-Mercaptopurine
Monoclonal antibodies
    Alemtuzamab
    Rituximab
Vinca alkaloids

5 seconds each. The jerking includes extension of the great toe, dorsiflexion of the ankle, and flexion of the knee and hip. It occurs more frequently in the first third of the sleep period but may last throughout the night. Seventeen percent of patients complaining of sleep maintenance insomnia and 11% of those complaining of daytime somnolence are afflicted with PLMD.[74] The frequency increases with age. Although no formal studies have evaluated the frequency of PLMD in cancer patients, one study documented an increased incidence of periodic limb movement in breast cancer patients complaining of insomnia.[8] Since the conditions associated with PLMD are found more frequently in the cancer population than the general population, however, it stands to reason that PLMD is also found more frequently among cancer patients.

PLMD is thought to be caused by a central dopamine problem. Since iron is required in the synthesis of dopamine, it makes sense that iron deficiency anemia is associated with PLMD. Other conditions associated with this condition include uremia, peripheral neuropathies, and electrolyte abnormalities. Evaluation of a person with suspected PLMD or RLS should include a check of electrolytes, including magnesium, iron, ferritin, vitamin B_{12}, and folate. PLMD is diagnosed only by NPSG; two-night NPSG is recommended.

Treatment of both RLS and PLMD focuses first on the underlying cause. Because caffeine, nicotine, fatigue, and extremes of temperatures are exacerbating factors for both RLS and PLMD, patients are first counseled to abstain from caffeine and nicotine. They are advised to do mental alerting activities during the times they normally would have symptoms. There is a circadian rhythm to these disorders in that there are several protected hours from around 5:00 to 9:00 am when patients are usually free of symptoms. If able, the patient can sleep later in the morning to obtain a full night's rest. Certain classes of medications, including serotonin reuptake inhibitors, neuroleptics, antiemetics, and antihistamines, can precipitate RLS and PLMD and may need to be limited.

Medications may be used in the treatment of RLS and PLMD (Table 5), although even these may have side effects. Augmentation is a side effect of dopaminergic agents in which symptoms worsen and require higher dosing of medications. This side effect is a particular problem for carbidopa/levodopa, which should be reserved for short-term use when there is a particular inciting event, such as a few days of bed rest in the hospital. Clonazepam is safe to use if the patient does not have a history consistent with OSA. If single agents alone are not successful, another class of agent or a combination of those listed can be tried.[75]

Other Causes of Excessive Daytime Somnolence

Somnolence syndrome, as described in the literature, is associated with hypersomnolence, extreme lethargy, and anorexia. It is seen in patients who have undergone radiation treatment of the brain and occurs as an early delayed reaction, meaning that it appears approximately 4 to 6 weeks after receiving brain irradiation, with a slow recovery.[76]

Some cancer treatment medications have somnolence as a side effect; these include narcotics, gabapentin, and seizure medications used for tumors involving the central nervous system. Specific biochemotherapeutic agents with this side effect are listed in Table 6.

A tumor involving the central nervous system can also cause hypersomnolence. Lesions in the hypothalamus or suprasellar regions can cause hypersomnia or even narcolepsy in some cases.[77] Narcolepsy is a sleep disorder that is characterized by REM sleep abnormalities with a tetrad of symptoms: hypersomnolence, cataplexy, sleep paralysis, and hypnagogic hallucinations. Diagnosing the cause of hypersomnolence requires an NPSG to evaluate for sleep-disordered breathing and PLMD. In some cases, a Multiple Sleep Latency Test is needed to evaluate for narcolepsy.

The first line of attack in treating hypersomnolence is to establish good sleep hygiene and to increase the level of daytime activity. Medications that may be causing this symptom should be limited. Stimulant medications (Table 7) may be prescribed to treat hypersomnolence not caused by sleep-disordered breathing or PLMD. The advantage of modafinil is that it is a centrally acting agent and lacks the peripheral side effects of the other stimulants. It also does not require triplicate prescriptions. There is a case report of improvement with donepezil for opioid-induced hypersomnolence.[78]

Chronobiology

The "circadian clock" that mediates sleep also plays a role in mediating hormones that influence the growth of cancer cells. For example, melatonin, which is released at the onset of darkness and triggers a temperature drop to signal sleep onset, is thought to have a mitigating effect on cancer cells. It has been found to reverse the tumorigenesis by carcinogens, to have antimitotic activity, and to modulate receptors in breast cancer cells. The addition of large doses of melatonin to chemotherapy or radiation therapy has improved survival.[79]

Conversely, the risk of developing cancer has also been linked to the circadian rhythm of hormone levels. Suppression of melatonin in those doing graveyard shift work has been associated with an increased risk of breast cancer,[80] although this is still under investigation. Also, the circadian rhythm of cortisol has also been used to predict survival in breast cancer patients as those with a flattened diurnal cortisol rhythm were found to have a higher mortality.[81] A higher amplitude in the cortisol diurnal rhythm is also associated with fewer sleep disturbances and improved quality of life.[82]

Table 6 Biochemotherapeutic Agents Associated with Somnolence

Ara-C
Alemtuzumab
Altretamine
Asparaginase
Benzamide ribose
Cladribine
Docetaxel
Interferon
Mechlorethamine
Methotrexate
Mitotane
Paclitaxel
Pentostatin
Rituximab
Thalidomide

Table 7 Stimulants for Hypersomnia

Medication	Dosing (mg daily)
Modafinil	200–400
Methylphenidate	15–100
Dextroamphetamine	15–100
Methamphetamine	15–80

Table 5 Medications for the Treatment of Restless Legs Syndrome and Periodic Limb Movement Disorder

Medication	Dosing
Pramipexole	0.125–2 mg, 2 h before bedtime
Ropinirole	0.25–2 mg, 2 h before bedtime
Carbidopa/levodopa	25/100, at bedtime
Clonazepam	0.5–2 mg at bedtime
Propoxyphene napsylate	100–200 mg
Tramadone	50–100 mg
Gabapentin	100–1,800 mg daily

Table 8 Circadian Timing of Chemotheratic Agents to Maximize Antitumor Effect and Minimize Side Effects

Agent	Administration	Circadian-Dependent Toxicities
Doxorubucin and etoposide	Midsleep	Marrow suppression, intestinal toxicity
Cisplatin and oxaliplatin	Late evening	Nephrotoxicity, marrow suppression, intestinal toxicity
5-FU and FUDR	Late evening	Leukopenia, intestinal toxicity
6-MP	Evening	Marrow suppression, intestinal toxicity
Methotrexate	evening	Marrow suppression, intestinal toxicity
Interferon	Evening	Flu-like symptoms, marrow suppression, renal and hepatic toxicity, somnolence

5-FU = 5-fluorouracil; FUDR = 5-fluorouracil deoxyribonucleoside; 6-MP = 6-mercaptopurine.

Chronotherapy

The idea of choosing a time within the circadian cycle that will maximize therapeutic effect and minimize side effects is called chronotherapy. There are circadian variations in tumor blood flow, corticosterone levels, tumor surface temperature, cell division, tumor markers, and enzyme levels.[83] There is also circadian variation in hepatic blood flow, enzymatic degradation, and elimination of drug products.[84] Because there appears to be a circadian rhythm in how tumors behave, it makes sense to tailor treatment to that rhythm. Table 8 summarizes the circadian timing of a few chemotherapeutic agents to maximize the antitumor effect and minimize side effects.[84,85]

Summary

Sleep medicine is a relatively new area of study in the field of oncology. Patients come with undiagnosed preexisting sleep disorders and develop sleep disturbances during cancer therapy. Cancer survivors also are at an increased risk of developing sleep disorders. Through the study of cancer-related sleep disturbances, we have an opportunity to improve patient outcomes and decrease the burden of symptoms. In the next few years, basic science and clinical research should bring new ways of managing our cancer patients who have sleep complaints.

REFERENCES

1. Anderson KO, Getto CJ, Mendoza TR, et al. Fatigue and sleep disturbance in patients with cancer, patients with clinical depression, and community-dwelling adults. J Pain Symptom Manage 2003;25:307–18.
2. Rosen RC, Rosekind M, Rosevear C, et al. Physician education in sleep and sleep disorders: a national survey of United States medical schools. Sleep 1993;16:249–54.
3. Sarna L. Correlates of symptom distress in women with lung cancer. Cancer Pract 1993;1:21–8.
4. Thomas C. Insomnia among individuals with cancer. Proc Oncol Nurs Soc 1986;13:63.
5. Derogatis LR, Feldstein M, Morrow G, et al. Survey of psychotropic drug prescriptions in an oncology population. Cancer 1979;44:1919–29.
6. Miaskowski C, Lee KA. Pain, fatigue, and sleep disturbances in oncology outpatients receiving radiation therapy for bone metastasis: a pilot study. J Pain Symptom Manage 1999;17:320–32.
7. Koopman C, Nouriani B, Erickson V, et al. Sleep disturbances in women with metastatic breast cancer. Breast J 2002;8:362–70.
8. Silberfarb PM, Hauri PJ, Oxman TE, Schnurr P. Assessment of sleep in patients with lung cancer and breast cancer. J Clin Oncol 1993;11:997–1004.
9. Cleeland CS, Mendoza TR, Wang XS, et al. Assessing symptom distress in cancer patients: the M. D. Anderson Symptom Inventory. Cancer 2000;89:1634–46.
10. McCorkle R. The measurement of symptom distress. Semin Oncol Nurs 1987;3:248–56.
11. Buysse DJ, Reynolds CF III, Monk TH, et al. The Pittsburgh Sleep Quality Index: a new instrument for psychiatric practice and research. Psychiatry Res 1989;28:193–213.
12. Beck SL, Schwartz AL, Towsley G, et al. Psychometric evaluation of the Pittsburgh Sleep Quality Index in cancer patients. J Pain Symptom Manage 2004;27:140–8.
13. Carpenter JS, Andrykowski MA. Psychometric evaluation of the Pittsburgh Sleep Quality Index. J Psychosom Res 1998;45:5–13.
14. Fortner BV, Stepanski EJ, Wang SC, et al. Sleep and quality of life in breast cancer patients. J Pain Symptom Manage 2002;24:471–80.
15. Owen DC, Parker KP, McGuire DB. Comparison of subjective sleep quality in patients with cancer and healthy subjects. Oncol Nurs Forum 1999;26:1649–51.
16. Hays RD, Martin SA, Sesti AM, Spritzer KL. Psychometric properties of the Medical Outcomes Study Sleep measure. Sleep Med 2005;6:41–4.
17. Hays RD, Shapiro MF. An overview of generic health-related quality of life measures for HIV research. Qual Life Res 1992;1:91–7.
18. Baumel MJ, Maislin G, Pack AI. Population and occupational screening for obstructive sleep apnea: are we there yet? Am J Respir Crit Care Med 1997;155:9–14.
19. Johns MW. Daytime sleepiness, snoring, and obstructive sleep apnea. The Epworth Sleepiness Scale. Chest 1993; 103:30–6.
20. Netzer NC, Stoohs RA, Netzer CM, et al. Using the Berlin Questionnaire to identify patients at risk for the sleep apnea syndrome. Ann Intern Med 1999;131:485–91.
21. Pradhan PS, Gliklich RE, Winkelman J. Screening for obstructive sleep apnea in patients presenting for snoring surgery. Laryngoscope 1996;106:1393–7.
22. Sadeh A, Hauri PJ, Kripke DF, Lavie P. The role of actigraphy in the evaluation of sleep disorders. Sleep 1995;18: 288–302.
23. Polysomnography Task Force, American Sleep Disorders Association Standards of Practice Committee. Practice parameters for the indications for polysomnography and related procedures. Sleep 1997;20:406–22.
24. Roth T, Drake C. Evolution of insomnia: current status and future direction. Sleep Med 2004;5 Suppl 1:S23–30.
25. Ford DE, Kamerow DB. Epidemiologic study of sleep disturbances and psychiatric disorders. An opportunity for prevention? JAMA 1989;262:1479–84.
26. Ohayon MM. Prevalence of DSM-IV diagnostic criteria of insomnia: distinguishing insomnia related to mental disorders from sleep disorders. J Psychiatr Res 1997;31: 333–46.
27. Davidson JR, MacLean AW, Brundage MD, Schulze K. Sleep disturbance in cancer patients. Soc Sci Med 2002;54: 1309–21.
28. Savard J, Simard S, Blanchet J, et al. Prevalence, clinical characteristics, and risk factors for insomnia in the context of breast cancer. Sleep 2001;24:583–90.

29. Engstrom CA, Strohl RA, Rose L, et al. Sleep alterations in cancer patients. Cancer Nurs 1999;22:143–8.
30. Chesson A Jr, Hartse K, Anderson WM, et al. Practice parameters for the evaluation of chronic insomnia. An American Academy of Sleep Medicine report. Standards of Practice Committee of the American Academy of Sleep Medicine. Sleep 2000;23:237–41.
31. Cleeland CS, Gonin R, Hatfield AK, et al. Pain and its treatment in outpatients with metastatic cancer. N Engl J Med 1994;330:592–6.
32. Gaston-Johansson F, Fall Dickson JM, Bakos AB, Kennedy MJ. Fatigue, pain, and depression in pre-autotransplant breast cancer patients. Cancer Pract 1999;7:240–7.
33. Grond S, Zech D, Diefenbach C, Bischoff A. Prevalence and pattern of symptoms in patients with cancer pain: a prospective evaluation of 1635 cancer patients referred to a pain clinic. J Pain Symptom Manage 1994;9:272–83.
34. Portenoy RK, Miransky J, Thaler HT, et al. Pain in ambulatory patients with lung or colon cancer. Cancer 1992; 70:1616–24.
35. Strang P. Emotional and social aspects of cancer pain. Acta Oncol 1992;31:323–6.
36. Derogatis LR, Morrow GR, Fetting J, et al. The prevalence of psychiatric disorders among cancer patients. JAMA 1983;249:751–7.
37. Massie MJ, Popkin MK. Depressive disorders. In: Holland JC, editor. Psycho-oncology. New York: Oxford University Press; 1998. p. 518–40.
38. Ginsburg ML, Quirt C, Ginsburg AD, Mackillop WJ. Psychiatric illness and psychosocial concerns of patients with newly diagnosed lung cancer. CMAJ 1995;152:701–8.
39. Morin CM, Culbert JP, Schwartz SM. Nonpharmacological interventions for insomnia: a meta-analysis of treatment efficacy. Am J Psychiatry 1994;151:1172–80.
40. Murtagh DR, Greenwood KM. Identifying effective psychological treatments for insomnia: a meta-analysis. J Consult Clin Psychol 1995;63:79–89.
41. Nowell PD, Mazumdar S, Buysse DJ et al. Benzodiazepines and zolpidem for chronic insomnia: a meta-analysis of treatment efficacy. JAMA 1997;278:2170–7.
42. Davidson JR, Waisberg JL, Brundage MD, MacLean AW. Nonpharmacologic group treatment of insomnia: a preliminary study with cancer survivors. Psychooncology 2001;10:389–97.
43. Shapiro SL, Bootzin RR, Figueredo AJ, et al. The efficacy of mindfulness-based stress reduction in the treatment of sleep disturbance in women with breast cancer: an exploratory study. J Psychosom Res 2003;54:85–91.
44. Simeit R, Deck R, Conta-Marx B. Sleep management training for cancer patients with insomnia. Support Care Cancer. 2004;12:176–83.
45. Ralph MR, Foster RG, Davis FC, Menaker M. Transplanted suprachiasmatic nucleus determines circadian period. Science 1990;247:975–8.
46. Regestein QR, Monk TH. Delayed sleep phase syndrome: a review of its clinical aspects. Am J Psychiatry 1995;152: 602–8.
47. Berger AM. Patterns of fatigue and activity and rest during adjuvant breast cancer chemotherapy. Oncol Nurs Forum 1998;25:51–62.
48. Mormont MC, dePrins J, Levi F. Assessment of activity circadian rhythms by wrist actigraphy: preliminary results in 30 patients with colorectal cancer. Pathol Biol (Paris) 1996;44:165–71.
49. Brown AC, Smolensky MH, Dalonzo GE, Redman DP. Actigraphy: a means of assessing circadian patterns in human activity. Chronobiol Int 1990;7:125–33.
50. Rosen GM, Bendel AE, Neglia JP, et al. Sleep in children with neoplasms of the central nervous system: case review of 14 children. Pediatrics 2003;112:E46–54.
51. Edgar DM, Dement WC, Fuller CA. Effect of SCN lesions on sleep in squirrel monkeys: evidence for opponent processes in sleep-wake regulation. J Neurosci 1993;13: 1065–79.
52. Chua W, Chediak AD. Obstructive sleep apnea: treatment improves quality of life—and may prevent death. Postgrad Med 1994;95:123–8.
53. Young T, Evans L, Finn L, Palta M. Estimation of the clinically diagnosed proportion of sleep apnea syndrome in middle-aged men and women. Sleep 1997;20:705–6.
54. Young T, Palta M, Dempsey J, et al. The occurrence of sleep-disordered breathing among middle-aged adults. N Engl J Med 1993;328:1230–5.
55. Johns MW. A new method for measuring daytime sleepiness: the Epworth Sleepiness Scale. Sleep 1991;14:540–5.

56. Hoijer U, Ejnell H, Hedner J. Obstructive sleep apnea in patients with pharyngeal tumours. Acta Otolaryngol (Stockh) 1992;112:138–43.

57. Friedman M, Landsberg R, Pryor S, et al. The occurrence of sleep-disordered breathing among patients with head and neck cancer. Laryngoscope 2001;111:1917–9.

58. Panje WR, Holmes DK. Mandibulectomy without reconstruction can cause sleep apnea. Laryngoscope 1984;94: 1591–4.

59. Rombaux P, Hamoir M, Plouin-Gaudon I, et al. Obstructive sleep apnea syndrome after reconstructive laryngectomy for glottic carcinoma. Eur Arch Otorhinolaryngol 2000; 257:502–6.

60. Chehal A, Haidar JH, Jabbour R, et al. Obstructive sleep apnea secondary to chronic lymphocytic leukemia. Ann Oncol 2002;13:1833.

61. Weil JV, McCullough RE, Kline JS, Sodal IE. Diminished ventilatory response to hypoxia and hypercapnia after morphine in normal man. N Engl J Med 1975;292: 1103–6.

62. Sullivan CE, Berthonjones M, Issa FG, Eves L. Reversal of obstructive sleep apnea by continuous positive airway pressure applied through the nares. Lancet 1981;1:862–5.

63. Kimura K, Adlakha A, Staats BA, Shepard JW. Successful treatment of obstructive sleep apnea with use of nasal continuous positive airway pressure in three patients with mucosal hemangiomas of the oral cavity. Mayo Clin Proc 1999;74:155–8.

64. Guilleminault C, Stoohs R, Schneider H, et al. Central alveolar hypoventilation and sleep: treatment by intermittent positive-pressure ventilation through nasal mask in an adult. Chest 1989;96:1210–2.

65. Sullivan CE, Kozar LF, Murphy E, Phillipson EA. Primary role of respiratory afferents in sustaining breathing rhythm. J Appl Physiol 1978;45:11–7.

66. Guilleminault C, Briskin JG, Greenfield MS, Silvestri R. The impact of autonomic nervous-system dysfunction on breathing during sleep. Sleep 1981;4:263–78.

67. White D, Miller F, Erickson R. Sleep apnea and nocturnal hypoventilation following western equine encephalitis. Am Rev Respir Dis 1983;127:132–3.

68. White DP. Central sleep apnea. In: Kryger MH, Roth T, Dement WC, editors. Principles and practice of sleep medicine. Philadelphia: Saunders; 2000. p. 827–39.

69. White DP, Zwillich CW, Pickett CK, et al. Central sleep apnea: improvement with acetazolamide therapy. Arch Intern Med 1982;142:1816–9.

70. Sin DD, Logan AG, Fitzgerald FS, et al. Effects of continuous positive airway pressure on cardiovascular outcomes in heart failure patients with and without Cheyne-Stokes respiration. Circulation 2000;102:61–6.

71. Hetzel MR, Clark TJH. Comparison of normal and asthmatic circadian rhythms in peak expiratory flow rate. Thorax 1980;35:732–8.

72. Shapiro CM, Catterall JR, Montgomery I, et al. Do asthmatics suffer bronchoconstriction during rapid-eye-movement sleep? Br Med J 1986;292:1161–4.

73. Bradley TD, Rutherford R, Grossman RF, et al. Role of daytime hypoxemia in the pathogenesis of right heart failure in the obstructive sleep apnea syndrome. Am Rev Respir Dis 1985;131:835–9.

74. Coleman RM, Pollak CP, Weitzman ED. Periodic movements in sleep nocturnal myoclonus: relation to sleep disorders. Ann Neurol 1980;8:416–21.

75. Silber MH, Ehrenberg BL, Allen RP, et al. An algorithm for the management of restless legs syndrome. Mayo Clin Proc 2004;79:916–22.

76. Faithfull S. Patients' experiences following cranial radiotherapy: a study of the somnolence syndrome. J Adv Nurs 1991;16:939–46.

77. Marcus CL, Trescher WH, Halbower AC, Lutz J. Secondary narcolepsy in children with brain tumors. Sleep 2002;25:435–9.

78. Bruera E, Strasser F, Shen L, et al. The effect of donepezil on sedation and other symptoms in patients receiving opioids for cancer pain: a pilot study. J Pain Symptom Manage 2003;26:1049–54.

79. Epstein FH. Mechanisms of disease: melatonin in humans. N Engl J Med 1997;336:186–95.

80. Davis S, Mirick DK, Stevens RG. Night shift work, light at night, and risk of breast cancer. J Natl Cancer Inst 2001;93:1557–62.

81. Sephton SE, Sapolsky RM, Kraemer HC, Spiegel D. Diurnal cortisol rhythm as a predictor of breast cancer. J Natl Cancer Inst 2002;94:532–3.

82. Mormont MC, Waterhouse J, Bleuzen P, et al. Marked 24-h rest/activity rhythms are associated with better quality of life, better response, and longer survival in patients with metastatic colorectal cancer and good performance status. Clin Cancer Res 2000;6:3038–45.

83. Mormont MC, Levi F. Circadian system alterations during cancer processes: a review. Int J Cancer 1997;70:241–7.

84. Wood PA, Hrushesky WJM. Circadian rhythms and cancer chemotherapy. Crit Rev Eukaryot Gene Expr 1996;6: 299–343.

85. Hrushesky WJM, Martynowicz M, Markiewicz M, et al. Chronotherapy of cancer: a major drug-delivery challenge. Adv Drug Deliv Rev 1992;9:1–83.

Nausea

John T. Patlan, MD

Nausea and vomiting, which are very common problems in cancer patients, may be due to the cancer itself or, quite often, the side effects of chemotherapy or radiotherapy. Nausea can be extremely debilitating and distressing and can significantly interfere with patients' quality of life. Patients rank nausea and vomiting among the most disturbing side effects of cancer therapy. Approximately 75% of cancer patients who receive chemotherapy experience treatment-induced nausea and vomiting; of these, 46% have thought about stopping their treatment.[1] Up to 50% of people with cancer may actually refuse or delay chemotherapy because they are afraid of the nausea and vomiting it may cause.[2] Even in the era of effective and well-tolerated antiemetics, patients still rank nausea and vomiting among the most significant adverse effects of cancer treatment.[3,4]

Clinical Manifestations

Nausea is difficult for some patients to describe, but clinicians define it as the unpleasant subjective sensation of being about to vomit or feeling a need to vomit. Nausea can occur alone or with vomiting (emesis), the forceful oral expulsion of gastric contents resulting from contractions of the gut and abdominal wall musculature, or with retching, the same forceful contractions without expulsion of upper gastrointestinal contents. It should be distinguished from regurgitation, the effortless passage of gastric or esophageal contents to the hypopharynx, which may be accompanied by rumination, or rechewing and reswallowing of these contents.[5]

Nausea often lasts longer than vomiting and may therefore be more distressing to patients and contribute to the cachexia seen in many cancer patients. In addition, vomiting or retching may exacerbate cancer-related headache or pain in the abdomen or back.

Protracted nausea and vomiting may also produce a number of complications, most often metabolic disturbances such as hypovolemia, hyponatremia, hypokalemia, hypochloremic metabolic alkalosis, and, importantly, malnutrition and failure to thrive owing to decreased caloric intake. Occasionally, forceful vomiting may cause gastrointestinal bleeding owing to esophageal Mallory-Weiss tears or esophageal rupture (Boerhaave's syndrome).

In addition, protracted nausea and vomiting and the subsequent malnutrition and electrolyte disturbances can lead to a decline in functional status, diminished cognitive ability, poor wound healing or dehiscence, and, as previously mentioned, withdrawal from potentially curative cancer therapy.

Pathophysiology

Nausea

The mechanisms of nausea are not well understood, but because it is a conscious perception and because some patients develop anticipatory nausea before chemotherapy, the development of nausea likely requires cerebral cortical mediation. Studies of induced motion sickness in humans have shown that the perception of nausea followed and was proportional to abnormal gastric myoelectric activity.[6]

Vomiting

The coordinated and stereotypic actions of vomiting are better understood. Pioneering studies by Borison and Wang in the 1950s identified two areas in the brainstem that control the emetic reflex.[7]

Emetic Center

Originally conceived as a single locus in the medullary reticular formation, the "vomiting center" is now recognized to consist of multiple parts. Several anatomically separate receptor and effector brainstem nuclei, most in the nucleus tractus solitarius, receive afferent input from a variety of sources and coordinate the efferent pathways associated with the act of vomiting (including the contraction of thoracic and abdominal wall muscles to produce high intra-thoracic and intra-abdominal pressures to propel the expulsion of gastric contents, the herniation of the gastric cardia across the diaphragm, and the upward movement of the larynx to promote oral propulsion of the vomitus). The emetic center is the final common pathway by which a variety of afferent stimuli can initiate vomiting.[8,9]

Chemoreceptor Trigger Zone

Located in the area postrema on the floor of the fourth ventricle, outside the blood-brain barrier, the chemoreceptor trigger zone (CTZ) is responsive to various chemical stimuli from the bloodstream and the cerebrospinal fluid. A number of metabolic derangements (such as uremia and diabetic ketoacidosis) and drugs (such as opiates, digitalis, and syrup of ipecac) stimulate the CTZ to cause vomiting. The CTZ is a major source of afferent input to the emetic center and an important site for a number of neurotransmitter receptors, as discussed below, which have provided targets for the development of antiemetic agents.[10]

Other sources of afferent input to the emetic center include higher brainstem and cortical structures. Input from the hypopharynx and the gastrointestinal tract is conveyed by the vagus and splanchnic nerves. Figure 1 shows the pathways by which chemotherapeutic drugs or other emetogenic stimuli may induce emesis.

A number of neurotransmitter receptors are found in the CTZ, the emetic center, and the gastrointestinal tract, and these receptors may play a role in stimulating vomiting. The three most clinically relevant neurotransmitters and their receptors are dopamine (D_2 receptors), serotonin or 5-hydroxytryptamine (5-HT_3 receptors), and substance P or neurokinin 1 (NK_1 receptors).

Medications designed to antagonize these neurotransmitters have been the major focus of the development of antiemetics, first with the development of antidopaminergic medications in the 1960s.[11] The relatively low efficacy and unfavorable side-effect profile (hypotension and extrapyramidal syndromes) of the antidopaminergic phenothiazines led to the search for other antiemetics. The development of high-dose metoclopramide improved the efficacy of nausea control but raised some questions. Since metoclopramide binds with high affinity to dopamine receptors, it appeared that low doses would saturate the available receptors. A new mechanism of action was postulated when it was discovered that metoclopramide blocks 5-HT_3 receptors, but with less affinity than D_2 receptors. This discovery led to the development of highly selective 5-HT_3 antagonists in the 1980s and 1990s.[12] Because of

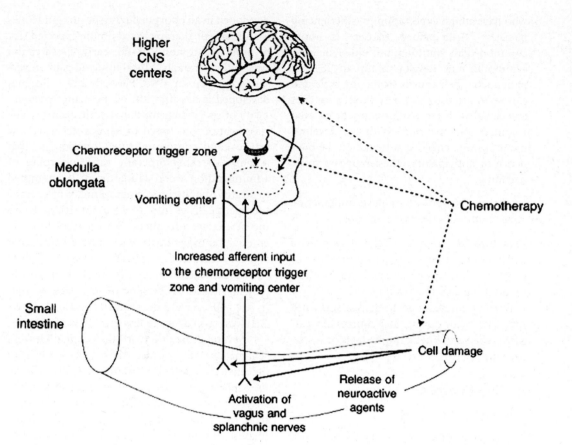

FIGURE 1 Chemotherapeutic agents may induce vomiting through cytotoxic effects in the gastrointestinal tract and stimulating vagal and splanchnic afferents, through direct effects on the chemoreceptor trigger zone, or through higher cortical responses (conditioned responses such as anticipatory nausea). Reproduced with permission from Grunberg SM, Hesketh PJ. Drug therapy: control of chemotherapy-induced emesis. N Engl J Med 1993;329:1790. CNS = central nervous system.

their efficacy and favorable side-effect profile, 5-HT$_3$ receptor antagonists have become the mainstay of antiemetic therapy for cancer patients. It was hypothesized that chemotherapy-induced emesis is mediated by serotonin itself and that chemotherapy may stimulate the liberation of endogenous serotonin from the small bowel, which might directly stimulate central nervous system 5-HT$_3$ receptors or act through vagal mediation to cause emesis. But the fact that 5-HT$_3$ antagonists at high doses cannot completely block emesis and the fact that nausea and vomiting are not prominent symptoms in carcinoid syndrome, where serotonin levels (as measured by 5-hydroxyindoleacetic acid excretion) are very high, led to the search for greater understanding of the neuropharmacology of emesis.[13] More recently, antagonists of substance P, which exerts its emetogenic effect by binding to the NK$_1$ receptor, have been shown to be potent antiemetics.[14] Other neuroreceptors in the central nervous system or vestibular system that may stimulate vomiting include the muscarinic acetylcholine receptors and receptors to corticosteroids, histamine, cannabinoids, and opiates.[15] Of these receptors, M$_1$ muscarinic antagonists (such as

scopolamine) and H$_1$ antihistamines (such as diphenhydramine or meclizine) are most useful in treating or preventing motion sickness but have limited utility in the treatment of cancer-related nausea and vomiting.

Etiology

Gastrointestinal Disorders

Cancer patients may experience nausea and vomiting owing to the same causes as any other patient would, and it should never be assumed that these symptoms are due to the cancer or its treatment. Gastroenteritis, biliary colic or acute cholecystitis, acute or chronic pancreatitis, and acute hepatitis are among the primary gastrointestinal disorders that may cause nausea and vomiting. In addition, patients may experience gastroparesis that is tumor induced or is secondary to medications (such as opiates) or some chemotherapeutic agents (such as vincristine).

Metabolic Causes

The metabolic causes of nausea and vomiting, which may merit special concern in cancer patients, include adrenal insufficiency owing to

metastatic involvement of the adrenal glands or to the use of corticosteroids in chemotherapeutic regimens. Uremia due to bilateral ureteral obstruction in pelvic tumors or to nephrotoxic agents may also occur. Hypercalcemia owing to osseous metastases or as a paraneoplastic syndrome is quite common and should be considered.

Medications

The side effects of nonchemotherapeutic medications may induce nausea and vomiting. Many antibiotics, digoxin, and oral contraceptives are associated with nausea. Because many cancer patients require regular use of narcotic analgesics for control of cancer-related pain, this class of medications deserves special mention. Any narcotic medication may induce nausea and should be suspected if the onset of symptoms coincides with the start of a new narcotic regimen. In addition, because narcotics slow gastrointestinal motility, they may cause constipation, adynamic ileus, or even colonic pseudo-obstruction.

Tumor Effects

The direct effects of tumors include nausea and vomiting. These symptoms may be a prominent feature of primary gastrointestinal cancers, such as esophageal, gastric, or colorectal malignancies. These symptoms can also occur by direct tumor extension or because of abdominal or peritoneal metastases of nongastrointestinal cancers. Nausea and vomiting can be due to mass effect and may be the presenting symptom of partial or complete bowel obstruction. In patients for whom metastatic disease is highly suspicious, brain metastases should always be considered, particularly if no other apparent gastrointestinal, metabolic, or medication-related cause is present.

Treatment-Related Causes

Radiotherapy

Nausea and vomiting after radiotherapy are fairly common but are less well understood than chemotherapy-induced emesis. Radiotherapy-induced emesis seems to be multifactorial and is related to the site treated, the size of the radiation field and dose delivered, overall patient metabolic status, concomitant use of chemotherapy (such as cisplatin in many head and neck malignancies), and other factors.

The cumulative incidence of radiotherapy-induced nausea and vomiting is about 33%.[16] The highest risk appears to be for patients who receive total-body, half-body, or abdominal radiotherapy. In patients who receive conventional fractionated radiotherapy (200 cGy per fraction) to the upper abdomen, half will experience radiation-induced nausea and vomiting within 2 to 3 weeks. It occurs more quickly and in more than 90% of patients who receive total-body irradiation before bone marrow transplantation.[17]

Chemotherapy

Chemotherapy-induced emesis is much better studied. Three distinct phases or patterns of chemotherapy-induced emesis have been identified:

1. Acute-onset emesis most commonly begins within 1 to 2 hours, peaks in the first 4 to 6 hours, and resolves within the first 24 hours. Exceptions to this temporal pattern include carboplatin and cyclophosphamide, which tend to cause later onset of nausea and vomiting in patients not given antiemetics, as late as 9 to 18 hours after chemotherapy. Acute emesis is the best studied and understood of the three emetic syndromes.
2. Delayed-onset emesis is somewhat arbitrarily defined as nausea and vomiting that occur more than 24 hours after chemotherapy. It was first recognized as a problem after effective antiemetics for acute emesis were developed but nausea and vomiting persisted for several days in some patients. This syndrome commonly develops after high-dose cisplatin but can also occur with carboplatin, cyclophosphamide, or doxorubicin.[18] Delayed emesis after cisplatin generally reaches maximal severity at 48 to 72 hours and then gradually subsides, and it can last 5 to 6 days. It is generally less severe than acute emesis and is not considered just a deferral of symptom onset.[19] Different patterns of vomiting beyond the initial period have been observed. In one study of patients treated with cisplatin who received metoclopramide, ondansetron, or placebo, there were two peak incidences of emesis, at 4 hours and 18 hours, with little vomiting between them, suggesting a bimodal incidence of vomiting.[18] In a later study of patients treated with high-dose cisplatin who received dexamethasone and serotonin antagonist antiemetics, there was a uniform distribution of vomiting during the study period.[20] Some authors have suggested reserving the term *delayed emesis* for the biphasic pattern of emesis after cisplatin therapy and using the term *prolonged emesis* for the late nausea and vomiting that occur after noncisplatin chemotherapy.[21]
3. Anticipatory emesis is defined as nausea or vomiting that begins before the administration of chemotherapy. It is believed to be a learned or conditioned response in patients who have had poor nausea control and acute or delayed emesis during previous chemotherapy. It has even been described in patients who have not yet received chemotherapy but who have a high expectation of experiencing nausea.[22] Anticipatory nausea is more common than vomiting, but either or both symptoms may develop in up to 25% of patients by their fourth treatment cycle and can be induced by a variety of sensory cues associated with receiving treatment or even cognitive anticipation.[23] With the development of more effective antiemetics, the incidence of anticipatory emesis appears to be declining.[23]

In the current era of modern antiemetics, two other syndromes deserve mention:

- Breakthrough emesis is defined as nausea and vomiting that occur despite the use of prophylactic treatment. Breakthrough emesis requires "rescue" medications.
- Refractory emesis refers to nausea and vomiting that occur during later courses of treatment when antiemetic prophylaxis or rescue has failed in earlier cycles.[24]

Predictive Factors

Patient-Related Factors

Some patient-related factors associated with increased risk of chemotherapy-induced nausea and vomiting are female gender, younger age, and a history of chemotherapy. A history of chronic heavy alcohol consumption seems to confer a lower risk of treatment-induced nausea.[25] This history may include a previous rather than a current history of high alcohol use, but a history of high alcohol use (eg, more than 100 g of alcohol or five mixed drinks per day for several years) seems to confer a lower risk of chemotherapy-induced emesis. Preexisting nausea and a low functional status or high fatigue score also seem to be correlated with a higher risk of nausea and vomiting.[26] If patients experienced nausea with previous chemotherapy, they are at higher risk of chemotherapy-induced emesis than treatment-naive patients are. Conversely, among patients who received prior chemotherapy but did not experience nausea or vomiting, the majority will remain free of chemotherapy-induced emesis during later treatments.[27] Anticipatory emesis occurs in patients who have had poorly controlled acute or delayed emesis and may be more likely to develop in patients who have a history of motion sickness.[28]

Acute Emesis

A number of treatment-related factors have been associated with the development of acute emesis, including chemotherapy dosage and the route and rate of administration.[29] But the most important factor by far is the intrinsic emetogenic potential of the specific chemotherapeutic agent. Several classification schemes have been developed in an effort to devise specific guidelines for antiemetic therapy based on the expected risk of emesis, but none of the early classification systems had enough clinical utility to gain universal acceptance. In 1997, Hesketh and colleagues developed a classification of the acute emetogenicity of specific chemotherapeutic agents.[30] The classification was based on clinical trials, review articles, and consensus expert opinion. In that scheme, the chemotherapy rate and route of administration were standardized. It attempted to stratify the intrinsic emetogenicity of chemotherapeutic drugs into five levels of risk based on the percentage of patients who developed acute emesis after receiving the chemotherapeutic agent and no antiemetic prophylaxis. Level 5 (highest risk) drugs caused emesis in more than 90% of patients, level 4 drugs in 60 to 90%, level 3 drugs in 30 to 60%, level 2 drugs in 10 to 30%, and level 1 (lowest risk) drugs in less than 10% of patients.

Several difficulties with the original Hesketh schema existed. Because of the relative lack of objective data, the classification relied heavily on the expert opinion of the authors. In addition, the scheme focused on acute emesis. Research studies tend to divide emesis into acute and delayed phases, but in clinical practice and from the patient's perspective, nausea and vomiting tend to occur on a continuum for several days after chemotherapy. Finally, with the growing use of oral cytotoxic agents for a period of days or weeks, the concept of acute versus delayed emesis loses some clinical relevance.

Consequently, in an effort to simplify the classification scheme and make it more straightforward and easier to use by practitioners in the everyday clinical setting, a new scheme was devised. It encompasses both the acute and the delayed risk of emesis owing to chemotherapy and the emetogenic potential of single oral chemotherapeutic agents (Table 1).

There is also a system with which to assess the emetic risk of combination chemotherapy. Hesketh and colleagues proposed an algorithm for assessing the relative contribution of combination therapy (Table 2).[30]

Delayed Emesis

The phenomenon of delayed emesis is less well studied and less well understood than acute emesis for several reasons: it is generally less severe than acute emesis, and it tends to occur when patients have left the clinic and are no longer being observed by their treating oncologist. Even experienced oncologists and oncology nurses tend to underestimate the incidence of delayed nausea after patients have left the hospital or clinic and are no longer directly observable.[4] Because cisplatin is so highly emetogenic and the risk of delayed emesis is highest with this drug than any other, most studies on delayed emesis

Table 1

High-risk drugs (level 5: > 90% frequency of emesis)
- Carmustine (> 250 mg/m^2)
- Cisplatin (> 50 mg/m^2)
- Cyclophosphamide (> 1,500 mg/m^2)
- Dacarbazine
- Dactinomycin
- Lomustine (> 60 mg/m^2)
- Mechlorethamine
- Streptozocin

Moderate-risk drugs (levels 3–4: 30–90% frequency of emesis)
- Amifostine (> 500 mg/m^2)
- Arsenic trioxide
- Busulfan (> 4 mg/d)
- Carboplatin
- Carmustine (< 250 mg/m^2)
- Cisplatin (< 50 mg/m^2)
- Cyclophosphamide (PO or < 1,500 mg/m^2)
- Cytarabine (> 1 g/m^2)
- Dactinomycin
- Doxorubicin
- Epirubicin
- Hexamethylmelamine (PO)
- Idarubicin
- Ifosfamide
- Interleukin-2 (> 12–15 million U/m^2)
- Irinotecan
- Melphalan (> 50 mg/m^2)
- Methotrexate (250–1,000 mg/m^2)
- Mitoxantrone (> 12 mg/m^2)
- Oxaliplatin (> 7 5mg/m^2)
- Procarbazine (PO)

Low-risk drugs (level 2: 10–30% frequency of emesis)
- Amifostine (< 300 mg/m^2)
- Asparaginase
- Bexarotene
- Capecitabine
- Cytarabine (100–200 mg/m^2)
- Docetaxel
- Doxorubicin (< 250 mg/m^2)
- Etoposide
- 5-Fluorouracil
- Gemcitabine
- Methotrexate (50–250 mg/m^2)
- Mitomycin
- Paclitaxel
- Pemetrexed
- Temozolomide
- Thiotepa
- Topotecan

Minimal-risk drugs (level 1: < 10% frequency of emesis)
- Alemtuzumab
- Bevacizumab
- Bleomycin
- Bortezomib
- Cetuximab
- Chlorambucil (PO)
- Cladribine
- Denileukin diftitox
- Dexrazoxane

Table 1 (Continued)

- Fludarabine
- Gefitinib
- Gemtuzumab ozogamicin
- Hydroxyurea
- Imatinib mesylate
- α-Interferon

- Melphalan (oral low dose)
- Methotrexate (< 50 mg/m^2)
- Pentostatin
- Rituximab
- Thioguanine (PO)
- Trastuzumab
- Valrubicin
- Vinblastine
- Vincristine
- Vinorelbine

Adapted from Koeller JM, et al. Antiemetic guidelines: creating a more practical treatment approach. Support Care Cancer 2002;10:519–22).
PO = orally.

Table 2 Combination Chemotherapy Algorithm

1. Identify the most emetogenic agent in the combination.
2. Assess the relative contribution of other agents to the emetic potential of the combination. When considering other agents, the following rules apply:
   a. Level 1 agents do not contribute to the emetogenicity of the regimen.
   b. Adding one or more level 2 agents increases the emetogenicity of the combination by one level greater than the most emetogenic agent in the combination.
   c. Adding level 3 or 4 agents increases the emetogenicity of the combination by one level per agent.

Adapted from Hesketh PJ, et al.[32]

have been done with patients treated with cisplatin-containing regimens. Without antiemetic pretreatment, the incidence of delayed emesis owing to cisplatin was between 60 and 90%. In these studies, the most significant risk factor for delayed emesis was a lack of emetic control during the first 24 hours.[31] In patients followed for three cycles of treatment, the rate of delayed vomiting in each cycle was related to the degree of control of acute emesis in the first 24 hours. The dose of cisplatin was also an important prognostic factor: patients who received less than 90 mg/m^2 had a 19 to 22% incidence of emesis, whereas patients who received more than 90 mg/m^2 had an incidence of 43 to 47%.[31]

Patients who receive moderately emetogenic chemotherapy are also at risk of delayed emesis. In a study of patients who received carboplatin, cyclophosphamide, doxorubicin, or epirubicin but no antiemetic prophylaxis after the first 24 hours, the incidence of delayed nausea and vomiting was 20 to 25%.[32] In these patients, as in cisplatin-treated patients, the most important prognostic factor was receiving effective antiemetic prophylaxis during the first 24 hours. In patients who had ineffective control and experienced acute nausea and vomiting after moderately emetogenic chemotherapy, the rate of delayed nausea and vomiting was 55 to 75%.[32]

Anticipatory Emesis

As described above, anticipatory emesis is usually a conditioned response in patients who have experienced nausea and vomiting with previous chemotherapy cycles. A number of studies have concluded that classic or Pavlovian conditioning contributes to the development of anticipatory emesis in cancer patients.[33] One of the most important prognostic factors, then, is the development of nausea and vomiting after previous chemotherapy. Other risk factors are age less than 50 years; "moderate, severe, or intolerable" nausea after the last cycle; a side effect of treatment as feeling "warm or hot all over"; susceptibility to motion sickness; diaphoresis with the previous cycle; and "generalized weakness" with the previous cycle.[34]

Diagnosis

The diagnosis of chemotherapy- or radiotherapy-induced emesis can usually be readily established by the appropriate history of recent treatment and the appropriate temporal relationship to the onset of symptoms. The caveat, of course, is that treatment-related nausea and vomiting are essentially a diagnosis of exclusion. Consideration should always be given to other non–treatment-related causes of nausea, and some screening by history and physical examination is essential to reasonably exclude other, potentially more serious or otherwise treatable conditions that occur with nausea.

Patients with prominent abdominal pain require some investigation for primary intra-abdominal causes of nausea, such as acute pancreatitis or renal or biliary colic. If there is abdominal distention along with pain, evaluation for partial or complete bowel obstruction is required.

Vomiting in a febrile patient may be a nonspecific symptom related to sepsis or, if it is accompanied by abdominal tenderness or signs of peritoneal irritation, suggests serious abdominal pathology (such as bowel perforation or acute appendicitis). Thorough evaluation, including surgical consultation, would be indicated.

Vomiting that is persistent but not in the time period expected in relation to chemotherapy or radiotherapy suggests some other cause, perhaps electrolyte disturbance (such as hypercalcemia) or cerebral metastases. A higher clinical suspicion for a central nervous system cause of nausea should exist, especially if there is headache, any neurologic signs or symptoms, or projectile or positional vomiting.

In addition to a history and a physical examination, an evaluation of serum chemistries in a patient with persistent vomiting is generally indicated to look for electrolyte disturbances, either as a cause or an effect of the vomiting. Obtaining plain radiographs, usually an abdominal series, is a good starting point if there is significant abdominal pain or distention to look for bowel obstruction or evidence of perforation.

Computed tomographic scans of the abdomen or brain should be obtained if there is sufficient suspicion of serious abdominal or central nervous system pathology as the cause of vomiting.

Treatment

Serotonin (5-HT$_3$) Receptor Antagonists

5-HT$_3$ receptor antagonists are the mainstay of therapy for the prevention and treatment of acute emesis in patients who receive high- or moderate-risk chemotherapy. In the 1980s, such patients were treated with high-dose metoclopramide usually along with steroids, which had between 40 and 60% efficacy in preventing emesis. Specific 5-HT$_3$ receptor antagonists developed later were more effective as single agents than high-dose metoclopramide and more effective when given with dexamethasone than was the combination of metoclopramide and steroids.[35] In addition to increased efficacy, 5-HT$_3$ receptor antagonists may be administered orally or intravenously, and they have a much lower incidence of unfavorable side effects. In the United States, currently four serotonin antagonists are approved for use: ondansetron (Zofran), granisetron (Kytril), dolasetron (Anzemet), and the newest member of the class, palonosetron (Aloxi).

Regarding the first three of those serotonin antagonists, a number of comparative trials have been performed. These trials have failed to show any clinically significant differences between them when used at appropriate doses.[36,37] In general, the 5-HT$_3$ antagonists are equally efficacious and have favorable side-effect profiles. The relatively mild side effects include headache in 15 to 20% of patients, asthenia and constipation in 5 to 10%, and dizziness in 5 to 10%.[38] There may also be mild transient elevation in transaminases or prolongation of cardiac intervals. Importantly, the extrapyramidal symptoms (such as dystonic reactions or akathisia) and limiting side effects of older antiemetics do not occur, even with

multiple doses on subsequent days.

Several clinically important points in the use of these drugs should be noted. First, they have good bioavailability (50–80%) and good oral absorption.[39] Oral administration appears to be as effective as intravenous administration in preventing emesis.[38] Oral administration may be particularly useful because there are so many 5-HT$_3$ receptors in the enterochromaffin cells in the gastrointestinal tract, which may be involved in stimulating nausea. Second, a single dose given before chemotherapy is as effective as multiple doses in preventing emesis.[40,41] For both oral and intravenous administration of serotonin antagonists, efficacy is increased when they are used with corticosteroids.[42] Finally, for each of the serotonin antagonists, there is a plateau of efficacy at a given dose level, beyond which increased dosing does not yield any clinical benefit, presumably because the relevant receptors are saturated.[39]

Palonosetron is pharmacologically distinct from the other three 5-HT$_3$ receptor antagonists and may offer some clinical advantages over them. It has an approximately 100-fold higher binding affinity for the 5-HT$_3$ receptor and a longer half-life (approximately 40 hours). In two studies, it was shown to have greater control of emesis in patients who received moderately emetogenic chemotherapy than did ondansetron or dolasetron when used as single agents.[43] In one study, a single dose of intravenous palonosetron was equivalent to a single dose of dolasetron in preventing acute emesis but was superior to dolasetron in preventing delayed chemotherapy-induced nausea and vomiting, perhaps because of the longer half-life.[44] In these trials, no significant differences in efficacy were found between the 0.25 and 0.75 mg doses of palonosetron. The drug was approved for use in the United States in 2003 with a recommended dose of 0.25 mg intravenously 30 minutes before the start of chemotherapy. Because of the long half-life, lack of additional benefit with a higher dose, and lack of safety or efficacy data with serial administration, repeated dosing within 7 days is not recommended.[45] The standard dosing of the 5-HT$_3$ antagonists is shown in Table 3.

Corticosteroids

Corticosteroids have a very high therapeutic index when used as antiemetics for chemotherapy-induced nausea. They have been studied extensively, both as single agents and as part of combination therapy. They are effective and well tolerated; insomnia, mood changes, and disturbance of glucose metabolism are among the most common side effects. The exact mechanism of action of corticosteroids is not completely understood. A variety of corticosteroids have been studied, but comparison trials are lacking. The most extensively studied steroid, dexamethasone,

has the advantage of being available in a number of dose formulations and as a low-cost generic formulation.

A meta-analysis of 32 randomized trials compared dexamethasone with no treatment, placebo, and metoclopramide. Dexamethasone was superior to no therapy and to placebo in preventing both acute and delayed emesis and was at least as good as metoclopramide in preventing acute emesis.[46] For more than 90% of patients receiving mildly or moderately emetogenic chemotherapy (level 2 agents, emetic risk 10–30%), dexamethasone is routinely used as a single-agent emesis prophylaxis.[47]

For patients receiving moderately or highly emetogenic chemotherapy (level 3–5 agents, emesis risk higher than 30%), single-agent corticosteroids do not reliably prevent emesis, but they are extremely useful when combined with 5-HT$_3$ antagonists. In a study of dexamethasone, granisetron, or both in patients who received moderately emetogenic chemotherapy, the combination therapy offered significantly better protection against emesis than either agent alone.[48] In an attempt to quantify the degree of benefit conferred by the addition of dexamethasone to serotonin antagonists, a meta-analysis looked at 22 randomized trials comparing combination therapy and single-agent 5-HT$_3$ antagonists or 5-HT$_3$ antagonist plus placebo and found that the addition of dexamethasone enhanced protection from vomiting by 25%.[46]

To find the optimal dose of dexamethasone in patients receiving highly emetic chemotherapy, a randomized trial was conducted in patients who received cisplatin (more than 50 mg/m^2). Single dexamethasone doses of 4, 8, 12, and 20 mg were studied, and all patients received standard dosing of ondansetron. The 20 mg dose provided the best protection against both nausea and vomiting, although the differences between the 12 and 20 mg doses were not statistically significant. No increase in adverse effects was seen at the 20 mg dose compared with the lower doses.

The results of other trials seem to indicate that single corticosteroid dosing is as effective as multiple dosing and that administration of corticosteroids immediately before chemotherapy is as effective as giving it the day before chemotherapy.[49] Consequently, a dose of 12 to 20 mg intravenously before highly emetogenic chemotherapy is generally recommended.

To compare single intravenous doses of 8 and 24 mg of dexamethasone before chemotherapy and a dexamethasone regimen of 8 mg intravenously before chemotherapy followed by 4 mg orally every 6 hours, a study was conducted using patients who received moderately or highly emetogenic chemotherapy (but no cisplatin) and a standard dosing of ondansetron.[50] No significant differences were found between the groups.

Table 3 Recommended Doses of Antiemetic Drugs

Drug	Dose range	Schedule	
		Acute emesis	Delayed emesis
5-HT3 receptor antagonists			
Ondansetron IV	8 mg or 0.15 mg/kg IV	Once, prechemotherapy	
Ondansetron PO	16–24 mg for acute emesis, 8 mg in delayed emesis	Once, prechemotherapy	BID x 2–3 days
Granisetron IV	1 mg or 0.010 mg/kg IV	Once, prechemotherapy	
Granisetron PO	2 mg PO	Once, prechemotherapy	
Dolasetron IV	100 mg or 1.8 mg/kg IV	Once, prechemotherapy	
Dolasetron PO	100 mg PO	Once, prechemotherapy	
Palonosetron	0.25 mg IV	Once, prechemotherapy	
Corticosteroids			
Dexamethasone IV	8 to 20 mg IV	Once, prechemotherapy	
Dexamethasone PO	Oral doses not well studied for acute emesis. For delayed emesis 4–8 mg PO		8 mg PO daily starting 24 hours after the start of chemotherapy for 4 days (cisplatin); 8 mg PO bid for 2 days (non-cisplatin)
Neurokinin 1 antagonists			
Aprepitant	125 mg PO prechemotherapy 80 mg PO postchemotherapy	125 mg once, prechemotherapy	80 mg PO daily for two days starting 24 hours after the start of chemotherapy
Dopaminergic antagonists			
Metoclopramide IV	2–3 mg/kg IV	Prechemotherapy and 2 hours post chemotherapy	
Metoclopramide PO	20 mg or 0.5 mg/kg PO in delayed emesis		QID starting 24 hours after the start of chemotherapy for 3–4 days
Prochlorperazine IV	10 mg IV	Q 3–4 hours PRN	
Prochlorperazine PO	10 mg PO	Q 3–4 hours PRN	

As effective as the combination of serotonin antagonists and corticosteroids is, many patients who receive highly emetogenic chemotherapy will still experience nausea and vomiting. In a study of patients who received cisplatin (more than 100 mg/m²), the combination of ondansetron and dexamethasone failed to prevent emesis in 39% of patients.[51]

NK1 Receptor Antagonists

As described previously, agents that block the binding of substance P at NK₁ receptors in the central nervous system are potent antiemetics and seem to provide a complementary mechanism of action to the blockade of 5-HT₃ or other emetogenic neuroreceptors. In 2003, the NK₁ receptor antagonist aprepitant (Emend) was approved for use in the United States by the Food and Drug Administration (FDA).

The use of aprepitant is best studied in the setting where best standard therapy fails a significant proportion of patients (such as patients who receive highly emetogenic chemotherapy, including cisplatin). Phase III trials have compared standard therapy with ondansetron and dexamethasone plus placebo versus standard therapy plus aprepitant in patients who received cisplatin-containing chemotherapy (>70 mg/m²). Aprepitant was given as 125 mg orally on day 1 and 80 mg orally on days 2 and 3. Compared with ondansetron and dexamethasone alone, aprepitant significantly reduced the incidence of both acute and delayed emesis.[52] Another study looked at the use of granisetron plus dexamethasone versus aprepitant plus dexamethasone versus the combination of all three agents in patients who received cisplatin-containing chemotherapy; the triple combination provided the best protection against both acute and delayed emesis.[53]

A recent study showed that the addition of aprepitant to standard antiemetic therapy in patients who received moderately emetogenic (non–cisplatin containing) chemotherapy enhanced the control of acute and delayed emesis. In this trial, breast cancer patients who received cyclophosphamide plus doxorubicin or epirubicin were treated with ondansetron and dexamethasone with or without aprepitant. A significantly higher percentage of patients in the aprepitant group achieved a complete response with no vomiting or use of rescue medications during both the acute and delayed phases.[54]

Dopamine (D₂) Receptor Antagonists

The oldest of the antiemetic classes and still widely used, there are three chemical subgroups of antidopaminergics that may be used in cancer patients.

Phenothiazines

Phenothiazines act primarily at D₂ receptors in the CTZ. The main drugs in current use are prochlorperazine (Compazine) and chlorpromazine (Thorazine). Prochlorperazine can be given orally, intravenously, or intramuscularly; is believed to be less effective than metoclopramide or dexamethasone; and is approximately equivalent in antiemetic efficacy to tetrahydrocannabinol (THC). It is useful in mildly and moderately emetogenic chemotherapy but not in highly emetic treatment.[55] Chlorpromazine is used less often as an antiemetic and is more often given for intractable hiccups. This agent is limited by the side effect of hypotension, which is more common in the elderly or when administered intravenously. Other side effects of chlorpromazine are the same as those of all of the dopamine receptor antagonists, namely extrapyramidal reactions such as dystonia or akathisia, which may be treated with anticholinergics such as benztropine (Cogentin) or diphenhydramine (Benadryl).

Butyrophenones

The butyrophenone neuroleptics droperidol (Inapsine) and haloperidol (Haldol) have some antiemetic effect, and no substantial difference in efficacy between the two has been documented. The half-life of haloperidol is 14 to 36 hours after a single dose, which can limit its use as an antiemetic because of prolonged side effects; the half-life of droperidol is shorter. These drugs, often called major tranquilizers, are quite sedating and have the same extrapyramidal side effects as other agents in this class, including the development of tardive dyskinesia if used chronically.[11]

Benzamides

As mentioned earlier, the benzamide metoclopramide (Reglan) causes central and peripheral antagonism of D₂ receptors at low doses and weaker 5-HT₃ antagonism at higher doses. It is a moderately effective antiemetic and has the effect of promoting gastric emptying and improving gastroparesis by stimulating the cholinergic receptors on gastric smooth muscle.[56] These effects make metoclopramide useful in alleviating the nausea and gastroparesis that often occur in cancer patients who require chronic narcotic analgesics. As an antiemetic, metoclopramide is less effective than serotonin antagonists and can produce the extrapyramidal side effects of other members of the class, so it has largely been replaced by serotonin antagonists. Dromperidone (Motilium) is a D_2 antagonist with selective activity in the upper gastrointestinal tract. It does not cross the blood-brain barrier and so does not produce extrapyramidal side effects, but it is not available for use in the United States.

Anticholinergics

The anticholinergic scopolamine (TransDerm Scop) is frequently used as an antiemetic to prevent motion sickness. It has not been demonstrated to be useful in treating or preventing chemotherapy-induced emesis. The major side effects of scopolamine are amnesia, dry mouth, urinary retention, and constipation.

Antihistamines

Promethazine (Phenergan) is the antihistamine medication most often used as an antiemetic in cancer patients. It is a phenothiazine derivative, but it has much less affinity for dopamine receptors than prochlorperazine does, and like the other members of this class, it also blocks H_1 and acetylcholine receptors. The other antihistamines commonly used as antiemetics, meclizine (Antivert) and diphenhydramine (Benadryl), are used primarily for motion sickness, but they can be useful in alleviating the extrapyramidal side effects of antidopaminergics (such as prochlorperazine and haloperidol) when they are used for antiemesis. The major side effects of this class of drugs are sedation and the anticholinergic side effects described above.

Benzodiazepines

The most common benzodiazepines used for cancer antiemesis are lorazepam (Ativan) and alprazolam (Xanax). They are not potent single-agent antiemetics but are most often given in combination therapy to help reduce anxiety and akathisia related to the use of corticosteroids and antidopaminergics.[57] Benzodiazepines may also be helpful in alleviating anticipatory emesis, as is described below. More recently, the thienobenzodiazepine olanzapine (Zyprexa), which has affinity for a number of receptors (including serotonin, dopamine, and histamine), was found in a phase II trial to be effective in preventing acute and delayed emesis in patients who received moderately or highly emetic chemotherapy.[58]

Cannabinoids

The medicinal use of cannabinoids has two aspects, scientific and political. The scientific interest in using cannabinoids arose because of anecdotal reports of an antiemetic effect by patients who used marijuana during chemotherapy. Studies of medicinal use of cannabinoids

have primarily used nabilone, a synthetic cannabinoid, or dronabinol (Marinol), a purified Δ9-THC. These two agents have been found to be superior to placebo and equivalent to or slightly more effective than prochlorperazine as antiemetics.[59] In a double-blind randomized trial of patients who received highly emetic chemotherapy, however, high-dose metoclopramide was three times more effective than dronabinol and had fewer side effects.[60] Whether inhaled marijuana is more effective than oral THC as an antiemetic has been addressed in a double-blind randomized crossover trial. Patients who received cisplatin or cyclophosphamide were given inhalant marijuana plus a placebo THC capsule or a THC capsule plus an inhalant placebo cigarette and were crossed over to the opposite treatment with the next course of treatment. Neither treatment was highly effective, and there was a trend toward patient preference for THC.[61] In all of the cannabinoid trials, side effects were prominent, including sedation, dry mouth, ataxia, dizziness, and mood alteration, either euphoria (feeling "high") or dysphoria.

Despite the findings that metoclopramide and the serotonin antagonists are more efficacious than cannabinoids and have fewer side effects, a systematic review of cannabinoid studies showed that in crossover studies, between 38 and 90% of patients preferred the cannabinoids.[62] Perhaps many of the side effects of cannabinoids, such as euphoria or even sedation or somnolence, could be viewed as favorable, especially when patients are experiencing many other unpleasant effects of their disease or its treatment.

Strong interest continues in the medicinal use of cannabinoids in the United States. In a 2004 poll commissioned by the American Association of Retired Persons, 72% of Americans aged 45 years and older thought that marijuana should be legal for medicinal purposes if recommended by a doctor. Currently, state laws that effectively remove criminal penalties for growing or possessing medical marijuana are in place in Alaska, California, Colorado, Hawaii, Maine, Maryland, Montana, Nevada, Oregon, Vermont, and Washington. However, in June 2005, the US Supreme Court ruled that physicians can be blocked from prescribing marijuana for patients even in states that have compassionate-use law. Currently, then, the political and legal status of medical marijuana is even murkier than its medical and scientific status.

Acupuncture

Interest in acupuncture as a nonpharmacologic and adjunctive therapy is based on its long history of use in the Far East and the speculation that it may modulate endogenous opiates, substance P, or serotonin. Data are conflicting regarding the efficacy of acupuncture as an antiemetic therapy, and much skepticism has been centered on a

possible placebo effect or differences related to the amount of clinician attention and treatment. To address these possibilities, a trial of 104 women who received myeloablative chemotherapy compared combination antiemetic therapy alone (prochlorperazine, lorazepam, and diphenhydramine) with the same pharmacotherapy plus electroacupuncture at classic antiemetic acupuncture points and with the same pharmacotherapy plus minimal needling at control points with mock electrostimulation. The median number of emesis episodes per patient over 5 days was lower in the electroacupuncture group (5 episodes) and the minimal needling group (10 episodes) than in the pharmacotherapy-alone group (15 episodes).[63] In a contrasting placebo-controlled study, however, no differences between treatment groups were observed when 80 patients who underwent high-dose chemotherapy received ondansetron plus either invasive acupuncture or non–skin-penetrating placebo acupuncture.[64]

Treatment Guidelines for the Prevention of Acute and Delayed Emesis

Antiemetic guidelines have been devised and published by a number of organizations.[24,65–67] These guidelines are not in universal agreement, and they differ somewhat in emesis risk stratification and in recommendations regarding specific antiemetic agents. Their differences may stem from the fact that newer guidelines reflect newer data, the interpretation of trial data, or the perceived relative importance of the pharmacoeconomics of treatment. The algorithm in Figure 2 is derived primarily from the National Comprehensive Cancer Network (NCCN) Practice Guidelines in Oncology regarding Antiemesis, version 1.2005.

Special Emetic Problems

Anticipatory Emesis

It is widely believed that the most effective means of preventing anticipatory nausea and vomiting is to ensure good control of acute and delayed nausea. Both the American Society of Clinical Oncology (ASCO) and the Multinational Association of Supportive Care in Cancer (MASCC) recommend that the best treatment for anticipatory emesis is the best possible control of acute and delayed emesis.[68] No formal prospective trial has been performed to compare levels of control of acute emesis and its effect on the development of anticipatory emesis. However, observational data showed that in patients given highly effective antiemetics (such as granisetron) in each cycle of chemotherapy, the incidence of anticipatory nausea was fairly low, at 10% per cycle, and the incidence of anticipatory vomiting was even lower, at 2%.[69] These rates compare favorably

EMETOGENIC POTENTIAL OF ANTINEOPLASTICS AGENTS

LEVEL	AGENT	
High emetic risk, level 5 (> 90 % frequency of emesis)*	• Carmustine > 250 mg/m² • Cisplatin ≥ 50 mg/m² • Cyclophosphamide > 1,500 mg/m² • Dacarbazine	• Mechlorethamine • Streptozocin • AC combination defined as either doxorubicin or epirubicin with cyclophosphamide
Moderate emetic risk, level 4 (60- 90 % frequency of emesis)*	• Amifostine > 500 mg/m² • Busulfan > 4 mg/d • Carboplatin • Carmustine ≤ 250 mg/m² • Cisplatin < 50 mg/m² • Cyclophosphamide > 750 mg/m² ≤ 1,500 mg/m²	• Cytarabine > 1 g/m² • Dactinomycin • Doxorubicin ≥ 60 mg/m² • Epirubicin > 90 mg/m² • Melphalan > 50 mg/m² • Methotrexate > 1,000 mg/m² • Procarbazine (oral)
Moderate emetic risk, level 3 (30-60 % frequency of emesis)*	• Amifostine > 300 - ≤ 500 mg/m² • Arsenic trioxide • Cyclophosphamide ≤ 750 mg/m² • Cyclophosphamide (oral) • Doxorubicin 20 - < 60 mg/m² • Epirubicin ≤ 90 mg/m² • Hexamethylmelamine (oral) • Idarubicin	• Ifosfamide • Interleukin-2 > 12-15 million units/m² • Irinotecan • Lomustine • Methotrexate 250-1,000 mg/m² • Mitoxantrone < 15 mg/m² • Oxaliplatin > 75 mg/m² Low emetic risk, level 2 (See AE-7) Minimal emetic risk, level 1 (See AE-7)

*Proportion of patients who experience emesis in the absence of effective antiemetic prophylaxis

Adapted with permission from Hesketh PJ, et al. Proposal for classifying the acute emetogenicity of cancer chemotherapy. J. Clin Onc 15: 103-9, 1997.

Note: All recommendations are category 2A unless otherwise indicated.
Clinical Trials: NCCN believes that the best management of any cancer patient is in a clinical trial. Participation in clinical trials is especially encouraged.

EMETOGENIC POTENTIAL OF ANTINEOPLASTICS AGENTS

LEVEL	AGENT	
Low emetic risk, level 2 (10-30 % frequency of emesis)*	• Amifostine ≤ 300 mg • Bexarotene • Cytarabine (low dose) 100-200 mg/m² • Capecitabine • Docetaxel • Doxorubicin (liposomal) • Etoposide • 5-Fluorouracil	• Gemcitabine • Methotrexate > 50 mg/m² < 250 mg/m² • Mitomycin • Paclitaxel • Pemetrexed • Temozolomide • Topotecan
Minimal emetic risk, level 1 (< 10 % frequency of emesis)*	• Alemtuzumab • Asparaginase • Alpha Interferon • Bevacizumab • Bleomycin • Bortezomib • Cetuximab • Chlorambucil (oral) • Cladribine • Dexrazoxane • Denileukin diftitox • Fludarabine • Gefitinib	• Gemtuzumab ozogamicin • Hydroxyurea • Imatinib mesylate • Melphalan (oral low-dose) • Methotrexate ≤ 50 mg/m² • Pentostatin • Rituximab • Thioguanine (oral) • Trastuzumab • Valrubicin • Vinblastine • Vincristine • Vinorelbine

*Proportion of patients who experience emesis in the absence of effective antiemetic prophylaxis

Adapted with permission from Hesketh PJ, et al. Proposal for classifying the acute emetogenicity of cancer chemotherapy. J. Clin Onc 15: 103-9, 1997.

Note: All recommendations are category 2A unless otherwise indicated.
Clinical Trials: NCCN believes that the best management of any cancer patient is in a clinical trial. Participation in clinical trials is especially encouraged.

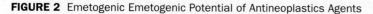

FIGURE 2 Emetogenic Emetogenic Potential of Antineoplastics Agents

with those from older studies using less effective antiemetics, for which the incidence of acute and delayed nausea and vomiting was very high, between 86 and 92%, that of anticipatory nausea was 31 to 33%, and that of anticipatory vomiting was 10 to 11%.[70]

Benzodiazepines

The use of benzodiazepines has been studied both as part of an antiemetic combination therapy to reduce the symptoms of acute, delayed, and anticipatory nausea and as an adjunct to a psychological support program to reduce the incidence of anticipatory nausea. In a randomized trial to evaluate the efficacy of lorazepam as part of an antiemetic regimen, patients who received high-dose cisplatin infusion received dexamethasone, metoclopramide, and either an antihistamine or lorazepam. The lorazepam group experienced significantly less acute and anticipatory nausea and fewer of the expected side effects of mild sedation and amnesia.[71] In a small, double-blind, placebo-controlled study of breast cancer patients who received adjuvant chemotherapy, the addition of low-dose alprazolam to a psychological support program including relaxation training significantly reduced the incidence of anticipatory nausea (0% with lorazepam and 18% with placebo) and the need for hypnotic therapy to control sleep disturbances associated with the cancer treatment.[72]

Behavioral and Psychological Interventions

Given that anticipatory nausea is viewed as primarily a psychological phenomenon, a variety of psychological and behavioral interventions have been studied to reduce symptoms, such as systematic desensitization, progressive muscle relaxation training, hypnosis, biofeedback, guided imagery, and music therapy. Two recent reviews of published studies concluded that such interventions are effective in reducing the incidence of anticipatory nausea in adult and pediatric patients receiving chemotherapy.[73,74] The evidence for the efficacy of behavioral interventions in controlling chemotherapy-induced nausea and vomiting is mixed. However, a recent study assessing the ability of progressive muscle relaxation training (PMRT) to prevent postchemotherapy emesis produced mixed results. Patients were randomly assigned to receive dexamethasone plus metoclopramide or the same two antiemetics along with PMRT (25-minute sessions along with guided imagery techniques) 1 hour before chemotherapy and then daily PMRT sessions for the next 5 days. PMRT decreased the duration of nausea and vomiting in the group that received PMRT, but there was no significant difference in the incidence of emesis or the intensity of symptoms between the two treatment groups.[75]

Multiple-Day Chemotherapy

Most antiemetic studies have been conducted using patients receiving single-day treatment with highly or moderately emetogenic agents. Fewer data are available regarding the management of patients receiving multiple-day chemotherapy (such as cisplatin combination chemotherapy in patients with germ cell tumors). The standard treatment for testicular cancer, for example, includes bleomycin, etoposide, and cisplatin (20 mg/m² for 5 consecutive days). Historically, patients who received this 5-day course of cisplatin had the most severe nausea and vomiting on day 1 and gradually diminishing emetic symptoms over the next several days. With the development of highly effective antiemetics such as the 5-HT$_3$ antagonists, the opposite pattern is now seen: there is often complete emetic control the first 1 to 2 days and then worsening nausea and some vomiting on days 3 to 5.[76]

Several studies have established the value of giving a repetitive dosing of 5-HT$_3$ antagonists on each day of cisplatin for the control of acute nausea and vomiting.[77] Control of later-onset symptoms has been the focus of discussion. There is disagreement regarding the dosing of dexamethasone. Concern has been expressed about the side effects of dexamethasone if given for all 5 days of cisplatin. One recommendation is to give oral dexamethasone as a single 20 mg dose on days 1 and 2 for control of acute emesis, then as an 8 mg dose twice daily on days 6 and 7, and finally as a 4 mg dose twice on day 8 for control of delayed symptoms.[76] The NCCN guidelines recommend that for multiple-day chemotherapy regimens, a 5-HT$_3$ receptor antagonist be administered before each day's first dose of highly or moderately emetogenic chemotherapy and that dexamethasone be administered daily during chemotherapy and then for 2 to 3 days afterward if the regimen is likely to cause delayed emesis.[24]

Palonosetron, the long-acting serotonin antagonist, has not been studied in multiple-day chemotherapy regimens. However, the long half-life and duration of action of this agent may make it particularly well suited to this situation. The NCCN guidelines offer that palonosetron may be used before the start of a multiple-day chemotherapy regimen. In the acute emesis guidelines, it is recommended as a single 0.25 mg dose to cover both the acute and delayed periods, but in multiple-day regimens, repeat dosing may be required. On the basis of results from a phase II trial in which doses up to 30 times the FDA-approved dose were administered and from several phase III trials in which a single dose of 0.75 mg was evaluated, repeated dosing of the 0.25 mg dose is likely to be safe.[24]

Aprepitant, the NK$_1$ antagonist, has not been studied in multiple-day chemotherapy regimens. The NCCN guidelines suggest that for multiple-day regimens with highly emetogenic chemotherapy, this agent may be administered as a 125 mg oral dose before chemotherapy on day 1 and then as an 80 mg oral dose on days 2 and 3, as one would do for highly emetogenic single-day chemotherapy. The guidelines further state that on the basis of phase II data, additional 80 mg oral doses can be safely administered on days 4 and 5 of a multiple-day regimen.[24] Data regarding the efficacy of additional dosing are not available.

High-Dose Chemotherapy

Treatment-related nausea and vomiting are especially difficult problems for patients receiving high-dose chemotherapy in association with a bone marrow or peripheral blood stem cell transplant. In addition to the use of highly and moderately emetogenic chemotherapy agents, there are a number of exacerbating factors, such as multiple-day administration, concurrent use of prophylactic antibiotics and narcotic analgesics, and the use of radiotherapy (including highly emetogenic total-body irradiation). There are very few studies regarding the use of antiemetics in patients receiving high-dose therapy; most are phase II studies of 5-HT$_3$ receptor antagonists, with or without dexamethasone. The efficacy of 5-HT$_3$ receptor antagonists has ranged from a low of 30% among breast cancer patients, who achieved complete or partial nausea protection from granisetron plus dexamethasone,[78] to a high of 98% among patients treated with high-dose cyclophosphamide and total-body irradiation, who achieved complete (50%) or partial (48%) emesis protection from granisetron plus dexamethasone.[79] In general, the antiemetic effects of current treatment appear to be less effective in this setting than in standard-dose highly emetogenic chemotherapy. The general consensus is that the standard of care should be a combination of a 5-HT$_3$ receptor along with dexamethasone.[80] Neither palonosetron nor aprepitant has been studied in this patient population.

Radiation-Induced Nausea

Similar to the risk stratification in chemotherapy-induced nausea, efforts have been make to predict the emetic risk of radiotherapy, based primarily on the site of irradiation. The following classification has been proposed[81]:

- Greater than 90% emetic risk: total-body or total-node irradiation
- A 60 to 90% emetic risk: upper hemibody, upper abdomen, or whole-abdomen irradiation
- A 30 to 60% emetic risk: lower hemibody irradiation, lower thoracic or pelvic region irradiation, craniospinal irradiation, or cranial radiosurgery
- Less than 30% emetic risk: irradiation of the head and neck, extremities, or extra-abdominal areas

For the high-risk category (>90% risk), MASCC and ASCO guidelines recommend prophylaxis with 5-HT$_3$ antagonists plus dexamethasone. For the moderate-risk category (60–90% risk), both guidelines recommend prophylaxis with a 5-HT$_3$ antagonist. For the low-risk category (30–60% risk), either prophylaxis or rescue with 5-HT$_3$ antagonists can be used. In the minimal-risk category (<30% risk), rescue with a dopamine receptor antagonist or a 5-HT$_3$ antagonist can be used.[82]

Several points about these guidelines deserve mention. First, few randomized trials have compared the efficacy of antiemetics in radiation-induced emesis; most included patients receiving total-body, upper hemibody, or upper abdominal irradiation because these treatments carry the highest risk of emesis. Second, although some trials have demonstrated the efficacy of 5-HT$_3$ antagonists and of dexamethasone over placebo in radiation-induced nausea, no trials have compared dexamethasone plus a 5-HT$_3$ antagonist against the use of 5-HT$_3$ antagonist alone in this setting. Recommendations regarding the use of both drugs together are based on data showing the efficacy of dexamethasone plus ondansetron versus placebo or ondansetron plus dexamethasone versus metoclopramide plus dexamethasone[83] and on some extrapolation from the data regarding the use of corticosteroids and serotonin antagonists in highly emetogenic chemotherapy. Finally, neither the MASCC nor the ASCO guidelines address the prevention of emesis when patients are receiving both chemotherapy and radiotherapy. In the NCCN guidelines, the emetic risk of patients receiving chemoradiation is determined by the emetogenic potential of the chemotherapy. Thus, the same antiemetic prophylaxis is used for patients receiving both chemotherapy and radiotherapy as that used for patients receiving chemotherapy alone.[24]

Breakthrough or Refractory Emesis

Despite the development of highly effective emetic prophylaxis, a significant number of patients will develop treatment-related nausea and vomiting. Antiemetic medications are effective at preventing the onset of nausea and vomiting, but once persistent emesis is established, pharmacologic intervention is much less effective.

When patients present with breakthrough emesis after chemotherapy, the management should be threefold. First, the clinician must try to discern whether the nausea and vomiting are due not to the chemotherapy but to some other cause (such as hypercalcemia), are a side effect of other medications (such as narcotics), are a manifestation of brain metastases, or are a primary gastrointestinal disorder (such as bowel obstruction). Second, the treating physician must ensure that the patient is receiving optimal antiemetic prophylaxis. Despite consensus guidelines regarding best-evidence management of any clinical problem, practice patterns are often slow to be adopted. As an example, a 2000 survey of Italian cancer centers after the promulgation of treatment guidelines for chemotherapy-induced emesis revealed that a significant number of patients received treatment that was considered suboptimal according to the new guidelines: 22% of the patients being treated with highly emetogenic chemotherapy received a 5-HT$_3$

antagonist and no dexamethasone during the acute emesis phase, and 41% of the patients received no antiemetic during the delayed emesis phase.[84]

Third, if a patient has received prophylaxis and still experiences nausea and vomiting, the general principle of breakthrough therapy is to add an additional agent from a different drug class. Since there are multiple neurotransmitter receptors in the important emetogenic pathways, blockade of an additional pathway might provide additional clinical benefit. And since oral medications cannot generally be tolerated in the presence of intractable vomiting, intravenous administration is generally necessary. If the patient seemed to have derived benefit from the original antiemetic regimen (such as a serotonin antagonist), then that regimen should be retained and an additional medication with a different mechanism of action (such as an antidopaminergic) should be added.[24] Multiple antiemetic agents on an alternating schedule may be necessary.

If a patient has received chemotherapy with a lower emetic potential and thus has received less aggressive emesis prophylaxis, the antiemetic therapy could be changed to a higher-level therapy typically used for a higher-risk group. For example, a patient who has received only dexamethasone for delayed symptoms may require the addition of a 5-HT_3 antagonist.

It has been assumed that because of their similar chemical structure, failure of one 5-HT_3 receptor antagonist predicts the failure of the entire class. However, there may be patient variability in response, and if a patient who has received a 5-HT_3 antagonist develops emesis, a different serotonin antagonist could be considered. In a double-blind trial of 40 patients who received ondansetron plus dexamethasone after highly emetogenic chemotherapy yet experienced nausea and vomiting in the first 24 hours, the patients were randomly assigned to continue the same therapy or to switch to granisetron plus dexamethasone. The rate of complete protection from emesis was significantly higher in the patients who switched to granisetron than in those who continued with the same regimen.[85] It should be noted that in that small study, a high dose of granisetron (3 mg) was compared with a relatively low dose of ondansetron (8 mg). There could be a lack of complete cross-resistance between the serotonin antagonists, or the recommended dosing may be inadequate for some patients.

Patients with Advanced Cancer

In contrast to the large number of trials designed to address the problem of chemotherapy-induced emesis, relatively few have been performed to study the clinical problem of nausea and vomiting not related to chemotherapy in patients with advanced cancer. Yet the symptoms are very common in both patient groups and very vexing in patients with advanced cancer: 60% experience nausea and 30% complain of vomiting.[86] The list of potential causes of nausea and vomiting in this population is long, and often these symptoms are multifactorial. Palliative care specialists may use a "mechanistic" approach to treat nausea and attempt to deduce the pathophysiologic mechanism of emesis from their clinical evaluation and administer treatment accordingly, or they may use an "empiric" approach and use antiemetics until they find one that is effective. Favoring the mechanistic approach, a randomized controlled trial found that metoclopramide was 75% effective in relieving symptoms of cancer-related dyspepsia thought to be due to a gastroparetic mechanism.[87]

Patients with inoperable malignant bowel obstruction represent a special clinical scenario that may result in nausea and vomiting. For palliative care patients, the relief of symptoms of colicky abdominal pain and vomiting is paramount. Although nasogastric tube decompression of the gastrointestinal tract is standard care for such patients, it is very uncomfortable. Placement of a draining gastrostomy tube is another option if the clinical situation is persistent and not likely to resolve. Corticosteroids such as intravenous dexamethasone are often used in palliative care practice to reduce the inflammation associated with a malignant lesion and thus relieve the obstruction. The results from several trials have suggested a trend toward a benefit from this therapy, although the advantages have been small and have not reached statistical significance.[88,89]

Regarding the use of 5-HT_3 antagonists in patients with advanced cancer, there has been some concern over the acquisition costs (eg, for patients in hospice care) and the side effects, such as constipation, for which this patient population is at high risk. One small study found a trend toward superiority of ondansetron over placebo in the treatment of opioid-induced nausea and vomiting, but this trend did not achieve statistical significance.[90] In another study, the serotonin antagonist tropisetron was significantly better than metoclopramide or chlorpromazine in patients with advanced cancer.[91]

Summary

More than 20 years ago, patients who received chemotherapy rated nausea and vomiting as the most distressing aspects of their treatment.[1] There have since been considerable advances in understanding the pathophysiology of nausea and vomiting, the predictive factors to stratify emetic risk, and the development of highly effective and well-tolerated antiemetic drugs. Complete prevention of chemotherapy-induced emesis is achievable with currently available therapy in most patients and should be the goal of all patients receiving treatment. To accomplish this objective, the following key facts should be kept in mind:

- Several neurotransmitter receptors in the CTZ are involved in triggering emesis, the most important of which are the D_2, 5-HT_3, and NK_1 receptors. These receptors are the targets of antiemetic drugs. Blockade of only one receptor class is often insufficient to completely prevent nausea and vomiting.

- Cancer patients should always be assessed for other causes of nausea and vomiting, such as electrolyte disturbances, medication side effects, and primary gastrointestinal disorders (such as bowel obstruction), before the emesis is attributed to chemotherapy side effects.

- The most important factor in assessing emetic risk is the intrinsic emetic potential of the chemotherapeutic agent. Antiemetic treatment should be guided by the predicted level of emetogenicity and by known patient factors.

- The risk of emesis for patients receiving moderate– to high–emetic risk chemotherapy lasts for 4 to 5 days; patients require preventive treatment for that entire period.

- Anticipatory nausea is a conditioned response occurring after poor control of acute or delayed emesis. The best treatment is to prevent acute or delayed symptoms in the first place by optimal antiemetic therapy during every cycle. Behavioral interventions or benzodiazepines may also be helpful.

- Prophylaxis for radiation-induced nausea and vomiting may be tailored according to the risk stratification based on the body site treated. Patients receiving concurrent chemotherapy should receive antiemetic treatment according to the emetogenic potential of their chemotherapy regimen.

- Breakthrough emesis is generally managed by adding an antiemetic agent from a different class or by stepping up therapy to that used for higher-risk chemotherapy.

- In patients with advanced cancer, nausea unrelated to chemotherapy may be multifactorial. A mechanistic approach to identify the pathophysiologic cause of emesis can guide therapy.

REFERENCES

1. Coates A, Abraham S, Kaye SB, et al. On the receiving end—patient perception of the side-effects of cancer chemotherapy. Eur J Cancer Clin Oncol 1983;19:203–8.
2. Jenns K. Importance of nausea. Cancer Nurs 1994;17: 488–93.
3. Griffin AM, Butow PN, Coates AS, et al. On the receiving end. V: patient perceptions of the side effects of cancer chemotherapy in 1993. Ann Oncol 1996;7:189.
4. Grunberg SM, Deuson RR, Mavros P, et al. Incidence of chemotherapy-induced nausea and emesis after modern antiemetics. Cancer 2004;100:2261–8.

5. Hasler WL, Chey WD. Nausea and vomiting. Gastroenterology 2003;125:1860.

6. Koch KL, Stern RM, Vasey MW, et al. Neuroendocrine and gastric myoelectrical responses to illusory self-motion in humans. Am J Physiol 1990;258:E304.

7. Borison HL, Wang SC. Physiology and pharmacology of vomiting. Pharmacol Rev 1953;5:193.

8. Carpenter DO. Neural mechanisms of emesis. Can J Physiol Pharmacol 1990;68:230.

9. Miller AD, Wilson VJ. 'Vomiting center' reanalyzed: an electrical stimulation study. Brain Res 1983;270:154.

10. Miller AD, Leslie RA. The area postrema and vomiting. Front Neuroendocrinol 1994;15:301.

11. Moertel CG, Reitemeier RJ, Gage R. A controlled clinical evaluation of antiemetic drugs. JAMA 1963;186:116–8.

12. Cubbedu LX, Hoffman IS, Fuenmayor NT, et al. Efficacy of ondansetron and the role of serotonin in cisplatin-induced nausea and vomiting. N Engl J Med 1990;322:810–6.

13. Gralla RJ. Antiemetic therapy. In: Kufe D, Pollock R, Weichselbaum R, et al, editors. Holland-Frei cancer medicine. 6th ed. Hamilton (ON): BC Decker; 2003.

14. Kris MG, Radford JE, Pizzo BA, et al. Use of an NK-1 receptor antagonist to prevent delayed emesis following cisplatin. J Natl Cancer Inst 1997;66:817–8.

15. Dodds LJ. The control of cancer chemotherapy-induced nausea and vomiting. J Clin Hosp Pharm 1985;3:1379–84.

16. Feyer P, Titlbach OJ, Wilkinson J, Budach V. Gastrointestinal reactions in radiotherapy. Support Care Cancer 1996;4:249.

17. Scarantino CW, Ornitz RD, Hoffman LG, Anderson RF. Radiation induced emesis: effects of ondanseton. Semin Oncol 1992;19(6 Suppl 15):38–43.

18. Kris MG, Gralla RJ, Clark RA, et al. Incidence, course, and severity of delayed nausea and vomiting following the administration of high-dose cisplatin. J Clin Oncol 1985;3:1379–84.

19. Kris MG, Gralla RJ, Tyson LB, et al. Controlling delayed vomiting: double-blind, randomized trial comparing placebo, dexamethasone alone, and metoclopramide plus dexamethasone in patients receiving cisplatin. J Clin Oncol 1989;7:108–14.

20. Italian Group for Antiemetic Research. Ondansetron vs granisetron, both combined with dexamethasone, in prevention of cisplatin-induced delayed emesis. J Clin Oncol 1995;6:805–10.

21. Martin M. The severity and pattern of emesis following different cytotoxic agents. Oncology 1996;53 Suppl 1:2–31.

22. Roscoe JA, Bushunow P, Morrow GR, et al. Patient expectation is a strong predictor of severe nausea after chemotherapy. Cancer 2004;101:2701–8.

23. Morrow GR, Roscoe JA, Kirshner JJ, et al. Anticipatory nausea and vomiting in the era of 5-HT3 antiemetics. Support Care Cancer 1998;6:244–7.

24. National Comprehensive Cancer Network. Guidelines for supportive care, antiemesis. Available at: http://www.nccn.org/professionals/physician_gls/f_guidelines.asp?button=I+Agree#care) (accessed 10-11 2005).

25. Pollera CF, Giannarelli D. Prognostic factors influencing cisplatin-induced emesis. Definition and validation of a predictive logistic model. Cancer 1989;64:1117.

26. Osoba D, Zee B, Warr D, et al. Quality of life studies in chemotherapy-induced emesis. Oncology 1996;53 Suppl:92–5.

27. Morrow GR, Roscoe JA, Hickok JT, et al. Initial control of chemotherapy-induced nausea and vomiting in patient quality of life. Oncology (Huntingt) 1998;12:32.

28. Morrow GR. The effect of a susceptibility to motion sickness on the side effects of cancer chemotherapy. Cancer 1985;55:2766.

29. Jordan NS, Schauer PK, Schauer A, et al. The effect of administration rate on cisplatin-induced emesis. J Clin Oncol 1985;3:559.

30. Hesketh PJ, Kris MG, Grunberg SM, et al. Proposal for classifying the acute emetogenicity of cancer chemotherapy. J Clin Oncol 1997;15:103–9.

31. Italian Group for Emetic Research. Cisplatin-induced delayed emesis: pattern and prognostic factors during three subsequent cycles. Ann Oncol 1994;5:585–9.

32. Italian Group for Emetic Research. Delayed emesis induced by moderately emetogenic chemotherapy: do we need to treat all patients? Ann Oncol 1997;8:561–7.

33. Stockhorst U, Klosterhalfen S, Klosterhalfen W, et al. Anticipatory nausea in cancer patients receiving chemotherapy: classical conditioning etiology and therapeutic implications. Integr Physiol Behav Sci 1993;28:177–81.

34. Morrow GR. Clinical characteristics associated with the development of anticipatory nausea and vomiting in cancer patients undergoing chemotherapy treatment. J Clin Oncol 1984;2:1170–6.

35. Heron JF, Goedhals L, Jordaan JP, et al. Oral granisetron alone and in combination with dexamethasone: a double-blind randomized comparison against high-dose metoclopramide plus dexamethasone in prevention of cisplatin-induced emesis. The Granisetron Study Group. Ann Oncol 1994;5:579.

36. del Giglio A, Soares HP, Caparroz C, Castro PC. Granisetron is equivalent to ondansetron for prophylaxis of chemotherapy-induced nausea and vomiting: results of a meta-analysis of randomized controlled trials. Cancer 2000;89:2301.

37. Hesketh PJ, Navari R, Grote T, et al. Double-blind, randomized comparison of the antiemetic efficacy of intravenous dolasetron mesylate and intravenous ondansetron in the prevention of acute cisplatin-induced emesis in patients with cancer. J Clin Oncol 1996;14:2242.

38. Perez EA, Hesketh PJ, Sandbach J, et al. Comparison of single-dose oral granisetron versus intravenous ondansetron in the prevention of nausea and vomiting induced by moderately emetogenic chemotherapy: a multi center, double-blind, randomized parallel study. J Clin Oncol 1998;16:754.

39. Gandara DR, Rollam F, Warr D, et al. Consensus proposal for 5HT3 antagonists in the prevention of acute emesis related to highly emetogenic chemotherapy. Dose, schedule, and route of administration. Support Care Cancer 1998;6:237.

40. Beck TM, Hesketh PJ, Madajewicz S, et al. Stratified, randomized, double-blind comparison of intravenous ondansetron administered as a multiple-dose regimen versus two single-dose regimens in the prevention of cisplatin-induced nausea and vomiting. J Clin Oncol 1992;10:1969.

41. Ettinger DS, Eisenberg PD, Fitts D, et al. A double-blind comparison of the efficacy of two dose regimens of oral granisetron in preventing acute emesis in patients receiving moderately emetogenic chemotherapy. Cancer 1996;78:144.

42. Roila F, Tonato M, Cognetti F, et al. Prevention of cisplatin-induced emesis: a double-blind multicenter randomized crossover study comparing ondansetron and ondansetron plus dexamethasone. J Clin Oncol 1991;9:675–8.

43. Gralla R, Lichinitser M, Van Der Vegt S, et al. Palonosetron improves prevention of chemotherapy-induced nausea and vomiting following moderately emetogenic chemotherapy: results of a double-blind randomized phase III trial comparing single doses of palonosetron with ondansetron. Ann Oncol 2003;14:1570–7.

44. Eisenberg P, Figueroa-Vadillo J, Zamora R, et al. Improved prevention of moderately emetogenic chemotherapy-induced nausea and vomiting with palonosetron, a pharmacologically novel 5-HT3 receptor antagonist: results of a phase III, single-dose trial versus dolasetron. Cancer 2003;98:2473–82.

45. "The pink sheet" FDC reports. Chevy Chase, MD. 2003;65(31):34.

46. Ioannidis JP, Hesketh PJ, Lau J. Contribution of dexamethasone to control of chemotherapy-induced nausea and vomiting: a meta-analysis of randomized evidence. J Clin Oncol 2000;18:3409.

47. Zagalama NE, Rosenblum SL, Sartiano GP et al. Single high-dose intravenous dexamethasone as an antiemetic in cancer chemotherapy. Oncology 1986;43:27.

48. Italian Group for Antiemetic Research. Dexamethasone, granisetron, or both for the prevention of nausea and vomiting during chemotherapy for cancer? N Engl J Med 1995;332:1.

49. Kris MG, Gralla RJ, Tyson LB, et al. Improved control of cisplatin-induced emesis with high-dose metoclopramide and with combinations of metoclopramide, dexamethasone and diphenhydramine. Cancer 1985;55:527–34.

50. Italian Group for Antiemetic Research. Randomized, double-blind, dose-finding study of dexamethasone in preventing acute emesis induced by anthracyclines, carboplatin, or cyclophosphamide. J Clin Oncol 2004;22:725.

51. Hesketh PJ, Harvey WH, Harker WG, et al. A randomized, double-blind comparison of intravenous ondansetron alone and in combination with intravenous dexamethasone in the prevention of nausea and vomiting associated with high-dose cisplatin. J Clin Oncol 1994;12:596.

52. Hesketh PJ, Grunberg SM, Gralla RJ, Warr DG. The oral neurokinin-1 antagonist aprepitant for the prevention of chemotherapy-induced nausea and vomiting: a multinational, randomized, double-blind, placebo-controlled trial in patients receiving high-dose cisplatin. The Aprepitant Protocol 052 Study Group. J Clin Oncol 2003;21:4112–9.

53. Campos D, Pereira JR, Reinhardt RR, et al. Prevention of cisplatin-induced emesis by the oral neurokinin-1 antagonist, MK-869, in combination with granisetron and dexamethasone or with dexamethasone alone. J Clin Oncol 2001;19:1759.

54. Warr DG, Hesketh PJ, Gralla RJ, et al. Efficacy and tolerability of aprepitant for the prevention of chemotherapy-induced nausea and vomiting in patients with breast cancer after moderately emetogenic chemotherapy. J Clin Oncol 2005;23:2822.

55. Gralla RJ, Itri LM, Pisko SE, et al. Antiemetic efficacy of high-dose metoclopramide: randomized trials with placebo and prochlorperazine in patients with chemotherapy-induced nausea and vomiting. N Engl J Med 1981;305:905–9.

56. Gralla RJ. Metaclopramide. A review of antiemetic trials. Drugs 1984;25 Suppl 1:63.

57. Bowcock SJ, Stockdale AD, Bolton JA, et al. Antiemetic prophylaxis with high dose metaclopramide or lorazepam in vomiting induced by chemotherapy. Br Med J (Clin Res Ed) 1984;288:1879.

58. Navari RM, Einhorn LH, Loehrer PH, et al. A phase II trial of olanzapine for the prevention of chemotherapy-induced nausea and vomiting. ASCO annual meeting proceedings. J Clin Oncol 2004;25:578–82.

59. Sallan SE, Cronin C, Zelen M, Zinberg NE. Antiemetics in patients receiving chemotherapy for cancer: a randomized comparison of delta-9 tetrahydrocannabinol and prochloroperazine. N Engl J Med 1980;302:135.

60. Gralla RJ, Tyson LB, Bordin LA, et al. Antiemetic therapy: a review of recent studies and a report of a random assignment trial comparing metoclopramide with delta-9 tetrahydrocannabinol. Cancer Treat Rep 1984;68:163–72.

61. Levitt M, Faiman C, Hawks R, et al. Randomized double-blind comparison of delta-9 tetrahydro-cannabinol (THC) and marijuana as chemotherapy antiemetics. Proc Am Soc Clin Oncol 1994;3:91.

62. Tramer MR, Carroll D, Campbell FA, et al. Cannabinoids for control of chemotherapy induced nausea and vomiting: quantitative systematic review. BMJ 2001;323:16–21.

63. Shen J, Wenger N, Glaspy J, et al. Electroacupuncture for the control of myeloablative chemotherapy-induced emesis: a randomized controlled trial. JAMA 2000;284:2755–61.

64. Streitberger K, Friedrich-Rust M, Bardenheuer H, et al. Effect of acupuncture compared with placebo-acupuncture at p6 as additional antiemetic prophylaxis in high-dose chemotherapy and autologous peripheral blood stem cell transplantation: a randomized controlled single-blind trial. Clin Cancer Res 2003;9:2538–54.

65. Antiemetic Subcommittee of the Multinational Association of Supportive Care in Cancer (MASCC). Prevention of chemotherapy- and radiotherapy-induced emesis: results of Perugia Consensus Conference. Ann Oncol 1998;9:811–9.

66. Gralla RJ, Roila F, Tonato M, et al. The 2004 Perugia Antiemetic Consensus guideline process: methods, procedures, and participants. Support Care Cancer 2005;13:77–9.

67. American Society of Health-System Pharmacists. ASHP therapeutic guidelines on the pharmacologic management of nausea and vomiting in adult and pediatric patients receiving chemotherapy or radiation therapy or undergoing surgery. Am J Health Syst Pharm 1999;56:729–64.

68. Aapro MS, Molassiotis A, Olver I. Anticipatory nausea and vomiting. Support Care Cancer 2005;13:117–21.

69. Aapro MS, Kirchner V, Terry JP. The incidence of anticipatory nausea and vomiting after repeat cycle chemotherapy: the effect of granisetron. Br J Cancer 1994;69:957–60.

70. Wilcox PM, Fetting JH, Nettesheim KM, Abeloff MD. Anticipatory vomiting in women receiving cyclophosphamide, methotrexate, and 5-FU (CMF) for breast carcinoma. Cancer Treat Rep 1982;66:1601–4.

71. Malik IA, Khan WA, Qazilbash M, et al. Clinical efficacy of lorazepam in prophylaxis of anticipatory, acute, and delayed nausea and vomiting induced by high doses of cisplatin. Am J Clin Oncol 1995;18:170–5.

72. Razavi D, Delvaux N, Farvacques C, et al. Prevention of adjustment disorders and anticipatory nausea secondary to adjuvant chemotherapy: a double-blind placebo-controlled study assessing the usefulness of alprazolam. J Clin Oncol 1993;11:1384–90.

73. Redd WH, Montgomery GH, DuHamel KN. Behavioral intervention for cancer treatment side effects. J Natl Cancer Inst 2001;93:810–23.

74. Mundy EA, DuHamel KN, Montgomery GH. The efficacy of behavioral interventions for cancer treatment-related side effects. Semin Clin Neuropsychiatry 2003;8:253–75.

75. Molassiotis A, Yung HP, Yam BM, et al. The effectiveness of progressive muscle relaxation training in managing chemotherapy-induced nausea and vomiting in Chinese breast cancer patients: a randomized controlled trial. Support Care Cancer 2002;10:237–46.

76. Einhorn LH, Rapoport B, Koeller J, et al. Antiemetic therapy for multiple day chemotherapy and high-dose chemotherapy with stem-cell transplant: review and consensus statement. Support Care Cancer 2005;13:112–6.

77. Baltzer P, Pisters KMW, Kris MG, et al. High dose ondansetron plus dexamethasone for the prevention of nausea and vomiting with multiple day cisplatin chemotherapy. Proc Am Soc Clin Oncol 1993;12:462.

78. Climent MA, Palau J, Ruiz A, et al. The antiemetic efficacy of granisetron plus dexamethasone haloperidol and lorazepam in breast cancer patients treated with high dose chemotherapy with peripheral blood stem cell support. Support Care Cancer 1998;6:287–90.

79. Abbott B, Ippoliti C, Bruton J, et al. Antiemetic efficacy of granisetron plus dexamethasone in bone marrow transplant patients receiving chemotherapy and total body irradiation. Bone Marrow Transplant 1999;23:265–9.

80. Gralla RJ, Osoba D, Kris MG, et al. Recommendations for the use of antiemetics: evidence-based, clinical practice guidelines. J Clin Oncol 1999;17:2971.

81. Tonini G, Vincenzi B, Santini D, et al. Prevention of radio-therapy-induced emesis. J Exp Clin Cancer Res 2003;22: 17–22.

82. Petra ChF, Maranzano E, Molossiotis A, et al. Radiotherapy-induced nausea and vomiting (RINV): antiemetic guidelines. Support Care Cancer 2005;13:122–8.

83. Italian Group for Antiemetic Research in Radiotherapy. Radiation-induced emesis: a prospective observational multicenter Italian trial. Int J Radiat Oncol Biol Phys 1999;44:619–25.

84. Roila F, De Angelis V, Patoia L, et al. Antiemetic prescriptions in 77 Italian oncological centers after the MASCC Consensus Conference. Support Care Cancer 2000;8:241.

85. De Wit R, de Boer AC, van der Linden GH, et al. Effective cross-over to granisetron after failure to ondansetron, a randomized double blind study in patients failing ondansetron plus dexamethasone during the first 24 hours following highly emetogenic chemotherapy. Br J Cancer 2001;85:1099–101.

86. Davis MP, Walsh D. Treatment of nausea and vomiting in advanced cancer. Support Care Cancer 2000;8:444–52.

87. Bruera ED, Belzile M, Neumann C, et al. A double blind crossover study of controlled release metoclopramide and placebo for the chronic nausea and dyspepsia of advanced cancer. J Pain Symptom Manage 2000;19:427–35.

88. Hardy J, Ling L, Mansi J, et al. Pitfalls in placebo-controlled trials in palliative care: dexamethasone for the palliation of malignant bowel obstruction. Palliat Med 1998;12: 437–42.

89. Laval G, Girardier J, Laussaniere JM, et al. The use of steroids in the management of inoperable intestinal obstruction in terminal cancer patients: do they remove the obstruction? Palliat Med 2000;14:3–10.

90. Hardy J, Daley S, McQuade B, et al. A double-blind, randomised parallel group, multinational, multicentre study comparing single dose ondansetron 24 mg p.o with placebo and metoclopramide 10 mg t.d.s. p.o in the treatment of opioid-induced nausea and emesis in cancer patients. Support Care Cancer 2002;10:231–6.

91. Mystakidou K, Befon S, Liossi C, Vlachose L. Comparison of the efficacy and safety of tropisetron, metoclopramide, and chlorpromazine in the treatment of emesis associated with far advanced cancer. Cancer 1998;83:1214–23.

Fever

Maria E. Cabanillas, MD
Ricardo H. Alvarez, MD

The past two decades have witnessed an increase in the number of patients who are immunocompromised as a consequence of primary or secondary immunodeficiency disorders or from the use of agents that depress one or more components of the immune system. Cancer patients are considered immunocompromised hosts who have an alteration in phagocytic, cellular, or humoral immunity. In this scenario, fever is a very common problem and can be secondary to infections, inflammation, transfusions, antineoplastics, antimicrobials, or tumor necrosis. Despite significant advancements in supportive care of patients with cancer, infections continue to be the major cause of morbidity and mortality in patients with cancer because of alterations in normal host defenses. This chapter reviews the potential causes and pathophysiologic mechanisms of fever in patients with cancer.

History

One of the first references about fever comes from the ancient Sumerian pictogram in the sixth century BC. Centuries later, Celso, a Roman writer of the first century AD, first listed the four cardinal signs of inflammation: redness, swelling, heat, and pain. In this description, fever was represented by local heat. Ultimately, Claude Bernard first recognized the metabolic process occurring within the body and the result of body heat. For many years, physicians monitored body temperature as a complementary diagnostic tool; however, the real impact in diagnosis was uncertain. The first scientific publication reported was in 1868 by Carl Reinhold August Wunderlich in a paper entitled "The Course of Temperature in Disease."[1] In his description, made after 1 million observations in 25,000 subjects, he put emphasis on the normal diurnal variation and posited 38°C (100.4°F) as the upper limit of the normal range. Most of his work was done using axillary measurement of temperature.

Definitions

One of the most common definitions of fever is promulgated by the International Union of Physiological Sciences Thermal Commission.[2] It defines fever as a state of elevated core temperature, which is often but not necessarily part of the defensive responses of multicellular organism (host) to the invasion of live (microorganism) or inanimate matter recognized as pathogenic or alien by the host. Fever develops when a pyrogen, a term used to describe any substance that causes fever, elevates the set point–determined core body temperature above normal. The genesis of fever requires the presence of an intact thermoregulatory mechanism.

With regard to the upper limit of the normal oral temperature, medical societies and modern textbooks differ in their definition. According to the 1977 guidelines from the Infectious Disease Society of America, fever is defined as a single oral temperature more than 38.3°C (101°F) or an elevation of 38°C (100.4°F) for at least 1 hour in the absence of obvious environmental causes.[3]

Unlike fever, hyperthermia represents a failure of thermoregulatory homeostasis in which cytokines are not involved and therapies with antipyretics are ineffective. Heat stroke is one example of hyperthermia and is defined as a body temperature > 40.5°C (105°F) with associated central nervous system (CNS) dysfunction, including seizure, delirium, and coma, in the setting of a large environmental heat load that cannot be dissipated. Hyperthermia is also caused by drugs in three different scenarios: neuroleptic malignant syndrome, malignant hyperthermia, and serotonin syndrome.[4]

The term *hyperpyrexia* denotes fever of more than 41.5°C (106.7°F) and occurs in patients with severe infections but most commonly occurs in patients with CNS hemorrhages.

Thermometric Variability

Thermometric measurements involve a number of basic technical details that are very important in the final temperature reading. Core body temperature refers to the temperature of the cranium, thorax, and abdominal cavities. The gold standard for core body temperature measurement is the pulmonary artery catheter, which approximates the temperature of the heart. However, because this method is invasive, it is not practical for use on all patients. Peripheral temperature measurements are only an estimate of the core temperature owing to compensatory mechanisms such as vasoconstriction, which can change the peripheral temperature in relation to the core temperature. Noninvasive sites, such as the tympanic membrane, posterior sublingual pocket (oral), rectum, and axilla, are the most commonly used.

The tympanic membrane is an ideal site for estimating the core temperature because the arterial irrigation of the tympanic membrane is in proximity to the artery supplying the hypothalamic area, and it is considered to be the closest body temperature to the thermoregulatory center. The accessibility is optimal; however, proper technique is a major factor influencing accuracy. When the probe is placed incorrectly, the temperature reading may be that of the skin, the external ear canal, or the cerumen instead of the tympanic membrane.[5] With proper training and use, this method can provide rapid and accurate measurements.

Oral temperature measurement is the most common site used because it is accessible and responds promptly to changes in the core temperature. The sublingual pocket is irrigated by a main artery, which is a branch of the external carotid artery. Several factors can alter the final reading of oral temperature. Mastication and smoking both cause significant and persistent increases in the oral temperature, whereas drinking ice beverages, mouth breathing, and aerosol treatments may cause transient decreases in the oral temperature. This method is convenient and reliable in proper candidates.

A rectal temperature reading provides higher levels than those obtained at other sites and is no longer considered the gold standard. This increased rectal temperature may be secondary to heat generated as a result of the metabolic activity of fecal bacteria. This site is used in the hospital setting; however, in patients with hemodynamic shock, the arterial perfusion of the rectum may be severely impaired. For this reason, this site provides a reliable approximation only in patients who have a thermal balance.

Although more convenient, axillary readings do not accurately reflect core body temperature and should be used only when it is impossible to obtain a temperature reading by any other means.[6–8]

Physiologic Variables

Several variables in body temperature registration change with regard to age, sex, and circadian rhythm. For many years, there was a tendency to believe that older people have lower body temperatures than their younger counterparts. However, a recent investigation showed that healthy elderly subjects (mean age 80.3 years; range 62–99 years) have the same average core temperature than healthy younger people.[9] Women exhibit increases in body temperature of about 0.5°C (0.9°F) at the time of ovulation. They have a slightly higher average oral temperature than men (36.9°C vs 36.7°C) but do not exhibit greater average diurnal temperature oscillations than their male counterparts (0.56°C vs 0.54°C).

Body temperature exhibits circadian rhythmicity that is associated with the sleep-wake cycle. During normal circadian cycle, the core temperature reaches its highest levels in the late afternoon or early evening and its nadir in the early morning. The adaptations to night shift work cause a reversal in this pattern. Therefore, when clinical thermometric measurements are made, it is important to consider not only the time and site of measurement but also the sleep-wake cycle of the subject being studied (Table 1).

Clinical Manifestations

Broadly defined, an immunocompromised host has an alteration in phagocytic, cellular, or humoral immunity that increases the risk of infectious complications or opportunistic infections. Fever is the principal, and sometimes the only, manifestation of serious infection in the cancer patient.

Fever has two components. One is objective and is represented by a temperature measurement above the normal range. The other component is subjective and is represented by a constellation of symptoms (chills, shivering, and sweating), which are produced by the elevation of core temperature. These two components are commonly defined as febrile response, which is the result of an innate physiologic reaction,

including cytokine production and activation of multiple endocrine, immunologic, and hematologic systems.

Although a number of fever patterns have been associated with various infectious or non-infectious illnesses, no pathognomonic pattern or degree of fever has been clearly associated with a specific infection in immunocompromised patients.

Febrile episodes are characterized by three different phases: initiation, steady state, and defervescent.[10] During initiation, a pyrogen elevates the thermoregulatory set point above normal. The individual experiences cutaneous vasoconstriction, which leads to heat retention, followed by shivering that generates additional heat to achieve the new set point. At steady state, heat production is equivalent to heat loss, and shivering stops. After lowering the set point, defervescence commences with cutaneous vasodilatation and sweating, which lead to radiant and evaporative heat loss, respectively.

Pathophysiologic Mechanism

The mechanism responsible for the body temperature is localized in the hypothalamus. The suprachiasmatic nuclei and the preoptic and anterior hypothalamus appear to be responsible for this exquisite thermoregulation. Several studies suggest that the preoptic region regulates body temperature by integrating thermal input signals from thermosensors in the skin and CNS. A variety of endogenous and exogenous pyrogens, including drugs, appear to affect temperature regulation by altering the activity of hypothalamic neurons. Exogenous pyrogens are, for the most part, microorganisms and toxin products of microbial origin. According to current concepts, exogenous pyrogens depend on their physiochemical structure and initiate fever by inducing the macrophages to produce endogenous pyrogens. These endogenous pyrogens, also called cytokines, cross the blood-brain barrier and activate thermosensitive neurons. Four major pyrogenic cytokines have been described: interleukin (IL)-1, tumor necrosis factor (TNF)α, (IL-6, and interferon (IFN)-γ-. In healthy subjects, the pyrogenic cytokines are undetectable in serum under basal conditions and have a very short intravascular half-life. Interestingly, the pyrogenic cytokines are pleiotropic, in that they interact with receptors present on many different types of host cells in picomolar quantities.

Acute-Phase Changes

Body temperature may change under several factors, such as infection, trauma, inflammatory process, and malignant disease. This physiologic response is nonspecific and is generally referred to as the acute-phase reaction, although it is seen in both chronic and acute inflammatory states.

The full spectrum of the response includes dramatic increases (ie, C-reactive protein, fibrinogen, and ferritin) or decreases (ie, albumin, transferrin, and transthyretin) in the synthesis of several hepatic proteins. Table 2 shows the list of important plasma proteins that increase during the acute-phase response.

One of the most important acute-phase proteins, C-reactive protein (CRP), is synthesized by the liver, mainly in response to IL-6. CRP is thought to activate the complement system by binding to polysaccharides present on bacteria, fungi, and parasites. In vitro, CRP activates neutrophils, promotes platelet degradation, and enhances natural killer cell activity. The secretion of CRP occurs rapidly after the stimulus and falls rapidly after the disappearance of the stimulus. Despite the lack of specificity, it is useful in clinical practice because it reflects the presence and intensity of the inflammatory process. It is also an inexpensive and widely available test.[11,12]

Fever may be present in conjunction with lethargy and increased sleep. Leukocytosis with immature neutrophils is also common. Dysfunction of the thyroid gland and abnormal glucose and lipid metabolism are frequently seen. Oligoelements such as zinc and serum iron are depressed. Another metabolic change related to the acute-phase reaction is an increase in liver gluconeogenesis, energy expenditure, and muscle proteolysis, all of which contribute to weight loss.

The most florid manifestation of the acute-phase response is observed in patients with acute

Table 1 Normal Variations in Temperature

Temperature Diurnal/Evening	Tympanic Membrane	Oral	Rectal
6:00 am	36.6°C (98°F)	37.2°C (98.9°F)	37.6°C (99.6°F)
4:00 pm	37.3°C (99°F)	37.7°C (99°F)	38.1°C (100.6°F)

Table 2 Plasma Proteins that Increase during the Acute-Phase Response

C-reactive protein
Serum amyloid A protein
α_1-Glycoprotein
Ceruloplasmin
α-Macroglobulins
Complement components
α_1-Antitrypsin
α_1-Antichymotrypsin
Fibrinogen
Prothrombin
Factor VIII
Plasminogen
Haptoglobin
Ferritin
Immunoglobulin
Lipoproteins

bacterial infection, extensive body surface area burns, or multiple and traumatic injuries. However, occult infections, chronic illnesses such as rheumatoid arthritis, Crohn's disease, and other autoimmune diseases also are characterized by acute-phase response elevation. In several cases, the acute-phase response serves as an indicator of silent disease in some cancers, particularly renal cell carcinoma and Hodgkin's disease.

Induction of the Acute-Phase Response

The initiation of the acute-phase response is linked to the production of cytokines elicited by infections, injuries, inflammation, and immunologic reactions. Cytokines are proteins produced by many cell types (principally activated lymphocytes and macrophages, but also endothelium, epithelium, and connective tissue cells) that modulate the function of other cell types. These proteins are pleotropic in that they can act on different cell types. Cytokine effects are often redundant and can influence the synthesis or action of other cytokines. They are multifunctional in that individual cytokines may have both positive and negative regulatory actions. Cytokines mediate their effects by binding to specific receptors on target cells. The expression of cytokine receptors can be regulated by a variety of exogenous and endogenous signals. For some responsive cells, cytokines stimulate cell proliferation, acting as traditional growth factors.

Cytokines can be grouped into five classes:

1. Cytokines that regulate lymphocyte function: these cytokines regulate lymphocyte activation, growth, and differentiation. IL-2 and IL-4 act in lymphocyte growth, as well as IL-10 and transforming growth factor β, which are negative regulators of immune responses.
2. Cytokines involved with natural immunity: these include two major inflammatory cytokines, TNF-α and IL-1β.
3. Cytokines that activate inflammatory cells: these cytokines activate macrophages during the cell-mediated immune response and include IFN-γ, TNF-α, TNF-β (lymphotoxin), IL-5, IL-10, and IL-12.
4. Chemokines: this group of cytokines is characterized by chemotactic activity for various leukocytes.
5. Cytokines that stimulate hematopoiesis: these mediate immature leukocyte growth and differentiation and include IL-3, IL-7, c-kit ligand, GSF, and granulocyte-macrophage colony-stimulating factor.

Several cytokines induce acute-phase changes: IL-1, TNF-α, IFN-γ, IL-6, leukemia inhibitory factor, ciliary neurotropic factor, oncostatin M, and IL-11.

The development of the acute-phase response in a patient with a localized bacterial infection starts 1 to 2 hours after blood monocytes and tissue macrophages become activated by phagocytosis or microorganism exposure to its products or toxins. These mediators enter the circulation and reach the brain, where they initiate fever. Within 8 to 12 hours after the onset of infection or trauma, the liver increases the synthesis of acute-phase proteins. In addition, several normal plasma proteins increase several-fold during the acute-phase response, including haptoglobin, certain protease inhibitors, complement components, ceruloplasmin, and fibrinogen.

Despite the anabolic processes of the liver, the acute-phase response is accompanied by marked catabolism of muscle protein associated with loss of body weight and overall negative nitrogen balance.

Etiology

Thirty percent of patients with cancer develop fever at some point during the course of their malignancy,[13] with the majority having an underlying infection. Infection, tumor, and drugs are among the most common causes of fever in patients with cancer (Figure 1). The major differential point in determining whether the fever is due to infection is the presence or absence of neutropenia. In patients with low white blood cell counts, infection causes more than two-thirds of all fevers, whereas patients with normal white blood cell counts are infected far less frequently. The wide variation in fever frequency reflected in Table 3 relates to differences in the definition of fever, the population studied, the primary tumor site, and medical advances during the period studied.[10]

There are two clinical conditions associated with a risk of life-threatening infections: severe neutropenia (ie, an absolute neutrophil count of less than 500/mm²) and a history of splenectomy. In both situations, rapidly progressive infections may be life-threatening if untreated.[14]

Fever Caused by Infection

Infection is a leading cause of fever in both the neutropenic and non-neutropenic patient. A risk stratification model was proposed in the cancer patient setting and is described in Table 4.[15] Patients with cancer have a perturbation in the host mechanism of defense. Usually, these patients have aberrations of skin and mucosa, with disorders of neutrophils, T lymphocytes, plasma cells, and complement system. These abnormalities will predispose patients to specific infections; therefore, the physician must identify the probable immune defect (often there will be more than one) in the febrile cancer patient.

Acute fever in non-neutropenic cancer patients, if clinical signs suggest infection, should be managed similarly to fever in patients without cancer. Special attention should be given to a possible cancer causing an obstruction in natural passages, for example, pneumonia in bronchial cancer, pyelitis in bladder or prostatic cancer, and cholangitis in pancreatic carcinoma. Obstruction is also frequently responsible for relapses of infection after successful therapy. *Streptococcus pneumoniae* remains a major pathogen in lung cancer patients, whereas *Escherichia coli* and *Streptococcus faecalis* are often isolated in patients with pancreatic and hepatobiliary tumors. Colon carcinomas are associated with an increased frequency of *Streptococcus bovis* bacteremia and endocarditis.

Central Nervous System

Infection of the CNS should be suspected in a febrile cancer patient with altered mental status. Common bacterial pathogens causing meningitis in patients with or without cancer include *S. pneumoniae* and *Neisseria meningitidis*. Patients who have undergone a neurosurgical procedure are at increased risk of meningitis caused by gram-negative bacilli. The incidence of *Listeria* meningitis is increased in the elderly and patients with decreased cell-mediated immunity. Patients with subcutaneous reservoirs and ventricular catheters (eg, Ommaya reservoir) are at increased risk of meningitis owing to *Pseudomonas*, *Propionibacterium acnes*, and staphylococci. Although *Coccidioides immitis*, *Histoplasma capsulatum*, and *Cryptococcus neoformans* are the major fungal CNS pathogens in the United States, the latter is the most common cause of meningitis in cancer patients. The onset is often insidious but may be more acute in patients receiving corticosteroids or another immunosuppressive therapy.

Indwelling Catheters

The use of indwelling intravenous catheters has become a commonplace source of infection in patients with cancer. Infectious complications are of two types: local infections involving the subcutaneous tunnel or exit site and such as bacteremia. Unfortunately, local signs and symptoms are unreliable indicators of catheter infections. Many catheters responsible for bacteremia appear to be totally innocuous, and this is particularly true for neutropenic patients. It became clear early in the use of indwelling central venous catheters that the treatment of catheter infections did not always require removal of the offending device. The gold standard for the diagnosis of a catheter-related infection has been the demonstration of ≥ 15 colony-forming units per catheter tip.[16] However, the success of treatment is dependent on the pathogenicity of the offending organism, and many authorities recommend removal of the

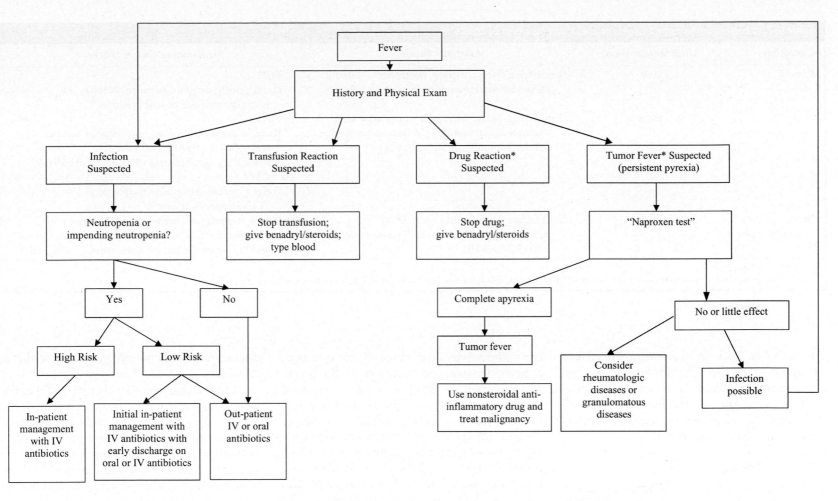

*Diagnosis of exclusion

FIGURE 1 Algorithm for cause of fever in cancer patients. IV = intravenous.

Table 3 Frequency and Cause of Fever in Cancer Patients					
Study	*Number of Patients*	*Fever (%)*	*Caused by Infection (%)*	*Caused by Tumor (%)*	*Comments*
Boggs and Frei[32]	9,532*	24[†]	44[‡]	56	Frequency of fever caused by tumor stable throughout illness; fever caused by infection increased in last quartile of illness
Briggs[33]	238	53	< 15[§]	53	Frequency similar in local and disseminated disease; fever most common in primary tumors of lung and pleura, liver and biliary tree, and head and neck
Browder et al[34]	343	70	38[‖]	5	Frequency similar in local and disseminated disease; infection increased in pelvic tumors
Fenster and Klatskin[35]	81	—	—	23	Fever presenting complaint in 7%
Klatersky et al[36]	47	100	57	38	Tumor-related fever most common in lymphomas (67%)
Reuben et al[24]	1,592	100	57	38	In terminally ill patients; the presence/absence of fever is not predictive of survival

Adapted from Zhukovsky DS.[10]
*Number of hospital days.
[†]Percentage of hospital days with fever.
[‡]Percentage of 193 febrile episodes in 86 patients.
[§]Infection and other complications.
[‖]infection, obstruction, postoperative complications.

Table 4 Risk Factors for Fever and Causes of Infectious Agents in Patients with Cancer

Condition	Risk Stratification	Major Risk Factor	Predominant Causes of Fever
Cancer	Low	Underlying disease, therapy, neutropenia < 10 d, altered mucosal immunity, indwelling catheter	FUO Gram-positive or gram-negative bacteria, respiratory viruses or herpesviruses
	High	Underlying disease, therapy, neutropenia > 10 d, altered mucosal immunity, defects in humoral or cellular immunity, indwelling catheter	FUO Bacteria: gram-positive or gram-negative aerobes, anaerobes at sites of mixed infection Viruses: RSV, parainfluenza virus, adenovirus, HSV, CMV Fungi: *Candida, Aspergillus, Cryptococcus, Trichosporon, Fusarium*
Bone marrow transplantation	High	Risk factors for high-risk cancer, plus immunosuppressive regimen, previous infection with CMV, GVHD	Similar to those with high-risk cancer; pattern of infection is influenced by time since transplantation and type of procedure (ie, autologous or allogeneic)

Adapted from Pizzo PA.[15]

CMV = cytomegalovirus; FUO = fever of unknown origin; GVHD = graft-versus-host disease; HSV = herpes simplex virus; RSV = respiratory syncytial virus.

catheter when *Staphylococcus aureus, Pseudomonas* sp, *Candida* sp, or polymicrobic infection are encountered. In addition, a consensus exists that the majority of exit-site infections can be treated with antibiotics alone, whereas tunnel infections often require catheter removal.

Skin

The differential diagnosis of fever in cancer patients with dermatologic signs is challenging. Numerous infections have been associated with skin lesions, but underlying malignancy and hypersensitivity drug reactions can involve the skin. Common dermatologic infections occurring in normal hosts, such as staphylococcal cellulitis, are readily diagnosed and treated. These infections are frequently caused by intravenous catheters, trauma, or other breaches of the skin. The morphology of the lesions may be atypical in the immunosuppressed host, and a new rash or nodule may be the earliest or the only warning sign of a serious systemic process. A prompt biopsy with histologic staining and culture for bacteria, mycobacteria, viruses, and fungi can provide prompt information on which to base treatment.

Gastrointestinal Tract

Infection can occur anywhere in the gastrointestinal tract, and the risk of gastrointestinal infections in cancer patients includes decreased cell-mediated immunity, radiation therapy, chemotherapy, and broad-spectrum antibiotics. The oral cavity is a common site of infection in cancer patients. In a classic prospective clinical study in hematologic cancer patients, 20% of patients had an acute oral infection without signs of an extraoral infection and two-thirds of patient had both oral and extraoral infections. The most common oral infection was *Candida*.[17] In the setting of

chemotherapy-induced mucositis, streptococci, enterobacteriacea, and anaerobes are the prevalent organisms. Esophagitis should be suspected in patients with odynophagia or dysphagia with fever. *Candida*, cytomegalovirus, and herpes simplex viruses are common causes of esophagitis in patients with acquired immune deficiency syndrome (AIDS), hematologic malignancies, and organ transplant. Esophagoscopy with biopsy and culture is required for a definitive diagnosis. The symptoms of pseudomembranous colitis caused by *Clostridium difficile* include a high fever, bloody diarrhea, and abdominal pain. One survey found *C. difficile* in the stool of up to 12% of asymptomatic leukemic patients compared with 5% of asymptomatic healthy volunteers.[18] Infection usually occurs during or following antibiotic therapy but can be secondary to chemotherapy agents as well.

Neutropenia predisposes the patient to severe and rapidly progressing infection by bacterial and fungal pathogens; therefore, empiric therapy has become an accepted practice and should be designed to cover the most likely pathogens, namely gram-negative rods, especially *Pseudomonas aeruginosa*.

Tumor Fever

In the absence of infection, it is thought that cancer cells can produce cytokines, which are responsible for tumor fever. Renal cell carcinoma is the most common cancer associated with fever, with fever occurring in up to half of patients.[19] Hepatoma patients develop fever one-third of the time.[20] Fever may play a role in the staging of some cancers. The Ann Arbor Staging System for Hodgkin's disease includes B symptoms such as persistent or recurrent fever, weight loss, or night sweats. Pel-Ebstein fever (persistent fever for days to weeks followed by afebrile intervals and then recurrent fever) is seen in patients with Hodgkin's

disease and is an important prognostic feature in the disease.

Clinical characteristics may be useful to distinguish between infectious and neoplastic fevers, but no one feature reliably differentiates them. Therefore, tumor fever is a diagnosis of exclusion, made after an exhaustive evaluation for infection and when exclusion of other causes of fever has been made. Diagnostic criteria for tumor fever are described in Table 5.

The infected patient is often ill, or even toxic, with chills, tachycardia, and possible hypotension. In the case of fever related to cancer, chills and tachycardia are lacking or minimal. Aspirin and acetaminophen have little effect on fever caused by a malignant tumor, whereas a dramatic response to nonsteroidal anti-inflammatory drugs occurs. Consequently, some investigators use the response to nonsteroidal anti-inflammatory drugs to differentiate fever caused

Table 5 Diagnostic Criteria for Neoplastic Fever

I.   Temperature over 37.8°C (100°F) at least once each day
II.   Duration of fever over 2 wk

III.   Lack of evidence of infection on
    A.   Physical examination
    B.   Laboratory examination, eg, cultures from sputum, blood, urine, bone marrow, spinal fluid, stool, pleural fluid, and skin lesions
    C.   Imaging studies

IV.   Absence of drug or transfusion reaction
V.   Lack of response of fever to empiric, adequate antibiotic therapy for at least 7 d
VI.   Prompt, complete resolution of fever by the naproxen test

Adapted from Zell JA and Chang JC.[33]

by infection from that caused by a tumor. In two separate studies, the response to indomethacin and naproxen was associated with a high incidence of tumor-related fever compared with infectious causes.[21,22] Based on these observations, the "naproxen test" (three doses of 375 mg of naproxen at 12-hour intervals) has been proposed for the diagnosis of cancer fever; it should result in complete resolution of pyrexia, and the patient should experience sustained normal temperature while receiving naproxen.

Fever Caused by Transfusion

Oncology patients, like other transfusion recipients, experience adverse reactions to blood components. Most reactions occur during or shortly after a blood transfusion, but reactions may present several hours to days later. Typically, febrile reactions are benign and rarely lead to serious sequelae, such as death. There are two categories of transfusion reactions: immunologic and nonimmunologic. Hemolytic and nonhemolytic reactions are included in the immunologic category, both of which involve antigen-antibody complex formation. Pseudohemolytic transfusion reactions are nonimmunologic reactions, whereby bacterial contamination of the blood product and disease transmission are the cause of fever.[23] Only transfusion reactions that lead to fever are discussed here.

Hemolytic Transfusion Reactions

Acute hemolytic transfusion reactions are reactions that result in the destruction of red blood cells and are caused by antigen-antibody interactions. The most common symptoms are fever and chills but also include chest pain, hypotension, nausea, flushing, dyspnea, anuria, and hemoglobinuria. Laboratory testing reveals anemia, elevation of indirect bilirubin, a positive Coombs' test, and decreased haptoglobin levels. Bleeding from disseminated intravascular coagulation, renal failure, and death are the most serious outcomes of hemolytic transfusion reactions. The most common cause of hemolytic transfusion reactions is human error as a result of misidentification of the recipient or of the patient sample, resulting in transfusion of incompatible blood. Other causes are technician failure to identify an antibody in the donor or recipient serum and the presence of antibodies that are not detectable by current testing methods. Therapy for hemolytic transfusion reactions involves stopping the transfusion and measures to maintain blood pressure and perfusion to the kidneys with intravenous fluids.[24] Use of furosemide and "renal dose" dopamine has been described in the literature.

Delayed hemolytic transfusion reactions involve the extravascular clearance of antibody-coated red blood cells by the reticuloendothelial system. The clinical course is benign, but severe reactions have been reported. These reactions occur in patients previously sensitized to red blood cell alloantigens but with levels too low to detect on screening. Thus, when the patient is reexposed to the antigen, an anamnestic response results in production of alloantibody that binds donor red blood cells. They typically occur 7 to 14 days after the transfusion but may occur earlier, within 2 to 4 days. Fever, jaundice, and hemoglobinuria are common symptoms. Laboratory testing reveals anemia, elevation of indirect bilirubin, and a normal haptoblobin level. When necessary, treatment with general support and transfusion of antigen-negative red cells should be provided.[23,25]

Nonhemolytic Reactions that Cause Fever

The febrile nonhemolytic reaction is the most common adverse reaction to blood transfusion and is presumably caused by antibodies (leukoagglutinins) in the recipient that are directed against human leukocyte antibody–specific or leukocyte-specific antigens, or both, on donor blood cells and platelets. It is related to previous exposure to foreign leukocyte antigens; therefore, patients have a history of multiple transfusions or pregnancy. Common symptoms include fever, chills, headache, myalgias, nausea, and nonproductive cough. Less commonly, hypotension, chest pain, vomiting, and dyspnea may occur. Premedication with antipyretics, such as acetaminophen, may minimize mild febrile nonhemolytic reactions. Antihistamines do not prevent or treat febrile nonhemolytic reactions, and corticosteroids can minimize it if they are administered several hours before the transfusion. Leukoreduction of blood components decreases but does not eliminate the frequency of febrile nonhemolytic reactions. Another way to prevent febrile nonhemolytic reactions is to use single donor platelets instead of pooled random donor platelets because the former may contain fewer leukocytes than the latter.[26]

Transfusion-associated graft-versus-host disease (TA-GVHD) is a fulminant and often fatal nonhemolytic reaction caused by the transfusion of viable donor lymphocytes into immunosuppressed patients. The transfused lymphocytes are able to proliferate, engraft, and recognize the recipient's tissue as foreign. Fever usually presents 7 to 10 days after transfusion, and death usually occurs 3 to 4 weeks after transfusion. In addition, depending on the organs involved, skin rash, diarrhea, hepatitis, bone marrow suppression, and infection may occur. The diagnosis is made by demonstrating donor cells in the involved tissue or circulating as peripheral blood chimerism. Irradiation of blood containing lymphocytes is the only effective means to prevent TA-GVHD.[27]

Pseudohemolytic Transfusion Reactions that Cause Fever

Transfusion of blood contaminated with bacteria, although rare, can be fatal, resulting in shock, disseminated intravascular coagulation, renal failure, and hemoglobinuria. Most commonly, endotoxin-producing gram-negative bacteria are involved. Treatment with antibiotics should be implemented early, and if clinical suspicion is high, the remaining untransfused blood product should be cultured.

The current risk of transmission of viral hepatitis, human immunodeficiency virus (HIV), and human T-lymphotrophic viruses is low. Advances in testing for viral proteins, antibody responses, and, more recently, viral nucleic acids have significantly reduced the risk.

Fever Caused by Drugs

Drugs used in cancer patients may cause fever. Bleomycin, daunorubicin, cisplatin, asparaginase, cyclophosphamide, cytarabine, vincristine, 5-fluorouracil, and methotrexate are the commonly used chemotherapeutic agents that have been found to elicit fever. Other drugs used in the cancer setting that commonly cause fever are monoclonal antibodies such as rituximab and alemtuzumab, growth factors such as filgrastim and sargramostim, and biologic agents such as IFN and IL-2.[28] Antibiotics such as amphotericin B, trimethoprim-sulfamethoxazole, ciprofloxacin, and rifampicin can also cause fever. Fever usually disappears after discontinuing the offending drug and may be attenuated with the use of acetaminophen, a nonsteroidal anti-inflammatory drug, and steroid premedication. Meperidine is commonly used as a premedication or for treatment of chills associated with drug fever.

More dramatic reactions occur in patients with neuroleptic malignant syndrome, which manifests with hyperthermia. This rare but potentially fatal syndrome is seen in patients receiving neuroleptic drugs. The manifestation is the presence of hyperthermia, and the pathogenesis of this event is related to an idiosyncratic reaction to antipsychotic agents such as piperazine, butyrophenones, and haloperidol. Neuroleptic malignant syndrome should be differentiated from malignant hyperthermia, characterized by a genetic predisposition that may be manifested after the administration of anesthetic agents such as succinylcholine and halothane. Clinical features include marked hyperthermia, muscle rigidity, hypotension, arrhythmias, and disseminated intravascular coagulation.

Other Causes of Fever

Radiation-induced fever, adrenal crisis, and central nervous system metastasis should be given consideration when evaluating an oncology patient with fever. Central nervous system metastasis may cause fever from hypothalamic involvement, meningeal leukemia, or meningeal carcinomatosis. Steroid withdrawal and metastasis or primary tumor involvement of the adrenal gland are possible causes of adrenal insufficiency. Primary adrenal non-Hodgkin's lymphoma is a rare and aggressive disease.[29] The most common cancers that cause metastasis to the adrenal glands are lung, esophageal, gastric, and liver or bile duct carcinomas.[30] Fever owing to radiation should be considered in patients receiving radiation alone, after infection has been ruled out. The fever usually presents hours after the initial treatment. In acute radiation pneumonitis, fever may be part of the syndrome, which includes dyspnea and nonproductive cough developing 2 to 3 months after radiation therapy.[31]

Other systemic illnesses that cause fever, such as rheumatoid arthritis and lupus erythematosus, may coexist in cancer patients. Careful review of the patient's symptoms and medical history are invaluable for diagnosing these diseases.[31]

REFERENCES

1. Wunderlich C. Das Verhalten der Eigenwarme in Krankenheiten. Leipzig: Otto Wigard; 1868.
2. IUPS Thermal Commission. Glossary of terms for thermal physiology. 2nd ed. Pflugers Arch 1987;410:567–87.
3. Hughes WT, Armstrong D, Bodey GP, et al. 1977 guidelines for the use of antimicrobial agents in neutropenic patients with unexplained fever. Clin Infect Dis 1977;25:551–73.
4. Braunwald E, Fauci AS, Kasper DL, et al. Harrison's principles of internal medicine, 15th ed. McGraw-Hill; 2001. p. 91–2.
5. Stanhope N. Temperature measurement in the phase I PACU. J Perianesth Nurs 2006;27–36.
6. Fulbrook P. Core temperature measurement in adults: a literature review. J Adv Nurs 1993;1451–60.
7. Fulbrook P. Core body temperature measurement: a comparison of axilla, tympanic membrane and pulmonary artery blood temperature. Intensive Crit Care Nurs 1977;266–72.
8. Falzon A, Grech V, Caruana B, et al. How reliable is axillary temperature measurement? Acta Paediatr 2003;309–13.
9. Jones SR. Fever in the elderly. In: Mackowiack PA, editor. Fever: basic mechanism and management. New York: Raven Press; 1991. p. 233–42.
10. Zhukovsky DS. Fever and sweats in the patient with advanced cancer. Hematol Oncol Clin North Am 2002;12:579–88.
11. Póvoa P. C-reactive protein: a valuable maker of sepsis. Intensive Care Med 2002;28:235–43.
12. Kushner I. Acute phase proteins. Up to date 2006. Available at: www.uptodate.com.
13. Greenberg SB, Taber L. Fever of unknown origin. In: Mackowiak PA, editor. Fever: basic mechanism in management. New York: Raven Press; 1991. p. 183.
14. Bodey GP, Buccley M, Sathe YS, et al. Quantitative relationships between circulating leukocytes and infection in patients with acute leukemia. Ann Intern Med 1966;64:328–40.
15. Pizzo PA. Fever in immunocompromised patients. N Engl J Med 1999;341:893–900.
16. Maki DG, Weise CE, Sarafin HW. A semiquantitative culture method for identifying intravenous-catheter-related infection. N Engl J Med 1977;296:1305.
17. Bergman OJ. Oral infections and fever in immunocompromised patients with hematologic malignancies. Eur J Clin Microbiol Infect Dis 1989;68:151.
18. Fekety R, Shah AB. Diagnosis and treatment of Clostridium difficile colitis. JAMA 1993;71:269.
19. Friocourt L, Jouquan J, Khoury S, et al. Fever in adult renal cancer. In: Renal tumors: proceedings of the First International Symposium on Kidney Tumors. New York: Alan R. Liss; 1982. p. 283.
20. Ashraf SJ, Arya SC, El-Sayed M, et al. A profile of primary hepatocellular carcinoma patients in the Gizan area of Saudi Arabia. Cancer 1986;58:2163.
21. Warshaw AL, Carey RW, Robinson DR. Control of fever associated with visceral cancers by indomethacin. Surgery 1981;89:414.
22. Chang JC, Gross HM. Utility of naproxen in the differential diagnosis of fever or undetermined origin in patients with cancer. Am J Med 1983;76:597.
23. Brzica SM. Complications of transfusion. Int Anesthesiol Clin 1982;20:171.
24. Reuben DB, Mor V, Hiris J. Clinical symptoms and length of survival in patients with terminal cancer. Arch Intern Med 1988;148:1586.
25. Braunwald E, Fauci AS, Kasper DL, et al. Harrison's principles of internal medicine. 15th ed. McGraw-Hill; 2001. p. 736–7.
26. Sloop GD, Friederg RC. Complications of blood transfusion. Postgrad Med 1995;98:159.
27. Higgins MJ, Blackall DP. Transfusion-associated graft-versus-host disease: a serious residual risk of blood transfusion. Curr Hematol Rep 2005;4:470.
28. Zell JA, Chang JC. Neoplastic fever: a neglected paraneoplastic syndrome. Support Care Cancer 2005;13:870.
29. Mantzios G, Tsirigotis P, Veliou F, et al. Primary adrenal lymphoma presenting as Addison's disease: case report and review of the literature. Ann Hematol 2004;83:460.
30. Lam KY, Lo CY. Metastatic tumours of the adrenal glands: a 30-year experience in a teaching hospital. Clin Endocrinol (Oxf) 2002;56:95.
31. Cleary JF. Fever and sweats: including the immunocompromised host. In: Berger A, Portenoy RK, Weissman DE, editors. Principles and practice of supportive oncology. Philadelphia: Lippincott-Raven; 1998. p. 119–31.
32. Boggs DR, Frei E. Clinical studies of fever and infection in cancer. Cancer 1960;13:1240.
33. Briggs LH. The occurrence of fever in malignant disease. Am J Med Sci 1923;166:846.
34. Browder AA, Huff JW, Petersdorf RG. The significance of fever in neoplastic disease. Ann Intern Med 1961;55:932.
35. Fenster LF, Klatskin G. Manifestations of metastatic tumor of the liver: a study of eighty-one patients subjected to needle biopsy. Am J Med 1961;31:238.
36. Klatersky J, Weerts D, Hensgens C, et al. Fever of unexplained origin in patients with cancer. Eur J Cancer 1973;9:649.

Imaging

William A. Murphy, Jr., MD

Gregory W. Gladish, MD

Sanjay Gupta, MD

Ashok J. Kumar, MD

Aurelio Matamoros, Jr., MD

Franklin C. Wong, MD, PhD, JD

Radiologic imaging services provided to patients with cancer go well beyond the diagnosis, staging, and treatment of the cancer(s) the patient may have. In addition to local relationships, proliferation, and metastasis, cancers affect the human body in many ways. Neoplasms may stimulate or elaborate biologically active substances that cause paraneoplastic syndromes. Solid tumors may create local mass effects on adjacent organs. Complications of tumors and therapy are many and include vascular problems, infection, induced necrosis, and organ failure. Imaging methods are often critical for elucidation of the specific clinical problem and provision of an interventional therapy.

The entire spectrum of imaging methods is required to manage accurate diagnosis and characterization of the problem(s) suffered by the patient with cancer. Conventional radiography is best suited to survey the chest, abdomen, and skeleton. Computed tomography (CT) provides detailed anatomic information about the brain, spine, thorax, abdomen, pelvis, and extremities. With the addition of appropriate contrast agents, CT is effective for assessment of the heart and pulmonary vasculature, as well as intra-abdominal organs and vessels. Magnetic resonance imaging (MRI) with or without gadolinium contrast enhancement is preferred for many central nervous system (CNS), cardiac, abdominal, and musculoskeletal soft tissue conditions. Conventional nuclear medicine methods, including single photon emission computed tomography (SPECT), positron emission tomography (PET), and combined CT-PET, are preferred for physiologic and functional imaging tasks. Scintigraphy provides qualitative answers to questions of whether there is normal or abnormal function of the brain, heart, blood elements, viscera, and vasculature. It answers quantitative questions of how well the organ works or how badly the organ

is damaged. Ultrasonography is employed for imaging solid organs, hollow organs, blood vessels, muscles, and masses of any origin. All of these technologies are available to interventional radiologists, who must perform biopsies and drainages and implant various devices within bronchial, ductular, and vascular structures. The partnership of diagnostic and interventional radiologists with internists, surgeons, pathologists, and other clinicians is required to achieve the most specific diagnosis; the most complete characterization of the problem, anatomy, and function; and the best minimally invasive diagnostic or therapeutic procedure for the individual patient. There is no substitute for teamwork based on reasonable knowledge of the expertise contributed by each member of the team.

Contemporary imaging is wholly digital and therefore able to be distributed in a timely fashion to all involved health care providers in a simultaneous manner, permanently and reliably stored and preserved, and easily duplicated into transferable formats for patients and distant providers.

Paraneoplastic Syndromes

Paraneoplastic syndromes are nonmetastatic clinical syndromes that accompany tumors but occur at a distance from the tumor. These conditions develop as a result of substances produced by the tumor or stimulated by the tumor but produced by other tissues. Fever is the most common clinical manifestation, but many other endocrine, rheumatologic, neurologic, dermatologic, cardiovascular, gastrointestinal, and renal symptom complexes occur. At times, the paraneoplastic syndrome precedes the discovery of the primary tumor, and recognition of the syndrome leads to a search for the tumor. Many times, the syndrome occurs concomitantly with the tumor. Sometimes

decreased or increased activity in the syndrome complex corresponds to changes in the primary or metastatic tumor burden. Although a complete exposition of paraneoplastic syndromes is outside the scope of this chapter, there are many instances in which imaging plays a role in syndrome verification and quantification.

Oncogenic (tumor-induced) osteomalacia is an example of an endocrine paraneoplastic syndrome.[1] Tumors elaborate a phosphaturic peptide that acts at the proximal renal tubule and causes phosphate wasting, with resultant hypophosphatemia. The serum calcium level is generally normal. The condition is usually caused by benign tumors, such as a hemangiopericytoma. The patient presents with debilitating osteomalacia and insufficiency fractures, both of which are evident on conventional radiographs (Figure 1). Recognition that a tumor is the cause and actual localization of the tumor may take many years. CT, MRI, and nuclear medicine tests are effective for tumor detection. Resection of the tumor commonly leads to reversal of the phosphaturic effect and remineralization of the skeleton, with regained muscle strength. Skeletal remineralization can be monitored by conventional bone surveys and by bone mineral mass (densitometry) tests.

Hypertrophic osteoarthropathy (HOA) is an example of a rheumatologic paraneoplastic syndrome manifested by swollen painful joints, clubbing of the fingers and toes, and symmetric periosteal reactions of the long bones and short tubular bones.[2] Humoral and neurogenic mechanisms have been theorized, but no etiologic agent has been proven. HOA occurs with a variety of conditions of the head and neck, thorax, and abdomen, including malignant and benign tumors, infections, and gastrointestinal inflammatory conditions. The most common association is with lung cancer. The HOA symptom complex may precede diagnosis of the cancer and

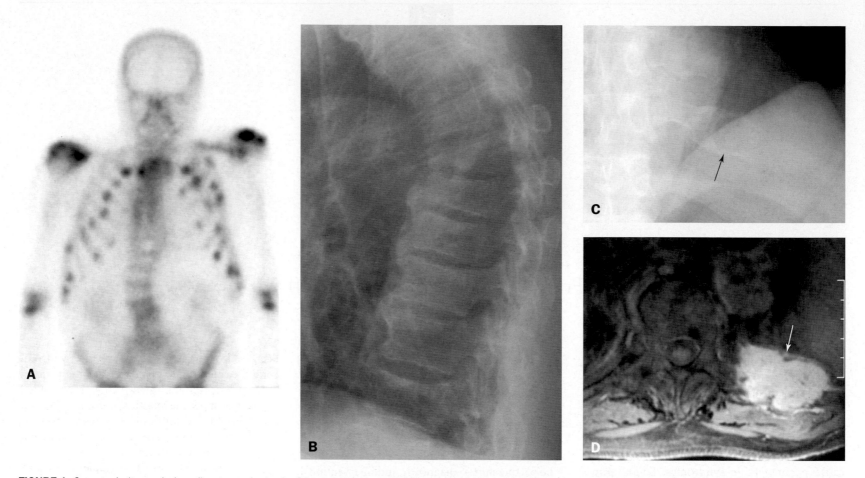

FIGURE 1 Oncogenic (tumor-induced) osteomalacia. An 80-year-old man, originally treated for B-cell lymphoma, presented with severe pain and progressively developed multiple insufficiency fractures of the ribs (*A*, detail from a radionuclide bone scan shows multiple bilateral rib fractures) and severe osteopenia with thoracic kyphosis owing to vertebral insufficiency fractures (*B*, detail from a lateral chest radiograph shows demineralized vertebral bodies with wedge deformities). Hypophosphatemic osteomalacia was diagnosed. Four years later, a rib lesion was detected (*C*, detail from a rib series shows a lytic, expansile lesion in the left tenth rib [*arrows*]) and shown to be a tumor by magnetic resonance imaging (*D*, detail from an axial section with contrast enhancement shows a soft tissue tumor [*arrow*]). After resection of a hemangiopericytoma, the skeleton remineralized, the rib fractures healed, and the pain abated.

be responsible for the search for the cancer. Clinical and radiologic manifestations vary from barely perceptible to severe. Hand involvement may seem like an intense flair of rheumatoid arthritis, with conventional films showing dramatic periarticular osteopenia in addition to thick immature periostitis (Figure 2). Radionuclide scintigraphy may show periostitis of all long bones and confirm generalized synovial joint inflammation. CT and MRI are used to detect and characterize the responsible malignant process in the head and neck, thorax, or abdomen. Sometimes resection of the primary tumor leads to total resolution of the HOA.

Paraneoplastic neurologic disease (PND) refers to central or peripheral nervous system syndromes that result from indirect effects of systemic cancer on the nervous system.[3] These syndromes can precede the detection of the primary cancer, and in the absence of any other cancer symptoms, the neurologic disability caused by the paraneoplastic syndrome is often profound. Treating the primary cancer can improve the

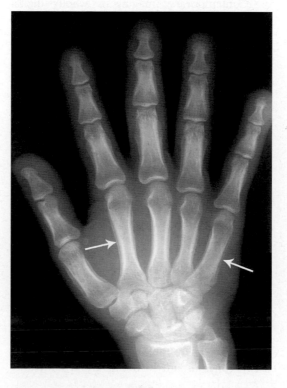

neurologic symptoms. The incidence of PND is less than 1% of patients with systemic cancer; higher incidences are reported when peripheral nerve and neuromuscular disorders are included. The first description, a peripheral neuropathy in a lung cancer patient, by Oppenheimer in 1888 was followed by descriptions of other PND syndromes: myasthenia gravis in association with thymic tumor, sensory neuropathy with lung cancer, subacute cerebellar degeneration associated with ovarian carcinoma and small cell lung carcinoma, myasthenic syndrome with small cell lung carcinoma, and cancer-associated retinopathy. The diagnosis of PND by neurologists is based primarily on the clinical presentation and

FIGURE 2 Hypertrophic osteoarthropathy. A 20-year-old man with lower extremity osteosarcoma metastatic to the lungs, mediastinum, and pericardium presented with arthritis. Posteroanterior radiograph of the right hand shows thick periostitis (*arrows*) and periarticular osteopenia.

lack of an alternative diagnosis. MRI is the imaging modality of choice for detection of pathologic processes within the brain and hence is used to detect abnormalities within the brain related to PND. Unfortunately, MRI-detectable brain and spinal cord alterations exist in only a few paraneoplastic neurologic conditions. These include paraneoplastic cerebellar degeneration, limbic encephalitis, brainstem encephalitis, and optic neuritis. PND-related spinal cord lesions detected by MRI include myelitis and necrotizing myelopathy. The discovery of serum autoantibodies that reacted with neurons offered initial insight to the pathogenesis of PND. Several PND autoantibodies and their associated antigens have been characterized.

Paraneoplastic cerebellar degeneration (PCD) was described in 1919. Serum anti–Purkinje cell antibody (anti-Yo) occurs with PCD in women in association with gynecologic malignancies, most commonly adenocarcinoma of the ovary, adnexa, endometrium, and breast. Anti-Yo is a polyclonal immunoglobulin G autoantibody that reacts primarily with Purkinje cell cytoplasm. Patients with Hodgkin's and non-Hodgkin's lymphoma may develop this syndrome but are negative for anti–Purkinje cell antibodies. Most males with PCD have either small cell lung carcinoma or lymphoma. Patients with small cell lung carcinoma or breast cancer may have anti-Hu antibodies. Patients can develop neurologic symptoms before or at the time of discovery of the neoplasm or during remission. Signs and symptoms include gait ataxia, nystagmus, dysarthria, and tremors. Pathologic findings include atrophy of the cerebellum secondary to loss of cerebellar Purkinje neurons and thinning of the granular neuronal layer. MRI can be normal in initial stages of the disease, but when cerebellar atrophy is prominent, MRI can easily detect the extent of vermian or cerebellar atrophy and resultant dilatation of cerebellar sulci.

Limbic encephalitis symptoms precede the discovery of tumor in more than half of patients. Associated tumor types are lung, testicular, and breast. Most patients have antineuronal antibodies: anti-Hu, anti-Ma, or anti-Ma2. Signs and symptoms of limbic encephalitis include personality changes that develop over days or weeks and are associated with severe impairment of recent memory, agitation, confusion, hallucinations, and seizures. Pathologic changes are usually restricted to the limbic and insular cortices, but deep gray matter and surrounding white matter may also be involved. Histologic findings include extensive loss of neurons with reactive gliosis, perivascular lymphocytic cuffing, and microglial proliferation. MRI can detect abnormal findings in one or both temporal lobes, particularly involving the region of the hippocampus and insular cortex. Imaging findings consist of abnormal hyperintensity on T_2-weighted sequences with or without abnormal enhancement following administration of a contrast agent.

Brainstem encephalitis can result in loss of cranial nerve function, with resultant diplopia, dysphagia, dysarthria, nystagmus, vertigo, and hearing loss. This condition is usually part of an encephalomyelitis or may present as an isolated finding. Patients with brainstem encephalitis usually have anti-Hu antibodies and small cell lung carcinoma. Pathologic findings include perivascular cuffing of lymphocytes and diffuse proliferation of microglial cells in the lower brainstem, particularly involving the inferior olives of the medulla. MRI can reveal generalized swelling of the brainstem with decreased signal on T_1-weighted images and increased signal on T_2-weighted images.

Myelitis, as a paraneoplastic lesion, is usually associated with a diffuse encephalomyelitis pattern. Paraneoplastic myelitis is most common with small cell lung carcinoma and is associated with anti-Hu antibody. Patients present with progressive weakness, lower motoneuron signs including fasciculations, sensory loss, and incontinence. Pathologic findings include inflammatory cells, demyelination, and neuronal loss. MRIs of the spinal cord can demonstrate the abnormality within the spinal cord with low signal intensity on T_1-weighted images and increased signal intensity on T_2-weighted images with or without contrast enhancement.

Gastrointestinal and genitourinary paraneoplastic syndromes are infrequently encountered by radiologists.[4,5] Excess prostaglandin production may produce malabsorption syndromes that are evaluated by conventional barium examinations or by abdominal CT. They have the nonspecific findings of sprue. Fever not associated with infection can occur in patients with hepatic metastases from gastrointestinal adenocarcinomas. Hepatomas have been associated with hypercalcemia, hypoglycemia, erythrocytosis, hypertension, and porphyria. Hypercalcemia as a paraneoplastic syndrome in gallbladder carcinoma has been reported. Nephrotic syndrome is sometimes encountered with lymphomas and solid tumors of the lung, colon, ovary, or pancreas. When nephrotic syndrome is considered, ultrasonography, CT, and nuclear medicine tests are employed as appropriate to the individual clinical situation. Rarely, paraneoplastic syndromes mimic pregnancy. Ultrasonography is particularly valuable to rule out intrauterine or ectopic pregnancy.

Pancreatic paraneoplastic syndromes are well known. Multiple syndromes are associated with the pancreas. Islet cell tumors can lead to hypoglycemia (insulinoma), Zollinger-Ellison syndrome (gastrinomas), glucagonomas, pancreatic cholera (Verner-Morrison syndrome), hypercalcemia, ectopic adrenocorticotropic hormone syndrome, syndrome of inappropriate antidiuretic hormone, hyperpigmentation, and systemic nodular panniculitis. Pancreatic cancer is also associated with migratory superficial thrombophlebitis (Trousseau's syndrome). The pancreas is initially imaged by ultrasonography, although the tail of the pancreas is not seen in a significant number of patients. Color Doppler evaluation can be used to assess the adjacent vasculature. Thin-slice multidetector CT scans with dedicated pancreatic protocols provide the best detail of the pancreas, adjacent and regional vasculature, and other solid and hollow viscera in the abdomen. MRI, magnetic resonance cholangiopancreatography, angiography, and nuclear medicine scintigraphy can also be used in the evaluation of pancreatic disease based on the clinical situation.

Direct Medical Complications of the Cancer

Clinicians and radiologists often encounter problems directly caused by the cancer that require accurate diagnosis, detailed characterization, and appropriate treatment for relief of the symptoms they cause. The local effect of a tumor mass on an adjacent structure is a prime example.

Superior vena cava syndrome (SVCS) is caused by obstruction of the superior vena cava (SVC) and/or brachiocephalic veins and can present with facial and arm swelling, chest pain, cough, proptosis, hoarseness, stridor, dyspnea, cyanosis, and symptoms of increased intracranial pressure, such as somnolence, syncope, convulsions, and visual disturbance. SVCS usually presents with slowly progressive symptoms but can present with an abrupt onset, constituting a true medical emergency. More than 80% of the cases result from malignant etiologies, with bronchogenic carcinoma, lymphoma, and metastatic carcinoma being the most common.[6]

In the most typical presentation of SVCS, the appearance of a large mediastinal mass at conventional chest radiography is usually adequate for the diagnosis of neoplastic obstruction, although infectious masses can also cause obstruction. Smaller masses or masses high in the thoracic inlet may not be visible by conventional radiography and require contrast-enhanced chest CT for adequate evaluation. Patients with radiographically obvious masses may also require CT for radiation therapy planning to relieve the obstruction. In the absence of a mass, SVC stenosis may cause the syndrome and be related to previous radiation therapy or thrombosis from long-term central venous catheter placement.[7] CT can provide excellent delineation of any mediastinal mass or vascular stenosis.

Although medical therapy with elevation of the affected extremities and head, along with anticoagulation, corticosteroids, and diuretics, may temporize the condition, short- and long-term results are poor. In SVCS caused by malignancy, radiotherapy and/or chemotherapy are considered the current standard for treatment, with resolution rates up to 90%; however, regression of symptoms occurs slowly (2–4 weeks) and may be incomplete. Symptoms recur in 10 to 30% of the patients. Moreover, response rates are highly dependent on tumor histology and radio- or chemosensitivity. Surgical bypass of the obstructed SVC is associated with a high rate of morbidity and mortality and often fails because of thrombosis of the graft.

Imaging-guided percutaneous endovascular techniques, such as transluminal angioplasty, thrombolysis, and stent implantation, used alone or in combination, have shown excellent short-term and midterm success in patients with SVCS secondary to malignancy.[8] Generally, percutaneous techniques have been used after failure of radiotherapy and/or chemotherapy. However, with the refinement of endovascular techniques, percutaneous stenting of the SVC is increasingly used as the primary treatment modality. Balloon angioplasty is used to assist stent deployment; although balloon angioplasty alone can cause immediate improvement in symptoms, short- and long-term vessel patency is poor. Intravascular metallic stent implantation provides significant resolution of symptoms in 70 to 100% of patients. In the majority of cases, a subjective improvement is noticed after a few hours and the soft tissue edema disappears in 24 to 72 hours. In patients with SVCS associated with acute thrombosis, local thrombolytic treatment by direct administration of fibrinolytic substances via an infusion catheter improves the results of stenting. Mechanical thrombectomy devices may be used to remove the thrombus in patients with significant clot burden or in patients who may not receive thrombolysis safely. Complications resulting from thrombolytic treatment or stent placement are infrequent. Stent migration, prosthesis breakage, cardiac arrhythmias, transient phrenic nerve paralysis, and bleeding have been reported.

Symptoms of SVCS recur in 4 to 45% of treated patients and are usually secondary to tumor ingrowth, extrinsic tumor compression, or thrombus formation. Recurrent obstruction can be treated with anticoagulation, angioplasty of the stented area, or repeat stenting. A covered stent may be used to retard tumor ingrowth; however, its efficacy is unproven.

Intrinsic venous stenosis secondary to venous thrombosis or thrombophlebitis owing to long-term central venous catheter placement for chemotherapy is usually asymmetric because the location of the stenosis typically develops before the confluence of brachiocephalic veins.[9] CT and digital venography are diagnostic tests. When the upper extremity edema is asymmetric, it is important that contrast media be administered through the edematous extremity. If central venous thrombosis is suspected, bilateral arm injection of contrast media can be performed.[10] Venous stenosis caused by long-term catheter placement or radiation therapy typically demonstrates a long segment of venous stenosis or complete obliteration of the involved vein, with no appreciable soft tissue mass. By comparison, thrombosis presents a well-defined filling defect within the vein and thrombophlebitis as a mildly enhancing, poorly defined tubular mass along the expected course of the vein (Figure 3). Flow artifacts from incomplete mixing of the contrast agent with the intravascular blood must be differentiated from true filling defects within the venous system. The continued presence of a central venous catheter can simulate contrast passing through a residual lumen of the occluded vessel, but the presence of extensive collateral venous drainage will confirm the severity of the stenosis. Anticoagulation or thrombolytic therapy is the usual treatment strategy.

Inferior vena cava (IVC) obstruction secondary to primary or secondary liver malignancies or other abdominal tumors presents with debilitating features such as leg edema, scrotal or vulvar edema, venous stasis ulceration, ascites, and anasarca below the diaphragm. CT and MRI are effective for the diagnosis and staging of this complication. Endovascular stent placement can be used to palliate symptoms related to malignant

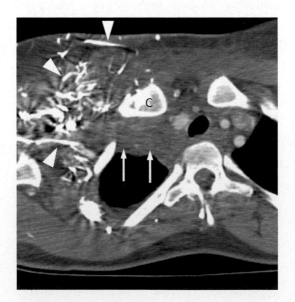

FIGURE 3 Subclavian vein thrombophlebitis. A 22-year-old woman with osteosarcoma had a right central venous catheter removed for infection. Computed tomography of the chest at the thoracic inlet demonstrates a poorly defined tubular mass (*arrows*) in the course of the right subclavian vein behind the right medial clavicular head (C). Note abundant collateral vein enhancement (*arrowheads*).

IVC obstruction. In a study involving 50 consecutive patients with malignant IVC syndrome who were treated with intrahepatic stent placement, Broutzos and colleagues reported primary and secondary patency rates of 59 and 100%, respectively, at 540 days.[11] All symptoms related to IVC obstruction were significantly improved after stent placement and, with the exception of ascites, remained significantly improved until the last follow-up. Even patients with a very short life expectancy benefited significantly from palliative stent placement.

Dysphagia owing to esophageal stricture in patients with inoperable primary or secondary esophageal malignancies is safely and effectively treated by fluoroscopic placement of self-expandable metal stents, such as the Gianturco Z stent, Wallstent, and Ultraflex stent. These stents successfully relieve esophageal obstruction and yield rapid relief of dysphagia and improved quality of life.[12] Esophageal stents can be inserted endoscopically without fluoroscopic guidance. However, use of fluoroscopic guidance and catheter guidewire technology is essential for crossing tight esophageal stenoses and for accurately positioning the metallic stents. Interventional radiologists are in the ideal position to perform these procedures safely and relatively easily. Stents should never be placed across the superior esophageal sphincter (C5–C6 level), and crossing the gastroesophageal junction with the stent should be avoided if possible. Covered stents appear to be efficacious for sealing malignant esophagorespiratory fistulae.

Other contemporary methods used for palliation of malignant esophageal strictures, such as surgical bypass, laser ablation, radiation therapy, and endoscopic alcohol injection, are associated with substantial morbidity and mortality. Although the complication rate of metallic stent placement is less than that of other palliative methods, complications such as chest pain, stent migration (0–35%), tumor ingrowth or overgrowth (5–50%), hemorrhage (0–10%), perforation or fistulization (0–8%), and food impaction (6%) have been reported.

Bowel obstruction or perforation is first evaluated with a conventional abdominal or obstructive series, although the imaging modality of choice is often a CT scan of the abdomen and pelvis with use of gastrointestinal and intravenous contrast (Figure 4). A CT scan gives a global view of the gastrointestinal tract and the solid viscera, vasculature, and lung bases. Ascites and suspected appendicitis can be evaluated by ultrasonography. A CT scan is a better study in difficult patients and can image the rest of the hollow organs and solid viscera for disease processes mimicking appendicitis.

Gastric outlet and duodenal obstructions in patients with primary or metastatic cancer are

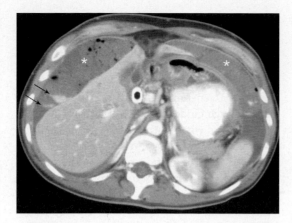

FIGURE 4 Small bowel perforation. Contrast-enhanced axial computed tomographic image of the upper abdomen shows free fluid and gas (*) secondary to the perforation. Wisps of extravasated gastrointestinal contrast agent are evident (*arrows*).

serious conditions causing nausea, vomiting, and abdominal distention that can lead to progressive deterioration in the patient's condition and quality of life. Surgical palliation may be associated with significant morbidity and mortality, with symptomatic improvement in only half of the cases. Laparoscopic gastroenterostomy can provide successful palliation with less morbidity and mortality; however, it still requires general anesthesia and may not be feasible in patients with ascites and/or peritoneal malignant disease. Fluoroscopically guided placement of a gastrostomy tube by an interventional radiologist is a simple, minimally invasive method for symptom palliation in patients with malignant gastroduodenal obstruction. Alternatively, a dual-lumen gastrojejunostomy catheter can be placed; the gastric (proximal) port provides drainage, and the jejunal (distal) port provides a conduit for alimentation. In spite of their effectiveness, these measures do not allow oral intake and the nausea and vomiting are not always resolved.

Self-expanding metal stents are increasingly placed for symptom palliation in patients with inoperable malignant gastroduodenal obstructions.[13] Both uncovered and covered metal stents have been used for this purpose, and both provide effective palliation. A metallic stent allows the patient to eat and improves quality of life. Recurrent obstruction secondary to tumor ingrowth through the openings between the wire filaments of uncovered stents remains a major problem; recurrent stenosis rates of 8 to 46% have been reported. The use of a covered stent decreases the rate of recurrent obstruction by preventing tumor ingrowth. However, because of the smooth surface of the stent covering, there is an increased risk of stent migration, seen in up to 26% of patients 1 to 4 days after placement. Further investigations are still needed to develop an ideal stent design that combines the advantages of

covered (low tumor ingrowth rate) and uncovered (low migration rate) stents. Recently, Lopera and colleagues described the use of a partially covered stent to overcome these limitations; a central covered portion prevents tumor ingrowth, and uncovered flared ends anchor the stent to the bowel mucosa to prevent migration.[14] Another technique involves placement of coaxial placement of an outer uncovered stent and an inner covered stent. Although initial results are promising, a larger group of patients is necessary to determine the effectiveness of these new techniques.

Biliary obstruction frequently complicates primary or secondary abdominal malignancy. Complications associated with obstructive jaundice, such as malabsorption, coagulopathy, hepatocellular dysfunction, disabling pruritus, and cholangitis, greatly interfere with a patient's quality of life. Endoscopic or percutaneous insertion of a biliary stent is a well-established method for palliation of inoperable malignant obstructive jaundice.[15,16] Although endoscopic placement of biliary stents is the preferred method for most biliary obstructions, percutaneous biliary drainage is used in situations when the endoscopic approach fails or when gastric outlet obstruction or partial gastrectomy makes endoscopic placement difficult or impossible. The percutaneous transhepatic approach is also preferred in patients with high obstructions and bilateral or multiple strictures.

Percutaneous biliary drainage can be of three types: external, combined external-internal, or internal (Figure 5). An external drainage catheter ends proximal to the obstruction, and the bile

drains into an external bag. An internal-external catheter extends across the level of obstruction, with the distal tip of the catheter in the duodenum and multiple side holes along the catheter shaft allowing internal drainage. Internal biliary drainage can be accomplished with the use of plastic or metal stents. Self-expanding metallic stents are associated with reduced reintervention rates, lower complication rates, and longer patency rates compared with plastic stents. Long-term patency remains an important problem with uncovered metal stents. Reobstruction rates varying from 5 to 100%, with a weighted mean of 22%. Proximal and distal tumor overgrowth, tumor ingrowth through the wire mesh, and encrustation and sludge formation are common causes of stent occlusion. Several investigators have described use of covered stents in an effort to improve the patency rates. Various prototype covered stents have been used for treatment of malignant biliary obstruction.[17] However, their occlusion rates remain high, varying from 0 to 37%, with a weighted mean of 14.7%. Also, fully or partially covered stents are prone to migration (3–11% of cases); use of anchoring fins at each end of the stent can reduce the risk of migration.

Ureteral obstruction is common in advanced pelvic malignancy, occurs with metastatic disease from nonpelvic malignancy, and may be related to iatrogenic causes, such as surgery and radiation. Ultrasonography is the study of choice to evaluate hydronephrosis, not only for obstruction but also to assess renal echogenicity, location, number, shape, size, calculi, and masses and with color Doppler evaluation to determine the status of the renal vasculature. Some tiny calculi

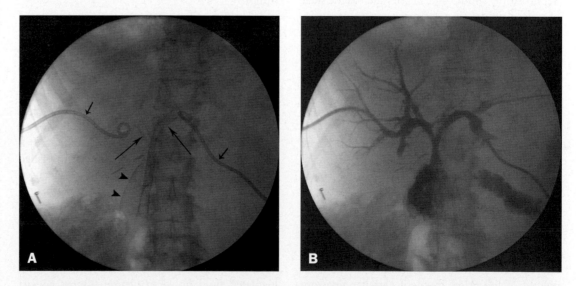

FIGURE 5 Biliary drainage. A 71-year-old man with inoperable pancreatic head carcinoma and hilar adenopathy presented with biliary obstruction. *A*, A spot abdominal radiograph shows percutaneously placed external biliary drainage catheters (*short arrows*) and internal metal stents in the right and left bile ducts (*long arrows*) and in the common duct. Note the presence of a duodenal stent (*arrowheads*), which was placed for duodenal obstruction. *B*, Contrast administration through the left and right external biliary drainage catheters shows adequate drainage through the biliary and duodenal stents and into the duodenum.

may not be seen by ultrasonography, especially in large patients. The full length of the ureters may not be completely visualized even though a distal obstruction with hydroureter(s) may be present. Dedicated CT urography, which does not require intravenous contrast, is available to evaluate renal colic. Routine CT scans can also evaluate hydronephrosis, masses, and disease within the abdomen and pelvis that can mimic renal colic. CT scans can also help identify the etiology and location of obstruction or source of hematuria. MRI can evaluate the kidneys especially when the patient is in renal failure or is allergic to iodinated intravenous contrast agents. The kidneys and collecting systems can also be evaluated using conventional radiography, intravenous urography, and scintigraphy.

Percutaneous nephrostomy (PCN) is a well-established safe and effective technique for the management of urinary obstruction.[18] In these patients, urinary diversion with PCN helps preserve renal function and allows institution of appropriate anticancer treatment. It is particularly important in patients whose therapeutic regimens will include agents that depend on renal excretion and are potentially nephrotoxic.

Many cancer patients presenting with ureteral obstruction may expect a reasonably good quality of life, and intervention is often warranted. However, the quality of life after palliative urinary diversion must be carefully examined. Patients who present with bilateral obstruction and uremia have a poor performance status and short life expectancy after ureteral decompression if their disease remains untreated. Many authors believe that nephrostomy is of little use in patients with advanced disease if no effective salvage therapy is available. Hence, selection of cancer patients for nephrostomy should take factors such as the stage of cancer, prognosis of primary cancer, prospects of further antineoplastic treatment, and quality of life into consideration before the PCN is created.

Major or minor complications may be seen in 10% of patients who undergo a PCN procedure.[18] Although transient hematuria is common, major hemorrhagic complications that require transfusion or intervention occur in only 1 to 3% of patients. Hydrothorax, hemothorax, and pneumothorax can also occur, and their prevalence increases when renal access is supracostal. The mortality rate for PCN is low (0.046–0.3%). Although initial PCN has a high technical success rate, long-term management of nephrostomy catheters is cumbersome and the presence of an external drainage bag and the need for daily catheter care substantially compromise the patient's quality of life. Also, frequent catheter revisions may be required.

Internal ureteral stenting is an alternative to external nephrostomy catheterization for provision of long-term urinary drainage.[19] Internal stents can be placed from either a retrograde approach via the bladder by cystoscopy or from the antegrade approach through the kidney following percutaneous access. Internal ureteral stents eliminate the need for external collection devices and improve patient independence. Internal stents need to be exchanged every 6 months; this is in contrast to external nephrostomy tubes, which often require exchange at 3-month intervals. Double-J plastic stents are the most commonly used ureteral stents. Metal stents have also been used in the treatment of malignant ureteral obstructions, with encouraging initial results. However, mid- and long-term outcomes are poor, with a primary patency rate of only 31% at 12 months. Newer stents with a biocompatible covering (stent grafts) may improve patency rates of metal stents.

Pleural effusions are a common consequence of pleural tumor or may result from therapy.[20] Large pleural effusions can cause significant respiratory impairment. Pleural effusion can typically be demonstrated with conventional radiography. For moderate-size effusions, lateral decubitus views may be helpful to demonstrate free flow or layering as distinct from loculation of the effusion. Contralateral decubitus views are helpful in distinguishing between compressive atelectasis and pulmonary consolidation that may be associated with the effusion. For very large effusions, decubitus views are unlikely to add much additional information. If the hemithorax is completely opacified, then CT or ultrasonography is useful in distinguishing effusion from the mass and to direct appropriate drainage therapy. Talc pleurodesis performed to treat chronic pleural effusion can result in abnormal uptake on fluorodeoxyglucose PET. Correlation with CT should allow this uptake to be differentiated from pleural tumor.[21]

Almost half of patients with disseminated cancer develop symptomatic malignant pleural effusion (MPE) during the course of their disease. The most common causative neoplasms are lung cancer, breast cancer, lymphoma, ovarian cancer, and gastric cancer. These patients face a dismal prognosis, with a median survival time of less than 6 to 12 months. MPEs are associated with significant morbidity because of resultant dyspnea, cough, chest discomfort, and diminished quality of life. Repeated thoracentesis can be used for management of MPE; however, it is uncomfortable, carries a 10% risk of pneumothorax, can contaminate the pleural space, and may provide only temporary symptom relief. Although thoracentesis can be performed in the clinic, image guidance may be necessary in patients with loculated fluid or when pleural tumors coexist with the effusion. The use of repeated thoracentesis is typically limited to symptomatic patients with an effusion expected to respond to systemic therapy or for patients with a very limited life expectancy.

Tube thoracostomy followed by chemical pleurodesis is the standard treatment for MPE. Although large surgical chest tubes traditionally are used for this purpose, smaller-caliber tubes placed by interventional radiologists are equally effective.[22] Generally, a 12F or 14F tube is placed under image guidance, and a sclerosing agent is administered when outputs drop to less than 150 to 300 mL/d and when chest imaging shows drainage of the fluid and reexpansion of the lung. The most commonly used sclerosing agents are tetracycline, doxycycline, bleomycin, and talc. Randomized trials have shown no significant differences among various agents.

Chemical pleurodesis may not be effective in patients with (1) persistent high-output effusion that prevents adequate apposition of the pleural layers; (2) the presence of a trapped lung from a pleural peel, endobronchial obstruction, or parenchymal lung disease; or (3) viscous or loculated fluid interfering with drainage. Administration of fibrinolytic agents through the catheter can be used to liquify viscous or loculated fluid. The major drawbacks of chemical pleurodesis are the need for 4 to 7 days of hospitalization, the presence of pain and discomfort associated with the procedure, and the occasional development of multiloculated fluid collections following treatment.

Recently, the use of an indwelling tunneled pleural catheter has been accepted as an effective alternative to chemical pleurodesis in managing MPE.[23] The Denver Pleurx catheter (Denver Biomaterials, Inc., Golden, CO) is a 15.5F soft silicone catheter with multiple distal side holes to enhance drainage, a polyester cuff along the proximal shaft to promote fibrosis in the subcutaneous tunnel, and a valve in its hub that prevents inadvertent entry of air or leakage of fluid. The drainage system consists of a vacuum bottle with a preconnected tube that has a dilator at its end to fit into the hub of the catheter. The system is commonly used in the outpatient setting by a visiting nurse, family members, or the patient. Drainage is performed at least every other day but can be done more frequently if necessary. This treatment achieves safe, long-term, outpatient control of MPE and related symptoms in 80 to 90% of patients. Also, the presence of the tube and intermittent complete aspiration of the fluid can cause pleurodesis in up to 50% of patients. Administration of a sclerosing agent through the tube may enhance the pleurodesis rates. Complications are uncommon but include sequestration of the catheter from the effusion caused by formation of a fibrotic sleeve, catheter occlusion, development of separate loculations, infection, and catheter fracture during removal.

Pericardial effusions owing to tumor or therapy are frequent. Cardiac tamponade is an uncommon complication of tumor involvement.[24] The relatively slow accumulation of pericardial fluid usually allows the pericardium to enlarge to accommodate the volume. Although conventional radiography may show cardiac silhouette enlargement, echocardiography or CT is needed to accurately distinguish effusion from cardiomegaly and may also demonstrate right atrial and right ventricular collapse resulting from tamponade (Figure 6).

Hemorrhage, occasionally life threatening, is a common problem in oncology patients that may be related to the tumor itself or may be encountered as a complication of thrombocytopenia, surgery, or radiotherapy. Technetium 99m (Tc 99m)-labeled sulfur colloid can localize the hemorrhage, with bleeding rates as low as 0.1 mL per minute.[25] However, because of the prompt trapping of the sulfur colloid by the reticuloendothelial system from the general circulation, Tc 99m sulfur colloid can detect active bleeding only during the first few minutes after injection. For more prolonged periods (several hours) of detection, Tc 99m–labeled red blood cells are preferred because they remain in the blood pool much longer. However, because of the high background circulating radioactivity, Tc 99m red blood cells detect bleeding that occurs only at rates above 1 mL per minute (Figure 7).[26] Angiographic methods may also be used to detect bleeding sites, particularly when interventional procedures are selected to control the hemorrhage.

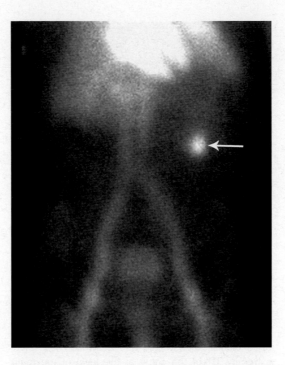

FIGURE 7 Red blood cell scan for gastrointestinal bleeding. A patient with bright red blood per rectum underwent a gastrointestinal bleeding scan using 20 mCi technetium 99m–labeled red blood cells. The scintigraphs were 1 minute apart, and abnormal focal tracer activity accumulated in the left upper quadrant. The activity subsequently localized in the small bowel (*arrow*).

Intra-arterial administration of embolic agents to induce vascular occlusion is a well-established technique used to arrest hemorrhage. Numerous devices or materials have been used as embolic agents. The choice of the embolic agent for a given case depends on the nature of the bleeding, the desired level and duration of occlusion, the availability of the particular agent, and the experience and preference of the interventional radiologist.

Pelvic bleeding from gynecologic and urologic tumors can present as chronic, intractable bleeding or occasionally as massive and potentially life-threatening hemorrhage. Although surgical ligation of internal iliac arteries has been used for management of pelvic bleeding, surgery may not be appropriate in many patients either because of the poor general condition of the patient or because of deformed, friable pelvic tissues owing to radiotherapy, previous surgery, or tumor recurrence. Percutaneous transcatheter arterial embolization of the anterior division of internal iliac artery results in complete control of bleeding in about 70% of pelvic malignancies.[27]

Endovascular techniques can also be used to manage iatrogenic pelvic bleeding. Hemorrhagic cystitis resulting from chemotherapy or following radiotherapy can present with intractable hematuria. Although simple bladder irrigation; cystodiathermy; oral, parenteral, and intravesical agents; hyperbaric oxygen therapy; or urinary

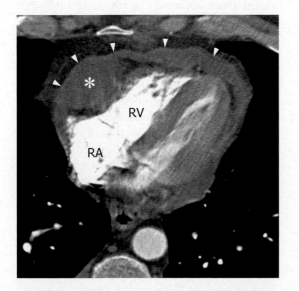

FIGURE 6 Malignant pericardial effusion. A 69-year-old man with lung cancer developed fatigue and dyspnea. Computed tomography of the chest at the level of the right atrium (RA) and right ventricle (RV) demonstrates low-attenuation pericardial thickening with enhancement of the parietal pericardium (*arrowheads*). A partly loculated portion of the effusion (*) is compressing the right ventricle. A pericardial window was performed to relieve the compression.

diversion can help control the bleeding in a majority of patients, bilateral internal iliac embolization has also been successful. Arterioureteral fistulae are uncommon causes of potentially life-threatening hemorrhage and can be seen after pelvic surgery for malignancy, often in association with irradiation and chronic indwelling ureteral stenting. Percutaneous embolization of the iliac artery followed by extra-anatomic arterial bypass has been successfully used to manage these cases. More recently, covered stents have been used to close the fistula while maintaining antegrade flow through the iliac artery.[28]

Head and neck hemorrhage in patients with head and neck cancer can be difficult to control because of postsurgical changes, fistulae, infection, radiation necrosis, or recurrent tumor. In these patients, hemorrhage usually results from erosion of vessels. Conventional noninvasive measures such as nasal packing and balloon tamponade often fail. Transcatheter arterial embolization is a safe and effective alternative treatment of severe epistaxis.[29] Diagnostic internal and external carotid artery angiography is performed to detect the source of bleeding and any possible anastomoses between the two arterial systems that might present a risk of embolization of non-target tissues. Superselective catheterization and embolization are then performed.

Rupture of the extracranial carotid arteries, the so-called carotid blowout, often results in catastrophic hemorrhage. Predisposing factors include radiation therapy, radical resection, flap necrosis, wound infection, pharyngocutaneous fistula, and recurrent or persistent carcinoma. Emergency surgical ligation of the common or internal carotid artery is associated with unacceptable rates of death and stroke. Endovascular occlusion with detachable balloons or coils after a balloon occlusion test to assess cross-circulation yields improved outcome; however, recurrent bleeding and delayed neurologic ischemic events may occur. More recently, covered stents have been used to exclude carotid pseudoaneurysms with parent vessel preservation.

Hemoptysis with bronchogenic carcinoma, pulmonary metastases, and postradiation bronchiectasis can be massive and recurrent. Conservative management of massive hemoptysis has a mortality of 50 to 100%, asphyxiation being the most common cause of death. Because of poor pulmonary reserve and other comorbid conditions, most cancer patients with massive hemoptysis are not surgical candidates. Transcatheter arterial embolization results in control of bleeding in 51 to 85% of patients, but recurrent bleeding requiring repeat embolization is seen in 16% of cases.[30] Major complications such as spinal cord injury related to invisible anastomotic connections between the bronchial circulation and the anterior spinal artery, transient thoracic pain, and bronchial, esophageal, pulmonary arterial, or aortic wall necrosis are rare.

Gastrointestinal hemorrhage can result from primary bowel neoplasms, direct invasion by adjacent tumors, or bowel metastases. Transcatheter arterial embolization can successfully control malignancy-related gastrointestinal hemorrhage in patients with inoperable cancer or to stabilize the patient prior to definitive surgery. Pseudoaneurysms involving the gastroduodenal artery or pancreaticoduodenal arteries can develop as a complication of pancreaticoduodenectomy for pancreatic cancer and can present with gastrointestinal bleeding. Transcatheter superselective arterial embolization is the preferred technique for control of bleeding in these patients.

Indirect Medical Complications of the Cancer

Pulmonary embolism (PE) remains a diagnostic challenge because it is often occult and because the results from physical examination, laboratory, and most radiologic tests are commonly nonspecific. The imaging evaluation of dyspnea, the most common presenting symptom, typically begins with a conventional chest radiograph. A number of radiographic signs have been associated with PE. These include a peripherally based, wedge-shaped pulmonary opacity known as a Hampton hump, decreased blood flow in the lung affected by PE known as Westermark's sign, and enlargement of the central pulmonary artery known as Fleischner's sign.[31] However, these signs are infrequently encountered and are neither sensitive nor specific for PE. In fact, the most common radiographic findings of PE include a normal-appearing chest radiograph or nonspecific pulmonary consolidation and pleural effusion.[32]

The traditional imaging test for a more sensitive and specific diagnosis of PE is ventilation-perfusion scintigraphy, which can be effective when there are no significant pulmonary abnormalities demonstrated by chest radiography. Ventilation-perfusion scanning effectively identifies patients with a very high or very low probability of PE, and this determination is sufficient for therapeutic management. However, many patients have intermediate or indeterminate-probability nuclear scans for PE and thus require further evaluation. Conventional pulmonary angiography emerged as the definitive imaging test in cases of indeterminate probability. However, its invasive nature, limited availability, and perceived risks discouraged its use.

More recently, CT pulmonary angiography has matured as a method to image PE (Figure 8).[33] Contemporary CT scanners allow rapid acquisition of thinly collimated images and provide a high-resolution direct assessment of the

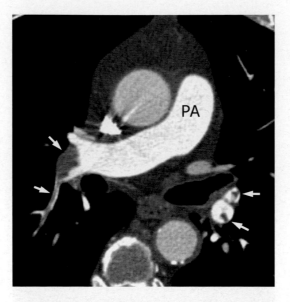

FIGURE 8 Pulmonary embolus by computed tomography (CT). A 73-year-old man with colon cancer developed pleuritic chest pain and a swollen left lower extremity. CT of the chest at the level of the main pulmonary artery (PA) demonstrates pulmonary emboli in the right pulmonary artery and branches of the left pulmonary artery (*arrows*). Notice how the emboli extend across the bifurcation of the right pulmonary artery and lie centrally in the left pulmonary artery branches.

pulmonary arterial tree. The accuracy of CT angiography has been validated through the demonstration of its negative predictive value. Several studies have shown absence of significant risk for future PE events in patients with a negative CT pulmonary angiographic study.[34–36] Because of its wide availability and confidence in its interpretation, CT pulmonary angiography has largely displaced other methods to detect pulmonary emboli. Additionally, CT pulmonary angiography provides prognostic information for those patients in whom PE is confirmed.[37] Evidence of right ventricular strain, including bowing of the septum toward the left ventricle and an increase in the right ventricle to left ventricle diameter ratio, is predictive of the need for intensive care unit admission.[38] An important feature of CT angiography is its ability to show features that indicate alternative diagnoses in the absence of PE. CT can identify independent causes of dyspnea, including atelectasis, pneumonia, effusion, pneumothorax, and other cardiovascular abnormalities.

The utility of CT pulmonary angiography can be enhanced with preexamination use of a D-dimer assay to exclude patients without evidence of intravascular thrombosis. This strategy reduces the number of negative examinations and prevents unnecessary radiation exposure.[39] However, because of its low specificity, a positive D-dimer assay alone is not justification for performing CT pulmonary angiography.

PE is estimated to result in 150,000 deaths per year in the United States. Standard management consists of anticoagulation with heparin and warfarin to prevent recurrence of PE; however, the 3-month mortality rate still ranges from 10 to 17.5%.[40] Also, anticoagulation alone may constitute sufficient therapy for massive PE. Systemic thrombolytic therapy and interventional procedures, including catheter-directed thrombolysis, percutaneous embolectomy, and percutaneous thrombus fragmentation techniques, are alternative treatment options. These aggressive measures are usually reserved for life-threatening massive PE associated with hemodynamic instability and cardiogenic shock.

There is no consensus regarding the indications for thrombolytic therapy in patients with a PE. Although several randomized controlled trials have shown that thrombolytic agents dissolve clot more rapidly than does heparin, reduced recurrence and mortality rates have been difficult to demonstrate. Nevertheless, since thrombolysis provides a rapid reduction in thrombus burden, allowing restoration of pulmonary blood flow, thrombolytic treatment is strongly recommended and can be lifesaving in patients with an acute massive PE associated with shock. More recently, based on studies showing that right ventricular hypokinesia, as demonstrated on the echocardiogram, is associated with decreased survival in these patients, thrombolytic therapy has been advocated in hemodynamically stable patients with right ventricular dysfunction. The usefulness of thrombolytic therapy in this subset of patients requires large, prospective, randomized, controlled trials. Currently available thrombolytic agents include urokinase, alteplase (tissue plasminogen activator), reteplase, and tenecteplase. There is no significant difference in the efficacy of these agents.

Percutaneous placement of a catheter within the pulmonary artery allows catheter-directed local delivery of a thrombolytic drug into the pulmonary circulation or into the thrombus itself. This strategy has been proposed as an alternative to systemic thrombolysis in patients with acute massive PE. Theoretically, local delivery should accelerate clot lysis and achieve more rapid reperfusion of the pulmonary circulation. In one report, catheter-directed thrombolysis with recombinant tissue plasminogen activator (rt-PA) resulted in rapid clot lysis in 94% of patients.[41] In another report, intrapulmonary infusion of rt-PA did not offer significant benefit compared with intravenous administration.[42] Further research is needed to define the role of catheter-directed thrombolysis in the management of these patients. Improvements in survival and long-term pulmonary perfusion will require consistent demonstration.

Thrombolytic therapy is associated with major bleeding events, the most feared of which is intracranial hemorrhage. A recent meta-analysis of available data demonstrated that thrombolysis is associated with an increased risk of bleeding (13.7%) compared with heparin (7.7%) in patients with an acute PE.[43] Although it has been suggested that catheter-directed thrombolysis could reduce the risk of hemorrhage, this remains to be proven. Any patient considered for thrombolytic treatment should be evaluated for contraindications such as recent cerebrovascular accident, intracranial surgery (< 2 months), active intracranial abnormality (neoplasm, aneurysm, or vascular malformation), or recent major hemorrhage.

Patients with massive PE and compromised hemodynamic status, in whom thrombolytic therapy is not effective or is contraindicated and who are not candidates for open surgery, can be treated with percutaneous interventional procedures such as embolectomy, clot fragmentation, and thrombectomy.[43] Percutaneous mechanical devices can fragment, macerate, aspirate, or remove clots. They can break the thrombus into smaller fragments that migrate into the peripheral pulmonary artery branches, opening up the central pulmonary arteries and improving perfusion. There is some evidence that redistribution of larger central clots into the peripheral pulmonary arteries may result in an acute reduction in pulmonary pressure and an increase in total pulmonary blood flow. These devices can be used as a complement to thrombolytic therapy. Fragmentation of the clot exposes fresh surfaces for infused thrombolytic drugs. Conversely, softening of the clot by a thrombolytic drug may facilitate debulking and fragmentation of occlusive clots.

Venous thrombosis is a common precursor to PE. Although anticoagulation remains the treatment of choice for venous thrombosis and PE, IVC filters provide a viable and effective alternative for reduction of PE (Figure 9). Absolute indications for IVC filter placement include (1) contraindication to anticoagulation; (2) failure of anticoagulation, such as recurrent PE despite adequate anticoagulation; (3) development of complication from anticoagulation therapy; and (4) inability to anticoagulate to a therapeutic range despite patient compliance with medication. Some relative indications include (1) a large free-floating thrombus in the IVC, (2) chronic untreated PE prior to pulmonary embolectomy, (3) thromboembolic disease with marginal cardiopulmonary reserve, (4) poor compliance with anticoagulant medication, and (5) thrombolysis of deep venous thrombophlebitis. The only absolute contraindications to IVC filter placement are chronic thrombosis of the IVC and a lack of venous access.

Vena cava filters are generally placed in the infrarenal IVC. Suprarenal placement of filters is

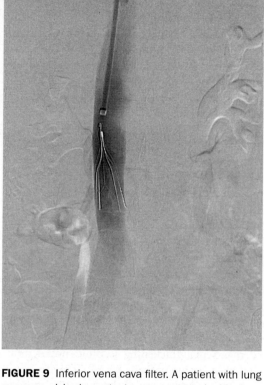

FIGURE 9 Inferior vena cava filter. A patient with lung cancer and brain metastases presented with deep venous thrombosis involving the right femoral vein. A cavogram through a transjugular sheath shows a filter deployed in the infrarenal portion of the inferior vena cava.

indicated in the following situations: infrarenal vena cava thrombosis precluding infrarenal placement, renal vein thrombosis, ovarian vein thrombosis, possible current or future pregnancy, and thrombus proximal to an infrarenal filter.

Most complications of IVC filter placement are minor in nature. The recurrent symptomatic PE rate is similar, with all available filters and ranges from 2 to 5%.[44] IVC thrombosis is seen in 2 to 30% of patients and although usually partial and asymptomatic can rarely become complete and cause phlegmasia cerulea dolens, necessitating thrombolysis. Other complications include recurrent deep venous thrombosis, filter migration and embolization, IVC penetration, filter fracture, venous insufficiency, guidewire entrapment, and access-site thrombosis.

Currently, 10 different filters approved by the Food and Drug Administration are available for use in the United States. Most filters are constructed of nonferromagnetic material and hence are considered safe during MRI and do not cause significant artifact on MRIs. Although safe, the stainless steel Greenfield filter and the Bird's Nest filter produce substantial artifact in MRIs. Even though MRI can be performed safely in patients with all types of IVC filters, a delay of

6 weeks between implantation and imaging is recommended.

Systemic Complications of Malignancy and Therapy

Neutropenic fever is a diagnostic challenge because the host lacks its usual responses to infection. The imaging evaluation typically begins with a chest radiograph.[45] The findings at chest radiography can be very minimal. In this clinical setting, subtle findings of linear atelectasis or small pleural effusions must be viewed with suspicion as they may be the only evidence of infection. CT can be effective in the evaluation of pulmonary infections in these patients as CT has a greater sensitivity to subtle alveolar filling and interstitial thickening. There is value in characterization of pulmonary infections with CT, although no findings are entirely specific for a particular infectious agent.[46] Because of the overlap in appearance between various infectious etiologies and with other lung diseases, other evaluations, such as bronchoscopy and culture, are usually necessary to direct therapy.

Other sources of infection are found throughout the body. Indium 111–labeled white blood cells (either autologous or from human leukocyte antigen–matched donors) can detect focal infectious sources with great sensitivity.[47] Osteomyelitis can also be detected by the three-phase bone scan in which all three phases will demonstrate abnormally elevated focal tracer distribution.[48] Both the indium 111 white blood cell and three-phase bone scans are partly limited by the use of antibiotics and the chronicity of the infection.

Renal infection and inflammation are initially evaluated by ultrasonography to determine the type of renal echogenicity, renal size, and the presence of focal lesions, which can be either unilateral or bilateral. The most common ultrasound finding in pyelonephritis is a normal scan. Multidetector contrast-enhanced CT scans are also valuable to identify acute pyelonephritis, pyonephrosis, renal abscess, and chronic infection.

Pulmonary infections are usually bacterial and present as single or multifocal areas of pulmonary consolidation and ground-glass opacity.[49] Nodular and cavitary lesions are suggestive of fungal infections or septic emboli (Figure 10).[50] However, bacterial infections can also have nodular or cavitary components. Branching tubular opacities with mucous plugging of the bronchial tree may be due to poor clearance of secretions or to infection, such as bronchopulmonary aspergillosis. Pulmonary nodules associated with invasive pulmonary aspergillosis may have a halo of ground-glass opacity.[51] Pulmonary infections that extend from the lung into the chest wall or into mediastinal structures are uncommon

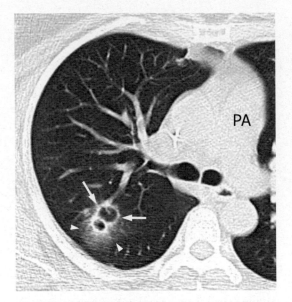

FIGURE 10 Septic pulmonary emboli by computed tomography (CT). A 49-year-old woman with breast cancer developed fever and new pulmonary nodules detected by chest radiography. CT of the chest at the level of the main pulmonary artery (PA) demonstrates cavitary nodules in the right upper lobe (*arrows*). Hemorrhage around the nodules causes the surrounding ground-glass attenuation halo (*arrowheads*). Blood cultures revealed *Staphylococcus aureus*, and the nodules resolved with antibiotic therapy.

and indicate an aggressive organism such as actinomycosis, nocardia, or mucormycosis.[52]

The pulmonary pattern most characteristic of viral infection is interstitial thickening, but nodules or consolidation is more frequently encountered.[53,54] Interstitial thickening is also seen in a variety of other pulmonary infections and in noninfectious lung disease. Tiny nodules can be seen along peripheral bronchovascular bundles and in the center of secondary pulmonary lobules in many early infections. Most often these are clustered in distribution. Although associated with *Mycobacterium avium* complex (MAC) infections, this pattern can be seen in virtually any early infection.[55] MAC infection frequently has a distribution involving the anterior middle lobe and lingula and often has bronchiectasis associated with the tiny nodules. Similar findings of clustered nodules and bronchiectasis can be seen in chronic aspiration, most often distributed dependently in the lower lobes. Thus, the combination of CT appearance and distribution of findings can be helpful in suggesting an infectious etiology.

Respiratory failure as a consequence of chemotherapy, surgery, or infection can evolve into a diffuse lung injury known as acute respiratory distress syndrome (ARDS).[56,57] The condition is most frequently imaged with portable chest radiography in an intensive care unit as patients are generally too unstable to be transported to the imaging department for a conventional chest radiograph or CT examination. By portable chest radiography, ARDS presents as heterogeneous opacification throughout both lungs, usually in a relatively symmetric distribution. The distribution can be asymmetric, with areas of sparing. The pulmonary pattern is difficult to distinguish from infection or pulmonary edema. The slowly changing relatively stable appearance can be suggestive of ARDS over the other possibilities.

Pulmonary edema can sometimes be distinguished from ARDS if there are other signs of volume overload, such as cardiomegaly or widening of the vascular pedicle, on serial radiographs.[58] However, the assessment is severely limited on the typical supine portable radiographs obtained in these patients. The supine position causes low lung volumes, which increases the apparent size of the heart and mediastinum. This is accentuated further by the anteroposterior orientation of the patient and short source-to-image distance for the examination. In addition, the low lung volumes cause indistinctness of the pulmonary vessels and redistribution of pulmonary blood flow, two features that are otherwise useful on upright radiography in identifying pulmonary edema. Septal thickening is often not demonstrated in supine patients because gravity causes dependent distribution of the interstitial fluid to the posterior portions of the lungs and away from the lateral portions of the lungs, where septal thickening is normally identified. The time course of changes in the radiographic findings may provide the most useful information as pulmonary edema is likely to respond relatively quickly to manipulations of fluid status.[59]

Metastatic disease in the chest is a concern as a differential possibility in evaluating pulmonary lesions identified on a chest radiograph or CT scan.[50,51] The pulmonary nodules typically seen in metastatic disease are usually more sharply demarcated than nodules of an infectious process. However, neoplasms with associated hemorrhage, such as choriocarcinoma, melanoma, or vascular neoplasms, may have poorly defined margins more typical of infection. Cavitary metastatic disease, in particular, can simulate fungal infection or septic emboli. These entities can most readily be distinguished with clinical information about signs and symptoms of infection and the time course of appearance of lesions.

In these extremely ill patients with multiorgan failure, appropriate assessment is dependent on integration of all medical information and the sequence of recent images.

Hepatic dysfunction is common in oncology patients who are subject to hepatic complications associated with therapy but who may also experience any of the broad spectrum of liver disorders that are independent of cancer. The hepatic parenchyma can be diffusely abnormal with infiltration, cirrhosis, passive congestion, portal hypertension, and hemochromatosis. Hepatic metastases can lead to hepatic dysfunction and an abnormal liver test profile. Imaging can identify a diffuse parenchymal pattern or a space-occupying lesion, the presence or absence of biliary ductal dilation, and the patency status of the intrahepatic vasculature. Ultrasonography with or without Doppler evaluation should be the initial study of choice. The ultrasound study can be performed at the bedside, is noninvasive and inexpensive, and involves no radiation but is operator dependent. The results are influenced by the patient's body habitus, with large patients and/or patients with fatty infiltrated livers being more difficult to study. Multidetector CT and MRI, with dedicated liver protocols, are alternative imaging modalities that can provide information not rendered by the ultrasound study.

Liver dysfunction is common in bone marrow transplant patients, the common etiologies being graft-versus-host disease; viral, bacterial, and fungal infections; drug- (cytotoxic or immunosuppressive drugs, antimicrobials, total parenteral nutrition) related hepatotoxicity; veno-occlusive disease; and iron overload. When the cause of liver dysfunction cannot be determined by noninvasive means, liver histology may suggest the correct diagnosis. Liver tissue for histologic analysis may be obtained by image-guided percutaneous liver biopsy or transjugular liver biopsy in patients with coagulopathy and thrombocytopenia.

Ultrasonography is the initial imaging modality of choice to evaluate conditions involving the gallbladder and biliary tree. These diseases include cholelithiasis, cholecystitis, choledocholithiasis, gallbladder polyps and masses. Alternative imaging modalities include CT, MRI, magnetic resonance cholangiopancreatography, hepatobiliary nuclear scintigraphy, and percutaneous transhepatic cholangiography.

Renal dysfunction can occur in patients with nonrenal carcinoma. Some of these complications include radiation nephritis, antineoplastic drug-induced toxicities, antibiotic-associated nephropathies, analgesic nephropathy, and contrast-associated nephropathy. Infiltration of the kidneys can occur with leukemia and lymphoma. Hypercalcemia, hypocalcemia, hyponatremia, and tumor lysis syndrome can also occur. Glomerular disease can be produced by membranous glomerulopathy associated with carcinomas of the lung, gastrointestinal tract, and breast; minimal change disease; amyloidosis; and consumptive coagulopathy.

Osteoporosis is a naturally occurring condition in humans that increases in severity with increasing age and therefore is a comorbid process in older persons with cancer. Osteoporosis in cancer patients worsens owing to therapeutic success in the treatment of cancer (increased longevity leads to increased osteopenia) and to the direct bone-resorptive effects of the cancer therapies themselves.[60] Thus, osteoporosis increases with increased patient age, progressive stage of disease, and duration of specific therapy. With lengthened survival, this comorbid condition emerges as a more important determinant of both morbidity (quality of life) and mortality, primarily owing to fractures. The goal is to control bone mineral density and to effectively treat osteoporosis to reduce its affect on morbidity and mortality. Several bone mineral measurement methods are available for the detection of osteoporosis, for prediction of fracture risk, and for determination of therapeutic success. These tests include quantitative CT of the spine, dual x-ray absorptiometry of the spine and femoral neck, quantitative ultrasonography of the calcaneus, and others. Unfortunately, agreement among the tests is poor.[61]

Chronic back pain diminishes the quality of life for many oncology patients. Imaging is a critical component of the diagnostic assessment. Radionuclide bone scans localize metabolically active lesions. The pattern may indicate the presence of metastatic disease, but often the pattern is nonspecific or nondiagnostic. Conventional radiography of the spine often improves specificity by revealing features diagnostic of metastasis, degenerative disk disease, apophyseal joint osteoarthritis, or osteoporosis. Commonly, some combination of conditions exists or the radiographs do not provide a satisfactory correlate for the symptoms. MRI is more sensitive and specific for detection of metastases, for differentiation of acute and chronic vertebral fractures, and for differentiation of osteoporotic fractures from metastatic fractures.[62]

Percutaneous vertebroplasty may be used for treating refractory vertebrogenic pain from malignant vertebral body fractures in patients with myeloma, lymphoma, leukemia, and metastases and provides rapid pain relief and significantly improved mobility and quality of life. The results in patients with metastatic fractures indicate similar levels of symptom control as in those with osteoporotic fractures. Sixty to 85% of patients with neoplastic vertebral collapse experience a marked reduction in narcotic requirements or complete relief within 72 hours.[63] Vertebroplasty palliates pain through the solidification of the osteolytic lesion and provides structural stability to the spine. Although it has been suggested that a direct cytotoxic effect alone or in combination with a thermal reaction resulting from the cement injection may have a tumoricidal effect, this remains unproven.

Although radiotherapy is widely used for pain control of malignant vertebral lesions, radiotherapy alone may not be effective when the pain is primarily mechanical, such as with wedge fracture or vertebral collapse. Vertebroplasty is complementary to radiotherapy in these patients. Vertebroplasty is a preferred treatment when immediate pain relief is required; radiotherapy requires around 1 to 2 weeks for pain relief.

Vertebroplasty is generally performed under fluoroscopic guidance, although CT guidance may be used for needle placement for certain cervical or thoracic vertebrae. A large-bore needle is advanced into the anterior portion of the vertebral body, frequently by a transpedicular approach. Once the needle position is confirmed, polymethylmethacrylate, an acrylic polymer noted for its excellent compressive strength, is injected under direct fluoroscopic visualization. Potential complications include bleeding; infection; trauma to the nerve roots or spinal cord; fracture of a lamina, pedicle, or rib; and cement extravasation into the epidural, paravertebral, foraminal, or disk spaces. The incidence of complications is quite low.

CNS malfunction can be a significant issue during the life of oncology patients. Radionuclide tests may provide qualitative information as an aid in these situations. Changes in mental status may result from the use of oncologic drugs, including interferons. Specific patterns of hypoperfusion of the temporal and parietal lobes as confirmed by SPECT or PET (for glucose hypometabolism) can distinguish Alzheimer's dementia from other causes of dementia or delirium.[64] Other cancer-related CNS diseases, such as cerebrospinal fluid (CSF) block or iatrogenic CSF leakage, can be confirmed with scintigraphy using indium 111–labeled diethylenetriaminepentaacetic acid (DTPA). Fast clearance or abnormal appearance of indium 111 DTPA after intrathecal injection indicates extrathecal activities or CSF leakage.[65] Slow clearance of indium 111 DTPA from the CSF or abrupt cessation of flow indicates CSF block, which in cases of leptomeningeal metastasis may show flow improvement and symptomatic relief on focal external beam irradiation.[66]

One of the most crucial questions of patient care is whether the patient is alive. Even though the consensus from the president's commission and the Harvard criteria is that the final diagnosis of brain death must be made by specialty-trained physicians, including a neurologist, an anesthesiologist, or a neurosurgeon, radionuclide cerebral blood flow determination remains the most important ancillary and objective test for that assessment.[67,68]

Chemotherapy-Induced Toxicity

Chemotherapy-induced toxicity of the brain is relatively uncommon and presents in a nonspecific fashion with seizures, altered mental status, and motor deficit.

Methotrexate toxicity results when this common chemotherapeutic agent is used for the treatment of leptomeningeal metastases (involvement of pia and arachnoid mater that envelops the brain and spinal cord) from lymphoma, leukemia, and lung and breast cancers. Common CNS tumors that invade the leptomeninges are glioblastoma, medulloblastoma, ependymoma, and primitive neuroectodermal tumors. Methotrexate does not penetrate the blood CSF barrier in systemic therapeutic doses given orally or parenterally. To provide more uniform distribution of the drug through CSF and better penetration into brain parenchyma and perivascular spaces, methotrexate is used as a high-dose chemotherapeutic agent. In the treatment and prevention of leptomeningeal metastasis secondary to leukemia or lymphoma, methotrexate is commonly administered via lumbar puncture into the lumbar subarachnoid space. Intraventricular injection of methotrexate though an Ommaya reservoir is performed to treat leptomeningeal metastasis secondary to primary CNS solid tumors because intrathecal chemotherapy via the lumbar route is less effective and also circumvents the problems of local subdural or epidural injection of the chemotherapeutic agent when a lumbar route is employed. Methotrexate-induced leukoencephalopathy is a chronic, progressive demyelinating encephalopathy that can appear months to years after treatment. The encephalopathy gives rise to headaches, seizures, drowsiness, blurred vision, and dysarthria and can even lead to dementia. MRI readily demonstrates the toxic effects of methotrexate on the white matter as large areas of T_2-weighted hyperintensity, particularly involving the periventricular white matter and the region of the centrum semiovale. Periventricular white matter is preferentially involved. Because of local concentration differences, methotrexate-induced leukoencephalopathy is more common with intraventricular and intrathecal chemotherapy than with systemic therapy. MRI can also detect methotrexate-induced necrosis of the brain occurring as a result of accidental leakage of methotrexate into the brain substance during intraventricular chemotherapy installation, a rare complication. MRI findings of necrotizing leukoencephalopathy of the brain owing to a chemotherapeutic agent consist of a focal area of abnormal contrast enhancement with surrounding edema and can be mistaken for a metastatic lesion. The area of abnormal enhancement occurring along the path of the ventricular catheter particularly close to the entrance of the catheter into the ventricle should suggest the current diagnosis of chemotherapy-induced necrosis (Figure 11).

Tacrolimus (Prograf) toxicity results when this potent immunosuppressive agent is used for the prophylaxis of organ rejection in kidney, liver,

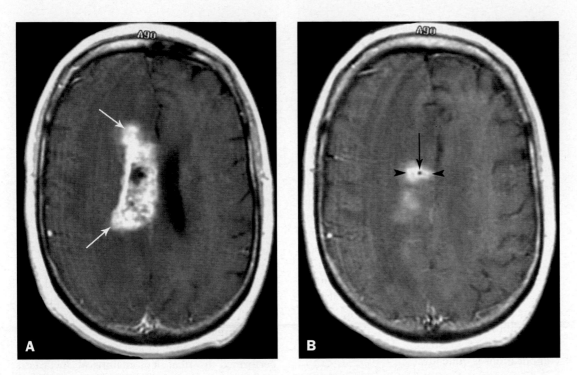

FIGURE 11 Cytarabine-induced necrotizing leukoencephalopathy after intraventricular therapy for acute myelogenous leukemia. *A*, Axial postcontrast T$_1$-weighted magnetic resonance image (MRI) demonstrates abnormal contrast enhancement involving the lateral ventricular walls (*arrows*). *B*, Adjacent MRI shows abnormally enhanced supraventricular white matter (*arrowheads*) surrounding the catheter (*arrow*).

heart, and bone marrow transplants. It is associated with a posterior reversible encephalopathy syndrome (PRES) in about 2% of treated patients.[69] The diagnosis is made by characteristic clinical findings consisting of headache, a change in mental status, seizures, visual abnormalities, and/or focal neurologic deficits. The median patient age is about 35 years, and the median time to the onset of PRES is about 60 days from institution of tacrolimus. Imaging findings in PRES consist of parieto-occipital hypodensity on CT images, an area of low signal intensity on T$_1$-weighted MRIs, and hyperintensity on fluid attenuated inversion recovery (FLAIR) T$_2$-weighted MRIs. The abnormality involves the subcortical white matter and adjacent cortex, with a predilection for areas supplied by the posterior circulation, namely the occipital, parietal, and temporal lobes and cerebellum.

In 1996, Hinchey and colleagues described a clinicoradiologic condition named posterior reversible leukoencephalopathy syndrome, which is characterized by visual disorders, seizures, and altered mental status, with changes in the subcortical white matter of the temporoparieto-occipital lobes detected in neurologic images.[70] These clinical manifestations were associated with arterial hypertension. Although the precise pathogenesis is not known, the striking similarities of the symptoms and the imaging findings among patients with tacrolimus toxicity and those with hypertensive encephalopathy, cyclosporine toxicity, and eclampsia of pregnancy suggest a common mechanism. Tacrolimus and cyclosporine both

cause inhibition of neuronal and endothelial nitric oxide synthase activity. Inhibition of nitric oxide results in vasodilatation, and fluid extravasation has been suggested as the cause of eclamptic encephalopathy. The loss of autoregulation presumed to occur in PRES results in blood barrier disruption and leads to interstitial fluid accumulation in the subcortical white matter and the cortex. This vasogenic edema accounts for the abnormal findings seen in brain imaging. Magnetic resonance FLAIR imaging is particularly sensitive for detection of early edema seen with this syndrome.

Clinical symptomatology and MRI findings of PRES can be mistaken for acute infarction. MRI findings of acute infarction consist of cortical swelling, gyral enhancement, abnormal hyperintensity on FLAIR images, and restricted diffusion, producing bright signal intensity on diffusion-weighted images. Diffusion-weighted imaging improves acute stroke detection by 95%. PRES can be differentiated from acute stroke with an appropriate clinical history and recognition of MRI findings of bilateral vasogenic edema primarily involving the subcortical white matter and with no evidence of restricted diffusion. Drug-induced encephalopathy is usually reversible when the drug is discontinued or the dose is reduced (Figure 12). Drug toxicity can lead to acute infarction with or without hemorrhage if early signs are not recognized.

Cardiac toxicity results in decreased cardiac function manifest as decreased ejection fraction and stroke volume.[71] These changes can be

demonstrated at radionuclide ventriculography, echocardiography, or cardiac MRI. The multigated cardiac radionuclide ventriculogram radionuclide test using Tc 99m–labeled red blood cells remains the most reliable method to measure cardiac function before and after chemotherapy. In general, left ventricular ejection fraction below 45% or an interval decrease of more than 15% implies impending cardiotoxicity.[72] In compensation for decreased contractility, the ventricles become dilated. This dilation may be apparent at conventional radiography or may be demonstrated at CT or echocardiography.[73] Eventually, the heart can no longer compensate for the decreased contractility, and cardiac failure results.

Acute cardiac failure is best demonstrated with conventional chest radiography, the typical findings of which include bilateral perihilar opacity, indistinct pulmonary vessels, and peripheral interlobular septal thickening.[59] Pleural effusions may also be present. Widening of the vascular pedicle, the mediastinal structures above the aortic arch, to more than 74 mm indicates volume overload or congestive heart failure.[74] At CT, dilated cardiac chambers and increased pulmonary attenuation owing to fluid filling the interstitium and alveoli are seen in cardiac failure. There may be an increase in the prominence and attenuation of mediastinal soft tissues.[75] Contrast material administered through the upper extremity venous system may reflux into the IVC and hepatic veins owing to poor cardiac function. A congestive pattern may also be seen in the liver as patchy increased attenuation centered on the hepatic veins. Cardiac failure can also result in enlargement of mediastinal lymph nodes, simulating adenopathy.[76] Enlarged nodes that develop in this setting should be reevaluated after resolution of cardiac failure rather than be accepted as recurrent or metastatic tumor.

Pulmonary toxicity secondary to chemotherapeutic agents typically presents as diffuse pneumonitis or bronchiolitis obliterans organizing pneumonia.[77] The radiographic appearance can range from air trapping, demonstrated as mosaic attenuation in the lungs that is accentuated on expiratory imaging, to nodular or patchy areas of consolidation or poorly defined ground-glass opacities (Figure 13).[78] Although the pattern of involvement is usually diffuse throughout the lungs, it may be asymmetric or even unilateral. This appearance may be very difficult to distinguish from pulmonary infection. Pulmonary fibrosis that results from chemotherapy-induced pulmonary toxicity is a less common presentation. It has the typical appearance of fibrosis, with basilar distribution of interstitial thickening, a subpleural honeycomb pattern, and decreased total lung volume. PE may also be seen as a consequence of chemotherapy, particularly with thalidomide.

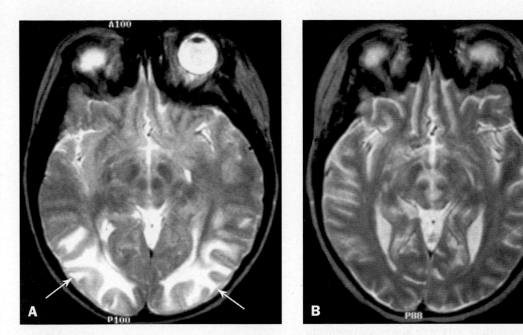

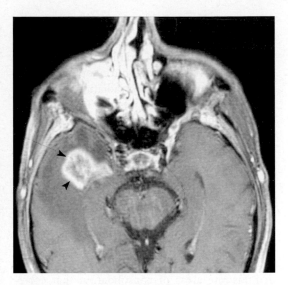

FIGURE 14 Radiation necrosis involving the right temporal lobe 2 years after receiving radiation therapy for nasopharyngeal carcinoma. Axial postcontrast T₁-weighted magnetic resonance image shows focal enhancement (*arrowheads*) with central necrosis.

FIGURE 12 Cyclosporine-induced posterior reversible encephalopathy syndrome.. *A,* A T₂-weighted image shows bilateral abnormally increased signal intensity involving the cortex/subcortical white matter of the occipital lobes (*arrows*). *B,* A follow-up magnetic resonance examination 8 months later reveals complete resolution of the abnormal findings after cessation of cyclosporine therapy.

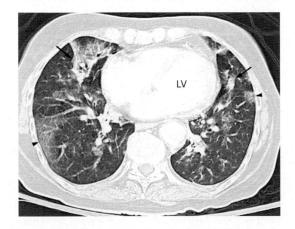

FIGURE 13 Pulmonary toxicity owing to carmustine. A 66-year-old woman with glioblastoma multiforme developed dyspnea after carmustine chemotherapy. Computed tomography of the chest at the level of the left ventricle (LV) demonstrates symmetric distribution of patchy areas of consolidation (*arrows*) and ground-glass attenuation (*arrowheads*). No infectious etiology was demonstrated at bronchoscopy. The patient's symptoms improved after withholding further carmustine treatments.

Radiation-Induced Toxicity

Radiation-induced neurotoxicity is postulated to derive from the combined effects of vascular injury, glial and white matter damage, and alterations in the fibrinolytic enzyme system. Vascular injury consists of endothelial damage, vascular ectasia, and telangiectasia, all of which result in increased capillary permeability, with resultant cytotoxic and vasogenic edema. Progressive vascular changes include vessel wall thickening

caused by hyalinization, with consequent thrombosis, infarction, and necrosis. Oligodendrocytes are extremely sensitive to radiation, and their destruction is associated with demyelination. Metabolic changes in irradiated cells reduce glycolysis and glucose consumption and result in decreased glucose and oxygen use observed on PET scans. Necrotic brain tissue shows absent tissue plasminogen activator and excess urokinase plasminogen activator, a combination that contributes to cytotoxic edema and tissue necrosis. Radiation necrosis most commonly develops around blood vessels within the white matter and is manifested as fibrinoid necrosis of the blood vessel wall with surrounding perivascular parenchymal coagulative necrosis. Confluence of multifocal perivascular necrotic zones results in larger zones of parenchymal necrosis. Clusters of abnormally dilated thin-walled telangiectasias are common. Late vascular changes include vessel wall thickening caused by hyalinization, with resultant luminal narrowing. White matter changes include focal and diffuse demyelination.

Radiation necrosis may develop months to years after completion of radiation therapy and is frequently irreversible and often progressive. Radiation necrosis most commonly occurs at the site of maximum radiation delivery, typically in the immediate vicinity of a surgical cavity following partial or total resection of tumor. It is important to recognize the spectrum of MRI features of radiation necrosis because the tissue damage can mimic other pathologic processes.[79] The typical MRI finding in radiation necrosis is an enhancing mass with central necrosis (Figure 14). Other, less common patterns may be observed, including (1)

multiple lesions, (2) lesions in the contralateral hemisphere, and (3) lesions arising remotely from a primary cerebral site, such as in the cerebellum or brainstem. Each pattern can be mistaken for a different pathologic process. For example, radiation necrosis occurring at the site of the resected primary tumor easily can be mistaken for recurrent tumor. Necrosis occurring distant from the site of the primary tumor may mimic multifocal glioma. Contralateral hemisphere involvement can be diagnosed as multicentric glioma. Multiple foci can resemble multiple metastases. Periventricular white matter involvement may mimic tumefactive multiple sclerosis. Radiation-induced necrotic lesions can also spread subependymally and mimic subependymal tumor spread.

The incidence of radiation necrosis after conventional radiation therapy ranges from 5 to 24%, with higher rates at autopsy. The interval from completion of radiation therapy to histopathologic confirmation varies from 3 to 48 months, mostly occurring between 7 and 24 months. The use of platinum-based chemotherapy drugs, such as cisplatin and carboplatin, combined with radiation therapy may contribute to the development of radiation-induced necrosis. It is important to recognize that radiation-induced necrosis is a dynamic pathophysiologic process with several possible clinical outcomes. Although continued growth with attendant cytolytic edema and mass effect is commonly seen, lethal progression is not inevitable in all cases. Some lesions will stabilize, whereas others will regress. Surgery may be required to reduce the mass effect and edema. Despite advancements in special imaging techniques, biopsy may be needed to establish an accurate histopathologic diagnosis.

Radiation-induced cranial neuropathy is relatively rare. Radiation-induced optic neuropathy can occur when focused radiation is delivered to tumors in the perioptic regions. The pathologic process of this neuropathy consists of optic pathway vasculopathy with secondary hemorrhage, reactive gliosis, necrosis, and atrophy.

Radiation-induced brain atrophy can also occur, with shrinkage of the white matter and cortex.

Radiation-induced pneumonitis and pulmonary fibrosis can be a significant cause of respiratory compromise and can present a diagnostic challenge. Conventional radiography and CT demonstrate areas of consolidation that correspond to the radiation ports used for therapy.[80] The acute phase of pneumonitis presents as focal consolidation with obscuration of the underlying pulmonary vessels and bronchi at CT. As the process progresses to fibrosis, the air space consolidation may clear or may become more sharply demarcated. Typically, the involved area decreases in volume, with resulting traction on adjacent mediastinal and pulmonary structures. Within the area of involvement, the bronchi become distorted and ectatic. The process often stabilizes within 9 to 12 months but rarely may continue to evolve over more than 2 years. In cases with slower evolution, new areas of involvement do not emerge after about 1 year, but consolidation and volume loss progress in the involved area. The fibrotic process does not cause filling of the bronchi. Bronchial filling that develops after radiation fibrosis has begun to mature should be regarded as evidence of recurrent tumor or superimposed infection.[81]

Radiation-induced pleural and pericardial effusions most often emerge about 3 to 9 months after therapy. Radiation therapy to involved mediastinal lymph nodes typically reduces the size of the nodes and may induce calcification within the nodes. In addition, radiation can cause increased attenuation of the mediastinal fat and blurring of soft tissue borders within the mediastinum. In radiation-induced esophagitis, the esophageal walls become thickened and the borders of the esophagus become poorly defined. As with radiation pneumonitis, radiation-induced esophagitis may cause increased metabolic activity on PET scans.[82] This metabolic activity limits the value of early follow-up with PET. Pleural scarring related to radiation fibrosis or radiation-induced pleural effusion can result in traction on the underlying lung causing focal areas of rounded atelectasis, which can simulate infection or a mass lesion. Because the scarring may be related to the resolution of the effusion rather than being directly due to radiation therapy, it can occur outside the original radiation field.

The important feature for identification of radiation-induced pneumonitis and fibrosis is detection of the limits of the radiation port. The port borders are typically linear and do not correspond to normal anatomic boundaries. Commonly observed radiation injury patterns include involvement of the anterior subpleural lung from tangential breast radiation, involvement of the lung apices from cervical lymph node radiation, and paramediastinal involvement from mediastinal lymph node radiation (Figure 15).[83]

Radiation therapy to the primary lung tumor is also common. When conventional radiation therapy is used, a significant portion of lung may be irradiated. Ensuing radiation fibrosis will have the linear, nonanatomic borders seen with mediastinal and tangential radiation. The use of three-dimensional conformal radiation therapy can complicate the identification of radiation fibrosis. Because multiple exposure ports are used, the pattern of lung injury is more complex (Figure 16). Consolidation can develop outside the usual anteroposterior and posteroanterior ports used for conventional radiation therapy. Conformal radiation therapy also results in a less linear appearance to the boundaries of radiation fibrosis.[84]

Intensity-modulated radiation therapy (IMRT) is a method of delivering conformal radiation therapy with nonuniform beams of radiation energy and also induces radiation injury in a pattern different from conventional radiation therapy. For example, in IMRT treatment of mesothelioma, the therapeutic dose contour is matched to the pleural surface and chest wall. The radiation injury therefore involves less of the underlying pulmonary parenchyma. Because the

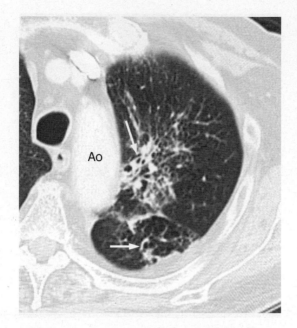

FIGURE 16 Pulmonary radiation effect from conformal radiotherapy. A 75-year-old man with stage I lung cancer was not a surgical candidate owing to poor cardiac function. Computed tomography of the chest at the level of the aortic arch (Ao) 8 months after the completion of therapy demonstrates bronchiectasis (*arrows*) and surrounding consolidation and ground-glass attenuation. The area of involvement has poorly defined borders and does not have the typical linear margins seen with conventional radiation therapy, as seen in Figure 13-15.

radiation ports include the upper aspect of the liver, low attenuation can be induced in the periphery of the liver and should not be confused with recurrent tumor or infection.

Radiation-induced skeletal changes include growth disturbances, focal osteopenia, osteoradionecrosis, and induced benign or malignant neoplasms.[85] Growing bone is sensitive to radiation, and the growing physis is most sensitive, with damage roughly proportional to the amount of radiation absorbed. Radiography shows metaphyseal sclerosis and fraying with physeal plate widening. A transient dense metaphyseal band may develop as healing commences, giving way to normal bone remodeling. Scoliosis may develop secondary to asymmetric irradiation of the spine. Mature bone and cartilage are very radioresistant. However, focal osteopenia and cortical thinning may follow long bone irradiation. Osteoradionecrosis is the result of vascular damage and osteoblast death. It is most prevalent in the mandible but also occurs in the clavicle, shoulders, ribs, pelvis, sacrum, and knees. The typical radiographic features begin with subtle osteopenia or osteosclerosis, eventually leading to fragmentation or disintegration of the irradiated bone. The involved bone segments are subject to fracture and infection. Conventional radiography is usually sufficient for diagnosis of the condition and for assessment of complications. CT and MRI

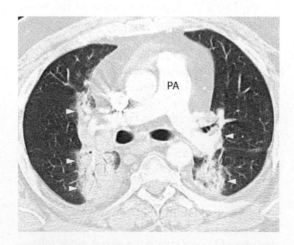

FIGURE 15 Pulmonary radiation fibrosis from conventional radiotherapy. A 40-year-old man with lymphoma received conventional mantle radiation therapy. Computed tomography of the chest at the level of the pulmonary artery (PA) 2 months after the completion of therapy reveals bilateral paramediastinal consolidation (*arrowheads*) with linear lateral margins confined to the radiation ports.

are effective in areas of complex anatomy or in difficult diagnostic situations.

Osteocartilaginous exostoses are the most frequent benign radiation-induced tumors of bone. They typically develop in growing bones and may occur in any location in any irradiated bone. Osteosarcoma is the most common radiation-induced malignant tumor of bone. Radiation-induced bone sarcomas have an imaging appearance similar to those that spontaneously occur. Radiographic features are generally sufficient for diagnosis, and CT and MRI are effective for characterization and staging.

Surgically Induced Conditions in Patients with Cancer

Postoperative alterations of the thorax can cause diagnostic dilemmas in subsequent evaluation of thoracic disease. Small pneumothoraces are routinely present after pulmonary and esophageal resections. These are usually satisfactorily managed with drainage catheters placed at the time of surgery. Pneumothoraces that persist or enlarge despite catheter drainage suggest air leak and may need surgical management. Postoperative pleural infections typically require catheter drainage and may also require surgical débridement.[86] After pneumonectomy, there is a shift of mediastinal structures into the pneumonectomy space, and the space slowly fills fluid over about 3 to 4 weeks. The absence of any mediastinal shift over the first few postoperative days could indicate the presence of tension pneumothorax. If the pleura fills with fluid much more rapidly than expected, hemothorax and empyema are considerations. In the setting of extrapleural pneumonectomy, the pneumonectomy space will fill with fluid more rapidly than with simple pneumonectomy. As with many major surgical procedures, PE is a concern after lung resection. The postpneumonectomy syndrome is a late complication owing to chronic tracheobronchial narrowing resulting from marked shift of mediastinal structures.[87]

Anastomotic leaks are a concern following several types of surgery. After esophagectomy with gastric pull-up or bowel interposition, leaks present as a collection of fluid alongside the anastomotic site, sometimes separated from the anastomosis by a short distance.[88] Communication of the fluid collection with the bowel lumen can be demonstrated with use of oral contrast agents either at fluoroscopy or with CT. To prevent bronchopleural fistula formation after lung resection and in the treatment of known bronchopleural fistula or an anastomotic leak from esophageal resection, a variety of vascular flaps are used to provide additional soft tissue coverage.[89] These can alter the radiographic appearance and simulate recurrent tumor or infection. Many flaps are predominantly fat and therefore easy to identify,

but muscular flaps are more difficult to assess. Muscular flaps should have some linear areas of fat attenuation on CT, even shortly after operation. They also may have linear calcifications. These features allow muscular flaps to be distinguished from soft tissue masses of more concern.

Abscess formation following surgery remains a serious and potentially fatal complication, with mortality rates up to 30%. Image-guided percutaneous catheter drainage (PCD) of abscesses offers a less invasive alternative to open surgical drainage and has become the procedure of choice in this group of patients.[90] Postoperative abscesses in various locations, such as the peritoneal space, retroperitoneum, viscera, pelvis, mediastinum, and extremities, are amenable to PCD. PCD is most effective in patients with unilocular abscesses, with cure rates up to 95%. Several recent studies have shown that PCD is also very successful (80–90% cure) with complex postoperative abscesses (ie, loculated, poorly defined collections, abscesses communicating with enteric fistulae, and interloop abscesses). In patients with abscesses associated with enteric fistulae, PCD, along with concomitant enteric decompression and diversion of bowel contents with nasoenteric tubes, allows spontaneous closure of the fistulae in 57 to 88% of cases.

Either ultrasonography or CT may be used for guidance during the PCD procedure. The main advantages of ultrasound guidance include real-time imaging and portability, allowing a bedside procedure in critically ill patients. Combining fluoroscopy with ultrasonography allows for precise positioning of the catheter. Ultrasonography is commonly used for superficial and unilocular abscesses. Endocavitary ultrasonography is also used for transrectal or transvaginal drainage of deep pelvic abscesses. However, ultrasonography is of limited use in obese patients, in the presence of intra-abdominal free air, when bowel gas interferes with sonographic visualization, and in patients with open surgical wounds or dressings overlying the abscess. Because of the deep location of many abscesses and the frequent presence of free air in postoperative tissues, CT is commonly the imaging modality of choice for PCD guidance.

Lymphoceles of the pelvis or abdomen are a complication of radical lymphadenectomy performed for prostatic or gynecologic malignancy and are believed to result from surgical transection or inadequate ligation of lymphatic vessels during lymph node dissection. Most lymphoceles are small and asymptomatic and eventually resolve spontaneously. Large lymphoceles can cause abdominal distention, hydronephrosis, bladder dysfunction, constipation, and thrombosis of iliac vessels, or they may become infected and present with fever, chills, and sepsis. Large or infected lymphoceles require treatment. Surgical

treatment is successful in up to 90% of cases but is associated with mortality and morbidity and requires hospitalization. Simple needle aspiration is safer than surgery, but repeated procedures are necessary in 80 to 90% of patients. PCD is a safe and effective treatment for symptomatic lymphoceles, with success rates ranging from 50 to 87% in most series.[91] In patients with pronged drainage, transcatheter sclerotherapy with tetracycline, doxycycline, povidone-iodine, or alcohol results in improved success rates of 79 to 93%.

Urinoma may be secondary to iatrogenic ureteral injury following genitourinary, retroperitoneal, or gynecologic surgeries or following manipulation during endourologic procedures, or it may be due to an anastomotic leak following ureteral diversion procedures. Interventional management of ureteral injuries requires combined use of PCD of the urinoma along with a PCN to divert the urine away from the leak. Placement of a J stent or a nephroureteral stent across the site of ureteral injury for 4 to 8 weeks permits regrowth of uroepithelium over the site of injury.

Biloma formation may complicate hepatobiliary and pancreatic surgery. PCD of the biloma in conjunction with percutaneous biliary drainage is a safe and effective minimally invasive technique for management of this complication. Placement of a percutaneous transhepatic biliary catheter extending across the site of leak prevents further leakage of bile and allows the anastomosis to heal.

Summary

Patients with cancer typically have comorbidity that complicates their general medical care and the care of their specific cancers.[92] In fact, the comorbid conditions increase in number and severity, with increased number and intensity of the therapies the patients undergo in the treatment of their cancers. Thus, the bulk of imaging resources consumed by patients with cancer are not used for diagnosis and staging but rather are expended in the management of comorbid conditions.

REFERENCES

1. Schapira D. Tumor-induced osteomalacia. Semin Arthritis Rheum 1995;25:35–46.
2. Pineda C. Diagnostic imaging in hypertrophic osteoarthropathy. Clin Exp Rheumatol 1992;10 Suppl 7:27–33.
3. Jaeckle KA. Paraneoplastic neurologic disease. In: Levin VA, editor. Cancer in the nervous system. New York: Oxford University Press; 2002. p. 423–37.
4. Rosenthal PE. Paraneoplastic and endocrine syndromes. In: Leonard RE, Osteen RT, Gansler T, editors. Clinical oncology. Atlanta: American Cancer Society; 2001. p. 725–6.
5. John WJ, Foon KA, Patchell RA. Paraneoplastic syndromes. In: DeVita VT Jr, Hellman S, Rosenberg SA, editors. Cancer: principles and practice of oncology. 5th ed. Philadelphia: Lippincott-Raven; 1997. p. 2397–422.
6. Morales M, Comas V, Trujillo M, Dorta J. Treatment of catheter-induced thrombotic superior vena cava

syndrome: a single institution's experience. Support Care Cancer 2000;8:334–8.
7. Gonsalves CF, Eschelman DJ, Sullivan KL, et al. Incidence of central vein stenosis and occlusion following upper extremity PICC and port placement. Cardiovasc Intervent Radiol 2003;26:123–7.
8. Lanciego C, Chacon JL, Julian A, et al. Stenting as first option for endovascular treatment of malignant superior vena cava syndrome. AJR Am J Roentgenol 2001;177:585–93.
9. Otten TR, Stein PD, Patel KC, et al. Thromboembolic disease involving the superior vena cava and brachiocephalic veins. Chest 2003;123:809–12.
10. Qanadli SD, El Hajjam M, Bruckert F, et al. Helical CT phlebography of the superior vena cava: diagnosis and evaluation of venous obstruction. AJR Am J Roentgenol 1999;172:1327–33.
11. Brountzos EN, Binkert CA, Panagiotou IE, et al. Clinical outcome after intrahepatic venous stent placement for malignant inferior vena cava syndrome. Cardiovasc Intervent Radiol 2004;27:129–36.
12. Therasse E, Oliva VL, Lafontaine E, et al. Balloon dilation and stent placement for esophageal lesions: indications, methods, and results. Radiographics 2003;23:89–105.
13. Jung GS, Song HY, Seo TS, et al. Malignant gastric outlet obstructions: treatment by means of coaxial placement of uncovered and covered expandable nitinol stents. J Vasc Interv Radiol 2002;13:275–83.
14. Lopera JE, Alvarez O, Castano R, et al. Initial experience with Song's covered duodenal stent in the treatment of malignant gastroduodenal obstruction. J Vasc Interv Radiol 2001;12:1297–303.
15. Morgan RA, Adam AN. Malignant biliary disease: percutaneous interventions. Tech Vasc Interv Radiol 2001;4: 147–52.
16. Lee MJ, Dawson SL, Mueller PR, et al. Percutaneous management of hilar biliary malignancies with metallic endoprostheses: results, technical problems, and causes of failure. Radiographics 1993;13:1249–63.
17. Miyayama S, Matsui O, Akakura Y, et al. Efficacy of covered metallic stents in the treatment of unresectable malignant biliary obstruction. Cardiovasc Intervent Radiol 2004;27: 349–54.
18. Farrell TA, Hicks ME. A review of radiologically guided percutaneous nephrostomies in 303 patients. J Vasc Interv Radiol 1997;8:769–74.
19. Seymour H, Patel U. Ureteric stenting-current status. Semin Interv Radiol 2000;17:351–65.
20. Barton JC, Jones SC, Lamberth WC, et al. Cardiac tamponade associated with imatinib mesylate therapy of chronic myelogenous leukemia. Am J Hematol 2002;71:139–40.
21. Murray JG, Patz EF Jr, Erasmus JJ, Gilkeson RC. CT appearance of the pleural space after talc pleurodesis. AJR Am J Roentgenol 1997;169:89–91.
22. Patz EF Jr. Malignant pleural effusions: recent advances and ambulatory sclerotherapy. Chest 1998;113 Suppl 1:74S–7S.
23. Pollak JS, Burdge CM, Rosenblatt M, et al. Treatment of malignant pleural effusions with tunneled long-term drainage catheters. J Vasc Interv Radiol 2001;12:201–8.
24. Cullinane CA, Paz IB, Smith D, et al. Prognostic factors in the surgical management of pericardial effusion in the patient with concurrent malignancy. Chest 2004;125: 1328–34.
25. Alavi A, Ring EJ. Localization of gastrointestinal bleeding: superiority of Tc99m sulfur colloid compared with angiography. AJR Am J Roentgenol 1981;137:741–8.
26. Dusold R, Burke K, Carpenter W, et al. The accuracy of technetium-99m labeled red cell scintigraphy in localizing gastrointestinal bleeding. Am J Gastroenterol 1994;89: 345–8.
27. Schwartz PE, Goldstein HM, Wallace S, Rutledge FN. Control of arterial hemorrhage using percutaneous arterial catheter techniques in patients with gynecologic malignancies. Gynecol Oncol 1975;3:276–88.
28. Madoff DC, Gupta S, Toombs BD, et al. Arterioureteral fistulas: a clinical, diagnostic, and therapeutic dilemma. AJR Am J Roentgenol 2004;182:1241–50.
29. Morrissey DD, Andersen PE, Nesbit GM, et al. Endovascular management of hemorrhage in patients with head and neck cancer. Arch Otolaryngol Head Neck Surg 1997; 123:15–9.
30. Yu-Tang Goh P, Lin M, Teo N, En Shen Wong D. Embolization for hemoptysis: a six-year review. Cardiovasc Intervent Radiol 2002;25:17–25.
31. Fraser RS, Muller NL, Colman N, Paré PD. Thrombosis and thromboembolism. In: Fraser RS, Muller NL, Colman N, Paré PD, editors. Fraser and Paré's diagnosis of diseases of the chest. 4th ed. Philadelphia: W.B. Saunders; 1999. p. 1773–843.
32. Light RW. Pleural effusion due to pulmonary emboli. Curr Opin Pulm Med 2001;7:198–201.
33. Schoepf UJ, Costello P. CT angiography for diagnosis of pulmonary embolism: state of the art. Radiology 2004; 230:329–37.
34. Kavanagh EC, O'Hare A, Hargaden G, Murray JG. Risk of pulmonary embolism after negative MDCT pulmonary angiography findings. AJR Am J Roentgenol 2004;182: 499–504.
35. Lombard J, Bhatia R, Sala E. Spiral computed tomographic pulmonary angiography for investigating suspected pulmonary embolism: clinical outcomes. Can Assoc Radiol J 2003; 54:147–51.
36. Tillie-Leblond I, Mastora I, Radenne F, et al. Risk of pulmonary embolism after a negative spiral CT angiogram in patients with pulmonary disease: 1-year clinical follow-up study. Radiology 2002;223:461–7.
37. Wu AS, Pezzullo JA, Cronan JJ, et al. CT pulmonary angiography: quantification of pulmonary embolus as a predictor of patient outcome: initial experience. Radiology 2004;230:831–5.
38. Araoz PA, Gotway MB, Trowbridge RL, et al. Helical CT pulmonary angiography predictors of in-hospital morbidity and mortality in patients with acute pulmonary embolism. J Thorac Imaging 2003;18:207–16.
39. Abcarian PW, Sweet JD, Watabe JT, Yoon HC. Role of a quantitative D-dimer assay in determining the need for CT angiography of acute pulmonary embolism. AJR Am J Roentgenol 2004;182:1377–81.
40. Goldhaber SZ, Visani L, De Rosa M. Acute pulmonary embolism: clinical outcomes in the International Cooperative Pulmonary Embolism Registry (ICOPER). Lancet 1999;353:1386–9.
41. Goldhaber SZ, Markis JE, Meyrovitz MF, et al. Acute pulmonary embolism treated with tissue plasminogen activator. Lancet 1986;2:886–9.
42. Verstraete M, Miller GA, Bounameaux H, et al. Intravenous and intrapulmonary recombinant tissue-type plasminogen activator in the treatment of acute massive pulmonary embolism. Circulation 1988;77:353–60.
43. Uflacker R. Interventional therapy for pulmonary embolism. J Vasc Interv Radiol 2001;12:147–64.
44. Kinney TB. Update on inferior vena cava filters. J Vasc Interv Radiol 2003;14:425–40.
45. Navigante AH, Cerchietti LC, Costantini P, et al. Conventional chest radiography in the initial assessment of adult cancer patients with fever and neutropenia. Cancer Control 2002;9:346–51.
46. Maschmeyer G. Pneumonia in febrile neutropenic patients: radiologic diagnosis. Curr Opin Oncol 2001;13:229–35.
47. Goodwin DA. Clinical use of In-111 leukocyte imaging. Clin Nucl Med 1983;8:36–8.
48. Holder LE. Clinical radionuclide bone imaging. Radiology 1990;176:607–14.
49. Fraser RS, Muller NL, Colman N, Paré PD. Bacteria other than mycobacteria. In: Fraser RS, Muller NL, Colman N, Paré PD, editors. Fraser and Paré's diagnosis of diseases of the chest. 4th ed. Philadelphia: W.B. Saunders; 1999. p. 734–97.
50. Lee KH, Lee JS, Lynch DA, et al. The radiologic differential diagnosis of diffuse lung diseases characterized by multiple cysts or cavities. J Comput Assist Tomogr 2002;26: 5–12.
51. Gaeta M, Blandino A, Scribano E, et al. Computed tomography halo sign in pulmonary nodules: frequency and diagnostic value. J Thorac Imaging 1999;14:109–13.
52. Fraser RS, Muller NL, Colman N, Paré PD. Fungi and actinomyces. In: Fraser RS, Muller NL, Colman N, Paré PD, editors. Fraser and Paré's diagnosis of diseases of the chest. 4th ed. Philadelphia: W.B. Saunders; 1999. p. 875–978.
53. Oikonomou A, Muller NL, Nantel S. Radiographic and high-resolution CT findings of influenza virus pneumonia in patients with hematologic malignancies. AJR Am J Roentgenol 2003;181:507–11.
54. Gasparetto EL, Ono SE, Escuissato D, et al. Cytomegalovirus pneumonia after bone marrow transplantation: high resolution CT findings. Br J Radiol 2004;77:724–7.
55. Maycher B, O'Connor R, Long R. Computed tomographic abnormalities in Mycobacterium avium complex lung disease include the mosaic pattern of reduced lung attenuation. Can Assoc Radiol J 2000;51:93–102.
56. Alpard SK, Duarte AG, Bidani A, Zwischenberger JB. Pathogenesis and management of respiratory insufficiency following pulmonary resection. Semin Surg Oncol 2000;18:183–96.
57. Kirch C, Blot F, Fizazi K, et al. Acute respiratory distress syndrome after chemotherapy for lung metastases from non-seminomatous germ-cell tumors. Support Care Cancer 2003;11:575–80.
58. Ely EW, Haponik EF. Using the chest radiograph to determine intravascular volume status: the role of vascular pedicle width. Chest 2002;121:942–50.
59. Chen JT. Radiographic diagnosis of heart failure. Heart Dis Stroke 1992;1:58–63.
60. Pfeilschifter J, Diel IJ. Osteoporosis due to cancer treatment: pathogenesis and management. J Clin Oncol 2000;18: 1570–93.
61. Grampp S, Genant HK, Mathur A, et al. Comparisons of noninvasive bone mineral measurements in assessing age-related loss, fracture discrimination, and diagnostic classification. J Bone Miner Res 1997;12:697–711.
62. Jung H-S, Jee W-H, McCauley TR, et al. Discrimination of metastatic from acute osteoporotic compression spinal fractures with MR imaging. Radiographics 2003;23: 179–87.
63. Zoarski GH, Stallmeyer MJ, Obuchowski A. Percutaneous vertebroplasty: A to Z. Tech Vasc Interv Radiol 2002;5:223–38.
64. Newberg A, Alavi A. Role of positron emission tomography in the investigation of neuropsychiatric disorders. In: Sandler MP editor. Diagnostic nuclear medicine. 4th ed. Philadelphia: Lippincott, Williams and Wilkins; 2003. p. 783–819.
65. Wong, FC, Podoloff DA. Evaluation of ventricular shunts and pumps via radionuclide technique. In: Khalkhali I, Maublant J, Goldsmith S, editors. Nuclear oncology. Philadelphia: Lippincott, Williams & Wilkins; 2001. p. 183–6.
66. Chamberlain MC, Corey-Bloom J. Leptomeningeal metastasis: indium-DTPA CSF flow studies. Neurology 1991;41: 1765–9.
67. Laurin NR, Driedger AA, Hurwitz GA, et al. Cerebral perfusion imaging with technetium 99m HMPAO in brain death and severe central nervous system injury. J Nucl Med 1989;30:1627–35.
68. Speith MD, Ansari AN, Kawada TK, et al. Direct comparision of Tc99m DTPA and Tc 99m-HMPAO for the evaluating brain death. Clin Nucl Med 1994;19:867–972.
69. Wong R., Beguelin GZ, de Lima M, et al. Tacrolimus-associated posterior reversible encephalopathy syndrome after allogeneic haematopoietic stem cell transplantation. Br J Haematol 2003;122:128–34.
70. Hinchey J, Chaves C, Appignani, et al. A reversible posterior leukoencephalopathy syndrome. N Engl J Med 1996;334: 494–500.
71. Nousiainen T, Jantunen E, Vanninen E, Hartikainen J. Early decline in left ventricular ejection fraction predicts doxorubicin cardiotoxicity in lymphoma patients. Br J Cancer 2002;86:1697–700.
72. Anderlini P, Benjamin RS, Wong FCL, et al. Idarubicin cardiotoxicity: a retrospective study in acute myeloid leukemia and myelodysplasia. J Clin Oncol 1995;13: 2827–34.
73. Ernst ER, Shub C, Bailey KR, et al. Radiographic measurements of cardiac size as predictors of outcome in patients with dilated cardiomyopathy. J Card Fail 2001;7:13–20.
74. Pistolesi M, Milne EN, Miniati M, Giuntini C. The vascular pedicle of the heart and the vena azygos. Part II: acquired heart disease. Radiology 1984;152:9–17.
75. Miller JA, Contractor S, Maldjian P, Wolansky L. Transient mediastinal enlargement: an unusual computed tomographic manifestation of pulmonary venous hypertension and congestive heart failure. Respiration 2000;67:216–8.
76. Erly WK, Borders RJ, Outwater EK, et al. Location, size, and distribution of mediastinal lymph node enlargement in chronic congestive heart failure. J Comput Assist Tomogr 2003;27:485–9.
77. Kalambokis G, Stefanou D, Arkoumani E, et al. Fulminant bronchiolitis obliterans organizing pneumonia following 2 days of treatment with hydroxyurea, interferon-alpha and oral cytarabine ocfosfate for chronic myelogenous leukemia. Eur J Haematol 2004;73:67–70.
78. Erasmus JJ, McAdams HP, Rossi SE. High-resolution CT of drug-induced lung disease. Radiol Clin North Am 2002; 40:61–72.
79. Kumar AJ, Leeds NE, Fuller GN et al. Malignant gliomas: MR imaging spectrum of radiation therapy—chemotherapy-induced necrosis of the brain after treatment. Radiology 2000;217:377–84.

80. Libshitz HI, Shuman LS. Radiation-induced pulmonary change: CT findings. J Comput Assist Tomogr 1984;8:15–9.

81. Libshitz HI, Sheppard DG. Filling in of radiation therapy-induced bronchiectatic change: a reliable sign of locally recurrent lung cancer. Radiology 1999;210:25–7.

82. Bhargava P, Reich P, Alavi A, Zhuang H. Radiation-induced esophagitis on FDG PET imaging. Clin Nucl Med 2003;28:849–50.

83. Park KJ, Chung JY, Chun MS, Suh JH. Radiation-induced lung disease and the impact of radiation methods on imaging features. Radiographics 2000;20:83–98.

84. Aoki T, Nagata Y, Negoro Y, et al. Evaluation of lung injury after three-dimensional conformal stereotactic radiation therapy for solitary lung tumors: CT appearance. Radiology 2004;230:101–8.

85. Mitchell M, Logan PM. Radiation-induced changes in bone. Radiographics 1998;18:1125–36.

86. Kacprzak G, Marciniak M, Addae-Boateng E, et al. Causes and management of postpneumonectomy empyemas: our experience. Eur J Cardiothorac Surg 2004;26:498–502.

87. Kelly RF, Hunter DW, Maddaus MA. Postpneumonectomy syndrome after left pneumonectomy. Ann Thorac Surg 2001;71:701–3.

88. Alanezi K, Urschel JD. Mortality secondary to esophageal anastomotic leak. Ann Thorac Cardiovasc Surg 2004;10:71–5.

89. Klepetko W, Taghavi S, Pereszlenyi A, et al. Impact of different coverage techniques on incidence of postpneumonectomy stump fistula. Eur J Cardiothorac Surg 1999;15:758–63.

90. van Sonnenberg E, Wittich GR, Goodacre BW, et al. Percutaneous abscess drainage: update. World J Surg 2001;25:362–9; discussion 370–2.

91. Caliendo MV, Lee DE, Queiroz R, Waldman DL. Sclerotherapy with use of doxycycline after percutaneous drainage of postoperative lymphoceles. J Vasc Interv Radiol 2001;12:73–7.

92. Piccirillo JF, Tierney RM, Costas I, et al. Prognostic importance of comorbidity in a hospital-based cancer registry. JAMA 2004;291:2441–7.

Laboratory Investigation

Beverly C. Handy, MD, MS

Cancer Center Laboratory

Laboratory support for the oncology patient typically encompasses two discreet yet interdependent functions. Being subject to the same non–cancer-related conditions prevalent in the general population of similar demographic makeup, in addition to those that are directly or indirectly cancer related, patients require a range of testing services that sufficiently meet both needs. Reflecting these dual functions, the organization of a cancer center laboratory optimally includes clinical chemistry, hematology, microbiology, and transfusion services that offer expanded testing options to support the diagnosis, staging, and monitoring of malignancies, cancer-related conditions, and cancer therapy–associated conditions. Included are bone marrow evaluation, hematology, and flow cytometry functions for diagnosis and monitoring, along with extended transfusion medicine and apharesis services to support bone marrow and peripheral blood stem cell transplantation. Tumor-related or treatment-related blood component deficiencies must also be addressed. A full range of microbiology laboratory services is also needed to address the needs of the immunosuppressed patient, as well as a clinical chemistry laboratory that offers tumor marker and other biochemical testing required for the confirmation of a diagnosis of a malignancy, monitoring of treatment response, and detection of cancer-related or therapy-associated conditions. Additional services are also commonly available, such as those provided by molecular diagnostic and human leukocyte antigen laboratories.

In general, a substantial volume of testing typically reflects the diagnostic and follow-up needs of a patient population receiving somewhat longer-term or chronic care, with a lesser volume devoted to acute, short-term, emergency services. In this population, several types of aberrant laboratory results are encountered frequently and often necessitate further investigation. Some of these are discussed in this chapter.

Laboratory Issues in the Oncology Patient Population

Test Result Validity

A substantial portion of the testing performed in the cancer center clinical laboratory typically involves the use of immunoassays. These provide relatively sensitive, accurate assays that are well adapted for high-volume testing and serial monitoring. Interferences in these methodologies, however, can occur. These can be patient independent, such as those that are caused by the use of inappropriate anticoagulant or specimen tube type, medications, hemolysis, hyperlipidemia, and other factors that either degrade specimen integrity or interfere with the test methodology, and are seen in any clinical laboratory. A common example is the background interference found with hyperlipidemic sera when immunoglobulins or other protein concentrations are measured using nephelometry-based testing. These are generally predictable and are avoided by adhering to published specimen collection requirements. Others are patient specific and are caused by either unexpected antibodies within the sample that effectively interfere with the activity of test kit reagent antibodies or are due to ectopic production of the substance of interest, such as a hormone by tumor. Patients with malignancies are at particular risk of having human antimouse antibodies (HAMAs),[1] autoantibodies,[2–7] and ectopic hormone production. Consequently, laboratories serving a cancer patient population frequently have protocols in place to evaluate suspect samples when it appears that patient-specific factors are impacting test results. Expedient resolution is usually required to avoid unnecessary delays in treatment. For example, elevated serum or urine β-human chorionic gonadotropin (hCG) concentrations can be seen owing to ectopic production by nontrophoblastic tumors. This can be found with a diverse variety of cancers, including carcinomas of the breast, liver, and gastrointestinal tract; melanoma; and multiple myeloma,[8–13] and can serve as a source of confusion when performing routine pregnancy testing prior to administration of chemotherapy or radiation treatment. It has been estimated that up to 30% of cancers in general can be associated with increased serum β-hCG levels.[2] Similarly, the production of HAMAs is known to be an occasional consequence of exposure to mouse monoclonal antibodies used in cancer treatment or imaging studies.[1,14] Their presence or absence, however, cannot be predicted in individual patients.[15] Consequently, in this setting, requests for the

laboratory to review results can be helpful when they appear to be inconsistent with previous results or when they are incompatible with observed clinical findings. The laboratory's role involves a step-by-step process to rule out or identify potential sources of interference. This typically includes comparing results from analyzers that use different methodologies, assessing the reproducibility of results at differing concentrations, using antibody-blocking reagents, and assessing the ability to obtain expected results from known quantities of the substance in question.[16] Given the large volume of testing performed in the typical cancer center laboratory, detectable interference from HAMAs, heterophiles, or other antibodies appears to be relatively infrequent, although it can potentially affect virtually any immunoassay. Table 1, although not all-inclusive, illustrates that a broad range of routine testing is commonly performed using immunoassays. Other patient-specific factors can also affect non–immunoassay-based testing. These include pseudohyperkalemia owing to marked leukocytosis or thrombocytosis,[17] artifactually abnormal cell counts owing to large amounts of white blood cell fragmentation found with some leukemias,[18] platelet satellitism or clumping, or the presence of cold agglutinins,[18–21] among others. Laboratory review, again, is usually helpful in clinically suspicious cases.

The clinical laboratory also serves a role as a direct source of information on specific test performance characteristics. For those providing service to cancer centers, questions not uncommonly arise concerning the optimum use of tumor markers and other assays performed for serial monitoring, in particular. Interpretation of temporal changes in laboratory values is dependent on the ability to discriminate clinically relevant changes from those that are due to biologic or

Table 1 Tests that Are Frequently Performed by Immunoassay
Cardiac marker testing
Cytokine measurement
Hormone level assessment
Infectious disease screening
Therapeutic drug monitoring
Tumor marker measurement

random variation. Knowledge of physiologic factors, such as diurnal variation and method of clearance, that specifically affect the substance of interest and the individual test kit characteristics are both key to an accurate interpretation of both baseline values and serial changes. Some of these are listed in Table 2.

Serum Proteins

Confirmation of and/or establishing a diagnosis of malignancy and monitoring for treatment response, disease recurrence, or treatment side effects together encompass a substantial portion of the chemistry testing.

Serum protein concentration abnormalities are not uncommon, whether they consist of a relatively mild, moderate, or severe hypogammaglobulinemia or, alternately, an increased total protein of varying proportions. Hypogammaglobulinemia, with its extensive list of potential causes, some of which work in concert, can require additional evaluation. A consequence of deficient immunoglobulin production, enhanced loss, or both, treatment, when necessary, will focus on amelioration of the underlying cause.[22] In the setting of cancer, etiologies can include gastrointestinal or renal protein loss but also frequently involve immunologic mechanisms that are as yet poorly understood and do not appear to be readily reversible.[23–25] Infectious complications can be a significant cause of morbidity and mortality, particularly for patients with hematologic malignancies, and not uncommonly, these are associated with a hypogammaglobulinemia.[23,26–28] When it is the presenting feature, serum immunoglobulin quantitation, serum immunofixation, serum free light chain assessment, and Bence Jones protein studies with urine immunofixation are helpful in ruling out the presence of a monoclonal protein as the cause. Determining prealbumin concentrations along with those of albumin can be useful adjuncts to the clinical history and physical examination in the assessment of nutritional status; however, levels of both can be unreliable in the presence of acute inflammation.[29–31]

Because an increased serum total protein in the absence of a known infectious, inflammatory, or other benign etiology, like a hypogammaglobulinemia, may also herald an underlying malignancy, serum protein electrophoretic studies and quantitation of immunoglobulins are usually helpful initial aids in distinguishing polyclonal from monoclonal immunoglobulin production. If the results are indicative of or the clinical suspicion remains high for the presence of a monoclonal gammopathy, further laboratory investigation includes immunofixation, Bence Jones protein studies, and serum free light chain concentration assessments, as were discussed previously for the evaluation of patients with low gammaglobulin levels. In addition, when the constellation of clinical findings includes the cerebral, cardiovascular, pulmonary, renal, or bleeding abnormalities suggestive of microcirculatory insufficiency, this may raise a suspicion that hyperviscosity syndrome is present and prompt the measurement of serum viscosity.[32,33] Onset of symptoms can occur acutely or manifest slowly over prolonged periods of time and can consist of headache, altered mental status, disturbance of gait, mucosal bleeding including the gastrointestinal or the urinary tract, cardiac failure, visual changes, papilledema, or retinal hemorrhage.[34–36] The presence or absence of symptoms cannot be readily predicted by serum protein concentrations alone as other factors influence blood protein–protein interactions, such as polymerization tendency, the effects of pH and temperature, and protein size and shape.[32] As a result, patients with relatively modest levels of a monoclonal protein component may present with a severity of symptoms that are seemingly out of proportion to its concentration, whereas others with high levels can appear to be surprisingly unaffected.[32,35] Table 3 lists conditions that have been associated with hyperviscosity syndrome. Most commonly, it occurs as a complication of hematologic malignancies, which have resulted in excessive immunoglobulin or blood component production, although it can occasionally be found with benign conditions or, even rarely, with malignancies that are nonhematopoietic in origin.[33–35,37–50] Cryoglobulinemia, in particular, is one disorder commonly associated with increased viscosity that can be considered in a symptomatic patient with a monoclonal gammopathy. Consisting of cold precipitable proteins, which are most often immunoglobulins, they are estimated to be present in up to 20% of patients with Waldenström's macroglobulinemia and up to 10% of patients with multiple myeloma.[51] Generally categorized into three types, type 1 is due to an isolated monoclonal immunoglobulin, type 2 (mixed) involves a monoclonal immunoglobulin (frequently IgM) with activity against polyclonal immunoglobulins (often IgG), and type 3 involves polyclonal proteins (frequently IgM and IgG).[51,52] Type 1 is characteristically found in patients with multiple myeloma, Waldenström's macroglobulinemia, or other lymphoproliferative disorders, whereas type 2 can be found in lymphoproliferative disorders, autoimmune diseases, and infections (especially with hepatitis C virus).[51,53] Although often asymptomatic, patients can present with a variety of manifestations, including skin changes (purpura, uticaria, Raynaud's phenomenon), arthralgias, peripheral neuropathy, and organ dysfunction (hepatic, pulmonary, renal).[51,53] Symptoms are the result of either the occlusion of small blood vessels or vasculitis associated with immune complex deposition.[51,53] When the clinical suspicion is high that a cryoglobulin may be present, it is helpful to maintain close communication with the clinical laboratory as special specimen handling (maintenance at 37°C) is necessary for accurate diagnosis,[54] as well as the fact that the presence of a cryoglobulin in a blood sample can interfere with the results of other laboratory tests.

Electrolytes

Electrolytes are routinely monitored closely as cancer patients have an increased risk of experiencing fluid or electrolyte imbalances during the course of their disease, either directly as a tumor-related effect or secondarily as a side effect of treatment.[55,56] Some can be anticipated based on tumor type or a known treatment complication, whereas others appear to be patient dependent. Although abnormalities of sodium, potassium, and phosphate, among others, are not uncommon, assessment for possible hypomagnesemia or hypercalcemia is of particular interest in patients with malignancies.

It has been suggested that hypomagnesemia may be present in a substantial portion of patients seen in general clinical practice but often goes unrecognized.[57] It has been estimated to occur in

---

Table 2 Factors Important in the Evaluation of Baseline and Serial Values

Clearance rate: How is it influenced by hepatic, renal, or other diseases?

Specificity of test: What other substances or conditions can give positive results?

Sensitivity of test: What is the smallest amount that can be reliably measured?

Potential interferences in test method

Physiologic variability: How much variation can occur with no real change in disease status?

Analytic variability: How much variability is inherent in the laboratory measurement?

Table 3 Conditions that Have Been Associated with Hyperviscosity Syndrome

Monoclonal hematopoietic disorders
  Waldenström's macroglobulinemia
  Multiple myeloma (most often immunoglobulin A or G)
  Leukemias
  Polycythemia vera
Nonhematopoietic malignancies
  Ovarian carcinoma
  Metastatic breast carcinoma
Polyclonal gammopathies
  Rheumatoid arthritis
  Sjögren's syndrome
  Systemic lupus erythematosus
  Human immunodeficiency virus (HIV) infection
Other conditions
  Cryoglobulinemia
  Iatrogenic

approximately 10% of patients hospitalized for various reasons[58] and over 17% of patients hospitalized for cancer.[59] Causes include insufficient dietary intake, losses through the kidneys or gastrointestinal tract or as a secondary effect of treatment, particularly with cisplatin-containing regimens.[57,60,61] Obvious signs and symptoms are usually absent or are nonspecific and are attributed to either depression or the primary disease, leading to underrecognition.[62,63] These vary from subtle to clinically acute. They range from headache, general apathy, or other seemingly psychiatric-based behavioral changes or other associated electrolyte deficiencies to neuromuscular hyperexcitability, cardiac arrhythmias, and even coma.[63,64] Measurement of serum total, ionized, intracellular, and urinary magnesium concentrations have all been employed, in addition to the use of the magnesium loading test in the evaluation of patients with magnesium abnormalities. Optimum test selection, at this time, appears to be situation dependent.[65,66]

In clinical practice, hypercalcemia is most often caused by either primary hyperparathyroidism or malignancy.[67] It has been estimated to be found in up to 20% of patients with malignant neoplasms overall, although the actual prevalence varies by tumor type.[56,68–70] Known mechanisms include tumor cell cytokine production promoting local osteolysis and the activity of parathyroid hormone–related protein and other humoral factors that promote skeletal resorption and renal tubular calcium reabsorption.[56,71] Similar to patients with hypomagnesemia, the presentation can consist of only vague or essentially nonspecific complaints. Depending on the rapidity of onset and the severity of the abnormality, symptoms range from general feelings of fatigue, lethargy, or anorexia through muscular, gastrointestinal, cardiovascular, renal, and neurologic manifestations.[56,72] Given the common occurrence of this electrolyte disturbance in the cancer patient population and its diverse clinical presentation, serum calcium levels are routinely measured to confirm the presence of normocalcemia.

Organ Systems

Central Nervous System

Although cerebrospinal fluid (CSF) is obtained in general, for several well-established clinical indications, including the diagnosis of demyelinating disorders, central nervous system (CNS) infections, and subarachnoid hemorrhage,[73,74] in the cancer center, it is often obtained to evaluate for CNS involvement by either primary or metastatic tumor. Neurologic symptoms range from relatively subtle to overt and include headache, cranial nerve palsy, seizures, and coma.[75] Findings of CNS involvement can occasionally be the initial

evidence that a patient has a malignancy.[75,76] Macroscopically observable and chemically measurable CSF characteristics can be associated with the presence of tumor, including xanthochromia,[73] increased cell counts,[73] abnormal total protein concentrations,[73,75] and decreased glucose concentrations.[73] The diagnosis, however, is dependent on the cytologic identification of malignant cells. A positive cytology confirms tumor involvement of the leptomeninges or the ventricles.[77] Evidence suggests that the test performance is enhanced by the use of immunocytochemistry[77,78] and, if necessary, repeat sampling.[78] Electrophoresis with immunofixation to detect the presence of an M-protein within the CSF can also be helpful if a plasma cell–derived malignancy is suspected. Several specimen collection–related factors have been identified that help minimize the occurrence of false-negative results.[79] These consist of immediate sample processing, collecting the specimen from a known area of leptomeningeal involvement, ensuring an adequate sample volume, and, again, obtaining a repeat sample if the first result was negative despite a high level of clinical suspicion.[79]

Cardiac

In addition to the degree of risk for cardiovascular disease prevalent in individuals of similar background, patients with malignancies can be exposed to tumor or treatment-related effects that negatively impact cardiac function.[80] Tumor-associated conditions include compression of the heart or large blood vessels by masses, the presence of pericardial effusions, and the production of substances such as catecholamines by the malignant cells that either have cardiotoxic properties or promote arrhythmias.[80] Among the treatment side effects are chemotherapy-associated cardiac failure, myocarditis, pericarditis, and coronary artery spasms.[80] Measurement of either brain natriuretic peptide or pro–brain natriuretic peptide serves as a fast, easily performed, and economical blood test to assist in the assessment of suspected heart failure or, when appropriate, the clinical evaluation of patients prior to surgery or administration of cardiotoxic chemotherapy. Cardiac marker tests such as cardiac troponin I or T, creatine kinase MB, and myoglobin are useful adjuncts to the electrocardiogram in the assessment of chest pain. Because the predictive value of these tests varies by time since onset of the cardiac event, measurement of an "early" marker, such as myoglobin, is frequently combined with that of a "late" marker, such as cardiac troponin I or T. Serial measurements (typically three or four) are obtained over a 24-hour period to detect the expected changes in values over time characteristic of cardiac injury. Increased cardiac marker values can also be found in conditions other than acute myocardial infarction that are commonly

seen in patients hospitalized with cancer. These include renal failure, pulmonary emboli, myocarditis, pericarditis, sepsis, and heart failure.[81] As a result, clinical correlation is important, especially when evaluating the clinically ill, hospitalized patient to ensure the accurate interpretation of results.

Gastrointestinal Tract

Clostridium difficile is a common cause of hospital-acquired diarrhea in patients treated with antibiotics and, consequently, is a source of treatment-related complications in the oncology patient as treatment with antibiotics usually occurs sometime during the course of the disease.[82] Although a cytotoxin-mediated diarrhea is frequently the only overt symptom, an increase in the white blood cell count, an elevated temperature, or even toxic megacolon can also be present.[82] Rarely, the organism can be associated with other findings, such as abscess formation, peritonitis, and other infections.[83] A pseudomembranous colitis is the classic finding, although the diagnosis is often made clinically when cytotoxin is detected in individuals who are also symptomatic.[82] It should be noted, however, that asymptomatic colonization is estimated to occur in approximately 3% of healthy adults,[83] and these do not require treatment.[82]

Skin

Ancillary laboratory studies can be useful in the evaluation of skin lesions when malignancy is suspected and the diagnosis will be aided by additional confirmatory evidence. Such studies are most often helpful when tumors are hematopoietic in origin. An example is the assessment of patients for a possible diagnosis of mycosis fungoides. Biopsy of the skin typically shows an atypical dermal lymphoid infiltrate. Additional complementary studies include immunohistochemical stains that provide evidence of T-cell lineage (CD3$^+$, CD4$^+$) while simultaneously ruling out the presence of B-cell, myeloid, or other tumor cell types. T-cell receptor gene rearrangement studies are useful to confirm the presence of monoclonality, whereas flow cytometry analysis performed on a blood sample can evaluate for the presence of an aberrant T-cell population within the patient's peripheral blood. Use of immunohistochemistry, flow cytometry, and molecular analysis can particularly enhance the ability to discriminate benign, inflammatory skin lesions from true clonal expansions, as well as to identify the specific cell type of origin in malignant skin tumors that are hematopoietic in nature. As such, these studies can provide invaluable confirmatory information in these types of cases.

Hematology

Cancer has a well-recognized association with the presence of coagulopathies, although the underlying mechanisms are still under investigation. It is estimated that thrombosis may be the most common complication experienced by cancer patients and the second most common cause of mortality.[84] Symptoms associated with cancer-related hypercoagulability range from ischemic strokes[85] to recurrent episodes of thromboembolism.[85] Symptoms and laboratory evidence of a coagulation disorder, including thrombocytopenia and increased D-dimer levels,[86,87] can be the first manifestation of a previously undetected malignancy.[86]

Summary

Patients with cancer are at risk of both disease-related and treatment-related complications. These include electrolyte disturbances, serum protein abnormalities, coagulation disorders, cardiac manifestations, and infection. A broad range of testing services are necessary to provide the needed level of support for diagnosis and treatment.

REFERENCES

1. Reinsberg J. Interference by human antibodies with tumor marker assays. Hybridoma 1995;14:205–8.
2. Bar-Dayan Y, Kaveri SV, Kazatchkine MD, Shoenfeld Y. Is cancer an autoimmune process dependent on anti-apoptotic autoantibodies? Med Hypotheses 2000;55:103–8.
3. Lucchinetti CF, Kimmel DW, Lennon VA. Paraneoplastic and oncologic profiles of patients seropositive for type 1 antineuronal nuclear autoantibodies. Neurology 1998;50:652–7.
4. Thirkill CE. Lung cancer-induced blindness. Lung Cancer 1996;14:253–64.
5. Sokol RJ, Booker DJ, Stamps R. Erythrocyte autoantibodies, autoimmune haemolysis, and carcinoma. J Clin Pathol 1994;47:340–3.
6. Gray ES, McLay AL, Thompson WD, et al. Non-organ specific autoantibodies in malignant diseases. Scott Med J 1976;20:203–8.
7. Wasserman J, Glas U, Blomgren H. Autoantibodies in patients with carcinoma of the breast. Correlation with prognosis. Clin Exp Immunol 1975;19:417–22.
8. Halim AM, Barakat M, el-Zayat AM, et al. Urinary beta-hCG in benign and malignant urinary tract diseases. Disease Markers 1995;12:109–15.
9. AIA-Pack beta-hCG [package insert]. Tokyo: TOSOH Corporation; July 1995.
10. Braunstein GD. Placental proteins as tumormarkers. In: Herberman RB, Mercer DW, editors. Immunodiagnosis of cancer. New York: Marcel Dekker. 1991;673–701.
11. ICON® II HCG ImmunoConcentration™ Assay [package insert]. Fullerton (CA): Beckman Coulter; March 2001.
12. Hussa RO. Human chorionic gonadotropin, a clinical marker. Review of its biosynthesis. Ligand Rev 1981;3:6.
13. Hussa RO. The clinical marker hCG. Praeger Publishers; New York. 1987.
14. Preissner CM, Dodge LA, O'Kane DJ, et al. Prevalence of heterophilic antibody interference in eight automated tumor marker immunoassays. Clin Chem 2005;51:208–10.
15. Emerson JF, Ngo G, Emerson SS. Screening for interference in immunoassays. Clin Chem 2003;49:1163–9.
16. Klee GG. Interferences in hormone immunoassays. Clin Lab Med 2004;24:1–18.
17. Handy BC, Shen Y. Evaluation of potassium values in a cancer patient population. Lab Med 2005;36:95–7.
18. Morris MW, Davey FR. Basic examination of blood. In: Henry JB, editor. Clinical diagnosis and management by laboratory methods. 20th ed. Philadelphia: W.B. Saunders; 2001. p. 479–519.
19. Ahmed P, Minnich V, Michael JM. Platelet satellitosis with spurious thrombocytopenia and neutropenia. Am J Clin Pathol 1978;69:473.
20. Lombarts AJ, deKieviet W. Recognition and prevention of pseudothrombocytopenia and concomitant pseudoleukoctosis. Am J Clin Pathol 1988;89(5):634–9.
21. Hattersley PG, Gerard PW, Caggniano V, Nash DR. Erroneous values on the Model S Coulter due to high titer cold agglutinins. Am J Clin Pathol 1971;55:422.
22. Makhoul I, Ballard J, Makhoul H. Hypogammaglobulimenia. Available at: http://www.emedicine.com/med/topic1/12/06.htm.
23. O'Brian SN, Blijlevens NMA, Mahfouz TH, Anaisse EJ. Infections in patients with hematologic cancer: recent developments. Hematology 2003;1:438–72.
24. Verne GN, Amann ST, Cosgrove C, Cerda JJ. Chronic diarrhea associated with thymoma and hypogammaglobulinemia (Good's syndrome). South Med J 1997;90:444–6.
25. Waldmann TA, Broder S, Krakauer R, et al. The role of suppressor cells in the pathogenesis of common variable hypogammaglobulinemia and the immunodeficiency associated with myeloma. Fed Proc 1976;35:2067–72.
26. Perkins JG, Flynn JM, Howard RS, Byrd JC. Frequency and type of serious infections in fludarabine-refractory B-cell chronic lymphocytic leukemia and small lymphocytic lymphoma: implications for clinical trials in this patient population. Cancer 2002;94:2033–9.
27. Reaman G, Zeltzer P, Bleyer WA, et al. Acute lymphoblastic leukemia in infants less than one year of age: a cumulative experience of the Children's Cancer Study Group. J Clin Oncol 1985;3:1513–21.
28. Leikin S, Miller D, Sather H. Immunologic evaluation in the prognosis of acute lymphoblastic leukemia. A report from the Children's Cancer Study Group. Blood 1981;58:501–8.
29. Sarhill N, Mahmoud FA, Christie R, Tahir A. Assessment of nutritional status and fluid deficits in advanced cancer. Am J Hosp Palliat Care 2003;20:465–73.
30. Bernstein LH, Ingelbleek Y. Transthyretin: its response to malnutrition and stress injury. Clinical usefulness and economic implications. Clin Chem Lab Med 2002;40:1344–8.
31. Johnson AM, Rohifs EM, Silverman LM. Proteins. In: Burtis CA, Ashwood ER, editors. Tietz textbook of clinical chemistry. 3rd ed. Philadelphia: W.B. Saunders; 1999. p. 477–540.
32. Coppell J. Consider "hyperviscosity syndrome" in unexplained breathlessness. Acta Hematol 2000;104:52–3.
33. Somer T. Rheology of paraproteinaemias and the plasma hyperviscosity syndrome. Baillieres Clin Hematol 1987;1:695–723.
34. Frewin R, Henson A, Provan D. ABC of clinical haematology: haematological emergencies. BMJ 1997;314:1333.
35. Winters JL, Pineda AA. Hemapheresis. In: Henry JB, editor. Clinical diagnosis and management by laboratory methods. 20th ed. Philadelphia: W.B. Saunders; 2001. p. 776–805.
36. Foerster J. Plasma cell dyscrasias: general considerations. In: Lee GR, Bithell TC, Foerster J, editors. Wintrobe's clinical hematology. 9th ed. Philadelphia: Lea and Febiger; 1993. p. 2202–18.
37. Baer MR, Stein RS, Dessypris EN. Chronic lymphocytic leukemia with hyperleukocytosis. The hyperviscosity syndrome. Cancer 1985;56:2865–9.
38. Hild DH, Myers TJ. Hyperviscosity in chronic granulocytic leukemia. Cancer 1980;46:1418–21.
39. Chae SW, Cho JH, Lee JH, et al. Sudden hearing loss in chronic myelogenous leukemia implicating hyperviscosity syndrome. J Laryngol Otol 2002;116:291–3.
40. Oh KT, Boldt HC, Danis RP. Iatrogenic central retinal vein occlusion and hyperviscosity associated with high-dose intravenous immunoglobulin administration. Am J Ophthalmol 1997;124:416–8.
41. Rampling MW. Hyperviscosity as a complication in a variety of disorders. Semin Thromb Hemost 2003;29:459–65.
42. Ambrus JL, Ambrus CM, Dembinsky W, et al. Thromboembolic disease susceptibility related to red cell membrane fluidity in patients with polycythemia vera and effect of phlebotomies. J Med 1999;30:299–304.
43. Zakzook SI, Yunus MB, Mulconrey DS. Hyperviscosity syndrome in rheumatoid arthritis with Felty's syndrome: case report and review of the literature. Clin Rheumatol 2002;21:82–5.
44. Simon JA, Lazo-Langer A, Duarte-Rojo A, et al. Serum hyperviscosity syndrome responding to therapeutic plasmapheresis in a patient with primary Sjogren's syndrome. J Clin Apher 2002;17:44–6.
45. Garderet L, Fabiani B, Lacombe K, et al. Hyperviscosity syndrome in an HIV-1-positive patient. Am J Med 2004;117:891–3.
46. Martin CM, Matlow AG, Chew E, et al. Hyperviscosity syndrome in a patient with acquired immunodeficiency syndrome. Arch Intern Med 1989;149:1435–6.
47. Jara LJ, Capin NR, Lavalle C. Hyperviscosity syndrome as the initial manifestation of systemic lupus erythematosus. J Rheumatol 1989;16:225–30.
48. von Tempelhoff GF, Heilmann L, Hommel G, et al. Hyperviscosity syndrome in patients with ovarian carcinoma. Cancer 1998;82:1104–11.
49. Grigg AP, Allardice J, Smith IL, et al. Hyperviscosity syndrome in disseminated breast adenocarcinoma. Pathology 1994;26:65–8.
50. Della Rossa A, Tavoni A, Bombardieri S. Hyperviscosity syndrome in cryoglobulinemia: clinical aspects and therapeutic considerations. Semin Thromb Hemost 2003;29:473–7.
51. Mohamed K, Rehman HU. Cryoglobulinemia. Acta Med Austriaca 2003;30:65–8.
52. Brouet JC, Clauvel JP, Danon F, et al. Biological and clinical significance of cryoglobulins. A report of 86 cases. Am J Med 1974;57:775–88.
53. Dispenzieri A, Gertz MA. Cryoglobulinemia, heavy chain diseases, and monoclonal gammopathy-associated disorders. In: Greer JP, Rodgers GM, Foerster J, et al. editors. Wintrobe's clinical hematology. 11th ed. Philadelphia: Lippincott Williams & Wilkins; 2004. p. 2683–94.
54. Bakker AJ, Slomp J, de Vries T, et al. Adequate sampling in cryoglobulinaemia: recommended warmly. Clin Chem Lab Med 2003;41:85–9.
55. Kapoor M, Chan GZ. Fluid and electrolyte abnormalities. Crit Care Clin 2001;17:503 29.
56. Flombaum CD. Metabolic emergencies in the cancer patient. Semin Oncol 2000;27:322–34.
57. Iannello S, Belfiore F. Hypomagnesemia. A review of the pathophysiological, clinical and therapeutical aspects. Panminerva Med 2001;43:177–209.
58. Abbott LG, Rude RK. Clinical manifestations of magnesium deficiency. Miner Electrolyte Metab 1993;19:314–22.
59. D'Erasmo E, Celi FS, Acca M, et al. Hypocalcemia and hypomagnesemia in cancer patients. Biomed Pharmacother 1991;45:315–7.
60. Kelepouris E, Agus ZS. Hypomagnesemia: renal magnesium handling. Semin Nephrol 1998;18:58–73.
61. Lajer H, Daugaard G. Cisplatin and hypomagnesemia. Cancer Treat Rev 1999;25:47–58.
62. Rasmussen HH, Mortensen PB, Jensen IW. Depression and magnesium deficiency. Int J Psychiatry Med 1989;19:57–63.
63. Flink EB. Magnesium deficiency. Etiology and clinical spectrum. Acta Med Scand Suppl 1981;647:125–37.
64. Mauskop A, Altura BT, Cracco RQ, Altura BM. Intravenous magnesium sulfate rapidly alleviates headaches of various types. Headache 1996;36:154–60.
65. Saur P, Niedmann PD, Brunner E, Kettler D. Do intracellular, extracellular or urinary magnesium concentrations predict renal retention of magnesium in critically ill patients? J Anesthesiol 2005;22:148–53.
66. Sanders GT, Huijgen HJ, Sanders R. Magnesium in disease: a review with special emphasis on the serum ionized magnesium. Clin Chem Lab Med 1999;37:1011–33.
67. Pecherstorfer M, Brenner K, Zojer N. Current management strategies for hypercalcemia. Treat Endocrinol 2003;2:273–92.
68. Mundy GR, Guise TA. Hypercalcemia of malignancy. Am J Med 1997;103:134–45.
69. Warrel RP Jr. Metabolic emergencies. In: DeVita VT, Hellman S, Rosenberg SA, editors. Cancer: principles and practices of oncology. Vol 2, 5th ed. Philadelphia: Lippincott-Raven; 1997. p. 2486–500.
70. Bajorunas DR. Disorders of endocrine function. In: Groeger JS, editor. Critical care of the cancer patient. 2nd ed. St Louis: Mosby Year Book; 1991. p. 192–225.
71. Esbrit P. Hypercalcemia of malignancy—new insights into an old syndrome. Clin Lab 2001;47:67–71.
72. Tattersall MH. Hypercalcaemia: historical perspectives and present management. Support Care Cancer 1993;1:19–25.

73. Smith GP, Kjeldsberg CR. Cerebrospinal, synovial, and serous body fluids. In: Henry JB, editor. Clinical diagnosis and management by laboratory methods. 20th ed. Philadelphia: W.B. Saunders; 2001. p. 403–24.

74. American College of Physicians. The diagnostic spinal tap. Ann Intern Med 1986;104:880.

75. Glosova L, Dundr P, Effler J, Ruzickova M. Gallbladder carcinoma cells in cerebrospinal fluid as the first manifestation of a tumor. A case report. Acta Cytol 2003;47: 1087–90.

76. Perez-Jaffe LA, Salhany KE, Green RJ, et al. Cerebral spinal fluid involvement by Hodgkin's disease diagnosed by CSF cytology and immunocytochemistry. Diagn Cytopathol 1999;20:219–23.

77. Gupta RK, Naran S, Lallu S, Fauck R. Cytodiagnosis of neoplasms of the central nervous system in cerebrospinal fluid samples with an application of selective immunostains in differentiation. Cytopathology 2004;15:38–43.

78. Thomas JE, Falls E, Velasco ME, Zaher A. Diagnostic value of immunocytochemistry in leptomeningeal tumor dissemination. Arch Pathol Lab Med 2000;124:759–61.

79. Glantz MJ, Cole BF, Glantz LK, et al. Cerebrospinal fluid cytology in patients with cancer: minimizing false-negative results. Cancer 1998;82:733–9.

80. Keefe DL. Cardiovascular emergencies in the cancer patient. Semin Oncol 2000;27:244–55.

81. Roongsritong C, Warraich I, Bradley C. Common causes of troponin elevations in the absence of acute myocardial infarction: incidence and clinical significance. Chest 2004; 125:1877–84.

82. Quadri TL, Brown AE. Infectious complications in the critically ill patient with cancer. Semin Oncol 2000;27: 335–46.

83. Reisner BS, Woods GL. Medical bacteriology. In: Henry JB, editor. Clinical diagnosis and management by laboratory methods. 20th ed. Philadelphia: W.B. Saunders; 2001. p. 1088–118.

84. De Lucia D, De Francesco F, Marotta R, et al. Phenotypic APC resistance as a marker of hypercoagulability in primitive cerebral lymphoma. Exp Oncol 2005;27: 159–61.

85. Jovin TG, Boosupalli V, Zivkovic SA, et al. High titers of CA-125 may be associated with recurrent ischemic strokes in patients with cancer. Neurology 2005;64:1944–5.

86. Borowski A, Ghodsizad A, Gams E. Stroke as a first manifestation of ovarian cancer. J Neurooncol 2005;71:267–9.

87. Sase T, Wada H, Yamaguchi M. Haemostatic abnormalities and thrombotic disorders in malignant lymphoma. Thromb Haemost 2005;93:153–9.

Risk Assessment and the Management of Neutropenia and Fever

Kenneth V. I. Rolston, MD

The relationship between neutropenia and the frequency and severity of infection was first described by Bodey and colleagues four decades ago.[1] Febrile neutropenic patients can develop rapidly progressive infections and serious medical comorbidity, necessitating aggressive antimicrobial therapy and supportive care, including close monitoring in the hospital.[2] It has long been recognized, however, that not all neutropenic patients have the same risk of developing serious infections and/or complications. Our ability to reliably identify such patients early in the course of a febrile episode was quite limited until very recently, leading to the uniform policy of administering hospital-based empiric antibiotic therapy to all febrile neutropenic patients.[3] As our understanding of the syndrome of "febrile neutropenia" has grown, it has become possible to identify low-risk patients with reasonable accuracy at the onset of a febrile episode.[4] Several risk assessment schemes are available, including statistically derived and validated risk prediction rules and clinical criteria developed primarily at The University of Texas M. D. Anderson Cancer Center (MDACC).[4–8] Improvements in supportive care, including drug development and delivery systems and the ability to manage substantial numbers of patients in an ambulatory setting, have enabled clinicians to consider not only the nature of empiric antibiotic therapy in febrile neutropenic patients (eg, combination regimens vs monotherapy) but the route of administration (parenteral, sequential, or oral), and the treatment setting (hospital, ambulatory treatment center, home) as well. This chapter focuses on risk assessment in neutropenic patients, the various choices available to treat low-risk patients, and the infrastructure necessary to develop and maintain a successful program of outpatient therapy. Many of the principles that are discussed were developed at MDACC, where outpatient antibiotic therapy in low-risk febrile neutropenic patients has been practiced safely since the late 1980s.

Historical Perspective

The development of chemotherapy represented a significant step in the fight against cancer. Most chemotherapeutic regimens caused some degree of myelosuppression, leading to the two most common complications associated with chemotherapy: bleeding owing to thrombocytopenia and infection secondary to neutropenia. In neutropenic patients, fever is almost always the result of an infection and is often the only manifestation of infection, although, occasionally, noninfectious causes, such as tumor fever or drug fever, might be present.[9] Approximately 15 to 50% of patients with a solid tumor and > 80% of patients with hematologic malignancies will develop at least one episode of fever.[10] Early autopsy studies demonstrated that, particularly in patients with hematologic malignancies, infections were among the most frequent causes of death.[11,12] Often these infections were unrecognized and untreated, negating the potential benefit of antineoplastic therapy on the underlying neoplastic disorder. These data led to the concept of administering "empiric" antimicrobial therapy to neutropenic patients before documenting a specific infection.[13]

Early empiric therapy consisted of agents such as oxacillin, nafcillin, and vancomycin for gram-positive coverage and aminoglycosides such as gentamicin for gram-negative coverage.[13] These regimens had a significant impact on gram-positive infections, but aminoglycosides were associated with treatment failures despite in vitro susceptibility of gram-negative bacilli, such as *Escherichia coli* and *Pseudomonas aeruginosa*, to them.[14] The first major advance in the treatment of gram-negative infections was the development of the antipseudomonal agent penicillin-carbenicillin, which, when combined with an aminoglycoside or used as a single agent in high doses, was successful in treating many gram-negative bacteremic infections.[15,16] Further refinements, such as the addition of a cephalosporin to the empiric regimen to cover *Klebsiella* species and to enhance gram-positive coverage, led to

regimens that were associated with response rates of 60 to 75%.[17–20]

All early empiric regimens were administered parenterally. The first experience with oral antibiotic therapy in hospitalized patients was the use of trimethoprim-sulfamethoxazole (TMP-SMX) for infections that were refractory to other antibiotic regimens.[21] With the subsequent development of the fluoroquinolones, particularly ciprofloxacin (which had potent activity against most gram-negative organisms, including *P. aeruginosa*), sequential (ie, intravenous → oral) or oral antibiotic therapy for the entire febrile episode became a viable option.[22,23,24] Economic pressures led to the development of home health care agencies, which shifted the focus away from hospital-based care. Many institutions invested in the infrastructure necessary to maintain ambulatory or home health care programs as part of a comprehensive health care plan. All of these developments have had an impact on the management of febrile neutropenic patients.

Risk Assessment Strategies

Several investigators have attempted to devise risk prediction rules since the late 1980s. Talcott and colleagues at the Dana-Farber Cancer Institute identified four subsets among febrile neutropenic patients in a deviation study.[5] Group 1 consisted of patients primarily with hematologic malignancies and substantial medical comorbidities, who were already in hospital when they developed their febrile episode (Table 1). This group had a complication rate of 34% and a mortality rate of 23%. The three remaining groups were not hospitalized when their febrile episodes developed. Group 2 consisted of outpatients with concurrent medical comorbidity (eg, volume depletion, nausea or vomiting, pain). Of the patients in group 2, serious complications occurred in 55% and 14% died. Group 3 contained outpatients without concurrent comorbidity but whose cancer was uncontrolled. Major complications occurred in 31% of these patients and 15% died. None of these three groups were

Table 1 Outcomes Related to Risk Groups among Febrile Neutropenic Patients*

Risk Group	Number of Patients (%)	Serious Complications (%)	Deaths (%)
Group 1 (inpatients)	369 (52)	128 (37)	48 (13)
Group 2 (outpatients with concurrent comorbidity)	65 (9)	26 (40)	8 (12)
Group 3 (outpatients with uncontrolled cancer)	55 (8)	14 (25)	8 (15)
Group 4 (low-risk outpatients)	216 (31)	7 (3)	0 (0)
All patients	705 (100)	175 (25)	64 (9)

*Combined data from Talcott and colleagues' derivation and validation studies.[5,6]

considered to be low risk. Group 4 consisted of patients with no comorbidity and responsive tumors, that is, uncomplicated fever and neutropenia. The complication rate in this group was 3%, and there were no deaths. These patients were considered to be low risk. These findings were later validated in a two-center validation study and formed the basis for some initial studies of early discharge or outpatient treatment of low-risk febrile neutropenic patients.[6,25] Interestingly, the presence of a hematology malignancy or a bloodstream infection did not appear to portend a poor outcome in the analysis.

Several years later, an international collaborative study conducted through the Multinational Association for Supportive Care in Cancer (MASCC) established and validated a scoring system to identify low-risk febrile neutropenic patients at the time of presentation.[7] Integer weights were assigned to seven different characteristicsr to develop a risk index score (Table 2). These characteristics included the extent of illness, hypotension, lung disease, solid tumor or absence of fungal infection, no dehydration, outpatient status, and age < 60 years (children were excluded). A score of 21 or greater identified low-risk patients with a positive predictive value of 91%. This MASCC risk index has been internationally accepted and endorsed by societies such as the Infectious Diseases Society of America

Table 2 MASCC Risk Index Scoring System for Identification of Low-Risk Neutropenic Patients*

Characteristic	Score
Burden of illness (no symptoms or mild symptoms)	5
No hypotension	5
No COPD	4
Solid tumor or no previous fungal infection	4
No dehydration	3
Burden of illness (moderate symptoms)	3
Outpatient status at onset of fever	3
Age < 60 yr	2

COPD = chronic obstructive pulmonary disease; MASCC = Multinational Association for Supportive Care in Cancer.

*Highest score possible is 26. A score of ≥ 21 indicates strong likelihood of low-risk status.[7]

(IDSA) and the National Comprehensive Cancer Network (NCCN).[26,27]

Before the development and validation of these risk assessment rules, several institutions, including the National Cancer Institute (NCI), the European Organisation for Research and Treatment of Cancer (EORTC), and MDACC, used clinical criteria to identify low-risk patients for clinical trials.[8,28,29] These criteria included hemodynamic stability, outpatient status, expected duration of neutropenia ≤ 7 to 10 days, and absence of a significant medical comorbidity, such as abdominal pain, bleeding, mental status changes, suspected serious catheter-related infection, or a new pulmonary infiltrate. Some centers do not consider patients with hematologic malignancies to be low risk, regardless of other clinical characteristics.[8,30] These clinical criteria might be more practical to use in busy clinical practices, whereas the MASCC risk index is recommended when conducting clinical trials to ensure uniformity in patient selection and interpretation of study data.[31]

Most risk assessment rules have been derived and validated in adult oncology patients. One study from the Memorial Sloan-Kettering Cancer Center evaluated 161 pediatric oncology patients with 509 episodes of fever and neutropenia and determined that children who initially lack signs of sepsis, are afebrile, and have an absolute neutrophil count (ANC) of 100 or higher after 48 hours are at low risk of complications and could be selectively discharged on antimicrobial agents after a 48-hour period of hospitalization.[32] These and other criteria are now being used to identify low-risk pediatric oncology patients for outpatient antibiotic therapy from the onset of a febrile episode.[33]

Epidemiology of Infection

The epidemiology of infection in neutropenic patients undergoes periodic change and is often subject to geographic and institutional factors. Nevertheless, certain general trends are consistently observed. Approximately half the number of patients with fever and neutropenia will have episodes of "unexplained fever," that is, a clinical course consistent with infection but with no clinical microbiologic or serologic documentation of infection.[9] Approximately 20 to 30% will have "clinically documented infections," that is, a clinical site such as cellulitis or pneumonia, but negative cultures. Only 25 to 30% will have a "microbiologically documented infection," that is, positive cultures from a normally sterile site, such as blood or urine (Figure 1). A very small proportion of patients, generally less than 5%, will have noninfectious causes of fever, such as tumor fever or drug fever.

Among patients with documented infections, the most common sites are the bloodstream, urinary tract, respiratory tract, skin and skin structure, and gastrointestinal tract.[9] Approximately 50% of microbiologically documented infections are caused by gram-positive organisms, predominantly *Staphylococcus* species, various streptococci, and *Enterococcus* species (Table 3).[34,35] If only bloodstream infections are considered, the proportion of gram-positive infections is even higher (70–75%).[36] Gram-negative organisms cause 20 to 25% of microbiologically documented infections, and a similar number are polymicrobial.[37] Anaerobes are isolated very infrequently. Fungal and viral infections occur much later in the course of a neutropenic episode, and some viral infections are seasonal (eg, community respiratory viruses). These infections are dealt with in Viral Infections (Chapter 17) and Fungal Infections (Chapter 18). The frequency of infection in low-risk patients is approximately 20 to 30%. The spectrum is different from that seen in high-risk patients, with very few infections caused by viridans group streptococci, *Enterococcus* species, *P. aeruginosa*, *Stenotrophomonas maltophilia*, and other multidrug-resistant bacteria being seen in this patient subset.[38]

Risk-Based Therapy

There is uniform agreement that patients who are not classified to be low risk should receive hospital-based, parenteral, broad-spectrum empiric antibiotic therapy.[39] The various benefits of this approach and the many treatment options (including combination regimens and monotherapy) are discussed in detail in Chapter 19. In

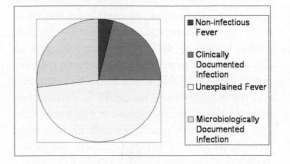

FIGURE 1 Nature of febrile episodes in neutropenic patients.

Table 3 Common Bacterial Pathogens in Neutropenic Patients	
Pathogen	*Comments*
Gram positive	
Coagulase-negative staphylococci	> 90% methicillin resistant
Staphylococcus aureus	> 50% MRSA
Viridans group streptococci	{223} 20% penicillin resistant
Enterococcus species	{223} 30% VRE
Bacillus species	10% vancomycin resistant
Streptococcus pyogenes	
Streptococcus pneumoniae	~ 20% penicillin resistant
Steptococcus groups B, C, G	Penicillin/vancomycin tolerant
Corynebacterium species	
Stomatococcus mucilaginosus	Frequently causes meningitis
Gram negative	
Enterobacteriaceae	ESBL producers
Pseudomonas aeruginosa	Multidrug-resistant strains
Pseudomonas (nonaeruginosa) species	
Stenotrophomonas maltophilia	Multidrug-resistant strains
Acinetobacter species	

ESBL = Extended spectrum beta-lactarmase; MRSA = methicillin-resistant *Staphylococcus aureus*; VRE = vancomycin-resistant enterococci.

general, empiric therapy should take into consideration local epidemiology and susceptibility or resistance patterns. It is probably not advisable to have one standard regimen for use in such patients since this hastens the development of resistance.[40] Using various options based on patient type and the nature and site of infection (termed antibiotic heterogeneity) is probably a better approach, although there are no randomized trials comparing these two approaches. The remainder of this discussion focuses on the various options available to treat low-risk, febrile neutropenic patients.

Antibiotic Therapy in Low-Risk Patients

The various treatment options for low-risk febrile neutropenic patients are listed in Tables 4 and 5. Each option is discussed separately with appropriate background information.

Hospital-Based Oral Antibiotic Therapy

Despite the development of reasonably accurate risk prediction rules, the availability of oral antimicrobial agents (eg, the fluoroquinolones)

Table 4 Treatment Options for Low-Risk Febrile Neutropenic Patients
Hospital-based oral antibiotic therapy
Initial parenteral therapy in hospital, followed by early discharge on outpatient parenteral or oral antibiotics, when stable
Outpatient parenteral, sequential (intravenous → oral), or oral antibiotic therapy for the entire febrile episode

with a broad spectrum of activity, including potent gram-negative activity, and the emergence of home health care agencies, many clinicians and investigators did not feel comfortable with the concept of oral outpatient antibiotic therapy for low-risk febrile neutropenic patients. Consequently, they chose to evaluate oral therapy in hospitalized low-risk patients, making the assumption that the hospital was the safest place to treat such patients. Two large prospective randomized trials compared oral antibiotics with standard parenteral regimens in hospitalized low-risk patients. The International Antimicrobial Therapy Cooperative Group of EORTC compared intravenous ceftriaxone plus amikacin with oral ciprofloxacin plus amoxicillin-clavulanate and found these two regimens to be equivalent (84% vs 86% success rate). The frequency of adverse events, including death (related or unrelated to infection), was also found to be similar for both regimens.[28]

Table 5 Common Therapeutic Regimens in Low-Risk Febrile Neutropenic Patients
Parenteral regimens
Aztreonam + clindamycin
Ciprofloxacin + clindamycin
Ceftriaxone + amikacin
Ceftazidime or cefepime
Oral regimens
Ciprofloxacin + clindamycin
Ciprofloxacin + amoxicillin-clavulanate
Gatifloxacin or moxifloxacin*
Ofloxacin, levofloxacin†

*Only pilot data are available. No randomized studies yet. (Gatifloxacin not available in U.S.)
†Not recommended as monotherapy.

Investigators from the NCI and allied institutions compared oral ciprofloxacin plus amoxicillin-clavulanate with intravenous ceftazidime monotherapy.[29] Although both regimens were again found to be equivalent (success rates of 71% and 67%, respectively), the response rates achieved with both regimens were lower than expected. Also, there was a high rate of intolerance of the oral regimen (16%) in comparison with the intravenous regimen (1%). Nevertheless, there were no deaths in either regimen, and more than 90% of patients were afebrile by day 5 of therapy.

The success of oral antibiotic regimens demonstrated in these and other smaller trials may have significant implications for the management of neutropenic patients with fever, particularly in countries with limited resources.[41] In the United States and other nations with similar reimbursement and legal systems, hospital-based oral antibiotic therapy will probably not enjoy widespread use. In reality, most low-risk patients who are able to tolerate oral therapy can probably be discharged from the hospital and treated as outpatients. A small number may need to be hospitalized for reasons not related to their febrile episode or might live alone and be unable to adequately care for themselves. Such patients might benefit from hospital-based oral therapy.

Early Discharge on Parenteral or Oral Antibiotics

Another approach in low-risk febrile neutropenic patients is initial treatment in hospital, followed by early discharge (after approximately 48 hours of hospitalization) on oral or parenteral antibiotics. Several trials have evaluated this approach. Shortly after developing their risk prediction rule, Talcott and colleagues conducted a pilot study to test the feasibility of this approach.[25] Low-risk patients who had evidence of a significant source of infection, including an infiltrate on a chest radiograph or bacterial growth from initial blood cultures, and those who were 65 years or older were excluded to reduce the risk to patients further. All patients received "standard" parenteral regimens for 48 hours in a hospital and were then discharged on the same regimen for home antibiotic therapy. The regimens included ceftazidime as monotherapy or mezlocillin + gentamicin as a combination regimen.

The results of this trial were disappointing. Of the 30 patients treated on this trial, 9 (30%) required readmission to the hospital. Four of these had medical complications (hypotension, renal failure, persistent fever, development of new infections, including mucormycosis), and five required changes to their antibiotic regimen after discharge. It was notable that 75% of serious complications occurred in patients with > 7 days of neutropenia. These results brought into question Talcott and colleagues' criteria for the identification of low-risk patients, particularly the inclusion of patients with leukemia with the potential to develop prolonged neutropenia.

Better results were achieved by investigators from the United Kingdom, who modified Talcott and colleagues' criteria for patient selection (excluding patients with documented infections and only enrolling patients with solid tumors or lymphomas and an anticipated duration of neutropenia of 7 days of less).[42] Early discharge on oral ciprofloxacin and amoxicillin-clavulanate was associated with a much lower readmission rate (7.6%), the regimen was well tolerated, and there were no deaths associated with this approach.[43]

In a similar study, children presenting with fever and neutropenia at six hospitals in Santiago, Chile, were randomly assigned to receive ambulatory antibiotic treatment after 24 to 36 hours of hospital-based therapy if categorized to be low risk.[33] Initial parenteral therapy consisted of intravenous teicoplanin and ceftriaxone followed by oral cefuroxine on early discharge. Seventy-four (95%) of 78 patients treated in this manner had a positive response. Three recovered completely after therapeutic modifications. One developed fulminant infection owing to *P. aeruginosa* and died within 96 hours. Although the results of this trial are encouraging, they do highlight the fact that, occasionally, fulminant infections do occur even in patients considered to be low risk. Notably, neither regimens used in this study (intravenous or oral) had adequate antipseudomonal coverage.

Ambulatory Management of the Entire Febrile Episode

A significant proportion of patients cared for at MDACC come from other countries, are uninsured, and/or pay out of pocket. In the early 1980s, approximately 50 patients with solid tumors who developed fever and neutropenia while receiving outpatient chemotherapy refused hospital admission and were treated with oral antibiotic regimens (primarily TMP-SMX + rifampin or clindamycin) without hospitalization. Most of these patients responded to oral, outpatient therapy, with no serious complications and no deaths (K. Rolston, 1988). This experience served as pilot data for formal trials of outpatient antibiotic treatment of febrile neutropenic patients at this institution. To date, three randomized trials have evaluated this approach at MDACC, and a few other trials have been conduced at other institutions as well. A recently published meta-analysis of these trials concluded that "oral antibiotics may be safely offered to neutropenic patients with fever who are at low risk for mortality.[44] The results of four trials (and outcomes of patients treated on MDACC

institutional outpatient pathways) conducted at MDACC are summarized in Table 6. These results demonstrate that both parenteral and oral regimens are safe and effective in low-risk febrile neutropenic patients. The response rates associated with these regimens ranged from 80 to 95%. Many patients not responding to the initial regimen responded to alternative outpatient regimens. Among the few patients requiring hospital admission, none had serious complications, none required care in the intensive care unit, and there were no infection-related deaths.[8,45–48]

All of the therapeutic approaches discussed above for the treatment of low-risk febrile neutropenic patients have now been accepted and endorsed by the IDSA and the NCCN as the standard of care.[26,27,39] Some important issues regarding risk-based therapy are discussed below.

Risk-Based Therapy: General Issues

The above discussion has summarized progress that has been made over several decades but particularly during the past 15 years. This progress is the result of several factors, including

– Increased understanding of the syndrome of "febrile neutropenia"

Technological advances in vascular access, infusion therapy, and outpatient monitoring

– The availability of potent oral antimicrobial agents that are easy to administer and are associated with very few adverse events
– Improved microbiologic techniques
– The current climate of the health care industry, which has provided much of the impetus for evaluating nontraditional methods and sites of care
– The "team approach" to management, which includes the patients and their families

It must be remembered that most of the strategies discussed above have been developed and tested in large tertiary care hospitals and/or comprehensive cancer centers, with a particular interest and substantial experience and expertise in caring for cancer patients. The ability to create and maintain an infrastructure that can handle these strategies and the complicated logistics involved in large numbers of patients is critical to the success of such programs, and may not be available at many institutions. This infrastructure includes health care providers from various disciplines—physicians, nurses, pharmacists, vascular access and infusion therapy teams, home health care personnel, and patients and their caregivers—all acting in concert to ensure that

Table 6 Results of Trials of Outpatient Antibiotic Therapy in Low-Risk Patients with Fever and Neutropenia Conducted at The University of Texas M. D. Anderson Cancer Center

Author	Reference	Type of Study and Patient Population	Antibiotic Regimen(s)	% Response to Initial Regimen
Rubenstein et al	8	Randomized trial of outpatient regimens, all adults, 83 episodes	IV, aztreonam 2 g q8h + clindamycin 600 mg q8h vs	95
			PO, ciprofloxacin 750 mg q8h + clindamycin 600 mg q8h	88
Rolston et al	45	Randomized trial of outpatient regimens in adults, 179 episodes	IV, aztreonam 2 g q8h + clindamycin 600 mg q8h vs	87
			PO, ciprofloxacin 500 mg q8h + amoxicillin-clavulante 500 mg q8h	90
Mullen et al	46	Randomized trial of outpatient regimens in pediatric patients, 75 episodes	IV, ceftazidime 50 mg/kg/q8h vs	94
			PO, ciprofloxacin 12.5 mg/kg/q12h	80
Rolston et al	47	Open-label trial of quinolone monotherapy in adults, 40 episodes	PO, gatifloxacin 400 mg once daily	95
Escalante et al	48	Patients enrolled on institutional outpatient pathway, 257 episodes	IV, ceftazidime 2 g q8h + clindamycin 600 mg q8h vs	80*
			PO, ciprofloxacin 500 mg q8h + amoxicillin-clavulanate 500 mg q8h	
Rolston, et al	49	Open label trial of quinolone monotherapy in adults, 21 episodes	PO/IV moxifloxacin, 400 mg once daily	95

IV = intravenous; PO = oral.
*Combined response rate for parenteral and oral regimens as individual response rates are not mentioned.

the best supportive care is delivered as efficiently and safely as possible (Table 7). At institutions in which such an infrastructure does not exist, standard hospital-based care should continue to be provided to low-risk patients.

Risk-Based Therapy: Advantages and Disadvantages

Standard, hospital-based antibiotic treatment of the febrile neutropenic patient has been extremely successful in reducing the mortality and improving the overall outcome of such patients, particularly high-risk patients prone to developing serious complications.[39] It is, however, not necessary or even beneficial in all febrile neutropenic patients. Risk-based therapy is associated with several benefits, which are outlined in Table 8.

Data presented at the Fourth Decennial International Conference on Nosocomial and Healthcare-Associated Infections (Atlanta, GA, 2002) documented that each year approximately

---

Table 7 Requirements for a Successful Program of Outpatient Antibiotic Therapy

Institutional infrastructure/support
Dedicated team of health care personnel
Local microbiologic data (epidemiology, resistance rates)
Selection of appropriate treatment regimens (based on local epidemiology/susceptibility patterns)
Adequate monitoring and follow-up of nonhospitalized patients
Motivated, compliant patients and family or other support personnel
Adequate transportation and communication facilities
24 h/d access to a management team (eg, hotline number) and proximity to the primary health care facility

---

Table 8 Pros and Cons of Risk-Based Therapy

Advantages
 Reduced rate of "health care–associated" infections
 Avoidance of iatrogenic hazards
 Lower costs/better resource use
 Improved quality of life (patients)
 Increased conveniences (family/other caregivers)
Disadvantages
 Needs dedicated team and infrastructure
 Potential for serious complications in an unsupervised setting
 Potential for noncompliance or issues with vascular access
 Potential for litigation (?)

---

2 million patients in the United States develop infections while hospitalized for other conditions.[51] These infections cost 4.6 billion dollars to treat and result in 88,000 deaths. Additionally, more than 70% of these infections are caused by organisms resistant to at least one antibiotic (many are multidrug resistant) generally used to treat such infections. Such infections are much more common in a hospital or long-term care setting than in a home care setting. Studies done in the 1960s demonstrated that patients acquired "hospital flora" 5 to 7 days after hospitalization. Consequently, early discharge from hospital to a home health care setting or total ambulatory care substantially reduces the frequency of resistant nosocomially acquired infections, particularly in patients who are otherwise at very low risk of developing serious complications or mortality.

As mentioned previously, many clinicians assumed that the hospital is the safest place to deliver health care and that care delivered at other sites must be shown to be "as safe as" hospital-based care. This assumption was brought into serious question in a disturbing report entitled "To Err Is Human," produced by the Institute of Medicine.[50] This report focuses on several studies conducted across the United States and points out that the frequency of adverse events in US hospitals ranges between 2.9 and 3.7% of hospitalizations. Furthermore, between 8.8 and 13.6% of these events lead to death, and over half of these adverse events are due to medical errors that are considered to be preventable. When extrapolated to the 37 million annual admissions to US hospitals, these studies imply that between 44,000 and 98,000 patients die each year as a result of medical errors. Although medical errors (preventable or otherwise) occur in all health care settings, this report also points out that four of five such events occur in the hospital. These data strongly suggest that the hospital may not be the safest place to deliver health care. The low complication and death rates associated with outpatient therapy seem to support the findings of this important report. Governmental and nongovernmental organizations responsible for developing policies for the delivery of health care need to take these outcomes into consideration.

Several studies have demonstrated the positive economic benefits of early discharge and/or outpatient antibiotic therapy compared with hospital-based therapy.[8,25,33,47] Studies have also documented significant improvements in the quality of life of patients receiving risk-based therapy (particularly outpatient therapy) and increased convenience for their families or other caregivers as well.[8,25,44] This aspect does not receive much mention in today's "outcomes" and financially focused health care environment. It is, however, an extremely important consideration

in the overall care of the cancer patient and should not be ignored.

There are some potential disadvantages of risk-based (particularly oral, outpatient) therapy. Low risk does not mean "no risk," and the potential for developing serious complications, such as septic shock, severe bleeding, or seizures, in a relatively unsupervised environment does exist. Careful patient selection and close monitoring of patients generally prevent but do not eliminate the occurrence of such events or enable one to manage them promptly should they occur. The potential for litigation might be a bit higher since hospital-based mishaps appear to be better accepted than those that occur outside the hospital. Additionally, some patients, particularly those on oral therapy, might not be fully compliant. Maintaining adequate vascular access can also occasionally become a problem that might be difficult to deal with immediately in an ambulatory or home care setting. Finally, patients might develop a false sense of security regarding their febrile episode since it did not require hospitalization and may ignore early signs or symptoms of progressive infection or other complications. It is imperative that patients be given very specific, written instructions regarding follow-up and monitoring. Some institutions might be unwilling or unable to invest in the infrastructure necessary to maintain these standards and requirements.

Future Considerations

Current risk assessment strategies are reasonably accurate. However, misclassification of patients does occur. This can have serious consequences when high-risk patients are misclassified as low risk. Further refinements in risk prediction rules that increase sensitivity and specificity and reduce the misclassification rate might increase the safety of this approach and perhaps make it applicable even in institutions that lack the infrastructure required currently.

The duration of neutropenia following the development of an episode of neutropenic fever is a critical determinant of low risk. Our ability to predict the duration of neutropenia has improved, but studies are under way to develop prediction rules that are more accurate. The impact of hematopoietic growth factors (granulocyte colony-stimulating factor and granulocyte-macrophage colony-stimulating factor) on the risk and duration of neutropenia also needs to be fully investigated.

As the epidemiology of infection and susceptibility or resistance patterns change (eg, the startling increase in community-acquired methicillin-resistant *Staphylococcus aureus*) and as newer antimicrobial agents become available, newer treatment and preventive regimens and strategies will need to be developed.

Summary

The use of empiric antibiotic therapy in neutropenic patients with fever has been a very successful strategy that has dramatically improved the overall survival of such patients. The recent recognition of distinct risk groups among febrile neutropenic patients has led to the development of newer treatment strategies for low-risk patients instead of the uniform strategy of hospital-based parenteral antibiotic therapy for all patients. Newer options include hospital-based oral antibiotic therapy for a selected group of patients, early discharge on parenteral or oral regimens after initial hospitalization, and ambulatory (clinic, office, home) management of the entire febrile episode. The advantages of risk-based therapy currently far outweigh the potential disadvantages. Newer challenges and newer opportunities will undoubtedly arise as future changes occur in the treatment of cancer patients.

REFERENCES

1. Bodey GP, Buckley M, Sathe YS, Freireich EJ. Quantitative relationships between circulating leukocytes and infection in patients with acute leukemia. Ann Intern Med 1966;64:328–40.
2. Hughes WT, Armstrong D, Bodey GP, et al. Guidelines for the use of antimicrobial agents in neutropenic patients with unexplained fever. J Infect Dis 1990;161:381–96.
3. Hughes WT, Armstrong D, Bodey GP, et al. 1997 Guidelines for the use of antimicrobial agents in neutropenic patients with fever. Clin Infect Dis 1997;25:551–73.
4. Rolston K. New trends in patient management: risk-based therapy for febrile patients with neutropenia. Clin Infect Dis 1999;29:515–21.
5. Talcott JA, Finberg R, Mayer RJ, Goldman L. The medical course of cancer patients with fever and neutropenia. Clinical identification of a low-risk subgroup at presentation. Arch Intern Med 1988;148:2561–8.
6. Talcott JA, Siegel RD, Finberg R, Goldman L. Risk assessment in cancer patients with fever and neutropenia: a prospective, two-center validation of a prediction rule. J Clin Oncol 1992;10:316–22.
7. Klastersky J, Paesmans M, Rubenstein E, et al. The MASCC risk index: a multinational scoring system to predict low-risk febrile neutropenic cancer patients. J Clin Oncol 2000;18:3038–51.
8. Rubenstein EB, Rolston K, Benjamin RS, et al. Outpatient treatment of febrile episodes in low risk neutropenic cancer patients. Cancer 1993;71:3640–6.
9. Rolston KVI, Bodey GP. Infections in patients with cancer. In: Holland JF, Frei E, editors. Cancer medicine. 6th ed. Hamilton (ON): BC Decker; 2003. p. 2633–58.
10. Bodey GP. Antibiotics in patients with neutropenia. Arch Intern Med 1984;144:1845–51.
11. Hersh EM, Bodey GP, Nies BA, Freireich EJ. Causes of death in acute leukemia. A ten year study of 414 patients from 1954-1963. JAMA 1965;193:105–9.
12. Feld R, Bodey GP, Rodriguez V, Luna M. Causes of death in patients with malignant lymphoma. Am J Med Sci 1974;268:97–106.
13. Frei E III, Levin RH, Bodey GP, et al. The nature and control of infections in patients with acute leukemia. Cancer Res 1965;25:1511–5.
14. Bodey GP, Middleman E, Umsawasdi T, Rodriguez V. Intravenous gentamicin therapy for infections in patients with cancer. J Infect Dis 1971 124 Suppl:S174–9.

15. Bodey GP, Rodriguez V, Luce JK. Carbenicillin therapy of gram-negative bacilli infections. Am J Med Sci 1969;257:408–14.
16. Bodey GP, Feld R, Burgess MA. Beta-lactam antibiotics alone or in combination with gentamicin for therapy of gram-negative bacillary infections in neutropenic patients. Am J Med Sci 1976;71:179–86.
17. Valdivieso M, Bodey GP, Burgess MA, Rodriguez V. Therapy of infections in neutropenic patients—results with gentamicin in combination with cephalothin or chloramphenicol. Med Pediatr Oncol 1976;2:99–108.
18. Bodey GP, Valdivieso M, Feld R, et al. Carbenicillin plus cephalothin or cefazolin as therapy for infections. Am J Med Sci 1977;273:309–18.
19. Bodey GP, Ketchel SJ, Rodriguez V. Carbenicillin plus cefamandole in the treatment of infections in patients with cancer. J Infect Dis 1978;137 Suppl:S139–43.
20. Keating MJ, Bodey GP, Valdivieso M, Rodriguez V. A randomized comparative trial of three aminoglycosides—comparison of continuous infusions of gentamicin, amikacin and sisomicin combined with carbenicillin in the treatment of infections in neutropenic patients with malignancies. Medicine 1979;58:159–70.
21. Bodey GP, Grose WE, Keating MJ. Use of trimethoprim-sulfamethoxazole for treatment of infections in patients with cancer. Rev Infect Dis 1982;4:579–81.
22. Haron E, Rolston KVI, Cunningham C, et al. Oral ciprofloxacin therapy for infections in cancer patients. J Antimicrob Chemother 1989;24:955–62.
23. Rolston KVI, Haron E, Cunningham C, Bodey GP. Intravenous ciprofloxacin for infections in cancer patients. Am J Med 1989;87 Suppl 5A:261S–5S.
24. Malik IA, Khan WA, Karim M, et al. Feasibility of outpatient management of fever in cancer-patients with low-risk neutropenia: Results of a prospective randomized trial. Am J Med 1995;98:224–31.
25. Talcott JA, Whalen A, Clark J, et al. Home antibiotic therapy for low risk cancer patients with fever and neutropenia: a pilot study of 30 patients based on a validated prediction rule. J Clin Oncol 1994;12:107–14.
26. Rolston KVI. The Infectious Diseases Society of America 2002 guidelines for the use of antimicrobial agents in patients with cancer and neutropenia: salient features and comments. Clin Infect Dis 2004;39 (Suppl 1):S44–8.
27. Freifeld AG, Brown AE, Elting L, NCCN Fever and Neutropenia Panel Members. Fever and neutropenia NCCN clinical practice guidelines in oncology. J Natl Compr Cancer Netw 2004;2:390–432.
28. Freifeld A, Marchigiani D, Walsh T, et al. A double-blind comparison of empirical oral and intravenous antibiotic therapy for low-risk febrile patients with neutropenia during cancer chemotherapy. N Engl J Med 1999;341:305–11.
29. Kern WV, Cometta A, DeBock R, et al. Oral versus intravenous empirical antimicrobial therapy for fever in patients with granulocytopenia who are receiving cancer chemotherapy. N Engl J Med 1999;341:312–8.
30. Rolston KVI. Prediction of neutropenia. Int J Antimicrob Agents 2000;16:113–5.
31. Feld R, Paesmans M, Freifeld AG, et al. Methodology for clinical trials involving patients with cancer who have febrile neutropenia: updated guidelines of the immunocompromised host society/multinational association for supportive care in cancer, with emphasis on outpatient studies. Clin Infect Dis 2002;35:1463–8.
32. Lucas KG, Brown AE, Armstrong D, et al. The identification of febrile, neutropenic children with neoplastic disease at low risk for bacteremia and complications of sepsis. Cancer 1996;77:791–8.
33. Santolaya ME, Alvarez AM, Aviles CL, et al. Early hospital discharge followed by outpatient management versus continued hospitalization of children with cancer, fever, and neutropenia at low risk for invasive bacterial infection. J Clin Oncol 2004;22:3784–9.
34. Yadegarynia D, Tarrand J, Raad I, Rolston K. Current spectrum of bacterial infections in cancer patients. Clin Infect Dis 2003;37:1144–5.

35. Wisplinghoff H, Seifert H, Wenzel RP, Edmond MB. Current trends in the epidemiology of nosocomial bloodstream infections in patients with hematological malignancies and solid neoplasms in hospitals in the United States. Clin Infect Dis 2003;36:1103–10.
36. Zinner SH. Changing epidemiology of infections in patients with neutropenia and cancer: emphasis on gram-positive and resistant bacteria. Clin Infect Dis 1999;29:490–4.
37. Adachi JA, Yadegarynia D, Rolston K. Spectrum of polymicrobial bacterial infection in patients with cancer, 1975–2002 [abstract]. American Society for Microbiology. Polymicrobial Diseases; 2003 Oct 19–23; Lake Tahoe, NV.
38. Kamana M, Escalante E, Mullen C, et al. Spectrum of bacterial infection in low-risk patients with fever and neutropenia [abstract]. 41st Annual Meeting of the Infectious Diseases Society of America; 2003 Oct 9–12; San Diego, CA.
39. Hughes WT, Armstrong D, Bodey GP, et al. 2002 guidelines for the use of antimicrobial agents in neutropenic patients with cancer. Clin Infect Dis 2002;34:730–51.
40. Rolston KVI. Challenges in the treatment of infections caused by gram-positive and gram-negative bacteria in neutropenic cancer patients. Clin Infect Dis 2005; 40(Suppl 4):S246–52.
41. Safdar A, Torres I, Cleeland C, Rolston K. Antimicrobial availability for oncology patients with advanced malignancy in Latin America: WHO/PAHO Medical Oncology Survey Report 2000-2002 [abstract]. The 14th European Congress of Clinical Microbiology and Infectious Diseases (ECCMID); Clinical Microbiology and Infection [oral presentation]. 2004 May 1–4; Prague, Czech Republic.
42. Innes HE, Smith DB, O'Reilly SM, et al. Oral antibiotics with early hospital discharge compared with in-patient intravenous antibiotics for low-risk febrile neutropenia in patients with cancer: a prospective randomized controlled single centre study. Br J Cancer 2003;89:43–9.
43. Rolston KVI. Oral antibiotic administration and early hospital discharge is a safe and effective alternative for treatment of low-risk neutropenic fever. Cancer Treat Rev 2003;29:551–4.
44. Vidal L, Paul M, Ben dor I, et al. Oral versus intravenous antibiotic treatment for febrile neutropenia in cancer patients: a systematic review and meta-analysis of randomized trials. J Antimicrob Chemother 2004;54:29–37.
45. Rolston KR, Rubenstein EB, Elting L, et al. Ambulatory management of febrile episodes in low-risk neutropenic patients [abstract]. 35th Interscience Conference on Antimicrobial Agents and Chemotherapy; 1995 Sept 17–20; San Francisco, CA.
46. Mullen CA, Petropoulos D, Roberts WM, et al. Outpatient treatment of febrile neutropenia in low risk pediatric cancer patients. Cancer 1999;86:126–34.
47. Rolston, Frisbee-Hume S, Manzullo E, et al. Once daily, oral, outpatient, quinolone monotherapy for low-risk, febrile neutropenic patients (FNP) [abstract]. 41st Annual Meeting of the Infectious Diseases Society of America; 2003 Oct 9–12; San Diego, CA.
48. Escalante CP, Weiser MA, Manzullo E, et al. Outcomes of treatment pathways in outpatient treatment of low risk febrile neutropenic cancer patients. Support Care Cancer 2004;12:657–62.
49. Rolston KVI, Manzullo EF, Elting LS, et al. Once daily, oral, outpatient quinolone monotherapy for low-risk cancer patients with fever and neutropenia. Cancer 2006;106:2489–94.
50. Gerberding JL. Preventing antimicrobial-resistance healthcare infections: beyond 2000. Clinical updates in infectious diseases. National Foundation for Infectious Diseases, Bethesda, MD. Vol V, Issue 2. August 2000.
51. Kohn L, Corrigan J, Donaldson M, editors, Committee on Quality of Health Care in America. To err is human: building a safer health system. Institute of Medicine report. Washington (DC): National Academy Press; 2000.

Bacterial Infectious Disease Issues: Catheter-Related Infections

Issam I. Raad, MD

Hend Hanna, MD, MPH

Dennis G. Maki, MD

The management and care of patients with cancer and critically ill patients have, no doubt, been revolutionized by the technologic advances in medical devices, including the availability of central venous catheters (CVCs). Patients with cancer often need these devices, particularly long-term Silastic catheters, to receive chemotherapy, antibiotics, blood products, and intravenous hyperalimentation. CVCs are vascular access devices that are made of soft flexible biocompatible polymers. After being inserted into a large vein of the vascular system, such as the subclavian or internal jugular vein, they are advanced until the tip of the catheter is resting in the superior vena cava.

Prior to the advent of central catheterization, patients with cancer received intravenous chemotherapeutic agents, including vesicant agents through small peripheral venous catheters. This process was often complicated by extravasation and thrombosis of peripheral veins, which often interfered with anticancer chemotherapy administration. CVCs allowed for the safe and extended use of anticancer agents and the appropriate use of total parenteral nutrition, such as for patients with short bowel syndrome, as well as blood products and intravenous therapeutic agents. Similarly, patients requiring hemodialysis are in need of CVC as either an interim access during maturation of a graft or fistula or as a permanent vascular access for patients who may have failing arteriovenous fistulae or shunts. Therefore, it is no surprise that health care organizations purchase millions of intravascular catheters annually.

CVCs are not, however, without risk, and their use puts patients at potential risk of infections, both local and systemic. Infectious complications associated with the use of CVCs include local site infection, catheter-related bloodstream infection (CRBSI), septic thrombophlebitis, and other metastatic infections, such as endocarditis, osteomyelitis, endophthalmitis, and occasional organ abscesses.

Epidemiology and Impact

Hospitals and clinics in the United States purchase annually more than 150 million intravascular devices to administer various intravenous medications, blood products, and parenteral nutrition fluids; to provide hemodialysis; and to monitor hemodynamic status.[1] Although the majority of these devices are peripheral catheters, still, each year, over 5 million CVCs are inserted. More than 200,000 health care–related bloodstream infections (BSIs) occur in the United States per year, where most of these infections are associated with the use of CVCs, with the rates of BSIs being higher among patients with CVCs than among those without these devices.[1] The incidence of CRBSIs depends on the type, material, and site of the catheter; how often the catheter is manipulated and accessed; the patient's underlying disease; the acuity of the illness; and the type of drug injected through the catheter. According to recommendations from the Centers for Disease Control and Prevention (CDC) and the Joint Commission on Accreditation of Healthcare Organizations (JCAHO), the rates of CRBSIs are better expressed as the number of BSIs per 1,000 catheter-days.[2,3] Reporting the rate of infection in such a manner accounts for the BSI over time, adjusting the risk of the infection to the number of days the catheter is in use, and, hence, is at risk of infection.

Since the 1970s, the CDC established a National Nosocomial Infection Surveillance (NNIS) system to collect data on hospital-acquired infections and their etiology and incidence, including BSIs associated with the use of CVCs. The NNIS data are collected from more than 300 participating hospitals in the United States, and the rates of CRBSI vary, depending on the size of the hospital, the particular service or unit at the hospital, the type of intensive care unit (ICU), and the type of catheter used.[3] According to NNIS data, from January 1995 through June 2003, the rates of CRBSI, ranged from 2.9 (in cardiothoracic ICU) to 10.6 (in a neonatal nursery for infants weighing $\leq 1,000$ g) BSIs per 1,000 catheter-days.[3]

The problem of CVC-associated infections creates an undeniable substantial burden, both to the patient, in terms of morbidity and mortality, and to the economy, in terms of cost of care. It is estimated that about 80,000 CRBSIs occur annually in ICUs in the United States.[4] The magnitude of this problem among these patients was estimated with the aid of a computer model that was based on American Hospital Association data. According to this model, Mermel estimated that an average of 5.3 CRBSIs per 1,000 catheter-days occur annually, which accounts for around 80,000 CRBSIs per year and approximately 2,400 to 20,000 deaths owing to CRBSIs.[5,6] The model also helped estimate that the annual management of these ICU patients with CRBSIs could cost from $296 million to $2.3 billion.[5,6] In addition to these critically ill and hospitalized patients, many patients are discharged with central venous lines in place while they continue their intravenous therapy on an outpatient basis. This patient group is also at risk of acquiring catheter-related infections. When the entire health care–related services (not only ICUs) are considered, it is estimated that about 250,000 cases of CRBSIs occur annually. These infections are associated with prolongation of hospital stay and attributable mortality that range from 12 to 25%, with a cost of care that is estimated to be from $34,508 to $56,000 per each episode of infection, and the yearly cost of managing and caring for patients with CRBSIs was found to range from $296 million to $2.3 billion.[1,3,6–10]

Pathophysiology and Risk Factors

A thorough understanding of the pathogenesis of catheter-related infections is an important prerequisite for accurate diagnosis, effective prevention, and successful management of these infections. Catheter-related infections are often caused by organisms that are resistant to many available antimicrobial agents and hence are difficult to treat. For the CVC to be inserted into the blood vessel, the integrity of the skin has to be broken to allow for the introduction and advancement of the device into the vascular system. Indwelling catheters connect a sterile environment, namely, the interior of the blood vessel, with the nonsterile skin surface at the catheter insertion site, allowing organisms, commonly colonizing the skin surface, to migrate along the catheter surface.

Sources of Infections and Microbiologic Characteristics

Once the catheter is inserted, it becomes at risk of being colonized with microorganisms that eventually may lead to catheter-related infections. Microorganisms that are able to colonize the surface of the catheter may originate from different sources through any of the following mechanisms (Figure 1):

Organisms colonizing the skin are able to invade the percutaneous tract around the catheter insertion site, colonizing the catheter surface, particularly the extraluminal. This can occur either at the time of catheter insertion, especially when maximal sterile barrier precautions are not being thoroughly practiced, as during an emergent insertion of a catheter, or afterward during the catheter dwelling.[11] Short-term, nontunneled, and noncuffed catheters are often colonized through this route, whereby organisms migrate along the external surface of the catheter, colonizing the catheter tip, which may eventually lead to BSI.[12–14]

As the catheter hub is accessed and manipulated during the catheter use (such as for blood drawing, intermittent medication administration, or flushing), microorganisms from the hands of health care personnel may contaminate the catheter hub and lumen, causing intraluminal colonization of the catheter. This route of contamination is more relevant for long-term tunneled silicone catheters, such as Hickman or Broviac, or long-term totally implantable catheters, such as ports, where the lumen of the hub or the bell of the port, as they are accessed for use, becomes the major source of colonization, which may eventually lead to infection.[15,16]

Catheters can also be colonized during the flow of contaminated infusate, as shown by reports of several epidemics of infusion-related bacteremia; however, this mechanism for catheter-related pathogenesis is not very common.[17,18] Whereas *Staphylococcus* and *Candida* are responsible for most other CRBSIs, infusion-related sepsis is often caused by gram-negative bacilli, with *Enterobacter*, *Pseudomonas*, *Citrobacter*, and *Serratia* species being the most commonly seen. In addition, it is known that parenteral nutrition solutions and lipid emulsions promote the growth of certain bacteria and fungi, such as *Candida parapsilosis* and *Malassezia furfur*.[19–21]

Microorganisms originating from an infected site elsewhere in the body, such as pneumonia, urinary tract infection, or gastrointestinal infection, may be carried through the blood, hematogenously, and ultimately adhere to the surface of the inserted catheter, colonizing it (Figure 1). Although hematogenous seeding of the CVC has been suggested,[22,23] its role in catheter colonization and subsequent infection is rarely demonstrated. A study that used electron microscopy in studying catheters that were removed from patients with gram-negative or fungal BSI failed to show evidence of catheter seeding with organisms responsible for the bacteremias that preceded the removal of the catheters.[24]

Because the skin of the patient and the hands of health care workers are the main sources of the contamination of the indwelling catheter, the organisms that are commonly found to be colonizing the CVCs are the ones found to be skin colonizers. Staphylococci, particularly coagulase-negative staphylococci (such as *Staphylococcus epidermidis*) and *Staphylococcus aureus*, are the leading causes of CRBSIs.[14,25–28] Catheters may also become colonized by gram-negative bacilli, mostly nonenteric, originating from the hospital's environment, such as *Pseudomonas*, *Stenotrophomonas*, and *Acinetobacter* species.[25–31] In addition, the hands of medical personnel could also be colonized by yeast, such as *Candida albicans* and *C. parapsilosis*,[32] which are also known to be associated with the use of total parenteral nutrition and infusions containing glucose and, hence, could be responsible for CRBSIs.[24,25] Less commonly, gram-positive bacilli, such as *Corynebacterium* species, although rarely do they colonize the skin or the catheter hub, can sometimes cause catheter-related infections.[25–28,33,34]

Pathogenesis and Biofilm Formation

The interaction between microorganisms, the medical device itself, and the patient as a host results in the occurrence of catheter-related infections. Microorganisms are able to colonize the catheter because of their ability to attach themselves to the surface of the polymer and synthesize or produce a hydrated extracellular polymeric exopolysaccharide, creating a complex matrix in which they aggregate, forming a biofilm.[35] Virtually all indwelling CVCs become colonized by microorganisms that become embedded in the biofilm matrix, as was shown by scanning and transmission electron microscopy.[36] On catheter insertion, platelets, plasma, and a variety of host tissue proteins, such as fibronectin, fibrinogen, fibrin, collagen, thrombospondin, and laminin, act as mediators of bacterial adherence to the surface of the catheter.[36–41] Different organisms adhere differently to these host tissue proteins; for example, coagulase-negative staphylococci, as well as *C. albicans*, have the ability to adhere to fibrin,[42] whereas *S. aureus* is able to strongly adhere to fibronectin and laminin.[38,39]

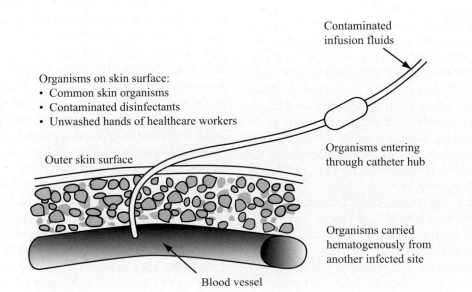

FIGURE 1 Pathogenesis of catheter-related bloodstream infections and possible sources of infection.

The presence of platelets, even in small numbers, was found to greatly enhance the adherence of both streptococci and staphylococci to the fibrin matrix.[37] Raad and colleagues showed that although the biofilm formation on CVC surfaces was universal, its extent and its location depended on the duration of catheterization.[14] Raad and colleagues found that biofilm formation was greater on the external surface of the catheter for short-term catheters that remained in place > 10 days, whereas long-term catheters, with at least 30 days of dwell time, had more biofilm formation on the inner lumen of the catheter. Furthermore, the type of fluid being infused through the CVC may also influence microbial growth; for example, gram-negative organisms, such as *Pseudomonas aeruginosa*, *Klebsiella*, *Enterobacter*, *Pantoea*, and *Serratia* species, grew well in intravenous fluids, whereas gram-positive *S. epidermidis* and *S. aureus* did not.[1,43,44]

During the process of catheter colonization, staphylococci produce significant amounts of extracellular slime, in which these organisms are embedded and covered (Figure 2). This slimy material acts to protect the microorganisms against the host defense mechanisms and antimicrobial agents.[45] Microorganisms within the biofilm are known to behave differently from free-floating or suspended organisms, also known as planktonic organisms. Anwar and colleagues showed that organisms in biofilm are more resistant to antimicrobial treatment, where the cell count of *P. aeruginosa* in biofilm was reduced by about two logs, after treatment with levels of piperacillin plus tobramycin that far exceeded its minimum inhibitory concentration, whereas the same dosage of the antibiotics produced more than an eight-log decrease in the planktonic *P. aeruginosa*.[46] Their study suggested that young biofilm cells of mucoid *P. aeruginosa* could be effectively eradicated with the combination of piperacillin and tobramycin, whereas old biofilm cells were very resistant to these antibiotics and eradication of old biofilm cells was not achievable.

Risk Factors

The risk of catheter-related infections varies according to several factors (Table 1). Prolonged

Table 1 Types of Central Venous Catheters and Rates of Infection Associated with Each

Type of Vascular Device	Exit Site	Length (cm)	Rate of CRBSI per 1,000 Catheter-Days, Pooled Mean (95% CI)*	Estimated Cost of Insertion at MDACC ($)
Peripheral venous catheter	Peripheral veins of forearm or hand	< 7	0.6 (0.3–1.2)	< 1,000
Arterial catheter	Major artery: radial, femoral, axillary, dorsalis, pedis, or brachial	< 7 cm	2.9 (1.8–4.5)	≈ 1,300
Nontunneled CVC	Subclavian, internal jugular, or femoral	25–40	2.3 (2.0–2.4)	≈ 1,300
Pulmonary artery catheter	Swan-Ganz: subclavian, internal jugular, or femoral	Up to 110	5.5 (3.2–12.4)	≈ 1,300
Peripherally inserted central catheter	Basilic, cephalic, or brachial veins into superior vena cava	40–60	0.4 (0.2–0.7)	≈ 1,000
Tunneled venous catheter	Surgically implanted into subclavian, internal jugular, or femoral vein	> 8	1.2 (1.0–1.3)	≈ 6,500
Hemodialysis catheter Noncuffed		> 8		
	Surgically implanted into subclavian, internal jugular, or femoral vein		2.8 (2.3–3.1)	
Cuffed			1.1 (0.7–1.6)	≈ 6,500
Port, implanted	Surgically implanted subclavian or internal jugular	> 8	0.2 (0.1–0.2)	≈ 7,000

Adapted from Crnich CJ and Maki DG[103] and Schinabeck MK and Ghannoum MA.[104]

CI = confidence interval; CRBSI = catheter-related bloodstream infection; CVC = central venous catheter; MDACC = M. D. Anderson Cancer Center.

*Based on 206 published prospective studies.

duration of catheterization has been found, by several studies, to be a major risk factor for infections associated with the use of venous and arterial vascular catheters.[13,47–50] Because catheter colonization involves microbial adherence to the catheter surface, the polymer material that catheters are made of may also play an important role in promoting thrombogenesis and adherence of organisms. Linder and colleagues demonstrated that catheters made of polyurethane and flexible silicone were less thrombogenic than catheters made of polyvinyl chloride and hence

are associated with fewer infections.[51] Furthermore, staphylococci and fungi adhere better to polyvinyl chloride surfaces than to Teflon.[52,53] Numerous studies, mostly nonrandomized and retrospective in nature, suggest that the risk of infection seems to be higher among catheters with triple lumens than among those with a single lumen.[54–59] Triple-lumen catheters are more likely to be manipulated and accessed more often than single-lumen ones. However, triple-lumen catheters tend to be used more frequently in sicker patients than single-lumen catheters. Prospective randomized trials that included sicker patients at higher risk of developing catheter-related infections failed to show a difference in infection rates, based on the number of lumens.[60–62] The location of the catheter could also influence the risk of catheter-related infection. CVCs have been found to be associated with higher infection rates than arterial catheters or short peripheral catheters. In a review by Hampton and Sherertz, in which they evaluated 30 prospective studies, the daily risk of infection per day of catheterization was found to be 1.3% per day for peripheral venous catheters, 1.9% per day for peripheral arterial catheters, and 3.3% per day for CVCs.[63]

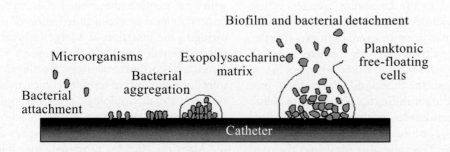

FIGURE 2 Biofilm formation on catheter surface.

Catheters inserted into internal jugular veins were found to be at higher risk of infection than those inserted into subclavian veins, as in the study by Mermel and colleagues, in wihch catheters inserted into an internal jugular vein were associated with a higher risk of infection (relative risk 4.3, $p < .01$).[13] On the other hand, Senagore and colleagues did not find such an association, and they concluded that using a standard, sterile-insertion technique and a catheter maintenance protocol yielded a low risk of insertion and infectious complications at either the internal jugular or the subclavian site.[64] In a prospective randomized trial, patients in the ICU were randomized to receive either femoral or subclavian CVCs. Femoral catheterization was found to be associated with a higher incidence rate of overall infectious complications (20% vs %, $p < .001$) and thrombotic complications (22% vs 2%, $p < .001$). Femoral catheterization was the only factor associated with infectious complications in that study (hazard ratio 4.8, 95% confidence interval [CI] 1.96–11.93, $p < .001$).[65]

The type of dressing applied to the catheter insertion site has also been studied in terms of its impact on the risk of catheter-related infection. In one prospective randomized study, patients with CVCs for 3 or more days were prospectively randomized to receive an occlusive transparent or gauze dressing and the incidences of insertion-site colonization, local catheter-related infection, and CRBSI were compared.[66] After 48 hours, transparent dressings were associated with significantly increased rates of insertion-site colonization ($p \le .009$), local catheter-related infection ($p = .002$), and CRBSI ($p = .015$) in patients with long-term CVCs.[66] Occlusive dressing tends to create a warm, moist atmosphere at the insertion site, where microbial growth would be favorable, and, hence, the risk of catheter colonization and infection. Craven and colleagues confirmed these findings in a study in which, by multiple logistic regression analysis, catheter-tip colonization was found to be associated with the summer season (odds ratio 3.0, 95% CI 1.4–6.2) and transparent polyurethane dressings (odds ratio 1.8, 95% CI 1.1–3.2).[67] In addition, Hoffmann and colleagues performed a meta-analysis of all studies published in the English literature, including abstracts, letters, and reports that examined the infection risks associated with transparent compared with gauze dressings for use on central and peripheral venous catheters.[68] The results demonstrated a significantly increased risk of catheter-tip colonization with the use of transparent compared with gauze dressings when used with either central or peripheral catheters. An increased risk of CRBSI associated with the use of transparent compared with gauze dressings was also suggested by the findings of the study, although not confirmed.

Other risk factors that have been observed by investigators include multiple catheter manipulations, the inexperience of some inserters, and violations of aseptic techniques.[63]

Types of Intravascular Devices

A number of different CVCs are available with varying insertion techniques, sizes, and catheter materials. CVCs may be single-lumen or multilumen, double or triple (Table 1).

Nontunneled Percutaneously Inserted Catheters

These may be made of silicone or polyurethane materials, and they are inserted into either the peripheral venous system (subclavian vein) or in the neck (jugular vein), through a percutaneous stick, where the catheter tip is advanced until it rests into the superior vena cava. These catheters can be placed in outpatient nonsurgical settings and can be exchanged over a guidewire, at the onset of catheter-related infection. An example of these catheters is the Hohn catheter.

Tunneled Catheters

These catheters are tunneled surgically under the skin for several inches to the cannulated vein. In 1973, Dr. John W. Broviac designed an intravenous catheter that provided access for patients who required prolonged parenteral alimentation.[69]

Dr. Robert Hickman altered Broviac's prototype in 1979 for patients with leukemia who required chemotherapy.[70] His modified catheter had a larger lumen that facilitated the drawing of blood and the infusion of chemotherapeutic agents, blood, and intravenous fluids. After the catheter is inserted, its distal tip is advanced to just above the right atrium. The proximal end exits via a subcutaneous tunnel from the lower anterior chest wall. A felt Dacron cuff is used to anchor the catheter in place subcutaneously, where eventually it becomes enmeshed with fibrous tissues, allowing the catheter to become securely anchored and, hence, rendering it more stable and less likely to be pulled out accidentally. The cuff also creates a tissue interface that acts as a barrier against the migration of microorganisms. A further modification of these tunneled catheters led to the Groshong catheter, which, unlike the traditional open-ended catheters, has a rounded closed tip, with an adjacent two-slit valve that remains closed unless the catheter is in use. Because the valve remains closed when not in use, it literally seals the fluid inside the catheter, preventing it from getting in contact with the patient's blood and hence reducing the risk of intraluminal blood clotting or infusion of air when the catheter is not in use. The valve also eliminates the need for routine clamping of the catheter.

Implantable Ports

Ports are totally implantable vascular access devices that are made of plastic or titanium material and are inserted completely beneath the skin, connected to the catheter tube.[71] Ports are surgically placed as either a central subclavian port, which is placed in the subcutaneous pocket of the upper chest wall, or as a peripheral port, which is placed in the antecubital fossa of the arm. Ports are available as single- or double-lumen catheters, with or without the Groshong valve.

Peripherally Inserted Central Venous Catheters

The use of peripherally inserted central venous catheters (PICCs) has gained acceptance as a method for long-term venous access. A PICC is a catheter made of silicone or polyurethane material and may or may not have the Groshong valve. It is inserted peripherally at or above the antecubital space into the cephalic, basilic, medial cephalic, or medial basilic vein, after which it is advanced into the superior vena cava above the right atrium. These catheters are usually placed in a nonsurgical outpatient setting, under local anesthesia, and may be placed by a skilled and trained infusion therapy nurse. At The University of Texas M. D. Anderson Cancer Center, PICCs were shown to be safe, with a mean duration of dwell of 87 days, and associated with a low rate of infection and a low cost of insertion.[72]

Manifestations and Definitions

Local Catheter Infection

Local signs and symptoms of infection may indicate catheter-related infections. Local infection may exist alone, in the absence of BSI, at the catheter exit site, tunnel, or port pocket. It may be manifested by clinical signs of inflammation and/or infection, such as erythema, swelling, pain, or purulent exudates in the immediate proximity of the catheter insertion site. However, this local inflammatory reaction may be absent, especially in immunocompromised neutropenic patients who lack those inflammatory cells. Clinical evidence of local infection at an exit site, tunnel, or port pocket may suggest that the catheter is the source of a BSI. However, this is not always the case. For example, PICC lines may be associated with local aseptic catheter-site inflammation, secondary to local mechanical irritation of the vein owing to the insertion of a large catheter in the relatively small cephalic or basilic veins.[72] Therefore, it is important to define local catheter-related infections, not only in terms of clinical manifestations but also microbiologic evidence implicating the catheter as the source of the infection. The guidelines from the Infectious Diseases Society of America (IDSA) proposed the following definitions of local catheter infections[73]:

- *Exit-site infection.* Clinically, it could be manifested by erythema, induration, and/or tenderness within 2 cm of the catheter exit site. These manifestations may be associated with other signs and symptoms of infection, such as fever or purulent discharge oozing from the exit site, in the presence or absence of concomitant BSI. Microbiologically, a culture of the exudate or purulent discharge at the catheter exit site may yield a microorganism, with or without concomitant BSI.
- *Pocket infection.* Purulent exudates in the subcutaneous pocket of a totally implantable intravascular device, containing the reservoir of the port, often in the presence of local tenderness, erythema, and/or induration over the pocket, usually indicate pocket infection. Necrosis of the overlying skin or spontaneous rupture and drainage may also occur, with or without concomitant BSI.
- *Tunnel infection.* Clinical signs and symptoms of infection, such as tenderness, erythema, and induration more than 2 cm from the catheter exit site or along the subcutaneous tract of tunneled catheters, such as Broviac or Hickman catheters, in the presence or absence of BSI.[74,75]

Systemic Catheter Infection

Probable CRBSI consists of bacteremia or fungemia in a patient with a CVC and one or more positive cultures of blood samples (preferably from the peripheral vein) in the presence of signs and symptoms of infection, such as fever, chills, and hypotension, and no apparent source for the BSI, other than the catheter. In addition, documented or definite CRBSI requires further confirmation through one of the following:

1. Positive result of semiquantitative (≥ 15 colony-forming units [CFU]/catheter segment) or quantitative ($\geq 10^2$ CFU/catheter segment) catheter culture, whereby the culture yields the same organism (identical species and antibiogram) isolated from the peripheral blood sample
2. Quantitative cultures of blood samples, drawn simultaneously through the CVC and via a peripheral vein, with a ratio of $\geq 5:1$ (CVC vs peripheral)
3. Differential time to positivity, whereby the culture of blood drawn through the CVC becomes positive and yields the same microorganism, at least 2 hours before the culture of blood drawn simultaneously from a peripheral vein

Most CRBSIs are uncomplicated. However, some virulent microorganisms, such as *S. aureus*, *C. albicans*, and *P. aeruginosa*, may be associated with complicated deep-seated infections, including catheter-related septic thrombosis, whereby the CRBSI is associated with an infected thrombus.[76–78] Septic thrombosis is characterized by occasional swelling above the site of the thrombotic vein and persistent BSI in spite of appropriate antimicrobial therapy and the removal of the catheter. CRBSI may also become disseminated to another anatomic site, causing deep-seated infections, such as endocarditis, osteomyelitis, organ abscesses, and retinitis.[76,77] Signs and symptoms of such deep-seated infections depend on the site affected by the infection.

Diagnosis

Catheter-related infections are often misdiagnosed, resulting in wasteful removal of catheters and unnecessary administration of antimicrobial agents. Clinical manifestations of sepsis, with no obvious cause other than the presence of a CVC, usually lead to suspecting CRBSI; however, signs and symptoms of sepsis, such as fever, chills, or hypotension, are nonspecific and may be caused by a myriad of etiologic factors, other than an infected catheter. Catheter-related BSIs are occasionally associated with local signs and symptoms at the catheter exit site, such as erythema, tenderness, warmth, and lymphangitis. However, these clinical manifestations of local inflammatory signs have poor correlation with catheter-related infections because although their presence has a highly predictive value for infection, their absence has a very poor negative value.[79] Safdar and Maki recently evaluated short-term catheters for CRBSIs, using insertion-site inflammation as the diagnostic indicator.[80] Their study yielded sensitivity $\leq 3\%$, indicating that insertion-site inflammation is not predictive of CRBSI. Therefore, signs of local infection should be evaluated carefully when diagnosing CRBSI, and it is important to use microbiologic techniques to identify catheter colonization or infection.

Furthermore, as infections in immunocompromised patients increase in number and complexity, laboratory diagnosis of catheter-related infections in this patient population presents the following challenges: (1) clinical presentation of the infection is often muted or delayed and nonpecific, (2) frequent blood drawing for cultures should be done judiciously, especially for pancytopenic patients, and (3) careful consideration should be given to the decision of catheter removal and insertion of new catheter at a different site, especially in thrombocytopenic patients with poor vascular access, and, hence, the critical need for diagnosing catheter-related infections before removing the catheter.

It is important to accurately diagnose CRBSIs based not only on clinical findings but also on reliable microbiologic results. In the following section, we review two major diagnostic approaches based on whether the diagnosis of the catheter-related infection is achieved while the suspected catheter is still in place or after the catheter is removal.

Diagnostic Techniques without Catheter Removal

Ideally, diagnosing CRBSIs needs to be done before removing the catheter, to avoid the needless removal of catheters not responsible for the infection. A good diagnostic method would accomplish this early diagnosis without compromising its accuracy.

Cultures of Blood Drawn Percutaneously or through the Catheter

According to this method, patients with suspected CRBSI have two sets of blood cultures done, in which at least one set is drawn through a peripheral venipuncture. Single blood cultures, quantitative or qualitative, according to which blood is drawn only through the CVC, have low positive predictive values as they do not compare the results of these cultures with the results of peripheral blood cultures and hence are not reliable. In a study of hospitalized hematology-oncology patients, culture of blood drawn through either the central catheter or peripheral vein showed excellent negative predictive value (99% and 98%, respectively), whereas culture of blood drawn through an indwelling CVC had low positive predictive value (63%), apparently less than from a peripheral venipuncture (73%).[81] The study suggested that the use of a catheter to obtain blood for culture may be an acceptable method for ruling out BSIs. However, a positive culture of blood drawn through a catheter would require further clinical interpretation.

Partial Simultaneous Quantitative Cultures of Peripheral and Catheter Blood Samples

This technique relies on the results of quantitative cultures of simultaneously drawn blood samples, in which one is drawn via a peripheral vein and the other through the CVC. Studies suggest that when quantitative cultures of blood drawn through the CVC yield at least fivefold the colony count (CFU) of blood drawn simultaneously through the peripheral vein, this finding is predictive of CRBSI.[82–85] However, studies differ in regard to the exact cutoff point for this ratio, where it was found to be between $\geq 4:1$[84] and 10:1.[85] Nonetheless, this test was shown to be 94% sensitive and 100% specific.[84] Recently, Franklin and colleagues suggested a method for diagnosing CRBSI when a peripheral culture is unavailable.[86] They defined CRBSI as a fivefold or greater difference in CFU/mL between the two catheter lumens in pediatric patients, with sensitivity, specificity, a positive predictive value, and a likelihood ratio of 62%, 93%, 92%, and 9.2, respectively.

Endoluminal Brush Technique

This technique involves introducing a nylon brush through the catheter hub and into the lumen, brushing its interior wall. The brush is withdrawn and immediately placed into a buffered container that is sonicated, and the solution is cultured onto a blood agar plate, with counts > 100 CFU/mL considered positive. This technique was found to have sensitivity of 95% and specificity of 84% by Kite and colleagues, who found the technique to be easy, with no adverse effects,[87] contrary to another study in which it was associated with arrhythmia and embolization.[79] The method is also criticized for being impractical and unreliable and may result in subsequent bacteremia owing to the brush's entry into the lumen, which may introduce microorganisms into the catheter or may lodge them further. The brush may even disrupt any existent biofilm, releasing organisms into the bloodstream.

Skin and Hub Cultures

There is no standard method for culturing the skin around the insertion site and no agreed on criteria for positive quantitative cultures. Basically, the area chosen for culture, either the skin at the catheter exit site or the interior of the catheter hub, is swabbed and then the swab is streaked onto an agar plate to be cultured semiquantitatively.[88] Skin culturing, as a diagnostic test for CRBSI, was found to have ≤ 61% sensitivity, 72% specificity, and 62% positive predictive value.[89] However, when infection is suspected, sensitivity rises to 75%, specificity to > 90%, and the positive predictive value to 100%.[90] Skin culturing at the catheter exit site has been studied, with varied results, which may be attributed to surface contamination.

Cultures of the hub alone still have a low sensitivity of 61%.[89] However, when both the skin and the hub were cultured together, sensitivity improved to 86%, although specificity and the positive predictive value remain low. An alternative combination of superficial cultures is taking a culture of the hub and subcutaneous catheter segment, which slightly boosts the specificity to 82% and the positive predictive value to 78%, whereas the sensitivity remains at 84%.

Differential Time to Positivity

In the presence of CRBSI, blood drawn through the catheter hub would turn positive much more quickly than blood drawn through a peripheral vein. This method relies on the availability of an automated blood culture system that records the time at which a culture turns positive. Recent studies suggest that if the difference in the time it takes for the culture of blood drawn through the CVC and a culture drawn simultaneously from a peripheral vein to become positive is at least 120 minutes, then it is highly suggestive of a CRBSI.[91,92]

This has been shown in a study involving 235 neutropenic patients with febrile neutropenia, in which the differential time to positivity had 82% sensitivity and 88% specificity in diagnosing CRBSI.[93] Although the differential time to positivity could not be verified as a diagnostic method among intensive care patients,[94] recently, Raad and colleagues found it to be diagnostic in 191 cases of BSI.[95] The patient pool was subanalyzed for short-term catheterization (< 30 days) and long-term catheterization (≥ 30 days), and the study reported 81% sensitivity with 92% specificity and 93% sensitivity with 75% specificity, respectively. Furthermore, receiver operating characteristic curve analysis showed that the ≥ 120-minute cutoff optimizes sensitivity and specificity. However, interpretation of this diagnostic method could become complicated when antibiotics are given intraluminally at the time of drawing blood cultures through the catheter, in which case, colonized catheters may become falsely negative and sensitivity can be compromised.[95] The technique is also limited in that it does not evaluate cases with negative peripheral blood cultures in the presence of positive central blood cultures, a combination indicative of possible CRBSI catheter colonization.

Diagnostic Techniques Requiring Catheter Removal

Quantitative Catheter Culture

According to this technique, the removed catheter tip is immersed in broth, which is then cultured, and any growth is considered significant.[96] This method lacks sufficient quantitation, and at the present time, its use is limited owing to its low specificity and high frequency of contamination.

Semiquantitative Roll Plate Catheter Culture

After the catheter is removed, its intravascular tip is cut and rolled four times, back and forth, on an agar plate. The microorganisms are retrieved only from the external surface of the catheter, and after being cultured on the agar plate, the colonies are counted. Catheters are considered to be colonized if at least 15 CFU/catheter-tip segment are grown.[97] If the same microorganism is isolated from both the catheter tip, at the quantitative level that defines colonization, and the bloodstream, the diagnosis of CRBSI is established. This method is limited in that it retrieves free-floating (nonbiofilm) microorganisms only from the external surface of the catheter and therefore misses culturing organisms colonizing the intraluminal surface of the catheter, such as with long-term catheters.

Quantitative Catheter Culture

Several methods, such as centrifugation, vortexing, and sonication, are used to retrieve microorganisms from both the external and the internal surfaces of the catheter. The catheter is said to be colonized when at least 1,000 CFU/catheter-tip segment are retrieved. If the same organism colonizing the catheter tip also grows from a peripheral blood culture, in the presence of signs and symptoms of infection and in the absence of other sources for the infection, the diagnosis of CRBSI is established.[98] A recent meta-analysis showed that quantitative catheter culture was a more sensitive diagnostic method than the semiquantitative catheter culture method.[99]

Stain and Microscopy Rapid Diagnostic Techniques

Staining of the removed catheter segments and subsequent microscopy have been suggested as a simple and immediate diagnostic method. Cooper and Hopkins explored the use of direct Gram staining of the catheters for diagnosis.[100] After being cultured, the catheters were immediately stained, and extraluminal organisms were identified under the oil immersion objective. The cutoff value of one organism per 20 oil immersion fields indicates that the catheter is colonized. Cooper and Hopkins reported 100% sensitivity, 97% specificity, a positive predictive value of 84%, and a negative predictive value of 100%, but the results were not reproduced in another study.[101] In a similar technique, acridine orange staining has been used for diagnosis, in which fluorescence is indicative of positivity.[102] In addition to achieving a sensitivity of 84% and a specificity of 99%, acridine orange staining perhaps may be more easily performed than Gram staining, although microscopic techniques as a whole are labor intensive.

Preventive Strategies

Because CRBSIs are associated with serious morbidity and mortality and because of the difficulty and complexity of its diagnosis and its management, particularly in immunocompromised patients, major effort should be exerted in trying to prevent these infections (Table 2).[103,104]

Successful preventive strategies should aim at carefully controlling all factors that could lead to the colonization of the CVC by microorganisms. Evidence-based guidelines and preventive measures have been published to provide health care practitioners with background information and specific recommendations aimed at reducing the incidence of intravascular CRBSIs (Table 2). The published guidelines represent the recommendations of the Healthcare Infection Control Practices Advisory Committee (HICPAC) and other professional organizations, including the IDSA, Society for Healthcare Epidemiology of America (SHEA), and American Society of Critical Care Anesthesiologists (ASCCA), among others.[105] In the next section, we review major

Table 2	Strategies for the Prevention of Catheter-Related Bloodstream Infection
Strategies during CVC insertion
Maximal sterile barrier precautions[11]
Using an expert infusion therapy team[108,109]
Use of antiseptics at CVC exit site[27,127]
Device-related strategies
Select the least number of lumens needed[54–59]
Antimicrobial coating of CVC[117–122]
CVCs with silver cuff[128–130]
Tunneled CVC[26]
Implantable port[70]
Strategies during CVC dwell period
Avoid needless manipulation of CVC[63]
Use of nonocclusive dressing[66]
Topical antiseptics or antibiotics[27,126,127]
Anticoagulant and antimicrobial flush solution[123–125]
CVC = central venous catheter.

strategies for prevention of catheter-related infections.

Specialized Infusion Therapy Team

Well-organized programs that help health care workers provide, monitor, and evaluate care given to patients and that facilitate patient education and continuous education to physicians, fellows, and medical students are critical for a successful preventive strategy. Risk of infection is known to decline following standardization of aseptic care.[106–108] When medical centers used the services of experienced infusion therapy teams, for the insertion and maintenance of catheters, including dressing changes, catheter-associated infection rates decreased five- to eightfold.[109,110] At M. D. Anderson Cancer Center, where an experienced infusion therapy team is available, the infection rates of nontunneled, noncuffed, Silastic catheters were found to be 0.13 infections per 100 catheter-days, comparable to the low rates of the tunneled Hickman catheters.[72]

Maximal Sterile Barriers

The insertion of some types of catheters, such as implantable ports and tunneled catheters, requires involved surgical procedures; therefore, these types are usually inserted in the operating room. On the other hand, nontunneled catheters and PICCs are usually inserted elsewhere; hence, their insertion may not be subject to the same stringently sterile atmosphere of an operating room. However, a prospective randomized clinical trial succeeded in proving that the use of maximal sterile barrier precautions during the insertion of nontunneled long-term silicone catheters in the subclavian vein and PICCs resulted in a significant reduction in infections associated with these devices.[11] The devices had a mean dwell time of 70 days, and the rate of CRBSI dropped from

0.5/1,000 catheter-days to 0.02/1,000 catheter-days. Maximal sterile barrier precautions involved wearing a sterile gown, gloves, and a cap and using a large drape, during the insertion of catheters, similar to the drapes used in operating rooms.

Tunneling

These catheters are buried under the skin in a subcutaneous tunnel and a felt Dacron cuff is used to anchor the catheter subcutaneously in place. The cuff eventually becomes enmeshed with fibrous tissues, allowing the catheter to become securely anchored, and it also creates a tissue interface that acts as a barrier against the migration of microorganisms. A prospective randomized study found that CRBSI occurred more frequently and more rapidly in the nontunneled than in the tunneled group, in which catheters were tunneled into the internal jugular vein ($p = .02$, log rank test), with an infection rate of 1.9 per 100 catheter-days in the nontunneled group and 0.7 per 100 catheter-days in the tunneled group.[26] The study demonstrated that subcutaneous tunneling of internal jugular CVCs reduced by at least fourfold the risk of CRBSI in critically ill patients. However, another prospective randomized study of tunneled silicone catheters inserted in the subclavian vein in immunocompromised patients failed to demonstrate the efficacy of subcutaneous tunneling, in which the infection rate among the patients with tunneled catheters was 0.22/100 catheter-days and among the nontunneled catheters was 0.20/100 catheter-days.[111] Nonetheless, the main issue here is whether tunneling is cost effective since the surgery required for the procedure may cost an additional $2,500, and other, more cost-effective alternatives could be as efficacious in reducing the rate of catheter-related infections.

Antimicrobial Coating of Catheters

A newer approach to prevention of CRBSI is the coating of the catheter surface with antimicrobial agents to prevent the initial biofilm formation. This method allows sustained and slow release of the antimicrobial agents, with virtually undetectable serum levels. First-generation catheters impregnated with chlorhexidine and silver sulfadiazine (CHX-SSD) lowered the rate of CRBSIs from 7.6 per 1,000 catheter-days to 1.6 per 1,000 catheter-days ($p = .03$).[12] A cost-effectiveness analysis concluded that using these catheters in patients at high risk of catheter-related infections reduces the incidence of CRBSI and death and provides significant saving in costs estimated to be $196 per catheter inserted.[112] These first-generation CHX-SSD catheters were coated only on the external surface, and the catheters in the study were cultured by the roll plate technique, retrieving microorganisms only from the outer surface of the catheter. This may explain the failure

of three subsequent studies to reproduce the results of Maki and colleagues,[12] especially when both catheter surfaces were cultured by sonication.[113–115] Mermel estimated the effect of this device on CRBSI and showed that the CHX-SSD catheter reduces the risk of infection in short-term catheterization but is not effective for catheters placed for an average of 3 weeks, probably owing to the reduction in its antimicrobial activity over time.[4] Mermel also attributed the lack of long-term efficacy to the fact that only the outer surface of the catheter was impregnated; therefore, there was no protection against luminal colonization. A second-generation CHX-SSD catheters impregnated on both surfaces is now available. However, the zones of inhibition produced by this second-generation catheters were shown to decrease to less than 10 mm in only 3 days.[116] This second-generation CHX-SSD catheters were tested in a prospective randomized study in patients from 14 ICUs of university hospitals in France. Although the use of the CHX-SSD catheters decreased the catheter colonization significantly from 11/1,000 catheter-days (13%) to 3.6/1,000 catheter-days (3.7%), $p = .01$, they failed to decrease the rate of CRBSI.[117]

Raad and colleagues and Darouiche and colleagues developed commercially available polyurethane catheters impregnated intraluminally and extraluminally with minocycline and rifampin, and they were more efficacious when compared, in prospective, randomized, double-blind, controlled studies, with uncoated catheters and with catheters impregnated with CHX-SSD.[118,119] In comparison with first-generation CHX-SSD catheters, the catheters impregnated with minocycline and rifampin were 12-fold less likely to be associated with CRBSI (relative risk 0.1, 95% CI 0.0–0.6) and 3-fold less likely to be colonized. In a review for the CDC, Wenzel and Edmond estimated that 4,745 to 9,450 lives would be saved with the use of catheters impregnated with minocycline and rifampin according to varying attributable mortality rate estimates.[120] The use of minocycline and rifampin catheters, in medical and surgical intensive care units, was associated with a significant decrease in nosocomial BSIs, including vancomycin-resistant enterococci (VRE) bacteremia, catheter-related infections, and lengths of hospital and ICU stay.[121] The risk of developing resistnace after prolonged use of these antimicrobially coated catheters was investigated in a retrospective evaluation of 4-year clinical use of minocycline and rifampin–impregnated catheters in bone marrow transplantation patients. The study found no evidence of development of staphylococcal resistance to the antibiotics coating the catheters.[122] A recent prospective randomized study evaluated long-term nontunneled silicone CVCs impregnated with minocycline and rifampin and found them to also be significantly more efficacious than control uncoated catheters in reducing CRBSIs in cancer patients.[123]

Anticoagulant and Antimicrobial Lock Solutions

This technique is particularly useful for long-term catheters, in which hub contamination is the main source of catheter colonization and, ultimately, CRBSI.[15] According to this method, the catheter lumen is flushed and then filled with 2 to 3 mL of anticoagulant in combination with an antimicrobial agent. Heparin as an anticoagulant, alone or in combination with vancomycin, has been used to lock the catheter lumen. Heparin interferes with the thrombin sheath formation on the catheter surface and was shown, alone and combined with vancomycin, to reduce catheter-tip colonization.[124,125] However, using vancomycin prophylactically should be avoided to minimize the risk of emergence of vancomycin-resistant organisms. Also, there is a potential for a superinfection with gram-negative bacilli and *Candida* because vancomycin has an antimicrobial spectrum limited to gram-positive bacteria. Raad and colleagues prevented recurrent CRBSI by using a lock solution of 3 mg minocycline and 30 mg ethylenediaminetetraacetic (EDTA) as prophylaxis in three patients.[126] The combination of minocycline and EDTA showed synergistic activity against methicillin-resistant staphylococci, gram-negative bacilli, and *C. albicans* and a cidal effect on bacteria in the biofilm.[127–129]

Topical Antiseptics or Antibiotics

Topical antibiotics, such as polymixin-neomycin-bacitracin, significantly decrease the risk of catheter-related infections but may increase the risk of fungal colonization and infection.[130] Maki and colleagues compared the effectiveness of 70% alcohol, 10% povidone-iodine, and 2% chlorhexidine gluconate and the rate of CRBSI was almost fourfold lower in the chlorhexidine arm than in the other two arms.[27] A meta-analysis evaluated the efficacy of skin disinfection with chlorhexidine gluconate compared with povidone-iodine solution in preventing CRBSI and found that chlorhexidine gluconate reduced the risk of CRBSI by 49%.[131]

Silver Cuff

A collagen cuff impregnated with silver and connected to the catheter is placed subcutaneously to act as a mechanical barrier against migrating organisms. The device failed to reduce the rates of CRBSI when used with long-term catheters,[132,133] possibly owing to the biodegradable nature of the collagen since it degrades within a week. However, in critically ill patients with short-term catheters, it was shown to reduce infections.[134] The silver cuff is rarely used in the United States.

Management

The management of CRBSI involves making decisions related to (1) whether the CVC should be removed, (2) the type of antimicrobial therapy, based on the type of organism and its resistance pattern, and (3) the duration of antimicrobial therapy. Such decisions depend on two factors. The first is the type of organism and whether this organism has a high tendency to be associated with deep-seated complications and a high rate of relapse. Second is whether there are clinical manifestations suggestive of a complicated source, such as the persistence of fever and bacteremia or fungemia after catheter removal and initiation of appropriate antimicrobial therapy.

Given that the CVC is an identifiable, removable source of the infection, there is a tendency to consider all patients with a CVC and an associated BSI to represent a catheter-related infection. Indiscriminate removal of the CVC in this situation would result in an unnecessary, wasteful, and highly expensive practice. Therefore, it is important for the clinician to carefully determine whether the catheter is the source of the BSI prior to making management decisions as to the need for CVC removal and the duration of antimicrobial therapy. Hence, simultaneous blood cultures need to be drawn at the time of presentation of the patient, and the internist should make determinations on the diagnosis of CRBSI based on the differential time to positivity[91–95] or the differential quantitative blood cultures,[82–86] as outlined in the Diagnosis section of this chapter (Figure 3). Because management decisions as to whether the CVC should be removed and the duration and type of therapy depend on the type of organism causing CRBSI, we discuss such organisms below.

Coagulase-Negative *Staphylococcus*

These organisms are considered to be the most likely cause of CRBSI.[26–28] Since these organisms, which include *S. epidermidis*, are usually skin organisms, they are often the cause of contaminated blood cultures. Therefore, a single blood culture drawn from the CVC and subsequently found to be positive for coagulase-negative staphylococci could reflect hub or intraluminal colonization of the catheter rather than a true bacteremia.[135] To ascertain the diagnosis of bacteremia, at least two blood cultures, including a positive blood culture drawn from a peripheral vein, are necessary. When quantitative blood cultures are used, a colony count of > 15 CFU of coagulase-negative staphylococci isolated from a blood sample drawn through the CVC is highly suggestive of true bacteremia.[136]

Although catheter removal was once thought to be necessary, most (almost 80%) of the CRBSI caused by coagulase-negative staphylococci could

be treated with glycopeptide antibiotics, such as vancomycin, without catheter removal. However, if the CVC is not removed, there is a 20% chance that the bacteremia will recur.[137] This is compared with only a 3% risk of recurrence if the catheter is removed ($p < .005$). Because this organism is associated with low virulence and a low tendency for metastatic deep-seated infections (such as endocarditis), the IDSA guidelines on management suggested that the catheter associated with CRBSI caused by coagulase-negative staphylococci could be salvaged through antibiotic lock therapy.[73] Hence, if the CVC is to be retained, a longer duration of therapy consisting of 10 to 14 days (rather than 5 to 7 days if the CVC is removed) is to be considered with antibiotic lock therapy. Alternatives to vancomycin are available for the treatment of coagulase-negative staphylococcal bacteremia. These include dalbavancin, which is a long-acting glycopeptide given once per week. Dalbavancin was recently shown to be superior to vancomycin in the treatment of CRBSI caused by coagulase-negative staphylococci and *S. aureus*.[138] The high frequency of infections caused by methicillin-resistant *S. aureus*, including coagulase-negative staphylococci, has been the driving force for the wide use of glycopeptide antibiotics, which, in turn, has resulted in higher rates of VRE. Other alternative antibiotics with an activity against VRE are also available. These include linezolid and daptomycin.[139,140]

S. aureus

The CVC is the leading source of *S. aureus* bacteremia in the cancer patient.[141] *S. aureus* is associated with a high rate of deep-seated metastatic infections, including endocarditis, particularly in the nonthrombocytopenic solid tumor patient. Deep-seated infections, including septic thrombosis and endocarditis, have been reported in 33 to 35% of non-neutropenic, nonthrombocytopenic patients with solid tumor.[76,141] The associated overall mortality was reported as 38%.[141] In contrast, thrombocytopenic and neutropenic patients with underlying hematologic malignancy and *S. aureus* bacteremia have a very low rate of metastatic infection (< 3%), with an overall mortality of 11%.[142] This difference could be attributed to several factors. First, nonthrombocytopenic cancer patients with a solid tumor have a high prevalence of cardiac valve lesions and nonbacterial thrombotic vegetations of the valve associated with thromboembolism.[143] This serves as a substrate for a higher rate of infective bacterial endocarditis in the setting of *S. aureus* bacteremia.

Second, an important factor in the development of infective endocarditis is the formation of platelet bacterial thrombi on the surface of the valve.[144,145] *S. aureus* cells have been shown to form

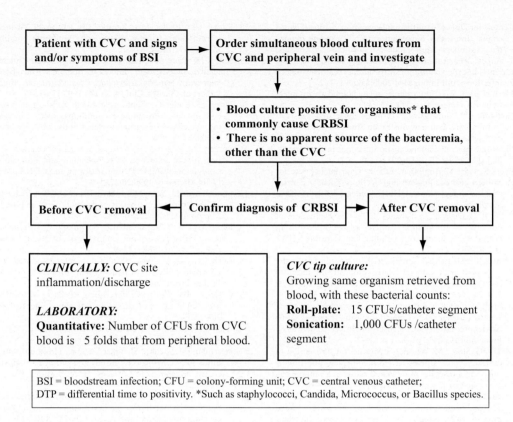

```
┌──────────────────────────┐     ┌──────────────────────────────────┐
│ Patient with CVC and signs│────▶│ Order simultaneous blood cultures from│
│ and/or symptoms of BSI    │     │ CVC and peripheral vein and investigate│
└──────────────────────────┘     └──────────────────────────────────┘
```

• **Blood culture positive for organisms* that commonly cause CRBSI**
• **There is no apparent source of the bacteremia, other than the CVC**

Before CVC removal ◀── **Confirm diagnosis of CRBSI** ──▶ **After CVC removal**

CLINICALLY: CVC site inflammation/discharge

LABORATORY:
Quantitative: Number of CFUs from CVC blood is 5 folds that from peripheral blood.

CVC tip culture:
Growing same organism retrieved from blood, with these bacterial counts:
Roll-plate: 15 CFUs/catheter segment
Sonication: 1,000 CFUs /catheter segment

BSI = bloodstream infection; CFU = colony-forming unit; CVC = central venous catheter; DTP = differential time to positivity. *Such as staphylococci, Candida, Micrococcus, or Bacillus species.

FIGURE 3 Algorithm for the diagnosis of catheter-related bloodstream infection (CRBSI). BSI = bloodstream infection; CFU = colony-forming unit; CVC = central venous catheter; DTP = differential time to positivity. *Such as staphylococci, *Candida*, *Micrococcus*, or *Bacillus* species.

platelet aggregations through fibronectin-binding proteins, leading to platelet bacterial valvular thrombi and vegetation formation.[145] Hence, the thrombocytopenia could be a protective factor against the formation of the platelet bacterial valvular thrombi.

Three observational prospective studies have demonstrated that removal of the CVC in *S. aureus* CRBSI (including the uncomplicated cases) has been associated with a more rapid response to therapy and a lower relapse rate.[146–148] In a subset of thrombocytopenic patients with hematologic malignancy and a surgically implantable catheter with no other available vascular access, consideration should be given to catheter salvage and antibiotic lock therapy.[73,126] This consists of filling the lumen of the catheter with 2 mL of an antibiotic combination, often mixed with an anticoagulant. Vancomycin in combination with heparin or minocycline and vancomycin in combination with EDTA are some of the options to be considered.[125–127] Combinations could be alcohol based, consisting of 25% ethanol solution.[149]

The type of antibiotics used should be based on the susceptibility of *S. aureus*. For methicillin-sensitive *S. aureus*, a semisynthetic antistaphylococcal penicillin or first-generation cephalosporin is the first choice.[73] For methicillin-resistant *S. aureus*, several options can be considered, including vancomycin, linezolid, daptomycin, or even

dalbavancin.[138–140] The duration of therapy should be based on the likelihood of deep-seated complications. For uncomplicated *S. aureus* CRBSI, a 10-day to 2-week course is acceptable if the CVC is removed.[73] Raad and colleagues showed in several studies including patients with underlying cancer that the persistence of fever and bacteremia for more than 72 hours after antibiotic initiation and catheter removal is highly suggestive of a complicated course associated with deep-seated infections, including septic thrombosis and endocarditis.[76,150] These findings were further supported by a large prospective observational study that included 720 consecutive adults with *S. aureus* bacteremia.[151] The strongest predictor of *S. aureus* bacteremia was the persistence of fever and/or bacteremia for more than 72 hours. In this subpopulation of *S. aureus* CRBSI with persisting fever and bacteremia, strong consideration should be given to transesophageal echocardiography to rule out endocarditis and the treatment duration should be expanded to at least 4 weeks.[73] In uncomplicated cases of *S. aureus* CRBSI, consideration should be given to the use of an oral antibiotic combination beyond 7 days of parenteral antibiotic treatment. Recent studies have suggested that a combination of quinolones plus rifampin active against *S. aureus* could be useful in patients who are allergic to β-lactam antibiotics, including those patients with staphylococcal CRBSI.[152]

Gram-Negative Bacilli

Gram-negative bacillary bacteremia usually emerges from a non–catheter-related source, such as nosocomial urinary tract infection, nosocomial pneumonia, or intra-abdominal infection. However, gram-negative bacillary CRBSI caused by organisms such as *Klebsiella pneumoniae*, *Enterobacter* species, *Pseudomonas* species, *Acinetobacter* species, and *Stenotrophomonas maltophilia* have been reported.[29,30,78] Elting and Bodey reported on 149 episodes of bacteremias caused by *S. maltophilia* and other non-*aeruginosa Pseudomonas* species in which the CVC was the most common source of the BSI.[30] Failure to remove the catheter in this cancer patient population was associated with a significantly higher rate of treatment failure and bacteremia recurrence. In another study involving cancer patients from Memorial Sloan-Kettering Cancer Center, catheter-related infections caused by *Pseudomonas* species were associated with a higher rate of treatment failure unless the catheter was removed.[78] A more recent study by Hanna and colleagues demonstrated that documented CRBSIs caused by gram-negative bacilli were associated with a high frequency of relapse if the CVC was retained, whereas CVC removal was associated with only a 1% risk of relapse ($p < .001$).[153] Therefore, if the gram-negative bacillary bacteremia is judged to be CRBSI, then it is prudent to remove the CVC in cancer patients and treat with a 1-week course of appropriate broad-spectrum anti-bacillary antibiotics (Figure 3).[73]

Candida Species

Catheter-related candidemia may be associated with serious complications, such as septic thrombosis and endocarditis.[154,155] In a multivariate analysis of nosocomial BSIs, *Candida* species were the only organisms independently predictive of a poor outcome.[156–170] Fourteen studies evaluated the impact of CVC removal on the outcome of candidemia. All five prospective studies have demonstrated that CVC removal was associated with improved outcome.[157–161] These included large studies in which multivariate analysis showed that catheter retention proved to be a significant independent risk factor for the persistence of candidemia and was associated with higher mortality.[157] Of the nine retrospective studies, eight have demonstrated an improved outcome with CVC removal.[162–169] In cancer patients, catheter removal improved outcome independent of persistent neutropenia and vascular catheter retention proved to be an independent risk factor for the persistence of candidemia.[158,162,169] Nucci and colleagues prospectively analyzed the risk factors for death among 145 patients with nosocomial candidemia.[158] Catheter retention was found to be an independent variable for increased risk of death in multivariate analysis independent of persistent neutropenia. In a retrospective study, Anaissie and colleagues reviewed 416 patients with cancer and underlying candidemia and showed that the catheter retention was associated with poor outcome, death, and persistence of the infection compared with the outcome of patients who underwent guidewire exchange or removal of the catheter ($p = .002$), independent of the severity of the illness and the persistence of the neutropenia.[162] In a recent retrospective study involving 404 cancer patients with candidemia and an indwelling CVC, Raad and colleagues determined by multivariate analysis that CVC retention for more than 72 hours is associated with a poor outcome (decreased response to antifungal agents, morbidity, and mortality) in patients with *Candida* CRBSI.[169] In that study, CVC removal did not have any impact on improving outcome in patients with non–catheter-related secondary candidemia. Therefore, in cancer patients, the CVC should be removed early within 72 hours in patients with suspected or documented catheter-related candidemia. According to the study by Raad and colleagues, patients with previous chemotherapy or high-dose steroids are more prone to have their candidemia emerging from a noncatheter source and, hence, may not benefit from the early CVC removal.[169]

Rex and colleagues demonstrated that fluconazole has comparable efficacy to amphotericin B in the treatment of candidemia (71% of the cases were considered to be catheter related), with a significantly better safety profile in favor of fluconazole.[171] Echinocandins (caspofungin and micafungin) were demonstrated through prospective randomized trials to be equivalent to amphotericin B or liposomal amphotericin B respectively in the treatment of candidemia with an improved safety profile. A recent multicenter study showed that anidulafungin (another echinocandins) is equivalent to and possibly superior to fluconazole in the treatment of invasive candidiasis. Therefore, in patients with catheter-related candidemia, fluconazole or echinocandins should be considered efficacious and safer alternatives to amphotericin B. In a center in which there are higher rates of fluconazole-resistant *Candida glabrata* and *Candida krusei*, echinocandins should serve as a better alternative to fluconazole.[173,174] The duration of therapy for uncomplicated catheter-related candidemia has been suggested to be 2 weeks from the last positive blood culture, according to the IDSA guidelines.[73]

REFERENCES

1. Maki DG, Mermel LA. Infections due to infusion therapy. In: Bennett JV, Brachman PS, editors. Hospital infections. 4th ed. Philadelphia: Lippincott-Raven; 1998. p. 689–724.
2. Joint Commission on the Accreditation of Healthcare Organizations. Accreditation manual for hospitals. Chicago: Joint Commission on the Accreditation of Healthcare Organizations; 1994.
3. Centers for Disease Control and Prevention. National Nosocomial Infections Surveillance (NNIS) system report, data summary from January 1992-June 2003, issued August 2003. Am J Infect Control 2003;31:481–98.
4. Mermel LA. Prevention of intravascular catheter-related infections. Ann Intern Med 2000;132:391–402.
5. Mermel LA. Correction: catheter-related bloodstream infections. Ann Intern Med 2000;133:395.
6. Collignon PJ. Intravascular catheter associated sepsis: a common problem. The Australian Study on intravascular catheter associated sepsis. Med J Aust 1994;161:374–8.
7. Pittet D. Nosocomial bloodstream infections in the critically ill. JAMA 1994;272:1819–20.
8. Byers K, Adal K, Anglim A, Farr B. Case fatality rate for catheter-related bloodstream infections (CRBSI): a meta-analysis. Infect Control Hosp Epidemiol 1995;16(Pt 2 Suppl):23.
9. Rello J, Ochagavia A, Sabanes E, et al. Evaluation of outcome of intravenous catheter-related infections in critically-ill patients. Am J Respir Crit Care Med 2000; 162:1027–30.
10. Dimick JB, Pelz RK, Consunji R, et al. Increased resource use associated with catheter-related bloodstream infection in the surgical intensive care unit. Arch Surg 2001;136:229–34.
11. Raad II, Hohn DC, Gilbreath B, et al. Prevention of central venous catheter-related infections using maximal sterile barrier precautions during insertion. Infect Control Hosp Epidemiol 1994;15:231–8.
12. Maki DG, Stolz SM, Wheeler S, Mermel LA. Prevention of central venous catheter-related bloodstream infection by use of an antiseptic impregnated catheter: a randomized controlled trial. Ann Intern Med 1997;127:257–66.
13. Mermel LA, McCormick RD, Springman SR, Maki DG. The pathogenesis and epidemiology of catheter-related infection with pulmonary artery Swan-Ganz catheters: a prospective study utilizing molecular subtyping. Am J Med 1991;91 Suppl 3B:197S–205S.
14. Raad I, Costerton W, Sabharwal U, et al. Ultrastructural analysis of indwelling vascular catheters: a quantitative relationship between luminal colonization and duration of placement. J Infect Dis 1993;168:400–7.
15. Stiges-Serra A, Puig P, Linares J, et al. Hub colonization as the initial step in an outbreak of catheter-related sepsis due to coagulase negative staphylococci during parenteral nutrition. JPEN J Parenter Enteral Nutr 1984;8:668–72.
16. Salzman MB, Isenberg HD, Shapiro JF, et al. A prospective study of the catheter hub as the portal of entry for microorganisms causing catheter-related sepsis in neonates. J Infect Dis 1993;167:487–90.
17. Centers for Disease Control and Prevention. Nosocomial bacteremia associated with intravenous fluid therapy. MMWR Morb Mortal Wkly Rep 1971;20 Suppl 9:S1–2.
18. Maki DG, Rhame FS, Mackel DC, et al. Nation-wide epidemic of septicemia caused by contaminated intravenous products. Am J Med 1976;60:471–85.
19. Jarvis WR, Highsmith AK. Bacterial growth and endotoxin production in lipid emulsion. J Clin Microbiol 1984;19:17–20.
20. Danker WM, Spector SA, Fierer J. Malassezia fungemia in neonates and adults: complication of hyperalimentation. Rev Infect Dis 1987;9:743–837.
21. Plouffe JF, Brown DG, Silva J, et al. Nosocomial outbreak of Candida parapsilosis fungemia related to intravenous infusions. Arch Intern Med 1977;137:1686–99.
22. Kovacevich DS, Faubion WC, Bender JM, et al. Association of parenteral nutrition catheter sepsis with urinary tract infections. JPEN J Parenter Enteral Nutr 1986;10:639–41.
23. Pettigren RA, Lang DSR, Haycock DA, et al. Catheter-related sepsis in patients on intravenous nutrition: a prospective study of quantitative catheter cultures and guideline changes for suspected sepsis. Br J Surg 1985;72:52–5.
24. Anaissie E, Samonis G, Kontoyiannis D, et al. Role of catheter colonization and infrequent hematogenous seeding in catheter-related-infections. Eur J Clin Microbiol Infect Dis 1995;14:134–7.
25. Cobb DK, High KP, Sawyer RG, et al. A controlled trial of scheduled replacement of central venous and pulmonary artery catheters. N Engl J Med 1991;327:1062–8.
26. Timsit J-F, SabilleV, Farkas J-C, et al. Effect of subcutaneous tunneling on internal jugular catheter-related sepsis in critically ill patients: a prospective randomized multicenter study. JAMA 1996;276:1416–20.
27. Maki DG, Ringer M, Alvarado CJ. Prospective randomized trial of povidone-iodine, alcohol, and chlorhexidine for prevention of infection associated with central venous and arterial catheters. Lancet 1991;338:339–43.
28. Kamal GD, Pfaller MA, Remple LE, Jebson PJ. Reduced intravascular catheter infection by antibiotic bonding. JAMA 1991;265:2364–8.
29. Seifert H, Strate A, Schultz A, Pulvere G. Vascular catheter-related bloodstream infection due to Acinetobacter johnsonii (formerly Acinetobacter calaoceticus var. lwoffi). Report of 13 cases. Clin Infect Dis 1993;17:632–6.
30. Elting LS, Bodey GP. Septicemia due to Xanthomonas species and non-aeruginosa Pseudomonas species: increasing incidence of catheter-related infections. Medicine 1990;69:196–206.
31. Reagan DR, Pfaller MA, Hollis RJ, Wenzel RP. Characterization of the sequence of colonization and nosocomial candidemia using DNA fingerprinting and a DNA probe. J Clin Microbiol 1990;28:2733–8.
32. Strausbaugh LJ, Sewell DL, Ward TT, et al. High frequency of yeast carriage on hands of hospital personnel. J Clin Microbiol 1994;32:2299–300.
33. Reibel W, Frantz N, Adelstein D, Spagnuolo PJ. Corynebacterium JK: a cause of nosocomial device-related infection. Rev Infect Dis 1986;8:42–9.
34. Saleh RH, Schorin MA. Bacillus sp. sepsis associated with Hickman catheters in patients with neoplastic diseases. Pediatr Infect Dis 1987;6:851–6.
35. Costerton JW, Stewart PS, Greenberg EP. Bacterial biofilms: a common cause of persistent infections. Science 1999;284:1318–22.
36. Raad I. Intravascular-catheter-related infections. Lancet 1998;351:893–8.
37. Herrmann M, Suchard SJ, Boxer LA, et al. Thrombospondin binds to Staphylococcus aureus and promotes staphylococcal adherence to surfaces. Infect Immun 1991;59:279–88.
38. Hawiger J, Timmons S, Strong DD, et al. Identification of a region of human fibrinogen interacting with staphylococcal clumping factor. Biochemistry 1982;21:1407–13.
39. Kuusela P. Fibronectin binds to Staphylococcus aureus. Nature 1978;276:718–20.
40. Lopes JD, Dos Reis M, Brentani RR. Presence of laminin receptors in Staphylococcus aureus. Science 1985;229:275–7.
41. Vaudaux P, Pittet D, Haeberli A, et al. Host factors selectively increase staphylococcal adherence on inserted catheters: a role for fibronectin and fibrinogen or fibrin. J Infect Dis 1989;160:865–75.
42. Bouali A, Robert R, Tronchin G, Senet JM. Characterization of binding of human finbrinogen to the surface of germtubes and mycelium of Candida albicans. J Gen Microbiol 1987;133:454–551.
43. Maki DG, Martin WT. Nationwide epidemic of septicemia caused by contaminated infusion products. IV growth of microbial pathogens in fluids for intravenous infusion. J Infect Dis 1975;131:267–72.
44. Anderson RL, Highsmith AK, Holland BW. Comparison of the standard pour plate procedure and the ATP and limulus amoebocyte lysate fluids. J Clin Microbiol 1986;23:465–8.
45. Chrisensen GD, Simpson WA, Bisno AI, Beachey EH. Adherence of slime producing strains of Staphylococcus epidermidis to smooth surfaces. Infect Immun 1982;17:318–26.
46. Anwar H, Strap JL, Chen K, Costerton JW. Dynamic interactions of biofilms of mucoid Pseudomonas aeruginosa with tobramycin and piperacillin. Antimicrob Agents Chemother 1992;36:1208–14.
47. Band JD, Maki DG. Infections caused by arterial catheters used for hemodynamic monitoring. Am J Med 1979; 67:735–41.
48. Shinozaki T, Deane RS, Mazuzan JE Jr, et al. Bacterial contamination of arterial lines. JAMA 1983;249:223–5.
49. Thomas F, Burke JP, Parker J, et al. The risk of infection related to radial vs femoral sites for arterial catheterization. Crit Care Med 1983;11:807–12.
50. Michel L, Marsh M, McMichan JC, et al. Infection of pulmonary artery catheters in critically ill patients. JAMA 1981;245:1032–6.
51. Linder LE, Curelaru I, Gustavsson B, et al. Material thrombogenecity in central venous catheterization: a comparison between soft, antebrachial catheters of silicone elastomer and polyurethane. JPEN J Parenter Enteral Nutr 1984;8:399–406.
52. Sheth NK, Franson TR, Rose HD, et al. Colonization of bacteria on polyvinyl chloride and Teflon intravascular catheter in hospitalized patients. J Clin Microbiol 1983;18:1061–3.
53. Rotrosen D, Calderone RA, Edwards JE Jr. Adherence of Candida species to host tissues and plastic surfaces. Rev Infect Dis 1986;8:73–85.

54. Wolfe BM, Ryder MA, Nishikawa RA, et al. Complications of parenteral nutrition. Am J Surg 1986;152:93–9.

55. Pemberton LB, Lyman B, Lauder V, et al. Sepsis from triple vs single-lumen catheters during total parenteral nutrition in surgical or critically ill patients. Arch Surg 1986; 121:591–4.

56. Appelgran KN. Triple-lumen catheters: technological advance or setback? Arch Surg 1987;53:113–6.

57. Hilton E, Haslett TM, Borenstein MT, et al. Central catheter infections: single vs triple-lumen catheters; influence of guidelines on infection rates when used for replacement of catheters. Am J Med 1988;84:667–72.

58. Yeung C, May J, Hughes R. Infection rate for single-lumen vs triple-lumen subclavian catheters. Infect Control Hosp Epidemiol 1988;9:154–8.

59. Mantese VA, German DS, Kruminski DL, et al. Colonization and sepsis from triple-lumen catheters in critically ill patients. Am J Surg 1987;154:579–601.

60. Powell C, Fabri PJ, Kudsk KA. Risk of infection accompanying the use of single-lumen vs double-lumen subclavian catheters: a prospective randomized study. JPEN J Parenter Enteral Nutr 1988;12:127–9.

61. MacCarthy MC, Shivers JK, Robinson RJ, et al. Prospective evaluation of single and triple lumen catheters in total parenteral nutrition. JPEN J Parenter Enteral Nutr 1987;11:259–62.

62. Farkas JC, Liu N, Bleriot JP, et al. Single versus triple-lumen central catheter-related sepsis: a prospective randomized study in critically ill population. Am J Med 1992;93: 277–82.

63. Hampton AA, Sherertz RJ. Vascular-access infections in hospitalized patients. Surg Clin North Am 1988;68:57–71.

64. Senagore A, Waller JD, Bonnell BW, et al. Pulmonary artery catheterization: a prospective study of internal jugular and subclavian approaches. Crit Care Med 1987;15:35–7.

65. Merrer J, De Jonghe B, Grolliot F, et al. Complications of femoral and subclavian evenous catheterization in critically ill patients: a randomized controlled trial. JAMA 2001;286:700–7.

66. Conly JM, Grieves K, Peters B. A prospective, randomized study comparing transparent and dry gauze dressings for central venous catheters. J Infect Dis 1989;159:310–9.

67. Craven DE, Lichtenberg DA, Kunches LM, et al. A randomized study comparing a transparent polyurethane dressing to a dry gauze dressing for peripheral intravenous catheter sites. Infect Control 1985;6:361–6.

68. Hoffmann KK, Weber DJ, Samsa GP, Rutala WA. Transparent polyurethane film as an intravenous catheter dressing. A meta-analysis of the infection risks. JAMA 1992;267:2072–6.

69. Broviac JW, Cole JJ, Scribner GH. A silicone rubber arterial catheter for prolonged parenteral alimentation. Surg Gynecol Obstet 1973;136:602.

70. Hickman RO, Buckner CD, Clift RA, et al. A modified right arterial catheter for access to the venous system in marrow transplant recipients. Surg Gynecol Obstet 1979;148:871.

71. Goodman MS, Wickman R. Venous access devices: an overview. Oncol Nurs Forum 1984;11:16–23.

72. Raad I, Davis S, Becker M, et al. Low infection rate and long durability of nontunneled silastic catheters: a safe and cost-effective alternative for long-term venous access. Arch Intern Med 1993;153:1791–6.

73. Mermel LA, Farr BM, Sheretz RJ, et al. Guidelines for the management of intravascular catheter-related infections. Clin Infect Dis 2001;32:1249–72.

74. Greene JN. Catheter-related complications of cancer therapy. Infect Dis Clin North Am 1996;10:255–95.

75. Engelhard D, Elishoov H, Strauss N, et al. Nosocomial coagulase-negative staphylococcal infection in bone marrow transplantation recipients with central vein catheter. A 5-year prospective study. Transplantation 1996;61: 430–4.

76. Raad I, Narro J, Khan A, Tarrand J, et al. Serious complications of vascular catheter-related *Staphylococcus aureus* bacteremia in cancer patients. Eur J Clin Microbiol Infect Dis 1992;11:675–82.

77. Striden WD, Helgerson R, Maki DG. Candida septic thrombosis of the great central veins associated with central catheters. Ann Surg 1985;202:653–8.

78. Benezra D, Kiehn TE, Gold GWM, et al. Prospective study of infection in indwelling central venous catheters using quantitative blood cultures. Am J Med 1988;85:495–8.

79. Bouza E, Burillo A, Munoz P. Catheter-related infections: diagnosis and intravascular treatment. Clin Microbiol Infect 2002;8:265–74.

80. Safdar N, Maki DG. Inflammation at the insertion site is not predictive of catheter-related bloodstream infection with short-term, noncuffed central venous catheters. Crit Care Med 2002;30:2632–5.

81. DesJardin JA, Falagas ME, Ruthazer R, et al. Clinical utility of blood cultures drawn from indwelling central venous catheters in hospitalized patients with cancer. Ann Intern Med 1999;131:641–7.

82. Wing EJ, Norden CW, Shadduck RK, Winkelstein A. Use of quantitative bacteriologic techniques to diagnose catheter-related sepsis. Arch Intern Med 1979;139:482–3.

83. Flynn PM, Shenep JL, Barrett FF. Differential quantitation with a commercial blood culture tube for diagnosis of catheter-related infection. J Clin Microbiol 1988;26: 1045–6.

84. Capdevila JA, Planes AM, Palomar M, et al. Value of differential quantitative blood cultures in the diagnosis of catheter-related sepsis. Eur J Clin Microbiol Infect Dis 1992;11:403–7.

85. Raucher HS, Hyatt AC, Barzilai A, et al. Quantitative blood cultures in the evaluation of septicemia in children with Broviac catheters. J Pediatr 1984;104:29–33.

86. Franklin JA, Gaur AH, Shenep JL, et al. In situ diagnosis of central venous catheter-related bloodstream infection without peripheral blood culture. Pediatr Infect Dis J 2004;23:614–8.

87. Kite P, Dobbins BM, Wilcox MH, et al. Evaluation of a novel endoluminal brush method for in situ diagnosis of catheter related sepsis. J Clin Pathol 1997;50:278–82.

88. Fan ST, Teoh-Chan CH, Lau KF, et al. Predictive value of surveillance skin and hub cultures in central venous catheters sepsis. J Hosp Infect 1988;12:191–8.

89. Fortun J, Perez-Molina JA, Asensio A, et al. Semiquantitative culture of subcutaneous segment for conservative diagnosis of intravascular catheter-related infection. JPEN J Parenter Enter Nutr 2000;24:210–4.

90. Raad II, Baba M, Bodey GP. Diagnosis of catheter-related infections: the role of surveillance and targeted quantitative skin cultures. Clin Infect Dis 1995;20:593–7.

91. Blot F, Schmidt E, Nitenberg G, et al. Earlier positivity of central-venous- versus peripheral-blood cultures is highly predictive of catheter-related sepsis. J Clin Microbiol 1998;36:105–9.

92. Blot F, Nitenberg G, Chachaty E, et al. Diagnosis of catheter-related bacteremia: a prospective comparison of the time to positivity of hub-blood versus peripheral blood cultures. Lancet 1999;354:1071–7.

93. Seifert H, Cornely O, Seggewiss K, et al. Bloodstream infection in neutropenic cancer patients related to short-term nontunneled catheters determined by quantitative blood cultures, differential time to positivity, and molecular epidemiological typing with pulsed-field gel electropgoresis. J Clin Microbiol 2003;41:118–23.

94. Rijnders BJ, Verwaest C, Peetermans WE, et al. Difference in time to positivity of hub-blood versus nonhub-blood cultures is not useful for the diagnosis of catheter-related bloodstream infection in critically ill patients. Crit Care Med 2001;29:1399–403.

95. Raad I, Hanna HA, Alakech B, et al. Differential time to positivity: a useful method for diagnosing catheter-related bloodstream infections. Ann Intern Med 2004;140: 18–25.

96. Druskin MS, Siegel PD. Bacterial contamination of indwelling intravenous polyethylene catheters. JAMA 1963;185: 966–8.

97. Maki DG, Weise CE, Sarafin HW. A semiquantitative culture method for identifying intravenous-catheter-related infection. N Engl J Med 1977;296:1305–9.

98. Cleri DJ, Corrado ML, Seligman SJ. Quantitative culture of intravenous catheters and other intravascular inserts. J Infect Dis 1980;141:781–6.

99. Veenstra DL, Saint S, Lumley T, Sullivan SD. Efficacy of antiseptic-impregnated central venous catheters in preventing catheter-related bloodstream infection. A meta-analysis. JAMA 1999;281:261–7.

100. Cooper GL, Hopkins CC: Rapid diagnosis of intravascular catheter-associated infection by direct Gram staining of catheter segments. N Engl J Med 1985;312:1142–7.

101. Spencer RC, Kristinsson KG. Failure to diagnose intravascular-associated infection by direct Gram staining of catheter segments. J Hosp Infect 1986;7:305–6.

102. Zufferey J, Rime B, Francioli P, Bille J. Simple method for rapid diagnosis of catheter-associated infection by direct acridine orange staining of catheter tips. J Clin Microbiol 1988;26:175–7.

103. Crnich CJ, Maki DG. The promise of novel technology for the prevention of intravascular device-related bloodstream infection. I. Pathogenesis and short-term devices. Clin Infect Dis 2002;34:1232–42.

104. Schinabeck MK, Ghannoum MA. Catheter-related infection: diagnosis, treatment, and prevention. Clin Microbiol Newslett 2003;25:113–8.

105. Centers for Disease Control and Prevention. Guidelines for the prevention of intravascular catheter-related infections. MMWR Morb Mortal Wkly Rep 2002; 51(RR-10):1–36.

106. Sherertz RJ, Ely EW, Westbrook DM, et al. Education of physicians-in-training can decrease the risk for vascular catheter infection. Ann Intern Med 2000;132:641–8.

107. Murphy LM, Lipman TO. Central venous catheter care in parenteral nutrition: a review. JPEN J Parenter Enteral Nutr 1987;11:190–201.

108. Eggimann P, Harbarth S, Constantin MN, et al. Impact of a prevention strategy targeted at vascular access care on incidence of infections acquired in intensive care. Lancet 2000;355:1864–8.

109. Faubion WC, Wesley JR, Khalidi N, et al. Total parenteral nutrition catheter sepsis: impact of the team approach. JPEN J Parenter Enteral Nutr 1986;10:642–5.

110. Nelson DB, Kien CL, Mohr B, et al. Dressing changes by specialized personnel reduce infection rates in patients receiving central venous parenteral nutrition. JPEN J Parenter Enteral Nutr 1986;10:220–2.

111. Andrivet P, Bacquer A, Ngoc CV, et al. Lack of clinical benefit from subcutaneous tunnel insertion of central venous catheters in immunocompromised patients. Clin Infect Dis 1994;18:199–206.

112. Veenstra DL, Saint S, Sullivan SD. Cost-effectiveness of antiseptic-impregnated central venous catheters for the prevention of catheter-related bloodstream infection. JAMA 1999;282:554–60.

113. Heard SO, Wagle M, Vijayakumar E, et al. Influence of triple-lumen central venous catheters coated with chlorhexidine and silver sulfadiazine on the incidence of catheter-related bacteremia. Arch Intern Med 1998;158: 81–7.

114. Ciresi D, Albrecht RM, Volkers PA, et al. Failure of an antiseptic bonding to prevent central venous catheter-related infection and sepsis. Am Surg 1996;62:641–6.

115. Pemberton LB, Ross V, Cuddy P, et al. No difference in catheter sepsis between standard and antiseptic central venous catheters: a prospective randomized trial. Arch Surg 1996;131:986–9.

116. Bassetti S, Hu J, D'Agostino RB, et al. Prolonged antimicrobial activity of a catheter containing chlorhexidine-silver sulfadiazine extends protection against catheter infections in vivo. Antimicrob Agents Chemother 2001; 45:1535–8.

117. Brun-Buisson C, Doyon F, Sollet JP, et al. Prevention of intravascular catheter-related infection with newer chlorhexidine-silver sulfadiazine-coated catheters: a randomized controlled trial. Intensive Care Med 2004;30: 837–43.

118. Raad I, Darouiche R, Dupuis J, et al. Central venous catheters coated with minocycline and rifampin for the prevention of catheter-related colonization and bloodstream infections: a randomized, double-blind trial—The Texas Medical Center Study Group. Ann Intern Med 1997; 127:267–74.

119. Darouiche RO, Raad II, Heard SO, et al. Comparison of two anti-microbial impregnated central venous catheters. N Engl J Med 1999;340:1–8.

120. Wenzel RP, Edmond MB. The impact of hospital-acquired bloodstream infections. Emerg Infect Dis 2001;7:174–7.

121. Hanna HA, Raad II, Hacket B, et al. Antibiotic-impregnated catheters associated with significant decrease in nosocomial and multidrug-resistant bacteremias in critically ill patients. Chest 2003;124:1030–8.

122. Chatzinikolaou I. Hanna H, Graviss L, et al. Clinical experience with minocycline and rifampin-impregnated central venous catheters in bone marrow transplantation recipients: efficacy and low risk of developing staphylococcal resistance. Infect Control Hosp Epidemiol 2003;24: 961–3.

123. Hanna H, Benjamin R, Chatzinikolaou I, et al. Long-term silicone central venous catheters impregnated with minocycline and rifampin decrease rates of catheter-related bloodstream infection in cancer patients: a prospective randomized clinical trial. J Clin Oncol 2004;22:3163–71.

124. Bailey MJ. Reduction of catheter-associated sepsis in parenteral nutrition using low-dose intravenous heparin. Br Med J 1979;1:1671–3.

125. Schwartz C, Henrickson KJ, Roghmann K, Powell K. Prevention of bacteremia attributed to luminal colonization of tunneled central venous catheters with vancomycin-susceptible organisms. J Clin Oncol 1990;8:591–7.

126. Raad I, Buzaid A, Rhyne J, et al. Minocycline and ethylenediaminetetraacetate for the prevention of recurrent vascular catheter infections. Clin Infect Dis 1997;25:149–51.

127. Raad I, Hachem R, Tcholakian RK, et al. Efficacy of minocycline and EDTA lock solution in preventing catheter-related bacteremia, septic phlebitis, and endocarditis in rabbits. Antimicrob Agents Chemother 2002;46:327–32.

128. Chatzinikolaou I, Zipf TG, Hanna H, et al. Minocycline-ethylenediamine tetraacetate lock solution for the prevention of implantable port infections in children with cancer. Clin Infect Dis 2003;36:116–9.

129. Bleyer A, Mason I, Raad I, et al. A randomized, double-blind trial comparing minocycline/EDTA vs. heparin as flush solutions for hemodialysis catheters. Infect Control Hosp Epidemiol 2000;21:100–1.

130. Maki DG, Band JD. A comparative study of polyantibiotic and iodophor ointments in prevention of vascular catheter-related infection. Am J Med 1981;70:739–44.

131. Chaiyakunapruk N, Veenstra DL, Lipsky BA, Saint S. Chlorhexidine compared with povidone-iodine solution for vascular catheter-site care: a meta analysis. Ann Intern Med 2002;136:792–801.

132. Maki DG, Cobb L, Garman JK, et al. An attachable silver-impregnated cuff for prevention of infection with central venous catheters: a prospective randomized multicenter trial. Am J Med. 1988;85:307–14.

133. Groeger JS, Lucas AB, Coit D, et al. A prospective randomized evaluation of silver-impregnated subcutaneous cuffs for preventing tunneled chronic venous access catheter infections. Ann Surg 1993;218:206–10.

134. Flowers RH III, Schwenzer KJ, Kopel RF, et al. Efficacy of an attachable subcutaneous cuff for the prevention of intravascular catheter-related infection. JAMA 1989;261:878–83.

135. Bryant JK, Strand CL. Reliability of blood cultures collected from intravascular catheter versus venipuncture. Am J Clin Pathol 1987;88:113–6.

136. Chatzinikolaou I, Hanna H, Darouiche R, et al. Prospective study of the value of quantitative culture of organisms from blood collected through central venous catheters in differentiating between contamination and bloodstream infection. J Clin Microbiol. 2006;44:1834–5.

137. Raad I, Davis S, Khan A, et al. Catheter removal affects recurrence of catheter-related coagulase-negative staphylococci bacteremia (CRCNSB). Infect Control Hosp Epidemiol 1992;13:215–21.

138. Raad I, Darouiche R, Vazquez J, et al. Efficacy and safety of weekly dalbavancin in the treatment of catheter-related bloodstream infections due to gram-positive pathogens. Clin Infect Dis 2005;40:374–80.

139. Birmingham MC, Rayner CR, Meagher AK, et al. Linezolid for the treatment of multidrug-resistant, gram-positive infections: experience from a compassionate-use program. Clin Infect Dis 2003;36:159–68.

140. Carpenter CF, Chambers HF. Daptomycin: another novel agent for treating infection due to drug-resistant gram-positive pathogens. Clin Infect Dis 2004;38:994–1000.

141. Gopal AK, Fowler VG, Shah M, et al. Prospective analysis of Staphylococcus aureus bacteremia in nonneutropenic adults with malignancy. J Clin Oncol 2000;28:1110–5.

142. Venditti M, Falcone M, Micozzi A, et al. Staphylococcus aureus bacteremia in patients with hematologic malignancies: a retrospective case-control study. Haematologica 2003;88:923–30.

143. Edoute Y, Haim N, Rinkevich D, et al. Cardiac valvular vegetations in cancer patients: a prospective echocardiograhic study of 200 patients. Am J Med 1997;102:252–8.

144. O'Brien L, Kerrigan SW, Kaw G, et al. Multiple mechanisms for the activation pf human platelet aggregation by Staphylococcus aureus: roles of the clumping factors ClfA and ClfB, the serine-aspartate repeat protein SdrE and protein A. Mol Microbiol 2002;44:1033–44.

145. Heilmann C, Niemann S, Sinha B, et al. Staphylococcus aureus fibronectin-binding protein (FnBP)-mediated adherence to platelets, and aggregation of platelets induced by FnBPA but not by FnBPB. J Infect Dis 2004;190:321–9.

146. Dugdale DC, Ramsey P. Staphylococcus aureus bacteremia in patients with Hickman catheters. Am J Med 1990;89:137–41.

147. Malanoski G, Samore M, Pefanis A, et al. Staphylococcus aureus bacteremia: minimal effective therapy and unusual infectious complications associated with arterial sheath catheters. Arch Intern Med 1995;155:1161–6.

148. Fowler VG, Sanders LL, Sexton DJ, et al. Outcome of Staphylococcus aureus bacteremia according to compliance with recommendations of infectious disease specialists: experience with 244 patients. Clin Infect Dis 1998;27:478–86.

149. Metcalf SC, Chambers ST, Pithie AD. Use of ethanol locks to prevent recurrent central line sepsis. J Infect Dis 2004;49:20–2.

150. Raad I, Sabbagh M. Optimal duration of therapy for catheter related Staphylococcus aureus bacteremia: a study of 55 cases and review. Clin Infect Dis 1992;14:75–82.

151. Fowler VG Jr, Olsen MK, Corey R, et al. Clinical identifiers of complicated Staphylococcus aureus bacteremia. Arch Intern Med 2003;163:2066–71.

152. Schrenzel J, Harbarth S, Schockmel G, et al, Swiss Staphylococcal Study Group. A randomized clinical trial to compare fleroxacin-rifampicin with flucloxacillin or vancomycin for the treatment of staphylococcal infections. Clin Infect Dis 2004;39:1285–92.

153. Hanna H, Afif C, Alakech B, et al. Central venous catheter-related bacteremia due to gram-negative bacilli: significance of catheter-removal in preventing relapse. Infect Control Hosp Epidemiol 2004;25:646–9.

154. Strinden WD, Helgerson RB, Maki DG. Candida septic thrombosis of the great central veins associated with central catheters: clinical features and management. Ann Surg 1985;202:653–8.

155. Leung W-H, Lau C-P, Tai Y-T, et al. Candida right ventricular mural endocarditis complicating indwelling right atrial catheter. Chest 1990;97:1492–3.

156. Pittet D, Li N, Woolson RF, Wenzel RP. Microbiological factors influencing the outcome of nosocomial bloodstream infections [abstract 79]. Infect Control Hospital Epidemiol 1996;17 Suppl:29.

157. Nguyen MH, Peacock JE Jr, Tanner DC, et al. Therapeutic approaches in patients with candidemia: evaluation in a multicenter, prospective observational study. Arch Intern Med 1995;155:2429–35.

158. Nucci M, Colombo AL, Silveira F, et al. Risk factors for death in patients with candidemia. Infect Control Hosp Epidemiol 1998;19:846–50.

159. Hung C-C, Chen Y-C, Chag S-C, et al. Noscomial candidemia in a university hospital in Taiwan. J Formos Med Assoc 1996;95:19–28.

160. Rex JH, Bennett JE, Sugar AM, et al. Intravascular catheter-exchange and duration of candidemia. Clin Infect Dis 1995;21:995–6.

161. Karkowicz MG, Hashimoto LN, Kelly RE, Buescher ES. Should central venous catheters be removed as soon as candidemia is detected in neonates? Pediatrics 2000;106:E63.

162. Anaissie EJ, Rex JH, Uzun O, Vartivarian S. Predictors of adverse outcome in cancer patients with candidemia. Am J Med 1998;104:238–45.

163. Luzzati R, Amalfitano G, Lazzarine L, et al. Nosocomial candidemia in non-neutropenic patients at an Italian tertiary care hospital. Eur J Clin Microbiol Infect Dis 2000;19:602–7.

164. Girmenia C, Martino P, Bernardis FD, et al. Rising incidence of Candida parapsilosis in patients with hematologic malignancies: clinical aspects, predisposing factors, and differential pathogenicity of the causative strains. Clin Infect Dis 1996;23:506–14.

165. Stamos JK, Rowley AH. Candidemia in a pediatric population. Clin Infect Dis 1995;20:571–5.

166. Dato VM, Dajani AS. Candidemia in children with central venous catheters: role of catheter removal and amphotericin B therapy. Pediatr Infect Dis J 1990;9:309–14.

167. Eppes SC, Troutman JL, Gutman LT. Outcome of treatment of candidemia in children whose central catheters were removed or retained. Pediatr Infect Dis J 1989;8:99–104.

168. Lecciones JA, Lee FW, Navarro EE, et al. Vascular catheter-associated fungemia in patients with cancer: analysis of 155 episodes. Clin Infect Dis 1992;14:875–83.

169. Raad I, Hanna H, Boktour M, et al. Management of central venous catheters in patients with cancer and candidemia. Clin Infect Dis 2004;38:1119–27.

170. Goodrich JM, Reed EC, Mori M, et al. Clinical features and analysis of risk factors for invasive candidal infection after marrow transplantation. J Infect Dis 1991;164:731–40.

171. Rex JH, Bennett JE, Sugar AM, et al. A randomized trial comparing fluconazole with amphotericin B for the treatment of candidemia in patients without neutropenia. N Engl J Med 1994;331:1325–30.

172. Mora-Duarte J, Betts R, Rotstein C, et al. Comparison of caspofungin and amphotericin B for invasive candidiasis. N Engl J Med 2002;347:2020–9.

173. Kuse ER, Chetchotisakd P, da Cunha CA, et al. Micafungin versus liposomal amphotericin B for candidemia and invasive candidosis: a phase III randomized double-blind trial. Lancet 2007;369:1519–27.

174. Reboli AC, Rotstein C, Pappas PG, et al. Anidulafungin versus fluconazole for invasive candidiasis. N Engl J Med 2007;356:2472–82.

Viral Infections

Harrys A. Torres, MD

Michael Boeckh, MD

Roy F. Chemaly, MD, MPH

Viruses have been implicated in the pathogenesis of several malignancies. In addition, viral infections are common complications among cancer patients and are associated with considerable morbidity and mortality, especially in those with hematologic malignancies and those who have undergone hematopoietic stem cell transplantation (HSCT). For example, herpes viruses are common pathogens in these patient populations, especially herpes simplex virus, varicella-zoster virus, and cytomegalovirus (CMV) and, to a lesser extent, Epstein-Barr virus (EBV), and human herpesvirus (HHV)-6. Other common viruses in these immunocompromised patients are community-acquired respiratory viruses (CRVs), including respiratory syncytial virus (RSV), influenza virus, and parainfluenza virus (PIV), which produce upper respiratory tract infections (URIs) that can potentially progress to severe lower respiratory tract infections (LRIs). Other, less common viruses that can cause serious illness in cancer patients and HSCT recipients include hepatitis viruses, polyomaviruses, picornaviruses, rhinoviruses, coronaviruses, enteroviruses, adenoviruses, and metapneumoviruses. In this chapter, we review the potential role of viruses as causative agents of cancer and cover relevant issues on viral infections affecting both patients with cancer and HSCT recipients.

Viral Infections as Causes of Cancer

Several viruses, including herpesviruses, hepatitis viruses, retroviruses, and polyomaviruses, have been implicated in the pathogenesis of various malignancies (Table 1).[1-7] Such an association has been supported by the oncogenic properties of these viruses in animal models or cell cultures, and epidemiologic evidence is mounting. Tumor viruses might drive the malignant growth or modify the tumor phenotype. Viral carcinogenicity is cell type specific, multifactorial, and influenced by cofactors; the interaction between viral and chemical carcinogens may explain the cause of several cancers (see Table 1). For example, cervical cancer, hepatocellular carcinoma (HCC),

and Kaposi's sarcoma (KS) may be the result of the virus-chemical interaction.

EBV was the first human virus associated with carcinogenesis, specifically to the origin of B-cell lymphomas.[8] To date, a variety of EBV-related tumors, such as Hodgkin's disease and nasopharyngeal cancer, have been described (see Table 1).

HHV-8 has been suggested as the etiologic agent for KS, with deoxyribonucleic acid (DNA) sequences of this herpesvirus isolated in KS tissues.[9] Hence, this virus is also termed Kaposi's sarcoma–associated herpesvirus (KSHV).[10] The pathogenesis of human immunodeficiency virus (HIV)-associated KS appears to be multifactorial. For instance, the use of nitrite inhalants and exposure to wet clay soils or other environmental sources appear to be linked to the unique epidemiology of HIV-associated KS.[11,12]

Hepatitis B (HBV) and C (HBC) viruses have also been associated with the development of HCC, and their interaction with chemical carcinogens such as aflatoxin exposure, heavy alcohol consumption, inorganic arsenic ingestion, radioactive thorium dioxide exposure, iron overload, oral contraceptive use, and anabolic steroid use appears to be important in the pathogenesis of HCC.[6,13,14] HCV might also have a role as an etiologic agent in non-Hodgkin's B-cell lymphoma,[15,16] although this association may have some geographic variations.[17]

Human papillomavirus (HPV) has been associated with a variety of cancers, and its interaction with cofactors (eg, smoking, oral contraceptives, high parity) may play a carcinogeneic role.[18] Virtually all cases of cervical cancer are due to a subset of HPV types, of which the most important are HPV-16, HPV-18, and HPV-45.[1] HPV has also been associated with the development of penile, anal, or vulvar cancers, as well as with pulmonary adenocarcinoma, head and neck squamous cell carcinoma, laryngeal squamous cell carcinoma, and ovarian cancer.[1,5,19-22] Polyomaviruses such as JC virus and simian virus 40 (SV40) could also contribute to the pathogenesis of cancer, especially those affecting the central nervous system and the skin.[3,23]

Human T-cell leukemia virus type 1 has been identified as the causative agent of T-cell leukemia or lymphoma.[1] Unlike other retroviruses that have direct oncogenic properties, HIV is thought to facilitate—through the suppression of the immune system—the occurrence of several cancer types caused by other infectious agents,[24] although recent data indicate that HIV-1 infection may actively promote cancer growth, based on the evidence that the HIV-1–encoded Tat protein can directly induce tumor angiogenesis and enhance transmission of KSHV to target cells.[10]

The importance of detecting viruses as causes of cancer has enormous implications for public health. Such infectious agents constitute an identifiable and possibly preventable cause of cancer, and treatment options to prevent infection with or to eradicate these viruses could diminish the incidence of cancer. For example, HBV's association with HCC and HPV's association with cervical cancer have led to trials of vaccines for preventing cancer; encouraging results have been reported.[25,26]

Viral Hepatitis

The existence of more than 400 million people chronically infected with HBV and another 170 million individuals chronically infected with HCV makes these two infections a serious global public health problem.[27-29] More than 25% of people with chronic hepatitis B infection will die of liver disease, and more than 1 million deaths result from this infection annually.[28] Likewise, chronic hepatitis C is a major cause of chronic liver disease and death throughout the world, with approximately 280,000 deaths attributable to this infection annually.[29]

HBV Infection

Clinical Manifestations

For adults, the risk of the HBV infection becoming chronic (ie, carriage of HBV surface antigen [HBsAg] for at least 6 months) is less than 5%.[30] Chronic HBV infection can cause hepatic cirrhosis and cancer.[28]

Table 1 Association between Viruses and Various Cancers

Virus Family	Type of Association and Cancer	Other Factors Associated with These Cancers
Herpesviridae		
EBV	Proven: Burkitt's lymphoma, Hodgkin's disease, non-Hodgkin's lymphoma, AIDS-associated lymphomas, nasopharyngeal cancer, post-transplantation lymphoproliferative disorders	Burkitt's lymphoma: malaria, nitrosamines Non-Hodgkin's lymphoma: polychlorinated biphenyls, pesticides, hair dyes
	Controversial: breast cancer, gastric cancer, leiomyosarcomas	
HHV-8 (KSHV)	Proven: Kaposi's sarcoma, primary effusion lymphoma	HIV, nitrite inhalants, immunosuppressants, water and/or volcanic soils, nitrosamines
Hepadnaviridae		
HBV	Proven: hepatocellular carcinoma	Dietary aflatoxins, alcohol
Flaviviridae		
HCV	Proven: hepatocellular carcinoma	Alcohol
	Potential: non-Hodgkin's lymphoma	
Papovaviridae		
Polyomaviruses		
JC virus	Potential: human brain tumors and non-neural tumors	No data
Simian virus 40	Potential: mesothelioma, brain tumors	Mesothelioma: asbestos, tobacco
Papillomaviruses		
HPV	Proven: cervical cancer, oropharyngeal cancer	Cervical cancer: HSV-2 coinfection, tar-based vaginal douches, tobacco, wood smoke, oral contraceptives, high parity, tobacco
	Potential: penile cancer, squamous cell skin cancer, pulmonary adenocarcinoma, laryngeal squamous cell carcinoma, esophageal squamous cell carcinoma	Oropharyngeal cancer: alcohol, tobacco
	Controversial: colorectal tumors	
Retroviridae		
HTLV-1	Proven: adult T-cell leukemia	No data

EBV = Epstein-Barr virus; HBV = hepatitis B virus; HCV = hepatitis C virus; HHV-8 = human herpesvirus 8; HIV = human immunodeficiency virus; KSHV = Kaposi's sarcoma–associated herpesvirus; HPV = human papillomavirus; HSV-2 = herpes simplex virus type 2; HTLV-1 = human T-cell leukemia virus type 1.

HBV infection can produce a high incidence of hepatic complications during therapy for cancer.[31] Acute hepatitis owing to HBV reactivation is a complication observed in up to 67% of HBsAg-positive patients undergoing chemotherapy.[32–34] In most cases, the reactivation of HBV is asymptomatic, with mild and transient elevations of alanine aminotransferase levels. Some patients may have more severe flare-ups; massive necrosis and liver failure are associated with a mortality rate of 5 to 40%.[31,35,36] Therefore, the possibility of HBV reactivation should be considered in patients with a history of HBV infection who develop liver dysfunction following chemotherapy.

Pathophysiologic Mechanisms

In reactivation of HBV or HCV, chemotherapy depresses the immune system, leading to enhanced viral replication and an increase in the number of infected hepatocytes.[34,35] In both infections, hepatocellular damage appears to be mediated primarily by host cellular immune responses, and the clinical signs of acute hepatitis are usually manifested at reconstitution of circulating lymphocytes. After discontinuation of chemotherapy and restoration of the individual's immune system, T cells directed at HBV or HCV antigens press on hepatocytes, potentiate inflammation, and can initiate hepatocyte lysis and progression to fibrosis.[32,35,37,38]

Diagnosis

HBV reactivation in cancer patients appears to be more common in male subjects, of young age, who have a diagnosis of lymphoma or breast cancer, positive results for hepatitis B early antigen (HbeAg), a high prechemotherapy HBV viral load, and previous exposure to anthracyclines and/or corticosteroids.[31,33,39,40] The presence of corticosteroids in the chemotherapy regimens is considered one of the most important risk factors for chemotherapy-induced HBV reactivation.[34,39] HBV contains a corticosteroid-responsive element that is an HBV enhancer.[38] Other chemotherapeutic agents or immunosuppressive drugs, apart from anthracyclines or corticosteroids,

that have been linked to the reactivation of HBV include vincristine, bleomycin, etoposide, methotrexate, actinomycin D, mercaptopurine, azauridine, chlorambucil, cytosine arabinoside, leukovorin, cisplatin, and gemcitabine[39] and the newer chemotherapeutic drugs fludarabine[32] and rituximab.[41]

Patients previously infected with HBV and undergoing HSCT are also at higher risk of hepatitis-related morbidity and mortality.[27,40] Nevertheless, the presence of chronic hepatitis B or C infection before transplantation should not be an absolute contraindication to HSCT, particularly in patients with normal serum aminotransferases and patients without marked hepatic fibrosis or cirrhosis.[27,40]

Patients should be screened routinely for HBsAg in endemic areas of chronic HBV infection before they undergo cytotoxic treatment.[36] Enzyme-linked immunosorbent assays are used to test for the presence of HBsAg, HBeAg, and antibodies against HBeAg. Patients who have positive results and are suspected to be having an HBV reactivation should have HBV-DNA levels measured for confirmation.[32,36] In addition, during chemotherapy and immunosuppressive therapy, serologic antibody markers of hepatitis may be negative, thus making HBV-DNA monitoring by polymerase chain reaction (PCR) useful.[42] Reactivation of HBV infection can occur with either HBeAg-positive or HBeAg-negative/anti–HBe-positive cancer patients.[34,39] Similarly, reactivation can occur despite the presence of HBV surface antibody following HSCT.[43] Pretransplantation liver biopsy to assess for the presence of fibrosis or cirrhosis is recommended in patients with abnormal serum aminotransferases or clinical manifestations of chronic liver disease.[37]

Chemotherapy regimens in individuals with HBV reactivation are usually discontinued and restarted several months after the acute event, when liver function test results normalize and HBV-DNA levels become undetectable.[38] Reactivation-related acute hepatitis can also cause delays and necessitate reductions in chemotherapy, reducing the chance of cancer remission and increasing the mortality rate.[34,44]

Treatment

The two modes of treatment for hepatitis B infection are viral suppression (eg, with nucleoside analogues such as lamivudine or adefovir dipivoxil) and immunomodulation (eg, with interferon-α) (Table 2).[28,45–50] Lamivudine has been successfully used for the treatment of acute HBV reactivation in cancer patients undergoing chemotherapy.[38,51] In these patients, treatment of HBV infection may be indicated when a high risk of hepatic disease progression is documented during or at the end of chemotherapy.[27] In cancer

Table 2 Antiviral Agents Used for Treating Hepatitis B and C Viral Infections

Antiviral Agent	Mechanism of Action	FDA-Approved Indication	Reported Adverse Effects
Lamivudine	Inhibition of reverse transcriptase and incorporation into viral DNA, which halts the DNA synthesis of HBV	Chronic hepatitis B infection	Fatigue, headache, rashes, insomnia, myalgias, arthralgias, decreased appetite, diarrhea, nausea, vomiting, hepatomegaly with steatosis, pancreatitis, fat redistribution, lactic acidosis, death
Adefovir dipivoxil (oral prodrug of adefovir)	Inhibition of DNA synthesis of HBV through competitive inhibition of reverse transcriptase and incorporation into viral DNA	Chronic hepatitis B infection	Headache, asthenia, abdominal pain, diarrhea, dyspepsia, flatulence, nausea, pruritus, rash, renal failure
Interferon-α	The precise mechanism of action has not been determined; thought to be related to altered synthesis of RNA and DNA, enhanced phagocytic activity of macrophages, and augmented specific cytotoxicity of lymphocytes for target cells	Chronic viral hepatitis caused by either HBV (interferon-α-2b, peginterferon α-2a and α-2b) or HCV (interferon-α-2a or -2b or alphacon 1, peginterferon α-2a and α-2b)	Influenza-like symptoms (eg, fever, chills, fatigue, headache, malaise, myalgia, and arthralgia), alopecia, anorexia, nausea, vomiting, diarrhea, dizziness, hypersensitivity, pruritis, aplastic anemia, hepatotoxicity, liver enzyme elevations, nephrotic syndrome, neutropenia, thrombocytopenia, pancreatitis, impaired concentration, severe somnolence, depression, suicidal ideation, anxiety, psychosis, pneumonitis, renal insufficiency/failure, retinal hemorrhages, cotton-wool spots, retinal artery/vein obstruction, thyroid and liver function test abnormalities
Ribavirin	Still unclear; may act at several sites, including cellular enzymes, to interfere with viral nucleic acid synthesis	Chronic hepatitis C infection with compensated liver disease (in combination with interferon-α-2b, peginterferon α-2a and α-2b)	Fatigue, headache, anorexia, dyspepsia, nausea, rash, lethargy, increased concentrations of serum bilirubin, pruritus, conjunctivitis, headache, hemolytic anemia, pancreatitis, bronchospasm, worsening respiratory status, cardiac arrest, hypotension, bradycardia, death

DNA = deoxyribonucleic acid; FDA = US Food and Drug Administration; HBV = hepatitis B virus; HCV = hepatitis C virus; RNA = ribonucleic acid.

and HSCT patients, nucleoside analogues are preferable because they do not cause substantial myelosuppression, a possible complication of interferon-α therapy.[35,40] Liver transplantation is also effective and should be considered in patients with end-stage disease that does not respond to medical therapy.[28] In children undergoing chemotherapy or HSCT, the criteria to start treatment must be the same as those used in children with chronic hepatitis, such as disease lasting for at least 6 months with abnormal transaminase levels and HBV-DNA positivity.[27]

Primary prophylactic therapy using lamivudine is well tolerated and effective in reducing the incidence of HBV reactivation in chronic HBsAg carriers undergoing chemotherapy.[34,38,52] Lamivudine treatment should continue for 6 to 12 months following the last dose of immunosuppressive treatment.[38] Prophylactic use of nucleoside analogues such as lamivudine or famciclovir may also result in a significant decrease in the incidence and severity of HBV reactivation after HSCT.[40,53] However, limiting the use of prophylactic antiviral agents to patients who are at the highest risk of developing HBV reactivation may reduce the potential complication of emergence of mutant viruses.[39]

Besides the prophylactic use of nucleoside analogues in HBsAg-positive patients, other strategies to reduce the risk of reactivation of HBV in patients with HBV infection and cancer who receive cytotoxic chemotherapy include the use of less aggressive and less immunosuppressive chemotherapy protocols in HBsAg-positive patients, close monitoring every 1 to 3 weeks throughout the course of chemotherapy, and early intervention during reactivation.[34,44] To date, insufficient information exists to allow recommendation of antiviral prophylaxis for the population that has been exposed to HBV but tests negative for HBsAg.[35]

HCV Infection

Clinical Manifestations

Acute HCV infection is generally benign in less than one-third of patients and tends to become chronic in more than 70% of them, at which stage it can induce cirrhosis, end-stage disease, liver failure, and liver cancer.[29,54] Several factors are clearly associated with the rate of fibrosis progression, including a low CD4 count.[29]

Pathophysiologic Mechanisms

These are described in the section on HBV infection.

Diagnosis

HCV infection may be diagnosed using serologic assays for antibodies and molecular tests for viral particles. Antibodies against HCV are detected by enzyme immunoassays that are very sensitive and very specific. However, cancer patients, especially those with hematologic malignancies, can have false-negative results. In these patients, the conventional detection of anti-HCV antibodies is not sufficient for diagnosis, thus necessitating PCR determination of HCV–ribonucleic acid (RNA).[27,29,55,56] Knowledge of the viral load is also helpful for predicting treatment response and relapse.[29] Liver biopsy should be considered in patients with clinical manifestations of cirrhosis, patients with chronic HCV infection and elevated serum aminotransferase levels, and patients with HCV who have a history of excessive alcohol intake. Patients with marked hepatic fibrosis or cirrhosis should not proceed to high-dose myeoloablative therapy and HSCT because of the high risk of complications and death from HCV infection.[37]

It seems that HCV has a lower reactivation rate than HBV has following chemotherapy, but when it occurs, it can be fatal.[32,34]

Treatment

The combination of pegylated interferon and ribavirin can eradicate HCV in more than 50% of patients (see Table 2). Combination antiviral therapy has been more effective than monotherapy with either agent and has a higher rate of sustained response.[48] Combination therapy should be considered for patients with decompensated but stable chronic HCV liver disease.[57]

These antiviral treatments reduce the progression of liver fibrosis and can reverse cirrhosis.[29] Liver transplantation is the primary treatment option for patients with decompensated cirrhosis.[29] A high viral load degree and the presence of genotype 1 are predictors of poor outcome in the general population.[27]

Ribavirin, administered during conditioning and after transplantation in HCV-infected patients requiring HSCT, appears to be safe and can result in clearance of HCV-RNA.[58]

High alcohol consumption must be avoided[59] and metabolic disorders (eg, diabetes, overweight) improved.[60] Superinfection with hepatitis A virus in patients with chronic HCV infection can result in severe acute or even fulminant hepatitis. Therefore, hepatitis A vaccine should be recommended for individuals with HCV infection and evidence of chronic liver disease.[61] Based on limited data, hepatitis A vaccination can be used among HSCT recipients 24 months or older at least 12 months after HSCT.[62]

Cytomegalovirus

CMV is a ubiquitous herpesvirus that infects 40 to 100% of adults.[63] CMV infection is a considerable problem in patients who have undergone allogeneic or autologous HSCT,[64,65] and it is an emerging infection with significant morbidity and mortality among patients with leukemia[66] and lymphoma.[67,68]

Clinical Manifestations

The most common forms of infection in patients with hematologic malignancies and in HSCT recipients are CMV infection (antigenemia) and CMV disease (end-organ disease). Pneumonia and gastrointestinal disease are the most common manifestations of CMV disease in these patient populations; other manifestations, such as myocarditis, hepatitis, adrenalitis, thyroiditis, pancreatitis, nephritis, and encephalitis, are less common.[64,66,67,69,70] Retinitis, a common manifestation of CMV disease in acquired immune deficiency syndrome (AIDS) patients,[71] is rare in cancer patients and those who have undergone HSCT.[63,67,72,73]

The mortality rate from CMV pneumonia varies according to the underlying malignancy, reported as 30% in patients with lymphoma, 57% in those with leukemia, and up to 90% in those who have undergone HSCT.[64,66,74,75] With current treatment regimens consisting of ganciclovir and intravenous immunoglobulin (IVIG), the mortality rate is approximately 60% for pneumonia.[74] In patients with CMV pneumonia, the presence of lymphopenia in leukemia patients[66] and a high APACHE II score and development of antiviral toxicity in lymphoma patients are predictors of poor outcome.[67]

Development of either CMV infection or CMV disease in cancer patients has been associated with the use of corticosteroids[68,70] and new chemotherapeutic agents such as, alemtuzumab, and fludarabine.[66,76,77] Potential risk factors for the development of CMV disease in HSCT recipients include pretransplantation CMV seropositivity, transplantation of hematopoietic stem cells from a matched unrelated donor or a mismatched related donor, use of T cell–depleted marrow, severe graft-versus-host disease, previous use of tacrolimus, and administration of prophylactic ganciclovir only three times per week.[63–65,78,79]

Pathophysiologic Mechanisms

CMV remains latent in tissues after a patient's recovery from the initial infection.[63] Lymphocytes, particularly cytotoxic T cells, play a crucial role in maintaining CMV in the latent stages and in controlling CMV infection[80]; thus, their impairment may contribute to the development of CMV infection or CMV disease in cancer patients or those who have undergone HSCT.[67,81] CMV also exerts an immunomodulatory role, which predisposes patients to fungal infections.[82] For instance, patients with hematologic malignancies and HSCT who develop either CMV infection or CMV pneumonia commonly have concomitant *Pneumocystis jiroveci* (formerly *Pneumocystis carinii*) pneumonia and an increased risk of subsequent development of invasive pulmonary aspergillosis.[83,84]

Diagnosis

Early detection of CMV infection is critical to its optimal management.[66] Conventional viral culturing has been the gold standard for diagnosing CMV to date but is limited by its poor predictive value, lack of quantitation, false-negative results, and up to 6 weeks' turnaround time.[85–88] Rapid viral culturing using the shell vial method, a modification of conventional culturing, has reduced the diagnosis time to approximately 2 days and has a sensitivity of 68 to 100% compared with conventional culturing.[85,87,89] The CMV pp65 antigenemia assay using peripheral blood leukocytes is another reliable, rapid, and sensitive test. Similarly, the CMV pp67–messenger RNA assay appears to be a promising diagnostic tool with high specificity for the diagnosis of CMV infection, comparable to that of the quantitative pp65-antigenemia assay.[90,91] In patients who have undergone HSCT, the presence of antigenemia is a predictor of the development of CMV pneumonia,[79,85,92] although no correlation between CMV antigenemia and the development of CMV pneumonia has been observed in patients with lymphoma.[67] Real-time PCR for detection of CMV-DNA in the blood is an alternative that is also rapid and sensitive for diagnosing active

disease and monitoring the response to therapy; additionally, it appears to be more sensitive than the identification of antigenemia in detecting CMV reactivation in patients with lymphoid malignancies and after HSCT.[93,94] Virus quantitation can be used to risk-stratify patients and to monitor treatment.[94] CMV in tissue and bronchoalveolar lavage specimens may also be identified by cytology, histopathologic examination for viral inclusions, or immunohistochemical staining.[67,85,89]

A definitive diagnosis of CMV pneumonia depends on the detection of the virus in lung tissue.[85] However, lung biopsies are rarely performed in patients with cancer because of the morbidity (eg, bleeding) associated with this procedure.[85] Detection of CMV in bronchoalveolar lavage samples correlates highly with detection in lung biopsies[95] and is therefore presently the preferred method of diagnosis. Therefore, most cases of CMV pneumonia in cancer patients are diagnosed by the presence of both clinical and radiographic evidence of pneumonia and the isolation of CMV in respiratory samples obtained by noninvasive procedures (eg, bronchoalveolar lavage samples or sputum). The clinical manifestations and radiologic appearances of CMV pneumonia are indistinguishable from those of other causes of pneumonia in patients with cancer and after HSCT (Figure 1). Consequently, establishing the diagnosis by bronchoalveolar lavage samples is critical in these patients.

The second most common presentation of CMV disease in cancer patients is gastrointestinal infection (Figure 2).[69] Gastrointestinal CMV disease mainly involves the stomach (41%) and

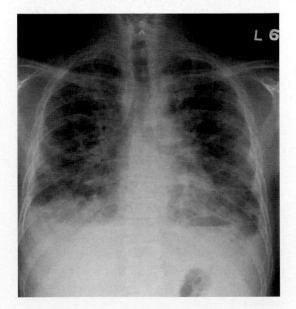

FIGURE 1 Cytomegalovirus pneumonia in a patient with lymphoma. Chest radiograph shows bilateral interstitial and alveolar infiltrates along with right pleural effusion.

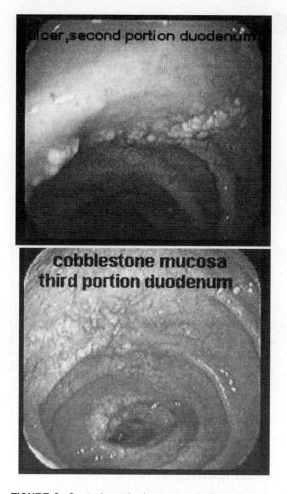

FIGURE 2 Gastrointestinal cytomegalovirus disease in a patient with cancer. Esophagogastroduodenoscopy showing cytomegaloviral infection associated with ulcer, granulation tissue, and edema.

colon (28%) and may be associated with a high attributable mortality rate (42%) among patients with cancer, particularly those with disseminated CMV disease or AIDS.[69] We previously reported that the presentation of gastrointestinal CMV disease varies according to the type of cancer and is influenced by the HIV serostatus.[69] More specifically, upper gastrointestinal tract CMV disease is more common in patients with hematologic malignancies than in those with solid tumors. Even more, cancer patients with AIDS are more likely than those without AIDS to have colonic involvement, whereas cancer patients without AIDS are more likely than those with AIDS to have gastric involvement.[69] Thus, gastrointestinal CMV disease should be suspected even in non-HSCT patients to initiate treatment before dissemination occurs.

Therapy

The use of antiviral agents affects the outcome of cancer patients with CMV infection or CMV disease (Table 3).[46,48,49,66–69,96–98] Therapy for CMV infection consists of intravenous administration of ganciclovir with or without IVIG for CMV

pneumonia. The use of ganciclovir is limited by the associated development of neutropenia, however, which can increase the risk of superinfections, and the emergence of ganciclovir-resistant CMV infection.[99] Foscarnet is used in patients who experience severe myelosuppression during ganciclovir therapy. This agent does not cause neutropenia but is associated with nephrotoxicity and electrolyte imbalances. Valganciclovir is an oral prodrug of ganciclovir with a 10-fold greater bioavailability than oral ganciclovir's and has the potential to replace intravenous drug treatment in cancer patients who can take oral medication.[96] Cidofovir can also be used for treatment, but like foscarnet, it causes nephrotoxicity and occasionally neutropenia.[97] CMV infections refractory to sequential therapy with foscarnet and cidofovir have been reported.[99]

Combinations of antiviral agents against CMV disease have not been systematically evaluated in cancer patients. Although combination therapy with ganciclovir and high-dose IVIG appears to be more effective than therapy with ganciclovir alone in the treatment of CMV pneumonia in patients who have undergone HSCT,[75] no randomized trials have been done comparing these two treatment modalities.

Thus, to date, therapy for CMV disease in cancer or HSCT patients is suboptimal, and more effective and less toxic antiviral agents are urgently needed. However, preventing CMV infection has been more successful. It can be prevented in CMV-negative HSCT recipients by using bone marrow and screened blood products from donors who are also seronegative for CMV. Because of the high risk of CMV infection in seropositive HSCT recipients or those whose donors are seropositive, instituting measures to prevent CMV disease is important. Two strategies are used to prevent CMV infection in seropositive patients who are at risk of reactivation. One is the prophylactic administration of ganciclovir (foscarnet can be used as an alternative); valganciclovir may be useful in some high-risk patients. The second strategy involves early or preemptive therapy for subclinical CMV infection, based on positive surveillance testing (ie, antigenemia or PCR) for CMV from blood or the fluid obtained during bronchoalveolar lavage.[88] Each of these strategies has limitations, but both prophylactic and preemptive therapies are effective for preventing CMV disease.[65,78] Novel strategies include the use of donor-derived CMV-specific T cells.[62,100,101]

HIV/AIDS-Related Cancers

Immunodeficiency, whether congenital or acquired (eg, HIV infection, drug or transplant related), increases the risk of certain types of cancers.[102,103] Patients with AIDS have an increased

incidence of certain cancers, some of them with unusual spectra and manifestations.[24,103–105] AIDS patients have a definite increased incidence of five cancers: KS; non-Hodgkin's lymphoma (NHL), including primary central nervous system lymphoma (PCNSL); squamous cell carcinoma of the conjunctiva; Hodgkin's disease; and childhood leiomyosarcoma.[102] Most of these cancers are known to be associated with specific herpesviruses and HPV coinfections.[10,102,103]

Kaposi's Sarcoma

HHV-8, also known as KSHV, has been suggested as the causative agent of KS.[9,10] The distribution of KS appears to have geographic variations, at least partially related to the effect of the use of highly active antiretroviral therapy (HAART). For example, KS is relatively common in parts of Africa,[24] whereas it is rare in the United Kingdom.[102] In Africa, a steady increase in the incidence of KS has been observed over the last several years, and its occurrence in women has increased.[104,106] An increase in childhood KS has also been noted.[106] In developed countries, the incidence of KS has declined since the introduction of HAART, but this cancer is still a problem for AIDS patients in these countries.[107,108] This is probably because KS manifests less aggressively in patients receiving HAART, although the natural history and outcome do not appear to be influenced by the use of this therapy.[109]

The skin is the most common site of KS, with painless, slightly raised nodular tumors or plaque-like lesions, although, rarely, it can manifest in skeletal muscle and bone.[108] HIV-associated KS often manifests as multiple lesions affecting both the skin and internal organs.[102] HIV-infected patients with KS should be treated with HAART.[108] Identification of the optimal chemotherapy or immunotherapy against KS as well as antiviral therapy is the subject of continuous investigations.

Non-Hodgkin's Lymphoma

NHL is a relatively late complication of HIV infection, and the incidence increases with the duration of infection.[105] The effect of HAART in HIV-associated NHL is mixed. For example, the incidence of systemic NHL has decreased[110,111] but to a lesser extent than the incidence of other AIDS-defining malignancies, such as KS and PCNSL.[107,111] Moreover, the prognosis of NHL has improved,[110,112] but it is still the most frequent cause of death among AIDS patients,[111,112] even in the era of HAART.[111] Roughly half of all cases of systemic NHL related to AIDS are linked to EBV infection.[103]

HIV-associated systemic NHL exhibits pleomorphic features, has a range of subtypes, and can have an aggressive clinical course.[102] The vast

Table 3 Systemic Antiviral Agents Used for Treating Cytomegalovirus Infection or Disease

Antiviral Agent	Mechanism of Action	Indication	Reported Adverse Effects
Ganciclovir	Guanosine analogue; inhibits DNA synthesis by suppressing DNA chain elongation	CMV prophylaxis and treatment*; CMV infections, particularly CMV retinitis in immunocompromised (eg, AIDS) patients (treatment and prophylaxis)	Anemia, neutropenia, thrombocytopenia, hypersensitivity (eg, fever, skin rash), phlebitis, anorexia, nausea or vomiting, eosinophilia, increased levels of creatinine or blood urea nitrogen, central nervous system effects (eg, mood or other mental changes, nervousness, tremor, seizures, confusion, encephalopathy), increased liver function test results
Foscarnet	Pyrophosphate analogue that acts by inhibiting DNA polymerase during the DNA polymerization process	CMV retinitis,* CMV prophylaxis and treatment	Anemia, fever, headache, diarrhea, nausea, vomiting, nephrotoxicity, seizures, electrolyte disturbances (eg, hypocalcemia, hypophosphatemia, hyperphosphatemia, hypomagnesemia, hypokalemia)
Valganciclovir	Prodrug of ganciclovir, then acts as described for ganciclovir	CMV retinitis in AIDS patients* and CMV disease prophylaxis (heart, kidney, kidney-pancreas transplantation)*; therapy and prophylaxis of CMV infection	Headache, insomnia, pyrexia, anemia, neutropenia, thrombocytopenia, abdominal pain, diarrhea, nausea, vomiting
Cidofovir	Inhibition of viral DNA polymerase by its diphosphorylated metabolite	CMV retinitis in patients with AIDS*; may be effective in the treatment and prophylaxis of CMV infection	Nausea, vomiting, headache, rash, severe nephrotoxicity, metabolic acidosis, ocular hypotony, anterior uveitis, iritis, neutropenia, thrombocytopenia

AIDS = acquired immune deficiency syndrome; CMV = cytomegalovirus; DNA = deoxyribonucleic acid.
*Indication approved by the US Food and Drug Administration.

majority of systemic AIDS-related NHLs belong to the three high-grade B-cell lymphomas: Burkitt's lymphoma, immunoblastic lymphoma, and large cell lymphoma. Among the less common types are primary effusion lymphoma and multicentric Castleman's disease–associated NHLs.[10] Most NHLs are of nodal origin (71%),[106] but HIV-associated NHL is characterized by widespread disease involving extranodal sites such as the bone marrow, gastrointestinal tract, central nervous system, ovary, and skin.[102,106,113] In Africa, a significant increase in the incidence of NHLs in women has been reported.[104] The response to HAART remains an important prognostic factor in patients with NHL.[112] Standard chemotherapies similar to those used for systemic NHL in non–HIV-infected patients have also been used for those infected with HIV.[112]

Primary Central Nervous System Lymphoma

PCNSL is an aggressive cancer in AIDS patients. More than 95% of cases are of B-cell origin, with microscopic and immunologic features similar to those of systemic NHL, including its association with EBV infection.[110,114] However, PCNSL is rarely accompanied by lymphoma outside the central nervous system. PCNSL occurs most often in the advanced stages of AIDS, typically observed in HIV-infected patients who have CD4+ cell counts below 50/mm³.[110,114] The incidence of PCNSL has dropped since the introduction of HAART.[112,114]

These patients have constitutional symptoms, altered mental status, seizures, and multiple irregular or ring-shaped enhancing lesions on magnetic resonance images.[114] PCNSL must be differentiated from a more common AIDS-defining illness, cerebral toxoplasmosis. In the absence of a response to a trial of antitoxoplasmosis therapy, cytologic examination of the cerebrospinal fluid and EBV-DNA detection or a stereotactic biopsy are required to confirm the diagnosis of PCNSL. The median survival rate is poor, and the optimal therapy against PCNSL is not well defined. Local radiotherapy is favored over chemotherapy, and the combination of radiotherapy and HAART improves patients' survival rate.[110]

Hodgkin's Disease

The risk of developing Hodgkin's disease is high after the onset of AIDS.[103] Like systemic NHL and PCNSL, most HIV-associated Hodgkin's disease tumors are also linked to EBV infection.[103] Among HIV-infected individuals, Hodgkin's disease is clinically unusual, generally presenting at a late stage with extranodal dissemination and an atypical, aggressive clinical course.[102,113] The predominant histologic subtypes are mixed cellularity and lymphocyte depletion, which are relatively rare in HIV-negative patients.[102] The effect of HAART on the epidemiology of HIV-associated Hodgkin's disease remains unclear.[107]

Other Cancers

A dramatic increase in the incidence of eye tumors, particularly of squamous cell tumors of the conjunctiva, has been observed in Africa, one of the regions most affected by the AIDS epidemic.[104,106] Similarly, HIV-infected children have been observed to have a high risk of developing leiomyosarcoma.[115] Increases in oral, testicular, skin, brain, lung, breast, and thyroid cancers have been linked to HIV infection, although further research is needed to clarify such associations.[102]

The incidence of cervical cancer remains very high, and it is the most common cancer among women with AIDS.[104] However, there has been no suggestion that the natural history of cervical cancer has been affected by HIV.[104,106] HIV infection appears to increase the risk of low-grade cervical lesions but not the risk of invasive cervical cancer.[102] Furthermore, there is no evidence that the oncogenic role of HPV is different in HIV-infected women than it is in HIV-noninfected women.[10] Similarly, in no study has an increase in the relative risk of HCC been observed in HIV-seropositive subjects.[102]

Community-Acquired Respiratory Viruses

CRVs can produce severe infections in both community and hospital settings.[116–118] These viruses frequently cause respiratory illnesses that are associated with high morbidity and mortality rates among cancer patients and HSCT recipients.[116–125] For instance, among adult HSCT recipients in 1997 at The University of Texas M. D. Anderson Cancer Center, CRV infection was the major cause of death, second only to *Aspergillus* infection.[126] However, there are seasonal differences in the intensity and virulence of the epidemics in the communities and between regions; thus, the impact of CRV infections in HSCT recipients varies between centers.

The CRVs include some virulent and highly contagious viruses, the most common of which include RSV, the influenza viruses, and PIV[122,127–129]; there are two subtypes of RSV (A and B), three types of influenza viruses (A, B, and C), and four types of PIV (1 through 4, with serotype 3 the most common). Picornavirus, rhinovirus, coronavirus, adenovirus, and enterovirus are less common respiratory viruses.[116,121,129–131]

CRV infections in HSCT recipients have been extensively studied, and their characteristics are summarized in Table 4.[117,119–121,126–129,132–135] Overall, they occur in up to 36% of all adult HSCT recipients.[120,126,127] The risk from CRV infection is higher in allogeneic HSCT recipients than in autologous HSCT recipients.[119,126,127]

In the case of hematologic malignancies, especially leukemia, CRV infections occur in up to 33% of affected patients; the characteristics of those infections in this subset of patients are summarized in Table 5.[123–125,130,131,136,137]

Of note is that the incidence of RSV, influenza, or PIV infection varies between different series of HSCT recipients and patients with hematologic malignancies. These differences might result from the CRV infection rates in the community and/or differences in the diagnostic methods and infection control measures used in the different centers.

Clinical Manifestations

RSV and influenza infections are observed in seasonal patterns. In the United States, most RSV infections occur during November and May,[116] although, rarely, cases have been reported at different times throughout the year, including the summer months.[138] The start of influenza season typically follows that of the RSV season, and most cases are reported during the winter months. The seasonal prevalence of influenza infections in patients with hematologic malignancies and in HSCT recipients parallels their prevalence in the general community.[117,118] On the other hand, PIVs, rhinoviruses, and adenoviruses are prevalent throughout the year.[128–131]

Immunocompromised patients with CRV infections usually display a more prolonged duration of infection and viral shedding and have more varied initial manifestations of symptoms than normal CRV hosts do.[116] Cancer patients may present with mild to moderate URIs, such as pharyngitis or laryngitis, or with potentially lethal LRIs, such as tracheobronchitis, bronchiolitis, or pneumonia.[116] The most common signs and symptoms of CRV infections are cough, fever, sputum, rhinorrhea, sinus congestion, sore throat, rales, or rhonchi.[133,134] It is interesting that in HSCT recipients with CRV infection, alveolar condensation is the most common abnormality, followed by the presence of an interstitial infiltrate.[133] An association of CRV infections with late airflow obstruction has recently been described.[139]

Up to 80% of CRV-associated URIs in HSCT recipients and patients with hematologic malignancies may progress to LRIs; however, in the majority of studies, progression occurs in 30 to 50% for RSV and 25 to 30% for PIV.[117,118,124,126,133] Progression usually occurs within 2 weeks of the diagnosis of a URI (median 7 days), with

certain variations observed according to the virus involved, and it appears to be more commonly produced by RSV than by an influenza virus or PIV (see Table 4 and Figure 3). Allogeneic HSCT recipients appear to have a higher risk of developing LRIs than autologous HSCT recipients do.[127] Progression from influenza URI to pneumonia has been reported in HSCT recipients given amantadine or rimatadine but not in those given osetalmivir or zanamivir.[117] Influenza in patients treated with corticosteroids, antiviral agents, or both is less likely to progress to an LRI than it is in untreated HSCT patients.[117] The strongest risk factors for progression to LRIs in HSCT recipients are older age, lymphopenia in patients with RSV infection, and use of systemic corticosteroids and lymphopenia in patients with PIV infection.[128]

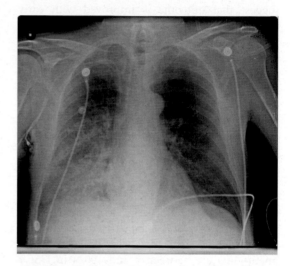

FIGURE 3 Respiratory syncytial virus pneumonia in a patient with chronic myeloid leukemia. Chest radiograph shows airspace disease in the right lower lobe.

Table 4 Characteristics of the Most Common Community-Acquired Respiratory Virus Infections in Hematopoietic Stem Cell Transplant Recipients

Virus	Incidence (%)	Risk Factors for Infection	Progression from URI to LRI (%)	Risk Factors for Progression to LRI	Median Days (range) to Progression to LRI	Shedding Duration, d (range)	Treatment	Mortality Rate* (%)
RSV	5–10	Male sex	27–80	Older age, stem cells from mismatched or unrelated donor, pre-engraftment period, lymphopenia	4–7 (0–7)	10–16 (1–30)	RSV-IVIG plus aerosolized ribavirin	7–100
Influenza	1	Female sex, advanced disease	7–32	Lymphopenia, less exposure to corticosteroids, autologous HSCT	11 (4–14)	7 (2–37)	Oseltamivir appears to be more effective than rimantadine	10–57
PIV	2–7	Use of unrelated stem cell donor	0–27	Use of high-dose corticosteroids	3 (0–30)	No data	Aerosolized ribavirin with or without IVIG	0–75

HSCT = hematopoietic stem cell transplantation; IVIG = intravenous immunoglobulin; LRI = lower respiratory tract infection; PIV = parainfluenza virus; RSV = respiratory syncytial virus; URI = upper respiratory tract infection.
*Mainly due to LRI.

Risk factors for progression of CRV-associated URIs to LRIs in patients with hematologic malignancies include inpatient status at the onset of infection, lymphopenia, and CRV infection caused by RSV.[118]

In HSCT recipients, prolonged shedding of CRVs may occur for all species (see Table 4). Influenza virus shedding has a longer duration in allogeneic recipients, those given higher doses of corticosteroids, or those who have not received antiviral therapy.[117]

The most common periods during which CRV infections occur are in the first 30 days and 90 days after HSCT.[119,133] Patients who develop CRV pneumonia before engraftment are at the greatest risk of death, with a reported mortality rate of up to 80%.[116,121] However, the outcome of infection in such a patient population varies with the type of infection and the virus involved (see Table 4), and the results from recent studies suggest that outcome is improved with early institution of therapy.[140]

Notable geographic and probably center-to-center differences occur in the outcome of CRV infections in HSCT recipients. For example, in the United States, the highest mortality rate observed in this patient population appears to occur in those with RSV infection,[117] whereas in Brazil, influenza A infection accounts for most fatal cases.[133] Furthermore, in Europe, the mortality rate associated with RSV infection appears to be higher in allogeneic than in autologous recipients, whereas the mortality rate associated with influenza infection seems to be similar in the two groups of HSCT recipients.[127] Overall, the mortality rates associated with CRV-associated pneumonia are between 7 and 100% in HSCT recipients[118,123,124,126] and 5 and 83% in patients with leukemia (see Tables 4 and 5).[118,123] These differences are likely due to differences in the definition of LRIs, underlying immunosuppression, the presence of copathogens, and the timing and type of treatment regimens.

Pathophysiologic Mechanisms

In immunocompromised patients, URIs caused by CRVs can spread to the lower respiratory tract. For example, RSV, influenza viruses, and PIV may predispose cancer patients and HSCT recipients to serious secondary bacterial or fungal infections.[116–118,123,127,129,133] Additionally, coinfection with more than one of these CRVs has been reported in 3 to 7% of HSCT recipients and in 12 to 50% of patients with hematologic malignancies.[118,119,125,127,137] It is interesting that RSV infections were also associated with delayed engraftment following transplantation in one study.[141]

Diagnosis

Prompt and accurate diagnosis of CRV infections allows early treatment, possibly delays the

Table 5 Characteristics of the Most Common Community-Acquired Respiratory Virus Infections in Patients with Leukemia

Virus	Incidence (%)	Predominant Leukemia	Frequency of LRI (%)	Treatment	Mortality Rate* (%)
RSV	10	Acute and chronic myeloid	59–67	Aerosolized ribavirin plus RSV-IVIG	53–83
Influenza	33	Acute and chronic lymphoid	35–80	Oseltamivir, zanamivir, amantadine, rimantadine, aerosolized ribavirin	5–43
PIV	3	Acute and chronic lymphoid	55–67	Aerosolized ribavirin	15–66

IVIG = intravenous immunoglobulin; LRI = lower respiratory tract infection; PIV = parainfluenza virus; RSV = respiratory syncytial virus.
*Mainly due to LRI.

necessity for chemotherapy and transplantation, and permits rapid initiation of infection control measures.[120,126,128,133] Methods used for diagnosing CRVs include viral culture, enzyme-linked immunosorbent assays for antigen detection, direct or indirect immunofluorescence assays with monoclonal antibodies, PCR amplification, and chemical reactions for enzyme detection.[116,122,129,133] PCR testing also allows virus quantitation. Histopathologic examination of lung tissue with immunohistochemical staining has also been used for diagnosing CRV infections.[125,134]

In patients who have rhinorrhea, nasal or sinus congestion, otitis media, pharyngitis, and/or cough without hypoxemia or infiltrates on chest radiography, CRV-associated URIs are usually diagnosed when a CRV is microbiologically isolated in a specimen from the upper respiratory tract. However, CRV-associated LRIs are diagnosed when a CRV is either microbiologically isolated from a lower respiratory tract sample or identified during histopathologic examination of lung tissue in the presence of symptoms and radiographic findings compatible with a diagnosis of a viral LRI.[117,130,134,142]

Therapy

Without treatment, the mortality rate associated with RSV LRIs may be as high as 100%,[116,120,127] although recent reports also suggest that some RSV-infected patients may have a good outcome without treatment.[141] The results with the use of antiviral therapy against RSV URIs in HSCT recipients (mainly autologous recipients) and patients with multiple myeloma have been conflicting.[127,138,141] The reasons for these differences are poorly understood but are likely due to the immunosuppressive state of the patient.

The experience from several transplantation centers suggests that the patients at highest risk of severe RSV disease are those whose transplants have not yet fully engrafted; therefore, treatment should be initiated early in the pre-engraftment period.[126,134,135] At M. D. Anderson Cancer Center

and the Fred Hutchinson Cancer Research Center, our current practice is to individualize care for HSCT recipients with a postengraftment RSV-associated URI based on the presence of risk factors for progression to severe disease, such as the presence of lymphopenia.[134,135]

To date, the only available antiviral therapy for RSV infection is aerosolized ribavirin.[49,116] RSV-IVIG is derived from pooled adult plasma containing high titers of neutralizing antibodies against RSV. Monotherapy with RSV-IVIG may modify RSV infections.[126] In recent years, the use of aerosolized ribavirin plus RSV-IVIG has been associated with better outcomes than available previously in patients with RSV LRIs, especially when treatment is initiated early during the infection; however, these results were not obtained in randomized trials.[116,120,126,134,135] For HSCT recipients, the prompt use of this combination approach resulted in a dramatic decrease in the overall mortality rate from 100% to less than 40%.[116,126,143] However, the benefit of combining aerosolized ribavirin with IVIG in HSCT recipients remains to be elucidated in prospective controlled clinical trials, as does the benefit of using standard IVIG preparations rather than antibody preparations containing high titers of RSV-neutralizing antibody or RSV-specific monoclonal antibody.[135,140]

Initial treatment options for uncomplicated influenza A viral infection include amantadine, rimantadine, oseltamivir, and zanamivir. Amantadine and rimantadine are chemically related antiviral drugs with the same target (M2) and are effective in the treatment of influenza A infection.[96,116] Oseltamivir and zanamivir belong to a new class of antiviral agents, the neuraminidase inhibitors, which are active against both influenza A and B viruses and are approved for the treatment of influenza infections.[96,116] Treatment options for uncomplicated influenza B viral infections include oseltamivir and zanamivir. The results of noncontrolled studies have shown that oseltamivir might be more effective than rimantadine for the treatment of influenza virus–associated URIs and LRIs.[117] Ribavirin is a broad-spectrum antiviral agent with activity against RNA and DNA viruses, including influenza A and B viruses, PIV, and RSV.[48] Few clinical studies exist on ribavirin in treating influenza infection.

The idea of combination antiviral therapy for treatment of severe influenza infections has not been explored in controlled trials.[116] Combination therapy of M2 and neuraminidase inhibitors can be considered for severe disease; however, published data are limited.[117] Compared with single agents, combinations of ribavirin with amantadine or rimantadine have shown enhanced antiviral activity in vitro and in animal models of influenza A infection.[144] Ribavirin could be used in combination with neuraminidase inhibitors for life-threatening influenza B infections. Antiviral therapy against influenza virus infections should be administered for at least 5 days in patients with hematologic malignancies because a shorter duration of therapy might be associated with progression to an LRI in high-risk patients.[142]

Currently, no licensed antiviral therapy is available for treating severe PIV infections. Ribavirin is active against PIV in vitro but possesses only marginal activity in vivo.[116,124] Several investigators have reported that successful outcomes with ribavirin depended on early initiation of therapy, that is, when the virus was confined to the upper respiratory tract.[116,145] However, PIV infections appear to be less responsive than RSV infections to treatment with aerosolized ribavirin.[128] Ribavirin has also failed to shorten the time for PIV shedding in HSCT recipients.[129] Although the combination of IVIG and ribavirin has also been used to treat PIV-associated LRIs, the results have been inconclusive.[116,129]

In the absence of optimal therapy against CRV infections in HSCT recipients and cancer patients, preventing such infections is of the utmost importance. RSV-IVIG has been used for prevention of severe RSV-associated LRIs in children with chronic lung disease or a history of premature birth.[116] The development of palivizumab, a monoclonal antibody directed against RSV, has provided another option for preventing RSV infection.[116] The mainstay of influenza prophylaxis in the general population is the inactivated influenza vaccine.[116] Prophylactic oral antiviral therapy against influenza viruses may be warranted for patients in high-risk groups if vaccination is contraindicated or if supplies of vaccine are insufficient.[116] Antiviral drugs currently approved for influenza chemoprophylaxis include amantadine, rimantadine, and oseltamivir.[116] Amantadine and rimantadine are equally effective in preventing influenza A infection, with efficacy rates of 70 to 90% in controlled trials.[116] Neuraminidase inhibitors are highly effective in prophylaxis[146]; the side-effect profile appears to be more favorable than that of M2 inhibitors. Surveillance, vaccination of contacts, and preemptive antiviral therapy might also minimize the effect of influenza infection in HSCT recipients.[62,117]

Finally, the use of infection control measures is important and has dramatically reduced the incidence of CRV infections.[126] At M. D. Anderson Cancer Center and the Fred Hutchinson Cancer Research Center, patients are screened for CRV infections before they undergo stem cell transplantation if they are symptomatic, and transplantation is delayed if a URI is present.[62,147] Whether all transplants must be delayed (including autologous transplants for multiple myeloma) remains controversial,[138] and more research is needed to identify patients who can safely be transplanted. PCR testing might prove useful in this regard in future. Meanwhile, we favor delaying transplantation in patients with URI. Patients are encouraged to wash their hands frequently, visits to patients are limited, and both visitors and staff must wear masks and gloves when entering the rooms of patients with URI symptoms.[126] Whether a general mask policy (even during contact with uninfected patients) is effective remains controversial. Contact of family members, visitors, and staff with uncontrolled respiratory secretions should be minimized. In addition, patients should be placed in respiratory isolation conditions until they are symptom free and respiratory samples yield negative microbiologic results.[117,126]

Summary

Clinical and epidemiologic studies have suggested that many viruses may be associated with carcinogenesis. In addition, viral infections are important causes of morbidity and mortality in HSCT recipients and patients with hematologic malignancies. Less is known about the effect of these infections on other subsets of cancer patients. The risk factors for developing a severe viral infection need better definition to permit identification of high-risk patients who may benefit from preventive measures and/or early diagnosis and therapy. Because of the suboptimal response of these infections to the currently available antiviral therapies, new antiviral agents are needed. Finally, prevention remains the most important approach in this patient population, and infection control measures are of paramount importance.

REFERENCES

1. Kinlen L. Infections and immune factors in cancer: the role of epidemiology. Oncogene 2004;23:6341–8.
2. Carbone M, Klein G, Gruber J, Wong M. Modern criteria to establish human cancer etiology. Cancer Res 2004;64:5518–24.
3. Khalili K, Del Valle L, Otte J, et al. Human neurotropic polyomavirus, JCV, and its role in carcinogenesis. Oncogene 2003;22:5181–91.
4. Thompson MP, Kurzrock R. Epstein-Barr virus and cancer. Clin Cancer Res 2004;10:803–21.
5. Chen YC, Chen JH, Richard K, et al. Lung adenocarcinoma and human papillomavirus infection. Cancer 2004;101:1428–36.
6. Haverkos HW. Viruses, chemicals and co-carcinogenesis. Oncogene 2004;23:6492–9.
7. Butel JS. Viral carcinogenesis: revelation of molecular mechanisms and etiology of human disease. Carcinogenesis 2000;21:405–26.
8. Epstein MA, Achong BG, Barr YM. Virus particles in cultured lymphoblasts from Burkitt's lymphoma. Lancet 1964;15:702–3.
9. Chang Y, Cesarman E, Pessin MS, et al. Identification of herpesvirus-like DNA sequences in AIDS-associated Kaposi's sarcoma. Science 1994;266:1865–9.
10. Aoki Y, Tosato G. Neoplastic conditions in the context of HIV-1 infection. Curr HIV Res 2004;2:343–9.
11. Haverkos HW, Kopstein AN, Wilson H, Drotman P. Nitrite inhalants: history, epidemiology, and possible links to AIDS. Environ Health Perspect 1994;102:858–61.
12. Ziegler JL, Simonart T, Snoeck R. Kaposi's sarcoma, oncogenic viruses, and iron. J Clin Virol 2001;20:127–30.
13. Beasley RP, Hwang LY, Lin CC, Chien CS. Hepatocellular carcinoma and hepatitis B virus. A prospective study of 22 707 men in Taiwan. Lancet 1981;2:1129–33.
14. Colombo M, Kuo G, Choo QL, et al. Prevalence of antibodies to hepatitis C virus in Italian patients with hepatocellular carcinoma. Lancet 1989;2:1006–8.
15. Vallisa D, Berte R, Rocca A, et al. Association between hepatitis C virus and non-Hodgkin's lymphoma, and effects of viral infection on histologic subtype and clinical course. Am J Med 1999;106:556–60.
16. de Sanjose S, Nieters A, Goedert JJ, et al. Role of hepatitis C virus infection in malignant lymphoma in Spain. Int J Cancer 2004;111:81–5.
17. Isikdogan A, Ayyildiz O, Dursun M, et al. Hepatitis C virus in patients with non-Hodgkin's lymphoma in southeastern Anatolia region of Turkey: a prospective case-control study of 119 patients. Leuk Lymphoma 2003;44:1745–7.
18. Castellsague X, Munoz N. Cofactors in human papillomavirus carcinogenesis—role of parity, oral contraceptives, and tobacco smoking. J Natl Cancer Inst Monogr 2003;31:20–8.
19. Almeida G, do Val I, Gondim C, et al. Human papillomavirus, Epstein-Barr virus and p53 mutation in vulvar intraepithelial neoplasia. J Reprod Med 2004;49:796–9.
20. Hafkamp HC, Manni JJ, Speel EJ. Role of human papillomavirus in the development of head and neck squamous cell carcinomas. Acta Otolaryngol (Stockh) 2004;124:520–6.
21. Wu QJ, Guo M, Lu ZM, et al. Detection of human papillomavirus-16 in ovarian malignancy. Br J Cancer 2003;89:672–5.
22. Almadori G, Cadoni G, Cattani P, et al. Human papillomavirus infection and epidermal growth factor receptor expression in primary laryngeal squamous cell carcinoma. Clin Cancer Res 2001;7:3988–93.
23. Carbone M, Pass HI, Miele L, Bocchetta M. New developments about the association of SV40 with human mesothelioma. Oncogene 2003;22:5173–80.
24. Serraino D. The spectrum of AIDS-associated cancers in Africa. AIDS 1999;13:2589–90.
25. Chang MH, Chen CJ, Lai MS, et al. Universal hepatitis B vaccination in Taiwan and the incidence of hepatocellular carcinoma in children. Taiwan Childhood Hepatoma Study Group. N Engl J Med 1997;336:1855–9.
26. Galloway DA. Papillomavirus vaccines in clinical trials. Lancet Infect Dis 2003;3:469–75.
27. Gigliotti AR, Fioredda F, Giacchino R. Hepatitis B and C infection in children undergoing chemotherapy or bone marrow transplantation. J Pediatr Hematol Oncol 2003;25:184–92.
28. Lai CL, Ratziu V, Yuen MF, Poynard T. Viral hepatitis B. Lancet 2003;362:2089–94.
29. Poynard T, Yuen MF, Ratziu V, Lai CL. Viral hepatitis C. Lancet 2003;362:2095–100.
30. Hyams KC. Risks of chronicity following acute hepatitis B virus infection: a review. Clin Infect Dis 1995;20:992–1000.
31. Liang RH, Lok AS, Lai CL, et al. Hepatitis B infection in patients with lymphomas. Hematol Oncol 1990;8:261–70.

32. Picardi M, Pane F, Quintarelli C, et al. Hepatitis B virus reactivation after fludarabine-based regimens for indolent non-Hodgkin's lymphomas: high prevalence of acquired viral genomic mutations. Haematologica 2003; 88:1296–303.

33. Yeo W, Chan PK, Zhong S, et al. Frequency of hepatitis B virus reactivation in cancer patients undergoing cytotoxic chemotherapy: a prospective study of 626 patients with identification of risk factors. J Med Virol 2000;62: 299–307.

34. Ozguroglu M, Bilici A, Turna H, Serdengecti S. Reactivation of hepatitis B virus infection with cytotoxic therapy in non-Hodgkin's lymphoma. Med Oncol 2004;21:67–72.

35. Keeffe EB. Hepatitis B virus reactivation with chemotherapy: diagnosis and prevention with antiviral prophylaxis. Rev Gastroenterol Disord 2004;4:46–8.

36. Steinberg JL, Yeo W, Zhong S, et al. Hepatitis B virus reactivation in patients undergoing cytotoxic chemotherapy for solid tumours: precore/core mutations may play an important role. J Med Virol 2000;60:249–55.

37. Strasser SI, McDonald GB. Hepatitis viruses and hematopoietic cell transplantation: a guide to patient and donor management. Blood 1999;93:1127–36.

38. Idilman R, Arat M, Soydan E, et al. Lamivudine prophylaxis for prevention of chemotherapy-induced hepatitis B virus reactivation in hepatitis B virus carriers with malignancies. J Viral Hepat 2004;11:141–7.

39. Yeo W, Zee B, Zhong S, et al. Comprehensive analysis of risk factors associating with hepatitis B virus (HBV) reactivation in cancer patients undergoing cytotoxic chemotherapy. Br J Cancer 2004;90:1306–11.

40. Lau GK, Leung YH, Fong DY, et al. High hepatitis B virus (HBV) DNA viral load as the most important risk factor for HBV reactivation in patients positive for HBV surface antigen undergoing autologous hematopoietic cell transplantation. Blood 2002;99:2324–30.

41. Dervite I, Hober D, Morel P. Acute hepatitis B in a patient with antibodies to hepatitis B surface antigen who was receiving rituximab. N Engl J Med 2001;344:68–9.

42. Ishiga K, Kawatani T, Suou T, et al. Fulminant hepatitis type B after chemotherapy in a serologically negative hepatitis B virus carrier with acute myelogenous leukemia. Int J Hematol 2001;73:115–8.

43. Senecal D, Pichon E, Dubois F, et al. Acute hepatitis B after autologous stem cell transplantation in a man previously infected by hepatitis B virus. Bone Marrow Transplant 1999;24:1243–4.

44. Yeo W, Chan PK, Hui P, et al. Hepatitis B virus reactivation in breast cancer patients receiving cytotoxic chemotherapy: a prospective study. J Med Virol 2003;70:553–61.

45. Noble S, Goa KL. Adefovir dipivoxil. Drugs 1999;58:479–87; discussion 488–9.

46. De Clercq E. Antiviral drugs in current clinical use. J Clin Virol 2004;30:115–33.

47. Papatheodoridis GV, Hadziyannis SJ. Review article: current management of chronic hepatitis B. Aliment Pharmacol Ther 2004;19:25–37.

48. Keating MR. Antiviral agents for non-human immunodeficiency virus infections. Mayo Clin Proc 1999;74: 1266–83.

49. De Clercq E. Antivirals and antiviral strategies. Nat Rev Microbiol 2004;2:704–20.

50. Matthews SJ, McCoy C. Peginterferon alfa-2a: a review of approved and investigational uses. Clin Ther 2004;26: 991–1025.

51. Maguire CM, Crawford DH, Hourigan LF, et al. Case report: lamivudine therapy for submassive hepatic necrosis due to reactivation of hepatitis B following chemotherapy. J Gastroenterol Hepatol 1999;14:801–3.

52. Heider U, Fleissner C, Zavrski I, et al. Treatment of refractory chronic lymphocytic leukemia with Campath-1H in combination with lamivudine in chronic hepatitis B infection. Eur J Haematol 2004;72:64–6.

53. Lau GK, Liang R, Wu PC, et al. Use of famciclovir to prevent HBV reactivation in HBsAg-positive recipients after allogeneic bone marrow transplantation. J Hepatol 1998;28: 359–68.

54. Zein NN. The epidemiology and natural history of hepatitis C virus infection. Cleve Clin J Med 2003;70 Suppl 4: S2–6.

55. Locasciulli A, Testa M, Pontisso P, et al. Prevalence and natural history of hepatitis C infection in patients cured of childhood leukemia. Blood 1997;90:4628–33.

56. Pawlotsky JM. Use and interpretation of virological tests for hepatitis C. Hepatology. 2002 Nov; 36:(5 Suppl 1): S65–73.

57. Smith AD, Rockey DC. Viral hepatitis C. Lancet 2004; 363:661.

58. Ljungman P, Andersson J, Aschan J, et al. Oral ribavirin for prevention of severe liver disease caused by hepatitis C virus during allogeneic bone marrow transplantation. Clin Infect Dis 1996;23:167–9.

59. Corrao G, Arico S. Independent and combined action of hepatitis C virus infection and alcohol consumption on the risk of symptomatic liver cirrhosis. Hepatology 1998;27:914–9.

60. Heathcote J. Weighty issues in hepatitis C. Gut 2002;51:7–8.

61. Mascitelli L, Pezzetta F. Viral hepatitis C. Lancet 2004;363: 661.

62. Centers for Disease Control and Prevention. Guidelines for preventing opportunistic infections among hematopoietic stem cell transplant recipients: recommendations of CDC, the Infectious Disease Society of America, and the American Society of Blood and Marrow Transplantation. MMWR Morb Mortal Wkly Rep 2000;49:1–128.

63. Stocchi R, Ward KN, Fanin R, et al. Management of human cytomegalovirus infection and disease after allogeneic bone marrow transplantation. Haematologica 1999;84: 71–9.

64. Konoplev S, Champlin RE, Giralt S, et al. Cytomegalovirus pneumonia in adult autologous blood and marrow transplant recipients. Bone Marrow Transplant 2001;27: 877–81.

65. Nguyen Q, Champlin R, Giralt S, et al. Late cytomegalovirus pneumonia in adult allogeneic blood and marrow transplant recipients. Clin Infect Dis 1999;28:618–23.

66. Nguyen Q, Estey E, Raad I, et al. Cytomegalovirus pneumonia in adults with leukemia: an emerging problem. Clin Infect Dis 2001;32:539 45.

67. Chemaly RF, Torres HA, Hachem RY, et al. Cytomegalovirus pneumonia in patients with lymphoma. Cancer. 2005;104: 1213–20

68. Torres HA, Kontoyiannis DP, Aguilera EA, et al. Cytomegalovirus infection in patients with lymphoma: an important cause of morbidity and mortality. Clin Lymphoma Myeloma. 2006;6:393–8.

69. Torres HA, Kontoyiannis DP, Bodey GP, et al. Gastrointestinal cytomegalovirus disease in patients with cancer: a two decade experience in a tertiary care cancer center. Eur J Cancer. 2005;41:2268–79

70. Bodey GP, Wertlake PT, Douglas G, Levin RH. Cytomegalic inclusion disease in patients with acute leukemia. Ann Intern Med 1965;62:899–906.

71. Gallant JE, Moore RD, Richman DD, et al. Incidence and natural history of cytomegalovirus disease in patients with advanced human immunodeficiency virus disease treated with zidovudine. The Zidovudine Epidemiology Study Group. J Infect Dis 1992;166:1223–7.

72. Crippa F, Corey L, Chuang EL, et al. Virological, clinical, and ophthalmologic features of cytomegalovirus retinitis after hematopoietic stem cell transplantation. Clin Infect Dis 2001;32:214–9.

73. Ljungman P. Cytomegalovirus infections in transplant patients. Scand J Infect Dis Suppl 1996;100:59–63.

74. Ljungman P. Cytomegalovirus pneumonia: presentation, diagnosis, and treatment. Semin Respir Infect 1995;10: 209–15.

75. Crumpacker C, Marlowe S, Zhang JL, et al. Treatment of cytomegalovirus pneumonia. Rev Infect Dis 1988;10 Suppl 3:S538–46.

76. Lundin J, Hagberg H, Repp R, et al. Phase 2 study of alemtuzumab (anti-CD52 monoclonal antibody) in patients with advanced mycosis fungoides/Sezary syndrome. Blood 2003;101:4267–72.

77. Nguyen DD, Cao TM, Dugan K, et al. Cytomegalovirus viremia during Campath-1H therapy for relapsed and refractory chronic lymphocytic leukemia and prolymphocytic leukemia. Clin Lymphoma 2002;3:105–10.

78. Maltezou H, Whimbey E, Abi-Said D, et al. Cytomegalovirus disease in adult marrow transplant recipients receiving ganciclovir prophylaxis: a retrospective study. Bone Marrow Transplant 1999;24:665–9.

79. Meyers JD, Ljungman P, Fisher LD. Cytomegalovirus excretion as a predictor of cytomegalovirus disease after marrow transplantation: importance of cytomegalovirus viremia. J Infect Dis 1990;162:373–80.

80. Salomon N, Perlman DC. Cytomegalovirus pneumonia. Semin Respir Infect 1999;14:353–8.

81. Riddell SR. Pathogenesis of cytomegalovirus pneumonia in immunocompromised hosts. Semin Respir Infect 1995;10: 199–208.

82. Rook AH. Interactions of cytomegalovirus with the human immune system. Rev Infect Dis 1988;10 Suppl 3:S460–7.

83. Marr KA, Carter RA, Boeckh M, et al. Invasive aspergillosis in allogeneic stem cell transplant recipients: changes in epidemiology and risk factors. Blood 2002;100:4358–66.

84. Torres HA, Chemaly RF, Storey R, et al. Influence of type of cancer and hematopoietic stem cell transplantation on clinical presentation of Pneumocystis jiroveci pneumonia in cancer patients. Eur J Clin Microbiol Infect Dis. 2006 Jun;25(6):382–8.

85. de la Hoz RE, Stephens G, Sherlock C. Diagnosis and treatment approaches of CMV infections in adult patients. J Clin Virol 2002;25 Suppl 2:S1–12.

86. Goldstein LC, McDougall J, Hackman R, et al. Monoclonal antibodies to cytomegalovirus: rapid identification of clinical isolates and preliminary use in diagnosis of cytomegalovirus pneumonia. Infect Immun 1982;38:273–81.

87. Gleaves CA, Smith TF, Shuster EA, Pearson GR. Comparison of standard tube and shell vial cell culture techniques for the detection of cytomegalovirus in clinical specimens. J Clin Microbiol 1985;21:217–21.

88. Nicholson VA, Whimbey E, Champlin R, et al. Comparison of cytomegalovirus antigenemia and shell vial culture in allogeneic marrow transplantation recipients receiving ganciclovir prophylaxis. Bone Marrow Transplant 1997; 19:37–41.

89. Emanuel D, Peppard J, Stover D, et al. Rapid immunodiagnosis of cytomegalovirus pneumonia by bronchoalveolar lavage using human and murine monoclonal antibodies. Ann Intern Med 1986;104:476–81.

90. Gerna G, Baldanti F, Lilleri D, et al. Human cytomegalovirus pp67 mRNAemia versus pp65 antigenemia for guiding preemptive therapy in heart and lung transplant recipients: a prospective, randomized, controlled, open-label trial. Transplantation 2003;75:1012–9.

91. Blank BS, Meenhorst PL, Pauw W, et al. Detection of late pp67-mRNA by NASBA in peripheral blood for the diagnosis of human cytomegalovirus disease in AIDS patients. J Clin Virol 2002;25:29–38.

92. Boeckh M, Bowden RA, Goodrich JM, et al. Cytomegalovirus antigen detection in peripheral blood leukocytes after allogeneic marrow transplantation. Blood 1992;80: 1358–64.

93. Ikewaki J, Ohtsuka E, Kawano R, et al. Real-time PCR assay compared to nested PCR and antigenemia assays for detecting cytomegalovirus reactivation in adult T-cell leukemia-lymphoma patients. J Clin Microbiol 2003;41: 4382–7.

94. Boeckh M, Boivin G. Quantitation of cytomegalovirus: methodologic aspects and clinical applications. Clin Microbiol Rev 1998;11:533–54.

95. Crawford SW, Bowden RA, Hackman RC, et al. Rapid detection of cytomegalovirus pulmonary infection by bronchoalveolar lavage and centrifugation culture. Ann Intern Med 1988;108:180–5.

96. Reusser P. Management of viral infections in immunocompromised cancer patients. Swiss Med Wkly 2002;132: 374–8.

97. Lalezari JP, Stagg RJ, Kuppermann BD, et al. Intravenous cidofovir for peripheral cytomegalovirus retinitis in patients with AIDS. A randomized, controlled trial. Ann Intern Med 1997;126:257–63.

98. Ljungman P, Deliliers GL, Platzbecker U, et al. Cidofovir for cytomegalovirus infection and disease in allogeneic stem cell transplant recipients. The Infectious Diseases Working Party of the European Group for Blood and Marrow Transplantation. Blood 2001;97:388–92.

99. Avery RK, Bolwell BJ, Yen-Lieberman B, et al. Use of leflunomide in an allogeneic bone marrow transplant recipient with refractory cytomegalovirus infection. Bone Marrow Transplant 2004;34:1071–5.

100. Boeckh M, Nichols WG, Papanicolaou G, et al. Cytomegalovirus in hematopoietic stem cell transplant recipients: current status, known challenges, and future strategies. Biol Blood Marrow Transplant 2003;9:543–58.

101. Einsele H, Hebart H. CMV-specific immunotherapy. Hum Immunol 2004;65:558–64.

102. Beral V, Newton R. Overview of the epidemiology of immunodeficiency-associated cancers. J Natl Cancer Inst Monogr. 1998;23:1–6.

103. Goedert JJ, Cote TR, Virgo P, et al. Spectrum of AIDS-associated malignant disorders. Lancet 1998;351:1833–9.

104. Chokunonga E, Levy LM, Bassett MT, et al. AIDS and cancer in Africa: the evolving epidemic in Zimbabwe. AIDS 1999;13:2583–8.

105. Moore RD, Kessler H, Richman DD, et al. Non-Hodgkin's lymphoma in patients with advanced HIV infection treated with zidovudine. JAMA 1991;265:2208–11.

106. Parkin DM, Wabinga H, Nambooze S, Wabwire-Mangen F. AIDS-related cancers in Africa: maturation of the epidemic in Uganda. AIDS 1999;13:2563–70.

107. Gates AE, Kaplan LD. AIDS malignancies in the era of highly active antiretroviral therapy. Oncology (Huntingt) 2002;16:657–65; 668–70.

108. Pantanowitz L, Dezube BJ. Advances in the pathobiology and treatment of Kaposi sarcoma. Curr Opin Oncol 2004;16:443–9.

109. Nasti G, Martellotta F, Berretta M, et al. Impact of highly active antiretroviral therapy on the presenting features and outcome of patients with acquired immunodeficiency syndrome-related Kaposi sarcoma. Cancer 2003;98:2440–6.

110. Newell ME, Hoy JF, Cooper SG, et al. Human immunodeficiency virus-related primary central nervous system lymphoma: factors influencing survival in 111 patients. Cancer 2004;100:2627–36.

111. Lewden C, Salmon D, Morlat P, et al. Causes of death among human immunodeficiency virus (HIV)-infected adults in the era of potent antiretroviral therapy: emerging role of hepatitis and cancers, persistent role of AIDS. Int J Epidemiol. 2005;34(1):121–30.

112. Noy A. Update in HIV-associated lymphoma. Curr Opin Oncol 2004;16:450–4.

113. Knowles DM, Chamulak GA, Subar M, et al. Lymphoid neoplasia associated with the acquired immunodeficiency syndrome (AIDS). The New York University Medical Center experience with 105 patients (1981-1986). Ann Intern Med 1988;108:744–53.

114. Batara JF, Grossman SA. Primary central nervous system lymphomas. Curr Opin Neurol 2003;16:671–5.

115. Chadwick EG, Connor EJ, Hanson IC, et al. Tumors of smooth-muscle origin in HIV-infected children. JAMA 1990;263:3182–4.

116. Hicks KL, Chemaly RF, Kontoyiannis DP. Common community respiratory viruses in patients with cancer: more than just "common colds." Cancer 2003;97:2576–87.

117. Nichols WG, Guthrie KA, Corey L, Boeckh M. Influenza infections after hematopoietic stem cell transplantation: risk factors, mortality, and the effect of antiviral therapy. Clin Infect Dis 2004;39:1300–6.

118. Martino R, Ramila E, Rabella N, et al. Respiratory virus infections in adults with hematologic malignancies: a prospective study. Clin Infect Dis 2003;36:1–8.

119. Machado CM, Boas LS, Mendes AV, et al. Low mortality rates related to respiratory virus infections after bone marrow transplantation. Bone Marrow Transplant 2003;31:695–700.

120. Whimbey E, Champlin RE, Couch RB, et al. Community respiratory virus infections among hospitalized adult bone marrow transplant recipients. Clin Infect Dis 1996;22:778–82.

121. Bowden RA. Respiratory virus infections after marrow transplant: the Fred Hutchinson Cancer Research Center experience. Am J Med. 1997;102(3A):27–30.

122. Ison MG, Hayden FG, Kaiser L, et al. Rhinovirus infections in hematopoietic stem cell transplant recipients with pneumonia. Clin Infect Dis 2003;36:1139–43.

123. Gonzalez Y, Martino R, Rabella N, et al. Community respiratory virus infections in patients with hematologic malignancies. Haematologica 1999;84:820–3.

124. Whimbey E, Englund JA, Couch RB. Community respiratory virus infections in immunocompromised patients with cancer. Am J Med 1997;102:10–8.

125. Whimbey E, Couch RB, Englund JA, et al. Respiratory syncytial virus pneumonia in hospitalized adult patients with leukemia. Clin Infect Dis 1995;21:376–9.

126. Champlin RE, Whimbey E. Community respiratory virus infections in bone marrow transplant recipients: the M.D. Anderson Cancer Center experience. Biol Blood Marrow Transplant 2001;7 Suppl:8S–10S.

127. Ljungman P, Ward KN, Crooks BN, et al. Respiratory virus infections after stem cell transplantation: a prospective study from the Infectious Diseases Working Party of the European Group for Blood and Marrow Transplantation. Bone Marrow Transplant 2001;28:479–84.

128. Nichols WG, Gooley T, Boeckh M. Community-acquired respiratory syncytial virus and parainfluenza virus infections after hematopoietic stem cell transplantation: the Fred Hutchinson Cancer Research Center experience. Biol Blood Marrow Transplant 2001;7 Suppl:11S–5S.

129. Nichols WG, Corey L, Gooley T, et al. Parainfluenza virus infections after hematopoietic stem cell transplantation: risk factors, response to antiviral therapy, and effect on transplant outcome. Blood 2001;98:573–8.

130. Marcolini JA, Malik S, Suki D, et al. Respiratory disease due to parainfluenza virus in adult leukemia patients. Eur J Clin Microbiol Infect Dis 2003;22:79–84.

131. Couch RB, Englund JA, Whimbey E. Respiratory viral infections in immunocompetent and immunocompromised persons. Am J Med 1997;102:2–9; discussion 25–6.

132. Ljungman P. Respiratory virus infections in bone marrow transplant recipients: the European perspective. Am J Med 1997;102:44–7.

133. Raboni SM, Nogueira MB, Tsuchiya LR, et al. Respiratory tract viral infections in bone marrow transplant patients. Transplantation 2003;76:142–6.

134. Ghosh S, Champlin RE, Englund J, et al. Respiratory syncytial virus upper respiratory tract illnesses in adult blood and marrow transplant recipients: combination therapy with aerosolized ribavirin and intravenous immunoglobulin. Bone Marrow Transplant 2000;25:751–5.

135. Ghosh S, Champlin RE, Ueno NT, et al. Respiratory syncytial virus infections in autologous blood and marrow transplant recipients with breast cancer: combination therapy with aerosolized ribavirin and parenteral immunoglobulins. Bone Marrow Transplant 2001;28:271–5.

136. Elting LS, Whimbey E, Lo W, et al. Epidemiology of influenza A virus infection in patients with acute or chronic leukemia. Support Care Cancer 1995;3:198–202.

137. Yousuf HM, Englund J, Couch R, et al. Influenza among hospitalized adults with leukemia. Clin Infect Dis 1997;24:1095–9.

138. Anaissie EJ, Mahfouz TH, Aslan T, et al. The natural history of respiratory syncytial virus infection in cancer and transplant patients: implications for management. Blood 2004;103:1611–7.

139. Chien JW, Martin PJ, Gooley TA, et al. Airflow obstruction after myeloablative allogeneic hematopoietic stem cell transplantation. Am J Respir Crit Care Med 2003;168:208–14.

140. Boeckh M, Berrey MM, Bowden RA, et al. Phase 1 evaluation of the respiratory syncytial virus-specific monoclonal antibody palivizumab in recipients of hematopoietic stem cell transplants. J Infect Dis 2001;184:350–4.

141. Abdallah A, Rowland KE, Schepetiuk SK, et al. An outbreak of respiratory syncytial virus infection in a bone marrow transplant unit: effect on engraftment and outcome of pneumonia without specific antiviral treatment. Bone Marrow Transplant 2003;32:195–203.

142. Aguilera EA, Torres HA, Gonzalez VR, et al. The impact of influenza epidemic with a predominant mismatched circulating strain with the vaccine strain on patients with hematologic malignancies during winter 2003-2004 [abstract]. In: Abstracts of the 1st Meeting on Internal Medicine & The Cancer Patient. Houston; 2004.

143. Whimbey E, Champlin RE, Englund JA, et al. Combination therapy with aerosolized ribavirin and intravenous immunoglobulin for respiratory syncytial virus disease in adult bone marrow transplant recipients. Bone Marrow Transplant 1995;16:393–9.

144. Hayden FG. Combination antiviral therapy for respiratory virus infections. Antiviral Res 1996;29:45–8.

145. Hohenthal U, Nikoskelainen J, Vainionpaa R, et al. Parainfluenza virus type 3 infections in a hematology unit. Bone Marrow Transplant 2001;27:295–300.

146. Cooper NJ, Sutton AJ, Abrams KR, et al. Effectiveness of neuraminidase inhibitors in treatment and prevention of influenza A and B: systematic review and meta-analyses of randomised controlled trials. BMJ 2003;326:1235.

147. Peck AJ, Corey L, Boeckh M. Pretransplantation respiratory syncytial virus infection: impact of a strategy to delay transplantation. Clin Infect Dis 2004;39:673–80.

Fungal Infections in Immunocompromised Hosts with Cancer

Dimitrios P. Kontoyiannis, MD, ScD

Russell E. Lewis, Pharm D

T. J. Walsh, MD

For many years, the major focus of attention in the study of infectious complications of cancer was on bacterial infections. In recent years, however, with the use of more aggressive therapies, widespread use of human stem cell transplantation, and the ability to control most bacterial infections, fungal infections have emerged as serious and frequently fatal complications in patients with cancer, especially those with acute leukemia and recipients of human stem cell transplants (HSCTs).[1-4] This chapter provides an overview of modern antifungal agents and the current issues regarding the most important mycoses that internists encounter in patients with cancer.

Overview of Antifungal Agents

Until the early 1990s, treatment of life-threatening invasive fungal infections was essentially limited to the use of only one antifungal agent, amphotericin B (AMB) deoxycholate (AMB-d).[5] The introduction of several new antifungal agents with activity against opportunistic yeasts and molds has provided new treatment options, however.[2,6,7] Currently, 13 antifungals are licensed for the treatment of invasive mycoses. These drugs belong principally to four classes: polyenes, pyrimidines, azoles, and echinocandins (Table 1). No ideal antifungals for the treatment of deep mycoses have been identified, and the drug of choice is influenced by many factors, such as the specific type of fungal infection, its site, and the presence of comorbidities (Table 2). Consequently, selection of antifungal therapy should be an individualized process with careful consideration of the disease severity, potential for organ toxicity, and drug interactions.

Amphotericin B

For decades, conventional AMB has been considered the gold standard for the treatment of deeply invasive fungal infections.[5] However, the significant toxic effects of the conventional AMB formulation, which include infusion-related fever, rigors, headache, dose-limiting nephrotoxicity, and anemia, often limit the effectiveness of this agent in severely ill patients.[5] Consequently, lipid-based formulations of AMB (eg, AmBisome, Abelcet, Amphotec) that offer the advantages of fewer infusion-related side effects and reduced nephrotoxicity were developed.[6,8] The dose equivalency of these formulations differs from that of conventional AMB-d, with the requirement of lipid formulation doses three- to five-fold higher (in mg/kg) for similar efficacy.[6,8] When AMB is incorporated into a lipid carrier, the pharmacokinetics of the drug change depending on the particle size of the formulation. The larger-particle formulations (Abelcet and Amphotec) are rapidly removed from the bloodstream by macrophages and other cells of the reticuloendothelial system and deposited into deep tissue sites such as the liver, spleen, and lung, resulting in more rapid clearance from the bloodstream relative to the standard AMB formulation.[6] In contrast, the smaller-particle liposomal AMB formulation (AmBisome) circulates in the bloodstream for longer periods before being sequestered into deep tissue sites.[6] Therefore, clearance of this formulation and the volume of its distribution are lower than those of AMB.[6] The clinical impact of these pharmacokinetic differences between different AMB formulations is unclear.[8] All three lipid formulations accumulate to a lesser degree in the kidneys when compared with the standard AMB formulation, however, which accounts for their reduced rates of nephrotoxicity.

Despite the improved therapeutic index of these lipid formulations of AMB, there are still relatively few data from prospective clinical trials suggesting that these considerably more expensive formulations are more effective than conventional AMB. Moreover, the 10- to 20-fold higher acquisition cost of the lipid formulations has required many institutions to restrict their use to patients with preexisting renal failure or those at high risk of nephrotoxicity while receiving AMB (eg, patients receiving concomitant nephrotoxic drugs). Currently, there is no consensus regarding the clinical or pharmacoeconomic threshold for using lipid AMB formulations as first-line therapy for most invasive mycoses in patients with cancer. Cost-effective use of these formulations relies on institution-specific factors, including their acquisition (primary) costs and secondary costs (eg, increased length of stay; use of a pharmacy, blood bank, laboratory, and radiology services) associated with managing the additional toxic effects of the standard AMB formulation.

The most common acute toxic effects of all AMB formulations are infusion-related reactions, which are characterized by fever, chills, rigors, anorexia, nausea, vomiting, myalgia, arthralgia, and headache.[5] Hypotension, flushing, and dizziness are less common, but bronchospasm and true anaphylactic reactions have been reported with both the conventional and lipid formulations of AMB. Severe hypokalemia and cardiac arrhythmia have also been reported in patients with a central venous catheter in place who received a rapid infusion or excessive dose of the conventional AMB formulation.[5] Therefore, slower infusion rates (more than 4–6 hours) and electrocardiogram monitoring should be considered for patients with underlying cardiac conduction abnormalities. Because thrombophlebitis is a common local side effect with infusion into a peripheral vein, use of a central venous catheter is required if AMB will be administered for more than 1 week.[5] Slower infusion rates, rotation of infusion sites, application of hot packs, use of low-dose heparin, and avoidance of AMB concentrations greater than 1 g/L can minimize thrombophlebitis.

Table 1 Systemic Antifungal Therapies

Antifungals	Trade Name(s)	Usual Adult Dose	Mechanism of Action	Toxic Effects	Spectrum/Comments
Polyenes AMB Lipid formulations of AMB Liposomal AMB ABLC ABCD	Fungizone AmBisome, Abelcet, Amphotec	0.25–1.50 mg/kg IV q24h 3–10 mg/kg/q24h 5 mg/kg/q24h 3–4 mg/kg/q24h	Binds to ergosterol and intercalates the fungal cell membrane, resulting in increased membrane permeability to univalent and divalent cations Delayed: azotemia (26%), tubular acidosis, hypokalemia, hypomagnesemia, anemia	Acute: fever, chills, rigor, arthralgia with infusion Thrombophlebitis, dyspnea (rare), arrhythmia (rare)	Drug of choice for severe infections caused by endemic dimorphic fungi, most *Candida* spp, and common α-hylohyphomycetes (*Aspergillus, Zygomycetes*) Nephrotoxicity is the dose-limiting side effect, which is reduced with lipid AMB formulations and saline before and after hydration Infusion-related reactions: AmBisome < Abelcet < Amphotec AmBisome is considered the preferred formulation for central nervous system mycoses
Fluoropyrimidines Flucytosine (5-FC)	Ancobon	100 mg/kg/d PO divided q6h Dosage adjustment required in renal impairment	Drug is transported into susceptible fungi by cytosine permease and then deaminated to active form (5-fluorouracil) by cytosine deaminase where the drug interferes with DNA/RNA synthesis	Increase in serum transaminase levels (7%); nausea and vomiting (5%); diarrhea, abdominal pain, rash, enterocolitis (rare) Less common: leukopenia, thrombocytopenia, anemia	Narrow spectrum for deep mycoses: *Candida* and *C. neoformans* only. Resistance is common when used as monotherapy. Typically administered in combination with AMB for cryptococcal meningitis. Risk of bone marrow suppression is increased with persistent flucytosine levels >100 µg/mL. Careful dosage adjustment is required for patients with renal dysfunction.
Azoles Ketoconazole	Nizoral	200–800 mg PO q24h Divided doses recommended at doses of 400 mg/d or greater	Inhibition of cytochrome P-450 14-α-demethylase decreased production of ergosterol, accumulation of lanosterol leading to perturbation of fungal cell membrane, fungistasis	Gastrointestinal (20–50%) including nausea and vomiting, anorexia, rash (2%), transient increases in hepatic enzyme levels, severe hepatotoxicity (rare), alopecia, inhibition of adrenal steroid synthesis (especially at dosages > 600 mg/d)	Oral formulation only. Inconsistencies in oral absorption/poor gastrointestinal tolerance limits use for treatment of deep mycoses Potent inhibition of mammalian cytochrome P-450 can lead to potentially severe drug interactions when administered concomitantly with other P-450-metabolized drugs

Table 1 Continued

Antifungals	Trade Name(s)	Usual Adult Dose	Mechanism of Action	Toxic Effects	Spectrum/Comments
Itraconazole	Sporanox	200–400 mg PO q24h, IV 200–400 mg q12h, and then q24h Divided doses recommended at ≥ 400 mg/d	Similar to ketoconazole but more selective for fungal P-450 demethylase	Gastrointestinal (20%) including nausea and vomiting, diarrhea, rash (2%), taste disturbance (oral solution), transient increases in hepatic enzymes, severe hepatotoxicity (rare), alopecia, inhibition of adrenal steroid synthesis (especially at dosages > 600 mg/d) Accumulation of hydroxypropyl-β-cyclodextran vehicle in patients with creatine clearance < 30 mL/min (intravenous formulation); consider switch to oral therapy if possible Congestive heart failure (rare)	Spectrum similar to fluconazole with enhanced activity against C. krusei and Aspergillus. Not active against Fusarium or Zygomycetes. Drug of choice for mild to moderate infections caused by endemic dimorphic fungi. Bioavailability of oral solution is improved over capsules by 30% under fed conditions and 60% under fasting conditions. Potent inhibitor of mammalian cytochrome P-450 enzymes. Serum level monitoring is occasionally recommended; trough levels measured by high-performance liquid chromatography should exceed 0.5 μg/mL.
Fluconazole	Diflucan	100–800 mg PO/IV q24h Dosage adjustment required for renal impairment	Similar to ketoconazole but a more selective inhibitor of cytochrome P-450 enzyme 14-β-demethylase	Gastrointestinal (5–10%), rash, headache, transient increases in hepatic enzyme levels, hepatotoxicity (rare), alopecia	Spectrum includes most Candida spp. C. neoformans, and endemic dimorphic fungi. Less active against C. glabrata. C. krusei is intrinsically resistant. Not clinically active for deep mycoses caused by invasive molds. Best tolerated of the azoles. Higher daily dosages are recommended (eg, 12 mg/kg/d) for critically ill patients or in institutions where C. glabrata infection is common (> 10% of all Candida spp). Inhibitor of mammalian cytochrome P-450 enzymes
Voriconazole	Vfend	6 mg/kg IV q12h for two doses and then 4 mg/kg q12h 200 mg PO q12h if ≥ 40 kg, 100 mg PO q12h if < 40 kg	Similar to fluconazole but with greater affinity for fungal cytochrome P-450 enzyme 14-α-demethylase	Transient visual disturbances (reported up to 30%), rash, hallucinations (2%), transient increases in hepatic enzyme levels, severe hepatotoxicity (rare) Accumulation of sulfobutyl ester cyclodextran vehicle may occur in patients with CrCl < 50 mL/min receiving intravenous formulation	Spectrum similar to itraconazole with enhanced activity against Aspergillus, Fusarium, and Scedosporium apiospermum. Retains activity against some fluconazole-resistant C. glabrata, but cross-resistance is possible. Considered by many experts as the initial drug of choice for invasive aspergillosis Inhibitor of mammalian cytochrome P-450 enzymes

Table 1 Continued

Antifungals	Trade Name(s)	Usual Adult Dose	Mechanism of Action	Toxic Effects	Spectrum/Comments
Posaconazole	Noxafil	200 mg PO q6h for 7 d and then 400 mg q12h / Dose-proportional saturable oral absorption	Similar to voriconazole	Gastrointestinal (5–15%), fever, headache, musculoskeletal pain (5%)	Spectrum similar to voriconazole with enhanced activity against *Fusarium, Zygomycetes,* and black molds (phaeohyphomycetes) molds (phaeohyphomycetes) Inhibitor of mammalian cytochrome P-450 3A4
Echinocandins					
Caspofungin	Cancidas	70 mg IV on day 1 and then 50 mg q24h	Inhibition of cell wall glucan synthesis leading to osmotic instability of fungal cell	Fever, chills, phlebitis/thrombophelibitis (peripheral line), rash; drug concentrations decrease with P-450 3A4 inducers; decreases tacrolimus blood levels by 25%; increases liver toxicity with cyclosporine?	Spectrum includes most *Candida* spp, including fluconazole-resistant *C. krusei* and *C. glabrata.* Higher dosages may be required for *C. parapsilosis.* Active against *Aspergillus* spp. Not active against *C. neoformans, Fusarium, Zygomycetes,* or black molds (phaeohyphomycetes)
Micafungin	Mycamine	50–100 mg IV q24h	Similar to caspofungin	Similar to caspofungin	Similar to caspofungin
Anidulafungin	Eraxis	200 mg IV on day 1 and then 100 mg/d	Similar to caspofungin	Similar to caspofungin	Similar to caspofungin

ABCD = amphotericin B cholesterol dispersion; ABLC = amphotericin B lipid complex; AMB = amphotericin B; DNA = deoxyribonucleic acid; IV = intravenously; PO = orally; q6h = every 6 hours; q12h = every 12 hours; q24h = every 24 hours; RNA = ribonucleic acid.

Table 2 Common Mycoses and Treatment

Mycoses	Recommended Therapy*	Alternative Therapies	Comment
Primary mycoses			
Histoplasmosis*			
Mild to moderate	Observation or itraconazole 200 mg PO daily for 6–12 wk	Itraconazole 200 mg PO daily for 6–12 weeks or IV 200 mg q12h for 1 d and then 200 mg q24h (non-CNS disease only) or fluconazole 800 mg PO daily for 6–12 wk	Itraconazole is not effective for CNS infections Fluconazole is less effective but better tolerated than itraconazole
Severe, including CNS disease or immunocompromised host	AMB 0.7 mg/kg/d IV or L-AMB 3 mg/kg/d for 12 wk or until clinically stable	AMB 0.7 mg/kg/d IV or L-AMB 3 mg/kg/d until clinically stable	Lipid formulations may be more effective than conventional formulations, especially for CNS disease. Once the patient is clinically stable, he or she can be transitioned to itraconazole or fluconazole. Corticosteroid therapy should be considered for hypoxic patients with acute pulmonary infection
Blastomycosis*			
Mild to moderate	Itraconazole 200 mg PO daily × 6 mo	Ketoconazole 400–800 mg PO daily or fluconazole 400–800 mg PO daily; L-AMB formulations	Relapses are common in immunocompromised hosts. Suppressive therapy with itraconazole 200 mg PO/d or fluconazole 800 mg PO/d is recommended.
Severe, including CNS or immunocompromised host	AMB 0.7 mg/kg/d IV until patient is clinically stable and then itraconazole (non-CNS) or fluconazole 800 mg PO daily for 6 mo		

Table 2 Continued

Mycoses	Recommended Therapy*	Alternative Therapies	Comment
Coccidioidomycosis*			
Mild to moderate	Observation or itraconazole 200 mg PO twice daily for 6–8 mo	Fluconazole 400–800 mg PO daily or L-AMB formulations	Itraconazole demonstrated a trend toward superiority over fluconazole in a randomized controlled trial for progressive, nonmeningeal coccidioidomycosis; however, fluconazole is better tolerated than itraconazole
Diffuse pneumonia or disseminated infection	AMB 1.0–1.5 mg/kg/d with dose and frequency decreased as improvement occurs		Fluconazole 800–1,000 mg/d may be preferred for meningitis
Opportunistic mycoses			
Candidiasis*			
Catheter related and acute hematogenous	Two weeks of antifungal therapy: AMB 0.7 mg/kg/d IV or fluconazole 400–800 mg IV q24h or caspofungin 70 mg IV for 1 and then 50 mg q24h or AMB plus fluconazole	L-AMB formulations or AMB 0.5–0.7 mg/kg/d plus flucytosine 100 mg/kg/d PO divided q6h or voriconazole 6 mg/kg q12h for 1 d and then 3–4 mg/kg q12h; itraconazole 200 mg q12h for 2 d and then 200 mg IV q24h	Patients can be switched to oral fluconazole when clinically stable if isolate is susceptible. Caspofungin and AMB are the preferred agents for fluconazole-resistant species. Voriconazole appears to be effective against fluconazole-resistant *Candida krusei*.
Empiric therapy in neutropenic patients	Fluconazole 400–800 mg/d (low risk) or AMB 0.7 mg/kg/d IV or itraconazole 200 mg q12h for 2 d and then 200 mg IV q24h or L-AMB 3 mg/kg q24h	Caspofungin 70 mg IV for 1 d and then 50 mg q24h or voriconazole 6 mg/kg q12h for 1 d and then 3–4 mg/kg q12h	Antifungals with coverage of *Aspergillus* should be used in higher-risk patients and those with prolonged neutropenia (> 2 wk)
Urinary candidiasis	Fluconazole 200 mg IV or PO for 7–14 d	AMB 0.3 mg/kg/d IV for 1–7 d; AMB bladder irrigation effective only for infection in the bladder	Asymptomatic candiduria does not require therapy. However, treatment is recommended for neutropenic, low birth weight infants and patients undergoing urologic manipulation or with renal allografts.
Cryptococcosis*			
Pulmonary, isolated	Fluconazole 200–400 mg/d IV or PO for 6–12 mo	AMB 0.7–1.0 mg/kg/d plus flucytosine 100 mg/kg/d PO divided for 6–10 wk	L-AMB was shown to produce faster sterilization of CSF when compared with conventional AMB-d and was less nephrotoxic
Severe or disseminated disease, including CNS	Induction: AMB 0.7–1.0 mg/kg/d plus flucytosine 100 mg/kg/d PO divided q6h for 2 wk; Consolidation: fluconazole 400–800 mg/d for 10 wk	AMB 0.7–1.0 mg/kg/d for 6–10 wk; L-AMB 5 mg/kg/d for 6–10 wk	
Invasive aspergillosis†	Voriconazole 6 mg/kg q12h for 1 d and then 4 mg/kg q12h	L-AMB or AMB 1.0–1.5 mg/kg/d or caspofungin 70 mg IV for one dose and then 50 mg IV q12h or posaconazole§ 200 mg PO QID × 14 d and then 200 mg PO q12h or combination therapy	Voriconazole can be administered as oral therapy in patients taking oral medications. Because of the high dosages and prolonged treatment courses, lipid formulations are preferred for AMB-based therapy. Preclinical studies suggest mold-active azoles plus echinocandins have enhanced activity against *Aspergillus*
Invasive fusariosis†	L-AMB or voriconazole 6 mg/kg q12h for 1 d and then 4 mg/kg q12h	Posaconazole§ 200 mg PO QID for 14 d and then 200 mg PO q12h or combination therapy	Activity of AMB and voriconazole is decreased versus *Aspergillus* spp. Higher doses or combination therapy may be indicated for more refractory cases.
Invasive zygomycosis†	High-dose L-AMB (eg, 7.5–10.0 mg/kg/d)	Posaconazole§ 200 mg PO QID for 14 d and then 200 mg PO q12h or combination therapy	Prompt diagnosis and surgical débridement are essential for successful outcome. High dosages of L-AMB are required. Posaconazole is the only azole with activity against zygomycoses.

AMB = amphotericin B; AMB-d = amphotericin B deoxycholate; CNS = central nervous system; CSF = cerebrospinal fluid; IV = intravenously; L-AMB = lipid formulation of amphotericin B; PO = orally; q6h = every 6 hours; q12 = every 12 hours; q24 = every 24 hours..

*Based on guidelines published by the Infectious Diseases Society of America.

†Not part of the guidelines of the Infectious Diseases Society of America.

‡Lipid formulations of AMB (L-AMB, 3–5 mg/kg IV q24h; AMB lipid complex, 5 mg/kg IV q24h; or AMB cholesterol dispersion, 3–4 mg/kg IV q24h).

§Investigational.

Acute reactions to AMB generally subside over time and with subsequent infusions of it. Use of lipid formulations reduces, to varying degrees, the incidence of infusion-related reactions. Interestingly, the concentration of each AMB formulation (% weight/volume) may play a role in the incidence of infusion reactions. AmBisome (10% w/v) has the lowest incidence of reactions, followed by Abelcet (34% w/v) and conventional AMB-d (35% w/v). The cholesterol dispersion lipid formulation of AMB (Amphotec) has both the highest concentration of AMB (50% w/v) and the highest reported rates of infusion-related reactions. Lipid AMB formulations have also been associated with a unique triad of acute infusion-related reactions, including dyspnea; severe abdominal, flank, and/or leg pain; and flushing and urticaria. Most of these reactions can be effectively managed by administration of diphenhydramine and interruption of the lipid AMB infusion. In the past, administration of a test dose of AMB-d (eg, 1–5 mg) was recommended prior to initiating therapy, but this is no longer considered useful for screening patients for hypersensitivity reactions. Premedication with agents such as low-dose hydrocortisone (1 mg/kg), diphenhydramine, meperidine (0.5 mg/kg), and nonsteroidal anti-inflammatory agents may be performed prior to AMB infusions to blunt symptoms of acute reactions, although the data from organized clinical trails supporting their routine use are limited. Premedication should also be considered with the use of lipid AMB formulations, even though their infusion reactions are somewhat less severe (formulation dependent) when compared with those of the conventional AMB formulation.

Nephrotoxicity is the most significant delayed toxic effect of AMB and can be classified by glomerular and tubular mechanisms.[5] AMB directly constricts the afferent arteriole, resulting in a decrease in both renal blood flow and glomerular filtration (increased serum creatinine), eventually leading to azotemia (increased blood urea nitrogen). AMB-induced azotemia can be delayed by ensuring that patients are well hydrated prior to starting therapy and sodium loading (intravenously administering 0.5–1.0 L of normal saline before and after infusing AMB) to maintain renal blood flow and adequate glomerular filtration pressure. Although the exact amount of sodium needed to reduce nephrotoxicity is unknown, studies in human adults receiving AMB-d have examined the use of 85 to 600 mg/d of sodium before AMB administration.[5] Although several recent uncontrolled studies have suggested that administration of AMB-d by continuous infusion can delay glomerular toxic effects, this dosing approach is not widely recommended. Azotemia with AMB administration is generally reversible, although 5 to 10% of patients may have persistent renal impairment after discontinuation of therapy.

Distal tubular membrane damage caused by AMB leads to Fanconi-like syndrome with impaired urinary acidification, defective urinary concentrating ability, and potassium and magnesium wasting.[5] Hypokalemia in particular is common in patients receiving either conventional or lipid formulations of AMB and may require the administration of up to 15 mEq of supplemental potassium per hour. Hypokalemia and hypomagnesemia frequently precede decreases in glomerular filtration (increased serum creatinine level), especially in patients who are adequately hydrated or receiving lipid formulations of AMB. However, continued tubular damage eventually results in decreases in renal blood flow and glomerular filtration through tubuloglomerular feedback mechanisms that constrict the afferent arteriole. Therefore, renal protective measures, such as sodium loading, should still be considered for patients receiving lipid AMB formulations.

Prolonged courses of treatment with AMB may result in normochromic, normocytic anemia owing to the inhibitory effects of AMB on renal erythropoietin synthesis.[1,2] Patients with diseases other than cancer may experience decreases in hemoglobin of 15 to 35% below baseline that will return to normal within several months of discontinuation of the drug; these decreases may be even more severe in patients with cancer. Administration of recombinant erythropoietin has been suggested for patients with symptomatic anemia during AMB administration.

5-Flucytosine

Flucytosine is the fluoropyrimidine approved for the treatment of invasive fungal infections and is available only as an oral capsule formulation.[6] The usefulness of flucytosine in treating invasive mycoses is hampered by its relatively narrow spectrum, high rates of acquired resistance in common pathogens (ie, *Candida* spp), and significant potential for toxic effects. Thus, flucytosine is not used as monotherapy and has a narrowly defined role in the treatment of most mycoses. Because flucytosine is widely distributed throughout the body, including the cerebrospinal fluid (CSF), after oral administration, it is a useful adjuvant to antifungals with slow or minimal distribution into anatomically privileged sites, such as the meninges.

Flucytosine was originally developed as an antitumor chemotherapeutic agent before it was discovered to have antifungal activity against common yeast.[6] Not surprisingly, its most common side effects are nausea and vomiting, increases in serum transaminase levels, and bone marrow suppression.[6] The risk of bone marrow suppression can be reduced if serum levels are maintained at less than 100 μg/mL. Because flucytosine is eliminated unchanged through the kidneys, serum level monitoring and dosage adjustment are required for patients receiving flucytosine in combination with AMB or other nephrotoxic agents.

Azole Antifungals

The availability of azole antifungals, particularly the oral triazoles itraconazole, fluconazole, and, most recently, voriconazole, fulfills a critical need for effective and better tolerated alternatives to AMB.[2,6,7] Fluconazole, itraconazole, and voriconazole have proven to be valuable agents in the prevention and treatment of both primary and opportunistic mycoses. All three triazoles are available in tablet or capsule form, oral solution or suspension, and intravenous formulations, providing clinicians with added flexibility in therapy selection. Because all azoles are potentially teratogenic, their use should be avoided in pregnant women.

Fluconazole

Of the triazoles, fluconazole (Diflucan) is clearly the best tolerated and has the most desirable pharmacologic properties, including high bioavailability, high water solubility, a low degree of protein binding, linear pharmacokinetics, and a wide volume of distribution, including the CSF, eye, and urine.[6,7] Fluconazole has a more limited spectrum of activity than itraconazole does, including most *Candida* spp (except *Candida krusei* and, in certain cases, *Candida glabrata*) and *Cryptococcus neoformans*, and it is a second-line agent for *Histoplasma capsulatum*, *Blastomyces dermatitidis*, and *Coccidioides immitis*. Fluconazole[6,7] does not have clinically useful activity against molds such as *Aspergillus*. Unlike other azoles, fluconazole is eliminated primarily unchanged through the kidneys and is less susceptible to clinically significant drug interactions through mammalian cytochrome P-450 enzymes at standard dosages used to treat superficial (100–200 mg/d) or systemic (400–800 mg/d) infections. However, administration of higher dosages of fluconazole (eg, 800 mg/d) may result in more pronounced cytochrome P-450 inhibition.

Itraconazole

Itraconazole (Sporanox) was introduced in the early 1990s as a capsule formulation that was effective against superficial fungal infections and mild to moderately severe endemic mycoses. However, its erratic absorption in critically ill patients limited its effectiveness against opportunistic mycoses. The subsequent reformulation of itraconazole into an oral and intravenous solution with hydroxy-β-propyl cyclodextran significantly improved the blood levels of the agent that could be obtained in critically ill and immunocompromised patients. Specifically, administration of the oral liquid formulation results in a 30% higher area under the curve (AUC) over 24 hours under fed conditions and 60% higher AUC under fasting conditions. Itraconazole is a relatively broad-spectrum triazole with activity against many common fungal pathogens, including most *Candida* spp, *Cryptococcus*, endemic dimorphic fungi (*H. capsulatum*, *B. dermatitidis*, and *C. immitis*), and *Aspergillus* spp.[6,7] This drug is lipophilic and highly protein bound and has a long half-life, nonlinear pharmacokinetics, and limited distribution into some body fluids, including the CSF and urine. Itraconazole is metabolized in the liver and, to a lesser extent, the gut into more hydrophilic metabolites, one of which (hydroxyitraconazole) retains potent antifungal activity.

The most common adverse effects of oral itraconazole therapy are gastrointestinal effects, rash, and asymptomatic increases in hepatic transaminase levels. Cases of severe idiosyncratic hepatitis have been reported infrequently in patients receiving itraconazole therapy. Prolonged therapy with itraconazole can be associated with metabolic disturbances (suppression of adrenal steroid synthesis) and increased risk of congestive heart failure. Itraconazole is a substrate and potent inhibitor of mammalian cytochrome P-450 enzymes and is therefore susceptible to a number of clinically significant drug interactions (see Azole Drug Interactions). When administered as an oral solution, the cyclodextran vehicle used to dissolve itraconazole is passed through the gastrointestinal tract with minimal metabolism.[7] In the intravenous formulation, however, cyclodextran must be cleared through the kidneys. This vehicle may accumulate in patients with moderate to severe renal dysfunction (eg, estimated creatinine clearance of < 30 mL/min), which in animal studies has been associated with toxic effects in the bladder epithelium.[7] Although these effects have not been observed in humans, patients with poor renal function who are candidates for itraconazole should be preferentially given the oral formulation of itraconazole unless the potential benefits of the intravenous formulation high blood levels) outweigh the theoretical risk.

Voriconazole

Voriconazole (Vfend) is a methylated analogue of fluconazole with enhanced activity against yeast and important opportunistic molds, including *Aspergillus* and *Fusarium* spp.[6,7] Voriconazole is not active, however, against *Zygomycetes*. In terms of its clinical pharmacology, voriconazole has characteristics of both fluconazole and itraconazole. Like fluconazole, voriconazole is well absorbed orally, has limited protein binding, and is distributed widely throughout the body, including the CSF. Like itraconazole, intravenous voriconazole is formulated in a cyclodextran solution (sulfobutylether cyclodextran) and has nonlinear pharmacokinetics and similar precautions for its use in patients with marked renal dysfunction. Voriconazole is metabolized into inactive metabolites through the liver and is an inhibitor of mammalian cytochrome P-450 enzymes. In addition to the common adverse effects seen with other triazoles (gastrointestinal effects, rash, increases in hepatic enzyme levels), voriconazole causes transient visual disturbances in 15 to 30% of patients, manifesting as photophobia, perception of blinking or flashing lights (even with the eyes closed), and, occasionally, hazy or blurred vision. These side effects tend to occur during the first week of therapy and disappear with continued therapy in most patients. Occasionally, visual disturbances are intensified by hallucinations, a separate side effect seen in 2 to 8% of patients receiving voriconazole (often with concomitant benzodiazepines and narcotic analgesic therapy). These visual disturbances are thought to result from temporary alterations in electrical conduction of photoreceptors in the rods and cones of the retina, which revert to normal once therapy is stopped. No permanent damage to the retina has been noted in human or animal studies of voriconazole.

The dose-limiting toxicity of voriconazole, like that of most azole antifungals, is hepatic toxicity that initially presents with asymptomatic increases in serum transaminase levels. Generally, these increases are reversible and transient and do not require discontinuation of therapy. However, serious hepatic reactions during treatment with voriconazole and other azoles have been reported, including clinical hepatitis, cholestasis, and fulminant hepatic failure. These reactions often occur when an azole is administered concomitantly with other hepatotoxic drugs. Liver function tests should be evaluated at the start of and during the course of azole therapy. Abnormal elevations in liver function should be routinely monitored, and azole therapy should be discontinued if severe hepatic impairment develops.

Posaconazole

Posaconazde (Noxafil) is a recently approved oral triazole for the treatment and prevention of invasive fungal intections. This agent has a very broad spectrum of activity against yeasts and molds, including the Zygomycetes[7]. Posaconazole is given orally 2–4 times a day. It is widely distributed in the Body metabolized by the liver, and well tolerated, even in long-term.

Azole Drug Interactions

An inherent limitation of azole pharmacology is that the target of their antifungal activity, the cytochrome P-450 enzyme 14-α-demethylase, shares considerable homology with mammalian cytochrome P-450 enzymes involved in drug metabolism.[5] Thus, azole antifungals are both substrates and inhibitors of cytochrome P-450 systems in humans. Not surprisingly, these drugs have many interactions with the metabolism of other drugs; many of these interactions have the potential to result in severe clinical outcomes if not detected early. Cytochrome P-450 3A4 inducers increase the metabolism of all azoles to varying degrees depending on their lipophilicity. Coadministration of rifampin, for example, can reduce fluconazole serum concentrations by approximately 50% and itraconazole, voriconazole, and posaconazole concentrations by up to 90%. When possible, azole antifungal therapy should be avoided during high-dose conditioning chemotherapy prior to hematopoietic cell transplantation owing to an increased risk of acute hepatotoxicity and accumulation of toxic chemotherapy metabolites.

Echinocandins

With the introduction of caspofungin (Cancidas) in 2001, the echinocandins became the first truly novel class of antifungal agents to be introduced in more than 40 years.[6] Echinocandins disrupt the integrity of the fungal cell wall by disturbing the synthesis of β-(1,3)-glucan polymers, which are critical cross-linking structural components in the cell wall of *Candida* and *Aspergillus* spp and the mycelial forms of some endemic fungi. Although echinocandin resistance appears to be rare, some *Candida* spp (*C. parapsilosis* and *C. guilliermondii*) may be inherently less susceptible to lower echinocandin concentrations than other species candida due to subtle differences in their β-(1,3)-D-glucan synthase structure. Also, echinocandins have no clinically effective activity against *C. neoformans*. They also appear to have suboptimal in vitro activity against endemic fungi. In most cases, differences in fungal cell wall construction appear to define the spectrum of these agents. For example, the cell walls of *Zygomycetes* spp are constructed primarily of chitin and chitosan polymers, with relatively fewer β-(1,3)-D-glucan synthases, glucuronomannoproteins, and matrix components. Not surprisingly, echinocandins are not effective against *Zygomycetes*.[6]

One echinocandin, caspofungin, has been approved for the treatment of infections by *Candida* and *Aspergillus* spp. Two other echinocandins, micafungin and anidulafungin, were recently approved. Despite some modest differences in pharmacokinetics and potency, the echinocandins are pharmacologically similar and probably interchangeable. All three of these agents are available only as intravenous formulations, have predominantly linear pharmacokinetics, have relatively high tissue concentrations (except in the CSF, eyes, and urine), have a prolonged elimination half-life, and are metabolized mostly through chemical degradation followed by secondary hepatic metabolism (caspofungin and micafungin). Caspofungin dosage adjustment is recommended for patients with severe hepatic dysfunction (Child-Pugh score 7–9). All three echinocandins were well tolerated in phase II and III clinical trials, with the most common adverse effects being phlebitis or venous irritation, headache, fever, and rash. Infusion-related reactions analogous to the ones seen with vancomycin have been described with caspofungin because of its potential to cause histamine release from mast cells. The most common adverse effects reported with echinocandin therapy in the laboratory are transient elevations in serum transaminase and alkaline phosphatase levels. The echinocandins are neither substrates nor inhibitors of cytochrome P-450 enzymes of P-glycoprotein enzymes. For reasons not completely understood, coadministration of echinocandins with inducers of cytochrome P-450 3A4 (eg, rifampin, phenytoin) results in modest (25–50%) decreases in the AUC of these antifungals, which can be overcome with increased dosages. Furthermore, caspofungin modestly (20%) decreases the AUC of concomitant tacrolimus therapy. Coadministration of caspofungin and cyclosporine in early phase I and II trials resulted in increased cyclosporine levels and elevated serum transaminase levels. Although this interaction was not observed in subsequent clinical trials or with other echinocandins, current caspofungin labeling does not recommend coadministration of the drug with cyclosporine unless the benefits outweigh the potential risk of increased hepatotoxicity.

Pathogenesis of Fungal Infections

Multiple, frequently interrelated factors impact the susceptibility of patients with cancer to a variety of fungal infections (Table 3).[3,9,10] *Candida* spp are often part of the patient's endogenous flora,[9] whereas opportunistic molds (eg, *Aspergillus* and *Fusarium* spp) are ubiquitous in the environment.[1,10,11] Although symptoms of infection with these organisms usually develop while the patient is in the hospital, except during periods of

Table 3 Overview of Risk Factors for Candidiasis in Patients with Cancer

Nosocomial factors
  Broad-spectrum antibiotics
  Chemotherapy-induced mucositis
  Central venous catheters
  Systemic corticosteroids
  Major surgery, especially intra-abdominal
  Length of intensive care unit stay
  Total parenteral nutrition
Underlying conditions/comorbidities
  Neutropenia
  Hematologic malignancy
  Diabetes mellitus
  Solid tumors with necrosis
  Pancreatitis
  Chronic renal failure

hospital construction or faulty air handling, most infections are community acquired.[11] Most serious fungal infections occur in patients with cancer who have prolonged, severe neutropenia.[3,9–11] This is not surprising as neutrophils are capable of ingesting and killing *Candida* spp, and neutrophils were found to be the primary defense against the hyphae of *Aspergillus* spp in animal studies.[3,9–11] Administration of high doses of adrenal corticosteroids, especially for protracted periods, predisposes patients to mycoses, especially to aspergillosis and other mold infections.[12] The alveolar macrophages ingest and kill *Aspergillus* spores, and corticosteroids interfere with the fungicidal activity of macrophages.[12] In addition, disruption of mucocutaneous barriers predisposes patients to fungal infections. Furthermore, candidemia[3] and, rarely, *Fusarium* fungemia[13] are associated with the use of intravascular catheters. Local *Aspergillus*[11] and *Zygomycetes* infections[14] have occurred at catheter insertion sites, often leading to disseminated infection. Disseminated fusariosis[13,15] occasionally arises from paronychia caused by skin trauma adjacent to sites of onychomycosis.[13,15] Other sites of tissue damage may also facilitate fungal infections. For example, leukemic infiltrates and chemotherapy-induced ulcerations of the oropharynx and gastrointestinal tract may be sites of origin for disseminated candidiasis.[3,9] Different types of defects in cellular immunity, such as decreased numbers of CD4 T lymphocytes and defects in T-cell signaling, play an important role in predisposing patients to certain fungal infections, such as oropharyngeal candidiasis,[3] cryptococcosis, reactivation of histoplasmosis, and coccidioidomycosis.

Broad-spectrum antibiotic therapy has been associated with fungal infections, especially candidiasis.[3,9] This may be due to suppression of the normal flora, allowing for fungal overgrowth, as has been shown with *Candida* spp in the oropharynx and gastrointestinal tract. Antibacterial and antifungal prophylaxis also may be associated with fungal infections, the latter of which facilitates acquisition of fungi resistant to antifungal agents. For example, fluconazole prophylaxis has been associated with increased colonization and, in some studies, infection with fluconazole-resistant non-*albicans Candida* spp, such as *C. krusei* and *C. glabrata*.[16–20]

Candidiasis

Candidiasis is the most common mycosis in patients with cancer, although its frequency has decreased in recent years because of the widespread use of antifungal prophylaxis, especially with fluconazole, in highly susceptible populations.[16,21] Multiple risk factors predispose patients with cancer to candidiasis (see Table 3). The spectrum of infections caused by *Candida* spp in

cancer patients is broad. Hence, *Candida* spp can cause a range from mild yet uncomfortable superficial infections to major organ and widely disseminated infections.[3]

Although *C. albicans* has accounted for more than 50% of systemic infections for some time, other *Candida* spp that are frequently resistant to fluconazole have emerged as relatively common pathogens in patients with cancer.[16–20] For example, *Candida tropicalis* mimics acute bacterial sepsis in neutropenic patients with leukemia,[22] is more likely to cause the characteristic skin lesions associated with disseminated candidiasis, and occasionally causes a syndrome of skin lesions and painful myositis. *C. glabrata* has variable susceptibility to fluconazole, and increased colonization and infection with this species have been associated with fluconazole prophylaxis.[23] Also, *C. parapsilosis* has been associated with parenteral alimentation and use of intravascular catheters.[3] Finally, *C. krusei* is inherently resistant to fluconazole and has been isolated with increasing frequency of colonization and infection in institutions that use fluconazole prophylactically.[17–19]

Oral Candidiasis

The most common superficial *Candida* infection in patients with cancer who are not receiving prophylaxis is acute pseudomembranous candidiasis of the oropharynx (thrush).[3] This infection occurs following mucosal damage by chemotherapy or radiotherapy, such as patients with head and neck cancer who undergo chemoradiation. The lesions associated with it are creamy, whitish, curd-like plaques or pseudomembranes on the buccal mucosa, palate, or tongue, the exposed base of which is erythematous and painful and may bleed. These lesions may be associated with fissures in the angles of the mouth. Rarely, patients with cancer who have clinically significant thrush also have esophageal involvement manifesting with only mild or moderate odynophagia.

Diagnosis of oral candidiasis is confirmed by the presence of yeasts and pseudohyphae on scraping of an infected area and in culture analysis.[3] Recovery of *Candida* spp from a culture alone is insufficient evidence because these fungi are commonly found as colonies in the oropharyngeal mucosal surfaces, especially in patients who are receiving antibiotics. The most effective therapy for oral candidiasis has been fluconazole, which is well absorbed from the gastrointestinal tract, easy to take, and well tolerated. Some patients have a response to topical agents; however, these agents are not palatable (eg, nystatin, clotrimazole).

Candida Esophagitis

Patients with cancer are also susceptible to esophageal candidiasis.[3] Symptoms of esophageal candidiasis include dysphasia, retrosternal pain, and odynophagia. This infection, if left undetected, can have serious complications, including chronic esophageal strictures, bronchoesophageal fistulae, and mediastinitis. Approximately 70% of patients with *Candida* esophagitis also have thrush; hence, the diagnosis is usually easy to suspect. A barium contrast roentgenogram may show peristaltic abnormalities, spasm, shaggy ulcerations, and a moth-eaten appearance of the mucosa. It is important to recognize, however, that esophagitis in cancer patients has other causes, such as herpes simplex virus and cytomegalovirus. Thus, esophagoscopy with brushing, biopsy, and culture analysis is the only way to confirm the diagnosis of *Candida* esophagitis.[3] Because *Candida* spp are the most common causes of infectious esophagitis, it is usually appropriate to initiate therapy empirically with an antifungal agent and reserve esophagoscopy for patients who do not have a response after several days of therapy, However, esophagitis in cancer patients who have been receiving antifungal prophylaxis should lower the threshold for early esophagoscopy. Fluconazole is the optimal agent for most cases of esophageal candidiasis because it can be initially administered intravenously if necessary and then be administered orally. Caspofungin has been shown to be as effective as fluconazole in acquired immune deficiency syndrome (AIDS) patients, but its use results in slightly higher rates of relapse. Furthermore, caspofungin is available only as an intravenous formulation. Oral itraconazole and intravenous AMB are occasionally indicated for these infections.

Urinary Candidiasis

Primary infections of the urinary tract can develop in patients with cancer if they have a urinary obstruction or a urinary catheter in place.[3] Discriminating between colonization and infection on the basis of quantitative cultures is difficult as no culture density suggests infection. *Candida* casts in the urine are diagnostic but are found infrequently. In addition to cystitis, a *Candida* sp may migrate through the urethra to the renal pelvis in some patients (especially those with diabetes mellitus) and cause a urinary obstruction owing to fungus ball formation or necrotizing papillitis. Candiduria in a febrile neutropenic patient may be a manifestation of a disseminated infection. Fluconazole is the most appropriate agent for this infection.

Disseminated Candidiasis

Disseminated candidiasis usually originates from lesions of the oropharynx or gastrointestinal tract or from intravenous catheters.[3] Sites usually involved include the kidney, heart, muscle, gastrointestinal tract, lung, liver, and spleen. Most patients with cancer who have disseminated candidiasis have no unique signs or symptoms that would differentiate it from other infections. Patients usually are debilitated, have experienced a previous or concomitant bacterial infection, and have persistent or recurrent fever that may be associated with pulmonary infiltrates or deteriorating liver or renal function. Some patients present with acute onset of fever and hypotension, which is suggestive of endotoxic shock.

Eye lesions suggestive of disseminated candidiasis may develop. Therefore, a careful ophthalmologic examination should be performed when this infection is suspected.[3] Typical eye lesions are single or multiple whitish, fluffy exudates with indistinct margins that are sometimes associated with hemorrhaging and borders covered by a vitreous haze. Patients often have no symptoms, although some complain of ocular pain, blurred vision, scotoma, or photophobia. These lesions are rarely found in neutropenic patients because these patients are unable to mount an adequate inflammatory reaction.

Characteristic skin lesions have been described in about 10% of patients with disseminated candidiasis. These lesions may be generalized or localized to the extremities and may be numerous or few.[3] They are nontender, firm, raised nodules that are pink to red in color and do not blanch under pressure. Some patients with these lesions have myositis (usually associated with *C. tropicalis* infection) that manifests as diffuse severe muscle tenderness, which is most pronounced in the legs. *Candida* spp can be identified in the dermis and cultured from about half of biopsy specimens.

Diagnosis of disseminated candidiasis may be difficult as the organism was not isolated from multiple blood culture specimens obtained from up to 40% of patients with widespread infection demonstrated at autopsy examination in previous studies.[3,24] The use of lysis centrifugation and high-volume sensitive culture systems (eg, the BacT/ALERT system, which monitors CO_2 production via infrared detection) has improved the yield of positive blood cultures. A variety of methodologies have been developed to detect circulating *Candida* antigens or metabolites (eg, mannan), including polymerase chain reaction, but none have been entirely satisfactory. Also, the ability to culture *Candida* spp from multiple nonsterile sites (eg, sputum, urine, feces) does not establish the diagnosis of candidiasis. Because the diagnosis may be difficult to establish, empiric administration of antifungal therapy is often appropriate for colonized neutropenic patients who do not have a response to broad-spectrum antibacterial agents, especially if they have not received antifungal prophylaxis.

Chronic Disseminated Candidiasis

A distinct syndrome known as chronic disseminated candidiasis has been described almost exclusively in patients with acute leukemia.[3,25] Typically, these patients have fever that is unresponsive to broad-spectrum antibacterial agents after prolonged periods of neutropenia. After neutropenia is resolved, the patient remains febrile; experiences anorexia, progressive debilitation, and weight loss; and may have hepatosplenomegaly or pain in the right upper quadrant. Also, the patient's alkaline phosphatase level is usually greatly elevated, whereas transaminases and total bilirubin are only mildly elevated. Multiple small lesions can be detected in the liver and spleen by magnetic resonance imaging (MRI), computed tomography (CT), or ultrasonography. The disease can persist for several months despite therapy and interfere with subsequent administration of cytotoxic chemotherapy. The diagnosis of chronic disseminated candidiasis can be confirmed by visualizing hyphae on liver biopsy specimens, but the organism is cultured from only 50% of biopsy specimens. Occasionally, patients may have hypersplenism. This form of candidiasis is rarely seen in leukemic patients receiving treatment at institutions where fluconazole prophylaxis is used routinely.

Candida Pneumonia

Although the lung is usually involved in disseminated *Candida* infections, primary *Candida* pneumonia occurs infrequently in patients with cancer.[3,26] However, aspiration of *Candida*-containing oral secretions and pneumonia may develop in some patients. Isolation of *Candida* spp in clinical specimens from a patient with a pulmonary infiltrate does not establish the diagnosis of *Candida* pneumonia, however. A recent autopsy study of patients with cancer demonstrated that whereas many patients with pneumonia had *Candida* spp cultured from sputum and bronchoalveolar lavage specimens, the specificity and positive predictive value of the cultures were low.[26] Only histopathologic evidence is confirmatory, although it is often impossible to obtain for many patients. Empiric antifungal therapy may be indicated for high-risk patients with cancer who have *Candida*-positive sputum cultures and/or cytology and progressive pulmonary infiltrates despite undergoing broad-spectrum antibacterial therapy.

Candida Meningitis

Multiple small abscesses may be present in the brain in patients with disseminated candidiasis; however, they usually do not have any symptoms.[3] *Candida* meningitis occurs infrequently and is associated with disseminated infection in the majority of cases or the use of ventricular shunts.

There are no specific clinical signs or symptoms that discriminate *Candida* meningitis from bacterial meningitis. Examination of CSF specimens from patients with *Candida* meningitis reveals decreased glucose and elevated protein concentrations and lymphocytosis. *Candida* spp are rarely visualized by direct microscopic examination of CSF, however.

Treatment and Supportive Care

Mortality rates for candidemia and disseminated candidiasis are especially high in patients with cancer and recipients of HSCTs.[27,28] The mortality rates approach 70% in patients who receive AMB-d. Few neutropenic patients survive their infection unless their neutrophil counts recover. AMB-d has been compared with fluconazole in several prospective randomized trials, most of which have excluded neutropenic patients.[29,30] All of these studies showed these two drugs to be essentially equally efficacious, although fluconazole was substantially less toxic. In one study that included patients with neutropenia at the onset of their infection, the response rate for fluconazole was significantly higher, although the number of patients was not large. Whether fluconazole is superior to AMB-d in patients with persistent neutropenia is not certain, but it is unlikely to be worse as few of these patients have a response to AMB-d. Lipid formulations of AMB are less nephrotoxic than AMB-d, but there is no convincing evidence that they are more effective for invasive candidiasis. Because prolonged antifungal therapy is not required for most cases of acute candidiasis, however, the use of these more expensive lipid preparations might not be justified. Finally, the value of routine in vitro susceptibility testing as a guide for selecting antifungal therapy for invasive candidiasis has not been convincingly demonstrated in this population.[31,32]

Given the broad-spectrum activity of caspofungin against *Candida* spp, it would appear to be an ideal agent for treatment of severe *Candida* infections, particularly in patients with preexisting risk factors or underlying renal dysfunction owing to treatment with AMB.[5] Caspofungin, an echinocandin with broad-spectrum fungicidal activity against *Candida* spp,[6] has been compared with AMB-d in therapy for systemic *Candida* infections, 90% of which were candidemia; few neutropenic patients were included in this trial. Caspofungin was found to be at least as effective as AMB-d and considerably less toxic; thus, it has promise in the treatment of candidiasis.[33,34]

Therapy for chronic disseminated candidiasis is often difficult to perform, and the response to it has often been unsatisfactory.[3,25] However, one small study showed that a lipid formulation of AMB was effective against it.[21] A larger study indicated that fluconazole was effective, even in patients who did not have a response to treatment with AMB-d.[25] Evidence of response may require several weeks of therapy. The duration of therapy should be determined according to the rapidity of clinical improvement and resolution of lesions in roentgenographic examinations, ideally, 2 to 6 months.[25] Patients may have residual lesions in the liver and spleen because of scarring.

A controversial issue is whether indwelling intravascular catheters should be removed routinely from patients with candidemia.[35–38] Use of these catheters is often vital to the management of seriously ill patients, and there is considerable expense in removing and replacing surgically implanted catheters. Nevertheless, some but not all studies have shown that catheter removal shortens the duration of candidemia and improves the rate of response to antifungal therapy.[35–38] This is especially true if the infecting organism is *C. parapsilosis*; in such cases, fungemia can persist for more than a week despite the use of appropriate therapy if the catheter is not removed. In vitro studies have shown that caspofungin is more active than azoles or AMB against *Candida* spp growing in biofilm, which characteristically forms on catheters.[39] The clinical significance of this is unclear, however. Figure 1 outlines the general principles of management of acute candidiasis in patients with cancer.

Aspergillosis

Invasive aspergillosis has emerged as an important and significant infection, accounting for 20 to 40% of systemic fungal infections in patients with acute leukemia, 10 to 20% in recipients of bone marrow transplants (BMTs), and 5 to 15% in recipients of solid organ transplants.[1,11,40] On the other hand, this infection is rare in patients with solid tumors.[41] In view of the decreased incidence of candidiasis in the era of azole prophylaxis, this mycosis has emerged as a leading cause of death in patients with leukemia and/or recipients of BMTs.[16,42] Most cases of invasive aspergillosis occur in patients with neutropenia or who are receiving adrenal corticosteroids, which interfere with macrophage function. *Aspergillus fumigatus* is responsible for most of these infections,[1,11] although the frequency of aspergillosis caused by more resistant *Aspergillus* spp, such as *Aspergillus terreus*, may be increasing.[43] In most cases, the infection is acquired by inhalation of spores, and epidemics have occurred in hospitals undergoing construction within the facility itself or in adjacent areas. *Aspergillus* spp invade blood vessels, causing thrombosis and infarction, and can erode through facial planes, cartilage, and bone.

Over 70% of *Aspergillus* infections involve the lung, and some patients may present with symptoms suggestive of pulmonary embolism, such as sudden onset of pleuritic pain, fever, hemoptysis, and a pleural friction rub.[1,11,42] Other patients may present with fever unresponsive to antibacterial agents and may not initially have any abnormalities on chest roentgenograms. A few patients have acute pulmonary hemorrhage that is fatal.

The earliest-appearing abnormality on chest roentgenograms in patients with aspergillosis is

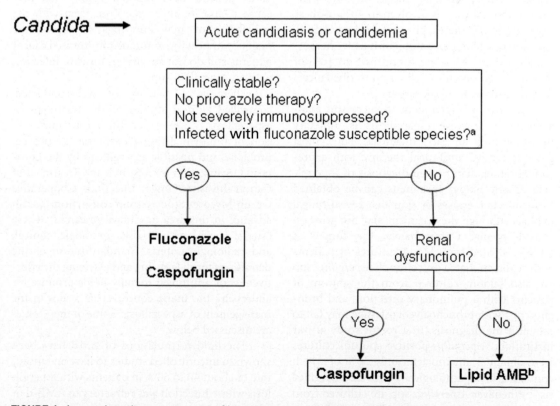

FIGURE 1 Approach to the management of hematogenous candidiasis in the high risk cancer patient.

a single or multiple nodular lesions.[1,11,42] As the infection progresses, wedge-shaped infarcts, necrotizing bronchopneumonia, lobar consolidation, or diffuse infiltrates may be found. Patients with normal roentgenograms should undergo a CT scan, which will usually reveal a nodular infiltrate surrounded by a halo of low attenuation. If the infection is controlled, one or several cavitations usually develop, which often contain a fungus ball.

Approximately 15 to 20% of *Aspergillus* infections in neutropenic patients involve the sinuses.[1] Signs and symptoms include fever, headache, retro-orbital erythema, swelling, and rhinorrhea. Usually, a necrotic lesion can be found on the nose or palate. A CT scan or MRI will show opacification of the sinuses and bony obstructions. As the infection progresses, it causes proptosis, ophthalmoplegia, endophthalmitis, and cerebral infarction. Invasive oral infections involving the gingiva and spreading to facial muscle and bone have been described in patients with leukemia.

Primary invasive cutaneous *Aspergillus* infections have been observed, usually associated with venous access devices.[11] Deposition of *Aspergillus* spores may occur during catheter insertion or subsequent dressing with contaminated materials. The lesions in these cases begin as erythematous or violaceous plaques that progress to necrotic ulcers covered by black eschars.

Hematogenous dissemination occurs in 30 to 40% of *Aspergillus* infections.[1,4,21] The central nervous system is a common site of involvement, resulting in cerebral infarction, which causes neurologic defects, seizures, stupor, or coma. The gastrointestinal tract is involved in 40% of these cases, especially the esophagus and large bowel, which may lead to perforation or massive hemorrhaging. Skin lesions are found in 5 to 10% of patients and evolve into well-circumscribed ulcers that are covered by black eschars.

One major impediment to successful management of invasive aspergillosis is difficulty in establishing an early diagnosis. Thus, most patients receive antifungal therapy with a presumed rather than proven diagnosis of aspergillosis. Tissue biopsy specimens can be obtained from infected sinuses or skin that reveal fungal hyphae, although the organism may not grow on culture media. Unfortunately, the fungus is seldom isolated from blood cultures of patients with a disseminated infection.[44] *Aspergillus* spp are also seldom cultured from the sputum of patients with a pulmonary infection, and bronchoscopy with bronchoalveolar lavage may fail to establish the diagnosis. In a recent study at our institution, *Aspergillus*-positive sputum cultures were obtained antemortem, only 30% of which contained histopathologically proven aspergillosis.[45] Whenever *Aspergillus* spp are cultured from respiratory secretions of susceptible patients, they are either already infected or likely to become infected in the near future.

A variety of noncultural methods have been used to improve early diagnosis of invasive aspergillosis, but most of them have not been entirely satisfactory.[46–49] Serologic methods designed to detect circulating free antigens or immune complexes have been developed by using enzyme-linked immunosorbent assay and radioimmunoassay techniques.[46–51] These procedures have focused on detecting galactomannan and β-(1,3)-D-glucan.[46–52] These tests might underperform in the setting of *Aspergillus*-active antifungal prophylaxis[52] and false-positive reactions with too commonly used antibiotics, such as piperacillin-tazobactan, in patients with cancer.[53] Despite these limitations, attempts have been made to select patients for preemptive therapy who are at high risk of invasive aspergillosis based on antigen detection and imaging techniques. Molecular approaches such as polymerase chain reaction are also promising as diagnostic tools.[46–49,54,55] The role of these newer, non–culture-based methods for therapeutic monitoring in aspergillosis is not clear at present.

Interpreting the results of therapy for aspergillosis is difficult.[56–58] Many patients do not receive treatment until they have advanced disease, whereas others receive treatment for probable or possible but not proven infection. The status of the patient's host defenses is critical to his or her therapeutic response.[58] Neutropenic patients do not have a response unless their neutrophil count recovers during therapy, a factor that is not often reported in the clinical literature. Some patients have residual lesions that may cause relapse of their infection. Even with the availability of new antifungal therapies, the majority of heavily immunocompromised cancer patients still do not survive an invasive infection with an *Aspergillus* spp.

There is a paucity of well-conducted, controlled clinical studies of the treatment of aspergillosis.[56–58] However, the recent introduction of uniform diagnostic criteria for proven, probable, and possible aspergillosis by the European Organization for Research and Treatment of Cancer Invasive Fungal Infections Cooperative Group/Mycoses Study Group consortium was an advance in this area of clinical research.[59] These criteria consist of host-risk, mycologic, clinical, and radiologic criteria. Standardization of the definitions for diagnosing and assessing the effectiveness of antifungal therapy holds promise for addressing the many controversial issues in the management of aspergillosis. Some of these issues are discussed below.

The lipid formulations of AMB have been shown in uncontrolled studies to have an efficacy rate of about 40 to 60% in patients with aspergillosis whose infection was refractory to AMB-d or who could not tolerate it.[8,60] There is a consensus that use of the lipid formulations of AMB decreases nephrotoxicity and infusion-related toxicity,[5] but the daily acquisition prices of these products are much higher than those of AMB-d.[8] The nephrotoxicity in these cases frequently appears to be clinically significant, especially in the most heavily immunosuppressed patients.[61] An even more controversial issue is whether there are clinically meaningful differences in the various lipid formulations of AMB.[8,56] Most of the available data on this have been derived from indirect comparisons and suggest that all of the lipid formulations of AMB, when given at the standard dosage of 5 mg/kg/d, appear to have comparable efficacy.

Although itraconazole has been approved for the treatment of aspergillosis, its role in primary therapy remains to be clarified. In most of the published reports of the efficacy of oral itraconazole, it was administered only to less heavily immunosuppressed patients with aspergillosis[62] as the use of intravenous itraconazole was only recently approved. Therapeutic serum levels of itraconazole can be achieved rapidly and reliably by using the intravenous preparation of the drug. Recent encouraging data from a small open-label multicentered study of aspergillosis indicate that administration of intravenous itraconazole followed by oral itraconazole is safe and reliably results in therapeutic levels of the drug and good response rates.[63] Intravenous itraconazole could be a viable option for primary therapy for aspergillosis, especially in slightly immunosuppressed cancer patients who have a stable clinical picture. However, if there is concern about the bioavailability of itraconazole because of interactions with other concomitantly administered medications, another agent should be used, even in stable patients, unless the itraconazole serum level[5] can be routinely monitored in a timely fashion.

A major advance in the treatment of aspergillosis has been the arrival of new antifungals with improved activity against *Aspergillus* spp, such as voriconazole and caspofungin.[64–67] The new triazoles show impressive in vitro activity in animal models of aspergillosis, and their availability in oral form allows their use in long-term therapy.[6,7] Early clinical experience suggested that they are also active in humans in both salvage therapy and primary therapy for aspergillosis.[64–66] Recently, a large randomized multicenter study comparing treatment with voriconazole and AMB-d followed by other licensed antifungal therapy showed a survival advantage in patients randomized to receive voriconazole.[64] The superiority of voriconazole over the other agents tested was consistent in all of the subgroups studied. Voriconazole likely will become the preferred agent for the majority of cases of documented aspergillosis. Echinocandins are static drugs in vitro against *Aspergillus* spp, but their activity in animal models and selected groups of patients with aspergillosis refractory to or intolerant of other antifungals appears to be promising.[67]

The lack of effective treatment of aspergillosis and availability of new antifungal agents has made the concept of combination therapy for aspergillosis theoretically appealing.[68] To date, no clinical studies have convincingly determined whether therapy with antifungal combinations is more beneficial than that of monotherapy in aspergillosis. For instance, our recent experience suggests that combinations of itraconazole[69] or caspofungin[70] with lipid formulations of AMB are not beneficial. In contrast, a recent small study suggested that the combination of caspofungin and voriconazole is beneficial as salvage therapy for refractory aspergillosis.[71]

The optimal duration of therapy for aspergillosis is uncertain.[56] Such therapy should be highly individualized with respect to resolution of all of the symptoms and signs of the infection, radiologic near-normalization, *Aspergillus*-negative cultures, and, ideally, restoration of the impaired immune defenses.

Pulmonary infarcts and tissue sequestration are common causes of antifungal therapy failure and fatal hemorrhage. Also, the role of adjunctive surgery in the management of aspergillosis has not been addressed in a conclusive way. Early detection of *Aspergillus* lesions by chest CT combined with aggressive combined antifungal and surgical treatment appears to confer a survival advantage,[72] and resection of infected pulmonary tissue has been shown to be beneficial in some patients.[73] After successful antifungal therapy, the presence of residual cavitary lesions, especially those containing fungus balls, may cause late exsanguinating hemorrhage or reactivation of the infection during subsequent myelosuppressive chemotherapy. Removal of these lesions when surgically feasible should be considered and may provide a survival benefit.[73] Surgical intervention may be lifesaving for patients with acute pulmonary hemorrhage, even when performed early in the disease process.

Finally, the role of immunomodulators in the management of aspergillosis remains unresolved.[1,56] As is the case with the other refractory opportunistic mycoses, the beneficial adjunctive role of immunomodulation with cytokines or infusion of immune effector cells in various combinations (eg, granulocyte-macrophage colony-stimulating factor [GM-CSF], granulocyte colony-stimulating factor, interferon-α, GM-CSF-primed white cell transfusions) in cases of refractory or recurrent aspergillosis has been suggestive only in anecdotal clinical reports. However, substantial preclinical evidence supports the role of immunomodulation in the control of *Aspergillus* spp. Further studies are needed in this important area of clinical investigation. Figure 2 outlines the general principles of the management of acute aspergillosis in patients with cancer.

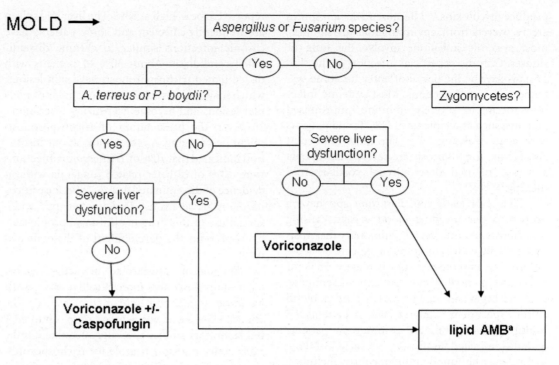

FIGURE 2 Approach to the management of invasive mold infection in the high risk cancer patient.

Zygomycosis

Zygomycosis refers to infections caused by a variety of molds of the order *Mucorales*. These molds are widely distributed in the environment and are usually acquired by inhalation of spores but occasionally are acquired by contamination of open skin lesions or ingestion.[14] Like *Aspergillus* spp, these fungi invade blood vessels, causing thrombosis and infarcts. The types of zygomycosis are rhinocerebral, pulmonary, sinusitis, gastrointestinal cutaneous, and disseminated.[14,74] Sinopulmonary is the most common type of zygomycosis in cancer patients.[74]

Pulmonary macrophages and neutrophils are important host defenses against these infections. Cancer patients susceptible to zygomycosis include recipients of BMTs; patients with acute leukemia, malnutrition, or diabetes mellitus; and patients receiving treatment with adrenal corticosteroids or undergoing hemodialysis and receiving deferoxamine. The presentations of zygomycosis are similar to those of aspergillosis. Although it occurs less frequently than aspergillosis does, zygomycosis appears to be on the rise in patients with cancer.[74,75] Importantly, the increasing use of agents with good activity against *Aspergillus* but no activity against *Zygomycetes* (eg, voriconazole, echinocandins) may increase the incidence of zygomycosis as a breakthrough infection.[76]

The mortality rate of zygomycosis is high in patients with hematologic malignancies. More specifically, the 3-month mortality rate was 71% in a recent unselected cohort of 24 patients with cancer who had definite or probable zygomycosis at The University of Texas M. D. Anderson Cancer Center.[74] The attributable mortality rate in these patients was 92%, and 75% of those who died did so within 4 weeks from the onset of their symptoms. Finally, the outcome of disseminated zygomycosis in the setting of continuous immunosuppression, such as in patients with refractory neutropenia, has been almost uniformly fatal despite the use of aggressive antifungal therapy.

The optimal management of zygomycosis has not been well defined as no prospective studies have evaluated the management of this uncommon infection. The introduction of the lipid formulations of AMB, which have improved the therapeutic index and allow for the delivery of higher daily dosages of the agent,[60] as well as posaconazole, a broad-spectrum triazole with promising preclinical activity against the *Zygomycetes*,[77] has renewed interest in studying new therapeutic strategies for this devastating mycosis. Proper management of ketoacidosis in diabetic patients and use of "radical" surgery with extensive débridement of all necrotic areas is important to recovery from zygomycosis.

The widespread use of voriconazole, a triazole with no inherent activity against the Zygomycetes has been recently associated with a rise in incidence of Zygomywsis in high risk hematology patients.

Fusariosis

Fusarium spp are found in the air and soil throughout the world and are common plant pathogens.[13,15,78] Several of these species have been recognized as human pathogens, including *Fusarium solani*, *Fusarium moniliforme*, *Fusarium oxysporum*, and *Fusarium dimerum*. Some species produce mycotoxins.[13,15] Because *Fusarium* spores are recovered from environmental air samples, most systemic infections involve the lung or sinuses. Chronic superficial infection of the skin or nails may be the portal of entry for some systemic *Fusarium* infections. Most systemic infections occur in severely immunocompromised patients, such as recipients of HSCTs and patients with acute leukemia.[13,15,78] The most important risk factors for fusariosis are severe neutropenia and use of high-dose adrenal corticosteroid therapy.[13,15,78,79]

Like *Aspergillus* spp, *Fusarium* spp have a propensity for invading blood vessels, causing thrombosis and infarcts.[13,15] Pulmonary fusariosis may present with symptoms suggesting an acute pulmonary embolism. Approximately 75% of infections in neutropenic patients disseminate, and the organism can be isolated from blood culture specimens in about 70% of patients.[13,15] Multiple skin lesions are common in patients with disseminated fusariosis.[13,15] A variety of these lesions may be found simultaneously, including red or gray macules, papules (some with central necrosis or an eschar), and pustules.[80] Some patients experience significant myalgia or painful subcutaneous lesions.[15] Occasionally, patients with less severely compromised host defenses may have only localized infections of the skin, such as paronychia, erythematous nodules, hemorrhagic bullae, and tender, progressive necrotic lesions at sites of previous trauma.

The susceptibility of *Fusarium* spp to antifungal agents in vitro has been variable, but, overall, it has been mediocre.[15] Some *Fusarium* isolates are susceptible to new triazoles, such as voriconazole and posaconazole.[6,7] In fact, voriconazole was shown to be active as salvage therapy in a small series of patients with fusariosis.[66] At the present time, no antifungal agent is reliably effective in neutropenic patients with fusariosis, and most patients receive high doses (≥ 5 mg/kg/d) of a lipid formulation of AMB with or without voriconazole. However, in neutropenic patients, recovery of neutrophil production is the most critical factor for a successful outcome.

Trichosporonosis

Trichosporon asahii (*beigelii*) and the related yeast *Blastoschizomyces capitatus* are widely distributed in air, soil, and decaying fruit.[81,82] Infections with these fungii occur predominantly in patients with acute leukemia and recipients of HSCTs. These infections can cause endophthalmitis, meningitis, pneumonia, and osteomyelitis, but more than 80% of the infections are disseminated.[81,82] The organisms can be isolated from blood culture specimens obtained from about 80% of patients with a disseminated infection. The mortality rate in patients with disseminated trichosporonosis who have persistent neutropenia has been

reported to be as high as 80%. The liver and spleen are frequently infected, and some patients have chronic infections similar to chronic disseminated candidiasis. About 30% of patients with disseminated trichosporonosis have skin lesions, which may begin as small maculopapular or nodular lesions and become necrotizing ulcerations. However, the presentation of trichosporonosis might be changing. A recent study at our institution indicated that 70% of *Trichosporon* infections were cases of catheter-related fungemia without evidence of disseminated disease.[83] Because fluconazole is active against *Trichosporon* spp,[5] widespread use of this drug in antifungal prophylaxis likely prevents the development of disseminated infection.

Fluconazole appears to be active against trichosporonosis and more effective than AMB based on animal and human studies.[5,81,82,84] The clinical experience with voriconazole is limited,[85] but laboratory studies have suggested that it is the most active available triazole for trichosporonosis. Animal studies have suggested that combination therapy with AMB plus an azole is the optimal therapy for disseminated trichosporonosis.[84]

Overview of Endemic Mycoses and Cryptococcosis

Endemic mycoses and cryptococcosis are relatively less common causes of morbidity and mortality in patients with cancer, particularly those with chronic deficits in cell-mediated immunity. There is a significant spectrum of manifestations and severity of these infections, ranging from asymptomatic lung nodules to fulminant disseminated infection. Most of these infections occur in patients with hematologic malignancies, especially those with severely suppressed T-cell function.[86–89] These patients are also susceptible to reactivation of latent infections acquired prior to the development of their malignancy. The therapeutic options for endemic mycoses include AMB-d, lipid formulations of AMB (3–5 mg/kg/d),[90–92] and intravenous itraconazole (200 mg given twice daily for 2 days and then once daily). Caspofungin has limited activity, and the experience with voriconazole is very limited at present. AMB-based therapy is preferred for severely ill patients with systemic mycoses who have pneumonia, meningitis, or disseminated infection. Once the patient has improved substantially and is clinically stable, liquid itraconazole (200 mg/d)[89] may be given orally. Therapy should be administered for at least 3 to 6 months or until immunosuppression abates.

Histoplasmosis

Most cases of histoplasmosis in patients with hematologic malignancies are disseminated

infections.[87] Physical findings may include hepatosplenomegaly, mucocutaneous ulcerations (especially in the oral cavity), and signs of central nervous system involvement.[87] *Histoplasma* is visualized or cultured from infected tissues, respiratory secretions, or blood specimens.[87]

Coccidioidomycosis

C. immitis may cause fulminant pneumonia in immunocompromised hosts with high fever, hypoxemia, and diffuse pulmonary infiltrates.[86] Often these patients have a disseminated infection that may involve the skin, bones, and meninges. Skin lesions in cases of coccidioidomycosis may be papular, pustular, nodular, or ulcerative. Although serologic tests are often positive for coccidioidomycosis, the fulminant nature of the infection usually requires a more aggressive diagnostic approach with examination and culture of tissue specimens, sputum, or CSF.

Cryptococcosis

C. neoformans has tropism toward the central nervous system and is a well-known cause of meningitis and disseminated infection in patients with AIDS.[93] Patients with cancer who have a lymphoid malignancy or T-cell dysfunction secondary to systemic corticosteroid use are at high risk of cryptococcosis.[88] However, recent studies have increasingly identified this infection in patients with solid tumors as routine fluconazole prophylaxis is performed less often in these patients.[88] Pulmonary cryptococcosis is the most common presentation of this infection, which often is asymptomatic and could mimic pulmonary malignancy.[88] AMB-d and lipid formulations of AMB (with or without 5-flucytosine) and fluconazole have clinical activity against cryptococcosis.[5,88,93]

Empiric Antifungal Treatment

In autopsy studies of neutropenic patients with cancer who had prolonged fever, 40 to 69% had evidence of an invasive fungal infection.[4] This high incidence, along with the high mortality rate associated with fungal infections (approaching 90% in selected patient groups); difficulties in reliable, timely diagnosis; and a lack of clinical signs and symptoms at the initial stages of the infection in neutropenic patients, led to the introduction of empiric antifungal therapy in the 1980s. Most experts recommend introducing an antifungal drug for patients who remain febrile for 5 or more days despite undergoing an appropriate initial regimen and in whom resolution of neutropenia is not imminent. Some authors prefer to institute antifungal therapy earlier (day 3) or even include antifungals up-front for high-risk patients because of the poor prognosis for infections when treatment is delayed.[94,95]

Regardless, physicians should make individualized decisions about the perceived risk of fungal sepsis and timing and type of antifungals to be administered.[94] For example, for a patient with leukemia and a history of invasive pulmonary aspergillosis, the threshold for initiating antifungal therapy should be very low early on in the setting of febrile neutropenia.[94]

The optimal duration of empiric antifungal treatment in patients with no clinical or microbiologic documentation of an invasive fungal infection has not been established.[94] Again, the key factor is resolution of neutropenia. If neutropenia has resolved and the patient is clinically well, antifungal administration can be discontinued. If neutropenia persists despite defervescence and repeated workup shows no suspicious lesions, antifungal administration can be stopped after 2 weeks. In unstable patients with persistent fever and neutropenia, antifungal treatment should be continued for the entire febrile episode, probably at a more intense level.

For some time, AMB has been the only drug available for antifungal therapy, but its efficacy has been limited by significant nephrotoxicity and infusion-related toxic effects. Thus, efforts have been made to develop new, effective, less toxic antifungal drugs. Lipid formulations of AMB have been introduced and proven to be as effective as AMB, with fewer renal and infusion-related toxic effects in empiric antifungal therapy.[96] However, these formulations are far more expensive than the parent drug, making the pharmacoeconomic threshold for their use unclear in neutropenic patients with persistent fever.

Second- and third-generation triazoles, such as fluconazole,[97] itraconazole,[98] and voriconazole,[99] are frequently used as empiric antifungal treatment regimens. Fluconazole has proven to be an acceptable alternative to AMB provided that the probability of infection with *Aspergillus* or resistant *Candida* spp is low. Patients in this group include those without high-risk leukemia and/or any BMTs, sinusitis, pneumonia, or previous prophylactic or empiric use of fluconazole.[97] Additionally, itraconazole and voriconazole have been found to have similar efficacy but lower toxicity when compared with AMB. In a recently completed large, multi-institutional, prospective, randomized study, caspofungin was compared with liposomal AMB in persistently febrile neutropenic patients. Caspofungin was found to be more efficacious and less toxic than liposomal AMB.[100]

Given the growing number of treatment options for fungal infections, the question is which agent is best for empiric antifungal therapy? In the future, with the introduction of non–culture-based diagnostic methods, such as polymerase chain reaction and antigen detection, empiric antifungal therapy will likely evolve to preemptive antifungal therapy.

Conclusions

Despite the major progress that has been made in the management of mycoses in patients with cancer over the past decade, major challenges remain. The goals for future research include the development of new effective antifungals to overcome the emerging resistant fungal pathogens, refinement of the existing models for risk stratification to reliably identify best therapeutic strategies, and introduction of new non–culture-based modalities for early detection of fungal infection, which will lead to the replacement of empiric therapy with pathogen-specific preemptive therapy.

REFERENCES

1. Wiederhold N, Lewis RE, Kontoyiannis DP. Invasive aspergillosis in patients with hematologic malignancies. Pharmacotherapy 2003;23:1592–610.
2. Kontoyiannis DP, Mantadakis E, Samonis G. Systemic mycoses in the immunocompromised host: an update in antifungal therapy. J Hosp Infect 2003;53:243–58.
3. Bodey GP. Hematogenous and major organ candidiasis. In: Bodey, editor. Candidiasis: pathogenesis, diagnosis and treatment. 2nd ed. New York: Raven Press; 1993. p. 279–329.
4. Bodey G, Bueltmann B, Duguid W, et al. Fungal infections in cancer patients. Eur J Clin Microbiol Infect Dis 1992;11:99–109.
5. Gallis HA, Drew RH, Pickard WW. Amphotericin B: 30 years of experience. Rev Infect Dis 1990;12:308–29.
6. Groll AH, Pitscitelli SC, Walsh TJ. Clinical pharmacology of systemic antifungal agents: a comprehensive review of agents in clinical use, current investigational compounds, and putative targets for antifungal drug development. Adv Pharmacol 1998;44:343–500.
7. Sheehan DJ, Hitcock CA, Sibley CM. Current and emerging azole antifungal agents. Clin Microbiol Rev 1999;12:40–79.
8. Wingard JR. Lipid formulations of amphotericins: are you a lumper or a splitter? Clin Infect Dis 2002;35:891–5.
9. Cole GT, Halawa AA, Anaissie EJ. The role of the gastrointestinal tract in hematogenous candidiasis: from the laboratory to the bedside. Clin Infect Dis 1996;22:S73.
10. Fleming RV, Walsh TJ, Anaissie EJ. Emerging and less common fungal pathogens. Infect Dis Clin North Am 2002;16(4):915–33.
11. Latgé JP. *Aspergillus fumigatus* and aspergillosis. Clin Microbiol Rev 1999;12:310–50.
12. Lionakis MS, Kontoyiannis DP. Glucocorticoids and invasive fungal infections. Lancet 2003;62:1828–38.
13. Nelson PE, Dignani MC, Anaissie EJ. Taxonomy, biology, and clinical aspects of *Fusarium* species. Clin Microbiol Rev 1994;7(4):479–504.
14. Ribes JA, Vanover-Sams CL, Baker DJ. *Zygomycetes* in human disease. Clin Microbiol Rev 2000;13:236–301.
15. Torres H, Kontoyiannis DP. In: Dismukew W, Pappas P, Sobel J, editors. Hyalohyphomycoses. Oxford textbook of clinical mycology. New York: Oxford University Press; 2003. p. 252–70.
16. van Burik JA, Leisenring W, Myerson D, et al. The effect of prophylactic fluconazole on the clinical spectrum of fungal diseases in bone marrow transplant recipients with special attention to hepatic candidiasis. Medicine 1998;77:246–54.
17. Wingard JR. Importance of *Candida* species other than *C. albicans* as pathogens in oncology patients. Clin Infect Dis 1995;20:115–25.
18. Abbas J, Bodey GP, Hanna HA, et al. *Candida krusei* fungemia: an escalating serious infection in immunocompromised patients. Arch Intern Med 2000;160:2659–64.
19. Kontoyiannis DP, Reddy BT, Hanna H, et al. Breakthrough candidemia in cancer patients differs from de novo candidemia in host factors and *Candida* species but not intensity. Infect Control Hosp Epidemiol 2002;542–5.
20. Abi-Said D, Anaissie E, Uzun O, et al. The epidemiology of hematogenous candidiasis caused by different *Candida* species. Clin Infect Dis 1997;24:1122–8.
21. Groll AH, Shah PM, Menzel C, et al. Trends in the postmortem epidemiology of invasive fungal infections at a university hospital. J Infect 1996;33:23–32.
22. Kontoyiannis DP, Vaziri I, Hanna H, et al. Risk factors for *Candida tropicalis* fungemia in patients with cancer. Clin Infect Dis 2001;33:1676–81.
23. Bodey GP, Mardani M, Hanna HA, et al. The epidemiology of *Candida glabrata* and *Candida albicans* fungemia in immunocompromised patients with cancer. Am J Med 2002;112:380–5.
24. Walsh TJ, Pizzo PA. Laboratory diagnosis of candidiasis. In: Bodey GP, editor. Candidiasis: pathogenesis, diagnosis and treatment. New York: Raven Press; 1993. p. 109.
25. Kontoyiannis DP, Luna MA, Samuels BI, Bodey GP. Hepatosplenic candidiasis: a manifestation of chronic disseminated candidiasis. Infect Dis Clin North Am 2000;14:721–39.
26. Kontoyiannis DP, Reddy BT, Torres H, et al. Pulmonary candidiasis in patients with cancer: an autopsy study. Clin Infect Dis 2002;34:400–3.
27. Anaissie E, Rex J, Uzun O, Vartivarian S. Predictors of adverse outcome in cancer patients with candidemia. Am J Med 1998;104:238–2458.
28. Uzun O, Anaissie EJ. Problems and controversies in the management of hematogenous candidiasis. Clin Infect Dis 1996;22 Suppl 2:S95–101.
29. Anaissie EJ, Darouiche RO, Abi-Said D, et al. Management of invasive candidal infections: results of a prospective, randomized, multicenter study of fluconazole versus amphotericin B and review of the literature. Clin Infect Dis 1996;23:964–72.
30. Anaissie EJ, Vartivarian SE, Abi-Said D, et al. Fluconazole versus amphotericin B in the treatment of hematogenous candidiasis: a matched cohort study. Am J Med 1996;101:170–6.
31. Antoniadou A, Torres H, Lewis RE, et al. In vitro susceptibility of bloodstream candidiasis in cancer patients: correlation with outcome of antifungal therapy. Medicine 2003;82:309–21.
32. Kontoyiannis DP, Lewis RE. Antifungal drug resistance of pathogenic fungi. Lancet 2002;359:1135–44.
33. Mora-Duarte J, Betts R, Rotstein C, et al, Caspofungin Invasive Candidiasis Study Group. Comparison of caspofungin and amphotericin B for invasive candidiasis. N Engl J Med 2002;347:2020–9.
34. Pappas PG, Rex JH, Sobel JD, et al. Guidelines for treatment of candidiasis. Clin Infect Dis 2004;38:161–89.
35. Rex JH. Editorial response. Catheters and candidemia. Clin Infect Dis 1996;22:467–70.
36. Raad I, Hanna H, Boktour M, et al. Management of central venous catheters in patients with cancer and candidemia. Clin Infect Dis 2004;38:1119–27.
37. Rex JH, Bennett JE, Sugar AM, et al. Intravascular catheter exchange and duration of candidemia. Clin Infect Dis 1995;21:994–6.
38. Lecciones JA, Lee JW, Navarro EE, et al. Vascular catheter-associated fungemia in patients with cancer: analysis of 155 episodes. Clin Infect Dis 1992;14:875–83.
39. Ramage G, VandeWalle K, Bachmann SP, et al. In vitro pharmacodynamic properties of three antifungal agents against preformed *Candida albicans* biofilms determined by time-kill studies. Antimicrob Agents Chemother 2002;46:3634–6.
40. Patterson TF, Kirkipatrick WR, White M, et al. Invasive aspergillosis: disease spectrum, treatment practices, and outcomes. Medicine 2000;79:250–60.
41. Ohmagari N, Raad II, Hachem R, Kontoyiannis DP. Invasive aspergillosis in cancer patients with solid tumors. Cancer 2004;101:2300–2.
42. Kontoyiannis DP, Bodey GP. Invasive aspergillosis in 2002: an update. Eur J Clin Microbiol Infect Dis 2002;21:161–72.
43. Hachem R, Kontoyiannis DP, Boktour M, et al. *Aspergillus terreus*: an emerging amphotericin B resistant opportunistic mold in patients with hematologic malignancy. Cancer 2004;101:1594–600.
44. Kontoyiannis DP, Sumoza D, Tarrand J, et al. The significance of aspergillemia in patients with cancer: a 10-year study. Clin Infect Dis 2000;31:188–9.
45. Tarrand JT, Lichterfeld M, Warraich I, et al. Diagnosis of invasive septate mold infections. A correlation of microbiological culture and histologic or cytologic examination. Am J Clin Pathol 2003;119:854–8.
46. Richardson MD, Kokki MH. New perspectives in the diagnosis of systemic fungal infections. Ann Med 1999;31:327–35.

47. Erjavec Z, Verweij PE. Recent progress in the diagnosis of fungal infections in the immunocompromised host. Drug Resist Update 2002;5:3–10.

48. Stevens DA. Diagnosis of fungal infections: current status. J Antimicrob Chemother 2002;49:11–9.

49. McLintock LA, Jones BL. Advances in the molecular and serological diagnosis of invasive fungal infection in haemato-oncology patients. Br J Haematol 2004;126: 289–97.

50. Maertens J, Verhaegen J, Demuynck H, et al. Autopsy-controlled prospective evaluation of serial screening for circulating galactomannan by a sandwich enzyme-linked immunosorbent assay for hematological patients at risk for invasive aspergillosis. J Clin Microbiol 1999;37: 3223–8.

51. Odabasi Z, Mattiuzzi G, Estey E, et al. Beta-D-glucan as a diagnostic adjunct for invasive fungal infections: validation, cutoff development, and performance in patients with acute myelogenous leukemia and myelodysplastic syndrome. Clin Infect Dis 2004;39:199–205.

52. Marr KA, Balajee SA, McLaughlin L, et al. Detection of galactomannan antigenemia by enzyme immunoassay for the diagnosis of invasive aspergillosis: variables that affect performance. J Infect Dis 2004;190:641–9.

53. Walsh TJ, Shoham S, Petraitiene R, et al. Detection of galactomannan antigenemia in patients receiving piperacillin-tazobactam and correlations between in vitro, in vivo, and clinical properties of the drug-antigen interaction. J Clin Microbiol 2004;42:4744–8.

54. Hebart J, Löffler J, Meisner C, et al. Early detection of *Aspergillus* infection after allogeneic stem cell transplantation by polymerase chain reaction screening. J Infect Dis 2000;181:1713–9.

55. Pham AS, Tarrand JJ, May GS, et al. Diagnosis of invasive mold infection by real-time quantitative PCR. Am J Clin Pathol 2003;119:38–44.

56. Kontoyiannis DP. A clinical perspective for the management of invasive fungal infections: focus on IDSA guidelines. Pharmacotherapy 2001;21:175S–87S.

57. Chiller TM, Stevens DA. Treatment strategies for *Aspergillus* infections. Drug Resist Update 2000;3:89–97.

58. Lin SJ, Schranz J, Teutsch SM. Aspergillosis case-fatality rate: systematic review of the literature. Clin Infect Dis 2001; 32:358–66.

59. Ascioglu S, Rex JH, de Pauw B, et al. Defining opportunistic invasive fungal infections in immunocompromised patients with cancer and hematopoietic stem cell transplants: an international consensus. Clin Infect Dis 2002; 34:7–14.

60. Walsh TJ, Hiemenz JW, Seibel NK, et al. Amphotericin B lipid complex for invasive fungal infections: analysis of safety and efficacy in 556 cases. Clin Infect Dis 1998; 26:1383.

61. Wingard JR, Kubilis P, Lee L, et al. Clinical significance of nephrotoxicity in patients treated with amphotericin B for suspected or proven aspergillosis. Clin Infect Dis 1999;29:1402–7.

62. Stevens DA, Lee JY. Analysis of compassionate use itraconazole therapy for invasive aspergillosis by the NIAID mycoses study group criteria. Arch Intern Med 1997; 157:1857–62.

63. Caillot D, Bassaris H, McGeer A, et al. Intravenous itraconazole followed by oral itraconazole in the treatment of invasive pulmonary aspergillosis in patients with hematologic malignancies, chronic granulomatous disease, or AIDS. Clin Infect Dis 2001;33:e83–90.

64. Herbrecht R, Denning DW, Patterson TF, et al. Voriconazole versus amphotericin B for primary therapy of invasive aspergillosis. N Engl J Med 2002;347:408–15.

65. Denning DW, Ribaud P, Milpied N, et al. Efficacy and safety of voriconazole in the treatment of acute invasive aspergillosis. Clin Infect Dis 2002;15:1273–5.

66. Perfect JR, Marr KA, Walsh TJ, et al. Voriconazole treatment for less-common, emerging, or refractory fungal infections. Clin Infect Dis 2003;36:1122–31.

67. Maertens J, Raad I, Petrikkos G, et al. Efficacy and safety of caspofungin for treatment of invasive aspergillosis in patients refractory to or intolerant of conventional antifungal therapy. Clin Infect Dis 2004;39:1563–71.

68. Kontoyiannis DP, Lewis RE. Towards more effective antifungal therapy: the prospects for combination therapies. Br J Haematol 2004;126:165–75.

69. Kontoyiannis DP, Boktour M, Hanna H, et al. Itraconazole added to a lipid formulation of amphotericin B does not improve outcome of primary treatment of invasive aspergillosis. Cancer 2005;103(11):2334–7.

70. Kontoyiannis DP, Hachem R, Lewis RE, et al. Efficacy and toxicity of caspofungin in combination with liposomal amphotericin B as primary or salvage treatment of invasive aspergillosis in patients with hematologic malignancies. Cancer 2003;98:292–9.

71. Marr KA, Boeckh M, Carter RA, Kim HW. Combination antifungal therapy for invasive aspergillosis. Clin Infect Dis 2004;39:797–802.

72. Caillot D, Casasnovas O, Bernard A, et al. Improved management of invasive pulmonary aspergillosis in neutropenic patients using early thoracic computed tomographic scan and surgery. J Clin Oncol 1997;15:139–47.

73. Yeghen T, Kibbler CC, Prentice HG, et al. Management of invasive pulmonary aspergillosis in hematology patients: a review of 87 consecutive cases at a single institution. Clin Infect Dis 2000;31:859–68.

74. Kontoyiannis DP, Wessel VC, Bodey GP, Rolston KVI. Zygomycosis in the 1990s in a tertiary care cancer center. Clin Infect Dis 2000;30:851–6.

75. Marr KA, Carter RA, Crippa F, et al. Epidemiology and outcome of mould infections in hematopoietic stem cell transplant recipients. Clin Infect Dis 2002;34:909–17.

76. Kontoyiannis DP, Lionakis MS, Lewis RE, et al. Zygomycosis in a tertiary-care cancer center in the era of Aspergillus-active antifungal therapy: a case-control observational study of 27 recent cases. J Infect Dis 2005;191(8): 1350–60.

77. Greenberg RN, Anstead G, Herbrecht R, et al. Posaconazole as salvage treatment for zygomycosis. Antimicrob Agents Chemother 2006;50(1):126–30.

78. Boutati EI, Anaissie EJ. *Fusarium*, a significant emerging pathogen in patients with hematologic malignancy: ten years' experience at a cancer center and implications for management. Blood 1997;90(3):999–1008.

79. Kontoyiannis DP, Hanna H, Hachem R, et al. Risk factors of poor outcome of fusariosis in a tertiary care cancer center. Leuk Lymphoma 2004;45:141–3.

80. Bodey GP, Boktour M, Mays S, et al. Skin lesions associated with *Fusarium* infection. J Am Acad Dermatol 2002;47: 659–66.

81. Walsh TJ. Trichosporonosis. Infect Dis Clin North Am 1989;3:43–52.

82. Walsh TJ, Melcher GP, Rinaldi MG, et al. *Trichosporon beigelii*, an emerging pathogen resistant to amphotericin B. J Clin Microbiol 1990;28:1616–22.

83. Kontoyiannis DP, Torres HA, Chagua M, et al. Trichosporonosis in a tertiary care cancer center: risk factors, changing spectrum and determinants of outcome. Scand J Infect Dis 2004;36:564–9.

84. Anaissie EJ, Hachem R, Karyotakis NC, et al. Comparative efficacies of amphotericin B, triazoles, and combination of both as experimental therapy for murine trichosporonosis. Antimicrob Agents Chemother 1994;38:2541–4.

85. Fournier S, Pavageau W, Feuillhade M, et al. Use of voriconazole to successfully treat disseminated *Trichosporon asahii* infection in a patient with acute myeloid leukaemia. Eur J Clin Microbiol Infect Dis 2002;21:892–6.

86. Stevens DA. Coccidioidomycosis. N Engl J Med 1995; 332:1077–82.

87. Wheat LJ. Histoplasmosis. Infect Dis Clin North Am 1988; 2:841–59.

88. Kontoyiannis DP, Peitsch KW, Reddy B, et al. Cryptococcosis in patients with cancer. Clin Infect Dis 2001;32: 145–50.

89. Torres H, Rivero G, Kontoyiannis DP. Endemic mycoses in a cancer hospital. Medicine 2002;81:201–12.

90. Wheat J, Sarosi G, McKinsey D, et al. Practice guidelines for the management of patients with histoplasmosis. Clin Infect Dis 2000;30:688–95.

91. Galgiani JN, Ampel NM, Catazaro A, et al. Practice guidelines for the treatment of coccidioidomycosis. Clin Infect Dis 2000;30:658–61.

92. Galgiani JN, Gatanzaro A, Cloud GA, et al. Comparison of oral fluconazole and itraconazole for progressive, non-meningeal coccidioidomycosis. Ann Intern Med 2000; 133:676–86.

93. Saag MS, Graybill RJ, Larsen RA, et al. Practice guidelines for the management of cryptococcal disease. Clin Infect Dis 2000;30:710–8.

94. Bodey GP, Kontoyiannis DP, Lewis R. Empiric antifungal therapy for persistently febrile neutropenic patients. Curr Opin Infect Dis 2002;4:521–33.

95. Goldstone AH, O'Driscoll A. Early AmBisome in febrile neutropenia in patients with haematological disorders. Bone Marrow Transplant 1994;14 Suppl 5:S15–7.

96. Walsh TJ, Finberg RW, Arndt C, et al. Liposomal amphotericin B for empirical therapy in patients with persistent fever and neutropenia. N Engl J Med 1999;340:764–71.

97. Winston DJ, Hathorn JW, Schuster MG, et al. A multi-center randomized trial of fluconazole versus amphotericin B for empirical antifungal therapy of febrile neutropenic patients with cancer. Am J Med 2000;108:282–9.

98. Boogaerts M, Winston DJ, Bow EJ, et al. Intravenous and oral itraconazole versus intravenous amphotericin B deoxycholate as empirical antifungal therapy for persistent fever in neutropenic patients with cancer who are receiving broad-spectrum antibacterial therapy: a randomized, controlled trial. Ann Intern Med 2001;135: 412–22.

99. Walsh TJ, Pappas P, Winston DJ, et al. Voriconazole compared with liposomal amphotericin B for empirical antifungal therapy in patients with neutropenia and persistent fever. N Engl J Med 2002;346:225–34.

100. Walsh TJ, Teppler H, Donowitz GR, et al. Caspofungin versus liposomal amphotericin B for empirical antifungal therapy in patients with persistent fever and neutropenia. N Engl J Med 2004;351:1391–402.

Parasitic Disease Issues in Cancer Patients

Javier A. Adachi, MD

Herbert L. DuPont, MD

Parasitic diseases in patients with underlying malignancies are uncommon infectious problems in the United States, a direct reflect of the very low prevalence of parasitic infections in the general population in this country.[1,2] In contrast, parasitic infections are relatively more frequent in cancer patients in other areas of the world, especially in those with higher prevalence of gastrointestinal parasitic infections (such as cryptosporidiosis, strongyloidiasis), blood-borne parasitic infections (malaria) and central nervous system parasitic infections (toxoplasmosis, cysticercosis).

The objective of this chapter is to review the epidemiology, clinical presentation, diagnosis, treatment and prevention of *Pneumocystis jiroveci* pneumonia (formerly known as *Pneumocystis carinii* pneumonia [PCP]) and *Toxoplasma gondii* infections in cancer patients, follow by a short review of other miscellaneous parasitic infections.

Pneumocystis jiroveci Infection

Introduction

P. carinii was first identified in 1909–1910 by Chagas and by Carini[3,4] and was recently renamed *P. jiroveci*.[1,5] The first description of PCP was in 1952.[6] Although, initially classified as a protozoan, more recent molecular genetic studies have demonstrated that *P. jiroveci* may be considered an atypical fungus,[2,5,7,8] consisting in multiple strains, each one restricted to infecting a single host species.[5,7] The life cycle and the origin of infection (de novo or reactivation) are still unknown.[2,5]

In 1976, Hughes and colleagues[9] found an incidence of 22 to 45% of PCP in children with acute lymphoblastic leukemia, depending on the stage and the chemotherapy used. Later on, the same author demonstrated that trimethoprim-sulfamethoxazole (TMP-SMX) was an effective prophylaxis,[10] and its routine use has resulted in a decrease of the incidence to 0%.[5,11–13] Since the

1980s, PCP is a well-known life-threatening opportunistic infection in patients with impaired cellular immunity, such as patients with AIDS, hematological malignancies, recipients of transplant, severe malnutrition, congenital T-cell deficiencies, or those receiving high-dose systemic steroids or other immunosuppressive agents.[2,5,14]

Epidemiology

The incidence of PCP without TMP-SMX prophylaxis varies by the type of cancer and the use of immunosuppressive therapy. Patients with hematologic malignancies (leukemia and lymphoma) have a higher incidence (between 22% and 67%)[2,5,9,14,15] than the incidence among patients with solid tumors, usually taking immunosuppressive therapy (1.3 to 34%)[2,5,16,17]. Recipients of hematopoietic stem cell transplantation (HSCT) or solid organ transplantation (especially those post-lung transplant, who also have a high incidence of PCP [from 5% to more than 25%]).[2,5] The majority of patients was found to have lymphopenia (< 1,000 lymphocytes/mL) at the onset of infection.[15]

Clinical Presentation

The clinical presentation of PCP in cancer patients is characterized by the presence of fever (86%), dyspnea (75 to 78%) and non-productive cough (70%).[2,5,15] Compared to HIV-positive patients,[18] cancer patients with PCP have shorter median duration of symptoms (28 vs. 5 days, respectively) and lower median arterial oxygen tension at room air (69 vs. 55 mm Hg, respectively), with a high rate of admission to the intensive care unit (41 to 60%) and of use of mechanical ventilation (30 to 41%).[14,15,18,19] Coinfection with other opportunistic infections is also commonly found.[15]

Diagnosis

The diagnosis of PCP is based on the detection of the organism in a clinical specimen using colorimetric (Gomori's methanemine silver stain

or Giemsa stain) or immunofluorescent stain (using monoclonal antibody 2G2), the latter being more sensitive and specific.[5] Bronchoalveolar lavage specimens from cancer patients have a higher yield for PCP, compared to lung tissue or induced sputum specimens.[2,5,15] It has been reported in the literature that the *P. jiroveci* load seen on microscopic examination of respiratory specimens is lower in cancer patients.[5] PCP shows an acellular intra-alveolar eosinophilic exudate in histopathologic studies.[5]

Recent studies using molecular-based methods have been shown to be more sensitive than the stains for detection of PCP and have also demonstrated the presence of asymptomatic colonization.[5,20,21]

The characteristic radiographic findings of PCP are bilateral interstitial infiltrates, which progress to alveolar infiltrates. However, up to 10% of patients may have normal chest radiograph.[5,15,18,22] The computed tomography of the chest usually demonstrates a characteristic ground glass opacity pattern.[5]

Treatment and Clinical Outcome

The treatment of PCP has remained basically the same since the 1970s. TMP-SMX is the first-line therapy against PCP in any kind of patient, including cancer patients,[2,5] Patients intolerant of TMP-SMX could be treated with one of the alternative therapies summarized in Table 1. Although in-vitro–resistant mutations have been demonstrated, there is no correlation between these mutations and clinical resistance to TMP-SMX.[23]

The duration of therapy for cancer patients with PCP was established to be 2 weeks, unless the PCP is severe, the clinical response is not optimal, or further immunosuppressive therapy is given.[2,5]

Although no adequate clinical trials have been done testing the possible benefit of adjuvant steroids therapy in HIV-negative patients with PCP, it is recommended to follow the same indications for adding steroids to the regimen as

Table 1 Treatment Regimens of *Pneumocystis Jiroveci* Pneumonia

Drug	Dose
TMP-SMX *	2 tablets double-strength oral every 8h
TMP-SMX	5 mg/kg of TMP every 8h
Alternatives	
TMP + Dapsone	320 mg oral q8h + 100 mg daily
Atovaquone	750 mg oral twice daily
Clindamycin + primaquine	300 to 450 mg oral/IV every 6h + 15 to 30 mg oral daily
Pentamidine	4 mg/kg IV daily
Trimetrexate + leucovorin	45 mg/m² IV daily + 20 mg/m² oral/IV every 6h
Adjunctive Therapy	
Prednisone	(if PaO₂ at room air < 70 mm Hg)

IV = intravenous; SMX = sulfamethoxazole; TMP = trimethoprim

Table 2 Prophylactic Regimens of *Pneumocystis Jiroveci* Pneumonia

Drug	Dose
TMP-SMX *	1 tablet double-strength oral daily
	1 tablet single-strength oral daily
Alternatives	
TMP-SMX	1 tablet double-strength oral 3 times/week
Dapsone	100 mg oral daily
Aerosolized Pentamidine	300 mg via nebulizer monthly
Atovaquone	1,500 mg oral daily

SMX = sulfamethoxazole; TMP = trimethoprim

were established for patients with AIDS and PCP.[24]

Survival rates vary based on the population at risk, with cancer patients showing the worst rates.[2,5,15,25] Recent data have shown that the survival rate associated with PCP in AIDS patients has declined noticeably during the last decade, in contrast to the little improvement of survival of HIV-negative patients with PCP.[2,5]

Reported poor prognostic factors in cancer patients with PCP were prolonged steroid therapy (> 15 days), diffuse lung involvement, mechanical ventilation, an elevated serum lactate dehydrogenase level and elevated C-reactive protein.[14,15,25]

Prevention

Since TMP-SMX prophylaxis was demonstrated to be effective prophylactic therapy by Hughes and colleagues,[10] this antimicrobial is the preferred prophylactic agent in any patient population. However, its associated adverse effects, mainly myelotoxicity, have been the driving force behind the use of alternative prophylactic agents, as shown in Table 2. The optimal duration of prophylaxis remains to be determined.

Summary

In conclusion, PCP is still an uncommon, but life-threatening pulmonary infection in cancer patients. The type of cancer, history of transplant and the use of immunosuppressive therapy influence the clinical presentation and outcome of this infection. In contrast to PCP in HIV-positive patients, there have not been any improvements

in mortality rate for PCP in HIV-negative patients. Early diagnosis, identification of risk factors and prompt and better therapy of this infection among cancer patients should improve the clinical outcome.

Toxoplasma gondii Infection

Introduction

T. gondii is an intracellular protozoan parasite that infects humans and animals. Seroprevalence of toxoplasmosis in the general population varies between geographic areas, from 14 to 40% in the United States to 50 to 90% in continental Europe and Latin America, and increases with age.[26–29] Most infections are asymptomatic, but symptomatic infection may present with a mononucleosis-like picture, chronic infection with chorioretinitis, acute disseminated infection, and single-organ disease (encephalitis or pneumonitis).[26,27,29] Transmission may occur transplacentally, by ingestion of undercooked infested meat or by exposure to oocysts in contaminated soil.

Most of the epidemiology, clinical manifestations, and the outcome, treatment, and prevention of toxoplasmosis in immunosuppressed cancer patients comes from the studies of toxoplasmosis in patients with AIDS.[27] A first-class study contrasting the characteristics of toxoplasmosis in HIV-infected patients with HIV-negative patients is still waiting to be done.

Epidemiology

Toxoplasmosis occurs frequently in severe immunosuppressed patients—mainly patients with AIDS. It is a rare, but important and often devastating parasitic infection in patients undergoing hematopoietic stem cell transplantation.[27,30,31] Disseminated toxoplasmosis apparently results from reactivation of a latent infection associated with cellular immunodeficiency.[26,27] One recent

European study reported 41 cases of toxoplasmosis after HSCT. Most patients (94%) were seropositive for *T. gondii* before the HSCT, and 73% developed moderate to severe graft-versus-host disease prior to developing the infection.[28]

Clinical Presentation

Encephalitis is the most common type of infection in cancer patients post-HSCT with toxoplasmosis (60 to 80%), followed by pulmonary involvement in up to 41% of the cases reported.[28,30,31] These patients, like any other immunosuppressed patients, may present with non-specific clinical manifestations (fever, headaches, lymphadenopathy, myalgia, or anorexia) or with more specific ones (confusion, drowsiness, meningism or seizures)[28]

Diagnosis

The presumptive diagnosis of toxoplasmosis in immunocompromised patients is based on the detection of IgG to *Toxoplasma* in serum and radiologic findings compatible. Diagnosis of acute infection could be established by the simultaneous detection of serum IgG and IgM to *Toxoplasma*[26–28] Determination of IgG titers in cerebral-spinal fluid (CSF) may be useful to help identify the infection[27]

Immunohistochemistry or conventional histology examination with identification of parasites in tissue samples are definitive diagnostic tests but are not convenient daily clinical practice.[26,27]

The identification of genetic material of the parasite is under investigation in HSCT recipients, testing blood samples or CSF samples,[27,32] with controversial results.

Imaging studies (computed tomography of the head or magnetic resonance imaging of the brain) could demonstrate focal or multifocal abnormalities in the central nervous system (CNS). However, these findings are not pathognomonic. Radiologic studies are important in order to assess the response to therapy.[26–28]

Treatment and Clinical Outcome

Table 3 shows the treatment regimens available for acute toxoplasmosis in immunocompromised patients. Combination therapy with pyrimethamine and sulfadiazine, complemented with leucovorin is the first choice.[26,27]

The mortality rate of toxoplasmosis in post-HSCT patients is around 60 to 70%, apparently higher than for AIDS patients, with an elevated number of cases diagnosed post-mortem.[26–28]

In contrast to toxoplasmosis in AIDS, which could be a subacute medical problem, this parasitic infection could be rapidly fatal in patients post-HSCT if they are not treated without delay. Appropriate antimicrobial therapy was identified

Table 3 Treatment Regimens Of Toxoplasmosis

Drug	Dose
Pyrimethamine	200 mg oral follow by 75 to 100 mg oral daily
+ sulfadiazine	+ 1 to 1.5 gm oral every 6h
+ leucovorin	+ 10 to 15 mg oral daily
TMP-SMX *	5 mg/kg of TMP every 12h
Alternatives	
Pyrimethamine	
+ leucovorin	(As above)
+ clindamycin	+ 600 mg oral/IV every 6h
or + clarithromycin	or + 1.0 gm oral daily
or + azithromycin	or + 1.2 to 1.5 gm oral daily
or + dapsone	or + 100 mg oral daily

IV = intravenous; SMX = sulfamethoxazole; TMP = trimethoprim

Table 4 Prophylactic Regimens Of Toxoplasmosis

Drug	Dose
TMP-SMX *	1 tablet double-strength oral daily 1 tablet single-strength oral daily
Alternatives	
Dapsone	50 mg oral daily
+ pyrimethamine	+ 50 mg oral weekly
+ leucovorin	+ 25 mg oral weekly
Atovaquone	1,500 mg oral daily

TMP = trimethoprim; SMX = sulfamethoxazole

as the most important survival factor.[28,29] Therefore, a presumptive diagnosis of CNS toxoplasmosis should prompt the immediate treatment. The optimal duration and role of suppressive therapy needs to be studied.

Prevention

In AIDS patients, the prophylaxis for PCP is also effective for toxoplasmosis (Table 4). In cancer patients, the use of prophylaxis in seropositive patients after HSCT is apparently justified.[26,33] However, further studies are necessary to confirm this postulate, to determine the role of secondary prophylaxis, and to define the optimal duration of prophylactic regimen.

Summary

In conclusion, toxoplasmosis is an uncommon, but life-threatening infection in immunocompromised patients with cancer, especially to those post-HSCT. Additional studies should be done to determine the importance of the type of cancer, history of transplant, and the use of immunosuppressive therapy in the clinical presentation and outcome of this infection. Early diagnosis, identification of risk factors, and prompt and better therapy of this infection among cancer patients should improve the clinical outcome.

Miscellaneous Parasitic Infections

Strongyloides stercoralis

Strongyloides is an uncommon helminth that can produce a wide variety of clinical syndromes in cancer patients, based on the immunologic status of the host. It could remain localized in patients with solid tumors, or develop a hyperinfection syndrome with gastrointestinal manifestations, diffuse pneumonitis and respiratory failure, usually together with gram-negative sepsis, described most often in patients with hematological

malignancies or post-HSCT.[30,34,35] Apparently, the patients with the disseminated disease do not have a good response to any antimicrobial therapy (thiabendazole or ivermectin), unless there is a recovery of the immune status.

Schistosoma species

Infection by this trematode is associated with development of cystitis, intestinal and vesical ulcerations, hepatic fibrosis, portal hypertension and bladder cancer. This parasite infection is endemic in tropical and subtropical countries, but there have not been any native reported cases in the United States.[36,37]

Intestinal Protozoan Infections

Although *Giardia, Cryptosporidium, Isospora, Cyclospora, Microsporida* and *Entamoeba histolytica*, have been associated with chronic infectious diarrhea in AIDS patients, there are very low incidences in infectious enterocolitis in patients with an underlying malignancy in the United States.[38,39,40] Routine microbiology tests for these enteric parasites, as well as for all "classic" enteropathogenic bacteria (*Salmonella, Shigella, Campylobacter, Yersinia, Aeromonas, Plesiomonas* and *Vibrio*) should not be recommended as routine tests in cancer patient with acute uncomplicated diarrhea or without a identified epidemiological risk factor.[38,39] The detection of *Clostridium difficile* toxin in stools of cancer patients with acute diarrhea is the only exception, because of the high prevalence of this infection in cancer patients, especially those with hematological malignancies.[41,42]

REFERENCES

1. Protozoal diseases. In: Mandell GL, Bennett JE, Dolin R; editors. Principles and practice of infectious diseases. 6th ed. New York: Churchill Livingstone; 2004.
2. Sepkowitz KA. Opportunistic infections in patients with and patients without Acquired Immunodeficiency Syndrome. Clin Infect Dis 2002;34:1098–107.
3. Chagas C. Nova tripanomiaze humana. Estudos sobre a morfolojia e o ciclo evolutivo do Schizotrypanum cruzi n.

gen., n. sp., ajente etiolojico de nova entidade morbida do homen. Mem Inst Oswaldo Cruz 1909;1:159–218.
4. Carini A. Formas des eschizogonia do trypanosoma lewisii. Arch Soc Med. CI Sao Paulo 1910;38:204.
5. Kovacs JA, Gill VJ, Meshnick S, Masur H. New insights into transmission, diagnosis, and drug treatment of *Pneumocystis carinii* pneumonia. JAMA 2001;286:2450–60.
6. Vanek J, Jirovek O. Parasitare Pneumoniae "Interstitielle" Plasmazellenpneumoniae der Fruhgeborenen, verursacht durch *Pneumocystis carinii*. Zentralb Bakteriol [Orig A] 1952;158:120–7.
7. Stringer JR. *Pneumocystis carinii*: what is it, exactly? Clin Microbiol Rev 1996;9:489–98.
8. Roux P, Latouche S. Molecular epidemiology of human pneumocystosis. Medecine et maladies infectieuses 1999;29:733–8.
9. Hughes WT. Protozoan infections in haematological diseases. Clin Haematol 1976;5:329–45.
10. Hughes WT, Kuhn S, Chaudhary S, et al. Successful chemoprophylaxis for *Pneumocystis carinii* pneumonitis. N Engl J Med 1977;297:1419–26.
11. Walzer PD, Perl DP, Krogstad DJ, et al. *Pneumocystis carinii* pneumonia in the United States. Epidemiologic, diagnostic, and clinical features. Ann Intern Med 1974;80:83–93.
12. McNeil MM, Nash SL, Hajjeh RA, et al. Trends in mortality due to invasive mycotic diseases in the United States, 1980–1997. Clin Infect Dis 2001;33:641–7.
13. Pagano L, Fianchi L, Mele L, et al. A *Pneumocystis carinii* pneumonia in patients with malignant haematological diseases: 10 years' experience of infection in GIMEMA centres. Br J Haematol 2002;117:379–86.
14. Roblot F, Le Moal G, Godet C et al. *Pneumocystis carinii* pneumonia in patients with hematologic malignancies: a descriptive study. J Infect 2003;47:19–27.
15. Torres H, Chemaly RF, Storey R, et al. *Pneumocystis jiroveci* pneumonia in cancer patients: influence of type of cancer, hematopoietic stem cell transplantation and acquired immune deficiency syndrome to presentation and outcome. Clin Infect Dis.[Submitted].
16. De la Horra C, Varcla JM, Fernandez-Alonso J, et al. Association between human-pneumocystis infection and small-cell lung carcinoma. Eur J Clin Invest 2004;34: 229–35.
17. Mahindra AK, Grossman SA. *Pneumocystis carinii* pneumonia in HIV negative patients with primary brain tumors. J Neurooncol 2003;63:263–70.
18. Kovacs JA, Hiemenz JW, Macher AM, et al. *Pneumocystis carinii* pneumonia: a comparison between patients with the acquired immunodeficiency syndrome and patients with other immunodeficiencies. Ann Intern Med 1984; 100:663–71.
19. Zahar JR, Robin M, Azoulay E, et al. *Pneumocystis carinii* pneumonia in critically ill patients with malignancy: a descriptive study. Clin Infect Dis 2002;35:929–34.
20. Lu JJ, Chen CH, Bartlett MS, et al. Comparison of six different PCR methods for detection of *Pneumocystis carinii*. J Clin Microbiol 1995;33:2785–8.
21. Sing A, Trebesius K, Roggenkamp A, et al. Evaluation of diagnostic value and epidemiological implications of PCR for *Pneumocystis carinii* in different immunosuppressed and immunocompetent patient groups. J Clin Microbiol 2000;38:1461–7.
22. Opravil M, Marcineck B, Fuchs WA, et al. Shortcomings of chest radiography in detecting *Pneumocystis carinii* pneumonia. J Acquir Immune Defic Syndr Hum Retrovirol 1994;7:39–45.
23. Helweg-Larsen J, Benfield TL, Eugen-Olsen J, et al. Effects of mutations in *Pneumocystis carinii* dihydropteroate synthase gene on outcome of AIDS-associated *P. carinii* pneumonia. Lancet 1999;354:1347–51.
24. Bozzette SA, Sattler FR, Chiu J, et al. A controlled trial of early adjunctive treatment with corticosteroids for *Pneumocystis carinii* pneumonia in the acquired immunodeficiency syndrome. California Collaborative Treatment Group. N Engl J Med 1990;323:1451–7.
25. Roblot F, Godet C, Le Moal G, et al. Analysis of underlying diseases and prognosis factors associated with *Pneumocystis carinii* pneumonia in immunocompromised HIV-negative patients. Eur J Clin Microbiol Infect Dis 2002; 21:523–31.
26. Israelki D, Remington J. Toxoplasmosis in the non-AIDS immunocompromised host. In: Remington J, Schwartz M, editors. Current clinical topics in infectious diseases. Vol 13. Boston: Blackwell Scientific; 1993. p. 322–56.
27. Hill D, Dubey JP. *Toxoplasma gondii*: transmission, diagnosis and prevention. Clin Microbiol Infect 2002; 8:634–40.

28. Martino R, Maertens J, Bretagne S, et al. Toxoplasmosis after hematopoietic stem cell transplantation. Clin Infect Dis 2000;31:1188–95.

29. Ruskin J, Remington JS. Toxoplasmosis in the compromised host. Ann Intern Med 1976;84:193–9.

30. Rolston KV. The spectrum of pulmonary infections in cancer patients. Curr Opin Oncol 2001;13:218–23.

31. Maschke M, Dietrich U, Prumbaum M, et al. Opportunistic CNS infection after bone marrow transplantation. Bone Marrow Transplant 1999;23:1167–76.

32. Held TK, Kruger D, Switala AR, et al. Diagnosis of toxoplasmosis in bone marrow transplant recipients: comparison of PCR-based results and immunohistochemistry. Bone Marrow Transplant 2000;25:1257–62.

33. Peacock JE Jr, Greven CM, Cruz JM, Hurd DD. Reactivation toxoplasmic retinochoroiditis in patients undergoing bone marrow transplantation: is there a role for chemoprophylaxis? Bone Marrow Transplant 1995;15:983–7.

34. Safdar A, Malathum K, Rodriguez SJ, et al. Strongyloidiasis in patients at a comprehensive cancer center in the United States. Cancer 2004;100:1531–6.

35. Orlent H, Crawley C, Cwynarski K, et al. Strongyloidiasis pre and post autologous peripheral blood stem cell transplantation. Bone Marrow Transplant 2003;32:115–7.

36. Richter J. The impact of chemotherapy on morbidity due to schistosomiasis. Acta Trop 2003;86:161–83.

37. Badawi AF, Mostafa MH, Probert A, O'Connor PJ. Role of schistosomiasis in human bladder cancer: evidence of association, aetiological factors, and basic mechanisms of carcinogenesis. Eur J Cancer Prev 1995;4:45–59.

38. Gorschluter M, Marklein G, Hofling K, et al. Abdominal infections in patients with acute leukaemia: a prospective study applying ultrasonography and microbiology. Br J Haematol 2002;117:351–8.

39. Rotterdam H, Tsang P. Gastrointestinal disease in the immunocompromised patient. Hum Pathol 1994;25:1123–40.

40. Bodey GP, Fainstein V. Infections of the gastrointestinal tract in the immunocompromised patient. Annu Rev Med 1986;37:271–81.

41. Blot E, Escande MC, Besson D, et al. Outbreak of Clostridium difficile-related diarrhoea in an adult oncology unit: risk factors and microbiological characteristics. J Hosp Infect 2003;53:187–92.

42. Gorschluter M, Glasmacher A, Hahn C, et al. Clostridium difficile infection in patients with neutropenia. Clin Infect Dis 2001;33:786–91.

Mycobacterial Infections in Patients with Cancer

Amar Safdar, MD
Donald Armstrong, MD

Tuberculosis has a substantial impact on global public health; nearly 8 million new cases of *Mycobacterium tuberculosis* are estimated to occur yearly, adding to the existing burden of 1,700 million cases worldwide.[1,2] In 1993, the World Health Organization declared tuberculosis a public health emergency because 3 million patients were expected to die annually owing to complications arising from tuberculosis, making it the most frequent cause of death due to an infectious organism.[3] Humans are the only known reservoir of *M. tuberculosis*, and nearly one-third of the world's population is now estimated to be infected with this potentially devastating infection. Public health measures, including bacilli Calmette-Guérin vaccination, improved living standards, especially among the inhabitants of inner cities has resulted in marked reduction in the infection rates in populations of the developed regions of the world, although the tuberculosis attack rate remains undeterred in underdeveloped and developing countries.

In the United States, reported cases of tuberculosis consistently declined during the 20th century until 1985. The unanticipated sudden increase in the newly diagnosed cases of tuberculosis between 1985 and 1992 in United States were attributed to the epidemic of human immunodeficiency virus (HIV), acquired immunodeficiency syndrome (AIDS), illicit drug use, homelessness, and ineffective tuberculosis control programs in large urban centers.[4,5] The decline in tuberculosis since 1992 was attributed to re-implementation of effective tuberculosis control programs with emphasis on early diagnosis to interrupt spread in the community, directly observed therapy that ensured compliance of adequate anti-tuberculosis therapy, and a number of other preventive measures. They were all creditedwith establishing in 1997 the lowest ever number of new recorded cases.[6]

Most *M. tuberculosis* infections occur in patients with no known immune defects, although inadequate adaptive cellular immune response substantially increases the risk of both new infection and reactivation of remotely acquired disease. The host factors that promote tuberculosis include protein-calorie malnutrition and residing in communities with inadequate sanitation, poor ventilation, and overcrowding. In developed regions of the world, homelessness, illicit drug use, incarceration in correctional facilities, prolonged use of systemic corticosteroids and tumor necrosis factor inhibitor therapy has been associated with increased risk of tuberculosis.[7,8] Since the introduction of effective antiretroviral therapy (ART) and ART-related cellular immune reconstitution, patients with HIV-AIDS are less susceptible to developing active tuberculosis.[9]

Patients with an underlying malignancy, Hodgkin's diseases, gastric, head and neck cancers were considered a susceptible population.[10,11] One report said most cases of active tuberculosis in HIV-negative cancer patients receiving care at a comprehensive cancer center in the United States were noted in patients with hematologic malignancies, including acute and chronic myelogenous leukemia, and non-Hodgkin's lymphoma.[12] Tuberculosis has also been reported in the recipients of hematopoietic stem cells, although the infection rate (despite severe cellular immune dysfunction) has remained low in the residents of North America and Europe.[13] Recipients of organ transplantation, however, appear to have a higher rate of developing active tuberculosis.[14] This discrepancy is less obvious in patients undergoing hematopoietic stem cell transplantation in the areas of high *M. tuberculosis* endemicity.[15–17] In the United States, reactivation of *M. tuberculosis* remains a concern in foreign-born cancer patients who have increased risk of infection reactivation during antineoplastic-therapy–induced severe immune suppression.[12,18,19]

In this chapter, we provide a brief introduction of hosts' immune resistance against mycobacterial pathogens and immune defects that promote systemic disease due to mycobacteria. The clinical spectrum of disease and antituberculous therapies are discussed under two sections: Tuberculosis and Nontuberculous Mycobacteriosis.

Antimycobacterial Immune Defense

Intact reticuloendothelial systems provide the bases of innate immune defense against the invading virulent *M. tuberculosis* as well as most non-virulent environmental mycobacterial species other than *M. tuberculosis*. However, it is the adaptive cellular immune response that provides effective containment and elimination of intracellular mycobacteria residing within the mononuclear cells.[20] All components of T-lymphocytes including γ δ cells play a role, although CD4 cells are the dominant α β lymphocytes that provide the backbone of a host's immune response against mycobacterial infections.[21,22] Interferon-γ (IFN-γ) is the most important proinflammatory cytokine secreted by primed T-helper type-1 (T_H1) lymphocytes, which activates fixed tissue macrophages, recruits peripheral mononuclear cells to the site of infection and sets the stage for granuloma formation.[23] The granuloma 1) serves as a physical barrier for mycobacterial propagation, 2) promotes unfavorable oxygen and micronutrient-deficient environments and 3) most importantly, creates a milieu in which various components of the immune cells and extracellular cytokines and chemokines interact to enhance effector-cell–mediated mycobacterial cell death.[24,25]

The delayed-type hypersensitivity reaction against the invading mycobacterial infection on one hand is critical in effective containment of infection, and on the other hand, via calcification of granulomas, large quantities of caseation necrosis and formation of pulmonary cavities paradoxically enable the intracellular mycobacteria to evade the host's immune surveillance.[26] The cytokines that play an important role in antimycobacterial immune defense cascade other than IFN-γ include interleukin 12, T-cell-derived tumor necrosis factor alpha (TFN-α) and the expending family of TNF-related immuno-active peptides.[27–29]

Immune Defects

The host's immune defects, in the light of earlier discussion, mostly involve dysregulation of cellular adaptive immune response. A complicated cascade of events are set into effect following exposure to mycobacterial antigens, and organism-specific antigen-primed T-cells at the infection site orchestrate events leading to cell death of these intracellular pathogens.

Defects in the protagonist T_H1 cytokine, IFN-γ may present as a deficiency in cytokine production. Dysfunctional cytokine specific receptors (IFN-γ) have been shown to increase difficult-to-treat systemic mycobacteriosis.[30–33] Furthermore, defects in post-receptor cytoplasmic signaling pathways such as signal transducer and activator of transcription 1 (STAT1), signal transducing molecule, nuclear factor (NF)$_\kappa$β essential modulator (NEMO), or ancillary cytokines including interleukin-12, interleukin-18, and TNF-α can also lead to enhanced risk of severe disseminated infection due to otherwise non-virulent mycobacteria.[20,23,27]

At present, the consensus to undertake an immunologic work is warranted in only HIV-negative patients who present with refractory mycobacterial infections or those with recurring pulmonary nontuberculous mycobacteriosis with no known underlying predisposing conditions. Most patients with *M. tuberculosis* do not have a known immune defect, and for most patients, appropriate antimycobacterial therapy alone results in good sustained response. Nontuberculous mycobacteriosis, even due to organisms with low disease-causing potential, are often in the setting of immunologically intact host, and an extensive immunologic workup at present may not yield clinically relevant information. In a select group of patients with unresponsive mycobacterial infection, immunologic investigation may be undertaken in consultation with Infectious Diseases.

Tuberculosis

Among the four species of *M. tuberculosis* complex, *M. tuberculosis* and *M. bovis* are associated with the most cases of tuberculosis in humans. Of infections due to the other two species, *M. africanum* causes rare tuberculosis-like illness in Africa and *M. microti*, an agent associated with devastating infection among rodents, leads to rare, accidental infection in humans.

Acute Infection and Risk of Disease

As humans are the only reservoir of *M. tuberculosis*, infection is spread from person to person, and the most common method of transmission is via inhalation of aerosolized respiratory secretions from an infected individual. Exposure to patients with acid-fast bacilli (AFB) positive sputum smear have a 25 to 50% risk of acquiring infection. In certain situations such as close, prolonged exposure (especially in overcrowded situations), the attack rate may be as high as 80%.[34] Interestingly, in patients with smear-negative active pulmonary infection, risk of transmission to a non-infected person is not significantly higher than the risk of infection acquisition in the community at large.[35] Nursing home residents are at a higher risk of infection, which may present several predisposing risks, including prolonged close exposures to other individuals compounded by age-associated senescence of adaptive cellular immune response.[36] Other settings that may increase the risk of spreading tuberculosis include shelters for the homeless and correctional facilities. However, it is important to state that only a fraction of patients, after *M. tuberculosis* infection, will go on to develop clinical tuberculosis, and the lifetime risk in the general population varies from 5% to 15%. In contrast, individuals with severe immune suppression have a very high risk of developing active disease following acute infection. Patients with renal failure, alcoholism, malnutrition, underlying malignancy, prolonged systemic corticosteroid use, stem cell and organ transplantation, and especially AIDS, have a nearly 8% to 10% per year lifetime risk of developing tuberculosis after acute infection.[37]

Pulmonary Tuberculosis

This by far is the most common presentation of tuberculosis. Most pulmonary infections present as reactivation of remotely acquired infection, although in the developed countries, a substantial proportion of pulmonary infection represents recently acquired infection, especially in the non-immigrant native population.

Primary Pulmonary Tuberculosis

In contrast to young individuals, adults are immunologically better equipped to handle acute *M. tuberculosis* infection; most infections remains localized to lungs; systemic dissemination seldom occurs; regional lymphadenopathy, if present, is modest, and erythema nodosum or phlyctenular (vesicular) keratoconjunctivitis are not often seen. Pulmonary infiltrates remain localized, with minimal clinical signs and symptoms, especially in patients with ineffective immune defenses, which leads to delay in diagnosis and institution of appropriate therapy, and potentially increases the community- and hospital-based risk of spread of infection to other susceptible individuals.

Post-primary Pulmonary Tuberculosis

This is the prevalent form of disease worldwide. Infection is often asymmetrical and involves apices of lungs and/or the apex of the lower lobes. Focal pneumonitis leads to caseous necrosis that drains in the bronchial tree to form a cavity and which remains patent due to fibrosis and inelasticity of the infected non-necrotic surrounding lung tissue. The caseous drainage in the bronchial tree leads to bronchogenic spread of tuberculosis to other patients with unaffected lungs, and also extends to the trachea, larynx and oropharynx. Along with bronchogenic spread, the organism-rich caseous drainage (via aerosolized respiratory droplets) plays a central role in person-to-person transmission of infection. Infections in this setting are often limited to lungs, and hematogenous spread is kept in check for the most part due to hypersensitivity-induced thrombosis of the involved pulmonary parenchyma. In contrast to primary pulmonary tuberculosis, lymphadenopathy and calcification of paratracheal and mediastinal lymph nodes is not present.

The pulmonary cavities, especially those with thick walls, remain patent for extended periods after completion of effective anti-tuberculosis therapy. These patent cavities provide favorable milieu for secondary superinfections due to *Aspergillus* spp and other nontuberculous mycobacteria. Patients may present with new-onset hemoptysis without the evidence of recurrent tuberculosis. In most cases, this represents locally angioinvasive *Aspergillus* superinfection. This clinical presentation should be considered in the background of more ominous *M. tuberculosis*-associated erosion of pulmonary artery (Rasmussen's aneurysm), which may result in serious hemoptysis, exsanguinations, and death.

In elderly patients, post-primary tuberculosis of the lung may present as a chronic infection that spears upper lobes and that is difficult to distinguish from other infectious causes of chronic pneumonia. A high level of suspicion is needed to attempt an early diagnostic intervention in elderly patients in whom what appears to be bacterial pneumonia fails to responds to appropriate broad-spectrum antimicrobial therapy.

Constitutional symptoms such as loss of appetite, low-grade late-afternoon fever, night sweats, and weight loss are classically described in patients with post-primary tuberculosis, although in patients with cancer or recipients of transplantation, these symptoms do not help in diagnosis of tuberculosis. Cough is invariably present, although in chronic cases, cough may be well compensated. Occasional hemoptysis is also suggestive of tuberculosis, although in cancer patients with severe thrombocytopenia, this important feature becomes subdued as a cardinal sign of advancing pulmonary tuberculosis. Serofibrinous pleural effusion may accompany a long-standing untreated infection, and true plural tuberculous empyema are seldom seen in the post-anti-tuberculous chemotherapy era.

In patients with advancing pulmonary tuberculosis, the upper respiratory tract may be involved, including the well-described (although now seldom seen) laryngeal disease. Most laryngeal infection now represents hematogenous seeding rather than what used to be an extension of pulmonary tuberculosis via bronchogenic spread. Nevertheless, patients with untreated laryngeal tuberculosis pose a serious public health risk, as they are able to aerosolize a large number of viable infectious organisms leading to high rate of disease transmission. Laryngeal infections are often pleomorphic, and ulcerative or exophytic lesions may be mistaken for cancer.

Diagnosis

A high level of suspicion is central in the early diagnosis of tuberculosis. Early-morning sputum, or gastric aspirates in patients who do not produce sputum may provide diagnosis in the majority of patients with pulmonary disease. Although AFB-negative sputum does not eliminate the possibility of *M. tuberculosis* infection, especially in immunosuppressed cancer patients, diagnostic bronchoalveolar lavage via fiberoptic bronchoscopy, with or without transbronchial biopsy, may be able to enhance diagnostic yield. Percutaneous fine-needle aspiration or video-assisted thoracotomy may be undertaken to obtain samples of lung, pleura, and lymph nodes in patients suspected of cryptic tuberculosis if other less invasive procedures fail to provide conclusive results.

Treatment

Prior to the availability of effective antituberculosis therapy, disease progressed in three out of four patients, despite various now-antiquated methods, including iatrogenic collapse of the affected lung. This changed dramatically with the availability of streptomycin and, more importantly, isoniazid and rifampin making sanatorium-based treatment obsolete. The post-antibiotic era, however, has become marred with the emergence and global spread of *M. tuberculosis* strains that are resistant to the bactericidal drugs isoniazid and rifampin (strains known as multi-drug resistant tuberculosis (MDR-TB).

For infections due to drug-sensitive *M. tuberculosis*, the duration of therapy is suggested as 6 to 9 months, although shorter courses have been tried with variable success. The recommended four first-line drug regimen includes a combination of isoniazid, rifampin plus pyrazinamide for the first 8 weeks; ethambutol hydrochloride is included in most regimens, along with pyrazinamide, for the first 2 months of therapy. Patients receiving the ethambutol-based regimen should have visual examinations at frequent intervals to detect ocular toxicity before the patient become symptomatic.

Other anti-tuberculosis agents include streptomycin and levofloxacin, which are regarded as first-line agents, although they are not recommended in the initial choice of drug combinations for the patient who tolerates the suggested 3- or 4-drug combination. Agents known as second-line drugs are ethionamide, cycloserine, kanamycin, capreomycin, para-aminosalicylic acid, and clofazamine. These antimicrobials are reserved for patients who are either intolerant to the first-line drugs, or more importantly, in the treatment of infections due to MDR-TB.

Systemic corticosteroids may be used cautiously in patients who are on effective anti-tuberculosis therapy. Indications for a limited systemic steroid use include patients who are severely debilitated with serous anemia, hypoalbuminemia, protracted hectic fevers, and those with refractory life-threatening hypoxia.

Extrapulmonary Tuberculosis

M. tuberculosis can infect almost any body site. Extrapulmonary tuberculosis is considered an infection involving a non-pulmonary end-organ site, and, at present, bloodstream invasion is the most common method of tuberculosis systemic spread. Bronchogenic spread of tuberculosis to the upper respiratory tract or larynx, or contiguous spread to the pleural space or to the chest wall are discussed elsewhere.

Tuberculous Lymphadenitis

Scrofula is the predominant form of extrapulmonary tuberculosis; the cervical lymph node chain along the anterior border of the sternocleidomastoid muscle is commonly involved. Infection is often unilateral with minimum constitutional symptoms. Excisional lymph node biopsy is diagnostic, although precautions are needed to present post-surgical fistula tract formation. In patients with bilateral, or multicentric tuberculous lymphadenitis, evaluation for an underlying HIV-associated immune suppression is warranted, as widespread tuberculous lymphadenitis represents more severe systemic disease; patients in this setting often have systemic symptoms and are ill-appearing.[38] In localized cervical infection, a short course (6 months) of therapy may be adequate in patients with drug-susceptible strains of *M. tuberculosis*. A paradoxical lymph node enlargement, pain, or fistula formation during or after completion of antituberculous therapy represent the hosts' inflammatory response, which may be treated with a short course of systemic corticosteroids, especially in patients with a clinically disabling paradoxical reaction. This, however, must not be confused with immune reconstitution syndrome noted in patients with highly active antiretroviral-therapy–induced immune reconstitution.

Miliary Tuberculosis

The current description of miliary tuberculosis is hematogenous dissemination of *M. tuberculosis* via the bloodstream to remote body sites. Miliary tuberculosis may either present as an acute or cryptic form of disease. In the post-antibiotic era, miliary tuberculosis is most frequently reported in patients with cancer, those receiving antineoplastic therapy, chronic alcoholism, cirrhosis of the liver, and patients with rheumatologic diseases.[39–41] Secondary foci of infection include the meninges, peritoneum, liver, adrenals, kidneys, and pleura. In the lungs, a miliary radiographic pattern may help in establishing the correct diagnosis, although lymphangitic spread of solid-organ cancer, widespread pulmonary lymphoma, and invasive fungal infections can present a miliary pattern, which is difficult to distinguish from tuberculosis. Rapid diagnosis is imperative, as is a biopsy of either enlarged lymph nodes or a scrotal mass; the finding of caseating granulomas on liver or bone marrow biopsy should alert the healthcare provider to the possibility of disseminated tuberculosis and to the prompt institution of combination therapy, including isoniazid, rifampin and pyrazinamide. In patients with severe hypoxemia refractory to supplemental oxygen therapy or patients with evidence of disseminated intravascular coagulation, adjuvant systemic corticosteroid therapy is suggested.

Skeletal Tuberculosis

In the developed countries, tuberculous spondylitis (or Pott's disease) involves elderly rather than young adults as it does in regions of endemic tuberculosis. This potentially devastating disease of the spine originates as either due to a remotely acquired infection via hematogenous route or, less likely, extension from pleural or peritoneal tuberculosis, and rarely via lymphatic spread. The primary site of infection is intervertebral disc space; adjoining vertebral bones become involved as the infection progresses. In nearly half the patients, at the time of diagnosis, infection may involve paraspinal space, and if unchecked, the paraspinal abscess may lead to fistula formation. Compromise of motor functions is a serious concern in patients with paraspinal abscess. Any sign of lower-extremity weakness, loss of sensation, or paresthesia must be investigated with a contrast-enhanced MRI scan to evaluate possible nerve root or spinal cord compromise, which, if untreated, will result in devastating paralysis. In some instances, paralysis may develop after anti-tuberculosis treatment has commenced; this paradoxical reaction may warrant emergent laminectomy to relieve pressure and prevent spinal cord damage.

Similarly, osteoarticular tuberculosis is a disease of the elderly; multiple joints may be involved with periarticular abscess formation. In one study, the shoulder joint was the most frequently involved joint, in contrast with monarthric disease of the past, which usually involved knee or hip joints.[42,43] Patients may also present with tuberculous tenosynovitis in the hand. A patient with chronic wrist joint tuberculous may seek medical attention due to carpal tunnel syndrome.

Genitourinary Tuberculosis

Most patients with renal tuberculosis have either a history of, or ongoing, active pulmonary tuberculosis. Rarely, patients with cryptic, slowly progressive miliary (hematogenous) tuberculosis may develop features of renal mycobacterial disease. Papillary necrosis, urethral strictures, scarring-related asymmetrical hydronephrosis, cavitary lesions in the renal cortex, and focal renal calcifications are all seen with, and considered, features of renal tuberculosis. Diagnostic workup consists of first-of-the-day voided urine sample, AFB stain, and mycobacterial cultures. An intravenous pyelogram may show the collection channel abnormalities mentioned above. In selected cases, renal biopsy may be undertaken to establish appropriate diagnosis. Renal function is often preserved, although compromised renal function and hypertension are the hallmarks of the rarely seen tuberculous interstitial nephritis.

Female genital tract tuberculosis starts as hematogenous seeding of the endosalpinx; infection then spreads to the endometrium, ovaries, and cervix; the vagina is rarely involved. Most patients are diagnosed during workup for infertility, although menstrual irregularities and dull lower abdominal discomfort are not uncommon. Cervical and endometrial tuberculosis may present as an ulcerative mass that is frequently mistaken for cancer; similarly, patients with ovarian tuberculosis may receive a misdiagnosis of malignancy. Those with tuberculous peritonitis have been incorrectly diagnosed with metastatic ovarian cancer with carcinomatosis.[44,45]

Gastrointestinal Tuberculosis

In the era prior to the availability of effective anti-tuberculosis therapy, a large proportion of patients with active pulmonary disease would have concomitant gastrointestinal (GI) tract tuberculosis. Any part of GI tract may be involved, although the ileocecal area is the most frequent site of GI tuberculosis, presenting as chronic weight loss, anorexia, diarrhea, intestinal obstruction, and bleeding. In chronic untreated cases, patients may present with a palpable, soft, non-tender, lower abdominal mass. Other features of enteric tuberculosis include intestinal obstruction, perforation, and fistula formation between the bowel loops and/or small intestinal lumen and skin (enterocutaneous fistula).

Hepatic and biliary tract tuberculosis has prominent obstructive patterns; alkaline phosphatase levels are disproportionately high compared with often normal levels of transaminase and bilirubin. Pancreatic tuberculosis presents as a mass in the epigastric retroperitoneal region, and is difficult to distinguish form cancer.

Tuberculous Peritonitis

Of the two varieties of peritoneal tuberculosis, the "serous" variety is common, whereas the "plastic" form, which presents as a "doughy abdomen" on examination, is seldom seen. Patients present with chronic weight loss, and have dull abdominal pain, recurring fever, and occasionally, clinical presentation may mimic acute bacterial peritonitis, especially in patients with end-stage cirrhosis of the liver. Similar to pleural tuberculosis, peritoneal fluid is often non-diagnostic. Biopsy of the involved peritoneum and/or direct peritoneal fluid polymerase chain reaction may improve probability of correct diagnosis. Treatment is same as that for pulmonary infection, and we recommend against the use of adjuvant corticosteroids to prevent intestinal obstruction, which may occur either during or after completion of anti-tuberculosis therapy.

Aural Tuberculosis

Aural tuberculosis is a rare infection and often misdiagnosed as a refractory bacterial otitis media, or otitis externa; in most patients, the only symptom is painless otorrhea. Infection leads to gradual loss of hearing, and granulomatous inflammation is in abundance. If unchecked, infection can lead to extensive destruction of mastoid and temporal bones. In some cases, caseation necrosis may extend into intracranial cavity and present as new onset seizures and with other neurological abnormalities.[46] Clinical worsening after institution of anti-tuberculosis therapy similar to tuberculous cervical lymphadenitis, or tuberculous meningitis may represent paradoxical reaction resulting from uncontrolled inflammatory response. In these select patients, a short course of systemic corticosteroids may ameliorate symptoms, while effective combination anti-tuberculosis therapy is continued.

Cutaneous Tuberculosis

Skin involvement may result from either direct inoculation, or extension from an infected underlying structure such as bone, joint, or lymph node. In patients with severe immune dysfunction, hematogenous dissemination may lead to skin lesions that are often multiple, asymmetrical, and widespread. In general, cutaneous tuberculosis can mimic a variety of cutaneous disorders; nodular lesions with underlying induration or necrotic ulceration are prominent findings.

Diagnosis requires full-thickness skin biopsy. Treatment depends on the underlying primary site of infection. In patients with hematogenous disseminated disease, treatment is the same as that for miliary tuberculosis.

Tuberculosis Mimicking Tumor

Tuberculosis can imitate clinical and radiographic features of various diseases; as mentioned earlier, abdominopelvic tuberculosis may be misinterpreted as cancer—especially infections involving the peritoneum, ovaries, uterus, and pancreas.[43,44,47] In patients with chronic, slowly progressive, indolent pulmonary tuberculosis may be mistaken for lung cancer.[48] In one study, nearly 60% of patients with focal pulmonary tuberculosis were referred to a comprehensive cancer for treatment of presumed lung cancer.[12] It is also important to realize that certain malignancies may be mistaken for tuberculosis, especially bronchoalveolar carcinoma, and pulmonary non-Hodgkin's lymphoma.[49,50]

In patients with an underlying malignancy, the risk of tuberculosis reactivation is higher than in the general population.[51] Therefore, a high suspicion that tuberculosis may coexist with an undiagnosed cancer, or (in patients with known malignancies) that tuberculosis may develop concurrently, may help in early identification and institution of appropriate therapy.[52–54] A diagnostic attempt may include fiberoptic bronchoscopic evaluation, transthoracic fine-needle aspiration, or evaluation of surgically obtained lung tissue, which may provide timely diagnosis in a select group of patients in whom the probability of concurrent cancer and tuberculosis may coexist.[55–58]

Nontuberculous Mycobacteriosis

The scope of mycobacterial infections due to species other than M. tuberculosis have expanded near-exponentially in the recent past. In part, this increase is attributed to the widespread availability of newer molecular identification methods.[59] Most nontuberculous mycobacteria (NTM) are ubiquitous in nature, and unlike M. tuberculosis, person-to-person spread is not a significant means of transmission of infection. Isolation of these low-virulence mycobacteria is not uncommon, and, in immunologically intact, non-susceptible individuals, they frequently represent either laboratory/environmental contaminant or non-disease associated colonization of respiratory, orointestinal or genitourinary tracts. In patients with severe adaptive cellular immune defects, these mycobacteria may pose a serious threat.

Another feature that distinguishes these organisms from M. tuberculosis is that they exhibit variable antimicrobial susceptibility profiles and they are often not susceptible to the first-line anti-tuberculosis agents. The NTM are discussed under two broad headings based on the time needed for them to grow in the laboratory. Slow-growing mycobacteria (SGM) are somewhat similar to *M. tuberculosis* and take between 4 to 8 weeks to grow in enriched culture medium, whereas in the case of rapidly growing mycobacteria (RGM) growth becomes evident within 7 days.

Slow-Growing Mycobacteria

Mycobacterium avium-intracellulare

M. avium and *M. intracellulare* were originally differentiated on the bases of virulence to chickens and rabbits, respectively. Human infections were reported in 1943, and during the 1980s and 1990s, increased appreciation of diseases associated with MAC has been attributed in part due to the HIV epidemic, although a higher number of HIV-negative patients have also been described as having infection diseases due to these NTMs.

Pulmonary infections are most common, and isolation of MAC in respiratory tract samples, including tracheal aspirate, or bronchial samples, by itself is not diagnostic of pulmonary MAC infection. Diagnosis requires presence of a radiographic and clinical disease that is compatible with MAC infection. The radiographic feature suggestive of pulmonary NTM includes small, multicentric nodules, tree-in-bud appearances, and/or small thin-walled cavitary lesions. Cough is the most prominent symptom; sputum production is relatively minimal, except in patients with severe cystic bronchiectasis. Chronic lung disease is a well-recognized predisposing factor in non-immunosuppressed patients, including patients with silicosis, chronic bronchitis, emphysema, and cystic fibrosis. Patients with healed fibrocavitary tuberculosis remains at risk for secondary *M. avium-intracellulare* infection.

Since the 1980s, an increasing number of MAC-associated pulmonary NTM cases have been noted in middle-aged and elderly women with no obvious immune defects. The most common feature of this illness is chronic cough, fatigue, inability to gain weight, depression, and, in advanced cases, multicentric, cystic bronchiectatic pulmonary lesions; fever and night sweats are often not present. Some authors described an underlying defect in IFN-γ production in patients who were initially mischaracterized as having Lady Windermere syndrome.[30,31] This defect in the critical cytokine pathway has led to otherwise healthy patients to develop indolent, locally destructive pulmonary lesions due to environmental mycobacteria with low disease-causing potential in otherwise healthy individuals.

MAC infections are difficult to treat owing to resistance to several antimicrobial agents; therapeutic regimens comprise three to four drugs to which clinical isolates are susceptible; rifampin, ethambutol, macrolide derivatives such as azithromycin and clarithromycin, plus a quinolone (like ciprofloxacin) are often used. Clofazimine-based regimens are not suggested owing to unacceptable drug toxicity and high mortality seen in HIV-seropositive patients with disseminated MAC. The duration of therapy is longer than that for patients with pulmonary tuberculosis. Most patients are treated for 18 to 24 months; in those with extrapulmonary disease, duration may be extended to 36 months.

Mycobacterium kansasii

M. kansasii is antigenically related to *M. tuberculosis* and may be associated with false positive PPD due to antigenic cross-reactivity. Most infections in the United States are seen in urban centers situated in the southeast and Midwestern parts of the country. As animal studies suggest, presence of dust by unexplained mechanisms enhances disease-causing potential of *M. kansasii*[60]; it is not surprising that patients with pneumoconiosis are more susceptible to *M. kansasii* lung infection compared to the general population; infections are fourfold higher in men compared to women. Similarly, infections tend to be common with certain occupations that involve chronic exposure to dust. These include miners, welders, sandblasters, and painters.

Pulmonary infections are slowly progressive, although, unlike MAC, *M. kansasii* leads to lung involvement difficult to distinguish from tuberculosis. Infections frequently involve the upper lung lobes, and thin-wall cavities are seen routinely in patients with *M. kansasii* pulmonary nontuberculous mycobacteriosis. Treatment is rifampin-based, although rifampin-resistant strains are on the rise, especially in patients with AIDS receiving rifampin prophylaxis.[61,62] *M. kansasii* is intrinsically resistant to pyrazinamide,[63] and a large study has shown that isoniazid can be excluded for antimicrobial regimen.[64] Clarithromycin is often added with rifampin plus ethambutol, while awaiting rifampin susceptibility results.[65] Duration of therapy is 12 to 18 months.

Other Slow-Growing Mycobacteria

M. ulcerans, M. marinum, M. genavense M. haemophilum, and *M. simiae* are occasionally associated with infection in human.

M. haemophilum was almost exclusively seen in patients with severe immune dysfunction, either due to AIDS[66] or in recipients of hematopoietic stem cell transplantation.[67] Disseminated infections were common, and predilection for tendon sheaths, bone, and joints was similar to infection seen with RGM.

M. simiae complex includes *M. simiae, M. lentiflavum,* and *M. triplex;* like *M. kansasii,* these SGMs lead to pulmonary disease that is difficult to distinguish from tuberculosis. However, nearly three-quarters of clinical isolates may be associated with no discernable disease.[68,69] In certain regions of the United States, it has become the second most frequent NTM.[69] Infections tend to be more refractory to antimicrobial therapy, and high frequency of drug resistance further complicates options for effective drug regimen. Clarithromycin, quinolones, ethambutol, cycloserine, and ethionamide show favorable in vitro activity.[70]

Rapidly Growing Mycobacteria

These organisms exhibit prominent growth on solid culture medium within 7 days after incubation. The most recent distribution of pathogenic species includes *M. fortuitum* complex, which besides *M. fortuitum, M. mucogenicum,* and *M. septicum,* now also incorporates formerly known species of *M. chelonae* complex (*M. chelonae* and *M. abscessus*). *M. smegmatis* forms the newly described second group, including *M. smegmatis, M. wolinskyi,* and *M. goodii*.[71]

Pneumonia

In patients with pulmonary nontuberculous mycobacteriosis in the United States, RGM are the third most common cause of NTM after MAC and *M. kansasii,* respectively. *M. abscessus* is associated with most pulmonary infections in the RGM group, whereas infections due to *M. fortuitum,* sub. sp. *fortuitum, M. smegmatis* sub. sp. *smegmatis,* and *M. goodii* are less frequent.[72] *M. goodii* has been mostly isolated in patients with aspiration lipoid pneumonia. Similar to SGM, isolation of RGM from respiratory tract samples is not sufficient to make a diagnosis of RGM infection; as in most cases, these organisms may represent either colonization or environmental contamination.

To establish an RGM's link to pulmonary disease, microbiologic isolation should be accompanied with radiographic and clinically compatible disease.[73] Clinical symptoms of pulmonary NTM, which at best are non-specific of mycobacterial infection, include chronic, minimally productive cough, low-grade fever, weight loss, and, in severe cases, hemoptysis may occur.[73]

Clinical and microbiological response to antimicrobial therapy for RGM pulmonary mycobacteriosis is less encouraging compared to treatment response in patients with SGM infections.[74] Drug combination including clarithromycin, high-dose cefoxitin plus amikacin have been associated with good clinical response, albeit microbiologically refractory *M. abscessus* infections are not uncommon.

Skin and Soft Tissue Infection

M. fortuitum is the most common RGM that is often associated with skin and soft tissue infection in immunologically competent patients; most infections occur due to accidental inoculation, such as stepping on a nail. Whereas most infections due to *M. chelonae* is seen in patients with a underlying predisposing condition, such as chronic corticosteroid use, rheumatoid arthritis, lupus, and cancer.[73,75]

Health-related infections occur sporadically and have been seen in patients after deep intramuscular injection, sternal wound infection following cardiac surgery, and after a variety of reconstructive and plastic surgical procedures, including augmentation mammaplasty and chest wall reconstruction after tumor resection.[76]

Catheter-Related Infections

These infections have become the most common health care-related infections due to RGM; most infections involve patients with long-term indwelling intravascular catheters, and often catheter-insertion sites are involved. In cancer patients, *M. chelonae* and *M. abscessus* are by far the most common in this setting.[77] Recently identified RGM species are increasingly reported in patients with cancer with catheter-related infection. They include *M. smegmatis*,[78] *M. neoaurum*,[79] *M. aurum*,[80] *M. lacticola*,[81] and *M. brumae*.[82]

It is important to emphasize the fact that RGM are frequently isolated in hospital and laboratory water supplies, and a number of pseudo-outbreaks involving contaminated blood culture materials and fiberoptic bronchoscope sterilizing machine contamination have been described.[83,84] Therefore, a strict criteria must be instituted before attributing catheter infection to these low-virulence ubiquitous nontuberculous mycobacteria.[85] Treatment includes prompt removal of infected devices, and systemic combination antimicrobial therapy for 6 to 12 weeks. Selection of antimicrobials depends on RGM species; as a general rule, RGM are resistant to most antituberculosis agents with the exception of ethambutol. In patients with *M. chelonae-M. abscessus* infections, selection of appropriate drug therapy is even more limited due to high-level intrinsic drug resistance. Clarithromycin-based regimens are currently recommended, although so are newer fluoroquinolones, such as gatifloxacin and moxifloxacin; linezolid in vitro profile also appears promising, although further clinical experience is needed before such treatment is recommended. Other agents under investigation includes tigecycline, a new glycocycline that shows promising activity against most clinical isolates of *M. abscessus*.[86]

Summary

M. tuberculosis has become a rare infection in patients receiving antineoplastic therapy in the United States and tends to be prominent in non-native, foreign-born patient population. In recent years, a change in the underlying malignancy has also been noted as patients with leukemia and non-Hodgkin's lymphoma have overshadowed head and neck and gastric cancers. Most cancer patients have a favorable response to therapy, and multi-drug resistant strains are seldom encountered in this patient population.

The spectrum of non-tuberculosis mycobacteria is changing rapidly, as the immunopathogenesis of SGM continues to improve. In recent years, difficult-to-treat infections due to RGM are on the rise; this may, in part, reflect newer molecular identification methods, but a rise in the susceptible immunosuppressed patient population and the frequent use of indwelling prosthetic devices are also important contributors in this trend. Despite resistance to a number of available antimicrobials, newer agents may provide the much-needed treatment options for high-risk cancer patients with mycobacterial infection-disease.

REFERENCES

1. Kochi A. The global tuberculosis situation and the new control strategy of the World Health Organization. Tubercle 1991;72:1–6.
2. Sudre P, Ten Dam G, Kochi A. Tuberculosis: a global overview of the situation today. Bull World Health Organ 1992;70:149–59.
3. Bloom BR. Tuberculosis—the global view. N Engl J Med 2002;346:1434–5.
4. World Health Organization report on the tuberculosis epidemic, 1997. Geneva, Switzerland.
5. Centers for Disease Control and Prevention. Tuberculosis morbidity – United States, 1997. MMWR Morb Mortal Wkly Rep 1998;47:253–7.
6. Kaplan JE, Masur H, Holmes KK. Guidelines for preventing opportunistic infections among HIV-infected persons—2002. Recommendations of the U.S. Public Health Service and the Infectious Diseases Society of America. MMWR Recomm Rep 2002;51(RR-8):1–52.
7. Keane J, Gershon S, Wise RP, et al. Tuberculosis associated with infliximab, a tumor necrosis factor α-neutralizing agent. N Engl J Med 2001;345:1098–104.
8. Gomez-Reino JJ, Carmona L, Valverde VR, et al. Treatment of rheumatoid arthritis with tumor necrosis factor inhibitors may predispose to significant increase in tuberculosis risk: a multicenter active-surveillance report. Arthritis Rheum 2003;48:2122–7.
9. American Thoracic Society. Control of tuberculosis in the United States. Am Rev Respir Dis 1992;146:1623–33.
10. Kaplan MH, Armstrong D, Rosen P. Tuberculosis complicating neoplastic disease. A review of 201 cases. Cancer 1974;33:850–8.
11. Safdar A, Armstrong D. Infectious morbidity in critically ill patients with cancer. Crit Care Clin 2001;17:531–70.
12. De La Rosa GR, Jacobson KL, Rolston KV, et al. *Mycobacterium tuberculosis* at a comprehensive cancer center: active disease in patients with underlying malignancy during 1990–2000. Clin Microbiol Infect Dis 2004;10:749–52.
13. Roy V, Weisdorf D. Mycobacterial infections following bone marrow transplantation: a 20 year retrospective review. Bone Marrow Transplant 1997;19:467–70.
14. Singh N, Paterson DL. *Mycobacterium tuberculosis* infection in solid-organ transplant recipients: impact and implications for management. Clin Infect Dis 1998;27:1266–77.
15. Yuen KY, Woo PC. Tuberculosis in blood and marrow transplant recipients. Hematol Oncol 2002;20:51–62.
16. Mohite U, Das M, Saikia T, et al. Mycobacterial pulmonary infection post allogeneic bone marrow transplantation. Leuk Lymphoma 2001;40:675–8.
17. George B, Mathews V, Sirvastava A, Chandy M. Infections among allogeneic bone marrow transplant recipients in India. Bone Marrow Transplant 2004;33:311–5.
18. Talbot EA, Moore M, McCray E, Binkin NJ. Tuberculosis among foreign-born persons in the United States, 1993–1998. JAMA 2000;284:2894–900.
19. Weis SE, Moonan PK, Pogoda JM, et al. Tuberculosis in the foreign-born population of Tarrant county, Texas by immigration status. Am J Respir Crit Care Med. 2001; 164:953–957.
20. Flynn JL, Chan J. Immunology of tuberculosis. Annu Rev Immunol 2001;129:93–129.
21. Flynn JL, Goldstein MM, Triebold KJ, et al. Major histocompatibility complex class I-restricted T cells are required for resistance to *Mycobacterium tuberculosis* infection. Proc Natl Acad Sci USA 1992;89:12013–7.
22. D'Souza CD, Cooper AM, Frank AA, et al. An anti-inflammatory role for gamma delta T lymphocytes in acquired immunity to *Mycobacterium tuberculosis*. J Immunol 1997;158:1217–21.
23. Murray HW. Interferon-gamma and host antimicrobial defense: current and future clinical applications. Am J Med 1994;97:459–67.
24. Algood HMS, Chan J, Flynn JL. Chemokines and tuberculosis. Cytokine Growth Factor Rev 2003;14: 467–77.
25. Patarroyo M. Adhesion molecules mediating recruitment of monocytes to inflamed tissue. Immunobiology 1994;191: 474–7.
26. Kobayashi K, Kaneda K, Kasama T. Immunopathogenesis of delayed-type hypersensitivity. Microsc Res Tech 2001;53: 241–5.
27. Dorman SE, Holland SM. Interferon-γ and interleukin-12 pathway defects and human disease. Cytokine Growth Factor Rev 2000;11:321–33.
28. Saunders BM, Briscoe H, Britton WJ. T cell-derived tumor necrosis factor is essential, but not sufficient, for protection against *Mycobacterium tuberculosis* infection. Clin Exp Immunol 2004;137:279–87.
29. Ehlers S, Hölscher C, Scheu S, et al. The lymphotoxin β receptor is critically involved in controlling infections with the intracellular pathogens *Mycobacterium tuberculosis* and *Listeria monocytogenes*. J Immunol 2003;170: 5210–8.
30. Safdar A, White DA, Stover D, et al. Profound interferon gamma deficiency in patients with chronic pulmonary nontuberculous mycobacteriosis. Am J Med 2002;113: 756–9.
31. Safdar A, Armstrong D, Murray HW. A novel defect in interferon-gamma secretion in patients with refractory nontuberculous pulmonary mycobacteriosis. Ann Intern Med 2003;138:521.
32. Holland SM, Eisenstin EM, Kuhns DB, et al. Treatment of refractory disseminated nontuberculous mycobacterial infection with interferon gamma. N Engl J Med 1994; 330:1348–55.
33. Dorman SE, Picard C, Lammas D, et al. Clinical features of dominant and recessive interferon gamma receptor 1 deficiencies. Lancet 2004;364:2113–21.
34. Stead WW. Tuberculosis among elderly persons: an outbreak in a nursing home. Ann Intern Med 1981;94:606–10.
35. Stylbo K. Recent advances in epidemiological research in tuberculosis. Adv Tuberc Res 1980;20:1.
36. Stead WW, Lofgren JP, Warren E, Thomas C. Tuberculosis as an endemic and nosocomial infection among the elderly in nursing homes. N Engl J Med 1985;312: 1483–7.
37. Selwyan PA, Hartel D, Lewis VA, et al. A prospective study of the risk of tuberculosis among intravenous drug users with human immunodeficiency virus infection. N Engl J Med 1989;320:545–55.
38. Hewlett D Jr, Duncanson FP, Jagadha V, et al. Lymphadenopathy in an inner city population consisting principally of intravenous drug abusers with suspected acquired immunodeficiency syndrome. Am Rev Respir Dis 1988; 137:1275–9.
39. Kim JH, Langston AA, Gallis HA. Miliary tuberculosis: epidemiology, clinical manifestations, diagnosis, and outcome. Rev Infect Dis 1990;12:583–90.
40. Martens G, Willcox PA, Benatar SR. Miliary tuberculosis: rapid diagnosis, hematologic abnormalities, outcome in 109 treated adults. Am J Med 1990;89:291–6.
41. Munt PW. Milliary tuberculosis in the chemotherapy era: with a clinical review in 69 American adults. Medicine 1972;51:139–55.
42. LiZares LF, Valcarcel A, Del Castillo JM, et al. Tuberculous arthritis with multiple joint involvement. J Rheumatol 1991;18:635–6.

43. Garrido G, Gomez-Reino JJ, Fernandez-Dapica P, et al. A review of peripheral tuberculous arthritis. Semin Arthritis Rheum 1988;18:142–9.

44. Mahdavi A, Malvija VK, Herschman BR. Peritoneal tuberculosis disguised as ovarian cancer: an emerging clinical challenge. Gynecol Oncol 2002;84:167–70.

45. Protopapas A, Milingos S, Diakomanolis E, et al. Miliary tuberculous peritonitis mimicking advanced ovarian cancer. Gynecol Obstet Invest 2003;56:89–92.

46. Safdar A, Brown AE, Kraus DH, Malkin M. Paradoxical reaction syndrome complicating aural infection due to *Mycobacterium tuberculosis* during therapy. Clin Infect Dis 2000;30:625–7.

47. Kouraklis G, Glinavou A, Karayiannakis A, Karatzas G. Primary tuberculosis of the pancreas mimicking a pancreatic tumor. Int J Pancreatol 2001;29:151–3.

48. Rolston KVI, Rodriguez S, Dholakia N, et al. Pulmonary infections mimicking cancer: a retrospective, three-year review. Support Care Cancer 1997;5:90–3.

49. Chandrasekhar HR, Shashikala P, Murthy BN, et al. Bronchioloalveolar carcinoma mimicking miliary tuberculosis. J Assoc Physicians India 2001;49:281–2.

50. Miyake S, Yoshizawa Y, Ohkouchi Y, et al. Intern Med 1997;36:420–3.

51. Karnak D, Kayacan O, Beder S. Reactivation of pulmonary tuberculosis in malignancy. Tumori 2002;88:251–4.

52. Rybacka-Chabros B, Mandziuk S, Berger-Lukasiewicz A, et al. The coexistence of tuberculosis infection and lung cancer in patients treated in pulmonary department of Medical Academy in Lublin during last ten years (1990–2000). Folia Histochem Cytobiol 2001;39(Suppl2):73–4.

53. Saygili U, Guclu S, Altunyurt S, et al. Primary endometrioid adenocarcinoma with coexisting endometrial tuberculosis. A case report. J Reprod Med 2002;47:322–4.

54. Inadome Y, Ikezawa T, Oyasu R, Noguchi M. Malignant lymphoma of bronchus-associated lymphoid tissue (BALT) coexistent with pulmonary tuberculosis. Pathol Int 2001;51:807–11.

55. Chan HS, Sun AJ, Hoheisel GB. Bronchoscopic aspiration and bronchoalveolar lavage in the diagnosis of sputum smear-negative pulmonary tuberculosis. Lung 1990;168:215–20.

56. Baughman RP, Dohn MN, Loudon RG, Frame PT. Bronchoscopy with bronchoalveolar lavage in tuberculosis and fungal infections. Chest 1991;99:92–7.

57. White DA, Wong PW, Downey R. The utility of open lung biopsy in patients with hematologic malignancies. Am J Respir Crit Care Med 2000;161:723–9.

58. Wong PW, Stefanec T, Brown K, White DA. Role of fine-needle aspirates of focal lung lesions in patients with hematologic malignancies. Chest 2002;121:527–32.

59. Han XY, Pham AS, Tarrand JJ, et al. Rapid and accurate identification of mycobacteria by sequencing hypervariable regions of the 16S ribosomal RNA gene. Am J Clin Pathol 2002;118:796–801.

60. Geruez-Rienx C, Tacquet A, Devulder B. Experimental study of interactions of pneumoconiosis and mycobacterial infections. Ann N Y Acad Sci 1972;200:106.

61. Klein JL, Brown TJ, French GL. Rifampin resistance in *Mycobacterium kansasii* is associated with rpoB mutations. Antimicrob Agents Chemother 2001;45:3056–8.

62. Wallace RJ Jr, Dunbar D, Brown BA, et al. Rifampin-resistant *Mycobacterium kansasii*. Clin Infect Dis 1994;18:736–43.

63. Sun Z, Zhang Y. Reduced pyrazinamidase activity and the natural resistance of *Mycobacterium kansasii* to the antituberculosis drug pyrazinamide. Antimicrob Agents Chemother 1999;43:537–42.

64. Research Committee, British Thoracic Society. *Mycobacterium kansasii* pulmonary infection: a prospective study of the results of nine months of treatment with rifampin and ethambutol. Thorax 1994;49:442–5.

65. Yew WW, Piddock LJ, Li MS, et al. In-vitro activity of quinolones and macrolides against mycobacteria. J Antimicrob Chemother 1994;34:343–51.

66. Lerner C, Safdar A, Coppel S. *Mycobacterium haemophilum* infection in AIDS. Infect Dis Clin Practice 1995;4:233–6.

67. White MH, Papadopoulos EB, Small TN, et al. *Mycobacterium haemophilum* infections in bone marrow transplant recipients. Transplantation 1995;15:957–60.

68. Rynkiewicz DL, Cage GD, Butler WR, Ampel NM. Clinical and microbiological assessment of *Mycobacterium simiae* isolates from a single laboratory in Southern Arizona. Clin Infect Dis 1998;26:625–30.

69. Valero G, Paters J, Jorgensen JH, Graybill JR. Clinical isolates of *Mycobacterium simiae* in San Antonio, Texas. An 11-yr review. Am J Respir Crit Care Med 1995;152:1555–7.

70. Valero G, Moreno F, Graybill JR. Activity of clarithromycin, ofloxacin, and clarithromycin plus ethambutol against *Mycobacterium simiae* in murine model of disseminated infection. Antimicrob Agents Chemother 1994;38:2676–7.

71. Brown BA, Springer B, Steingrube VA, et al. Description of *Mycobacterium wolinskyi* and *Mycobacterium goodii* two new rapidly growing species related to *Mycobacterium smegmatis* and associated with human wound infections: a cooperative study from the International Working Group on Mycobacterial Taxonomy. Int J Syst Bacteriol 1999;49:1493–511.

72. Griffith DE, Girard WM, Wallace RJ Jr. Clinical features of pulmonary disease caused by rapidly growing mycobateria: an analysis of 154 patients. Am Rev Respir Dis 1993;147:1271–8.

73. Jacobson K, Garcia R, Libshitz H, et al. Clinical and radiological features of pulmonary disease caused by rapidly growing mycobacteria in cancer patients. Eur J Clin Microbiol Infect Dis 1998;17:615–21.

74. Wallace RJ Jr, Cook JL, Glassroth J, et al. Diagnosis and treatment of disease caused by nontuberculous mycobacteria. American Thoracic Society Statement. Am J Respir Crit Care Med 1997;156(Suppl 1):1–25.

75. Wallace RJ Jr, Brown BA, Onyi GO. Skin, soft tissue, and bone infections due to *Mycobacterium chelonae chelonae*: importance of prior corticosteroid therapy, frequency of disseminated infections, and resistance to oral antimicrobials other than clarithromycin. J Infect Dis 1992;166:405–12.

76. Safdar A, Bains M, Polsky B. Clinical microbiological case: refractory chest wall infection following reconstructive surgery in a patient with relapsed lung cancer. Clin Microbiol Infect 2001;7:563–4, 577–9.

77. Engler HD, Hass A, Hodes DS, Bottone EJ. *Mycobacterium chelonei* infection of a Broviac catheter insertion site. Eur J Clin Microbiol Infect Dis 1989;8:521–3.

78. Skiest DJ, Levi ME. Catheter-related bacteremia due to *Mycobacterium smegmatis*. South Med J 1998;91:36–7.

79. Woo PC, Tsoi HW, Leung KW, et al. Identification of *Mycobacterium neoaurum* isolated from a neutropenic patient with catheter-related bacteremia by 16S rRNA sequencing. J Clin Microbiol 2000;38:3515–7.

80. Koranyi KI, Ranalli MA. *Mycobacterium aurum* bacteremia in an immunocompromised child. Pediatr Infect Dis 2003;22:1108–9.

81. Kiska DL, Turenne CY, Dubansky AS, Domachowske JB. First case report of cathter-related bacteremia due to "*Mycobacterium lacticola*". J Clin Micrbiol 2004;42:2855–7.

82. Lee SA, Raad II, Adachi JA, Han XY. Catheter-related bloodstream infection caused by *Mycobacterium brumae*. J Clin Microbiol 2004;42:5429–31.

83. Ashford DA, Kellerman S, Yakrus M, et al. Pseudo-outbreak of septicemia due to rapidly growing mycobacteria associated with extrinsic contamination of culture supplement. J Clin Microbiol 1997;35:2040–2.

84. Fraser VJ, Jones MJ, Murray PR, et al. Contamination of flexible fiberoptic bronchoscopes with *Mycobacterum chelonae* linked to an automated bronchoscope disinfection machine. Am Rev Respir Dis 1992;145:853–5.

85. Safdar A, Raad II. Management and treatment. In: O'Grady NP, Pittet D, editors. Catheter-related infections in the critically ill. 1st ed. Boston: Kluwer Academic Publishers; 2004. p. 99–112.

86. Wallace RJ, Brown-Elliott BA, Crist CJ, et al. Comparison of the in vitro activity of the glycylcycline tigecycline (formerly GAR-939) with those of tetracycline, minocycline, and doxycycline against isolates of nontuberculous mycobacteria. Antimicrob Agents Chemother 2002;46:3164–7.

Hypercalcemia of Malignancy

Gregory A. Clines, MD, PhD
Theresa A. Guise, MD

Malignancy is the most common cause of hypercalcemia in the hospitalized patient, and malignancy-associated hypercalcemia is one of the more common paraneoplastic syndromes. Up to 30% of patients with cancer may develop hypercalcemia during the course of their disease.[1] Generally, the cancer is well advanced when hypercalcemia occurs, and the prognosis is poor.[2] Survival beyond six months is uncommon.[3] The relative frequencies of malignancies associated with hypercalcemia are listed in Table 1.[4]

Symptoms of Hypercalcemia

Symptoms of hypercalcemia (Table 2) may vary in individual patients and are related both to the absolute concentration of serum calcium and to the rate of rise in serum calcium.[5] Nonspecific gastrointestinal symptoms of anorexia, constipation, nausea, and vomiting may predominate. Optimal neurological function is dependent on extracellular calcium level and symptoms can range from subtle neuropsychiatric manifestations, such as irritability and depression, to muscle weakness, delirium, and even coma. Cardiovascular manifestations of hypercalcemia include arrhythmias and hypertension. Hypercalcemia causes an impaired ability of the distal nephron to concentrate urine, resulting in polyuria and polydipsia. The hypercalcemic effects of anorexia, nausea, vomiting, and impaired renal concentrating ability lead to dehydration and, subsequently, altered mental status. This, in turn, may promote immobilization and lead to worsening hypercalcemia.

Table 1 Malignancies Associated with Hypercalcemia

Malignancy	Frequency (%)
Lung	35
Breast	25
Hematologic	14
Head and neck	6
Renal	3
Prostate	3
Unknown primary	7
Others	7

Reproduced with adapted from Mundy GR and Martin TJ.[4]

Table 2 Clinical Features of Hypercalcemia

Neurologic and psychiatric	Lethargy, drowsiness
	Confusion, disorientation
	Disturbed sleep, nightmares
	Irritability, depression
	Hypotonia, decreased deep tendon reflexes
	Stupor, coma
Gastrointestinal	Anorexia, vomiting
	Constipation
	Peptic ulceration
	Acute pancreatitis
Cardiovascular	Arrhythmias
	Synergism with digoxin
	Hypertension
Renal	Polyuria, polydipsia
	Hypercalciuria
	Nephrocalcinosis
	Impaired glomerular filtration

Humoral Mediators of Hypercalcemia of Malignancy

Hypercalcemia occurring in the setting of malignancy may be due to (1) humoral factors secreted by tumors that act systemically on target organs of bone, kidney, and intestine to disrupt normal calcium homeostasis; (2) local factors secreted by tumors in bone, either metastatic or hematologic, which directly stimulate osteoclastic bone resorption; and (3) coexisting primary hyperparathyroidism (1°HPT). The first two of these situations should be viewed as opposite ends of a continual spectrum, rather than as completely unrelated pathologies. Clearly the pathophysiology of hypercalcemia in patients with solid tumors and no bone metastases at one end of the spectrum, and myeloma associated with extensive local bone destruction adjacent to the tumor cells at the other, is very different. However, in between these extremes are hypercalcemic patients with squamous cell carcinomas in which hypercalcemia may occur with some, but not extensive, osteolytic bone metastases, and hypercalcemic patients with advanced breast carcinoma in which hypercalcemia almost never occurs in the absence of extensive osteolytic bone destruction. Separating hypercalcemia into subcategories based on the assumption that the underlying mechanisms are distinct is not entirely satisfactory. This is because the mediators may be identical, except that in one situation it is a local mediator, while in another it is a humoral mediator. Additionally, if the tumor burden in bone is great, local tumor-produced mediators of bone resorption may be produced in sufficient quantities to have systemic effects. Although this review will discuss the effects of cancer on bone organized into such categories, it is important to understand that a significant portion of cancer patients will fall into the middle of this spectrum, having both humoral and local effects of tumor on bone.

Parathyroid Hormone-Related Protein

Hypercalcemia has been associated with malignancy since the development of serum calcium assays in the 1920s. Only in 1941, however, did Fuller Albright advance the hypothesis that parathyroid hormone (PTH) is ectopically produced by certain tumor types. Over the subsequent five decades, investigators determined that PTH was not, in fact, the cause of humoral hypercalcemia of malignancy (HHM), but that a "PTH-like factor" was responsible for most cases. In 1987, this PTH related-protein (PTHrP) was purified from human lung cancer,[6] breast cancer,[7] and renal cell carcinoma[8] simultaneously by several independent groups and cloned shortly thereafter.[9]

PTHrP shares 70% sequence homology with PTH over the first 13 amino acids at the N-terminus. Beyond the initial amino-terminal sequence, the protein is unique and shows no further sequence homology with PTH. The cloned PTHrP protein is larger than PTH and three distinct isoforms of 139, 141, and 173 amino acids have been demonstrated. Similarly, the human PTHrP gene is much larger and more complex than the parathyroid hormone gene, spanning 15 kilobase of genomic deoxyribonucleic acid (DNA) and having nine exons and three promoters. Despite these differences, both PTH and PTHrP bind to a common PTH/PTHrP receptor[10] and share similar biologic activities.[11]

PTHrP has been detected in a variety of tumor types as well as in normal tissue.[12,13] The widespread expression of PTHrP in normal tissue was the first evidence that the hormone had a role in normal physiology. In addition to the PTH-like effects, emerging work testifies to the fact that PTHrP plays a role in the (1) regulation of cartilage differentiation and bone formation[14]; (2) the growth and differentiation of skin,[15] mammary gland,[16] and teeth[17]; (3) cardiovascular function[18]; (4) transepithelial calcium transport in mammary epithelia and placenta[19,20]; (5) relaxation of smooth muscle in the uterus, bladder, arteries, and ileum[21–24]; and (6) host immune function.[25,26] Normal subjects do not have detectable circulating levels of PTHrP, suggesting that, in normal physiology, PTHrP acts as a local regulator or cytokine in the tissues where it is produced.

Approximately 80% of hypercalcemic patients with solid tumors have detectable or increased plasma concentrations of PTHrP.[7] In addition to the diverse normal physiologic functions of PTHrP, it has a multifunctional role in cancer as well. Such identified functions include (1) mediating hypercalcemia; (2) aiding in the development and progression of osteolytic bone metastasis, as will be discussed in subsequent sections; (3) regulating growth of cancer cells[27–29]; and (4) acting as a cell survival factor.[30] The first identified consequence of PTHrP in cancer was the humoral hypercalcemia of malignancy syndrome.

Humoral Hypercalcemia of Malignancy versus 1°HPT

Despite similarities between the syndromes of HHM and 1°HPT and the similar biologic activities of PTHrP and PTH, respectively, unexplained differences between these syndromes exist. First, patients with PTHrP-mediated HHM have low 1,25-dihydroxyvitamin D3 (1,25-$(OH)_2D_3$) levels compared to patients with 1°HPT, even though both hormones stimulate 1α-hydroxylase activity.[31] Moreover, infusion of PTH or PTHrP in healthy volunteers over a 48-hour period increased plasma 1,25-$(OH)_2D_3$ levels; however, PTH was more effective than PTHrP.[32] Second, while both syndromes have marked increases in osteoclastic bone resorption, many patients with HHM do not have the normally coupled increase in osteoblastic activity experienced by those with 1°HPT. Studies using either serum markers of bone turnover[33] or quantitative bone histomorphometry[34] have demonstrated this uncoupling of bone resorption from bone formation. Finally, unlike the metabolic acidosis seen in patients with 1°HPT, patients with HHM often have a metabolic alkalosis with a low plasma chloride and high plasma bicarbonate concentration. Although many explanations have been postulated for the discrepancies between HHM and 1°HPT, such as the pulsatile secretion of PTH and the apparent continuous secretion of PTHrP and biologically active PTHrP fragment,[35] and suppression of bone formation and 1α-hydroxylase activity by other tumor-associated factors, the reasons for these differences have not been adequately elucidated.

PTHrP in Hypercalcemia Associated with Breast Cancer

The role of PTHrP in breast cancer–associated hypercalcemia deserves special consideration. Breast cancer predominantly affects bone through metastatic mechanisms, typically with lytic deposits in the skeleton. Approximately 10% of women with breast cancer will have hypercalcemia as a complication at some point in the disease. The association of hypercalcemia with extensive osteolytic lesions in breast cancer is so strong that the presentation of hypercalcemia without bone metastases should suggest the presence of coexistent primary hyperparathyroidism.[36] Based on this association, it was long held that breast cancer–associated hypercalcemia results from excessive reabsorption of bone around tumor deposits. However, clinical studies[3] failed to demonstrate any relationship between the extent of bone metastasis and serum calcium levels. Conversely, studies exploring the potential role for a humoral mediator of hypercalcemia in breast cancer clearly demonstrated altered renal handling of calcium and phosphate, as well as increased nephrogenous cyclic adenosine monophosphate (cAMP), suggesting that 10 to 60% of hypercalcemic patients with breast cancer had a circulating factor with PTH-like properties. The identification of PTHrP as this factor is hardly surprising when it is recalled that PTHrP appears to play an important role in normal breast physiology. In the case of breast cancer, PTHrP appears to have both paracrine and endocrine actions.

PTHrP was detected by immunohistochemical staining in 60% of 102 invasive breast tumors removed from normocalcemic women, but not in normal breast tissue.[37] At least four other studies have confirmed these percentages, and one of these demonstrated immunoreactive PTHrP within the cytoplasm of lobular and ductal epithelial cells in normal and fibrocystic breast tissues.[38–41] Furthermore, 65 to 92% of hypercalcemic breast cancer patients (with and without bone metastasis) had detectable plasma PTHrP concentration by radioimmunoassay similar to those documented in patients with humoral hypercalcemia of malignancy due to non-breast tumors.[38,42] PTHrP is an important mediator of hypercalcemia in breast cancer. It also plays a significant role in the pathophysiology of breast cancer metastasis to bone, as evidenced by clinical studies indicating that PTHrP expression by primary breast cancer is more commonly associated with the development of bone metastasis and hypercalcemia.[39]

PTHrP in Hypercalcemia Associated with Hematologic Malignancies

Hypercalcemia associated with hematologic malignancies results both from systemic effects of tumor-produced factors such as 1,25-$(OH)_2D_3$ (discussed below), and from secretion of local bone-active cytokines, such as interleukin-6 (IL-6), IL-1, and lymphotoxin or TNFβ, from tumor in bone. PTHrP has been demonstrated to be an important pathogenic factor in the development of hypercalcemia in some patients with hematologic malignancies. In a clinical study of 76 patients with various hematologic malignancies, 50% of the 14 hypercalcemic patients had significant increases in plasma PTHrP concentrations.[43] Of these, five had non-Hodgkin's lymphoma, one had Hodgkin's disease, and one had multiple myeloma. The serum 1,25-$(OH)_2D_3$ concentrations, when measured, were low in the hypercalcemic non-Hodgkin's lymphoma patients who had increased plasma PTHrP concentrations. Also of interest in this study is the fact that several normocalcemic patients with non-Hodgkin's lymphoma, Hodgkin's lymphoma, multiple myeloma, and Waldenström's macroglobulinemia had increased plasma PTHrP concentrations as measured by an amino-terminal PTHrP assay. Using a sensitive, two-site immunoradiometric assay, other investigators have noted increased plasma PTHrP concentrations in patients with adult T cell leukemia and B cell lymphoma.[44] Finally, in separate studies, circulating concentrations of PTHrP (comparable to those in HHM) were present in two of four hypercalcemic patients with non-Hodgkin's lymphoma, in three of nine with myeloma, and in a patient with myeloid blast crisis of chronic myeloid leukemia.[45,46] Thus, the humoral mediators in the hypercalcemia associated with hematologic malignancies include both 1,25-$(OH)_2D_3$ and PTHrP.

1,25-Dihydroxyvitamin D

Under normal physiologic conditions, serum calcium concentration and levels of 1,25-$(OH)_2D_3$ are inversely related. In the setting of hypercalcemia, serum 1,25-$(OH)_2D_3$ concentrations are suppressed unless there is persistent stimulation of 1α-hydroxylase activity from an autonomous source of PTH, such as with primary hyperparathyroidism. Outside of this situation, lack of 1,25-$(OH)_2D_3$ suppression indicates abnormal regulation of 1,25-$(OH)_2D_3$ synthesis and further suggests extra-renal production such as that observed with granulomatous disease. In granulomatous disease, activated macrophages within the granuloma synthesize 1,25-$(OH)_2D_3$.[47–49] Similarly, a major mediator of hypercalcemia in Hodgkin's disease, non-Hodgkin's lymphoma, and other hematologic malignancies appears to be an extra-renal production of 1,25-(OH)$_2$D$_3$.[50] The mechanism is similar to that observed in granulomatous disease. In this scenario, hypercalcemic patients have increased plasma 1,25-(OH)$_2$D$_3$ concentrations with low or normal plasma PTH and urinary cAMP concentrations,[51] without the presence of bone involvement. Affected patients have also been shown to have increased fasting urinary calcium excretion[51] as well as increased intestinal calcium (^{47}Ca) absorption.[52] Increased 1,25-(OH)$_2$D$_3$ concentrations were noted in 12 of 22 hypercalcemic patients with non-Hodgkin's lymphoma. In addition, 71% of 22 normocalcemic patients with non-Hodgkin's lymphoma were hypercalciuric, and 18% had increased serum 1,25-(OH)$_2$D$_3$ concentrations. These findings led the investigators to conclude that disregulated 1,25-(OH)$_2$D$_3$ production was common in patients with diffuse large cell lymphoma.[50] The low serum PTH and urinary cAMP concentrations indicated that neither PTH nor PTHrP mediated the hypercalcemia in this setting. Prostaglandins, when measured, have been low, and selected patients had no calcium-lowering effect from indomethacin therapy.[45]

Thus, the mechanisms responsible for hypercalcemia in this setting appear to be multifactorial and include 1,25-(OH)$_2$D$_3$–mediated increases in intestinal absorption of calcium and osteoclastic bone resorption. Additionally, many of the reported patients had altered renal function, a finding that suggests that impaired renal calcium clearance may also be contributing to the hypercalcemia in certain patients. It is likely that the lymphoma tissue itself hydroxylates 25-hydroxyvitamin D to the active 1,25-(OH)$_2$D$_3$ similar to the situation in hypercalcemia associated with granulomatous disease. One α-hydroxylase activity has been demonstrated in human T cell lymphotrophic virus type-I-transformed lymphocytes as well as in other extrarenal tissues.[53,54] None of the reported patients with 1,25-(OH)$_2$D$_3$-mediated hypercalcemia had concomitant granulomatous disease; and hypercalcemia often improved with medical or surgical therapy that resulted in a decrease in serum 1,25-(OH)$_2$D$_3$ concentration. Recurrence of hypercalcemia and increased plasma 1,25-(OH)2D3 concentrations has been documented with recurrence of disease.[55]

Parathyroid Hormone

For many years after Fuller Albright's observations in 1941, malignancy-associated hypercalcemia was attributed to ectopic-tumor–produced PTH. It is now clear that PTHrP is responsible in the great majority of cases of HHM. There have been rare cases, however, of authentic-tumor–produced PTH causing hypercalcemia. Specifically, ectopic PTH production has been documented in a small cell carcinoma of the lung,[56] a squamous cell carcinoma of the lung,[57] an ovarian cancer,[58] a widely metastatic primitive neuroectodermal tumor,[59] a papillary adenocarcinoma of the thyroid[60] and a thymoma.[61] Molecular analysis of the ovarian carcinoma revealed both DNA amplification and rearrangement in the upstream regulatory region of the PTH gene. Interestingly, the primitive neuroectodermal tumor produced both PTH and PTHrP that resulted in severe hypercalcemia. These reported patients did not have coexisting primary hyperparathyroidism since the parathyroid glands were normal at the time of neck exploration or at autopsy in all cases. However, the fact remains that ectopic production of PTH is a rare event, and it is clearly documented that most patients with malignancy-associated hypercalcemia have suppressed plasma PTH concentrations.[62] It should be emphasized that the most likely cause of hypercalcemia in the setting of malignancy that is associated with a normal or increased serum PTH concentration is co-existing hyperparathyroidism.

Other Tumor-Associated Factors

There is accumulating evidence that solid tumors may produce other humoral factors, either alone or in combination with PTHrP, that have the capacity to stimulate osteoclastic bone resorption and cause hypercalcemia. These factors include IL-1, IL-6, transforming growth factor α (TGFα), tumor necrosis factor (TNF) and granulocyte colony-stimulating factor (G-CSF). Administration of IL-1 injections to mice caused a mild hypercalcemia,[63,64] which has been effectively blocked by the IL-1 receptor antagonist.[65] Mice bearing Chinese hamster ovarian tumors transfected with the complementary DNA for IL-6 developed mild hypercalcemia,[66] as did mice bearing a renal carcinoma that cosecreted IL-6 and PTHrP.[67] High serum levels of IL-6 in patients with humoral hypercalcemia of malignancy have also been reported.[68,69]

Human TGFα and TNFα stimulated osteoclastic bone resorption in vitro and resulted in hypercalcemia in vivo.[70–72] TNFα also caused hypercalciuria, without an increase in nephrogenous cAMP, and increased osteoclastic bone resorption in vivo in a mouse model.[73] In addition, as noted in the previous section, some of these factors have been shown to modulate the end-organ effects of PTHrP on bone and kidney. In some instances, factors such as TGFα, IL-1, IL-6, and TNF enhanced the hypercalcemic effects of PTHrP. The ability of IL-6 to enhance PTHrP-mediated hypercalcemia appeared to be due to increased production of the early osteoclast precursors by IL-6 (as measured by granulocyte macrophage colony forming units), in combination with increased production of the more committed osteoclast precursors by PTHrP.[74]

Prostaglandins of the E series are powerful stimulators of bone resorption,[75] although their role in bone destruction associated with malignancy remains unclear.[76] Some of the effects of cytokines on bone may be mediated in part through prostaglandins. Indomethacin, a prostaglandin synthesis inhibitor, and has been shown to block part of the osteoclast-stimulatory effects of IL-1 in vivo.[63,64] Although prostaglandins have been demonstrated to be produced by cultured tumor cells in vitro, indomethacin treatment of malignancy-associated hypercalcemia is only occasionally effective.[77] Thus, it is unlikely that prostaglandins have a major causal role in hypercalcemia associated with malignancy.

Treatment of Hypercalcemia of Malignancy

The ultimate treatment of malignancy-associated hypercalcemia is eradication of the underlying cancer. However, cure is frequently not possible, and in patients with symptomatic or life-threatening hypercalcemia, therapy must be aimed specifically against the mediating mechanisms. Increased osteoclastic bone resorption is present in essentially every patient with hypercalcemia of malignancy and is, therefore, a key target for treatment and prevention of hypercalcemia. Two of these mechanisms in particular, increased osteoclastic bone absorption and increased renal tubular calcium reabsorption, are common to most patients with hypercalcemia of malignancy, even those cases not associated with PTHrP production.[78] Medical therapy is therefore aimed at inhibiting bone resorption and promoting renal calcium excretion.

Because many hypercalcemic patients are dehydrated at presentation, the latter can be effectively addressed with intravenous administration of isotonic saline. This first step of therapy serves to rehydrate the patient while enhancing calciuresis by increasing the glomerular filtration rate and reducing the fractional reabsorption of calcium and sodium. The use of loop diuretics, such as furosemide, to enhance calcium excretion is frequently overemphasized in clinical practice. These agents may exacerbate fluid loss; therefore their use should be limited to the volume-repleted patient and only then with close monitoring of volume status.[79] Hydration alone rarely results in full resolution of hypercalcemia,[80] however, and more aggressive therapies are usually needed.

Bisphosphonates are currently the mainstay for long-term treatment of hypercalcemia and osteolytic bone disease. They have an affinity for bone surfaces undergoing active resorption and are released in the bone microenvironment during remodeling. These compounds decrease osteoclastic bone resorption by two described mechanisms. First, the nitrogen-substituted bisphosphonates, such as alendronate, risedronate and zoledronic acid, are potent inhibitors of the enzyme farnesyl diphosphate synthase, thereby blocking protein isoprenylation. It is believed that the prenylation of small GTP-binding proteins is important for structural integrity of the osteoclast; without it, the osteoclasts undergo apoptosis. Second, the non-nitrogen containing bisphosphonates, clodronate and etidronate, are less potent and also induce osteoclastic apoptosis but by a different mechanism. These bisphosphonates are metabolically incorporated into nonhydrolyzable ATP analogs that inhibit ATP-dependent intracellular enzymes. The bisphosphonates have been known to inhibit osteoclastic bone resorption for over 30 years.

There are also several lines of evidence that suggest bisphosphonates affect osteoclastic bone resorption indirectly through actions on osteoblasts. For example, bisphosphonates have previously been shown to have multiple actions on osteoblasts such as (1) modulation of proliferation and differentiation[81]; (2) prevention of apoptosis[82]; (3) modulation of extracellular matrix protein production[83,84]; (4) regulation of the expression and excretion of IL-6[85,86]; and (5) decrease of angiogenesis.[87,88] Recently, Viereck and colleagues presented in vitro evidence that bisphosphonates act directly on human osteoblasts to increase the production of both osteoprotegerin (OPG) messenger ribonucleic acid (mRNA) and protein.[89] Clearly, the implication is that by increasing OPG expression, the receptor activator of NF-κB ligand (RANKL)-mediated stimulation of osteoclasts can be neutralized.

The various bisphosphonates available on the market vary in potency, but all are poorly absorbed from the gut and are most effective for treatment of hypercalcemia when used intravenously. Intravenous etidronate, the least potent of its class, normalized calcium concentration in 30 to 40% of patients when given in doses of 7.5 mg/kg on three consecutive days.[90–92] Oral etidronate, at dosages of 25 mg/kg/d for more than 6 months can cause bone mineralization defects.[93] Pamidronate, alternatively, combines high potency with low toxicity and has become the agent of choice for the treatment of hypercalcemia of malignancy. When used in the recommended doses of 30 to 90 mg intravenously over 4 to 24 hours, it is highly effective in normalizing serum calcium concentrations and is not associated with mineralization defects. The onset of clinically apparent action is somewhat delayed with the bisphosphonates. Clinical studies using a 90-mg infusion of pamidronate over 4 hours indicate that the mean time to achieve normocalcemia is approximately 4 days, while the mean duration of normocalcemia is 28 days.[94] An effective method for achieving a rapid and sustained reduction in serum calcium concentration is to use pamidronate in combination with calcitonin. The combined use of a bisphosphonate with calcitonin lowers serum calcium levels more rapidly and effectively than either alone.[95]

Zoledronic acid, the most potent bisphosphonate available, is very effective for the treatment of hypercalcemia of malignancy. At doses of 4 mg and 8 mg, this bisphosphonate was compared to a single 90-mg infusion of pamidronate in patients with hypercalcemia of malignancy. Zoledronic acid was superior in respect to response rates, time to calcium normalization, and response duration.[96] The 4-mg dose is FDA-approved, as renal dysfunction occurred with the 8-mg dose.

Inhibiting osteoclastic bone resorption and renal tubular calcium reabsorption within minutes of administration, calcitonin also makes an excellent agent for the acute treatment of hypercalcemia. Unfortunately, tachyphylaxis frequently develops within 48 hours as a result of down-regulation of the calcitonin receptor. Concomitant use of glucocorticoids, however, can prolong the effective time of treatment.[97] This effect appears to result from a glucocorticoid mediated up-regulation of cell-surface calcitonin receptors and increased de novo production of calcitonin receptors in the osteoclast.[98] Calcitonin can be administered every 6 to 12 hours in doses of 4 to 8 U/kg. Human calcitonin is available, but salmon calcitonin is generally used. If salmon calcitonin is used, then a test dose of 1 unit should be administered first, since rare anaphylactic reactions have been reported.

Two antineoplastic agents have been used effectively for the treatment of malignancy-associated hypercalcemia, but are rarely used now. Plicamycin, formerly called mithramycin, is an inhibitor if DNA-dependent RNA synthesis and a potent inhibitor of bone resorption. The dosage used to treat hypercalcemia (25 mcg/kg) is one-tenth the usual chemotherapeutic dose and should be infused over 4 hours. It has considerable side effects of nephrotoxicity, hepatotoxicity, thrombocytopenia, nausea, and vomiting. Gallium nitrate is another antineoplastic agent with calcium-lowering effects. It also has serious nephrotoxicity and is somewhat inconvenient to use as it is administered over a continuous 5-day infusion. Use of these antineoplastic agents should be reserved for cases of hypercalcemia that are unresponsive to maximum doses of bisphosphonates.

Finally, about 30% of patients treated with glucocorticoids for malignancy-associated hypercalcemia respond with a fall in serum calcium concentration. Glucocorticoids are most likely to have clinical effect in the setting of hypercalcemia associated with multiple myeloma or hematologic malignancies associated with 1,25-$(OH)_2D_3$. In these situations, glucocorticoids inhibit osteoclastic bone resorption by decreasing tumor production of locally active cytokines, in addition to having direct tumorolytic effects.[99] Glucocorticoids, in dosage equivalents of 40 to 60 mg of prednisone daily, should be given. If no appreciable response is observed within 10 days, then glucocorticoid therapy should be discontinued.

In conclusion, hypercalcemia of malignancy is due to a heterogeneous group of tumor-derived factors that disrupt normal calcium homeostasis. Regardless of the pathophysiology, in most instances, the central mediator of this process is the osteoclast. The standard of care for this complication of malignancy is now bisphosphonate treatment, which is effective in most cases. However, the possibility of bisphosphonate resistance has emerged. Thus, future therapeutic options should address this issue. Possible alternative therapies include inhibitors of the RANKL pathway or neutralizing antibodies to PTHrP. The latter would also reverse the increased renal tubular reabsorption of calcium caused by increased PTHrP concentrations. Clinical trials, in progress, should determine if these modalities will be as effective or complementary to bisphosphonate treatment.

REFERENCES

1. Grill V, Martin TJ. Hypercalcemia of malignancy. Rev Endocr Metab Disord 2000;1:253–63.
2. Stewart AF. Hypercalcemia associated with cancer. N Engl J Med 2005;352:373–9.
3. Ralston SH, Gallacher SJ, Patel U, et al. Cancer-associated hypercalcemia: morbidity and mortality. Clinical experience in 126 treated patients. Ann Intern Med 1990;112:499–504.
4. Mundy GR, Martin TJ. The hypercalcemia of malignancy: pathogenesis and management. Metab Clin Exp 1982;31:1247–77.
5. LeBoff MS, Mikulec KH. Hypercalcemia: clinical manifestations, pathogenesis, diagnosis, and management. In: Favus MJ, editor. Primer on the metabolic bone diseases and disorders of mineral metabolism. 5th ed. Washington (DC): American Society for Bone and Mineral Research; 2003. p. 225–9.
6. Moseley JM, Kubota M, Diefenbach-Jagger H, et al. Parathyroid hormone-related protein purified from a human lung cancer cell line. Proceedings of the National Academy of Sciences of the United States of America 1987;84:5048–52.
7. Burtis WJ, Brady TG, Orloff JJ, et al. Immunochemical characterization of circulating parathyroid hormone-related protein in patients with humoral hypercalcemia of cancer. N Engl J Med 1990;322:1106–12.
8. Strewler GJ, Stern PH, Jacobs JW, et al. Parathyroid hormone-like protein from human renal carcinoma cells. Structural and functional homology with parathyroid hormone. J Clin Invest 1987;80:1803–7.
9. Suva LJ, Winslow GA, Wettenhall RE, et al. A parathyroid hormone-related protein implicated in malignant hypercalcemia: cloning and expression. Science 1987;237:893–6.
10. Abou-Samra AB, Juppner H, Force T, et al. Expression cloning of a common receptor for parathyroid hormone and parathyroid hormone-related peptide from rat osteoblast-like cells: a single receptor stimulates intracellular accumulation of both cAMP and inositol trisphosphates and increases intracellular free calcium. Proceedings of the National Academy of Sciences of the United States of America 1992;89:2732–6.
11. Horiuchi N, Caulfield MP, Fisher JE, et al. Similarity of synthetic peptide from human tumor to parathyroid hormone in vivo and in vitro. Science 1987;238:1566–8.

12. Asa SL, Henderson J, Goltzman D, Drucker DJ. Parathyroid hormone-like peptide in normal and neoplastic human endocrine tissues. J Clin Endocrinol Metab 1990;71: 1112–8.
13. Danks JA, Ebeling PR, Hayman J, et al. Parathyroid hormone-related protein: immunohistochemical localization in cancers and in normal skin. J Bone Miner Res 1989; 4:273–8.
14. Minina E, Wenzel HM, Kreschel C, et al. BMP and Ihh/PTHrP signaling interact to coordinate chondrocyte proliferation and differentiation. Development 2001;128: 4523–34.
15. Wysolmerski JJ, Broadus AE, Zhou J, et al. Overexpression of parathyroid hormone-related protein in the skin of transgenic mice interferes with hair follicle development. Proceedings of the National Academy of Sciences of the United States of America 1994;91:1133–7.
16. Wysolmerski JJ, Philbrick WM, Dunbar ME, et al. Rescue of the parathyroid hormone-related protein knockout mouse demonstrates that parathyroid hormone-related protein is essential for mammary gland development. Development 1998;125:1285–94.
17. Philbrick WM, Dreyer BE, Nakchbandi IA, Karaplis AC. Parathyroid hormone-related protein is required for tooth eruption. Proceedings of the National Academy of Sciences of the United States of America 1998;95: 11846–51.
18. Schluter KD, Piper HM. Cardiovascular actions of parathyroid hormone and parathyroid hormone-related peptide. Cardiovasc Res 1998;37:34–41.
19. Wysolmerski JJ, Carucci JM, Broadus AE, Philbrick WM. PTH and PTHrP antagonize mammary gland growth and development in transgenic mice. J Bone Miner Res 1994;9: 121.
20. Kovacs CS, Lanske B, Hunzelman JL, et al. Parathyroid hormone-related peptide (PTHrP) regulates fetal-placental calcium transport through a receptor distinct from the PTH/PTHrP receptor. Proceedings of the National Academy of Sciences of the United States of America 1996;93: 15233–8.
21. Thiede MA, Daifotis AG, Weir EC, et al. Intrauterine occupancy controls expression of the parathyroid hormone-related peptide gene in preterm rat myometrium. Proceedings of the National Academy of Sciences of the United States of America 1990;87:6969–73.
22. Yamamoto M, Harm SC, Grasser WA, Thiede MA. Parathyroid hormone-related protein in the rat urinary bladder: a smooth muscle relaxant produced locally in response to mechanical stretch. Proceedings of the National Academy of Sciences of the United States of America 1992;89: 5326–30.
23. Pirola CJ, Wang HM, Strgacich MI, et al. Mechanical stimuli induce vascular parathyroid hormone-related protein gene expression in vivo and in vitro. Endocrinology 1994;134:2230–6.
24. Botella A, Rekik M, Delvaux M, et al. Parathyroid hormone (PTH) and PTH-related peptide induce relaxation of smooth muscle cells from guinea pig ileum: interaction with vasoactive intestinal peptide receptors. Endocrinology 1994;135:2160–7.
25. Funk JL, Shigenaga JK, Moser AH, et al. Cytokine regulation of parathyroid hormone-related protein messenger ribonucleic acid levels in mouse spleen: paradoxical effects of interferon-gamma and interleukin-4. Endocrinology 1994;135:351–8.
26. Funk JL, Lausier J, Moser AH, et al. Endotoxin induces parathyroid hormone-related protein gene expression in splenic stromal and smooth muscle cells, not in splenic lymphocytes. Endocrinology 1995;136:3412–21.
27. Luparello C, Ginty AF, Gallagher JA, et al. Transforming growth factor-beta 1, beta 2, and beta 3, urokinase and parathyroid hormone-related peptide expression in 8701-BC breast cancer cells and clones. Differentiation 1993;55: 73–80.
28. Luparello C, Burtis WJ, Raue F, et al. Parathyroid hormone-related peptide and 8701-BC breast cancer cell growth and invasion in vitro: evidence for growth-inhibiting and invasion-promoting effects. Mol Cell Endocrinol 1995; 111:225–32.
29. Li H, Seitz PK, Selvanayagam P, et al. Effect of endogenously produced parathyroid hormone-related peptide on growth of a human hepatoma cell line (Hep G2). Endocrinology 1996;137:2367–74.
30. Chen HL, Demiralp B, Schneider A, et al. Parathyroid hormone and parathyroid hormone-related protein exert both pro- and anti-apoptotic effects in mesenchymal cells. J Biol Chem 2002;277:19374–81.
31. Schilling T, Pecherstorfer M, Blind E, et al. Parathyroid hormone-related protein (PTHrP) does not regulate 1,25-dihydroxyvitamin D serum levels in hypercalcemia of malignancy. J Clin Endocrinol Metab 1993;76:801–3.
32. Horwitz MJ, Tedesco MB, Sereika SM, et al. Direct comparison of sustained infusion of human parathyroid hormone-related protein-(1-36) [hPTHrP-(1-36)] versus hPTH-(1-34) on serum calcium, plasma 1,25-dihydroxyvitamin D concentrations, and fractional calcium excretion in healthy human volunteers. J Clin Endocrinol Metab 2003;88:1603–9.
33. Nakayama K, Fukumoto S, Takeda S, et al. Differences in bone and vitamin D metabolism between primary hyperparathyroidism and malignancy-associated hypercalcemia. J Clin Endocrinol Metab 1996;81:607–11.
34. Stewart AF, Vignery A, Silverglate A, et al. Quantitative bone histomorphometry in humoral hypercalcemia of malignancy: uncoupling of bone cell activity. J Clin Endocrinol Metab 1982;55:219–27.
35. Plawner LL, Philbrick WM, Burtis WJ, et al. Cell type-specific secretion of parathyroid hormone-related protein via the regulated versus the constitutive secretory pathway. J Biol Chem 1995;270:14078–84.
36. Fierabracci P, Pinchera A, Miccoli P, et al. Increased prevalence of primary hyperparathyroidism in treated breast cancer. J Endocrinol Invest 2001;24:315–20.
37. Southby J, Kissin MW, Danks JA, et al. Immunohistochemical localization of parathyroid hormone-related protein in human breast cancer. Cancer Res 1990;50:7710–6.
38. Bundred NJ, Ratcliffe WA, Walker RA, et al. Parathyroid hormone related protein and hypercalcaemia in breast cancer. BMJ 1991;303:1506–9.
39. Bundred NJ, Walker RA, Ratcliffe WA, et al. Parathyroid hormone related protein and skeletal morbidity in breast cancer. Eur J Cancer 1992;28:690–2.
40. Kohno N, Kitazawa S, Fukase M, et al. The expression of parathyroid hormone-related protein in human breast cancer with skeletal metastases. Surg Today 1994;24: 215–20.
41. Liapis H, Crouch EC, Grosso LE, et al. Expression of parathyroid-like protein in normal, proliferative, and neoplastic human breast tissues. Am J Pathol 1993;143: 1169–78.
42. Grill V, Ho P, Body JJ, et al. Parathyroid hormone-related protein: elevated levels in both humoral hypercalcemia of malignancy and hypercalcemia complicating metastatic breast cancer. J Clin Endocrinol Metab 1991;73:1309–15.
43. Kremer R, Shustik C, Tabak T, et al. Parathyroid-hormone-related peptide in hematologic malignancies. Am J Med 1996;100:406–11.
44. Ikeda K, Ohno H, Hane M, et al. Development of a sensitive two-site immunoradiometric assay for parathyroid hormone-related peptide: evidence for elevated levels in plasma from patients with adult T-cell leukemia/lymphoma and B-cell lymphoma. J Clin Endocrinol Metab 1994;79:1322–7.
45. Firkin F, Seymour JF, Watson AM, et al. Parathyroid hormone-related protein in hypercalcaemia associated with haematological malignancy. Br J Haematol 1996;94: 486–92.
46. Seymour JF, Grill V, Martin TJ, et al. Hypercalcemia in the blastic phase of chronic myeloid leukemia associated with elevated parathyroid hormone-related protein. Leukemia 1993;7:1672–5.
47. Gkonos PJ, London R, Hendler ED. Hypercalcemia and elevated 1,25-dihydroxyvitamin D levels in a patient with end-stage renal disease and active tuberculosis. N Engl J Med 1984;311:1683–5.
48. Mason RS, Frankel T, Chan YL, et al. Vitamin D conversion by sarcoid lymph node homogenate. Ann Intern Med 1984;100:59–61.
49. Adams JS, Sharma OP, Gacad MA, Singer FR. Metabolism of 25-hydroxyvitamin D3 by cultured pulmonary alveolar macrophages in sarcoidosis. J Clin Invest 1983;72: 1856–60.
50. Seymour JF, Gagel RF, Hagemeister FB, et al. Calcitriol production in hypercalcemic and normocalcemic patients with non-Hodgkin lymphoma. Ann Intern Med 1994;121: 633–40.
51. Rosenthal N, Insogna KL, Godsall JW, et al. Elevations in circulating 1,25-dihydroxyvitamin D in three patients with lymphoma-associated hypercalcemia. J Clin Endocrinol Metab 1985;60:29–33.
52. Breslau NA, McGuire JL, Zerwekh JE, et al. Hypercalcemia associated with increased serum calcitriol levels in three patients with lymphoma. Ann Intern Med 1984;100:1–6.
53. Fetchick DA, Bertolini DR, Sarin PS, et al. Production of 1,25-dihydroxyvitamin D3 by human T cell lymphotrophic virus-I-transformed lymphocytes. J Clin Invest 1986;78:592–6.
54. Zehnder D, Bland R, Williams MC, et al. Extrarenal expression of 25-hydroxyvitamin d(3)-1 alpha-hydroxylase. J Clin Endocrinol Metab 2001;86:888–94.
55. Mercier RJ, Thompson JM, Harman GS, Messerschmidt GL. Recurrent hypercalcemia and elevated 1,25-dihydroxyvitamin D levels in Hodgkin's disease. Am J Med 1988;84:165–8.
56. Yoshimoto K, Yamasaki R, Sakai H, et al. Ectopic production of parathyroid hormone by small cell lung cancer in a patient with hypercalcemia. J Clin Endocrinol Metab 1989;68:976–81.
57. Nielsen PK, Rasmussen AK, Feldt-Rasmussen U, et al. Ectopic production of intact parathyroid hormone by a squamous cell lung carcinoma in vivo and in vitro. J Clin Endocrinol Metab 1996;81:3793–6.
58. Nussbaum SR, Gaz RD, Arnold A. Hypercalcemia and ectopic secretion of parathyroid hormone by an ovarian carcinoma with rearrangement of the gene for parathyroid hormone. N Engl J Med 1990;323:1324–8.
59. Strewler GJ, Budayr AA, Clark OH, Nissenson RA. Production of parathyroid hormone by a malignant nonparathyroid tumor in a hypercalcemic patient. J Clin Endocrinol Metab 1993;76:1373–5.
60. Iguchi H, Miyagi C, Tomita K, et al. Hypercalcemia caused by ectopic production of parathyroid hormone in a patient with papillary adenocarcinoma of the thyroid gland. J Clin Endocrinol Metab 1998;83:2653–7.
61. Rizzoli R, Pache JC, Didierjean L, et al. A thymoma as a cause of true ectopic hyperparathyroidism. J Clin Endocrinol Metab 1994;79:912–5.
62. Stewart AF, Horst R, Deftos LJ, et al. Biochemical evaluation of patients with cancer-associated hypercalcemia: evidence for humoral and nonhumoral groups. N Engl J Med 1980;303:1377–83.
63. Sabatini M, Boyce B, Aufdemorte T, et al. Infusions of recombinant human interleukins 1 alpha and 1 beta cause hypercalcemia in normal mice. Proceedings of the National Academy of Sciences of the United States of America 1988;85:5235–9.
64. Boyce BF, Aufdemorte TB, Garrett IR, et al. Effects of interleukin-1 on bone turnover in normal mice. Endocrinology 1989;125:1142–50.
65. Guise TA, Garrett IR, Bonewald LF, Mundy GR. Interleukin-1 receptor antagonist inhibits the hypercalcemia mediated by interleukin-1. J Bone Miner Res 1993;8: 583–7.
66. Black K, Garrett IR, Mundy GR. Chinese hamster ovarian cells transfected with the murine interleukin-6 gene cause hypercalcemia as well as cachexia, leukocytosis and thrombocytosis in tumor-bearing nude mice. Endocrinology 1991;128:2657–9.
67. Weissglas M, Schamhart D, Lowik C, et al. Hypercalcemia and cosecretion of interleukin-6 and parathyroid hormone related peptide by a human renal cell carcinoma implanted into nude mice. J Urol 1995;153:854–7.
68. Ueno M, Ban S, Nakanoma T, et al. Hypercalcemia in a patient with renal cell carcinoma producing parathyroid hormone-related protein and interleukin-6. Int J Urol 2000;7:239–42.
69. Barhoum M, Hutchins L, Fonseca VA. Intractable hypercalcemia due to a metastatic carcinoid secreting parathyroid hormone-related peptide and interleukin-6: response to octreotide. Am J Med Sci 1999;318:203–5.
70. Ibbotson KJ, Twardzik DR, D'Souza SM, et al. Stimulation of bone resorption in vitro by synthetic transforming growth factor-alpha. Science 1985;228:1007–9.
71. Yates AJ, Boyce BF, Favarato G, et al. Expression of human transforming growth factor alpha by Chinese hamster ovarian tumors in nude mice causes hypercalcemia and increased osteoclastic bone resorption. J Bone Miner Res 1992;7:847–53.
72. Bertolini DR, Nedwin GE, Bringman TS, et al. Stimulation of bone resorption and inhibition of bone formation in vitro by human tumour necrosis factors. Nature 1986; 319:516–8.
73. Johnson RA, Boyce BF, Mundy GR, Roodman GD. Tumors producing human tumor necrosis factor induced hypercalcemia and osteoclastic bone resorption in nude mice. Endocrinology 1989;124:1424–7.
74. Hulter HN, Halloran BP, Toto RD, Peterson JC. Long-term control of plasma calcitriol concentration in dogs and humans. Dominant role of plasma calcium concentration

in experimental hyperparathyroidism. J Clin Invest 1985;76:695–702.

75. Klein DC, Raisz LG. Prostaglandins: stimulation of bone resorption in tissue culture. Endocrinology 1970;86: 1436–40.

76. Mundy GR. Hypercalcemia. In: Mundy GR, editor. Bone remodeling and its disorders. London: Martin Dunitz; 1995. p. 88–103.

77. Mundy GR, Wilkinson R, Heath DA. Comparative study of available medical therapy for hypercalcemia of malignancy. Am J Med 1983;74:421–32.

78. Tuttle KR, Kunau RT, Loveridge N, Mundy GR. Altered renal calcium handling in hypercalcemia of malignancy. J Am Soc Nephrol 1991;2:191–9.

79. Suki WN, Yium JJ, Von Minden M, et al. Actue treatment of hypercalcemia with furosemide. N Engl J Med 1970;283: 836–40.

80. Hosking DJ, Cowley A, Bucknall CA. Rehydration in the treatment of severe hypercalcaemia. Q J Med 1981;50: 473–81.

81. Reinholz GG, Getz B, Pederson L, et al. Bisphosphonates directly regulate cell proliferation, differentiation, and gene expression in human osteoblasts. Cancer Res 2000; 60:6001–7.

82. Plotkin LI, Weinstein RS, Parfitt AM, et al. Prevention of osteocyte and osteoblast apoptosis by bisphosphonates and calcitonin. J Clin Invest 1999;104:1363–74.

83. Klein BY, Ben-Bassat H, Breuer E, et al. Structurally different bisphosphonates exert opposing effects on alkaline phosphatase and mineralization in marrow osteoprogenitors. J Cell Biochem 1998;68:186–94.

84. Giuliani N, Pedrazzoni M, Negri G, et al. Bisphosphonates stimulate formation of osteoblast precursors and mineralized nodules in murine and human bone marrow cultures in vitro and promote early osteoblastogenesis in young and aged mice in vivo. Bone 1998;22:455–61.

85. Giuliani N, Pedrazzoni M, Passeri G, Girasole G. Bisphosphonates inhibit IL-6 production by human osteoblast-like cells. Scand J Rheumatol 1998;27:38–41.

86. Tokuda H, Kozawa O, Harada A, Uematsu T. Tiludronate inhibits interleukin-6 synthesis in osteoblasts: inhibition of phospholipase D activation in MC3T3-E1 cells. J Cell Biochem 1998;69:252–9.

87. Wood J, Bonjean K, Ruetz S, et al. Novel antiangiogenic effects of the bisphosphonate compound zoledronic acid. J Pharmacol Exp Ther 2002;302:1055–61.

88. Green JR, Clezardin P. Mechanisms of bisphosphonate effects on osteoclasts, tumor cell growth, and metastasis. Am J Clin Oncol 2002;25:3–9.

89. Viereck V, Emons G, Lauck V, et al. Bisphosphonates pamidronate and zoledronic acid stimulate osteoprotegerin production by primary human osteoblasts. Biochem Biophys Res Commun 2002;291:680–6.

90. Singer FR, Ritch PS, Lad TE, et al. Treatment of hypercalcemia of malignancy with intravenous etidronate. A controlled, multicenter study. The Hypercalcemia Study Group [comment] [published erratum appears in Arch Intern Med 1991;151:2008]. Arch Intern Med 1991;151: 471–476.

91. Gucalp R, Ritch P, Wiernik PH, et al. Comparative study of pamidronate disodium and etidronate disodium in the treatment of cancer-related hypercalcemia. J Clin Oncol 1992;10:134–42.

92. Kanis JA, Urwin GH, Gray RE, et al. Effects of intravenous etidronate disodium on skeletal and calcium metabolism. Am J Med 1987;82:55–70.

93. Fleisch H. Bisphosphonates. Pharmacology and use in the treatment of tumour-induced hypercalcaemic and metastatic bone disease. Drugs 1991;42:919–44.

94. Purohit OP, Radstone CR, Anthony C, et al. A randomised double-blind comparison of intravenous pamidronate and clodronate in the hypercalcaemia of malignancy. Br J Cancer 1995;72:1289–93.

95. Thiebaud D, Jacquet AF, Burckhardt P. Fast and effective treatment of malignant hypercalcemia. Combination of suppositories of calcitonin and a single infusion of 3-amino 1-hydroxypropylidene-1-bisphosphonate. Arch Intern Med 1990;150:2125–8.

96. Major P, Lortholary A, Hon J, et al. Zoledronic acid is superior to pamidronate in the treatment of hypercalcemia of malignancy: a pooled analysis of two randomized, controlled clinical trials. J Clin Oncol. 2001;19:558–67.

97. Binstock ML, Mundy GR. Effect of calcitonin and glutocorticoids in combination on the hypercalcemia of malignancy. Ann Intern Med 1980;93:269–72.

98. Wada S, Yasuda S, Nagai T, et al. Regulation of calcitonin receptor by glucocorticoid in human osteoclast-like cells prepared in vitro using receptor activator of nuclear factor-kappaB ligand and macrophage colony-stimulating factor. Endocrinology 2001;142:1471–8.

99. Mundy GR, Rick ME, Turcotte R, Kowalski MA. Pathogenesis of hypercalcemia in lymphosarcoma cell leukemia. Role of an osteoclast activating factor-like substance and a mechanism of action for glucocorticoid therapy. Am J Med 1978;65:600–6.

Endocrine Paraneoplastic Syndromes

Mimi I. Hu, MD

Sai-Ching Jim Yeung, MD, PhD

Robert F. Gagel, MD

Paraneoplastic syndromes are cancer-associated clinical syndromes caused by biologic or humoral factors, including hormones, cytokines, and immunoglobulins. In this chapter, we focus on the endocrine paraneoplastic syndromes, also known as ectopic hormone syndromes, other than hypercalcemia of malignancy, which is discussed in Chapter 23, "Endocrine Neoplastic Syndromes."

Early awareness of a paraneoplastic syndrome is important clinically. An occult malignancy may initially manifest as a paraneoplastic syndrome, which can allow for early detection and treatment and potential cure. Treatment of the effects of the syndrome can be palliative even if a cure for the tumor is implausible. When a paraneoplastic syndrome mimics the effects of metastatic disease, however, a patient may be mistakenly considered an inappropriate candidate for potentially curative treatments. Development of the syndrome can also be used as a marker of tumor recurrence or to signify a poor prognosis. Autocrine growth hormones (GHs) causing the syndrome are potential therapeutic targets.

The mechanisms underlying ectopic hormone production may vary between different tumors. In some examples, the tumor cells may have produced the hormone during an earlier stage in their development. For example, parathyroid hormone–related protein, the cause of hypercalcemia of malignancy, is normally expressed in actively differentiating squamous cells but is expressed at low levels or not at all in completely differentiated squamous epithelium.[1] In addition, the production of hormone precursors and peptides that may be normally produced by nonendocrine tissues can increase with neoplastic transformation.[2,3] In other cases, the synthesizing machinery of a hormone-producing cell is coopted to produce a different hormone. Production of peptides by neuroendocrine tumors is the most common ectopic hormone mechanism of this type. Neuroendocrine cells are dispersed through nearly all organs: lung, gastrointestinal tract, pancreas, thyroid gland, adrenal medulla, breast, prostate, and skin. These neural crest–derived cells may produce biogenic amines and a long list of polypeptide hormones, including adrenocorticotropic hormone (ACTH), corticotropin-releasing hormone (CRH), growth hormone–releasing hormone (GH-RH), calcitonin, vasoactive intestinal peptide, and pancreatic polypeptide.

Ectopic Adrenocorticotropic Hormone Syndrome

Ectopic ACTH secretion causing Cushing's syndrome was the second hormonal syndrome —after hypercalcemia of malignancy—to be associated with cancer in 1928.[4] Tumoral production of CRH is a rare cause of paraneoplastic Cushing's syndrome.

Tumors

Among all patients with Cushing's syndrome, 40% have an obvious pituitary tumor causing Cushing's syndrome, 28% have a nonvisible pituitary source, 17% have adrenal hypersecretion of cortisol, and 15% have ectopic ACTH secretion from an underlying tumor.[5] Extrapituitary tumors that produce ACTH are classically lung cancers, particularly of the small cell type, and comprise 50% of all tumors causing ectopic adrenocorticotropic hormone syndrome (EAS) (Table 1). However, only 0.4 to 2% of all lung cancers and 2 to 5% of small cell lung carcinomas are associated with ectopic ACTH production.[4–6] Recent reports have noted a greater association between benign tumors, such as carcinoids, and EAS. EAS tumors can be grouped into two histologic categories: carcinoid-oat cell and pheochromocytoma-neuroblastoma.[5,7]

Tumors can also produce CRH, the peptide normally produced by the hypothalamus that stimulates pituitary ACTH production and secretion, with or without ACTH.[5] Neoplasms that produce CRH include medullary thyroid carcinoma,[8] ganglioneuroblastoma,[9] and prostate cancer.[10]

Carcinomas of the liver, prostate, and breast have been documented to produce ACTH. Some malignancies can concomitantly produce ACTH and CRH.[11,12] Sarcomas have not been associated with EAS.[6]

Pathophysiology

All tissues in the body make pro-opiomelanocortin-derived peptides, albeit in smaller amounts than that produced in the pituitary gland; tumors or carcinomas can produce excessive quantities of it.[6] Pro-ACTH, or "big" ACTH, a prohormone by-product of pro-opiomelanocortin, can be enzymatically cleaved into multiple biologically active peptides: ACTH (leading to adrenal gland stimulation and cortisol secretion), melanocyte-stimulating hormone (effecting skin hyperpigmentation), and β-endorphin and metenkephalin (which have opiate-like activity).

Clinical Manifestations

Ectopic ACTH secretion leads to bilateral adrenal hyperplasia (as does a pituitary source) and many of the classic findings of hypercortisolism (Table 2). A review of 90 patients by the National Institutes of Health found that the three most common signs and symptoms of EAS were proximal muscle weakness (92%), hypertension (78%), and menstrual irregularity (78%).[3] Because the adrenal glands are stimulated to produce excessive amounts of 11-deoxycorticosterone and cortisol, which have mineralocorticoid and glucocorticoid

Table 1 Tumors Causing Ectopic Adrenocorticotropic Hormone Syndrome

Lung cancer—50%
Carcinoid tumors—25%
  Bronchus
  Thymus
  Small intestine
Neural crest tumors—15%
  Pheochromocytoma
  Neuroblastoma
  Medullary carcinoma of the thyroid
Thymoma—10%
Carcinoma of breast, gastrointestinal tract, ovary, cervix, prostate—rare

Table 2 Clinical Manifestations of Ectopic Adrenocorticotropic Hormone Syndrome

Proximal muscle weakness
Hypertension
Mentrual irregularity
Hirsutism
Osteopenia/osteoporosis
Fracture
Hypokalemia
Hyperglycemia
Edema
Weight loss
Psychiatric disorder (depression, psychosis)
Ecchymosis
Infection

effects, edema, metabolic alkalosis, and hypokalemia are more prominent features of EAS than they are of Cushing's syndrome from other causes.[6] Centripetal obesity, purplish abdominal/axillary striae, moon facies, a dorsocervical fat pad, and hyperpigmentation of the buccal mucosa are not typical signs when there is an underlying malignant tumor, such as oat cell carcinoma of the lung; these are more frequently seen with indolent tumors.

Occasionally, especially with slow-growing disseminated neuroendocrine tumors, the onset of Cushing's syndrome may occur many years after the diagnosis of a tumor. Some tumors, such as thymic or bronchial carcinoids, may not cause any clinical manifestations of ACTH production because they do not produce a sufficient amount of the peptide. Highly aggressive malignancies, however, usually cause rapid development of Cushing's syndrome.

Occult tumors producing hypercortisolemia are defined as undetectable tumors of nonpituitary origin that produce excessive ACTH or CRH for more than 4 to 6 months before tumor identification.[13] A review conducted at the National Institutes of Health found that patients with unidentifiable primary tumors causing EAS survived longer than those with known tumors.[3] Of the identifiable tumors, primary pulmonary tumors, with the exception of small cell lung carcinomas, were associated with longer survival periods than other tumor types. The average survival time after diagnosis of an overt tumor was 24 months.[3]

Diagnosis

The keys to diagnosing EAS are having clinical suspicion and conducting a rational, systematic series of biochemical tests prior to obtaining imaging studies. A typical clinical scenario that raises concern for the presence of EAS involves a patient with a known tumor who experiences weight loss, unexplained hypokalemic alkalosis, and abnormal glucose tolerance.

First, screening for hypercortisolism should be performed with a 24-hour urine collection for free cortisol (UFC), a low-dose overnight dexamethasone (DXM) suppression test, or a midnight salivary cortisol test. The 24-hour UFC test has a 100% sensitivity and 98% specificity for Cushing's syndrome and can distinguish hypercortisolism from obesity.[6,14] An elevated 24-hour UFC level (> 4 times the normal reference range) with a simultaneously elevated ACTH level (> 10 pg/mL) is highly suggestive of EAS.[15] Three different urine collections on separate days may be needed because cortisol production is variable. A low-dose overnight DXM suppression test consists of 1 mg of DXM given orally at 11 pm followed by a blood sample drawn at 8 am to determine the serum cortisol level. A suppressed cortisol level of < 1.8 µg/dL rules out hypercortisolemia, but a level of > 14.3 µg/dL confirms the presence of Cushing's syndrome from any source (pituitary, adrenal, or ectopic).[15,16] A midnight salivary cortisol test is simple and noninvasive, but the results are highly variable, depending on the laboratory. A salivary cortisol level of > 0.55 µg/dL is a good screen for Cushing's syndrome: this cutoff value identified 93% of patients with Cushing's syndrome and excluded 100% without it.[17]

After one confirms the presence of hypercortisolism, an ACTH level (with a two-site immunoradiometric assay) should be evaluated to determine whether the Cushing's syndrome is dependent on ACTH (ie, pituitary adenoma or EAS) or independent from ACTH (ie, primary adrenal disease). A plasma ACTH concentration > 20 pg/mL suggests an ACTH-dependent process, whereas an ACTH level of < 10 pg/mL is consistent with an adrenocortical process (adrenal adenoma or carcinoma).[16] Although a serum ACTH level of > 200 pg/mL is suggestive of EAS, bronchial and thymic carcinoids and occult tumors may exhibit lower levels of ACTH, serum cortisol, and UFC than aggressive or overt tumors do.[6] If the ACTH level is within the range of 10 to 20 pg/mL, further dynamic testing with CRH stimulation (as described below) will be needed.

Identifying the source of ACTH (pituitary vs ectopic tumor producing ACTH vs ectopic tumor producing CRH) in ACTH-dependent Cushing's syndrome is one of the most difficult diagnostic evaluations in endocrinology (Figure 1). DXM suppression of cortisol and CRH stimulation of ACTH are tests that help distinguish the source of excessive ACTH. With EAS tumors, plasma cortisol is resistant to exogenous glucocorticoid suppression, and the ACTH level usually does not rise in response to CRH stimulation. One exception to this observation is that in the presence of a CRH-producing tumor, since the hypothalamic-pituitary axis is essentially intact, the clinical presentation is similar to that of a classic pituitary ACTH-producing tumor. In addition, in 30% of occult EAS tumors and 41% of thoracic carcinoids, cortisol can be suppressed with DXM. Alternatively, in 9 to 25% of cases of pituitary-dependent Cushing's syndrome, DXM will fail to suppress cortisol production (Table 3).[6]

The response to dexamethasone is observed with the high-dose dexamethasone suppression test (HDDST), which can be performed in various ways. The 2-day HDDST consists of 2 mg of DXM given orally every 6 hours for 48 hours, with 24-hour urine specimens collected at baseline and after days 1 and 2 of DXM administration for determination of the UFC level. A decrease in the UFC level of > 90% from the baseline level is suggestive of a pituitary source of ACTH. The overnight HDDST is performed by giving 8 mg of DXM orally once at 11 pm with an evaluation of the plasma cortisol level at 8 am the following day. A decline in plasma cortisol of > 50% from the baseline level or a level of < 5 µg/dL suggests a pituitary tumor. The overnight HDDST is more sensitive and accurate than the 2-day HDDST for pituitary ACTH production.[6]

A CRH stimulation test is performed by administering 1 µg/kg (maximum dose 100 µg) of synthetic ovine CRH intravenously and evaluating the plasma ACTH and cortisol levels at baseline and every 15 minutes after the injection for 60 minutes. EAS tumors will respond with stable or only minimally increased ACTH and cortisol levels. With pituitary tumors, ACTH and cortisol levels will rise > 50% (sensitivity 86%, specificity 90%) and 20% (sensitivity 91%, specificity 95%), respectively, from baseline levels.[18] A combination of the 2-day HDDST and CRH stimulation tests, the DXM-CRH test, will increase the sensitivity and specificity of the evaluation for pituitary Cushing's syndrome.[19]

In the absence of an obvious pituitary tumor or other neoplasm, bilateral inferior petrosal sinus sampling (IPSS) should be done in patients with ACTH-dependent Cushing's syndrome to determine the source of the ACTH because the pituitary circulation drains directly into the inferior petrosal sinuses (IPSs). Simultaneous blood samples for ACTH from the bilateral IPSs and peripheral (P) circulation will reveal an IPS to P ratio of ≥ 3 after CRH stimulation in the presence of a pituitary tumor.[20] The sensitivity and specificity of IPSS for diagnosing pituitary Cushing's syndrome are about 94%.[7] IPSS is especially helpful in differentiating occult EAS from pituitary Cushing's syndrome because occult EAS tumors can respond to the previously described dynamic tests similarly to the way pituitary tumors do. The limitations of IPSS arise from technical inexperience, high cost, and rare neurologic and thromboembolic complications.

Other diagnostic modalities include radiologic studies or tumor markers. Chest radiography and computed tomography or magnetic resonance imaging of the neck, chest, and/or

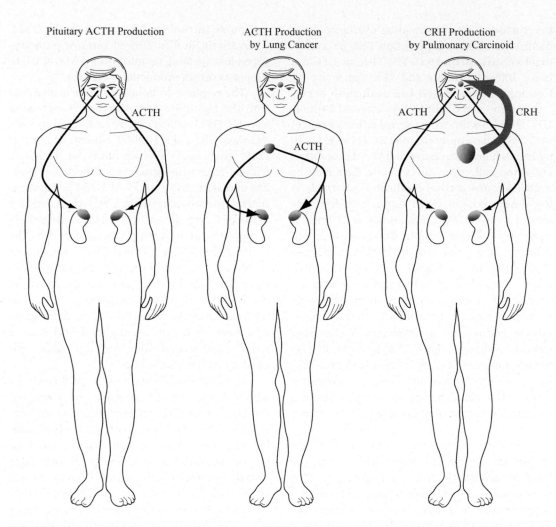

Pituitary ACTH Production ACTH Production by Lung Cancer CRH Production by Pulmonary Carcinoid

FIGURE 1 Sources of adrenocorticotropic hormone (ACTH)-dependent Cushing's syndrome. It is difficult to differentiate between a pituitary (*left panel*) and an ectopic (*middle panel*) source of ACTH, the most common causes of ACTH-dependent Cushing's syndrome. To differentiate with certainty, placement of catheters in veins draining the pituitary gland (inferior petrosal sinuses) combined with stimulation by exogenous corticotropin-releasing hormone (CRH) permits differentiation with certainty. Ectopic CRH production by a tumor results in increased ACTH production by the pituitary gland (*right panel*). It is difficult to differentiate between ectopic CRH production and pituitary gland–dependent Cushing's syndrome, necessitating the measurement of CRH in peripheral blood to make the diagnosis with certainty. Malignant tumors occasionally produce both CRH and ACTH, further complicating the diagnostic evaluation.

Table 3 Differences between Ectopic Adrenocorticotropic Hormone Syndrome and Cushing's Disease

Laboratory Finding	Ectopic ACTH Syndrome	Cushing's Disease (Pituitary Source)
Hypokalemia	Common	Rare
Serum or urinary cortisol	Markedly elevated	Modestly high, high normal
Serum ACTH	High	Inappropriately "normal" or slightly high
High-dose dexamethasone suppression of urinary cortisol	Unusual	Usual
Rise in serum ACTH or cortisol with CRH administration	Unusual	Usual

ACTH = adrenocorticotropic hormone; CRH = corticotropin-releasing hormone.

abdomen are ordered to evaluate patients for pulmonary, thymic, or abdominal tumors. The use of OctreoScan with indium [111] pentetreotide (Mallinckrodt, Inc., St. Louis, MO) can identify neuroendocrine tumors that can express somatostatin receptors. Ninety percent of occult EAS tumors are neuroendocrine in nature; thus, neuron-specific enolase or chromogranins can be useful tumor markers.

Treatment

As with most paraneoplastic syndromes, the most definitive therapy for EAS is to treat the underlying tumor with surgery, chemotherapy,

or radiotherapy. However, a study at the Mayo Clinic on 106 patients with EAS showed only a 12% cure rate after surgical excision of the primary tumor,[2] and the National Institutes of Health showed a 29% curative rate with surgical removal.[3] Surgical excision of benign tumors (such as bronchial carcinoids or pheochromocytomas) causing EAS is associated with higher rates of cure.[6]

For incurable tumors producing EAS, pharmacologic agents can be used to inhibit adrenal production of cortisol; however, their use is often limited by their adverse side-effect profiles. In addition, hypoadrenalism and adrenal crises need to be avoided by using supplemental glucocorticoid and mineralocorticoid therapy. Mitotane, a derivative of the insecticide dichlorodiphenyltrichloroethane (DDT) that was found to cause necrosis and atrophy of the adrenal cortex, was the first adrenolytic used. Maximal benefit occurs after 4 to 6 months of continued use; however, the side effects of nausea, vomiting, diarrhea, and depression often become intolerable, causing most patients to discontinue therapy prematurely. Aminoglutethimide inhibits cholesterol processing, which disrupts the production of cortisol and aldosterone and androgens. Metyrapone, an 11-β-hydroxylase inhibitor, prevents cortisol synthesis. Increasing ACTH in response to decreasing cortisol levels does not overcome the adrenolytic effects of metyrapone. The combination of metyrapone and aminoglutethimide can be used to lower the individual dosages needed. Ketoconazole is an antimycotic agent that inhibits P-450-dependent enzymes involved with adrenal and gonadal steroid production and prevents cortisol from binding to glucocorticoid receptors. Octreotide, a somatostatin analogue, and RU-486, a glucocorticoid antagonist used in investigational protocols, have been used with variable efficacy.

At times when the primary tumor or ACTH excess cannot be treated, bilateral adrenalectomy may be an option.[21] The risk of developing Nelson's syndrome, hyperpigmentation secondary to pituitary hyperplasia and increased ACTH production, is 47%.[15] There is limited clinical experience with selective adrenal arterial embolization in patients who are poor surgical candidates and fail medical therapy.

Patients with rapidly progressive small cell lung carcinoma and EAS form a unique subset of patients because of the need to initiate chemotherapy on a timely basis. Unfortunately, these patients are also highly susceptible to opportunistic infections, and initiation of therapy will often lead to death or serious morbidity related to infection.[22] Adrenolytic agents may be required in these patients to control the hypercortisolemia with the goal of normalizing the serum cortisol for a period of 1 to 2 weeks or longer. Although this may correct the immune status, it can cause an unacceptable delay in the initiation of chemotherapy from an oncologic perspective. Prophylactic therapy for opportunistic infections caused by *Pneumocystis carinii* or other fungi is recommended during chemotherapy after normalization of the serum cortisol level.

Non–Islet Cell Tumor Hypoglycemia

Tumor-induced hypoglycemia is an uncommon but challenging and serious complication for cancer patients. Hypoglycemia in association with an underlying tumor can occur in a variety of situations, three of which are endocrine related (Table 4). First, excessive insulin can be produced by an islet cell tumor or insulinoma. Second, involvement of the hepatic parenchyma by primary or metastatic lesions can lead to "liver failure" and insufficient gluconeogenesis from hepatic destruction or cytokine activity with tumor necrosis factor α and interleukins 1 and 6. These cytokines have been shown to produce hypoglycemia in animal models.[23] Third, a tumor can secrete an aberrant form of insulin-like growth factor (IGF) type 2, which can mediate hypoglycemic effects by binding to insulin receptors. This process produces the endocrine paraneoplastic syndrome of non–islet cell tumor hypoglycemia (NICTH). NICTH is reported to be 25% as common as insulinomas, although this is most likely an underestimation.[23] Since the assays for IGF-1 and IGF-2 were established in 1990, more than 120 cases of NICTH were documented in just one region of the United Kingdom by 2004.[24]

Tumors

NICTH is most commonly seen in patients with mesenchymal tumors such as fibromas and fibrosarcomas, which constitute about half of all tumors associated with NICTH. Tumors with epithelial and hematopoietic origins also have been seen with NICTH. About half of the epithelial tumors consist of hepatocellular carcinomas.[25–27] Overall, NICTH is associated with a wide range of tumors (Table 5).[23,28] Large fibrosarcomas usually arise in the thoracic or retroperitoneal spaces. NICTH-associated tumors are typically large and slow-growing.

Pathophysiology

Aberrantly processed IGF-2 produced by tumor cells was first observed by Daughaday and colleagues in 1988 in a patient with leiomyosarcoma and recurrent hypoglycemia.[29] This abnormal IGF-2 was termed "big" IGF-2 because it has a higher molecular weight than normal mature IGF-2, indicating incomplete processing of pro–IGF-2 peptides. After tumor resection, big IGF-2 was nearly undetectable.[29] Lowe and colleagues found increased amounts of messenger ribonucleic acid in tumor tissue from patients with NICTH, thus establishing the role of big IGF-2 in this syndrome.[30]

In normal physiology, mature IGF-2 (molecular weight 7.5 kDa) is produced from a series of biochemical alterations of pre-pro-IGF-2, a 17 kDa molecule produced by the liver. IGF-1 and mature IGF-2 competitively bind to insulin-like growth factor binding protein type 3 (IGFBP-3) and other subtypes of IGFBPs. This IGF-IGFBP

complex then binds to a molecule called acid-labile subunit (ALS). More than 98% of mature IGF-2 is bound to IGFBPs, with the majority associated with the large ternary complex of mature IGF (1 or 2)/IGFBP-3/ALS (total molecular weight 150 kDa). Less than 2% of mature IGF-2 is free in the circulation and can readily cross the capillary barrier.[27] The ternary complex is too large to cross the capillary membrane into the interstitium.[23,27,31,32] The normal ratio of IGF-2 to IGF-1 in plasma is 3:1, with individual concentrations significantly greater than that of insulin. However, because of their formation of the large ternary complexes, which cannot access the insulin or IGF receptors in the interstitium, and the very small amount of free IGF-2 that can access the receptors, the IGFs are unable to exert any clinically relevant insulin-like effects.[23]

In the setting of NICTH, the tumor produces excessive amounts of IGF-2, which is primarily (60–77%) composed of the subgroup of big IGF-2 (10–15 kDa), which is unable to effectively form the ternary complex with ALS.[29,32,33] In addition, the high levels of big IGF-2 give negative feedback to the pituitary to cause a decrease in GH production, which, in turn, leads to decreased production of IGF-1, IGFBP-3, and ALS.[25] Alternatively, GH-independent IGFBP-2 will increase in response to hypoglycemia.[34] In the end, IGF-2 (normal and big) and the small amounts of IGF-1 present will be sequestered into binary complexes (molecular weight 50 kDa) with IGFBP-2 or IGFBP-3 rather than the larger ternary complexes. These smaller binary complexes, as well as free IGF-2, readily cross the capillary membrane, thus allowing IGF-2 to cross-react with insulin receptors in the interstitium (Figure 2).[23] The resultant

Table 4 Causes of Hypoglycemia in Cancer Patients
Sepsis
Renal failure
Liver failure
Adrenal insufficiency
Isolated growth hormone deficiency
Hypopituitarism
Starvation
Excessive insulin or sulfonylurea in the following settings:
Total parenteral nutrition with insulin therapy
Renal insufficiency
Factitious hypoglycemia
Drugs
Pentamidine for *Pneumocystis* pneumonia
Trimethoprim-sulfamethoxazole and renal failure
Quinine
Haloperidol
Salicylates
Insulinoma
Non–islet cell tumor hypoglycemia

Table 5 Tumors Causing Non–Islet Cell Tumor Hypoglycemia
Mesenchymal tumors
Fibromas and fibrosarcomas—50%
Mesothelioma
Hemangiopericytoma
Neurofibroma
Leiomyosarcoma
Sarcoma of kidney
Epithelial tumors
Liver—50%
Lung
Pancreas
Stomach
Adrenal gland
Kidney
Esophagus
Ovary
Prostate
Breast
Larynx
Bladder (transitional cell carcinoma)
Neuroendocrine tumors
Carcinoid
Unknown

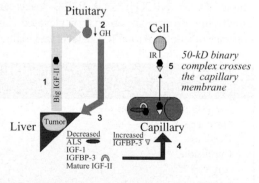

FIGURE 2 Pathophysiologic mechanism of non–islet cell tumor hypoglycemia (NICTH). (1) Excessive levels of big insulin-like growth factor (IGF)-2 (*black hexagon*) produced by the tumor is released into the circulation and negatively feeds back on pituitary growth hormone (GH) secretion. (2 and 3) Decreased levels of GH lead to decreased hepatic production of acid-labile subunit (ALS) (*green oval*), IGF-1, insulin-like growth factor binding protein (IGFBP)-3 (*blue semicircle*), and mature IGF-2. IGFBP-2 (*yellow inverted triangle*) production increases in response to hypoglycemia. (4) Increased concentrations of binary complexes (big IGF-2 + IGFBP-2) cross the capillary membrane. (5) IGF-2 binds to insulin receptors, causing hypoglycemia. IR = insulin receptor.

hypoglycemia is mediated through increased glucose consumption in skeletal muscle, suppressed hepatic glucose production, and suppressed lipolysis in adipose tissue.

In response to the hypoglycemia, insulin levels decrease and insulin receptors are up-regulated.[35] Thus, patients with NICTH may have an increased sensitivity to insulin-like peptides.

Clinical Manifestations

Neuroglycopenic and autonomic symptoms can occur anytime during the day but usually are associated with normal periods of fasting, that is, early morning and before meals. Recovery of neurologic function with administration of glucose or glucagon supports the diagnosis of symptomatic hypoglycemia. Occasionally, acromegaloid features may develop because of the actions of IGFs on GH receptors (Table 6).[36]

It is interesting that hypoglycemia can occur at any time during the course of the malignancy. In patients with NICTH treated with surgical excision or other antineoplastic therapy who have complete resolution of hypoglycemic episodes, production of big IGF-2 and hypoglycemia may not return with tumor recurrence for unclear reasons.[37]

Diagnosis

The keys to differentiating NICTH from an insulinoma or hepatic destruction as a cause of hypoglycemia are to recognize the symptoms and to conduct the correct biochemical tests at the time of hypoglycemia. These tests include determining the levels of glucose, insulin, proinsulin, C-peptide, IGF-1, IGFBP-3, GH, IGF-2, and ketones (Table 7). In NICTH, total IGF-2 levels are usually inappropriately normal or elevated. The presence of a normal total IGF-2 level is explained

Table 6 Clinical Manifestations of Non–Islet Cell Tumor Hypoglycemia

Neuroglycopenic symptoms
 Headache
 Dizziness
 Confusion
 Amnesia
 Seizure
 Lethargy or somnolence
 Diminished motor activity
 Stupor
 Coma
Autonomic symptoms
 Diaphoreses
 Palpitations
 Tachycardia
Acromegaloid signs
 Jaw prognathism
 Enlarged nose
 Acral swelling
 Skin tags
 Nuchal hyperpigmentation

Table 7 Distinction between Non–Islet Cell Tumor Hypoglycemia, Insulinoma, and Hepatic Tumor Burden

Laboratory Finding	NICTH	Insulinoma	Hepatic Tumor Burden
Insulin	Low	High	Low
C-peptide, proinsulin	Low	High	Low
GH	Low	Normal–high	Normal–high
IGF-1	Low	Normal	Normal
IGF-2	Normal–high	Normal	Normal
IGFBP-3	Low	Normal	Normal
β-Hydroxybutyrate	Low	Low	High

GH = growth hormone; IGF = insulin-like growth factor; IGFBP = insulin-like growth factor binding protein; NICTH = non–islet cell tumor hypoglycemia.

by two findings: the elevation of big IGF-2 levels is compensated for by a decrease in the normal IGF-2 level, and big IGF-2, which cross-reacts with the IGF-2 radioimmunoassay, is incompletely recognized by the assay.[27,37] Thus, an IGF-2 to IGF-1 ratio of >10 is more sensitive than an IGF-2 level alone for diagnosing NICTH.[23]

A glucagon stimulation test (1 mg of glucagon administered intravenously over 2 minutes with blood drawn at 0, 15, 30, and 45 minutes after administration to test for glucose level) performed during a hypoglycemic episode can be useful in distinguishing whether the hypoglycemia is insulin mediated (insulinoma or NICTH). This test takes advantage of glucagon's gluconeogenic action on the liver to stimulate glycogen breakdown into glucose. An increase in glucose by > 30 mg/dL from baseline is consistent with either insulinoma or NICTH as the glycogen stores are maintained in these pathologic conditions because of the antiglycogenolytic effects of insulin.[38]

Localization of the primary tumor with radiologic imaging is not difficult because the tumors associated with NICTH are often large.

Treatment

Surgical excision, chemotherapy, and radiotherapy to reduce tumor mass are the mainstays of treatment of the primary tumor and hypoglycemic effects. However, when a patient is unable to undergo surgical or chemoradiotherapy, palliative measures can be taken to control the hypoglycemic episodes. Glucose infusions (20% or 50% dextrose) can acutely manage hypoglycemia, and frequent small meals can prevent hypoglycemic episodes. Eventually, however, the progressive nature of the underlying malignancy will cause the hypoglycemia to become resistant to these conservative therapies.

Continuous infusion with glucagon has been described to maintain normoglycemia for a few months to allow for palliation or improvement of clinical performance status so that possible antineoplastic therapies can be provided in the future.[38] Unfortunately, the adverse side-effect profile and cost of the medication often limit its prolonged use.[39]

Glucocorticoids are also effective in the management of NICTH. A patient treated with prednisolone (30 mg/d) demonstrated increased IGF-1, IGFBP-3, and ALS levels but decreased IGF-2 levels, leading to an overall increase in the amount of ternary complexes and resolution of hypoglycemia.[26] Because IGF-2 may act as an autocrine growth factor for the primary tumor, control of IGF-2 levels with glucocorticoid therapy may stabilize tumor progression.[40] Glucocorticoids may decrease IGF-2 levels through a variety of mechanisms. They may induce enzymes to convert pro-IGF-2 into the mature form or increase clearance and/or suppress tumor production of big IGF-2.[41] Unfortunately, glucocorticoid therapy appears to be reversible and dose dependent, requiring prednisone equivalents of >20 mg/d.

GH therapy has also been used, although with less efficacy. Relief of hypoglycemia is possible with high doses of GH daily (4 U/d); however, its prolonged use can lead to adverse side effects, such as arthritis from acral edema and other acromegaloid features. Its therapeutic effect does not appear to be sustained despite continuous treatment.[23,26] Additionally, the theoretical potential for GH to stimulate tumor growth raises concern about its use as a treatment of choice.[28]

Syndrome of Inappropriate Antidiuretic Hormone

Hyponatremia was first associated with lung cancer in 1938, but its association with inappropriate secretion of an antidiuretic hormone (ADH)-like substance was made in 1957 by Schwartz and colleagues.[5,42] This report was followed by the finding of an ADH-like substance in lung carcinoma extract in 1963.[43]

Tumors

Syndrome of inappropriate antidiuretic hormone (SIADH) is most commonly associated with small cell lung carcinoma and carcinoid tumors. Forty percent of patients with small cell lung carcinoma have high ADH levels, but only about 15% manifest SIADH.[4,44,45] Rarely, SIADH has been seen with other tumor types:

prostate carcinoma, breast carcinoma, adreno-cortical carcinoma, esophageal carcinoma, pancreatic carcinoma, other gastrointestinal carcinomas, thymomas, Hodgkin's lymphoma, non-Hodgkin's lymphoma, and head and neck carcinomas.[4] One case of an immature teratoma was reported to cause SIADH (Table 8).[46]

Pathophysiology

Under normal conditions, serum osmolality is maintained in a narrow range between 280 and 295 mOsm/kg by ADH (also known as arginine vasopressin), which is produced by the supraoptic and paraventricular nuclei in the hypothalamus. Although serum osmolality is the most important stimulus for ADH secretion, arterial underfilling, nausea, hypothyroidism, hypocortisolism, and various medications also stimulate its release.[47,48]

ADH binds to its receptor on the collecting duct of the renal system to allow for intracellular aquaporin 2 channels to be fused to the luminal membrane, thus permitting the flow of water from the lumen into the cell and then into the interstitium. Natriuresis is likely facilitated by the decreased action of the renin-angiotensin-aldosterone system caused by the increase in blood volume accompanying water retention.[48]

ADH, oxytocin, and their binding proteins, neurophysins, can be produced by tumors. ADH production by tumors is not suppressed by hypo-osmolality. Besides inappropriate ADH secretion, there is some speculation that atrial and brain natriuretic peptides play a role in cancer-associated hyponatremia. Elevated atrial natriuretic peptide levels may cause hyponatremia in patients who have normal ADH levels.[44,49–51]

Clinical Manifestations

Most patients who develop SIADH are asymptomatic, with only mild hyponatremia, especially when the hyponatremia evolves slowly. The patients are euvolemic. When the serum sodium concentration falls below 120 mEq/L, however, 27 to 44% of patients may develop severe neurologic symptoms and signs (Table 9).[44] Focal neurologic disturbances can occur even in the absence of space-occupying lesions in the brain. In particular, premenopausal women who develop

Table 8 Tumors Causing SIADH

Small cell lung carcinoma
Pancreatic
Duodenal
Prostatic
Bladder
Urethral
Lymphoma
Olfactory neuroblastoma
Thymoma

SIADH = syndrome of inappropriate antidiuretic hormone.

Table 9 Clinical Manifestations of Hyponatremia

Neurologic
　Altered mental status (confusion, lethargy, psychotic behavior)
　Headache
　Focal neurologic deficits or abnormalities
　Seizure
　Coma
Gastrointestinal
　Anorexia
　Nausea or vomiting
　Abdominal cramps
Pulmonary
　Respiratory arrest
　Noncardiogenic pulmonary edema

hyponatremia may develop profound cerebral edema and are at greater risk than men or postmenopausal women for severe neurologic symptoms and residual complications.[52]

Diagnosis

The finding of hyponatremia should initiate a systematic investigation for the cause, which first entails an assessment of the tonicity. If the assessment reveals hypotonic hyponatremia, a distinction based on the patient's overall volume status can be made (Table 10).

Finding hyponatremia with serum hypo-osmolality and relative urinary hyperosmolality (usually serum osmolality <280 mOsm/kg and urinary osmolality >500 mOsm/kg) after excluding the presence of adrenal insufficiency or hypothyroidism supports the diagnosis of SIADH.

The urinary sodium level will be inappropriately elevated (urinary sodium >20 mEq/L), in the absence of diuretics and renal dysfunction, for the level of hyponatremia (Table 11). SIADH owing to an underlying tumor or other causes (eg, pulmonary disease, central nervous system disorder) is difficult to distinguish by biochemical workup alone. Clinical correlation will assist with diagnosis.

ADH levels can be measured by radioimmunoassay, but their clinical significance is unclear because ADH values do not correlate with the clinical presentation of hyponatremia.

Treatment

Aside from treating the underlying tumor with surgery or chemoradiotherapy, SIADH can usually be managed with free water restriction (ie, <500 mL/24 h or replacement of the urine output by 50%); this can correct the hyponatremia slowly, over 7 to 10 days. In critically ill (eg,

Table 11 Diagnostic Criteria for SIADH

Hyponatremia
Inappropriately high urine osmolality
Inappropriately high urinary sodium excretion
　(>20 mEq/L)
Euvolemia
Normal renal function
No diuretic use
Normal thyroid function
Normal adrenal function

SIADH = syndrome of inappropriate antidiuretic hormone.

Table 10 Causes of Hypotonic Hyponatremia

Volume Status	Laboratory Finding	Cause
Hypovolemic	Renal sodium loss (>20 mEq/L)	Diuretics
		Solute diuresis (glucose, mannitol)
		Salt-wasting nephropathy (chronic interstitial nephropathy, polycystic kidney disease, obstructive uropathy, Bartter's syndrome)
		Mineralocorticoid deficiency (Addison's disease)
		Cerebral salt wasting (post-traumatic)
	Nonrenal sodium loss (<20 mEq/L)	Gastrointestinal (diarrhea, vomiting, pancreatitis)
		Skin (sweating, burns)
		Blood loss
Euvolemic	Urine sodium >40 mEq/L	SIADH
		Tumors
		Central nervous system disorders (tumor, infection, trauma)
		Pulmonary diseases
		Drugs (alcohol, cisplatin, cyclophosphamide, vincristine, melphalan, morphine)
		Idiopathic
		Hypothyroidism
		Hypocortisolism
		Primary polydipsia
Hypervolemic		Renal failure (nephrotic syndrome)
		Congestive heart failure
		Cirrhosis

SIADH = syndrome of inappropriate antidiuretic hormone.

comatose) patients, more aggressive therapy with hypertonic saline and furosemide may be used with extreme caution to elicit a net fluid loss. The serum sodium level should be monitored closely for a rise of about 0.5 mEq/L/h to avoid central pontine myelinolysis or brain osmotic demyelination syndrome, which occurs with overly rapid correction of hyponatremia. Adrogue studied 62 patients with hyponatremia (sodium <110 mEq/L) and found that a higher risk of neurologic complications occurred with correction rates of >0.55 mEq/L/h.[53]

Demeclocycline is an antibiotic in the tetracycline family that blocks ADH-induced cyclic adenosine monophosphate formation in the renal tubules. This medication, given as 600 to 1,200 mg/d divided into three or four doses, leads to a decline in intracellular aquaporin 2 channel phosphorylation, which prevents the channel from inserting into the luminal membrane. Demeclocycline takes from 4 to 21 days to work but is preferable to other therapies for long-term treatment of SIADH.[44] Lithium is also used sometimes, but it is less effective than demeclocycline and has an inferior adverse side-effect profile.[54]

Urea, given at a dosage of 40 g dissolved in 100 to 150 mg of normal saline every 8 hours along with a normal saline infusion (60–100 mg/h) for 1 to 2 days, can correct the salt-losing tendency in SIADH without the need for water restriction since it induces osmotic diuresis. Rapid water shifts do not usually occur with this treatment, as they do with mannitol, thus limiting the risk of cardiac failure.[55]

Vasopressin receptor type 2 antagonists are currently being studied in animal and clinical trials.[56] These agents are especially promising because they directly block the action of ADH on the receptors on the renal tubules without worsening renal function and with minimal adverse side effects.

Resolution of SIADH correlates well with tumor regression in response to chemoradiotherapy. With tumor recurrence, 60 to 70% of patients will also have a recurrence of SIADH. However, the presence or absence of SIADH does not affect the prognosis of patients with small cell lung carcinoma.[44]

Tumor-Induced Osteomalacia

Oncogenic osteomalacia–rickets was first described by McCance in 1947,[57] but Prader and colleagues were the first to attribute it to the presence of tumor in 1959.[58] It has also been referred to as tumor-induced hypophosphatemic rickets, oncogenous osteomalacia, and tumor-induced osteomalacia (TIO).[59] TIO is a rare condition characterized by bone mineralization disease, hypophosphatemia, renal phosphate wasting, impaired calcitriol (1,25-dihydroxyvitamin D_3,

the active form of vitamin D) synthesis, fractures, and resolution of all of these abnormalities after removal of an underlying tumor.

Tumors

Only approximately 120 cases of TIO have been reported in the literature, although this may not reflect its true prevalence. Most tumors that cause TIO are mesenchymal in origin and are usually benign, although malignant types and other histologic types of tumors have been reported (Table 12).[59,60] The mesenchymal tumors can be further classified into the following four histologic subgroups[61]:

1. Phosphaturic mesenchymal tumor (PMT), mixed connective tissue type, is the most common of the subtypes, making up about 70% of the mesenchymal tumors associated with TIO[62]
2. Osteoblastoma-like PMT
3. Ossifying fibroma–like PMT
4. Nonossifying fibroma–like PMT

TIO tumors are often small and slow-growing and present in obscure areas, which makes them extremely difficult to locate; thus, clinicians must conduct long-term follow-up and surveillance in patients with TIO. Often tumors are found within bone, especially in the craniofacial regions and extremities (eg, nasopharynx, mandible, sinus, femur, tibia). Occasionally, they are located in the brain or in the popliteal, inguinal, or suprapatellar areas. In a review of 100 cases, 87% of TIO tumors were benign, 50% were vascular in origin, and 50% were located in skeletal tissues.[63]

Pathophysiology

Before discussing the pathophysiology involved with TIO, normal phosphate homeostasis should be reviewed briefly. A low serum phosphate level stimulates renal 25-hydroxyvitamin D_1-α-hydroxylase (1-α-hydroxylase) activity, which converts 25-hydroxyvitamin D into 1,25-

dihydroxyvitamin D_3 (calcitriol). Calcitriol, in turn, increases calcium and phosphorus absorption by the intestine and enhances their mobilization from the bone. The resulting increase in calcitriol and calcium levels will decrease parathyroid hormone secretion, which increases renal calcium excretion and phosphorus reabsorption. In addition, hypophosphatemia itself will stimulate renal reabsorption of phosphate.

In TIO, tumors highly express one or more hormones (phosphatonins) that demonstrate phosphaturic activity and inhibit 1-α-hydroxylase activity in cultured kidney cells.[64–67] The fibroblast growth factor 23 gene (FGF23), although expressed in low levels in normal tissue, is highly expressed in tumors associated with TIO.[68–70] It is also expressed in X-linked hypophosphatemia and has a role in autosomal dominant hypophosphatemic rickets.[71,72] FGF23 decreases expression of renal sodium–phosphorus cotransporters, which normally mediate phosphorus reabsorption, leading to hypophosphatemia. Excessive FGF23 levels will also down-regulate 1-α-hydroxylase activity to cause decreased levels of calcitriol, contributing to the hypophosphatemia.[66]

Secreted frizzled-related protein type 4 and matrix extracellular phosphoglycoprotein are other phosphatonins cloned from TIO-associated tumors.[73,74] No assays for these are currently commercially available.[75]

The cause of hypophosphatemia in TIO is distinct from that seen in light-chain nephropathy associated with hematogenous malignancies, in which renal phosphate wasting is mediated by light-chain proteinuria.[76]

Clinical Manifestations

Chronic hypophosphatemia causes inadequate mineralization of the osteoid, a condition called osteomalacia. Patients have long-term symptoms of bone and muscle pain. The poor quality of the bones will lead to recurrent fractures of the long bones, vertebral bodies, and ribs. In younger patients, growth retardation and bowing of the lower extremities can occur (Table 13).[59]

Patients typically have symptoms long before a diagnosis of TIO or identification of a tumor is

Table 12 Tumors Causing Tumor-Induced Osteomalacia

Mesenchymal tumors
  Sclerosing angioma
  Benign angiofibroma
  Hemangiomas
  Hemangiopericytoma
  Chondrosarcoma
  Primitive mesenchymal tumor
  Chondroma-like tumor
  Giant cell tumor of bone
Breast carcinoma
Prostate carcinoma
Small cell lung carcinoma
Multiple myeloma
Chronic lymphocytic leukemia

Table 13 Clinical Manifestations of Tumor-Induced Osteomalacia

Arthralgia
Myalgia
Proximal muscle weakness
Fatigue
Recurrent fractures
Chest wall abnormalities (restrictive respiratory problems)
Gait disturbances
Growth retardation (in younger patients)
Bowing of lower extremities

made. A review of the 120 published cases showed symptomatic periods ranging from 2.5 months to 19 years (average >2.5 years) before the diagnosis was made. In most patients, it was diagnosed in the sixth decade of life (range 1–74 years old), and only 15% were younger than 20 years old.[60]

Diagnosis

The list of possible underlying causes of hypophosphatemia far surpasses that of osteomalacia (Tables 14 and 15). The workup for hypophosphatemia should include determinations of fasting serum phosphorus, serum calcium,

alkaline phosphatase (bone specific), creatinine, intact parathyroid hormone, 25-hydroxyvitamin D, and calcitriol levels and a 24-hour urine collection for assessing phosphorus, creatinine, amino acids, and glucose levels. TIO is characterized by very low serum phosphorus (range 0.7–2.4 mg/dL) and normal serum calcium and 25-hydroxyvitamin D but low or normal calcitriol levels (Table 16). The presence of aminoaciduria and glucosuria reflect the proximal renal tubular defect caused by TIO, as in Fanconi's syndrome.

The results of biochemical testing for TIO are indistinguishable from those for X-linked hypophosphatemia and autosomal dominant hypophosphatemic rickets, but the clinical context of the abnormalities will help differentiate between these three disease states (Table 17). Most notably, patients with TIO will not have a family history of hypophosphatemia or bone disorders.[66] X-linked hypophosphatemia can be evaluated with genetic testing to detect a mutation of the *PHEX* gene (phosphate-regulating gene with homologies to endopeptidases on the X chromosome). Autosomal dominant hypophosphatemic rickets is associated with a mutation of the *FGF23*

gene. Resection of the tumor in TIO will reverse the biochemical abnormalities, which is the most definitive diagnostic criterion.

Radiographs of bones reveal osteopenia, pseudofractures, and coarsened trabeculae, and children will have wide epiphyseal plates. Bone scans yield findings typical of osteomalacia (eg, diffuse skeletal uptake, focal uptake at fracture sites) but are nonspecific for the cause.

Bone biopsies with tetracycline labeling can reveal a mineralization defect with increased mineralization lag time (reduced distance between tetracycline labels) and excessive unmineralized bone (osteoid).

Localization of the causative tumor may take years of surveillance and can exhaust biochemical and radiologic modalities. Besides computed tomographic, magnetic resonance, and positron emission tomographic scans, an indium 111 pentetreotide (octreotide) scan may be helpful because some mesenchymal tumors express somatostatin receptors.[77]

Treatment

Therapy for TIO is first directed toward complete resection of the tumor; typically, that is curative. However, when complete resection of the causative tumor is unsuccessful or impossible, correction of the two major biochemical abnormalities (hypophosphatemia and calcitriol deficiency) will often lead to clinical improvement. The therapeutic goals are to improve the patient's symptoms, maintain a low or normal fasting phosphorus level, normalize the alkaline phosphatase level, and avoid hypercalcemia and hypercalciuria.

Oral or intravenous phosphate supplementation combined with calcitriol therapy is usually effective. In general, oral phosphate therapy is well tolerated, although 5 to 10% of treated patients develop dose-related adverse gastrointestinal side effects, with symptoms including nausea, vomiting, diarrhea, or abdominal pain.

Table 14 Conditions to Rule Out as Causes of Hypophosphatemia

Decreased gastrointestinal absorption
   Inadequate dietary intake
   Antacids with aluminum or magnesium
     (phosphate binders)
   Chronic diarrhea, steatorrhea, or
     malabsorption
   Vitamin D deficiency
   Vomiting
Increased renal loss
   Primary hyperparathyroidism
   Vitamin D deficiency
   Fanconi's syndrome
   Polyostotic fibrous dysplasia
   Neurofibromatosis
   Kidney transplant
   Recovery from hemolytic-uremic syndrome
   X-linked hypophosphatemic rickets
   Autosomal dominant hypophosphatemic
     rickets
   Hereditary hypophosphatemic rickets with
     hypercalciuria (autosomal recessive)
   Tumor-induced osteomalacia
   Osmotic diuresis
   Diuretics acting on proximal tubules
   Hyperaldosteronism or mineralocorticoid
     administration or licorice ingestion
   Volume expansion
   SIADH
   Corticosteroid
   Aminophylline
   Cisplatin
Intracellular redistribution
   Insulin
   Respiratory alkalosis
   Hungry bone syndrome
   Recovery from hypothermia

SIADH = syndrome of inappropriate antidiuretic hormone.

Table 15 Conditions to Rule Out as Causes of Osteomalacia

Abnormal vitamin D metabolism
Abnormal bone matrix
Enzyme deficiencies (hypophosphatasia)
Mineralization inhibitors (aluminum, fluoride, bisphosphonates)
Calcium or phosphorus deficiency
Renal phosphate wasting

Table 16 Biochemical Tests in Tumor-Induced Osteomalacia

Study	Laboratory Value
Serum	
Phosphorus	Low
Calcium	Normal
25-Hydroxyvitamin D	Normal
1,25-Dihydroxyvitamin D (calcitriol)	Low or inappropriately normal
Intact parathyroid hormone	Normal–high
Alkaline phosphatase (bone)	High
Urine	
Phosphorus	High
Glucose	High
Amino acids	High

Table 17 Comparison of Tumor-Induced Osteomalacia, X-Linked Hypophosphatemic Rickets, Autosomal Dominant Hypophosphatemic Rickets, and Hereditary Hypophosphatemic Rickets with Hypercalciuria

Feature	TIO	XLH	ADHR	HHRH
Inheritance	None (acquired)	X-linked dominant	Autosomal dominant	Autosomal recessive
Tumor	Yes	No	No	No
Onset	Variable	After birth	Variable	Variable
Bone disease	Fractures	LE deformity Short stature	LE deformity Short stature	Variable
Biochemical tests				
Phosphorus	Very low	Very low	Very low	Mildly low
Calcitriol	Low–normal	Low–normal	Low–normal	High
Urine calcium	Normal	Normal	Normal	High
Genetic mutation	None	*PHEX*	*FGF23*	*SLC34A3*

ADHR = autosomal dominant hypophosphatemic rickets; HHRH = hereditary hypophosphatemic rickets with hypercalciuria; LE = lower extremity; TIO = tumor-induced osteomalacia; XLH = X-linked hypophosphatemic rickets.

Overreplacement of phosphate could lead to hypocalcemia from binding effects. Together, the hyperphosphatemia and hypocalcemia can lead to secondary hyperparathyroidism or parathyroid autonomy. Intravenous phosphate therapy has been given for extended periods when oral administration was not tolerated or there were concerns about metastatic calcification, hypocalcemia, cardiac arrhythmia, or unmanageable electrolyte disturbances.[78]

Calcitriol administration can improve the biochemical abnormalities and bone lesions, but care must be taken to avoid hypercalcemia, nephrolithiasis, or nephrocalcinosis.[79]

The data on treatment of TIO with octreotide, a somatostatin-receptor analogue, are limited and demonstrate mixed results.[80] Currently, its use is not recommended unless all other treatment modalities have failed.

Ectopic GH-RH Syndrome

Acromegaly owing to elevated GH and IGF-1 production is rare (38–69 cases/million population), with an annual incidence of 2.8 to 4 cases per million. Most cases are due to excessive GH secretion from a functional pituitary adenoma. GH-RH is normally produced by the hypothalamus to regulate pituitary GH production. Ectopic GH-RH-secreting tumors account for 1% of cases of acromegaly, although only about 50 cases have been reported in the literature. The true prevalence and incidence are unknown.[81] The infrequency of this paraneoplastic syndrome may be partly attributable to the misdiagnosis of pituitary GH adenoma since chronically elevated GH-RH will produce somatotropic hyperplasia.[82]

Tumors

Among the cases of ectopic GHRH syndrome reported, carcinoid tumors, primarily of the bronchial and intestinal regions, are the most common (about 60%). Pancreatic islet cell tumors are the next most common,[81] but other neuroendocrine tumors and malignancies have also been associated with this syndrome (Table 18).

Pathophysiology

In 1982, there were reports of three different forms of GH-RH produced by pancreatic islet cell

Table 18 Tumors Causing Ectopic Growth Hormone–Releasing Hormone Syndrome

Carcinoid (bronchial, intestinal)—60%
Pancreatic islet cell tumor
Pheochromocytoma
Retroperitoneal paraganglioma
Lung adenocarcinoma
Gastric adenocarcinoma

tumors: GH-RH(1-44)-NH$_2$, GH-RH(1-40)-OH, and GH-RH(1-37)-NH$_2$.[83,84] However, the full biologic activity is seen with a fragment as short as GH-RH(1-29).[82]

Clinical Manifestations

The ectopic GH-RH syndrome occurs predominantly in female patients. Patients with lung tumors usually have a longer duration of symptoms of the syndrome before tumor diagnosis than do those with pancreatic endocrine tumors (10.6 vs 5.3 years). The signs and symptoms are similar to those of GH-producing pituitary adenomas, although hyperprolactinemia is seen more frequently with ectopic GH-RH syndrome. In addition, these patients have symptoms directly caused by the underlying tumor (Table 19).[82]

Diagnosis

The initial evaluation for diagnosis of ectopic GHRH syndrome begins with checking the serum IGF-1 level. If IGF-1 is high, an oral glucose tolerance test (75 g) should be done to evaluate for physiologic suppression of GH levels. In normal subjects, the GH level (measured using sensitive immunoradiometric or immunochemiluminescence assays) will fall below 0.3 ng/mL within 2 hours of the glucose challenge.[85]

Next, the source of the excessive GH should be evaluated using magnetic resonance imaging of the pituitary gland since most cases are due to a functional pituitary adenoma. If the pituitary gland appears diffusely enlarged or does not show a clear adenoma, the clinician should evaluate for a source of ectopic GH-RH secretion. Imaging of other areas of the body may be needed to search for an underlying tumor.[82]

Table 19 Clinical Manifestations of Ectopic Growth Hormone–Releasing Hormone Syndrome

Macrognathia
Macroglossia
Acral swelling and overgrowth
Paresthesias of hands or feet
Coarsened facial features
Skin
   Thickened skin
   Skin tags
   Hyperhidrosis
   Increased hair growth or hirsutism
Impaired glucose tolerance or diabetes mellitus
Cardiovascular
   Hypertension
   Left ventricular hypertrophy
   Diastolic cardiomyopathy
Tumor related
   Cough
   Hemoptysis
   Recurrent pneumonia
   Abdominal mass

Serum GH-RH is not a widely available test, but when measured by a reliable laboratory, the level of GH-RH has been 100 to 1,000 times the normal reference range in all reported cases.[82]

Treatment

If the primary tumor causing ectopic GH-RH syndrome is not amenable to or fails surgical resection or chemoradiotherapy, the GH hypersecretion and its effects can be treated with a somatostatin analogue, such as octreotide. Octreotide can decrease the pituitary's secretion of GH, the size of the hyperplastic pituitary gland, and the growth of most neuroendocrine tumors.[86,87] Continuous infusion of octreotide may have greater efficacy than intermittent injections. If the pituitary enlargement causes compression on the optic chiasm or other serious effects, resection of the pituitary gland may be required; however, GH hypersecretion often persists because of residual pituitary tissue. Dopaminergic drugs are usually ineffective.

Human Chorionic Gonadotropin Syndrome

Many common tumors produce human chorionic gonadotropin (hCG), which may or may not lead to clinical sequelae. Because the level of hCG is often associated with disease status, it can serve as a useful marker of the tumor's response to treatment.

Tumors

Excessive production of hCG and gynecomastia are most commonly found in gestational trophoblastic tumors (eg, choriocarcinomas, hydatidiform moles), germ cell tumors of the testis or ovary (eg, seminomas, testicular embryonal carcinomas), and adenocarcinoma of the lung.[88] Fifteen percent of patients with lung cancer have detectable levels of β-hCG,[89] and 6 to 13% of patients with carcinomas of lung, stomach, colon, and pancreas have excessive β-hCG levels.[90] Rarely, hCG is produced by hepatoblastomas in children and by pancreatic adenocarcinomas in adults.

Pathophysiology

Two different protein subunits encoded by separate genes form hCG. The α subunit is homologous to that of all members of the pituitary glycoprotein hormone family (luteinizing hormone, follicle-stimulating hormone, and thyroid-stimulating hormone). The β subunit is unique to each of these hormones and confers biologic specificity. The homology of the α subunit in hCG with these hormones allows for cross-reactivity on their respective receptors, thus mediating the clinical manifestations of the syndrome.

Clinical Manifestations

The signs and symptoms of excessive gonadotropin activity by hCG differ depending on the age and sex of the patient. In preadolescent children, precocious puberty with premature development of sexual characteristics, accelerated skeletal growth, and prostatic hyperplasia will be the predominant features. Premenopausal women may experience oligomenorrhea or menometrorrhagia, abdominal discomfort from development of ovarian cysts, and false-positive pregnancy tests.[91] Men can develop gynecomastia, which may be painful.[92] Increased aromatase activity within a tumor (eg, hepatoma or sarcoma) may contribute to gynecomastia because the enzyme metabolizes androgen precursors (dehydroepiandrosterone or testosterone) into estradiol.[4] Testicular atrophy can also be seen in men with excessive hCG syndrome.[93]

Hyperthyroidism, either overt (high free thyroxine level with symptoms) or subclinical (normal free thyroxine level), with suppressed thyroid-stimulating hormone levels may develop from an interaction of hCG with the thyroid-stimulating hormone receptor, particularly when the level of β subunit is extremely high. A thyroid goiter can be noted on physical examination.

Diagnosis

A male patient with unexplained gynecomastia should undergo evaluation of serum β-hCG level by radioimmunoassay, a physical examination of the testes, and radiographic studies of the chest and mediastinum.

Treatment

Targeting therapy to the underlying tumor is the most effective therapy for clinical manifestations of excessive β-hCG production. Gynecomastia can regress with treatment of the causative tumor; its return can signify tumor recurrence.[94] Hyperthyroidism can be treated short term with thionamide therapy (ie, methimazole or propylthiouracil) if chemotherapy or other strategies to treat the underlying malignancy are likely to be effective; otherwise, thyroidectomy or radioactive iodine may be required.

Miscellaneous Ectopic Paraneoplastic Syndromes

Ectopic Renin Production

Renin production other than by the juxtaglomerular apparatus of the kidney is extremely rare. Production of renin by nonrenal tumors has been seen with lung cancer,[95] pancreatic carcinoma,[96] liver hamartoma,[97] leukemia,[98] Hodgkin's disease,[99] ovarian carcinomas,[100] and ileal carcinoma.[101] Ectopic renin produces a clinical syndrome characterized by hypertension,

hypokalemia, and metabolic alkalosis. These patients have evidence of hyperaldosteronism, but the renin activity levels are inappropriately elevated. The level of prorenin, the renin precursor, is also increased. Therapy with spironolactone, angiotensin-converting enzyme inhibitors, or angiotensin receptor antagonist inhibitors may lower the blood pressure and normalize electrolyte abnormalities in the patient whose tumor cannot be resected.

Ectopic Prolactin Production

Ectopic prolactin production is rare but has been found in gonadoblastoma,[102] lymphoma,[103] leukemia,[104] renal cell carcinoma,[105] uterine cervical carcinoma,[106] and colorectal cancer.[107] The prolactin level may have prognostic value for colorectal cancer because it correlates with disease activity.[107] The clinical syndrome includes galactorrhea and amenorrhea in women and hypogonadism in men. Dopamine agonists such as bromocriptine and cabergoline, which are effective for treatment of pituitary prolactinomas, are generally ineffective for treatment of ectopic prolactin production. Treatment of the primary tumor offers the best chance for reversal of hyperprolactinemia and its effects.

Ectopic Calcitonin Production

Excessive calcitonin production other than by thyroid C cells has been seen in some malignancies, such as lung carcinoma.[108] However, no known clinical syndrome is associated with ectopic calcitonin secretion.[109]

REFERENCES

1. Maioli E, Fortino V. The complexity of parathyroid hormone-related protein signalling. Cell Mol Life Sci 2004;61:257–62.
2. Aniszewski JP, Young WF Jr, Thompson GB, et al. Cushing syndrome due to ectopic adrenocorticotropic hormone secretion. World J Surg 2001;25:934–40.
3. Ilias I, Torpy DJ, Pacak K, et al. Cushing's syndrome due to ectopic corticotropin secretion: twenty years' experience at the National Institutes of Health. J Clin Endocrinol Metab 2005;90:4955–62.
4. Odell WD. Paraneoplastic syndromes. In: Bast RC, Holland JF, Frei E, editors. Cancer medicine. 5th ed. Hamilton (ON): BC Decker; 2000. p. 777–89.
5. Arnold SM, Patchell R, Lowy AM, Foon KA. Paraneoplastic syndromes. In: DeVita VT, Hellman S, Rosenberg SA, editors. Cancer: principles and practice of oncology. 6th ed. Philadelphia: Lippincott Williams & Wilkins; 2001. p. 2511–36.
6. Wajchenberg BL, Mendonca BB, Liberman B, et al. Ectopic adrenocorticotropic hormone syndrome. Endocr Rev 1994;15:752–87.
7. Skrabanek P, Powell D. Unifying concept of non-pituitary ACTH-secreting tumors: evidence of common origin of neural-crest tumors, carcinoids, and oat-cell carcinomas. Cancer 1978;42:1263–9.
8. Tagliabue M, Pagani A, Palestini N, et al. Multiple endocrine neoplasia (MEN IIB) with Cushing's syndrome due to medullary thyroid carcinoma producing corticotropin-releasing hormone. Panminerva Med 1996;38:41–4.
9. Zangeneh F, Young WF Jr, Lloyd RV, et al. Cushing's syndrome due to ectopic production of corticotropin-releasing hormone in an infant with ganglioneuroblastoma. Endocr Pract 2003;9:394–9.
10. Rickman T, Garmany R, Doherty T, et al. Hypokalemia, metabolic alkalosis, and hypertension: Cushing's syndrome in a patient with metastatic prostate adenocarcinoma. Am J Kidney Dis 2001;37:838–46.
11. Borrero CG, McCook B, Mountz JM. Indium-111 pentetreotide imaging of carcinoid tumor of the thymus. Clin Nucl Med 2005;30:218–21.
12. O'Brien T, Young WF Jr, Davila DG, et al. Cushing's syndrome associated with ectopic production of corticotrophin-releasing hormone, corticotrophin and vasopressin by a phaeochromocytoma. Clin Endocrinol (Oxf) 1992; 37:460–7.
13. Doppman JL. The search for occult ectopic ACTH-producing tumors. Endocrinologist 1992;2:41–6.
14. Mengden T, Hubmann P, Muller J, et al. Urinary free cortisol versus 17-hydroxycorticosteroids: a comparative study of their diagnostic value in Cushing's syndrome. Clin Investig 1992;70:545–8.
15. Nieman LK. Evaluation and treatment of Cushing's syndrome. Am J Med 2005;118:1340–6.
16. Arnaldi G, Angeli A, Atkinson AB, et al. Diagnosis and complications of Cushing's syndrome: a consensus statement. J Clin Endocrinol Metab 2003;88:5593–602.
17. Papanicolaou DA, Mullen N, Kyrou I, Nieman LK. Nighttime salivary cortisol: a useful test for the diagnosis of Cushing's syndrome. J Clin Endocrinol Metab 2002; 87:4515–21.
18. Kaye TB, Crapo L. The Cushing syndrome: an update on diagnostic tests. Ann Intern Med 1990;112:434–44.
19. Grossman AB, Howlett TA, Perry L, et al. CRF in the differential diagnosis of Cushing's syndrome: a comparison with the dexamethasone suppression test. Clin Endocrinol (Oxf) 1988;29:167–78.
20. Oldfield EH, Doppman JL, Nieman LK, et al. Petrosal sinus sampling with and without corticotropin-releasing hormone for the differential diagnosis of Cushing's syndrome. N Engl J Med 1991;325:897–905.
21. Li H, Yan W, Mao Q, et al. Role of adrenalectomy in ectopic ACTH syndrome. Endocr J 2005;52:721–6.
22. Dimopoulos MA, Fernandez JF, Samaan NA, et al. Paraneoplastic Cushing's syndrome as an adverse prognostic factor in patients who die early with small cell lung cancer. Cancer 1992;69:66–71.
23. Marks V, Teale JD. Tumours producing hypoglycaemia. Endocr Relat Cancer 1998;5:111–29.
24. Baxter RC. The role of insulin-like growth factors and their binding proteins in tumor hypoglycemia. Horm Res 1996;46:195–201.
25. Kuenen BC, van Doorn J, Slee PH. Non-islet-cell tumour induced hypoglycaemia: a case report and review of literature. Neth J Med 1996;48:175–9.
26. Baxter RC, Holman SR, Corbould A, et al. Regulation of the insulin-like growth factors and their binding proteins by glucocorticoid and growth hormone in nonislet cell tumor hypoglycemia. J Clin Endocrinol Metab 1995; 80:2700–8.
27. Zapf J, Futo E, Peter M, Froesch ER. Can "big" insulin-like growth factor II in serum of tumor patients account for the development of extrapancreatic tumor hypoglycemia? J Clin Invest 1992;90:2574–84.
28. Ford-Dunn S, Smith A, Sykes N. Tumour-induced hypoglycaemia. Palliat Med 2002;16:357–8.
29. Daughaday WH, Emanuele MA, Brooks MH, et al. Synthesis and secretion of insulin-like growth factor II by a leiomyosarcoma with associated hypoglycemia. N Engl J Med 1988;319:1434–40.
30. Lowe WL Jr, Roberts CT Jr, LeRoith D, et al. Insulin-like growth factor-II in nonislet cell tumors associated with hypoglycemia: increased levels of messenger ribonucleic acid. J Clin Endocrinol Metab 1989;69:1153–9.
31. Daughaday WH, Trivedi B, Baxter RC. Serum "big insulin-like growth factor II" from patients with tumor hypoglycemia lacks normal E-domain O-linked glycosylation, a possible determinant of normal propeptide processing. Proc Natl Acad Sci U S A 1993;90:5823–7.
32. Bond JJ, Meka S, Baxter RC. Binding characteristics of pro-insulin-like growth factor-II from cancer patients: binary and ternary complex formation with IGF binding proteins-1 to -6. J Endocrinol 2000;165:253–60.
33. Daughaday WH, Wu JC, Lee SD, Kapadia M. Abnormal processing of pro-IGF-II in patients with hepatoma and in some hepatitis B virus antibody-positive asymptomatic individuals. J Lab Clin Med 1990;116:555–62.
34. Daughaday WH, Kapadia M. Significance of abnormal serum binding of insulin-like growth factor II in the development of hypoglycemia in patients with non-islet-cell tumors. Proc Natl Acad Sci U S A 1989;86:6778–82.

35. Stuart CA, Prince MJ, Peters EJ, et al. Insulin receptor proliferation: a mechanism for tumor-associated hypoglycemia. J Clin Endocrinol Metab 1986;63:879–85.

36. Trivedi N, Mithal A, Sharma AK, et al. Non-islet cell tumour induced hypoglycaemia with acromegaloid facial and acral swelling. Clin Endocrinol (Oxf) 1995;42:433–5.

37. Teale JD. Non-islet cell tumour hypoglycaemia. Clin Endocrinol (Oxf) 1999;51:147.

38. Hoff AO, Vassilopoulou-Sellin R. The role of glucagon administration in the diagnosis and treatment of patients with tumor hypoglycemia. Cancer 1998;82:1585–92.

39. Case CC, Vassilopoulou-Sellin R. Reproduction of features of the glucagonoma syndrome with continuous intravenous glucagon infusion as therapy for tumor-induced hypoglycemia. Endocr Pract 2003;9:22–5.

40. Thompson MA, Cox AJ, Whitehead RH, Jonas HA. Autocrine regulation of human tumor cell proliferation by insulin-like growth factor II: an in-vitro model. Endocrinology 1990;126:3033–42.

41. Teale JD, Wark G. The effectiveness of different treatment options for non-islet cell tumour hypoglycaemia. Clin Endocrinol (Oxf) 2004;60:457–60.

42. Schwartz WB, Bennett W, Curelop S, Bartter FC. A syndrome of renal sodium loss and hyponatremia probably resulting from inappropriate secretion of antidiuretic hormone. Am J Med 1957;23:529–42.

43. Amatruda TT Jr, Mulrow PJ, Gallagher JC, Sawyer WH. Carcinoma of the lung with inappropriate antidiuresis. Demonstration of antidiuretic-hormone-like activity in tumor extract. N Engl J Med 1963;269:544–9.

44. Mazzone PJ, Arroliga AC. Endocrine paraneoplastic syndromes in lung cancer. Curr Opin Pulm Med 2003;9:313–20.

45. Flombaum CD. Metabolic emergencies in the cancer patient. Semin Oncol 2000;27:322–34.

46. Lam CM, Yu VS. SIADH associated with ovarian immature teratoma: a case report. Eur J Gynaecol Oncol 2004;25:107–8.

47. Sorensen JB, Andersen MK, Hansen HH. Syndrome of inappropriate secretion of antidiuretic hormone (SIADH) in malignant disease. J Intern Med 1995;238:97–110.

48. Verbalis JG. Disorders of body water homeostasis. Best Pract Res Clin Endocrinol Metab 2003;17:471–503.

49. Kamoi K, Ebe T, Hasegawa A, et al. Hyponatremia in small cell lung cancer. Mechanisms not involving inappropriate ADH secretion. Cancer 1987;60:1089–93.

50. Chute JP, Taylor E, Williams J, et al. A metabolic study of patients with lung cancer and hyponatremia of malignancy. Clin Cancer Res 2006;12:888–96.

51. Johnson BE, Damodaran A, Rushin J, et al. Ectopic production and processing of atrial natriuretic peptide in a small cell lung carcinoma cell line and tumor from a patient with hyponatremia. Cancer 1997;79:35–44.

52. Ayus JC, Wheeler JM, Arieff AI. Postoperative hyponatremic encephalopathy in menstruant women. Ann Intern Med 1992;117:891–7.

53. Adrogue HJ. Consequences of inadequate management of hyponatremia. Am J Nephrol 2005;25:240–9.

54. Miyagawa CI. The pharmacologic management of the syndrome of inappropriate secretion of antidiuretic hormone. Drug Intell Clin Pharm 1986;20:527–31.

55. Reeder RF, Harbaugh RE. Administration of intravenous urea and normal saline for the treatment of hyponatremia in neurosurgical patients. J Neurosurg 1989;70:201–6.

56. Kazama I, Arata T, Michimata M, et al. Lithium effectively complements vasopressin V2 receptor antagonist in the treatment of hyponatraemia of SIADH rats. Nephrol Dial Transplant 2007;22:68-76.

57. McCance RA. Osteomalacia with Looser's nodes (milkman's syndrome) due to a raised resistance to vitamin D acquired about the age of 15 years. Q J Med 1947;16:33–46.

58. Prader A, Illig R, Uehlinger E, Stalder G. [Rickets following bone tumor]. Helv Paediatr Acta 1959;14:554–65.

59. Drezner MK. Tumor-induced osteomalacia. Rev Endocr Metab Disord 2001;2:175–86.

60. Jan de Beur SM. Tumor-induced osteomalacia. In: Favus MJ, editor. Primer on the metabolic bone diseases and disorders of mineral metabolism. 6th ed. Washington (DC): American Society for Bone and Mineral Research; 2006. p. 345–51.

61. Weidner N, Santa Cruz D. Phosphaturic mesenchymal tumors. A polymorphous group causing osteomalacia or rickets. Cancer 1987;59:1442–54.

62. Folpe AL, Fanburg-Smith JC, Billings SD, et al. Most osteomalacia-associated mesenchymal tumors are a single histopathologic entity: an analysis of 32 cases and a comprehensive review of the literature. Am J Surg Pathol 2004;28:1–30.

63. Crouzet J, Mimoune H, Beraneck L, Juan LH. Hypophosphatemic osteomalacia with plantar neurilemoma. A review of the literature (100 cases). Rev Rhum Engl Ed 1995;62:463–6.

64. Jonsson KB, Mannstadt M, Miyauchi A, et al. Extracts from tumors causing oncogenic osteomalacia inhibit phosphate uptake in opossum kidney cells. J Endocrinol 2001;69:613–20.

65. Yoshikawa S, Nakamura T, Takagi M, et al. Benign osteoblastoma as a cause of osteomalacia. A report of two cases. J Bone Joint Surg Br 1977;59:279–86.

66. Jan de Beur SM. Tumor-induced osteomalacia. JAMA 2005;294:1260–7.

67. Miyauchi A, Fukase M, Tsutsumi M, Fujita T. Hemangiopericytoma-induced osteomalacia: tumor transplantation in nude mice causes hypophosphatemia and tumor extracts inhibit renal 25-hydroxyvitamin D 1-hydroxylase activity. J Clin Endocrinol Metab 1988;67:46–53.

68. Fukumoto S, Yamashita T. Fibroblast growth factor-23 is the phosphaturic factor in tumor-induced osteomalacia and may be phosphatonin. Curr Opin Nephrol Hypertens 2002;11:385–9.

69. Shimada T, Mizutani S, Muto T, et al. Cloning and characterization of FGF23 as a causative factor of tumor-induced osteomalacia. Proc Natl Acad Sci U S A 2001;98:6500–5.

70. Imel EA, Peacock M, Pitukcheewanont P, et al. Sensitivity of fibroblast growth factor 23 measurements in tumor induced osteomalacia. J Clin Endocrinol Metab 2006 91:2055-61.

71. Yamazaki Y, Okazaki R, Shibata M, et al. Increased circulatory level of biologically active full-length FGF-23 in patients with hypophosphatemic rickets/osteomalacia. J Clin Endocrinol Metab 2002;87:4957–60.

72. Jonsson KB, Zahradnik R, Larsson T, et al. Fibroblast growth factor 23 in oncogenic osteomalacia and X-linked hypophosphatemia. N Engl J Med 2003;348:1656–63.

73. Berndt T, Craig TA, Bowe AE, et al. Secreted frizzled-related protein 4 is a potent tumor-derived phosphaturic agent. J Clin Invest 2003;112:785–94.

74. Rowe PS, Kumagai Y, Gutierrez G, et al. MEPE has the properties of an osteoblastic phosphatonin and minhibin. Bone 2004;34:303–19.

75. Ito N, Fukumoto S, Takeuchi Y, et al. Comparison of two assays for fibroblast growth factor (FGF)-23. J Bone Miner Metab 2005;23:435–40.

76. Rao DS, Parfitt AM, Villanueva AR, et al. Hypophosphatemic osteomalacia and adult Fanconi syndrome due to light-chain nephropathy. Another form of oncogenous osteomalacia. Am J Med 1987;82:333–8.

77. Jan de Beur SM, Streeten EA, Civelek AC, et al. Localisation of mesenchymal tumours by somatostatin receptor imaging. Lancet 2002;359:761–3.

78. Yeung SJ, McCutcheon IE, Schultz P, Gagel RF. Use of long-term intravenous phosphate infusion in the palliative treatment of tumor-induced osteomalacia. J Clin Endocrinol Metab 2000;85:549–55.

79. Drezner MK, Feinglos MN. Osteomalacia due to 1alpha,25-dihydroxycholecalciferol deficiency. Association with a giant cell tumor of bone. J Clin Invest 1977;60:1046–53.

80. Seufert J, Ebert K, Muller J, et al. Octreotide therapy for tumor-induced osteomalacia. N Engl J Med 2001;345:1883–8.

81. Altstadt TJ, Azzarelli B, Bevering C, et al. Acromegaly caused by a growth hormone-releasing hormone-secreting carcinoid tumor: case report. Neurosurgery 2002;50:1356–59; discussion 1360.

82. Losa M, von Werder K. Pathophysiology and clinical aspects of the ectopic GH-releasing hormone syndrome. Clin Endocrinol (Oxf) 1997;47:123–35.

83. Guillemin R, Brazeau P, Bohlen P, et al. Growth hormone-releasing factor from a human pancreatic tumor that caused acromegaly. Science 1982;218:585–7.

84. Rivier J, Spiess J, Thorner M, Vale W. Characterization of a growth hormone-releasing factor from a human pancreatic islet tumour. Nature 1982;300:276–8.

85. Freda PU, Post KD, Powell JS, Wardlaw SL. Evaluation of disease status with sensitive measures of growth hormone secretion in 60 postoperative patients with acromegaly. J Clin Endocrinol Metab 1998;83:3808–16.

86. Faglia G, Arosio M, Bazzoni N. Ectopic acromegaly. Endocrinol Metab Clin North Am 1992;21:575–95.

87. Drange MR, Melmed S. Long-acting lanreotide induces clinical and biochemical remission of acromegaly caused by disseminated growth hormone-releasing hormone-secreting carcinoid. J Clin Endocrinol Metab 1998;83:3104–9.

88. Rudnick P, Odell WD. In search of a cancer. N Engl J Med 1971;284:405–8.

89. Marcillac I, Troalen F, Bidart JM, et al. Free human chorionic gonadotropin beta subunit in gonadal and nongonadal neoplasms. Cancer Res 1992;52:3901–7.

90. Braunstein GD, Vaitukaitis JL, Carbone PP, Ross GT. Ectopic production of human chorionic gonadotrophin by neoplasms. Ann Intern Med 1973;78:39–45.

91. Sagaster P, Zojer N, Dekan G, Ludwig H. A paraneoplastic syndrome mimicking extrauterine pregnancy. Ann Oncol 2002;13:170–2.

92. Yaturu S, Harrara E, Nopajaroonsri C, et al. Gynecomastia attributable to human chorionic gonadotropin-secreting giant cell carcinoma of lung. Endocr Pract 2003;9:233–5.

93. Metz SA, Weintraub B, Rosen SW, et al. Ectopic secretion of chorionic gonadotropin by a lung carcinoma. Pituitary gonadotropin and subunit secretion and prolonged chemotherapeutic remission. Am J Med 1978;65:325–33.

94. Nishiyama T, Washiyama K, Tanikawa T, et al. Gynecomastia and ectopic human chorionic gonadotropin production by transitional cell carcinoma of the bladder. Urol Int 1992;48:463–5.

95. Genest J, Rojo-Ortega JM, Kuchel O, et al. Malignant hypertension with hypokalemia in a patient with renin-producing pulmonary carcinoma. Trans Assoc Am Physicians 1975;88:192–201.

96. Ruddy MC, Atlas SA, Salerno FG. Hypertension associated with a renin-secreting adenocarcinoma of the pancreas. N Engl J Med 1982;307:993–7.

97. Cox JN, Paunier L, Vallotton MB, et al. Epithelial liver hamartoma, systemic arterial hypertension and renin hypersecretion. Virchows Arch A Pathol Anat Histol 1975;366:15–26.

98. Wulf GG, Jahns-Streubel G, Strutz F, et al. Paraneoplastic hypokalemia in acute myeloid leukemia: a case of renin activity in AML blast cells. Ann Hematol 1996;73:139–41.

99. Singh AP, Charan VD, Desai N, Choudhry VP. Hypertension as a paraneoplastic phenomenon in childhood Hodgkin's disease. Leuk Lymphoma 1993;11:315–7.

100. Stephen MR, Lindop GB. A renin secreting ovarian steroid cell tumour associated with secondary polycythaemia. J Clin Pathol 1998;51:75–7.

101. Saito T, Fukamizu A, Okada K, et al. Ectopic production of renin by ileal carcinoma. Endocrinol Jpn 1989;36:117–24.

102. Hoffman WH, Gala RR, Kovacs K, Subramanian MG. Ectopic prolactin secretion from a gonadoblastoma. Cancer 1987;60:2690–5.

103. Arbaiza D, Noriega K, Marcial J, et al. Ectopic production of prolactin in an infant with non-Hodgkin lymphoma. Med Pediatr Oncol 1999;32:311–2.

104. Hatfill SJ, Kirby R, Hanley M, et al. Hyperprolactinemia in acute myeloid leukemia and indication of ectopic expression of human prolactin in blast cells of a patient of subtype M4. Leuk Res 1990;14:57–62.

105. Turkington RW. Ectopic production of prolactin. N Engl J Med 1971;285:1455–8.

106. Hsu CT, Yu MH, Lee CY, et al. Ectopic production of prolactin in uterine cervical carcinoma. Gynecol Oncol 1992;44:166–71.

107. Bhatavdekar JM, Patel DD, Chikhlikar PR, et al. Ectopic production of prolactin by colorectal adenocarcinoma. Dis Colon Rectum 2001;44:119–27.

108. Zajac JD, Martin TJ, Hudson P, et al. Biosynthesis of calcitonin by human lung cancer cells. Endocrinology 1985;116:749–55.

109. Ray DW. Ectopic hormone syndromes. In: DeGroot LJ, Jameson JL, editors. Endocrinology. 5th ed. Philadelphia: Elsevier Saunders; 2006. p. 3585–95.

Endocrine Neoplastic Syndromes

S. Jim Yeung, MD, PhD

Robert F. Gagel, MD

Neoplastic diseases of endocrine tissues can lead to the dysregulated secretion of hormones that are normally produced by the endocrine tissue and thus to clinical syndromes caused by an excess of the hormones. Severe dysregulation of hormones may lead to abnormal bodily function or biochemistry, with significant morbidity or even mortality. In this chapter, we focus on the endocrine neoplastic syndromes owing to neoplastic diseases of endocrine tissues.

Hyperparathyroidism

Parathyroid hormone (PTH) plays a major role in calcium homeostasis. Normally, secretion of PTH is regulated by negative feedback: when serum calcium levels rise, PTH production by the parathyroid cells decreases. In primary hyperparathyroidism, PTH secretion is dysregulated, leading to hypercalcemia.

Most cases of primary hyperparathyroidism are caused by benign parathyroid adenomas. Parathyroid carcinoma is a rare cause of hyperparathyroidism, accounting for less than 1% of the cases (Figure 1A). The pathogenesis of parathyroid carcinoma is largely unknown, but mutations of the hyperparathyroidism type 2 tumor suppressor gene, *HRPT2*, have been found in most parathyroid carcinomas.[1]

Parathyroidectomy with ipsilateral hemithyroidectomy and lymph node dissection may reduce the risk of local tumor recurrence,[2] but en bloc resection at the time of initial surgery may offer the best chance of cure. Distinguishing between adenomas and carcinomas can be difficult, and in some patients, the appearance of metastatic disease is the first sign that the previously resected parathyroid tumor was malignant.[3] The time between the initial diagnosis and the discovery of metastatic disease varies widely and may be as long as 20 years.[4] Resection of metastases should be attempted whenever possible because parathyroid carcinomas are usually slow-growing and resection can effectively control of hyperparathyroidism. Surgery followed by external beam radiation therapy may increase long-term survival compared with surgery alone. The results of the limited experience with adjuvant chemotherapy suggest that its benefits are modest and short-lived.[5] Some patients may have extended survival despite the presence of metastatic disease.[5]

Patients with parathyroid carcinoma have severe hypercalcemia and extremely high PTH levels, but the basic strategy of clinical management for hypercalcemia remains unchanged. Initial management should focus on the reversal of dehydration, which is common in hypercalcemic patients, by infusion of a normal saline solution at rates between 100 and 300 mL/h. Hydration will commonly lower the serum calcium concentration by 10% over 6 to 12 hours. Patients with severe hypercalcemia (defined as a serum calcium concentration > 13 mg/dL [3.25 mmol/L]), altered mental status, or evidence of renal dysfunction attributable to hypercalcemia should be treated with either intravenous pamidronate (60–90 mg over 4 hours), zoledronate (4 mg over 30 minutes) (Figure 1B),[6] glucocorticoids (40 to 60 mg/d prednisone equivalent), or gallium nitrate (200 mg/m^2/d, infused daily for 7 days).[7,8]

Salmon calcitonin may lower the serum calcium concentration by 1 to 2 mg/dL early in the treatment course but rarely has long-term effectiveness. These drugs are often used in combination or sequentially in patients who do not respond well to only one treatment.

A new class of drugs known as calcimimetics has been used effectively in some patients to control the symptoms of severe hypercalcemia in a palliative setting.[1] Cinacalcet, a second-generation calcimimetic, is effective and well tolerated in the treatment of refractory hypercalcemia owing to parathyroid carcinoma.[9] Patients with parathyroid cancer should start cinacalcet therapy at a dosage of 30 mg twice daily. The US Food and Drug Administration–approved labeling recommends adjusting the cinacalcet dosage every 2 to 4 weeks to bring the serum calcium concentration into the normal range, 8.4 to 10.6 mg/dL. A maximum dosage of 90 mg four times daily is recommended in the package insert, although that dosage may be insufficient to normalize the serum calcium level in patients with parathyroid cancer.

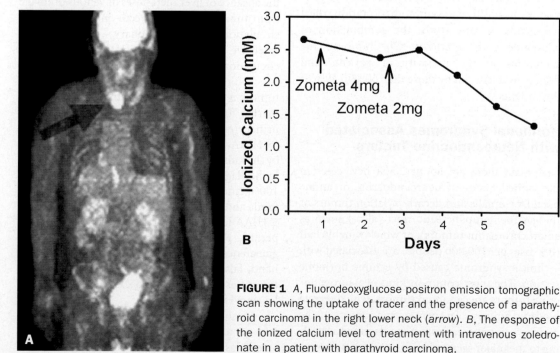

FIGURE 1 *A*, Fluorodeoxyglucose positron emission tomographic scan showing the uptake of tracer and the presence of a parathyroid carcinoma in the right lower neck (*arrow*). *B*, The response of the ionized calcium level to treatment with intravenous zoledronate in a patient with parathyroid carcinoma.

Calcitonin Syndrome

Patients with advanced medullary thyroid carcinoma have high levels of calcitonin, which causes calcitonin syndrome, characterized by diarrhea, flushing, and fatigue. Medullary thyroid carcinoma originates from the C cells of the thyroid gland. Four-fifths of medullary thyroid carcinomas are sporadic, and the remaining familial forms are familial medullary thyroid cancer and multiple endocrine neoplasia (MEN) types IIA and IIB. The *RET* proto-oncogene is responsible for all known forms of heritable medullary thyroid carcinoma and may also be seen in some sporadic cases. This gene is located on the long arm of chromosome 10 and encodes a protein, tyrosine kinase.

Calcitonin is used to detect and confirm medullary carcinoma of the thyroid and is a tumor marker that increases as the disease progresses. Pentagastrin and calcium infusions are used as provocative challenge tests for diagnosis of C-cell hyperplasia or malignancy, and in medullary carcinoma of the thyroid gland, levels of calcitonin greater than 1,000 pg/mL are often seen. Although calcitonin inhibits osteoclastic activity and increases renal excretion of calcium, its overall effect is to compensate for hypercalcemia; elevated calcitonin does not cause hypocalcemia, and its absence does not cause hypercalcemia. No definitive imaging study has been established for medullary thyroid carcinoma, but ^{131}I-metaiodobenzylguanidine (MIBG) and ^{99}Tc-octreotide scanning may be useful.

The management of calcitonin syndrome includes reducing the tumor bulk when possible. Depending on the location of metastatic disease, surgical tumor bulk reduction, chemoembolization, or other palliative approaches may be considered. In addition to symptomatic antidiarrheal treatments, in one study, the combination of lanreotide with interferon-α2b improved the symptoms in the majority of patients and decreased calcitonin by more than 50% in 40% of the patients.[10]

Hormonal Syndromes Associated with Neuroendocrine Tumors

Each year, there are about 2,500 new cases in the United States of neuroendocrine or amine precursor uptake and decarboxylation tumors of the gastroenteropancreatic tract (also known as enterochromaffin tumors), of which roughly half (0.2 cases per 100,000 people) are associated with a clinical syndrome caused by ectopic hormone section. The most common kind of neuroendocrine tumors are carcinoid tumors, which secrete biogenic amines. Neuroendocrine tumors of the gastroenteropancreatic tract are classified according to the major secreted hormone as gastrinoma,

VIPoma, insulinoma, glucagonoma, somatostatinoma, and others.[11] Calcitonin-secreting neuroendocrine tumors are extremely rare, and they usually cosecrete vasoactive intestinal peptide (VIP), somatostatin, or pancreatic polypeptide. Neuroendocrine tumors vary in their clinical courses and in their clinical endocrine syndromes. For example, insulinomas cause hypoglycemia; gastrinomas cause Zollinger-Ellison syndrome; VIPomas cause watery diarrhea, hypokalemia, achlorhydria (WDHA) syndrome; and glucagonomas cause glucagonoma syndrome. Among these tumors, gastrinoma is the most common malignant tumor and insulinoma is the most common benign tumor.

Carcinoid Syndrome

Carcinoid syndrome is caused by the release of a number of bioactive substances, but detailed knowledge of the pharmacologic mechanisms is still lacking. The most typical clinical manifestations of carcinoid syndrome are cutaneous flushing and diarrhea. Serotonin and biogenic amines cause the flushing, and motilin and substance P increase the motility of the small bowel and colon and cause the diarrhea. Other clinical manifestations of the syndrome include bronchoconstriction, telangiectasia, and cardiac valvular lesions (carcinoid heart disease).

Carcinoid tumors are the most common neuroendocrine tumors (estimated 7 to 13 cases per 1 million people per year). Carcinoid tumors can be part of MEN type I. Carcinoid tumors occur most commonly in the gastrointestinal tract and the lung. Most patients with carcinoid tumors are asymptomatic; only about 10% manifest carcinoid syndrome. Because the liver can metabolize and inactivate vasoactive amines efficiently, carcinoid syndrome rarely occurs in the absence of liver metastases or venous drainage from tumors entering directly into the systemic circulation (eg, pulmonary carcinoids or extensive bone metastases) instead of the portal circulation.

A biochemical tumor marker for carcinoid tumors is serum chromogranin A, and a specific marker for carcinoid syndrome is the increased urinary excretion of 5-hydroxyindoleacetic acid (5-HIAA, a liver metabolite of serotonin excreted by the kidneys). The specificity of urinary 5-HIAA in the diagnosis of carcinoid syndrome approaches 100% after excluding the ingestion of certain foods and medications that are known to elevate 5-HIAA levels (eg, avocados, bananas, kiwi fruit, pecans, plantains, pineapples, plums, walnuts, guaiafenesin, and acetaminophen). On the other hand, false-negative tests can result from ingestion of aspirin or levodopa, either of which can lower 5-HIAA levels.

In some patients with carcinoid syndrome and normal urinary 5-HIAA, documenting elevated plasma or platelet serotonin concentrations

or plasma histamine and peptide hormone levels may establish the diagnosis. Imaging studies to localize carcinoid tumors include abdominal ultrasonography (US), computed tomography (CT), magnetic resonance imaging (MRI), abdominal angiography, indium ^{111}In pentetreotide scintigraphy, [123]I- or ^{131}I-MIBG scintigraphy, and carbon ^{11}C serotonin positron emission tomography. Endoscopy, with or without endoscopic US, or videocapsule endoscopy may help localize carcinoid tumors in the intestinal tract.

Treatment

Surgical resection is the standard treatment modality for carcinoid tumors. If no metastatic disease is detectable and the primary carcinoid tumor is resectable, 5-year survival rates are 70 to 90%. Therapies for carcinoid syndrome are aimed at reduction of tumor bulk and inhibition of hormone secretion. To reduce tumor bulk, surgery, radiotherapy, hepatic artery embolization (chemo- or radiotherapy), alcohol sclerotherapy for liver metastases, radiofrequency ablation of liver metastases, cryosurgery for liver metastases, radioisotope-coupled somatostatin analogue (^{131}I-MIBG) administration for targeted delivery of a treatment radiation dose to the tumor, and occasionally chemotherapy may be considered. Somatostatin analogues (eg, octreotide) are effective in inhibiting hormone secretion. Symptoms in patients with carcinoid syndrome can usually be palliated by subcutaneous injections of octreotide (50–200 μg) two to three times a day. Pegylated-octreotide depot formulations for intramuscular injection can be administered once a month with equivalent efficacy. Some patients benefit from the use of interferon-α. Anecdotal reports of biologic activity indicate that some patients may respond to combined octreotide and interferon-α treatment.[12]

Insulinoma-Induced Hypoglycemia

Found in only 1.5% of detailed autopsies, islet cell tumors are uncommon cancers (200–1,000 new cases per year in the United States). About 85% of patients with MEN type 1 have pancreatic islet cell tumors. Insulinoma is the most common islet cell tumor. Over 90% of insulinomas are benign and solitary, and about 10% are malignant, with metastasis to the lymph nodes or liver. Whereas benign insulinomas can be cured by surgical resection, metastatic malignant insulinoma is not curable, and the clinical course of malignant insulinoma is often indolent owing to the relatively slow growth rate of these cancers.[13]

Diagnosis

The dysregulated release of insulin that occurs in insulinoma leads to fasting hypoglycemia, producing neuroglycopenic symptoms of confusion, loss of consciousness, coma, or seizures. Hypoglycemia can also activate the sympathetic nervous system to release catecholamines, producing tachycardia, tremulousness, and diaphoresis.[13]

The following is the differential diagnosis of hypoglycemia in patients with cancer: liver failure, starvation, hypopituitarism, hypoadrenalism, sepsis, insulin overdose, sulfonylurea overdose, insulinoma, and non–islet cell tumor–induced hypoglycemia. Diagnosis of insulinoma requires the presence of Whipple's triad: symptoms of hypoglycemia, glucose level below 50 mg/dL, and relief of symptoms after administration of glucose. The glucagon stimulation test is a simple and fast evaluation that can clarify the etiology of hypoglycemia and guide effective long-term strategies for control of hypoglycemia.[14] The differential diagnosis of fasting hypoglycemia may include an insulinoma, a non–islet cell tumor secreting insulin-like hormone, exogenous insulin, or stimulated release of insulin by secretagogues. Measurements of C-peptide and insulin levels, sulfonylurea and meglitinide levels, and insulin-like growth factor 2 levels help determine the correct diagnosis. C-peptide and insulin levels will be higher than normal in cases of insulinoma or after administration of an insulin secretagogue, whereas in factitious hypoglycemia owing to exogenous insulin, insulin levels will be higher than normal, but C-peptide levels will be lower than normal because exogenous insulin contains no C-peptide. The different hormonal profiles in insulinoma-induced hypoglycemia and non–islet cell tumor–induced hypoglycemia are shown in Table 1.

Treatment

Surgical resection is the treatment of choice for insulinomas. In the absence of preoperative localization and intraoperative detection of an insulinoma, blind pancreatic resection is not recommended.[15] Intraoperative US can be combined with other preoperative imaging modalities to improve tumor detection. Endoscopic US-guided ablation may be a minimally invasive alternative.[16] Glucocorticoid therapy can increase insulin resistance, reduce glucose use, increase hepatic glucose production, and impair insulin secretion and is a valid option for the control of insulinoma-induced hypoglycemia.[17] Other options for control of hypoglycemia include oral intake of carbohydrate, glucagon, or diazoxide and glucose infusion. The use of continuous infusion of glucagons to treat tumor-induced hypoglycemia may lead to side effects that resemble the symptoms of glucagonoma.[18] Octreotide or lanreotide has been tried in patients with insulin-producing islet cell tumors, generally without success. The lack of success may relate to the fact that the somatostatin analogues currently available are more effective for inhibiting glucagon than insulin secretion.

Glucagonoma Syndrome

Glucagonoma syndrome consists of a venous thromboembolism, necrolytic migratory erythema (Figure 2), and angular cheilitis. Glucagon-induced hyperglycemia is transient because a glucagon-induced increase in glycogenolysis does not persist; during sustained hyperglucagonemia, gluconeogenesis increases progressively. The transient glycogenolytic response to sustained hyperglucagonemia is not the result of glycogen depletion but the result of induction of counterregulatory hormones, such as insulin.

Glucagonoma has been reported in association with MEN type 1. A fasting plasma glucagon level of more than 1,000 ng/L establishes the diagnosis. More modest elevations of plasma glucagon levels may occur in diabetic ketoacidosis, renal failure, hepatic failure, sepsis, prolonged fasting, and gluten-sensitive enteropathy. Hypocholesterolemia and hypoaminoacidemia (ie, alanine, glycine, and serine levels <25% of normal) are common. Glucagonoma may be distinguished from other hyperglucagonemic states by the failure of glucose to suppress serum glucagon levels and the failure of arginine to enhance serum glucagon levels. To localize glucagonomas, angiography, CT, or MRI may be used. Glucagonomas are hypervascular and can be localized together with hepatic metastases by selective angiographic study of the celiac tripod. The CT and MRI studies of the pancreas may demonstrate the precise location of the tumor (in the tail of the pancreas in almost 90% of cases). Islet cell tumors have a marked increased signal intensity on T_2-weighted MRIs, and gadolinium enhancement in the non-necrotic areas of the tumor will allow differentiation of islet cell tumors from pancreatic adenocarcinoma. Other imaging methods, such as MIBG scintigraphy, positron emission tomography, or scintigraphic study with ^{111}In octreotide or with ^{11}C levodopa, may be used in the early localization of the tumor.

Treatment

Octreotide causes symptom regression in some patients. Administering the long-acting somatostatin analogue may be the first step of a multimodal therapeutic strategy, which almost always includes surgical resection of the primary tumor.

Table 1 Hormone Profiles of Tumor-Induced Hypoglycemia

Hormone	Change Compared with Normal	
	Non–Islet Cell	Insulinoma
IGF-1	Equivocal	Equivocal
IGF-2	Increased	Equivocal
IGFBP-3	Decreased	Equivocal
Insulin	Decreased	Increased
Glucose	Decreased	Decreased
Growth hormone	Decreased	Increased
β-Hydroxybutyrate	Decreased	Decreased

IGF = insulin-like growth factor; IGFBP = insulin-like growth factor binding protein.

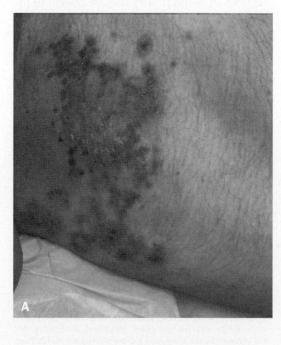

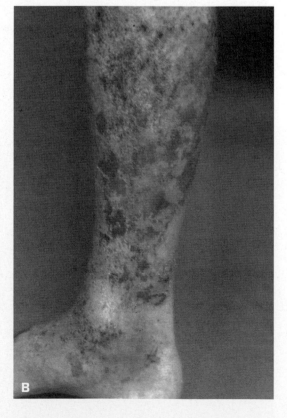

FIGURE 2 Necrolytic migratory erythema. *A,* Left inner upper thigh. *B,* Right leg.

Liver metastases may be treated by partial hepatectomy, hepatic arterial chemoembolization, and streptozocin-based systemic chemotherapy (doxorubicin plus streptozocin or 5-fluorouracil plus streptozocin).[19]

WDHA Syndrome

VIPoma causes a clinical syndrome characterized by watery diarrhea, hypokalemia, and achlorhydria. The diagnosis is based on clinical features and hormonal profiles demonstrating high serum VIP levels and the dominance of VIP over other pancreatic hormones. VIP levels at the time of diagnosis are more than three times the upper normal limit in the majority of cases.

To localize the primary lesion, CT, MRI, endoscopic US, angiography, or octreotide scintigraphy may be used. In about two-thirds of the cases of WDHA syndrome, the primary lesion is located in the pancreas, whereas in the rest of the cases, it is in the duodenum or retroperitoneum. Surgical resection is feasible in about two-thirds of the cases. For metastatic disease or poorly differentiated tumors, treatment with octreotide and chemotherapy should be offered. Reduction of tumor burden by surgery or chemoembolization in combination with administration of octreotide or chemotherapy may prolong survival in patients with advanced disease.[20] Because VIPomas usually have a slow rate of growth, unlike more aggressive malignancies, it is recommended that patients with advanced and incurable VIPomas receive palliative treatment. These patients appear to survive longer when they are treated proactively with sequential multimodality treatments.[21]

Zollinger-Ellison Syndrome

Neuroendocrine tumors associated with Zollinger-Ellison syndrome often cause gastric hydrochloric acid hypersecretion and upper gastrointestinal ulcer disease, which is often severe. Gastrin levels > 500 pg/mL in patients with basal acid hypersecretion are often indicative of gastrinoma, but gastrin levels > 500 pg/mL can also occur in patients with antral G-cell hyperplasia and hyperchlorhydria. Other conditions associated with moderately elevated gastrin levels include gastric ulcers, chronic renal failure, hyperparathyroidism, pyloric obstruction, carcinoma of the stomach, vagotomy without gastric resection, retained gastric antrum, and short bowel syndrome. If gastrinoma is likely but fasting gastrin levels are not diagnostic, the secretin test is the provocative test of choice. Intravenous secretin normally diminishes gastrin, but in gastrinomas, the gastrin level will be increased.

Gastrinoma-associated gastric acid hypersecretion is treated with antacids, proton pump inhibitors, and histamine receptor type 2 antagonists, and resectable gastrinoma is treated primarily with surgery. Gastrinoma can be staged by TNM criteria into four stages with different survival curves, with tumor size and distant metastases being statistically significant predictors of survival.[22] Patients with sporadic gastrinoma have a longer disease-free survival time than do patients with MEN type 1, although gross complete removal of the tumor improves survival in both types of patients.[22] Other disease complications that may require surgical intervention include a perforated viscus, acute gastrointestinal hemorrhage secondary to refractory peptic ulcer disease, and gastric outlet obstruction.

Somatostatinoma Syndrome

Somatostatinoma is a rare tumor (1 case per 40 million people annually). Excess somatostatin causes a clinical syndrome of diabetes mellitus, steatorrhea, and cholelithiasis.[23] Other complications, such as diabetic ketoacidosis[24] and relapsing cholangitis,[25] have also been reported to be associated with somatostatinoma. Tumors of the pancreas and gastrointestinal tract that secrete excess somatostatin are classified as somatostatinomas, although 10% of such tumors also secrete other humoral factors, including glucagon, gastrin, VIP, insulin, calcitonin, and adrenocorticotropic hormone.[26–28] Somatostatinomas are typically large, solitary, malignant tumors arising from the head of the pancreas and are often metastatic to the lymph nodes or liver at the time of diagnosis or surgery. They may be located in the pancreas (56%) or extrapancreatic sites (duodenum, ampulla, jejunum, or cystic duct). Duodenal somatostatinomas are often asymptomatic or only local symptoms rather than the clinical syndrome of excess somatostatin production.[29]

Like other tumors of the gastroenteropancreatic tract, somatostatinomas should be managed by surgery whenever possible. Palliative treatments and chemotherapy for progressive metastatic disease have been discussed for neuroendocrine tumors collectively,[30] but the literature on the management of specific types of advanced neuroendocrine tumors is lacking.

REFERENCES

1. Rodgers SE, Perrier ND. Parathyroid carcinoma. Curr Opin Oncol 2006;18:16–22.
2. Cheah WK, Rauff A, Lee KO, Tan W. Parathyroid carcinoma: a case series. Ann Acad Med Singapore 2005;34:443–6.
3. Busaidy NL, Jimenez C, Habra MA, et al. Parathyroid carcinoma: a 22-year experience. Head Neck 2004;26:716–26.
4. Wynne AG, van Heerden J, Carney JA, Fitzpatrick LA. Parathyroid carcinoma: clinical and pathologic features in 43 patients. Medicine (Baltimore) 1992;71:197–205.
5. Shane E. Clinical review 122: parathyroid carcinoma. J Clin Endocrinol Metab 2001;86:485–93.
6. Body JJ, Bartl R, Burckhardt P, et al. Current use of bisphosphonates in oncology. International Bone and Cancer Study Group. J Clin Oncol 1998;16:3890–9.
7. Chisholm MA, Mulloy AL, Taylor AT. Acute management of cancer-related hypercalcemia. Ann Pharmacother 1996;30:507–13.
8. Apseloff G. Therapeutic uses of gallium nitrate: past, present, and future. Am J Ther 1999;6:327–39.
9. Dong BJ. Cinacalcet: an oral calcimimetic agent for the management of hyperparathyroidism. Clin Ther 2005;27:1725–51.
10. Vitale G, Tagliaferri P, Caraglia M, et al. Slow release lanreotide in combination with interferon-alpha2b in the treatment of symptomatic advanced medullary thyroid carcinoma. J Clin Endocrinol Metab 2000;85:983–8.
11. Pearse AG. The APUD cell concept and its implications in pathology. Pathol Annu 1974;9:27–41.
12. Frank M, Klose KJ, Wied M, et al. Combination therapy with octreotide and alpha-interferon: effect on tumor growth in metastatic endocrine gastroenteropancreatic tumors. Am J Gastroenterol 1999;94:1381–7.
13. Vazquez Quintana E. The surgical management of insulinoma. Bol Asoc Med P R 2004;96:33–8.
14. Hoff AO, Vassilopoulou-Sellin R. The role of glucagon administration in the diagnosis and treatment of patients with tumor hypoglycemia. Cancer 1998;82:1585–92.
15. Tucker ON, Crotty PL, Conlon KC. The management of insulinoma. Br J Surg 2006;93:264–75.
16. Jurgensen C, Schuppan D, Neser F, et al. EUS-guided alcohol ablation of an insulinoma. Gastrointest Endosc 2006;63:1059–62.
17. Novotny J, Janku F, Mares P, Petruzelka L. Symptomatic control of hypoglycaemia with prednisone in refractory metastatic pancreatic insulinoma. Support Care Cancer 2005;13:760–2.
18. Case CC, Vassilopoulou-Sellin R. Reproduction of features of the glucagonoma syndrome with continuous intravenous glucagon infusion as therapy for tumor-induced hypoglycemia. Endocr Pract 2003;9:22–5.
19. El Rassi Z, Partensky C, Valette PJ, et al. Necrolytic migratory erythema, first symptom of a malignant glucagonoma: treatment by long-acting somatostatin and surgical resection. Report of three cases. Eur J Surg Oncol 1998;24:562–7.
20. Nikou GC, Toubanakis C, Nikolaou P, et al. VIPomas: an update in diagnosis and management in a series of 11 patients. Hepatogastroenterology 2005;52:1259–65.
21. Warner RR. Enteroendocrine tumors other than carcinoid: a review of clinically significant advances. Gastroenterology 2005;128:1668–84.
22. Ellison EC, Sparks J, Verducci JS, et al. 50-year appraisal of gastrinoma: recommendations for staging and treatment. J Am Coll Surg 2006;202:897–905.
23. Krejs GJ, Orci L, Conlon JM, et al. Somatostatinoma syndrome. Biochemical, morphologic and clinical features. N Engl J Med 1979;301:285–92.
24. Kim DM, Ahn CW, Kim KR, et al. Duodenal somatostatinoma associated with diabetic ketoacidosis presumably caused by somatostatin-28 hypersecretion. J Clin Endocrinol Metab 2005;90:6310–5.
25. Marakis G, Ballas K, Rafailidis S, et al. Somatostatin-producing pancreatic endocrine carcinoma presented as relapsing cholangitis—a case report. Pancreatology 2005;5:295–9.
26. Konomi K, Chijiiwa K, Katsuta T, Yamaguchi K. Pancreatic somatostatinoma: a case report and review of the literature. J Surg Oncol 1990;43:259–65.
27. Wynick D, Williams SJ, Bloom SR. Symptomatic secondary hormone syndromes in patients with established malignant pancreatic endocrine tumors. N Engl J Med 1988;319:605–7.
28. Anene C, Thompson JS, Saigh J, et al. Somatostatinoma: atypical presentation of a rare pancreatic tumor. Am J Gastroenterol 1995;90:819–21.
29. O'Brien TD, Chejfec G, Prinz RA. Clinical features of duodenal somatostatinomas. Surgery 1993;114:1144–7.
30. Brentjens R, Saltz L. Islet cell tumors of the pancreas: the medical oncologist's perspective. Surg Clin North Am 2001;81:527–42.

Diabetes and the Cancer Patient

Pankaj Shah, MD

Naifa L. Busaidy, MD

Jane M. Geraci, MD, MPH

Melissa Hamilton, RD

Mary Ann Weiser, MD, PhD

The prevalence of diabetes mellitus has more than doubled in the United States since 1980; currently, an estimated 20.8 million people living in the United States have diabetes, and for every two persons with diagnosed diabetes, there is one to two with undiagnosed diabetes.[1] Based on hospital records, it is estimated that approximately 20% of patients with various cancers are known to have diabetes.[2] It is well known that hospital records underreport the prevalence of diabetes mellitus.[3,4]

The prevalence of diabetes and cancer increases with age; there may be common risk factors for diabetes and some cancers; diabetes may predispose patients to certain cancers; and cancers and cancer therapies may worsen or precipitate diabetes. Cancer prognosis may be affected by glycemic status. Acute hyperglycemic complications of diabetes may interfere with timely cancer therapy, including surgery and chemotherapy. In a person with uncontrolled diabetes, the risks of infections may be higher and wound healing impaired. Cancer patients with diabetes may be at a higher risk of developing certain complications of cancer chemotherapy.

Timely diagnosis of diabetes is a prerequisite for its optimal management. Fasting plasma glucose is sufficient to screen for diabetes mellitus. A fasting plasma glucose ≥ 126 mg/dL following at least 8 hours (overnight) without caloric intake or a casual or nonfasting plasma glucose concentration ≥ 200 mg/dL with symptoms of diabetes clinches the diagnosis of diabetes, if confirmed on another day by at least one of the two tests. Some of the classic symptoms of diabetes, such as unexplained weight loss, may be confounded by the presence of the cancer.

Randomized controlled clinical trials in both type 1 and type 2 diabetes have conclusively demonstrated that tight blood glucose control reduces the risk of long-term complications of diabetes.[5–7] Tight blood glucose control with intensive insulin

therapy has also been shown to reduce morbidity and mortality among critically ill patients.[8] In contrast to the large evidence base that guides optimal diabetes management, there is very little research into effective management approaches and associated outcomes for patients with both cancer and diabetes mellitus. In this chapter, we review (1) the pathophysiology of both diseases, highlighting common pathways; (2) the available evidence indicating that hyperglycemia affects some cancer and cancer treatment outcomes; (3) what is known about the effect of cancer therapy on diabetes; and (4) management of diabetes in a cancer patient, including nutrition therapy and the care of diabetics with advanced cancer.

Diabetes and Cancer Outcomes

There is increasing evidence that patients with diabetes or impaired glucose tolerance may be at an increased risk of cancer, cancer recurrence, cancer-related mortality, and all-cause mortality.[9–11] Specifically in large cohort studies, pancreatic, colon, breast, liver, and endometrial cancers have been shown to occur more frequently in patients with a history of diabetes mellitus. For certain malignancies, the presence of diabetes and/or impaired glucose tolerance may also adversely affect the response to cancer treatment. Patients with stage II–III colon cancer treated with adjuvant chemotherapy had a lower 5-year survival rate if they had diabetes.[12] Diabetes was found to be an independent risk factor for a shorter overall (19.8 vs 29.2 months) and disease-free survival (11.3 vs 17.2 months) in patients with resectable pancreatic cancer receiving adjuvant or neoadjuvant treatment, in addition to surgery.[13] Patients with acute lymphocytic leukemia treated with hyper-CVAD (fractionated cyclophosphamide, vincristine, Adriamycin, and dexamethasone) ($N = 278$) had a shorter median remission duration and (24 vs 52 months) overall survival (29 vs 88 months) when they had diabetes or hyperglycemia.[14]

Chemotherapy and radiotherapy may be more toxic in people with diabetes. It is believed that diabetes predisposes patients to neuropathy induced by chemotherapies.[15] Likewise, late-radiation toxicities are higher in people with diabetes.[16]

There is a lack of randomized trials investigating if optimal treatment of diabetes affects cancer outcomes. It is likely that the targets of therapy and optimal choice for diabetes treatment may well be cancer type, site, and stage dependent, with a great deal of individualization when life expectancy is very short.

Insulin, which is typically elevated in the early stages of type 2 diabetes, is a potential growth factor for malignancies. Insulin reduces sex hormone–binding globulin levels, thereby increasing concentration of free estradiol, which may play a role in inducing neoplasia of the breast, endometrium, and ovary. Insulin cross-reacts with the insulin-like growth factor 1 (IGF-1) receptor; the latter activates intracellular tyrosine kinase activity, which stimulates cell growth. In cell culture, growth of virtually all cell lines is stimulated by insulin and IGF-1. Tumor cells may also lose their ability to down-regulate insulin-binding sites and become more sensitive to the stimulatory effects of insulin.[17] In vitro insulin may also inhibit the apoptotic effects of certain antineoplastic therapies, such as anti–epidermal growth factor receptor monoclonal antibody.[18] However, the concentration of insulin used in in vitro models is several orders of magnitude higher than the prevailing insulin concentrations in patients with diabetes. In vivo insulin has been shown to ameliorate enhanced tumor growth in a streptozocin-induced diabetic hamster model.[19] Therefore, whether insulin promotes cancer growth in vivo is still an open question.

Hyperglycemia may also directly affect tumor cell biology. Tumor cells tend to exhibit increased glycolytic metabolism.[20] Glycolysis per se may promote carcinogenesis.[21] Hyperglycemia may also reduce the sensitivity of certain tumor cell lines to certain types of chemotherapy.

Wound Healing and Diabetes

Uncontrolled diabetes is associated with more frequent infections and a tendency toward more complicated infections.[22] Poor control of diabetes is associated with impaired white blood cell function,[23] and infection rates have been decreased with more aggressive control of blood glucose.[24] Significant hyperglycemia is associated with poor collagen content and wound healing.[25]

Pathophysiology of Diabetes in Cancer

Certain neoplasms may produce hormones with counterinsulin (eg, glucagon, adrenocorticotropic hormone [ACTH], cortisol, catecholamine) or insulin-suppressant (somatostatin) actions. Diabetes may be one of the characteristics of these syndromes.[26–29] Acute diabetic complications have been reported with several of these tumors (glucagonoma,[30] ACTH-producing tumors,[31] and pheochromocytoma).[32] More commonly, on the other hand, malignancies not typically associated with secretion of the hormones mentioned above are associated with a new diagnosis of diabetes,[33] best exemplified for pancreatic cancer.

Systemic Factors

Prevailing plasma glucose concentrations are a result of the balance of the amount of glucose entering the circulation and the amount leaving. Increased glucose entering, reduced leaving, or both can cause hyperglycemia. Cancers are associated with increased glucose production and gluconeogenesis[34,35] and decreased glucose uptake.[36] Cancers, cancer therapies, and concurrent infections are associated with elevated free fatty acids.[37,38] Elevated free fatty acid concentration has been shown to be associated with reduced glucose use and increased glucose production, with increased gluconeogenesis.[39–41] Many malignancies and several chemotherapies are associated with catabolic states and with elevated lactic acid concentrations.[42,43] Elevated lactic acid concentrations, in turn, promote hepatic gluconeogenesis and ketogenesis.[44]

Cytokines and other substances released from the cancers[45] can cause hyperglycemia by inducing insulin resistance. Certain infections may be associated with increased cancer and diabetes occurrence; for example, hepatitis C infection is associated with both (hepatocellular) cancer and diabetes mellitus.[46] Plasma cortisol and glucagon concentrations in patients with malignant tumors are significantly increased when compared with patients with benign surgical disorders,[47,48] causing anorexia, enhanced tumor protein synthesis, stimulated tumor growth,[49] and an increased rate of appearance of glucose in the blood.

Effects of Cancer Treatment on Diabetes Mellitus

As summarized in Table 1, several drugs used for cancer may have adverse effects on glycemic control. Glucocorticoids used as antitumor agents or for symptom relief and prevention of hypersensitivity reactions worsen glycemic control in people with established diabetes and may precipitate diabetes, especially in people predisposed to type 2 diabetes. In our experience, this is related to the dose and potency of the glucocorticoid. The mechanisms are multiple, including increased hepatic glucose output and decreased peripheral glucose use, in addition to reduced insulin secretion.[50] Interferon-α2 is used to treat chronic myelogenous leukemia and melanoma; hyperglycemia is one of the main side effects of this drug. Some patients who develop interferon-alpha2 induced hyperglycemia require insulin for therapy. Therefore it is believed that Interferon-alpha 2 induced hyperglycemia may be immune mediated.[51] L-Asparaginase is used to treat acute leukemia and lymphoma; it is thought to cause hyperglycemia through inhibition of insulin activity or receptor synthesis.[51] Octreotide is a synthetic long-acting somatostatin analogue; it inhibits secretion of several hormones, including insulin,[52] and can cause hyperglycemia. Tacrolimus is an immunosuppressive drug used in both solid organ and stem cell transplantation. Hyperglycemia requiring insulin treatment has been observed in 5% of patients receiving it for graft-versus-host disease.[53]

Imatinib (Gleevec) binds to the BCR-ABL gene at the adenosine triphosphate binding site. This results in an inhibition of the activity of BCR-ABL gene and elimination of these BCR-ABL gene (Philadelphia chromosome) positive cells.[54] Imatinib may decrease blood glucose in patients with known diabetes, sometimes in a dramatic fashion,[55] by an as yet unknown mechanism.

Specific surgical procedures (pancreatectomy for pancreatic and gastrointestinal cancers) and radiotherapy to the abdominal region may also be associated with new-onset diabetes mellitus.[56]

Lifestyle Changes and Diabetes

Cancer-related fatigue, weakness, decreased muscle strength, anxiety, depression, and changes in body image are associated with decreased physical activity and can reduce insulin sensitivity.[57] Cancer patients have been advised to rest by the family and physicians, despite the benefits of regular physical acivity.[58] Prolonged decreased physical activity can cause disuse muscle atrophy and a further decline in activity.

Cachexia

Malignancies are associated with varying degrees of cachexia, with pancreatic and gastric cancer causing it most often. Unlike weight loss induced by regular exercise and dietary intervention, cachexia-associated muscle wasting leads to muscle weakness and fatigue, resulting in decreased physical activity and reduced glucose use. Infections are also common in cachectic persons because of poor immune function, complicating the insulin resistance of cachexia.

Nutrition Supplements

Nutritional supplements, including tube feeding and intravenous parenteral nutrition, can increase plasma glucose concentrations, especially if the

---

Table 1 Pharmacologic Agents in Oncology that May Affect Blood Glucose

Agent	Current Uses	Side Effect	Possible Mechanisms
Glucocorticoids	Chemotherapy for acute leukemia, lymphoma; symptomatic brain metastasis, nausea and vomiting, pain; premedication for taxanes and many other regimens	Hyperglycemia	Increased hepatic glucose production; decreased peripheral glucose use; decreased insulin effectiveness Decreased insulin secretion
Interferon-α2	Metastatic melanoma	Hyperglycemia	Immune mediated
L-Asparaginase	Acute leukemia	Hyperglycemia	Inhibition of insulin or insulin receptor synthesis
Octreotide (Sandostatin)	Carcinoid, pituitary tumors and VIP-secreting tumors	Hyperglycemia	Inhibition of insulin secretion
Tacrolimus (Prograf)	GVHD	Hyperglycemia and new-onset insulin-requiring DM	Inhibition of insulin secretion, peripheral insulin resistance
Imatinib (Gleevec)	CML; GIST	Improvement of hyperglycemia	Unknown; possibly reduced insulin resistance

CML = chronic myelogenous leukemia; DM = diabetes mellitus; GIST = gastrointestinal stromal tumor; GVHD = graft-versus-host disease; VIP = vasoactive intestinal peptide.

amount of glucose delivered is more than the body's ability to use it. Provision of extra insulin may not be able to compensate if overwhelming excess calories are provided to these patients with low muscle mass and diminished ability to use glucose.

Managing Diabetes in Patients with Cancer

Treating diabetes in a person with active cancer is often complicated by the very presence of cancer, cancer therapies, and treatment side effects, such as anorexia, nausea, and weight loss. Acute complications of diabetes and urgency of treating severe hyperglycemia often delay the treatment of cancer. The presence of diabetes increases the stress of cancer and cancer management.

The goals of diabetes management have become more stringent, with rapidly accumulating evidence of the benefits of tight glycemic control in preventing chronic complications from diabetes. However, in the presence of a severe illness, such as cancer, undergoing active therapy, the benefits of tight glycemic control are not clear. Extrapolating from the data, one could argue that glycemic control should be targeted to as close to normal as possible, without increasing hypoglycemic events or adding significant stress to the patient. Plasma glucose concentrations should be kept below 200 mg/dL (blood glucose below 180 mg/dL) since concentrations higher than that increase the risks of infection, poor healing, and possibly the risks of acute hyperglycemic complications.

Diabetes Education

Diabetes mellitus should not be labeled as "hyperglycemia" unless the specific or another cause of hyperglycemia is not likely to recur. Even if hyperglycemia is apparently attributable to a specific medication or stress, patients and their physicians should realize that such situations can and possibly will arise again during the subsequent treatment cycles. It is safer if a patient believes that she or he has "diabetes" and continues to monitor periodically and more frequently when ill. In this way, severe hyperglycemia is prevented by early recognition and intervention. Family and caregivers should understand that adequate diabetes education and management facilitate timely evaluation and treatment of the cancer and reduce the risk of infection, poor wound healing, and unplanned hospitalizations and doctors' visits. Skills learned during this time would be helpful for a healthy life after cancer.

It is ideal that patients and their family members acquire the skills of diabetes self-management. These include blood glucose monitoring, techniques of insulin injection, knowledge and skills of correcting the insulin dose for blood glucose, and self-adjustment of insulin doses based on a pattern emerging from a few days of monitoring. Hypoglycemia prevention and management plans (including glucagon injection technique if appropriate) and management plans for the days when sick, traveling, or fasting for tests should be in place for the patient. An identification card listing the current medicines and simple instructions for what to do when the patient is found with an altered mental status should be carried by patients taking agents that can cause hypoglycemia.

Nutrition

Medical nutrition therapy plays a central role in the treatment of diabetes mellitus. Medical nutrition therapy involves a comprehensive nutrition assessment to evaluate current nutritional status. In addition to the diet history, the nutrition assessment should include the patient's medical history, social history, physical data including height and weight, and laboratory data.[59]

In a cancer patient, the nutrition assessment should also consider cancer treatment modalities (such as surgery, chemotherapy, and radiation) and management of their side effects. In general, the overall goal for a person with diabetes and cancer is to maintain optimal metabolic control and achieve a weight that is appropriate for the patient.[59,60] Some patients with cancer and diabetes are overweight and are advised to lose weight, so caloric restriction may be appropriate for them. Others may be losing too much weight or losing weight too quickly, and in such situations, weight maintenance or improvement may be a nutritional management goal. Therefore, these patients require oral nutritional supplements in addition to a healthy diet.

A registered dietitian plays an important role in making recommendations that are specific to the individual and should provide a strategy for achieving a healthy diet and lifestyle.[60] The dietitian should participate in monitoring patient progress in establishing a healthy diet, maintaining a healthy weight, and achieving adequate glycemic control. If established goals have been met, then there may be no need for further change.

In general, carbohydrate and monounsaturated fat should provide 60 to 70% of estimated energy requirements, protein should be approximately 15 to 20% of total caloric intake (1–1.5 g/kg body weight), and fat should be limited to less than 30% of total caloric intake, with less than 10% of total caloric intake from saturated fat. Diets such as those that are "low sugar" or "sugar free" or have "no concentrated sweets" are not synonymous with medical nutrition therapy for diabetes and are not indicated for glycemic control. Sucrose does not increase glycemia to a greater extent than isocaloric amounts of starch. Therefore, sucrose and sucrose-containing foods do not need to be restricted by people with diabetes and should be eaten in the context of a healthy diet.[60]

If diabetes is being treated with sulfonylurea, other insulin secretagogues, or intermediate-acting or mixed insulin, the timing of meal and distribution of carbohydrate intake through the day are important, with the aim of preventing both significant hyper- and hypoglycemias. Spacing of meals, increasing fiber intake, and not skipping meals are critical. When actively treated cancer patients have anorexia, nausea, dysphagia, or other complications preventing timely food intake, they are encouraged to consume culturally appropriate foods that can be easily swallowed, retained, and digested. In such a setting, oral nutritional supplements may be most convenient. Alternatively, they may also need a change in their pharmacologic treatment of diabetes to avoid hypoglycemia.

If a person with diabetes needs intensive insulin therapy, prandial (meal related) insulin may need to be titrated to the total carbohydrate intake in the meal rather than the source or the type of carbohydrate. Initially, it may be convenient to teach the patient and the family to keep the carbohydrate content of each meal consistent, and this can be achieved by learning basic carbohydrate counting and meal exchanges. In this way, insulin doses can be titrated quickly. If required, later they can learn and work with the carbohydrate to insulin ratio.

Use of nutritional support may necessitate changes in the therapeutic regimen for diabetes. For example, patients being tube-fed overnight may need "prandial" insulin before their tube feeds in the form of Neutral Protamine Hagedorn (NPH). An enteral or parenteral nutritional supplement provides calories through an unphysiologic route and pattern, without a concomitant increase in incretin hormones; therefore, inadequate insulin concentrations in relation to the carbohydrates are provided. This, along with insulin resistance and relative insulin deficiency induced by sickness, cancer, and cancer therapies, necessitates careful calorie assessment and judicious provision of insulin. Broadly, wherever possible, regular food taken by mouth is better than enteral tube feeding, and the latter is better than parenteral nutrition. Parenteral nutrition should be restricted to situations with proven benefits or in a clinical trial setting. Parenteral feeding should be ramped down quickly whenever enteral or oral feeding can be resumed.

In-Patient Diabetes Management

Insulin is the mainstay of therapy in the hospital. Unpredictable oral intake makes use of insulin secretagogues best avoided in the inpatient setting (Table 2). Nausea from other medications

Table 2 Types of Oral Glucose-Lowering Medications

Class name	Generic Name (Brand Names)	Primary Action	Contraindications	Adverse Effects	Benefits	Implications for Actively Treated Cancer Patients
Biguanides	Metformin (generic, Glucophage, Glucophage XR)	Decreases hepatic glucose production, reduces appetite, improves glucose uptake by muscles and fat	Renal dysfunction (high creatinine), cardiovascular shock, acute myocardial infarction, septicemia, congestive heart failure, acute or chronic metabolic acidosis	Nausea, diarrhea, weight loss	Modest weight loss	May cause confusion: GI side effects and weight loss can be confused as the effect of cancer or its therapy. Shown in correlative and animal studies to be associated with possible cancer prevention. Often stopped for ≈48 hours before contrast radiography
Thiazolidinediones	Pioglitazone (Actos) Rosiglitazone (Avandia)	Increases glucose uptake by muscle and fat and reduces glucose production by the liver.	Heart failure (especially NYHA grade III and IV)	Water retention, anemia, weight gain	Does not cause hypoglycemia	Weight gain—may be desirable in some. Heart failure and fluid retention may be confused as the effects of cancer therapy. Actively being investigated for anticancer properties for several cancers
α-glucosidase inhibitors	Acarbose (Precose/Glucobay) Miglitol (Glyset)	Inhibits enzyme that facilitates the breakdown of complex sugars to glucose in the small intestine; causes carbohydrate malabsorption	Chronic intestinal disorders, severe renal impairment (creatinine clearance <25 mL/min)	Flatulence, abdominal bloating, diarrhea	Hypoglycemia does not occur when used alone	GI side effects and weight loss confused with cancer or therapy. Treat hypoglycemia with glucose, not sucrose or other carbohydrates
Sulfonylureas and other insulin secretagogues	Glyburide (generic, Glynase, DiaBeta, Micronase) Glipizide (generic, Glucotrol, Glucotrol XL), glimepiride (Amaryl) Nateglinide (Starlix) Repaglinide (Prandin)	Enhances insulin secretion	Most contraindicated in significant renal and hepatic diseases	Hypoglycemia: repaglinide, nateglinide, and glipizide least likely to cause hypoglycemia; chlorpropamide, glyburide most likely. Hyponatremia: chlorpropamide, glyburide	Most accumulated experience	May be difficult to use during cancer therapy: nausea and anorexia may cause erratic intake, and predisposition to hypoglycemia. In vitro studies imply anticancer action of some compounds and their derivatives

GI = gastrointestinal; NYHA = New York Heart Association.
Combination pills: metformin + glyburide (generic, Glucovance); metformin + rosiglitazone (Avandamet); metformin + glipizide (Metaglip).

and the risks of lactic acidosis in the inpatient setting with hypoxia, hypoperfusion, and renal insufficiency increase the risk of adverse events with metformin use (see Table 2). Oral medications take a long time to have a full effect, are titrated upward slowly, and have a slow onset of action, especially with thiazolidinediones (TZDs). Therefore, oral drugs are not the best option for most patients with hyperglycemia or diabetes during hospitalization.

There is increasing evidence that near-normoglycemia in the hospital has the potential for improved mortality and morbidity and decreased health care costs. Insulin therapy itself may have direct beneficial effects independent of its effect on blood glucose.[61] In December 2003, the American Association of Clinical Endocrinology together with the American Diabetes Association held a consensus conference on the management of the hyperglycemic patient in the hospital.[62] Target blood glucose levels were determined from the available literature to be the following: on the inpatient wards, target plasma glucose levels are < 110 mg/dL preprandially, with a maximum glucose of 180 mg/dL at any time. In the intensive care unit (ICU) setting, a goal of near-normoglycemia has been set to 80 to 110 mg/dL. Recently, the American Diabetes Association, American College of Endocrinology, American Association of Clinical Endocrinologists, and other organizations came together and produced a document highlighting the importance of implementation of optimal diabetes management for inpatients.[63]

In general, hospitalized diabetic patients require both basal and prandial (mealtime or bolus) insulin coverage, just as in the outpatient setting. Sliding scale insulins are to be avoided and actually increase the risk of hypoglycemia and hyperglycemia compared with basal and prandial insulin.[64–66]

Insulin needs to be adjusted once or twice daily to account for the rapid changes that occur in the hospital. Nausea, vomiting, changes in oral intake, intermittent enteral tube feeding, intravenous fluids, use of glucocorticoids, and parenteral nutrition all necessitate frequent reassessment of the doses. Illness-related insulin requirements are high at the onset of an illness and decrease as the illness improves (see Table 3 for the timing of insulin delivery).

In the mechanically ventilated surgical ICU patient, intensive glycemic control with a target glucose of 110 mg/dL with intravenous insulin has been shown to decrease mortality and morbidity.[8] Evidence strongly supports the use of intravenous insulin for patients in diabetic ketoacidosis and hyperosmolar coma. In addition, we use intravenous insulin therapy during cardiovascular surgery; after a stroke, myocardial infarction, or organ transplantation; and for many other patients who are difficult to control with other regimens. An appropriate transition protocol off the intravenous insulin drip to subcutaneous insulin should be in place in the hospital to avoid worsened hyperglycemia after the drip is turned off. Various insulin protocols have been published.[67,68] Often endocrinologists, intensivists, internists, and nutritionists need to work in close collaboration with the primary team for the management of the diabetic patient admitted to the hospital.

Outpatient Diabetes Management

Insulin

Insulin is indicated in all patients with uncontrolled diabetes for whom oral drugs are contraindicated (see Table 2). In addition, because of immediate onset of action, it is the most appropriate mode for quick control of severely uncontrolled diabetes, for example, glucose > 350 mg/dL or > 250 mg/dL with ketonuria. Treating outpatients with insulin using a "sliding scale" is also inappropriate.

Most patients needing insulin will at least require basal insulin; this can be in the form of two doses of NPH or one to two doses of glargine or detemir insulin. Many others will require splitting the dose, especially if the requirements are higher than 30 U/d. Premixed insulins are handy for brief therapies, such as the postprandial hyperglycemia induced by glucocorticoids. Ideally, patients with poor beta cell reserve should be treated with a combination of basal long-acting insulin (detemir or glargine, to supply basal needs) with rapid-acting insulin boluses (aspart or lispro for prandial needs), a regimen called basal-bolus or MDI (multiple daily injection of insulin).

Adjustments of insulin doses are based on the expected physiologic action of the insulin and determination of the glucose pattern before changing the doses. By definition, the basal insulin dose is intended to keep glucose stable when no food, intravenous glucose, or other form of insulin is given. Too often long-acting insulin (detemir or glargine) is being used to control both basal and prandial glycemia. This can lead to serious hypoglycemia if scheduled nutrition is interrupted.

Oral Antidiabetics

Sulfonylurea drugs are the least expensive but can precipitate hypoglycemia if food intake is erratic. Some, especially chlorpropamide and glyburide, can cause hyponatremia. These are used with caution in the elderly, those with liver and kidney diseases, and patients with erratic oral intake. Metformin is an underused drug but cannot be used in patients with liver, kidney, or heart failure. Metformin and drugs that prevent conversion of sucrose and starch to glucose (acarbose and miglitol) can cause gastrointestinal symptoms, which can be confused with complication of cancer or its therapies. Peroxisome Proliferator-Activated Receptors-gamma (PPAR-γ) receptor agonists (rosiglitazone and pioglitazone) can cause fluid retention and weight gain. All oral drugs are equally effective in bringing down

Table 3 Insulin				
Duration of Action	Subcutaneous Insulin			
	Rapid	*Short*	*Intermediate*	*Long*
Common names	Aspart (Novolog), lispro (Humalog), glulisine (Apidra)	Regular (Novolin R, Humulin R)	NPH (Novolin N, Humulin N)	Glargine (Lantus), detemir (Levemir)
Onset of insulin action	15 min	30 min to 1 h	2–4 h	2–4 h
Peak time of insulin action	1–2 h	2–3 h	4–10 h	Peakless
Duration of insulin action	3–4 h	3–6 h	10–16 h	20–24 h
Recommended administration of insulin	Usually taken immediately before or after eating	Usually taken 30–60 min before eating	Taken once or twice daily	Usually taken twice or once daily
Visual appearance	Clear	Clear	Cloudy	Clear
Implications for cancer patients	Best insulin when intake is unreliable; can be given after meal, based on food (carbohydrate) intake. Safety in cancer patients not studied.	Only form approved for IV use	Most accumulated experience	Glargine binds avidly to IGF-1 receptor. Implications not clear. Detemir more reliably absorbed. Safety in cancer patients not studied

IGF-1 = insulin-like growth factor 1; IV = intravenous; NPH = Neutral Protamine Hagedorn.

Table 4 New Antidiabetic Classes

Class	Generic Names (Brand Names)	Mechanism of Action	Contraindications	Indications	Major Adverse Effects	How Used	Implications for Cancer Patients
Glucagon-like peptide 1 analogues	Exenatide (Byetta)	Increases insulin and reduces glucagon response to glucose; reduces gastric emptying, reduces appetite and weight	Gastroparesis	Type 2 diabetes adjunctive with metformin, a sulfonylurea, or a combination of the two	Nausea, vomiting, diarrhea, feeling jittery, dizziness, headache, dyspepsia	Subcutaneous 5 µg twice a day with meals, increased to 10 µg twice a day after 4 wk, as tolerated	Weight loss may be confusing "Benign thyroid C-cell adenomas" in rats May promote islet differentiation May inhibit apoptosis of certain cell types Safety in cancer patients not studied
Amylin analogue	Pramlintide (Symlin)	Reduced gastric emptying; prevention of the postprandial rise in plasma glucagon; improved satiety and potential weight loss. Suppresses glucagon and stimulates insulin secretion.	Gastroparesis; hypoglycemia unawareness	Type 1 diabetes, adjunct for mealtime insulin therapy Type 2 diabetes, adjunct for mealtime insulin with or without a concurrent sulfonylurea agent and/or metformin	Nausea, headache, anorexia, vomiting, abdominal pain, fatigue, dizziness, coughing, pharyngitis	Subcutaneous Type 1 diabetes: 15 µg before each major meal, increased by 15 µg to 30 or 60 µg/dose, as tolerated Type 2 diabetes on insulin: 60 µg before each major meal, increased to 120 µg/dose, as tolerated	Weight loss may be confusing Safety in cancer patients not studied

hemoglobin A_{1c} (HbA_{1c}) on an average by 1 percentage point (except acarbose, miglitol, nateglinide, and repaglinide being slightly less effective, bringing down HbA_{1c} by 0.5 percentage point).

For the management of diabetes in a patient with cancer, usually metformin is the first-line oral drug for obese individuals and glipizide for nonobese individuals. Often TZDs are started as the primary agent. Metformin can be combined with glipizide or TZDs if either of them is not effective alone. Often the most difficult problem is to make sure that the adverse symptoms from cancer or its therapies are not compounded by the medications. Constant surveillance of the contraindications is also required while using these drugs in a cancer patient.

Newer Diabetes Treatments

Inhaled insulin, glucagon-like peptide 1 analogue, and amylin analogue were recently added to the options for diabetes management (Table 4). As with the newer subcutaneous insulin analogues, there are no good studies investigating the safety and utility of these drugs in cancer patients.

Management of Glucocorticoid-Induced Diabetes

There are no large studies investigating the options for management of glucocorticoid-induced diabetes. TZDs may be effective in preventing and treating diabetes in such patients. However, if hyperglycemia is significant, insulin is invariably required. It is generally believed that larger doses of prandial than basal insulin

are required for such patients, but not uncommonly, patients have very high fasting glucose concentrations that will necessitate increasing basal insulin doses. Management requires self-monitoring of blood glucose to identify the pattern of hyperglycemia and assess the treatment regimen.

Management of Diabetes during Tube Feeding

If the G-tube feedings are being given by gravity three to four times a day, subcutaneous regular insulin before each tube feeding may be sufficient, in addition to a basal insulin. However, if tube feeding is being provided using a pump over a length of time, we give NPH insulin before each tube feeding. In addition, long-acting insulin may also be given, for the basal insulin needs, based on changes in blood glucose during the time there is no tube feeding and no NPH insulin. Administration of subcutaneous insulin should be tapered off before feeding finishes to avoid hypoglycemia.

Management of Diabetes during Parenteral Nutrition

Insulin is often added to the parenteral nutrition solution, providing usually 1 unit per 10 g of glucose (range 0.5–2 U/g glucose) in the parenteral nutrition bag. This may not be sufficient to control glucose, and extra regular insulin is given intravenously or subcutaneously as needed. In patients with known diabetes and/or high insulin requirements, many people will provide a small dose of long-acting insulin subcutaneously. This

prevents onset of hyperglycemia if and when the parenteral nutrition is interrupted. Whenever diabetes is difficult to control and/or requires high doses of insulin, the amount of total calorie intake should be reassessed. Beyond a certain limit, excess calories cannot be compensated by extra insulin. This limit is often reached quickly in an insulin-resistant sick person, especially on unphysiologic nutritional support. Reassessment of nutritional support may require indirect calorimetric measurement of basal energy expenditure.

Management of Diabetes in a Person with a Very Short Life Expectancy

When life expectancy with terminal cancer is brief, diabetes management is not aimed at preventing chronic complications. It has been suggested that dietary restrictions should be relaxed and that blood glucose monitoring should be performed only if the patient is conscious and symptom control requires it.[69,70] Insulin and other diabetes medications should be reduced with reducing appetite and intake and with the sole aim of controlling symptoms to make the person comfortable. Specialist input should be sought for pain control, comfort care, and family counseling.

REFERENCES

1. Harris MI, Flegal KM, Cowie CC, et al. Prevalence of diabetes, impaired fasting glucose, and impaired glucose tolerance in U.S. adults. The Third National Health and Nutrition Examination Survey, 1988-1994. Diabetes Care 1998;21:518–24.

2. Fleming ST, Pursley HG, Newman B, et al. Comorbidity as a predictor of stage of illness for patients with breast cancer. Med Care 2005;43:132–40.

3. Carral F, Olveira G, Aguilar M, et al. Hospital discharge records under-report the prevalence of diabetes in inpatients. Diabetes Res Clin Pract 2003;59:145–51.

4. Leslie PJ, Patrick AW, Hepburn DA, et al. Hospital in-patient statistics underestimate the morbidity associated with diabetes mellitus. Diabet Med 1992;9:379–85.

5. Effect of intensive blood-glucose control with metformin on complications in overweight patients with type 2 diabetes (UKPDS 34). UK Prospective Diabetes Study (UKPDS) Group. Lancet 1998;352:854–65.

6. Intensive blood-glucose control with sulphonylureas or insulin compared with conventional treatment and risk of complications in patients with type 2 diabetes (UKPDS 33). UK Prospective Diabetes Study (UKPDS) Group. Lancet 1998;352:837–53.

7. Diabetes Control and Complications Trial Research Group. The effect of intensive treatment of diabetes on the development and progression of long-term complications in insulin-dependent diabetes mellitus. N Engl J Med 1993;329:977–86.

8. van den Berghe G, Wouters P, Weekers F, et al. Intensive insulin therapy in the critically ill patients. N Engl J Med 2001;345:1359–67.

9. Gapstur SM, Gann PH, Lowe W, et al. Abnormal glucose metabolism and pancreatic cancer mortality. JAMA 2000;283:2552–8.

10. Saydah SH, Loria CM, Eberhardt MS, Brancati FL. Abnormal glucose tolerance and the risk of cancer death in the United States. Am J Epidemiol 2003;157:1092–100.

11. Verlato G, Zoppini G, Bonora E, Muggeo M. Mortality from site-specific malignancies in type 2 diabetic patients from Verona. Diabetes Care 2003;26:1047–51.

12. Meyerhardt JA, Catalano PJ, Haller DG, et al. Impact of diabetes mellitus on outcomes in patients with colon cancer. J Clin Oncol 2003;21:433–40.

13. Busaidy NL, Yazbeck CF, Shah P, et al. Survival of resectable pancreatic cancer patients with diabetes. Journal of Clinical Oncology 2006;24(Part 1 Suppl. S):202S-202S 4098.

14. Weiser MA, Cabanillas ME, Konopleva M, et al. Relation between the duration of remission and hyperglycemia during induction chemotherapy for acute lymphocytic leukemia with a hyperfractionated cyclophosphamide, vincristine, doxorubicin, and dexamethasone/methotrexate-cytarabine regimen. Cancer 2004;100:1179–85.

15. Quasthoff S, Hartung HP. Chemotherapy-induced peripheral neuropathy. J Neurol 2002;249:9–17.

16. Herold DM, Hanlon AL, Hanks GE. Diabetes mellitus: a predictor for late radiation morbidity. Int J Radiat Oncol Biol Phys 1999;43:475–9.

17. Benson EA, Holdaway IM. Regulation of insulin binding to human mammary carcinoma. Cancer Res 1982;42:1137–41.

18. Wu V, Fan Z, Masui H, et al. Apoptosis induced by an anti-epidermal growth factor receptor monoclonal antibody in a human colorectal carcinoma cell line and its delay by insulin. J Clin Invest 1995;95:1897–905.

19. Fisher WE, Boros LG, Schirmer WJ. Reversal of enhanced pancreatic cancer growth in diabetes by insulin. Surgery 1995;118:453–7; discussion 457–8.

20. Andreeff M, Jiang S, Zhang X, et al. Expression of Bcl-2-related genes in normal and AML progenitors: changes induced by chemotherapy and retinoic acid. Leukemia 1999;13:1881–92.

21. Ashrafian H. Cancer's sweet tooth: the Janus effect of glucose metabolism in tumorigenesis. Lancet 2006;367:618–21.

22. Joshi N, Caputo GM, Weitekamp MR, Karchmer AW. Infections in patients with diabetes mellitus. N Engl J Med 1999;341:1906–12.

23. Bagdade JD, Stewart M, Walters E. Impaired granulocyte adherence. A reversible defect in host defense in patients with poorly controlled diabetes. Diabetes 1978;27:677–81.

24. Van den Berghe G, Wilmer A, Hermans G, et al. Intensive insulin therapy in the medical ICU. N Engl J Med 2006;354:449–61.

25. Yue DK, Swanson B, McLennan S, et al. Abnormalities of granulation tissue and collagen formation in experimental diabetes, uraemia and malnutrition. Diabet Med 1986;3:221–5.

26. van Beek AP, de Haas ER, van Vloten WA, et al. The glucagonoma syndrome and necrolytic migratory erythema: a clinical review. Eur J Endocrinol 2004;151:531–7.

27. Miehle K, Tannapfel A, Lamesch P, et al. Pancreatic neuroendocrine tumor with ectopic adrenocorticotropin production upon second recurrence. J Clin Endocrinol Metab 2004;89:3731–6.

28. Tong C, England P, de Crespigny PC, et al. Diabetes mellitus as the only manifestation of occult phaeochromocytoma prior to acute haemorrhage in pregnancy. Aust N Z J Obstet Gynaecol 2005;45:91–2.

29. Marakis G, Ballas K, Rafailidis S, et al. Somatostatin-producing pancreatic endocrine carcinoma presented as relapsing cholangitis—a case report. Pancreatology 2005;5:295–9.

30. Fenkci SM, Fidan Yaylali G, Sermez Y, et al. Malign cystic glucagonoma presented with diabetic ketoacidosis: case report with an update. Endocr Relat Cancer 2005;12:449–54.

31. Uecker JM, Janzow MT. A case of Cushing syndrome secondary to ectopic adrenocorticotropic hormone producing carcinoid of the duodenum. Am Surg 2005;71:445–6.

32. Ishii C, lnoue K, Negishi K, et al. Diabetic ketoacidosis in a case of pheochromocytoma. Diabetes Res Clin Pract 2001;54:137–42.

33. Chari ST, Leibson CL, Rabe KG, et al. Probability of pancreatic cancer following diabetes: a population-based study. Gastroenterology 2005;129:504–11.

34. Leij-Halfwerk S, van den Berg JW, Sijens PE, et al. Altered hepatic gluconeogenesis during L-alanine infusion in weight-losing lung cancer patients as observed by phosphorus magnetic resonance spectroscopy and turnover measurements. Cancer Res 2000;60:618–23.

35. Dagnelie PC, Sijens PE, Kraus DJ, et al. Abnormal liver metabolism in cancer patients detected by (31)P MR spectroscopy. NMR Biomed 1999;12:535–44.

36. Yoshikawa T, Noguchi Y, Doi C, et al. Insulin resistance was connected with the alterations of substrate utilization in patients with cancer. Cancer Lett 1999;141:93–8.

37. Sauerwein HP, Pesola GR, Godfried MH, et al. Insulin sensitivity in septic cancer-bearing patients. JPEN J Parenter Enteral Nutr 1991;15:653–8.

38. Russell DM, Shike M, Marliss EB, et al. Effects of total parenteral nutrition and chemotherapy on the metabolic derangements in small cell lung cancer. Cancer Res 1984;44:1706–11.

39. Shah P, Basu A, Rizza R. Fat-induced liver insulin resistance. Curr Diab Rep 2003;3:214–8.

40. Shah P, Vella A, Basu A, et al. Effects of free fatty acids and glycerol on splanchnic glucose metabolism and insulin extraction in nondiabetic humans. Diabetes 2002;51:301–10.

41. Shah P, Vella A, Basu A, et al. Elevated free fatty acids impair glucose metabolism in women: decreased stimulation of muscle glucose uptake and suppression of splanchnic glucose production during combined hyperinsulinemia and hyperglycemia. Diabetes 2003;52:38–42.

42. Nishijima T, Nishina M, Fujiwara K. Measurement of lactate levels in serum and bile using proton nuclear magnetic resonance in patients with hepatobiliary diseases: its utility in detection of malignancies. Jpn J Clin Oncol 1997;27:13–7.

43. van Beek AP, de Haas ER, van Vloten WA, et al. The glucagonoma syndrome and necrolytic migratory erythema: a clinical review. Eur J Endocrinol 2004;151:531–7.

44. Exton JH, Corbin JG, Harper SC. Control of gluconeogenesis in liver. V. Effects of fasting, diabetes, and glucagon on lactate and endogenous metabolism in the perfused rat liver. J Biol Chem 1972;247:4996–5003.

45. Risch HA. Etiology of pancreatic cancer, with a hypothesis concerning the role of N-nitroso compounds and excess gastric acidity. J Natl Cancer Inst 2003;95:948–60.

46. Davila JA, Morgan RO, Shaib Y, et al. Diabetes increases the risk of hepatocellular carcinoma in the United States: a population based case control study. Gut 2005;54:533–9.

47. Schaur RJ, Semmelrock HJ, Schauenstein E, Kronberger L. Tumor host relations. II. Influence of tumor extent and tumor site on plasma cortisol of patients with malignant diseases. J Cancer Res Clin Oncol 1979;93:287–92.

48. Knapp ML, al-Sheibani S, Riches PG, et al. Hormonal factors associated with weight loss in patients with advanced breast cancer. Ann Clin Biochem 1991;28:480–6.

49. Hartl WH, Demmelmair H, Jauch KW, et al. Effect of glucagon on protein synthesis in human rectal cancer in situ. Ann Surg 1998;227:390–7.

50. Besse C, Nicod N, Tappy L. Changes in insulin secretion and glucose metabolism induced by dexamethasone in lean and obese females. Obes Res 2005;13:306–11.

51. Yeung SC, Chiu AC, Vassilopoulou-Sellin R, Gagel RF. The endocrine effects of nonhormonal antineoplastic therapy. Endocr Rev 1998;19:144–72.

52. Lamberts SW, van der Lely AJ, de Herder WW, Hofland LJ. Octreotide. N Engl J Med 1996;334:246–54.

53. Jacobson P, Uberti J, Davis W, Ratanatharathorn V. Tacrolimus: a new agent for the prevention of graft-versus-host disease in hematopoietic stem cell transplantation. Bone Marrow Transplant 1998;22:217–25.

54. Cortes J, Kantarjian H. New targeted approaches in chronic myeloid leukemia. J Clin Oncol 2005;23:6316–24.

55. Veneri D, Franchini M, Bonora E. Imatinib and regression of type 2 diabetes. N Engl J Med 2005;352:1049–50.

56. Billings BJ, Christein JD, Harmsen WS, et al. Quality-of-life after total pancreatectomy: is it really that bad on long-term follow-up? J Gastrointest Surg 2005;9:1059–67.

57. Marat D, Noguchi Y, Yoshikawa T, et al. Insulin resistance and tissue glycogen content in the tumor-bearing state. Hepatogastroenterology 1999;46:3159–65.

58. Curt GA, Breitbart W, Cella D, et al. Impact of cancer-related fatigue on the lives of patients: new findings from the Fatigue Coalition. Oncologist 2000;5:353–60.

59. Mahan L, Escott-Stump S. Krause's food nutrition and diet therapy. 11th ed. Philadelphia: Saunders; 2003.

60. Franz MJ, Bantle JP, Beebe CA, et al. Nutrition principles and recommendations in diabetes. Diabetes Care 2004;27 Suppl 1:S36–46.

61. Dandona P, Aljada A, Bandyopadhyay A. The potential therapeutic role of insulin in acute myocardial infarction in patients admitted to intensive care and in those with unspecified hyperglycemia. Diabetes Care 2003;26:516–9.

62. Clement S, Braithwaite SS, Magee MF, et al. Management of diabetes and hyperglycemia in hospitals. Diabetes Care 2004;27:553–91.

63. Task Force on Inpatient Diabetes: American College of Endocrinology and American Diabetes Association Consensus Statement on Inpatient Diabetes and Glycemic Control. Diabetes Care 2006;29:1955–62.

64. Queale WS, Seidler AJ, Brancati FL. Glycemic control and sliding scale insulin use in medical inpatients with diabetes mellitus. Arch Intern Med 1997;157:545–52.

65. Gearhart JG, Duncan JL III, Replogle WH, et al. Efficacy of sliding-scale insulin therapy: a comparison with prospective regimens. Fam Pract Res J 1994;14:313–22.

66. Walts LF, Miller J, Davidson MB, Brown J. Perioperative management of diabetes mellitus. Anesthesiology 1981;55:104–9.

67. Metchick LN, Petit WA Jr, Inzucchi SE. Inpatient management of diabetes mellitus. Am J Med 2002;113:317–23.

68. Furnary AP, Wu Y, Bookin SO. Effect of hyperglycemia and continuous intravenous insulin infusions on outcomes of cardiac surgical procedures: the Portland Diabetic Project. Endocr Pract 2004;10 Suppl 2:21–33.

69. Poulson J. The management of diabetes in patients with advanced cancer. J Pain Symptom Manage 1997;13:339–46.

70. Ford-Dunn S, Smith A, Quin J. Management of diabetes during the last days of life: attitudes of consultant diabetologists and consultant palliative care physicians in the UK. Palliat Med 2006;20:197–203.

25

Obesity and Cancer

Robert H. Lustig, MD
H. Leon Bradlow, PhD

One of the unmistakable features of cancer is the cachexia and weight loss associated with both tumor presentation and treatment. However, the relation between cancer and energy balance is much more complex. Obesity appears to be a risk factor for the development of certain cancers; in particular, reproductive cancers. Conversely, the sequelae of therapy of certain cancers lead to long-term cachexia, while the sequelae of others lead to long-term obesity. This chapter will explore the biochemical relations between excessive energy storage and risk for cancer, and the mechanism and treatment of disorders of positive energy storage in the aftermath of cancer treatment.

Obesity as a Risk Factor for Cancer

Epidemiology

For a long time, obesity was considered to be a relatively harmless condition without serious side effects, and indeed a measure of prosperity in some cultures. Gradually over a period of years, it became generally recognized among scientists, and indeed the general public, that obesity was an important risk factor in cardiovascular disease, hypertension, lipid disorders, and Type 2 diabetes (collectively known as the Metabolic Syndrome),[1,2] although the endocrine role of fat had not yet been recognized.

Following the discovery of leptin as a specific cytokine released by adipocytes,[3] a spate of other adipose tissue-derived cytokines (resistin, adiponectin, TNF-α, and acylation stimulating protein) were characterized, and fat was recognized as a true endocrine organ.[4,5] In addition to being the source of adipocytokine synthesis and secretion, fat serves as a major source of circulating estrogen derived by the aromatization of androgens to estrogens,[6] particularly in postmenopausal women. All of these fat-derived hormones and cytokines are known to have powerful effects on the immune system and bone, and presumably other organs as well.[7,8]

Despite all the intimations about the potential biologic role of fat, the concept that obesity was a risk factor for cancer was slow to be accepted by the scientific community, and even slower by the general public. More attention has been paid to specific macronutrients and to toxins ingested in the diet as potential carcinogens, rather than total body fat itself. However, the role of obesity as a primary risk factor for certain cancers is now clear. As an example, the role of obesity in promoting colon cancer in rats proved to be independent of the type of diet on which the animals were maintained, with obese rats developing more colon cancer than thin rats.[6] The site of the fat appears to be important, with visceral fat rather than subcutaneous fat being responsible for cancer risk.[9–11]

Although computerized tomography and magnetic resonance imaging (MRI) can distinguish between subcutaneous fat and visceral fat, both of these are too expensive and impractical for large-scale studies. Therefore, investigators have turned to the low-budget measurement of body mass index (BMI; weight (kg) ÷ height (m)^2) to quantitate obesity in epidemiologic studies.[12] Although BMI is an accurate assessment of adiposity for most adults, it is not valid for well-trained athletes with a large muscle mass, nor is it valid for the elderly where there is a shift in body composition. Lastly, BMI does not distinguish between subcutaneous and visceral fat. Some studies have suggested that the waist-hip ratio or the waist circumference is a better measure for the determination of cancer risk.[13,14] This fits well with the putative primary role of visceral fat. Recent World Health Organization studies have also found that there are ethnic differences as to the BMI values that portend medical risk. For example, Chinese subjects are obese at lower levels of BMI than Caucasians,[15] while African-Americans at equal levels of BMI to Caucasians manifest a lower incidence of the Metabolic Syndrome.[16]

Examination of the literature reveals that there are two different comparisons that have been employed in estimating cancer risk, which in some cases lead to very different conclusions. One can compare degree of obesity against the risk of cancer incidence, or against the risk of cancer mortality. For example, in the case of prostate cancer, obesity shows no increased risk of cancer incidence and perhaps even a slight protective effect[17,18]; while obesity is a very significant risk factor for advanced disease in prostate cancer.[19] How much of this is biologic, as opposed to other factors (eg, socioeconomic status) has yet to be elucidated.

Although, in general, no association has been found between prior obesity and cancer risk, several studies have reported that increased birth weight may be associated with increased risk for breast cancer and prostate cancer.[20–23]

Initially, a series of small studies showed that obesity conferred an increased risk for various cancers,[24–28] but because the sample sizes were relatively small, the results were not convincing. Large-scale studies (Table 1) began in earnest with the work of Garfinkel on a cohort of 750,000 persons followed for 12 years, which showed an increased risk of cancer in both men and women who were more than 40% overweight, although the relative risk was still lower than that of cardiovascular sequelae.[29] A series of prospective studies on large populations, which were analyzed for all cancers in the United States, Canada, parts of Europe, and Japan,[30–34] showed an overall increase in the incidence of most types of cancer in obese subjects (Table 2). Examination of studies focusing on specific cancers also showed an increased risk in obese subjects, with a particularly high incidence for those with BMI levels greater than 35 kg/m^2 (Table 3).[35–44] In general, the relative risk of obesity in cancer appears to be higher in women than in men. Again, it is not clear if biologic or sociologic determinants are responsible.

Support for this hypothesis of increased cancer risk with obesity is not universal. In a meta-analysis, McGee concluded that the increased cancer risk due to obesity was quite small and less than the risks for other obesity-associated conditions.[45] Although most studies report a positive relationship between obesity and colon cancer, there are occasional studies that fail to find an association.[46] Somewhat surprisingly, Lukanova and colleagues found that the incidence of ovarian cancer is inversely related to obesity,[47] disagreeing with earlier reports of a positive correlation. The interpretation of many studies relating cancer incidence to obesity are often confusing in that they often fail to adjust for

Table 1 Overall Cancer Risk with Obesity

Authors	Population Size	Overall Cancer Risk	
		Men	Women
Calle et al.[34]	900,000	RR = 1.52	RR = 1/62
Garfinkel[29]	750,000	RR = 1.33	RR = 1.55
Pan et al.[33]	26,000	1.34	
Wolk et al.[30]	28,000	25% excess	37% excess
Kuriyama et al.[32]	27,500	1.46	1.75
Saminic et al.[193]	4,500,000	1.42WH, 1.77 BL	
Okasha et al.[194]	8600	1.36*	1.80*
Inoue et al.[195]	88,900	1.33	

In all cases, BMI >35 vs. <35.
BL = African American; RR = relative risk; WH = white.
*Excluding deaths from lung cancer.

Table 2 Individual Relative Risks for Different Cancers Based on Obesity in Men

Author	Prostate	Colon	Lymphoma	Esophagus	Stomach	Liver	Pancreas	Kidney	Leukemia
Calle et al.[34]	1.34	1.84	1.49	1.63	1.94	4.52	1.49	1.70	1.70
Porter and Stanford[196]	Incid.77								
Babagas et al.[197]									
Bianchini et al.[31]									
Pan et al.[33]	1.27	1.93	1.46				1.51	2.74	1.61
Moller et al.[198]	1.3						1.7		
Michaud et al.[37]							1.72		
Wolk et al.[30]			3.3						

Table 3 Incidence of Obesity in Cancer Survivors

Authors	Patient Population (n)	Percent Obese, Definition	Risk Factors, Comments
Sainsbury et al.[93]	ALL (86)	Increased weight/height within 1 year of therapy.	Did not standardize for treatment, CrXRT, steroids.
Zee and Chen[94]	ALL (414)	30% with BMI > 80th percentile.	Correlated with CrXRT. No controls.
Schell et al.[95]	ALL (91)	38% obesity by adulthood.	Correlated with CrXRT, younger age at diagnosis. No controls.
Odame et al.[96]	ALL (40)	57% for girls, BMI > 2 SD.	Especially in females. Age-matched controls.
Didi et al.[91]	ALL (114)	46% with BMI > 85th percentile.	Especially in females, correlation with chemotherapy, CrXRT 18 vs. 24 Gy no difference. No controls.
Craig et al.[97]	ALL (298)	12% for girls, 10% for boys, BMI z-score > 2.	Severe obesity only in females. CrXRT 18-20 Gy worse than 22-24 Gy. Used chemo only as controls.
Nysom et al.[99]	ALL (95)	Direct body fat (BF) measurments. 26% had BF above 90th percentile.	Correlated with CrXRT, GH deficiency. Used local controls.
Sklar et al.[98]	ALL (126)	40% with BMI > 85th percentile.	CrXRT 24 Gy worse than 18 Gy. Used chemo only as controls.
Stahnke et al.[106]	Craniopharyngioma (10)	80% obese at 1 year.	No controls.
Sorva[107]	Craniopharyngioma (22)	27% obese preop, 67% obese 1 year post-op.	No controls.
Pinto et al.[108]	Craniopharyngioma (17)	30% with BMI > 2 SD preop, 77% 1 year post-op.	Change in fasting insulin correlated with BMI change. No controls.

Reproduced with permission from Lustig RH.[110]
ALL = acute lymphoblastic leukemia; CrXRT = cranial irradiation; BMI = body mass index; SD = standard deviation; Gy = Gray; GH = growth hormone.

multiple risk factors or for indirect associations. For example, examination of the role of obesity regarding the risk of lung cancer in the general population suggests that there is no association. But if one instead restricts the analysis to non-smokers only, then there is a direct positive association.[48] Presumably smoking tends to decrease food consumption, which limits weight gain and protects against obesity, while ex-smokers tend to gain weight immediately after stopping smoking. Similarly, the overall association between obesity and cervical cancer is inconclusive; however, if one controls for human papilloma virus (HPV) infection, a twofold increase is then noted.

Unlike the positive association between obesity and endometrial and breast cancer, there are others like Giovanucci, who was concerned about the absence of mechanism and the failure to fulfill Koch's postulate by showing that weight loss reduces cancer risk.[49] This concern has recently been answered by an Iowa study showing that women who deliberately lost weight and kept it off for some years had a decreased incidence of cancer relative to those controls who did not lose weight.[50] Women who did not lose weight deliberately (but, rather, for other reasons) showed no such benefit. The paucity of studies correlating weight loss with decreased cancer incidence reflects in large part the failure of most previously obese subjects to maintain the weight loss. The typical pattern is an inexorably slow regain of the weight lost, plus extra.[51] For this reason, the cost of carrying out such a study in order to retain a sufficient number of reduced-weight subjects would be enormous.

Putative Mechanisms by Which Obesity Promotes Cancer

Oxidative Stress and Adipocytokine Production

In looking for a mechanism or mechanisms, one must keep in mind that fat is an important endocrine organ. As recently noted by a Japanese group,[52] fat tissue is a major source of reactive oxygen species (ROS) in the body due to oxidative stress in this tissue; indeed the obese exhibit significantly higher levels of 8-isoprostanes, a ROS-metabolite of arachidonic acid.[53,54] Aside from the possibility of direct DNA damage due to ROS, the oxidative stress results in dysregulation of the synthesis and release of adipocytokines, decreasing the formation of protective factors like adiponectin, and increasing the formation of NADP oxidase levels and risk-promoting cytokines like plasminogen activation inhibitor-1 (PAI-1), tumor necrosis factor-α (TNF-α), vascular endothelial growth factor, hepatocyte growth factor, heparin-binding epidermal growth factor-like growth factor, and interleukin-6.[55] Many of these promote angiogenesis, which may explain increased invasiveness and poor prognosis of cancer in the obese. Lastly, the adipocytokine leptin appears to have an important relationship with cancer. As an example, in a case-control study, Stattin and colleagues found a threefold increase in cancer incidence with increasing concentrations of leptin,[56] and Skibola and colleagues found a positive association between BMI, leptin receptor polymorphisms, and lymphoma.[57] Leptin, similar to obesity in general, correlates with increased prostate cancer mortality.[58] Again, while these circulating factors have not yet been directly implicated in carcinogenesis, they clearly have effects on immunomodulatory system function, which may contribute indirectly to cancer initiation or tumor promotion, and mortality.

Estrogen Synthesis and Metabolism

Breast, endometrial, and cervical cancer are examples of estrogen-dependent cancers, which increase their rate of growth in response to circulating estrogen levels.[59,60] Body fat, particularly postmenopausally, is a major source of estrogen derived by the aromatization of androstenedione to estrone (Figure 1).[61] Thus in obese women, increased amounts of estrogen substrate are manufactured, and the total estrogen burden is markedly increased over the lifetime of the individual. Indeed, Key and colleagues[62] suggested that the increased formation of estrone in adipose tissue is a significant factor in the increased rate of breast cancer observed in obese postmenopausal women. Once formed, estrogen can be metabolized either by hepatic 2-hydroxylation to the inactive 2-hydroxy- or catechol estrogens; or by 16α-hydroxlation within the breast tissue itself to the reactive species 16α-hydroxyestrone, which circulates and is finally cleared by the liver and 17β-oxidated to the final metabolite estriol, which is excreted in the urine. Obesity alters the metabolism of estrogen by decreasing the formation of 2-hydroxyestrone and increasing the amount of circulating active estrogen. This has been demonstrated by Schneider and colleagues both

in vitro[63] and in vivo.[64] Therefore, obese subjects have higher circulating levels of active estrogen in the forms of estradiol, estrone, and 16α-hydroxyestrone, which theoretically promote tumor progression. In addition, in vitro studies by Bradlow and colleagues have shown that adipocytes secrete a protein that inhibits 2-hydroxylation of estrogen in MCF-7 cells in culture.[65] The level of active estrogens is further increased by a decrease in the synthesis in the liver of sex hormone binding globulin (SHBG), which normally avidly binds sex hormones; thus potentiating levels of circulating free hormone in the obese, in order to promote increased cell proliferation.

The human papilloma virus (HPV), associated with most cervical cancers, is unusual in that the virus is estrogen-sensitive, with 16α-hydroxyestrone promoting viral proliferation, while the alternative metabolite 2-hydroxyestrone inhibits exons E6 and E7 resulting in inhibition of the virus[66] and causing remissions in children with laryngeal papillomatosis and cervical dysplasia.[67,68]

Hyperinsulinemia, Insulin-like Growth Factor-1, and Insulin-like Growth Factor–Binding Protein-1

Obesity is also associated with hyperinsulinemia, although there is still some controversy as to whether the obesity causes the hyperinsulinemia or vice versa.[69,70] The hyperinsulinemia and insulin resistance of obesity clearly plays a role in the promotion of the Metabolic Syndrome.[71–74] In addition, the hyperinsulinemia of obesity may also indirectly play a role in tumor promotion. A putative role for hyperinsulinemia also comes from studies in Type 2 diabetes, which is associated with an increased incidence of colorectal cancer.[75]

The hormone insulin-like growth factor-1 (IGF-1) has been implicated in numerous cancers, including colon, breast, and prostate cancer.[76] IGF-1 is a primary signal for mitogenesis, by directly binding to the IGF-1 receptor on the cell

surface, and inducing cells to progress from the G1 to the S phase of the cell cycle. IGF-1 has been shown to be a proliferating agent and an inhibitor of apoptosis in tumor cells,[77] while IGF-1 deficiency has been shown to reduce and delay tumorigenesis in knockout mice.[78] States of increased IGF-1 synthesis, such as acromegaly, are known to predispose one to colorectal carcinoma.[79] Insulin increases the availability of IGF-1 to induce mitogenesis by reducing hepatic production of IGF-binding protein-1 (IGFBP-1), the primary carrier protein of IGF-1 in the circulation. Conversely, the tumor suppressor p53 increases the level of another protein, IGFBP-3, in the circulation, effectively clearing free IGF-1.[80] As a result, in the obese hyperinsulinemic state, there is increased free IGF-1 at the target cell to stimulate cellular proliferation. It should be noted that there is no clear relationship between total circulating levels of IGF-1 and the degree of adiposity, which makes epidemiologic associations between obesity, IGF-1, and cancer difficult to interpret.

The role of IGF-1 in breast cancer is mixed since there are papers by the same authors reporting a positive relationship[43,81] and the absence of a relationship.[82] Stattin and colleagues found that higher IGF-1 levels increased prostate cancer mortality. Similar to the situation with estrogens, there is some confusion caused by the failure to always measure free IGF-1 rather than total IGF-1.[41]

Adipose Tissue as a Storehouse for Toxins

There are a variety of toxins [PCBs (polychlorinated biphenyls), Dioxins, PAHs (polycyclic aromatic hydrocarbon), etc] and estrogen modulators and synthetic estrogens [bisphenol A, nonylphenol, DDT (Dichlorodiphenyltrichloroethane), o,p-DDE (ortho, para-Dichlorodiphenyldichloroethylene), etc.] which are lipophilic and can accumulate in body fat for long periods of time. These compounds are released during weight loss[83] and during lactation.[84,85] These toxins and endocrine disruptors can be measured in mother's milk,[86] where these compounds could be potentially harmful to the nursing infant, although there is no evidence that their concentrations reach harmful levels.

Attempts to estimate static prior concentrations of these compounds from current levels in body fat have been unsuccessful. One problem is that many women engage in yo-yo dieting in which they lose body fat and subsequently regain it. In the course of this decrease in body fat, lipophilic compounds are flushed from the adipose tissue depot and cleared from the body. Following several such cycles the amounts of these compounds remaining in the body fat depot will be significantly reduced, blocking any attempts to use static measurements to estimate what was present back at the time when the

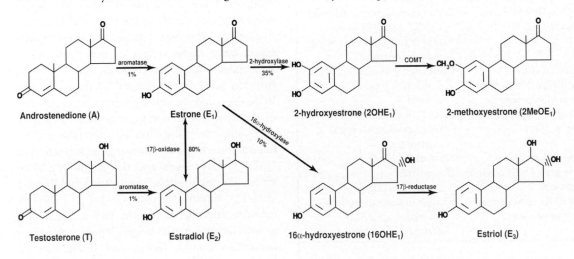

FIGURE 1 Pathways of human estrogen metabolism in humans. Percentages refer to enzyme activity as measured by radiometric assay (efficacy of conversion of tritiated precursor to tritiated water).

tumors were initiated. In addition, because of current legal restrictions on the use of many of these compounds, current exposure has greatly diminished, so any attempts to calculate differences between cancer patients and controls would be extremely difficult.

Presumably, the concentration of these compounds in the lipid droplets of the adipocytes is in equilibrium with what is free in the rest of the cell and in the circulation. It is these latter two pools that would be the active sites for these compounds. There have been no good studies on this equilibrium, or what concentrations would have to be achieved to reach toxic levels.

Summary

Obesity facilitates the production and availability of numerous mitogenic agents, (including estrogen and IGF-1), immune modulators (including leptin and IL-6), and angiogenic factors (including vascular endothelial growth factor and hepatocyte growth factor) to susceptible target cells throughout the body. These factors may be working at different levels of tumorigenesis in different tissues, thus a unifying hypothesis of obesity and cancer may not be forthcoming. Nonetheless, the epidemiologic and mechanistic data presented here implicate the process of obesity in an adjunct, if not a primary role, in carcinogenesis and mortality.

Obesity after Cancer Therapy

Epidemiology

Although cancer, its therapy, and its aftermath are routinely associated with cachexia, one unexpected outcome can be the development of obesity with all of its pathophysiologic sequelae.[87–89] This phenomenon has been noted primarily in the Acute Lymphoblastic Leukemia (ALL) and brain tumor survivor populations. A report from the Childhood Cancer Survivors Study documents an increased risk for BMI less than 18 (cachexia) in adult survivors of most childhood tumors, while the ALL survivor population demonstrates the opposite.[90] The incidence of obesity in adult survivors of ALL is 18.5% in females and 16.5% in males; while the odds ratio for developing obesity is 1.5 in females and 1.2 in males.

Several reviews document an increased prevalence of obesity in survivors of childhood ALL.[91–100] These evaluations have been retrospective, and suffer from several difficulties, including lack of control populations, variability of chemotherapeutic treatment, inclusion of patients who relapse, the use and dose of cranial irradiation, and the dose and type of long-term steroid use as a complicating variable. In addition, the literature questions the possible psychosocial etiologies of weight gain, particularly with respect to parental leniency and aggressivity regarding food availability and food choice in this vulnerable population (ie, since the presenting cachexia signified illness, the manifestation of increased caloric intake may be misconstrued by parents as a sign of health). Nonetheless, the majority of these studies document an abnormal increase in BMI long after tumor therapy has been discontinued, suggesting dysregulation of energy balance.

Similarly, long-term survivors of brain tumors have also been shown to be at risk for the development of obesity. This phenomenon has been documented both in the pediatric[90,101,102] and adult brain tumor populations.[103] Again, these studies have been retrospective; and it is not entirely clear from these studies whether the obesity is due to the tumor, the surgery, and/or the cranial irradiation that such patients inevitably receive.

Risk Factors for the Development of Obesity after Cancer Therapy

In the childhood ALL survivor population, the prevalence of adult obesity has been reported anywhere between 20 and 44%. Since these studies are retrospective, and it is difficult to compare specific treatment paradigms for risk, most of these analyses instead use multivariate linear regression analyses to extract specific risk factors for the development of obesity (see Table 3). In many of these studies, age at diagnosis, female gender, and the presence of cranial radiation have been found to be important risk factors for the development of obesity.

In the brain tumor population, the development of obesity appears to be restricted to involvement of the posterior fossa, and in particular, the hypothalamus. Since 50% of childhood tumors (while only 10 to 20% of adult brain tumors) involve the posterior fossa, the development of obesity after brain tumor therapy is most commonly manifest in the pediatric population. The phenomenon of obesity is most evident in children with craniopharyngioma (see Table 3). However, this is by no means exclusive to children; about 10% of craniopharyngiomas occur in late adulthood,[104] and a recent report demonstrates increased weight gain and BMI after brain tumor therapy in adults as well.[105]

A multivariate linear regression analysis of the BMI curves of children with brain tumors who survived longer than 5 years post-therapy determined risk factors for the development of obesity.[101] Five parameters were cited as being predictive. First, age at diagnosis and treatment was negatively correlated with risk for obesity; in other words, the younger at diagnosis, the more likely the subject would be obese as an adult. Second, those with tumors localized to the hypothalamus or thalamus, along with those originating in the temporal lobe (due to stereoscopic position of the hypothalamus during radiation for this area) gained weight much more rapidly than those with tumors in the rest of the posterior fossa or other hemispheric areas. Third, those with tumor histologies routinely localized to the diencephalon (ie, craniopharyngioma, germinoma, optic glioma, prolactinoma, hypothalamic astrocytoma) also gained weight more rapidly.[106–108] Fourth, those with quantitative direct radiation exposure of the hypothalamus of greater than 51 gray gained weight twice as rapidly after the completion of tumor therapy, even after those with hypothalamic or thalamic lesions were removed from the analysis. Finally, those with some other form of permanent hypothalamic endocrinopathy (ie, GH deficiency, hypothyroidism, precocious or delayed puberty, ACTH deficiency, diabetes insipidus) exhibited a rapidly escalating BMI curve. Thus, those risk factors linked to hypothalamic damage or dysfunction were ominous in terms of obesity.

Hypothalamic Obesity due to Central Nervous System Insult

Clinical Presentation and Manifestations

Damage to the hypothalamus, either due to tumor, surgery, or radiation, appears to be the primary etiologic factor in weight gain in cancer survivors. This phenomenon is clearly established with the syndrome of "hypothalamic obesity".[109,110] Originally described by Babinski and Frohlich, hypothalamic obesity is a testament to the primary role of the hypothalamus in the regulation of energy balance.[111,112]

The hypothalamus is the control center for several homeostatic hormonal systems, in which the pituitary is the primary effector. They include the GHRH (growth hormone releasing hormone)/SRIF (somatostatin)-Growth Hormone-IGF-1, TRH (thyrotropin releasing hormone)-TSH (thyroid stimulating hormone)-thyroid hormone, GnRH (gonadotropin releasing hormone)-gonadotropin-sex hormone, and CRF (corticotropin releasing factor)-ACTH (adrenocorticotropic hormone)-cortisol axes. In each case, the peripheral hormone product provides an afferent feedback signal, which binds to specific receptors within the ventromedial hypothalamus (VMH) to regulate efferent hypothalamic hormonal output. In addition, a fifth system, the AVP(arginine vasopressin)-water balance axis, is also controlled by the supraoptic and paraventricular nuclei of the hypothalamus, and in which the posterior pituitary is the storage site for AVP secretory vesicles. Here, the afferent inputs are osmoreceptors for sodium and baroreceptors for blood pressure, rather than a specific hormonal substrate.

The last 10 years has witnessed the documentation of yet another hypothalamic feedback system, in which the adipocyte hormone leptin, the β-cell hormone insulin, the gastric hormone ghrelin, and the intestinal hormone Peptide YY[3–36,113–116] bind to specific receptors within the

VMH to form the afferent arm of an axis that regulates energy balance (Figure 2).[117] Indeed, genetic abnormalities in leptin or its hypothalamic receptor,[118,119] or the hypothalamic melanocortin-4 receptor[120] which processes this information, have been shown to exhibit obese phenotypes, suggesting hypothalamic dysregulation of energy balance signal transduction. However, the efferent arm of this axis is extremely

complex, involving appetite/satiety, autonomic, hormonal, thermogenic, and motor effectors.[117,121,122] Presumably patients with hypothalamic obesity exhibit abnormal signaling within both arms.

In humans, hypothalamic obesity is the manifestation of hypothalamic damage from tumor, surgery, and/or radiation, resulting in an intractable weight gain, which is not amenable to

caloric restriction or exercise.[123] Craniopharyngioma accounts for half of the reported cases, with other posterior fossa tumors contributing smaller numbers. However, the syndrome has also been reported in cases of pseudotumor cerebri, trauma, and infiltrative or inflammatory diseases of the hypothalamus.[124]

Aside from the symptoms of tumor-induced increased intracranial pressure, patients with hypothalamic obesity classically exhibit signs of limbic system involvement, such as hypogonadism, somnolence, rage and hyperphagia[125]; however, such classic presentations are actually rare.[109] The majority of patients actually exhibit normal or only slightly increased daily caloric intake. Indeed, caloric restriction of either VMH-lesioned animals or humans with hypothalamic obesity rarely attenuates the weight gain, suggesting that energy expenditure is also affected.[126]

Examination of the German craniopharyngioma database[127] demonstrates that children with craniopharyngioma already manifest an increased BMI for age by the time of diagnosis, suggesting that the tumor itself alters energy balance. However, after surgery and/or radiation, they can accelerate their weight gain even more rapidly. Most of these patients have other cranial endocrinopathies,[101] and require growth hormone, thyroxine, and hydrocortisone, sex hormone, and desmopressin replacement therapy due to GHRH/GH, TRH/TSH CRF/ACTH, GnRH/gonadotropin, and AVP (antidiuretic hormone) deficiencies, respectively. In some cases, lack of appreciation of the syndrome of hypothalamic obesity by physicians has led them to incorrectly deduce that the hydrocortisone dosage is contributing to the patient's weight gain, leading to well-meaning but potentially dangerous reductions of hydrocortisone dosage below 10 mg/m^2/d. This accentuates the symptoms of malaise and lethargy exhibited by these patients.

Patients with hypothalamic obesity may also suffer from sequelae normally associated with exogenous obesity. These patients have been shown to have an increased incidence of the Metabolic Syndrome[88] and nonalcoholic fatty liver disease.[89] Furthermore they appear to have an increased risk for angina pectoris and other cardiovascular disease.[87,102] In addition to their obesity, the concomitant growth hormone deficiency that these patients manifest may also contribute to their adverse metabolic sequelae.[128]

Pathophysiologic Mechanisms

It is well known that bilateral electrolytic lesions or deafferentation of the VMH in rats leads to intractable weight gain,[109,129–132] even upon food 'restriction.[133] Originally, the obesity was felt to be due to damage to a "satiety" center, which promoted hyperphagia and increased energy storage.[134] However, we now recognize that the

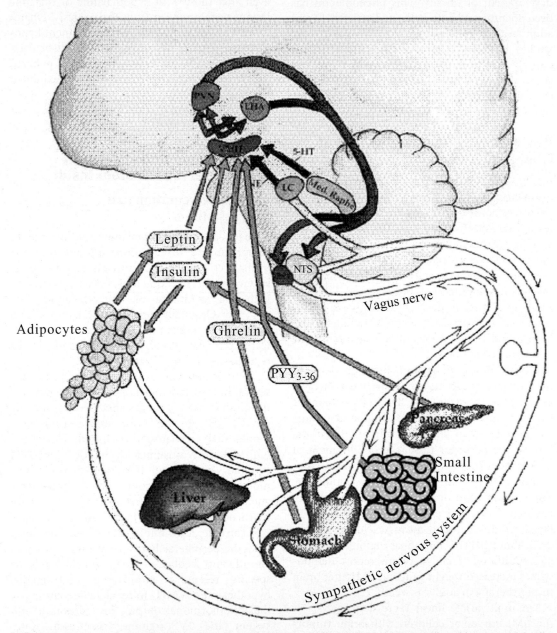

FIGURE 2 The negative feedback pathway of energy balance. Afferent neural (eg, vagal) and hormonal (ghrelin, insulin, leptin, PYY$_{3-36}$) signals are generated from the liver, gut, pancreas, and adipose. In addition, norepinephrine from the locus coeruleus and serotonin (5-HT) from the median raphe are elaborated. These signals of satiety versus hunger, and thinness versus fatness are interpreted by the nucleus tractus solitarii (NTS) and the hypothalamic gated neural network in the ventromedial hypothalamus (VMH). The peptides α-melanocyte stimulating hormone (α-MSH) and cocaine-amphetamine regulated-transcript are anorexigenic, while the peptides neuropeptide Y and agouti-related protein are orexigenic. These signals are integrated in the paraventricular nucleus (PVN) and lateral hypothalamus (LHA), through stimulation or inhibition of melanocortin receptors 3 and 4. Efferent signals from these areas in turn stimulate either the sympathetic nervous system to expend energy by activating β$_3$-adrenergic receptors and uncoupling proteins in the adipocyte, which releases energy the form of lipolysis, heat or physical activity; or stimulate the parasympathetic nervous system (efferent vagal) to increase insulin secretion, with resultant lipogenesis and energy storage. Reprinted with permission from Lustig RH, et al.[199]

HT = ; LC = ; DMV = ; Med. Raphe = ; PYY = ; NE = norephinephrine.

weight gain in this syndrome is actually secondary to: (1) inability to transduce peripheral hormonal energy balance signals; (2) overactivation of the parasympathetic nervous system, which promotes an obligate insulin hypersecretion and energy storage; and (3) defective activation of the sympathetic nervous system which retards lipolysis and energy expenditure.'

Defective Peripheral Hormonal Signal Transduction in the VMH

The negative feedback energy balance pathway (see Figure 2) is interesting in that the hormone insulin is a component of both the afferent and efferent limbs of the axis. In the afferent pathway, insulin conveys information about nutrients and energy balance to the hypothalamus, which limits food intake.[135] Insulin secreted by the pancreas in response to a meal provides blood-borne afferent information on nutrient intake and absorption to the VMH. A subpopulation of VMH neurons possesses insulin receptors,[136] and there is coordinated transport of insulin across the blood-brain barrier.[137] In experimental animals, acute and chronic ICV (intracerebroventricular) insulin infusions decrease feeding behavior and induce satiety.[138–140] The importance of central nervous system (CNS) insulin action was recently underscored by the construction of a brain/neuron-specific insulin receptor knockout (NIRKO) and an insulin receptor substrate 2 knockout mouse, which cannot transduce the CNS insulin signal.[141,142] They become hyperphagic, obese, and infertile, with high peripheral insulin levels. These mice suggest that peripheral insulin mediates a signal within the VMH to help control energy balance and other hypothalamic functions.[114,143]

Normally, in the fed state, both insulin and leptin levels are increased, which increase the synthesis and processing of hypothalamic pro-opiomelanocortin (POMC) to its component peptides, including α-melanocyte stimulating hormone (α-MSH), which along with its co-localized neuromodulator cocaine-amphetamine regulated transcript (CART), act at the lateral hypothalamic area (LHA) and paraventricular nucleus (PVN) to alter melanocortin-4 receptor (MC₄R) occupancy, which decreases appetite and food intake.[113,135,144,145] Insulin and leptin also directly inhibit the release of neuropeptide Y (NPY) and agouti-related protein (AgRP), further limiting feeding and providing for unantagonized MC₄R (melanocortin-4 receptor) occupancy.[146] Furthermore, PYY₃₋₃₆ (peptide YY₃₋₃₆) levels are elevated, and this hormone binds to the Y₂ receptor in the VMH, activating γ-aminobutyric acid (GABA), which inhibits the orexigenic signal transduction of neuropeptide Y.[147] Conversely, in the fasting state, gastric secretion of ghrelin is increased,[148,149] while leptin,

insulin, and PYY₃₋₃₆ levels are low, which leads to stimulation of hypothalamic NPY/AgRP and antagonism of α-MSH/CART. The resultant lack of anorexigenic pressure on the MC₄R results in increased feeding behavior and energy efficiency (with reduced fat oxidation), in order to store energy substrate as fat. In the syndrome hypothalamic obesity, hypothalamic damage prevents integration of these peripheral energy and adiposity signals; thus, the VMH cannot transduce these signals into a state of energy sufficiency sense a subjective sense of satiety.[132,150]

Vagally-Mediated Insulin Hypersecretion and Increased Energy Storage

Normally, excess blood-borne energy substrates (glucose, fatty acids) which are not utilized immediately by other tissues are stored in adipose tissue via the lipogenic effects of insulin. In the efferent pathway, insulin is responsible for shunting blood-borne nutrients into adipose for storage. The amplitude and duration of pancreatic insulin secretion, and the activity of the insulin molecule at the adipose insulin receptor, play integral roles in the genesis of lipogenesis and weight gain. Although there are numerous factors that promote lipolysis, the primary signal for lipogenesis is insulin.[151] Within the adipocyte, insulin increases: (1) Glut4 expression; (2) acetyl-CoA carboxylase; (3) fatty acid synthase; and (4) lipoprotein lipase.[152] Thus, the net effect of insulin on the adipocyte is the rapid clearance and storage of circulating glucose and lipid.

The LHA and PVN send efferent projections residing in the medial longitudinal fasciculus to the dorsal motor nucleus of the vagus (DMV).[153] The DMV, in turn, sends efferent projections throughout the alimentary system, including the β-cells of the pancreas.[154] This pathway is responsible for the "cephalic" or preabsorptive phase of insulin secretion, which is glucose-independent and can be blocked by atropine.[155] VMH lesions damage this pathway, leading to an increase in vagal firing rate.[156] For example, rats with VMH lesions exhibit both increased insulin levels and food intake; however, this can be prevented by pancreatic vagotomy.[129,157,158] Overactive vagal neurotransmission increases insulin secretion from β-cells through three distinct but overlapping mechanisms (Figure 3):[159]

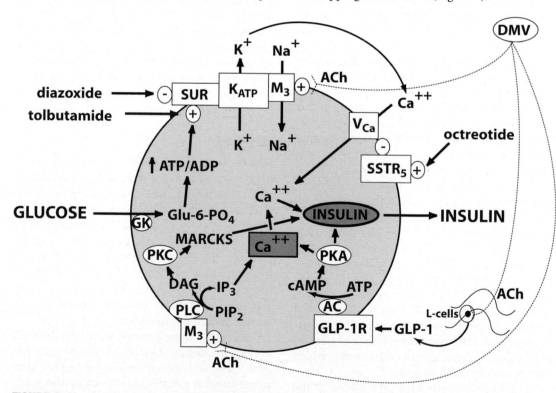

FIGURE 3 Vagal augmentation of insulin hypersecretion. (1) M₃ activation of a Na+ channel augments β-cell depolarization, which augments calcium influx. (2) M₃ activation increases phospholipases A₂, C, and D, which hydrolyze phosphatidylinositol (PIP₂) to diacylglycerol (DAG) and inositol 1,4,5-triphosphate (IP₃). DAG stimulates of protein kinase C (PKC) which phosphorylates myristoylated alanine-rich C kinase substrate (MARCKS), which binds actin-calcium-calmodulin, and induces vesicular exocytosis. IP₃ potentiates intracellular calcium release. (3) Release of glucagon-like peptide-1 (GLP-1) from intestinal L-cells. GLP-1 receptor activation induces adenyl cyclase, increasing cAMP, activating protein kinase A (PKA) potentiates intracellular calcium release. Reprinted with permission from Lustig RH.[200]

AC = adenyl cyclase; Ach = acetylcholine; ADP = adenosine diphosphate; ATP = adenosine triphosphate; Ca++ = ionized calcium; cAMP = cyclic adenosine monophosphate; DMV = dorsal motor nucleus of the vagus; GLP-1 = glucagon-like peptide-1; GLP-1R = glucagon-like peptide-1 receptor; Glu = glucose; K = potassium; L-cells = L-cells; M = muscarinic; Na = sodium; PLC = phospholipase C; PO = I don't see a PO; SUR = sulfonylurea receptor; VCa = voltage-gated calcium channel.

Vagal firing increases acetylcholine availability and binding to the M_3 muscarinic receptor, which is coupled to a sodium channel within the pancreatic β-cell membrane.[160] Under resting conditions, the ATP(adenosine triphosphate)-dependent potassium channel within the β-cell membrane remains open, and leads to a negative β-cell resting membrane potential of approximately −70 millivolts (mV), with essentially no insulin release. In this state, activation of the sodium channel by acetylcholine only minimally increases β-cell resting membrane potential to −65 mV, and has relatively minimal effects on insulin secretion and peripheral insulin levels. This phenomenon is responsible for the vagally mediated "cephalic" or preabsorptive phase of insulin secretion, which is glucose-independent and can be blocked by atropine.[155] As glucose enters the β-cell after ingestion of a meal, the enzyme glucokinase will phosphorylate glucose to form glucose-6-phosphate. This increases the generation of intracellular ATP, which induces closure of the β-cell's ATP-dependent potassium channel. Upon channel closure, the β-cell experiences an ATP-concentration–dependent β-cell depolarization,[161,162] and the opening of a separate voltage-gated calcium channel within the membrane. Intracellular calcium influx increases acutely, which results in rapid insulin vesicular exocytosis. Concomitant opening of the sodium channel by acetylcholine binding to the M_3 receptor augments the β-cell depolarization which, in turn, augments the intracellular calcium influx and results in insulin hypersecretion.[129,130,163] Conversely, knockout of the M_3 receptor in mice reduces vagal-mediated insulin secretion, and results in a hypophagic and lean phenotype.[164]

Vagally mediated acetylcholine increases phospholipases A_2, C, and D within the β-cell, which hydrolyze intracellular phosphatidylinositol to diacylglycerol (DAG) and inositol 1,4,5-triphosphate (IP_3).[159] DAG is a potent stimulator of protein kinase C (PKC)[165] which phosphorylates myristoylated alanine-rich protein kinase C substrate [MARCKS(myristoylated protein kinase C substrate)], which then binds actin and calcium-calmodulin, and induces insulin vesicular exocytosis.[166] IP_3 potentiates release of calcium within β-cells from intracellular stores, which also promotes insulin secretion.[167]

The vagus also stimulates the release of the peptide glucagon-like peptide-1 (GLP-1) from intestinal L-cells, which circulates and binds to a GLP-1 receptor within the β-cell membrane. Activation of this receptor induces a calcium-calmodulin–sensitive adenyl cyclase, with conversion of intracellular ATP to cAMP (cyclic adenosine monophosphate), which then activates protein kinase A (PKA). PKA causes both the release of intracellular calcium stores, and the phosphorylation of vesicular proteins, each contributing to an increase in insulin exocytosis.[168,169]

Decreased Sympathetic Responsiveness, Physical Activity, and Energy Expenditure

The adipocyte also responds to sympathetic nervous system activation to promote lipolysis and thermogenesis.[122] The most prominent and concerning complaints in patients with hypothalamic obesity is persistent fatigue, lack of energy, and lack of physical activity. This generalized malaise is not due to hypopituitarism, as it persists even after full hormonal replacement. Harz and colleagues showed that the voluntary energy expenditure of patients with craniopharyngioma, as measured by accelerometry, was significantly decreased compared to BMI-matched obese, but otherwise healthy, controls.[170] This decrease in energy expenditure may be mediated through defects in the regulation of the sympathetic nervous system. Two reports demonstrate an impaired ability of such patients to mount an epinephrine response to insulin-induced hypoglycemia,[171,172] and document decreased 24-hour epinephrine excretion,[172] although norepinephrine excretion was similar to controls. It is thought that this malaise and decrease in sympathetic tone may account for decreased rates of lipolysis through the adipocyte $β_3$-adrenergic receptor,[173] which result in decreased resting and voluntary energy expenditure. Thus, the mechanisms of lipogenesis in this syndrome are due to autonomic endocrinopathy; a combination of parasympathetic hypertransmission and sympathetic hypotransmission secondary to VMH damage.

Diagnosis

Patients with hypothalamic obesity gain weight despite attempts at diet and exercise. Indeed, Bray and colleagues showed that long-term caloric restriction was ineffective in modulating the weight gain in these patients,[109,123] attesting to the "obligate" nature of the weight gain in these patients. He and Gallagher also noted insulin hypersecretion in subjects with hypothalamic obesity.[123] Their results suggest that such patients exhibit a metabolic priority toward energy storage instead of expenditure.

Although some patients with hypothalamic obesity are already obese upon clinical presentation, most are normal weight-for-height. After surgery and/or radiation, their weight gain accelerates rapidly, usually at a rate of 1 kg/month or greater. Despite the high incidence of GH deficiency, most of these patients continue to exhibit normal linear growth,[174] probably due to insulin's effects on the IGF-1 receptor.[175] Most of these patients have other cranial endocrinopathies and require hormonal replacement. In some cases, lack of appreciation of the syndrome of hypothalamic obesity by physicians has led to the incorrect deduction that the hydrocortisone dosage was contributing to the patient's weight gain, resulting in well-meaning, but potentially dangerous, reductions of hydrocortisone dosage below 10 mg/m²/d. This accentuates the symptoms of malaise and lethargy exhibited by these patients.

The insulin excursion to oral glucose tolerance testing (OGTT) defines the syndrome. Two prospective studies of children with hypothalamic obesity revealed only minimally elevated fasting insulin concentrations of 22.7 ± 1.3 µU/mL, as compared to 36.3 ± 5.7 µU/mL for an age- and BMI-matched group of subjects with obesity, insulin resistance, and acanthosis nigricans.[176,177] However, these patients demonstrated accentuated early insulin responses to OGTT, which were elevated in comparison to their degree of obesity. Peak insulin levels were reached by 60 minutes, and were 281 ± 47 µU/mL, as compared to normal adolescents, whose peak insulin concentrations are routinely 100 to 150 µU/mL. The fall to baseline was reasonably rapid, suggesting that these patients did not exhibit defective insulin clearance, as is usually seen in insulin resistance. One report documents that the insulin hypersecretion in this disorder is primary, as controlling for the degree of insulin resistance did not reduce the statistical significance of the hypersecretion.[178]

Treatment

Numerous therapies have been attempted in the treatment of hypothalamic obesity. The appreciation of the role of dysfunctional vagal tone and insulin hypersecretion in the pathogenesis of hypothalamic obesity originally led to anecdotal case reports of successful treatment with pancreatic vagotomy.[179] However, subsequent experience with the procedure was inconsistent, and it fell out of favor.[180] Several trials of anorectic medication have been attempted,[181,182] with temporizing, but not long-term, efficacy.

We have attempted to inhibit this insulin hypersecretion pharmacologically. Although diazoxide, an oral β-cell potassium channel opener, is routinely used to treat hypoglycemia due to hyperinsulinism,[183] this drug suppresses insulin secretion globally, such that the possibility of hyperglycemia or frank diabetes exists.[184,185] Furthermore, we wished to antagonize insulin secretion at a point downstream of the sodium channel activity (Figure 3). The voltage-gated calcium channel is coupled to a somatostatin ($SSTR_5$) receptor.[186,187] Treatment with the somatostatin agonist octreotide limits the opening of this channel and the amount of insulin released acutely for any specific amount of glucose.[188,189] In an open-labeled pilot trial,[176] eight patients received subcutaneously administered octreotide for six months, at a dose of 5 µg/kg/d (in total, divided, tid), escalating in monthly 5 µg/kg/d increments to a maximum of 15 µg/kg/d (in total, divided, tid) by the third month. Insulin responses to glucose were normalized over 6 months. Of the eight patients, three lost substantial weight, two lost moderate amounts of weight, and three stabilized their weight. The degree of weight loss correlated both with changes in insulin response and with changes in leptin levels. The weight loss also appeared to correlate with decreases in appetite, and caloric intake in this cohort decreased by approximately 700 kilocalories per day. The lack of leptin negative feedback by the damaged VMH was not critical, as these patients responded with both weight loss, decreased caloric intake, and decreased leptin levels. In fact, an unexpected, but very welcome, side effect of the treatment was the resumption of normal physical activity by four patients, including vigorous exercise. A double-blind, placebo-controlled, six-month trial of octreotide in 18 subjects with hypothalamic obesity followed.[177] Prior to treatment, annualized weight gain in this population was 15.9 ± 2.9 kg/yr. Although the weight loss in this trial was not as pronounced as in the pilot (probably due to a delay in achieving maximum dosage until the fifth month), octreotide was effective in stabilizing weight ($+1.6 \pm 0.6$ kg) and BMI (-0.1 ± 0.1 kg/m^2), as compared to placebo (change in weight $+9.2 \pm 1.5$ kg, BMI $+2.3 \pm 0.5$ kg/m^2). Insulin secretion during the first 60 minutes was clearly suppressed by octreotide. Lastly, the Pediatric Cancer Quality of Life-32 (PCQL-32),[190] a validated instrument to measure improvements in quality of life in children, demonstrated marked improvements in physical activity as compared with those treated with placebo, and the improvement in quality of life correlated with the degree of insulin suppression. These findings suggested that insulin hypersecretion was responsible not only for weight gain in these patients, but for their lack of physical activity, which can be improved by normalizing their insulin response. Anecdotally, patients noted normal hunger at the time of meals, but noted the lack of drive to continue to eat past their first serving, or for snacking between meals. They also noted more interest in their schoolwork and in their social contacts. Treatment of those initially assigned to placebo in the second 6 months also resulted in stabilization of weight and improved quality of life. Studies of the long-acting somatostatin analog octreotide-LAR (octreotide long-acting release) are ongoing in this patient population.

Perhaps the best treatment for this syndrome is prevention. It is very clear that the hypothalamus represents the biologic seat of both food intake and energy balance in humans. Risk assessment of hypothalamic damage can be undertaken based on MRI, portal radiation dosimetry, and endocrinologic testing. In this way, oncologists can assess the risk for future development of obesity in populations with CNS insult so that clear explanation to patients and families, close follow-up, and early preventive measures can be instituted. Finally, the sensitivity of the hypothalamus to both surgical trauma and/or external beam radiation cannot be underestimated. Neurosurgeons and neuro-oncologists must incorporate these risk factors when making a therapeutic plan to limit long-term morbidity and mortality in such patients.[191,192]

Summary

The syndrome of hypothalamic obesity is the most obvious example of the organicity of obesity in a specific population. Prior to their cranial insult, these patients are completely normal, but afterward, they exhibit signs of hypothalamic dysfunction, including anterior pituitary endocrinopathy (hypopituitarism), posterior pituitary endocrinopathy (diabetes insipidus), and autonomic endocrinopathy (hypothalamic obesity). From combined data in rat and human, the primary etiologies appear to be defective insulin and leptin signal transduction at the level of the hypothalamus, increased vagal modulation, and decreased sympathetic modulation, leading to insulin hypersecretion with increased lipogenesis and decreased lipolysis. Diagnosis rests on documentation of accentuated early responses to OGTT, and at least one potentially beneficial therapeutic strategy involves suppression of the early insulin response.

REFERENCES

1. Formiguera A, Canton A. Obesity: epidemiology and clinical aspects. Balliere's Best Pract Res Clin Gastroenterol 2004;18:1125–46.
2. Pan WH, Flegal KM, Chang HY, et al. Body mass index and obesity related metabolic disorders in Taiwanese and US whites and blacks: implication for definitions of overweight and obesity for Asians. Am J Clin Nutr 2004;79:31–9.
3. Friedman JM, Halaas JL. Leptin and the regulation of body weight in mammals. Nature 1998;395:763–70.
4. Martin-Du Pan RC, Giusti V. Adipose tissue: a real endocrine gland synthesizing hormones and cytokines: clinical implications. Rev Med Suisse Romande 2004;124:171–5.
5. Pantanetti P, Garrapa GG, Mantero F, et al. Adipose tissue as an endocrine organ? A review of recent data related to cardiovascular complications of endocrine dysfunctions. Clin Exp Hypertens 2004;26:387–98.
6. Kirschner MA, Samojlik E. Sex hormone metabolism in upper and lower body obesity. Int J Obes 1991;15(Suppl 2):101–8.
7. Simpson ER. Sources of estrogen and their importance. J Steroid Biochem Mol Biol 2003;86:225–30.
8. Chehab FF, Qiu J, Ogus S. The use of animal models to dissect the biology of leptin. Recent Prog Horm Res 2004;59:245–66.
9. Ballard-Barbash R, Schatzkin A, Carter CL, et al. Body fat distribution and breast cancer in the Framingham Study. J Natl Cancer Inst 1990;82:1943–4.
10. Shapira DV, Kumar NB, Lyman GH. Obesity, body fat distribution, and sex hormones in breast cancer patients. Cancer 1991;67:2215–8.
11. Weber RV, Stein DE, Kral JG. Obesity potentiates AOM-induced colon cancer. Dig Sis Sci 2000;45:890–5.
12. Kuczmarski RJ, Carrol MD, Flegal KM, Troiano RP. Varying body mass index cut-off points to describe overweight prevalence among U.S. adults: NHANES III (1988 to 1994). Obes Res 1997;5:542–8.
13. Bigaard J, Frederiksen K, Tjonneland A, et al. Waist and hip circumferences and all-cause mortality: usefulness of the waist-to-hip ratio? Int J Obes 2004;28:741–7.
14. Gill T, Chittleborough C, Taylor A, et al. Body mass index, waist hip ratio, and waist circumference: which measure to classify obesity? Soz Praventivmed 2003;48:191–200.
15. WHO specialty consultation. Appropriate body-mass index for Asian populations and its implications for policy and intervention strategies. Lancet 2004;363(9403):157–63.
16. Park YW, Zhu S, Palaniappan L, et al. The metabolic syndrome: prevalence and associated risk factor findings in the US population from the Third National Health and Nutrition Examination Survey, 1988-1994. Arch Intern Med 2003;163:427–6.
17. Giovannucci E, Rimm EB, Stampfer MJ, et al. Height, body weight, and risk of prostate cancer. Cancer Epidemiol Bimarkers Prev 1997;6:557–63.
18. Presti JC. Obesity and prostate cancer. Curr Opin Urol 2005;15:13–6.
19. Irani J, Lefebvre O, Murat F, et al. Obesity in relation to prostate cancer risk: comparison with a population having benign prostatic hyperplasia. Brit J Urol Int 2003;91:482–4.
20. Ahlgren M, Sorenesen T, Wohlfarht J, et al. Birth weight and risk of breast cancer in a cohort of 106,504 women. Int J Cancer 2003;107:997–1000.
21. Vatten LJ, Maehle BO, Lund Nilsen TI, et al. Birth weight as a predictor of breast cancer. Brit J Cancer 2002;86:89–92.
22. Michels KB, Tricoupoulos D, Robins JM, et al. Birth weight as a risk factor for breast cancer. Lancet 1996;348:1542–5.
23. Tibblin G, Eriksson M, Cnattingius S, Ekbom A. High birth weight as a predictor of prostate cancer risk. Epidemiology 1995;6:423–4.
24. Freedland SJ, Aronson WJ, Kane CJ, et al. Impact of obesity on biochemical control after radical prostatectomy for clinically localized prostate cancer: a report by the Shared Equal Access Regional Cancer Hospital Database Study Group. J Clin Oncol 2004;22:446–53.
25. Lissner L, Kroon UB, Bjorntorp P, et al. Adipose tissue fatty acids and dietary fat sources in relation to endometrial cancer: a retrospective study of cases in remission, and population-based controls. Acta Obstet Gynecol Scand 1993;72:481–7.
26. Folsom AR, Kushi LH, Anderson KE, et al. Associations of general and abdominal obesity with multiple health outcomes in older women. Arch Int Med 2000;160:2117–28.
27. Cohen P. Serum insulin-like growth factor-I levels and prostate cancer risk—interpreting the evidence. J Natl Cancer Inst 1998;90:876–9.
28. Rodriquez C, Patel AV, Calle EE, et al. Body mass index, height, and prostate cancer mortality in two large cohorts of adult men in the United States. Cancer Epidemiol Biomarkers Prev 2001;10:345–53.
29. Garfinkel L. Variations in mortality by weight among 750,000 men and women. Ann Int Med 1985;103:1034–6.
30. Wolk A, Gridley G, Svensson M, et al. A prospective study of obesity and cancer risk (Sweden). Cancer Causes Control 2001;12:13–21.
31. Bianchini F, Kaaks R, Vainio H. Overweight, obesity, and cancer risk. Lancet Oncol 2002;9:565–74.
32. Kuriyama S, Tsubini Y, Hozawa A, et al. Obesity and risk of cancer in Japan. Int J Cancer 2005;113:148–57.
33. Pan SY, Johnson KC, Ugnat AM, et al. Association of obesity and cancer risk in Canada. Am J Epidemiol 2004;159:259–68.
34. Calle EE, Rodriguez C, Walker-Thurmond K, Thun MJ. Overweight, obesity, and mortality, from cancer in a prospectively studied cohort of U.S. adults. N Engl J Med 2003;348:1625–38.
35. Berrington de Gonzalez A, Sweetland S, Spencer EA. A meta-analysis of obesity and the risk of pancreatic cancer. Br J Cancer 2003;89:519–23.
36. Gapstur SM, Gann PH, Lowe W, et al. Abnormal glucose metabolism and pancreatic cancer mortality. JAMA 2000;283:2553–8.
37. Michaud DS, Giovannucci E, Willett WC, et al. Physical activity, obesity, and height, and the risk of pancreatic cancer. JAMA 2001;286:921–9.
38. Suadicane P, Hein O, Gyntelberg F. Height, weight, and the risk of colorectal cancer. An eighteen year followup in a cohort of 5249 men. Scand J Gastroenterol 1993;28:285–8.
39. Andersson SO, Wolk A, Bergstrom R, et al. Body size and prostate cancer: a 20-year follow-up study among 13500 Swedish construction workers. J Natl Cancer Inst 1997;89:385–9.
40. Amlin CL, C.J. K, Riffenburgh R, H., et al. Relationship between obesity and race in predicting adverse pathologic variables in patients undergoing radical prostatectomy. Urology 2003;58:723–8.
41. Stattin P, Bylund A, Rinaldi S, et al. Plasma insulin-like growth factor-1, insulin-like growth factor-binding

proteins, and prostate cancer risk: a prospective study. J Natl Cancer Inst 2000;92:1910–7.

42. Kaaks R, Lukanova A, Kurzer MS. Obesity, endogenous hormones, and endometrial cancer risk. Cancer Epidemiol Biomarkers Prev 2002;11:1531–43.

43. Kaaks R, Toniolo P, Akhmedkhanov A, et al. Serum c-peptide, insulin-like growth factor (IGF-1), IGF-binding proteins, and colorectal cancer risk in women. J Natl Cancer Inst 2000;92:2692–700.

44. Weiderpass E, Brismar K, Bellocco R, et al. Serum levels of insulin-like growth factor-1, IGF-binding proteins 1 and 3, and insulin and endometrial cancer risk. Br J Cancer 2003;89:1697–704.

45. McGee DL. Body mass index and mortality: a meta-analysis based on person-level data from twenty-six observational studies. Ann Epidemiol 2005;15:87–97.

46. Wiseman RA. Breast cancer: critical data analysis concludes that estrogens are not the cause, however lifestyle changes can alter risk rapidly. J Clin Epidemiol 2004;57:766–72.

47. Lukanova A, Toniolo P, Lundin E, et al. Body mass index in relation to ovarian cancer: a multi-center nested case-control study. Int J Cancer 2002;99:603–8.

48. Rauscher GH, Mayne ST, Janerich DT. Relation between body mass index and lung cancer risk in men and women never and former smokers. Am J Epidemiol 2000;152:506–13.

49. Giovannucci E. Insulin and colon cancer. Cancer Causes Control 1995;6:164–79.

50. French SA, Folsom AR, Jeffery RW, Williamson DF. Prospective study of intentionality of weight loss and mortality in older women: The Iowa Women's Health Study. Am J Epidemiol 1999;149:504–14.

51. Hill JO, Wyatt HR, Reed GW, Peters JC. Obesity and the environment: where do we go from here? Science 2003; 299:853–855.

52. Furukawa S, Fujita T, Shimabukuro M, et al. Increased oxidative stress in obesity and its impact on metabolic syndrome. J Clin Invest 2004;114:1752–61.

53. Morrow JD. Quantification of isoprostanes as indices of oxidant stress and the risk of atherosclerosis in humans. Arterioscler Thromb Vasc Biol 2005;25:1–18.

54. Bartsch H, Nair J. Oxidative stress and lipid peroxidation-derived DNA-lesions in inflammation driven carcinogenesis. Cancer Prev Detect 2004;28:385–391.

55. Rose DP, Komninou D, Stephenson GD. Obesity, adipocytokines, and insulin resistance in breast cancer. Obes Rev 2004;5:153–65.

56. Stattin P, Lukanova A, Biessy C, et al. Obesity and colon cancer: does leptin provide a link? Int J Cancer 2004; 109:149–52.

57. Skibola CF, Holly EA, Forrest MS, et al. Body mass index, leptin and leptin receptor polymorphisms, and non-Hodgkin lymphoma. Cancer Epidemiol Biomarkers Prev 2004;13:779–86.

58. Stattin P, Soderberg S, Hallmans G, et al. Leptin is associated with increased prostate cancer risk: a nested case-control reference study. J Clin Endocrinol Metab 2001;86:1341–5.

59. Pike M, Spicer DV. Endogenous estrogen and progesterone as the major determinants of breast cancer risk: prospects for control by "natural" and "technological" means. In: Li JJ, Nandi S, Li SA, editors. Hormonal carcinogensis. New York: Springer-Verlag; 1992. pp. 209–16.

60. Marshall E. Epidemiology. Search for a killer: focus shifts from fat to hormones. Science 1993;259:618–21.

61. Lustig RH, Hershcopf RJ, Bradlow HL. The effects of body weight and diet on estrogen metabolism and estrogen-dependent disease. In: Frisch RE, editor. Adipose tissue and reproduction. Basel: Karger; 1990. p. 107–24.

62. Key TJ, Appleby PN, Reeves GK, et al. Body mass index, serum sex hormones, and breast cancer risk in postmenopausal women. J Natl Cancer Inst 2003;95:1218–25.

63. Schneider J, Huh MM, Bradlow HL, Fishman J. Antiestrogen action of 2-hydroxyestrone on MCF-7 human breast cancer cells. J Biol Chem 1983;259:4840–5.

64. Schneider J, Bradlow HL, Strain G, et al. Effects of obesity on estradiol metabolism: decreased formation of nonuterotropic metabolites. J Clin Endocrinol Metab 1983;56:973–8.

65. Bradlow HL, Tiwari R, Sepkovic DW, Telang NT. The role of adipocytes as a breast cancer risk factor. In: *In vivo* submitted.

66. Yuan F, Chen DZ, Liu K, et al. Anti-estrogenic activities of indole-3-carbinol in cervical cells: implication for prevention of cervical cancer. Anticancer Res 1999;19:1673–80.

67. Bell MC, Crowley-Nowack P, Bradlow HL, et al. Placebo controlled trial of indole-3-carbinol in the treatment of cervical dysplasia. Gynecol Oncol 1999;78:123–9.

68. Rosen CA, Thompson JW, Woodson GE, Bradlow HL. Preliminary results of the use of indole-3-carbinol for recurrent respiratory papillomatosis. Otolaryngology 1998;118:810–5.

69. Sims EAH. Insulin resistance is a result, not a cause of obesity: Socratic debate: the con side. In: Angel A, Anderson H, Bouchard C, et al, editors. Progress in obesity research. London: Libbey; 1996. p. 587–92.

70. Ravussin E, Swinburn BA. Insulin resistance is a result, not a cause of obesity: Socratic debate: the pro side. In: Angel A, Anderson H, Bouchard C, et al, editors. Progress in obesity research. London: Libbey; 1996. p. 173–8.

71. Barakat HA, Mooney N, O'Brien K, et al. Coronary heart disease risk factors in morbidly obese women with normal glucose tolerance. Diabetes Care 1993;16:144–9.

72. Haffner SM, D'Agostino R, Saad MF, et al. Increased insulin resistance and insulin secretion in non-diabetic African-Americans and Hispanics compared with non-Hispanic whites: the insulin resistance atherosclerosis study. Diabetes 1996;45:742–8.

73. Ruige JB, Assendelft WJ, Dekker JM, et al. Insulin and risk of cardiovascular disease: a meta-analysis. Circulation 1998; 97:996–1001.

74. Despres JP, Lamarche B, Mauriege P, et al. Hyperinsulinemia as an independent risk factor for ischemic heart disease. N Engl J Med 1996;334:952–7.

75. Saydah SH, Platz EA, Rifai N, et al. Association of markers of insulin and glucose control with subsequent colorectal cancer risk. Cancer Epidemiol Biomarkers Prev 2003; 12:412–8.

76. Patel AC, Nunez NP, Perkins SN, et al. Effects of energy balance on cancer in genetically altered mice. J Nutr. 2004 Dec;134(12 Suppl):3394S-3398S

77. Grimberg A, Cohen P. Role of insulin-like growth factors and their binding proteins in growth control and carcinogenesis. J Cell Physiol 2000;183:1–9.

78. Yakar S, Liu JL, Stannard B, et al. Normal growth and development in the absence of hepatic insulin-like growth factor 1. Proc Natl Acad Sci USA 1999;96:7324–9.

79. Renehan AG, O'Connell J, O'Halloran D, et al. Acromegaly and colorectal cancer: a comprehensive review of epidemiology, biological mechanisms, and clinical implications. Horm Metab Res 2003;35:712–25.

80. Buckbinder L, Talbott R, Velasco-Miguel S, et al. Induction of the growth inhibitor IGF-binding protein 3 by p53. Nature 1995;377:646–9.

81. Kaaks R, Lukanova A. Energy balance and cancer: the role of insulin and insulin-like growth factor-1. Proc Nutr Soc 2001;60:91–106.

82. Kaaks R, Lundin E, Manjer J, et al. Prospective study of IGF-1, IGF-binding proteins, and breast cancer risk in northern and southern Sweden. Cancer Causes Control 2002;13:307–16.

83. Jandacek RA, Anderson N, Liu M, et al. Effects of yo-yo diet, caloric restriction, and olestra on tissue distribution of hexachlorobenzene. Am J Phys Gastrointest Liver Physiol 2005;288:G292–G9.

84. Steingraber S. To breastfeed or not to breastfeed is not the question: why risk-benefit analysis is the wrong way to look at the problem of breast milk contamination. The Ribbon 2003;8:4–5.

85. Harris CA, Woolridge MW, Hay AW. Factors affecting the transfer of organochlorine pesticide residues to breast milk. Chemosphere 2001;43:243–56.

86. Villa R, Bonetti E, Penza ML, et al. Target-specific action of organochlorine compounds in reproductive and non-reproductive tissues of estrogen-reporter male mice. Toxicol Appl Pharmacol 2004;201:137–48.

87. Heikens J, Ubbink MC, Van Der Pal HP, et al. Long term survivors of childhood brain cancer have an increased risk for cardiovascular disease. Cancer 2000;88:2116–21.

88. Srinivasan S, Ogle GD, Garnett SP, et al. Features of the metabolic syndrome after craniopharyngioma. J Clin Endocrinol Metab 2004;89:81–6.

89. Adams LA, Feldstein A, Lindor KD, Angulo P. Nonalcoholic fatty liver disease among patients with hypothalamic and pituitary dysfunction. Hepatology 2004;39:909–14.

90. Meacham LR, Gurney JG, Mertens AC, et al. Body mass index in long-term adult survivors of childhood cancer: a report of the Childhood Cancer Survivors Study (CCSS). Cancer. 2005 Apr 15;103(8):1730–9.

91. Didi M, Didcock E, Davies HA, et al. High incidence of obesity in young adults after treatment of acute lymphoblastic leukemia of childhood. J Pediatr. 1995;127:63–7.

92. Mayer EI, Reuter M, Dopfer RE, Ranke MB. Energy expenditure, energy intake, and prevalence of obesity after therapy for acute lymphoblastic leukemia during childhood. Hormone Research 2000;53:193–9.

93. Sainsbury CPQ, Newcombe RG, Hughes IA. Weight gain and height velocity during prolonged first remission from acute lymphoblastic leukaemia. Arch Dis Child 1985; 60:832–6.

94. Zee P, Chen CH. Prevalence of obesity in children after therapy for acute lymphoblastic leukemia. Am J Pediatr Hematol Oncol 1986;8:294–9.

95. Schell MJ, Ochs JJ, Schriock EA, Carter M. A method of predicting adult height and obesity in long-term survivors of childhood acute lymphoblastic leukemia. J Clin Oncol. 1992;10:128–33.

96. Odame I, Reilly JJ, Gibson BES, Donaldson MDC. Patterns of obesity in boys and girls after treatment for acute lymphoblastic leukaemia. Arch Dis Child 1994;71:147–9.

97. Craig F, Leiper AD, Stanhope R, et al. Sexually dimorphic and radiation dose dependent effect of cranial irradiation on body mass index. Arch Dis Child 1999;81:500–4.

98. Sklar CA, Mertens AC, Walter A, et al. Changes in body mass index and prevalence of overweight in survivors of childhood acute lymphoblastic leukemia: role of cranial irradiation. Med Pediatr Oncol 2000;35:91–5.

99. Nysom K, Holm K, Michaelsen KF, et al. Degree of fatness after treatment for acute lymphoblastic leukemia in childhood. J Clin Endocrinol Metab 1999;84:4591–6.

100. Ross JA, Oeffinger KC, Davies SM, et al. Genetic variation in the leptin receptor gene and obesity in survivors of childhood acute lymphoblastic leukemia: a report from the Childhood Cancer Survivor Study. J Clin Oncol 2004; 22:3558–62.

101. Lustig RH, Post SM, Srivannaboon K, et al. Risk factors for the development of obesity in children surviving brain tumors. J Clin Endocrinol Metab 2003;88:611–6.

102. Gurney JG, Kadan-Lottick NS, Packer RJ, et al. Endocrine and cardiovascular late effects among adult survivors of childhood brain tumors: Childhood Cancer Survivor Study. Cancer 2003;97:663–73.

103. Daousi C, Dunn AJ, Foy PM, et al. Endocrine and neuroanatomic predictors of weight gain and obesity in adult patients with hypothalamic damage. Am J Med 2005 Jan;118(1):45-50

104. Fahlbusch R, Honegger J, Paulus W, et al. Surgical treatment of craniopharyngioma: experience with 168 patients. J Neurosurgery 1999;90:237–50.

105. Pinkney J, Wilding J, Williams G, MacFarlane I. Hypothalamic obesity in humans: what do we know and what can be done? Obes Rev 2002;3:27–34.

106. Stahnke N, Grubel G, Lagenstein I, Willig RP. Long-term follow-up of children with craniopharyngioma. Eur J Pediatr 1984;142:179–85.

107. Sorva R. Children with craniopharyngioma: early growth failure and rapid post-operative weight gain. Acta Pediatrica Scandanavica 1988;77:587–92.

108. Pinto G, Bussieres L, Recasens C, et al. Hormonal factors influencing weight and growth pattern in craniopharyngioma. Horm Res 2000;53:163–9.

109. Bray GA, Inoue S, Nishizawa Y. Hypothalamic obesity. Diabetologia 1981;20:366–77.

110. Lustig RH. Hypothalamic obesity: the sixth cranial endocrinopathy. Endocrinologist 2002;12:210–7.

111. Babinski MJ. Tumeur du corps pituitaire san acromegalie et avec arret de developpement des organes genitaux. Rev Neurol 1900;8:531–3.

112. Frohlich A. Ein fall von tumor der hypophysis cerebri ohne akromegalie. Weiner Klin Rdsch 1901;15:883–6.

113. Elmquist JK, Elias CF, Saper CB. From lesions to leptin: hypothalamic control of food intake and body weight. Neuron 1999;22:221–32.

114. Schwartz MW, Figlewicz DP, Baskin DG, et al. Insulin and the central regulation of energy balance: update 1994. Endocrine Reviews 1994;2:109–13.

115. Kojima M, Hosoda H, Date Y, et al. Ghrelin is a growth-hormone-releasing acylated peptide from stomach. Nature 1999;402:656–60.

116. Batterham RL, Cowley MA, Small CJ, et al. Gut hormone PYY$_{3-36}$ physiologically inhibits food intake. Nature 2002; 418:650–4.

117. Lustig RH. The neuroendocrinology of obesity. Endocrinol Metab Clin North Am 2001;30:765–85.

118. Montague CT, Farooqi IS, Whitehead JP, et al. Congenital leptin deficiency is associated with severe early-onset obesity in humans. Nature 1997;387:903–8.

119. Clement K, Vaisse C, Lahlou N, et al. A mutation in the human leptin receptor gene causes obesity and pituitary dysfunction. Nature 1998;392:398–401.

120. Vaisse C, Clement K, Durand E, et al. Melanocortin-4 receptor mutations are a frequent and heterogeneous cause of morbid obesity. J Clin Invest 2000;106:253–62.

121. Boss O, Bachman E, Vidal-Puig A, et al. Role of the β_3-adrenergic receptor and/or a putative β_3-adrenergic receptor on the expression of uncoupling proteins and peroxisome proliferator-activated receptor-γ coactivator-1. Biochem Biophys Res Commun 1999;261:870–6.
122. Lowell BB, Spiegelman BM. Towards a molecular understanding of adaptive thermogenesis. Nature 2000;404: 652–60.
123. Bray GA, Gallagher TF. Manifestations of hypothalamic obesity in man: a comprehensive investigation of eight patients and a review of the literature. Medicine 1975; 54:301–33.
124. Bray GA. Syndromes of hypothalamic obesity in man. Pediatr Ann 1984;13:525–36.
125. Reeves AG, Plum F. Hyperphagia, rage, and dementia accompanying a ventromedial hypothalamic neoplasm. Arch Neurol 1972;20:616–24.
126. Bray GA, York DA. Hypothalamic and genetic obesity in experimental animals: an autonomic and endocrine hypothesis. Physiol Rev 1979;59:719–809.
127. Muller HL, Emser A, Faldum A, et al. Longitudinal study of growth and body mass index before and after diagnosis of childhood craniopharyngioma. J Clin Endocrinol Metab 2004;89:3298–305.
128. Murray RD, Adams JE, Shalet SM. Adults with partial growth hormone deficiency have an adverse body composition. J Clin Endocrinol Metab 2004;89:1586–91.
129. Berthoud HR, Jeanrenaud B. Acute hyperinsulinemia and its reversal by vagotomy following lesions of the ventromedial hypothalamus in anesthetized rats. Endocrinology 1979;105:146–51.
130. Rohner-Jeanrenaud F, Jeanrenaud B. Consequences of ventromedial hypothalamic lesions upon insulin and glucagon secretion by subsequently isolated perfused pancreases in the rat. J Clin Invest 1980;65:902–10.
131. Jeanrenaud B. An hypothesis on the aetiology of obesity: dysfunction of the central nervous system as a primary cause. Diabetologia 1985;28:502–13.
132. Satoh N, Ogawa Y, Katsura G, et al. Pathophysiological significance of the obese gene product, leptin in ventromedial hypothalamus (VMH)-lesioned rats: evidence for loss of its satiety effect in VMH-lesioned rats. Endocrinology 1997;138:947–54.
133. Bray GA, Nishizawa Y. Ventromedial hypothalamus modulates fat mobilization during fasting. Nature 1978; 274:900–2.
134. Sklar CA. Craniopharyngioma: endocrine sequelae of treatment. Pediatr Neurosurg 1994;21:120–3.
135. Schwartz MW, Woods SC, Porte D, et al. Central nervous system control of food intake. Nature 2000;404:661–71.
136. Baskin DG, Wilcox BJ, Figlewicz DP, Dorsa DM. Insulin and insulin-like growth factors in the CNS. Trends Neurosci 1988;11:107–11.
137. Baura GD, Foster DM, Porte D, et al. Saturable transport of insulin from plasma into the central nervous system of dogs in vivo: a mechanism for regulated insulin delivery to the brain. J Clin Invest 1993;92:1824–30.
138. VanderWeele DA. Insulin is a prandial satiety hormone. Physiol Behav 1994;56:619–22.
139. Woods SC, Lotter EC, McKay LD, Porte D. Chronic intracerebroventricular infusion of insulin reduces food intake and body weight of baboons. Nature 1979;282:503–5.
140. McGowan MK, Andrews KM, Grossman SP. Role of intrahypothalamic insulin in circadian patterns of food intake, activity, and body temperature. Behav Neurosci 1992; 106:380–5.
141. Brüning JC, Gautam D, Burks DJ, et al. Role of brain insulin receptor in control of body weight and reproduction. Science 2000;289:2122–5.
142. Lin X, Taguchi A, Park S, et al. Dysregulation of insulin receptor substrate 2 in β-cells and brain causes obesity and diabetes. J Clin Invest 2004;114:908–16.
143. Moran TH, Ladenheim EE. Identification of receptor populations mediating the satiating actions of brain and gut peptides. In: Smith GP, editor. Satiation: from gut to brain. New York: Oxford; 1998. p. 126–63.
144. Kalra SP, Dube MG, Pu S, et al. Interacting appetite-regulating pathways in the hypothalamic regulation of body weight. Endocr Rev 1999;20:68–100.
145. Lustig RH. The neuroendocrinology of childhood obesity. Pediatr Clin North Am 2001;48:909–30.
146. Elmquist JK, Ahima RS, Elias CF, et al. Leptin activates distinct projections from the dorsomedial and ventromedial hypothalamic nuclei. Proc Natl Acad Sci 1998; 95:741–6.
147. Small CJ, Bloom SR. Gut hormones and the control of appetite. Trends Endocrinol Metab 2004;15:259–63.
148. Kamegai J, Tamura H, Shimizu T, et al. Central effect of ghrelin, an endogenous growth hormone secretagogue, on hypothalamic peptide gene expression. Endocrinology 2000;141:4797–800.
149. Tschöp M, Smiley DL, Heiman ML. Ghrelin induces adiposity in rodents. Nature 2000;407:908–13.
150. Thornton JE, Cheung CC, Clifton DK, Steiner RA. Regulation of hypothalamic proopiomelanocortin mRNA by leptin in ob/ob mice. Endocrinology 1997;138:5063–6.
151. Marin P, Russeffé-Scrive A, Smith J, Bjorntorp P. Glucose uptake in human adipose tissue. Metabolism 1988;36: 1154–64.
152. Ramsay TG. Fat cells. Endocrinol Metab Clin North Am 1996;25:847–70.
153. Powley TL, Laughton W. Neural pathways involved in the hypothalamic integration of autonomic responses. Diabetologia 1981;20:378–87.
154. D'Alessio DA, Kieffer TJ, Taborsky GJ, Havel PJ. Activation of the parasympathetic nervous system is necessary for normal meal induced-insulin secretion in rhesus macaques. J Clin Endocrinol Metab 2001;86:1253–9.
155. Ahren B, Holst J. The cephalic insulin response to meal ingestion in humans is dependent on both cholinergic and noncholingergic mechanisms and is important for postprandial glycemia. Diabetes 2001;50:1030–8.
156. Lee HC, Curry DL, Stern JS. Direct effect of CNS on insulin hypersecretion in obese Zucker rats: involvement of vagus nerve. Am J Physiol 1989;256:E439–E44.
157. Tokunaga K, Fukushima M, Kemnitz JW, Bray GA. Effect of vagotomy on serum insulin in rats with paraventricular or ventromedial hypothalamic lesions. Endocrinology 1986;119:1708–11.
158. Inoue S, Bray GA. The effect of subdiaphragmatic vagotomy in rats with ventromedial hypothalamic lesions. Endocrinology 1977;100:108–14.
159. Gilon P, Henquin JC. Mechanisms and physiological significance of the cholinergic control of pancreatic β-cell function. Endocr Rev 2001;22:565–604.
160. Miura Y, Gilon P, Henquin JC. Muscarinic stimulation increases Na^+ entry in pancreatic β-cells by a mechanism other than the emptying of intracellular Ca^{2+} pools. Biochem Biophys Res Commun 1996;224:67–73.
161. Zawalich WS, Zawalich KC, Rasmussen H. Cholinergic agonists prime the β-cell to glucose stimulation. Endocrinology 1989;125:2400–6.
162. Nishi S, Seino Y, Ishida H, Seno M, Taminato T, Sakurai H, et al. Vagal regulation of insulin, glucagon, and somatostatin secretion in vitro in the rat. J Clin Invest 1987; 79:1191–6.
163. Komeda K, Yokote M, Oki Y. Diabetic syndrome in the Chinese hamster induced with monosodium glutamate. Experientia 1980;36:232–4.
164. Yamada M, Miyakawa T, Duttaroy A, et al. Mice lacking the M3 muscarinic acetylcholine receptor are hypophagic and lean. Nature 2001;410:207–12.
165. Tian YM, Urquidi V, Ashcroft SJH. Protein kinase C in β-cells: expression of multiple isoforms and involvement in cholinergic stimulation of insulin secretion. Mol Cell Endocrinol 1996;119:185–93.
166. Arbuzova A, Murray D, McLaughlin S. MARCKS, membranes, and calmodulin: kinetics of their interaction. Biochimica et Biophysica Acta 1998;1376:369–79.
167. Blondel O, Bell GI, Moody M, et al. Creation of an inositol 1,4,5-triphosphate-sensitive Ca^{2+} store in secretory granules of insulin-producing cells. J Biol Chem 1994;269: 27167–70.
168. Rocca AS, Brubaker PL. Role of the vagus nerve in mediating proximal nutrient-induced glucagon-like peptide-1 secretion. Endocrinology 1999;140:1687–94.
169. Kiefer TJ, Habener JF. The glucagon-like peptides. Endocr Rev 1999;20:876–913.
170. Harz KJ, Muller HL, Waldeck E, et al. Obesity in patients with craniopharyngioma: assessment of food intake and movement counts indicating physical activity. J Clin Endocrinol Metab 2003;88:5227–31.
171. Schofl C, Schleth A, Berger D, et al. Sympathoadrenal counterregulation in patients with hypothalamic craniopharyngioma. J Clin Endocrinol Metab 2002;87:624–9.
172. Coutant R, Maurey H, Rouleau S, et al. Defect in epinephrine production in children with craniopharyngioma: functional or organic origin? J Clin Endocrinol Metab 2003; 88:5969–75.
173. al-Adsani H, Hoffer LJ, Silva JE. Resting energy expenditure is sensitive to small dose changes in patients on chronic thyroid hormone replacement. J Clin Endocrinol Metab 1997;82:1118–25.
174. Geffner ME. The growth without growth hormone syndrome. Endocrinol Metab Clin North Am 1996;25: 649–63.
175. Olney RC, Mougey EB. Expression of the components of the insulin-like growth factor axis across the growth plate. Mol Cell Endocrinol 1999;156:63–71.
176. Lustig RH, Rose SR, Burghen GA, et al. Hypothalamic obesity in children caused by cranial insult: altered glucose and insulin dynamics, and reversal by a somatostatin agonist. J Pediatr 1999;135:162–8.
177. Lustig RH, Hinds PS, Ringwald-Smith K, et al. Octreotide therapy of pediatric hypothalamic obesity: a double-blind, placebo-controlled trial. J Clin Endocrinol Metab 2003;88:2586–92.
178. Preeyasombat C, Bacchetti P, Lazar AA, Lustig RH. Racial and etiopathologic dichotomies in insulin secretion and resistance in obese children. Journal of Pediatrics. J Pediatr 2005;146:474–81.
179. Smith DK, Sarfeh J, Howard L. Truncal vagotomy in hypothalmic obesity. Lancet 1983;1:1330–1.
180. Fobi MA. Operations that are questionable for the control of obesity. Obes Surg 1993;3:197–200.
181. Mason PW, Krawiecki N, Meacham LR. The use of dextroamphetamine to treat obesity and hyperphagia in children treated for craniopharyngioma. Arch Pediatr Adolesc Med 2002;156:887–92.
182. Molloy PT, Berkowitz R, Stallings VA, et al. Pilot study of evaluation and treatment of tumor-related obesity in pediatric patients with hypothalamic/chiasmatic gliomas and craniopharyngiomas. International Pediatric Oncology Meeting 1998;Rome, Italy:156.
183. Grant DB, Dunger DB, Burns EC. Long-term treatment with diazoxide in childhood hyperinsulinism. Acta Endocrinologica 1986;279:340–5.
184. Tabachnick IA, Gulbenkian A, Seidman F. The effect of a benzothiadiazine, diazoxide, on carbohydrate metabolism. Diabetes 1964;13:408–18.
185. Kvam DC, Stanton HC. Studies on diazoxide hyperglycemia. Diabetes 1964;13:639–44.
186. Hsu WH, Xiang HD, Rajan AS, et al. Somatostatin inhibits insulin secretion by a G-protein-mediated decrease in Ca^{2+} entry through voltage-dependent Ca^{2+} channels in the beta-cell. J Biol Chem 1991;266:837–43.
187. Mitra SW, Mezey E, Hunyady B, et al. Colocalization of somatostatin receptor sst5 and insulin in rat pancreatic β-cells. Endocrinology 1999;140:3790–6.
188. Lamberts SWJ, Van Der Lely AJ, De Herder WW, Hofland LJ. Drug therapy: octreotide. N Engl J Med 1996;334: 246–54.
189. Bertoli A, Magnaterra R, Borboni P, et al. Dose-dependent effect of octreotide on insulin secretion after OGTT in obesity. Hormone Research 1998;49:17–21.
190. Varni J, Katz E, Seid M, et al. The Pediatric Cancer Quality of Life Inventory-32 (PCQL-32). Cancer 1998;82:1184–96.
191. Sanford RA. Craniopharyngioma: results of survey of the American Society of Pediatric Neurosurgery. Pediatric Neurosurgery 1994;21(Suppl):39–43.
192. Eisenstat DD. Craniopharyngioma. Curr Treat Options Neurol. 2001 Jan;3(1):77–88.
193. Saminic C, Gridley G, Chow WH. Obesity and cancer risk among white and black United States veterans. Cancer Causes Control 2004;15:35–44.
194. Okasha M, McCarron P, McEwen J, Smith GD. Body mass index in young adulthood and cancer mortality: a retrospective cohort study. J Epidemiol Comm Health 2002;56: 780–4.
195. Inoue M, Sobue T, Tsugane S, JPHC Study Group. Impact of body mass index on the risk of total cancer incidence and mortality among middle-aged Japanese: data from a large-scale population-based cohort study—the JPHC study. Cancer Causes Control 2004;15:671–80.
196. Porter MP, Stanford JL. Obesity and the risk of prostate cancer. Prostate 2004;62:316–21.
197. Babagas JR, Lopez-Garcia E, Gutierrez-Fisac JL, et al. A simple estimate of mortality attributable to excess weight in the European Union. Eur J Clin Nutr 2003;57:201–8.
198. Moller H, Mellengaard A, Lindvig K, Olsen JH. Obesity and cancer risk: a Danish record-linkage study. Eur J Cancer 1994;30A:344–50.
199. Lustig RH, Preeyasombat C, Lazar AA, Bacchetti P. Insulin hypersecretion vs. insulin resistance in obese children: categorization by race and etiopathogenesis, and implications for therapy. Soc Pediatr Res 2004.
200. Lustig RH. Autonomic dysfunction of the β-cell and the pathogenesis of obesity. Rev Endocr Metab Disord 2003; 4:23–32.

Thyroid Disorders in Cancer Patients

Steven I. Sherman, MD

As observed by Osler, "the thyroid gland supplies some essential secretion of first importance,"[1] and knowledge of the normal and diseased functions of the thyroid is essential in the care of the cancer patient. Disorders of the thyroid gland occur commonly in an oncology practice, with the potential for confounding diagnostic evaluation of the malignant disease, for complicating antineoplastic treatments, and for increasing mortality in cancer patients.[2] Similarly, abnormalities of the thyroid are common consequences of cancer or the treatment of cancer. These effects on the thyroid often develop years and decades after cure of the malignant disease, necessitating long-term follow-up and awareness of the risk for thyroid abnormalities by the treating oncologist and subsequent care providers.

Physiology of the Hypothalamic-Pituitary-Thyroid Axis

The primary role of the thyroid gland is to produce thyroxine (T_4) and triiodothyronine (T_3), hormones that influence a broad variety of metabolic processes throughout the body. The synthesis of T_4 and T_3 begins with the active transport of iodide into the cell via an intrinsic plasma membrane sodium-iodide symporter.[3] Following oxidation by thyroid peroxidase, the iodide moiety is covalently attached to tyrosyl residues of thyroglobulin, and the resulting iodotyrosines are coupled and cleaved from thyroglobulin to form T_4 and T_3, normally in a 10:1 ratio.[4] This process results in the total daily output of 80 to 100 µg of T_4. In contrast, only 20% of circulating T_3 is produced by the thyroid, the remaining 80% deriving from the enzymatic outer-ring or 5'-monodeiodination of T_4 in extrathyroidal tissues such as the liver, kidney, brain, muscle, and skin.[5] Removal of the inner-ring 5-iodine of T_4 forms the inactive metabolite reverse T_3 (rT_3). Similar to hepatic drug disposal mechanisms, other thyroid hormone inactivating pathways include glucuronidation, sulfation, deamination, and cleavage.[6]

In serum, at least 99.95% of T_4 and 99.5% of T_3 molecules are bound by the transport proteins thyroxine-binding globulin (TBG), transthyretin (thyroxine-binding prealbumin), and albumin.[7]

Although TBG is present in lower concentration than either transthyretin or albumin, its greater affinity for thyroid hormones makes it the predominant serum carrier of T_4 and T_3. This large pool of protein-bound hormone provides a stable reservoir that maintains the supply of free, unbound hormone available for transport into the cells. Once within target cells, T_4 is converted by the enzyme 5'-deiodinase to T_3, which in the nucleus binds to a heterodimerized thyroid hormone receptor, modulating transcription of thyroid hormone-responsive genes and producing the clinical effects recognized as the metabolic effects of thyroid hormones.

The primary regulatory influence on thyroid gland function is the circulating level of thyrotropin (thyroid stimulating hormone [TSH]). Produced by thyrotroph cells of the anterior pituitary, TSH is a two-subunit glycoprotein, the specificity of which is conferred by its β-subunit; the α-subunit is structurally similar to that of follicle stimulating hormone, luteinizing hormone, and human chorionic gonadotropin. Negative feedback by T_4 and T_3 influences TSH synthesis and release, yielding a log-linear relationship between the serum concentrations of TSH and free T_4.[8,9] The hypothalamic tripeptide thyrotropin-releasing hormone (TRH) stimulates TSH secretion and modulates thyrotroph response to altered thyroid hormone levels. In conjunction with the suppressive effects of dopamine, corticosteroids, somatostatin, androgens, and endogenous opioids, TRH may be responsible for establishing the set-point for the negative feedback loop that controls thyroid hormone levels. Hypothalamic production of TRH itself is regulated by circulating thyroid hormones, as well as by multiple central nervous system factors.

TSH also functions as a trophic hormone for thyroid follicular cells. By binding to its cognate receptor on the plasma membrane, TSH triggers activation of multiple downstream signaling cascades through G-protein–linked adenylyl cyclases, phospholipases, phosphatidylinositol-3-kinases, and small GTPases. Downstream effectors of the actions of TSH include mitogen-activated protein kinases (MAPKs), c-jun N-terminal kinases (JNKs), and extracellular signal-regulated kinases (ERKs), which subsequently regulate thyrocyte proliferation, differentiation, and apoptosis.[10]

Hypothyroidism

Hypothyroidism is the clinical state resulting from an insufficient amount of circulating thyroid hormone to support normal body functions. Gull first described the adult form of hypothyroidism, referring to it as "a cretinoid state supervening in adult life."[11] That hypothyroidism occurs more commonly in women or is increasingly prevalent with advancing age did not escape Gull, or Vanderpump and Tunbridge . The prevalence of overt hypothyroidism, defined as the combination of clinical and biochemical findings of hypothyroidism, is approximately 1 to 2% in the general population and is about 10 times higher in women than in men.[12] Subclinical hypothyroidism, generally defined as a serum TSH between 5 and 20 mU/L in asymptomatic patients, occurs with a frequency of 2.5 to 10% but rises as high as 20% in women over age 70.[13,14]

Clinical Manifestations

The clinical signs and symptoms of hypothyroidism occur as a result of deficient thyroid hormone actions. Because chronic primary hypothyroidism usually develops over a span of years, the clinical features may develop insidiously and not be readily noticed. In contrast, severe hypothyroidism occurring following thyroid resection, thyroiditis, or pituitary resection is usually associated with a more subacute onset of symptoms. Complicating the recognition of hypothyroidism is the non-specific nature of symptoms, likely to be even more confusing in cancer patients. Among patients in a general medical practice presenting with the most common symptoms of hypothyroidism (constipation, weight gain, menstrual irregularities, fatigue, depression, cold intolerance, and galactorrhea), only 4% will actually be hypothyroid, and fewer than 2% will have a TSH level at least 5 mU/L more than normal.[15] In studies of patients with either solid or hematologic malignancies, the high prevalence of fatigue correlates poorly with biochemical evidence of hypothyroidism.[16,17] Even among long-term survivors of Hodgkin's disease, of whom the majority develop hypothyroidism, there is little evidence of an association between fatigue and the diagnosis of untreated hypothyroidism.[18,19] In contrast, symptoms and signs (including slow movements, coarse skin, decreased sweating, hoarseness, paresthesia, cold intolerance, periorbital edema, and delayed deep tendon reflex relaxation) may be more specific but have not been evaluated for their diagnostic value in cancer patients.

Nonetheless, an appreciation of the clinical manifestations of hypothyroidism is necessary to provide a degree of clinical suspicion for the diagnosis. Several manifestations of particular note in patients with cancer are discussed below.

The Neuromuscular System

Myopathies associated with malignancies, such as polymyositis and myasthenia gravis, may also be seen more commonly in hypothyroidism. The association of myasthenia gravis and hypothyroidism, may be of particular relevance in evaluating patients with thymoma.[20,21] Increased serum levels of creatine kinase (CK) are frequently found in hypothyroidism, regardless of the presence of overt myopathy. Fractionation studies revealed a preponderance of the MM isotype.[22] The elevated CK level is likely related to both a decrease in the enzyme clearance rate in hypothyroidism and sarcoplasmic damage. Aldolase, aspartate transaminase, and lactate dehydrogenase levels are also elevated, but are less sensitive or specific indicators of muscle dysfunction. Neuropathic symptoms such as paresthesia, painful dysesthesia, focal muscle weakness, and deafness can all result from compression of peripheral nerves. Central nervous system dysfunction in hypothyroidism can cause a wide variety of signs and symptoms that are also seen as a consequence of malignant disease and therapy. Typical encephalopathic findings in severe hypothyroidism include lethargy, depression, and impairment of memory without other evidence of intellectual deficits. Cerebellar ataxia can occur, characterized by gait disturbance, dysarthric speech, intention tremors, dysmetria and poor coordination.

The Cardiovascular System

Patients with thyroid hormone deficiency commonly present with inotropic and chronotropic cardiac abnormalities, including bradycardia and congestive failure. Reversible dilated cardiomyopathy can rarely be secondary to hypothyroidism.[23] Care must be exercised in the use of digitalis glycosides, as clearance is slowed and toxicity more likely. Pericardial effusion can contribute to enlargement of the cardiac silhouette in hypothyroid patients, although the development is sufficiently slow that tamponade is rarely observed. Increased systemic vascular resistance is commonly seen, along with diastolic hypertension. The cardiovascular effects of hypothyroidism can occur acutely, especially when thyroid cancer patients are withdrawn from their thyroxine therapy in anticipation of radioactive iodine treatment.[24]

The Respiratory System

Both hypoxic and hypercapnic ventilatory drives are impaired, leading to alveolar hypoventilation.[25] Pleural effusions are occasionally found in hypothyroidism, although usually in association with pericardial and peritoneal effusions.[26,27] As a result of increased capillary permeability, hypothyroid pleural effusates have moderate protein elevation. The volume of effusion is generally small, and the patients asymptomatic.

The Gastrointestinal System

Constipation, obstipation, or even megacolon due to decreased gut motility may be the cardinal presenting feature of hypothyroidism, with increased sensitivity to the effects of opiate analgesics.[28–30] Intestinal absorption is generally normal in hypothyroidism, although myxedematous infiltration of intestinal mucosa can rarely cause malabsorption. Patients with autoimmune thyroiditis are at increased risk for the development of pernicious anemia and achlorhydria due to atrophic gastritis. Aspartate transaminase levels may be increased due to impaired metabolic clearance of the muscle-derived enzyme.[31] The yellowish appearance that may be noted in the skin of hypothyroid patients, due to hypercarotenemia, should not be confused with jaundice; scleral and mucous membranes are generally anicteric.

The Integumentary System

The hypothyroid skin is generally pale with a tinge of yellowish discoloration, owing to the combined effects of elevated serum and tissue carotene levels (a consequence of the decrease in carotene metabolism), anemia, alopecia, and decreased cutaneous blood flow. It is also accompanied by non-pitting edema, secondary to increased accumulation of mucopolysaccharides and fluids in the dermis. Typically, this swelling is most marked around the eyes and hands. The skin also feels dry and cool, related to the decrease in eccrine and apocrine secretion. Peripheral vasoconstriction contributes to the cool sensation of the skin.[32]

The Hematopoietic System

Mild anemia is a common feature in hypothyroidism, occurring in about 25% of untreated patients.[33,34] Although decreased plasma volume may mitigate the reduction in total red cell mass, normochromic normocytic anemia is a consequence of decreased erythropoietin synthesis.[34] In general, red cell survival appears to be normal in hypothyroidism. Except for iron deficiency due to hypothyroidism-induced hypermenorrhea, thyroid hormone deficiency rarely affects serum ferritin, iron, or total iron binding capacity.[33] Macrocytic anemia can result from

malabsorption of either folate or vitamin B_{12}. As many as 10% of patients with hypothyroidism due to autoimmune thyroiditis have pernicious anemia.[34,35] Hypothyroid dyslipidemia can lead to increased membrane lipid content, also causing macrocytosis.

White blood cell and platelet counts are usually normal in hypothyroidism, unless there is coexistent pernicious anemia or folate deficiency causing low cell counts. Despite reports of decreased platelet adhesiveness, few hypothyroid patients abnormal bleeding times.[36] Similarly, decreased levels of factors VIII, IX, XI, and XII may be seen as a result of the general decrease in protein synthesis.[36,37] Fibrinolytic activity is also decreased.[37] However, clinically significant bleeding is infrequent.

Endocrine and Metabolic Systems

Hyperprolactinemia is common in primary hypothyroidism, due to stimulation of the lactotroph by thyrotropin-releasing hormone, and occasionally leading to galactorrhea. In severe cases of primary hypothyroidism, thyrotroph hyperplasia may occur, misidentified in sellar imaging as a mass lesion.

Despite delayed cortisol clearance in hypothyroidism, cortisol production rates and circadian rhythmicity remain essentially normal.[38] Direct stimulation of adrenal glands with adrenocorticotropic hormone (ACTH) frequently yields normal cortisol responses.[39] However, cortisol response to insulin-induced hypoglycemia may be subnormal, indicating slightly impaired hypothalamic-pituitary control over cortisol production.[40]

Hypothyroidism can be a cause of euvolemic hyponatremia, even in patients otherwise at risk for the syndrome of inappropriate antidiuretic hormone. Free water clearance is often decreased, which can be demonstrated by delayed water excretion following an acute water loading test.[41] Urine osmolality is inappropriately elevated for the degree of plasma hypo-osmolality. Although increased antidiuretic hormone secretion has been reported, vasopressin response to a saline-loading test is generally normal.[42] Postoperative hyponatremia occurs more commonly in unsuspected hypothyroid patients.[43]

Hypothyroidism leads to decreased oxygen consumption and carbon dioxide production, yielding a decreased basal metabolic rate. Substrate catabolism is reduced, and weight gain can be secondary to increased fat stores as well as fluid retention.

Altered pharmacokinetics of many medications occurs in hypothyroidism, including impaired metabolic clearance due to decreased hepatic levels of P450 and P450-reductase.[44] Studies of primary hepatocytes demonstrate that thyroid hormone negatively regulates the transcription of CYP3A4 and may increase expression of CYP1A2 , changes which, in theory, could affect metabolism of drugs such as paclitaxel, docetaxel, tamoxifen, flutamide, vincristine, vinblastine, doxorubicin, and etoposide.[45,46] Of particular importance is delayed clearance of drugs with a narrow therapeutic range, such as digoxin, theophylline, and phenytoin. Because catabolism of vitamin K–dependent clotting factors is decreased, warfarin requirements may be paradoxically increased in hypothyroidism, and doses may need to be reduced following thyroid hormone replacement therapy.[47] Although studies have not been published detailing the effect of hypothyroidism on the metabolism of specific chemotherapies in cancer patients, it is nonetheless reasonable to ensure that patients participating in pharmacokinetic studies of drugs metabolized by either CYP3A4 or CYP1A2 have hypothyroidism excluded or treated first.

Etiology and Pathophysiology

Primary hypothyroidism, due to direct impairment of the gland's capacity to produce thyroid hormone, constitutes the great majority of the cases. In iodine-replete regions, autoimmune thyroid diseases and thyroablative therapy cause the majority of cases of primary hypothyroidism. Although most patients with chronic hypothyroidism are treated with thyroid hormone replacement therapy, regardless of the etiology, the cause of hypothyroidism should be determined in each patient. This is especially true in cases of secondary or tertiary hypothyroidism, in which concomitant hormonal insufficiencies may also require therapy. Reversible hypothyroidism may also occur due to transient thyroiditis, or drugs and food with antithyroid effects.

Autoimmune Thyroid Disease

Both humoral and cell-mediated immune mechanisms have been implicated in the pathogenesis of autoimmune thyroiditis, the primary cause of chronic primary hypothyroidism. Circulating antibodies to thyroid peroxidase (TPO) and thyroglobulin are present in up to 95% and 70%, respectively,[48] of patients with chronic autoimmune thyroiditis, but they are not likely to be pathogenetic despite the ability of anti-TPO antibodies to fix complement.[49] However, significant titers of these antibodies may identify euthyroid patients at risk of developing overt thyroid failure.[50] Uncommonly, antibodies that interfere with binding of TSH to its receptor on the follicular cell can block physiologic thyroid stimulation.[51]

In contrast, cell-mediated immunity due to failure of T cell tolerance is the predominant mechanism leading to chronic autoimmune thyroiditis. Under stimulation from interferon-γ-containing T cells, thyrocytes in autoimmune thyroiditis express antigen-presenting MHC class II molecules that can then bind to T cell receptors to induce activation of CD4 T cells.[52] The thyroid gland is infiltrated by lymphocytes characterized by Th1 differentiation. A variety of secreted cytokines directly affect thyroid follicular cells, including expression of Fas stimulated by interleukin-1 (IL-1); inhibition of the sodium-iodine symporter by interferon-γ, IL-1, and tumor necrosis factor; and expression of intercellular adhesion molecule-1 which can then trigger binding to lymphocyte function-associated antigen-1 and increased T cell-mediated cytotoxicity.[53,54] The key role of the immune system in chronic thyroiditis is underscored by reports of passage of thyroid autoimmunity from donor to recipients of marrow and stem cell transplantation.[55,56] Once initiated, the rate of decline of thyroid function in patients with chronic autoimmune thyroiditis is typically slow, with only about 5% of affected women developing overt hypothyroidism yearly.[50] Acute exposure to large amounts of stable iodine, such as following infusion of iodinated radiographic contrast media containing 150 to 500 mg iodine per milliliter, can produce transient hypothyroidism, especially in patients with euthyroid autoimmune thyroiditis.[57,58]

Transient hypothyroidism may occur as part of the course of silent thyroiditis, typically of autoimmune etiology, and granulomatous subacute thyroiditis.[59] These disorders are characterized by subacute development of thyroid inflammation, typically without death of follicular cells. The initial inflammatory phase may produce thyrotoxicosis due to release of preformed thyroid hormone from disrupted follicles. Because the hyperthyroid phase is often clinically overlooked, patients frequently present during the hypothyroid phase that develops in 50 to 75% of patients, lasting up to several months. However, about 5% develop permanent hypothyroidism.

Both transient and chronic hypothyroidism occur frequently in patients treated with various cytokines for malignancy. An association between therapy with interferon-α (IFN-α) and thyroiditis was first recognized in patients treated for carcinoid tumors and breast cancer.[60,61] Because of overlapping symptomatology between hypothyroidism and interferon toxicity, such as fatigue, hair loss, myalgia, and weight gain, the diagnosis of hypothyroidism is often overlooked. IFN-induced thyroiditis can be autoimmune, similar to Hashimoto's disease and silent thyroiditis, as well as non-autoimmune, subacute thyroiditis.[62] Although the frequency of IFN-induced thyroiditis is highest in patients treated for hepatitis C rather than cancer, risk factors for developing hypothyroidism include female gender, longer duration of IFN-α therapy, and older age. Preexisting autoimmune thyroiditis, evidenced by the presence of anti-TPO antibodies before IFN therapy, increases the risk of thyroid dysfunction to 60% from 3 to 6%.[63]

Treatment with IL-2 is associated with a significant risk of hypothyroidism—up to 35% during therapy and 14% permanently.[64,65] Cumulative dose and duration of therapy with IL-2, along with female gender and preexisting autoimmune thyroid disease, increase the risk of subsequent thyroid dysfunction.[66] In patients treated with both IL-2 and IFN-α, the risk of thyroid abnormalities, primarily transient biphasic thyroiditis, can approach 90%. Thyroiditis leading to hypothyroidism has also been described in a significant proportion of patients treated with low-dose IL-2 combined with peptide vaccines for advanced melanoma, along with a wide variety of other autoimmune phenomena.[67] Use of monoclonal antibodies directed against the immunomodulatory protein CTLA-4 has also been associated with developing autoimmune thyroiditis.[68,69] Recently, transient fulminant thyroiditis leading to hypothyroidism was reported in patients with mycosis fungoides treated with denileukin diftitox, a novel fusion protein comprised of the cytotoxic diphtheria toxin and the ligand binding domain of IL-2.[70]

Postablative Hypothyroidism

Transient hypothyroidism can occur in patients who undergo surgical resection of a single thyroid lobe for nodular disease. Permanent hypothyroidism occurs in up to 25% of cases, especially if autoimmune thyroiditis is also present.[71,72] Following radioiodine therapy for Graves' disease, most patients eventually develop permanent postablative hypothyroidism.

External beam radiotherapy for lymphoma or head and neck carcinomas are usually given in doses of more than 20 gray (Gy) (2,000 rad). Thyroidal exposure is sufficient to produce hypothyroidism even in patients treated with total body irradiation before marrow transplantation, and the risk of eventual hypothyroidism increases with higher doses.[73–75] The frequency of hypothyroidism may be as high as 65% if laryngectomy or partial thyroidectomy is also performed.[76] As with other causes of postablative hypothyroidism, subclinical hypothyroidism may be present for many years before disease becomes symptomatic. In survivors of childhood Hodgkin's disease treated with radiotherapy, the relative risk of developing hypothyroidism within 20 years was 17, compared with sibling controls.[77] In addition to external radiotherapy, internal radiation emitters, such as (131)I-MIBG used in treatment of neuroblastoma or pheochromocytoma, can cause long-term hypothyroidism in a majority of patients, despite pretreatment prophylaxis with potassium iodide.[78]

Central Hypothyroidism

Owing to the trophic and regulatory effects of TSH on the thyroid gland, disorders of TSH production or function can cause hypothyroidism. However, even in the absence of TSH, a basal level of thyroid hormone synthesis persists. Therefore, circulating T_4 and T_3 levels are typically not as low in central hypothyroidism as they are in primary thyroidal failure.[79]

More common causes of central hypothyroidism are acquired destructive processes affecting the pituitary gland. These generally produce multiple pituitary hormone deficiencies, although any combination is possible. Neoplastic diseases such as pituitary adenoma, craniopharyngioma and metastatic disease to the pituitary (eg, renal cell cancer, leukemia, and breast cancer) may cause acquired TSH deficiency. These mass lesions either destroy normal pituicytes or compress the pituitary stalk, thereby disrupting the portal supply of trophic factors from the hypothalamus. Patients with plurihormonal deficiency exhibit features of hypothyroidism as well as that of gonadotropin, ACTH and growth hormone deficiencies.

Disorders of hypothalamic function can affect the pituitary production of TSH by altered synthesis or release of trophic factors, particularly TRH. Neoplastic diseases such as germinomas, craniopharyngiomas or meningiomas often cause defective TRH secretion. Diabetes insipidus is a frequent feature due impairment of vasopressin production and release. Cranial or head and neck irradiation in cancer patients can also lead to hypothalamic hypothyroidism.[80] Because dopamine transport to the pituitary is frequently affected, mild hyperprolactinemia is commonly seen in these patients.

Reversible central hypothyroidism occurs as a dose-dependent complication of therapy with bexarotene, a retinoid X receptor (RXR)-selective drug used in the treatment of mycosis fungoides and cutaneous T cell lymphoma.[81] Studies suggest that the mechanism of RXR-mediated hypothyroidism is suppression of transcription of the TSH β subunit gene, independent of the role of thyroid hormone receptors, and reduction of TSH concentrations can be seen within hours of a single oral dose of the drug.[81–83] Additional evidence suggests that the drug also accelerates thyroid hormone metabolic clearance, leading to markedly higher doses of thyroid hormone needed to treat the hypothyroid patient.[84]

Miscellaneous Etiologies of Hypothyroidism

Damage to the thyroid can occur as a result of diffuse infiltration of the gland. Amyloidosis of various etiologies, including secondary to multiple myeloma, often produces asymptomatic infiltration and goiter, with hypothyroidism seen in as many as 15% of patients.[85] Gammopathy-associated hypothyroidism can also be seen as a "minor" diagnostic criterion in the POEMS or Crow-Fukase syndrome, although cytokine-induced autoimmunity has been postulated.[86] Thalidomide has also been implicated to cause mild to severe hypothyroidism in up to 20% of treated myeloma and renal cell carcinoma patients, of uncertain etiology.[87,88] Aminoglutethimide has been associated with the development of hypothyroidism of uncertain etiology in prostate and breast cancer patients.[89] Exacerbation of preexisting hypothyroidism and increasing levothyroxine dose requirements have been described in cancer patients treated with numerous medications, including imatinib, bexarotene, estrogens, tamoxifen citrate, mitotane, fluorouracil, and methadone, likely due either to increased metabolic clearance of the hormone or altered serum transport proteins.[84,90–92] Increased metabolism of T_4 and "consumptive hypothyroidism" has been reported in patients with tumors that express high levels of the type III deiodinase, including massive hemangiomas, hemangiomepithelioma , and a malignant solitary fibrous tumor.[93,94]

Diagnosis

Clinical manifestations, hypothyroxinemia, and an elevated serum TSH establish the diagnosis of overt primary hypothyroidism, and therefore first-line laboratory testing for suspected hypothyroidism should be measurement of the serum concentration of TSH, with abnormal results followed by measurement of free T_4.[95] Due to the greater sensitivity of TSH measurements, the presence of an elevated TSH with a free T_4 level in the lower portion of the reference range would be consistent with subclinical primary hypothyroidism. In rare patients with central hypothyroidism, the serum TSH will generally not be elevated, but the diagnosis would be suggested by an inappropriately low free T_4. If pituitary or hypothalamic disease is suspected, other abnormalities of anterior pituitary function are often found (eg, inappropriately normal gonadotropin levels in a postmenopausal woman). Radiologic imaging of the sella is also often indicated. Additional tests can occasionally be helpful in establishing the diagnosis and cause of hypothyroidism. The diagnosis of autoimmune thyroiditis, either chronic or transient, is confirmed by the presence of serum anti-TPO antibodies.

Hypothyroxinemia and hypotriiodothyroninemia are common findings in patients with nonthyroidal illness.[8,96] In addition to deficiency of albumin and transthyretin, other proposed mechanisms include inhibition of hormone binding to TBG, perhaps due to free fatty acids released from damaged tissues or cytokines such as tumor necrosis factor.[97] Numerous medications interfere with thyroid hormone binding to serum proteins, including diphenylhydantoin, furosemide, heparin, sertraline, and certain anti-inflammatory agents.[98] L-asparaginase causes frank reduction in TBG concentrations. Inhibition of 5′-monodeiodinase activity in extrathyroidal tissues, probably related to increased levels of interleukin-6 and TNF-α, reduces production of T_3, reduces clearance of rT_3, and accelerates clearance of T_4 through non-deiodinative mechanisms, thus contributing to reduced levels of T_4 and T_3 but increased rT_3.[6] Medications such as glucocorticoids, amiodarone, oral radiocontrast agents, gold, and high dose propranolol and propylthiouracil (PTU) also inhibit T_4 deiodination to T_3; however, clinical signs of hypothyroidism are unlikely to develop. Pituitary TSH production is suppressed by endogenous and/or exogenous glucocorticoids, dopamine, somatostatin, and endorphins, and may also be mediated by reduced hypothalamic TRH secretion.[99] Alteration of TSH sialylation and bioactivity may occur in critical illness as well.[100] Mild illness is typically accompanied by reductions in T_4 to T_3 conversion, resulting in a low T_3 state; similar changes have been reported after intravenous chemotherapy administration.[101] With increasing severity of nonthyroidal illness, all of the proposed mechanisms presumably result in a low T_4, low T_3 state. These laboratory abnormalities reverse with recovery from the nonthyroidal illness or discontinuation of the interfering medication.

The sequence of thyroid hormone changes in nonthyroidal illness has been studied in considerable detail in patients undergoing bone marrow transplantation. During the first several weeks following transplant, T_4, T_3, and TSH levels all markedly decline, inversely proportional to rises in serum levels of IL-6 and TNF-α.[102–104] In one study, one-year mortality due to transplant complications was sixfold higher in patients whose serum total T_4 levels fell below 4 mcg/dL, consistent with the proposition that the severity of hypothyroxinemia correlates with the severity of the underlying nonthyroidal illness as suggested in studies of critically ill patients.[102]

Although most of the effects of nonthyroidal illness may represent energy-conserving adaptive mechanisms, the traditional view of these patients as being "euthyroid" is not universally held.[105,106] However, no survival benefit from thyroid hormone supplementation has ever been demonstrated in clinical trials in severely or critically ill patients, and increased catabolism and protein wasting have been reported. In this context, it is important to emphasize that diagnosis of nonthyroidal illness is a clinical diagnosis that does not require laboratory testing, such as measurement of rT_3 levels, for identification; the challenge, instead, is to determine whether there is any reason to suspect a preexisting thyroid disease underlying the changes that are superimposed by nonthyroidal illness. Therefore, judicious therapy is suggested only in patients with evidence of elevated TSH levels despite acute illness.[106]

Treatment

The goal of therapy for overt hypothyroidism is to make the patient clinically and biochemically euthyroid, which is usually associated with normalization of the serum TSH level. The treatment of choice to accomplish this is oral synthetic levothyroxine sodium, which is available in 12 individual dose strengths. For individuals under age 60 with overt and symptomatic disease, full hormone replacement requires an average of 1.7 mcg/kg daily, although there is considerable variation around this mean. Owing to the long half-life of the hormone and the gradual rise in serum concentration over several weeks after initiating daily oral treatment, most of these patients can be started directly on this full replacement dose without toxicity. However, in older patients and those with known or suspected cardiovascular disease, even this gradual rise is too rapid, inducing anginal symptoms or palpitations in a small proportion. Thyroid hormone does improve the efficiency of myocardial contractility and is a potent vasodilator, and thus an equivalent proportion of patients may instead experience an improvement in their angina.

Whether patients with subclinical or mild hypothyroidism absolutely require supplemental doses of levothyroxine to normalize their laboratory tests remains controversial. However, patients with active autoimmune disease or who have radiation-induced hypothyroidism are very likely to progress to overt disease, thereby justifying earlier intervention to prevent development of symptomatic hypothyroidism. Low doses of hormone, 50 to 100 mcg daily, are usually sufficient to normalize the TSH.

When levothyroxine sodium is administered daily by mouth, decreasing serum TSH concentrations plateau within 4 to 6 weeks, and measurement of the TSH level should await this new equilibrium. Patients with persistently elevated serum TSH levels generally require an increased dose of levothyroxine, whereas those patients with a low serum TSH concentration usually require a decrease in dose. Serum T_4 and T_3 levels are usually normal during therapy, although mild hyperthyroxinemia can occur in as many as 20% of patients who are otherwise euthyroid. Once a hypothyroid patient becomes euthyroid, follow-up evaluation should be performed after several months, given the gradual increase of T_4 clearance that occurs in these patients. Subsequent evaluations generally are required only annually. To monitor therapy in patients with secondary or tertiary hypothyroidism, the patient's clinical status and serum free T_4 levels should be assessed.

The goal of therapy should be attainment of a clinically euthyroid state, with normal or high-normal free T_4 levels since the serum TSH concentration is not a reliable indicator of thyroid hormone status in this setting.[107]

In cancer patients, the routine approach to oral hormone replacement therapy is occasionally inadequate. As described previously, several medications appear to increase metabolic clearance of levothyroxine, therefore leading to increased dose requirements. Patients who require enteral administration through a feeding jejunostomy may also require considerable increase in their hormone dose, a problem that is apparently avoided by administration of the drug into the stomach first.[108] High thyroid hormone dose requirements can sometimes be a clue to the presence of a broader malabsorption condition, such as short bowel syndrome or Whipple's disease.[109]

Patients receiving therapy with T_3-containing preparations, which are shorter acting than levothyroxine alone, may be more difficult to monitor. Individuals who take desiccated thyroid or other formulations containing triiodothyronine are likely to have variable T_3 levels during the day. Most recent placebo-controlled studies have demonstrated that there is no significant measurable benefit accrued to patients when treated with combination formulations of varying ratios of T_4 and T_3, compared with T_4 alone.[110]

Thyrotoxicosis

Thyrotoxicosis refers to the clinical state of increased metabolism due to increased serum concentrations of T_4 and/or T_3. Whereas hyperthyroidism defines the forms of thyrotoxicosis secondary to increased synthesis of thyroid hormones, other etiologies can include thyroiditis and excessive ingestion of thyroid hormone. The prevalence of thyrotoxicosis, including both mild and overt disease, is only about 1% in the United States, but is generally more common in women than men.[14] Thyrotoxicosis as a consequence of cancer or its treatment is also considerably less frequent than similarly caused hypothyroidism.

Clinical Manifestations

Thyrotoxicosis is generally more likely to be more symptomatic, even in its mild forms, than hypothyroidism. A common constitutional symptom is fatigue, often misconstrued to indicate hypothyroidism. Weight loss is generally secondary to increased metabolic rate, despite increased appetite and food intake, but occasionally weight gain can be seen as well. Organ system-specific manifestations are addressed below.

The Neuromuscular System

Multiple neuromuscular abnormalities result from thyrotoxicosis. A majority of patients experience proximal muscle weakness and tremor, often a presenting symptom of the patient's thyroid disease. Less common manifestations include bulbar weakness and fasciculations that can be mistaken for amyotrophic lateral sclerosis. Increased protein catabolism is a key contributory factor, along with depletion of glycogen and ATP.[111] A common autoimmune pathophysiology links thyrotoxic Graves' disease and myasthenia gravis, and 5 to 10% of patients with myasthenia have coexistent Graves' disease; thymic hyperplasia, however, is a common finding in thyrotoxic patients even in the absence of myasthenia.[112,113] Recurrent episodes of severe muscle weakness associated with marked hypokalemia characterizes thyrotoxic periodic paralysis, but unlike familial periodic paralysis, the relation between potassium channel function and thyrotoxicosis is unknown.[114,115] Neuropsychiatric consequences of thyrotoxicosis are common, including anxiety, irritability, emotional lability and difficulty concentrating.

The Cardiovascular System

A complex web of direct and indirect effects converge on the cardiovascular system, leading to a broad variety of symptoms and abnormalities, including palpitations, tachycardia, and increased "cardiac awareness."[116] Increased metabolism leading to increased oxygen demand contributes to tachycardia, along with direct stimulation of the sinus node pacemaker.[117] Perhaps secondary to increased nitric oxide production by vascular endothelial cells, systemic vascular resistance can decrease by as much as 70% in thyrotoxicosis, causing decreased diastolic blood pressure, activation of the renin/angiotensin/aldosterone system, sodium retention, and eventual increased preload. Combined with enhanced calcium release and reuptake by myocardial sarcoplasmic reticulum, these peripheral hemodynamic effects lead to increased myocardial contractility and output; however, heart failure has been reported in patients who experience a disproportionate rise in systemic vascular resistance associated with exercise.[118] Beyond sinus tachycardia, atrial fibrillation occurs three times as frequently in older patients with suppressed TSH levels compared with euthyroid controls, with less frequent spontaneous cardioversion and possibly a higher rate of thromboembolic complications.[119,120]

The Respiratory System

Patients with thyrotoxicosis demonstrate various respiratory abnormalities, many arising due to increased metabolic demand for oxygen. Oxygen consumption and carbon dioxide production are invariably increased, leading to tachypnea and increased minute ventilation. Although airway resistance is typically normal, chronic thyrotoxicosis can lead to respiratory myopathy and possibly alterations in lung compliance.[121] In contrast with hypothyroidism, ventilatory responses to hypercapnia and hypoxia may be enhanced.[122] Patients with concurrent lung disease are therefore more likely not to be able to meet their demand for increased gas exchange and become symptomatic.

Substernal goiter can lead to upper airway compression, which in the thyrotoxic patient can exacerbate the respiratory consequences. About 15% of patients with substernal goiter have symptoms to suggest upper airway obstruction, including exertional dyspnea. On pulmonary function testing, flow volume loops tend to be flattened. If the obstruction is extrathoracic, the changes occur primarily on inspiratory airflow, whereas intrathoracic obstruction causes expiratory flattening.

The Gastrointestinal System

The common manifestations of thyrotoxicosis in the gastrointestinal tract include increased gut motility, rapid transit, and hyper-defecation. Despite increased esophageal peristalsis, dysphagia can occasionally result from pharyngeal and esophageal myopathy.[123] Due to overlapping autoimmune conditions, antiparietal cell antibodies, vitamin B_{12} malabsorption, and pernicious anemia are considerably more common. Cases of extreme fat malabsorption have also been described, but whether due simply to increased motility or due to thyroid hormone effects on small bowel lining function is controversial.[124] Hepatic function is frequently altered in thyrotoxicosis, with increased hepatic oxygen consumption. However, arterial blood flow to the liver is generally not increased, and therefore centrizonal necrosis has been reported in severe cases. Splenomegaly, previously a common finding in thyrotoxic patients, is now rarely seen.[125]

The Integumentary System

Direct skin effects of thyroid hormones are experienced by both the epidermis and dermis as well as cutaneous appendages. The skin is generally thin but without atrophy, perhaps secondary to inhibition of dermal fibroblasts.[126] Thyroid hormone also affects the transcription of numerous genes involved in keratin synthesis. Although it has been reported that surgical wound healing might be delayed in hypothyroidism, thyrotoxicosis does not appear to accelerate healing.[127,128] Hair and nail changes include increased hair growth rate, leading to fine and soft hair, and soft nails with distal onycholysis. Increased transcutaneous heat loss and erythema of face and palms accompanies peripheral vasodilatation. Due to exaggerated adrenergic responsiveness, hyperhidrosis is commonly experienced.

A characteristic autoimmune dermopathy can be seen in thyrotoxicosis due to Graves' disease. Skin thickening because of glycosaminoglycan deposition can vary from a localized "peau d'orange" appearance to a rare generalized infiltration.[129] Typically, the affected skin is raised, waxy, slightly hyperpigmented, and rarely pruritic. Thyroid acropachy is characterized by clubbing, soft tissue swelling of hands and feet, and periosteal new bone formation. Both dermopathy and acropachy are also seen more commonly in patients with severe orbital complications of Graves' disease. Other autoimmune cutaneous phenomena are more common as well, including alopecia, bullous disorders, and urticaria.

The Hematopoietic System

Erythropoiesis is stimulated in thyrotoxic patients, with increased levels of erythropoietin likely due to alterations in tissue oxygen demand.[130] In bone marrow, erythroid hyperplasia can be seen, provided no nutritional deficiencies coexist.[131] However, increased plasma volume can result in normochromic, normocytic anemia in up to 25% of thyrotoxic patients.[132] Ferritin levels are generally increased, due to direct stimulation of ferritin synthesis by thyroid hormones.[133] Mild granulocytopenia and lymphocytosis can occur, of uncertain etiology. Both granulocytopenia and thrombocytopenia can be related to autoimmune destruction, but increased reticuloendothelial consumption has also been reported. The clearance of various clotting factors is increased, but clinical measures of coagulation tend to be normal. However, thyrotoxic patients are more sensitive to the anticoagulant effects of warfarin owing to increased clotting factor clearance and possible decreased plasma protein binding.[134]

Endocrine and Metabolic Systems

Thyrotoxicosis leads to increased transcription and secretion of growth hormone and prolactin, but clinical consequences are uncommon.[135,136] Metabolic clearance of cortisol is augmented, causing increased production of ACTH and consequently cortisol itself.

As thyrotoxicosis stimulates osteoblast and osteoclast activity, bone turnover is accelerated, leading to increased calcium efflux from the bone, hypercalciuria, and often hypercalcemia with parathyroid hormone suppression.[137] Hypomagnesemia occurs secondary to increased renal magnesium wasting, which also contributes to parathyroid suppression, and can exacerbate hypomagnesemia from platinum chemotherapy.[138] Other less frequent abnormalities of relevance in cancer patients include hyperuricemia, hypophosphatemia, and hypokalemia.[139]

Little is known about the impact of thyrotoxicosis on the pharmacokinetics of drugs used in the treatment of cancer. However, hepatic microsomal enzyme activity is likely to be enhanced in thyrotoxic patients, as suggested by the reduction in the serum half-life and area under the concentration-time curve of antipyrine.[140]

Etiology and Pathophysiology

The causes of thyrotoxicosis include increased thyroid hormone production (hyperthyroidism), accelerated release of previously synthesized hormone, and excessive exogenous hormone administration. Hyperthyroidism can result from excessive stimulation of follicular cells through their TSH receptors to produce hormone, or TSH-independent autonomously hyperfunctioning neoplasms.

Graves' Disease and TSH Receptor-Mediated Hyperthyroidism

The most common etiology of hyperthyroidism is Graves' disease, an autoimmune condition in which immunoglobulins interact with and stimulate the TSH receptor. As postulated for autoimmune thyroiditis leading to hypothyroidism, class II-expressing thyroid follicular cells in Graves' disease likely acquire the capacity to present autoantigens to intrathyroidal CD4-expressing lymphocytes. In animal models, immunization with human TSH receptor, in the presence of class II antigens, can induce the production of immunoglobulins directed against the TSH receptor, often capable of stimulating receptor function and downstream signaling.[141,142] Modest associations exist between HLA alleles -DR3, -DR4, and -DR5 and Graves' disease, but a stronger association has been recently identified with polymorphisms of CTLA-4 in a variety of populations.[143,144]

Similar to autoimmune thyroiditis, patients exposed to a variety of treatments for cancer have increased risk for developing Graves' disease, especially IFN-α and IL-2.[62,65,66] However, Graves' disease has been reported as a potential adverse event of treatment with IL-4, GM-CSF, and possibly denileukin diftitox.[70,145,146] Hyperthyroidism clinically consistent with Graves' disease was reported to be eightfold more common in survivors of childhood Hodgkin's disease treated with irradiation than in their siblings.[77] However, other malignancies treated with irradiation are not associated with such a degree of risk for Graves' disease, suggesting to some that an underlying immune dysregulation may be responsible.[147]

A distinguishing feature of Graves' disease is that the ophthalmopathy coexists in about one-third of patients. Likely due to an autoantigen or epitope that is shared between thyroid follicular cells and orbital tissues, Graves' ophthalmopathy is characterized by a broad variety of clinical abnormalities, ranging from minimal exophthalmos, lid retraction, and retrobulbar discomfort to restrictive strabismus, corneal damage, and sight loss. An increased frequency of phthalmopathy has been reported in Hodgkin's disease survivors who develop Graves' disease.[148] Rarely, lymphoma, myeloma, and other malignancies have been reported to present with similar findings of ophthalmopathy, and therefore, the clinician should carefully evaluate the patient with orbital complaints for a variety of etiologies.

Although not autoimmune, other etiologies can be responsible for hyperthyroidism mediated through the TSH receptor but would not produce ophthalmopathy. About 1 to 2% of pituitary adenomas secrete bioactive TSH, often producing severe hyperthyroidism. Most will present with a large pituitary mass, and often, findings include visual field deficits and headache .

Although capable of interacting with the TSH receptor, the thyroid stimulating activity of one unit of hCG is equivalent to only 1×10^{-9} units of TSH. Nonetheless, hydatidiform moles, choriocarcinomas, and other germ cell tumors can often secrete sufficiently large amounts of hCG to produce hyperthyroidism that generally improves with aggressive treatment of the underlying neoplasm.[149,150]

Toxic Nodular Disease

Solitary and multiple adenomas of the thyroid can develop with autonomous, TSH-independent thyroid hormone production. Most such neoplasms can be found to harbor constitutively activating mutations of the TSH receptor or the α subunit of the receptor-coupled stimulatory guanine nucleotide-binding protein that signals through cyclic adenosine monophosphate , but other downstream mutations are likely to be identified as well.[151] Neoplastic autonomy is more common in areas of relative iodine deficiency, with evidence suggesting a progression from hyperplasia to frank neoplastic hyperthyroidism following acquisition of constitutive, growth-stimulating mutations.[152] Rarely, malignant follicular tumors can also produce sufficient amounts of hormone to yield hyperthyroidism, but these typically are associated with a large metastatic burden.[153]

Transient Thyroiditis

Destructive inflammation of the thyroid can cause either thyrotoxicosis or hypothyroidism (as described previously), and commonly both can occur sequentially. During the thyrotoxic phase, rapid tissue injury leads to disruption of follicular structure and proteolysis of thyroglobulin, resulting in elevated levels of free T_4 and T_3. Mild symptoms typical of thyrotoxicosis can be seen, including fatigue, nervousness, and tachycardia. Thyrotoxicosis can last up to three months but is typically shorter.

Evidence for an autoimmune basis for silent thyroiditis includes (1) increased frequency of personal or family history of autoimmunity; (2) increased frequency of HLA-DR3 and –DR5 haplotypes; and (3) presence of intrathyroidal T cells similar in phenotype to chronic autoimmune thyroiditis. Initiating factors include treatment with amiodarone (type I thyrotoxicosis), lithium, IL-2, IFN-α, granulocyte colony-stimulating factor, and leuprolide acetate, and the disease has been associated with thymomas.[154–157]

Subacute thyroiditis, in contrast, is not a primary autoimmune disease, although thyroid autoimmunity may appear due to sensitization to thyroid antigens during inflammation. Instead, subacute thyroiditis typically occurs following an upper respiratory infection with adenovirus, coxsackievirus, Epstein-Barr virus, and influenza virus.[156] It has also been reported in patients treated with interferon and ribavirin therapy for hepatitis C. Genetic susceptibility is associated with HLA-Bw35 antigen. Acute suppurative thyroiditis is a rare cause of thyrotoxicosis and has usually been reported from bacterial or opportunistic infections, particularly in immunosuppressed hosts. Radiation injury to the thyroid can trigger release of thyroglobulin and transient thyroiditis, lasting for up to 3 months after thyroid exposure to at least 40 Gy.[158] A non-autoimmune destructive thyroiditis is also associated with amiodarone therapy (type II thyrotoxicosis).

Diagnosis

Clinical manifestations, elevated serum thyroid hormone concentrations, and a subnormal serum TSH level typically establish the diagnosis of thyrotoxicosis. In hyperthyroidism, the ratio of serum T_3:T_4 levels tends to be increased, reflecting relatively greater production of T_3 in these states; conversely, in transient thyroiditis, release of previously formed hormone is typically associated with lower T_3:T_4 ratios. Patients with T_3 toxicosis due to mild or recurrent Graves' disease or hyperfunctioning adenomas can present with normal or occasionally low serum free T_4, and the diagnosis of hyperthyroidism may be missed by not measuring T_3 levels in patients with suspected thyrotoxicosis as well.

Measurement of free T_4 levels is critical to distinguish the patient with true thyrotoxic hyperthyroxinemia from euthyroid hyperthyroxinemia owing to increased hormone binding to serum proteins. Most commercially available, free T_4 assays can account for the common hormone-binding abnormalities, such as those due to excess levels of TBG in patients with hyperestrogenemia or being treated with tamoxifen, raloxifene, or methadone. But, paraneoplastic production of transthyretin in pancreatic and hepatic neoplasms leading to increased serum hormone binding may not be readily identified, and documentation of a normal TSH is often necessary to distinguish from thyrotoxicosis.[159,160]

Unfortunately, most commercially available free T_3 assays are unreliable, and total T_3 levels must suffice instead.

Additional tests are occasionally useful in establishing the diagnosis and etiology of thyrotoxicosis. In a patient with a tender goiter and hyperthyroidism of short duration, an elevated erythrocyte sedimentation rate is characteristic of subacute thyroiditis. An elevated radioiodine uptake is typically found in Graves' disease and hyperfunctioning nodular disease, but is not seen in subacute or silent thyroiditis. Similarly, the serum thyroglobulin and radioiodine uptake are typically low in factitious and iatrogenic thyrotoxicosis. Testing for TPO antibodies or thyroid stimulating immunoglobulins may assist in the discrimination between Graves' disease and toxic multinodular goiter. Radiologic imaging of the sella and a serum α-subunit level would be indicated in the evaluation of the patient with TSH-mediated hyperthyroidism.

Treatment

Treatment of hyperthyroidism relies upon use of therapies directed toward (1) reduction in production of thyroid hormones, and (2) amelioration of the symptoms of thyroid hormone excess. Whereas the latter approach is also of value in the symptomatic patient with destructive thyroiditis, treatment to reduce hormone production is only of value in hyperthyroidism.

Antithyroid drugs have been a mainstay of treatment of hyperthyroidism for six decades. Thionamides, including propylthiouracil (PTU) and methimazole available in the United States and carbimazole elsewhere, work by a variety of intrathyroidal mechanisms, including inhibition of iodine oxidation, organification, iodotyrosine coupling, and possibly thyroglobulin synthesis and function. Outside the follicular cell, PTU at high doses inhibits the type 1 deiodinase, thus blocking T_4 to T_3 conversion. Immunosuppressive actions have been attributed to thionamides as well that could be of benefit in treatment of Graves' disease, but it remains unclear whether clinically achieved concentrations produce these effects. Because methimazole is more potent, has a longer half-life, and has better patient compliance with once-daily dosing, methimazole therapy is more effective at reducing serum T_4 and T_3 levels.[161] Daily starting doses of methimazole range from 10 to 40 mg, higher doses being required for patients with more severe hyperthyroxinemia; the typical initial dose of PTU is 100 mg three times daily.[162] With gradual normalization of thyroid hormone levels, doses can typically be reduced by about half. Toxicities commonly include urticarial rash, arthralgias, mild granulocytopenia, and fever. More serious and less common side effects include an autoimmune agranulocytosis (in 0.2 to 0.5%

of treated patients), aplastic anemia, fulminant hepatitis, and vasculitis. Because the typical presentation of thionamide-induced agranulocytosis is a gram-positive pharyngitis, patients are instructed to discontinue their medication and contact their physician when developing fever and a sore throat. Antibiotics and, when necessary, G-CSF therapy allow for rapid recovery from this consequence.

Definitive therapy of hyperthyroidism usually requires either radioiodine ablation or surgical resection of the overactive gland. Treatment with 131-I delivering 50 to 150 Gy to the thyroid gland induces acute and chronic radiation necrosis, eventually leading to hypothyroidism in most patients with Graves' disease. Long-term safety of this treatment is excellent, with only case reports linking radioiodine treatment of Graves' disease with increased risk of secondary malignancies. Thus, except in children for whom long-term follow-up data are more sparse, radioiodine therapy is the most commonly applied definitive treatment for hyperthyroid Graves' disease. In contrast, recent data suggest an increased risk for developing thyroid carcinoma in patients with toxic nodular disease treated with 131-I, likely due to sublethal and mutagenic radiation doses absorbed by the paranodular thyroid cells.[163] Thyroidectomy remains an excellent treatment option for hyperthyroidism, particularly for those patients with severe Graves' ophthalmopathy (which can acutely worsen following radioiodine administration), for younger patients with toxic nodular goiters, and for patients with large obstructing goiters.

Symptoms of thyrotoxicosis are generally ameliorated with therapy with β-adrenergic receptor blockers. In the patient who cannot tolerate this treatment, calcium channel antagonists can also be of benefit. In anticipation of surgery for the hyperthyroid patient, combined administration of β-adrenergic receptor blockers and thionamides are generally necessary to lower hormone levels toward normal and reduce the risk for decompensated thyrotoxicosis or thyroid storm; addition of large doses of inorganic, stable iodine for no more than 10 to 14 days can also accelerate presurgical preparation.

Because normalization of the serum TSH concentration may lag behind thyroid hormone levels by several months, initial therapy should be directed to reducing thyroid hormone levels. Once the TSH level is detectable, it is again a sensitive indicator of thyroid hormone status. Given the increased $T_3:T_4$ ratio typical of increased glandular synthesis of hormone, the T_4 level may become normal or even low while the T_3 level remains elevated, producing persistent T_3-toxicosis. In addition, an elevated T_3 level may be the earliest sign of recurrent hyperthyroidism. Thus, both the T_3 and free T_4 levels should be monitored during treatment of hyperthyroidism. In patients with TSH-mediated hyperthyroidism, clinical assessment and thyroid hormone levels are the only measures of use, as the serum TSH level does not reflect thyroid hormone status.

Thyroid Neoplasia

Clinical Manifestations

Thyroid nodules are approximately four times more common in women than in men. These nodules increase in frequency throughout life, reaching a prevalence of about 5% in the US population aged 50 years and older. Nodules are even more prevalent when the thyroid gland is examined at autopsy or surgery, or when using ultrasonography; as many as 67% of thyroids so studied have nodules, which are almost always benign.[164] New nodules develop at a rate of about 0.1% per year, beginning in early life, but they develop at a much higher rate (about 2% per year) after exposure to head and neck irradiation.

About 5% of all incident nodules prove to be malignant, mostly being primary carcinomas of the thyroid gland (papillary, follicular, medullary, and anaplastic). Like thyroid nodules, thyroid neoplasia occurs two to three times more often in women than in men. With the incidence increasing by 4% per year, thyroid cancer is currently the seventh most common malignancy diagnosed in women.[165] Among persons aged 15 to 24 years, thyroid cancer accounts for 7.5% to 10% of all diagnosed malignancies. The disease is also diagnosed more often in white Americans than in African Americans. Although thyroid carcinoma can occur at any age, the peak incidence was around age 50 to 54 in women and 65 to 69 in men for the period 1996 to 2000.

Nonthyroidal malignancies can occasionally metastasize to the thyroid gland, and are often detected many years after the initial disease diagnosis. The most common primary sites for metastatic disease to the thyroid include kidney, breast, colon, lung, esophagus, and uterus.[166,167] Metastatic melanoma may be disproportionately more commonly found at autopsy and less commonly seen clinically. Conversely, metastatic thyroid carcinoma is occasionally identified in patients undergoing treatment for other head and neck malignancies; in these patients, the thyroid cancer is rarely clinically significant or a cause of subsequent morbidity or mortality.[168]

With increasingly sensitive radiologic and scintigraphic technologies used to follow patients with cancer, new clinical syndromes are identified due to incidental discovery of unanticipated abnormalities. Thus, ultrasound reports of the neck commonly comment on incidental thyroid nodules being detected. Recently, the incidental "PEToma" has been described as focal uptake of 18-F-deoxyglucose in the thyroid in patients undergoing positron emission tomography (PET). Between 1 and 4% of patients undergoing FDG-PET or FDG-PET-computed tomography (CT) studies for evaluation of malignancy have been reported to have such incidental thyroid findings.[169–171] Of those patients subsequently evaluated cytologically, 30 to 40% were found to have malignant disease, perhaps best predicted by low attenuation characteristics on the accompanying CT images and minimal degrees of FDG uptake.[169]

Etiology

The only well-established risk factor for papillary thyroid cancer is radiation exposure, especially during infancy.[172] External radiation, delivered therapeutically decades ago for benign conditions, such as thymic and tonsillar enlargement, and currently for malignant diseases, such as Hodgkin's lymphoma and before bone marrow transplantation, is associated with an excess relative risk for thyroid malignancy of 3 to 9 per Gy. The risk of radiation-induced thyroid carcinoma is greater in females, certain Jewish populations, and patients with a family history of thyroid carcinoma. Exposure to internal sources of radiation after the Chernobyl nuclear accident led to a three- to 75-fold increase in the incidence of papillary carcinoma, the highest risks seen in younger children.[173] Although nuclear weapon testing and other sources of radiation fallout have affected large areas of the United States, follow-up studies have yet to identify definite evidence of increased rates of thyroid cancer.[174,175]

Differentiated (papillary or follicular) carcinoma is a component of several inherited syndromes, including familial adenomatous polyposis, Gardner's syndrome, Cowden disease, Turcot's syndrome, and Carney's complex. Familial non-medullary carcinoma, described in families with at least two first-degree relatives with the disease, has been reported in 5% of all papillary carcinoma patients, and may portend a more-aggressive disease course. Medullary carcinoma can occur in a variety of familial syndromes, including multiple endocrine neoplasia (MEN) types IIa and IIb and isolated familial medullary thyroid carcinoma. Patients with MEN syndromes may often be identified on the basis of the nonthyroidal tumors, parathyroid adenomas and pheochromocytomas, but increasingly, these patients are identified by prospective familial screening programs.

Diagnosis

The primary method for evaluating a thyroid nodule is fine needle aspiration, often guided by ultrasonography.[176] Ultrasonographic criteria that increase the likelihood of malignancy include the presence of microcalcifications, hypoechogenicity, and increased intranodular vascularity.[177] In the setting of an unsuppressed serum TSH concentration, thyroid ultrasonography followed by cytologic examination of a fine-needle aspirate (FNA) of solitary nodules at least 1 cm in size is the most appropriate diagnostic procedure; in the setting of multiple nodules, those with suspicious ultrasonographic appearances should be preferentially aspirated.[178] Papillary, medullary, and anaplastic carcinomas can be readily diagnosed on the basis of cytologic criteria. However, the distinction between follicular carcinoma and benign follicular adenoma requires histologic demonstration of either invasion through the tumor capsule or vascular invasion. Hence, follicular adenomas and carcinomas are grouped together cytologically as indeterminate or suspicious follicular neoplasms. Up to 25% of aspirations are inadequate or nondiagnostic, largely because of aspiration of cystic, hemorrhagic, or hypocellular colloid nodules.[179] The false-positive and false-negative rates for nodules characterized as "malignant" and "benign," respectively, are less than 5%.[180] For suspicious follicular lesions, the overall rate of carcinoma is approximately 20%, with higher rates associated with larger nodule size, older age, and male gender.[181–183] Intraoperative frozen section evaluation adds little to the evaluation of follicular neoplasms, but may occasionally be helpful to confirm the diagnosis of cytologically suspected papillary carcinoma.[184,185] For nodules in which fine-needle aspiration yields inadequate diagnostic material, repeat aspiration, particularly with ultrasonography guidance, can augment the accuracy of the procedure.[186]

By radionuclide scanning, malignant thyroid lesions are usually hypofunctioning or "cold," but this finding is both nonspecific and nondiagnostic. In contrast, a "hot" hyperfunctioning nodule causing thyrotoxicosis is highly likely to be a benign follicular adenoma. Thus, only patients with a suppressed TSH should undergo radioiodine scanning to determine the function of significant nodules, and FNA only performed for nonfunctioning lesions. Other imaging procedures, such as CT, magnetic resonance imaging (MRI), and PET have no role in the routine diagnostic evaluation of thyroid nodules.

Treatment

Patients with benign thyroid nodules rarely require therapy for an asymptomatic neoplasm. In iodine-sufficient populations, there is little evidence of significant clinical benefit from use of thyroid hormone suppression therapy for euthyroid benign nodular disease.[176,187] As discussed for the management of thyrotoxicosis, surgical resection is often the preferred approach to treatment of the toxic follicular adenoma. The management

of patients with thyroid carcinoma is the subject for other treatises.[176,188,189]

As for patients with isolated metastatic disease to the thyroid gland, long-term benefit can result from thyroidectomy.[190] However, in the setting of disseminated metastases, appropriate diagnosis of an intrathyroidal metastasis can permit avoidance of unnecessary thyroidectomy and instead lead to consideration of systemic interventions.[166,167]

REFERENCES

1. Osler W. The principles and practice of medicine. New York: D. Appleton and Company; 1892.
2. Tammemagi CM, Neslund-Dudas C, Simoff M, Kvale P. Impact of comorbidity on lung cancer survival. Int J Cancer 2003;103:792–802.
3. Dai G, Levy O, Carrasco N. Cloning and characterization of the thyroid iodide transporter. Nature 1996;379:458–60.
4. Kopp P. Thyroid hormone synthesis. In: Braverman LE, Utiger RD, editors. Werner & Ingbar's The Thyroid. 9th ed. Philadelphia: Lippincott Williams & Wilkins; 2005. p. 52–76.
5. Bianco AC, Salvatore D, Gereben B, et al. Biochemistry, cellular and molecular biology, and physiological roles of the iodothyronine selenodeiodinases. Endocr Rev 2002;23:38–89.
6. Wu SY, Green WL, Huang WS, et al. Alternate pathways of thyroid hormone metabolism. Thyroid 2005;15:943–58.
7. Schussler GC. The thyroxine-binding proteins. Thyroid 2000;10:141–9.
8. Fliers E, Alkemade A, Wiersinga WM. The hypothalamic-pituitary-thyroid axis in critical illness. Best Pract Res Clin Endocrinol Metab 2001;15:453–64.
9. Spencer CA, Schwarzbein D, Guttler RB, et al. Thyrotropin (TSH)-releasing hormone stimulation test responses employing third and fourth generation TSH assays. J Clin Endocrinol Metab 1993;76:494–8.
10. Vandeput F, Perpete S, Coulonval K, et al. Role of the different mitogen-activated protein kinase subfamilies in the stimulation of dog and human thyroid epithelial cell proliferation by cyclic adenosine 5′-monophosphate and growth factors. Endocrinology 2003;144:1341–9.
11. Gull WW. On a cretinoid state supervening in adult life in women. Trans Clin Soc London 1874;7:180–5.
12. Vanderpump MP, Tunbridge WM. Epidemiology and prevention of clinical and subclinical hypothyroidism. Thyroid 2002;12:839–47.
13. Canaris GJ, Manowitz NR, Mayor G, Ridgway EC. The Colorado thyroid disease prevalence study. Arch Intern Med 2000;160:526–34.
14. Hollowell JG, Staehling NW, Flanders WD, et al. Serum TSH, T(4), and thyroid antibodies in the United States population (1988 to 1994): National Health and Nutrition Examination Survey (NHANES III). J Clin Endocrinol Metab 2002;87:489–99.
15. Schectman JM, Kallenberg GA, Shumacher RJ, Hirsch RP. Yield of hypothyroidism in symptomatic primary care patients. Arch Intern Med 1989;149:861–4.
16. Dimeo F, Schmittel A, Fietz T, et al. Physical performance, depression, immune status and fatigue in patients with hematological malignancies after treatment. Ann Oncol 2004;15:1237–42.
17. Shafqat A, Einhorn LH, Hanna N, et al. Screening studies for fatigue and laboratory correlates in cancer patients undergoing treatment. Ann Oncol 2005;16:1545–50.
18. Ng AK, Li S, Recklitis C, et al. A comparison between long-term survivors of Hodgkin's disease and their siblings on fatigue level and factors predicting for increased fatigue. Ann Oncol 2005;16:1949–55.
19. Knobel H, Havard Loge J, Brit Lund M, et al. Late medical complications and fatigue in Hodgkin's disease survivors. J Clin Oncol 2001;19:3226–33.
20. Cojocaru IM, Cojocaru M, Musuroi C. Study of anti-striational and anti-thyroid antibodies in patients with myasthenia gravis. Rom J Intern Med 2000;38–39:111–20.
21. Marino M, Ricciardi R, Pinchera A, et al. Mild clinical expression of myasthenia gravis associated with autoimmune thyroid diseases. J Clin Endocrinol Metab 1997;82:438–43.

22. Beyer IW, Karmali R, Demeester-Mirkine N, et al. Serum creatine kinase levels in overt and subclinical hypothyroidism. Thyroid 1998;8:1029–31.
23. Ladenson PW, Sherman SI, Baughman KL, et al. Reversible alterations in myocardial gene expression in a young man with dilated cardiomyopathy and hypothyroidism [published erratum appears in Proc Natl Acad Sci U S A 1992;89:8856]. Proc Natl Acad Sci U S A 1992;89:5251–5.
24. Regalbuto C, Alagona C, Maiorana R, et al. Acute changes in clinical parameters and thyroid function peripheral markers following L-T4 withdrawal in patients totally thyroidectomized for thyroid cancer. J Endocrinol Invest 2006;29:32–40.
25. Zwillich C, Pierson D, Hofeldt F, et al. Ventilatory control in myxedema and hypothyroidism. N Engl J Med 1975;292:662–5.
26. Gottehrer A, Roa J, Stanford G, et al. Hypothyroidism and pleural effusions. Chest 1990;98:1130–2.
27. Sachdev Y, Hall F. Effusions into body cavities in hypothyroidism. Lancet 1975;1:564–5.
28. Miller L, Gorman C, Go V. Gut-thyroid interrelationships. Gastroenterology 1978;75:901–11.
29. Shafer R, Prentiss R, Bond J. Gastrointestinal transit in thyroid disease. Gastroenterology 1984;86:852–5.
30. Patel R, Hughes RWJ. An unusual case of myxedema megacolon with features of ischemic and pseudomembranous colitis. Mayo Clin Proc 1992;67:369–72.
31. Babb R. Associations between diseases of the thyroid and the liver. Am J Gastroenterol 1984;79:421–3.
32. Feingold K, Elias P. Endocrine-skin interactions: cutaneous manifestations of pituitary disease, thyroid disease, calcium disorders, and diabetes. J Am Acad Dermatol 1987;17:921–40.
33. Fein H, Rivlin R. Anemia in thyroid diseases. Med Clin N Amer 1975;59:1133–45.
34. Green S, Ng J. Hypothyroidism and anaemia. Biomed Pharmacother 1986;40:326–31.
35. Horton L, Coburn J, England J, Himsworth R. The haematology of hypothyroidism. Q J Med 1975;45:101–24.
36. Edson JR, Fecher DR, Doe RP. Low platelet adhesiveness and other hemostatic abonormalities in hypothyroidism. Ann Intern Med 1975;82:342–6.
37. Rennie J, Bewsher P, Murchison L, Ogston D. Coagulation and fibrinolysis in thyroid disease. Acta Haemat 1978;59:171–7.
38. Iranmanesh A, Lizarralde G, Johnson M, Veldhuis J. Dynamics of 24-hour endogenous cortisol secretion and clearance in primary hypothyroidism assessed before and after partial thyroid hormone replacement. J Clin Endocrinol Metab 1990;70:155–61.
39. Havard C, Saldanha V, Bird R, Gardner R. Adrenal function in hypothyroidism. Br Med J 1970;1:337–9.
40. Lessof M, Lyne C, Maisey M, Sturge R. Effect of thyroid failure on the pituitary-adrenal axis. Lancet 1969:642–3.
41. Derubertis FR, Michelis M, Bloom ME, et al. Impaired water excretion in myxedema. Am J Med 1971;51:41–53.
42. Hochberg Z, Benderly A. Normal osmotic threshold for vasopressin release in the hyponatremia of hypothyroidism. Hormone Res 1983;17:128–33.
43. Ladenson PW, Levin AA, Ridgway EC, Daniels GH. Complications of surgery in hypothyroid patients. Am J Med 1984;77:261–6.
44. Hasler JA, Estabrook R, Murray M, et al. Human cytochromes P450. Mol Aspects Med 1999;20:1–137.
45. Sarlis NJ, Gourgiotis L. Hormonal effects on drug metabolism through the CYP system: perspectives on their potential significance in the era of pharmacogenomics. Curr Drug Targets Immune Endocr Metabol Disord 2005;5:439–48.
46. Liddle C, Goodwin BJ, George J, et al. Separate and interactive regulation of cytochrome P450 3A4 by triiodothyronine, dexamethasone, and growth hormone in cultured hepatocytes. J Clin Endocrinol Metab 1998;83:2411–6.
47. Van Oosterom A, Kerkhoven P, Veltkamp J. Metabolism of the coagulation factors of the prothrombin complex in hypothyroidism in man. Thrombos Haemostas 1979;41:273–85.
48. Murakami Y, Takamatsu J, Sakane S, Kuma K. Serum levels of antibodies against thyroglobulin and microsomes in relation to thyroid function in patients with Hashimoto thyroiditis: analysis with various antibody measurement. In: Nagataki S, Mori T, Torizuka K, editors. 80 years of hashimoto disease. Amsterdam: Elsevier Science Publishers B.V.; 1993. p. 235–9.

49. Chiovato L, Bassi P, Santini F, et al. Antibodies producing complement-mediated thyroid cytotoxicity in patients with atrophic or goitrous autoimmune thyroiditis. J Clin Endocrinol Metab 1993;77:1700–5.

50. Vanderpump MP, Tunbridge WM, French JM, et al. The incidence of thyroid disorders in the community: a twenty-year follow-up of the Whickham Survey. Clin Endocrinol (Oxf) 1995;43:55–68.

51. Konishi J, Iida Y, Endo K, et al. Inhibition of thyrotropin-induced adenosine 3'5'-monophosphate increase by immunoglobulins from patients with primary myxedema. J Clin Endocrinol Metab 1983;57:544–9.

52. Weetman AP. Autoimmune thyroid disease: propagation and progression. Eur J Endocrinol 2003;148:1–9.

53. Hammond LJ, Palazzo FF, Shattock M, et al. Thyrocyte targets and effectors of autoimmunity: a role for death receptors? Thyroid 2001;11:919–27.

54. Ajjan RA, Watson PF, Findlay C, et al. The sodium iodide symporter gene and its regulation by cytokines found in autoimmunity. J Endocrinol 1998;158:351–8.

55. Tauchmanova L, Selleri C, De Rosa G, et al. Endocrine disorders during the first year after autologous stem-cell transplant. Am J Med 2005;118:664–70.

56. Au WY, Lie AK, Kung AW, et al. Autoimmune thyroid dysfunction after hematopoietic stem cell transplantation. Bone Marrow Transplant 2005;35:383–8.

57. Gartner W, Weissel M. Do iodine-containing contrast media induce clinically relevant changes in thyroid function parameters of euthyroid patients within the first week? Thyroid 2004;14:521–4.

58. Woeber KA. Iodine and thyroid disease. Med Clin North Am 1991;75:169–78.

59. Nikolai TJ, Brosseau J, Kettrick MA. Lymphocytic thyroiditis with spontaneously resolving hyperthyroidism (silent thyroiditis). Arch Intern Med 1980;140:478–82.

60. Burman P, Totterman TH, Oberg K, Karlsson FA. Thyroid autoimmunity in patients on long term therapy with leukocyte-derived interferon. J Clin Endocrinol Metab 1986;63:1086–90.

61. Fentiman IS, Thomas BS, Balkwill FR, et al. Primary hypothyroidism associated with interferon therapy of breast cancer. Lancet 1985;1:1166 .

62. Monzani F, Caraccio N, Dardano A, Ferrannini E. Thyroid autoimmunity and dysfunction associated with type I interferon therapy. Clin Exp Med 2004;3:199–210.

63. Koh LK, Greenspan FS, Yeo PP. Interferon-alpha induced thyroid dysfunction: three clinical presentations and a review of the literature. Thyroid 1997;7:891–6.

64. Vassilopoulou-Sellin R, Sella A, Dexeus FH. Acute thyroid dysfunction (thyroiditis) after therapy with interleukin-2. Horm Metab Res 1992;24:434–8.

65. Krouse RS, Royal RE, Heywood G, et al. Thyroid dysfunction in 281 patients with metastatic melanoma or renal carcinoma treated with interleukin-2 alone. J Immunother Emphasis Tumor Immunol 1995;18:272–8.

66. Vialettes B, Guillerand MA, Viens P, et al. Incidence rate and risk factors for thyroid dysfunction during recombinant interleukin-2 therapy in advanced malignancies. Acta Endocrinol (Copenh) 1993;129:31–8.

67. Chianese-Bullock KA, Woodson EM, Tao H, et al. Autoimmune toxicities associated with the administration of antitumor vaccines and low-dose interleukin-2. J Immunother 2005;28:412–9.

68. Ribas A, Camacho LH, Lopez-Berestein G, et al. Antitumor activity in melanoma and anti-self responses in a phase I trial with the anti-cytotoxic T lymphocyte-associated antigen 4 monoclonal antibody CP-675,206. J Clin Oncol 2005;23:8968–77.

69. Attia P, Phan GQ, Maker AV, et al. Autoimmunity correlates with tumor regression in patients with metastatic melanoma treated with anti-cytotoxic T-lymphocyte antigen-4. J Clin Oncol 2005;23:6043–53.

70. Ghori F, Polder KD, Pinter-Brown LC, et al. Thyrotoxicosis following denileukin diftitox therapy in patients with mycosis fungoides. J Clin Endocrinol Metab 2006 .

71. Geerdsen JP, Frolund L. Thyroid function after surgical treatment of nontoxic goiter. A randomized study of postoperative thyroxine administration. Acta Med Scand 1986;220:341–5.

72. Miller FR, Paulson D, Prihoda TJ, Otto RA. Risk factors for the development of hypothyroidism after hemithyroidectomy. Arch Otolaryngol Head Neck Surg 2006;132:36–8.

73. Grande C. Hypothyroidism following radiotherapy for head and neck cancer: mutivariate analysis of risk factors. Radiother Oncol 1992;25:31–6.

74. Berger C, Le-Gallo B, Donadieu J, et al. Late thyroid toxicity in 153 long-term survivors of allogeneic bone marrow transplantation for acute lymphoblastic leukaemia. Bone Marrow Transplant 2005;35:991–5.

75. Boulad F, Bromley M, Black P, et al. Thyroid dysfunction following bone marrow transplantation using hyper-fractionated radiation. Bone Marrow Transplant 1995;15:71–6.

76. Garcia-Serra A, Amdur RJ, Morris CG, et al. Thyroid function should be monitored following radiotherapy to the low neck. Am J Clin Oncol 2005;28:255–8.

77. Sklar C, Whitton J, Mertens A, et al. Abnormalities of the thyroid in survivors of Hodgkin's disease: data from the Childhood Cancer Survivor Study. J Clin Endocrinol Metab 2000;85:3227–32.

78. van Santen HM, de Kraker J, van Eck BL, et al. High incidence of thyroid dysfunction despite prophylaxis with potassium iodide during (131)I-meta-iodobenzylguanidine treatment in children with neuroblastoma. Cancer 2002;94:2081–9.

79. Ferretti E, Persani L, Jaffrain-Rea ML, et al. Evaluation of the adequacy of levothyroxine replacement therapy in patients with central hypothyroidism. J Clin Endocrinol Metab 1999;84:924–9.

80. Samaan NA, Schultz PN, Yang KP, Vassilopoulou-Sellin R. Endocrine complications after radiotherapy for tumors of the head and neck. J Lab Clin Med 1987;109:364–72.

81. Sherman SI, Gopal J, Haugen BR, et al. Central hypothyroidism associated with retinoid X receptor-selective ligands. N Engl J Med 1999;340:1075–9.

82. Macchia PE, Jiang P, Yuan YD, et al. RXR receptor agonist suppression of thyroid function: central effects in the absence of thyroid hormone receptor. Am J Physiol Endocrinol Metab 2002;283:E326–31 .

83. Golden WA, Weber KB, Hernandez TL, et al. Single-dose rexinoid rapidly and specifically suppresses serum TSH in normal subjects. J Clin Endocrinol Metab.[submitted]

84. Sherman SI. Etiology, diagnosis, and treatment recommendations for central hypothyroidism associated with bexarotene therapy for cutaneous T-cell lymphoma. Clin Lymphoma 2003;3:249–52.

85. Kimura H, Yamashita S, Ashizawa K, et al. Thyroid dysfunction in patients with amyloid goitre. Clin Endocrinol (Oxf) 1997;46:769–74.

86. Dispenzieri A, Kyle RA, Lacy MQ, et al. POEMS syndrome: definitions and long-term outcome. Blood 2003;101:2496–506.

87. Badros AZ, Siegel E, Bodenner D, et al. Hypothyroidism in patients with multiple myeloma following treatment with thalidomide. Am J Med 2002;112:412–3.

88. Amato RJ, Morgan M, Rawat A. Phase I/II study of thalidomide in combination with interleukin-2 in patients with metastatic renal cell carcinoma. Cancer 2006;106:1498–506.

89. Figg WD, Thibault A, Sartor AO, et al. Hypothyroidism associated with aminoglutethimide in patients with prostate cancer. Arch Intern Med 1994;154:1023–5.

90. Gittoes NJ, Franklyn JA. Drug-induced thyroid disorders. Drug Saf 1995;13:46–55.

91. de Groot JW, Zonnenberg BA, Plukker JT, et al. Imatinib induces hypothyroidism in patients receiving levothyroxine. Clin Pharmacol Ther 2005;78:433–8.

92. Arafah BM. Increased need for thyroxine in women with hypothyroidism during estrogen therapy. N Engl J Med 2001;344:1743–9.

93. Ruppe MD, Huang SA, Jan de Beur SM. Consumptive hypothyroidism caused by paraneoplastic production of type 3 iodothyronine deiodinase. Thyroid 2005;15:1369–72.

94. Huang SA, Fish SA, Dorfman DM, et al. A 21-year-old woman with consumptive hypothyroidism due to a vascular tumor expressing type 3 iodothyronine deiodinase. J Clin Endocrinol Metab 2002;87:4457–61.

95. Baloch Z, Carayon P, Conte-Devolx B, et al. Laboratory medicine practice guidelines. Laboratory support for the diagnosis and monitoring of thyroid disease. Thyroid 2003;13:3–126.

96. Umpierrez GE. Euthyroid sick syndrome. South Med J 2002;95:506–13.

97. Feelders RA, Swaak AJ, Romijn JA, et al. Characteristics of recovery from the euthyroid sick syndrome induced by tumor necrosis factor alpha in cancer patients. Metabolism 1999;48:324–9.

98. Harel Z, Biro FM, Tedford WL. Effects of long term treatment with sertraline (Zoloft) simulating hypothyroidism in an adolescent. J Adolesc Health 1995;16:232–4.

99. Fliers E, Guldenaar SE, Wiersinga WM, Swaab DF. Decreased hypothalamic thyrotropin-releasing hormone gene expression in patients with nonthyroidal illness. J Clin Endocrinol Metab 1997;82:4032–6.

100. Magner J, Roy P, Fainter L, et al. Transiently decreased sialylation of thyrotropin (TSH) in a patient with the euthyroid sick syndrome. Thyroid 1997;7:807–8.

101. Nellen Hummel H, Gutierrez Espindola G, Talavera J, et al. Effect of chemotherapy on thyroid hormone concentration in patients with malignant hematologic diseases. Arch Med Res 1997;28:215–7.

102. Lee WY, Kang MI, Oh KW, et al. Relationship between circulating cytokine levels and thyroid function following bone marrow transplantation. Bone Marrow Transplant 2004;33:93–8.

103. Vexiau P, Perez-Castiglioni P, Socie G, et al. The 'euthyroid sick syndrome': incidence, risk factors and prognostic value soon after allogeneic bone marrow transplantation. Br J Haematol 1993;85:778–82.

104. Wehmann RE, Gregerman RI, Burns WH, et al. Suppression of thyrotropin in the low-thyroxine state of severe nonthyroidal illness. N Engl J Med 1985;312:546–52.

105. DeGroot LJ. "Non-thyroidal illness syndrome" is functional central hypothyroidism, and if severe, hormone replacement is appropriate in light of present knowledge. J Endocrinol Invest 2003;26:1163–70.

106. Stathatos N, Wartofsky L. The euthyroid sick syndrome: is there a physiologic rationale for thyroid hormone treatment? J Endocrinol Invest 2003;26:1174–9.

107. Carrozza V, Csako G, Yanovski JA, et al. Levothyroxine replacement therapy in central hypothyroidism: a practice report. Pharmacotherapy 1999;19:349–55.

108. Smyrniotis V, Vaos N, Arkadopoulos N, et al. Severe hypothyroidism in patients dependent on prolonged thyroxine infusion through a jejunostomy. Clin Nutr 2000;19:65–7.

109. Sherman SI, Malecha SE. Absorption and malabsorption of levothyroxine. Am J Ther 1995;2:814–8.

110. Escobar-Morreale HF, Botella-Carretero JI, Gomez-Bueno M, et al. Thyroid hormone replacement therapy in primary hypothyroidism: a randomized trial comparing L-thyroxine plus liothyronine with L-thyroxine alone. Ann Intern Med 2005;142:412–24.

111. Alshekhlee A, Kaminski HJ, Ruff RL. Neuromuscular manifestations of endocrine disorders. Neurol Clin 2002;20:35–58, v–vi.

112. Budavari AI, Whitaker MD, Helmers RA. Thymic hyperplasia presenting as anterior mediastinal mass in 2 patients with Graves' disease. Mayo Clin Proc 2002;77:495–9.

113. Nicolle MW. Pseudo-myasthenia gravis and thymic hyperplasia in Graves' disease. Can J Neurol Sci 1999;26:201–3.

114. Schalin-Jantti C, Laine T, Valli-Jaakola K, et al. Manifestation, management and molecular analysis of candidate genes in two rare cases of thyrotoxic hypokalemic periodic paralysis. Horm Res 2005;63:139–44.

115. Kung AW, Lau KS, Cheung WM, Chan V. Thyrotoxic periodic paralysis and polymorphisms of sodium-potassium ATPase genes. Clin Endocrinol (Oxf) 2006;64:158–61.

116. Klein I. Thyroid and the heart. Thyroid 2002;12:439 .

117. Sun ZQ, Ojamaa K, Nakamura TY, et al. Thyroid hormone increases pacemaker activity in rat neonatal atrial myocytes. J Mol Cell Cardiol 2001;33:811–24.

118. Graettinger JS, Muenster JJ, Selverstone LA, Cambell JA. A correlation of clinical and hemodynamic studies in patients with hyperthyroidism with and without congestive heart failure. J Clin Invest 1959;38:1316–27.

119. Sawin CT, Geller A, Wolf PA, et al. Low serum thyrotropin concentrations as a risk factor for atrial fibrillation in older persons. N Engl J Med 1994;331:1249–52.

120. Shimizu T, Koide S, Noh JY, et al. Hyperthyroidism and the management of atrial fibrillation. Thyroid 2002;12:489–93.

121. Mier A, Brophy C, Wass JA, et al. Reversible respiratory muscle weakness in hyperthyroidism. Am Rev Respir Dis 1989;139:529–33.

122. Pino-Garcia JM, Garcia-Rio F, Diez JJ, et al. Regulation of breathing in hyperthyroidism: relationship to hormonal and metabolic changes. Eur Respir J 1998;12:400–7.

123. Meshkinpour H, Afrasiabi MA, Valenta LJ. Esophageal motor function in Graves' disease. Dig Dis Sci 1979;24:159–61.

124. Goswami R, Tandon RK, Dudha A, Kochupillai N. Prevalence and significance of steatorrhea in patients with active Graves' disease. Am J Gastroenterol 1998;93:1122–5.

125. O'Reilly RA. Splenomegaly in 2,505 patients in a large university medical center from 1913 to 1995. 1913 to 1962: 2,056 patients. West J Med 1998;169:78–87.
126. Safer JD, Crawford TM, Fraser LM, et al. Thyroid hormone action on skin: diverging effects of topical versus intraperitoneal administration. Thyroid 2003;13:159–65.
127. Cannon CR. Hypothyroidism in head and neck cancer patients: experimental and clinical observations. Laryngoscope 1994;104:1–21.
128. Safer JD, Crawford TM, Holick MF. A role for thyroid hormone in wound healing through keratin gene expression. Endocrinology 2004;145:2357–61.
129. Fatourechi V. Pretibial myxedema: pathophysiology and treatment options. Am J Clin Dermatol 2005;6:295–309.
130. Brenner B, Fandrey J, Jelkmann W. Serum immunoreactive erythropoietin in hyper- and hypothyroidism: clinical observations related to cell culture studies. Eur J Haematol 1994;53:6–10.
131. Das KC, Mukherjee M, Sarkar TK, et al. Erythropoiesis and erythropoietin in hypo- and hyperthyroidism. J Clin Endocrinol Metab 1975;40:211–20.
132. Ford HC, Carter JM. The haematology of hyperthyroidism: abnormalities of erythrocytes, leucocytes, thrombocytes and haemostasis. Postgrad Med J 1988;64:735–42.
133. Kubota K, Tamura J, Kurabayashi H, et al. Evaluation of increased serum ferritin levels in patients with hyperthyroidism. Clin Investig 1993;72:26–9.
134. Chute JP, Ryan CP, Sladek G, Shakir KM. Exacerbation of warfarin-induced anticoagulation by hyperthyroidism. Endocr Pract 1997;3:77–9.
135. Cooper DS, Ridgway EC, Kliman B, et al. Metabolic clearance and production rates of prolactin in man. J Clin Invest 1979;64:1669–80.
136. Valcavi R, Dieguez C, Zini M, et al. Influence of hyperthyroidism on growth hormone secretion. Clin Endocrinol (Oxf) 1993;38:515–22.
137. Pantazi H, Papapetrou PD. Changes in parameters of bone and mineral metabolism during therapy for hyperthyroidism. J Clin Endocrinol Metab 2000;85:1099–106.
138. Elin RJ. Magnesium metabolism in health and disease. Dis Mon 1988;34:161–218.
139. Lin SH. Thyrotoxic periodic paralysis. Mayo Clin Proc 2005;80:99–105.
140. Nayak VK, Desai NK, Kshirsagar NA, et al. Antipyrine and doxycycline pharmacokinetics in patients with thyroid disorders. J Postgrad Med 1991;37:5–8.
141. Kohn LD, Shimojo N, Kohno Y, Suzuki K. An animal model of Graves' disease: understanding the cause of autoimmune hyperthyroidism. Rev Endocr Metab Disord 2000;1:59–67.
142. Ando T, Imaizumi M, Graves P, et al. Induction of thyroid-stimulating hormone receptor autoimmunity in hamsters. Endocrinology 2003;144:671–80.
143. Simmonds MJ, Gough SC. Unravelling the genetic complexity of autoimmune thyroid disease: HLA, CTLA-4 and beyond. Clin Exp Immunol 2004;136:1–10.
144. Ban Y, Concepcion ES, Villanueva R, et al. Analysis of immune regulatory genes in familial and sporadic Graves' disease. J Clin Endocrinol Metab 2004;89:4562–8.
145. Weiss GR, Fehrenkamp SH, Tokaz LK, Sunderland MC. Vitiligo and Graves' disease following treatment of malignant melanoma with recombinant human interleukin 4. Dermatology 1996;192:283–5.
146. Locker GJ, Steger GG, Gnant MF, et al. Induction of immunomediated diseases by recombinant human granulocyte-macrophage colony-stimulating factor during cancer treatment? J Immunother 1999;22:85–9.
147. Jereczek-Fossa BA, Alterio D, Jassem J, et al. Radiotherapy-induced thyroid disorders. Cancer Treat Rev 2004;30:369–84.
148. Hancock SL, R.S. C , McDougall IR. Thyroid diseases after treatment of Hodgkin's disease. N Engl J Med 1991;325:599–605.
149. Hershman JM. Physiological and pathological aspects of the effect of human chorionic gonadotropin on the thyroid. Best Pract Res Clin Endocrinol Metab 2004;18:249–65.
150. Giralt SA, Dexeus F, Amato R, et al. Hyperthyroidism in men with germ cell tumors and high levels of beta-human chorionic gonadotropin. Cancer 1992;69:1286–90.
151. Arturi F, Scarpelli D, Coco A, et al. Thyrotropin receptor mutations and thyroid hyperfunctioning adenomas ten years after their first discovery: unresolved questions. Thyroid 2003;13:341–3.
152. Laurberg P, Pedersen KM, Hreidarsson A, et al. Iodine intake and the pattern of thyroid disorders: a comparative epidemiological study of thyroid abnormalities in the elderly in Iceland and in Jutland, Denmark. J Clin Endocrinol Metab 1998;83:765–9.
153. Als C, Gedeon P, Rosler H, et al. Survival analysis of 19 patients with toxic thyroid carcinoma. J Clin Endocrinol Metab 2002;87:4122–7.
154. Kasayama S, Miyake S, Samejima Y. Transient thyrotoxicosis and hypothyroidism following administration of the GnRH agonist leuprolide acetate. Endocr J 2000;47:783–5.
155. Mandac JC, Chaudhry S, Sherman KE, Tomer Y. The clinical and physiological spectrum of interferon-alpha induced thyroiditis: toward a new classification. Hepatology 2006;43:661–72.
156. Pearce EN, Farwell AP, Braverman LE. Thyroiditis. N Engl J Med 2003;348:2646–55.
157. Hoekman K, von Blomberg-van der Flier BM, Wagstaff J, et al. Reversible thyroid dysfunction during treatment with GM-CSF. Lancet 1991;338:541–2.
158. Nishiyama K, Kozuka T, Higashihara T, et al. Acute radiation thyroiditis. Int J Radiat Oncol Biol Phys 1996;36:1221–4.
159. Bartalena L, Robbins J. Variations in thyroid hormone transport proteins and their clinical implications. Thyroid 1992;2:237–45.
160. Rajatanavin R, Liberman C, Lawrence GD, et al. Euthyroid hyperthyroxinemia and thyroxine-binding prealbumin excess in islet cell carcinoma. J Clin Endocrinol Metab 1985;61:17–21.
161. Nicholas WC, Fischer RG, Stevenson RA, Bass JD. Single daily dose of methimazole compared to every 8 hours propylthiouracil in the treatment of hyperthyroidism. South Med J 1995;88:973–6.
162. Cooper DS. Antithyroid drugs. N Engl J Med 2005;352:905–17.
163. Ron E, Doody MM, Becker DV, et al. Cancer mortality following treatment for adult hyperthyroidism. Cooperative Thyrotoxicosis Therapy Follow-up Study Group. JAMA 1998;280:347–55.
164. Tan GH, Gharib H. Thyroid incidentalomas: management approaches to nonpalpable nodules discovered incidentally on thyroid imaging. Ann Intern Med 1997;126:226–31.
165. Jemal A, Siegel R, Ward E, et al. Cancer statistics, 2006. CA Cancer J Clin 2006;56:106–30.
166. Nakhjavani MK, Gharib H, Goellner JR, van Heerden JA. Metastasis to the thyroid gland. A report of 43 cases. Cancer 1997;79:574–8.
167. Mirallie E, Rigaud J, Mathonnet M, et al. Management and prognosis of metastases to the thyroid gland. J Am Coll Surg 2005;200:203–7.
168. Vassilopoulou-Sellin R, Weber RS. Metastatic thyroid cancer as an incidental finding during neck dissection: significance and management. Head Neck 1992;14:459–63.
169. Choi JY, Lee KS, Kim HJ, et al. Focal thyroid lesions incidentally identified by integrated 18F-FDG PET/CT: clinical significance and improved characterization. J Nucl Med 2006;47:609–15.
170. Chu QD, Connor MS, Lilien DL, et al. Positron emission tomography (PET) positive thyroid incidentaloma: the risk of malignancy observed in a tertiary referral center. Am Surg 2006;72:272–5.
171. Kim TY, Kim WB, Ryu JS, et al. 18F-fluorodeoxyglucose uptake in thyroid from positron emission tomogram (PET) for evaluation in cancer patients: high prevalence of malignancy in thyroid PET incidentaloma. Laryngoscope 2005;115:1074–8.
172. Rubino C, Cailleux AF, De Vathaire F, Schlumberger M. Thyroid cancer after radiation exposure. Eur J Cancer 2002;38:645–7.
173. Pacini F, Vorontsova T, Demidchik EP, et al. Post-Chernobyl thyroid carcinoma in Belarus children and adolescents: comparison with naturally occurring thyroid carcinoma in Italy and France. J Clin Endocrinol Metab 1997;82:3563–9.
174. Gilbert ES, Tarone R, Bouville A, Ron E. Thyroid cancer rates and 131I doses from Nevada atmospheric nuclear bomb tests. J Natl Cancer Inst 1998;90:1654–60.
175. Burke JP, Hay ID, Dignan F, et al. Long-term trends in thyroid carcinoma: a population-based study in Olmsted County, Minnesota, 1935-1999. Mayo Clin Proc 2005;80:753–8.
176. Cooper DS, Doherty GM, Haugen BR, et al. Management guidelines for patients with thyroid nodules and differentiated thyroid cancer. Thyroid 2006;16:109–42.
177. Papini E, Guglielmi R, Bianchini A, et al. Risk of malignancy in nonpalpable thyroid nodules: predictive value of ultrasound and color-Doppler features. J Clin Endocrinol Metab 2002;87:1941–6.
178. Ravetto C, Colombo L, Dottorini ME. Usefulness of fine-needle aspiration in the diagnosis of thyroid carcinoma: a retrospective study in 37,895 patients. Cancer 2000;90:357–63.
179. Cochand-Priollet B, Guillausseau PJ, Chagnon S, et al. The diagnostic value of fine-needle aspiration biopsy under ultrasonography in nonfunctional thyroid nodules: a prospective study comparing cytologic and histologic findings. Am J Med 1994;97:152–7.
180. Gharib H. Fine-needle aspiration biopsy of thyroid nodules: advantages, limitations, and effect. Mayo Clin Proc 1994;69:44–9.
181. Tyler DS, Winchester DJ, Caraway NP, et al. Indeterminate fine-needle aspiration biopsy of the thyroid. Identification of subgroups at high risk for invasive carcinoma. Surgery 1994;116:1054–60.
182. Tuttle RM, Lemar H, Burch HB. Clinical features associated with an increased risk of thyroid malignancy in patients with follicular neoplasia by fine-needle aspiration. Thyroid 1998;8:377–83.
183. Baloch ZW, Fleisher S, LiVolsi VA, Gupta PK. Diagnosis of "follicular neoplasm": a gray zone in thyroid fine-needle aspiration cytology. Diagn Cytopathol 2002;26:41–4.
184. Udelsman R, Westra WH, Donovan PI, et al. Randomized prospective evaluation of frozen-section analysis for follicular neoplasms of the thyroid. Ann Surg 2001;233:716–22.
185. Roach JC, Heller KS, Dubner S, Sznyter LA. The value of frozen section examinations in determining the extent of thyroid surgery in patients with indeterminate fine-needle aspiration cytology. Arch Otolaryngol Head Neck Surg 2002;128:263–7.
186. Cramer H. Fine-needle aspiration cytology of the thyroid: an appraisal. Cancer 2000;90:325–9.
187. Castro MR, Caraballo PJ, Morris JC. Effectiveness of thyroid hormone suppressive therapy in benign solitary thyroid nodules: a meta-analysis. J Clin Endocrinol Metab 2002;87:4154–9.
188. Sherman SI. Thyroid carcinoma. Lancet 2003;361:501–11.
189. Sherman SI, Angelos P, Ball DW, et al. Thyroid carcinoma. J Natl Compr Canc Netw 2005;3:404–57.
190. Chen H, Nicol TL, Udelsman R. Clinically significant, isolated metastatic disease to the thyroid gland. World J Surg 1999;23:177–80; discussion 81.

Pituitary and Adrenal Complications in Cancer Patients

Sai-Ching Jim Yeung, MD, PhD

Robert F. Gagel, MD

Cancer and its treatment can lead to endocrine dysfunction and to clinical and laboratory abnormalities that obscure or mimic endocrine diseases. The pituitary is the "master" gland in the body; among the various endocrine axes regulated by the hypothalamic-pituitary system, the hypothalamic-pituitary-adrenal axis is one of the vital hormonal systems, severe dysfunction of which can lead to death. In this chapter, we focus on the impact of cancer and cancer treatments on the hypothalamus, pituitary gland, and adrenal glands.

Hypothalamic-Pituitary Dysfunction

Radiotherapy is a common cause of hypothalamic and pituitary dysfunction in cancer patients. In contrast, there is no strong direct evidence to implicate chemotherapy as a cause of permanent hypothalamic or pituitary dysfunction. (Glucocorticoid-induced hypoadrenalism and targretin-induced central hypothyroidism are reversible after cessation of the drugs.) Metastasis to the hypothalamic region or the pituitary gland is uncommon,[1] and clinical manifestations of endocrine dysfunction owing to metastatic disease in this region are even rarer. However, benign tumors, such as pituitary tumors and craniopharyngiomas, frequently affect this anatomic region and cause endocrine dysfunction.

Radiation-induced anterior pituitary hormone deficiencies are irreversible and progressive. Although the hypothalamus is the the regional structure most affected by radiation damage, hypothalamic damage can lead to pituitary atrophy over time owing to the lack of hypothalamic trophic factors. The pituitary gland may also be directly damaged by radiation. The severity, frequency, and timing of onset of hypothalamic and pituitary hormone deficiencies correlate with the total dose and fraction size of radiation in the hypothalamic-pituitary area and previous pituitary compromise by tumor and/or surgery and correlate inversely with the age of the patient at the time of radiotherapy.

The development of radiation-induced hypothalamic dysfunction is usually insidious; hormone deficiencies can manifest clinically years after radiation exposure. There is considerable variation in the sequence and frequency of hormonal dysfunctions among the several axes of hypothalamic-pituitary function. The somatotropic axis appears to be the most sensitive to radiation. Growth hormone (GH) deficiency typically occurs in isolation following exposure of the hypothalamic-pituitary area to less than 30 Gy of radiation; with higher levels of radiation exposure (30–50 Gy), the frequency of GH deficiency substantially increases to as high as 50 to 100%. The thyrotropic axis appears to be the least sensitive to radiation (Figure 1).[2–5] Abnormalities in gonadotropin secretion are dose dependent: precocious puberty owing to dysregulation of gonadotropin secretion can occur after radiation doses less than 30 Gy in girls and after doses of 30 to 50 Gy in boys and girls. Gonadotropin deficiency occurs infrequently and is usually a long-term complication following a radiation dose of 30 Gy or more. Much higher incidences of gonadotropin, adrenocorticotropic hormone (ACTH or corticotropin), and thyroid-stimulating hormone (TSH or thyrotropin) deficiencies (30–60% after 10 years) occur after the more intensive irradiation typically used for nasopharyngeal carcinomas and tumors of the skull base (> 70 Gy) and for pituitary tumors (30–50 Gy). In a recent study, 41% of adult patients treated with cranial irradiation for primary nonpituitary brain tumors had hypopituitarism, which was time and dose dependent.[6]

The diagnosis of hypothalamic-pituitary dysfunction requires vigilance by the physician because most of the presenting symptoms are nonspecific and can easily be attributed to other causes. For example, fatigue and weakness, symptoms of pituitary dysfunction, are common among cancer patients. Regular screening examinations and testing are required to ensure timely diagnosis and early hormone replacement therapy to prevent short stature and ill health in children cured of cancer and to prevent ill health, sexual dysfunction, and osteoporosis and improve the quality of life in adults. An initial diagnostic evaluation for hypothalamic and pituitary dysfunction may include serum GH and insulin-like growth factor 1 (IGF-1) measurements and evaluation for gonadal failure. Signs of overt hypopituitarism include hypoglycemia, hypotension, and hypothermia.

In children and teenagers, evaluation of sexual development is a useful diagnostic tool. The investigation should include staging of sexual development according to the Tanner staging criteria, examination of pubic and axillary hair, and review of menstrual history in girls and penile or testicular size in boys. In children who have had cranial irradiation, height and growth velocity should be measured at 6-month intervals. In children treated with spinal or craniospinal irradiation, local rather than general growth abnormalities may be present and, if so, require further specific evaluation. Foot size is a reliable indicator of growth that can be measured on a routine clinic visit.[7] A child whose growth rate is not within the limits of a normal growth curve should be evaluated for GH deficiency, hypothyroidism, and adrenal insufficiency. If the initial evaluation of GH, IGF-1, TSH, and free thyroxine levels and radiographic bone age reveals abnormalities, then detailed dynamic testing to evaluate secretion of GH, ACTH, and gonadotropin-releasing hormone should be performed (Table 1).

In adults who have received cranial or head and neck irradiation, detection of hypothalamic-pituitary abnormalities is more challenging. One strategy to detect hypothalamic-pituitary abnormalities in adults consists of routine screening for abnormal GH and IGF-1 levels and gonadal failure, the most sensitive indicators of radiation-induced hypothalamic-pituitary damage. It is recommended that measurements of IGF-1 and testosterone levels in men and documentation of menstrual history in women be performed

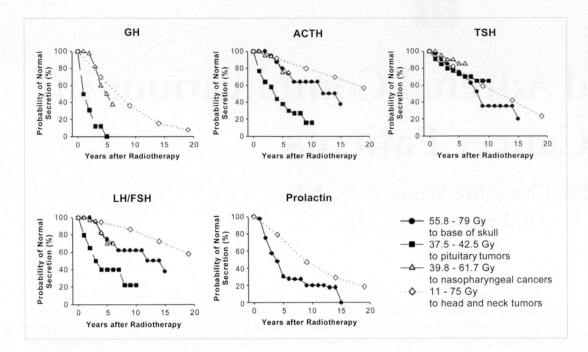

FIGURE 1 Probability of normal pituitary hormone secretion over time after exposure of the hypothalamic-pituitary area to radiation. Data from four studies are plotted. In the study by Pai and colleagues (*closed circles*), patients received 55.8 to 79 Gy to the base of the skull.[3] In the study by Shalet and colleagues (*solid squares*), patients with pituitary tumors received 37.5 to 42.5 Gy.[32] In the study by Lam and colleagues (*open triangles*), patients with nasopharyngeal carcinoma received 39.8 to 61.7 Gy.[2] In the study by Samaan and colleagues (*open diamonds*), patients with head and neck tumors received 11 to 75 Gy.[4] ACTH = adrenocorticotropic hormone; GH = growth hormone; LH/FSH = luteinizing hormone/follicle-stimulating hormone; TSH = thyroid-stimulating hormone.

annually for the first 5 years and then at 5-year intervals for the next 10 years. Any abnormalities noted should be pursued with further dynamic testing to evaluate all of the axes of hypothalamic-pituitary function (see Table 1).

Once specific hormonal deficiencies are diagnosed, hormone replacement therapy is quite straightforward, except for GH. GH therapy in cancer patients is an extremely controversial issue because of the association between GH and cancer. Experimental data have shown that GH and IGF-1 promote cancer cell survival and proliferation, and epidemiologic studies of patients with acromegaly indicate an increased risk of colorectal cancer. Although IGF-1 replacement to levels within the normal range is expected to have the same risk as the general population, GH therapy may result in a small increase in cancer risk compared with untreated patients with GH deficiency. The risk of tumor progression needs to be weighed against the known morbidity of GH deficiency and potential benefits in terms of improvement in quality of life.[8]

Pituitary apoplexy is a potentially life-threatening medical emergency with acute symptoms of headache, nausea, vomiting, visual field changes, ptosis, and diplopia owing to acute pituitary hemorrhage. In addition to the mass effect and resulting neurologic symptoms and sequelae, pituitary apoplexy can lead to adrenocortical insufficiency. A wide variety of conditions related to cancer and its treatment can trigger pituitary apoplexy, such as pituitary irradiation, general anesthesia, pituitary stimulatory tests, and medications such as bromocriptine and cabergoline, used in the treatment of prolactinoma. In men with locally advanced prostate cancer who are prescribed leuprolide, the initial stimulatory effects of this gonadotropin-releasing hormone analogue may induce pituitary apoplexy if an unrecognized or asymptomatic gonadotroph adenoma is present.[9] Tumors in the sphenoid sinus with extension into the sella turcica can cause symptoms similar to those of pituitary apoplexy.[10] Patients with pituitary apoplexy with acute neuro-ophthalmologic signs may need neurosurgical intervention, and those patients who do not have neuro-ophthalmologic signs or progressive clinical signs can be managed conservatively in the acute stage with monitoring for subsequent development of hypopituitarism.[11]

Adrenal Diseases

Adrenal Metastasis

Hematogenous metastasis to the adrenal glands is common, with the adrenal glands being the fourth most frequent site of hematogenous metastasis after the lungs, liver, and bones.[12] Autopsy studies have documented that 9 to 27% of patients who died of malignant diseases had adrenal metastasis, with bilateral involvement in half to two-thirds of affected patients. Ninety percent of adrenal metastases are carcinomas, and 60% of these are adenocarcinomas.[12] The primary tumors that most commonly metastasize to the adrenal glands are, in order of decreasing frequency, cancers of the lungs, stomach, esophagus, and liver or bile duct.[13] Many adrenal metastases are discovered shortly (about 7 months) after the diagnosis of the primary cancer.

The presence of adrenal metastasis may have important implications for diagnostic and therapeutic planning. When patients with cancer have an adrenal mass but no evidence of metastasis elsewhere, it is vital to determine whether the mass is a metastatic deposit or a separate, unrelated adrenal lesion. Recent advances in imaging techniques have allowed the identification of adrenal lesions as part of the tumor staging evaluation. The location of the adrenal glands in the perinephric fat allows the detection of almost all normal glands and contour-deforming masses as small as 5 mm. Computed tomography (CT) is sensitive and specific in the detection of adrenal masses. CT characteristics that suggest adrenal metastasis rather than primary adrenal disease include heterogeneity, contrast enhancement, bilaterality, and size greater than 3 cm.

Without other evidence of metastatic disease, whether an adrenal mass is actually a metastatic tumor is critical information in determining the appropriate cancer therapy. Evaluation of a patient who is suspected of having an adrenal metastasis should include a history and physical examination to elicit evidence of adrenal insufficiency, Cushing's syndrome, mineralocorticoid excess, or pheochromocytoma. Biochemical assessment should include a short ACTH stimulation test to rule out adrenal insufficiency. A 24-hour urine collection should be obtained to measure urinary free cortisol, aldosterone, catecholamines, and metanephrines. Pheochromocytoma must be excluded, especially if the patient has hypertension or an operative procedure of any type is contemplated. It has been reported that half of patients who had a clinically unsuspected pheochromocytoma and underwent a non–adrenal gland–related surgical procedure had clinical deterioration or even died immediately following surgery.[14]

If the biochemical assessment for pheochromocytoma is negative, CT-guided fine-needle aspiration should be considered. This procedure has a sensitivity of 85% in detecting malignant diseases in the adrenal glands.[15] Magnetic resonance imaging (MRI) also may be helpful in the diagnosis of adrenal lesions. Functional scintigraphy using 6-[131I]iodomethyl-19-*nor*-cholesterol (NP-59) may be used in conjunction with CT and

Table 1 Dynamic Testing of Hypothalamic-Pituitary Function

Test	Method	Interpretation
Insulin tolerance test	Position patient recumbent for 30 min prior to rapid IV injection of regular insulin, 0.10 U/kg. Collect samples at baseline, 30, 60, and 90 min for glucose, GH, ACTH, and cortisol. Monitor blood glucose levels at bedside. Adequate pituitary stimulation is evident when the patient becomes symptomatic (sweating or tremor) and/or when the glucose level drops below 45 mg/dL within 30 min. May give additional insulin at 30 min if these criteria are not met. In this case, collect an additional (120 min) sample.	Peak cortisol >20 µg/dL suggests that the hypothalamic-pituitary-adrenal axis is intact. GH and ACTH levels 3–5 times higher than baseline reflect normal pituitary secretion of GH and ACTH, respectively.
GH-RH + arginine test[33]	Give GH-RH, 1.0 µg/kg IV bolus, and arginine hydrochloride, 0.5 g/kg IV, over 30 min. Collect samples for GH at baseline and 30, 60, 90, and 120 min.	The lower the peak GH responses to this test, the more severe is the degree of hypopituitarism[33]
GH-RH stimulation	Give GH-RH, 1.0 µg/kg IV bolus. Collect samples for GH at baseline and 30, 60, 90, and 120 min.	GH levels 5–10 times higher than baseline indicate normal pituitary GH secretion
Arginine stimulation	Give arginine hydrochloride, 0.5 g/kg IV over 30 min. Exercise (10–15 min) may be added to potentiate the response. Collect samples for GH at baseline and 30, 60, 90, and 120 min.	Peak GH >7 ng/mL or increase of more than 5 ng/mL above baseline indicates normal GH secretion
Metyrapone stimulation test, overnight	At 11 pm, patient takes metyrapone (30 mg/kg, maximum 3 g) orally with a snack to prevent gastric irritation. At 8 am next day, collect blood sample for cortisol and 11-deoxycortisol.	11-Deoxycortisol >7 µg/dL indicates normal function of the hypothalamic-pituitary-adrenal axis
GH suppression test	Should be performed after an overnight fast with the patient maintained at bedrest. The patient should drink a solution of 100 g of glucose. Collect samples for GH at baseline and 90 and 120 min.	Suppression of GH to <5 ng/mL indicates the absence of acromegaly
Gn-RH stimulation test	Give Gn-RH, 100 µg IV. Collect samples for serum LH at baseline and 40 min.	LH level 2–5 times higher than baseline indicates normal responses of the gonadotropic axis
High-dose dexamethasone test, 48 h	Collect samples for serum cortisol at 9 am. Give dexamethasone (2.0 mg; 50 µg/kg in children) immediately afterward and again every 6 h for 8 doses. Collect second sample for serum cortisol at 9 am, 6 h after the last dexamethasone dose.	Patients with functional adrenal adenomas show no suppression of cortisol levels in the 48 h sample relative to the initial (baseline) sample. Seventy-eight percent of patients with a pituitary source of excess ACTH show $>50\%$ suppression of plasma cortisol, whereas only 11% of patients with an ectopic source of excess ACTH have $>50\%$ suppression.
Low-dose dexamethasone test, overnight	Based on the principle that the sensitivity of the pituitary is greatest at night. Give dexamethasone orally (1.0 mg; 20 µg/kg in children) between 11 pm and midnight. Collect sample for serum cortisol at 8–9 am the next morning.	Cortisol level <1.8 µg/dL essentially excludes Cushing's syndrome
ACTH stimulation test, 48 h	Beginning at 9 am, obtain 24 h urine for 17-OHCS and creatinine for baseline. The next day beginning at 9 am, give 250 µg cosyntropin in 250 mL normal saline IV every 8 h for 48 h. Alternatively, 40 IU of depot formulation of purified bovine ACTH in gelatin can be injected IM every 12 h for 48 h. Repeat 24 h urine collections.	>18 µg/dL or 2–5 times over basal values higher than baseline indicates adequate response of the adrenal glands to ACTH
ACTH stimulation test, 1 h	Draw blood for baseline cortisol with or without aldosterone. Inject 250 µg cosyntropin IM or IV (if IV, dilute cosyntropin in 2–5 mL of sterile saline and inject over 2 min). Draw blood for cortisol (with or without aldosterone) at 30 and 60 min.	Cortisol >18 µg/dL indicates adequate adrenal gland function, and central adrenal insufficiency is unlikely

ACTH = adrenocorticotropic hormone; GH = growth hormone; GH-RH = growth hormone–releasing hormone; Gn-RH = gonadotropin-releasing hormone; IM = intramuscularly; IV = intravenously; LH = luteinizing hormone; 17-OHCS = 17-hydroxycorticosteroids.

MRI to aid in the diagnosis of a unilateral adrenal mass greater than 2 cm.[16] [^{18}F]Fluorodeoxyglucose positron emission tomography can accurately characterize adrenal lesions and is informative in about half of cancer patients with inconclusive adrenal lesions on CT. Image-guided fine-needle aspiration biopsy in conjunction with MRI (as the sole imaging modality) is cost-effective in the management of patients with an adrenal lesion and may be the strategy of choice to distinguish between benign and malignant nonfunctioning adrenal masses larger than 2 cm in diameter.[17]

Adrenal metastasis in the absence of extra-adrenal metastases is rare, and the use of surgery, especially laparoscopic adrenalectomy, is controversial in the management of adrenal metastasis. Although laparoscopic adrenalectomy for adrenal metastasis is feasible, similar to the case of primary adrenal malignancy, the procedure should be performed with special care to avoid the dissemination of tumor cells in the surgical cavity. When laparoscopic surgery is performed for adrenal tumors larger than 6 cm or for tumors that are considered potentially malignant after preoperative imaging or endocrine studies, the operation should be performed only by a highly skilled laparoscopic surgeon, who should immediately switch to open surgery if the laparoscopic surgery becomes difficult.[18] In a retrospective study, laparoscopic adrenalectomy achieved an acceptable 5-year overall survival rate, comparable to that with open surgery.[19]

Adrenal Hemorrhage

Spontaneous massive retroperitoneal hemorrhage from an adrenal gland is rare,[20] although the risk factors of coagulopathy and thrombocytopenia are frequently present in cancer patients. Hemodynamically unstable patients who experience an adrenal hemorrhage may require transfusions and hemodynamic support in the intensive care unit, embolization if deemed feasible, or urgent surgical exploration. In patients with active bleeding, angiography with arterial embolization is a valuable therapeutic option to achieve hemostasis and allow for further evaluation of the adrenal tumor to plan the subsequent surgical resection. Emergency surgical removal of a malignant adrenal tumor within a large retroperitoneal hematoma should be avoided because optimal oncologic resection may not be possible under emergency situations.

Adrenal Insufficiency

Despite the relatively high prevalence of adrenal infiltration by many common cancers, clinically evident adrenal hypofunction occurs infrequently in cancer patients, except when both adrenal glands are affected by metastatic disease.[21] It is estimated that more than 80% of adrenal tissue must be destroyed before corticosteroid production, under both basal and stress conditions, is impaired.[22] Only about 1% of patients with adrenal metastases have adrenal insufficiency.[13]

The clinical manifestations of adrenal insufficiency are nonspecific and overlap with other common findings in cancer patients. For example, the cachexia and weakness that often occur gradually in patients with adrenal insufficiency can mimic the general wasting seen in patients with extensive metastatic disease; and electrolyte abnormalities can easily be explained by poor intake, malnutrition, the side effects of chemotherapeutic agents, or paraneoplastic syndromes. Therefore, a high index of suspicion is required to detect adrenal insufficiency.

Adrenal insufficiency will develop in 20 to 30% of patients with bilateral adrenal metastasis.[21] Measurements of plasma ACTH and serum cortisol in simultaneous samples can be useful in the differential diagnosis of a variety of adrenal disorders (Table 2). Patients with suspected adrenal insufficiency should all be evaluated by an ACTH stimulation test and should receive glucocorticoid and mineralocorticoid replacement therapy when adrenal insufficiency is suspected and until normal adrenal function is documented.

Table 2 Typical Adrenocorticotropic Hormone and Cortisol Levels in Various Clinical States		
Disease	*ACTH Level*	*Plasma Cortisol Level*
Cushing's syndrome	Elevated to high-normal	Elevated
Ectopic ACTH syndrome	Markedly elevated	Elevated
Adrenal carcinoma or adenoma	Low to undetectable	Elevated
Addison's disease	Consistently elevated	Decreased
Nelson's disease	Consistently elevated	Decreased
Adrenogenital syndrome	Elevated	Decreased

ACTH = adrenocorticotropic hormone.

Patients who are stable should receive 20 mg of hydrocortisone in the morning and 10 mg in the early afternoon. In the event of circulatory instability, sepsis, emergency surgery, or other major complications, stress dosages of a parenteral glucocorticoid should be given (eg, 100 mg of hydrocortisone succinate intravenously every 8 hours).

Other causes of primary adrenal insufficiency in cancer patients include autoimmune adrenalitis, adrenal hemorrhage, and granulomatous diseases. In immunocompromised cancer patients, particularly patients with leukemia or lymphoma and patients who have undergone bone marrow transplantation, infection of the adrenal glands by cytomegalovirus, mycobacteria, or fungi may lead to adrenal insufficiency.

Adrenal insufficiency also may be drug-induced. Etomidate,[21] a common intravenous anesthetic, and ketoconazole, an antifungal drug, both inhibit the production of cytochrome P-450–dependent enzymes in the glucocorticoid synthesis pathway, leading to low levels of glucocorticoids. Aminoglutethimide and metyrapone are drugs that inhibit enzymes in steroidogenesis, and both may cause adrenal insufficiency when used in the treatment of prostate, breast, and adrenocortical cancers. Mitotane, structurally related to the insecticide dichlorodiphenyltrichloroethane (DDT), has selective toxicity for normal and neoplastic adrenocortical cells. Adrenal insufficiency is common after mitotane is administered in the doses necessary to treat adrenocortical cancer; glucocorticoid replacement therapy is mandatory in such patients.[23] Increased protein binding may lead to an increased daily requirement of glucocorticoid dosages during replacement therapy. Suramin, recently proposed as an anticancer agent based on its activity against the tumor growth factors, also may cause adrenal insufficiency.

Secondary adrenal insufficiency owing to metastasis to the pituitary or hypothalamus may also occur. The most common cause of secondary adrenal hypofunction, however, is exogenous glucocorticoid therapy that suppresses the hypothalamic-pituitary adrenal axis. A prolonged course of therapy may lead to hypothalamic-pituitary suppression lasting for many months.

Short periods of steroid therapy (ie, 1–4 weeks) in patients with leukemia and lymphoma suppress adrenal function for 2 to 4 days beyond the end of therapy in most patients but for longer in some patients. In patients who have received glucocorticoids for more than 2 weeks, a tapering period of 10 to 14 days should be considered. This is especially true for patients who receive chemotherapy regimens that include high-dose glucocorticoids, such as regimens for acute leukemia and lymphoma. Using low-dose (1 µg) cosyntropin stimulation tests, high-dose glucocorticoid therapy can cause adrenal suppression lasting more than 1 week in children with acute lymphoblastic leukemia, even after tapering the dose.[24] Researchers have reported that adrenocortical insufficiency occurs and may persist for several months in children with acute lymphoblastic leukemia after treatment with high doses of prednisolone or dexamethasone.[25] Furthermore, glucocorticoid replacement during stress episodes is indicated within 1 to 2 months after discontinuation of a short course of high-dose glucocorticoid therapy and thereafter based on selective testing of adrenal function in accordance with symptoms. In addition, patients who have been treated within the past year with prolonged glucocorticoid therapy should receive stress dosages of glucocorticoid if acute medical or surgical complications occur (eg, neutropenic fever with hypotension, acute typhlitis).

Megestrol acetate, a progesterone analogue used as a palliative therapy for breast and endometrial cancers and as an appetite stimulant for cancer-related cachexia, has weak glucocorticoid activity that can also lead to secondary adrenal suppression.[26–29] Megestrol (800 mg for 12 weeks) can decrease TSH, luteinizing hormone, ACTH, and cortisol and increase prolactin and estradiol.[30]

Another cause of secondary adrenal insufficiency is irradiation of the hypothalamic-pituitary region. ACTH deficiency and secondary adrenal insufficiency occur in 19 to 42% of patients who receive this therapy[2,3,4,32] (see Figure 1). In a retrospective review of 310 childhood cancer survivors referred for evaluation of slow growth, fatigue, or abnormal pubertal timing, ACTH deficiency was diagnosed by low response to metyrapone and/or low-dose ACTH testing in 18%.[31]

Several diagnostic approaches have been used to evaluate secondary adrenal insufficiency, including basal 8 am serum cortisol measurements and dynamic tests with 1 μg of cosyntropin (synthetic $ACTH_{(1-24)}$), insulin-induced hypoglycemia, or metyrapone (see Table 1). Pituitary and adrenal complications of cancer and its treatment usually have non-specific signs and symptoms, making it challenging for the clinicians to diagnose. Once diagnosed, the management of these complications are relatively straight forward.

REFERENCES

1. Fassett DR, Couldwell WT. Metastases to the pituitary gland. Neurosurg Focus 2004;16:E8.
2. Lam KS, Tse VK, Wang C, et al. Effects of cranial irradiation on hypothalamic-pituitary function—a 5-year longitudinal study in patients with nasopharyngeal carcinoma. Q J Med 1991;78:165–76.
3. Pai HH, Thornton A, Katznelson L, et al. Hypothalamic/pituitary function following high-dose conformal radiotherapy to the base of skull: demonstration of a dose-effect relationship using dose-volume histogram analysis. Int J Radiat Oncol Biol Phys 2001;49:1079–92.
4. Samaan NA, Schultz PN, Yang KP, et al. Endocrine complications after radiotherapy for tumors of the head and neck. J Lab Clin Med 1987;109:364–72.
5. Shalet SM. Disorders of the endocrine system due to radiation and cytotoxic chemotherapy. Clin Endocrinol (Oxf) 1983;19:637–59.
6. Agha A, Sherlock M, Brennan S, et al. Hypothalamic-pituitary dysfunction after irradiation of nonpituitary brain tumors in adults. J Clin Endocrinol Metab 2005;90:6355–60.
7. Vassilopoulou-Sellin R, Klein MJ. Physical growth parameters in children treated for malignant diseases. Int J Hematol Oncol 1996;3:213–9.
8. Eiser C, Vance YH, Glaser A, et al. Growth hormone treatment and quality of life among survivors of childhood cancer. Horm Res 2005;63:300–4.
9. Davis A, Goel S, Picolos M, et al. Pituitary apoplexy after leuprolide. Pituitary 2006;9:263-5.
10. Sani S, Smith A, Leppla DC, et al. Epidermoid cyst of the sphenoid sinus with extension into the sella turcica presenting as pituitary apoplexy: case report. Surg Neurol 2005;63:394–7; discussion 397.
11. Sibal L, Ball SG, Connolly V, et al. Pituitary apoplexy: a review of clinical presentation, management and outcome in 45 cases. Pituitary 2004;7:157–63.
12. Abrams H, Spiro R, Goldstein N. Metastasis in carcinoma—one thousand autopsied cases. Cancer 1950;3:74.
13. Lam KY, Lo CY. Metastatic tumours of the adrenal glands: a 30-year experience in a teaching hospital. Clin Endocrinol (Oxf) 2002;56:95–101.
14. Platts JK, Drew PJ, Harvey JN. Death from phaeochromocytoma: lessons from a post-mortem survey. J R Coll Physicians Lond 1995;29:299–306.
15. Katz RL, Patel S, Mackay B, Zornoza J. Fine needle aspiration cytology of the adrenal gland. Acta Cytol 1984;28:269–82.
16. Francis IR, Smid A, Gross MD, et al. Adrenal masses in oncologic patients: functional and morphologic evaluation. Radiology 1988;166:353–6.
17. Lumachi F, Basso SM, Borsato S, et al. Role and cost-effectiveness of adrenal imaging and image-guided FNA cytology in the management of incidentally discovered adrenal tumours. Anticancer Res 2005;25:4559–62.
18. Tsuru N, Ushiyama T, Suzuki K. Laparoscopic adrenalectomy for primary and secondary malignant adrenal tumors. J Endourol 2005;19:702–8; discussion 708–9.
19. Sebag F, Calzolari F, Harding J, et al. Isolated adrenal metastasis: the role of laparoscopic surgery. World J Surg 2006;30:888-92.
20. Hendrickson RJ, Katzman PJ, Queiroz R, et al. Management of massive retroperitoneal hemorrhage from an adrenal tumor. Endocr J 2001;48:691–6.
21. Redman BG, Pazdur R, Zingas AP, Loredo R. Prospective evaluation of adrenal insufficiency in patients with adrenal metastasis. Cancer 1987;60:103–7.
22. Cedermark BJ, Sjoberg HE. The clinical significance of metastases to the adrenal glands. Surg Gynecol Obstet 1981;152:607–10.
23. van Seters AP, Moolenaar AJ. Mitotane increases the blood levels of hormone-binding proteins. Acta Endocrinol (Copenh) 1991;124:526–33.
24. Rix M, Birkebaek NH, Rosthoj S, Clausen N. Clinical impact of corticosteroid-induced adrenal suppression during treatment for acute lymphoblastic leukemia in children: a prospective observational study using the low-dose adrenocorticotropin test. J Pediatr 2005;147:645–50.
25. Petersen KB, Muller J, Rasmussen M, Schmiegelow K. Impaired adrenal function after glucocorticoid therapy in children with acute lymphoblastic leukemia. Med Pediatr Oncol 2003;41:110–4.
26. Meacham LR, Mazewski C, Krawiecki N. Mechanism of transient adrenal insufficiency with megestrol acetate treatment of cachexia in children with cancer. J Pediatr Hematol Oncol 2003;25:414–7.
27. Ozguroglu M, Yildiz O, Turna H, Kadioglu P. Megestrol acetate induced hypoadrenalism with cushingoid phenotype in endometrial cancer. Gynecol Oncol 2006;101:183.
28. Orme LM, Bond JD, Humphrey MS, et al. Megestrol acetate in pediatric oncology patients may lead to severe, symptomatic adrenal suppression. Cancer 2003;98:397–405.
29. Chidakel AR, Zweig SB, Schlosser JR, et al. High prevalence of adrenal suppression during acute illness in hospitalized patients receiving megestrol acetate. J Endocrinol Invest 2006;29:136–40.
30. Bodenner DL, Medhi M, Evans WJ, et al. Effects of megestrol acetate on pituitary function and end-organ hormone secretion: a post hoc analysis of serum samples from a 12-week study in healthy older men. Am J Geriatr Pharmacother 2005;3:160–7.
31. Rose SR, Danish RK, Kearney NS, et al. ACTH deficiency in childhood cancer survivors. Pediatr Blood Cancer 2005;45:808–13.
32. Shalet SM, Clayton PE, Price DA. Growth and pituitary function in children treated for brain tumours or acute lymphoblastic leukaemia. Hormone Res 1988;30:53–61.
33. Aimaretti G, Corneli G, Di Somma C, et al. Different degrees of GH deficiency evidenced by GHRH+arginine test and IGF-I levels in adults with pituritary disease. J Endocrinol Invest 2005;28:247–52.

Hypogonadism and Hormone Replacement in Men with Cancers

Christine Lee, MD

Shehzad Basaria, MD

Adrian S. Dobs, MD, MHS

Hypogonadism, regardless of its etiology, results in decreased sex hormone production from the gonad. There is a well-known association between increasing age and incidence of hypogonadism in men. In a longitudinal study of 890 men from ages 22 to 91, followed over a 40-year period, the incidence of hypogonadism diagnosed by free testosterone index was 9%, 34%, 68%, and 91% at for men in their 50s, 60s, 70s, and 80s, respectively.[1] With subgroup analysis of chronic illnesses within this population, only cancer was associated with a greater decrease in testosterone levels than the decline occurring with aging alone. In a retrospective analysis, hypogonadism was found to be present in 50 to 59% of 122 men with malignant lung cancer compared to 10% of 106 normal men.[2] Patients with cancer have a variety of etiologies that may lead to the development of hypogonadism, including cancer cachexia. In this chapter, we will discuss various etiologies, clinical manifestations, and diagnosis and treatment of men with cancer who develop hypogonadism. Since cancer cachexia itself is a known cause of hypogonadism, and hypogonadism itself may be responsible for wasting, this entity is discussed in even greater detail.

Normal Physiology of the Hypothalamic-Pituitary-Gonadal Axis

Gonadotropin-releasing hormone (GnRH) is secreted from the arcuate nucleus of the hypothalamus in a pulsatile fashion and targets the gonadotrophs in the anterior pituitary via the portal venous system. When stimulated by GnRH, the gonadotrophs synthesize and secrete luteinizing hormone (LH) and follicle-stimulating hormone (FSH). In males, LH acts on the Leydig cells in the testes to produce testosterone. FSH targets the Sertoli cells (which results in the production of inhibin) and seminiferous tubules to stimulate spermatogenesis.[3] Both testosterone

and inhibin cause negative inhibition of LH and FSH, respectively.

Total testosterone levels in postpubertal males range between 300 to 1,000 ng/dL. Although there is some debate on the definition of the normal range, total testosterone levels below 300 ng/dL in conjunction with symptoms of low androgen levels constitutes male hypogonadism. Signs and symptoms of hypogonadism in adult males include reductions in libido, erectile function, body hair, testicular size, muscle mass, bone density, prostate size, energy level and a sense of well-being. Women will commonly present with irregular menses, amenorrhea, infertility, vasomotor instability, decreased libido and reduced bone density.

Differential Diagnosis of Hypogonadism in Cancer Patients

The classical approach to hypogonadism is to classify it into primary, secondary, and tertiary disease based on the site of defect along the hypothalamic-pituitary-gonadal axis attributing for decreased sex hormone levels (Table 28-1).

Primary Hypogonadism

In primary hypogonadism, the defect is located in the testis or ovaries, resulting in the classically laboratory finding of low serum testosterone and elevated gonadotropins. Examples of primary hypogonadism include Klinefelter's syndrome, anorchism, gonadal dysgenesis, aplastic Leydig cells, testicular trauma, and orchitis. Primary hypogonadism also occurs in patients with testicular, ovarian or hematologic malignancies treated by cytotoxic chemotherapy and radiation. The most gonadotoxic chemotherapeutic drugs are alkylating agents, such as cyclophosphamide, chlorambucil, mustine, melphalan, busulfan, carmustine and lomustine. Other agents (eg, cytarabine, vinblastine, cisplatin, and procarbazine)

Table 1 Causes of Hypogonadism
Primary Hypogonadism
Klinefelter's syndrome
Noonan's syndrome
Anorchism
Gonadal dysgenesis
Aplastic Leydig cells
Testicular trauma
Orchiectomy
Cytotoxic chemotherapy (Cyclophosphamide, chlorambucil, melphalan)
Testicular/Pelvic irradiation
Chronic Illnesses (Renal failure, Cirrhosis, COPD, AIDS)
Infiltrative diseases (sarcoidosis, hemochromatosis)
Secondary Hypogonadism
Prolactinoma
Pituitary macroadenomas
Pituitary apoplexy
Post-surgical pituitary damage
Infiltrative diseases (sarcoidosis, hemochromatosis)
Cerebral trauma
Cranial irradiation
Medications (glucocorticoids, GnRH agonists)
Tertiary Hypogonadism
Kallmann's syndrome
Prader-Labhart-Willi syndrome
Laurence-Moon-Bardet-Biedl syndrome
Infiltrative diseases (sarcoidosis, hemochromatosis)
Trauma
Anorexia/weight loss
Critical Illness
Vascular Insufficiency
Cranial irradiation
Post-surgical hypothalamic damage
Medications (Opioids, GnRH analogs)
AIDS = acquired immunodeficiency syndrome; COPD = chronic obstructive pulmonary disease; GnRH = gonadotropin-releasing hormone.

are also known to cause gonadal dysfunction. These drugs predominantly affect germinal epithelium and spermatogenesis more than Leydig cells. Patients with lymphoma treated with chemotherapy tend to develop azoospermia, high FSH and LH, and normal or low-normal testosterone levels. Use of cyclophosphamide along with procarbazine results in permanent azoospermia as well as Leydig cell damage. Radiation to the testis or surrounding tissues also results in damage to sensitive germinal epithelium. Transient azoospermia and oligospermia may result from doses as low as 0.1 gray (Gy).[4] Leydig cell damage is more commonly seen at high-dose treatments of 20 to 30 Gy.

In addition to chemotherapy and radiotherapy, malignancy itself, by a poorly understood mechanism, may result in primary hypogonadism. Patients with bronchial carcinoma were found to have lower testosterone—but elevated LH—levels compared to healthy controls.[5] Furthermore, testosterone levels were significantly lower in patients with metastases. Elevated levels of circulating cytokines may be responsible for the impaired production/secretion of testosterone.

Secondary Hypogonadism

In secondary hypogonadism, there is inadequate or lack of secretion of LH/FSH from the anterior pituitary. Causes of secondary hypogonadism include medications (glucocorticoids), tumor infiltration of the pituitary, trauma, radiation, pituitary macroadenomas, pituitary apoplexy, infiltrating diseases (sarcoidosis, hemochromatosis) or hyperprolactinemia (of any etiology).[3] The induction of secondary hypogonadism, with leuprolide, goserelin, or abarelix, is used therapeutically in patients with prostate cancer. The first two are GnRH analogs that cause an initial surge in gonadotropins and testosterone after binding to the GnRH receptors on the anterior pituitary. However, over time, they result in a decrease in secretion of gonadotropins via invagination of the GnRH receptors. Abarelix is a GnRH antagonist that immediately suppresses gonadotropin and testosterone levels.

Tertiary Hypogonadism

Low-level, or absence of, GnRH secretion from the hypothalamus results in tertiary hypogonadism. In cancer patients, this can result from cranial irradiation, trauma, tumor, infiltration, anorexia, drugs, infection, vascular insufficiency, and extreme stress (see Table 28-1). As noted above, patients with intracranial neoplasms may develop tertiary hypogonadism if they undergo cranial irradiation or resection that may result in damage to the hypothalamus. Medications can also result in tertiary hypogonadism. Cancer patients on chronic high-dose opioids may be at

increased risk for central hypogonadism. Both intrathecal and oral opioids have led to central hypogonadism with low LH and testosterone levels, likely by inhibiting GnRH secretion via opioid receptors located in the hypothalamus. Another possibility is opioid-induced hyperprolactinemia that, in turn, causes suppression of GnRH synthesis. However, this hyperprolactinemia is transient.[6] Cancer patients in general may also develop tertiary hypogonadism in the setting of critical illness. A transient hypogonadal state has been noted in critically ill patients (patients with sepsis or burns) and patients undergoing surgery. More importantly, weight loss can result in a hypothalamically mediated GnRH suppression, likely due to increased production of cytokines or CRH, both of which can suppress GnRH.[7] The amount of weight required to result in hypothalamic deficiencies is unclear, but is likely due to reductions in body fat. Cancer cachexia is mentioned here as a cause of hypogonadism but, in turn, can be a result of the low testosterone as well.

Consequences and Clinical Manifestations of Hypogonadism

If hypogonadism is left untreated, the sequelae of androgen and estrogen insufficiency can cause significant morbidity and mortality. The most significant effects of untreated hypogonadism include cachexia, anemia, osteoporosis, and depression. It is crucial to make the diagnosis, since the clinical effects of low testosterone or estrogen may not be appreciated and simply attributed to the malignancy itself.

Cachexia

Although cachexia is not a common occurrence in conventional hypogonadism, it can contribute to cancer cachexia, similar to the well-described acquired immunodeficiency syndrome (AIDS) wasting syndrome. Weight loss in cancer patients is associated with increased morbidity and mortality. The weight loss in this population is multifactorial due to decreased caloric intake from anorexia, mechanical obstruction of the alimentary tract, and nausea as a result of chemotherapy. Moreover, there are a variety of disturbances in glucose, lipid, and muscle metabolism that occur in and contribute to cachexia in cancer patients. Significant muscle wasting, weight loss, and nutritional deficiencies are associated with poor outcomes. In the Eastern Cooperative Oncology Group study, patients with more wasting and weight loss had a poor prognostic response to chemotherapy, decreased performance status, and decreased survival.[8] With loss of muscle mass and strength, patients become more debilitated and ultimately lose

independence and become bed-bound. This increases the risk of complications such as bedsores, deep venous thrombosis formation and even pulmonary embolism. Decreased mobility itself also perpetuates the cycle of muscle wasting.

Mechanism of Cachexia

Changes in Fuel Metabolism   In cancer cachexia, there are specific alterations in the metabolism of glucose, lipids and protein. Cancer patients have a state of glucose intolerance which results in increased serum glucose levels. The consequence of this hyperglycemic state is decreased glucose storage and oxidation. The increased hepatic gluconeogenesis utilizes peripheral lean tissue mass, contributing to muscle wasting.[9] Peripheral muscle wasting is not only due to increased peripheral muscle catabolism, but also decreased muscle protein synthesis. Increased serum levels of glycerol and free fatty acids are seen in cancer patients and suggest increased lipolysis. These provide substrate for gluconeogenesis and possibly for tumor growth.[10]

Role of Cytokines   Researchers have investigated the role of various cytokines in contributing to cancer cachexia and anorexia. Tumor necrosis factor-α (TNF-α) and interleukin-1 (IL-1) have been found to act directly on the brain to cause anorexia. However, there is no convincing evidence that either one is responsible for the cachectic. IL-6 has been shown to directly cause muscle protein catabolism in vitro and has also been found at increased levels in both animal and humans with cancer cachexia.[11]

Role of Catabolic Factors   Increased catabolic factors may contribute to weight loss. Skeletal muscle catabolism in cancer cachexia may be mediated through proteolysis-inducing factor (PIF). Elevated levels of this factor have been isolated in both animals and humans with cancer and wasting. In vivo studies show that PIF may cause protein degradation by stimulating ubiquitin-proteosome pathway in skeletal muscle. Lipolysis may be induced from a lipid-mobilizing factor (LMF) that has been identified in animal and human models of cancer cachexia. This factor targets adipocytes and stimulates lipolysis via cyclic adenosine monophosphate. LMF has been isolated in cachexia-inducing murine tumor (MAC16) and has also been found in the urine of cachectic patients with pancreatic carcinoma.[11]

Hormonal Factors   Hormonal changes also contribute to cachexia. Muscle breakdown in cancer cachexia results from decreased anabolism and increased catabolism. Factors that play a role in decreased anabolism include decreased insulin-like growth factor (IGF) or resistance to IGF-1, decreased androgenic steroids, and decreased growth hormone. Increased catabolism in cancer cachexia may also be mediated by an increase in serum glucagon and cortisol levels. In a study from the Netherlands, 10 newly-diagnosed, untreated lung cancer patients with > 10% decrease in body weight were compared to those patients losing < 10% of body weight.[12] There was a statistically significant decrease in testosterone, IGF-1 and albumin levels in patients with > 10% weight loss. This does not, however, explain causality, since weight loss can cause depression in hormones, or the hormonal deficiency can decrease anabolism.

Treatment of Cachexia

Prior efforts in treating cancer cachexia due to anorexia have focused on agents that increase weight and appetite. Corticosteroids, progestational agents and cannabinoids have all been used in the past to meet these goals. However, corticosteroids are catabolic and use of corticosteroids or progestational agents result in weight gain primarily by increasing fat mass. Based on the understanding of mechanisms driving cancer cachexia, studies have used anti-inflammatory agents such as omega-3 fatty acids, cyclooxygenase-2 inhibitors, nonsteroidal anti-inflammatory drugs, anticytokine antibodies and thalidomide to treat cachexia.[13] Supplementing anabolic hormones in cachectic patients has also been studied. Unfortunately, in cancer patients, growth hormone and IGF-1 are contraindicated since they promote tumor growth.[14] In contrast, anabolic-androgenic steroids have been used to help build lean body mass (LBM) in cachectic patients with human immunodeficiency virus (HIV), renal disease, and, more recently, cancer patients.[15]

Testosterone and anabolic steroids improve muscle mass in cachectic patients by countering abnormalities in the endocrine system, in fuel metabolism, and in cytokine concentration. Testosterone is a lipophilic molecule that traverses cell membranes via diffusion and binds to a steroid hormone receptor within the cell. This complex acts as a transcription factor to up-regulate or inhibit transcription of DNA within the cell.[16] Studies have shown that testosterone increases skeletal muscle protein synthesis by up-regulating androgen receptors in muscle cells.[17,18] Further anabolic effects of testosterone may be due to its effects on growth hormone and IGF-1. Both growth hormone (GH) and IGF-1 increase skeletal muscle protein synthesis. Androgen administration increases pituitary release of GH, skeletal muscle IGF-1 production, and

hepatic synthesis of IGF-1.[19,20] With the exception of possibly stimulating the growth of prostate cancer, there are no data to implicate testosterone in the induction or spread of cancer. Testosterone also counters catabolic effects of glucocorticoids on a molecular level through competitive inhibition of the intracellular glucocorticoid receptor and by impeding various hormone response elements in the glucocorticoid signaling pathway.[21] Finally, as noted above, TNF-α and IL-1 have been implicated in cancer anorexia, and IL-6 has been shown to correlate with protein catabolism and cachexia. Testosterone has been found to decrease production of these cytokines in vitro and in vivo.[22,23] Therefore, based on these studies, it may be reasonable to treat cancer cachexia and anorexia with testosterone.

The use of anabolic-androgenic agents was first adopted by the athletic community for building muscle mass. This prompted studies on the action of testosterone on muscle. Testosterone supplementation in hypogonadal men was shown to improve muscle mass.[24] Further studies have found that testosterone replacement in men with HIV and hypogonadal elderly men also results in increased muscle mass and strength.[25–27] Given the correlation between hypogonadism and more profound cachexia in cancer patients, it seems intuitive to supplement these patients with testosterone.[12] Unfortunately, the use of androgen replacement in cancer cachexia has not been extensively studied. A study in mice with poorly differentiated sarcoma was performed to study both tumor growth and cachexia with and without administration of intraperitoneal nandrolone.[28] This study showed increased weight in the mice treated with nandrolone; however, the weight gain was felt to be due primarily to water because there was no significant increase in protein mass. Furthermore, muscle enzyme activity measured in muscle biopsies appeared equal in both groups. There was no change in tumor weight, size, or overall mortality between the two groups. A 4-week, randomized, placebo-controlled trial of weekly nandrolone 200 mg intramuscularly (IM) versus placebo in 37 patients with unresectable non-small cell lung cancer on chemotherapy showed decreased weight loss and improved survival in the nandrolone group.[29] However, the difference in weight loss between the two groups was not statistically significant. Oxandrolone has also been studied in cancer cachexia. Boughton reported on 131 patients with various cancers treated with oxandrolone 20 mg daily over a 4-month period.[30] By the end of the study, 80% of the patients gained weight or maintained the same body weight. There was an average 4-pound increase in LBM. Furthermore, there was an improvement in physical function.

Further large-scale studies of cancer cachexia need to be performed with use of testosterone and

other anabolic agents measuring functional status, mortality, muscle mass, strength, testosterone, GH, IGF-1, cortisol, and cytokine levels to aid in the understanding and treatment of cancer cachexia.

Anemia

Anemia is commonly encountered in cancer patients. A retrospective study found that patients with lymphoma had the highest incidence of anemia on presentation (82%), followed by those with colon cancer (71%), lung cancer (70%), ovarian cancer (68%), and breast cancer (44%).[31] While anemia in cancer patients can be a result of nutritional deficiencies, blood loss, immune-mediated hemolysis or myelofibrosis, many cancer patients develop an anemia that resembles an anemia of chronic disease. Furthermore, anemia in cancer patients may be due to a relative deficiency of erythropoietin as well as suppression of CFU-E formation by inflammatory cytokines.[32] Hypogonadism in cancer patients may also contribute to anemia. Studies in eunuchoid men have demonstrated erythrocytopenia and anemia, which improve with administration of androgens. Similarly, men with prostate cancer who have undergone castration are anemic compared to eugonadal men.[33] Furthermore, treatment of 68 women with advanced breast cancer with androgens has shown an improvement in hemoglobin and hematocrit.[34]

Prior to the discovery of recombinant human erythropoietin, anemia of chronic disease, especially in patients with chronic renal disease, were treated primarily with blood transfusions, nutritional supplements and androgen therapy. There are few trials showing improvement in hemoglobin with the use of testosterone enanthate in patients with chronic renal insufficiency.[35,36]

Many studies have also been performed using alkylated androgens to treat anemia in this population. Seventeen patients in one double-blind crossover study were noted to have a mean rise in hematocrit from 23 to 27% while on the anabolic steroid nandrolone, with no improvements seen on placebo.[37] Another double-blinded, placebo-controlled study yielded similar results.[38] With the introduction of recombinant human erythropoietin, androgen use in anemia of chronic disease lost popularity. However, recently, a randomized prospective study was conducted comparing recombinant human erythropoietin with nandrolone in patients on peritoneal dialysis. Both resulted in a statistically significant rise in hematocrit of approximately 8%. The added benefits of nandrolone were increases in weight, body mass index, triceps skinfold, mid-arm circumference, mid-arm muscle circumference, total protein, albumin, prealbumin, and transferrin.[39] The mechanism by which nandrolone raises red cell mass is not completely known. Hypotheses include increasing the responsiveness of erythroid progenitors to erythropoietin, aiding in red blood cell survival, or possibly affecting erythropoietic precursors directly in their maturation process.[40]

At this time, only recombinant human erythropoietin and epoetin alfa can be recommended to treat cancer-related anemia. However, if a man is found to be hypogonadal, testosterone replacement therapy can provide an added benefit of producing an erythropoietic effect, while being more economical.[41]

Reduced Bone Density

Osteoporosis predisposes to increased risk of fracture; hypogonadism is a known risk factor for osteopenia and osteoporosis. Androgen receptors are found on epiphyseal chondrocytes, stromal cells, osteoblasts, and osteoclasts. Thus, decreased bone mineral density could result directly from the absence of testosterone or indirectly via a deficiency in testosterone's aromatization to stradiol. In addition, androgens also work indirectly again by stimulating the growth hormone/IGF-I axis.[42]

Most of the cancer literature has focused on men rendered hypogonadal by medical or surgical castration for the treatment for prostate cancer. Androgen deprivation therapy (ADT) is usually employed in men with metastatic or recurrent prostate cancer. In one study, men lost an average of 2.4% and 10% of bone mineral density after one and two years following surgical castration, respectively. Those who had medical castration lost an average 3.4% and 6.5% of bone mineral density after one and two years, respectively, following initiation of therapy.[43] Similarly, men treated with orchiectomy have a twofold risk of fractures compared with controls.[44] Not only do men on ADT suffer from decreased bone mineral density, but they are also at greater risk for increased morbidity from fractures. Several other studies on ADT in men with prostate cancer have reported similar findings.[45,46]

Further evidence supporting the relation between hypogonadism and osteoporosis exists in studies of hypogonadal men who have improvements in bone mineral density with testosterone repletion. Spinal bone mineral density was measured in 36 hypogonadal men and 44 eugonadal men at baseline. The hypogonadal men then received testosterone supplementation at 100 mg/wk and had bone mineral density measurements taken up to 18 weeks out. Hypogonadal men had a significantly lower bone mineral density than eugonadal men. Furthermore, there was a statistically significant increase in spinal bone mineral density among the hypogonadal patients receiving testosterone supplementation. In this situation, markers of bone formation increase, and markers of bone resorption decrease.[47] Similar findings were reported with transdermal testosterone preparations.[48,49]

There have been no studies evaluating the benefits of testosterone replacement in male cancer patients. One could assume that the effects would be similar to those in men without cancers. Thus, men who are at increased risk of developing osteoporosis (eg, from glucocorticoid treatment, immobility, nutritional deficiency, and hypogonadism) should undergo a DEXA scan. Supplementation with calcium and vitamin D should be recommended for most patients, assuming no contraindications (eg, hyperparathyroidism). Testosterone replacement should be offered to men with osteopenia and hypogonadism. Bisphosphonates should be considered for subjects diagnosed with osteoporosis.

Depression

Depression in cancer patients is often unrecognized and untreated. This may be in part due to difficulty in diagnosing major depression with coexisting somatic symptoms. However, in epidemiologic studies, major depression has been found in approximately 25% of cancer patients. If depression in this population is left untreated, it can predispose the patient to decreased quality of life, increased pain, non-compliance with treatment, a depressed immune system, lower life expectancy and even suicide.[50,51] In cases where hypogonadism exists in the cancer patient, a low testosterone level may contribute to depression.

Hypogonadal men have a significantly increased rate of depression (21.7%) versus eugonadal men (7.1%).[52] Men with prostate cancer who are rendered hypogonadal with ADT show higher depressive and anxiety scores.[53] Similar associations between low testosterone levels and depression have been seen in non-cancer patients. For example, hypogonadal men with HIV show improvement in depression scores on testosterone replacement.[54]

There have been limited studies to investigate the effects of hypogonadism and androgen replacement at the cellular level in the brain. When male rats are castrated, $5HT_{2A}R$ sites in the frontal, cingulated, piriform cortex, olfactory tubercle and nucleus accumbens were significantly decreased compared to normal male rats. The brains of castrated rats supplemented with testosterone proprionate were also studied and found to have increased $5HT_{2A}R$ sites in the regions mentioned above that were comparable to or greater than those in normal male rats.[55] In humans, increased blood perfusion has been documented on single photon emission computed tomography images in the midbrain, superior frontal gyrus, and cingulate gyrus in hypogonadal older men receiving testosterone replacement. While this study did not use formal mood or psychiatric assessment to correlate the findings with testosterone replacement, the authors did note an increased sense of well-being and social interactions based on questionnaire data.[56] Testosterone may be affecting mood by modulating serotonin activity in these areas of the brain.

Although there have been no studies evaluating hormone replacement in cancer patients, there may be some improvement in mood. This symptom should be distinguished from clinical depression, in which antidepressants would be needed. Depression and the resulting effect on decreased quality of life need to be treated appropriately.

Cognitive Dysfunction

Hormones have been known to influence memory. Castrated male rats show decreased performance in visuospatial tasks.[57] Since there is also growing concern that hypogonadal elderly males may be more prone to developing cognitive difficulties and dementia, more clinical studies have been targeted at this group. However, it would be important to also be aware of potential cognitive impairments that may also develop in cancer patients as a result of coexisting hypogonadism. Of particular concern in this patient population is the potential to have impaired decision-making skills and decreased activating brain function, which may impact on quality of life and medical decision-making.

Studies on cognition in hypogonadal males have focused on elderly men and men undergoing androgen suppression therapy for prostate cancer. Because most studies examining cognition were designed from previous studies noting a cognitive difference in men and women (with men having better visuospatial ability and women scoring better on tests of verbal fluency), there was an underlying hypothesis in these studies that hypogonadal men would experience reduced visuospatial ability compared to eugonadal men or men receiving testosterone supplementation. The studies primarily used a block design test to evaluate visuospatial organization. To test verbal measures, the vocabulary subsets of the Wechsler Adult Intelligence Scale were often used. Several studies incorporated the Mini-mental Status Exam (MMSE) or Cambridge Examination for Mental Disorders of the Elderly (CAMCOG) to test changes in general cognitive function.

Two large cohort studies were performed in elderly men to examine whether varying levels of testosterone would correlate with cognitive functioning. In one cohort of 547 men aged 59 to 89 years, there was a positive correlation of long-term memory, mental control, and verbal memory with age- and education-adjusted testosterone levels.[58] Another longitudinal cohort of 407 men aged 50 to 91 years showed that high levels of free testosterone were associated with a decreased rate of visual memory. The data in this cohort was also analyzed to compare hypogonadal men with eugonadal men. When controlled for age, the hypogonadal men had lower cognitive scores on tests of visual memory, verbal memory, and visuospatial skills.[59] Both of these studies imply that higher levels of testosterone in elderly men are associated with less cognitive decline, and the latter study suggests that lower testosterone levels correlate with some degree of decreased cognitive skills.

Two studies evaluating cognitive function in men prior to, during, and after treatment with flutamide and leuprolide had varied results. One found no significant change in any tests of cognitive function, but did note improvement in CAMCOG and one of the verbal tests with cessation of anti-androgen treatment.[53] The other study also did not find a significant change in the tests during the treatment phase, but noted improvement of verbal memory and decline in spatial rotation once the treatment was stopped.[60]

There are also studies testing cognitive function in hypogonadal men before and during treatment with testosterone replacement and comparing them with eugonadal men with and without testosterone supplementation. One study found that all groups of men had improvements in cognitive tests on verbal ability, visuospatial ability, and perceptual speed. Hypogonadal men were found to have significantly lower cognitive skills in verbal ability, compared to the eugonadal men at baseline, which improved with testosterone replacement.[61] Another similar study found no significant change in performance on tests of auditory verbal learning, perceptual motor speed, manual dexterity, and verbal intellectual functioning in all groups. There was a small improvement in word fluency and decrease in visuospatial skills among eugonadal men treated with testosterone. Hypogonadal men were also noted to have lower verbal intellectual functioning and perceptual motor speed at baseline compared to eugonadal men.[62]

Overall, the studies on cognition in various groups of hypogonadal men, with and without testosterone supplementation, are inconsistent. Some studies, which appear to show improved cognitive functioning on testosterone replacement, may actually be reflecting improved scores from retesting with the same test. Nevertheless, the studies seem to suggest that hypogonadal men score lower on various aspects of cognitive testing in comparison with eugonadal men. This needs to be investigated in a cancer population. At this point, there is not enough evidence to define the type of cognitive dysfunction in hypogonadal cancer patients or support the use of testosterone supplementation in improving any cognitive dysfunction.

Sexual Dysfunction

Hypogonadism results in erectile dysfunction and a decrease in libido and can be treated well with replacement therapy. In a study of 32 hypogonadal men, sexual dysfunction was evaluated at baseline and during testosterone replacement. Men experienced significant improvement in their libido and potency on testosterone replacement compared to baseline.[63] Another study used more objective measures to evaluate erectile dysfunction due to low testosterone levels. In this study, 15 hypogonadal men had erectile function evaluated with penile color duplex ultrasound, nocturnal penile tumescence, and visually stimulated erection evaluation before and after testosterone supplementation. Hypogonadal men had a significantly decreased number of nocturnal erections, lower cavernous arterial inflow and resistive index by duplex Doppler, and impaired visually stimulated and pharmacologically stimulated erections compared with healthy controls. After 6 months of a testosterone 5 mg patch daily, there were significant improvements in all of these measures.[64]

The data in young, hypogonadal men may not be applicable to older men or men with chronic diseases, such as cancer. In the latter situation, vascular insufficiency, depression, or non-specific fatigue may explain a large proportion of the sexual dysfunction. Therefore, testosterone therapy may not completely alleviate the problem, but rather it may be used in combination with PDE-5 inhibitors.

Laboratory Diagnosis of Male Hypogonadism

Currently, there are no guidelines for screening and diagnosing hypogonadism in cancer patients. A morning serum testosterone level (to take into account the circadian rhythm of the androgen) should be obtained in all men with cancer who have any of the signs and symptoms mentioned above (ie, weight loss, anemia, osteoporosis, depression, fatigue or sexual dysfunction). If total testosterone is between 200 and 400 ng/dL, a measure of free testosterone should be done (bioavailable or free testosterone level by free dialysis method), since many of these patients are malnourished and may have reduced sex hormone binding globulin (SHBG) synthesis.[65] The free testosterone value can be measured by free dialysis method or calculated from serum total testosterone and SHBG levels.

Once hypogonadism is confirmed, LH, FSH, and prolactin levels should be checked to distinguish between primary and secondary mechanisms. Pituitary magnetic resonance imaging (MRI) should be performed in those subjects without a known etiology for central hypogonadism such as irradiation, (especially with serum total testosterone levels <150 ng/dL) to rule out

a mass lesion. However, it is important to be cognizant of the fact that, even if the patient has primary hypogonadism, the gonadotropins levels may not be appropriately elevated in these patients since increased corticotrophin-releasing hormone may suppress GnRH secretion during illness.[7] Patients with history of cranial irradiation, surgical resection of pituitary tumors, treatment with high-dose glucocorticoids, or GnRH analogues will likely have secondary hypogonadism and low gonadotropin levels. In such patients with known etiology of secondary hypogonadism, there is no need for MRI.

Treatment Options for Hypogonadal Men with Cancer

Testosterone replacement therapy is absolutely contraindicated in patients with prostate or breast cancer since there is a risk of growth/recurrence of the cancer. Various modalities of testosterone replacement therapy are currently available (Table 28-2).

Esterified forms of testosterone have been used the longest and are associated with a longer half-life. Testosterone enanthate, testosterone cypionate and testosterone propionate are all derived from esterification of the 17β hydroxyl group of testosterone. Testosterone enanthate is the most commonly used of the three preparations, given as 200 mg IM every 2 weeks. The maximum concentration is reached in approximately 10 hours, and the half-life is 4 to 5 days.[66] There are multiple studies showing the use of testosterone enanthate in treating anemia in patients with chronic renal insufficiency[35,36] and for treating osteoporosis, depression, and erectile dysfunction in hypogonadal men.[47,66,67] Testosterone enanthate has also been shown to increase muscle mass in elderly men, hypogonadal AIDS patients, and chronic obstructive pulmonary disease patients.[25,26,68]

There are very few studies specifically evaluating cancer patients. In hypogonadal elderly males and in men rendered hypogonadal after high-dose chemotherapy for hematologic malignancies, testosterone cypionate has been shown to improve libido and erectile performance.[69,70] Men with HIV and hypogonadal symptoms were found to have improved libido, energy, mood, and muscle mass on testosterone cypionate.[71]

Testosterone scrotal patches were developed and had to be worn over 24 hours delivering approximately 4 to 6 mg/d with peak levels obtained after 2 to 4 hours.[72] Scrotal patches are no longer available in the United States. Androderm is another transdermal testosterone preparation that is applied to non-scrotal skin. Typically, 5-mg patches are applied on non-scrotal skin over 24 hours with peak concentrations at 8 hours.[73] It has been shown to maintain mood and sexual function in hypogonadal men

Table 2 Modalities of Testosterone Replacement

Testosterone

Drug	Route of delivery	Dosage
Testosterone Esters		
Testosterone propionate	IM	10–25 mg 2 to 3 times/wk
Testosterone enanthate	IM	200 mg every 2–4 wks
Testosterone cypionate	IM	200 mg every 2–4 wks
Testosterone undecanoate	IM	1000 mg every 12 wks
Testosterone patch Androderm	Topical	5 mg/d
Testosterone gel Androgel, Testim	Topica	5 g/d l
Buccal Testosterone Striant	Buccal	30 mg twice a day

IM = intramuscularly

while delivering testosterone levels that are within the physiologic range. However, there is a fairly high incidence of skin irritation (33%).[74] Transdermal testosterone gel (Androgel and Testim) have recently become available. It is applied in 5 to 10 mg doses daily. In hypogonadal males, this form of testosterone replacement has been shown to improve sexual function, mood, bone mineral density, and hematocrit. It has also been shown to increase lean body mass, but did not result in statistically significant increase in muscle strength.[75]

The newest form of testosterone delivery has been developed in a buccal mucoadhesive testosterone preparation. A 30-mg twice daily buccal administration dose of testosterone was studied and shown to elevate testosterone levels into the normal range. It did not cause significant polycythemia or prostate enlargement. The primary side effect of this preparation is buccal mucosa irritation.[76]

Oral free testosterone should not be used owing to insufficient serum levels from hepatic inactivation and side effects of hepatotoxicity.

Alkylated androgens have also been studied for treatment of many clinical symptoms of hypogonadism. These androgens were formulated by the addition of an alkyl group to the 17α position of testosterone. Examples of the alkylated androgens include methyltestosterone, fluoxymesterone, oxymetholone, oxandrolone, ethylestrenol, stanozolol, methandrostenolone, norethandrolone, and danazol. Nandrolone has been found to increase muscle mass and muscle strength in HIV patients and patients on chronic glucocorticoid therapy.[77,78] It has also been shown to be comparable to recombinant human erythropoietin in peritoneal dialysis and hemodialysis patients.[40,79] The data on its use for osteoporosis is conflicting. When studied in men on chronic steroids, there seems to be no change in bone mineral density[78]; however, multiple studies in post-menopausal

women suggest that nandrolone increases bone mineral density.[80–82] While there is evidence in the use of nandrolone for increasing muscle mass, hematocrit, and bone mineral density, there are no direct studies on its use for improving mood, sexual dysfunction, or cognition. Oxandrolone has been studied for improving muscle mass in cancer patients, pediatric burn patients, HIV patients, and elderly men.[30,83–85] While there is convincing evidence for the use of oxandrolone to increase muscle mass and treat cachexia, it is associated with liver function abnormalities. At this point, there would be no indication to used alkylated products for treatment of male hypogonadism.

Summary/Recommendations

Hypogonadism may be under-recognized and under-diagnosed in cancer patients. Cancer patients who are most predisposed to hypogonadism include those who have testicular cancers or hematologic malignancies treated with gonadotoxic chemotherapeutic agents and those undergoing cranial irradiation. Patients who are critically ill and treated with opioids also develop hypogonadism. However, since malignancies in general may predispose patients to lower testosterone levels via Leydig cell dysfunction and reduced gonadotropins secretion, any cancer patient who present with symptoms of hypogonadism, including cachexia, anemia, decreased bone mineral density, depression, sexual dysfunction and cognitive dysfunction, should be screened for hypogonadism.

There are different types of androgens and delivery modalities to use for replacement therapy. Currently, there is good evidence for the use of testosterone supplementation to improve sexual function, mood, bone mineral density, hematocrit, and lean body mass in hypogonadism. Testosterone preparations with shorter

half-lives (gel and patches) may mimic physiologic levels more accurately than esterified testosterone preparations with longer half-lives. Alkylated androgens such as oxandrolone and nandrolone have been shown to be good agents in treating anemia and cancer cachexia; due to potential hepatotoxicity, negative effect on plasma lipids, and a lack of benefit in terms of sexual function, however, we recommend testosterone replacement in this patient population as the first-line therapy. While data from these studies can likely be extrapolated and applied to hypogonadal patients with cancer, there is great need for larger scale studies on the effects of androgen and testosterone preparations on muscle mass, mortality, anemia, bone mineral density, quality of life, mood, cognitive function, and sexual function to be performed directly in cancer patients with hypogonadism.

REFERENCES

1. Harman SM, et al. Longitudinal effects of aging on serum total and free testosterone levels in healthy men. Baltimore Longitudinal Study of Aging. J Clin Endocrinol Metab 2001;86:724–31.
2. Blackman MR, et al. Comparison of the effects of lung cancer, benign lung disease, and normal aging on pituitary-gonadal function in men. J Clin Endocrinol Metab 1988;66:88–95.
3. Warren MP, Vu C. Central causes of hypogonadism—functional and organic. Endocrinol Metab Clin North Am 2003;32:593–612.
4. Howell S, Shalet S. Gonadal damage from chemotherapy and radiotherapy. Endocrinol Metab Clin North Am 1998;27:927–43.
5. Taggart DP, et al. Serum androgens and gonadotrophins in bronchial carcinoma. Respir Med 1993;87:455–60.
6. Roberts LJ, et al. Sex hormone suppression by intrathecal opioids: a prospective study. Clin J Pain 2002;18:144–8.
7. Spratt DI. Altered gonadal steroidogenesis in critical illness: is treatment with anabolic steroids indicated? Best Pract Res Clin Endocrinol Metab 2001;15:479–94.
8. Dewys WD, et al. Prognostic effect of weight loss prior to chemotherapy in cancer patients. Eastern Cooperative Oncology Group. Am J Med 1980;69:491–7.
9. Younes RN, Noguchi Y. Pathophysiology of cancer cachexia. Rev Hosp Clin Fac Med Sao Paulo 2000;55:181–93.
10. Tisdale MJ. Cancer cachexia: metabolic alterations and clinical manifestations. Nutrition 1997;13:1–7.
11. Tisdale MJ. Cancer anorexia and cachexia. Nutrition 2001; 17:438–42.
12. Simons JP, et al. Weight loss and low body cell mass in males with lung cancer: relationship with systemic inflammation, acute-phase response, resting energy expenditure, and catabolic and anabolic hormones. Clin Sci (Lond) 1999;97:215–23.
13. MacDonald N, et al. Understanding and managing cancer cachexia. J Am Coll Surg 2003;19:143–61.
14. Thordarson G, et al. Mammary tumorigenesis in growth hormone deficient spontaneous dwarf rats; effects of hormonal treatments. Breast Cancer Res Treat 2004;87: 277–90.
15. Basaria S, Wahlstrom JT, Dobs AS. Clinical review 138: anabolic-androgenic steroid therapy in the treatment of chronic diseases. J Clin Endocrinol Metab 2001;86: 5108–17.
16. Beato M, Klug J. Steroid hormone receptors: an update. Hum Reprod Update 2000;6:225–36.
17. Sheffield-Moore M, et al. Short-term oxandrolone administration stimulates net muscle protein synthesis in young men. J Clin Endocrinol Metab 1999;84:2705–11.
18. Doumit ME, Cook DR, Merkel RA. Testosterone upregulates androgen receptors and decreases differentiation of porcine myogenic satellite cells in vitro. Endocrinology 1996;137:1385–94.
19. Veldhuis JD, Iranmanesh A. Physiological regulation of the human growth hormone (GH)-insulin-like growth

factor type I (IGF-I) axis: predominant impact of age, obesity, gonadal function, and sleep. Sleep 1996;19 (10 Suppl):221–4.

20. Mauras N, et al. Testosterone deficiency in young men: marked alterations in whole body protein kinetics, strength, and adiposity. J Clin Endocrinol Metab 1998; 83:1886–92.

21. Hickson RC, et al. Glucocorticoid antagonism by exercise and androgenic-anabolic steroids. Med Sci Sports Exerc 1990;22:331–40.

22. D'Agostino P, et al. Sex hormones modulate inflammatory mediators produced by macrophages. Ann N Y Acad Sci 1999;876:426–9.

23. Malkin CJ, et al. The effect of testosterone replacement on endogenous inflammatory cytokines and lipid profiles in hypogonadal men. J Clin Endocrinol Metab 2004;89: 3313–8.

24. Brodsky IG, Balagopal P, Nair KS. Effects of testosterone replacement on muscle mass and muscle protein synthesis in hypogonadal men—a clinical research center study. J Clin Endocrinol Metab 1996;81:3469–75.

25. Bhasin S, et al. Testosterone replacement and resistance exercise in HIV-infected men with weight loss and low testosterone levels. JAMA 2000;283:763–70.

26. Grinspoon S, et al. Effects of androgen administration in men with the AIDS wasting syndrome. A randomized, double-blind, placebo-controlled trial. Ann Intern Med 1998;129:18–26.

27. Ferrando AA, et al. Testosterone administration to older men improves muscle function: molecular and physiological mechanisms. Am J Physiol Endocrinol Metab 2002;282:E601–E607.

28. Lyden E, et al. Effects of nandrolone propionate on experimental tumor growth and cancer cachexia. Metabolism 1995;44:445–51.

29. Chlebowski RT, et al. Influence of nandrolone decanoate on weight loss in advanced non-small cell lung cancer. Cancer 1986;58:183–6.

30. Boughton B. Drug increases lean tissue mass in patients with cancer. Lancet Oncol 2003;4:135.

31. Tas F, et al. Anemia in oncology practice: relation to diseases and their therapies. Am J Clin Oncol 2002;25:371–9.

32. Moliterno AR, Spivak JL. Anemia of cancer. Hematol Oncol Clin North Am 1996;10:345–63.

33. Basaria S, et al. Long-term effects of androgen deprivation therapy in prostate cancer patients. Clin Endocrinol (Oxf) 2002;56:779–86.

34. Kennedy BJ, Gilbertsen AS. Increased erythropoiesis induced by androgenic-hormone therapy. N Engl J Med 1957;256: 719–26.

35. Schustack A, et al. Intramuscular iron replenishment and replacement combined with testosterone enanthate in maintenance hemodialysis anemia: a follow-up of up to 8 years on 16 patients. Clin Nephrol 1985;23:303–6.

36. Neff MS, et al. A comparison of androgens for anemia in patients on hemodialysis. N Engl J Med 1981;304:871–5.

37. Hendler ED, et al. Controlled study of androgen therapy in anemia of patients on maintenance hemodialysis. N Engl J Med 1974;291:1046–51.

38. Williams JS, Stein JH, Ferris TF. Nandrolone decanoate therapy for patients receiving hemodialysis. A controlled study. Arch Intern Med 1974;134:289–92.

39. Navarro JF, et al. Randomized prospective comparison between erythropoietin and androgens in CAPD patients. Kidney Int 2002;61:1537–44.

40. Ferrario E, et al. Treatment of cancer-related anemia with epoetin alfa: a review. Cancer Treat Rev 2004;30:563–75.

41. Navarro JF. In the erythropoietin era, can we forget alternative or adjunctive therapies for renal anaemia management? The androgen example. Nephrol Dial Transplant 2003;18:2222–6.

42. Vanderschueren D, et al. Androgens and bone. Endocr Rev 2004;25:389–425.

43. Daniell HW, et al. Progressive osteoporosis during androgen deprivation therapy for prostate cancer. J Urol 2000;163: 181–6.

44. Dickman PW, et al. Hip fractures in men with prostate cancer treated with orchiectomy. J Urol 2004;172(6 Part 1 of 2):2208–12.

45. Deng JH, et al. Effect of androgen deprivation therapy on bone mineral density in prostate cancer patients. Asian J Androl 2004;6:75–7.

46. Wei JT, et al. Androgen deprivation therapy for prostate cancer results in significant loss of bone density. Urology 1999;54:607–11.

47. Katznelson L, et al. Increase in bone density and lean body mass during testosterone administration in men with acquired hypogonadism. J Clin Endocrinol Metab 1996;81:4358–65.

48. Wang C, et al. Effects of transdermal testosterone gel on bone turnover markers and bone mineral density in hypogonadal men. Clin Endocrinol (Oxf) 2001;54: 739–50.

49. Snyder PJ, et al. Effects of testosterone replacement in hypogonadal men. J Clin Endocrinol Metab 2000;85: 2670–7.

50. Valente SM, Saunders JM, Cohen MZ. Evaluating depression among patients with cancer. Cancer Pract 1994;2:65–71.

51. Reiche EM, Nunes SO, Morimoto HK. Stress, depression, the immune system, and cancer. Lancet Oncol 2004;5: 617–25.

52. Shores MM, et al. Increased incidence of diagnosed depressive illness in hypogonadal older men. Arch Gen Psychiatry 2004;61:162–7.

53. Almeida OP, et al. One year follow-up study of the association between chemical castration, sex hormones, beta-amyloid, memory and depression in men. Psychoneuroendocrinology 2004;29:1071–81.

54. Grinspoon S, et al. Effects of hypogonadism and testosterone administration on depression indices in HIV-infected men. J Clin Endocrinol Metab 2000;85:60–5.

55. Fink G, et al. Androgen actions on central serotonin neurotransmission: relevance for mood, mental state and memory. Behav Brain Res 1999;105:53–68.

56. Azad N, et al. Testosterone treatment enhances regional brain perfusion in hypogonadal men. J Clin Endocrinol Metab 2003;88:3064–8.

57. Adler A, et al. Gonadectomy in adult life increases tyrosine hydroxylase immunoreactivity in the prefrontal cortex and decreases open field activity in male rats. Neuroscience 1999;89:939–54.

58. Barrett-Connor E, Goodman-Gruen D, Patay B. Endogenous sex hormones and cognitive function in older men. J Clin Endocrinol Metab 1999;84:3681–5.

59. Moffat SD, et al. Longitudinal assessment of serum free testosterone concentration predicts memory performance and cognitive status in elderly men. J Clin Endocrinol Metab 2002;87:5001–7.

60. Cherrier MM, Rose AL, Higano C. The effects of combined androgen blockade on cognitive function during the first cycle of intermittent androgen suppression in patients with prostate cancer. J Urol 2003;170:1808–11.

61. Alexander GM, et al. Androgen-behavior correlations in hypogonadal men and eugonadal men. II. Cognitive abilities. Horm Behav 1998;33:85–94.

62. O'Connor DB, et al. Activational effects of testosterone on cognitive function in men. Neuropsychologia 2001;39: 1385–94.

63. Mulhall JP, et al. Effect of testosterone supplementation on sexual function in hypogonadal men with erectile dysfunction. Urology 2004;63:348–52.

64. Foresta C, et al. Role of androgens in erectile function. J Urol 2004;171 (6 Pt 1):2358–62.

65. Morley JE, Patrick P, Perry HM III. Evaluation of assays available to measure free testosterone. Metabolism 2002; 51:554–9.

66. Amory JK, et al. Exogenous testosterone or testosterone with finasteride increases bone mineral density in older men with low serum testosterone. J Clin Endocrinol Metab 2004;89:503–10.

67. Dobs AS, et al. Pharmacokinetics, efficacy, and safety of a permeation-enhanced testosterone transdermal system in comparison with bi-weekly injections of testosterone enanthate for the treatment of hypogonadal men. J Clin Endocrinol Metab 1999;84:3469–78.

68. Casaburi R, et al. Effects of testosterone and resistance training in men with chronic obstructive pulmonary disease. Am J Respir Crit Care Med 2004;170:870–8.

69. Hajjar RR, Kaiser FE, Morley JE. Outcomes of long-term testosterone replacement in older hypogonadal males: a retrospective analysis. J Clin Endocrinol Metab 1997; 82:3793–6.

70. Chatterjee R, et al. Management of erectile dysfunction by combination therapy with testosterone and sildenafil in recipients of high-dose therapy for haematological malignancies. Bone Marrow Transplant 2002;29:607–10.

71. Rabkin JG, Wagner GJ, Rabkin R. A double-blind, placebo-controlled trial of testosterone therapy for HIV-positive men with hypogonadal symptoms. Arch Gen Psychiatry 2000;57:141–7.

72. Zitzmann M, Nieschlag E. Hormone substitution in male hypogonadism. Mol Cell Endocrinol 2000;161(1–2): 73–88.

73. Behre HM, et al. Long-term effect of testosterone therapy on bone mineral density in hypogonadal men. J Clin Endocrinol Metab 1997;82:2386–90.

74. Bhasin S, et al. Testosterone replacement and resistance exercise in HIV-infected men with weight loss and low testosterone levels. JAMA 2000;283:6:763–70.

75. Wang C, et al. Long-term testosterone gel (AndroGel) treatment maintains beneficial effects on sexual function and mood, lean and fat mass, and bone mineral density in hypogonadal men. J Clin Endocrinol Metab 2004; 89:2085–98.

76. Wang C, et al. New testosterone buccal system (Striant) delivers physiological testosterone levels: pharmacokinetics study in hypogonadal men. J Clin Endocrinol Metab 2004;89:3821–9.

77. Sattler FR, et al. Effects of pharmacological doses of nandrolone decanoate and progressive resistance training in immunodeficient patients infected with human immunodeficiency virus. J Clin Endocrinol Metab 1999; 84:1268–76.

78. Crawford BA, et al. Randomized placebo-controlled trial of androgen effects on muscle and bone in men requiring long-term systemic glucocorticoid treatment. J Clin Endocrinol Metab 2003;88:3167–76.

79. Gascon A, et al. Nandrolone decanoate is a good alternative for the treatment of anemia in elderly male patients on hemodialysis. Geriatr Nephrol Urol 1999;9:67–72.

80. Passeri M, et al. Effects of nandrolone decanoate on bone mass in established osteoporosis. Maturitas 1993;17: 211–9.

81. Hassager C, et al. Nandrolone decanoate treatment of post-menopausal osteoporosis for 2 years and effects of withdrawal. Maturitas 1989;11:305–17.

82. Gennari C, et al. Effects of nandrolone decanoate therapy on bone mass and calcium metabolism in women with established post-menopausal osteoporosis: a double-blind placebo-controlled study. Maturitas 1989;11: 187–97.

83. Fox-Wheeler S, et al. Evaluation of the effects of oxandrolone on malnourished HIV-positive pediatric patients. Pediatrics 1999;104:e73.

84. Wolf SE, et al. Improved net protein balance, lean mass, and gene expression changes with oxandrolone treatment in the severely burned. Ann Surg 2003;237:801–10.

85. Schroeder ET, et al. Treatment with oxandrolone and the durability of effects in older men. J Appl Physiol 2004; 96:1055–62.

Gastroesophageal Issues

Alexander A. Dekovich, MD

Primary and metastatic tumors of the aerodigestive tract themselves and the modalities of surgery or radiation used to treat these cancers can result in mechanical obstructions that require treatment or palliation to restore function. Because eating is a social event, the loss of the ability to ingest a meal in the usual manner leads to a great decrease in the quality of life, even if alternative means for maintenance of hydration and nutrition such as hyperalimentation or enteral tube feeding can be provided. The goal of intervention is to restore this function to as close to the original physiology as possible for as long as possible and, therefore, to allow for a better quality of life. Palliation of obstruction of the gastrointestinal and biliary tract has improved considerably over the past 25 years by the introduction of percutaneous endoscopic gastrostomy (PEG) for enteral feeding, thermal and chemical tumor ablative procedures, and the evolution of stents for the biliary tract, esophagus, duodenum and colon.

Esophageal Obstruction

Esophageal obstruction results most often from primary cancer of the esophagus, although cancer in the mediastinum can often lead to esophageal obstruction due to extrinsic compression. Obstruction due to strictures resulting from primary treatment (surgery or radiation) and tumor recurrence is also frequently encountered.

Squamous cell carcinoma and adenocarcinoma together comprise 90% of esophageal cancers. Rarely, other cancers (including metastatic malignant melanoma, metastatic breast cancer, leiomyosarcoma, lymphoma, and other more rare tumors) may develop in the esophagus.[1] Worldwide, squamous cell carcinoma of the esophagus is still the predominant cancer. In the United States, adenocarcinoma of the esophagus and gastric cardia has rapidly increased in incidence during the latter part of the twentieth century, primarily in the white male population. This is thought to be, in part, due to a number of factors, among them the aging of the population coupled with a change in diet (leading to an increase in obesity and gastroesophageal reflux) and the general decrease in cigarette smoking that contributes both to the decline of squamous cell cancer of the esophagus and to the increase in adenocarcinoma.[2,3] Adenocarcinoma now comprises at least 50% of all esophageal cancers[4] diagnosed in the United States and is usually found in the mid to distal esophagus and rarely involves the more proximal esophagus. Although the overall 5-year survival rate for esophageal cancer is low, 15.8% for the period 1995 to 2000,[5] it has improved from the 4% overall survival rate reported for the period 1950 to 1954. More favorable 5-year survival is dependent on discovery and treatment of the esophageal cancer at an earlier stage. Patients with metastatic disease at diagnosis and treated with palliative chemotherapy or irradiation have a median survival of less than one year.[6]

Dysphagia to a normal solid food diet is generally not present until the esophageal lumen has been reduced to less than or equal to 13 mm in diameter. Some dietary adjustment is necessary when the lumen is reduced to approximately 18 mm—a reduction to 70% of the normal lumen diameter.[7] This accommodation by the esophagus to the growing tumor coupled with delay in seeking medical evaluation that is prompted by improvement of symptoms with modification of diet and denial leads to progression and spread of the disease, so that, unfortunately, more than 50% of patients with esophageal cancer, at presentation are unresectable.[6] Palliation becomes the primary goal in these patients as amelioration or relief of anorexia, dysphagia, nausea, vomiting, and pain adds greatly to the quality of remaining life.[4] Although the anorexia and pain are more difficult to treat successfully, there are multiple modalities and combinations of modalities available for the palliation of dysphagia.

Chemo-Radiation

Although both adenocarcinomas and squamous cell carcinomas are responsive to chemotherapy and external beam radiation therapy, palliation occurs in only about 40 to 60% of cases, is short-lived, and may take 2 to 8 weeks for dysphagia to improve. It appears that chemotherapy is as effective as radiation for palliation of dysphagia.[6] The combination of chemotherapy and radiotherapy is associated with significant morbidity. In a study of 121 patients reported by Herskovic and colleagues,[8] the combination of chemotherapy and radiation therapy alleviated dysphagia in 58% of their patients and was more effective than radiation alone, but life-threatening complications occurred in 20% of the patients, and serious complications occurred in 44%. In a retrospective study of 57 patients with T_3 or T_4 squamous cell cancer of the esophagus, Kaneko and colleagues reported that 90% of their patients had grade 3 or 4 dysphagia prior to chemoradiotherapy but following definitive chemoradiotherapy, 70% of these patients downgraded their dysphagia scores to 0 or 1.[9]

Dilatation

Dilatation of a benign stricture of the esophagus encountered in the post-esophagectomy patient can be accomplished with balloons or bougies, usually with good overall results and low complication rates.[10–12] Although dilatation of radiation-induced strictures of the esophagus can generally be accomplished with adequate palliation in the majority of patients, it is more difficult to perform and may be associated with more complications.[13] The esophageal lumen needs to be dilated to a diameter greater than 13 mm for solid food dysphagia to be partially relieved, and preferably to a 16 to 17 mm diameter for solid food dysphagia to be adequately palliated. The frequency of dilatation depends on the recurrence of dysphagia. Early dilatation, shortly after recurrence of symptoms, is preferable to late dilatation after near obstruction of the esophageal lumen has recurred.

Dilatation of the esophageal lumen obstructed with tumor can also be accomplished with balloons or bougies and has been shown to be safe for procedure related needs.[14,15] However, patients treated with dilatation primarily for malignant obstruction have a higher incidence of perforation (5% to 10%), and the perforations tend to be more severe. The resulting palliation from dilatation is usually very short-lived.[16–18] In a small series of 20 patients with obstruction due to esophagogastric junction cancer, Ko and colleagues showed that balloon dilatation of the stricture followed immediately by chemotherapy and/or radiation therapy was effective in improving dysphagia in 15 of the 20 patients (75%) reported, and 7 of the 15 responders (35% of the total group) did not require any further intervention.[19] Although esophageal luminal dilatation can be accomplished in patients with obstruction due to a malignant tumor, on average, the palliation is short-lived (sometimes for only a few days), and with continued attempts at dilatation, the procedure becomes more difficult and more likely to result in serious complication. Fortunately, other modes for the palliation of dysphagia exist.

Thermal and Other Ablative Techniques

Other palliative modalities for the restoration of a tumor obstructed esophageal lumen are thermal tumor ablation techniques utilizing the laser or argon plasma coagulator, injection of absolute alcohol into the tumor substance, and photodynamic therapy. Experience in the application and availability of these modalities is variable. When properly applied, all these modalities can palliate dysphagia but have not been consistently associated with prolonged survival. These modalities can be used in various combinations depending on the nature of the particular clinical problem at hand. Ultimately deployment of a self-expanding metal stent can be considered.

Laser

Tumor ablation using the neodymium:yttrium-aluminum-garnet (Nd:YAG) laser is not widely available, probably due to the cost of the apparatus, maintenance requirements of the equipment and fibers, need for a dedicated operating room, laser precautions, and time needed for therapy. The introduction of self-expandable metal stents (SEMS) has led to the supplanting of laser as well as other ablative modalities for the treatment of malignant luminal obstruction.[20] Three to five treatment sessions using the laser are needed initially to achieve palliation, and the interval between interventions is usually short—on the order of 3 to 4 weeks.[21] The application of the high power laser is usually done retrograde using the non-contact method after pre-dilation of the lumen, when necessary, in order to lessen the possibility of perforation. But sometimes the pre-dilation itself can cause perforation.[21] Wu and colleagues reported similar good results with the use of the low-power contact laser passed in the antegrade manner.[22] Complication rates increase and laser ablation becomes more difficult[23] with increasing frequency of application, serious complications ranging from 4 to 9%.[24–26]

Use of the Nd:YAG laser can be limited by the location and growth characteristics of the tumor and the need for accurate aiming of the laser beam, which can be obscured by the smoke generated during application. Laser therapy is best applied to exophytic mid-esophageal tumors where the lumens are not too long or tortuous.[27]

It cannot be used for the treatment of flat tumors invading the wall of the esophagus or for the relief of obstruction due to extrinsic compression.

Alexander and colleagues reported a series of 29 patients with locally advanced esophageal cancer who underwent laser debulking of their tumors with good results in the relief of dysphagia and, when coupled with aggressive multimodality therapy, an improved survival when compared to historical controls.[28] Although placement of an esophageal stent is associated with fewer interventions and a more immediate relief of dysphagia, the overall costs of the two procedures are not markedly different, and laser therapy may have a survival advantage and may be associated with fewer significant complications.[29,30]

Argon Plasma Coagulation

Argon Plasma Coagulation (APC) is a non-contact diathermy-based technique that uses an electrosurgery frequency current to ionize a cloud of argon gas in order to propagate a spark to the nearest tissue contact, inducing electrocoagulation necrosis. The tissue injury occurring as a consequence of APC is seldom deep enough to cause perforation, penetrating the tissues less than 2.5 mm.[31,32] APC is useful to control tumor bleeding, to recanalize tumor obstructed stents, and to control small or non-circumferential cancers of the esophagus. Although some have reported very good palliation with effectiveness and complications comparable to Nd:YAG laser,[33] APC is unlikely to restore adequate luminal patency to the esophagus obstructed by large tumors.[34]

Absolute Ethanol Injection

The injection of absolute ethanol into an exophytic tumor of the esophagus in order to induce chemical tumor necrosis is less widely practiced than other ablative procedures. It has been shown to be effective in palliating dysphagia[35,36] and has been found to be equivalent to Nd:YAG laser therapy.[37] Ethanol injection is inexpensive and the expertise for delivery is more readily available. However, diffusion of the ethanol into the tissues of the esophageal wall is difficult to control, leading to worries about perforation. Significantly more post-procedure pain requiring narcotic analgesia occurs in patients treated with ethanol injection as compared to laser therapy.[37]

Photodynamic Therapy

Photodynamic therapy for tumor ablation utilizes a photosensitizing agent—porfimer sodium (Photofrin II), injected intravenously 40 to 50 hours before the endoscopically guided placement of a diffusing tip fiber to deliver non-thermal 630 nm (red) light from a tunable dye laser. The Photofrin accumulates in the substance of the tumor in greater proportion than in normal

tissue—at least in a 2:1 ratio. When cancer cells containing the Photofrin II are exposed to the 630 nm (red) light, a cytotoxic superoxide is formed causing oxidation of cellular components such as tumor cell nuclei and mitochondria leading to cell death.[38,39] Because the patient is likely to remain photosensitive for at least 4 to 6 weeks, the patient must be warned to avoid bright direct and indirect light, whether indoors or out, and to wear protective clothing when venturing out of doors. Conventional sunscreens that block ultraviolet rays do not protect patients who have been injected with porfimer sodium because activation of the drug is by visible light. Severe erythema and edema of the skin can occur upon light exposure outdoors, even on cloudy days. Once the patient has been injected with a photosensitizer, there is no antidote.

Very good palliation of dysphagia was reported by Litle and colleagues in a series of 215 patients.[40] She found that the ideal patient for photodynamic therapy was one with an obstructing esophageal cancer. She noted effective palliation in 85% of treatment courses with a 2% incidence of perforation, 2% incidence of stricture and 1.8% procedure-related mortality with a mean dysphagia-free interval of 66 days. As with all palliative modalities, the longer the patient survives, the greater the chances that the palliation becomes less effective due to significant complications. Careful evaluation and recommendation for the application of specific palliative measures is very important in the satisfactory management of these unfortunate patients. Frequent trips to the hospital to undergo potentially dangerous procedures are a true burden to patients with a limited time to live.

Self-expandable Metal Stents

Ultimately, a stent can be placed to palliate esophageal luminal obstruction when other modalities have failed or the circumstances, such as stage of the disease and life expectancy, dictate that stent placement is the most likely modality to effectively and quickly palliate dysphagia. Palliation of dysphagia with patients able to tolerate at least liquids or a soft diet occurs almost immediately or within 24 to 48 hours after successful deployment of an esophageal stent.[41] Stent placement can be accomplished in an outpatient setting.

Over the years, stents have evolved from the rigid plastic type that necessitated dilation of the lumen to a diameter greater than 16 mm to the modern self-expandable metal stents which most often do not require dilation of the lumen at all, or only minimally. They are much easier to place and are associated with fewer immediate complications—particularly perforation. Other advantages of metal stents over plastic stents are the greater internal diameter, once deployed, and the ability to span more complicated stenoses due to their more flexible nature and thinner delivery systems.[42] For all these reasons, plastic stents have been supplanted by the self-expandable metal stents. Although the initial cost of self-expandable metal stents is higher than the cost of the plastic stents, the lower serious and life-threatening complication rate, fewer endoscopic re-interventions, and less need for hospitalization makes them a safe and cost-effective alternative to plastic esophageal stents.[42] Some manipulation of the self-expandable stent can be accomplished immediately after deployment (some stents are better than others in this regard). For all intents and purposes, however, once the stent is deployed, it cannot be removed. Therefore, careful evaluation and pre-procedure planning are necessary to ensure the intended palliation post-procedure with the least possibility of complication.

The most common indications for stenting the esophagus are dysphagia for liquids and saliva, treatment of tracheoesophageal fistula and, occasionally, control of tumor bleeding.[41] Probably, the successful treatment of a tracheoesophageal fistula, either with primary esophageal stenting or in conjunction with endotracheal or endobronchial stenting, may be the only instance in which esophageal stents can be said to not only improve the quality of life but to actually prolong it.[43,44]

The average survival of patients after esophageal stent placement, whether using the old plastic stents or the newer self-expandable metal stents, ranges from three to six months.[7,45,46] As with other palliative treatments, tumors in the mid-esophagus are more amenable to stenting with fewer resultant problems.[44] Stenting tumors of the distal esophagus can result in severe gastroesophageal reflux, which for the most part, can be treated by anti-reflux measures and proton pump inhibitors. A stent with a sleeve at the distal end has been designed in an effort to lessen gastroesophageal reflux. This type of stent may present additional deployment problems and does not seem greatly effective in eliminating reflux.[47] Stenting tumors of the proximal esophagus, if too close to the cricopharyngeus, can result in intractable pain, tracheal compression, proximal migration and foreign body sensation although some have reported satisfactory results even when the stent bridges the cricopharyngeus. But more usually, stents can be deployed through lesions close to the cricopharyngeus safely with low rates of difficulty if close attention to detail is paid in the selection of the stent and preventing the stent from migrating proximal to the cricopharyngeus.[48]

Stent deployment in the esophagus commonly results in chest pain most likely due to the expansion of the stent. This pain usually responds to narcotic analgesics and usually improves after several days.[49] If a bulky tumor is located in the proximal esophagus, one must always anticipate that expansion of the stent may lead to compression of the tracheal lumen leading to respiratory embarrassment. Patients with an esophageal tumor proximal to the level of the left main stem bronchus should have bronchoscopy to determine tracheal compromise prior to esophageal stent deployment[7] and, choosing a stent of a lesser diameter for placement, when available, would be prudent in this situation. A barium esophagogram prior to any interventional palliative procedure for dysphagia is recommended, not only for planning purposes prior to the procedure but for follow-up as well.[7]

Most stents deployed in the esophagus today are of the covered variety, with short segments of the proximal and distal ends left uncovered to help control the tendency for these covered stents to migrate. The coated portion of the stent is designed to impede ingrowth of the tumor into the mesh of the stent and thereby delay occlusion of the stent lumen. Stenosis of the lumen due to proximal and distal tumor ingrowth and overgrowth into the uncovered portion of the stent occurs over time, as well as luminal stenosis or occlusion consequent to exuberant growth of granulation tissue in response to the irritation caused by the uncovered portions of the stent. These problems are such that treatment with laser, argon plasma coagulation, débridement with a snare, endoscopic adjustment of position, or telescoping placement of another stent may be necessary to relieve renewed dysphagia.[50]

Palliation of dysphagia due to compression of the esophagus by an extrinsic tumor or metastatic deposit can be accomplished by SEMS and cannot easily be accomplished by any other means. The palliation of dysphagia is not as good in this situation as it is in those patients with an intrinsic esophageal lesion.[51]

The ideal stent has not been created, but a new generation of plastic stent has become available lately in the United States. It is a self-expandable plastic stent (the Polyflex stent) which is made of a polyester mesh covered with a silicone membrane. The inside of the stent is smooth and the outside is slightly textured. The proximal portion of the stent is slightly flared, whereas the middle and distal portions are not.[52] The major advantage of this stent is that it can be removed even several months after deployment, but the major disadvantage is that the esophageal lumen must be dilated to at least 1 mm larger than the application device, which is 12 or 14 mm in diameter, depending on the size of the stent itself, in order for the delivery system to pass through the tumor lumen and allow stent deployment.[53] Because the delivery system is thicker than the delivery systems of the self-expandable metal stents, it is, therefore, stiffer and more difficult to pass and position. Because of this stiffer delivery system and need to dilate the esophageal stricture

prior to deployment, there is a higher failure rate on initial deployment of the Polyflex stent.[52] Unlike the metal stents, the Polyflex stent must be loaded into the delivery system just prior to insertion, which sometimes may result in the flared end being improperly oriented in the delivery system and which would not be apparent until deployment.

The Polyflex stent has been used in the esophagus in all situations that metal stents have been used[54]; but, because it induces only minimal tissue reaction and granulation tissue formation, it does not become incorporated into the substance of the esophagus, and therefore, has a role in the management of benign but recalcitrant strictures of the esophagus.[55] The stent can be used as a scaffold for the remodeling of the stricture, and subsequently, it can be removed, resulting (it is to be hoped) in dysphagia-free swallowing. The Polyflex stent is cheaper than its metal counterparts in Europe but comparable in price to metal stents in the United States.

Gastric Outlet Obstruction

Severe nausea, regurgitation, vomiting, bloating, abdominal pain, and distention associated with a succussion splash leading to severe esophagitis, malnutrition and dehydration, and electrolyte imbalance are the common signs and symptoms of gastric outlet obstruction. These all lead to debilitation and a markedly decreased quality of life. Prior to the advent of H_2 blockers, complicated peptic ulcer disease was the most common cause for gastric outlet obstruction. Today, however, malignancy is the primary cause of gastric outlet obstruction and is encountered in more than 50% of cases.[56,57] Cancers of the pancreas, duodenum, ampulla, stomach, and biliary tree, as well as metastatic disease from other organ sites, can all lead to gastric outlet obstruction. Locally advanced pancreatic cancer, however, is the most common cause of malignant gastric outlet obstruction. In approximately 90% of patients with malignant gastric outlet obstruction the pylorus and the first and second part of the duodenum are the most common sites of obstruction. The distal portion of the duodenum is infrequently involved.[58,59] Ten to 20% of patients with pancreatic carcinoma develop gastric outlet obstruction late in the course of their disease.[60]

Although nausea, vomiting and weight loss are common presenting features of patients with pancreatic cancer, mechanical gastric outlet obstruction due to tumor ingrowth is present in only 5% of these patients.[61] True gastric outlet obstruction is due to invasion by tumor into the pylorus or duodenum, leading to stenotic mechanical obstruction. One must demonstrate this obstruction to be indeed mechanical by various diagnostic modalities such as endoscopy, upper gastrointestinal barium contrast study, or abdominal CT because up to 60% of patients with pancreatic cancer have slowed gastric emptying without evidence of gastroduodenal tumor invasion.[62] Pancreatic carcinoma has been shown to induce changes in the gastric myoelectric activity, usually bradygastria, leading to symptomatic decrease in the emptying of solids and liquids without actual mechanical obstruction.[63]

Consequent to gastric outlet obstruction, malnutrition, weight loss, dehydration, and electrolyte abnormalities develop, leading to poor performance status and a decreased quality of life. Malignant gastric outlet obstruction is often considered a pre-terminal event.[64]

By the time that mechanical gastric outlet obstruction occurs, treatment options for control of the primary cancer have usually been exhausted. The primary goal of palliative treatment should be to relieve symptoms by means that have minimal morbidity so as to improve or maintain the quality of the short remaining life.[65] In patients with good performance status, surgical bypass of biliary and duodenal obstruction and splanchnicectomy for the control of pain has been advocated.[66] However, in patients with advanced disease, associated malnutrition, limited life span, and poor tolerance for surgery, the choices remaining for palliation of these patients are limited.

Laparotomy/Laparoscopic Surgery

Laparotomy to relieve mechanical gastric outlet obstruction has been the most common treatment modality employed in the past.[66] However, it has been reported that the greater the need for gastrojejunostomy palliation of pancreatic cancer, the less likely is a favorable outcome.[67,68] For those patients who are taken to surgery with curative resection in mind but who are found to be unresectable because of locally advanced disease (major blood vessel involvement), palliation by gastrojejunostomy is advocated if there is not widespread metastatic disease. Prognosis is more favorable in those patients with locally advanced disease than in those with more widely metastatic disease, and thus, the likelihood for late gastric outlet obstruction is greater.[69]

Today, in the era of minimally invasive procedures, palliation of the obstructed duodenum can be accomplished not only by laparotomy but also by laparoscopic surgery, and more recently, by a novel application of self-expandable metal stents. Espat and colleagues reported that, if staging laparoscopy revealed advanced or metastatic pancreatic cancer, then routine prophylactic biliary and duodenal bypass procedures were not necessary in 152 of 155 patients studied,[70] that surgical biliary bypass should only be advocated in those patients in whom endoscopic biliary stenting has failed, and that gastroenterostomy should be reserved to those patients with

confirmed gastric outlet obstruction. However, Lillemoe and colleagues reported that, in their prospective randomized trial, prophylactic gastrojejunostomy significantly decreased the incidence of late gastric outlet obstruction—0% in the prophylactic group versus 19% in those not so treated.[71] Shyr and colleagues concurred in advocating prophylactic gastrojejunostomy in addition to biliary bypass in patients with unresectable periampullary carcinoma because of the high incidence of late gastric outlet obstruction in those patients not initially treated by gastrojejunostomy.[72] Palliation of biliary and gastric outlet obstruction can be accomplished by laparoscopic construction of a cholecystojejunostomy (if the cystic duct enters the common bile duct at a point distant from the tumor) and gastroenterostomy. In a small series reported by Nagy and colleagues of 10 patients with gastric outlet obstruction (9 due to malignancy), there were no operative deaths, and the most significant postoperative complication was delayed gastric emptying with mean time to regain gut function of 10 days.[73] Twenty percent of Nagy's laparoscopic surgeries had to be converted to the open procedure. In another small study, Alam and colleagues reported that there were no perioperative complications in 8 patients with malignancy-induced gastric outlet obstruction treated with laparoscopic gastrojejunostomy.[74] The median time to solid food intake was 4 days, and the median postoperative stay was 7 days. Choi also reported better tolerance for laparoscopic gastrojejunostomy versus open gastrojejunostomy with fewer postoperative complications and better postoperative hormonal and immune function, which may be responsible for the more rapid recovery and decreased pain in the laparoscopic group.[75]

Self-expandable Metal Stents

In the quest for a less invasive means to palliate malignant gastric outlet obstruction, the use of SEMS is evolving into the preferred method for palliation in all but perhaps the most medically fit patients for whom surgical palliation may still hold some advantage.[76,77] Before deciding to place a SEMS to relieve gastroduodenal obstruction, adequate assessment of the site and length of stricture and assessment of the bowel distal to the obstruction must be made in order to increase confidence that placement of the stent will result in the desired palliation.[78] Simultaneous palliation of malignant biliary and duodenal obstruction with SEMS can be accomplished in the outpatient setting with a very high success rate, low morbidity, and no procedure-associated mortality, although endoscopic access to the papilla after stent deployment can be very difficult.[79] SEMS have been placed by radiologists[80] utilizing only fluoroscopic techniques and by gastroenterologists utilizing both endoscopic and

fluoroscopic methods.[59,79] It is intuitive that utilizing both endoscopic and fluoroscopic methods leads to a better success rate in more difficult circumstances, especially in the patient with a dilated stomach due to prolonged obstruction. Palliation is almost immediate, and the patient is able to at least take liquids shortly after the deployment of the stent[77] or, at most, within 4 days after stent placement.[81] This immediate relief of gastric outlet obstruction and resumption of oral intake, ranging from liquids to soft and pureed food to a regular diet, results in an improved sense of well being and an improved quality of remaining life. In a review of 32 studies relating to the use of SEMS in malignant gastric outlet obstruction, which was conducted by Dormann and colleagues, pooled results were calculated involving 606 patients.[81] Ninety-four percent of these patients were unable to take nourishment orally. Stent deployment and placement was successful in 97%. Of the group in which technical success was achieved, 89% achieved clinical success—defined as resolution of symptoms of gastric outlet obstruction and ability to take in an oral diet—representing 87% of the total group in which stent placement was attempted. There were no procedure-related deaths. Severe complications (bleeding and perforation) were seen in only 1.2%, and stent migration in an additional 5%. Stent obstruction occurred in 18% mainly due to tumor ingrowth. The mean survival period was 12.1 weeks. Fiori and colleagues reported a randomized prospective trial of surgical gastroenterostomy versus endoscopic stenting and found no statistical difference between the two procedures at 3 months but noted that endoscopic stenting was significantly more effective with respect to operative time, restoration of oral intake and length of hospital stay.[82] Based on these findings, it appears that duodenal stenting for relief of obstruction is a safe, effective, and maybe the preferred, treatment.

Although no specific study has been done to determine cost-effectiveness per se, several studies suggest that the deployment of SEMS is cost-effective when compared to surgical intervention. SEMS are expensive, but the deployment can be made on an outpatient basis without the additional expenses of the operating room and postoperative hospitalization.[66] Yim and colleagues reported that the median survival time for patients with pancreatic cancer who underwent stenting of gastric outlet obstruction, compared with those who underwent surgical gastrojejunostomy, was 94 and 92 days, respectively; charges were $9,921 and $28,173, and the duration of hospitalization was 4 and 14 days, respectively.[83] The use of SEMS in the setting of malignant gastroduodenal obstruction is proving to be a cost- and clinically effective palliative treatment for these unfortunate patients.

The two most significant problems, stent migration and tumor and/or granulation tissue ingrowth with re-obstruction of the gastric outlet, have been addressed, but a perfect solution has not emerged. As in the case of esophageal tumors, the placement of covered duodenal stents has been proposed. Good technical and clinical success rates with a low incidence of stent migration and stent-related biliary outflow obstruction at the papilla have been reported.[84-86] Jung and colleagues reported favorable results in decreasing the migration rate of covered duodenal stents and improving resistance to tumor ingrowth of uncovered stents by coaxial placement of a covered stent inside a previously deployed uncovered stent.[87]

Venting Gastrostomy

In patients with gastric outlet obstruction due to malignancy in whom all other modalities of palliative treatment have failed, a percutaneous palliative venting gastrostomy should be offered because nausea and vomiting may be effectively palliated in a high percentage of patients and may even restore some level of oral intake.[88] If feasible, the addition of a feeding jejunostomy may also be considered.

Gastroesophageal Reflux after Esophagectomy

Transhiatal esophagectomy (the Ivor-Lewis operation) is often employed as a curative procedure in the treatment of cancer of the distal esophagus. It is a major operation that is associated with significant morbidity, among which are dysphagia, early satiety, stricture and inflammation at the anastomosis, regurgitation, heartburn and emotional problems that impact quality of life. Although more than one-half of the patients studied by de Boer and colleagues still experienced some of these symptoms,[89] the overall conclusion was that the quality of life of long-term survivors (minimum follow-up of 2 years) was comparable with reference values for the same age group, and in some parameters (ie, emotional well-being) was even better than the reference group. It is interesting to note that in a study of quality of life in patients with various gastrointestinal conditions, patients with functional disorders displayed more emotional distress than did patients with organic disease.[90]

A high incidence of gastroesophageal reflux has been reported in patients treated for head and neck cancers[91,92] and in patients after esophagectomy for cancers of the esophagus.[93] Reflux after esophagectomy occurs because the normal antireflux mechanisms of the intact esophagus and lower esophageal sphincter, and the normal hiatal anatomy that contributes to normal lower esophageal sphincter function, have been disrupted by the resection. After resection and anastomosis,

a large portion of the stomach is in the thorax, where negative pressure predominates, and this (combined with the positive pressure of the abdominal cavity) leads to free reflux of gastric and duodenal contents across the anastomosis into the esophageal remnant. This, coupled with impaired gastric motility and the return of acid secretion by the gastric conduit, leads to heartburn, regurgitation, night-time aspiration, dysphagia, esophagitis, sleep disturbance and general decrease in the quality of life.[93]

For most patients, gastric emptying is delayed in the supine position and improved in the upright position for 3–12 months after esophagogastrectomy, but some 4 to 6% of patients have long-lasting chronic gastroparesis after esophagectomy.[94] The denervated stomach, whether used in whole or fashioned into a tube as an esophageal substitute, progressively recovers more and more motor activity, even displaying a real phase 3 motor pattern in patients followed for more than 3 years post-operation.[95] Motor recovery is much better when the stomach is maintained as a whole, rather than when a conduit is fashioned from the greater curvature.[96]

The colon, small bowel, and stomach have all been used as substitutes for the resected esophagus.[97] The creation of a gastric tube is favored because of the simplicity of the operation and the lower postoperative morbidity and mortality.[98] Because vagotomy is an inevitable consequence of esophagectomy there is loss or disruption of the normal physiology of the stomach, such as accommodation to meals, tonic motility, and neurohumoral enterogastric feedback leading to delayed gastric emptying of solids but more rapid emptying of semisolids and liquids.[99] The delay in gastric emptying contributes to reflux, among other symptoms.[100] This dysfunction of gastric emptying coupled with reflux of duodenal contents into the stomach can lead to pathologic exposure of the gastric and remnant esophageal mucosa to bile acids in the early post-vagotomy period,[101] perhaps leading to more severe esophagitis and its consequences, such as stricture and Barrett's epithelium.[102] Acid reflux is more likely to be symptomatic than bile reflux, but erosive esophagitis can occur in isolated bile reflux.[103] The study by Logeman and colleagues concludes that, by constructing a narrow gastric tube as an esophageal substitute, a small distal gastric remnant is created with low compliance leading to an increased pressure gradient between the stomach and the duodenum, therefore favoring gastric emptying in the face of pyloroplasty or pyloromyotomy.[100] In a study, reported by Finley and colleagues, of 249 cases of esophagectomy performed for the treatment of malignancy, the rate of gastric emptying was not dependent on whether or not a gastric drainage procedure was employed,[104] but it seemed that the construction

of a narrow gastric tube fixed in the posterior mediastinum as a substitute for the esophagus was associated with less delay in gastric emptying. As regards food intake and functional dysphagia following esophagectomy and reconstruction, fixing the esophageal substitute in the posterior mediastinum appears to be more physiologic and associated with fewer symptoms than fixing the gastric tube in the retrosternal space.[105] The gastric tube is not inert but produces phasic contractions on distention in response to feeding, and in time, after the operation, there is at least partial recovery of gastric tone.[100] A study reported by Walsh and colleagues in which the whole stomach was used as the conduit after esophagectomy, demonstrated that the stomach functions as a dynamic conduit, and that erythromycin, which appears to primarily directly effect motilin receptors but which may also effect cholinergic transmission, induces peristaltic activity in the vagally denervated stomach to a greater extent than in normal controls.[99]

Treatment

Treatment of gastroesophageal reflux following Ivor-Lewis esophagogastrectomy must take into consideration the alteration of normal esophagogastroduodenal physiology and the abolition of natural anti-reflux mechanisms. As has already been discussed, delayed gastric emptying plays an important role in the perpetuation of symptomatic reflux. Therefore alteration of the diet is important, particularly eating smaller, more frequent meals that are low in fat, maintaining a standing posture after meals, and avoiding large meals approaching bedtime. Elevation of the head of the bed on 4-inch to 6-inch blocks is advised. The use of proton pump inhibitors is always helpful as acid secretion by the intrathoracic stomach after truncal vagotomy and esophagectomy may be unchanged,[106] and erythromycin as a promotility agent, particularly in the early postoperative period, should be considered.[107] Several antireflux surgical procedures[93] have been described, such as the intercostal pedicle esophagogastropexy[108]; all have proved complex to create and have not met wide acceptance.

Tube Gastrostomy

Frequently, a patient with cancer (particularly cancer of the upper aero-digestive tract) will need enteral nutrition because of dysphagia due to tumor involvement of the pharynx or esophagus. Sometimes access to the gastrointestinal tract will be obtained in anticipation of complications due to chemotherapy and/or radiotherapy leading to severe oro-pharyngeal-esophageal mucositis precluding the ability to swallow. It has been shown that early nutritional intervention through PEG tube insertion and maintenance of nutrition and hydration in patients with head and neck and esophageal cancer leads to better tolerance of treatment, completion of treatment at recommended doses, and avoidance of hospitalization. PEG placement in these circumstances has been associated with a low morbidity and mortality. Rarely, metastasis of the primary tumor to the PEG site has been reported. PEG placement does not preclude the stomach from being used to construct a conduit as an esophageal replacement during resection of distal esophageal cancers, as some thoracic surgeons have feared.[109–111] In this last regard, however, it is best to ascertain the surgeon's preferences.

In cancer patients, nutritional deficiencies can be restored and the quality of life can be maintained or improved by appropriate placement of a PEG tube.[112] Although nasoenteric tubes and other methods have been used to provide enteral nutrition and hydration in times past and at present,[113] PEG tubes are preferred because they are socially and cosmetically better tolerated, better anchored and more comfortable for the patient, and easier for caregivers to manage. A PEG tube can be safely placed in the outpatient setting and full strength iso-osmolar formula feedings can be safely started as little as 3 hours after tube placement.[114,115] Because PEG tubes are more easily managed by caregivers, more feeding formula can be infused in a shorter period of time resulting in better nutrition and hydration for most patients and better productivity for nursing home personnel. Therefore, most nursing homes demand that patients needing feeding assistance have PEG tubes in place before admission to their facilities.

In contradistinction to nasoenteric tubes, a PEG tube in non-acutely ill patients is better tolerated over a longer period of time and is associated with improved survival, less aspiration, and is less likely to be pulled out. Achievement of overall nutritional status was similar in patients with a PEG tube as in patients with a nasogastric tube.[116,117] PEG tubes need to be exchanged only occasionally and, usually, this exchange can be accomplished easily at the bedside. A variety of modifications of the replacement PEG tube have been developed. A modified replacement tube can be used for the exchange and will provide a more comfortable gastrostomy with less patient and caregiver anxiety about accidental dislodgement.[118]

Whether in the cancer or non-cancer patient, one should consider the placement of a nasogastric-enteric feeding tube if the anticipated need for tube feedings will be 30 days or less. For long-term tube feeding (greater than 30 days), it has been shown that a PEG tube is better tolerated and results in a better quality of life for patients and caregivers alike.[116]

Whenever a decision regarding artificial enteral nutrition is made, ethical considerations enter into the picture. The anticipated benefits must outweigh the potential harm due to possible complications. Decision regarding the placement of a PEG tube is often made difficult by emotions and misconceptions surrounding the benefits and risks of the procedure and the uncertainty, in some cases, that the intervention will bring material long-term benefit. The decisions about offering or withdrawing artificial nutritional support should be considered in the same ethical light as any other medical treatment.[119] Even now, more than 25 years since the introduction of the PEG into clinical practice, physicians are struggling with understanding the proper role of PEG and long-term enteral nutrition in the management of patients at the end of life. Because a procedure is readily available and relatively easily performed by experienced operators, it does not mean that it should be employed in all circumstances without regard to ethical standards.

Percutaneous Endoscopic Gastrostomy

The first PEG was performed on a 4 ½-month old infant in June 1979. Gauderer and Ponsky first reported this technique, including an additional 11 pediatric patients, in 1980.[120] The germinal ideas, however, and the experimental demonstration for feasibility of percutaneous gastrostomy placement were reported in 1967 by both Jascalevich and Edlich and colleagues.[121,122] Since the introduction of PEG into clinical practice, it has become the procedure of choice to obtain enteral access in patients who for a variety of reasons have impaired swallowing but otherwise have a functioning upper gastrointestinal tract. It has virtually replaced open surgical gastrostomy because of lower morbidity and mortality rates, ease and speed of placement, avoidance of general anesthesia and lower cost.[113] Open gastrostomy is useful, however, when placed as an adjunct to an abdominal operation being done for some other reason.

In the setting of cancer management, PEG is most commonly placed in patients with oropharyngeal and esophageal malignancy before, during or after treatment with chemo-radiation or surgery.[123] Several techniques have been developed ranging from the original Ponsky-Gauderer 'pull' method,[120] the over the guide wire 'push' Sachs-Vine method,[124] the 'introducer-push' or Russell method,[125] and the fluoroscopic-assisted Seldinger technique.[126] Gastrostomy tubes can be placed by the interventional radiologist,[126] by the surgeon using either the open or laparoscopic technique,[127] or by the gastroenterologist.[128]

Patients needing a PEG should be carefully screened and a primary determination made as to whether the patient's condition is such that a life expectancy of at least 30 days is likely. When compared to a similar nursing home population, factors that adversely affect the 30- and 60-day mortality rates after PEG placement in hospitalized patients are a serum albumin < 3, chronic obstructive pulmonary disease, and diabetes mellitus.[129] The reported procedure-associated mortality and major complication rates are low, with minor complication rates around 13%. Early mortality (< 30 days) has ranged from 8 to 22%,[130–132] 30-day mortality is improved considerably if the PEG tube is not placed during hospitalization for an acute illness. Patients who had PEG tube insertion 30 days after discharge achieved a 40% lower 30-day mortality rate than patients who had PEG tubes placed while hospitalized.[133]

Complications can be modified or averted by paying meticulous attention to details before and after PEG placement, such as using pre-procedure antibiotics,[134] being aware of the contraindications to PEG tube placement, carefully selecting patients who are more likely to benefit from PEG placement,[135] and ascertaining that, post-procedure, the external bumper does not exert undue pressure on the gastric or abdominal wall.[136] If improvement in the patient's condition and nutritional state cannot be reasonably expected, then placement of a PEG tube should be avoided.[119]

The decision to place a PEG tube prior to therapy for head and neck cancer can be difficult. The consistency of the diet consumed by the patient prior to institution of treatment may be a guide. The less like a normal diet that a patient consumes, the more likely a PEG will be needed.[137] PEG tube placement can be safely accomplished with greater than a 90% success rate in head and neck cancer patients with a low complication rate, several days or weeks before the anticipated treatment, at the time of other associated operative interventions, or in the postoperative period.[123,138–140]

The "pull" percutaneous gastrostomy technique as described by Ponsky and Gauderer is most commonly employed because of its simplicity and relative ease of placement.[120,141] An unsedated transnasal approach to PEG tube placement using an ultrathin endoscope has recently been reported and may be useful in patients with nearly obstructing lesions of the pharynx and in patients with trismus.[142]

There may be advantages to placing a PEG tube using the Russell "push" technique,[125] relative to the incidence of rare PEG-site metastasis,[124] stomal infections, and other minor complications associated with the procedure.[143,144] The Russell procedure has not been widely practiced by gastroenterologists. The introduction and placement of the gastrostomy tube is more complicated and time-consuming, and the feeding tube is of a lesser diameter than can be placed by the pull technique. It is also associated with a greater incidence of major complications.[145] In patients with advanced head and neck cancer who are elderly and have comorbid medical conditions, it is prudent to plan placement of the PEG at the time of anticipated resection.[146]

Although the placement of PEG tubes for enteral feeding has been proven safe, with a low incidence of minor and major complications, there has been concern about the occurrence of metastatic tumor implantation in the PEG stoma site. There have been approximately 30 patients reported with metastatic tumor implantation at the PEG tube site since 1989.[147] The incidence of this complication is unknown but it has been variably estimated at less than 1% to as high as 3%. The exact mechanism for this complication is unknown, and various theories have been advanced. The mechanisms that have been proposed include the direct contamination with malignant cells of the PEG tube as it traverses the tumor in the "pull technique" and the hematogenous and lymphatic spread of circulating tumor cells to predisposed tissues, such as the fresh PEG tube stoma. The majority of patients reported had squamous cell cancer of the head and neck although esophageal tumors have also been reported to metastasize to the PEG stoma as well. The discovery of the metastatic deposit has occurred on average 7 to 9 months after PEG placement. The most common signs and symptoms in patients with this complication include stomal leakage, stomal induration, exuberant and friable soft tissue growth and abdominal wall pain. The continued presence of the PEG tube was not necessary for this complication to occur. Some of the PEG tubes had been removed several months prior to the discovery of PEG site metastases. The PEG tubes continued to function in the face of metastatic disease to the stoma. The majority of reports have been in patients with aggressive, advanced cancers (stage III and IV) who also had evidence of other distant metastasis. It appears that, since 1989, all the cases reported have been in patients who have had the PEG placed by the "pull technique."[148–150] This may be due to the fact that the "pull technique" is by far the most popular technique employed and not due to some inherent but undefined problem with the technique. Some authors have proposed that alternative methods be employed in the placement of PEG in these patients.[147]

Other Uses

Sometimes percutaneous endoscopic gastrostomy is employed not for establishment of nutrition but for palliation of intractable nausea and vomiting due to intestinal obstruction caused by inoperable intraluminal tumor or abdominal carcinomatosis. Intractable nausea and vomiting can be palliated in the majority of these patients, obviating admission to the hospital. Some may return to a clear liquid diet which can boost the quality of life. If feasible, the combination of venting gastrostomy and feeding jejunostomy may be considered.[88,151,152]

REFERENCES

1. Gregory Zuccaro, Jr. The esophagus. 4th ed. In: Castell DO, Richter JE, (eds). Lippincott Williams & Wilkins, 530 Walnut Street, Philadelphia, PA 19106 13:275–289.
2. Devesa SS, Blot WJ, Fraumeni JF. Changing patterns in the incidence of esophageal and gastric carcinoma in the United States. Cancer 1998;83:2049–53.
3. Brown LM, Devesa SS. Epidemiologic trends in esophageal and gastric cancer in the United States. Surg Oncol Clin N Am 2002;11:235–56.
4. DeMeester TR. Esophageal carcinoma: current controversies. Semin Surg Oncol 1997;13:217–33.
5. Table I3. Summary of changes in cancer incidence and mortality, 1950–2001 and 5-year relative survival rates 1950– 2000. Available at: http://seer.cancer.gov/csr/1975_2001/results_merged/topic_survival.pdf (accessed March 15, 2005).
6. Enzinger PC, Mayer RJ. Esophageal cancer [review article]. N Eng J Med 2003;349:2241–52.
7. Boyce, HW Jr. Palliation of dysphagia of esophageal cancer by endoscopic lumen restoration techniques. Cancer Control 1999;6:28–35.
8. Herskovic A, Martz K, Al-Sarraf M, et al. Combined chemotherapy and radiotherapy compared with radiotherapy alone in patients with cancer of the esophagus. N Engl J Med 1992;326:1593–8.
9. Kaneko K, Ito H, Konishi K, et al. Definitive chemoradiotherapy for patients with malignant stricture due to T3 or T4 squamous cell carcinoma of the esophagus. Br J Cancer 2003;88:18–24.
10. Honkoop P, Siersema PD, Tilanus HW, et al. Benign anastomotic strictures after transhiatal esophagectomy and cervical esophagogastrostomy: risk factors and management. J Thorac Cardiovasc Surg 1996;111:1141–6.
11. Petrin G, Ruol A, Battaglia G, et al. Anastomotic stenoses occurring after circular stapling in esophageal cancer surgery. Surg Endosc 200;14:670–4.
12. Pierie JP, de Graaf PW, Poen H, et al. Incidence and management of benign anastomotic stricture after cervical oesophagogastrostomy. Br J Surg 1993;80:471–4.
13. Swaroop VS, Desai DC, Mohandas KM, et al. Dilation of esophageal stricture induced by radiation therapy for cancer of the esophagus. Gastrointest Endosc 1994;40:311–5.
14. Wallace MB, Hawes RH, Sahai AV, et al. Dilation of malignant esophageal stenosis to allow EUS guided fine-needle aspiration: safety and effect on patient management. Gastrointest Endosc 200;51:309–13.
15. Pfau PR, Ginsberg GG, Lew RJ, et al. Esophageal dilation for endosonographic evaluation of malignant esophageal strictures is safe and effective. Am J Gastroenterol 2000;95:2813–5.
16. Aste H, Munizzi F, Martines H, et al. Esophageal dilation in malignant dysphagia. Cancer 1985;56:2713–5.
17. Lundell L, Leth R, Lind T, et al. Palliative endoscopic dilatation in carcinoma of the esophagus and esophagogastric junction. Acta Chir Scand 1989;155:179–84.
18. Clouse RE. Complications of endoscopic gastrointestinal dilation techniques. Gastrointest Endosc Clin N Am 1996;6:323–41.
19. Ko GY, Song HY, Hong HJ, et al. Malignant esophagogastric junction obstruction: efficacy of balloon dilation combined with chemotherapy and/or radiation therapy. Cardiovasc Intervent Radiol 2003;26:141–5.
20. Kozarek RA. Endoscopic palliation of esophageal malignancy Endoscopy 2003;35(8):9–13
21. Hurley JF, Cade RJ. Laser photocoagulation in the treatment of malignant dysphagia. Aust N Z J Surg 1997;67:800–3.
22. Wu KL, Tsao WL, Shyu RY. Low-power laser therapy for gastrointestinal neoplasia. J Gastroenterol 2000;35:518–23.
23. Rutgeerts P, Vantrappen G, Broeckaert L. Palliative Nd:YAG laser therapy for cancer of the esophagus and gastroesophageal junction: impact on the quality of remaining life. Gastrointest Endosc 1988;34:87–90.
24. Loizou LA, Grigg D, Atkinson M, et al A prospective comparison of laser therapy and intubation in endoscopic palliation for malignant dysphagia. Gastroenterology 1991;100:1303–10.
25. Hahl J, Salo J, Ovaska J, et al. Comparison of endoscopic Nd: YAG laser therapy and oesophageal tube in palliation of oesophagogastric malignancy. Scand J Gastroenterol 1991;26:103–08.
26. Tyrrell MR, Trotter GA, Adam A, et al. Incidence and management of laser-associated oesophageal perforation. Br J Surg 1995;82:1257–8.
27. Spinelli P, Dal Fante M, Mancini A. Endoscopic palliation of malignancies of the upper gastrointestinal tract using Nd: YAG laser: results and survival in 308 treated patients. Lasers Surg Med 1991;11:550–5.
28. Alexander P, Mayoral W, Reilly HF 3rd, et al. Endoscopic Nd:YAG laser with aggressive multimodality therapy for locally advanced esophageal cancer. Gastrointest Endosc 2002;55:674–9.
29. Dallal HJ, Smith GD, Grieve DC, et al. A randomized trial of thermal ablative therapy verses expandable metal stents in the palliative treatment of patients with esophageal carcinoma. Gastrointest Endosc 2001;54:549–57.
30. Sihvo EIT, Pentikainen T, Luostarinen ME, et al. Inoperable adenocarcinoma of the oesophagogastric junction: a comparative clinical study of laser coagulation versus self-expanding metallic stents with special reference to cost analysis. Eur J Surg Oncol 2002;28:711–5.
31. Watson JP, Bennett MK, Griffin SM, et al. The tissue effect of argon plasma coagulation on esophageal and gastric mucosa. Gastrointest Endosc 2000;52:342–5.
32. Johanns W, Janssen LW, Kahl S, et al. Argon plasma coagulation (APC) in gastroenterology: experimental and clinical experiences. Eur J Gastroenterol Hepatol 1997;9:581–7.
33. Heindorff H, Wojedemann M, Bisgaard T, et al. Endoscopic palliation of inoperable cancer of the oesophagus or cardia by argon electrocoagulation. Scand J Gastroenterol 1998;33:21–3.
34. Akhtar K, Byrne JP, Bancewicz J, et al. Argon beam plasma coagulation in the management of cancers of the esophagus and stomach. Surg Endosc 2000;14:1127–30.
35. Moreira LS, Coelho RC, Sadala RU, et al. The use of ethanol injection under endoscopic control to palliate dysphagia caused by esophagogastric cancer. Endoscopy 1994;26:311–4.
36. Chung SC, Leong HT, Choi CY, et al. Palliation of malignant esophageal obstruction by endoscopic alcohol injection. Endoscopy 1994;26:275–7.
37. Carazzone A, Bonavina L, Segalin A, et al. Endoscopic palliation of oesophageal cancer: results of a prospective comparison of Nd:YAG laser and ethanol injection. Eur J Surg 1999;165:351–6.
38. Janssen, WG. Photodynamic therapy: a guide to instrumentation and dosimetry calculations. Minim Invasive Surg Nurs 1996;10:105–108.
39. Lightdale, CJ. Palliative application of photodynamic therapy in esophageal cancer treatment [special report]. Gastroenterology & Endoscopy News 2002.
40. Litle, VR, Luketich, JD, Christie, NA, et al. Photodynamic therapy as palliation for esophageal cancer: experience in 215 patients. Ann Thorac Surg 2003;76:1687–93.
41. Tomaselli F, Maier A, Sankin O, et al. Ultraflex stent—benefits and risks in ultimate palliation of advanced, malignant stenosis in the esophagus. Hepatogastroenterology 2004;51:1021–6.
42. Knyrim K, Wagner H-J, Bethge N, et al. A controlled trial of an expansile metal stent for palliation of esophageal obstruction due to inoperable cancer. N Eng J Med 1993;329:1302–7.
43. van den Bongard HJGD, Boot H, Baas P et al. The role of parallel stent insertion in patients with esophagorespiratory fistulas. Gastrointest Endosc 2002;55:110–5.
44. Baron TH. Current concepts: expandable metal stents for the treatment of cancerous obstruction of the gastrointestinal tract. N Engl J Med 2001;344:1681–7.
45. Boyce, HW Jr. Stents for palliation of dysphagia due to esophageal cancer [editorial]. N Eng J Med 1993;329:1345–6.
46. Bethge N, Vakil N. A prospective trial of a new self-expanding plastic stent for malignant esophageal obstruction. Am J Gastro 2001;96:1350–4.
47. Homs MYV, Wahab PJ, Kuipers EJ, et al. Esophageal stents with antireflux valve for tumors of the distal esophagus and gastric cardia: a randomized trial. Gastrointest Endosc 2004;60:695–702.
48. Bethge N, Sommer A, Vakil N. A prospective trial of self-expanding metal stents in the palliation of malignant esophageal strictures near the upper esophageal sphincter. Gastrointest Endosc 1997;45:300–3.
49. Golder M, Tekkis PP, Kennedy C, et al. Chest pain following oesophageal stenting for malignant dysphagia. Clin Radiol 2001;56:202–5.

50. Homs MYV, Steyerberg EW, Kuipers EJ, et al. Causes and treatment of recurrent dysphagia after self-expanding metal stent placement for palliation of esophageal carcinoma. Endoscopy 2004;36:880–6.
51. Bethge N, Sommer A, Vakil N. Palliation of malignant esophageal obstruction due to intrinsic and extrinsic lesions with expandable metal stents. American J Gastroenterol 1998;93:1829–32.
52. Costamagna G, Shah SK, Tringali A, et al. Prospective evaluation of a new self-expanding plastic stent for inoperable esophageal strictures. Surg Endosc 2003;17:891–5.
53. Dormann AJ, Elsendrath P, Wigginhaus B, et al. Palliation of esophageal carcinoma with a new self-expanding plastic stent. Endoscopy 2003;35:207–11.
54. Radecke K, Gerken G, Treichel U. Impact of a self-expanding, plastic esophageal stent on various esophageal stenoses, fistulas, and leakages: a single-center experience in 39 patients. Gastrointest Endosc 2005;61:812–8.
55. Pungpapong S, Wallace MB, Woodward TA. Problematic esophageal stricture: an emerging indication for self-expandable silicone stents. Gastrointest Endosc 2004;60: 842–5.
56. Shone DN, Nikoomanesh P, Smith-Meek MM, et al. Malignancy is the most common cause of gastric outlet obstruction in the era of H2 blockers. Am J Gastroenterol 1995;90:1769–70.
57. Chowdhury A, Dhali GK, Banerjee PK. Etiology of gastric outlet obstruction. Am J Gastroent 1996;91:1679.
58. Kaw M, Singh S, Gagneja H, et al. Role of self-expandable metal stents in the palliation of malignant duodenal obstruction. Surg Endosc 2003;17:646–50.
59. Adler DG, Baron TH, Endoscopic palliation of malignant gastric outlet obstruction using self-expanding metal stents: experience in 36 patients. Am J Gastroent 2002; 97:72–8.
60. Egrari S, O'Connell TX. Role of prophylactic gastrojejunostomy for unresectable pancreatic cancer. Am Surg 1995;61:862–4.
61. Potts JR, Vogt DP, Broughan T, et al. Indications for gastric bypass in palliative operations for pancreatic carcinoma. Am Surg 1991;57:24–8.
62. Barkin JS, Goldberg RI, Sfakianakis GN, et al. Pancreatic carcinoma is associated with delayed gastric emptying. Dig Dis Sci 1986;31:265–7.
63. Thor PJ, Popiela T, Sobocki J, et al. Pancreatic carcinomainduced changes in gastric myoelectric activity and emptying. Hepatogastroenterology 2002;49:268–70.
64. Van Wagensveld BA, Coene PPLO, Van Gulik TM et al. Outcome of palliative biliary and gastric bypass surgery for pancreatic head carcinoma in 126 patients. Br J Surg 1997;84:1402–6.
65. Molinari M, Helton WS, Espat NJ. Palliative strategies for locally advanced unresectable and metastatic pancreatic cancer. Surg Clin North Am 2001;81:651–66.
66. Lillemoe KD, Pitt HA. Palliation. Surgical and otherwise. Cancer 1996;78(3 Suppl):605–14.
67. Weaver DW, Wiencek RG, Bouwman DL, et al. Gastrojejunostomy: is it helpful for patients with pancreatic cancer? Surgery 1987;102:608–13.
68. Fujino Y, Suzuki Y, Kamigaki T, et al. Evaluation of gastroenteric bypass for unresectable pancreatic cancer. Hepatogastroenterology 2001;48:563–8.
69. Di Fronzo, LA, Cymerman J, Egrari S, et al. Unresectable pancreatic carcinoma: correlating length of survival with choice of palliative bypass. Am Surg 1999;65:955–8.
70. Espat NJ, Brennan MF, Conlon KC. Patients with laparoscopically staged unresectable pancreatic adenocarcinoma do not require subsequent surgical biliary or gastric bypass. J Am Coll Surg 1999;188:649–57.
71. Lillemoe KD, Cameron JL, Hardacre JM, et al. Is prophylactic gastrojejunostomy indicated for unresectable periampullary cancer? Ann Surg 1999;230:322–30.
72. Shyr YM, Su CH, Wu CW, et al. Prospective study of gastric outlet obstruction in unresectable periampullary adenocarcinoma. World J Surg 2000;24:60–5.
73. Nagy A, Brosseuk D, Hemming A, et al. Laparoscopic gastroenterostomy for duodenal obstruction. Am J Surg 1995;169:539–42.
74. Alam TA, Baines M, Parker MC. The management of gastric outlet obstruction secondary to inoperable cancer. Surg Endosc 2003;17:320–3.
75. Choi, YB. Laparoscopic gastrojejunostomy for palliation of gastric outlet obstruction in unresectable gastric cancer. Surg Endosc 2002;16:1620–6.
76. Kozarek RA. Malignant gastric outlet obstruction: is stenting the standard? Endoscopy 2001;33:876–7.
77. Nassif T, Prat F, Meduri B, et al. Endoscopic palliation of malignant gastric outlet obstruction using self-expandable metallic stents: results of a multicenter study. Endoscopy 2003;35:483–9.
78. Razzaq R, Laasch H-U, England R, et al. Expandable metal stents for the palliation of malignant gastroduodenal obstruction. Cardiovasc Intervent Radiol 2001;24:313–8.
79. Kaw M, Singh S, Gagneja H. Clinical outcome of simultaneous self-expandable metal stents for palliation of malignant biliary and duodenal obstruction. Surg Endosc 2003; 17:457–61.
80. Profili S, Meloni GB, Bifulco V, et al. Self-expandable metal stents in the treatment of antro-pyloric and/or duodenal strictures. Acta Radiol 2001;42:176–80.
81. Dormann A, Meisner S, Verin N, et al. Self-expanding metal stents for gastroduodenal malignancies: systematic review of their clinical effectiveness. Endoscopy 2004;36:543–50.
82. Fiori E, Lamazza A, Volpino P, et al. Palliative management of malignant antro-pyloric strictures. Gastroenterostomy vs. endoscopic stenting. A randomized prospective trial. Anticancer Res 2004;24:269–71.
83. Yim HB, Jacobson MD, Saltzman JR, et al. Clinical outcome of the use of enteral stents for palliation of patients with malignant upper GI obstruction. Gastrointest Endosc 2001;53:329–332.
84. Lopera JE, Alvarez O, Castano R, et al. Initial experience with Song's covered duodenal stent in the treatment of malignant gastroduodenal obstruction. J Vasc Interv Radiol 2001;12:1297–303.
85. Jeong JY, Han JK, Kim AY, et al. Fluoroscopically guided placement of a covered self-expandable metallic stent for malignant antroduodenal obstructions: preliminary results in 18 patients. AJR 2002;178:847–52.
86. Park KB, Do YS, Kang WK, et al. Malignant obstruction of the gastric outlet and duodenum: palliation with flexible covered metallic stents. Radiology 2001;219:679–83.
87. Jung GS, Song HY, Seo TS, et al. Malignant gastric outlet obstructions: treatment by means of coaxial placement of uncovered and covered expandable nitinol stents. J Vasc Interv Radiol 2002;13:275–83.
88. Brooksbank MA, Game PA, Ashby MA. Palliative venting gastrostomy in malignant intestinal obstruction. Palliat Med 2002;16:520–6.
89. de Boer AGEM, Onorbe Genovesi PI, Sprangers MAG, et al. Quality of life in long-term survivors after curative transhiatal oesophagectomy for oesophageal carcinoma. Br J Surg 2000;87:1716–21.
90. Wiklund IK, Glise H. Quality of life in different gastrointestinal conditions. Eur J Surg 1998;164(Suppl 582):56–61.
91. Smit CF, Tan J, Mathus-Vliegen LMH, et al. High incidence of gastropharyngeal and gastroesophageal reflux after total laryngectomy. Head Neck 1998;20:619–22.
92. Biacabe B, Gleich LL, Laccourreye O, et al. Silent gastroesophageal reflux disease in patients with pharyngolaryngeal cancer: further results. Head Neck 1998;20: 510–4.
93. Aly A, Jamieson GG. Reflux after oesophagectomy. Br J Surg 2004;91:137–41.
94. Burt M, Scott A, Williard WC, et al. Erythromycin stimulates gastric emptying after esophagectomy with gastric replacement: a randomized clinical trial. J Thorac Cardiovasc Surg 1996;111:649–54.
95. Collard J-M, Romagnoli R, Otte J-B, et al. The denervated stomach as an esophageal substitute is a contractile organ. Ann Surg 1998;227:33–9.
96. Collard J-M, Romagnoli R, Otte J-B, et al. Erythromycin enhances early postoperative contractility of the denervated whole stomach as an esophageal substitute. Ann Surg 1999;229:337–43.
97. Gaissert HA, Mathisen DJ, Grillo HC, et al. Short-segment intestinal interposition of the distal esophagus. J Thorac Cardiovasc Surg 1993;106:860–6.
98. Visbal AL, Allen MS, Miller DL, et al. Ivor Lewis esophagectomy for esophageal cancer. Ann Thorac Surg 2001;71: 1803–8.
99. Walsh TN, Caldwell MT, Fallon C, et al. Gastric motility following oesophagectomy. Br J Surg 1995;82:91–4.
100. Logeman F, Roelofs JMM, Obertop H. Tonic motor activity of the narrow gastric tube used as an oesophageal substitute. Eur J Surg 2000;166:301–6.
101. Gutschow CA, Collard J-M, Romagnoli R, et al. Bile exposure of the denervated stomach as an esophageal substitute. Ann Thorac Surg 2001;71:1786–91.
102. Nehra D, Howell P, Pye JK, et al. Assessment of combined bile acid and pH profiles using an automated sampling device in gastro-oesophageal reflux disease. Br J Surg 1998;85:134–7.
103. Marshall REK, Anggiansah A, Owen WA, et al. Investigation of oesophageal reflux symptoms after gastric surgery with combined pH and bilirubin monitoring. Br J Surg 1999;86:271–5.
104. Finley RJ, Lamy A, Clifton J, et al. Gastrointestinal function following esophagectomy for malignancy. Am J Surg 1995;169:471–5.
105. Shiraha S, Matsumoto H, Terada M, et al. Motility studies of the cervical esophagus with intrathoracic gastric conduit after esophagectomy. Scandinavian J Thorac Cardiovasc Surg 1992;26:119–23.
106. Nishikawa M, Murakami T, Tangoku A, et al. Functioning of the intrathoracic stomach after esophagectomy. Arch Surg 1994;129:837–41.
107. Nakabayashi T, Mochiki E, Garcia M, et al. Gastropyloric motor activity and the effects of erythromycin given orally after esophagectomy. Am J Surg 2002;183:317–23.
108. Demos NJ, Kulkarni VA, Port A, et al. Control of post-resection gastroesophageal reflux: the intercostal pedicle esophagogastropexy experience of 26 years. Am Surg 1993;59:137–48.
109. Piquet MA, Ozsahin M, Larpin I, et al. Early nutritional intervention in oropharyngeal cancer patients undergoing radiotherapy. Support Care Cancer 2002;10:502–4.
110. Margolis M, Alexander P, Trachiotis G, et al. Percutaneous endoscopic gastrostomy before multimodality therapy in patients with esophageal cancer. Ann Thorac Surg 2003;76:1694–8.
111. Stockeld D, Fagerberg J, Granstrom L, et al. Percutaneous endoscopic gastrostomy for nutrition in patients with oesophageal cancer. Eur J Surg 2001;167:839–44.
112. Klose J, Heldwein W, Rafferzeder M, et al. Nutritional status and quality of life in patients with percutaneous endoscopic gastrostomy (PEG) in practice: Prospective one year follow up. Dig Dis Sci 2003;48:2057–63.
113. Pearce CB, Duncan HD. Enteral feeding. Nasogastric, nasojejunal, percutaneous endoscopic gastrostomy, or jejunostomy: its indications and limitations. Postgrad Med J 2002;78:198–204.
114. Choudry U, Bard CJ, Markert R, Gopalswamy N. Percutaneous endoscopic gastrostomy: a randomized prospective comparison of early and delayed feeding. Gastrointest Endosc 1996;44:164–7.
115. Mandal A, Steel A, Davidson AR. Day-case percutaneous endoscopic gastrostomy: a viable proposition? Postgrad Med J 2000;76:157–9.
116. Dwolatzky T, Berezovski S, Friedmann R, et al. A prospective comparison of the use of nasogastric and percutaneous endoscopic gastrostomy tubes for long-term enteral feeding in older people. Clin Nutr 2001;20:535–40.
117. Roche V. Percutaneous endoscopic gastrostomy: clinical care of PEG tubes in older adults. Geriatrics 2003;58: 22–9.
118. Gauderer MW. Percutaneous endoscopic gastrostomy and the evolution of contemporary long-term enteral access. Clin Nutr 2002;21:103–10.
119. Angus F, Burakoff R, MD. The percutaneous endoscopic gastrostomy tube: medical and ethical issues in placement. Am J Gastroenterol 2003;98:272–7.
120. Gauderer MW, Ponsky JL, Izant RJ. Gastrostomy without laparotomy: a percutaneous endoscopic technique. J Pediatr Surg 1980;15:872–5.
121. Jascalevich ME. Experimental trocar gastrostomy. Surgery 1967;62:452–3.
122. Edlich RF, Prevost MV, Tsung, MS, et al. Transilluminated distention gastrostomy: a preliminary report of a simplified method employing an illuminated gastric catheter. Surgery 1967;62:448–51.
123. Baredes S, Behin D, Deitch E, Percutaneous endoscopic gastrostomy tube feeding in patients with head and neck cancer. Ear Nose Throat J 2004;83:417–9.
124. Tucker AT, Gourin CG, Ghegan MD, et al. 'Push' versus 'Pull' percutaneous endoscopic gastrostomy tube placement in patients with advanced head and neck cancer. Laryngoscope 2003;113:1898–902.
125. Russell TR, Brotman M, Norris F. Percutaneous gastrostomy: a new simplified and cost effective technique. Am J Surg 1984;142:132–7.
126. Given MF, Lyon SM, Lee MJ. The role of the interventional radiologist in enteral alimentation. Eur Radiol 2004;14: 38–47.

127. Nagle AP, Murayama KM. Laparoscopic gastrostomy and jejunostomy. J Long Term Eff Med Implants 2004;14: 1–11.

128. The Standards of Practice Committee of the American Society for Gastrointestinal Endoscopy. Role of endoscopy in enteral feeding. Gastrointest Endosc 2002;55: 794–7.

129. Lang A, Bardan E, Chowers Y, et al. Risk factors for mortality in patients undergoing percutaneous endoscopic gastrostomy. Endoscopy 2004;36:522–6.

130. Malmgren A, Cederholm T, Faxen Irving G, et al. Percutaneous endoscopic gastrostomy (PEG) in elderly—indications and survival. Clin Nutr 2003;22(Suppl 1): 82–3.

131. Fernandez-Viadero C, Pena Sarabia N, Jimenez Sainz M, et al. Percutaneous endoscopic gastrostomy: better than nasoenteric tube? J Am Geriatr Soc 2002;50:199–200.

132. Skelly RH, Kupfer RM, Metcalfe ME, et al. Percutaneous endoscopic gastrostomy (PEG): change in practice since 1988. Clin Nutr 2002;21:389–94.

133. Abusksis G, Mor M, Plaut S, et al. Outcome of percutaneous endoscopic gastrostomy (PEG): comparison of two policies in a 4-year experience. Clin Nutr 2004;23:341–6.

134. Lockett MA, Templeton ML, Byrne TK, et al. Percutaneous endoscopic gastrostomy complications in a tertiary-care center. Am Surg 2002;68:117–20.

135. Kobayashi K, Cooper GS, Chak A, et al. A prospective evaluation of outcome in patients referred for PEG placement. Gastrointest Endosc 2002;55:500–6.

136. Lin HS, Ibrahim HZ, Kheng JW, et al. Percutaneous endoscopic gastrostomy: strategies for prevention and management of complications. Laryngoscope 2001;111: 1847–52.

137. Dawson FR, Jackson M, Macgregor CA, et al. An audit designed to assess the need for planned pretreatment PEG placement in patients with stage III & stage IV oral cancer. J Hum Nutr Diet 2004;17:575.

138. Hujala K, Sipila J, Pulkkinen J, et al. Early percutaneous endoscopic gastrostomy nutrition in head and neck cancer patients. Acta Otolaryngol 2004;124:847–50.

139. Riera L, Sandiumenge A, Calvo C, et al. Percutaneous endoscopic gastrostomy in head and neck cancer patients. J Otorhinolaryngol Relat Spec 2002;64:32–4.

140. Lloyd CJ, Penfold CN. Insertion of percutaneous endoscopic gastrostomy tubes by a maxillofacial surgical team in patients with oropharyngeal cancer. Br J Oral Maxillofac Surg 2002;40:122–4.

141. Ponsky JL, Gauderer MWL. Percutaneous endoscopic gastrostomy: a nonoperative technique for feeding gastrostomy. Gastrointest Endosc 1981;27:9–11.

142. Dumortier J, Lapulus MG, Pereira A, et al. Unsedated transnasal PEG placement. Gastrointest Endosc 2004;59: 54–7.

143. Akkersdijk WL, van Bergeijk JD, van Egmond T, et al. Percutaneous endoscopic gastrostomy (PEG): comparison of push and pull methods and evaluation of antibiotic prophylaxis. Endoscopy 1995;27:313–6.

144. Maetani I, Tada T, Inoue H, et al. PEG with introducer or pull method: a prospective randomized comparison. Gastrointest Endosc 2003;57:837–41.

145. Petersen TI, Kruse A. Complications of endoscopic gastrostomy. Eur J Surg 1997;163:351–6.

146. Cunliffe DR, Swanton C, White SR, et al. Percutaneous endoscopic gastrostomy at the time of tumour resection in advanced oral cancer. Oral Oncol 2000;36:471–3.

147. Hunter JG. Tumor implantation at PEG exit sites in head and neck cancer patients: how much evidence is enough? J Clin Gastroenterol 2003;37:280.

148. Cossentino MJ, Fukuda MM. Cancer metastasis to a percutaneous gastrostomy site. Head Neck 2001;23: 1080–3.

149. Maccabee D, Sheppard BC. Prevention of percutaneous endoscopic gastrostomy stoma metastases in patients with active oropharyngeal malignancy. Surg Endosc 2003;17:1678.

150. Pickhardt PJ, Rohrmann CA Jr, Cossentino MJ. Stomal metastases complicating percutaneous endoscopic gastrostomy: CT findings and the argument for radiologic tube placement. Am J Roentgenology 2002;179:735–9.

151. Jolicoeur L, Faught W. Managing bowel obstruction in ovarian cancer using a percutaneous endoscopic gastrostomy (PEG) tube. Can Oncol Nurs J 2003;13:212–9.

152. Scheidbach H, Hornbach T, Groitl H, Hohenberger W, Percutaneous endoscopic gastrostomy/jejunostomy (PEG/PEJ) for decompression in the upper gastrointestinal tract Surgical Endoscopy. 1999;13:1103–05.

Hepatobiliary and Pancreatic Disorders

John T. Mullen, MD

Eddie K. Abdalla, MD

For long-term cancer survivors, and especially for cancer patients receiving treatment, disorders of the liver, biliary tree, and pancreas are common. The goal of this chapter is to provide a framework for diagnosis and treatment of disorders of these organ systems in the context of the patient's treatment and cancer-related prognosis. Because of space constraints, this chapter will not discuss every hepatobiliary or pancreatic disorder that clinicians may confront.

For many of the disorders described herein, invasive or interventional tests are needed for the diagnostic work-up, requiring the expertise of radiologists, gastroenterologists, and surgeons. The referring oncologist provides a critical perspective on the underlying cancer and the patient's prognosis, and the work-up is modified on the basis of this background information. Every interventional test carries risks and must be applied judiciously—complications of the diagnostic work-up can have catastrophic consequences for patients and families if the individual patient circumstances are not taken into account. Thus, when interventions such as endoscopy or biopsy are suggested below, they are to be considered only when the clinical scenario is critically appraised in light of the underlying cancer diagnosis and prognosis by the consulting oncologist in concert with interventional radiologists, gastroenterologists, and surgeons. This chapter will address the most common hepatobiliary and pancreatic disorders seen in cancer patients: jaundice, hepatic toxic reactions due to anticancer therapies, cholecystitis, cholangitis, ascites, pancreatitis, and exocrine and endocrine pancreatic insufficiency.

Hepatobiliary Disorders

Jaundice

Jaundice, or icterus (yellow pigmentation of the skin and sclerae) is due to accumulation of bilirubin in the tissues. Causes of increased serum bilirubin levels include increased degradation of heme and impaired hepatic metabolism or excretion of bilirubin. The liver plays a central role in the metabolism of bilirubin. Hepatocytes take up unconjugated bilirubin, which is bound to albumin, conjugate the bilirubin to glucuronic acid, and then excrete the conjugated bilirubin into bile. This last step, bilirubin excretion, is the rate-limiting step and the step most likely to be impaired when hepatocytes are injured. After excretion into bile, conjugated bilirubin is transported through the bile ducts and into the duodenum to emulsify fatty foodstuffs and facilitate absorption; unabsorbed conjugated bilirubin is either excreted unchanged in the stool or metabolized by ileal and colonic bacteria to urobilinogen, which is absorbed by the intestinal mucosa to be either re-excreted into bile or filtered by the kidneys and excreted in the urine.

Causes of Jaundice

The first step in the evaluation of a patient with jaundice is to establish whether the jaundice is due to unconjugated or conjugated hyperbilirubinemia (Figure 1). Jaundice associated with unconjugated hyperbilirubinemia is most commonly seen in the setting of increased erythrocyte destruction, as occurs with intravascular hemolysis, massive transfusion, or resorption of a large hematoma. Less commonly, unconjugated hyperbilirubinemia is caused by decreased hepatic glucuronosyltransferase activity, such as occurs in end-stage hepatic failure or sepsis.

Jaundice associated predominantly with conjugated hyperbilirubinemia is generally caused by one of three groups of disorders: hepatocellular disease, intrahepatic biliary obstruction (cholestasis), or extrahepatic biliary obstruction. Hepatocellular diseases that can cause jaundice include viral hepatitis (see Chapter 17, "Viral Infections"), drug-induced (especially chemotherapy-induced) hepatocellular disease, and cirrhosis. Intrahepatic cholestasis can be caused by long-term administration of total parenteral nutrition, can occur after surgery, or can be caused by sepsis or drugs (eg, chemotherapy). Extrahepatic biliary obstruction can be classified as either benign or malignant. Benign causes include infections, gallstones, and strictures. Malignant causes include periampullary cancers, cholangiocarcinomas, lymphomas, and cancers metastatic to the portal lymph nodes.

In patients with jaundice due predominantly to conjugated hyperbilirubinemia, levels of the other liver enzymes, including the transaminases and alkaline phosphatase, may suggest either a hepatocellular disorder (transaminase elevation predominant) or biliary obstruction (alkaline phosphatase elevation predominant). If liver enzyme levels suggest a hepatocellular disorder, serologic tests for hepatitis infection should be performed, and then a liver biopsy should be performed as needed to obtain diagnostic information and for treatment planning. If biliary obstruction is suspected, abdominal ultrasonography should be performed. The remainder of this section will be devoted to the diagnosis and treatment of obstructive jaundice in the cancer patient.

Diagnosis and Treatment of Patients with Obstructive Jaundice

In patients with suspected biliary obstruction, abdominal ultrasonography should be the initial radiologic imaging study (Figure 2).[1] Abdominal ultrasonography is noninvasive, inexpensive, and accurate, and the equipment required is portable. The study first and foremost provides information about the caliber of the biliary ducts, confirming the presence or absence of intra- and extrahepatic biliary ductal dilatation. With rare exceptions, ductal dilatation is present in all cases of obstructive jaundice. Abdominal ultrasonography has a sensitivity of greater than 95% in detecting gallstones, which may be the source of ductal obstruction.[2] However, abdominal ultrasonography may have a sensitivity lower than 50% in detecting common bile duct stones.[1]

In the event of normal findings on abdominal ultrasonography, abdominal computed tomography (CT) is often helpful to evaluate the entire hepatobiliary tract. Cholangiography should be delayed until after CT unless cholangitis necessitates immediate intervention, because the endoscopic manipulation of the biliary tree can significantly reduce the sensitivity of CT to detect biliary and pancreatic pathology. Endoscopy facilitates biopsy of lesions that can be identified; when no lesions are found, a liver biopsy should be considered to define the cause of the obstructive jaundice (see Figure 2) if the results of such a biopsy would guide treatment.

If ultrasonography documents intra- and/or extrahepatic biliary ductal dilatation and gallstones in a candidate for surgery, consultations with a gastroenterologist and surgeon can help to determine the options for percutaneous, endoscopic, and surgical intervention.

If the patient has the cardinal manifestations of cholangitis—fever, right upper quadrant pain, and jaundice—or severe pancreatitis, endoscopic retrograde cholangiopancreatography (ERCP) should be urgently performed after fluid resuscitation and administration of intravenous antibiotics to cover gram-negative organisms and anaerobes. If common bile duct stones are found, the calculi should be cleared, and a sphincterotomy should be performed. The patient can then undergo semi-elective cholecystectomy after resolution of the inflammatory process, usually during the same hospitalization. If a biliary stricture is found, brushings should be obtained for cytologic evaluation, if indicated, and a plastic stent should be placed. If a skilled endoscopist is available, endoscopic

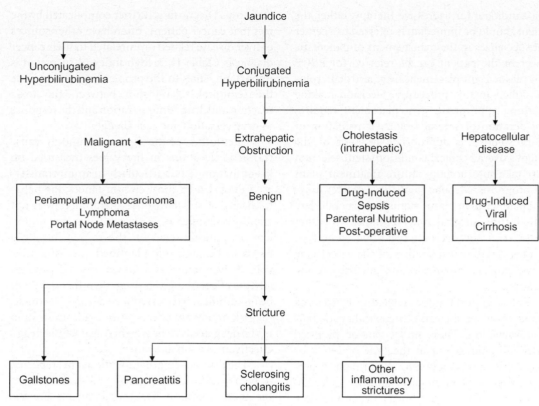

FIGURE 1 Flow diagram illustrating the causes of jaundice.

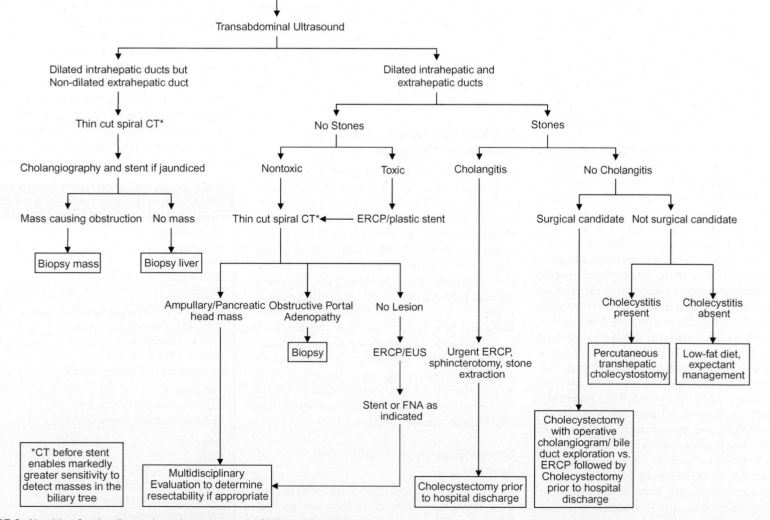

FIGURE 2 Algorithm for the diagnosis and management of biliary obstruction.

ultrasonography (EUS) can be performed to examine the head of the pancreas and bile duct wall for possible lesions. If lesions are detected, a needle biopsy is performed. Most patients with intra- or extrahepatic biliary stricture should be promptly referred to a specialized center experienced in the care of these patients after stent placement. A pathologic diagnosis is unnecessary, and repeated attempts to obtain sufficient tissue for diagnosis only result in delay of definitive treatment.

If the patient does not have cholangitis or severe pancreatitis, ERCP should not be the first course of action. Supportive measures should be instituted, and the patient should be observed. If the serum bilirubin level is elevated or cholangitis develops, ERCP should be considered; otherwise, if the patient is deemed to be a candidate for surgery, a cholecystectomy is appropriate. Indeed, several randomized trials have demonstrated improved outcomes with a surgical approach (cholecystectomy with or without common bile duct exploration) as the first intervention in uncomplicated choledocholithiasis.[3,4] This selective approach to the use of ERCP is cost-effective and spares the majority of patients without impacted or persistent common bile duct stones the risks of ERCP, including pancreatitis and duodenal perforation.[5] For patients who are not candidates for surgery and who have no evidence of cholecystitis, a low-fat diet and expectant management should be considered. In gravely ill patients with cholecystitis, a percutaneous cholecystostomy tube should be placed under ultrasound guidance, and the patient should be given supportive care and intravenous antibiotics. After recovery from systemic disease, cholecystectomy is indicated.

If abdominal ultrasonography shows dilated intra- and/or extrahepatic ducts in the absence of gallstones, especially if the patient has a bilirubin level greater than 10 mg/dL or symptoms suggestive of malignancy (ie, painless jaundice and weight loss), an abdominal CT scan should be obtained. CT enables the identification of mass lesions or adenopathy in the liver, porta hepatis, or pancreas and is more sensitive and specific than ultrasonography in diagnosing the etiology of extrahepatic biliary obstruction.[1] For patients whose underlying cancer diagnosis is not associated with a poor long-term prognosis, work-up for treatment of a periampullary neoplasm can be considered. If the underlying cancer diagnosis portends a low likelihood of long-term survival, the extensive work-up required for a potentially resectable periampullary neoplasm is not necessarily sensible, and management with plastic or metallic stents can be considered.

A hypodense lesion in the head of the pancreas on CT is suggestive of typical pancreatic ductal adenocarcinoma. If no lesion is seen on CT, ampullary and distal common bile duct lesions must be considered. If the patient would be a candidate for aggressive therapy, either the patient should be immediately referred to a center that specializes in the management of pancreatic cancer or the patient can be referred for ERCP with plastic stent placement by a gastroenterologist skilled in this procedure. Decision-making regarding appropriate stent placement requires consideration of several factors. If palliation of biliary stenosis is appropriate in light of the patient's overall clinical condition, stent selection must take into account future treatment plans and prognosis. Metallic stents have greater long-term patency than plastic stents but may interfere with future surgical interventions. In other words, even the decision regarding stent type requires careful consideration of the underlying disease process, prognosis, and potential future therapies.

Enlarged portal nodes related to lymphoma or metastatic disease can cause extrahepatic biliary obstruction. These nodes can be biopsied under CT guidance or at the time of ERCP or endoscopic ultrasonography. Treatment generally entails chemotherapy and/or radiation therapy, with or without biliary decompression. The preferred mode of biliary decompression is endoscopic, but when this route fails, transhepatic biliary drainage can be considered. Tube-free palliation can be achieved by internalizing external (transhepatic) stents at a second setting either by skilled interventional radiologists or by the endoscopist in concert with the radiologist. Such high level management of biliary obstruction requires close review of overall treatment plans, biliary anatomy and prognosis.

Hepatic Toxic Reactions Due to Anticancer Therapies

Hepatic toxic reactions are relatively common in patients receiving anticancer therapy. Toxic reactions range from mild, transient abnormalities on liver function tests with standard-dose chemotherapy to full-blown hepatic failure due to graft versus host disease (GVHD) or sinusoidal obstruction syndrome (SOS) after hematopoietic stem cell transplantation. Moreover, fulminant hepatic failure may be the presenting clinical feature in patients with Hodgkin's[6,7] or non-Hodgkin's lymphoma[7,8] and may develop from an exacerbation of underlying chronic hepatitis B virus (HBV) infection in patients on immunosuppressive cytotoxic therapy.[9,10] This section describes hepatic toxic reactions related to chemotherapy, bone marrow transplantation (BMT), and radiation therapy.

Chemotherapy-Induced Hepatic Toxic Reactions

The diagnosis of chemotherapy-induced hepatic toxic reactions is difficult as there are no biochemical or histologic features unique to this diagnosis. Diagnosis is further complicated by the fact that cancer patients often have other sources of liver disease related or unrelated to their cancer diagnosis (Table 1). A high index of suspicion is important. Clues to the proper diagnosis include the temporal relationship between the toxic reaction and drug administration and the response to drug cessation and rechallenge.

Chemotherapeutic agents commonly cause transient elevations in the values measured on liver function tests, particularly in aminotransferase values. Under most circumstances, the hepatotoxicity of standard-dose chemotherapy is not clinically significant. However, when hepatotoxicity is clinically evident, the responsible drug needs to be promptly identified and discontinued. If liver injury is a known dose-dependent adverse effect of a given drug, then that drug can be re-administered at a reduced dosage. Of course, the risk of adverse effects with re-administration of the drug needs to be weighed against the drug's effectiveness as an anticancer agent.

The list of chemotherapeutic agents reported to be hepatotoxic is extensive (Table 2). Some of the more common hepatotoxic agents are the alkylating agents cyclophosphamide (especially when given at a high dose and in conjunction with other agents),[11,12] busulfan,[13] and melphalan[14]; the antimetabolites methotrexate[15] and 6-mercaptopurine[16,17]; the hormones tamoxifen[18,19] and flutamide[20,21]; the cytokines interleukin-12 and interferon-alpha-2b[22]; and the monoclonal antibody gemtuzumab.[23]

Acute awareness of the potentially lethal complication of chemotherapy in hepatitis B carriers cannot be ignored. Viremia, acute fulminant hepatic failure, and death have been reported in patients receiving chemotherapy for solid tumors[9] as well as for hematologic malignancies,

Table 1 Causes of Hepatic Toxic Reactions in Cancer Patients
Chemotherapy
Alkylating agents
Antimetabolites
Hormones
Others
Hematopoietic stem cell transplantation
Sinusoidal obstruction syndrome
Graft vs. host disease
Induction chemotherapy
Immunosuppressive medications
Radiation
Radiation-induced liver disease
Radiation-induced biliary stenosis
Other
Sepsis
Parenteral nutrition
Infection (especially viral and fungal)
Parenchymal replacement by tumor
Budd-Chiari syndrome

Table 2 Chemotherapeutic Agents Known to Be Hepatotoxic

Drug	Type of Liver Injury
Cyclophosphamide[11,12]	SOS in high-dose conditioning regimens
Busulfan[13]	Cholestasis
Melphalan[14]	SOS in high-dose conditioning regimens
Methotrexate[15]	Steatohepatitis, fibrosis, cirrhosis
6-mercaptopurine[16,17]	Cholestasis
Cytarabine[81]	Cholestatic jaundice, hepatic failure
Dacarbazine[82]	SOS
Etoposide[11,12]	SOS and hepatic failure
Gemcitabine[83]	Severe cholestatic hepatitis, hepatic failure
Flutamide[20,21]	Severe cholestatic hepatitis, hepatic necrosis
Tamoxifen[18,19,84]	Steatosis, cirrhosis, hepatocellular cancer
Interferon alpha-2b[22,85]	Steatohepatitis
Interleukin-12[22]	Steatohepatitis
L-asparaginase[86]	Steatosis, hepatocyte necrosis, fulminant hepatic failure
Paclitaxel[87,88]	Hepatic failure
Oxaliplatin[89]	SOS
Gemtuzumab[23]	SOS and hepatic failure

@TF=SOS = sinusoidal obstruction syndrome.

and who are carriers of hepatitis B.[10] Viremia and subsequent lethal consequences can be completely obviated by prophylaxis with lamivudine, a highly effective nucleoside analogue against HBV, in all seropositive cancer patients receiving antineoplastic therapy.[10,24]

Hepatic Toxic Reactions Related to Hepatic Artery Infusional Chemotherapy

Infusion of chemotherapy directly into the hepatic artery was proposed in the 1960s[25,26] and has been promoted as a means to treat the liver with high-dose chemotherapy with minimal systemic toxicity.[27-31] Unfortunately, such regional therapy, particularly for colorectal liver metastases, has not improved survival but has generated a range of hepatic toxic reactions, from mild biochemical test abnormalities to lethal hepatic failure.[32]

The most common hepatic toxic reaction associated with hepatic artery infusional (HAI) chemotherapy is liver function test abnormalities, including a doubling of serum alkaline phosphatase levels in 29% of patients, a tripling of aminotransferase levels in 65%, and an increase in total

bilirubin levels to more than 3.0 mg/dL in nearly 20% of treated patients.[31,32] These liver function test abnormalities usually return to normal when the chemotherapy dose is lowered or when chemotherapy is discontinued. A less common but more significant, irreversible complication of HAI chemotherapy is biliary sclerosis, which may be mitigated by concurrent infusion of dexamethasone with chemotherapy.[33] Cholangiography should be performed in those patients who become jaundiced during the course of HAI chemotherapy. If there is a dominant biliary stricture, palliation can be achieved by placement of a biliary stent. Permanent biliary sclerosis with multiple strictures (9 to 17% of patients)[34,35] and death from fulminant hepatic failure (1%)[32,36] persist as dreaded complications of hepatic artery chemotherapy regardless of the infused chemotherapeutic agent. Other important hepatobiliary complications of HAI chemotherapy include hepatic artery thrombosis (6%),[32] which can be lethal or cause slow, progressive (untreatable) liver failure; catheter thrombosis (5%)[32]; catheter displacement (7%)[32]; and chemical cholecystitis, which occurs almost universally with HAI chemotherapy such that prophylactic cholecystectomy is now routinely performed at the time of infusion pump placement.[37,38]

Hepatic Toxic Reactions Related to Bone Marrow Transplantation

Hepatic toxic reactions occur in up to 70% of patients who undergo bone marrow transplantation (BMT); SOS and GVHD are the reactions associated with the highest morbidity and mortality.

SOS, formerly known as veno-occlusive disease, is a clinical syndrome characterized by jaundice, painful hepatomegaly, and fluid retention. The first signs of SOS are fluid retention and weight gain, which develop in the first 20 days after the pre-transplant chemotherapy regimen. Painful hepatomegaly and alterations in liver function tests occur later in the course of the disease. SOS is due to the synergistic toxicity of the high-dose chemotherapy and total-body irradiation that comprise the preparative regimen administered prior to BMT. The incidence of SOS is dependent on patient-related factors and the chemotherapy regimen, and ranges from less than 5% to as high as 70%.[39] The mortality rate from SOS varies from 20 to 50%.[39] Conditions that mimic SOS (including acute GVHD, sepsis with cholestasis, and heart failure) must be ruled out to establish the diagnosis. When the diagnosis is unclear, particularly in cases in which GVHD needs to be excluded, a liver biopsy should be performed. Percutaneous transjugular biopsy is preferred because procedure-related risks are extremely low, and this approach allows measurement of the hepatic venous pressure gradient,

which if greater than 10 mm Hg has a specificity of 90% in diagnosing SOS.[40] Histologic findings on liver biopsy in patients with SOS include sinusoidal congestion and fibrosis and hepatocyte necrosis.

The pathogenesis of SOS is not well understood but may be related to a disruption of the hepatic sinusoidal microcirculation. Treatment is largely supportive, including careful management of the patient's volume status. Mild to moderate SOS can typically be managed with diuretics, and complete recovery is the norm. Unfortunately, the majority of patients with severe SOS develop multisystem organ failure with hepatorenal syndrome, and the outcome is usually fatal.

The liver is the most common organ affected by GVHD after BMT; nearly 70% of patients with chronic GVHD exhibit hepatic involvement despite appropriate immunosuppression.[41] Hepatic GVHD typically develops 2 weeks after BMT and is characterized by a progressive rise in the values measured on liver function tests. Patients often have concomitant GVHD involving the intestine and skin, and the presence of these in conjunction with altered liver function tests should raise suspicion of hepatic GVHD. When the diagnosis is in doubt, a liver biopsy is diagnostic. The cornerstone of treatment is steroids; however, the majority of patients with acute GVHD of the liver go on to develop chronic GVHD.[42]

Radiation-Induced Liver Disease

Radiation-induced liver disease, or radiation hepatitis, is a dose-limiting complication of liver irradiation. The clinical syndrome consists of tender hepatomegaly without jaundice; ascites; and abnormal liver function tests, particularly an elevated serum alkaline phosphatase level. The syndrome is not unlike SOS seen in patients after BMT. In fact, the pathogenesis of radiation-induced liver disease is similar to that of SOS—radiation-induced liver disease is a veno-occlusive disease characterized histologically by marked venous congestion of the central portion of the hepatic lobule and sparing of the larger veins. The syndrome typically develops 2 weeks to 3 months after hepatic irradiation. The liver tolerates radiation poorly; radiation-induced liver disease is seen in 5 to 10% of patients treated with 30 to 35 gray of conventional radiation to the whole liver.[43] For this reason, radiation therapy has traditionally played a limited role in the treatment of hepatic malignancies.[44] Newer techniques of three-dimensional conformal radiation therapy enable the delivery of much higher doses of radiation to the affected liver while sparing an adequate volume of normal liver, thus substantially reducing the risk of radiation-induced liver disease. For patients who develop this disease, treatment is largely supportive and similar to that described for SOS. In severe cases, liver failure and death can ensue.[45]

Acute Cholecystitis

Symptoms and Diagnosis

Acute cholecystitis is a clinical diagnosis made upon analysis of the patient history and physical examination. Patients with acute cholecystitis typically present with a history of constant, dull right upper quadrant pain and tenderness that is localized and reproducible with palpation below the right subcostal margin. Treatment based solely on radiographic findings is problematic because gallstones and slight gallbladder wall thickening are commonly seen on imaging studies, even in asymptomatic individuals. A careful patient history and physical examination are thus critically important for the proper management of any patient with suspected gallbladder pathology.

Even in cancer patients receiving therapy, the vast majority of cases of acute cholecystitis (90 to 95%) result from gallstones. Stones obstruct the cystic duct, causing gallbladder distention, edema, and inflammation, with eventual progression to venous obstruction and necrosis of the gallbladder wall. In the majority of cases, however, the stone will dislodge from the cystic duct, and the inflammation will resolve spontaneously (biliary colic).

Acute cholecystitis may also occur in the absence of stones, in which case it is called acalculous cholecystitis. The cause of this type of cholecystitis is most likely ischemia and biliary stasis, which results in exposure of the gallbladder mucosa to stagnant bile. It is possible that gallbladder sludge resulting from biliary stasis serves to obstruct the cystic duct much as the stone does in the calculus variant. Acalculous cholecystitis is most commonly seen in patients who are severely ill, such as those with sepsis, with multisystem organ failure, or receiving prolonged parenteral nutrition.

Finally, cholecystitis can be the presenting diagnosis in patients with metastatic[46,47] and relapsing cancers[48] that infiltrate the gallbladder wall, and it can be caused by cancer therapies such as HAI chemotherapy, radiofrequency ablation[49] and percutaneous ethanol injection of liver tumors,[50] and preparative chemotherapeutic regimens for BMT.[51]

Onset of pain after a meal is a virtually universal symptom in patients with acute cholecystitis. Nausea and vomiting can occur, and often the symptoms subside after vomiting. If symptoms do subside, the diagnosis is not cholecystitis but rather biliary colic, which is managed nonemergently. If pain progresses and persists, sometimes with radiation to the right scapula or shoulder, acute cholecystitis should be considered. Acute cholecystitis may be associated with fever and anorexia, even in immunosuppressed patients. Jaundice is not a typical sign of acute cholecystitis unless complicated by common bile duct stones, although elevation in the bilirubin level to 2.0 to 2.5 mg/dL may occur in patients with uncomplicated acute cholecystitis. A bilirubin level higher than 3 mg/dL suggests common bile duct stones, while an elevated serum amylase level suggests pancreatitis. Pain radiating to the left side or to the back is more common with common bile duct stones than with cholecystitis alone. Mild leukocytosis (typically a leukocyte count of 12,000 to 15,000/mL) or a normal white blood cell count may be found, and mild liver function test abnormalities can occur. Some mild abdominal distention is common, and right subcostal tenderness to deep palpation is nearly universal. Occasionally, the gallbladder can be palpated.

Abdominal ultrasonography is the most sensitive (sensitivity ≈ 90%) and specific (specificity ≈ 80%) test to confirm cholecystitis when this diagnosis is suspected on the basis of clinical findings.[52] Typical findings on ultrasonography in patients with acute cholecystitis include gallstones, gallbladder wall thickening, pericholecystic fluid, and a ultrasonographic Murphy's sign. The gallbladder is dilated, not decompressed. Abdominal CT is much less sensitive and specific than ultrasonography and is usually not helpful in the clinical management of suspected acute cholecystitis. Functional nuclear studies such as a hepatobiliary technetium 99m-iminodiacetic acid scan can be helpful in rare circumstances, but if they are used without regard to clinical symptoms, they are generally not helpful in patient care.

Treatment

The initial management of acute cholecystitis (Figure 3) of any cause includes bowel rest, intravenous hydration, and intravenous broad-spectrum antibiotics tailored to the flora of the gastrointestinal tract. Definitive treatment is cholecystectomy, preferably performed by the laparoscopic approach.

The timing of cholecystectomy is largely based on the overall medical condition of the patient. For patients who are medically fit, cholecystectomy should be performed at onset of pain or, in severe cases, after symptoms regress and the clinical situation permits surgery—usually during the same hospitalization. For patients receiving chemotherapy or other immunosuppressive medications and for medically unfit patients, the acute attack is managed with supportive care as outlined in the preceding paragraph and with interval cholecystectomy as appropriate. Surgery should be delayed until the white blood cell count rebounds after chemotherapy (until the absolute neutrophil count exceeds 1000/mL and is rising).

Typically, acute *calculous* cholecystitis resolves with the aforementioned regimen of bowel rest, intravenous hydration, and intravenous broad-spectrum antibiotics; cholecystectomy is performed once therapy is completed and the bone marrow and immune system have recovered. If the patient fails to improve or deteriorates on this regimen, a percutaneous cholecystostomy tube can be placed under ultrasound guidance, even at the bedside if the patient is too ill to be transported to the radiology suite.[53] The cholecystostomy tube effectively drains the gallbladder and leads to clinical improvement in the majority of patients. Failure to see clinical improvement suggests a gangrenous gallbladder; in such cases, laparotomy with cholecystectomy may be necessary to avoid gallbladder perforation.

The treatment of acute *acalculous* cholecystitis is also tailored to the patient's medical condition (see Figure 3). Definitive treatment is cholecystectomy, but most patients with acalculous cholecystitis are too ill for an operation, so percutaneous cholecystostomy is the treatment of choice in most cases. The tube is left in place for at least 4 to 6 weeks to permit a mature fistula tract to form. A cholangiogram is obtained via the tube after this waiting period, and if it shows drainage into the biliary tree and duodenum, the tube is clamped and subsequently removed if the patient tolerates clamping. Elective cholecystectomy should be performed in medically fit patients with a reasonable prognosis (expected survival of more than 12 months) with respect to their cancer diagnosis.

Cholangitis

Cholangitis is a septic process of the biliary tree due to biliary tract obstruction and consequent overgrowth of bacteria that colonize the bile from duodenal reflux or from the systemic circulation. In the general population, cholangitis is most commonly due to common bile duct stones and benign strictures; in cancer patients, malignant biliary strictures and obstructed indwelling biliary stents are the most frequent causes. Patients typically present with fever and jaundice; abdominal pain, the symptom completing Charcot's triad, occurs in only about 20% of patients. Abdominal ultrasonography is the study of choice to document biliary ductal dilatation and gallstones. In patients known to have a biliary stricture or an indwelling biliary stent, one can proceed directly to ERCP, as it is both diagnostic and therapeutic.

The initial management of cholangitis includes aggressive fluid resuscitation and broad-spectrum intravenous antibiotics tailored to the likely gram-negative and anaerobic biliary pathogens. Definitive management requires adequate biliary drainage, and endoscopic drainage has been shown to be superior to emergent surgical

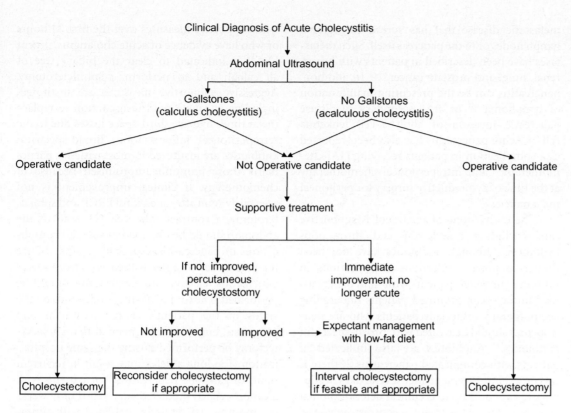

FIGURE 3 Algorithm for the diagnosis and management of acute cholecystitis.

drainage in terms of morbidity and mortality.[54] If common bile duct stones are present, they are cleared and a sphincterotomy is performed. Strictures are biopsied with brushings if a tissue diagnosis has not been established, and a stent is placed. Obstructed biliary stents are simply exchanged or removed. If endoscopic drainage is not available or technically feasible, the interventional radiologist can place a percutaneous transhepatic biliary drain. After the acute episode of cholangitis has resolved, efforts can be made to treat the underlying problem (eg, surgical resection of a biliary stricture).

Ascites

Ascites in cancer patients is most commonly a finding of end-stage disease secondary to peritoneal carcinomatosis. In this condition, metastatic tumor cells lining the peritoneum exude proteinaceous fluid. This form of ascites, referred to as malignant ascites, is seen most commonly in patients with breast, colon, gastric, and pancreatic cancers. Patients with ovarian and appendiceal malignancies often present with ascites as the first symptom of their disease. Ascites can also be caused by replacement of the liver parenchyma or compression of the portal vein by massive liver metastases, resulting in portal hypertension. Extrahepatic portal, superior mesenteric, and splenic vein obstruction can occur with pancreatic tumors, leading to portal hypertension and ascites. Of course, benign forms of ascites are seen in cancer patients as well, the most common of

which is ascites due to portal hypertension in patients with cirrhosis or, rarely, after treatment for portal vein obstruction.

The diagnosis of ascites is suggested by the characteristic symptoms of weight gain and increased abdominal girth and is confirmed by abdominal ultrasonography or CT. Paracentesis is used to obtain ascitic fluid for a cell count, albumin level measurement, gram stain and culture, and cytologic analysis as indicated. If the ascitic fluid appears milky, chyliform ascites is suggested, and triglyceride levels should be measured as well. Serum albumin should be measured at the same time to establish the serum-ascites albumin gradient (SAAG), which directly correlates with the portal pressure. The gradient is calculated by subtracting the albumin level of the ascites fluid from the albumin level of the serum. A SAAG ≥ 1.1 gm/dL (high SAAG) is diagnostic of portal hypertension; the most common causes include cirrhosis, Budd-Chiari syndrome, and cardiac ascites. A SAAG < 1.1 gm/dL (low SAAG) indicates a high concentration of protein in the ascitic fluid, as in peritoneal carcinomatosis.

The treatment of high-SAAG ascites includes diuretics and salt restriction; symptomatic patients with ascites refractory to diuretics may benefit from large-volume paracentesis. The treatment of low-SAAG ascites centers on treatment of the underlying cause. Peritoneal carcinomatosis secondary to the most common malignancies (ie, those of the breast, colon, pancreas, and lung) portends a dismal prognosis,

and so treatment is essentially palliative. Patients with carcinomatosis due to ovarian and appendiceal cancers may be candidates for aggressive surgical debulking and intraperitoneal chemotherapy and enjoy long-term survival. Peritoneo-venous shunting is contraindicated in virtually all cases of malignant ascites because the shunt would lead to continuous circulation of cancer cells from the peritoneum throughout the vascular system.

Pancreatic Disorders

Acute Pancreatitis

Acute pancreatitis is a complex disorder of the exocrine pancreas characterized by acinar cell injury and local and systemic inflammatory responses. In the vast majority of patients, acute pancreatitis is mild and self-limited, characterized by gland edema and perhaps a small peripancreatic fluid collection or phlegmon. This is referred to as simple, uncomplicated acute pancreatitis. In approximately 10% of patients, however, the disease is far more virulent and life-threatening and leads to complications, including pseudocysts, abscesses, ascites, and pancreatic necrosis. These patients may suffer significant physiologic derangements secondary to the inflammatory response, leading to sepsis, multisystem organ failure, and death.

The diagnosis of acute pancreatitis must be considered in patients with abdominal pain, especially pain in the epigastrium radiating to the back and associated with nausea and vomiting. The diagnosis is usually confirmed by elevated serum amylase and lipase values; occasionally only hyperamylasuria is found. Abdominal ultrasonography is the only radiologic imaging study necessary in the initial evaluation of a patient with mild acute pancreatitis. This study confirms or excludes gallstones or a retained common bile duct stone after previous cholecystectomy as the cause of the pancreatitis; abdominal ultrasonography is not obtained to study the pancreas, which is typically obscured by overlying bowel gas. The role of abdominal CT in the diagnosis and management of acute uncomplicated pancreatitis is limited (details below).

Even in patients receiving cancer treatment, the most common causes of acute pancreatitis—namely gallstones and alcohol abuse—must be ruled out prior to considering the diagnosis of drug-related (chemotherapy-related) pancreatitis. Abdominal ultrasonography can establish gallstones as the cause, and the patient history can establish alcohol abuse as a potential etiology. Acute pancreatitis also has innumerable other causes which will not be listed here. Rather, we will focus on the causes pertinent to the cancer patient (Table 3).

Acute, uncomplicated pancreatitis has been reported to occur as a complication of a number

Table 3 Causes of Acute Pancreatitis in Cancer Patients

Gallstones
Alcohol Abuse
Chemotherapy
Systemic
Intraperitoneal
Hepatic artery infusional

Hematopoietic stem cell transplantation
Induction chemotherapy
Graft vs. host disease
Immunosuppressive medications
Biliary sludge

Metastasis
To the pancreas
To regional lymph nodes

Ampullary neoplasm
Pancreatic
    Ductal adenocarcinoma
    Cystic neoplasm
    Neuroendocrine tumor
    Lymphoma
Distal bile duct adenocarcinoma
Ampullary carcinoma

Duodenal carcinoma

of different chemotherapeutic agents, including ifosfamide,[55,56] vinblastine,[57] L-asparaginase,[58] cisplatin,[59] capecitabine,[60] and paclitaxel (Table 4).[61] Attempts to administer the same chemotherapeutic agent(s) at a later time, even at a reduced dose, may result in a new episode of pancreatitis, necessitating a different antineoplastic regimen.[55] In addition, acute pancreatitis has been reported in 28% of BMT recipients at autopsy, although many of these cases were subclinical.[62] Although GVHD has been identified as a risk factor for the development of pancreatitis in BMT recipients, these patients also have a high incidence of other risk factors, including cytotoxic chemotherapy as part of the preparative regimen, prolonged treatment of GVHD with steroids and cyclosporine, and biliary sludge secondary to biliary stasis after BMT.[62]

In cancer patients, acute pancreatitis may result from ductal obstruction secondary to

Table 4 Chemotherapeutic Agents Known to Cause Pancreatitis

As Single Agents	*As Combination Therapy*
Azathioprine[90,91]	Methotrexate[92]
6-mercaptopurine[93]	Cyclophosphamide[94]
L-asparaginase[58]	Mitomycin-C[95]
Ifosfamide[55,56]	Vinblastine[96,97]
Prednisone[98]	5-fluorouracil[92]
Cytarabine[99]	Vincristine[92]
Capecitabine[60]	Cisplatin[95,100]
Paclitaxel[61]	Bleomycin[101]
	Thalidomide[102]

metastatic disease that has spread to regional lymph nodes or to the pancreas itself. Such metastases have been described in patients with breast, renal, lung, and prostate cancer.[63-65] In addition, pancreatitis can be the presenting manifestation of lymphoma[66,67] or arise secondary to diffuse pancreatic invasion of adult T-cell leukemia cells.[68] Acute pancreatitis has also been reported as a complication in patients receiving HAI chemotherapy[69] and intraperitoneal chemotherapy at the time of cytoreductive surgery for peritoneal malignancies.[70]

The cornerstone of treatment is supportive care, including bowel rest and intravenous hydration. Although antibiotics have not been shown to prevent infectious complications in immunocompetent patients with mild pancreatitis,[71] immunocompromised patients undergoing chemotherapy (especially patients who are neutropenic) should be treated with broad-spectrum antibiotics.[72] Antibiotics are also indicated in patients with complicated pancreatitis. If there is no clinical improvement after several days of supportive care or if there is clinical deterioration at any point during treatment, a contrast-enhanced abdominal CT scan should be obtained to rule out complicated pancreatitis. CT is not required in cases of uncomplicated pancreatitis because it does not predict the course of the disease; rather, CT is used selectively to guide the treatment of patients whose episode of pancreatitis is severe or complicated (below) or whose symptoms persist after several days of conservative treatment.

Complications of acute pancreatitis include pseudocyst, abscess, pancreatic ascites and/or effusion, fistula, and necrosis. These conditions may carry a much worse prognosis than simple, uncomplicated pancreatitis, so treatment should be tailored to each patient on the basis of the stage of disease and the cancer-related prognosis. Appropriate management of these problems requires close interaction between referring oncologists, gastroenterologists, interventional radiologists, and, occasionally, surgeons.

For cancer patients with gallstone pancreatitis, treatment is based on the severity of the pancreatitis and the health status of the patient with respect to the cancer diagnosis. Mild gallstone pancreatitis is generally a self-limited disease, and patients should be treated with supportive care as outlined above. With clinical improvement, a low-fat diet is instituted, and elective laparoscopic cholecystectomy is planned for when cell counts recover after chemotherapy. ERCP is not indicated for the routine treatment of mild gallstone pancreatitis and, in fact, is associated with increased costs and length of hospital stay in this setting.[73]

Severe gallstone pancreatitis can be life-threatening and demands skilled surgical and critical care. For patients who fail to improve

with supportive measures over the first 24 hours or who have evidence of acute cholangitis, urgent ERCP is indicated to clear the biliary tree of all calculi and to perform a sphincterotomy. Aggressive supportive measures are instituted, including adequate fluid resuscitation to replace the at times massive third-space losses due to the retroperitoneal inflammation. Broad-spectrum antibiotics are instituted in most patients, particularly those immunocompromised because of chemotherapy. If clinical improvement is not seen fairly soon after successful ERCP and sphincterotomy, a contrast-enhanced CT scan of the abdomen should be obtained to rule out complications of pancreatitis, especially necrosis. Once the patient has completely recovered from severe pancreatitis, elective cholecystectomy should be performed. The timing of surgery depends on the status of the patient's cancer treatment and prognosis, but it is recommended that cholecystectomy be performed during the same hospitalization. Too long a delay may result in recurrent bouts of gallstone pancreatitis. For patients with a cancer-related predicted survival of only weeks or months, particularly patients with intra-abdominal carcinomatosis/sarcomatosis and ascites, cholecystectomy is not indicated.

Pancreatic Exocrine Insufficiency

Exocrine insufficiency of the pancreas refers to impaired secretion of pancreatic enzymes via the pancreatic duct and consequent malabsorption of nutrients by the small intestine. This disorder manifests clinically as steatorrhea, increased stool frequency, crampy gas pains with meals, and weight loss. Pancreatic exocrine insufficiency is more common in diabetic patients, particularly those who are obese,[74] but the reason for the increased incidence in this population has yet to be elucidated. New-onset diabetes mellitus, especially in male smokers over the age of 70, should prompt consideration of pancreatic cancer. The mechanism by which pancreatic cancer can cause such findings is believed to be ductal obstruction by the pancreatic mass with distal gland atrophy. If data from the history and physical examination support a diagnosis of pancreatic cancer, a diagnostic work-up, including contrast-enhanced CT of the abdomen before endoscopy, should be considered.

There are no specific reports of pancreatic exocrine dysfunction secondary to chemotherapeutic agents. However, in patients who undergo hematopoietic stem cell transplantation, pancreatic exocrine insufficiency related to the preparative regimen can develop at any time after transplantation, though typically the condition develops within the first few years.[75] In addition, pancreatic exocrine insufficiency has been described in patients who develop either acute or chronic GVHD after allogeneic BMT.[76] Finally, short-term exocrine insufficiency is common after a pancreaticoduodenectomy or other major pancreatectomy, and long-term insufficiency may be present in as many as 40% of these patients.[77] In our patients who have undergone pancreatectomy, we routinely provide enzyme supplementation and follow patients closely in the clinic for signs and symptoms of persistent malabsorption.

The diagnosis of pancreatic exocrine insufficiency is typically made on clinical grounds, with the classic symptoms described above, and treatment can be initiated on this basis. A response to therapy can be regarded as confirmation of the diagnosis, although biochemical tests, including serum pancreatic enzyme and pancreatic elastase II levels, and fecal fat measurements, can be performed when the diagnosis is in doubt.

Treatment consists of three equally important measures: (1) dietary manipulation to achieve a reduction in fat intake to 25 to 30% of normal; (2) pancreatic enzyme supplementation, with supplements taken throughout the meal and in sufficient quantity to eliminate steatorrhea; and (3) adequate acid suppression with a proton-pump inhibitor or H_2-receptor antagonist to raise the intestinal pH to permit effective pancreatic enzyme activity and thus fat absorption.[78]

Pancreatic Endocrine Insufficiency

As mentioned above, in patients who develop new-onset diabetes mellitus, especially in association with pancreatic exocrine insufficiency, one must consider a diagnosis of pancreatic cancer. In fact, diabetes mellitus has been implicated as a predisposing factor in the development of pancreatic cancer.[79,80] In addition, diabetes mellitus develops during the course of chemotherapy in a significant percentage of patients—particularly those receiving corticosteroids in combination therapy regimens for the prevention of transplant rejection, for GVHD, and for the prevention of nausea and vomiting. (Please see Chapter 24, "Management of Diabetes Mellitus," for further detail about the management of diabetes mellitus in cancer patients.)

Summary

Disorders of the liver, biliary tree, and pancreas are common in cancer patients at presentation, during anticancer therapy, and long after curative treatment. Although cancer patients can develop biliary and pancreatic disorders unique to their cancer diagnosis and treatment, the most common causes of these disorders in cancer patients are the causes in non-cancer patients. However, perspective on the prognosis of the underlying cancer diagnosis guides not only treatment but also clinical decision-making regarding the appropriate use of interventional diagnostic modalities. Just as for decision-making regarding cancer therapy,

diagnostic and therapeutic decision-making for non-oncologic issues in complex cancer patients is optimal when oncologists and other specialists work together in a multidisciplinary setting.

REFERENCES

1. Blackbourne LH, Earnhardt RC, Sistrom CL, et al. The sensitivity and role of ultrasound in the evaluation of biliary obstruction. Am Surg 1994;60:683–90.
2. Cooperberg PL, Gibney RG. Imaging of the gallbladder, 1987. Radiology 1987;163:605–13.
3. Rhodes M, Sussman L, Cohen L, Lewis MP. Randomized trial of laparoscopic exploration of common bile duct versus postoperative endoscopic retrograde cholangiography for common bile duct stones. Lancet 1998;351:159–61.
4. Suc B, Escat J, Cherqui D, et al. Surgery vs endoscopy as primary treatment in symptomatic patients with suspected common bile duct stones: A multicenter randomized trial. French Associations for Surgical Research. Arch Surg 1998;133:702–8.
5. Urbach DR, Khajanchee YS, Jobe BA, et al. Cost-effective management of common bile duct stones—A decision analysis of the use of endoscopic retrograde cholangiopancreatography (ERCP), intraoperative cholangiography, and laparoscopic bile duct exploration. Surg Endosc 2001;15:4–13.
6. Vardareli E, Dundar E, Aslan V, Gulbas Z. Acute liver failure due to Hodgkin's lymphoma. Med Princ Pract 2004;13:372–4.
7. Thompson DR, Faust TW, Stone MJ, Polter DE. Hepatic failure as the presenting manifestation of malignant lymphoma. Clin Lymphoma 2001;2:123–38.
8. Lettieri CJ, Berg BW. Clinical features of non-Hodgkin's lymphoma presenting with acute liver failure: A report of five cases and review of published experience. Am J Gastroenterol 2003;98:1641–6.
9. Steinberg JL, Yeo W, Zhong S, et al. Hepatitis B virus reactivation in patients undergoing cytotoxic chemotherapy for solid tumours: precore/core mutations may play an important role. J Med Virol 2000;60:249–55.
10. Ozguroglu M, Bilici A, Turna H, Serdengecti S. Reactivation of hepatitis B virus infection with cytotoxic therapy in non-Hodgkin's lymphoma. Med Oncol 2004;21:67–72.
11. Ritchie DS, Szer J, Roberts AW, et al. A phase I dose-escalation study of etoposide continuous infusion added to busulphan/cyclophosphamide as conditioning prior to autologous or allogeneic stem cell transplantation. Bone Marrow Transplant 2002;30:645–50.
12. Kroger N, Zabelina T, Sonnenberg S, et al. Dose-dependent effect of etoposide in combination with busulfan plus cyclophosphamide as conditioning for stem cell transplantation in patients with acute myelogenous leukemia. Bone Marrow Transplant 2000;26:711–6.
13. Andersson BS, Thall PF, Madden T, et al. Busulfan systemic exposure relative to regimen-related toxicity and acute graft-versus-host disease: Defining a therapeutic window for IV BuCy2 in chronic myelogenous leukemia. Biol Blood Marrow Transp 2002;8:477–85.
14. Ayash LJ, Elias A, Wheeler C, et al. Double dose-intensive chemotherapy with autologous marrow and peripheral-blood progenitor-cell support for metastatic breast cancer: A feasibility study. J Clin Oncol 1994;12:37–44.
15. van Outryve S, Schrijvers D, van den Brande J, et al. Methotrexate-associated liver toxicity in a patient with breast cancer: Case report and literature review. Neth J Med 2002;60:216–22.
16. Laidlaw ST, Reilly JT, Suvarna SK. Fatal hepatotoxicity associated with 6-mercaptopurine therapy. Postgrad Med J 1995;71:639.
17. Schmiegelow K, Pulczynska M. Prognostic significance of hepatotoxicity during maintenance chemotherapy for childhood acute lymphoblastic-leukemia. Br J Cancer 1990;61:767–72.
18. Elefsiniotis IS, Pantazis KD, Ilias A, et al. Tamoxifen-induced hepatotoxicity in breast cancer patients with pre-existing liver steatosis: the role of glucose intolerance. Eur J Gastroenterol Hepatol 2004;16:593–8.
19. Oien KA, Moffat D, Curry GW, et al. Cirrhosis with steatohepatitis after adjuvant tamoxifen. Lancet 1999;353:36–37.
20. Cetin M, Demirci D, Unal A, et al. Frequency of flutamide induced hepatotoxicity in patients with prostate carcinoma. Hum Exp Toxicol 1999;18:137–40.
21. Wysowski DK, Fourcroy JL. Flutamide hepatotoxicity. J Urol 1996;155:1396.
22. Alatrash G, Hutson TE, Molto L, et al. Clinical and immunologic effects of subcutaneously administered interleukin-12 and interferon alfa-2b: phase I trial of patients with metastatic renal cell carcinoma or malignant melanoma. J Clin Oncol 2004;22:2891–900.
23. Amadori S, Suciu S, Willemze R, et al. Sequential administration of gemtuzumab ozogamicin and conventional chemotherapy as first line therapy in elderly patients with acute myeloid leukemia: a phase II study (AML-15) of the EORTC and GIMEMA leukemia groups. Haematologica 2004;89:950–6.
24. Rossi G. Prophylaxis with lamivudine of hepatitis B virus reactivation in chronic HbsAg carriers with hemato-oncological neoplasias treated with chemotherapy. Leuk Lymphoma 2003;44:759–66.
25. Clarkson B, Young C, Dierick W, et al. Effects of continuous hepatic artery infusion of antimetabolites on primary and metastatic cancer of the liver. Cancer 1962;15:472–88.
26. Sullivan RD, Norcross JW, Watkins E Jr. Chemotherapy of metastatic liver cancer by prolonged hepatic-artery infusion. N Engl J Med 1964;270 :321–7.
27. Lorenz M, Muller HH, Schramm H, et al. Randomized trial of surgery versus surgery followed by adjuvant hepatic arterial infusion with 5-fluorouracil and folinic acid for liver metastases of colorectal cancer. German Cooperative on Liver Metastases (Arbeitsgruppe Lebermetastasen). Ann Surg 1998;228:756–62.
28. Rudroff C, Altendorf-Hoffmann A, Stangl R, Scheele J. Prospective randomized trial on adjuvant hepatic-artery infusion chemotherapy after R0 resection of colorectal liver metastases. Langenbecks Arch Surg 1999;384:243–9.
29. Wagman LD, Kemeny MM, Leong L, et al. A prospective, randomized evaluation of the treatment of colorectal cancer metastatic to the liver. J Clin Oncol 1990;8:1885–93.
30. Kemeny MM, Adak S, Gray B, et al. Combined-modality treatment for resectable metastatic colorectal carcinoma to the liver: surgical resection of hepatic metastases in combination with continuous infusion of chemotherapy—an intergroup study. J Clin Oncol 2002;20:1499–505.
31. Kemeny N, Huang Y, Cohen AM, et al. Hepatic arterial infusion of chemotherapy after resection of hepatic metastases from colorectal cancer. N Engl J Med 1999;341:2039–48.
32. Barnett KT, Malafa MP. Complications of hepatic artery infusion: a review of 4580 reported cases. Int J Gastrointest Cancer 2001;30:147–60.
33. Kemeny N, Seiter K, Niedzwiecki D, et al. A randomized trial of intrahepatic infusion of fluorodeoxyuridine with dexamethasone versus fluorodeoxyuridine alone in the treatment of metastatic colorectal cancer. Cancer 1992;69:327–34.
34. Aldrighetti L, Arru M, Ronzoni M, et al. Extrahepatic biliary stenoses after hepatic arterial infusion (HAI) of floxuridine (FUdR) for liver metastases from colorectal cancer. Hepatogastroenterology 2001;48:1302–7.
35. Kemeny MM, Battifora H, Blayney DW, et al. Sclerosing cholangitis after continuous hepatic artery infusion of FUDR. Ann Surg 1985;202:176–81.
36. Nelson RL, Freels S. A systematic review of hepatic artery chemotherapy after hepatic resection of colorectal cancer metastatic to the liver. Dis Colon Rectum 2004;47:739–44.
37. Ottery FD, Scupham RK, Weese JL. Chemical cholecystitis after intrahepatic chemotherapy. The case for prophylactic cholecystectomy during pump placement. Dis Colon Rectum 1986;29:187–90.
38. Lafon PC, Reed K, Rosenthal D. Acute cholecystitis associated with hepatic arterial infusion of floxuridine. Am J Surg 1985;150:687–9.
39. Kumar S, Deleve LD, Kamath PS, Tefferi A. Hepatic veno-occlusive disease (sinusoidal obstruction syndrome) after hematopoietic stem cell transplantation. Mayo Clin Proc 2003;78:589–98.
40. Shulman HM, Gooley T, Dudley MD, et al. Utility of transvenous liver biopsies and wedged hepatic venous-pressure measurements in 60 marrow transplant recipients. Transplantation 1995;59:1015–22.
41. Chiba T, Yokosuka O, Kanda T, et al. Hepatic graft-versus-host disease resembling acute hepatitis: additional

treatment with ursodeoxycholic acid. Liver 2002;22: 514–7.

42. Martin PJ, Schoch G, Fisher L, et al. A retrospective analysis of therapy for acute graft-versus-host diseases—secondary-treatment. Blood 1991;77:1821–8.

43. Dawson LA, Normolle D, Balter JM, et al. Analysis of radiation-induced liver disease using the Lyman NTCP model. Int J Radiat Oncol Biol Phys 2002;53:810–21.

44. Dawson LA, Lawrence TS. The role of radiotherapy in the treatment of liver metastases. Cancer J 2004;10:139–44.

45. Lawrence TS, Robertson JM, Anscher MS, et al. Hepatic toxicity resulting from cancer treatment. Int J Radiat Oncol Biol Phys 1995;31:1237–48.

46. Goldin EG. Malignant melanoma metastatic to the gallbladder: case report and review of the literature. Am Surg 1990;56:369–73.

47. Guida M, Cramarossa A, Gentile A, et al. Metastatic malignant melanoma of the gallbladder: a case report and review of the literature. Melanoma Res 2002;12:619–25.

48. Hurley R, Weisdorf DJ, Jessurun J, et al. Relapse of acute-leukemia presenting as acute cholecystitis following bone-marrow transplantation. Bone Marrow Transplant 1992;10:387–9.

49. Chopra S, Dodd GD, Chanin MP, Chintapalli KN. Radiofrequency ablation of hepatic tumors adjacent to the gallbladder: feasibility and safety. AJR Am J Roentgenol 2003;180:697–701.

50. Memba R, Llado L, Lopez-Ben S, et al. Acute cholecystitis as a complication following percutaneous ethanol injection of a hepatocellular carcinoma. Rev Esp Enferm Dig 2003; 95:730–9.

51. Kuttah L, Weber F, Creger RJ, et al. Acute cholecystitis after autologous bone-marrow transplantation for acute myeloid-leukemia. Ann Oncol 1995;6:302–4.

52. Ralls PW, Colletti PM, Lapin SA, et al. Real-time sonography in suspected acute cholecystitis—prospective evaluation of primary and secondary signs. Radiology 1985;155: 767–71.

53. Sosna J, Copel L, Kane RA, Kruskal JB. Ultrasound-guided percutaneous cholecystostomy: update on technique and clinical applications. Surg Technol Int 2003;11:135–9.

54. Lai EC, Mok FP, Tan ES, et al. Endoscopic biliary drainage for severe acute cholangitis. N Engl J Med 1992;326: 1582–6.

55. Izraeli S, Adamson PC, Blaney SM, Balis FM. Acute pancreatitis after ifosfamide therapy. Cancer 1994;74:1627–8.

56. Gerson R, Serrano A, Villalobos A, et al. Acute pancreatitis secondary to ifosamide. J Emerg Med 1997;15:645–7.

57. Tester W, Forbes W, Leighton J. Vinorelbine-induced pancreatitis: a case report. J Natl Cancer Inst 1997;89: 1631.

58. Sahu S, Saika S, Pai SK, Advani SH. L-Asparaginase (Leunase) induced pancreatitis in childhood acute lymphoblastic leukemia. Pediatr Hematol Oncol 1998;15: 533–8.

59. Bunin N, Meyer WH, Christensen M, Pratt CB. Pancreatitis following cisplatin—a case-report. Cancer Treat Rep 1985;69:236–7.

60. Jones KL, Valero V. Capecitabine-induced pancreatitis. Pharmacotherapy 2003;23:1076–8.

61. Kumar DM, Sundar S, Vasanthan SA. A case of paclitaxel-induced pancreatitis. Clin Oncol 2003;15:35.

62. Ko CW, Gooley T, Schoch HG, et al. Acute pancreatitis in marrow transplant patients: prevalence at autopsy and risk factor analysis. Bone Marrow Transplant 1997;20: 1081–6.

63. Mountney J, Maury AC, Jackson AM, et al. Pancreatic metastases from breast cancer: an unusual cause of biliary obstruction. Eur J Surg Oncol 1997;23:574–6.

64. Law CH, Wei AC, Hanna SS, et al. Pancreatic resection for metastatic renal cell carcinoma: presentation, treatment, and outcome. Ann Surg Oncol 2003;10:922–6.

65. Z'graggen K, Fernandez-del Castillo C, Rattner DW, et al. Metastases to the pancreas and their surgical extirpation. Arch Surg 1998;133:413–6.

66. Bernardeau M, Auroux J, Cavicchi M, et al. Secondary pancreatic involvement by diffuse large B-cell lymphoma presenting as acute pancreatitis: Treatment and outcome. Pancreatology 2002;2:427–30.

67. Safadi R, Or R, Bar ZJ, Polliack A. Lymphoma-associated pancreatitis as a presenting manifestation of immunoblastic lymphoma. Leuk Lymphoma 1994;12:317–9.

68. Mori A, Kikuchi Y, Motoori S, et al. Acute pancreatitis induced by diffuse pancreatic invasion of adult T-cell leukemia/lymphoma cells. Dig Dis Sci 2003;48:1979–83.

69. Kern W, Beckert B, Lang N, et al. Phase I and pharmacokinetic study of hepatic arterial infusion with oxaliplatin in combination with folinic acid and 5-fluorouracil in patients with hepatic metastases from colorectal cancer. Ann Oncol 2001;12:599–603.

70. Park BJ, Alexander HR, Libutti SK, et al. Treatment of primary peritoneal mesothelioma by continuous hyperthermic peritoneal perfusion (CHPP). Ann Surg Oncol 1999;6:582–90.

71. Mayumi T, Ura H, Arata S, et al. Evidence-based clinical practice guidelines for acute pancreatitis: proposals. J Hepatobiliary Pancreat Surg 2002;9:413–22.

72. Sharma VK, Howden CW. Prophylactic antibiotic administration reduces sepsis and mortality in acute necrotizing pancreatitis: a meta-analysis. Pancreas 2001;22:28–31.

73. Chang L, Lo S, Stabile BE, et al. Preoperative versus postoperative endoscopic retrograde cholangiopancreatography in mild to moderate gallstone pancreatitis—a prospective randomized trial. Ann Surg 2000;231:82–7.

74. Nunes AC, Pontes JM, Rosa A, et al. Screening for pancreatic exocrine insufficiency in patients with diabetes mellitus. Am J Gastroenterol 2003;98:2672–5.

75. Sanders JE. Chronic graft-versus-host disease and late effects after hematopoietic stem cell transplantation. Int J Hematol 2002;76:15–28.

76. Maringhini A, Gertz MA, DiMagno EP. Exocrine pancreatic insufficiency after allogeneic bone-marrow transplantation. Int J Pancreatol 1995;17:243–7.

77. Huang JJ, Yeo CJ, Sohn TA, et al. Quality of life and outcomes after pancreaticoduodenectomy. Ann Surg 2000;231:890–6.

78. Sarner M. Treatment of pancreatic exocrine deficiency. World J Surg 2003;27:1192–5.

79. Chow WH, Gridley G, Nyren O, et al. Risk of pancreatic cancer following diabetes-mellitus—a nationwide cohort study in Sweden. J Natl Cancer Inst 1995;87:930–1.

80. Fisher WE. Diabetes: risk factor for the development of pancreatic cancer or manifestation of the disease? World J Surg 2001;25:503–8.

81. George CB, Mansour RP, Redmond J, III, Gandara DR. Hepatic dysfunction and jaundice following high-dose cytosine arabinoside. Cancer 1984;54:2360–2.

82. Johnson RO, Metter G, Wilson W, et al. Phase I evaluation of DTIC (NSC-45388) and other studies in malignant melanoma in the Central Oncology Group. Cancer Treat Rep 1976;60:183–7.

83. Robinson K, Lambiase L, Li J, et al. Fatal cholestatic liver failure associated with gemcitabine therapy. Dig Dis Sci 2003;48:1804–8.

84. Moffat DF, Oien KA, Dickson J, et al. Hepatocellular carcinoma after long-term tamoxifen therapy. Ann Oncol 2000;11:1195–6.

85. Jonasch E, Kumar UN, Linette GP, et al. Adjuvant high-dose interferon alfa-2b in patients with high-risk melanoma. Cancer J 2000;6:139–45.

86. Sahoo S, Hart J. Histopathological features of L-asparaginase-induced liver disease. Semin Liver Dis 2003; 23:295–9.

87. Oettle H, Arnold D, Esser M, et al. Paclitaxel as weekly second-line therapy in patients with advanced pancreatic carcinoma. Anticancer Drugs 2000;11:635–8.

88. Feenstra J, Vermeer RJ, Stricker BH. Fatal hepatic coma attributed to paclitaxel. J Natl Cancer Inst 1997;89: 582–4.

89. Rubbia-Brandt L, Audard V, Sartoretti P, et al. Severe hepatic sinusoidal obstruction associated with oxaliplatin-based chemotherapy in patients with metastatic colorectal cancer. Ann Oncol 2004;15:460–6.

90. Floyd A, Pedersen L, Nielsen GL, et al. Risk of acute pancreatitis in users of azathioprine: a population-based case-control study. Am J Gastroenterol 2003;98:1305–8.

91. Kawanishi H, Rudolph E, Bull FE. Azathioprine-induced acute pancreatitis. N Engl J Med 1973;289:357.

92. Newman CE, Ellis DJ. Pancreatitis during combination chemotherapy. Clin Oncol 1979;5:83–4.

93. Willert JR, Dahl GV, Marina NM. Recurrent mercaptopurine-induced acute pancreatitis: a rare complication of chemotherapy for acute lymphoblastic leukemia in children. Med Pediatr Oncol 2002;38:73–4.

94. Kroger N, Hoffknecht M, Hanel M, et al. Busulfan, cyclophosphamide and etoposide as high-dose conditioning therapy in patients with malignant lymphoma and prior dose-limiting radiation therapy. Bone Marrow Transplant 1998;21:1171–5.

95. Samel S, Singal A, Becker H, Post S. Problems with intraoperative hyperthermic peritoneal chemotherapy for advanced gastric cancer. Eur J Surg Oncol 2000;26: 222–6.

96. Kim KB, Eton O, East MJ, et al. Pilot study of high-dose, concurrent biochemotherapy for advanced melanoma. Cancer 2004;101:596–603.

97. Atkins MB, Gollob JA, Sosman JA, et al. A phase II pilot trial of concurrent biochemotherapy with cisplatin, vinblastine, temozolomide, interleukin 2, and IFN-alpha 2B in patients with metastatic melanoma. Clin Cancer Res 2002;8:3075–81.

98. Chrousos GA, Kattah JC, Beck RW, Cleary PA. Side effects of glucocorticoid treatment. Experience of the Optic Neuritis Treatment Trial. Jama 1993;269:2110–2.

99. McBride CE, Yavorski RT, Moses FM, et al. Acute pancreatitis associated with continuous infusion cytarabine therapy: a case report. Cancer 1996;77:2588–91.

100. Khuri FR, Rigas JR, Figlin RA, et al. Multi-institutional phase I/II trial of oral bexarotene in combination with cisplatin and vinorelbine in previously untreated patients with advanced non-small-cell lung cancer. J Clin Oncol 2001; 19:2626–37.

101. Socinski MA, Garnick MB. Acute pancreatitis associated with chemotherapy for germ cell tumors in two patients. Ann Intern Med 1988;108:567–8.

102. Rajkumar SV, Hayman S, Gertz MA, et al. Combination therapy with thalidomide plus dexamethasone for newly diagnosed myeloma. J Clin Oncol 2002;20:4319–23.

Disorders of the Digestive Tract and Nutrition: Intestinal Issues

John R. Stroehlein, MD

Gastrointestinal difficulties occur in most cancer patients. These problems are responsible for impairing quality of life and interfering with therapy. This chapter addresses important gastrointestinal issues in the cancer patient and focuses on evaluation and management of these problems.

Short Bowel Syndrome

One of the most severe and potentially catastrophic forms of malabsorption results from shortening of the absorptive surface of the small bowel owing to resection or bypass, which may be necessary in the management of intra-abdominal malignancies. In this context, intravenous and enteral nutritional support, diet modification with supplementation, and pharmacotherapy are critical to lessen the multiple consequences of short bowel syndrome (SBS). The provision of medications can also be a challenge for the clinician. Whenever possible, oral administration should be provided, recognizing that absorption needs to be monitored and that problems with absorption have been described.[1] Knowing the site of absorption and intraluminal requirements for absorption of specific medications is clinically very useful in planning the use of orally administered medications in the SBS patient. Fortunately, many, if not most, medications are absorbed from the proximal jejunum, which is often preserved in the SBS.[2]

Although SBS occurs when less than 200 cm of the small bowel remains, the severity of symptoms and the type of complications related to SBS are dependent on the extent and anatomic segment of small bowel resected or bypassed. The most critical portions of the small bowel to preserve include the terminal ileum and ileocecal valve, duodenum, and proximal jejunum. As a result of specialized functions, loss of the duodenum and/or ileum impairs critical components of absorption much more than other portions of the small bowel. Preservation of the colon also helps limit the severity of diarrhea and allows the colon to serve as a digestive organ for short-chain

fatty acids (SCFAs) in patients with SBS.[3] If the colon is preserved, carbohydrate malabsorption is of limited significance because up to 80% of calories can be absorbed as SCFAs after bacterial conversion from carbohydrates in the colon.[4]

An acute phase, an adaptive phase, and a maintenance phase of management have been described for patients with SBS.[5] During the acute phase, intravenous fluids and total parenteral nutrition (TPN) are required; however, oral or enteral intake of gradually increasing quantity, administered in small feedings or by continuous infusion, can usually be started on the fourth or fifth postoperative day and advanced to small frequent feedings of a high-fat, carbohydrate-supplemented diet to which a small amount of medium-chain triglycerides can be added.[5]

It has been known for many years that adaptation of the remaining small bowel resulting from hyperplasia and lengthening of the villi can help compensate for an otherwise decreased absorptive surface.[6–8] Adaptive processes mainly involve increasing the number of cells and cell surface since enterocytes do not improve their individual absorptive function, except for facilitated absorption of sodium and calcium.[9,10] It has been proposed that the release of glucagon-like peptides, peptide YY, and/or neurotensin from the ileum in response to luminal nutrients represents some of the trophic effects on the remaining small intestine.[11,12] The global clinical relevance of these observations is uncertain, as is the role of glutamine, which is a major source of energy for the enterocyte. Randomized studies have failed to demonstrate a positive adaptive effect of glutamine and a negative clinical effect when administered with growth hormone.[13,14] Although the basis of the hyperplastic adaptive response is incompletely understood, a trophic adaptive response is clearly linked to luminal contact with nutrients.[15,16]

Given that most patients with SBS will malabsorb approximately 30% of ingested nutrients, to achieve target absorption of 30 to 40 kcal/kg/d (ideal body weight), about 45 to 60 kcal/kg/d will need to be ingested.[5] Even if inadequate for energy

needs, oral or enteral feedings should be started as soon as possible to take advantage of adaptive changes. The value of modified enteral formulations designed to promote immunomodulation and decrease the propensity for bacterial translocation (considered to be an important source on sepsis in the critically ill patient) remains controversial.[17] Recent studies have demonstrated, for the first time, that high-fat enteral nutritional infusion increases plasma triacylglycerol and apolipoprotein B levels and decreases endotoxemia and bacterial translocation after hemorrhagic shock in the rat.[18]

Besides the development of nutritional deficiencies, patients with SBS frequently experience severe watery diarrhea and electrolyte losses, which can be modulated in several ways. These include treatment with histamine$_2$ (H2) or proton pump inhibitors, considered to have an effect similar to that of intravenous cimetidine, which was initially shown to significantly reduce diarrhea.[19] Although individuals with less than 100 cm of jejunum secrete more sodium and water than consumed orally, the use of glucose-polymer–based oral rehydration solutions (ORSs), which are commercially available or can be easily modified with additional sodium to achieve optimal concentration of at least 70 mmol/L, can substantially increase absorption of fluid and electrolytes if the proximal jejunum has been preserved.[2] To take advantage of this process, patients with SBS should not rely on water for thirst but be provided with an ORS, which can provide considerable benefit, which has been too frequently overlooked.[20]

Other practical aspects of dietary and pharmacotherapy of diarrhea in SBS include the use of antidiarrheal medications to decrease the volume and frequency of evacuation and urgency.[21,22] Octreotide is known to decrease intestinal secretions, prolong transit time, and improve quality of life in some patients with SBS; however, treatment is expensive and results in pancreatic insufficiency and increased incidence of gallstones.[23,24] In animal models, octreotide has been reported to impair postresection intestinal adaptation.

Effective pharmacotherapy also includes (1) treatment of bacterial overgrowth to lessen the adverse effect of intraluminal bacteria on bile acid concentration in the small bowel and competitors for nutrients; (2) use of pancreatic enzyme supplements to compensate for impaired synchrony of digestion; (3) calcium supplementation to compensate for malabsorption and decrease hyperoxaluria and nephrolithiasis; (4) supplementation with fat-soluble vitamins and trace minerals; and (5) correcting magnesium deficiency, which usually needs to be accomplished parenterally; however, magnesium gluconate added to a rice-based commercial oral rehydration formula has been shown to enhance magnesium absorption equivalent to bolus dosages.[25] Iron supplementation is usually needed in the setting of duodenal and/or gastric resection. Tables 1 and 2 summarize macro- and micronutrient recommendations, and Table 3 summarizes the pharmacotherapy for SBS.

Optimal administration of enteral nutrients may require continuous infusion via a nasoenteric tube, which can be placed by the patient for overnight infusion of nutrients, or via

Table 2 Vitamin Therapy for Short Bowel Syndrome*

Intervention	Basis	Comments
Vitamin B$_{12}$ (1,000 μg/mo)	Essential vitamin	Requires parenteral or intranasal route if ileal or gastric resection
Vitamin D (1,600 U/d)	Interruption of enterohepatic circulation contributes to deficiencies	Greater importance with ileal resection
Vitamin K (10 mg/wk)	Prevents deficiency if colon not preserved or antibiotic therapy needed	Uncommon in absence of jaundice and if colon is intact
Vitamin E (30 IU/d)	Deficiencies can cause hemolysis and neuromuscular disorders	Serum levels unreliable unless calculated as ratio to total serum lipid
Vitamin A (10,000–50,000 U/d)	Prevents ocular complications including visual loss and corneal ulceration	Use lower dose in presence of liver disease
Vitamin C (200–500 mg/d)	As precautionary measure	Deficiencies uncommon
Folic acid (1 mg/d)	Prevents anemia	More likely if proximal jejunum resected
Other water-soluble vitamins (minimum daily MDR)	As precaution to prevent deficiencies	Deficiencies uncommon Thiamine and biotin deficiency described

Adapted from Buchman AL et al.[2]

Table 1 Diet and Supplement Therapy of Short Bowel Syndrome

Intervention	Basis	Comments
Medium-chain triglycerides (if colon is present)	Micellar solubilization not required Can be absorbed from the colon Provide additional source of energy	May cause nausea vomiting or ketosis in high dosages
Carbohydrate (complex) (30–35 kcal/kg/d)	Usually well tolerated and may be converted to SCFAs and absorbed from the colon if present	Proximal jejunum where disaccharidases located usually preserved in SBS
Hig Fat diet (20–30% calories)	Increases available energy	Acceptable to have steatorrhea increased
Protein (intact) (1–1.5 g/kg/d)	Provides adequate nitrogen	Nitrogen absorption is least affected macronutrient by decreased absorptive surface
Soluble fiber (oats, psyllium, barley, some fruits and vegetables)	Conversion to SCFA energy source if colon is intact	Associated gaseousness and malodor of SCFA
Calcium (800–1,200 mg/d)	As calcium supplement Reduces oxalate absorption Compensates for intraluminal binding by fatty acids	As calcium carbonate Increased fat and ileal excreta described
Selenium (60–100 μg daily)	Compensates for increased loss in in SBS	Serum levels are reliable
Zinc sulfate (220–400 mg/d for deficiencies)	Deficiencies reported to cause growth abnormalities, delayed wound healing, and immune dysfunction	Use parenteral if needed Blood levels helpful but may be unreliable
Low-oxalate diet (40–50 mg/d)	Helps prevent nephrolithiasis	Completely avoid draft beer, juice with berries, cocoa, tea, lemonade or limeade, and tomato juice

Adapted from Buchman AL et al.[2]
SBS = short bowel syndrome; SCFA = short-chain fatty acid.

gastrostomy or enterostomy. Although continuous infusion of nutrients may lessen the symptoms of diarrhea, it is considered routine if using gastrostomy to initiate feedings with 100 cc full-strength bolus feeding followed by 50 cc water flush and advanced by 50 cc every 4 hours if there is no significant gastric residual.[26] After maximum volume is reached, the interval can be reduced to every 2 hours over a 12-hour interval. Tube feedings can be further fortified by the addition of safflower oil or polycose or switching to a higher–caloric density product.

When initiating intravenous nutritional support (TPN), 25 to 30 kcal/kg ideal body weight using standard formulas is recommended for normally nourished patients. Although most patients initially require TPN, many are able to be weaned and eventually rely exclusively on oral intake following adaptation. If maintenance TPN is required, it is important, for clinical reasons and factors related to reimbursement, to consider if (1) the condition is expected to persist for at least 90 days, (2) objective evidence supports the presence of gut dysfunction, and (3) attempts were made to improve nutritional status by enteral feedings, diet modification, and/or drug therapy, which are described above. Most patients who have at least 80 cm of remaining small bowel, including the ileocecal valve, and who have not had colonic resection can, after 6 to 12 months of adaptation, be maintained on oral nutrition alone. When maintenance intravenous nutritional support is necessary, enteral nutrition

Table 3 Pharmacotherapy of Short Bowel Syndrome

Intervention	Basis	Comments
Loperamide (4–16 mg/d)	Slow intestinal transit	No systemic side effects
Codeine (30 mg bid)	Slow intestinal transit	May have systemic effect Response less predictable
Pancreatic enzymes (25,000–40,000 U/meal)	Ensure adequate intraluminal enzyme concentrations	Almost always useful because of asynchrony
H_2 or PPI (equivalent to ranitidine 300 mg bid or omeprazole 40 mg/d)	Reduces gastric hypersecretion	Initiate in acute phase using parenteral or sublingual formulation; continue at least 6 mo
Cholestyramine (4–16 g/d)	Decreases bile acid–induced diarrhea	May worsen steatorrhea Not advised if extended ileal resection May impair vitamin absorption
Antibiotics (oral for 7 d) (doxycycline 100 mg bid, metronidazole 250 mg tid, or cefalosporin 250 mg qid	Treat bacterial overgrowth	Overgrowth predictable with ileocecal resection Retreatment usually needed every 6 wk
Octreotide (75 μg SC tid or 25 mg depo monthly)	Decreases secretions and prolongs intestinal transit	Expensive and concurrently decreases pancreatic secretions, may impair intestinal adaptation, and increases risk of cholelithiasis

bid = twice daily; H_2 = histamine$_2$; PPI = proton pump inhibitor; qid = four times daily; tid = three times daily; SC = subcutaneously.

should be concurrently provided to take advantage of the remaining small bowel and adaptive processes and to avoid cholestatic liver disease, which may be associated with chronic TPN. Transition from continuous to cycled TPN must be gradual to accommodate pancreatic insulin secretion in response to concentrated glucose load. Infusion of total TPN volume should be compressed by increments of 2 to 4 hours daily along with a 30- to 60-minute taper at the beginning and end of the infusion cycle until the total infusion period is 10 hours, which will be tolerated by most individuals in the absence of cardiac or renal disease.[2]

A variety of surgical procedures designed to slow intestinal transit have been selectively performed, with very little success.[2] Small bowel transplantation, which is rarely applicable to cancer patients, is usually performed in conjunction with liver transplantation and should be highly selective since it is associated with a 45% 5-year survival rate when performed alone and only 37% when performed as combined liver and small bowel transplantation.[2] The use of tissue-engineered small intestine (TESI) is an intriguing new development that has now been tested in a rat animal model. The making of TESI by the transplantation of organoid units derived from neonatal tissue containing a mesenchymal core surrounded by polarized intestinal epithelium on a biodegradable polymer scaffold was first reported in 1997.[27] Following improvement of the protocol to yield more organoid units in

shorter time, these investigators have provided the first report of a tissue-engineered vital organ functioning as salvage therapy in a replacement model.[28] The results included the observation that the TESI contained intact epithelial, muscular, vascular, and neural components and that having an attached segment of TESI reduced the overall period of weight loss from 14.6 to 7.7 days, maintained and regained higher percentages of weight than did animals who have massive small bowel resection alone, prolonged transit time, improved vitamin B_{12} absorption, and resulted in higher deoxyribonucleic acid (DNA) content of the native intestine.[28] The applicability of this to higher-order animals obviously remains uncertain but holds promise as a means to replace small intestine function without the morbidity and complications of other replacement techniques.

Malabsorption

Malabsorption of nutrients, which may be limited to a single constituent, implies an interruption of normal digestion and/or absorption. This may be the result of (1) a defective intraluminal phase of digestion owing to pancreatic exocrine insufficiency, impaired solubilization of fat caused by inadequate intraluminal bile acid concentration, or inaccessibility of nutrients for uptake and absorption illustrated by pernicious anemia; (2) defective intestinal or mucosal processing resulting from brush border enzyme deficiencies, loss of mucosal surface, or impaired absorption

by epithelial cells, as in the case of sprue; or (3) defective transport, which can occur with lymphatic obstruction. Many of these processes are interrelated as exemplified by decreased exocrine secretion resulting from decreased hormonal release in the presence of intestinal mucosal disease or the effect of bacterial overgrowth, which can decrease intraluminal bile acid concentration below a critical level needed for micellar solubilization of fats and also compete for nutrients, such as vitamin B_{12}.

Although the symptoms or signs of malabsorption often include diarrhea, weight loss, or the presence of bulky, foul-smelling stools, these more classic features are not essential for the diagnosis of malabsorption, which, as indicated, may be limited to a specific nutrient(s). As a general rule, when nutrient deficiencies, such as deficiency related to folate, iron, vitamin K, carotene, or vitamin D, are present, the pathophysiology usually involves the small bowel, whereas malabsorption owing to pancreatic exocrine insufficiency is more often characterized by greater amounts of steatorrhea without coexisting nutritional deficiency(s). The approach to malabsorption is highly dependent on the clinical setting, which often determines the presence of specific deficiencies. It is likewise clinically relevant that vitamin and macronutrient deficiencies take time to develop and acute or transient malabsorption is of limited clinical significance. It is likewise impossible in this section to cover all aspects of malabsorption. Therefore, those aspects considered to be more common in cancer patients are addressed.

One of the most predictable forms of maldigestion or malabsorption in cancer patients is the presence of pancreatic exocrine insufficiency in patients with cancer of the pancreas or following pancreaticoduodenectomy. The impact of impeded flow of pancreatic juice owing to mechanical obstruction is greatest when the head of the pancreas is involved. Weight loss in these patients can be temporarily prevented with enzyme supplements.[29] During long-term follow-up after pancreaticoduodenectomy, a predictable set of micronutrient deficiencies, including vitamins A, D, and E, selenium, zinc, and iron, have been reported and observed to be compounded by insufficient dietary intake.[30] The implications are obvious and include aggressive enzyme replacement, diet modification, and vitamin supplementation, with enzyme replacement being the most important.

Lactase deficiency and lactose intolerance are clinically benign but very common forms of malabsorption. Although often genetically determined, lactase deficiency determined by breath hydrogen has been reported in approximately 30% of individuals undergoing chemotherapy.[31–33] The development of lactose intolerance is not invariable, and lactose restriction is recommended only for symptomatic patients. A controversial aspect of lactose malabsorption involves the reported increased frequency of lactose malabsorption and possible galactose cytotoxicity in the pathogenesis of ovarian cancer.[34] The role of radiation in the development of lactose intolerance is debatable and likely related to the amount of bowel irradiated.[35,36] Iron deficiency occurs frequently after subtotal or extended gastric resection.[37] In this setting, atrophic gastritis and *Helicobacter pylori* involving the gastric stump seem to play an important role in the development of iron deficiency.[37] Iron deficiency is now also recognized as one of the most common manifestations of celiac disease (CD) in adults.[38]

Atrophic gastritis is also associated with vitamin B_{12} malabsorption and is reported to be associated with a higher risk of noncardia gastric neoplasia in cohort studies; however, data are lacking regarding the value of surveillance endoscopy in this setting.[39] A study of 152 residents of Rochester, Minnesota, with well-documented pernicious anemia during a 30-year interval were followed for more than 1,550 person-years, and only one gastric carcinoma was observed compared with an identical expected incidence.[40] Recent observation resulting from an average 7.1-year follow-up of 21,265 patients hospitalized between 1965 and 1999 unexpectedly revealed that the incidence of squamous cell carcinoma of the esophagus is increased threefold in the setting of pernicious anemia.[41] Although parenteral or intranasal administration of vitamin B_{12} is required for patients with pernicious anemia, those with food-cobalamin malabsorption may be effectively treated with crystalline cyanocobalamin 250 to 1,000 μg/d during clinical studies of 1-month duration.[42] In addition to more commonly recognized atrophic gastritis, ileal resection, and ileal disease, vitamin B_{12} malabsorption may occur as a sequela to pelvic irradiation. During prospective study, it has been observed that vitamin B_{12}, bile acids, and fat are malabsorbed as a consequence of radiation therapy.[43] Implications for therapy include administration of vitamin B_{12} and treatment with cholestyramine to control bile acid catharsis provided that there are no signs of intestinal obstruction.

Vitamin K deficiency is rare since it is derived from plant sources and gut microflora. Deficiencies can occur in patients on TPN without supplementation, on long-term antibiotics, and when fat is malabsorbed. This may result in clotting disorders and disordered bone mineralization wherein vitamin K is a cofactor.[44] The prevalence of vitamin K deficiency with elevated prothrombin time and coagulation disorders in subclinical CD is reported to be less than 1% and does not independently require screening for CD.[45]

Vitamin D deficiency has historically been considered to be a condition of the elderly and related to a combination of decreased intake, diminished absorption, and reduced exposure to sunlight; however, a study of 290 hospitalized patients found that 57% were vitamin D deficient and that 37% ingested amounts exceeding the recommended dietary allowance.[46] One condition to always consider in this setting is CD since 28% of newly diagnosed celiac patients have osteoporosis and may present with osteoporosis in the absence of other symptoms.[47] CD was once considered rare, but following the development of reliable serologic tests, it is now recognized to affect 1 in 120 to 300 in North American.[48] CD has great relevance to cancer medicine since it is a common cause of malabsorption that may be unmasked by cancer surgery or other insults to the small bowel and carries an increased risk of gastrointestinal cancer and lymphoma. Given that most adults with CD do not present with diarrhea, nutritional deficiencies should be considered a manifestation of CD. Immunoglobulin (Ig)A anti–endomysial antibody (EMA) carries a very high sensitivity and specificity for CD, with a reported sensitivity of 85 to 98% and a specificity of 97 to 100%.[38] Originally recognized to react with the endomysial lining of microfibrils using monkey esophagus or cultured human umbilical vein cells, it is now recognized that tissue transglutaminase (tTG) is the antigen to which EMA reacts. Anti-tTG has become the serologic test of choice since it is less expensive, easier to perform, and more sensitive.[49] It is relevant that IgG tTG appears to be almost as sensitive and specific as IgA tTG and can be used in IgA deficiency, which is not uncommon in sprue. Tests for antigliadin antibodies are not preferred since they are less specific and only moderately sensitive.[38]

Nausea and Vomiting

The management of nausea and vomiting in the cancer patient has been revolutionized by the development of antagonists to a 5-hydroxytryptamine (HT) neuronal mediator, 5-HT_3, and an antagonist to a neurokinin (NK), NK-1 receptor. Following our understanding of the pivotal role of 5-HT in the gut and NK receptors in the central nervous system and their relationship to nausea and vomiting, the development of these antagonists has markedly reduced the incidence of chemotherapy-induced nausea and vomiting (CINV) and radiation-induced nausea and vomiting (RINV).

The gut is the only organ that can display reflexes and integrative neuronal activity when isolated from the central nervous system, and it is now known that peristaltic and secretory reflexes are initiated by afferent neurons stimulated by 5-HT. Blocking the 5-HT_3 receptors can attenuate nausea and vomiting. 5-HT_3 not only mediates peristaltic and secretory reflexes, it also mediates signaling to the central nervous system, serotonergic transmission within the enteric nervous system, and activation of myenteric intrinsic pathways.[50] Meanwhile, blocking NK-1 receptors in the brain blocks the effect of this NK on substance P, the natural ligand in the central nervous system. This, in turn, helps control the development of CINV and augments the acute- and delayed-phase antiemetic effect of 5-HT_3 receptor antagonists.[51] Prior to the introduction of these newer agents, corticosteroids, adrenocorticotropic hormone, and metoclopramide were the primary mainstays to prevent or control CINV. As with all antiemetics, including the 5-HT_3 and NK-1 antagonists, they are more effective if given prophylactically, and it appears that a single dose given before chemotherapy is as effective as other dose schedules. Oral and intravenous formulations are equally effective, and one need give only the lowest dose needed to achieve a symptomatic effect. Five different 5-HT_3 receptor antagonists have now been developed and are often used in combination with steroids and NK-1 receptor antagonists in the control of CINV or the side effects of radiation therapy. CINV and RINV are covered in an earlier chapter and have been the subject of review articles and/or consensus reports.[50–56]

In addition to CINV, other causes of nausea and vomiting unique to cancer patients include the effects of graft-versus-host disease (GVHD) and abnormal motility that may result from a variety of retroperitoneal tumors that adversely affect gastric emptying without obstruction. Nausea and vomiting are a common occurrence when bone marrow transplantation is complicated by GVHD.[57] Involvement of the upper gastrointestinal tract with GVHD is being recognized more often since it was initially described in 1983.[58] It is characteristic for nausea and vomiting owing to GVHD (discussed in a separate chapter) to be associated with delayed gastric emptying and to respond to immunosuppressive therapy. When symptoms do not resolve, the probability of a coexisting infectious process such as cytomegalovirus or herpes simplex type 1 is more likely.[57]

The paraneoplastic syndrome of intestinal pseudo-obstruction has been associated with several types of malignancies, including small cell lung cancer, carcinoid, neuroblastoma, pancreatic adenocarcinoma, and retroperitoneal leiomyosarcoma.[59–62] Indeed, any process that causes myenteric ganglionitis may result in dysmotility and nausea and vomiting.[63] Although these conditions are rare, they are nonetheless important and should be considered when the cause of nausea and vomiting remains indeterminate. Gastroparesis with nausea and vomiting may also be iatrogenic from celiac block.[64] Paraneoplastic syndromes and dysmotility following celiac block may respond to prokinetic medications, the effect of celiac block usually improves with time, and delayed emptying from nonobstructing retroperitoneal tumors can be palliated with prokinetic medications.[65]

In addition to the CINV and nausea and vomiting associated with GVHD or radiation therapy, or as a paraneoplastic syndrome, which are all unique to cancer patients, nausea and vomiting have many other causes in the cancer patient that may or may not be related to cancer. These include but are not limited to the side effects of nonchemotherapy medications, gastroduodenal or other forms of intestinal obstruction, gastrointestinal motility disorders, gastric ulceration, dumping syndrome, pancreatitis, hepatitis, renal failure, and neurologic disorders. It is unrealistic to cover all of these topics; however, some salient points help to clinically determine the cause of nausea and vomiting. For example, when nausea and vomiting are caused by obstruction, vomiting is usually delayed following a meal, worsens during the course of the day, may contain food retained from a much earlier meal, usually worsens over time, and is typically associated with early satiety. With current imaging and endoscopy, it is easy to identify the presence of an obstruction. Management is understandably determined by the cause and extent of obstruction plus the patient's general condition. Whereas benign obstructive process are usually managed surgically, the use of endoscopically placed stents, described in a separate chapter, offers effective palliative management of obstruction owing to malignancy.

Treatment of motility disorders is, on the other hand, nonsurgical. These occur in the form of poorly understood gastroparesis, which may occur as a result of diabetes, as post-vagotomy syndrome, and as other causes of enteric neuropathy, including paraneoplastic syndrome and the result of retroperitoneal tumors, described above. Whether idiopathic or caused by diabetes, gastroparesis is a challenge to manage and is further complicated by the fact that modifiers of symptomatology and the severity of symptoms may not correlate with apparent pathophysiology. Furthermore, some diabetics have episodes of nausea and vomiting, whereas others may have delayed emptying with minimal symptoms and some experience more severe persistent symptoms.

There is poor correlation between improvement in the rate of gastric emptying and symptom relief.[66] In this context, other causes of vomiting need to be considered before embracing a diagnosis of gastroparesis. Uncertainties notwithstanding, when nausea and vomiting occur in the diabetic patient and are without another cause, it is quite reasonable to empirically initiate treatment with a prokinetic medication such as metoclopramide, erythromycin, or cisapride (the latter is available under special limited conditions from the manufacturer).[67] There is a dose-response relationship with the use of prokinetics; however, the incidence of side effects is likewise dose related and limits dosage escalation. The limited efficacy of these medications has prompted some investigators to take advantage of the role of pylorospasm, observed in association with diabetic gastroparesis, by using botulinum toxin injection of the pylorus, which has met with limited success in small open-label studies.[68] Attempts to address the putative pathophysiology are difficult, as is correlating symptoms with our very incomplete understanding of pathophysiology of gastric motility disorders. This is exemplified by the observation that sildenafil, known to induce pyloric relaxation, a major determinant of gastric emptying, did not improve gastric emptying in a study of 12 patients with end-stage renal disease.[69] Failure of medical therapy may lead to consideration of surgery, which is likewise poorly defined, reported as retrospective reviews or uncontrolled series, and should be approached with caution.[70]

Nausea and vomiting may be encountered as part of a dumping syndrome that results from osmotic fluid shifts, release of vasoactive neurotransmitters, and reactive hypoglycemia in the cancer and noncancer patient following gastric surgery. Up to 10% of patients have clinically significant symptoms, and up to 2% experience debility.[71] Measures to help achieve relief of symptoms should include minimizing ingestion of simple carbohydrates, excluding liquids with meals, and providing compounds such as pectin or guar to increase intraluminal viscosity and/or to give an α-glucosidase inhibitor, acarbose, to blunt the rapid absorption of glucose.[72] Pharmacotherapy for dumping has otherwise focused on the use of octreotide in an attempt to delay transit and decrease release of vasoactive mediators. Seven randomized controlled trials involving 63 patients with severe dumping alleviated symptoms with statistical significance.[73] For patients with dumping that does not respond to standard measures without pharmacotherapy, octreotide in a dosage of 50 to 100 μg subcutaneously or as a monthly depo intramuscular injection of 25 mg should be considered.

Constipation

Constipation, generally defined as decreased frequency of evacuation, abnormally hard stools, or the need to strain to complete bowel evacuation, is a very common problem that occurs in one-quarter to half of patients age 65 years and older.[74] It is even more common in the cancer patient population and may result from prolonged colonic transit, an abnormally firm consistency of stool, or an obstructive process. Although often multifactorial, determining the factors contributing to constipation is pivotal to selecting appropriate therapy. To prevent unnecessary suffering, a proactive approach is desirable in the management and prevention of constipation. The potential for proactive intervention has been demonstrated in hospitalized immobile vascular surgery patients in whom a protocol of dietary fiber, increased fluid, and hygiene measure over a 3-year period reduced the incidence of constipation from 59 to 9% and eliminated impaction.[75]

The clinical history is most important particularly as it pertains to (1) understanding the precise nature of the complaint, which may indicate an anorectal cause; (2) a history of constipation, which may indicate problems with gastrointestinal motility with colonic inertia or a history of laxative dependence; (3) the pattern of onset; (4) progression versus fluctuation of symptoms; (5) a history of neuromuscular and/or rheumatologic disorders; (6) relationship to medications, including over-the-counter and herbal medications; (7) the probability of an obstructive process; and (8) the presence of coexisting alarm symptoms, such as bleeding. Although the cause of constipation is often multifactorial, constipation most commonly occurs as a side effect of medications. This is not surprising when one considers the fact that 40% of patients reporting constipation defined by Rome II criteria were using medications known to cause constipation.[76] Of 392 patients in long-term care facilities, with a diagnosis of constipation and/or routine laxative use, over 72% had received at least one medication known to cause constipation.[77] The importance of constipation as an adverse drug reaction in a cancer patient population is underscored by the observation that constipation was the most common adverse drug reaction in a prospective study of 171 hospitalized oncology patients.[78] A list of medications commonly associated with constipation is summarized in Table 4. Although delayed transit secondary to medications is the most common

Table 4 Medication-Induced Constipation
Anticholinergics
Anticonvulsants
Antidiarrheal agents
Antihistamines
Calcium supplements
Calcium channel blockers
Cholestyramine
Diuretics
Iron supplements
Nonsteroidal anti-inflammatory drugs
Opioid analgesics
Tricyclic antidepressants

cause of constipation, it is likewise important to be reasonably confident that metabolic or endocrinologic causes of delayed transit or an obstructive process are not responsible for constipation. Laboratory tests, including complete blood count, serum electrolytes, calcium and phosphorus, thyroid-stimulating hormone, glucose, and creatinine, help exclude the former, whereas imaging studies (which should include decubitus views when doing a plain abdominal series, thus using air in the colon as a contrast medium) and/or endoscopy helpo exclude the latter. Provided that obstruction and reversible metabolic causes are excluded, empiric therapy can be pursued (Table 5 and Figure 1).

Medical management of constipation consists of increased water intake, fiber supplementation, stool softeners, osmotic products, stimulant laxatives, prostaglandin analogues or colchicine, enemas, and 5-HT$_4$ receptor agonists given alone or in combination. Medical therapy for constipation needs to be individualized and should be initiated early or prophylactically to prevent, as well as control, constipation. This is particularly relevant in that constipation has been observed to produce what has been described as a "complete person-experience" that particularly affects the

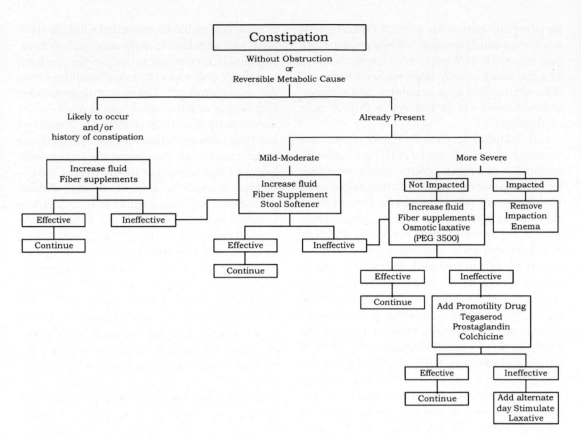

FIGURE 1 PEG = polyethylene glycol.

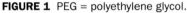

Table 5 Management of Constipation: Therapeutic Alternatives	
Fiber and bulk laxative	
Dietary fiber	20 g daily
Methylcellulose	1 tsp or 2 caplets with 6 oz water bid
Polycarbophil	1 to 2 tablets bid
Stool softeners	
Docusate	100–200 mg daily to bid
Mineral oil	15–45 mL daily
Osmotic products	
Lactulose	15–30 mL daily to bid
Sorbitol	15–30 mL daily to bid
Polyethylene glycol	8–32 oz daily with water
Glycerin suppository	1 daily
Stimulant laxative	
Bisacodyl suppository	10–20 mg daily every 2–3 d
Senna or cascara	2–4 tablets daily to bid
Promotility agents	
Tegaserod	2–6 mg bid
Misoprostol	200 μg daily; increase to qid
Colchicine	0.6 mg tid
Magnesium products	
Magnesium citrate	200 mL daily
Magnesium hydroxide	2 g daily

bid = twice daily; qid = four times daily; tid = three times daily.

cancer patient receiving palliative therapy by causing discomfort, mental preoccupation, a reminder of death, and social isolation.[79] Constipation, without the complications related thereto, is of limited direct clinical importance; however, the recognition that constipation causes significant impairment of quality of life has led to the recognition that constipation is clinically a serious condition for the majority of people afflicted.[80]

Cancer patients are often limited in their ability to pursue lifestyle changes that are considered to lessen constipation and that include increased physical activity, improved fiber intact or eating a breakfast meal on a regular basis, and sitting on the commode for several minutes after breakfast to take advantage of the gastrocolic reflex. Although these limitations may prevail, it is important to recognize that the effective management of constipation simply includes recognizing the merits of adequate water consumption. This is intuitive; however, studies have demonstrated that water supplementation enhances the effect of a high-fiber diet and laxative consumption in individuals with functional constipation.[81] This applies to all causes of constipation. Concurrently, minimizing caffeinated beverages is recommended to minimize their diuretic effect.

Because the patient population under discussion is often elderly and for other reasons may also not be able to consume adequate fiber as dietary fiber, supplements in the form of methylcellulose, psyllium, or polycarbophil are

often needed. Although fiber supplements may intensify symptoms of bloating and discomfort if constipation is more severe, they are useful as proactive intervention for less severe cases or prevention of constipation. Their slow onset of action and limited effect in more severe cases limit their use as single agents. Nonetheless, their efficacy in less severe cases of constipation or the prevention of constipation is well documented.[82–85]

The most commonly prescribed products to offset constipation are stool softeners.[86] Although frequently prescribed, their empiric use has been questioned.[87] Their efficacy, or lack thereof, may be, in part, related to the product used in that dioctyl calcium sulfosuccinate has been reported to increase the number of spontaneous bowel movements by 62%, whereas an increase of only 30% was observed with dioctyl sodium sulfosuccinate given once or twice daily in a homogeneous group of institutionalized patients.[88] Acute treatment with stimulant laxatives can be useful; however, long-term use is associated with a diminished colonic motor response to such agents.[89] These agents are therefore not preferable for long-term treatment; however, their use two to three times a week is not considered harmful.[89]

Since the introduction of polyethylene glycol (PEG) 3500, it has become a preferred osmotic laxative. Studies have demonstrated its effectiveness compared with placebo and with no clinically significant changes in blood chemistry, complete blood count, or urinalysis observed in a dosage of 17 g daily.[90,91] Like other osmotic products, PEG has no adverse effect on nerve and muscle cells in the colon and is better tolerated than poorly absorbed carbohydrates, such as lactulose or sorbitol, which cause more flatulence and abdominal distention.[92] If the desired effect is not achieved with 17 g PEG suspended in 6 oz water daily, the dosage can be safely increased to twice daily. Lactulose is preferable when using an osmotic product in the setting of hepatic encephalopathy. Sorbitol is a cost-effective alternative to lactulose in the treatment of chronic constipation.[93]

A novel approach in the treatment of constipation involves the use of misoprostol, a prostaglandin E_1 analogue, which is known to stimulate intestinal transit in healthy individuals and patients with chronic constipation. Although misoprostol is subject to causing cramping as a side effect and is not acceptable in young women who wish to become pregnant, it has a very high margin of safety and no significant drug-drug interactions. An initial short-term double-blind crossover study of nine patients with severe constipation and a subsequent long-term open-label trial of misoprostol in the treatment of chronic refractory constipation have demonstrated efficacy in the management of chronic refractory constipation.[94,95] To obviate cramping, starting at a dose of 200 µg every other day and gradually increasing, as tolerated, to three or four times daily has been advocated.[89] Colchicine is another drug known to stimulate motility in animal model studies and cause diarrhea as a side effect that has been used in a dosage of 0.6 mg orally three times daily for the treatment of chronic constipation.[96,97] There are no long-term studies of colchicine for chronic constipation, and its use is limited by side effects, including increased abdominal pain, during therapy.[97]

Although primarily investigated in the setting of constipation associated with an irritable bowel syndrome, tegaserod has been studied in two double-blind randomized placebo-controlled trials involving over 2,000 patients.[98,99] Response, defined by complete spontaneous evacuation, was significantly greater in patients treated with either tegaserod 2 (41%) or 6 (43%) mg twice daily compared with placebo (25%) in one study and significant improvement in subject global symptom assessment in the other randomized trial.[98,99] The effect of tegaserod is observed within the first week of treatment and is maintained over 12 weeks without significant side effects and the return of symptoms without rebound effect after withdrawal.

Enemas (tap water, oil retention, saline, soap suds, milk, and molasses) are often used for the acute management of constipation; however, they are not recommended in the treatment of chronic constipation. They must furthermore be used with caution since mucosal injury, bowel penetration, proctocolitis, and life-threatening metabolic complications can occur, particularly in patients with renal insufficiency and in the pediatric population.[100,101] Although adverse outcomes have been described much more often with preparations other than milk and molasses, even this preparation has been reported to result in severe complications.[102]

Acute colonic pseudo-obstruction often prompts emergency consultation and globally falls into the category of constipation. Unlike constipation, which is clinically defined as described above, pseudo-obstruction or Ogilvie's syndrome is determined by acute onset of colonic dilatation without obstruction, as documented on radiographs. Characteristically the result of a wide variety of associated medical or surgical conditions in hospitalized patients, the diagnosis is of concern because of the risk of perforation, which has been reported in 3% of cases when the cecal diameter reaches 12 cm.[103] Although most cases respond to conservative management, the risk of ischemia with increasing distention has prompted the use of colonoscopy for decompression in selected cases or more often medical intervention with 2 mg neostigmine given intravenously over 3 to 5 minutes with continuous cardiac monitoring and immediate availability of atropine to treat drug-induced bradycardia. This pharmacologic approach is predicated on the premise of ineffectual colonic motility caused by excessive sympathetic stimulation.

When neoplastic obstruction is the cause of constipation, an alternative to surgery, discussed in more detail in a following chapter, includes endoluminal stenting, which offers effective palliation for malignant obstruction. Stenting may also allow time to improve a patient's condition and permit definitive surgery or minimize the need for staged procedures. Although reported studies are retrospective, they are consistent in the observations that stenting offers a shorter hospital stay and effective palliation but does not otherwise prolong survival.[104,105] Although the overall technical success rate is reported to be 93%, with relief of obstruction in 80 to 92% cases, not all cases are suitable for stenting. Limitations include a tortuous delivery pathway and require advancing a guidewire across the obstruction.[106] The presence of a 3 cm segment of uncovered wire at the ends of the stent to enhance stabilization and minimize migration limits the use of stents for distal rectal obstruction. Restenosis owing to tumor ingrowth has been reduced by the use of covered stents; however, this remains a significant problem. To minimize intraluminal obstruction from fecal residue, a low-residue diet and use of stool softeners or osmotic laxative are routinely required. Endoscopic laser therapy can be useful in acutely relieving an obstruction and/or controlling bleeding from colorectal cancer.[107] Argon plasma coagulation and photodynamic therapy provide other endoscopic alternatives.[108] Unfortunately, ablation therapy is limited to the exophytic component of disease, whereas the process of obstruction, in the course of disease progression, usually becomes intramural or the result of extraluminal compression and limits the long-term efficacy of therapy using ablation techniques.

Diarrhea

Diarrhea is the result of excess water in stool and is defined as increased frequency or stools of loose consistency. The conditions that lead to diarrhea are so broad that recommending restricted investigative pathways and management is unrealistic; however, this does not preclude the fact that the probable pathophysiology is dependent on the pattern of diarrhea and the clinical setting in which it occurs. Considerations include but are not limited to an acute versus a chronic history of diarrhea, coexisting gastrointestinal disease, concurrent or recent drug therapy, immunodeficiency, the persistence of diarrhea when fasting, recent surgery or altered anatomy, a history of bone marrow transplantation, previous radiation therapy, malignancies known to cause secretory diarrhea, a history of diabetes, and the presence of systemic symptoms. A complete differential diagnosis of diarrhea is beyond the scope of this section; however, salient points relevant to the cancer patient will be considered and are summarized in Tables 5 and 6.

In the care of the cancer patient, it is readily recognized that many chemotherapeutic agents and abdominal or pelvic radiation frequently cause diarrhea, which is more likely when chemotherapy and radiation are combined.[109] If diarrhea, in this setting, is mild to moderate, as defined by the absence of systemic symptoms, severe cramping, neutropenia, or nausea / vomiting, management consists of intravenous or oral rehydration (including repletion of electrolytes) and loperamide 4 mg orally followed by 2 mg every 4 hours after every loose bowel movement (not to exceed 16 mg daily).[109] Revised guidelines for more severe diarrhea induced by chemotherapy or radiation recommend the use of octreotide 100 to 150 µg subcutaneously three times daily or 25 to 50 µg intravenously/hour, which has proven more effective than conventional antidiarrheal treatment in prospective studies.[109–112] The presence of severe diarrhea as defined above warrants withholding chemotherapy until the diarrhea has subsided for 24 hours. Octreotide, deodorized tincture of opium, paregoric, codeine, diphenoxylate with atropine, and loperamide also represent second-tier alternatives for persistent mild to moderate diarrhea. Sucralfate, a widely investigated agent used in an effort to prevent diarrhea, has not been shown to be effective in preventing diarrhea caused by chemotherapy or radiation.[109] Olsalazine, an anti-inflammatory medication used in the treatment of inflammatory bowel disease, is contraindicated during radiation therapy since it has been shown to increase diarrhea.[110] Chemotherapy- or radiation-induced diarrhea is usually self-limited; however, prolonged duration of radiation may cause persistent diarrhea and require the use of maintenance loperamide in a dosage up to 2 mg every 2 to 4 hours or the other second-tier medications described above. If diarrhea becomes chronic in the setting of pelvic radiation, bile acid malabsorption is a recognized pathophysiologic mechanism that has been reported in the majority of patients who experience chronic diarrhea after radiotherapy for gynecologic cancer, with bacterial overgrowth also reported in 45%.[113] Treatment with oral antibiotics and/or bile acid binding resins is reported to decrease the frequency of chronic diarrhea caused by radiation therapy.

In the management of all causes of diarrhea, it is important to remember that any agent that enhances fluid absorption in the intestine, regardless of the applicable mechanism, is potentially useful in counteracting diarrhea. The addition of glucose to ORSs can not only contribute significantly to the management of infectious diarrhea and SBS, as described in an earlier section of this chapter, it can also facilitate supportive care and rehydration in other cancer treatment–related diarrhea. Although the addition of glucose or free amino acids to ORSs does not necessarily inhibit a pathologic secretory process, they can facilitate the absorption of ingested electrolytes and water that otherwise would not be absorbed.[114] In the absence of secondary abnormalities that require diet modification, there is no need for specific dietary restrictions in the management of diarrhea.

If diarrhea is not directly the result of chemotherapy or radiation and particularly if it occurs in a hospital setting, *Clostridium difficile* diarrhea (CDAD) should be considered since this has become the most common cause of infectious diarrhea in hospitalized patients.[115] Although commonly associated with the use of broad-spectrum antibiotic therapy, the risk factors for CDAD or colitis also include bowel surgery, an immunocompromised state, and any process that suppresses the normal flora, including antifungal and chemotherapeutic agents. It has been documented that chemotherapy is a risk factor for the development of CDAD and augments the probability that antibiotic therapy will cause CDAD.[116] The diagnosis of CDAD consequently should be suspected when a patient without a primary gastrointestinal disease process develops diarrhea following treatment that can affect the normal

microflora. The confirmation of diagnosis is dependent on detection of *C. difficile* toxin in the stool or the presence of pseudomembranous colitis on endoscopy. It is important for clinicians to recognize the sensitivity and specificity of available tests and to know the limits of the tests that are used by a specific laboratory. Organism identification by culture or antigen is nonspecific since toxigenic and nontoxigenic strains are identified by these methods. Toxin A, an enterotoxin, and toxin B, a cytotoxin, may, however, be detected by tests using either latex agglutination, which actually detects glutamate dehydrogenase enzyme produced by *C. difficile*, enzyme immunoassays (EIAs) for toxins A and/or B, or tissue culture tests for toxin B. Latex agglutination and EIA are rapid and relatively inexpensive; however, the former is nonspecific and some of the EIA methods have limited sensitivity. Six commercially available rapid tests for direct detection of *C. difficile* and its toxins in fecal samples have been compared with fibroblast cytotoxicity assay.[117]

Mild cases of CDAD may resolve by discontinuing antibiotics, thus allowing reestablishment of colonic microflora, which is known to inhibit the growth of *C. difficile*. Metronidazole (250 mg four times daily to 500 mg three times daily for 10 to 14 days), given orally or intravenously, appears to be as effective as vancomycin (125 mg orally four times daily for 10 to 14 days) for mild to moderate cases.[118,119] Although debatable as first-line therapy, vancomycin given orally or by enema is the preferred treatment for more severe cases. The standard dose of vancomycin is 125 mg orally four times daily and appears to be comparable in efficacy to 500 mg orally four times daily.[119] Bacitracin given orally is a therapeutic alternative, and cholestyramine is a useful adjunct that may be used alone for mild cases.[115,119,121] The majority of patients with diarrhea or colitis caused by *C. difficile* respond to initial therapy; however, up to 20% experience relapse when treatment is discontinued and require repeat or prolonged therapy.[122,123] Since environmental contamination by *C. difficile* is common and may be carried by health care personnel, this illustrates yet another importance on hand washing to reduce the spread of nosocomial infection and is pivotal for optimal care of all cancer patients. Noninfectious nosocomial causes of diarrhea more commonly include the direct effect of medications or the ingestion of dietary products or medications that contain sorbitol or mannitol.

Other infectious causes of diarrhea cannot be discounted in the cancer patient but are more likely to occur in the setting of neutropenia, immunodeficiency related to human immunodeficiency virus (HIV), or bone marrow transplantation.[124,125] Although non–*C. difficile* infection is more common in association with

immunodeficiency, CDAD has been reported in 7% of all cycles of myelosuppressive chemotherapy on a retrospective review of almost 900 courses of treatment.[126] Diarrhea in the setting of neutropenia warrants broad-spectrum antibiotic therapy that includes metronidazole. Neither fecal leukocytes nor occult blood is predictive of the presence of CDAD.[127]

In the setting of acquired immune deficiency syndrome (AIDS), a potential infectious cause has been reported in at least one-third of cases of chronic, unexplained diarrhea.[128] The likelihood of an infectious process and the enhanced diagnostic yield of colonoscopy over sigmoidoscopy are greater when the CD4 count is below 100 cells/mm³.[128] Issues related to GVHD in bone marrow transplant patients are covered in a separate chapter. The management of secretory diarrhea caused by neuroendocrine tumors has been greatly enhanced with somatostatin, which has become the standard of care and has been summarized in review articles on this topic.[129–131] In the case of secretory diarrhea, fecal electrolytes account for most of the osmolality, whereas osmotic diarrhea is characterized by an osmotic gap that exceeds 50 to 100 mOsm/kg.[132] Taking a careful medication history, including the use of over-the-counter and alternative medications, determining if diarrhea persists during fasting, considering the common causes of nosocomial diarrhea, establishing risk factors for the probability of infectious diarrhea, performing stool examinations when symptoms are severe and/or pus and blood are present, doing diagnostic sigmoidoscopy when symptoms are persistent and colonoscopy if diarrhea is indeterminate in a patient with immune deficiency, establishing if malabsorption is present, and providing fluid and electrolyte repletion and symptomatic treatment for diarrhea will collectively facilitate management of this common problem..

Summary

In summary, recognition of important principles in the management of common gastrointestinal disorders can greatly facilitate care of the cancer patient. Some of these principles include (1) recognizing the value of supportive care and importance of enteral feedings in patients with SBS; (2) understanding the potential for malabsorption of specific nutrients and the probability of small bowel pathology when nutritional deficiencies are encountered; (3) providing exocrine pancreatic enzyme supplements in the presence of pancreatic disease; (4) knowing pharmacotherapy options in the management of nausea and vomiting; (5) appreciating the importance of constipation and the value of prevention and therapeutic options; and (6) recognition of the likely cause of diarrhea in various clinical settings and the importance of CDAD in the cancer patient. It is hoped that by applying basic principles, symptoms can be attenuated and cancer patient care can be enhanced.

Table 6 Diarrhea: Classification and Conditions Common to Cancer Patients

Osmotic
   Laxative use
   Carbohydrate malabsorption
Maldigestion
   Pancreatic insufficiency
      Resection
      Ductal obstruction
   Bile acid insufficiency (see below)
   Bacterial overgrowth
Malabsorption
   Short bowel
   Celiac disease
   Bacterial overgrowth
   Bile acid insufficiency
      Ileal disease
      Ileal resection
         Radiation therapy
Inflammatory
   Infectious nosocomial
      Clostridium difficile
   Infectious non-nosocomial (immunodeficiency associated)
      Bacterial
         Salmonella
         Shigella
         Escherichia coli 0157
         Yersinia
      Parasitic
         Amebiasis
         Strongyloides
      Ulcerating viral
         Cytomegalovirus
         Herpes
      Other
         Tuberculosis
   Bone marrow transplant
      GVHD
      Opportunistic infection
   Inflammatory bowel disease
      Ulcerative colitis
      Crohn's disease
      Microscopic colitis
Postoperative
   Pancreatic insufficiency
   Unmasked celiac
   Postvagotomy/dumping syndrome
   Short or bypassed bowel
Secretory
   Neuroendocrine
      Gastrinoma
      VIPoma
      Carcinoid
      Medullary cancer of the thyroid
      Somatostinoma
   Endocrine
      Hyperthyroidism
      Addison's disease

Table 6 Continued

Primary neoplastic
   Colon cancer
   Rectal villous adenoma
   Lymphoma
Pseudodiarrhea
   Fecal impaction
   Anorectal obstruction
Mixed inflammatory/secretory
   Chemotherapy induced
   Non–chemotherapy related
      NSAIDs
      Colchicine
      β-Adrenergic antagonists

GVHD = graft-versus-host disease; NSAID = nonsteroidal anti-inflammatory drug

REFERENCES

1. McFadden MA, Delegge MH, Kirby DF. Medication delivery in the short bowel syndrome. JPEN J Parenter Enteral Nutr 1993;17:180–6.
2. Buchman AL, Scolapio J, Fryer J. AGA technical review on short bowel syndrome and intestinal transplantation. Gastroenterology 2003;124:1111–34.
3. Nordgaard I, Hansen BS, Mortensen PB. Colon as a digestive organ in patients with short bowel syndrome. Lancet 1994;343:373–6.
4. Royall D, Wolever TM, Jeejeebhoy KN. Evidence for colonic conservation of malabsorbed carbohydrates in short bowel syndrome. Am J Gastroenterol 1992;87:751–6.
5. Keller J, Panter H, Layer P. Management of the short bowel syndrome after extensive small bowel resection. Best Pract Res Clin Gastroenterol 2004;18:977–92.
6. Weser E. Nutritional aspects of malabsorption. Am J Med 1979;67:1014–20.
7. Williamson RC. Intestinal adaptation (first of two parts). Structural, functional and cytokinetic changes. N Engl J Med 1978;298:1393–402.
8. Williamson RC. Intestinal adaptation (second of two parts). Mechanisms of control. N Engl J Med 1978;298:1444–50.
9. Schulzke JD, Fromm M, Bentzel CJ, et al. Ion transport in the experimental short bowel syndrome of the rat. Gastroenterology 1992;102:497–504.
10. Gouttebel MC, Saint AB, Colette C, et al. Intestinal adaptation in patients with short bowel syndrome. Measurement of calcium absorption. Dig Dis Sci 1989; 34:709–15.
11. Keller J, Runzi H, Goebell P, Layer P. Duodenal and ileal nutrient deliveries regulate human intestinal motor and pancreatic responses to a meal. Am J Physiol 1997;272: G632–7.
12. Layer P, Peschel S, Schlesinger T, Goebell H. Human pancreatic secretion and intestinal motility: effects of ileal nutrient perfusion. Am J Physiol 1990;258:G196–201.
13. Scolapio JS, Camilleri M, Fleming CR, et al. Effect of growth hormone, glutamine, and diet on adaptation in short-bowel syndrome: a randomized, controlled study. Gastroenterology 1997;113:1074–81.
14. Szkudlarek J, Jeppesen J, Mortensen PB. Effect of high dose growth hormone with glutamine and no change in diet on intestinal adsorption in short bowel patients: a randomized, double-blind, crossover, placebo-controlled study. Gut 2000;47:199–205.
15. Urban E, Weser E. Intestinal adaptation to bowel resection. Adv Intern Med 1980;26:265–91.
16. Weser E. Luminal nutrients and intestinal adaptation. J Pediatr Gastroenterol Nutr 1985;4:164–6.
17. Heyland DK, Samis A. Does immunonutrition in patients with sepsis do more harm than good? Intensive Care Med 2003;29:669–71.
18. Luyer MD, Jacobs, JA, Vreugdenhil AC, et al. Enteral administration of high-fat nutrition before and directly after hemorrhagic shock reduces endotoxemia and bacterial translocation. Ann Surg 2004;239:257–64.
19. Kato J, Sakamoto J, Teramukai S, et al. A prospective within-patient comparison clinical trial on the effect of parenteral cimetidine for improvement of fluid secretion
and electrolyte balance in patients with short bowel syndrome. Hepatogastroenterology 2004;51:1742–6.
20. Kelly DG, Nadeau J. Oral rehydration solution: a "low tech" oft neglected therapy. Pract Gastroenterol 2004;28: 51–62.
21. Kramer P Effect of antidiarrheal and antimotility drugs on ileal excreta. Am J Dig Dis 1977;22:327–32.
22. Rodrigues CA, Lennard-Jones JE, Thompson DG, Farthing MJ. The effects of octreotide, soy polysaccharide, codeine and loperamide on nutrient, fluid and electrolyte absorption in the short-bowel syndrome. Aliment Pharmacol Ther 1989;3:159–69.
23. Nightingale JM, Walker ER, Burnham WR, et al. Octreotide (a somatostatin analog) improves the quality of life in some patients with a short intestine. Aliment Pharmcol Ther 1989;3:367–73.
24. Nehra V, Camilleri M, Burton D, et al. An open trial of octreotide long-acting release in the management of short bowel syndrome. Am J Gastroenterol 2001;96:1494–8.
25. Chagas EH, Kelly DG, Camilleri M, Burritt MF. Oral magnesium gluconate increases urinary Mg 2+ in patient with short bowel syndrome. Gastroenterology 2003;124: A-430.
26. Mamel J. Percutaneous endoscopic gastrostomy. Am J Gastroenterol 1989;84:703–10.
27. Choi RS, Vacanti JP. Preliminary studies of tissue-engineered intestine using isolated epithelial organoid units on tubular synthetic biodegradable scaffolds. Transplant Proc 1997;29:848–51.
28. Grikscheit TC, Siddique ABA, Ochoa ER, et al. Tissue-engineered small intestine improves recovery after massive small bowel resection. Ann Surg 2004;240: 748–54.
29. Bruno MJ, Haverkort EB, Tijssen GP, et al. Placebo controlled trial of enteric coated pancreatin microsphere treatment in patients with unresectable cancer of the pancreatic head region. Gut 1998;42:92–6.
30. Armstrong T, Walters E, Varshney S, Johnson CD. Deficiencies of micronutrients, altered bowel function and quality of life during late follow-up after pancreaticoduodenectomy for malignancy. Pancreatology 2002;2:528–34.
31. Parnes HL, Fung E, Schiffer CA. Chemotherapy-induced lactose intolerance in adults. Cancer 1994;74:1629–33.
32. Osterlund P, Ruotsalainen T, Peuhkuri K, et al. Lactose intolerance associated with adjuvant 5-fluorouracil-based chemotherapy for colorectal cancer. Clin Gastroenterol Hepatol 2004;2:696–703.
33. Pearson AD, Craft AW, Pledger JV, et al. Small bowel function in acute lymphoblastic leukemia. Arch Dis Child 1984;59:460–5.
34. Meloni GF, Colombo C, LaVecchia C, et al. Lactose absorption in patients with ovarian cancer. Am J Epidemiol 1999;150:183–6.
35. Stryker JA, Bartholomew M. Failure of lactose-restricted diets to prevent radiation-induced diarrhea in patients undergoing whole pelvic irradiation. Int J Radiat Oncol Biol Phys 1986;12:789–92.
36. Weiss RG, Stryker JA. 14C-lactose breath tests during pelvic radiotherapy: the effect of the amount of small bowel irradiated. Radiology 1982;142:507–10.
37. Roviello F, Fotia G, Marrelli D, et al. Iron deficiency anemia after subtotal gastrectomy for gastric cancer. Hepatogastroenterology 2004;51:1510–4.
38. Farrell RJ, Kelly CP. Current concepts: celiac sprue. N Engl J Med 2002;346:180–8.
39. Bresky G, Mata A, Liach J, et al. Endoscopic findings in a biennial follow-up program in patients with pernicious anemia. Hepatogastroenterology 2003;50:2264–6.
40. Schafer LW, Larson DE, Melton LJ III, et al. Risk of development of gastric carcinoma in patients with pernicious anemia: a population-based study in Rochester, Minnesota. Mayo Clin Proc 1985;60:444–8.
41. Ye W, Nyren O. Risk of cancers of the oesophagus and stomach by histology or subsite in patients hospitalised for pernicious anemia. Gut 2003;52:939–41.
42. Andres E, Kaltenbach G, Noel E, et al. Efficacy of short-term oral cobalamin therapy for the treatment of cobalamin deficiencies related to food-cobalamin malabsorption: a study of 30 patients. Clin Lab Haematol 2003;25:161–6.
43. Yeoh E, Horowitz M, Russo A, et al. Effects of pelvic irradiation on gastrointestinal function: a prospective longitudinal study. Am J Med 1993;95:397–406.
44. Sharma N, Trope B, Lipman TO. Vitamin supplementation: what the gastroenterologist needs to know. J Clin Gastroenterol 2004;38:844–54.

45. Cavallaro R, Iovino P, Castiglione F, et al. Prevelance and clinical association of prolonged prothrombin time in adult untreated celiac disease. Eur J Gastroenterol Hepatol 2004;16:219–23.
46. Thomas MK, Lloyd-Jones DM, Thadhani RI, et al. Hypovitaminosis D in medical patients. N Engl J Med 1998; 338:777–83.
47. Bernstein CN, Leslie WD, Leboff MS. AGA technical review on osteoporosis in gastrointestinal diseases. Gastroenterology 2003;124:795–841.
48. Not T, Horvath K, Hill ID, et al. Celiac disease risk in the USA: high prevalence of antiendomysium antibodies in healthy blood donors. Scand J Gastroenterol 1998;33: 494–8.
49. Dieterich W, Laag E, Schopper H, et al. Autoantibodies to tissue transglutaminase as predictors of celiac disease. Gastroenterology 1998;115:1322–8.
50. Gershon MD. Review article: serotonin receptors and transporters—roles in normal and abnormal gastrointestinal motility. Aliment Pharmacol Ther 2004;7:3–14.
51. Dando TM, Perry CM. Aprepitant: a review of its use in the prevention of chemotherapy-induced nausea and vomiting. Drugs 2004;64:777–94.
52. Kris MG, Hesketh PJ, Herrstedt J, et al. Consensus proposals for the prevention of acute and delayed vomiting and nausea following high-emetic-risk chemotherapy. Support Care Cancer 2004;23. [Epub ahead of print]
53. Hesketh PJ. New treatment options for chemotherapy-induced nausea and vomiting. Support Care Cancer 2004; 12:550–4.
54. Grunberg SM. New developments in the management of chemotherapy-induced emesis: do they impact on existing guidelines? Oncology 2004;18:15–9.
55. Navari RM. Role of neurokinin-1 receptor antagonists in chemotherapy-induced emesis: summary of clinical trials. Cancer Invest 2004;22:569–76.
56. Haus U, Spath M, Farber L. Spectrum of use and tolerability of 5HT3 receptor antagonists. Scand J Rheumatol Suppl 2004;119:12–8.
57. Spencer GD, Hackman RC, McDonald GB, et al. A prospective study of unexplained nausea and vomiting after marrow transplantation. Transplantation 1986;42:602–7.
58. Weisdorf DJ, Snover DC, Haake R, et al. Acute upper gastrointestinal graft-versus-host disease: clinical significance and response to immunosuppressive therapy. Blood 1990; 76:624–9.
59. Lautenbach E, Lichtenstein GR. Retroperitoneal leiomyosarcoma and gastroparesis: a new association and review of tumor-associated intestinal pseudo-obstruction. Am J Gastroenterol 1995;90:1338–41.
60. Wildhaber B, Niggli F, Stallmach T, et al. Intestinal pseudoobstruction as a paraneoplastic syndrome in ganglioneuroblastoma. Eur J Pediatr Surg 2002;12: 429–31.
61. Chu G, Wilson PC, Carter CD, et al. Intestinal pseudo-obstruction, type 1 anti-neuronal nuclear antibodies and small-cell carcinoma of the lung. J Gastroenterol Hepatol 1993;8:604–6.
62. Barkin JS, Goldberg RI, Sfakianakis GN, et al. Pancreatic carcinoma is associated with delayed gastric emptying. Dig Dis Sci 1986;31:265–7.
63. De Giorgio R, Barbara G, Stangehellini V, et al. Idiopathic myenteric ganglionitis underlying intractable vomiting in a young adult. Eur J Gastroenterol Hepatol 2000;12: 613–6.
64. Iftikhar S, Loftus EV Jr. Gastroparesis after celiac block. Am J Gastroenterol 1998;93:2223–5.
65. Shivshanker K, Bennett R, Haynie TP. Tumor associated gastroparesis: correction with metoclopramide. Am J Surg 1983;145:221–5.
66. Talley N. Diabetic gastropathy and prokinetics. Am J Gastroenterol 2003;98:264–71.
67. O'Donovan D, Feinle-Bisset C, Jones K, Horowitz M. Idiopathic and diabetic gastroparesis. Curr Treat Options Gastroenterol 2003;6:299–309.
68. Lacy B, Crowell MD, Schettler-Duncan A, et al. The treatment of diabetic gastroparesis with botulinum toxin injection of the pylorus. Diabetes Care 2004;27:2341–7.
69. Dishy V, Cohen PM, Feldman L, et al. The effect of sildenafil on gastric emptying in patients with end-stage renal failure and symptoms of gastroparesis. Clin Pharmacol Ther 2004;76:281–6.
70. Jones MP, Maganti K. A systematic review of surgical therapy for gastroparesis. Am J Gastroenterol 2003;98:2122–9.
71. Scarpignato C. The place of octreotide in the medical management of the dumping syndrome. Digestion 1996;57: 114–8.
72. Hasler WL. Dumping syndrome. Curr Treat Options Gastroenterol 2002;5:139–45.
73. Li-Ling J, Irving M. Therapeutic value of octreotide for patients with severe dumping syndrome—a review of randomized controlled trials. Postgrad Med J 2001;77: 441–2.
74. DeLillo AR, Rose S. Functional bowel disorders in the geriatric patient: constipation, fecal impaction and fecal incontinence. Am J Gastroenterol 2000;95:901–5.
75. Hall GR, Karstens M, Rakel B, et al. Managing constipation using a research-based protocol. Med Surg Nurs 1995;4: 11–8.
76. Adeniji OA, Dipalma JA. Prevalence of medication-associated constipation. Am J Gastroenterol 2001;96: S140.
77. Phillips C, Polakoff D, Maue SK, Mauch R. Assessment of constipation management in long-term care patients. J Am Med Dir Assoc 2001;2:149–54.
78. Lau PM, Stewart K, Dooley M. The ten most common adverse drug reactions (ADRs) in oncology patients: do they matter to you? Support Care Cancer 2004;12: 626–33.
79. Friedrichsen M, Erichsen E. The lived experience of constipation in cancer patients in palliative hospital-based home care. Int J Palliat Nurs 2004;10:321–5.
80. Talley NJ. Definitions, epidemiology and impact of chronic constipation. Rev Gastroenterol Disord 2004;4:S3–10.
81. Anti M, Pignataro G, Armuzzi A, et al. Water supplementation enhances the effect of high-fiber diet on stool frequency and laxative consumption in adult patients with functional constipation. Hepatogastroenterology 1998;45: 727–32.
82. Graham D, Moser S, Estes M. The effect of bran on bowel function in constipation. Gastroenterology 1982;77: 599–603
83. Marlett JA, Li BU, Patrow CJ, Bass P. Comparative laxation of psyllium with and without senna in an ambulatory constipated population. Am J Gastroenterol 1987;82: 333–7.
84. Bass P, Clark C, DoPico GA. Comparison of the laxative efficacy and patient preference of calcium polycarbophil and psyllium suspension. Curr Ther Res Clin Exp 1988; 43:770–4.
85. Hamilton J, Wagner J, Burdick B, Bass P. Clinical evaluation of methylcellulose as a bulk laxative. Dig Dis Sci 1988;33: 993–8.
86. Phillips C, Polakoff D, Maue SK, Mauch R. Assessment of constipation management in long-term care patients. J Am Med Dir Assoc 2001;2:149–54.
87. Castle SC, Cantrell M, Israel DS, Samuelson MJ. Constipation prevention: empiric use of stool softeners questioned. Geriatrics 1991;46:84–6.
88. Fain AM, Susat R, Herring M, Dorton K. Treatment of Constipation in Geriatric and Chronically III Patients: A Comparison. South Med J 1978;71:677–80.
89. Wald A. Slow transit constipation. Curr Treat Options Gastroenterol 2002;5:279–83.
90. Cleveland MV, Flavin DP, Ruben RA, et al. New polyethelene glycol laxative for treatment of constipation in adults: a randomized, double-blind placebo-controlled study. South Med J 2001;94:478–81.
91. DiPalma JA, DeRidder PH, Orlando RC, et al. Am J Gastroenterol 2000;95:446–50.
92. Tiongco F, Tsand T, Pollack J. Use of oral GoLytely solution in relief of refractory fecal impaction. Dig Dis Sci 1997; 42:1454–7.
93. Lederle FA, Busch DL, Mattox KM, et al. Cost-effective treatment of constipation in the elderly: a randomized double-blind comparison of sorbitol and lactulose. Am J Med 1990;89:597–601.
94. Soffer EE, Metcalf A, Launspach J. Misoprostol is effective treatment for patients with severe chronic constipation. Dig Dis Sci 1994;39:929–33.
95. Roarty TP, Weber F, Soykan I, McCallum RW. Misoprostol in the treatment of chronic refractory constipation: results of a long-term open label trial. Aliment Pharmacol Ther 1997;11:1059–66.
96. Verne GN, Eaker EY, Davis RH, Sninsky CA. Colchicine is an effective treatment for patients with chronic constipation: an open label trial. Dig Dis Sci 1997;42:1959–63.
97. Verne GN, Davis RH, Robinson ME, et al. Treatment of chronic constipation with colchicine randomized double-blind, placebo controlled trial. Am J Gastroenterol 2003; 98:1112–6.
98. Johanson JF, Wald A, Tougas G, et al. Effect of tegaserod in chronic constipation: a randomized, double blind, controlled trial. Clin Gastroenterol Hepatol 2004;2: 796–805.
99. Novick J, Miner P, Krause R, et al. A randomized double-blind, placebo controlled trial of tegaserod in female patients suffering from irritable bowel syndrome with constipation. Aliment Pharmacol Ther 2002;16:1877–88.
100. Ismail EA, Al-Mutairi G, Al-Anzy H. A fatal small dose of phosphate enema in a young child with no renal or gastrointestinal abnormality. J Pediatr Gastroenterol Nutr 2000;30:220–1
101. Marraffa JM, Hui A, Stork CM. Severe hyperphosphatemia and hypocalcemia following the rectal administration of a phosphate-containing Fleet pediatric enema. Pediatr Emerg Care 2004;20:453–6.
102. Walker M, Warner BW, Brilli RJ, Jacobs BR. Cardiopulmonary compromise associated with milk and molasses enema use in children. J Pediatr Gastroenterol Nutr 2003; 36:144–8.
103. Vanek VW, Al-Salti M. Acute pseudo-obstruction of the colon (Ogilvie's syndrome): an analysis of 400 cases. Dis Colon Rectum 1986;29:203–10.
104. Carne PW, Frye JN, Robertson GM, Frizelle FA. Stents or open operation for palliation of colorectal cancer; a retrospective, cohort study of perioperative outsome and long-term survival. Dis Colon Rectum 2004;47:1455–61.
105. Johnson R, Marsh R, Corson J, Seymour K. A comparison of two methods of palliation of large bowel obstruction due to irremovable colon cancer. Ann R Coll Surg Engl 2004; 86:99–103.
106. Mauro MA, Koehler RE, Baron TH. Advances in gastrointestinal intervention: the treatment of gastroduodenal and colorectal obstructions with metallic stents. Radiology 2000;215:659–69.
107. Eckhauser ML, Mansour EG. Endoscopic laser therapy for obstructing and/or bleeding colorectal carcinoma. Am Surg 1992;58:358–63.
108. Ortner MA, Dorta G, Blum AL, Michetti P. Endoscopic intervention for preneoplastic and neoplastic lesions: mucosectomy, argon plasma coagulation, and photodynamic therapy. Dig Dis Sci 2002;20:167–72.
109. Benson AB, Ajani JA, Catalano RB, et al. Recommended guidelines for the treatment of cancer treatment-induced diarrhea. J Clin Oncol 2004;22:2918–26.
110. Martenson JA Jr, Hyland G, Moertel CG, et al. Olsalazine is contraindicated during pelvic irradiation therapy: results of a double-blind, randomized clinical trial. Int J Radiat Oncol Biol Phys 1996;35:299–303.
111. Yavuz MN, Yavuz AA, Aydin F, et al. The efficacy of octreotide in the therapy of acute radiation-induced diarrhea: a randomized controlled study. Int J Radiat Oncol Biol Phys 2002;54:195–202.
112. Gebbia V, Carreca I, Testa A, et al. Subcutaneous octreotide versus oral loperamide in the treatment of diarrhea following chemotherapy. Anticancer Drugs 1993;4: 443–5.
113. Danielsson A, Nyhlin H, Persson H, et al. Chronic diarrhea after radiotherapy for gynecological cancer: occurrence and etiology. Gut 1990;32:1180–7.
114. Carpenter CCJ. Clinical and pathophysiological features of diarrhea caused by *vibrio cholera* and *Escherichia coli*. In: Field M, Fordtran JS, Schultz SG, editors. Secretory diarrhea. Bethesda (MD): American Physiological Society; 1980. p. 67–83.
115. Kelly CP, Pothoulakis C, LaMont JT. Clostridium difficile colitis. N Engl J Med 1994;330:257–62.
116. Blot F, Escande MC, Besson D, et al. Outbreak of Clostridium difficile-related diarrhoea in an adult oncology unit: risk factors and microbiological characteristics. J Hosp Infect 2003;53:187–92.
117. Turgeon DK, Novicki TJ, Quick J, et al. Six rapid tests for direct detection of Clostridium difficile and its toxins in fecal samples compared with the fibroblast cytotoxicity assay. J Clin Microbiol 2003;41:667–70.
118. Teasley DG, Gerding DN, Olson MM, et al. Prospective randomized trial of metronidazole versus vancomycin for Clostridium-difficile-associated diarrhoea and colitis. Lancet 1983;2:1043–6.
119. Bartlett JG. Antibiotic-associated diarrhea. N Engl J Med 2002;346:334–9.
120. Fekety R, Silva J. Kauffman C, et al. Treatment of antibiotic-associated Clostridium difficile colitis with oral vancomycin: comparison of two dosage regimens. Am J Med 1989;86:15–9.

121. Chang TW, Gorbach SL, Bartlett JG, Saginur R. Bacitracin treatment of antibiotic-associated-colitis and diarrhea caused by Clostridium difficile toxin. Gastroenterology 1980;78:1584–6.

122. Fekety R, McFarland LV, Surawicz CM, et al. Recurrent Clostridium difficile diarrhea: characteristics of and risk factors for patients enrolled in a prospective, randomized, double-blinded trial. Clin Infect Dis 1997;24: 324–33.

123. Stroehlein J. Treatment of Clostridium difficile infection. Curr Treat Options Gastroenterol 2004;7:235–9.

124. Yolken RH, Bishop CA, Townsend TR, et al. Infectious gastroenteritis in bone-marrow transplant recipients. N Engl J Med 1982;306:1010–2.

125. El-Mahallawy HA, El-Din NH, Salah F, et al. Epidemiologic profile of symptomatic gastroenteritis in pediatric oncology patients receiving chemotherapy. Pediatr Blood Cancer 2004;42:338–42.

126. Gorschluter M, Glasmacher A, Hahn C, et al. Clostridium difficile infection in patients with neutropenia. Clin Infect Dis 2001;33:786–91.

127. Cirisano FD, Greenspoon JS, Stenson R, et al. The etiology and management of diarrhea in the gynecologic oncology patient. Gynecol Oncol 1993;50:45–8.

128. Bini EJ, Weinshel EH. Endoscopic evaluation of chronic human immunodeficiency virus related diarrhea: is colonoscopy superior to flexible sigmoidoscopy? Am J Gastroenterol 1998;93:56–60.

129. Degen L, Beglinger C. The role of octreotide in the treatment of gastroenteropancreatic endocrine tumors. Digestion 1999;60 Suppl 2:9–14.

130. Harris AG, O'Dorisio TM, Woltering EA, et al. Consensus statement: octreotide dose titration in secretory diarrhea. Diarrhea Management Consensus Development Panel. Dig Dis Sci 1995;40:1464–75.

131. Gorden P, Comi RJ, Maton PN, Go VL. NIH conference. Somatostatin and somatostatin analogue (SMS 201-995) in treatment of hormone-secreting tumors of the pituitary and gastrointestinal tract and non-neoplastic diseases of the gut. Ann Intern Med 1989;110:35–50.

132. Schiller LR. Chronic diarrhea. In: McNally PR, editor. GI/ liver secrets. 2nd ed. Philadelphia: Hanley & Belfus; 2002. p. 411.

Graft Versus Host Disease and the Immunologic Complications of Cancer

William A. Ross, MD, MBA

A wide spectrum of immunologic derangements are associated with cancer and its treatment. They range from immunosuppression to enhanced, albeit dysfunctional, performance. This chapter focuses on one such manifestation of immunologic dysfunction, namely graft-versus-host disease (GVHD) following allogeneic hematopoietic stem cell transplantation (HSCT). A brief discussion of three other dysfunctional immune responses concludes the chapter. The conditions discussed include two examples of constant antigenic stimulation resulting in cancer and an example of tumor-associated autoantibody production.

Graft-versus-Host Disease

GVHD is a frequent major complication of allogeneic HSCT. The likelihood of occurrence is directly related to the degree of human leukocyte antigen (HLA) incompatibility between donor and recipient. The pathogenesis is discussed in detail in Chapter 62. Briefly, three conditions must exist for GVHD to occur: (1) competent T cells are introduced with the graft, (2) antigenic differences between the host and the graft are sufficient to activate the donated T cells, and (3) the host immune response is insufficient to reject the graft.[1] GVHD prophylactic regimens are designed to suppress the donor-derived immune response without endangering the survival of the graft or putting the patient at too great a risk of infectious complications.[2] In addition, some aspects of the donor immune response manifesting as GVHD also account for the beneficial graft-versus-tumor effect seen after allogeneic HSCT.[3] The graft-versus-tumor effect probably accounts for the improved survival in patients with mild GVHD compared with those with no GVHD after allogeneic HSCT.[4] So a fine balancing act is required between donor and recipient immune systems as well as graft response to host-versus-tumor antigens.

Gastrointestinal (GI) tract damage during pretransplantation conditioning regimens plays a key role in GVHD development by creating a proinflammatory environment into which donor T cells are introduced.[5] The inflammatory cytokines activate donated T cells and stimulate them to multiply. These cells are attracted preferentially to the three organs that are involved in acute GVHD: the skin, liver, and gut. Acute GVHD is traditionally defined as onset in the first 100 days after transplantation. Chronic GVHD, traditionally defined as onset after the first 100 days, has a more diffuse organ system involvement. Whereas liver and oral cavity involvement is prominent in chronic GVHD, GI involvement is not.[6] Skin GVHD is discussed in Chapter 62. The focus of this chapter is on manifestations of GVHD in the liver, gut, and oral cavity.

Clinically significant acute GVHD is seen in 20 to 50% of patients following HLA-matched sibling HSCT. If the donor is unrelated or an HLA-mismatched sibling, then the incidence of significant GVHD increases to 60 to 80%.[7] The skin is the most commonly involved organ in acute GVHD, seen in 80 to 85% of patients.[8] GI tract involvement is seen in more than 50% of GVHD patients and is being increasingly recognized with more liberal use of endoscopy to evaluate GI complaints.[9] Liver involvement is seen in half of patients. Although initially felt to be rare in the absence of skin involvement, both gut and hepatic GVHD can present in lieu of any other organ involvement. Symptoms of GI involvement include diarrhea, abdominal pain, bleeding, nausea, and vomiting. Liver involvement is manifested primarily by cholestasis, with minimal hepatitis. Onset of acute GVHD is typically in the first 2 months post-transplantation. The differential diagnosis is extensive for both GI symptoms and abnormal liver function tests, with the after-effects of the conditioning regimen being a major concern, particularly in the first 2 or 3 weeks post-transplantation. Infections are high on the list owing to the neutropenic state that exists prior to engraftment and the frequent use of immunosuppressive therapy through the post-HSCT period. Drug toxicity remains on the differential diagnosis throughout the post-transplantation period.

Gastrointestinal GVHD

GI GVHD is readily diagnosed with endoscopic biopsy. The sine qua non is apoptosis, with an intracyptal location being the most specific.[10,11] However, apoptosis is not unique for GVHD and is associated with a number of drugs and infections common after HSCT. In the first 3 weeks post-HSCT, the conditioning regimen can account for apoptosis and complicate the evaluation in this early phase.[12] Cytomegalovirus can also cause apoptosis; however, its clinical significance has been much reduced with prophylactic use of antivirals.[13–15] More recently, *Cryptosporidium* has been described as causing apoptosis in an HSCT patient.[16] Drugs described as inducing apoptosis include cyclosporine, mycophenolate mofetil, ticlopidine, and nonsteroidal anti-inflammatory drugs.[17–20]

Diagnosis

There is some disagreement in the endoscopic literature as to what portion of the gut to biopsy for the highest diagnostic yield. Some argue that GVHD involves the entire gut and that the site of biopsy is not critical. The traditional approach has been to perform rectal biopsies. Early reports suggested good correlation with symptoms and more proximal intestinal disease.[21] However, later reports touted the utility of gastric biopsies even in those patients presenting with diarrhea.[22] The concept that GVHD represented a panintestinal process was challenged by data showing a lack of congruence between simultaneous rectal and gastric biopsies in 28% of patients.[23] Unlike early studies, endoscopic impressions and symptoms were found to correlate poorly with histology.[23] Although gastric biopsies were touted as the best approach, data existed suggesting a potential to underestimate the severity of more distal disease.[24] Reports of duodenal hematomas after biopsy in thrombocytopenic post-HSCT patients led to reluctance to biopsy the duodenum despite its endoscopically more impressive involvement.[22,24] However, others feel that duodenal biopsies produce the highest yield and are safe.[25,26]

Finally, some feel that the traditional approach to biopsy the rectum remains adequate.[27] The result is that no standard endoscopic approach to diagnosing gastrointestinal GVHD exists.[28] Our approach at The University of Texas M. D. Anderson Cancer Center is to biopsy the rectum, stomach, and duodenum in those patients referred for suspected GI GVHD.

The safety of endoscopic evaluation in this patient population has not been evaluated in a systematic fashion. Procedure-related mortality has been reported to be as high as 1.8%.[29] Our experience would argue for a much lower procedural mortality risk. Yet an ongoing concern in these frequently thrombocytopenic patients is bleeding from endoscopic biopsy. Reports on severe gastrointestinal bleeding following HSCT do not include any related to endoscopic biopsy.[30,31] However, colon perforation and duodenal hematomas have been described.[29,32] A platelet count of at least 50,000/cu mm is recommended by some authors prior to endoscopic biopsy.[24] Others feel that this threshold may be excessive, entailing unnecessary use of valuable blood products, and that a lower threshold would be equally efficacious.[28] There are few firm data to provide guidance. An ongoing review of our experience at M. D. Anderson may provide some insight on this question. Finally, the risk of infection in light of the prevalent neutropenia, particularly early after HSCT, is a concern. Again, the available published data are scanty and contradictory, with some reports showing increased risk of bacteremia and others finding none.[33,34] No specific recommendations regarding antibiotic prophylaxis for endoscopy exist for immunosuppressed patients, let alone those following HSCT.[35]

Clinical Manifestations

Diarrhea is a prominent symptom of gastrointestinal GVHD, and stool volume is the main parameter by which GI GVHD is graded (Table 1).[36] GVHD is the most frequent cause of diarrhea in allogeneic HSCT patients after the first 20 days post-transplantation.[22,37] The diarrhea is secretory and frequently refractory to antidiarrheals. Octreotide has been reported to be of benefit in some patients.[38]

Although GI complaints are frequent in patients with chronic GVHD, direct involvement of the gut by isolated chronic GVHD is felt to be rare.[6] Unresolved or recurrent acute GI GVHD accounts for the bulk of GI symptoms.[6] Some patients will develop de novo acute GI GVHD after day 100.[39] Other factors to consider are pancreatic insufficiency and infections in these immunosuppressed patients.[40] Weight loss and malnutrition are common in chronic GVHD patients, with 41% having a greater than 10% weight loss and 14% with a body mass index less than 18.5.[41,42] However, weight loss was not associated with gut GVHD, abdominal pain, dysphagia, or oral sensitivity. Weight loss and malnutrition were more likely in those patients with active chronic GVHD. Patients with extensive chronic GVHD have been shown to have increased resting energy expenditure compared with normal controls, which may contribute to weight loss.[43] The situation may be comparable to the cachexia seen in other chronic nonmalignant conditions and may not be related to gut dysfunction induced by GVHD.[44]

Oral GVHD

Oral mucositis occurs in two-thirds of patients in the first weeks following HSCT.[45] This early injury is secondary to the pretransplantation conditioning regiment, particularly if total-body radiation is employed.[45,46] Although allogeneic HSCT is a risk factor for oral mucositis in some reports, there appears to be no association between mucositis and subsequent acute GVHD.[45] Resolution is rapid and coincides with engraftment. If mucositis persists despite neutrophil counts exceeding 500/cu mm, then acute oral GVHD must be considered, although this is rare.[47]

However, oral lesions are a very frequent manifestation of chronic GVHD and are a major complaint of post-HSCT patients.[48–50] A composite score of oral abnormalities was correlated with decreasing performance status.[51] Some 60 to 80% of chronic GVHD patients will have oral involvement, with the skin being the only site more frequently involved.[49,50] The history and physical examination can be suggestive but are not diagnostic. Lichenoid lesions have a sensitivity of 61% and a specificity of 53%.[52] Salivary flow rates are diminished in chronic oral GVHD, but subjective xerostomia is a common complaint in HSCT patients with or without GVHD.[52,53] The histology of buccal mucosa or labial salivary glands is suggestive but not diagnostic.[52]

The best treatment is successful systemic therapy.[54] Case reports of resolution with various topical agents have appeared.[55] Long term, the risk of subsequent oral cancers is increased.[56]

Hepatic GVHD

GVHD involving the liver is just one of a number of potential etiologies of liver dysfunction following HSCT. The gambit of diseases was recently reviewed.[57] Acute hepatic GVHD typically presents as cholestasis, with very modest transaminase elevations in the first month or so after HSCT. However, abnormal liver function tests are very common after HSCT, being seen in up to 80% of patients.[57] The timing after HSCT can give some guidance as to probable etiologies. In the first few weeks following HSCT, the after-effects of the conditioning regimen must be considered. The first 3 weeks after HSCT is also prime time for veno-occlusive disease (VOD), which usually presents as cholestasis and right upper quadrant pain. After the initial 20 days of GVHD, drug toxicity and sepsis are the primary causes of abnormal liver tests.[58,59] In some patients, the cholestasis is multifactorial, with GVHD being the most prevalent in allogeneic HSCT and drug toxicity being the most common etiology after autologous HSCT.[58,60] The ability to test for hepatitis C virus (HCV) has simplified the picture by reducing its prevalence in HSCT patients.[60]

Cholestasis in the first few weeks associated with right upper quadrant pain, hepatomegaly, weight gain, and/or ascites makes VOD a prime consideration. Unfortunately, clinical criteria are not specific unless adhered to strictly, which decreases sensitivity to 56%.[61] Owing to the varying means of defining the diagnosis, the incidence is reported to be as low as 1% and up to 54%.[62–64] More recent reports tend to be at the lower end of this range.[65] Approximately one-quarter of affected patients will have severe VOD and be at high risk of fulminant hepatic failure.[63,65] Biopsy is useful in establishing a diagnosis, but thrombocytopenia early after HSCT dictates a transjugular approach.[61] The prognosis is dismal for severe

Table 1 Grading System for Acute Graft-versus-Host Disease			
Stage	*Skin*	*Liver*	*GI*
1	< 25% BSA	Bilirubin 2–3 mg/dL	Diarrhea 500–1,000 cc/d or persistent nausea
2	25–50% BSA	Bilirubin 3–6 mg/dL	Diarrhea 1–1.5 L/d
3	Generalized Erythroderma	Bilirubin 6–15 mg/dL	Diarrhea > 1.5 L/d
4	Desquamation	Bilirubin > 15 mg/dL	Severe abdominal pain or ileus

Grade	*Severity*	*Skin*		*Liver*		*Gut*
0	None	0		0		0
I	Mild	1–2		0		0
II	Moderate	3	*or*	1	*or*	1
III	Severe			2–3	*or*	2–3
IV	Life-threatening	4	*or*	4	*or*	4

BSA = body surface area; GI = gastrointestinal.

disease as effective therapeutic options are limited. Transjugular intrahepatic portosystemic shunt can reduce portal pressure but has not been shown to improve survival.[66] Defibrotide, a single-stranded polydeoxyribonucleotide with fibrinolytic, antithrombotic, and anti-ischemic properties, has some promise to help patients with severe VOD.[67]

Complicating the diagnosis of hepatic GVHD in some patients is the atypical presentation as an acute hepatitis.[59] In US reports, this presentation tends to be seen when immunosuppressive therapy is being tapered[68] or after donor lymphocyte infusions.[69] A different form was reported in a large series from Hong Kong, where 36% of all liver GVHD patients presented with an acute hepatitis picture.[59] There was no association with changes in immunosuppression or donor lymphocyte infusions as the onset of abnormal liver function tests was within days of that seen with the classic cholestasis picture. Peak bilirubin was the same in both types. However, mean peak transaminase levels were three to four times that seen in classic hepatic GVHD. Resolution with therapy took longer with the acute hepatitis–type presentation. Pathology shows more lobular hepatitis, with hepatocyte necrosis and acidophil bodies. Cholestasis and bile duct injury are less marked.[59,69]

A liver biopsy may clarify the situation in evaluating the HSCT patient with abnormal liver function tests, but it is rarely diagnostic in isolation and must be considered, along with clinical data. Many of the classic reports on liver pathology in HSCT were done prior to the ability to test for hepatitis C.[70,71] Retrospective analysis showed that HCV had a pretransplantation prevalence in a US center of 17%, which increased to 32% post-transplantation.[72] So some of the patients in these early reports on the pathology of hepatic GVHD probably had underlying HCV as well, making it difficult to distinguish the histologic changes unique to GVHD. Still, certain features are felt to be very suggestive of GVHD. These include prominent bile duct atypia with pleiomorphism and, in advanced cases, bile duct dropout. Endothelialitis was felt in early reports to be very suggestive of GVHD but not so in others.[70,71] Inflammatory infiltrates tend to be modest at this early stage of bone marrow reconstitution, and piecemeal necrosis is rare.[73] These changes take time to develop, so early biopsy, within 4 weeks of transplantation, can be unhelpful in establishing a diagnosis of GVHD.[70,71] If GHVD-induced jaundice has been present for 2 weeks or more, liver biopsy should contain findings suggestive of GVHD.[73,74] Unlike with early skin or gastrointestinal biopsies, there is no confusion with the hepatic effects of the preconditioning regimen.[75]

Chronic hepatic GVHD shows more extensive cholestasis with bile duct dropout and an increasing amount of periductal inflammatory infiltration as bone marrow function improves.[74] Portal fibrosis can be seen, but progression to cirrhosis is rare unless another disease process intervenes.[75] Changes among the hepatocytes are minimal.[73] Early surveys put liver involvement in chronic GVHD at 40 to 60%, but these may include chronic HCV patients.[49] More recent reports put the prevalence in the 30 to 40% range.[6,50] Although reports of development of cirrhosis in the setting of chronic GVHD exist, these are mostly prior to the ability to test for HCV.[76] So it is unclear if the cirrhosis is truly due to GVHD or from HCV. Another potential confounding factor is the high prevalence of iron overload in HCST patients owing to their transfusion requirements.[77] A report on 31 cases of cirrhosis in 3,721 HSCT patients who survived at least 1 year found no association with GVHD.[78] Data were collected from 1969 to 1995, when full viral serologic testing was available only in the later years. As a result, the hepatitis viruses played predominant roles in patients with cirrhosis. Twenty-five of the 31 cases had HCV, and 5 of these had hepatitis B virus coinfections. One case each could be attributed to autoimmune hepatitis and drug toxicity. Only one case had GVHD as the sole risk factor for liver disease. The authors felt that GVHD could accelerate liver injury in a patient with HCV but that GVHD alone was an extremely rare cause of cirrhosis.

Treatment for GVHD

The best management strategy is to minimize conditions that foster GVHD, namely HLA incompatibilities between donor and recipient. More sophisticated matching techniques have the potential to make unrelated donors as useful a source of stem cells as matched siblings.[79] Adding methotrexate to the prophylactic regimen with cyclosporine has helped reduce the incidence of GVHD.[80] Use of antithymocyte globulin (ATG) as part of the pretransplantation conditioning regimen in unrelated donor transplants can reduce both acute and chronic GVHD to levels seen with match-related donor transplants undergoing standard non-ATG containing preconditioning.[81] Despite the reduced incidence of GVHD, increases in long-term survival rates have been more difficult to demonstrate with prophylactic ATG.[82–84] This failure reflects a higher incidence of relapse and infectious complications at doses of ATG 10 mg/kg and greater.[84] However, too low a dose of ATG (eg, 4 mg/kg) has no effect on GVHD incidence. The question of the most appropriate dose was debated in recent reports.[85]

Systemic steroids are the first-line therapy for GVHD. Unfortunately, only half of patients respond, and there is no standard second-line therapy.[8] Acute hepatic GVHD is more refractory to treatment than skin or gut disease, with more patients progressing on therapy than responding.[8] This relative refractoriness for hepatic GVHD persists with second-line therapies as well.[86,87]

Although a wide range of agents have been tried in steroid-refractory GVHD, only recent reports are reviewed here. ATG has also been reported as a second-line therapy, with some series going back decades.[86,88] The results are mixed, with the group from Johns Hopkins University reporting extremely poor results, whereas the University of Minnesota group reported more favorable results.[88,89] Timing of the ATG administration may partially explain the disparity in the results as initiation soon after the diagnosis is associated with a better response.[90] The best long-term survival rate reported is 32%, with half of the survivors suffering from chronic GVHD.[89] Although the long-term survival rate was better in responders than nonresponders, the difference did not reach statistical significance. Two randomized trials in Italy compared 7.5 and 15 mg/kg of rabbit ATG with placebo.[82] The low-dose ATG group showed no reduction in GVHD, and survival was comparable to that of controls. The high-dose ATG group showed a significant decrease in GVHD, particularly grades III and IV. However, an increase in lethal infections and deaths from relapse negated any survival benefit. So ATG failed to show benefit in transplant-related mortality, relapse, or overall survival. Chronic GVHD was seen at comparable rates in the low-dose group and controls. Even when data were pooled from both dosage groups, the ATG group had a significantly lower incidence of chronic GVHD: 39% versus 62%. The authors recommended the use of low-dose ATG in pre-transplantation GVHD prophylaxis and early post-transplantation use, almost preemptively, in patients at high risk of GVHD. A report from the same group found that blood urea nitrogen > 21 mg/dL and total bilirubin > 0.9 mg/dL on day 7 post-transplantation stratified patients into low- and high-risk groups for transplant-related mortality.[91] Using data such as these could potentially identify groups most likely to benefit from early intervention. Unfortunately, ATG is a double-edged sword, with its immunosuppressive effects decreasing GVHD but increasing the risk of infection. Transplant-related mortality in the patients treated with ATG is divided almost evenly among GVHD, infection, and other etiologies (eg, multiorgan failure and leukemia).[82] This compares with controls, in whom GVHD accounts for two of every three deaths.

Infliximab, a monoclonal antibody to tumor necrosis factor, has been shown to lead to complete responses in 62% of 21 patients with steroid-resistant acute GVHD.[87] The responses in GI GVHD are particularly striking. However, the incidence of infectious complications was very high, with 81% having a bacteria infection, 90% a viral infection, and half a fungal infection. Only one death was attributable to infection, but eight patients died of chronic GVHD, in whom infections frequently contribute to death. The survival rate at 30 months was 35%, with all survivors suffering from chronic GVHD. Basiliximab, a monoclonal antibody to the alpha chain of the interleukin-2 receptor, has been shown to lead to complete response in over half of 17 patients with steroid-resistant GVHD.[92] Most patients went on to develop chronic GVHD. However, no bacterial or fungal infections were reported. CMV reactivation was seen in five. One-third of patients had survived for more than 1 year at the time of the report. Whereas the response to infliximab was not associated with survival, the response to basiliximab was strongly associated with survival.

Combining tacrolimus with ATG was reported in a series of 20 patients with steroid-resistant or -dependent acute GVHD.[93] There were complete responses in 40% and partial responses in another 30%. Infectious complications were seen in 80% despite viral and fungal prophylaxis. Infections were directly responsible for deaths in 15% and contributed to deaths in an additional 10%. The long-term survival rate was 35% and was associated with a response to tacrolimus and ATG.

Oral budesonide has been reported to be beneficial in patients with acute GI GVHD.[94,95] For difficult to treat hepatic GVHD, intra-arterial administration of methotrexate with steroids has been employed, with mixed results.[96,97]

Management of chronic hepatic GVHD involves long-term steroids that can be supplemented with cyclosporine.[57] Ursodeoxycholic acid can improve laboratory parameters, but the effect on outcomes is unclear.[57] Gastrointestinal complaints in long-term survivors should prompt evaluation for recurrent acute GVHD and other etiologies, such as pancreatic insufficiency or infections.

Other Tumor-Associated Immunologic Complications

Helicobacter pylori and Mucosa-Associated Lymphoid Tissue Lymphoma

Helicobacter pylori infection induces formation of mucosa-associated lymphoid tissue (MALT), a structure not normally found in the stomach. Part of this lymphoid tissue formation is the development of B-lymphocyte clones and increasing number of T helper cells.[98,99] The B-cell expansion is polyclonal and T cell dependent. In a small subset of patients, a single B-cell clone will expand and cause destruction of surrounding glands, forming the characteristic lymphoepithelial lesions of MALT lymphoma.[100] The mechanism

causing migration from a polyclonal to a monoclonal B-cell response is unclear. Attempts to correlate MALT lymphoma with bacterial virulence factors have not been fruitful.[101,102] The monoclonal expansion is initially dependent on T cells, and helper T cells are frequently seen infiltrating the tumor.[103] The type of T-cell response to *H. pylori* infection may dictate whether the outcome is chronic gastritis, peptic ulcer, or lymphoma.[104] Curiously, the expanding B-cell clone produces antibodies that are not reactive to *H. pylori* but rather act on various autoantigens of the gastric mucosa.[105] So this clonal expansion is not a functional response to the infection. Rather, the constant antigenic stimulation brings about a T cell–mediated dysfunctional immunologic response, leading to a B-cell malignancy in a subset of infected patients. Withdrawal of the antigen by eradication of the *H. pylori* can eliminate the MALT lymphoma but frequently not the MALT or B-cell clonal population.[99,106] In about half of patients with remission, the monoclonal tumor cells persist for years without histologic evidence of disease.[107] With time, these cells may disappear, but their persistence readily explains recurrence of lymphoma with reinfection by *H. pylori*.[108] Follow-up studies also document recurrence of MALT lymphoma without the need for reinfection with *H. pylori*.[109]

In a subset of MALT lymphomas, their expansion becomes independent of *H. pylori* and antibiotics fail to induce remission. Pretreatment endoscopic ultrasonography can help identify patients not likely to completely respond to eradication alone.[110] Lymphoma extending beyond the submucosa is unlikely to respond to antibiotics.[108] Whereas the optimal therapy remains unclear for those refractory to eradication of *H. pylori*, overall survival remains impressive with the various modalities employed.[105,111] For those patients who respond to eradication, follow-up is for an indefinite period as histologic demonstration of complete remission with biopsy material alone is problematic[108,112] and the significance of the persisting monoclonal populations remains unclear.[113] Finally, there is a risk of early gastric adenocarcinoma in patients after *H. pylori* eradication.[114]

Some MALT lymphomas can transform into a high-grade lymphoma that is histologically indistinguishable from a diffuse large B-cell lymphoma. There is molecular genetic evidence that the high-grade lymphoma evolves from a low-grade state.[115] MALT lymphomas with synchronous low- and high-grade components have been described with some frequency.[116] The exact mechanism of transformation is not defined. However, factors felt to be important for promoting growth in low-grade MALT, such as tumor-associated T cells and autoantibodies, are felt to play a diminished role as the tumor transforms

into a high-grade state.[105,117] The driving force behind the transformation appears to be the cumulative effect of various genetic abnormalities.[117] The average age of patients with high-grade lesions is 8 years older than that of those with low-grade lesions, suggesting a long course of evolution from one form to another.[118] Isolated case reports of a complete response to *H. pylori* eradication exist for high-grade lesions.[119,120] So for the patient with *H. pylori* infection, eradication should be a component of therapy.[99]

Enteropathy-Type Intestinal T-Cell Lymphoma

Constant antigenic stimulation from gluten in the diet leads to a fivefold increase in intraepithelial lymphocytes (IELs) in patients with celiac disease (CD).[121] In some patients, the usual polyclonal increase may evolve in which a single clone predominates. This is commonly seen in the rare entities refractory sprue and ulcerative ileojejunitis.[122] Curiously, the monoclonal population has different immunophenotypic markers from IELs in normal small bowel or those in other CD patients.[123] The same aberrant monoclonal type is seen in enteropathy-type intestinal T-cell lymphoma (EITCL), as well as in nonlymphomatous intestinal mucosa in EITCL patients.[124] This led to the proposal that these aberrant monoclonal cells represent a cryptic lymphoma in refractory sprue and ulcerative ileojejunitis.[125,126] As in *H. pylori*–induced MALT lymphoma, the immunologic response is dysfunctional, with expansion of a monoclonal population with no role in the response to the original inciting antigen.

Although the overall incidence of non-Hodgkin's lymphoma (NHL) is increasing, its presentation in extranodal sites, such as the GI tract, is increasing at an even faster rate.[113] The stomach is the most common extranodal site, with the small bowel being the primary site in less than 2% of NHL patients. Most gastrointestinal NHLs, like MALT lymphomas, are B cell derived, with the number of T-cell lymphomas making up only 12% of the total.[127] Patients with celiac sprue make up only 1% of NHL patients, and not all of their lymphomas are EITCL.[128] Conversely, although most patients with T-cell intestinal lymphoma have celiac sprue, it is not a universal finding.[129] The increased cancer risk in CD patients is almost exclusively due to NHL.[130] CD patients have an odds ratio of 3.1 for NHL, 16.9 for GI involvement, and 19.2 for T-cell lymphoma. CD patients have a mortality rate that is twice the expected rate in the first 3 years after diagnosis, and this is primarily due to NHL.[130] These deaths are primarily in patients with signs of malabsorption and not those with milder forms of the disease.

For EITCL, the lymphoma most specific to CD, the prognosis is poor. The EITCL is usually diagnosed prior to the CD.[131] The patients frequently present with major complications of the EITCL, such as obstruction or perforation.[131,132] Chemotherapy is complicated by poor nutritional status in many patients. The actuarial 5-year survival rate is 19.7%, but the disease-free survival rate is only 3.2%.[131] This limited prognosis is seen in intestinal T-cell lymphoma in a nonenteropathy setting as well.[132] Preliminary results with high-dose chemotherapy followed by autologous stem cell transplantation for EITCL have been disappointing, with high transplant-related mortality and universal relapse.[133] Other reports in abstract form are slightly more sanguine.[134]

Autoantibodies

The interactions between the immune system and cancer are complex. Although immunosuppressed states are associated with an increased risk of cancer development, cancer itself can induce immunologic dysfunction. This may take the form of immunosuppression or enhanced, albeit misdirected, function.[135,136] One manifestation of the latter is the formation of autoantibodies associated with cancer. These are felt to be antibodies directed at a tumor antigen that is shared by other tissues, usually neurologic.[137] They are associated with a number of solid tumors, especially lung cancer, but their clinical significance for the most part remains unclear.[138] A handful of autoantibodies are associated with various paraneoplastic neurologic syndromes (see Chapter 44 for further discussion).[139] Some are directly implicated in the pathogenesis of the neurologic syndrome and tend to be directed at peripheral nervous system antigens. Examples are myasthenia gravis and Eaton-Lambert syndrome. However, there are an increasing number of autoantibodies to central nervous system sites being described associated with many neurologic paraneoplastic syndromes that have an unclear role in pathogenesis.[140] Their number seems even larger as they are referred to in the literature by two parallel sets of nomenclature (Table 2).[141] These autoantibodies are most commonly seen with the following malignancies: small cell lung, breast, and ovarian cancers; Hodgkin's disease; and

thymoma.[142] Their presence or absence is not very sensitive or specific for any given neurologic syndrome or tumor type. Although some correlations exist, any given antibody can be associated with a number of different tumor types and neurologic syndromes. Conversely, a neurologic syndrome, such as cerebellar degeneration, can be associated with as many as nine different autoantibodies.[143] With no as yet defined role in pathogenesis, these autoantibodies may simply be an epiphenomenon and not involved in target tissue injury.[142]

The most common central nervous system autoantibody is anti-Hu (antineuronal nuclear antibody type 1 or ANNA-1). Anti-Hu is associated with multiple neurologic presentations, usually in patients with small cell lung cancer. Usually, the neurologic symptoms precede the diagnosis of the cancer. Cancer is ultimately diagnosed in 80 to 90% of patients with high titers (greater than 1:1,000 titers).[144] Low-titer anti-Hu is found in 16% of patients with small cell lung cancer without neurologic symptoms.[141] Although small cell lung cancer accounts for 90 to 95% of the associated cancers, cases are described with prostate, breast, GI, pancreatic, and bladder cancers; lymphomas; and thymomas and other lung cancers.[144–146] The most commonly associated neurologic symptoms are sensory neuropathy, limbic encephalitis, and cerebellar degeneration.[144] The antibody is also frequently found with paraneoplastic gut dysmotility most frequently associated with small cell lung cancer.[147] Gut dysmotility is the presenting symptom in up to 12% of anti-Hu patients.[145] The Hu antigen is made up of four different ribonucleic acid binding proteins, three of which are neuron specific. Antibodies to one of these, Hu-D, have been shown to induce apoptosis in neurons, suggesting that the antibody plays a direct role in the pathogenesis.[139]

Conclusions

The interactions between the graft and the host, dietary protein and the gut, bacteria and the stomach, and the tumor and the immune system described above demonstrate detrimental

immunologic responses. Our focused view has ignored other factors, such as the environment, that add to the milieu that influences the nature and outcome of immunologic response.[148] However, a better understanding of the immunologic role in pathogenesis helps explain various facets of the conditions under study and points the way to more effective prophylaxis of GVHD, control of *H. pylori*'s oncogenesis, treatment for CD, and limits on paraneoplastic syndromes.

REFERENCES

1. Billingham RE. The biology of graft-versus-host reactions. Harvard Lect 1966;62:21–78.
2. Vogelsang GB, Lee L, Bensen-Kennedy DM. Pathogenesis and treatment of graft-versus-host disease after bone marrow transplant. Annu Rev Med 2003;54:29–52.
3. Margolis J, Borrello I, Finn IW. New approaches to treating malignancies with stem cell transplantation. Semin Oncol 2000;27:524–30.
4. Gratwhol A, Hermans J, Apperley J, et al. Acute graft-versus-host disease: grade and outcome in patients with chronic myelogenous leukemia. Blood 1995;86:813–8.
5. Hill GR, Ferrara JLM. The primacy of the gastrointestinal tract as a target organ of acute graft-versus-host disease: rationale for the use of cytokine shields in allogenic bone marrow transplantation. Blood 2000;95:2754–9.
6. Akpek G, Chinratanalab W, Lee LA, et al. Gastrointestinal involvement in chronic graft-versus-host disease: a clinicopathologic study. Biol Blood Marrow Transplant 2003;9:46–51.
7. Tabbara IA, Zimmerman K, Morgan C, Nahleh Z. Allogenic hematopoietic stem cell transplantation. Arch Intern Med 2002;162:1558–66.
8. Martin PJ, Schoch G, Fisher L, et al. A retrospective analysis of therapy for acute graft-versus-host disease: initial treatment. Blood 1990;76:1464–72.
9. Martin PJ, McDonald GB, Sanders JE, et al. Increasingly frequent diagnosis of acute gastrointestinal graft-versus-host disease after allogenic hematopoietic cell transplantation. Biol Blood Marrow Transplant 2004;10:320–7.
10. Snover DC, Weisdorf SA, Vercellotti GM, et al. A histopathologic study of gastric and small intestinal graft-versus-host disease following allogenic bone marrow transplantation. Hum Pathol 1985;16:387–92.
11. Shidham VB, Chang C-C, Shidham G, et al. Colon biopsies for evaluation of acute graft-versus-host disease in allogenic bone marrow transplant patients. BMC Gastroenterol 2003;3:5.
12. Bombi JA, Nadal J, Carreras E, et al. Assessment of histopathologic changes in the colonic biopsy in acute graft-versus-host disease. Am J Clin Pathol 1995;103:690–5.
13. Snover DC. Mucosal damage simulating acute graft-versus-host reaction in cytomegalovirus colitis. Transplantation 1985;39:669–70.
14. Goodrich JM, Bowden RA, Fisher L, et al. Ganciclovir prophylaxis to prevent cytomegalovirus disease after allogenic marrow transplant. Ann Intern Med 1993;118:173–8.
15. Winston DJ, Ho WG, Bartoni K, et al. Ganciclovir prophylaxis of cytomegalovirus infection and disease in allogenic bone marrow transplant recipients. Ann Intern Med 1993;118:179–84.
16. Muller CI, Zeiser R, Grullich C, et al. Intestinal cryptosporidiosis mimicking acute graft-versus-host disease following matched unrelated hematopoietic stem cell transplantation. Transplantation 2004;77:1478–9.
17. Baron F, Gothot A, Salmon J-P, et al. Clinical course and predictive factors for cyclosporin-induced autologous graft-versus-host disease after autologous hematopoietic stem cell transplantation. Br J Haematol 2000;111:745–53.
18. Papadimitrious JC, Drachenberg LB, Beskow CO, et al. Graft-versus-host disease-like features in mycophenolate mofetil-related colitis. Transplant Proc 2001;33:2237–8.
19. Berrebi D, Sautet A, Fleejou J-F, et al. Ticlopidine induced colitis: a histopathological study including apoptosis. J Clin Pathol 1998;51:280–3.

Table 2 Autoantibodies for Neurologic Paraneoplastic Syndromes

Traditional Name	Alternate Name	Antigen Function	Associated Cancers
Anti-Hu	ANNA-1	RNA binding	SCLC
Anti-Ri	ANNA-2	RNA binding	Breast
ANNA-3		Unknown	SCLC
Anti-Yo	PCA-1	DNA binding	Breast, ovarian
Anti-PCA2		Unknown	Lung
Anti-CRMP5	Anti-CV2	Neuronal development	SCLC, thymoma
Anti-Ma		Unknown	Various
Anti-Tr	PCA-Tr	Unknown	Hodgkin's disease

ANNA = antineuronal nuclear antibody; DNA = deoxyribonucleic acid; RNA = ribonucleic acid; SCLC = small cell lung cancer.

20. Lee FD. Importance of apoptosis in the histopathology of drug-related lesions in the large intestines. J Clin Pathol 1993;46:118–22.
21. Sale GE, McDonald GB, Shulman HM, Thomas ED. Gastrointestinal graft-versus-host disease in man. Am J Surg Pathol 1979;3:291–9.
22. Cox GJ, Matsui SM, Lo RS, et al. Etiology and outcome of diarrhea after marrow transplantation: a prospective study. Gastroenterology 1994;107:1398–407.
23. Roy J, Snover D, Weisdorf S, et al. Simultaneous upper and lower endoscopic biopsy in the diagnosis of intestinal graft-versus-host disease. Transplantation 1991;51:642–6.
24. Ponec RJ, Hackman RC, McDonald GB. Endoscopic and histologic diagnosis of intestinal graft-versus-host disease after marrow transplantation. Gastrointest Endosc 1999;49:612–21.
25. Terdiman JP, Linker CA, Ries CA, et al. The role of endoscopic evaluation in patients with suspected intestinal graft-versus-host disease after allogenic bone marrow transplantation. Endoscopy 1996;28:680–5.
26. Daneshpouy M, Socie G, Lemann M, et al. Activated eosinophils in upper gastrointestinal tract of patients with graft-versus-host disease. Blood 2002;99:3033–40.
27. Schulenburg A Turetschek K, Wrba F, et al. Early and late gastrointestinal complications after myeloablative and nonmyeloablative allogenic stem cell transplantation. Ann Hematol 2004;83:101–6.
28. Igbal N, Salzman D, Lazenby AJ, Wilcox CM. Diagnosis of gastrointestinal graft-versus-host disease. Am J Gastroenterol 2000;95:3034–8.
29. Fallows G, Rubinger M, Bernstein CN. Does gastroenterology consultation change management of patients receiving hematopoietic stem cell transplantation? Bone Marrow Transplant 2001;28:289–94.
30. Kaur S, Cooper G, Fakult S, Lazarus HM. Incidence and outcome of overt gastrointestinal bleeding in patients undergoing bone marrow transplantation. Dig Dis Sci 1996;41:598–603.
31. Schwartz JM, Wolford JL, Thornquist MD, et al. Severe gastrointestinal bleeding after hematopoietic cell transplantation, 1987-97: incidence, causes, and outcome. Am J Gastroenterol 2001;96:385–93.
32. Murakami CS, Louie U, Chan GS, et al. Biliary obstruction I hematopoietic cell transplant recipients: an uncommon diagnosis with specific causes. Bone Marrow Transplant 1999;23:921–7.
33. Kaw M, Przepiorka D, Sekas G. Infectious complications of endoscopic procedures in bone marrow transplant recipients. Dig Dis Sci 1993;38:71–4.
34. Biano JA, Pepe MS, Higano C, et al. Prevalence of clinically relevant bacteremia after upper gastrointestinal endoscopy in bone marrow transplant recipients. Am J Med 1990;89:134–6.
35. Hirota WK, Petersen K, Baron TH, et al. Guidelines for antibiotic prophylaxis for gastrointestinal endoscopy. Gastrointest Endosc 2003;58:475–82.
36. Przepiorka D, Weisdorf D, Martin P, et al. Consensus conference on acute GVHD grading. Bone Marrow Transplant 1995;15:825–8.
37. van Kraaij MGJ, Dekker AW, Verdonck LF, et al. Infectious gastro-enteritis: an uncommon cause of diarrhea in adult allogenic and autologous stem cell recipients. Bone Marrow Transplant 2000;26:299–303.
38. Ippoliti C, Champlin R, Bugazia N, et al. Use of octreotide in the symptomatic management of diarrhea induced by graft-versus-host disease in patients with hematologic malignancies. J Clin Oncol 1997;15:3350–4.
39. Brand R, Pavletic, Lynch J, et al. Late acute graft-versus host disease of the gastrointestinal tract occurring after day 100: a new observation [abstract]. Blood 1999;94 Suppl 1:159a.
40. Akpek G, Valladares JL, Lee L, et al. Pancreatic insufficiency in patients with chronic graft-versus-host disease. Bone Marrow Transplant 2001;27:163–6.
41. Doherty J, Zahurak M, Margolis J, et al. Chronic GVHD and severe weight loss [abstract]. Blood 1999;94 Suppl 1:159a.
42. Jacobson DA. Margolis J, Doherty J, et al. Weight loss and malnutrition in patients with chronic graft-versus-host disease. Bone Marrow Transplant 2002;29:231–6.
43. Zauner C, Rabitsch W, Schneeweiss B, et al. Energy and substrate metabolism in patients with chronic extensive graft-versus-host disease. Transplantation 2001;71:524–8.
44. Witte KK, Clark AL. Nutritional abnormalities contributing to cachexia in chronic illness. Int J Cardiol 2002;85:23–31.
45. Robien K, Schubert MM, Bruemmer B, et al. Predictors of oral mucositis in patients receiving hematopoietic cell transplants for chronic myelogenous leukemia. J Clin Oncol 2004;22:1268–75.
46. Rapoport AP, Watelet LFM, Linder T, et al. Analysis of factors that correlate with mucositis in recipients of autologous and allogenic stem cell transplants. J Clin Oncol 1999;17:2446–53.
47. Woo S-B, Sonis ST, Monopolic MM, Sonis AL. A longitudinal study of oral ulcerative mucositis in bone marrow transplant recipients. Cancer 1993;72:1612–7.
48. Bellm LA, Epstein JB, Rose-Ped A, et al. Patient reports of complications of bone marrow transplantation. Support Care Cancer 2000;8:33–9.
49. Atkinson K. Chronic graft-versus-host disease. Bone Marrow Transplant 1990;5:69–82.
50. Arora M, Burns LJ, Davies SM, et al. Chronic graft-versus-host disease: a prospective cohort study. Biol Blood Marrow Transplant 2003;9:38–45.
51. Schubert MM, Sullivan KM, Morton TH, et al. Oral manifestations of chronic graft-versus-host disease. Arch Intern Med 1984;44:1591–5.
52. Nakamura S, Hiroki A, Shinohara M, et al. Oral involvement in chronic graft-versus-host disease after allogenic bone marrow transplantation. Oral Surg Oral Med Oral Pathol Oral Radiol Endod 1996;82:556–63.
53. Nagler R, Marmary Y, Krausz Y, et al. Major salivary gland dysfunction in human acute and chronic graft-versus-host disease. Bone Marrow Transplant 1996;17:219–24.
54. Majorana A, Schubert MM, Porta F, et al. Oral complications of pediatric hematopoietic cell transplantation: diagnosis and management. Support Care Cancer 2000;8:363–5.
55. Epstein JB, Nantel S, Sheoltch SM. Topical azathioprine in the combined treatment of chronic oral graft-versus-host disease. Bone Marrow Transplant 2000;25:683–7.
56. Abdelsayed RA, Sumner T, Allen CM, et al. Oral precancerous and malignant lesions associated with graft-versus-host disease: report of two cases. Oral Surg Oral Med Oral Pathol Oral Radiol Endod 2002;93:75–80.
57. Arai S, Lee LA, Vogelsang GB. A systematic approach to hepatic complications in hematopoietic stem cell transplantation. J Hematother Stem Cell Res 2002;11:215–29.
58. Kim BK, Chung KW, Sun HS, et al. Liver disease during the first post-transplant year in bone marrow transplantation: retrospective study. Bone Marrow Transplant 2000;26:193–7.
59. Ma SY, Au WY, Ng IOL, et al. Hepatitic graft-versus-host disease after hematopoietic stem cell transplantation: clinicopathologic features and prognostic implications. Transplantation 2004;77:1252–9.
60. Bertheau P, Hadengue A, Cazals-Hatem D, et al. Chronic cholestasis in patients after allogenic bone marrow transplantation: several diseases are often associated. Bone Marrow Transplant 1995;16:261–5.
61. Carreras E, Granena A, Navasa M, et al. On the reliability of clinical criteria for the diagnosis of hepatic veno-occlusive disease. Ann Hematol 1993;66:77–80.
62. Locasciulli A, Bacigalupo A, Alberti A, et al. Predictability before transplant of hepatic complications following allogenic bone marrow transplantation. Transplantation 1989;48:68–72.
63. McDonald GB, Hinds MS, Fisher LD, et al. Veno-occlusive disease of the liver and multiorgan failure after bone marrow transplantation: a cohort study of 355 patients. Ann Intern Med 1993;118:255–67.
64. Carreras E, Bertz H, Arcese W, et al. Incidence and outcome of hepatic veno-occlusive disease after blood or marrow transplantation: a prospective cohort study of the European Group for Blood and Marrow Transplantation. Blood 1998;92:3599–604.
65. Moscardo F, Urbano-Ispizua A, Sanz GF, et al. Positive selection for CD34+ reduces the incidence and severity of veno-occlusive disease of the liver after HLA-identical sibling allogenic peripheral blood stem cell transplantation. Exp Hematol 2003;31:545–50.
66. Azoulay D, Castaing D, Lemoine A, et al. Transjugular intrahepatic portosystemic shunt (TIPS) for severe veno-occlusive disease of the liver following bone marrow transplantation. Bone Marrow Transplant 2000;25:987–92.
67. Richardson PG, Murakami C, Zheghen J, et al. Multi-institutional use of defibrotide in 88 patients after stem cell transplantation with severe veno-occlusive disease and multisystem organ failure: response without significant toxicity in high risk population and factors predictive of outcome. Blood 2002;100:4337–43.
68. Strasser SI, Shulman HM, Flower ME, et al. Chronic graft-versus-host disease of the liver: presentation as an acute hepatitis. Hepatology 2000;32:265–71.
69. Akpek G, Boitnott JK, Lee LA, at al. Hepatitic variant of graft-versus-host disease after donor lymphocyte infusion. Blood 2002;100:3903–7.
70. Snover DC, Weisdorf SA, Ramsay NK, et al. Hepatic graft-versus-host disease: a study of the predictive value of liver biopsy in diagnosis. Hepatology 1984;4:123–30.
71. Shulman HM, Sharma P, Amos D, et al. A coded histologic study of hepatic graft-versus-host disease after human bone marrow transplantation. Hepatology 1988;8:463–70.
72. Strasser SI, Myerson D, Spurgeon CL, et al. Hepatitis C virus infection and bone marrow transplantation: a cohort study with 10-year follow-up. Hepatology 1999;29:1893–9.
73. Bombi JA, Palou J, Bruguera M, et al. Pathology of bone marrow transplantation. Semin Diagn Pathol 1992;9:220–31.
74. Liatsos C, Mehta AB, Potter M, Burroughs AK. The hepatologist in the haematologist's camp. Br J Haematol 2001;113:567–78.
75. Sloane JP, Norton J. The pathology of bone marrow transplantation. Histopathology 1993;22:201–9.
76. Knapp AB, Crawford JM, Rappeport JM, Gallan JL. Cirrhosis as a consequence of graft-versus-host disease. Gastroenterology 1987;92:513–9.
77. Strasser SI, Kowdley KV, Sale GE, McDonald GB. Iron overload in bone marrow transplant recipients. Bone Marrow Transplant 1998;22:167–73.
78. Strasser SI, Sullivan KM, Myerson D, et al. Cirrhosis of the liver in long-term marrow transplant survivors. Blood 1999;93:3259–66.
79. Flomenberg N, Baxter-Lowe LA, Confer D, et al. Impact of HLA class I and class II high resolution matching on outcomes of unrelated donor bone marrow transplantation: HLA-C mismatching is associated with a strong adverse effect on transplantation outcome. Blood 2004;104:1923–30.
80. Bruner RJ, Farag SS. Monoclonal antibodies for the prevention and treatment of graft-versus-host disease. Semin Oncol 2003;30:509–19.
81. Duggan P, Booth K, Chaudhry A, et al. Unrelated donor BMT recipients given pretransplant low dose antithymocyte globulin have outcomes equivalent to match sibling BMT. Bone Marrow Transplant 2002;30:681–6.
82. Bacigalupo A, Lamparelli T, Bruzzi P, et al. Antithymocyte globulin for graft-versus-host disease prophylaxis in transplants from unrelated donors: 2 randomized studies from Gruppo Italino Trapianti Midollo Osseo (GITMO). Blood 2001;98:2942–7.
83. Kroger N, Sabelina T, Kruger W, et al. In vivo T cell depletion with pretransplant anti-thymocyte globulin reduces graft-versus-host disease without increasing relapse in good risk myeloid leukemia patients after stem cell transplantation from matched related donors. Bone Marrow Transplant 2002;29:683–9.
84. Remberger M, Storer B, Ringden O, Anasetti C. Association between pretransplant thymoglobulin and reduced non-relapse mortality rate after marrow transplantation from unrelated donors. Bone Marrow Transplant 2002;29:391–7.
85. Remberger M, Svahn B-M, Mattsson J, Ringden O. Dose study of thymoglobulin during conditioning for unrelated donor allogenic stem cell transplantation. Transplantation 2004;78:122–7.
86. Remberger M, Aschan J, Barkholt K, et al. Treatment of severe acute graft-versus-host disease with anti-thymocyte globulin. Clin Transpl 2001;15:147–53.
87. Couriel D, Saliba R, Hicks K, et al. Tumor necrosis factor-alpha blockade for the treatment of acute GVHD. Blood 2004;104:649–54.
88. Arai S, Margolis J, Saburak M, et al. Poor outcome in steroid refractory graft-versus-host disease with antithymocyte globulin treatment. Biol Blood Marrow Transplant 2002;8:155–60.
89. MacMillan ML, Weisdorf DJ, Davies SM, et al. Early antithymocyte globulin therapy improves survival in patients with steroid-resistant acute graft-versus-host disease. Biol Blood Marrow Transplant 2002;8:40–6.

90. Graziani F, Van Lint MT, Dominietto A, et al. Treatment of acute graft-versus-host disease with low-dose, alternate-day antithymocyte globulin. Haematologica 2002;87:973–8.

91. Bacigalupo A, Oneto R, Bruno B, et al. Early predictors of transplant-related mortality (TRM) after allogenic bone marrow transplants (BMT): blood urea nitrogen (BUN) and bilirubin. Bone Marrow Transplant 1999;24:653–9.

92. Massenkeil G, Rackwitz S, Genvresse I, et al. Basiliximab is well tolerated and effective in the treatment of steroid refractory acute graft-versus-host disease after allogenic stem cell transplantation. Bone Marrow Transplant 2002;30:899–903.

93. Durrant S, Mollee P, Morton AJ, Irving I. Combination therapy with tacrolimus and anti-thymocyte globulin for the treatment of steroid-resistant acute graft-versus-host disease developing during cyclosporine prophylaxis. Br J Haematol 2001;113:217–23.

94. McDonald GB, Bouvier M, Hockenbery DM, et al. Oral beclomethasone dipropionate for treatment of intestinal graft-versus-host disease: a randomized, controlled trial. Gastroenterology 1998;115:28–35.

95. Bertz H, Afting M, Kreisel W, et al. Feasibility and response to budesonide as topical corticosteroid therapy for acute intestinal GVHD. Bone Marrow Transplant 1999;24:1185–9.

96. Shapira MY, Bloom AI, Or R, et al. Intra-arterial catheter directed therapy for severe graft-versus-host disease. Br J Haematol 2002;119:760–4.

97. Bloom AI, Shapira MY, Or R, et al. Intrahepatic arterial administration of low-dose methotrexate in patients with severe hepatic graft-versus-host disease: an open label, uncontrolled trial. Clin Ther 2004;26:407–14.

98. Bamford KB, Fan X, Crowe SE, et al. Lymphocytes in the human gastric mucosa during Helicobacter pylori have a T helper cell 1 phenotype. Gastroenterology 1998;114:482–92.

99. Wundisch T, Kim TD, Thiede C, et al. Etiology and therapy of Helicobacter pylori associated gastric lymphomas. Ann Hematol 2003;82:535–45.

100. Zucca E, Bertoni F, Roggero E, et al. Molecular analysis of the progression from Helicobacter pylori-associated chronic gastritis to mucosa-associated lymphoid tissue lymphoma of the stomach. N Engl J Med 1998;338:804–10.

101. Miehlke S, Yu J, Schuppler M, et al. Helicobacter pylori vac A, ice A, and cag A status and pattern of gastritis in patients with malignant and benign gastroduodenal disease. Am J Gastroenterol 2001;96:1008–13.

102. Lehours P, Menard A, Dupouy S, et al. Evaluation of the association of nine Helicobacter pylori virulence factors with strains involved in low-grade gastric mucosa-associated lymphoid tissue lymphoma. Infect Immun 2004;72:880–8.

103. Koulis A, Diss T, Isaacson PG, Dogan A. Characterization of tumor-infiltrating T-lymphocytes in B-cell lymphoma of mucosa-associated lymphoid tissue. Am J Pathol 1997;151:1353–60.

104. D'Elios MM, Amedei A, Del Prete G. Helicobacter pylori antigen-specific T-cell responses at gastric level in chronic gastritis, peptic ulcer, gastric cancer and low-grade mucosa-associated lymphoid tissue (MALT) lymphoma. Microbes Infect 2003;5:723–30.

105. Zucca E, Bertoni F, Roggero E, Cavalli F. The gastric marginal zone B cell lymphoma of MALT type. Blood 2000;96:410–9.

106. Steinbach G, Ford R, Glober G, et al. Antibiotic treatment of gastric lymphoma of mucosa-associated lymphoid tissue. Ann Intern Med 1999;131:88–95.

107. Thiede C, Wundisch T, Alpen B, et al. Long-term persistence of monoclonal B cells after cure of Helicobacter pylori infection and complete histologic remission in gastric mucosa-associated lymphoid tissue B-cell lymphoma. J Clin Oncol 2001;19:1600–9.

108. Stolte M, Bayerdorffer E, Morgner A, et al. Helicobacter and gastric MALT lymphoma. Gut 2002;50 Suppl III:iii19–24.

109. Fischback W, Goebeler-Kolve M-E, Dragosics B, et al. Long term outcome of patients with gastric marginal zone B cell lymphoma of mucosa associated lymphoid tissue (MALT) following exclusive Helicobacter pylori eradication therapy: experience from a large prospective series. Gut 2004;53:34–7.

110. Sackman M, Morgner A, Rudolph B, et al. Regression of gastric MALT lymphoma after eradication of Helicobacter pylori is predicted by endoscopic staging. Gastroenterology 1997;113:1087–90.

111. Du MQ, Isaacson PG. Gastric MALT lymphoma: from aetiology to treatment. Lancet Oncol 2002;3:97–104.

112. Ahmad A, Govil Y, Frank BB. Gastric mucosa-associated lymphoid tissue lymphoma. Am J Gastroenterol 2003;98:975–86.

113. Crump M, Gospodarowicz M, Shepherd FA. Lymphoma of the gastrointestinal tract. Semin Oncol 1999;26:324–37.

114. Morgner A, Miehlke S, Stolte M, et al. Development of early gastric cancer 4 and 5 years after complete remission of Helicobacter pylori associated gastric low grade marginal zone B cell lymphoma of the MALT type. World J Gastroenterol 2001;7:248–53.

115. Peng H, Du M, Diss TC, et al. Genetic evidence for a clonal link between low and high-grade components in gastric MALT B-cell lymphoma. Histopathology 1997;30:425–9.

116. Fischbach W, Dragosics B, Kolve-Goebeler ME, et al. Primary gastric B-cell lymphoma: results of a prospective multicenter study. Gastroenterology 200;119:1191–202.

117. Isaacson PG, Du MQ. MALT lymphoma: from morphology to molecules. Nat Rev Cancer 2004;4:644–53.

118. Yoshino T, Akagi T. Gastric low-grade mucosa-associated lymphoid tissue lymphomas: their histogenesis and high-grade transformation. Pathol Int 1998;48:323–31.

119. Ng WW, Lam CP, Chau WK, et al. Regression of high grade gastric mucosa-associated lymphoid tissue lymphoma with Helicobacter pylori after triple antibiotic therapy. Gastrointest Endosc 2000;51:93–6.

120. Morgner A, Mielke S, Fischbach W, et al. Complete remission of primary high-grade B cell gastric lymphoma after cure of Helicobacter pylori infection. J Clin Oncol 2001;19:2041–8.

121. Brousse N, Verkarre V, Patey-Mariaud de Serre N, et al. Is complicated celiac disease or refractory sprue an intestinal intra-epithelial cryptic T-cell lymphoma? Blood 1999;93:3154–5.

122. Carbonnel F, Grollet-Bioul L, Brouet JC, et al. Are complicated forms of celiac disease cryptic T-cell lymphoma? Blood 1998;92:3879–86.

123. Badgi E, Diss TC, Munson P, Isaacson PG. Mucosal intra-epithelial lymphocytes in enteropathy-associated T-cell lymphoma, ulcerative jejunitis, and refractory celiac disease constitute a neoplastic population. Blood 1999;94:260–4.

124. Ashton-Key M, Diss TC, Pan L, et al. Molecular analysis of T-cell clonality in ulcerative jejunitis and enteropathy-associated T-cell lymphoma. Am J Pathol 1997;151:493–8.

125. Ryan BM, Kelleher D. Refractory celiac disease. Gastroenterology 2000;119:243–51.

126. Daum S, Weiss D, Hummel M, et al. Frequency of clonal intraepithelial T-lymphocyte proliferations in enteropathy-type intestinal T-cell lymphoma, celiac disease and refractory sprue. Gut 2001;49:804–12.

127. Non-Hodgkin's Lymphoma Classification Project. A clinical evaluation of the International Lymphoma Study Group classification of non-Hodgkin's lymphoma. Blood 1997;89:3909–18.

128. Catassi C, Fabiani E, Corrao G, et al. Risk of non-Hodgkin's lymphoma in celiac disease. JAMA 2002;287:1413–9.

129. Chott A, Vesely M, Simonitsch I, et al. Classification of intestinal T-cell neoplasm and their differential diagnosis. Am J Clin Pathol 1999;111 Suppl:S68–74.

130. Corrao G, Corazza RG, Bagnardi V, et al. Mortality in patients with celiac disease and their relatives: a cohort study. Lancet 2001;258:356–61.

131. Gale J, Simmonds PD, Mead GM, et al. Enteropathy-type intestinal T-cell lymphoma: clinical features and treatment of 31 patients in a single center. J Clin Oncol 2000;18:795–803.

132. Daum S, Ullrich R, Heise W, et al. Intestinal non-Hodgkin's lymphoma: a multicenter prospective clinical study from the German Study Group on Intestinal Non-Hodgkin's Lymphoma. J Clin Oncol 2003;21:2740–6.

133. Jantunen E, Juvonen E, Wilund T, et al. High dose therapy supported by autologous stem cell transplantation in patients with enteropathy-associated T-cell lymphoma. Leuk Lymphoma 2003;44:2163–4.

134. Lennard AL, White J, Tiplady C. Prospective evaluation of a novel treatment protocol for intestinal T cell NHL. Ann Oncol 2002;13 Suppl:43.

135. Hadden JM. Immunodeficiency and cancer: prospect for correction. Int Immunopharmacol 2003;3:1061–71.

136. Chambers WH, Rabinowich H, Herbermann RB. Tumor-associated immunodeficiency and implications for tumor development and prognosis. In: Kufe DW, Pollack RE, Weichselbaum RR, et al, editors. Cancer medicine. 6th ed. Hamilton (ON): BC Decker; 2003. p. 229–40.

137. Posner JB. Immunology of paraneoplastic syndromes. Ann N Y Acad Sci 2003;998:178–86.

138. Tan EM, Shi FD. Relative paradigms between autoantibodies in lupus and autoantibodies in cancer. Clin Exp Immunol 2003;134:169–77.

139. DeGiorgio R, Guerrini S, Barbara G, et al. Inflammatory neuropathies of the enteric nervous system. Gastroenterology 2004;126:1872–83.

140. Vincent A, Honnorat J, Antoine JC, et al. Autoimmunity in paraneoplastic neurological disorders. J Neuroimmunol 1998;84:105–9.

141. Voltz R. Paraneoplastic neurological syndromes: an update on diagnosis, pathogenesis, and therapy. Lancet Neurol 2002;1:294–305.

142. Dropcho EJ. Neurologic paraneoplastic syndromes. Curr Oncol Rep 2004;6:26–31.

143. Shamsili S, Grefkens J, de Leeuw B, et al. Paraneoplastic cerebellar degeneration associated with antineuronal antibodies: analysis of 50 patients. Brain 2003;126:1409–18.

144. Graus F, Keime-Guibert F, Rene R, et al. Anti-Hu associated paraneoplastic encephalomyelitis: analysis of 200 patients. Brain 2001;124:1138–48.

145. Lucchineti CF, Kimmel DW, Lennon VA. Paraneoplastic and oncologic profiles of patients seropositive for type 1 antineuronal nuclear autoantibodies. Neurology 1998;50:652–7.

146. Vernino S, Eggenberger ER, Rogers LR, Lennon VA. Paraneoplastic neurological autoimmunity associated with ANNA-1 autoantibody and thymoma. Neurology 2002;59:929–32.

147. Lee HR, Lennon VA, Camilleri M, Prather CM. Paraneoplastic gastrointestinal motor dysfunction: clinical and laboratory characteristics. Am J Gastroenterol 2001;96:373–9.

148. Go MF. What are the host factors that place an individual at risk for Helicobacter pylori-associated disease? Gastroenterology 1997 Dec;113(Suppl):S15–20.

Interventional Gastroenterology

Jeffrey H. Lee, MD
William A. Ross, MD, MBA

Gastrointestinal malignancies are leading causes of cancer death throughout the world, and cure is largely dependent on surgical resection. Selection of appropriate treatment options depends on accurate diagnosis and staging. Recent developments in endoscopic technology have contributed to major improvements in early diagnosis and accurate staging. In addition, endoscopy plays an increasing role in the treatment and palliation of gastrointestinal malignancies. This chapter reviews advances in interventional endoscopy.

Endoscopic Ultrasonography

Endoscopic Ultrasonography in Esophageal Cancer

Adenocarcinoma of the esophagus has the highest increase in incidence of any cancer in the United States. It is a disease predominantly of white males with long-standing gastroesophageal reflux. The recognition of specialized columnar mucosa in Barrett's esophagus as a precursor for esophageal adenocarcinoma has provided a means to identify a patient group that may benefit from periodic endoscopic surveillance. Such surveillance leads to identification of lesions at an earlier asymptomatic stage. Accurate staging is critical in selecting the most appropriate therapy.

Evaluation by endoscopic ultrasonography (EUS) is an excellent tool to assess the depth of tumor (T) invasion and the status of regional lymph nodes (N) in patients with esophageal cancer. It also serves as a complementary imaging modality to assess the sites of distant metastases (M) of esophageal cancer (Table 1 and Figure 1). During an EUS examination, fine-needle aspiration (FNA) can be performed, using a 19- or 22-gauge needle, into the regional and/or celiac lymph nodes under ultrasound guidance with few risks of complication. All of these can be performed under conscious sedation.

Vazquez-Sequeiros and colleagues reported that helical computed tomographic (CT) scans with 5 to 7 mm cuts provide T-staging accuracy of 72% compared with 86% by EUS. For N staging, the accuracy of CT, EUS, and EUS-FNA was 61%, 81%, 87%, respectively.[1] EUS features of lymph nodes can help distinguish whether they

Table 1 System for Staging Esophageal Cancer	
Primary Tumor (T)	
Tx	Tumor limited to mucosa and muscularis mucosa
T0	Tumor limited to submucosa
T1	Tumor limited to muscularis propria
T2	Tumor infiltration to adventitia
T3	Tumor infiltration to adjacent organ
T4	Regional lymph nodes cannot be assessed
Regional Lymph Nodes (N)	
Nx	No regional lymph node metastasis
N1	Regional lymph node metastasis
Distant Metastasis (M)	
Mx	Distant metastasis cannot be assessed
M0	No distant metastasis
M1	Distant metastasis

The American Joint Committee on Cancer (AJCC), Manual for Staging of Cancer, 4th ed. 1992.

are benign or malignant. A modified set of seven EUS criteria for malignancy were described as hypoechoic, smooth border, round shape, width ≥ 5 mm, lymph node in celiac location, more than five lymph nodes identified, and T3 or T4 tumor on EUS. When three or more of the seven criteria were present, the accuracy of predicting malignancy was 88%. The presence of six or more criteria had a positive predictive value for malignancy of 100%.[2]

For patients who receive preoperative chemoradiation, repeat EUS staging is usually performed before planned surgery. In the postchemoradiation setting, however, the accuracy of EUS for T staging drops to 51% and for N staging to 49%.[3] Therefore it is necessary to sample the treatment site by endoscopic biopsy. When a suspicious lymph node is seen, FNA of the node should also be done to improve the accuracy of posttreatment staging.

EUS in Solid Tumors of the Pancreas

Eighty percent of pancreatic cancers present with metastatic disease. Only a subset of the remainder are felt to be true surgical candidates with resectable and, therefore, potentially curable disease. Given a 5-year survival rate of 4%, the emphasis has been on early detection and prompt management.[4] With improved imaging modalities such as helical CT and EUS, preoperative evaluations are more accurately staging patients, allowing a more select group of patients to undergo surgery. Pancreatic cancers can arise from both the exocrine and endocrine portions of the pancreas. Of pancreatic tumors, 95% develop from the exocrine portion of the pancreas, including the ductal epithelium, acinar cells, connective tissue, and lymphatic tissue. When a pancreatic mass is seen on a CT scan, the next step should be performing EUS-FNA to obtain local tumor staging and a tissue diagnosis (Table 2 and Figures 2 and 3). For pancreatic masses, the accuracy of EUS-FNA was reported to be 88%, with a sensitivity of 86%, a specificity of 94%, a positive

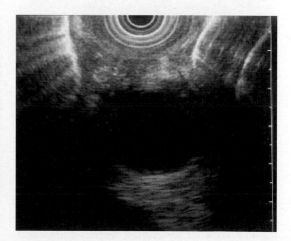

FIGURE 1 T4 esophageal cancer with a missing echoplane between the mass and the aorta.

Table 2 System for Staging of Pancreatic Adeno-carcinoma

T1	Tumor limited to pancreas
	Size <2 cm in greatest dimension
T2	Tumor limited to pancreas
	Size >2 cm in greatest dimension
T3	Tumor infiltration (extension) into duodenum, bile duct, papilla, or peripancreatic tissue
T4	Tumor infiltration (extension) into stomach, spleen, colon, or adjacent large vessels
Nx	Regional lymph nodes cannot be assessed
N0	No regional lymph node metastasis
N1	Regional lymph node metastasis
Mx	Distant metastasis cannot be assessed
M0	No distant metastasis
M1	Distant metastasis

The American Joint Committee on Cancer: AJCC Cancer Staging Manual. 5th ed. 1997

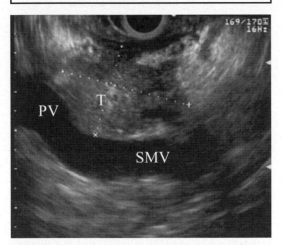

FIGURE 2 Endoscopic ultrasonographic view of a pancreatic head mass abutting the confluence of the portal vein and the superior mesenteric vein. PV = portal vein; SMV = superior mesenteric vein; T = tumor.

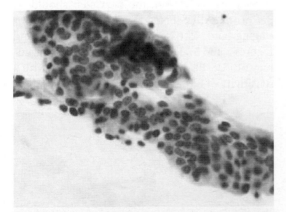

FIGURE 3 Fine-needle aspiration of pancreatic carcinoma: cytologic smear showing a fragment of ductal epithelium that displays atypical nuclear features that include focal enlargement, irregularity, hyperchromasia, crowding, and overlap. Nuclei are not evenly spaced, size (volume) ratios differ significantly from one nucleus to another, and areas of three-dimensionality are seen. These features taken together allow for a malignant diagnosis (Papanicolaou stain, medium power).

predictive value of 100%, and a negative predictive value of 86%.[5] When a mass is not visible on CT or magnetic resonance imaging (MRI) in patients presenting with obstructive jaundice, however, the sensitivity, specificity, positive predictive value, and negative predictive value of EUS-FNA are 47%, 100%, 100%, and 50%, respectively. In this setting, detection of mass, an irregular bile duct wall, or common bile duct wall thickness greater than 3 mm by EUS provides much improved sensitivity over FNA.[6]

The ability to detect pancreatic endocrine tumors (PENs) by conventional imaging studies such as transcutaneous ultrasonography, CT, and MRI is highly dependent on the size of the tumor. CT and MRI can localize fewer than 10% of PENs less than 1 cm in diameter, 30 to 40% of PENs 1 to 3 cm in size, and more than 50% of those more than 3 cm in diameter.[7–12] Intra-arterial secretin injection with portal venous sampling was shown in one study to have high positive and negative predictive values for the identification of gastrinoma.[13] However, this procedure is highly invasive and does not provide a tissue diagnosis. Zimmer and colleagues, however, reported a higher accuracy for EUS for localization of gastrinoma (79%) and insulinoma (93%).[14] In another study of 30 patients with suspected PEN, EUS-FNA had a sensitivity of 82.6%, a specificity of 85.7%, an accuracy of 83.3%, a positive predictive value of 95.0%, and a negative predictive value of 60.0%.[15]

EUS in a Bilroth II operation was once considered to be contraindicated. It is difficult to orient the anatomy owing to resection of the antrum and duodenal bulb and reconstruction. However, Pancreatic EUS following a Billroth II operation was once considered to be contraindicated. It is difficult to orient the anatomy owing to resection of the antrum and duodenal bulb and reconstruction. Linear-array echoendoscopes provide a more complete examination than radial echoendoscopes. Of note, the pancreatic neck may be difficult to visualize.[16]

When subtle pathologic conditions of the bile duct or pancreatic duct are suspected, intraductal ultrasonography can be performed by using a 12, 15, or 20 MHz, radial scanning ultrasound catheter probe (UM R-series, Olympus Optical Co, Tokyo, Japan). This requires cannulating either or both ducts using a duodenoscope and the probe.

EUS in Cystic Tumors of the Pancreas

Owing to better and more frequently used imaging studies, there has been an increase in the detection of cystic lesions in the pancreas. Cystic lesions represent less than 10% of pancreatic neoplasms. The most common pancreatic cystic lesion is a pseudocyst. When a pseudocyst is suspected, it is important to ask the patients whether they have a history of pancreatitis as

pseudocysts follow an episode of acute pancreatitis or occur in the setting of chronic pancreatitis. Cystic tumors could be benign, as in serous cystadenoma and pseudocyst, or malignant (or with malignant potential), as in mucinous cystic adenoma, intraductal mucinous papillary neoplasm (IPMN), or mucinous cystadenocarcinoma. EUS-FNA not only provides images to help distinguish benign from malignant cysts, it also allows aspiration of cystic content for fluid analysis (Figure 4). The benign EUS features include sunburst calcification with numerous microcysts resembling a honeycomb appearance, which suggests serous cystadenoma. The worrisome EUS features include intracystic growth or a solid mass associated with the cyst. The aspirated fluid is usually sent for cytology, carcinoembryonic antigen (CEA), cancer antigen (CA) 19-9, CA 125, CA 72-4, and amylase (Table 3). In a study by Brugge and colleagues, CEA was the most specific tumor marker for malignancy.[17] Using the CEA value of 192 ng/mL, the sensitivity for diagnosis of a mucinous cyst was 75%, with a specificity of 84% and an accuracy of 79%. In comparison, the accuracy of EUS morphology was 51% and cytology was 59%.

EUS can further characterize IPMN by visualizing the papillary growth along the duct. FNA enables obtaining tissue from the papillary growth and aspirating ductal contents for the presence of mucin and other studies.

EUS in Rectal Cancer

In a review of EUS accuracy in staging rectal cancer, in all published data between 1985 and 2003, EUS T-staging accuracy was reported in 40 studies and N-staging accuracy in 27 studies.[18] In 4,118 subjects, an overall mean T-staging accuracy was 85.2% (median 87.5%) and N-staging accuracy was 75.0% (median 76.0%). EUS staging of rectal cancer can facilitate appropriate employment of preoperative neoadjuvant therapy in those patients with advanced disease. However, EUS tends to overstage rectal cancers because

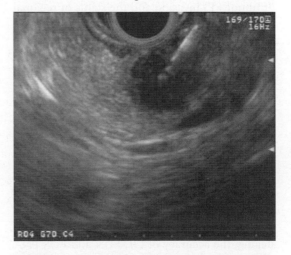

FIGURE 4 Endoscopic ultrasonography–fine-needle aspiration of a cystic lesion of the pancreas.

Table 3 Tumor Markers in Cystic Fluid in the Various Pancreas Cysts

Tumor Marker	SCA	MCA	MCAC	IPMN	Pseudocyst
CEA	Low	High	High	Variable	Low
CA 19-9	Variable	Variable	Variable	Variable	High
CA 15-3	Low	High	High	Low	Low
CA 72-4	Low	High	High	High	Low
CA 125	Low	Variable	Variable	Low	Low
Amylase	Low	Low	Low	High	High
Viscosity	Low	High	High	High	Low
Cytology	Glycogen	Mucin	Mucin	Mucin	Inflammatory

CA = cancer antigen; CEA = carcinoembryonic antigen; IPMN = intraductal papillary mucinous neoplasm; MCA = mucinous cystic adenoma; MCAC = mucinous cystadenocarcinoma.

high-resolution ultrasonography can detect, but not separate, hypoechoic inflammation around the malignancy from the tumor itself.[19]

EUS in T4 Lung Cancer

Nearly 30% of patients with lung cancer harbor mediastinal disease at presentation. Through the esophageal wall, EUS provides excellent access to the posterior mediastinum. In patients with lung cancer and posterior mediastinal adenopathy on CT, EUS-FNA was reported to be superior to CT for detection of malignancy, with a sensitivity of 90% and a specificity of 100%.[20–23] Although ultrasonography cannot penetrate air-filled structures such as the lungs, invasion of the mediastinum by lung cancer is suspected when there is a loss of interface between the mass and the soft tissue of the mediastinum, heart, great vessels, trachea, esophagus, or vertebral body. In a study of 175 patients with lung cancer who underwent EUS evaluation of the mediastinum, structures in the lateral mediastinum, such as upper paratracheal (2L/R) and lower paratracheal (4L/R) lymph nodes, were routinely imaged and sampled by EUS-FNA without difficulty. For detection of mediastinal invasion by lung cancer, EUS had a sensitivity of 87.5%, a specificity of 98%, a positive predictive value of 70%, and a negative predictive value of 99%, with no procedure-related complication.[24] Therefore, EUS-FNA is an accurate, safe, and cost-effective means of screening patients with lung cancer with possible mediastinal metastasis. However, T4 staging should be made by EUS only when invasion of great vessels or mediastinal organs (heart, spine, esophagus) is clearly evident or EUS-FNA confirms malignant pleural effusion. Loss of interface between the tumor and mediastinum detected by EUS should be further evaluated by other modalities before the tumor is considered unresectable.

Endoscopic Retrograde Cholangiopancreatography and Pancreatoscopy

The most common presenting symptom and sign of pancreatic cancer involving the head of the pancreas is painless obstructive cystic jaundice. There are many possible etiologies for obstructive jaundice, including benign and malignant conditions; among them are primary sclerosing cholangitis, chronic pancreatitis, cholangiocarcinoma, and pancreatic malignancies, including both solid and cystic tumors of the pancreas. The first step in management of obstructive jaundice in a suspected malignancy is obtaining a CT scan of the abdomen. If ascending cholangitis is suspected owing to biliary obstruction, the patient should be admitted for intravenous hydration and antibiotics. Charcot's triad of jaundice, fever, and right upper quadrant abdominal pain is seen in approximately 70% of the patients with ascending cholangitis. The antibiotics should be able to cover a broad spectrum, including *Escherichia coli*, *Enterococcus*, *Klebsiella*, and anaerobes. Following this, at the earliest possible time, endoscopic retrograde cholangiopancreatography (ERCP) should be performed to establish drainage of bile and pus. In severe asending cholangitis, a plastic biliary stent may not be sufficient to drain the large amount of viscous pus. A nasobiliary drainage that allows lavaging of the bile duct would be more effective in this setting. If ERCP is unsuccessful for technical or anatomic reasons, percutaneous drainage by an interventional radiology service should be performed.

In suspected pancreatic exocrine tumor presenting with obstructive jaundice, ERCP can be performed immediately following EUS-FNA to alleviate the symptoms of obstructive jaundice. During ERCP, the confirmation on tissue diagnosis on the cytology specimen obtained by EUS-FNA can be made by a cytopathologist. For biliary decompression in patients with resectable pancreatic cancers, traditionally, plastic stents were used for various presumed advantages over the metallic stents. However, Wasan and colleagues reported data on the utility of metal stents on resectable pancreatic cancer.[25] During the preoperative course, the incidence of cholangitis or cholecystitis was 15% in the metal stent group and 92% in the plastic stent group. In both groups, there were no stent-related intra- or postoperative complications. For both groups, the intraoperative time per patient was approximately 7 hours, with an intraoperative blood loss of 650 mL and length of hospital stay of 10.5 days. Overall, for the metal group, significantly fewer ERCP sessions were required, which more than compensated for the higher initial stent costs.[26]

For IPMN, the most common presenting symptom is abdominal pain. On ERCP, visualization of thick mucin extrusion from the widely open papilla is diagnostic of IPMN (Figure 5). Magnetic resonance cholangiopancreatography is a noninvasive imaging study that allows evaluation of the pancreatic duct, the presence or absence of a cyst, communication of cystic dilation with the main pancreatic duct, and the presence of side-branch IPMNs with minimal risk. A pancreatogram will frequently show multiple filling defects, ductal dilation, and, at times, cystic dilation of side branches. ERCP brushing and biopsy are not very sensitive, but intraoperative pancreatoscopy is highly sensitive and specific. Intraoperative pancreatoscopy also enables precise location of resection for clear surgical margins so that repetitive resection would not be needed.

Endoscopic Mucosal Resection

For selected patients with early esophageal or gastric cancer (T1a) who are poor or reluctant surgical candidates, endoscopic mucosal resection (EMR) should be considered. The first step in EMR is a conventional endoscopy to mark the periphery of the lesion and to inject saline solution into the submucosa. Next, the EMR cap (Olympus Optical Co., Ltd., Tokyo, Japan) is fitted at the tip of the endoscope. A crescent-shaped snare is then prelooped into the groove of the rim of the cap. The lesion is suctioned into the cap, and snare resection is performed. The two most common complications of EMR are perforation and bleeding. Most bleeding occurs within 24 hours, and the patients should be closely followed during this time. Bleeding occurring during EMR can usually be treated using a heater

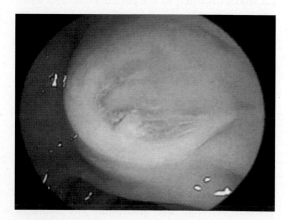

FIGURE 5 Mucin extrusion from a widely open papilla, diagnostic of intraductal mucinous papillary neoplasm.

probe, hemoclips, or other modalities. When the perforation is small and the patient is clinically stable, attempts to seal the perforation by endoscopic hemoclipping should be made if the area of perforation is easily accessible. When EMR is being considered rather than surgical resection for T1 lesions, it is important to be able to distinguish T1a (only mucosal and muscularis mucosal involvement) from T1b (submucosal involvement) by EUS as there is a higher rate of lymphatic invasion with T1b than with T1a. Post-EMR, close surveillance should be routine for early detection of recurrence. In the study published by Scotiniotis and colleagues, T1a could be separated from T1b with a sensitivity of 100%, a specificity of 94%, and a negative predictive value of 100% by EUS.[27] Kume and colleagues published new techniques of EMR using a soft, irrigation-prelooped hood. This technique allows effective irrigation, thus providing better visualization of the field. In this study, 15 patients (4 with early esophageal cancer, 11 with early gastric cancer) underwent successful EMR; the complications mentioned included 4 patients with limited bleeding, which was easily treated by endoscopic therapy. No perforation was observed.[28]

Endoscopic Ampullectomy

Patients with an ampullary adenoma frequently present with nondescript upper abdominal pain, jaundice, and/or gastrointestinal bleeding. Patients with familial adenomatous polyposis (FAP), including Gardner's variant, have an increased likelihood of papillary neoplasm and thus should undergo endoscopic surveillance.[29,30] CT is not sensitive for detection of ampullary tumors. To optimally visualize the ampulla, a side-viewing scope should be employed as the straight-viewing scope does not provide an accurate assessment of the ampulla. During the evaluation of the ampulla, biopsy specimens should be obtained from the ampulla if adenoma is suspected or routinely in the patients with FAP as an adenoma may be grossly evident or the ampulla may appear to be completely normal. If jaundice is present, ERCP should be performed with a biliary sphincterotomy to establish drainage and obtain biopsy specimens from the inner segment of the ampulla and a biliary stent should be placed if the stricture is still shown with poor drainage following biliary sphincterotomy. A cholangiogram should be obtained with brushing of the stricture. When the pathology results of ampullary biopsy confirm that it is an adenoma rather than a carcinoma, then EUS should be performed to stage the adenoma. The standard management for papillary neoplasms continues to be surgery, either local excision or pancreatico-duodenectomy. If an ampullary adenoma is confined within the mucosal or submucosal layer (confirmed by EUS), snare ampullectomy could be considered. Endoscopic ampullectomy can be performed in two ways. First, the ampulla can be snared off in one cut. The pancreatic duct needs to be found first so that it can be stented postampullectomy to prevent post-ERCP pancreatitis as the papillary edema could result in temporary blockage of the duct. Also, to prevent cholangitis, the bile duct should be cannulated and biliary sphincterotomy (with or without biliary stent placement depending on efficiency of bile drainage after sphicterotomy) should be performed. For ampullary tumors greater than 2 cm in size, alternatively, a pancreatic ductal stent can be inserted first and piecemeal ampullectomy can be performed. In this method, after ampullectomy is completed, thermal ablation of the base of the tumor could result in lower incidents of recurrence.

Only five studies have critically evaluated endoscopic ampullectomy. The success rates ranged from 60 to 90%, with complication rates ranging from 9.7 to 27%. The complications included acute pancreatitis, bleeding, cholangitis, duodenal perforation, and late papillary stenosis. Among all patients in reported series, there was only one death, which occurred as a result of severe necrotizing pancreatitis.[31–35] The largest one of the five studies had 103 patients. The long-term success rate was 80%, with a complication rate of 9.7%; complications included acute pancreatitis (5%), bleeding (2%), and late papillary stenosis (3%). By multivariate logistic analysis, predictors of successful endoscopic resection included age greater than 48 years ($p < .001$), lesion size of 24 mm or less ($p = .001$), and male gender ($p < .05$). Acute pancreatitis occurred more frequently in patients without pancreatic duct stents (17% vs 3.3%), and papillary stenosis also occurred more frequently in patients without pancreatic duct stents (8.3% vs 2.2%). The recurrence rate for papillary adenoma after ampullectomy was 20%. Significant risk factors for recurrence were larger size, genetic predisposition, younger age, and absence of adjuvant thermal ablation at the initial ampullectomy. For patients who have adenomas removed completely, endoscopic surveillance at 6-month intervals for a minimum of 2 years is recommended. For patients with FAP, more vigilant surveillance would be prudent.[35]

If the neoplasm is not completely removed at the initial procedure, ampullectomy and thermal ablation should be repeated at 2- to 3-month intervals until ablation is complete.

Photodynamic Therapy

Photodynamic therapy (PDT) with porfimer sodium has been used to treat patients with high-grade dysplasia (HGD) and early-stage esophageal cancer (T1). Patients receive an intravenous injection (2 mg/kg) of porfimer sodium (Photofrin, Axcan Pharma, Mont-Saint-Hilaire, QC). Three days after drug injection, 630 nm light from a potassium titanyl phosphate dye laser (Laserscope, San Jose, CA) is delivered by using a cylindrical diffuser inserted in a 20 nm-diameter reflective esophageal PDT balloon (Wilson-Cook Medical Inc., Winston-Salem, NC). Esophageal strictures can occur in 18 to 37% of patients after PDT for HGD in Barrett's esophagus.[36–39] Strictures occur within 3 to 4 weeks and require serial dilations. When different light doses were employed, the efficacy and stricture rate were different among them. In a study of 113 patients with Barrett's esophagus with HGD or T1 disease, residual HGD or T1 disease. After one treatment was seen in 17% of patients with a light dose of 115 J/cm, 33.3% with a light dose of 105 J/cm, 29.4% with a light dose of 95 J/cm, and 31.6% with a light dose of 85 J/cm. Complete ablation of Barrett's mucosa and total replacement of the treated area with squamous mucosa were achieved in 40.7% treated with a light dose of 115 J/cm, 35.3% of patients treated with a light dose of 105 J/cm, 33.3% of patients treated with a light dose of 95 J/cm, and 21% of patients treated with a light dose of 85 J/cm. 205 Although the overall rate of stricture formation was not directly correlated to the light dose, severe strictures requiring more than six dilations were seen in 15.3% with a light dose of 115 J/cm, 5.6% with a light dose of 105 J/cm, 5.9% with a light dose of 95 J/cm, and 5.3% with a light dose of 85 J/cm. Thus, decreasing the light dose below 115 J/cm reduced the rate of the stricture at the expense of efficacy. The optimal dose for treatment with PDT is yet to be established.[40]

Endoluminal Stenting

Esophageal Stents

Most esophageal cancer patients will present with unresectable disease, and treatment is limited to palliation.[41] Relief of dysphagia is a major focus, and this can be addressed with endoscopic measures, primarily self-expanding metallic stents (SEMSs). A subset of patients will develop tracheoesophageal fistulae (TEF) and be good candidates for a SEMS. Although other endoscopic modalities have been used in the past to reestablish esophageal lumen, SEMSs have become the primary endoscopic measure since their introduction in the early 1990s. Early studies showed a clear advantage over plastic stents.[42] Advantages over recanalization by laser therapy have been difficult to demonstrate.[43,44] PDT has not been shown to be more effective or safer than SEMSs.[45,46] Concerns about the high cost of SEMSs have been tempered by studies showing no cost disadvantage despite the high initial expense as patients palliated with SEMSs need fewer interventions than laser and have fewer complications than plastic stents.[47,48]

Placement of a SEMS is done with fluoroscopy and at some centers is performed by interventional radiology. A previous definition of the esophageal anatomy is desirable but not essential. The presence and location of a TEF should be confirmed by previous imaging or contrast injection at the time of stent placement. Most commercially available stents have a coating covering most, if not all, of the stent. Available lengths are typically 10 to 15 cm. The diameter of the delivery systems precludes through-the-scope placement. However, the relatively slim profile of some stents, such as the 18F diameter Wallstent II (Boston Scientific, Natick, MA), makes negotiation of strictures possible with little to no dilation. Antireflux valves are available with some stent designs for those patients prone to gastroesophageal reflux disease. Dilation of the stricture should be avoided or kept to a minimum to reduce the risk of perforation.[49] We use a small-caliber 5 mm in diameter scope (Pentax 1540, Pentax Inc. Montvale, NJ 1540) to facilitate passage through the stricture. A wire is placed into the stomach, and the scope is withdrawn after stricture length is determined. External metal markers are used to delineate the proximal and distal margins of the stricture. Alternatively, contrast material can be injected via a sclerotherapy needle into the submucosal layer at the margins. A stent length is chosen that will readily bridge the stricture, leaving 1 to 2 cm at either end to accommodate stent foreshortening and to avoid having the uncovered ends within the stricture. The stent is passed over the wire and into position. An endoscope can be introduced alongside to check proximal positioning. The stent is deployed slowly to allow an opportunity to make final adjustments in position prior to full release. The small-caliber endoscope is then reintroduced to assess stent patency and placement. Patients are allowed a liquid diet and are to advance their diet as tolerated as the stent expands over the next 48 hours. Proton pump blockers are routinely prescribed for those with a stent bridging the esophagogastric junction.

Dysphagia will improve in 80 to 90% of patients, although this may be modest.[50] At least 80% of TEF will close at least temporarily.[49,51] Despite less dysphagia, improvement in quality of life is not readily demonstrated.[44,52] Although the mainstay of endoscopic palliation, placement of a SEMS is a procedure plagued by a high complication rate.[53,54] A quarter to half of patients will suffer a major complication requiring another stent, endoscopy, admission, or a percutaneous endoscopic gastrostomy tube.[55–57] In addition, the operative mortality is 1 to 2%. Patient selection for SEMSs should be based on several factors. The presence of a TEF is the most clear-cut indication. The best timing of stent placement relative to other therapeutic interventions is debated. Whereas early reports suggested a higher

complication rate in those patients who have received chemoradiation, our experience and that of others have not shown such an increased risk.[58,59] On the other hand, there are reasons to defer stent placement prior to chemoradiation. First, chemoradiation may lead to improvement in dysphagia and that tumor regression can result in stent migration. In most cases of migration, the stents remain in the stomach, although some travel distally and can obstruct.[60,61] Stents designed for easy removal from the esophagus or stomach as chemoradiation is completed would effectively deal with this concern.[62] However, removal of a SEMS requires substantial technical expertise, with associated risk of bleeding and perforation.[63] Second, very high complication rates have been reported in patients with SEMSs who subsequently undergo radiation therapy.[64] High cervical lesions are problematic as there may be insufficient room proximally for stent placement without encroaching on the hypopharynx, and palliative benefit is limited.[65] Stents for tumors involving the esophagogastric junction can lead to reflux symptoms and have a higher rate of migration in some studies.[50] A stent with an antireflux valve is an option, although experience with them is mixed and the number of patients not responding to acid-suppressive therapy is small.[54,55,66,67]

So ideal timing of SEMS placement in the course of the patient's illness is unclear. Some authors argue for deferring SEMS placement until dysphagia proves refractory to all other modalities.[52] Prolonged patient survival with SEMS is associated with a higher risk of stent dysfunction.[68] Yet others argue that SEMSs should be reserved only for those with longer life expectancies.[43] The use of SEMSs has decreased over the years at our institution despite increasing numbers of esophageal cancer patients.[49,69] The limited benefits that SEMSs can offer, as well as an appreciation of their complication risks, have contributed to this decline. Other endoscopic modalities have not been substituted, nor are other services deploying SEMS. Rather, we have adopted a position of allowing sufficient time after chemoradiation for its benefits to be defined. In those patients who are not candidates for chemoradiation or who have completed radiation with recurrent dysphagia, SEMSs are placed if there is a reasonable life expectancy measured in weeks or months and the anatomy permits.

Enteral Stents

Gastric outlet obstruction can result from a primary or metastatic malignant process involving the distal stomach, duodenum, or periampullary region. The most common etiology is pancreatic adenocarcinoma.[70] The traditional approach has been surgical bypass, but SEMSs offer an alternative, with less morbidity and a faster return

to oral intake at a lower cost.[71–73] No control trials comparing the two approaches exist.

The technique is basically similar to that of esophageal stents, with the advantage that the slim delivery catheter allows through-the-scope placement. Previous barium studies are helpful to define the anatomy and to rule out additional distal strictures but are not necessary or at times possible owing to complete obstruction. Attempts at a barium study may complicate stent placement owing to retained barium hampering endoscopic and fluoroscopic views. A small-caliber scope may facilitate wire placement across the stricture. If the stricture is too tight for a scope, then advancing a biliary catheter into the stricture under fluoroscopy with intermittent injection of contrast can facilitate wire placement. A floppy wire may be required to traverse the stricture initially and can be replaced with a stiffer wire through the biliary catheter. The distal margin of the stricture should be carefully marked externally or, if possible, by an endoclip or submucosal injection of contrast. A typical stent has a delivery system 10F in diameter and can readily go through a 3.8 mm channel. Owing to its small caliber, dilation of the stricture is rarely required. If stent passage requires dilation, this should be kept to a minimum to attenuate the risk of perforation. Diameters of expanded stents are 20 to 22 mm, with lengths of 60 and 90 mm. Covered versions were found to migrate too readily and are no longer available.

Biliary ductal patency is a concern, and placement of a SEMS in the biliary tree prior to deployment of duodenal stents is desirable. The stents can be placed during the same procedure if the duodenoscope can be introduced.[74] However, a high failure rate has been reported in this setting even with stricture dilation to facilitate passage of the duodenoscope.[75] Dilation in this setting carries a 6% risk of perforation.[75] If biliary drainage cannot be achieved endoscopically, then a percutaneous approach with placement of the biliary SEMS through the sidewall of the duodenal SEMS is possible.[72]

Stricture length dictates placement of more than one stent in 7 to 18% of patients.[72,75–77] Two recent reviews found that technically adequate stenting is achieved in 94 to 97% of patients.[70,78] However, clinical success is not seen in 7 to 11% of those with adequate stent placement owing to dysmotility or distal disease.[70,78] As a result, the overall success rate is 87%. Data from five recent series show that resumption of a normal or soft diet is possible in 70% of patients.[71,72,75–77] Ten to 17% of stents will obstruct, usually with tumor ingrowth.[70,78] This compares with 10% of patients after bypass gastrojejunostomy who develop recurrent obstructive symptoms.[79] Migration is seen with 2.7% of uncovered stents.[78] Abdominal pain occurs in 2.5%.[70] Bleeding and perforation are seen in 1%.[70,78] Procedural mortality is not reported.[70] The median survival rate reported ranges from 7 to 14.5 weeks.[75–78,80] No improvement over historical median survival after surgical bypass is seen.[71]

In patients with incurable disease causing gastric outlet obstruction, SEMSs represent the best option for palliation, with an 87% likelihood of relieving symptoms and a 70% chance of resumption of a nearly normal diet. This intervention requires little, if any, hospital time versus a postgastrojejunostomy bypass recovery period of a median 14 to 17 days in patients with an average survival of only a few months.[73,79,81] The timing of stent placement should be dictated by symptoms, functional status, and available therapeutic options. Chemoradiation therapies should have been exhausted or have a low likelihood of producing major tumor regression to minimize the chances of distal migration or stent-induced perforation.[75]

Colonic Stents

Colonic obstruction can be the initial presentation of colon cancer or develop with recurrent or progressive disease. SEMSs offer an alternative to surgery for relieving the obstruction. As with enteral stents, no controlled trials comparing the two approaches exist.[82] A recent review involving 1,198 patients providessome perspective as to the role of SEMSs in this setting.[83] Two-thirds of stents were placed for palliation of recurrent or unresectable disease. The other third were placed for bridging the acutely obstructed patients to definitive resection, thereby forgoing an emergent decompressive colostomy. Eighty-six percent of the stents were for rectosigmoid disease. Eleven percent were for left colon obstruction. Two percent were deployed in the transverse colon and 0.5% in the ascending colon. Technical success is seen in 93% of patients, although this does not always equate with clinical success, which is seen in 88%.[83] Facilitating a single-stage surgery was possible in 72% in the "bridge to surgery" indication group. Migration is seen in 12%, with most occurring in the first week after deployment. The more proximal the stent, the higher the migration rate. Perforation is seen in 2.8% of patients not previously dilated. The perforation rate in those patients whose strictures were dilated prior to stent placement was almost six times higher. Perforations were responsible for five of seven procedure-related deaths, and procedure-related mortality was 0.58%. Reobstruction occurred in 7.8% of uncovered stents at a median time of 24 weeks. Additional complications seen are bleeding and migration in 5 and 10% of patients, respectively.[82] The need for surgical intervention for complications can be as high as 12.5%.[84] It is unclear if previous radiation therapy alters complication rates. [82]

As with other SEMSs, contrast studies are of limited utility in the acute setting and attempts at opacification can hinder subsequent endoscopic and fluoroscopic evaluation. Imaging studies such as CT or abdominal plain films to rule out perforation and give approximate location of stricture are vital. Colonoscopic evaluation of the stricture and its anatomy follows. A small-caliber scope can be critical to facilitate negotiation of the stricture and place a wire proximally. In those patients in whom endoscopic advance through the stricture is not possible, fluoroscopic guidance is sufficient for stent placement. Fluoroscopic images are easier to interpret with the patient in the supine position than the patient in the left lateral decubitus position. A biliary catheter can help with passage of the wire in those strictures too tight even for the small-caliber scopes. A wire with a floppy tip can help with initial passage. The biliary catheter can then be advanced through the stricture and a stiffer wire substituted to facilitate stent passage. Stents are identical to those used in the duodenum or are available from some vendors with slightly large diameters. Delivery catheter size in some versions allows passage through a therapeutic scope accessory channel, simplifying placement, particularly for proximal lesions.[82] All commercially available stents are uncovered owing to high migration rates with early covered versions. In those patients with fistulae, a covered esophageal stent can be deployed.[85] Present dilation is not advised as perforation rates are sharply increased. Prophylactic antibiotics are not routinely recommended yet may have a role in those patients with complete obstruction and marked colon dilation.[82]

Patients are advised to comply with a low-residue diet and adopt a bowel management regimen to avoid stool impaction in the stent.[82]

A small, randomized trial of left-sided partial obstruction treated with a SEMS versus colostomy showed better quality of life in the stent group, with comparable costs.[86] Using historical controls, Johnson and colleagues found comparable outcomes after SEMSs, despite a patient population with poorer performance status than surgical controls.[87] In an analysis of the bridge to surgery presentation, Targownik and colleagues found in a decision analysis that SEMSs followed by elective surgical resection had better outcomes at lower cost compared with emergent surgery with stoma formation or primary resection.[88] Stent placement in acute obstruction has no adverse effects on long-term prognosis compared with initial surgical decompression.[89]

Future in Interventional Gastroenterology

With ongoing development of new tools and technology, the future of endoscopic therapy of gastrointestinal malignancies has promising potential. Ideas that have been considered include EUS-guided radiofrequency ablation, EUS-guided PDT with probe insertion, EUS-guided alcohol injection into the solid tumors, including pancreatic cancer, and endoscopically delivered chemotherapy. We look forward to the results of further research in this exciting area.

REFERENCES

1. Vazquez-Sequeiros E, Wiersema MJ, Clain JE, et al. Impact of lymph node staging on therapy of esophageal carcinoma. Gastroenterology 2003;125:1626–35.
2. Vazquez-Sequeiros E, Levy MJ, Clain JE, et al. Routine versus selective EUS FNA approach for preoperative nodal staging of esophageal carcinoma [abstract]. Gastrointest Endosc 2002;55:AB227.
3. Kalha I, Kaw M, Fukami N, et al. The accuracy of endoscopic ultrasound for restaging esophageal carcinoma after chemoradiation therapy. Cancer 2004;101:940–7.
4. Ries, LAG, Kosarl CL, Hankey BF, et al. SEER cancer statistics review 1973–1996. Bethesda (MD): National Cancer Institute; 2000.
5. Wiersema MJ, Vilmann P, Giovannini M, et al. Endosonography-guided fine-needle aspiration biopsy: diagnostic accuracy and complication assessment. Gastroenterology 1997;112:1087–91.
6. Lee JH, Salem R, Aslanian H, et al. Endoscopic ultrasound and fine-needle aspiration of unexplained bile duct strictures. Am JGastroenterol 2004;99:1069–73.
7. Modlin IM, Tang LH. Approaches to the diagnosis of gut neuroendocrine tumors: the last word (today). Gastroenterology 1997;112:583–90.
8. Feldman M, Bruce FS., Marvin H. Sleisenger Jensen RT, Norton JA. Endocrine tumors of the pancreas. In: Sleisenger and Fordtran's gastrointestinal and liver disease: pathophysiology/diagnosis/management. 6th ed. Philadelphia: WB Saunders; 1998. p. 871.
9. Owen NJ, Sohaib SA, Peppercorn PD, et al. MRI of pancreatic neuroendocrine tumours. Br J Radiol 2001;74: 968–73.
10. Gunther RW, Klose KJ, Ruckert K, et al. Islet-cell tumors: detection of small lesions with computed tomography and ultrasound. Radiology 1983;148:485–8.
11. Stark DD, Moss AA, Goldberg HI, et al. CT of pancreatic islet cell tumors. Radiology 1984;150:491–4.
12. Frucht H, Doppman JH, Norton JA, et al. Gastrinoma: comparison of MR imaging with CT, angiography, and US. Radiology 1989;171:713–7.
13. Thom AK, Norton JA, Doppman JL, et al. Prospective study of the use of intraarterial secretin injection and portal venous sampling to localize duodenal gastrinomas. Surgery 1992;112:1002–8; discussion 1008–9.
14. Zimmer T, Stolzel U, Bader M, et al. Endoscopic ultrasonography and somatostatin receptor scintigrapy in the preoperative localization of insulinomas and gastrinomas. Gut 1996;39:562–8.
15. Ardengh JC, de Paulo GA, Ferrari AP. EUS-guided FNA in the diagnosis of pancreatic neuroendocrine tumors before surgery. Gastrointest Endosc 2004;60:378–84.
16. Lee JH, Topazian M. Pancreatic endosonography after Bilroth II gastrectomy. Endoscopy 2004;36:972–5.
17. Brugge WR, Lewandrowski K, Lee-Lewandrowski E, et al. Diagnosis of pancreatic cystic neoplasms: a report of the Cooperative Pancreatic Cyst Study. Gastroenterology 2004;126:1330–6.
18. Harewood GC. Assessment of publication bias in the reporting of EUS performance in staging rectal cancer. Am J Gastroenterol 2005;100:808–16.
19. Yamashita Y, Machi J, Shirouzu K, et al. Evaluation of endorectal ultrasound for the assessment of wall invasion of rectal cancer. Report of a case. Dis Colon Rectum 1998;31:617–23.
20. Gress FG, Savides TJ, Sandler A, et al. Endoscopic ultrasonography, fine needle aspiration biopsy guided by endoscopic ultrasonography, and computed tomography in the pre-operative staging of non-small cell lung cancer: a comparison study. Ann Intern Med 1997;127:604–12.
21. Silvestri GA, Hoffman BJ, Bhutani MS, et al. Endoscopic ultrasound with fine needle aspiration in the diagnosis and staging of lung cancer. Ann Thorac Surg 1996;61: 1441–6.

22. Wallace MB, Silvestri GA, Sahai AV, et al. Endoscopic ultrasound guided fine needle aspiration for staging patients with carcinoma of the lung. Ann Thorac Surg 2001; 72:1861–97.

23. Fritcher-Ravens A, Bohuslavizki KH, Brandt L, et al. Mediastinal lymph node involvement in potentially resectable lung cancer: comparison of CT, positron emission tomography, and endoscopic ultrasonography with and without fine-needle aspiration. Chest 2003;123:442–51.

24. Varadarajulu S, Schmulewitz N, Wildi S, et al. Accuracy of EUS in staging of T4 lung cancer. Gastrointest Endosc 2004;59:345–8.

25. Wasan SM, Ross W, Lee JH, et al. Use of expandable metallic biliary stents in resectable pancreatic cancer. Am J Gastroenterol 2005;100:1–6.

26. Wasan SM, Ross W, Lee JH, et al. Metal stents in surgically resectable pancreatic cancer. ACG Plenary Session 2004;105:3.

27. Scotiniotis IA, Kochman M, Lewis J, et al. Accuracy of EUS in the evaluation of Barrett's esophagus and high-grade dysplasia or intramucosal carcinoma. Gastrointest Endosc 2001;54:689–96.

28. Kume K, Yamasaki M, Kubo K, et al. EMR of upper GI lesions when using a novel soft, irrigation, prelooped hood. Gastrointest Endosc 2004;60:124–8.

29. Yao T, Iida M, Watanabe H. Duodenal lesions in familial polyposis of the colon. Gastroenterology 1977;73: 1086–92.

30. Jones TR, Nance FC. Periampullary malignancy in Gardner's syndrome. Ann Surg 1977;185:165–73.

31. Binmoeller KF, Boaventura S, Ramsperger K, et al. Endoscopic snare excision of benign adenomas of the papilla of Vater. Gastrointest Endosc 1993;39:127–31.

32. Norton ID, Gostout CJ, Baron TH, et al. Safety and outcome of endoscopic snare excision of the major duodenal papilla. Gastrointest Endosc 2002;56:239–43.

33. Greenspan AB, Walden DT, Aliperti G, et al. Endoscopic management of ampullary adenomas. A report of eight patients [abstract]. Gastrointest Endosc 1997;45:AB433.

34. Martin JA, Haber GB, Kortan PP, et al. Endoscopic snare ampullectomy for resection of benign ampullary neoplasms [abstract]. Gastrointest Endosc 1997;45: AB458.

35. Catalano MF, Linder JD, Chak A, et al. Endoscopic management of adenoma of the major duodenal papilla. Gastrointest Endosc 2004;59:225–32.

36. Overholt BF, Panjehpour M, Haydek JM, et al. Photodynamic therapy for Barrett's esophagus: follow-up in 100 patients. Gastrointest Endosc 1999;49:1–7.

37. Laukka MA, Wang KK. Initial results using low-dose photodynamic therapy in the treatment of Barrett's esophagus. Gastrointest Endosc 1995;42:59–63.

38. Overholt BF, Panjehpour M, Halberg DL. Photodynamic therapy for Barrett's esophagus with dysplasia and/or early stage carcinoma: long-term results Gastrointest Endosc 2003;58:183–8.

39. Overholt BF, Lightdale CL, Wang KK, et al. International multicenter, partially blinded, randomized study of the efficacy of photodynamic therapy using porfimer sodium for ablation of high-grade dysplasia in Barrett's esophagus: results of 24-month follow-up [abstract]. Gastroenterology 2003;124:A20.

40. Panjehpour M, Overholt BF, Phan MN, et al. Optimization of light dosimetry for photodynamic therapy of Barrett's esophagus: efficacy vs. incidence of stricture after treatment. Gastrointest Endosc 2005;61:13–8.

41. Enzinger PC, Mayer RJ. Esophageal cancer. N Engl J Med 2003;349:2241–52.

42. Knyrim K, Wagner H-J, Bethge N, et al. A controlled trial of an expansile metal stent for palliation of esophageal obstruction due to inoperable cancer. N Engl J Med 1993;329:1302–7.

43. Gevers AM, Macken E, Hiele M, et al. A comparison of laser therapy, plastic stents, and expandable metal stents for palliation of malignant dysphagia in patients without a fistula. Gastrointest Endosc 1998;48:383–8.

44. Dallal HJ, Smith GD, Grieve DC, et al. A randomized trial of thermal ablative therapy versus metal stents in the palliative therapy of patients with esophageal carcinoma. Gastrointest Endosc 2001;54:549–57.

45. Canto MI, Smith C, McClellend L, et al. Randomized trial of PDT vs. stent for palliation of malignant dysphagia: cost-effectiveness and quality of life. Gastrointest Endosc 2002;AB100.

46. Litle VR, Luketich JD, Christie NA, et al. Photodynamic therapy as palliation for esophageal cancer: experience in 215 patients. Ann Thorac Surg 2003;76:1687–93.

47. O'Donnell CA, Fularton GM, Watt E, et al. Randomized clinical trial comparing self-expanding metallic stents with plastic endoprosthesis in the palliation of oesophageal cancer. Br J Surg 2002;89:985–92.

48. Polinder S, Homs MYV, Siersema PD, et al. Cost study of metal stent placement vs single-dose brachytherapy in the palliative treatment of oesophageal cancer. Br J Cancer 2004;90:2067–72.

49. Raijman I, Siddique I, Ajani J, et al. Palliation of malignant dysphagia and fistulae with coated expandable metal stents: experience with 101 patients. Gastrointest Endosc 1998;48:172–9.

50. Christie NA, Buenaventura PO, Fernando HC, et al. Results of expandable metal stents for malignant esophageal obstruction in 100 patients: short-term and long-term follow-up. Ann Thorac Surg 2001;71:797–802.

51. Shin JH, Song H-Y, Ko G-Y, et al. Esophagorespiratory fistula: long-term results of palliative treatment with covered expandable metallic stents in 61 patients. Radiol 2004;232:252–9.

52. Homs MYV, Steyererg ELS, Eijkenboom WH-H, et al. Single-dose brachytherapy versus metal stent placement for palliation of dysphagia from oesophageal cancer: multicentre randomized trial. Lancet 2004;364:1497–504.

53. Jacobson BC, Hirota W, Baron TH, et al. The role of endscopy in the assessment and treatment of esophageal cancer. Gastrointest Endosc 2003;57:817–22.

54. Ramirez FC, Dennert B, Zierer ST, et al. Esophageal self-expandable metallic stents—indications, practice, techniques, and complications: results of a national survey. Gastrointest Endosc 1997;45:360–4.

55. Homs MYV, Wahab PJ, Kuipers EJ, et al. Esophageal stents with antireflux valve for tumors of the distal esophagus and gastric cardia: a randomized trial. Gastrointest Endosc 2004;60:695–702.

56. Thompson AM, Rapson T, Gilbert FJ, et al. Endoscopic palliative treatment for esophageal and gastric cancer. Surg Endosc 2004;18:1257–62.

57. Cwikiel W, Tranberg K-G, Cwikiel M, et al. Malignant dysphagia: palliation with esophageal stents—long-term results in 100 patients. Radiology 1998;207:513–8.

58. Raijman I, Siddique I, Lynch P. Does chemoradiation therapy increase the incidence of complications with self-expanding coated stents in the management of malignant esophageal strictures? Am J Gastroenterol 1997; 92:2192–6.

59. Homs MYV, Hansen BE, van Blankenstein M, et al. Prior radiation and/or chemotherapy has no effect on the outcome of metal stent placement for oesophagogastric carcinoma. Eur J Gastroenterol Hepatol 2004;16:163–70.

60. Thuraisingam A, Hughes ML, Smart HL. Down-staging of an advanced esophageal carcinoma with chemoradiotherapy leading to stent migration necessitating colectomy. Gastrointest Endosc 2004;90:457–60.

61. DePalma GD, Iovino P, Catanzano C. Distally migrated esophageal self-expanding metal stents: wait and see or remove? Gastrointest Endosc 2001;53:96–8.

62. Shin JH, Song H-Y, Kim JH, et al. Comparison of temporary and permanent stent placement with concurrent radiation therapy in patients with esophageal carcinoma. J Vasc Interv Radiol 2005;16:67–74.

63. Low DE, Kozarek RA. Removal of esophageal expandable metal stents: description of technique and review of potential applications. Surg Endosc 2003;17:990–6.

64. Nishimura Y, Nagata K, Katano S, et al. Severe complications in advanced cancer treated with radiotherapy after intubation of esophageal stents: a questionnaire survey of Japanese Society for Esophageal Diseases. Int J Radiat Oncol Biol Phys 2003;56:1327–32.

65. Conio M, Caroli-Bose F, Sorbi D, et al. Self-expanidng metal stents in the palliation of neoplasms of the cervical esophagus. Hepatogastroenterology 1999;46:272–7.

66. Sabharwal T, Hamady MS, Chui S, et al. A randomized prospective comparison of the Flamingo Wallstent and Ultraflex stent for palliation of dysphagia associated with lower third oesophageal carcinoma. Gut 2003;99:922–9.

67. Dua KS, Kozarek R, Kim J, et al. Self-expanding metal esophageal stent with anti-reflux mechanism. Gastrointest Endosc 2001;53:603–13.

68. Kozarek RA. Complications and lessons learned from 10 years of expandable gastrointestinal prosthesis. Dig Dis 1999;17:14–22.

69. Ross WA, Alkassab F, Lynch PM, et al. Evolving role of self-expanding metal stents in the treatment of malignant dysphagia and fistulas. Gastrointest Endosc 2007 Jan; 65(1):70–6

70. Dormann A, Meisner S, Verin N, et al. Self-expanding metal stents for gastroduodenal malignancies: systematic review of their clinical effectiveness. Endoscopy 2004;36:543–50.

71. Maetani I, Tada T, Ukita T, et al. Comparison of duodenal stent placement with surgical gastrojejunostomy for palliation in patients with duodenal obstructions caused by pancreaticobiliary malignancies. Endoscopy 2004; 36:73–8.

72. Adler DG, Baron TH. Endoscopic palliation of malignant gastric outlet obstruction using self-expanding metal stents: experience in 36 patients. Am J Gastroenterol 2002;97:72–8.

73. Yim HB, Jacobson BC, Saltzman JR, et al. Clinical outcome of the use of enteral stents for palliation of patients with malignant upper GI obstruction. Gastrointest Endosc 2001;53:329–32.

74. Kaw M, Singh S, Gagneja J. Clinical outcome of simultaneous self-expandable metal stents for palliation of malignant biliary and duodenal obstruction. Surg Endosc 2003;17:457–61.

75. Nassif T, Prat F, Meduri B, et al. Endoscopic palliation of malignant gastric outlet obstruction using self-expanding metallic stents: results of a multicenter study. Endoscopy 2003;35:483–9.

76. Kaw M, Singh S, Gagneja J, et al. Role of self-expandable metal stents in the palliation of malignant duodenal obstruction. Surg Endosc 2003;17:646–50.

77. Lindsay JO, Andreyev HJN, Vlavianos P, et al. Self-expanding metal stents for the palliation of malignant gastroduodenal obstruction in patients unsuitable for surgical bypass. Aliment Pharmacol Ther 2004;19:901–5.

78. Holt AP, Patel M, Ahmed MM. Palliation of patients with malignant gastroduodenal obstruction with self-expanding metallic stents: the treatment of choice? Gastrointest Endosc 2004;60:1010–7.

79. Van Wangensveld BA, Coene PPLO, Van Gulik TM, et al. Outcome of palliative biliary and gastric bypass surgery for pancreatic head carcinoma in 126 patients. Br J Surg 1997;84:1402–6.

80. Aviv RI, Shyamalan G, Khan FH, et al. Use of stents in the palliative treatment of malignant gastric outlet and duodenal obstruction. Clin Radiol 2002;57:587–92.

81. Wong YT, Brams DM, Munson L, et al. Gastric outlet obstruction secondary to pancreatic cancer. Surg Endosc 2002;16:310–2.

82. Baron TH, Kozarek RA. Endoscopic stenting of colonic tumours. Best Pract Res Clin Gastroenterol 2004;18: 209–29.

83. Sebastian S, Johnston S, Geoghegan T, et al. Pooled analysis of the efficacy and safety of self-expanding metal stenting in malignant colorectal obstruction. Am J Gastroenterol 2004;99:2051–7.

84. Raijman I, Linder J, Ami V, et al. Management of malignant colorectal obstruction with expandable stents: experience in 34 patients [abstract]. Gastrointest Endosc 1999;49: AB174.

85. Repici A, Reggio D, Saracco G, et al. Self-expanding covered esophageal Ultraflex stent for palliation of malignant colorectal anastomotic obstruction complicated by multiple fistulas. Gastrointest Endosc 2000;51:346–8.

86. Xinopoulos D, Dimitroulopoulos D, Theodosopoulos T, et al. Stenting or stoma creation for patients with inoperable malignant colonic obstructions? Results of a study and cost-effectiveness analysis. Surg Endosc 2004;18: 421–6.

87. Johnson R, Marsh R, Corson J, et al. A comparison of two methods of palliation of large bowel obsruction due to irremovable colon cancer. Ann R Coll Engl 2004;86: 99–103.

88. Targownik LE, Spiegel BM, Sack J, et al. Colonic stents vs. emergency surgery for management of acute left sided malignant colonic obstruction: a decision analysis. Gastrointest Endosc 2004;60:865–74.

89. Saida Y, Sumiyama Y, Nagao J, et al. Long-term prognosis of preoperative "bridge to surgery" expandable metallic stent insertion for obstructive colorectal cancer: comparison with emergency operation. Dis Colon Rectum 2003;46(Suppl 10):44–9.

Nutritional Issues in Cancer Patients

Yakir Muszkat, MD

Genetic predisposition and environmental factors play major roles in the etiology of cancer.[1,2] Dietary factors are among the most important environmental factors implicated in cancer development.[3] It has been estimated that approximately 35% (10–70%) of all cancers are attributable to diet.[4] Cancer is a multistage process that involves activation of a precarcinogen to an ultimate carcinogen, initiation of a tumor cell through oncogene expression, and, finally, promotion to clinical cancer. Nutritional factors can interact in all of these steps, both positively and negatively. Therefore, nutrients such as vitamins, minerals, or other food constituents may also function as chemopreventive agents that may help reverse, suppress, or prevent progression to invasive cancer.[5]

Although the role of diet in health and disease has been known since ancient times,[6] many of the current recommendations are based on evidence that is derived from more recent epidemiologic studies.[7] However, for a number of nutrients, well-designed dietary intervention studies have failed to demonstrate the anticipated protection against cancer.[8] A novel approach to understanding this discrepancy has been to study the response to a specific nutrient as determined by an individual's genotype. The great variability in the responses of subjects in nutritional intervention studies may be due to differences in study participants' genetic polymorphisms. This has led investigators to further define the role that nutrients play in influencing genetic processes involved in carcinogenesis, such as those that determine cellular metabolism, differentiation, and apoptosis. Therefore, even though genetic factors cannot be altered, making beneficial changes in nutritional habits may potentially decrease the risk of cancer substantially.[9]

Once cancer is diagnosed, up to 80% of patients will develop weight loss and malnutrition during the course of their illness.[10] Malnutrition in patients with cancer has been associated with longer hospital stays,[11] diminished tolerance of and responsiveness to both chemotherapy and radiotherapy,[10] increased perioperative morbidity,[12] increased cost,[13] worse performance status and quality of life, and decreased survival.[11] The etiology of malnutrition in such patients is multifactorial. The causes can be classified into two major categories: (1) anorexia, factors related to decreased food intake, and gastrointestinal dysfunction and (2) metabolic disturbances.[14,15] Although numerous techniques are available for the nutritional assessment of these patients, most of these methods are difficult to interpret in clinical practice and are poor indicators of response to therapy in patients with malignancy.[16]

Oral dietary therapy, oral supplements, and enteral or parenteral nutrition are all forms of nutritional therapy that can be used depending on the clinical circumstances.[17] It is important to clearly define the goals and objectives of therapy prior to initiating nutritional support and to limit the decision to initiate nutritional therapy to clinical situations in which the benefits outweigh the risks.[18] Cancer survivors may have persistent gastrointestinal failure secondary to the effects of previous radiation therapy or multiple surgical resections and may require long-term home enteral or total parenteral nutrition (TPN).[14]

Dietary Factors and Cancer

During the last few decades, increasing attention has been paid to various foods, nutrients, and dietary lifestyles as modifiers of cancer risk. Many hypotheses describing the effects of diet on cancer risk have been derived by analyzing the dietary patterns and cancer rates in different populations around the world. It was noted in the 1970s that developed Western countries have diets high in animal products, fat, and sugar and high rates of cancer of the colorectum, breast, and prostate. In contrast, developing countries typically have diets based on one or two starchy staple foods, low intakes of animal products, fat and sugar, low rates of 'Western'-type cancers, and higher rates of cancer of the esophagus, stomach, and liver. The international variations in diet and cancer rates suggest that diet is an important risk factor for many common cancers; therefore, cancer may be partially preventable by dietary changes.[19]

Epidemiologic Evidence

The great interest in diet and human cancer in the last several decades derives from the large variations in the rates of specific cancers among countries, changes in the incidence of certain types of cancer over a relatively short time span, and dramatic changes in cancer incidence among populations emigrating to regions with different cancer rates. More than 50 years ago, Burkitt and his associates noted a negligible risk of colon cancer among the indigenous populations of many African countries. The diets in these countries were quite similar: low in calories, low in fat and animal protein, high in fiber, and rich in vegetables, fruits, and cereal grains. Furthermore, over the past several decades, the incidence of stomach cancer in the United States has progressively declined. Similarly, 50 years ago, stomach cancer was the most prevalent malignancy in Japan and colorectal cancer was quite rare. Today, the incidence of stomach cancer is declining, whereas the rate of colon cancer is increasing. Finally, the incidence of breast cancer in Japan is much lower than in Japanese women from Hawaii. However, in one generation, Japanese women who move to Hawaii increase their risk of developing breast cancer, and in two generations, they develop the same risk as native-born Hawaiians.[1]

More recent studies have focused on the diet of individuals and the role of specific nutritional factors and the risk of developing cancer. The evidence linking nutritional factors to cancer is derived from many different lines of evidence of varying strengths. In vitro animal and epidemiologic studies have all contributed to understanding the relationship between nutrition and cancer. In vitro studies provide data on cellular mechanisms involving individual nutrients. Animal studies can test hypotheses and contribute causal inferences, but these may not be directly relevant to humans.[5] Epidemiologic studies such as case-control and prospective, observational studies have also greatly contributed to identifying risk factors and generating hypotheses, but these have their limitations. Case-control studies are useful for searching for possible dietary effects but cannot be relied on to establish moderate dietary associations because they are susceptible to both recall and selection bias. Accurate assessment of dietary intake through food records, food frequency questionnaires, and dietary recall can be problematic. Another limitation of case-control

Table 1 Dietary and Nutritional Factors and Cancer Risk[2,19]

Cancer Site	Probable		Possible	
	Harmful	**Protective**	**Harmful**	**Protective**
Oral cavity, pharynx, esophagus	Alcohol Obesity Hot drinks and food	Fruits and vegetables		Riboflavin Folate Vitamin C Zinc
Nasopharyngeal	Chinese style salted fish			
Stomach	Salted fish and meat Pickled vegetables Smoked foods High salt intake	Fruits and vegetables Vitamin C		ß-carotene Vitamin E Selenium
Colorectal	Obesity Red meat Smoked, salted & processed meat Total fat Saturated fat	Physical activity Folate Calcium		Fruits and vegetables Fiber
Liver	Alcohol Aflotaxin			
Pancreas	Obesity		Red meat	Vegetables
Lung	High intakes of ß-carotene			Fruits and vegetables
Breast	Obesity Alcohol	Physical activiy		
Endometrium	Obesity		Total fat Saturated fat	Fruits and vegetables
Cervix				Folate Carotenoids Fruits and vegetables
Prostate	Red meat Total fat	Physical activity Lycopene		Vitamin E Selenium Vegetables
Bladder				Fruits and vegetables
Kidney	Obesity		Meat and dairy products	Vegetables

studies is that healthy controls may not be fully representative of the base population. Although prospective cohort studies eliminate recall and selection bias, measurement errors and confounding factors must be considered when interpreting the results of these studies. In particular, it is difficult to sort out the independent effects of specific nutrients or foods among a myriad of potential confounders.[19,20]

In an ideal situation, dietary recommendations should be based on data from the most well-designed type of study, namely the randomized controlled trial. Randomized controlled trials eliminate both the biases and the confounding that can affect observational studies, and the results can therefore be confidently interpreted in terms of cause and effect. Within the field of diet and cancer, however, trials are limited by the difficulty of randomizing at the level of foods and by the constraints that only a small number of nutritional factors can be tested in each trial, usually for only a short period. In cases in which these trials do not show the desired effect, it remains

possible that an effect would have been seen at a different dose, at a different time in life, or if the duration of the trial had been longer. Another point that should be considered when interpreting the results of randomized controlled trials is the possibility that the effect of a dietary component on cancer risk may differ according to the characteristics of the population studied. For example, the effects of a multinutrient supplement could be more marked in a population with a low dietary intake of micronutrients than in a population with a high dietary intake of micronutrients.[19]

Energy Balance

Excessive energy intake in relation to requirements to maintain a normal body weight increases the risk of developing several common cancers.[21] Many studies, including retrospective and prospective studies, have found that a higher body mass index (BMI) is associated with an increased risk of colon cancer. An approximately twofold higher risk is typically observed in the 20% of

individuals with the highest BMI relative to those with the lowest 20%.[22] More recent evidence indicates that a tendency for central distribution of adiposity, also called visceral adiposity, increases the risk independently of the BMI.[23] A relationship also exists between positive caloric balance and the development of cancers of the esophagus, endometrium, kidney, and gallbladder.[21] The relationship between body adiposity and breast cancer is more complex. Prior to menopause, women with greater body fat have reduced risks of breast cancer, probably because of more anovulatory menstrual cycles in heavier women. After menopause, a positive, weak overall association with adiposity is seen, which is stronger for women who never used a hormone replacement.[21]

Whereas excess caloric intake appears to increase the risk of developing cancer, physical activity has been associated with a decrease in risk. Physical activity appears to decrease the risk of all-cancer mortality in men and women.[24] Colon cancer has been the most extensively

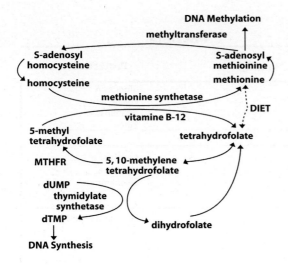

FIGURE 1 The pathways involved in the metabolism of folate and the production of methyl groups for deoxyribonucleic acid (DNA) methylation. Folate deficiency can induce DNA hypomethylation and lead to altered gene expression and increased risk of carcinogenesis. Cellular depletion of folate can also induce DNA damage by causing deoxyuridine (dUTP) instead of deoxythymidine (dTTP) to be incorporated into DNA. Methylene tetrahydrofolate reductase (MTHFR) converts 5,10-methylene tetrahydrofolate to 5-methyltetrahydrofolate. The methylene tetrahydrofolate pool is derived from folate and is required for the methylation of deoxyuridine monophosphate (dUMP) to deoxythymidine monophosphate (dTMP) by thymidylate synthetase. Folate deficiency decreases the amount of methylene tetrahydrofolate, causing dUTP to accumulate in DNA rather than dTTP, resulting in chromosomal breaks.[34,52,53]

studied site-specific cancer with regard to the impact of physical activity on the risk of cancer development. Over 50 studies in diverse populations show that more physically active individuals are at lower risk of colon cancer, although not for rectal cancer. An approximately 50% reduction in the incidence of colon cancer is observed among individuals with the highest level of physical activity. In spite of the wide variation in methodology among studies, including type of activity (leisure time or occupational) and method of assessment, a considerable protective effect persists.[22] With regard to breast cancer, there is also reasonably clear evidence that physically active women have about a 20 to 30% reduction in risk compared with inactive women. The data are less consistent with prostate and lung cancer.[25] Although the data are sparse, about 30 to 60 minutes per day of moderate to vigorous intensity physical activity is recommended to decrease the risk.[26] Several mechanisms by which increased physical activity and exercise can decrease the risk of cancer have been proposed. Exercise can improve T-cell function and natural killer cell activity. This enhanced immunity may increase resistance to the development of cancer. Increased physical activity can also attenuate the immune senescence that

normally occurs with aging and can enhance the body's natural free radical scavenger and antioxidant defense system. People who exercise more are also more likely to engage in other health-promoting behaviors. Other proposed mechanisms include exercise-induced reductions in serum iron levels and improved energy balance.[24]

Macronutrients

The question of whether individual energy-supplying macronutrients, independent of their contribution to energy intake, are related to cancer risk remains controversial. Studies between countries have shown a direct linear relationship between the amount of fat consumed and the incidence of both colon and breast cancer. Animal studies have also tended to show a direct correlation between fat content of the diet and the appearance of induced tumors.[21] However, evidence from longer-term randomized trials indicates that the fat composition of the diet has little, if any, relation to body fat and that excessive caloric intake from fat and carbohydrates similarly leads to weight gain and thus equally presents an increased risk for the development of cancer. Furthermore, as the findings from large prospective studies become available, support for the relationship between fat intake and several types of cancer has weakened considerably.[27]

On the other hand, some evidence suggests that the type of fat consumed may be important. In case-control studies conducted in Spain and Greece, women who used more olive oil had reduced risks of breast cancer.[28,29] Most prospective studies have shown an association between the intake of red meat, especially processed meat, and the risk of colorectal cancer.[30] In the Health Professionals Follow-up Study of 51,000 men, a positive association was seen with intake of red meat, total fat, and animal fat, which was largely limited to aggressive prostate cancers.[31] It is also possible that components of red meat other than fat may be responsible for the increased risk of cancer. Heme iron can act as a free radical catalyst, and heterocyclic amines formed from prolonged cooking of meat and nitrites in processed meat may also present carcinogenic risks in humans. Non-red sources of animal protein, including low-fat dairy products, fish, and poultry, have either not been associated with an increased risk or have even been related to a lower risk.[23]

Overconsumption of calories in general and a dietary pattern that includes high intakes of red and processed meats, high saturated and *trans* fat, and highly processed carbohydrates and sugars has also recently received some interest because of its hyperinsulinemic effect. There is increasing evidence to suggest that dietary patterns that induce hyperinsulinemia are associated with an increased risk of colon cancer.[22]

Fruits, Vegetables, and Dietary Fiber

Higher intake of fruits and vegetables has been associated with a reduced risk of cancers at many sites in numerous epidemiologic studies. The data were particularly strong for cancers of the lung and stomach. Inverse associations have also been observed in many studies of colon cancer. Other studies have also suggested possible inverse associations with cancers of the oral cavity, larynx, esophagus, endometrium, cervix, bladder, kidney, and breast.[21] At that time, however, the available literature was based largely on case-control studies, and subsequent prospective studies have not supported important protective effects for cancers of the lung and breast and have suggested that the reduction in risk of colorectal cancer may only be modest at best.[19] Although inverse associations have not been seen between overall fruit and vegetable consumption and the risk of prostate cancer, intake of tomato products, the primary source of the carotenoid lycopene, has been related to lower risk in case-control and prospective studies.[32]

Although support for a broad and strong protective effect of higher fruit and vegetable intake against cancer incidence has weakened with the results from recent studies, modest benefits of increasing fruit and vegetable intake have not been excluded and probably do exist. However, the exact constituents of these foods that are responsible for these reduced risks remain unclear. Fruits and vegetables contain many biologically active chemicals, including recognized nutrients and many more non-nutritive substances that could potentially reduce cancer incidence. Another complexity can arise when a particular nutrient can act as a chemopreventive agent only when it can interact with other nutrients present in foods or only when it is given as a supplement. Potentially protective factors include various carotenoids, folic acid, vitamin C, flavonoids, phytoestrogens, isothiocyanates, and fiber. The identification of specific protective constituents or a combination of constituents is often very difficult.[21]

Dietary fiber has been hypothesized to reduce the risk of colorectal cancer by diluting or adsorbing fecal carcinogens, reducing colonic transit time, altering bile acid metabolism, reducing colonic pH, and serving as the substrate for the generation of short-chain fatty acids that are the preferred substrate for colonic epithelial cells. Earlier studies suggested a 40 to 50% reduction in the risk of colon cancer; however, more recent evidence does not seem to support the hypothesis that higher consumption of grain fiber or fiber supplements can reduce the risk of colon cancer.[33]

Higher intake of fiber has also been hypothesized to reduce the risk of breast cancer by interrupting the enterohepatic circulation of estrogens.

Table 2 Current Guidelines on Diet, Nutrition, and Cancer Prevention[2,19,21,35,59]

- Maintain BMI between 18.5-25 kg/m².
- Keep physical activity to moderate intensity for at least 30 minutes on most days of the week.
- Limit consumption of alcoholic beverages.
- Minimize exposure of aflatoxin in foods.
- Chinese style salted fish and other salt-preserved foods and salt should be consumed in moderation.
- Eat at least 5 servings of fruits and vegetables daily.
- Eat plenty of whole grain and fiber rich foods; 20-30 g of fiber daily-wheat bran preferred.
- Limit red meat and preserved meat consumption.
- Reduce total fat intake to less than 25-30% of total calories and saturated fat to less than 10% of total calories.
- Do not consume foods or drinks when they are at a very hot temperature.

However, in prospective studies, little or no relationship has been observed between fiber intake and the risk of breast cancer.[34]

Vitamins, Minerals, and Trace Elements

Acute deficiencies of micronutrients are rare in developed countries, but suboptimal nutrient intake remains a widespread problem. Deficiencies in one aspect of the metabolic network can cause repercussions in many systems. Evidence of a link between various micronutrient deficiencies and deoxyribonucleic acid (DNA) damage has been accumulating in recent years. Optimizing vitamin and mineral intake by encouraging dietary change and multivitamin and multimineral supplementation when appropriate and fortifying foods might therefore help prevent cancer.[20]

Antioxidants

Antioxidants are compounds used by aerobic organisms for protection against oxidative stress induced by free radicals and active oxygen species. They exert their protective action either by suppressing the formation of free radicals or by scavenging free radicals. A wide range of biologic effects, established experimentally, may inhibit carcinogenesis. These include effects on tumor initiation, promotion, and progression; cell proliferation and differentiation; and DNA repair, cell membrane stability, and immune function. Diet-derived antioxidants such as carotenoids, vitamin C, vitamin E, and selenium have received much attention as potential cancer chemopreventive agents.[35]

Carotenoids are fat-soluble compounds classified as xanthophylls, carotenes, or lycopenes. Over 600 carotenoids occur in nature, and among them, the most commonly available in the human diet is β-carotene. β-Carotene is a naturally occurring precursor of vitamin A found in leafy green and yellow vegetables, carrots, and a variety of fruits. It has potent antioxidant properties and has been postulated to inhibit the process of carcinogenesis by preventing DNA damage directly induced by free radicals or by interfering with the metabolic activation of chemical carcinogens. Additionally, β-carotene is converted to vitamin A in the human body. The hormone-like effects of vitamin A on epithelial tissue cell growth and differentiation may antagonize the promotional stages of cancer development. β-Carotene and vitamin A both have immunomodulatory effects; increases in the humoral and cell-mediated immune response could potentially enhance immunosurveillance in carcinogenesis. Finally, β-carotene may modify enzymatic activation of carcinogens and enhance gap junction communication. Enhanced cell-to-cell communication would restrict clonal expansion of initiated cells, decreasing the likelihood of cancer occurring.[36]

Observational epidemiologic studies have indicated a protective effect of carotene-rich vegetables or β-carotene on cancers of the lung, esophagus, stomach, colorectum, cervix, oropharynx, and prostate. On the other hand, findings from several randomized clinical trials do not support the promising findings of observational studies. In three large randomized trials, β-carotene supplements did not reduce the risk of lung or other cancers.[21] Indeed, in two of these trials, the incidence of lung cancer was actually increased among those receiving β-carotene (in one of these studies, β-carotene was given in combination with vitamin A).[37,38]

Chemoprevention using vitamin A–related compounds in patients with oral leukoplakia, a precancerous lesion, has shown promising results. Trials using retinoic acid, isotretinoin, and vitamin A have reported decreased size or remission in patients assigned to these treatments compared with placebo. Studies using β-carotene have not shown as favorable results on leukoplakia.[5]

Lycopene is a carotenoid found primarily in tomatoes and tomato products; however, other sources include watermelon, pink grapefruit, and Japanese persimmons. Several studies have demonstrated a significant inverse association between the dietary intake of tomatoes and blood lycopene levels and the risk of prostate cancer. Lycopene is significantly taken up by prostate tissue and is associated with a reduction in DNA damage in both leukocytes and prostate epithelial cells. Lycopenes may exert protection against prostate cancer by decreasing plasma insulin-like growth factor 1 levels by a currently unknown mechanism.[39] In a prospective study of the biologic effects of lycopene in men with localized prostate cancer who subsequently underwent prostatectomy, men who received dietary lycopene supplementation after prostatectomy and over the 3-week period following prostatectomy had significantly smaller tumors, less involvement of the surgical margins, less diffuse involvement of the prostate by high-grade intraepithelial neoplasia, and lower serum mean prostate-specific antigen levels compared with men in the control group who did not receive lycopene supplementation.[40]

Vitamin C is another potent, naturally occurring antioxidant found in many fruits and vegetables. It is an important free radical scavenger in plasma and acts to regenerate active vitamin E in lipid membranes. Another postulated protective mechanism is the prevention of mutagenic nitrosamines in the stomach. In addition, vitamin C may also play an immune-enhancing role.[36]

Although several different factors in fruits and vegetables act jointly, the epidemiologic and biochemical evidence indicates an important role for vitamin C. The evidence for a protective effect of vitamin C is strongest for cancer of the stomach and upper aerodigestive tract and weaker for other forms of cancer.[21] However, randomized trials for vitamin C alone in the primary prevention of cancer are lacking. Another limitation in studying the relationship between vitamin C and cancer is that, in the absence of special preservation, vitamin C deteriorates rapidly during frozen storage. Thus, reliable assessments of blood vitamin C levels may be made only on fresh specimens or on samples that have been acid stabilized at −70°C.[36]

Vitamin E, a fat-soluble vitamin, is the major lipid-soluble antioxidant of the cell membrane. It acts as a free radical scavenger and inhibits peroxidation. It has also been postulated to be related to improved host immunity, inhibition of tumor initiators and promoters, activation of the *TP53* tumor suppressor gene, inhibition of tumor angiogenesis, reduction in DNA damage, alteration of in vitro cell signaling systems, and reduction in the effect of environmental carcinogens.

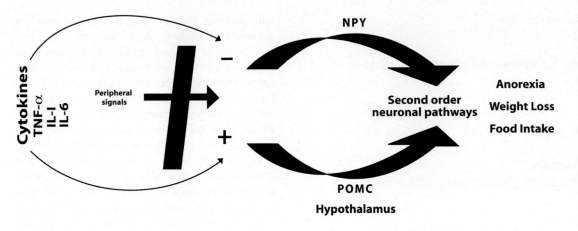

FIGURE 2 In cancer anorexia, increased expression of cytokines such as interleukin-1 (IL-1), interleukin-6 (IL-6), and tumor necrosis factor α (TNF-α) prevents the hypothalamus from appropriately responding to peripheral signals, causing hyperactivity of the pro-opiomelanocortin (POMC) system and inhibition of the neuropeptide Y (NPY) neuronal pathway. This leads to a strong negative influence on energy intake. Adapted from Laviano A et al.[65]

Reduction of the effect of carcinogens may occur through prevention of nitrosamine formation in the stomach, more rapid carcinogen metabolism, and prevention of conversion of carcinogens to their active form.[41] Rich sources of vitamin E include vegetable oils, margarine, nuts, seeds, cereal grains, and vegetables. Animal products such as milk fat, meat, poultry, and eggs also contain smaller amounts of this vitamin.[36]

In single studies, vitamin E supplements were associated with a reduced risk of oral cancer and colon cancer. In a large randomized trial conducted in Finland (α-Tocopherol, β-Carotene Cancer Prevention Study), men receiving vitamin E (50 IU/d) experienced reduced risk of prostate cancer.[37] Although statistically significant, this finding needs to be reproduced because it was not a previous hypothesis and many specific cancers were examined; chance remains a possible explanation.[21] In the Chinese Cancer Prevention Study, a randomized trial conducted in a region of China with very low consumption of fruits and vegetables, a supplement containing β-carotene, vitamin E, and selenium reduced the incidence of stomach cancer. Benefits began to emerge 1 to 2 years following initiation of vitamin supplementation.[42] A second randomized controlled trial also conducted in Linxian, China, compared a regimen of multiple vitamin-mineral supplementation that included vitamin E (as 60 IU/d of DL α-tocopherol acetate) with placebo in patients with esophageal dysplasia, a precursor of esophageal cancer. However, this trial failed to demonstrate a significant reduction in the incidence of stomach cancer, esophageal cancer, or cancer overall, and a reduction in cancer-specific mortality was not seen.[43]

Selenium is a trace element discovered by Berzelius in 1817. For a long time, selenium was considered more as an intriguing element in biochemistry rather than a truly relevant element in human biology. It is now recognized as an important essential micronutrient with the potential for chemoprevention.[44] Selenium appears to have two anticarcinogenic roles. When taken in doses of recommended dietary intake, selenium functions as an essential nutrient providing the catalytic centers of antioxidant enzymes such as glutathione peroxidase, thioredoxin reductase, iodothyronine 5′-deiodinase, and others. However, at supranutritional intakes, achievable only with dietary supplementation, certain chemical forms of selenium are metabolized to selenodiglutathione, hydrogen selenide, and methylselenol. These metabolites can directly affect tumorigenesis. Therefore, in selenium-deficient populations, the protective effect of selenium against cancer is derived mainly from its antioxidant activity through glutathione peroxidase and other selenoenzymes. On the other hand, in areas of supranutritional selenium exposures, the anticancer effects of selenium and its metabolites include enhancement of immune function, alteration in the metabolism of carcinogens, inhibition of tumor cell proliferation, enhancement of apoptosis, activation of the DNA repair response, and inhibition of tumor angiogenesis during tumor growth.[45]

Blood and tissue levels of selenium are often lower in cancer patients than in control subjects. However, this may be secondary to the malnutrition frequently seen in these patients.[46] There is also evidence from epidemiologic studies that high dietary selenium intakes and high selenium status in people are associated with lower cancer mortality.[46] A new impetus for the relationship between the dose and chemical form of selenium and cancer risk was provided by Clark and colleagues' study in 1996.[47] In a prospective, placebo-controlled, double-blind study conducted over about 4.5 years with more than 1,100 participants selected for a previous history of skin cancer,

these authors observed that selenium supplementation with 200 µg/d in the form of enriched yeast resulted in significantly lower incidences of various types of cancer (mainly of the lungs, prostate, and colorectum) and lower overall cancer mortality.

The selenium content of plants is dependent on the region of growth. For example, China has regions with both the lowest and the highest selenium-containing soil in the world.[44] Dietary selenium consists mainly of selenoamino acids and analogues such as L-selenomethionine from cereal grains or animal proteins or L-selenocysteine from animal meats, poultry, fish, and dairy products, with trace amounts of other selenium compounds, such as L-selenomethylcysteine. Alternatively, selenium supplements are available in both inorganic (selenite and selenate) and organic formulations, such as L-selenomethionine and selenium-enriched yeast, a less well-defined form of selenium. The adequate dose and optimal chemical form of selenium for nutritional or preventive and therapeutic purposes continue to be intensively investigated in a number of ongoing trials.[48]

Other Vitamins and Minerals

1,25-Dihydroxyvitamin D_3 is the active form of the fat-soluble vitamin D. Major dietary sources of vitamin D include liver, fatty saltwater fish, eggs, and fortified milk. Vitamin D functions in the regulation of calcium homeostasis. Vitamin D also inhibits proliferation and DNA synthesis, alters expression of several oncogenes, reduces lipid peroxidation and angiogenesis, and induces differentiation. Epidemiologic studies support an inverse relationship between vitamin D intake and colorectal cancer risk and have also shown that vitamin D_3 deficiency and low plasma levels of 1,25-dihydroxyvitamin D_3 increase the risk of prostate cancer. The overall evidence, however, remains insufficient.[35]

Several hypotheses have focused on the potential benefits of dietary calcium. Calcium has been proposed to reduce colorectal cancer risk by binding secondary bile acids and ionized fatty acids in the colonic lumen, thereby reducing the proliferative stimulus of these compounds on mucosal cells. Alternatively, calcium may have a direct beneficial influence on the proliferative activity of the colonic mucosa.[22] In a recently reported randomized trial, calcium supplements modestly reduced the recurrence of colonic adenomas.[49] However, in large prospective studies, only weak and nonsignificant inverse associations have been seen between calcium intake and the risk of colon cancer.[21] Calcium supplement use was also positively associated with the risk of prostate cancer in one study. Thus, avoidance of low intakes of calcium may be prudent, but the data do not currently support very high intakes of calcium for the purpose of cancer prevention.[21]

Table 3 Four-Step Pharmacologic Management for Cancer Anorexia and Cachexia[15,64]

History	Physical
• Weight change over past 6 months • Dietary intake and change relative to usual intake • Gastrointestinal symptoms persistent for at least 2 weeks • Functional capacity • Metabolic demand of underlying disease process	• Loss of subcutaneous fat • Muscle wasting • Ankle or sacral edema • Ascites • Mucosal lesions • Cutaneous and hair changes

Folate, a water-soluble B complex vitamin, is a major participant in the formation of purine and pyrimidine nucleotide precursors for DNA and ribonucleic acid, as well as in the formation of methionine, which is itself transformed to S-adenosylmethionine, a coenzyme needed for more than 100 transmethylation reactions in cells.[50] The richest sources of folate are green, leafy vegetables and, in the United States, fortified flour, cold cereal, and orange or grapefruit juice.[20,21]

There is much epidemiologic evidence indicating that low folate status increases the risk of many types of cancer.[20] The data are strongest for colorectal cancer. An increased occurrence of colorectal adenomas, precursors of colorectal cancer, has been observed fairly consistently among individuals with low circulating folate concentrations. In general, prospective studies also support an inverse association between low folate intake or circulating level and colon cancer risk.[22] Furthermore, a recent report indicated that the excess risk of colon cancer among women with a positive family history of colorectal cancer could be substantially reduced if they had high intakes of folate or took a multivitamin supplement.[51] Low folate status may be deleterious either by causing misincorporation of uracil into DNA and increased frequency of chromosomal breaks or by contributing to DNA hypomethylation.[52] Site-specific DNA methylation appears to control gene expression, and DNA hypomethylation can lead to dysregulated activation of proto-oncogenes involved in carcinogenesis. The finding that homozygotes with a variant form of methylenetetrahydrofolate reductase (MTHFR), the enzyme that regulates the conversion of 5,10-methylenetetrahydrofolate to 5-methyltetrahydrofolate, are at reduced risk of colon cancer further supports a role for folate. However, the protective effect of this genetic polymorphism may be lost in patients with a dietary deficiency of folate or with high alcohol consumption, which effectively impairs the absorption and use of folate.[53] Higher intakes of folic acid may also mitigate the elevated risks of breast cancer seen with daily alcohol consumption.[21]

Other Dietary Factors

There is considerable interest in the prevention of cancer by chemicals present in food plants that play no known nutritive role. These chemicals are often referred to as phytochemicals or nutraceuticals.[54] A number of animal studies have demonstrated that tea polyphenols can prevent induction of cancer of the lung, colon, esophagus, pancreas, and liver.[35] Epidemiologic studies suggest that soy proteins containing the isoflavone genistein can inhibit the growth of androgen-dependent and androgen-independent cell lines of prostate cancer. Genistein can also induce apoptosis, inhibit angiogenesis, and regulate transcription of the estrogen receptor.[35] A lot of evidence also suggests that soy consumption may decrease breast cancer risk; however, conflicting information that soy may be harmful for women with a history of breast cancer or who are at high risk makes it difficult to recommend soy consumption at this time.[55]

Aspirin and nonsteroidal anti-inflammatory drugs (NSAIDs) inhibit the enzyme cyclooxygenase (COX) involved in the metabolism of arachidonic acid and the production of prostaglandins. There are two recognized isoforms of COX. COX-1 is a constitutive isoform involved in a range of physiologic functions, whereas COX-2 is an inducible isoform expressed at sites of inflammation. There is growing evidence that the COX-2 isoform plays a key role in the early stages of intestinal polyp formation. A number of natural substances have been identified with COX-2 inhibitory properties. The natural COX-2 inhibitors identified include curcumin (the natural yellow pigment in tumeric), resveratol (a phytochemical found in grape skin), and the omega-3 fatty acids found in fish oil. Dietary supplementation with omega-3 fatty acids has been evaluated in several clinical trials, and the results suggest some benefits for cancer patients.[53]

On the other hand, some food substances and eating habits increase the risk of cancer. Aflatoxin in food causes liver cancer. Chinese-style salted fish increases the risk of nasopharyngeal carcinoma. Salt-preserved foods and high salt intake probably increase the risk of stomach cancer. Alcohol causes cancers of the oral cavity, pharynx, esophagus, and liver and a small increase in the risk of breast cancer. Very hot drinks and foods probably increase the risk of cancers of the oral cavity, pharynx, and esophagus; drinks and foods should not be consumed when they are scalding hot.[19]

Genetics and Nutrition

Inconsistencies between epidemiologic studies and randomized clinical trials have led to the development of a new discipline called nutritional genomics. Transforming nutrition and cancer research from a predominantly observational to a molecular approach offers exciting opportunities for truly identifying those who will and those who will not benefit from dietary intervention strategies.[8,56] Nutrients and genes can interact at two levels. Nutrients can induce gene expression, thereby altering individual phenotype. Conversely, genetic polymorphisms, in a range of genes important in inflammation and lipid metabolism, alter the bioactivity of important metabolic pathways and mediators and influence the ability of nutrients to interact with them.[57] Therefore, one can appreciate that the fundamental action of a nutrient is to serve as a regulator of gene expression and/or modulator of a gene product. Nutrients have specific sites of action, which can best be described as molecular targets. There is evidence that genetic polymorphisms can influence the dynamics between nutrients and molecular targets and thus contribute to the variation in response among individuals.[9] Current study of nutrient-modulated carcinogenesis involves exploring the effect of nutrients on DNA damage and repair mechanisms; DNA methylation, which influences gene expression and cellular phenotypes; antioxidant rearranging and oxidative stress; target receptors and signal transduction pathways; cell cycle controls and checkpoints; apoptosis; and antiangiogenic processes. The generation of this new knowledge on nutrient-gene interactions provides the justification for a research framework for diet and cancer prevention that is focused on identifying and developing new biomarkers as well as a novel and contemporary paradigm for dietary intervention.[58]

Table 4 Essential Features of the Subjective Global Assessment[77,78]

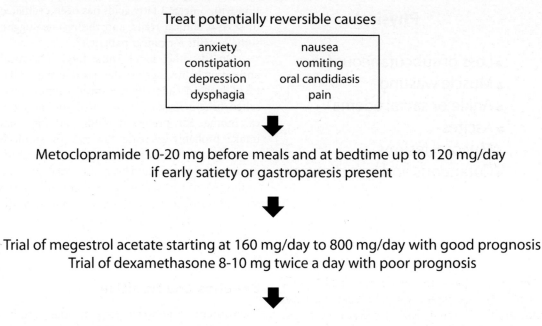

Treat potentially reversible causes

anxiety	nausea
constipation	vomiting
depression	oral candidiasis
dysphagia	pain

Metoclopramide 10-20 mg before meals and at bedtime up to 120 mg/day if early satiety or gastroparesis present

Trial of megestrol acetate starting at 160 mg/day to 800 mg/day with good prognosis
Trial of dexamethasone 8-10 mg twice a day with poor prognosis

Trial of Dronabinol 2.5 mg twice to three times daily, Thalidomide 100 mg at night, Eicosapentanoic acid 2-3 g/day or Melatonin 20-40 mg/day.

Current Dietary Recommendations

Dietary suggestions for cancer prevention by nutritional means should be based on the best available scientific research. Although many data have been presented, few dietary influences on cancer risk have been firmly established. Avoiding obesity, maintaining an ideal body weight, limiting alcohol intake to one drink a day for women and two drinks a day for men, and increasing physical activity to moderate to vigorous intensity for 30 minutes on most days will reduce cancer risk. Limiting consumption of Chinese-style salted fish and minimizing dietary exposure to aflatoxin will also reduce cancer risk in populations in which these dietary factors are important. Risk will probably be decreased by increasing the average intake of fruits and vegetables to five servings per day and by limiting the intake of preserved and red meat, salt-preserved foods and salt, and very hot drinks and foods. Consuming cereal products in a minimally refined whole-grain form and taking a multiple vitamin containing folic acid may also be of benefit.[2,3,5,19,21,59]

Malnutrition and Cancer

Nutritional decline is often accepted as part of the natural history of cancer and its treatment. The prevalence of weight loss and malnutrition in patients depends on the tumor type and stage, the organs involved, and the anticancer therapy. Weight loss and malnutrition in patients have been reported to range from 9% in breast cancer to 80% in patients with esophageal cancer. In addition, as many as 20% of patients with cancer die from the effects of malnutrition rather than the malignancy.[12] Patients with cancer of the pancreas, esophagus, or stomach have the highest frequency and severity of weight loss, whereas patients with breast cancer, leukemia, sarcoma, and lymphoma have the lowest risk of weight loss. Intermediate frequency of weight loss occurs in patients with colon, prostate, and lung cancers.[14] Among surgical patients in a Veterans Administration Hospital, 39% of those undergoing a major operation for cancer were malnourished, as judged by either a nutrition risk index or a combination of weight loss and low serum proteins.[60]

The presence of malnutrition in cancer patients has major prognostic significance. In a review of more than 3,000 cancer patients, DeWys and colleagues found better survival rates in those patients without weight loss compared with patients who had lost just 6% of their body weight.[61] Malnutrition not only affects morbidity and mortality but can also lead to a diminished quality of life and poor performance status.[10] Increased hospital stays,[11] unplanned hospitalizations, readmissions, and a greater incidence of postoperative complications result in higher health care costs.[13] Furthermore, the malnourished cancer patient has a poor response and diminished tolerance to antineoplastic treatments such as chemotherapy, radiotherapy, and surgery.[12] This highlights the need for early identification and treatment of malnourished cancer patients who could potentially benefit from nutritional intervention.

Etiology of Malnutrition

The cancer anorexia-cachexia syndrome results from progressive nutritional deterioration and is among the most debilitating and life-threatening aspects of cancer. Lean body mass wasting accounts for up to 30% of cancer-related deaths.[15] Cancer cachexia is clinically characterized by anorexia, early satiety, wasting, weight loss, anemia, weakness, fatigue, poor mental and physical performance, decreased capacity for wound healing, impaired immunologic function, and a compromised quality of life.[62] Cachexia should be expected if an involuntary or unexpected weight loss of greater than 5% has occurred within the previous 6-month period, especially when combined with muscle wasting. A weight loss of 10% or more indicates more severe depletion.[17]

Attempts to provide energy in patients with cancer cachexia often do not result in weight gain. One possible explanation is that the weight loss observed in cachexia is different from that seen in simple starvation or anorexia. The patient with cancer cachexia exhibits features of both starvation and injury. In cachexia, there is an accelerated loss of skeletal muscle in relation to adipose tissue. This contrasts with simple starvation, in which fat replaces glucose as the preferred fuel to spare lean body mass.[63]

The etiology of malnutrition in patients with cancer is multifactorial.[14] The causes can be classified into two major categories: (1) anorexia, factors related to decreased food intake, and gastrointestinal dysfunction and (2) metabolic disturbances.[15]

Pathophysiology of Anorexia

Appetite loss or anorexia is a substantial contributing factor to the malnutrition seen in cancer patients.[17] It can be caused by localized effects induced by the tumor itself or by systemic effects caused by metastasis or humoral factors produced by tumor cells.[12] Cancer patients may experience mechanical gastrointestinal obstruction, pain, constipation, maldigestion, malabsorption, debility, and the side effects of therapy, any of which can lead to decreased food intake. In some cases, the loss of appetite is due to depression or psychological stress.[64] Cancer patients may also develop anorexia secondary to food aversion learning after treatment with radiochemotherapy regimens.[65]

The pathogenesis of cancer-associated anorexia is related to disturbances of the central physiologic mechanisms controlling food intake. Convincing evidence suggests that cancer anorexia is brought about by the derangement of the hypothalamic system transducing peripheral signals into neuronal responses. Under normal conditions, peripheral signals (such as the hormone leptin produced by adipocytes exerting a strong

Table 5 Diets Commonly Prescribed for Cancer Patients

Postsupraglottic laryngectomy
- Solid, soft foods
- Avoid liquids

Esophageal strictures
- Soft foods
- Emphasize liquids or high calorie nutritional supplements

Gastric resection
- Five or six small meals per day
- Separate liquids from solids
- Limit mono-carbohydrates and lactose
- Supplement iron, and vitamin B_{12}, parenterally

Pancreatic insufficiency
- Limit fat
- Supplement pancreatic enzymes
- Medium-chain triglyerides

Short bowel
- Frequent, small meals
- Limit fat, fiber, mono-carbohydrates, and lactose
- Supplement calcium, magnesium, zinc, and vitamin B_{12} parenterally if terminal ileum resected

Chronic radiation enteritis
- Limit fat, fiber, and lactose

Adapted from Shike M.[14]

negative influence on food intake) interact with two separate neuronal populations within the arcuate nucleus of the hypothalamus, the neuropeptide Y neurons and the pro-opiomelanocortin neurons. These neurons constitute two pathways, the former stimulating and the latter inhibiting energy intake. In cancer anorexia, it appears that the hypothalamus is unable to respond appropriately to consistent peripheral signals owing to hyperactivation of the melanocortin system. Increased expression of cytokines by the tumor itself during tumor growth or by the host in response to the tumor inhibits the hypothalamus to appropriately respond to peripheral signals by persistently activating the melanocortin system and inhibiting the neuropeptide Y neuronal pathway.[65] Several cytokines have been proposed as possible mediators of the cachectic process. Elevated serum levels of tumor necrosis factor α, interleukin-1, and interleukin-6 have been found in some, but not all, cancer patients, and the serum levels of these cytokines seem to correlate with the progression of the tumor.[66] These cytokines and others may also produce long-term inhibition of appetite and feeding by stimulating the production and release of leptin and/or by mimicking the hypothalamic effect of excessive negative feedback signaling from leptin, leading to normal compensatory mechanisms for decreases in food intake and body weight.[15]

Another possible cause of anorexia is the increased serotoninergic activity within the central nervous system of patients with cancer cachexia, attributed to the enhanced availability of tryptophan to the brain. The fact that uptake of tryptophan into the brain is competitive with uptake of branched-chain amino acids has

suggested the use of branched-chain amino acids to decrease the incidence of anorexia in cachectic cancer patients.[64]

Gastrointestinal Dysfunction

Malignant disease and its treatment often lead to abnormalities in the mouth and elsewhere in the gastrointestinal tract and may interfere with the ingestion of food.[15] Altered taste and smell have been documented in about half of these patients. Changes in the recognition of sweet taste occur in approximately one-third of patients, whereas bitterness (responsible for meat aversion), sourness, and saltiness are less frequently affected. Many patients undergoing dose-intensive radiation and/or chemotherapy regimens experience reduced taste (hypogeusia) or altered taste (dysgeusia), which may have a significant impact on quality of life.[17]

Antineoplastic drugs that have been associated with taste changes include cisplatin, carboplatin, cyclophosphamide, doxorubicin, 5-fluorouracil, levamisole, and methotrexate.[67] In a study reported by Mattson and colleagues, 10 patients evaluated had dysgeusia during the aplastic phase of hematopoietic cell transplantation; the threshold for salt was most profoundly affected.[68] However, 1 year after transplantation, it was found that in 80% of them, taste acuity had normalized by the end of the year. Therefore, it seems that taste receptors have the capacity to regenerate and function can recover following injury.

Chemotherapy itself can also have an immediate effect on taste. Some patients will complain of a bitter or metallic taste during administration of the cytotoxic drug. This may occur because drugs pass into the saliva; hence, these drugs can be tasted or smelled once they enter the oral or nasal cavity. The etiology of taste disorders in the setting of chemotherapy is probably multifactorial and not merely due to damage to the taste receptors.[67] There have been reports in the literature linking hypogeusia to zinc deficiency. Some drugs that cause hypogeusia have a sulfhydryl group in their structures; the sulfhydryl group is known to bind and chelate heavy metal ions, including zinc.

Nonetheless, zinc supplementation rarely impacts on taste in these patients.[69]

Other drugs, such as some antibiotics, analgesics, bisphosphonates, antihypertensives and cardiac medications, bronchodilators, muscle relaxants, antidepressants, and anticonvulsants, can also alter taste. Agents that effect hormonal changes, such as tamoxifen, may also affect taste. Xerostomia is also a possible side effect of a number of medications, including antiemetics, antidepressants, and antihypertensives, and may contribute to taste changes. Damage to salivary glands may reduce the flow of saliva so that

tastants do not reach the receptor, rendering food tasteless. Changes in the oral flora; bacterial, viral, or fungal infections of the nasal or oral cavity; diseased teeth; dental caries; poor oral hygiene; and gastroesophageal reflux may also lead to altered taste.[68]

Considerable taste change also occurs during radiotherapy; however, unlike taste changes associated with chemotherapy, pretreatment taste sensation is usually not recovered. These taste complaints may be due to direct damage to taste receptors and to reduced saliva production and xerostomia, resulting in secondary infection and reduced delivery of tastants to receptor sites.[67]

Patients undergoing chemotherapy may also complain of smells during or after the administration of the drug, and some patients have a heightened sensitivity to odors. Olfactory hallucinations have also been reported, in which a patient may experience a chemical odor even when just thinking about previously administered therapy. Olfactory loss may also result from the direct toxic effects of radiation therapy; such effects may take over 6 months to resolve.[67]

Dysphagia and odynophagia are particularly marked in head and neck and esophageal cancer. Tumors elsewhere in the gastrointestinal tract and the hepatobiliary tract and metastatic tumors (such as ovarian cancer) causing extrinsic compression often lead to nausea, vomiting, and early satiety. Malabsorption with severe atrophy of the small bowel mucosa and exudative enteropathy have also been described. Furthermore, gastrointestinal dysmotility can lead to a sensation of early satiety, delayed digestion, and weight loss.[17]

Anticancer therapies are also a major cause of anorexia and weight loss.[14] Chemotherapy can cause nausea, vomiting, abdominal pain, mucositis, adynamic ileus, and malabsorption.[17] Surgery involving a segment of the gastrointestinal tract, such as the pharynx, esophagus, or stomach, can decrease the ability to ingest food. Extensive resections of the small bowel result in the short bowel syndrome characterized by malabsorption of nutrients and fluids. Pancreatic resections can result in pancreatic exocrine and endocrine insufficiency, creating major nutrition problems, such as steatorrhea and hyperglycemia. Major hepatic resections cause metabolic abnormalities in the immediate postoperative period.[32] Radiotherapy can induce acute and chronic complications that can interfere with the ingestion and absorption of nutrients. Edema and mucositis of the oropharynx and radiation esophagitis cause severe dysphagia and odynophagia, further compounding the swallowing difficulties imposed by the cancer itself. In the acute setting, patients receiving radiotherapy to the abdomen frequently experience self-limited nausea, vomiting, and diarrhea. However, chronic severe radiation enterocolitis is complicated by fistulae, complete obstruction

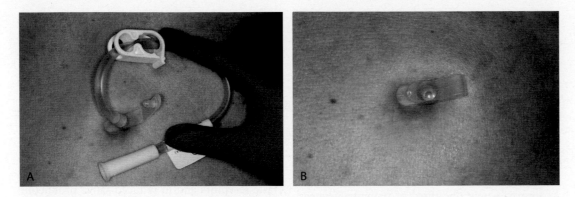

FIGURE 3 Patient with head and neck cancer on long-term enteral nutrition using a 24F 3.4 cm button gastrostomy tube. *A*, Feeding tube with extension tube attached; *B*, the closed feeding tube flap lies close to the skin and is less cumbersome between feedings.

secondary to strictures, or peritonitis, which may lead to prolonged nutritional support. Improved fractionation of radiation therapy and protective shielding of the intestines have considerably reduced such complications.[14]

Metabolic Disturbances

Inability to gain or maintain weight despite seemingly adequate nutrient intake may be due to increased metabolic needs generated by the accentuated nutritional demands of the semiautonomous tumor, generalized increased energy expenditure in the cancer patient, and failure of the cancer patient's host tissues to use the nutrients available in an efficient and effective manner to satisfy the energy requirements of the body.[14]

Malignant tumors are characterized by a high rate of growth. The tumor escapes all of the normal mechanisms of metabolic control. Most tumor tissue develops whatever the host's nutritional status and maintains a high level of metabolic activity at the expense of the host. Malignant cells have a high degree of anaerobic glycolysis and produce large amounts of lactate. An investigation of amino acid metabolism also showed net uptake of amino acids by human tumor tissue, suggesting that cachexia is at least partially caused by increased metabolic demands of the tumor.[17]

An increase in energy expenditure has been widely but not universally found in cancer patients.[14] Patients with newly diagnosed small cell lung cancer were shown to have a mean 37% increase in resting energy expenditure. Their food intake was not sufficient to meet the demands of the increased metabolic rate, resulting in a negative energy balance and weight loss. The high metabolic rate declined in patients who responded to chemotherapy.[70] Similar elevations in resting energy expenditure were reported in patients with gastric cancer,[71] sarcoma,[72] and a variety of other tumors.[73]

Maladaptive metabolism in cancer patients is associated with widespread metabolic derangements that decrease the efficiency of nutrient use and can affect the metabolism of carbohydrate, fat, protein, vitamins, and minerals.[74] Alterations in carbohydrate metabolism include the activation of low-efficiency biochemical cycles such as the Cori cycle, where lactate is converted to glucose in the liver, an increase in endogenous glucose production from alanine, glucose intolerance, and peripheral tissue insulin resistance.[63] The most consistent abnormalities of lipid metabolism involve increased mobilization of peripheral fat and excessive oxidation of fatty acids. This increase in endogenous lipolysis eventually leads to the depletion of lipid stores. Increased plasma concentrations of glycerol and free fatty acids reflect the mobilization of lipid stores and usually occur only in patients with malignant disease who develop weight loss. In healthy patients, a glucose infusion suppresses lipolysis but does not suppress lipolysis in cancer patients. Ultimately, the cancer patient depletes fat stores, develops hypertriglyceridemia, and manifests decreased lipoprotein lipase levels.[64] Protein metabolism is also altered in cancer patients. This is manifested by an increase in protein turnover, a reduction in muscle protein synthesis, an increase in inflammatory hepatic protein synthesis, increased muscle catabolism, and a progressive loss of body nitrogen with a negative nitrogen balance.[17] The cytokines tumor necrosis factor α and interleukin-1 produced by macrophages and interleukin-6 released by macrophages or by the tumor itself play important roles in the development of these metabolic disturbances.[65]

All of these metabolic abnormalities that occur in the cancer patient with cachexia point to a wasteful and inefficient metabolism in which the nutritional requirements of the tumor are selectively favored over those of the host. This makes it quite difficult to reverse malnutrition even with the highly sophisticated nutritional support techniques currently available.[14]

Diagnosis of Malnutrition

Nutritional assessment of the cancer patient is important to identify the subsets of patients who can potentially benefit from dietary counseling by a dietitian or other forms of nutritional intervention, as well as to determine the severity and causes of malnutrition, to identify patients at risk of complications from anticancer therapies, and to assess the efficacy of nutritional support.[17] Although many nutritional assessment techniques are available, each has its limitations.[75] Furthermore, the use of a single measurement in time provides an inaccurate assessment of an individual's nutritional status.[16] Therefore, an ideal evaluation for the clinician has been to shift nutritional assessment from a diagnostic to a prognostic instrument to identify patients who can benefit from nutritional therapy by decreasing the risk of malnutrition-associated medical complications.[76]

Nutritional status has been traditionally defined by body composition and anthropometric measurements, plasma protein concentrations, immunocompetence, and multivariate analysis of certain parameters.[62] Body composition analysis requires sophisticated equipment and is not always readily available.[77] Recent weight change is generally a good indicator of nutritional deficit. A weight loss of 10% or more within the previous 6 months or 5% or more within the previous month indicates severe malnutrition. However, weight changes do not always reflect nutritional deficits but can also occur secondary to changes in body fluid balance.[78] Subscapular and triceps skinfold thickness and midarm muscle circumference provide an estimate of body fat and fat-free mass, but values may vary with hydration status and are based on a standard that has not been validated in cancer patients. In addition, interobserver reproducibility is poor, even after several weeks of special training.[16] A strong relationship has been found between low albumin concentrations and poor outcome in cancer patients. However, many clinical conditions found in cancer patients can interfere with measurements of plasma protein concentrations. Serum albumin has a long half-life of 18 to 20 days and is severely depressed during stress, illness, infection, and states of overhydration and with hepatic and renal dysfunction. The use of other proteins with shorter half-lives, such as prealbumin, transferrin, and retinol binding protein, is also limited because those proteins are also affected by illness and hydration status.[77] Tests of immunocompetence, such as delayed cutaneous hypersensitivity, may indicate malnutrition but are also affected by infection, illnesses, medications, and medical procedures.[76] Absolute lymphocyte counts may be affected by infection and hematologic malignancy.[62] Creatinine height index measurements require accurate urine collections and are affected by alterations in protein intake, renal failure, sepsis, trauma, exercise, and steroid therapy.[76] Calculating nitrogen balance by obtaining a 24-hour urinary total or urea nitrogen has been used to determine the degree of protein catabolism present. However, many factors can affect this measurement, including the adequacy of collection, diuretics, renal function, and protein intake, so this test needs to be interpreted carefully.[79] Discriminant functional analysis of multiple nutritional parameters has been used by Buzby and colleagues to develop the prognostic nutrition index, which has been shown to provide a quantitative estimate of postoperative complications when applied prospectively to patients undergoing gastrointestinal surgery.[77] More recently, hand-grip strength and adductor pollicis relaxation rate have been shown to correlate with postoperative complications. Muscle function testing measures physiologic changes in malnutrition even before changes in body nitrogen or plasma protein concentration occur.[76] Bioelectrical impedance has also been used to evaluate nutritional status and to follow the effectiveness of nutrition support but requires specialized equipment and training.[78]

A clinical nutritional assessment was first developed by the Toronto group and has been termed subjective global assessment (SGA). The SGA combines elements from the history and physical examination and defines malnourished patients as those who are at increased risk of medical complications and who will presumably benefit from nutritional therapy. The SGA integrates five history and four physical examination findings to define nutritional status: weight loss pattern, change in dietary intake, gastrointestinal symptoms, the patient's functional status, the metabolic demand of the underlying disease, subcutaneous fat thickness, muscle wasting, the presence of edema and ascites, mucosal lesions, and skin and hair changes. The findings of the history and physical examination are used to categorize patients as well nourished (category A), moderately malnourished (category B), and severely malnourished (category C).[63,78] The SGA correlates closely with objective parameters, such as anthropometric measurements and serum protein levels, and accurately predicts clinical outcome after major surgery with 82% sensitivity and 72% specificity. Interobserver variability and reproducibility are satisfactory after a training period of a few days.[80]

In summary, the nutrition assessment of the cancer patient should initially include a careful history, a physical examination, and the SGA to identify patients who are at increased risk of malnutrition-associated complications, followed by appropriate laboratory testing to further evaluate considerations raised during the clinical examination. This will identify the patients who will most likely benefit from nutritional support.

Treatment of Malnutrition

Clearly, the most important treatment for the malnourished cancer patient would be the development of antineoplastic therapies that target and cure the underlying disease process. Until that goal is achieved, the adjunctive and palliative use of pharmacologic agents and unique nutritional formulations and therapies in an attempt to alter the course of progressive nutritional deterioration play significant roles in the treatment of the malnutrition frequently seen in cancer patients.[64]

Pharmacologic Treatment

Drugs that are directed toward improving functional status and quality of life in cancer patients have become an integral part of antineoplastic therapy. Symptomatic control of nausea, vomiting, mucositis, and gastrointestinal dysmotility can usually be accomplished. Several types of drugs have also been employed in an attempt to improve appetite, food intake, a sense of well-being, and body weight gain. These and other agents represent a new approach to management of the cancer anorexia-cachexia syndrome and an opportunity for combined therapeutic endeavors to improve the quality of life of these patients.[63]

Improvement of appetite in cancer patients also calls for treatment of other symptoms, such as pain, mucositis, depression, and the side effects of oncologic treatments.[17] Ondanestron and granisetron, which are often used as antiemetics during chemotherapy, are serotonin receptor antagonists that have also been used in cancer cachexia as antagonists to the satiating effects of serotonin. Although these agents failed to promote weight gain, treatment did improve the ability of patients to enjoy food. Cyproheptadine, another antiserotoninergic drug useful as an appetite stimulant in anorexia nervosa, also failed to prevent progressive weight loss in cancer patients. Metoclopramide has been used to ameliorate the emesis associated with chemotherapy and to treat patients with early satiety, delayed gastric emptying, and gastroparesis seen in advanced cancer.[64]

Megestrol acetate and medroxyprogesterone acetate are first-line therapy for cancer cachexia. Many randomized controlled trials have confirmed that progestational drugs can stimulate appetite, food intake, energy level, and significant weight gain in cancer patients.[81] The effect of megestrol acetate is dose related, ranging from 160 to 1,600 mg, with an optimal dose of 800 mg/d. In general, patients are started on the lowest effective dosage (160 mg/d) and the dose is increased according to the clinical response of the patient. The dose of medroxyprogesterone acetate is 500 mg twice daily.[63] Most of the weight gain obtained with progestational agents consists of fat

rather than lean body mass.[66] The effect of these drugs on appetite appears to be mediated by a down-regulation of the synthesis and release of cytokines, leading to an increase in neuropeptide Y hypothalamic levels.[65] The side effects of progestational agents include induction of thrombosis and thromboemboli, breakthrough uterine bleeding, hypertension, hyperglycemia, peripheral edema, alopecia, Cushing's syndrome, adrenal suppression, and adrenal insufficiency.[64] Side effects were seen in 10 to 30% of patients in clinical trials.[17] Caution must be taken in administering these drugs to patients with known thromboembolic disease, heart disease, or a high risk of fluid retention. Progestational agents are contraindicated in hormone-dependent tumors.[65]

Corticosteroids are frequently used as appetite stimulants in cancer patients. Although treated patients report an increased sense of well-being, there is no long-term benefit since any benefit is lost within a month of treatment. Dexamethasone's ability to stimulate appetite is equivalent to that of megestrol acetate but does not produce weight gain.[15]

The use of anabolic steroids in healthy people and athletes increases muscle mass, but this benefit has not been shown to occur in patients with gastrointestinal cancer. Only one small trial in lung cancer patients treated with nandrolone decanoate suggested benefit in attenuating weight loss.[82] Anabolic steroids are associated with some severe side effects, such as hepatotoxicity and endocrine effects.[74]

The metabolic inhibitor hydrazine sulfate inhibits an integral enzyme in gluconeogenesis, thereby interrupting the Cori cycle and normalizing carbohydrate metabolism. Unfortunately, several large studies have shown no significant impact on weight gain in cancer patients.[64]

Dronabinol, a commercially available cannabinoid, is an appetite stimulant that can promote minimal improvement in overall body weight. The usual dosage is 2.5 mg two to three times a day. Adverse effects include somnolence, confusion, and perceptual disturbances.[15]

Pentoxifylline is a methylxanthine-derived phosphodiesterase inhibitor that has been shown to decrease tumor necrosis factor α synthesis in cancer patients by decreasing gene transcription. In a randomized controlled trial in patients with advanced cancer, it failed to cause better appetite or body weight than placebo.[83]

Melatonin stimulates host immune defenses and inhibits tumor growth factor production. Studies in cancer patients using a dosage of 20 mg daily significantly lowered the percentage of treated patients who experienced a greater than 10% weight loss. More trials are needed before the widespread use of melatonin is recommended.[84]

β₂-Adrenergic receptor agonists can prevent muscle protein wasting in tumor-bearing rats. Tumor-bearing rats have an anabolic response with increases in muscle mass while receiving salbutamol, salmeterol, and clenbuterol. However, no controlled trials have been reported using these agents in cancer patients.[15]

Growth hormone increases lean body mass and protein synthesis and reduces urinary nitrogen excretion in patients in catabolic states. The use of recombinant growth hormone has not been studied in cancer cachexia.[64]

Eicosapentanoic acid, a polyunsaturated fatty acid, and NSAIDs inhibit COX. Diets rich in eicosapentanoic acid attenuate weight loss in patients with advanced pancreatic cancer.[85] Ibuprofen was shown to normalize protein kinetics in cachectic patients with colorectal cancer and stabilize weight while reducing resting energy expenditure and increasing quality of life in patients with pancreatic cancer.[86,87] Gastrointestinal side effects limit the use of NSAIDs.[54]

Thalidomide is a potent suppressor of tumor necrosis factor α production. It has been shown to improve insomnia, restlessness, and nausea in advanced cancer patients while improving appetite and a sense of well-being in a majority of patients studied. Side effects of thalidomide include fever, skin rash, and peripheral neuropathy in addition to its well-known teratogenic effect.[88]

A four-step pharmacologic management model has been proposed for the treatment of cancer cachexia. The first step includes the treatment of potentially reversible causes of anorexia, such as anxiety, constipation, depression, dysphagia, nausea, vomiting, oral candidiasis, or pain. If a patient has reduced appetite associated with early satiety or evidence of gastroparesis, a trial of metoclopramide 10 to 20 mg before meals and at bedtime up to 120 mg/d is a reasonable second step. If this fails, then a trial of megestrol acetate starting at 160 mg/d and increasing the dose up to 800 mg/d for patients with a relatively good prognosis or the use of dexamethasone 8 to 10 mg twice daily in patients with a poor prognosis is indicated. Megestrol acetate should not be combined with other chemotherapy agents. The fourth step is based on emerging evidence from clinical trials for dronabinol, thalidomide, eicosapentanoic acid, and melatonin. Dronabinol should be used 2.5 mg twice to three times daily, thalidomide at 100 mg per night, eicosapentanoic acid at 2 to 3 g/d, and melatonin at 20 to 40 mg/d.[15,64]

Use of Dietary Supplements during Cancer Therapy

Many cancer patients take nutritional supplements and herbs or start a special diet during or after conventional cancer treatment hoping to enhance the benefits of treatment, to alleviate side effects, and to maintain or improve general health and well-being.[89] Unfortunately, the use of dietary supplements during cancer treatment remains controversial.[56] Physicians should routinely ask their patients if they are taking any nutritional supplements or herbs, especially since patients often fail to inform their physician of their supplement use. Patients should also be cautioned not to substitute vitamin and mineral supplements for established medicine.[90]

Supplemental antioxidants remain one of the more popular nutritional supplements taken by cancer patients, often at doses higher than the recommended dietary allowances. The rationale for this practice is that antioxidants may improve the efficacy of cytotoxic therapies by selectively inhibiting the growth of tumor cells, inducing cellular differentiation, or altering the intracellular redox state.[91] Many oncologists, on the other hand, are reluctant to recommend antioxidant supplementation during treatment for fear that it will interfere with conventional therapy. Antioxidants may interfere with the oxidative breakdown of cellular DNA and cell membranes necessary for the agents to work. Furthermore, there is evidence to suggest that apoptotic breakdown of tumor cells is selectively increased by the presence of reactive oxygen species within the tissue. This cytotoxic process would most likely be slowed by an antioxidant-replete diet.[56] The American Institute for Cancer Research has concluded, based on current evidence, that supplementation of the diets of cancer patients undergoing active treatments with individual or combined antioxidants above their dietary reference intakes cannot be recommended as safe or effective. However, adding a daily multivitamin containing supplements at levels of the dietary reference intake can be done safely as part of a program of healthy nutrition including 5 to 10 servings of fruits and vegetables daily.[56]

The use of nonantioxidant supplements such as soy protein and isoflavones, herbal supplements, and special diets is not currently supported by substantial evidence. Potential drug interactions with other supplements, medications, and anticancer therapy and overlooking or misinterpreting the side effects of herbal supplements and possible contaminants can have serious consequences. It is important to establish efficacy, dosing timing, and duration of supplementation prior to recommending patient use. Recommendations should be based on sound scientific evidence.[90]

Nutritional Therapies

Nutrition screening should be performed as part of the initial assessment at the time of diagnosis. Options for nutrition intervention include oral supplements, hydration solutions, and dietary recommendations; enteral feeding with polymeric, monomeric, or specialized formulas; and TPN. Treatment should be individualized according to the needs of the patient.[17] It is important to define the goals of nutrition support on initiation of treatment. Nutritional therapy can be used as adjuvant treatment and support during anticancer therapy or as a means to provide long-term nutrient supplementation to patients with severely impaired gastrointestinal function who would not survive without intervention.[14]

Oral Dietary Therapy

Oral dietary therapy can improve nutrition in patients who are able to eat but require special diets because of gastrointestinal dysfunction. Simple dietary recommendations can significantly increase oral protein-energy intake by cancer patients in the course of treatment or in palliative care. Successful implementation of a diet requires instruction of the patient and family by a dietitian.[14] The dietitian should intervene as soon as possible after the diagnosis of cancer is made. The dietitian's role is to calculate food consumption and caloric requirements, develop meal plans, evaluate nutritional status, and anticipate the nutritional risks of both the cancer and its treatment. Regular monitoring and follow-up and close coordination with staff involved in patient care are important to alert the physician to the need for enteral or parenteral support.[17]

In addition to the diet, a variety of oral nutritional supplements are available. They vary according to the type of proteins, energy density, osmolarity, lactose, gluten and fiber content, commercial formulation (eg, liquid, powder, pudding, bar), and the range of flavors.[17] The main problem with the use of oral supplements is taste fatigue.[14] Nevertheless, such formulations can be an important source of nutrients in patients who are able to reach their caloric goals with oral intake alone.

Enteral Nutrition

Enteral feeding delivers nutrients to the gastrointestinal tract through tubes.[92] The enteral route is preferred over parenteral nutrition in the setting of a functional gastrointestinal tract.[93] Enteral feeding is more physiologic, preserves the gastrointestinal architecture, and prevents bacterial translocation from the gut.[75] Enteral nutrition solutions are easier to administer, have fewer complications, and are more cost effective. The rate of enteral feeding can be regulated to be delivered as a bolus or as a slow, continuous infusion to permit the optimal use of a limited small intestinal absorptive capacity. Enteral nutrition can bypass proximal obstruction or defects, overcome oropharyngeal dysphagia, or allow a gastrointestinal tract that has a limited absorptive capacity to be constantly bathed in nutrients.[11]

Once it has been decided to initiate enteral nutrition support, a choice of enteral access device must be made. Tubes may be placed through the nose or percutaneously, and the tip terminates in the stomach or small intestine. For patients for whom the anticipated duration of enteral support is less than 30 days, a nasogastric or nasoenteric tube is the best choice. These tubes are also useful to test for tolerance to enteral feeding before committing a patient to a percutaneous tube. Tubes typically range from 8F to 12F and have a mean durability of less than 10 days before they get clogged or dislodged.[11] A serious complication of transnasal tube placement is inadvertent placement into the lung or pleural cavity and the development of a pneumothorax. Radiographs or direct endoscopic visualization should be used to confirm the location of the tube prior to initiation of feeding.[93]

For patients who will require enteral nutrition for more than 4 weeks, a percutaneous feeding tube is indicated.[94] Surgical, radiologic, and endoscopic methods have been successfully used to place percutaneous feeding tubes in the stomach and small intestine.[92] Success rates of up to 99% with major complication rates of only 1.3% have made the placement of percutaneous endoscopic gastrostomy (PEG) tubes the most popular.[95] Commercially available PEG tubes are typically made of silicone or polyurethane and come in sizes ranging from 15F to 28F. These larger-bore tubes are associated with less frequent clogging than nasal tubes. With proper care, the average tube will last 1 to 2 years. In patients with cancer, PEG tubes have been shown to safely provide long-term enteral access, with few major complications. Complications of PEG placement include peritonitis, perforation, hemorrhage, and fasciitis.[11] In patients with head and neck cancer, metastases to the PEG stoma have been described. This may occur secondary to direct seeding of the stoma during PEG placement or by hematogenous or lymphatic spread.[96]

In general, gastric feeding is preferred. However, jejunal feeding is indicated in the presence of gastric outlet obstruction, gastroparesis, or proximal fistula or leak or if there is suspicion of aspiration of gastric contents.[97] Surgical jejunostomies are associated with significant morbidity and mortality, including intestinal obstruction and necrosis and the development of abscesses and fistulae, and carry a mortality rate of up to 10%.[98] Radiologically placed gastrojejunostomy tubes are safe and well tolerated.[99] There are two types of endoscopically placed jejunostomies: the jejunal extension tube (JET-PEG) and the direct percutaneous endoscopic jejunostomy (DPEJ). The JET-PEG is essentially a small-bore tube that is placed through a larger-bore PEG tube and endoscopically advanced to the jejunum. The small-bore extension tube often clogs or migrates

back into the stomach.[11] The placement of a DPEJ tube uses the same technique as PEG placement and has been performed by experienced endoscopists with success rates of 88% and complication rates of 3 to 7%.[100,101] DPEJ is particularly useful in patients who have had a previous esophagectomy or gastrectomy. Successful DPEJ placement has been shown to decrease dependence on TPN and simplify hospital discharge.[102,103] DPEJ tubes also last for 1 to 2 years before needing to be changed and can be safely used for long-term nutritional support if necessary. Whenever delivering nutrient solutions directly into the small intestine, a continuous infusion via a pump must be used. Bolus feedings are contraindicated. However, infusion rates of up to 180 mL/h are safe and can be tolerated.[11]

More than 100 different enteral feeding formulas are currently available. Formulas are classified as polymeric, monomeric, and disease specific. Polymeric formulas contain intact carbohydrate polymers, proteins, and triglycerides. They can be used safely in most patients. Monomeric formulas contain nutrients that have been partially or completely hydrolyzed and are therefore more easily absorbed if digestion is impaired. Proteins are present as short peptide chains or free amino acids, carbohydrates as oligosaccharides or maltodextrin, and fat as a mixture of long- and medium-chain triglycerides. They are indicated in patients with malabsorption. Disease-specific formulas are targeted toward patients with specific underlying conditions. Formulas have been developed for patients with diabetes mellitus, renal insufficiency, pulmonary insufficiency, and hepatic encephalopathy. Immune-enhancing formulas are also available for use in patients with acquired immune deficiency syndrome (AIDS), severe traumatic injury, or critical illness, as well as in cancer patients.[92]

There is no evidence to support the routine use of enteral feeding in well-nourished patients undergoing anticancer therapy.[62] On the other hand, patients with head and neck cancer represent a group of patients who benefit the most from placement of a PEG tube prior to the initiation of radiotherapy.[104] Enteral nutrition in these patients has been shown to prevent weight loss, treatment interruption, and hospitalization for dehydration. For malnourished patients undergoing resection of their tumor, 7 to 10 days of preoperative enteral nutrition support is associated with a 10% reduction in morbidity and improved quality of life.[105] In a prospective study of patients with esophageal cancer undergoing chemoradiation, enteral nutrition effectively prevented weight loss during therapy.[106] Placement of DPEJ tubes is useful in the management of complications after esophagectomy. Most patients will regain their ability to eat and can have the feeding tube removed. However, a

significant minority will become dependent on enteral nutrition and can be fed long term via a PEG tube, percutaneous endoscopic jejunostomy tube, or a button (skin level, low profile) gastrostomy or jejunostomy device with few complications.[11]

Immune-enhancing formulas contain substantial amounts of arginine, n-3 polyunsaturated fatty acids, nucleotides, and glutamine.[107] Studies using these specialized formulas in patients undergoing elective surgery for upper gastrointestinal or pharyngeal cancer show a consistent trend toward reduced infectious complications; however, none of them has demonstrated a statistically significant survival benefit. Furthermore, many of these studies have design flaws.[108] On the other hand, more recent evidence suggests that if an adequate volume of immunonutrition is delivered in advance of surgical insult, more impressive benefits can be appreciated. In a clinical trial by Braga and colleagues, 150 malnourished patients who were candidates for major elective surgery for malignancy of the gastrointestinal tract were randomly assigned to receive either postoperative enteral nutrition with a standard formula, 1 L/d for 7 days of immunonutrition formula preoperatively and standard enteral formula postoperatively, or immunonutrition formula 1 L/d for 7 days preoperatively and continued postoperatively.[109] Statistically significant reductions in infectious complications and in postoperative length of stay were noted in the groups receiving immunonutrition compared with the control group. Although more studies are needed before the routine use of immunonutrition is advocated, some practical strategies to maximize the success of these formulas have been suggested. Arginine should be at least 12 g/L; the duration should be at least 3 days; feeding goals should approach 25 kcal/kg and at least 800 mL/d; and enteral nutrition protocols should be more aggressive in feeding patients preoperatively and reaching enteral goals postoperatively.[108]

Total Parenteral Nutrition

TPN is an effective means of delivering hypertonic nutrient solutions via the central venous system into the general circulation and bypassing the gastrointestinal tract. In patients unsuitable for enteral nutrition support, parenteral nutrition remains an important option. Catheter-related complications include pneumothorax, venous thrombosis, arterial trauma, and sepsis. Metabolic and electrolyte abnormalities such as hypokalemia, hypophosphatemia, glucose intolerance, and noketotic hyperosmolar coma can also occur.[75] Many prospective randomized controlled studies have examined the role of TPN in the management of cancer patients. A clear benefit from nutritional support appears to be limited to a specific group of patients.[14]

Most studies reveal no benefits of specialized nutrition support during chemotherapy or radiation with regard to treatment tolerance, antitumor therapy side effects, or survival.[62] Furthermore, patients who receive TPN while undergoing chemotherapy have more infectious complications. However, in some of these studies, patients were not necessarily malnourished, and some had adequate oral intake and gastrointestinal function.[14] Therefore, patients who are severely malnourished or who develop prolonged gastrointestinal toxicity with treatment may be candidates for TPN.

A group of patients for whom prolonged gastrointestinal toxicity during treatment and poor tolerance to oral or enteral nutrition support is extremely common is in the setting of bone marrow transplantation.[62] The use of TPN has become routine practice to maintain body cell mass. Prophylactic TPN decreases the incidence of malignant relapse and improves survival in patients receiving bone marrow transplantation.[110] Studies using glutamine-supplemented parenteral nutrition solutions in bone marrow transplant recipients have also demonstrated a significant reduction in the incidence of clinical infections and the duration of hospital stay compared with those patients receiving standard TPN. However, there was no significant difference in the severity of mucositis, the incidence or severity of graft-versus-host disease, or inhospital mortality.[111,112] The role of glutamine-supplemented TPN needs more study prior to recommending its routine use.

The use of TPN during the perioperative period in malnourished cancer patients undergoing surgery has also been recommended.[10] Patients with gastrointestinal cancer who received TPN for 10 days before surgery had lower rates of postoperative wound infection, pneumonia, major complications, and mortality compared with patients on a regular hospital diet.[113] The Veterans Affairs Cooperative Study Group, in one of the largest clinical trials, randomly assigned 395 malnourished patients prior to surgery to receive TPN before and after surgery or no perioperative TPN. Approximately two-thirds of these patients had malignant disease. Although the overall incidence of infectious complications was higher in the group receiving TPN, the small subgroup of patients who were categorized as severely malnourished receiving TPN had fewer noninfectious complications and no concomitant increase in infectious complications compared with the control group.[60] The use of perioperative TPN in patients undergoing hepatectomy for hepatocellular carcinoma was also associated with a reduction in overall postoperative morbidity and diminished deterioration in postoperative liver function.[114] However, not all studies have demonstrated a clear benefit for the use of perioperative

TPN in cancer patients. In a randomized trial of 117 patients with pancreatic cancer who underwent major pancreatic resection, complications were significantly greater in the group receiving TPN postoperatively and were associated with an increase in the rate of intra-abdominal abscesses. The overall mortality rates were similar in the TPN and the control groups.[115] In a recent consensus conference sponsored by the National Institutes of Health, the American Society for Parenteral and Enteral Nutrition, and the American Society of Clinical Nutrition, 33 prospective randomized controlled trials, involving more than 2,500 surgical patients, were reviewed to evaluate perioperative nutrition support. The panel came to the following conclusions: (1) TPN given to malnourished patients (defined by weight loss, plasma proteins, or prognostic indices) with gastrointestinal cancer for 7 to 10 days before surgery reduces postoperative complications by 10%, (2) routine use of early postoperative TPN in malnourished general surgical patients who did not receive preoperative TPN increases postoperative complications by approximately 10%, and (3) postoperative nutritional support is necessary for patients unable to eat for prolonged periods after surgery (within 5 to 10 days after surgery) to prevent the adverse effects of starvation.[10]

Home Nutrition Support

Long-term home enteral nutrition and parenteral nutrition are tools that can be used by physicians in the appropriate clinical setting. Patients requiring home nutrition support fall into three general categories. The first group of patients are cancer survivors or patients with stable disease who develop gastrointestinal failure during the course of treatment. The second group of patients are moderately to severely malnourished and undergoing a defined curative or palliative oncologic intervention with anticipated side effects. The third group of patients are those with widely metastatic disease and little hope for cure who are being considered for palliative nutritional support.[62]

Patients with severe gastrointestinal failure secondary to massive small bowel resection or severe radiation enteritis usually require long-term home TPN.[14] In a published report, patients with intestinal failure secondary to therapy for malignancy received home TPN for an average of $1,092 \pm 867$ days.[116] Survival rates and TPN-related complications in such patients are comparable to those seen in patients with benign disease who require home TPN. Most deaths in patients on home TPN are secondary to progression of the primary disease process rather than TPN-related complications.[117]

In malnourished cancer patients with a defined treatment plan who are at high risk of

progressive nutritional deterioration secondary to therapy, enteral nutrition is the preferred treatment. Parenteral nutrition should be reserved for patients in whom enteral nutrition is contraindicated or not tolerated.[62] A review of the North American registry showed that 30% of patients on home enteral nutrition were able to resume oral intake and discontinue enteral feeding during the first year and 36% of all cancer patients on home enteral nutrition were alive after 1 year.[118] Home enteral nutrition is safe, with a hospitalization rate for complications owing to home enteral nutrition of fewer than 0.4 hospitalizations per patient per year.[118] Outpatient follow-up and repeated evaluations are necessary to determine whether patients enrolled in a home nutrition program require indefinite nutrition support or if they can eventually be transitioned to oral intake.[11]

Among patients with progressive disease despite specific treatments, home TPN offers little benefit.[14] Nevertheless, in the United States, cancer patients represent about one-third of patients receiving home TPN compared with about half in Italy. In addition, 50 to 75% of these patients have locoregional and/or metastatic progressive disease.[17] The 1-year survival rate in these conditions was 32% in the 1995 American survey, with preservation of satisfactory social and/or professional activity in 25% of the cases during the first year.[117] In the Italian study, the improvement in quality of life depended on functional status. Among patients with a Karnofsky index lower than 40, the average survival time was less than 3 months, and an improvement in the quality of life was found in only 9% of cases.[119] On the other hand, some investigators have advocated the use of selected immunonutrient formulas in palliative care. Significant weight gain and increases in oral food intake and functional status have been noted.[120] However, patients with widely metastatic disease usually already have available central access and are often reluctant to have a nasogastric tube or more permanent tube placed. They may also be intolerant of enteral feedings because of partial or complete bowel obstruction secondary to carcinomatosis and extrinsic compression.[17] The decision of whether to initiate home nutrition support in this clinical situation should also take into account patients' perceptions so that quality of life can be improved.[121] In a study aimed at assessing the life experience of patients with malignant bowel obstruction, it was determined that at that time, the most important issues confronting the patient were the inability to eat, alteration in physical activities, deterioration in mental abilities, social isolation, waiting for bowel movements to occur, and a lack of direction and personal inner reflection. However, if the patient had a goal, it meant that something was being done; regardless of whether that goal was palliative or active treatment, doing something appeared to be a way of maintaining hope, and doing nothing was seen as abandonment or desertion.[122]

Ultimately, the decision to initiate home nutrition support needs to be based on the ability of nutrition support to improve patients' clinical outcome and ethical principles that need to be interpreted and appropriately applied to each individual case. It is vital to maintain an open and honest relationship with patients and their families and to address these issues in a forum in which all parties concerned can effectively communicate their feelings, anxieties, and ethical principles.[121]

Home nutrition is no longer appropriate when a patient enters the terminal stages of the disease. Such patients usually have severely restricted oral intake or are dehydrated. Fluids or small amounts of food should be administered to alleviate hunger or thirst.[14,17]

Summary

The exact role that nutrients, dietary factors, and lifestyle changes play in cancer prevention remains elusive. However, as clinical breakthroughs are made with the performance of collaborative research involving larger and more well-designed studies and the development of the discipline of nutritional genomics, a deeper understanding of pathophysiologic mechanisms and nutrient-gene interactions can be achieved. Inevitably, this will lead to dietary and lifestyle recommendations based on a solid foundation of scientific evidence.

Malnutrition in cancer patients needs to be addressed early so that patients have the best chance of responding to anticancer therapy. Symptom control, pharmacologic therapies to improve appetite and food intake, dietary therapy, enteral and parenteral nutrition, and home nutrition support provide valuable adjuncts to treatment of the cancer patient. The study and development of immune-enhancing formulas for enteral and parenteral use and the role they have in preventing malnutrition-associated complications remain the focus of continued research in cancer patients.

REFERENCES

1. Winik M. Cancer and diet. Nutr Metab Cardiovasc Dis 1999;9(4 Suppl):52–5.
2. Cummings JH, Bingham SA. Diet and the prevention of cancer. BMJ 1998;317:1636–40.
3. Kim YI, Mason JB. Nutrition chemoprevention of gastrointestinal cancers: a critical review. Nutr Rev 1996;54:259–79.
4. Doll R, Peto R. The causes of cancer: quantitative estimates of avoidable risks of cancer in the United States today. J Natl Cancer Inst 1981;66:1191–265.
5. Hensrud DD, Heimburger DC. Diet, nutrients and gastrointestinal cancer. Gastroenterol Clin North Am 1998;27:325–46.
6. Berrino F, Krogh V, Riboli E. Epidemiology studies on diet and cancer. Tumori 2003;89:581–5.
7. Kritchevsky D. Diet and cancer: what's next? J Nutr 2003;133:3827S–9S.
8. Rennert G. Diet and cancer: where are we and where are we going? Proc Nutr Soc 2003;62:59–62.
9. Milner JA. Strategies for cancer prevention: the role of diet. Br J Nutr 2002;87:S265–72.
10. Wong PW, Enriquez A, Barrera R. Nutritional support in critically ill patients with cancer. Crit Care Clin 2001;17:743–67.
11. Schattner M. Enteral nutrition support of the patient with cancer. J Clin Gastroenterol 2003;36:297–302.
12. Capra S, Ferguson M, Ried K. Cancer: impact of nutrition intervention outcome-nutrition issues for patients. Nutrition 2001;17:769–72.
13. Reilly J, Hull S, Albert N, et al. Economic impact of malnutrition: a model system for hospitalized patients. JPEN J Parenter Enteral Nutr 1998;12:371–6.
14. Shike M. Nutrition therapy for the cancer patient. Hematol Oncol Clin North Am 1996;10:221–34.
15. Palesty JA, Dudrick SJ. What we have learned about cachexia in gastrointestinal cancer. Dig Dis 2003;21:198–213.
16. Brennan MF. Malnutrition in patients with gastrointestinal malignancy: significance and management. Dig Dis Sci 1986;31:77S–90S.
17. Nitenberg G, Raynard B. Nutritional support of the cancer patient: issues and dilemmas. Crit Rev Oncol Hematol 2000;34:137–68.
18. De Cicco M, Fantin D. Nutritional support. Tumori 2003;3:S63–7.
19. Key TJ, Schatzkin A, Willett WC, et al. Diet, nutrition and the prevention of cancer. Public Health Nutr 2004;7:187–200.
20. Ames BN, Wakimoto P. Are vitamin and mineral deficiencies a major cancer risk? Nat Rev 2002;2:694–704.
21. Willett WC. Diet and cancer. Oncologist 2000;5:393–404.
22. Giovannucci E. Diet, body weight, and colorectal cancer: a summary of the epidemiological evidence. J Womens Health 2003;12:173–82.
23. Giovannucci E. Modifiable risk factors for colon cancer. Gastroenterol Clin North Am 2002;31:925–43.
24. Kinigham RB. Physical activity and the primary prevention of cancer. Primary Care 1998;25:515–36.
25. Lee MI. Physical activity and cancer prevention—data from epidemiological studies. Med Sci Sports Exerc 2003;35:1823–7.
26. Friedenreich CM, Orenstein MR. Physical activity and cancer prevention: etiologic evidence and biological mechanisms. J Nutr 2002;3456S–64S.
27. Kushi L, Giovannucci E. Dietary fat and cancer. Am J Med 2002;113:63S–70S.
28. Martin-Moreno JM, Willett WC, Gorgojo L, et al. Dietary fat, olive oil intake and breast cancer risk. Int J Cancer 1994;58:774–80.
29. Trichopoulou A, Kaisouyanni K, Sniver S, et al. Consumption of olive oil and specific food groups in relation to breast cancer risk in Greece. J Natl Cancer Inst 1995;87:110–6.
30. Gatof D, Ahnen D. Primary prevention of colorectal cancer: diet and drugs. Gastroenterol Clin North Am 2002;31:587–623.
31. Giovannucci E, Rimm EB, Colditz GA et al. A prospective study of dietary fat and risk of prostate cancer. J Natl Cancer Inst 1993;85:1571–9.
32. Oh WK, Small EJ. Complementary and alternative therapies in prostate cancer. Semin Oncol 2002;29:575–84.
33. Fuchs CS, Colditz GA, Stampfer MJ, et al. Dietary fiber and the risk of colorectal cancer and adenoma in women. N Engl J Med 1999;340:169–76.
34. Willett WC, Hunter DJ, Stampfer MJ, et al. Dietary fat and fiber in relation to risk of breast cancer: an 8 year follow-up. JAMA 1992;268:2037–44.
35. Tamimi RM, Lagiou P, Adami HO, et al. Prospects for chemoprevention of cancer. J Intern Med 2002;251:286–300.
36. Lee IM. Antioxidant vitamins in the prevention of cancer. Proc Assoc Am Physicians 1999;111:10–5.
37. The α-Tocopherol β-Carotene Cancer Prevention Study Group. The effect of vitamin E and β-carotene on the incidence of lung cancer and other cancers in male smokers. N Engl J Med 1994;330:1029–35.
38. Omenn GS, Goodman GE, Thornquist MD, et al. Effects of a combination of {158}-carotene and vitamin A on lung cancer and cardiovascular disease. N Engl J Med 1996;334:1150–5.
39. Willis MS, Wians FH. The role of nutrition in preventing prostate cancer: a review of the proposed mechanism of action of various dietary substances. Clin Chim Acta 2003;330:57–83.
40. Kueuk O, Sarkar FH, Djuric Z, et al. Effects of lycopene supplementation in patients with localized prostate cancer. Exp Biol Med 2002;227:881–5.
41. Sung L, Greenberg ML, Koren G, et al. Vitamin E: the evidence for multiple roles in cancer. Nutr Cancer 2003;46:1–14.
42. Blot WJ, Li JY, Taylor PR, et al. Nutrition intervention trials in Linxian, China: supplementation with specific vitamin/mineral combinations, cancer incidence, and disease-specific mortality in the general population. J Natl Cancer Inst 1993;85:1483–92.
43. Li JY, Taylor PR, Li B, et al. Nutrition intervention trials in Linxian, China: multiple vitamin/mineral supplementation, cancer incidence, and disease-specific mortality among adults with esophageal dysplasia. J Natl Cancer Inst 1993;85:1492–8.
44. Whanger PD. Selenium and its relationship to cancer: an update. Br J Nutr 2004;91:11–28.
45. Combs GF. Considering the mechanisms of cancer prevention by selenium. Adv Exp Med Biol 2001;492:107–17.
46. Alaejos MS, Díaz-Romero FJ, Díaz-Romero C. Selenium and cancer: some nutritional aspects. Nutrition 2000;16:376–83.
47. Clark LC, Combs GF, Turnbull BW, et al. Effects of selenium supplementation for cancer prevention in patients with carcinoma of the skin: a randomized controlled trial. JAMA 1996;276:1957–63.
48. Nève J. Selenium as a 'nutraceutical': how to conciliate physiological and supra-nutritional effects for an essential trace element. Curr Opin Clin Nutr Metab Care 2002;5:659–63.
49. Baron JA, Beach M, Mandel JS, et al. Calcium supplements for the prevention of colorectal adenomas. N Engl J Med 1999;340:101–7.
50. Glynn SA, Albanes D. Folate and cancer: a review of the literature. Nutr Cancer 1994;22:101–19.
51. Fuchs CS, Willett WC, Colditz GA, et al. The influence of folate and multivitamin use on the familial risk of colon cancer in women. Cancer Epidemiol Biomarkers Prev 2002;11:227–34.
52. Giovannucci E. Epidemiologic studies of folate and colorectal neoplasia: a review. J Nutr 2002;132:2350S–55S.
53. Courtney EDJ, Melville DM, Leicester RJ. Review article: chemoprevention of colorectal cancer. Aliment Pharmacol Ther 2004;19:1–24.
54. Ferguson LR. Prospects for cancer prevention. Mutat Res 1999;428:329–38.
55. Norman HA, Butrum RR, Feldman E, et al. The role of dietary supplements during cancer therapy. J Nutr 2003;3794S–9S.
56. Milner JA, McDonald SS, Anderson DE, et al. Molecular targets for nutrients involved with cancer prevention. Nutr Cancer 2001;41:1–16.
57. Paoloni-Giacobino A, Grimble R, Pichard C, et al. Genetics and nutrition. Clin Nutr 2003;22:429–35.
58. Go VLW, Butrum RR, Wong DA. Diet, nutrition and cancer prevention: the postgenomic era. J Nutr 2003;133:3830S–6S.
59. Thomson CA, LeWinn K, Newton TR, et al. Nutrition and diet in the development of gastrointestinal cancer. Curr Oncol Rep 2003;5:192–202.
60. Veterans Affairs Total Parenteral Nutrition Cooperative Study Group. Perioperative total parenteral nutrition in surgical patients. N Engl J Med 1991;325:525–32.
61. DeWys WD, Begg C, Lavin PT, et al. Prognostic effect of weight loss prior to chemotherapy in cancer patients. Eastern Cooperative Oncology Group. Am J Med 1980;69:491–7.
62. Barrera R. Nutritional support in cancer patients. JPEN J Parenter Enteral Nutr 2002;26:S63–71.
63. Body JJ. The syndrome of anorexia-cachexia. Curr Opin Oncol 1999;11:255–60.
64. Davis MP, Dickerson D. Cachexia and anorexia: cancer's covert killer. Support Care Cancer 2000;8:180–7.
65. Laviano A, Meguid MM, Rossi-Fanelli F. Improving food intake in anorectic cancer patients. Curr Opin Clin Nutr Metab Care 2003;6:421–6.
66. Mantovani G, Macciò A, Lai P, et al. Cytokine activity in cancer-related anorexia/cachexia: role of megestrol acetate and medroxyprogesterone acetate. Semin Oncol 1998;25:45S–52S.
67. Comeau TB, Epstein JB, Migas C. Taste and smell dysfunction in patients receiving chemotherapy: a review of current knowledge. Support Care Cancer 2001;9:575–80.

68. Mattson T, Arvidson K, Heimdahl A, et al. Alterations in taste acuity associated with allogeneic bone marrow transplantation. J Oral Pathol Med 1992;21:33–7.

69. Lindsey A, Piper B. Anorexia, serum zinc, and immunologic response in small cell lung cancer patients receiving chemotherapy and prophylactic cranial radiotherapy. Nutr Cancer 1986;8:231–8.

70. Russell DM, Shike M, Marliss EB, et al. Effects of total parenteral nutrition and chemotherapy on the metabolic derangements in small cell lung cancer. Cancer Res 1984;44:1706–11.

71. Dempsey DT, Feuerer ID, Knox LS, et al. Energy expenditure in malnourished gastrointestinal cancer patients. Cancer 1984;53:1265–73.

72. Peacock JL, Inculet RI, Corsey R, et al. Resting energy expenditure and body cell mass alterations in noncachectic patients with sarcoma. Surgery 1987;102:465–72.

73. Hyltander A, Korner U, Lundholm KG. Evaluation of mechanisms behind elevated energy expenditure in cancer patients with solid tumors. Eur J Clin Invest 1993;23:46–52.

74. Lelli G, Montanari M, Gilli G, et al. Treatment of the cancer anorexia-cachexia syndrome: a critical reappraisal. J Chemother 2003;15:220–5.

75. Daly JM, Redmond HP, Lieberman MD, et al. Nutritional support of patients with cancer of the gastrointestinal tract. Surg Clin North Am 1991;71:523–36.

76. Klein S, Jeejeebhoy KN. The malnourished patient: nutritional assessment and management. In: Feldman M, Friedman LS, Sleisenger MH, editors. Sleisenger and Fordtran's gastrointestinal and liver disease: pathophysiology, diagnosis, management. 7th ed. Pennsylvania: Saunders; 2002. p. 265–85.

77. Jeejeebhoy KN. Nutritional assessment. Gastroenterol Clin North Am 1998;27:347–69.

78. Jeejeebhoy KN. Nutritional assessment. Nutrition 2000;16:585–90.

79. Hensrud DD. Nutrition screening and assessment. Med Clin North Am 1999;83:1525–46.

80. Baker JP, Detsky AS, Wesson DE, et al. Nutritional assessment: a comparison of clinical judgment and objective measurements. N Engl J Med 1982;306:969–72.

81. Ottery FD, Walsh D, Strawford A. Pharmacologic management of anorexia/cachexia. Semin Oncol 1998;25:S35–44.

82. Chlebowski R, Herrold J, Ali I. Influence of nandrolone decanoate on weight loss in advanced non-small cell lung cancer. Cancer 1986;58:183–6.

83. Goldberg R, Loprinzi C, Maillard J. Pentoxyfylline for treatment of cancer anorexia and cachexia? A randomized, double-blind, placebo-controlled trial. J Clin Oncol 1995;13:2856–9.

84. Gagnon B, Bruera E. A review of the drug treatment of cachexia associated with cancer. Drugs 1998;55:675–88.

85. Barber M, Ross J, Vossa C, et al. The effect of an oral nutritional supplement enriched with fish oil on weight loss in patients with pancreatic cancer. Br J Cancer 1999;81:80–6.

86. McMillan DC, Leen E, Smith J, et al. Effect of extended ibuprofen administration on the acute phase protein response in colorectal cancer patients. Eur J Surg Oncol 1995;21:531–4.

87. Wigmore SJ, Falconer JS, Plester CE, et al. Ibuprofen reduces energy expenditure and acute phase protein production

in cancer patients compared with placebo in pancreatic cancer patients. Br J Cancer 1995;72:185–8.

88. Bruera E, Neumann CM, Pituskin E, et al. Thalidomide in patients with cachexia due to terminal cancer: preliminary report. Ann Oncol 1999;10:857–9.

89. Ladas EJ, Jacobson JS, Kennedy DD, et al. Antioxidants and cancer therapy: a systematic review. J Clin Oncol 2004;22:517–28.

90. Jungi WF. Dangerous nutrition. Support Care Cancer 2003;11:197–8.

91. Prasad KN, Kumar A, Kochupillai V, et al. High doses of multiple antioxidant vitamins: essential ingredients in improving the efficacy of standard cancer therapy. J Am Coll Nutr 1999;18:13–25.

92. Kirby DF, Delegge MH, Fleming CR. American Gastroenterological Association medical position statement: guidelines for the use of enteral nutrition. Gastroenterology 1995;108:1280–301.

93. Haddad RY, Thomas DR. Enteral nutrition and enteral tube feeding: review of the evidence. Clin Geriatr Med 2002;18:867–81.

94. Delegge MH. Home enteral nutrition. JPEN J Parenter Enteral Nutr 2002;26:S4–7.

95. Grant JP. Percutaneous endoscopic gastrostomy: initial placement by a single endoscopic technique and long-term follow-up. Ann Surg 1993;217:168–74.

96. Schiano TD, Pfister D, Harrison L, et al. Neoplastic seeding as a complication of percutaneous endoscopic gastrostomy. Am J Gastroenterol 1994;89:131–3.

97. Shike M, Latkany L. Direct percutaneous endoscopic jejunostomy. Gastrointest Endosc Clin N Am 1998;8:569–80.

98. Tapia J, Murguia R, Garcia G, et al. Jejunostomy: techniques, indications, and complications. World J Surg 1999;23:596–602.

99. Lawrance JAL, Mais KL, Slevin NJ. Radiologically inserted gastrostomies: their use in patients with cancer of the upper aerodigestive tract. Clin Oncol 2003;15:87–91.

100. Shike M, Latkany L, Gerdes H, et al. Direct percutaneous endoscopic jejunostomies for enteral feeding. Gastrointest Endosc 1996;44:536–40.

101. Rumalla A, Baron TH. Results of direct percutaneous endoscopic jejunostomy: an alternative for providing jejunal feeding. Mayo Clin Proc 2000;75:807–10.

102. Bueno JS, Barrera R, Gerdes H, et al. Placement of direct percutaneous endoscopic jejunostomy in patients with complications following esophageal resection. Gastrointest Endosc 2001;53:AB209.

103. Barrera R, Schattner M, Nygard S, et al. Outcome of direct percutaneous endoscopic jejunostomy tube placement for nutritional support in critically ill mechanically ventilated patients. J Crit Care 2001;16:178–81.

104. Scolapio JS, Spangler PR, Romano MM, et al. Prophylactic placement of gastrostomy feeding tubes before radiotherapy in patients with head and neck cancer. J Clin Gastroenterol 2001;33:215–7.

105. Van Bokhorst-de Van der Schuer MA, Langendoen SI, Vondeling H, et al. Perioperative enteral nutrition and quality of life of severely malnourished head and neck cancer patients: a randomized clinical trial. Clin Nutr 2000;19:437–44.

106. Bozzetti F, Cozzaglio L, Gavazzi C, et al. Nutritional support in patients with cancer of the esophagus: impact on

nutritional status, patient compliance to therapy, and survival. Tumori 1998;84:681–6.

107. Alvarez W, Mobarhan S. Finding a place for immunonutrition. Nutr Rev 2003;61:214–8.

108. McCowen KC, Bistrian BR. Immunonutrition: problematic or problem solving? Am J Clin Nutr 2003;77:764–70.

109. Braga M, Gianotti L, Nespoli L, et al. Nutritional approach in malnourished surgical patients: a prospective randomized study. Arch Surg 2002;137:174–80.

110. Weisdorf SA, Lysne J, Wind D, et al. Positive effect of prophylactic total parenteral nutrition on long-term outcome of bone marrow transplantation. Transplantation 1987;43:833–8.

111. Ziegler TR, Young LS, Benfell K. Clinical and metabolic efficacy of glutamine-supplemented parenteral nutrition after bone marrow transplantation: a randomized, double-blind, controlled study. Ann Intern Med 1992;116:821–8.

112. Schloerb PR, Amare M. Total parenteral nutrition with glutamine in bone marrow transplantation and other clinical applications: a randomized, double-blind study. JPEN J Parenter Enteral Nutr 1993;17:407–13.

113. Bozzetti F, Gavazzi C, Miceli R. Perioperative TPN in malnourished, gastrointestinal cancer patients: a randomized, clinical trial. JPEN J Parenter Enteral Nutr 2000;24:7–14.

114. Fan ST, Lo CM, Lai ECS, et al. Perioperative nutritional support in patients undergoing hepatectomy for hepatocellular carcinoma. N Engl J Med 1994;331:1547–52.

115. Brennan MF, Pisters PWT, Posner M, et al. A prospective randomized trial of total parenteral nutrition after major pancreatic resection for malignancy. Ann Surg 1994;220:436–44.

116. Khvatyuk O, Simon N, Birch M, et al. Infectious complications in home parenteral nutrition patients: 30 years of experience at a comprehensive cancer center. Presented at the International Congress Centre Munich; 2001 Sep 9; Munich, Germany.
Klein S, Kinney J, Jeejeebhoy KN, et al. Nutritional support in clinical practice: review of published data and recommendation for future research directions. Am J Clin Nutr 1997;66:683–706.
Ottery FD. Nutritional consequences in reoperative surgery in recurrent malignancy. Semin Oncol 1993;20:528–37.

117. Howard L, Ament M, Fleming C, et al. Current use and clinical outcome of home parenteral and enteral nutrition therapies in the United States. Gastroenterology 1995;109:355–65.

118. Howard L, Patton L, Dahl RS. Outcome of long-term enteral feeding. Gastrointest Endosc Clin N Am1998;8:705–22.

119. Cozzaglio L, Balzola F, Cosentino F, et al. Outcome of cancer patients receiving home parenteral nutrition: Italian Society of Parenteral and Enteral Nutrition (SINPE). JPEN J Parenter Enteral Nutr 1997;21:339–42.

120. Barber MD, Fearon KC, Delmore G, et al. Should cancer patients with incurable disease receive parenteral or enteral nutrition support? Eur J Cancer 1998;34:279–85.

121. Echenique M, Correia MITD. Nutrition in advanced digestive cancer. Curr Opin Nutr Metab Care 2003;6:577–80.

122. Gwilliam B, Bailey C. The nature of terminal malignant bowel obstruction and its impact on patients with advanced cancer. Int J Palliat Nurs 2001;7:474–81.

Oral and Orofacial Considerations in Oncology

Mark S. Chambers, DMD, MS

Adam S. Garden, MD

Jack W. Martin, DDS, MS

Merrill S. Kies, MD

Randal S. Weber, MD

James C. Lemon, DDS

The care of cancer patients requires the combined efforts of a multidisciplinary team of health care providers whose collective goal is not only to cure patients of malignant disease but also to treat or prevent the morbid sequelae of oncologic treatment. In most cancer patients, problems in the oral cavity mirror those in the general population: moderate to advanced periodontal disease, poorly restored dentition, and associated soft tissue pathologies associated with tobacco use, alcohol use, nutritional neglect, general hygiene neglect, or a combination of these factors.[1,2] Evaluation, treatment, and prevention of any oral and dental preexisting pathology are important aspects of the overall treatment outcome for cancer patients.[1,2] Patients undergoing aggressive anticancer treatment encounter preventable, if not treatable, oral mucosal and dental sequelae that could produce morbid events.[3] Complications vary with each patient, depending on the individual's oral and dental status, the type of malignancy, and the therapeutic approach (ie, surgery, radiation therapy, chemotherapy, or a combination of these treatments).[4] Common and frequent treatment-limiting toxicities, such as mucositis, infection, and bleeding, can be minimized and in some cases eliminated if evaluated and treated early by an involved, trained dental health care team.

An oral and dental consultation before chemotherapy, radiation therapy, or head and neck surgery is extremely important in the oral management of cancer patients.[1,5-8] For patients receiving a tumor-ablative procedure involving the oral cavity, the treating physician should aim to control oral and dental problems before adjunct therapy and during the recovery phase. In the immediate postsurgical planning, the oral cavity should be prepared for appropriate prosthetic rehabilitation to correct postsurgical deficits. If radiation therapy, chemotherapy, or both are planned, the treating dental specialist should be aware that the resultant oral complications may be devastating; furthermore, the degree and type of oral sequelae may affect the patient's compliance with or continuance of cancer treatment.[9-12] Such complications may arise during cancer therapy and may result either from treatment (eg, chemotherapeutic complications related to myelosuppression, immunosuppression, or the direct cytotoxic effects of chemical agents on oral tissues) or from the malignant disease process.

A head and neck evaluation, an oral and dental clinical examination, and an intraoral radiologic evaluation should all be performed during the initial visit.[1] Selected dental radiographs are essential in evaluating potential areas of infection that are not obvious on clinical examination (eg, periodontal-periapical tooth pathology, residual cysts, and impacted or partially erupted exfoliating teeth). In addition, the oral health care provider should gather and record the patient's history of present illness, medical and dental histories, social history, review of systems, current medications, adverse drug reactions, and the anticipated cancer treatment plan. From this information, the dentist can plan oral treatment to control immediate needs. However, treatment of disease must always take priority over treatment of complications.[1,13] Dentists should communicate with the treating physicians to be aware of the diagnosis and staging of malignant disease, the goals of proposed therapy, the patient's prognosis, the type and dose of therapy to be administered, and the timing of treatment. If radiation therapy is to be used in the head and neck area, the dentist must know the volume of tissue to be radiated, treatment schedule, dosimetry, fractionation scheme, method of administration (eg, external beam radiation therapy or brachytherapy), type of energy (eg, photon, electron, or mixed beam), and total dose to be administered.[5,7,14-17]

The dentist's initial examination and early treatment of the patient are directed at documenting and reversing any preexisting acute or chronic pathologic conditions—such as dental abscesses, advanced periodontal disease, dental calculus causing gingivitis, partially erupted teeth with the potential for pericoronitis, or soft tissue tooth trauma—that may be factors in the selection of an overall cancer treatment strategy by the treating physician.[1,4] Even if the planned cancer treatment is not toxic to the mucosa and is not myelosuppressive (eg, hormonal therapy), the potential for infection remains even under "normal" circumstances. Additionally, the cancer may eventually progress, necessitating prompt and aggressive therapy; hence, the oral and dental status should be optimal to ensure minimal predictable complications. The periodontal status and degree of tooth decay are evaluated during the initial examination, as are the patient's ability and initiative to maintain optimal oral hygiene.[18] Patients must modify their oral care and hygiene techniques, if possible, to minimize the mucosal and gingival complications that are associated with their specific treatment.[10-20] Caries is another adverse condition resulting from increased caries-forming organisms and is in itself an important consideration in patients with drug- or radiation-induced xerostomia owing to potential pulpal involvement and subsequent periapical abscess formation.[4,18,21]

Oral Complications

Complications resulting from therapeutic administration of ionizing radiation to the head and neck and cytotoxic agents as treatment for cancer can be categorized as either acute (eg, mucositis, infectious stomatitis, alteration in taste or smell acuity, dermatitis, pain, inflammation, and difficulty swallowing) or chronic (eg, xerostomia, caries, abnormal development, fibrosis, trismus, photosensitivity, osteoradionecrosis [ORN], and pain).[1,21,22] The severity of treatment-induced morbidity depends on multiple factors, such as the radiation dose, volume of tissue treated, myelosuppressive treatment, pretreatment performance status, and pretreatment oral condition.[23] Complications arise primarily in three anatomic sites: the mucosa, periodontium, and teeth.[4]

The following is a discussion of five key oral complications: mucositis, xerostomia, ORN, oral infections, and caries. Included is a definition of each condition and information about the incidence and risk, etiology and pathophysiology, clinical features, and management of each entity.

Mucositis

Definition

The National Cancer Institute defines mucositis as a complication of some cancer therapies in which the lining of the digestive system becomes inflamed and, hence, sores develop in the mouth.[24] "Oral mucositis" generally indicates a nonhematologic complication of the aerodigestive tract secondary to chemotherapy or head and neck radiation therapy (Figure 1). The complicated sequelae of mucositis can be associated with odynophagia, dysphagia, infection, dehydration, malnutrition, dysgeusia, and other quality of life

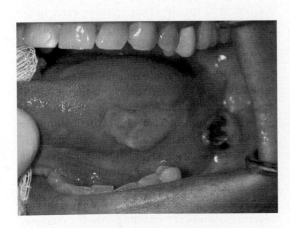

FIGURE 1 A patient undergoing external beam radiation therapy with localized backscatter mucositis.

challenges. This condition can be a significant risk factor for systemic infection, particularly for pancytopenic patients, and can result in increased therapeutic expenses.[25,26] In a study by Sonis and colleagues, severe mucositis was associated with increased fever and infection ($p < .01$), increased analgesia therapy ($p < .001$), a fourfold increase in mortality risk, and higher hospital charges, especially with ulcerative mucositis.[27]

The economic and clinical burden of mucositis was examined by Elting and colleagues reviewing a cohort of 599 patients with solid tumors or lymphoma who had a total of 1,236 chemotherapy cycles from 1994 to 1996 with reported thrombocytopenia.[25] This retrospective analysis assessed clinical outcomes (ie, hemorrhage, infection, oral and gastrointestinal mucositis, and death) and resource use (ie, hospitalization, emergency room visits, and antibiotic use). Mucositis was identified in 37% of the 1,236 cycles, with 11% representing grade 3 or 4 mucositis. The results of this trial revealed a significant correlation between mucositis and increased dose reduction or dose delay in the chemotherapeutic regimen, as well as increased infection, the need for nutritional support, the use of anti-infectives, hospitalization and opioid use, and mortality linked to infection.

Incidence and Risks

The incidence and severity of oral mucositis are influenced by the type of antineoplastic treatment administered and by patient-related factors.[26] Oral and gastrointestinal mucositis can affect up to 100% of patients undergoing high-dose chemotherapy and hematopoietic stem cell transplantation and up to 80% of patients with cancer of the head and neck receiving radiation therapy.[28] In one study, patients who had undergone bone marrow transplantation reported oral mucositis as the most debilitating side effect in comparison with nausea and vomiting, weakness, or diarrhea.[29]

The prevalence of oral mucositis is affected by a number of factors, including the patient's age (more common in the young), diagnosis (increased in patients with a hematologic malignancy), and preexisting oral health (increased in patients with poor oral health), as well as the intensity of antineoplastic therapy, that is, concomitant radiation and chemotherapy.[30] Localized oral infections can be transmitted into the bloodstream through the rich capillary beds that perfuse the mucosa with resultant septicemia. Studies have related septicemia to oral infections in up to 54% of neutropenic individuals.[31]

To improve the long-term disease-free survival rates for patients with head and neck cancer, more intensive regimens are being advocated. These include more aggressive radiation schedules and combining chemotherapy and

radiation. This has resulted in an increase in both the incidence of grade 3 mucositis and its duration. Fu and colleagues reported that patients treated with altered fractionation (hyperfractionation or accelerated fractionation) had a higher incidence of Radiation Therapy Oncology Group (RTOG) grade 3 or 4 mucositis versus standard fractionation (47% vs 25%; $p < .01$).[32] More recently, Forastiere and colleagues described the benefit of concurrent chemotherapy and radiotherapy for organ preservation in advanced laryngeal cancer in an RTOG study of 547 patients. With a median follow-up of 3.8 years, patients treated with radiation therapy with concurrent cisplatin had a higher larynx preservation rate but also a higher mucosal toxicity rate (grade 3 or 4; 43%) compared with patients treated with radiation alone or with induction chemotherapy.[33] Two additional phase III trials have demonstrated the benefit of concurrent postoperative radiation and chemotherapy for patients with advanced squamous cell carcinoma of the head and neck. Both randomized trials demonstrated that the addition of concurrent chemotherapy to radiation resulted in a greater disease-free survival but also contributed to higher mucosal toxicity.[34]

Considerable interpatient variability exists in the tolerance to chemotherapy regimens.[35] Treatment factors that influence the frequency and severity of oral mucositis include the chemotherapeutic agent used, dosage, delivery schedule, and combination with radiation therapy.[36] Other factors that may contribute to the severity of mucositis include smoking, use of over-the-counter mouthwashes, and the coexistence of collagen vascular diseases or human immunodeficiency virus (HIV) infection.[36]

Etiology and Pathophysiology

The etiology of mucositis is related to the direct and indirect effects of oncologic treatment and clinical factors, such as intercurrent illnesses. Mucosal injury is the cumulative result of a number of concurrent and sequential biologic processes. In general, oral mucositis is characterized by functional complaints, such as pain and dysphagia, and anatomic changes, such as edema, erythema, ulceration, pseudomembrane formation, alterations in mucus consistency, and xerostomia.[37]

Sonis and colleagues proposed a five-phase model to explain the pathophysiology of oral mucositis: initiation, up-regulation and message generation, signaling and amplification, ulceration, and healing.[38] Oral mucosal toxicity is initiated by chemotherapy and radiation therapy and is characterized by injury to the submucosal tissues. Early response genes are up-regulated, resulting in changes in the endothelium, connective tissue, and extracellular matrix, all mediated by the reactive oxygen species, ceramide pathway, and transcription factors.[38] This, in turn, causes a connective tissue breakdown, epithelial thinning, and initiation of a second set of genes, promoting early apoptosis of clonogenic stem cells in the basal epithelium. The molecules specific for signaling are proinflammatory cytokines derived from epithelial cells (ie, tumor necrosis factor [TNF]-α, interleukin [IL]-1β, and IL-6).[38–40] TNF-α causes local tissue damage, whereas IL-1β and IL-6 cause localized inflammation (increased vascularity). In addition, these molecules further amplify up-regulation of transcription factors, resulting in more elaboration of cytokines, tissue injury, and apoptosis. An unbalancing of apoptosis and necrosis exceeds the hyperproliferative rate and results in an ulcerative phase, with resultant mucosal damage.[30,38–40] This stage is complicated by bacterial colonization and intensifies the damage to the underlying submuscosa. The ulcers become colonized with gram-negative bacteria that produce endotoxins, which stimulate the release of cytokines and the production of nitric oxide.[38] The cytokines and nitric acid cause further local tissue damage and localized inflammation. Additional local responses are prompted, including angiogenesis. In the last phase, which is healing, epithelial integrity is stimulated by submucosal signaling and regenerative properties.[38]

Clinical Features

The most consistent symptom of mucositis is pain. The severity of the pain correlates directly with the severity of the mucositis.[41] The pain is typically constant and is aggravated by drinking, eating, and performance of oral hygiene measures. All intraoral sites may be affected, although nonkeratinized surfaces are most severely affected (mucosa of the lips, cheeks, floor of the mouth, ventral surface of the tongue, and soft palate). Erythema is the initial manifestation, followed by the development of white desquamative patches. Epithelial sloughing and fibrinous exudate lead to the formation of ulceration and a pseudomembrane.[36]

Definitions of the degree and intensity of mucositis vary. Numerous scoring systems, none universally accepted, have been proposed and are used in clinical trials.[28,41,42] The most common are the World Health Organization system, which considers subjective symptoms (dysphagia) into the scores, and the National Cancer Institute Common Toxicity Criteria system (version 3.0), a simple 0 to 4 scale based on the observed degree of mucositis.[1,28] The lack of uniformity in scoring and the question of the validity of these systems, despite their common use, further compound the difficulty in assessing trials exploring mucositis. In particular, the objections to systems that use observer scores alone argue that mucositis is not a problem but rather the subjective pain and dysphagia it causes, and evidence to correlate objective scores to degrees of subjective symptoms is lacking.

The complications of oral mucositis include dehydration, malnutrition, local infection, systemic infection, local hemorrhage, and interference with the cancer treatment regimen. The latter complication is particularly important because a delay in completing treatment or a reduction in the amount of treatment given may influence the eventual outcome of treatment. Oral mucositis is a self-limiting condition, with recovery occurring around 2 weeks after a course of chemotherapy and approximately 3 to 4 weeks after a course of radiation therapy.[30] Preexisting or predisposing factors that challenge wound healing can affect recovery from oral mucositis (eg, infection).[1,22,30]

Management

Mucositis management is primarily targeted to reduce symptomatology. The established or experimental prevention and treatment of oral mucositis focus on locally and systemically applied pharmacologic and nonpharmacologic methods.[26] There are multiple classes of agents for managing mucositis: anesthetics, antimicrobials, antioxidants, antiseptics, chemoprotectants, customized "cocktails," coating agents, cryotherapy, growth factors, immunomodulators, laser therapy, nutritional supplements, and others.[28] The majority of the agents used today fall into one of four categories: drugs designed to protect against damage to the proliferating cells, anti-inflammatories, antimicrobials, and drugs that provide anesthesia.

No standard therapy is universally accepted to be effective in the prevention of oral mucositis. Cryotherapy was the first mechanism-based therapy for mucositis demonstrating benefit of vasoconstriction.[28] A recent systematic review identified 21 interventions that had been evaluated in randomized controlled trials; only 9 of these interventions showed evidence of benefit.[44] The authors concluded that there was some ("sometimes weak") evidence to support the use of allopurinol, amifostine, antibiotics, granulocyte-macrophage colony-stimulating factor (GM-CSF), hydrolytic enzymes, ice chips, povidone, and oral care.[44] In many instances, evidence of the effectiveness of an intervention was based on studies performed in a specific patient or treatment groups. Similarly, no standard therapy is effective in the treatment or reversal of oral mucositis. In another systematic review, of six interventions evaluated in randomized controlled trials, evidence of benefit was found for only two.[45] The authors concluded that there was weak ("unreliable") evidence to support the use of allopurinol mouthwash and vitamin E. Considered together, these study results show that the primary objective in the treatment of mucositis should be palliation.

Management of pain related to oral mucositis is mainly treated with analgesics. In some cases, topical analgesics will control the pain. Nevertheless, in many cases, topical analgesics need to be supplemented or replaced by systemic analgesics. The principles of pain relief in this condition are the same as the general principles of pain relief in patients with cancer.[46] Patients often require opioids for moderate to severe pain; often these opioids must be given by transdermal administration, with a concomitant breakthrough in pain control.

Mucosal Protectors

Amifostine (WR-2721) is a phosphorylated aminothiol prodrug acting as a free radical scavenger (radioprotector).[47] The drug is currently approved by the US Food and Drug Administration (FDA) for the prevention of moderate to severe radiation-induced xerostomia and reducing the cumulative renal toxicity associated with repeated doses of cisplatin in patients with advanced ovarian cancer or non–small cell lung cancer. More recently, investigators have been interested in using this drug to prevent or reduce the severity of mucositis, but its effectiveness remains controversial. In a randomized clinical trial of over 300 patients with xerostomia, mucositis grade ≥ 3 occurred in 35% of the amifostine group and in 39% of the radiotherapy-alone patients.[48] The median duration of mucositis was 41 days versus 38 days, respectively.

Several smaller randomized trials have also investigated the role of amifostine for patients with head and neck cancer, with prevention of mucositis as a primary end point. Bourhis and colleagues randomized 26 patients treated with an accelerated course of radiation.[49] Patients randomized to amifostine had a lower incidence of grade 4 mucositis and needed feeding tubes for a shorter duration. Buntzel and colleagues investigated the role of amifostine with concurrent chemotherapy and radiation therapy.[50] Randomizing 28 patients, they reported a significant reduction in mucositis as none of the patients receiving amifostine had grade 3 or 4 mucositis compared with 86% of patients treated with radiation alone.

Growth factors and cytokines can either stimulate or suppress cell proliferation. Some, for example, IL-11,[40,51] transforming growth factor β_3,[38,51,52] and recombinant human keratinocyte growth factor (rHuKGF),[26,53] through a variety of mechanisms, may reduce mucositis by either interfering with epithelial proliferation or through other effects. Palifermin (rHuKGF) is indicated to decrease the incidence and duration of severe oral mucositis in patients with hematologic malignancies receiving myelotoxic therapy requiring hematopoietic stem cell support.[54] Keratinocyte growth factor (KGF) is another growth factor speculated to have a role in prevention of mucositis.[26,55] KGF has stem cell stimulatory properties. Clinical use of these agents for radiation-induced mucositis remains highly investigational.

Preclinical data have demonstrated that GM-CSF can influence the proliferation of keratinocytes.[56] Clinical observations that patients receiving GM-CSF with myeloablative chemotherapy for hematologic malignancies appeared to have a lower incidence of grade 3 and 4 mucositis compared with placebo controls[57] have also garnered interest. However, small trials using this agent via a subcutaneous route have been conducted and have not demonstrated a benefit with regard to mucositis reduction.[58,59] Topical administration of GM-CSF is also under investigation. Encouraging results have been reported in single-arm trials testing topical GM-CSF in patients receiving radiation for head and neck cancers.[60] However, a trial randomizing patients receiving chemoradiation to topical administration of GM-CSF or a control solution was discontinued when preliminary results did not demonstrate any benefit.[61]

Sucralfate, an agent that has little systemic absorption and adheres to ulcer bases, has been postulated to be of use in the prevention or amelioration of mucositis.[28] It is believed that the coating action provides some protection from injury and promotes healing. It is approved for the treatment of gastric ulceration. Numerous trials have investigated sucralfate rinses for oral mucositis secondary to radiation injury, and the results have been mixed.[26] However, the majority of studies, including double-blind, placebo-controlled, randomized trials, show little, if any, benefit of sucralfate in reducing radiation-induced oral side effects.[62–69]

Anti-inflammatory Agents

Steroid and nonsteroidal anti-inflammatory agents are not routinely used to treat mucositis.[26] Topical prostaglandins are believed to have anti-inflammatory properties that may benefit patients who will develop radiation-induced mucositis. However, both prostaglandin E_1 (misoprostol) and prostaglandin E_2 (prostin) have been evaluated in small trials, and neither has been demonstrated to prevent or reduce the severity of radiation-induced mucositis.[70,71]

Benzydamine hydrochloride is a topical agent that has been studied for preventing or alleviating radiation-induced mucositis. The primary mode of action is believed to be anti-inflammatory, and it has been demonstrated that benzydamine hydrochloride inhibits the production and effects of inflammatory cytokines, particularly TNF-α.[72] However, the drug has numerous other described properties, including analgesic, antimicrobial, and anesthetic properties.[28]

Epstein and colleagues conducted a randomized trial of nearly 150 patients, studying the efficacy of a 0.15% benzydamine rinse for the prevention of mucositis.[73] For conventionally fractionated radiation up to cumulative doses of 50 Gy, benzydamine significantly ($p = .006$) reduced erythema and ulceration by approximately 30% compared with the placebo and greater than 33% of benzydamine subjects remained ulcer free compared with 18% of placebo subjects ($p = .037$). However, benzydamine was not effective in subjects receiving accelerated radiation doses.

Currently, benzydamine is not approved for use in the United States. A large multicenter randomized trial is under way in the United States and will include patients treated with conventional and altered fractionation and patients treated with radiation alone or concurrent chemoradiation.

Decontamination

It has been theorized that the formation of ulcerative mucositis combined with changes in the pH of the oral cavity owing to the effects of radiation on salivary glands creates a favorable environment for microbial contamination and local infections; therefore, decontamination treatment may reduce this postradiation sequelae.[1,26] These infections create additional stress on the tissues and thereby intensify the severity of mucositis. Based on this theory, topical antimicrobials have been studied as a strategy to minimize mucositis. Numerous antimicrobials have been tested.[26,28]

Chlorhexidine, a broad-spectrum rinse effective against both gram-positive and gram-negative bacilli and yeast, has been tested in several randomized trials for preventing or alleviating oral mucositis. No trial has demonstrated it to be efficacious,[74,75] and Foote and colleagues concluded that not only was chlorhexidine not effective in preventing mucositis, it was even detrimental for their patients undergoing radiation for head and neck cancer.[76]

Several centers have studied rinses or pastilles using a combination of agents.[1,26] Typically, the combinations have included an antifungal (amphotericin B or clotrimazole) and antibacterials, particularly those to combat gram-negative organisms. PTA, a combination of polymyxin B, tobramycin, and amphotericin B,[77] has been tested in several centers as an antimicrobial strategy for mucositis prevention. PTA has been formulated into lozenges and administered several times per day during a course of radiation. Several randomized placebo-controlled trials have been conducted, and the results are mixed.

Okuno and colleagues found no differences in objective measures of mucositis in patients treated with an antibiotic lozenge compared with patients using a placebo lozenge, but patient-reported scores were better in patients treated with an active lozenge.[78] Symonds and colleagues similarly tested a PTA pastille.[79] There was no difference between the experimental and control arms for the study's primary end point, the incidence of thick pseudomembrane formation, but there were differences in several of the measured secondary end points, including a lower incidence of worse reported grade of mucositis, dysphagia, and weight loss in patients treated with the drug. Wijers and colleagues also tested a PTA paste in a randomized, placebo-controlled, double-blind study and did not find that PTA reduced the incidence of mucositis.[80] El-Sayed and colleagues randomized patients to either a lozenge of bacitracin, clotrimazole, and gentamicin or placebo and found no differences in the severity of mucositis in patients receiving conventionally fractionated radiation between the two groups.[81]

A trial investigating iseganan hydrochloride, a broad-spectrum antimicrobial rinse, randomized patients in a phase III multi-institutional trial to active drug, placebo rinse, or best standard of care. There was no benefit to the active drug compared with placebo, but, interestingly, patients using either active drug or placebo rinses fared better with respect to both objective and subjective measures compared with patients receiving standard care only.[82]

Anesthetics

The management of radiation-induced mucositis primarily involves managing pain. Mucositis that is not severe can be managed with topical agents, although their efficacy has not been proven.[26,28] Baking soda rinses with or without salt are advocated, although they, too, have not been proven to alleviate mucositis.[1,26] However, they are important in maintaining good oral hygiene.[1]

Lidocaine gel (2%) is occasionally useful, particularly for anterior oral sores. Diluting lidocaine in "magic mouthwashes" is a common practice. These mouthwashes combine an aluminum hydroxide antacid, diphenhydramine (Benadryl), and lidocaine. Although prophylactic antifungal agents are not needed, some practices include nystatin in the mouthwash. It should be emphasized that there are no significant evidence-based studies to support the use of these mouthwashes. Investigating magic mouthwash for chemotherapy-induced mucositis, Dodd and colleagues found that these mouthwashes were no more effective than salt and soda rinses.[83]

Other topical agents include aloe vera and Gelclair, both with soothing properties. Gelclair is a bioadherent gel that adheres to mucosal surfaces and protects overstimulated nerve endings by forming a protective barrier.[28] Neither aloe vera nor Gelclair has been shown in randomized phase III trials to benefit patients with radiation-induced mucositis.

Ultimately, mucositis is managed with analgesics. Early mucositis can be managed with acetaminophen or nonsteroidal anti-inflammatory agents, but as the severity of mucositis worsens, narcotics are often required.[1,28,84] Most pain regimens begin with codeine-based products. When patients breakthrough treatment progress to morphine-based products, primarily hydromorphone, morphine sulfate, or other narcotic products, such as methadone. Recently, fentanyl transdermal patches are effective for patients as they are long-acting and avoid contact with oral mucous membranes.

Xerostomia

Definition

Xerostomia is defined as a dryness of the mouth owing to salivary gland secretion dysfunction that can be caused by multiple conditions, for example, autoimmune disorders, medications, and oncologic treatments. Virtually all patients undergoing radiation therapy for head and neck cancers suffer from xerostomia, which causes oral discomfort and pain, increased dental caries and oral infection, and difficulty in speaking and swallowing. This significantly impairs quality of life and can compromise nutritional intake and continuity of cancer therapy.

Incidence and Risks

Salivary secretion may be decreased by a number of disease processes and other factors. Xerostomia has been estimated to affect 22 to 26% of the general population[85] but may occur more commonly in the elderly[86] and patients with advanced cancer (29–77%).[85] Radiation damage to the major glands results in either a transient or a permanent decrease in salivary flow. In a study of patients followed up to 25 years after radiation therapy, Liu and colleagues found that, compared with a nonirradiated group, patients who received bilateral ionizing radiation therapy involving the major salivary gland tissue exhibited, over time, mean decreases of 81% in stimulated and 78% in unstimulated salivary flow.[87] Patients who received unilateral radiation therapy involving only one parotid gland and one submandibular gland experienced mean decreases of 60% in stimulated and 51% in unstimulated salivary flow.[87] Patients who underwent cervical with supraclavicular radiation therapy (ie, mantle field treatment) experienced mean decreases of 43% in stimulated and 32% in unstimulated salivary flow.[87] Even low-dose total-body irradiation (as used in allogeneic bone marrow transplantation) may induce varying degrees of salivary hypofunction.[87–89]

Etiology and Pathophysiology

The most common cause of salivary gland dysfunction is drug treatment. Several medications can produce xerostomia, including chemotherapy agents (eg busulfan, procarbazine) and supportive care agents (eg analgesics, antidepressants, antiemetics).[90] Drug-induced salivary dysfunction is generally reversible, that is, discontinuation of the drug leads to resolution of the problem. Other medications associated with xerostomia include antihypertensives,[91] pain medications,[91] overactive-bladder agents,[92] and psychiatric agents.[92–94] Xerostomia has also been reported in association with some immunotherapies,[95] particularly involving the oral cavity or salivary glands.[96]

Salivary gland dysfunction is a predictable side effect of radiation therapy to the head and neck region.[97] It also occurs in patients who receive total-body irradiation as part of the conditioning regimen for a bone marrow transplant.[89] Radiation-induced xerostomia is generally irreversible. The severity of radiation-induced xerostomia is influenced by both the radiation therapy regimen (field, dose) and pretreatment salivary gland function (Figure 2).[97] In therapy for head and neck cancer, the appropriate daily and total radiation doses are based on tumor size and individual clinical situations.[97] Clinically, xerostomia has been reported with as little as two or three doses of 2 Gy, although many changes occurring with less than 60 Gy are reversible.[97] However, doses greater than 30 Gy can cause permanent xerostomia.[97,98]

Damage to the salivary glands results in reduced salivary flow, changes in the electrolyte and immunoglobulin composition of saliva, a reduction in salivary pH, and repopulation of the mouth by cariogenic microflora.[99] When the major salivary glands are included in the radiation field, salivary function often decreases by 50 to 60% in the first week, with basal salivary flow reaching a measurable minimum 2 to 3 weeks

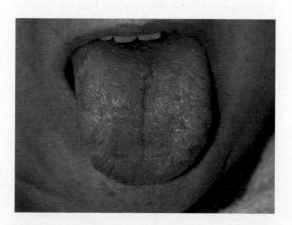

FIGURE 2 The patient received radiation therapy to the head and neck region involving the major salivary glands, resulting in post-treatment xerostomia. Note the fissuring of the dorsal tongue.

after 23 Gy of fractionated radiation therapy.[100,101] The extent of glandular change is generally directly related to the dose of radiation to the salivary glands, with the most severe and irreversible forms of salivary dysfunction resulting from damage to or loss of salivary acinar cells.[102]

Some workers have attributed the pathogenicity of radiation therapy administered to salivary glands to the atrophic effects of this treatment on the secretory cells of the glands.[103] Serous cells, found predominantly in the parotid glands, are extremely radiosensitive and undergo apoptosis when exposed to low doses of radiation.[104] Others have attributed salivary gland dysfunction to the direct effects of radiation on the vascular and connective tissues of the glands.[103,105] This may account for the effects on the submandibular glands, which have a high proportion of mucinous cells and are essential for resting saliva.

Clinical Features

Individuals with xerostomia can exhibit innumerable problems, including oral discomfort; taste disturbance; difficulty in chewing, swallowing, and speaking; dental caries; and other oral infections. Salivary gland dysfunction may intensify or prolong the process of oral mucositis.[106] These problems reflect the major functional roles of saliva: protection, early digestion, and lubrication.

Radiation-induced xerostomia can be an acute complication that improves with time but is often a permanent condition that seriously impairs the patient's well-being. Xerostomia predisposes patients to an altered oral microflora with increased virulent bacteria and fungal activity.[16] When not monitored and controlled, xerostomia may lead to accumulation of plaque and other debris on teeth and periodontal tissues.[106,107] Cariogenic plaque buildup on teeth may lead to tooth decay, gingivitis, and periodontitis. According to Berger and Kilroy,[108] elevated plaque matrix resulting from xerostomia may pose the greatest risk of ORN. Ill-fitting removable prostheses in patients with xerostomia, causing tissue irritation, can compound mucositis and result in fenestration of supporting mucosa and post-treatment ORN.[1]

Management

Current management strategies include stringent dental and oral hygiene, parotid gland–sparing radiation techniques to prevent or minimize xerostomia, and pharmacotherapies, such as salivary substitutes and sialogogues.[89] Future strategies may include salivary gland transfer, newer sialogogues, and gene therapy. To minimize the severity of xerostomia and oral complications, it is important to begin aggressive oral care before radiation therapy. Evaluation by a dental team experienced in oral oncology is essential to determine oral health status, perform necessary dental and oral interventions, and allow for healing from any invasive procedures required. Particulars that may require attention include mucosal lesions, dental caries and endodontic disease, periodontal disease, ill-fitting dentures, orthodontic appliances, temporomandibular dysfunction, and salivary abnormalities. A stringent oral hygiene program is critical and should be continued before, during, and after therapy.[1,17,107]

Amifostine is a cytoprotective agent used in the prevention of xerostomia in patients treated with radiation therapy for head and neck cancer.[108] This recommendation was based on the results of a phase III multi-institutional study reported by Brizel and colleagues.[48] Although randomized, the study was not blinded. The incidence of grade ≤ 2 chronic xerostomia was reduced from 57% in the control arm to 34% in patients receiving amifostine. There were no differences in survival or disease control, suggesting that amifostine protected salivary function without protecting the cancer. The recommended dose of amifostine is 200 mg/m²/d given as a slow intravenous push over 3 minutes, 15 to 30 minutes before each fraction of radiation therapy. Patients require close monitoring for side effects, including hypotension and nausea, and some patients may require antiemetics.[109] Investigations using a subcutaneous administration of amifostine are ongoing as this form of administration may be more practical and lower the toxicity of the drug.

The risk of complications of radiation therapy depends largely on the dose and the field. Devices and techniques such as interstitial implants, shrinking-field approaches, customized immobilization molds, and customized lead-alloy blocks are used to achieve safe and permanent control of larger lesions, shielding of peripheral tissues (ie, radiation stents), accurate and reproducible delivery, and protection of normal structures.[110–112]

An emerging parotid gland–sparing technique, three-dimensional intensity-modulated radiation therapy (IMRT), involves the manipulation of beam intensity across each treatment field, providing a dose distribution that conforms more accurately to the three-dimensional configuration of the target volume than conventional three-dimensional conformal radiation therapy.[89] This technique delivers a higher dose to the tumor target without increasing the dose to normal tissues, delivers a higher dose per fraction, and offers an improved physical and biologic therapeutic ratio.[98] IMRT can potentially deliver a lower dose of radiation to the parotid glands compared with conventional beam arrangements and thus offers the greatest potential for patients with mucosal primary tumors who require bilateral neck irradiation.[100,101]

Eisbruch and colleagues assessed long-term xerostomia in 84 patients with head and neck cancer who had undergone comprehensive bilateral neck radiation therapy using conformal and multisegmental IMRT to spare major salivary glands.[97] Xerostomia was assessed with a validated xerostomia-specific questionnaire. These researchers observed that, with these parotid gland–sparing techniques, xerostomia improved over time, with rising salivary production from the spared major salivary glands. In addition, the oral cavity mean radiation dose was found to be significantly correlated with xerostomia scores, indicating that it may be beneficial to spare the noninvolved oral cavity to further reduce xerostomia.

Chao and colleagues conducted a prospective clinical study to determine whether parotid gland–sparing techniques result in objective and subjective improvement in xerostomia.[100] Twenty-seven patients underwent inverse-planning IMRT and 14 received forward-planning three-dimensional radiation therapy, with attempts to spare the superficial lobe of the parotid glands. Dose-volume histograms were computed for each gland. Stimulated salivary flow 6 months after treatment was reduced exponentially, for each gland independently, at a rate of approximately 4% per Gy of mean parotid dose. Patients' answers to quality of life questions about eating and speaking function were also significantly correlated with salivary flow. In another study, Chao and colleagues concluded that the dosimetric advantage of IMRT conferred a significant reduction in late salivary toxicity, with no adverse impact on tumor control or disease-free survival.[101]

Although further study is needed, these and other emerging data indicate that IMRT and other new parotid gland–sparing techniques hold promise for the treatment of head and neck cancer, potentially offering reduced severity of xerostomia without compromised tumor control for appropriately selected patients.

Although the radiation ports used in treating head and neck cancer generally deliver 60 to 65 Gy to the major salivary glands, the submental region is regularly shielded, receiving only scatter radiation of 5% of the total dose.[17,97] Several animal studies have demonstrated the feasibility of microvascular autotransplantation of submandibular and parotid gland tissue.[113–115] In a recent human study, Seikaly and colleagues transferred the submandibular gland to the submental space in patients undergoing surgery and radiation therapy for head and neck cancer.[116] The glands survived transfer and continued to function after radiation therapy with appropriate shielding.

Emerging research and medical technology are providing specificity and sensitivity methods to determine the roles of human salivary components. Gene transfer may be potentially useful for treating inherited single-gene deficiency disorders and malignancies refractory to other therapies, as well as for repairing radiated salivary glands.[116,117] There are no published reports examining a prophylactic gene transfer approach to reducing or eliminating radiation damage of the salivary glands.[116] Translational studies involving plasmid-mediated gene transfer for reducing radiation-induced damage have been conducted, and the results of in vivo animal studies in lung and esophageal tissue are quite promising.[118,119] Research in nonviral gene-mediated therapeutics for restoring radiation-induced salivary gland dysfunction may prove beneficial.[120]

Current therapies for the pharmacologic management of radiation-induced xerostomia include the use of prescription fluoride agents to maintain optimal oral hygiene, antimicrobials to prevent dental caries and oral infection, saliva substitutes to relieve dryness, and sialogogic agents to stimulate saliva production from remaining intact salivary gland tissues.[1,22,89] Saliva substitutes containing hydroxyethyl-, hydroxypropyl-, or carboxymethylcellulose may be beneficial as palliative agents to relieve the discomfort of xerostomia by temporarily wetting the oral mucosa.[89] New saliva substitutes (moisturizing gels) with enzymatic and protein components (ie, glucose oxidase and lactoperoxidase), which present prospective antibacterial effectiveness and increased oral moisture, are under study.

For patients with residual salivary gland function, cholinergic agonists may produce symptomatic improvement.[1,89] Pilocarpine is currently the only sialogogic agent approved by the FDA for radiation-induced xerostomia. Pilocarpine functions primarily as a muscarinic-cholinergic agonist with mild β-adrenergic activity, which can increase secretion of exocrine glands, such as salivary and sweat glands, and the tone of smooth muscle in the gastrointestinal and urinary tracts. Studies have shown oral pilocarpine to have efficacy in patients with Sjögren's syndrome, radiation-induced xerostomia, and opioid-induced xerostomia, as well as increasing salivary flow and restoring salivary composition in those with graft-versus-host disease owing to allogeneic bone marrow transplantation.[102,121–127] LeVeque and colleagues conducted a randomized, placebo-controlled, dose-escalation study, and Johnson and colleagues a three-arm, randomized, placebo-controlled trial (placebo, pilocarpine 5 mg three times daily, and pilocarpine 10 mg three times daily).[122,128] In both studies, significantly more pilocarpine-treated patients than placebo recipients reported improvement in xerostomia. In addition, LeVeque and colleagues found that treatment with pilocarpine led to a significant decrease in the use of oral comfort agents, such as artificial saliva, hard candies, and water.[122]

Other cholinergic agents with sialogogic properties, such as cevimeline hydrochloride, may prove beneficial for cancer patients with xerostomia. Cevimeline is a newer muscarinic agonist that has been found to be safe and effective in treating xerostomia associated with Sjögren's syndrome and received FDA approval for that use.[89,129,130] It is currently under study for use in patients with head and neck cancer who have radiation-induced xerostomia. The most common drug-related side effects are excessive sweating, nausea, rhinitis, and diarrhea.[131]

Osteoradionecrosis

Definition

ORN has been defined as "radiological evidence of bone necrosis within the radiation field, where tumour recurrence has been excluded."[132] ORN is death of the bony tissues of the maxillae and mandible secondary to radiation therapy (Figure 3). ORN can be a debilitating condition that can occur either soon after a course of radiation therapy or months to years following treatment. It can be self-limiting, and in its most severe form, ORN is characterized by severe pain, trismus, fistula and cicatrix formation, pathologic fracture, and loss of soft and osseous tissues.[1]

ORN is not infection of compromised bone, as was previously believed. It is now understood to be a progressive avascular necrosis by the tissue effects of either external beam radiation therapy or brachytherapy. These tissue effects include hypocellularity, hypovascularity, and hypoxia and create a new composite tissue referred to as "three-H tissue."[133] ORN can occur spontaneously, but most commonly trauma to this three-H tissue creates further pathophysiologic changes that result in ORN.

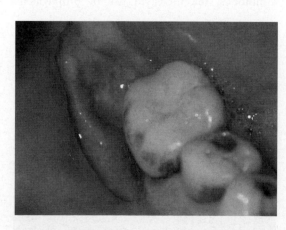

FIGURE 3 A patient who received induction chemotherapy followed by external beam radiation therapy with mandibular osteoradionecrosis. The patient will undergo hyperbaric oxygen therapy followed by surgical intervention.

Incidence and Risks

ORN is rare in patients who receive less than 60 Gy of radiation therapy. However, the frequency of ORN is uncertain because there is no standard mechanism for reporting the disease. The RTOG requests its members to report radiation toxicity, including ORN; however, universally, the condition is probably underreported. On average, ORN may occur within the first few years after radiation treatment and is not captured in most head and neck cancer longitudinal multicenter studies. Additionally, this late sequela of radiation is often reported as a crude incidence rather than an actuarial incidence, making the incidence fewer in frequency than it is in reality.

The mandible is much more susceptible to ORN than the maxilla. Patients with teeth are at greater risk of developing ORN than edentulous patients.[134] ORN may occur at any time following radiation therapy but commonly occurs within 3 years of the radiation therapy.[135] Cases have been reported describing ORN developing over 35 years after radiation therapy.[136]

Etiology and Pathophysiology

The underlying mechanisms of ORN relate to the "three-H principle" of irradiated tissue, that is, hypocellularity, hypovascularity, and hypoxia. In such tissue, the ability to replace normal cellular and collagen loss is severely compromised, with resultant necrosis occurring in relation to the rate of normal or induced cellular death and collagen lysis.[137] The risk of ORN following trauma or oral surgical procedures can be significant.

ORN can be either spontaneous (39% of cases) or the result of an insult (61% of cases).[133,137] Spontaneous ORN occurs when, in the process of otherwise normal turnover of bone, the degradative function exceeds new bone production. ORN develops following injury when the reparative capacity of bone within an irradiated field is insufficient to overcome an insult. Bone injury can occur through direct trauma (eg, tooth extraction [up to 84%], related tumor ablative surgery or biopsy [12%], frictional irritation [1%]) or exposure of the oral cavity to the environment secondary to overlying soft tissue necrosis.[133] The cumulative progressive endarteritis caused by radiation therapy results in insufficient blood supply and tissue oxygen delivery, with resultant poor wound-healing capacity.[137,138]

Clinical Features

The clinical features are influenced by the stage of ORN. Patients with early-stage necrosis may be relatively asymptomatic. In contrast, patients with advanced-stage ORN are often very symptomatic (eg, pain, discharge). The diagnosis of ORN is based on a combination of clinical and radiologic features.[135]

Store and Boysen proposed the following staging classification of ORN[132]:

- Stage 0: exposed bone; no radiologic signs
- Stage 1: mucosa intact; radiologic signs present
- Stage 2: exposed bone; radiologic signs present
- Stage 3: exposed bone; radiologic signs present; orocutaneous fistula; localized infection

In working up a patient with ORN, conventional laboratory studies and diagnostic imaging are ordered to rule out recurrence and second primary malignancy with a biopsy as indicated. Information pertaining to the volume of tissue irradiated can be obtained in radiation oncology treatment summaries to determine the method of treatment, dosimetry, and energy used.[1,22] Diagnostic imaging can include studies of plain radiographs of the mandible and maxillae, such as a panoramic radiograph, to determine gross areas of local decalcification or sclerosis. Plain radiographs can show decreased bone density and detect fractures. Magnetic resonance imaging (MRI) depicts ORN with reduced bone marrow signal intensity on T_1-weighted images and increased signal intensity on T_2-weighted images.[139] Absence of a marrow signal on MRI can be used to identify significant radiation injury in the mandible. Computed tomographic (CT) scans are excellent in identifying sites of significant bone injury and diagnosing ORN.[139] Alteration in trabeculation, cortical thinning, and sclerosis are common findings in sites of injury. Single-photon emission tomography may have a role in the future as more experience is gained with this modality.[139,140]

Management

The most important aspect of ORN-related treatment is prevention. ORN may be avoided if patients receive appropriate dental care prior to radiation therapy, maintain high standards of oral hygiene during and after radiation therapy, and avoid dental extractions and other types of oral surgery after radiation therapy. Strategies for preventing ORN include appropriate dental prophylaxis prior to, during, and following a course of treatment with radiation to the head and neck. Should ORN develop despite these measures, management will depend on the individual clinical status.

In most cases, the management of ORN is conservative and involves some or all of the following modalities: removal of loose bone fragments, gentle sequestration, irrigation, topical antiseptics, systemic antibiotics, and hyperbaric oxygen (HBO).[135] Other modalities that have been reported to be effective include pentoxyfilline and vitamin E, ultrasound therapy, and electromagnetic stimulation.[135]

In advanced cases (symptomatic), surgical intervention is required and involves either radical sequestration or hemimandibulectomy with reconstruction.[140,141] If oral surgical intervention is required after radiation therapy, then pre- and postoperative HBO therapy may increase the potential for healing and minimize the risk of ORN.[142] HBO therapy increases wound-healing capacity by stimulating osteogenesis and angiogenesis. It should be noted that many dental procedures can be safely done after radiation therapy, including routine restorative procedures, endodontic procedures, and prosthetic procedures.

Currently used HBO protocols by stage of disease are as follows:

Stage I. Perform 30 HBO treatments (one treatment per day, Monday–Friday) to 2.4 atmospheres for 90 minutes breathing 100% oxygen. The patient is closely monitored to evaluate decreased bone exposure, granulation tissue covering exposed bone, resorption of nonviable bone, and absence of inflammation and infection. For patients who respond favorably, continue treatment to a total of 40 or more treatments. For patients who are not responsive, advance to stage II.[133,143–147]

Stage II. Perform transoral sequestrectomy, attempting primary wound closure followed by continued HBO therapy to a total of 40 treatments. If wound dehiscence occurs, advance patients to stage III. Patients who present with orocutaneous fistula, pathologic fracture, or resorption to the inferior border of the mandible advance to stage III immediately after the initial 30 treatments.[146,147]

Stage III. Perform transcutaneous mandibular resection, wound closure, and mandibular fixation, that is, maxillomandibular fixation or reconstruction plating, followed by an additional 10 to 20 postoperative HBO treatments.[146,147]

Stage IIIR. Perform mandibular reconstruction 10 weeks after successful resolution of mandibular ORN. Marx advocates the use of autogenous cancellous bone within a freeze-dried allogeneic bone carrier and/or packed with plasma rich protein. Complete 10 to 20 additional postoperative HBO treatments.[146,147]

In addition to a staged therapy with HBO treatment, as described by Marx, microvascular free-tissue transfer reconstruction affords the clinician and patient another opportunity to correct ORN.[1,147–150] Excellent outcomes of immediate reconstruction of the mandible and maxillae following resection of ORN using free-tissue transfer techniques have been reported in the literature.[148–150]

Radiation can permanently destroy cellular elements of bone and thus limit the potential for wound maintenance and the ability to heal after infection or trauma (eg, dental extraction, alveoloplasty).[151,152] Further, the risk of complications following trauma or oral surgical procedures in an irradiated field can be highly significant, depending on a predetermined threshold of irradiation, and can result in ORN.[152–154] For these reasons, elective oral surgical procedures, such as extractions or soft tissue surgery, are contraindicated within an irradiated field owing to hypovascularity, hypocellularity, and hypoxia.[1] However, nonsurgical dental procedures that can be safely performed include routine restorative procedures, oral prophylaxis, radiography, and endodontic and prosthodontic procedures.[1,22]

Following initial recovery from radiation effects, nonsurgical periodontal therapy, usually with prophylactic antibiotic coverage, is appropriate for treatment of the periodontium within the radiation field. It is important to detect and treat dental caries or traumatic dental injury that could lead to pathosis. However, ORN can occur spontaneously if wound healing is compromised.[155–157] If postradiation extractions are necessary, HBO therapy, along with a specific oral care regimen, is indicated to augment wound healing. In such cases, tissues should be managed gently, and antibiotic coverage is required. Local anesthetics containing epinephrine should be avoided, when possible, to prevent further vascular constriction.[1,3] Workers have reported successful placement of endosseous implants in irradiated fields with a pretreatment regimen of HBO.[158,159] In contrast, ORN has been initiated by such an elective surgical intervention.[1,133,155,159]

Oral Infections

Definition

Oral infections are a common acute complication of chemotherapy and radiation therapy. The oral cavity is a complex environment composed of a myriad of commensal bacteria, fungi, and viruses that populate the oral mucosa, connective tissue, salivary glands, taste buds, bones, and teeth. Multiple factors predispose individuals to infections such as treatment-induced neutropenia, hypogammaglobulinemia, T-cell dysfunction, and mucosal damage.[37]

Incidence and Risks

Most of the patients treated for head and neck cancer and almost half of the patients receiving chemotherapy for non–head and neck cancer develop acute oral complications, that is, mucositis and/or infections (Figure 4).[160,161]

Etiology and Pathophysiology

The etiology of infections includes damage to the oral mucosa and systemic immunosuppression.[162] Oral infections usually occur in association with the hematologic nadir, although they may occur at other times in the chemotherapy cycle. For example, oral herpes simplex virus (HSV) infections can be seen early in the chemotherapy cycle. The treatment-induced mucosal barrier injury is a risk factor for severe infectious complications. The intact mucosa is the first defense against systemic infections. Compromise of the mucosal barrier can contribute to local invasion by colonizing microorganisms and eventual systemic infection.[37] Mucosal injury can lead to gram-positive infections, anaerobic infections, neutropenic enterocolitis, *Candida* infections, acute graft-versus-host disease, and malnutrition.[37] The risk of infection is directly related to the depth and length of neutropenia or lowered white blood cell count. More than 60% of patients with neutropenia will become infected. If the absolute neutrophil count is $<100/mm^3$, approximately 20% of febrile patients will have a documented bacteremia.[163–165] Most infections are due to bacteria, although fatal infections are usually due to fungal organisms.[163]

Clinical Features

Patients with cancer who undergo treatment with chemotherapy, radiation, or surgery are at significant risk of infection. This risk is related to compromised host defenses and sequelae of treatment owing to the absence of neutrophils, infection barrier disruption, and shifts in microbial flora. The mortality attributed to infections has decreased over the years because of the development of β-lactam and fluoroquinolone antibiotics, the increased use of prophylactic

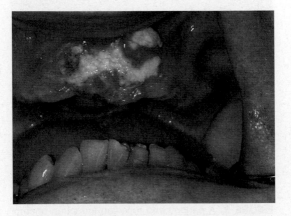

FIGURE 4 A patient with acute myelogenous leukemia undergoing therapy with a fungal infection at the edentulous premaxillae. The patient wears a maxillary complete denture.

antifungals and antivirals, and the use of colony-stimulating factors in selected patients.[163] The interaction of infection and mucosal barrier injury is well displayed in the third phase of a mucosal barrier injury of the gastrointestinal tract, as described by Blijlevens and colleagues, when necrosis and ulcerations occur with the translocation of resident microflora and their products (ie, endotoxin) into the bloodstream.[166] Damaged mucosa leads to significant morbidity and potential infection. Oropharyngeal candidiasis is a common infection in patients undergoing oncologic treatment. Oral mucosal colonization (up to 93%) and infection (ranging from 17 to 29%) with *Candida* are particularly common in patients receiving radiation therapy for head and neck cancer.[167] Although all patients with cancer who are undergoing chemotherapy are at risk of oral complications, some patients are at a greater risk than others, depending primarily on the type of malignancy and the aggressiveness of the cancer treatment. Patients with hematologic malignancies (eg, leukemia and lymphoma) have a greater risk than patients with solid tumors (eg, breast cancer, lung cancer, and sarcomas) because the protective elements that maintain bodily homeostasis are part of the malignant process of hematologic malignancies.[168,169]

Viral reactivitiation may lead to severe oral or disseminated infections during periods of myeloimmunosuppression. In particular, HSV infections are often associated with severe, painful, and prolonged ulcerations atypical of those found in immunocompetent hosts.[12,170-174] Suspected HSV lesions should be treated with antiviral agents such as acyclovir administered orally or intravenously and managed as described above for irradiated patients. The diagnosis should be established using viral cultures, direct immunofluorescence or other rapid diagnostic tests, and the lesions.[12,170-173,175,176]

Bacterial infections following chemotherapy can cause localized mucosal lesions, sialoadenitis, periodontal abscesses, pericoronitis, or acute necrotizing ulcerative gingivitis.[22,177] Because systemic infection is a serious complication in neutropenic patients, constant vigilance must be maintained to prevent or manage oral infections of any type.[1,21,22,175] Because antileukemic therapy is designed to achieve myelosuppression, this risk may be higher among patients with leukemia than among those with solid tumors.[175,178] Oral infections should be treated with selected antibiotic combinations (broad-spectrum antibiotics), including an agent effective against anaerobic gram-negative bacilli, such as *Pseudomonas*, *Klebsiella*, or enterobacteria, which are often found in the oral cavity of immunocompromised individuals.[21,22,177,179] Oral microbial culture testing should be used to ensure antibiotic sensitivity and resistance selection and to assist in identification of the causative organisms.[180]

Vascular endothelial damage can occur following stem cell transplantation or external beam radiation therapy with release of higher levels of proinflammatory cytokines and radiation-induced fibrosis of the vascular lining.[37] This cascading event can exacerbate multiple manifestations in the head and neck area, that is, graft-versus-host disease and ORN. A variety of different infections may occur in the oral cavity at separate or combined times, such as candidiasis, anaerobic infection, herpes simplex viral shedding, and caries. As previously described, the etiology of these infections includes damage to the oral mucosa and salivary gland dysfunction.[162] The chronic nature of these infections reflects the ongoing nature of hypovascularity and the salivary gland dysfunction.

Oral infections can cause morbidity per se, can aggravate oral mucositis, and can lead to systemic infections. The clinical features may be relatively specific or relatively nonspecific (ie, oral mucositis). Moreover, the clinical features may be typical or atypical, particularly in immunosuppressed patients. Thus, health care professionals should have a low threshold for screening for the presence of such oral infections.

Management

The management of upper aerodigestive tract infections relies on the identification of the patients at significant risk of life-threatening infections, initiation of appropriate clinical and diagnostic tests, and timely initiation of antimicrobial therapy, that is, broad-sprectrum antibiotics.[37] In response to more effective drug therapy, the types of infections have changed as resistant and opportunistic organisms emerge.[163] Strategies to minimize and prevent infection in patients with mild to moderate short-term neutropenia are generally successful. Prophylactic treatment of infection with oral antibiotics in neutropenic patients is now being widely used. However, complete prevention or elimination of infection has not been accomplished in high-risk patients, such as those undergoing stem cell transplantation or intensive chemotherapy.[163] Therefore, to minimize the risks of oral infection, it is important to develop simple and practical guidelines for maintaining periodontal health and for diagnosing, preventing, and treating periodontal infections during therapy.[1,22] Cancer patients should make regular dental visits for overall dental and periodontal assessment. Patients receiving chemotherapy can undergo a dental cleaning provided that they meet the following hematologic conditions: first, an absolute neutrophil count of approximately 1,000/mm³ (white blood cell count times the percentage of neutrophils equals the absolute neutrophil count), a level at which the risk of developing an infection is minimal, and second, a platelet count >50,000/mm³ with a

normal coagulation profile.[180] The administration of prophylactic antibiotics is essential owing to the induced bacteremia, immunocompromised status, and potential for hypofunctioning white blood cells introduced by chemotherapy.

Patients with an uninfected dentition and good periodontal health do not pose a diagnostic treatment challenge, nor do patients with advanced periodontal disease that mandates immediate surgical intervention. However, patients with increased loss of attachment with furcation involvement or periodontal pocket formation with furcation involvement pose a treatment dilemma.[22] Patients in whom the soft tissue parallels the bone loss and in whom pocket depth is normal can be treated with regular periodontal care and maintenance. Extraction should be considered only for patients with pathologic mobility of dentition or with a fulminant periapical abscess.[1,22] Patients with moderate to advanced periodontal disease present a greater challenge and would, under usual circumstances, receive instructions for infection prophylaxis and dental hygiene, as well as surgical correction. However, the feasibility of such comprehensive therapy during chemotherapy can be limited by several factors, including performance status, type of malignant disease, cycling of chemotherapy, and hematologic competence. The clinician should strive to provide a thorough scaling and to encourage maintenance through exceptional plaque control (ie, brushing, flossing, and use of chlorhexidine gluconate).[22,168,169] To reduce the risk of septic foci, extractions should be considered for patients with any exacerbated acute periodontal infection. This oral surgical correction should be performed at the appropriate time in the treatment cycle (at the beginning of the cycle or during the recovery phase with hematologic or chemistry stability) or when the patient's cancer is in complete remission. If chemotherapy is on hold, periodontal surgery could be considered provided that the hematologic status is appropriate. The dentist must discuss with the treating medical oncologist the patient's oral status, treatment plan, and contraindications to surgical intervention, as well as the appropriate timing of oral treatment intervention.[29,57,134]

Toothbrushing and flossing should be the standard of dental care for patients who routinely brush and floss. However, as in the general population, many patients with cancer either do not floss or floss infrequently. Thus, clinicians may either instruct patients to floss or may stress brushing techniques only. In most cases, patient factors and limited time parameters do not permit the patient to become proficient in flossing techniques. However, if the clinician identifies an area where food continually lodges, the patient should be encouraged to floss the area to reduce the risk of gingival inflammation.[21,22] Patients who floss on a regular basis are instructed to modify the flossing technique in certain clinical situations. First, patients are instructed to floss gently when the lining of the oral cavity starts to become sensitive to thermal changes or food substances, indicating mucosal thinning owing to the suppressive effects of chemotherapy on the normally proliferative epithelium.[38–40] Second, patients are instructed to floss only to the gingiva when the platelet count falls below 50,000/mm³. This technique removes most of the debris from this area.[22]

Oral lavage therapy, including toothbrushing, is imperative for plaque control. The patient should be instructed to brush after every meal. In certain clinical situations, such as increased mucosal sensitivity to food or thermal changes, increased sensitivity to toothbrush bristles, irritation of the gingival tissues by the toothbrush, or profound thrombocytopenia ($<20,000/mm^3$), patients should change from a soft to an ultra–soft-bristled or sensitive-bristled toothbrush.[1,21,22] In controlling plaque accumulation, it is important to minimize the risk of gingival inflammation, the oral bacterial load, and the potential for infection.[22] Along with routine brushing and flossing, rinsing with chlorhexidine gluconate should be initiated when patients begin chemotherapy. Such rinsing is an adjunct to ideal oral-periodontal care and can also be used when indications arise, such as oral mucosal changes secondary to chemotherapy and subsequent increased soft tissue sensitivity.[22,181–185] Patients undergoing chemotherapy should be encouraged to rinse with a dilute saline and sodium bicarbonate solution (5%) to reduce adherent mucoid debris on oral soft tissues, lubricate oral mucosal and oropharyngeal tissues, and elevate the pH of oral fluids.[21,22] Patients encountering nausea and anorexia should be encouraged to rinse with a sodium bicarbonate and salt water solution several times throughout the day to reduce oral acidity and minimize the mucosal insult.[1,22]

Caries

Definition

Dental caries is defined as a soft decayed area in a tooth. Progressive decay can lead to the death of a tooth.

Incidence and Risks

Tooth decay is one of the most common of all disorders, second only to the common cold. It usually occurs in children and young adults but can affect any person. It is the most important cause of tooth loss in humans. Dental caries is a common sequela of radiation and is often exacerbated by xerostomia.[1,22] Irradiation of major salivary glands leads to qualitative and quantitative changes in salivary secretions. This results in an increase in plaque and mucoid debris accumulation and a reduction in the salivary pH antimicrobial proteins and the buffering capacity of saliva.[186] This creates a cariogenic oral environment, particularly in patients ingesting a diet high in carbohydrates or sucrose.

Etiology and Pathophysiology

Dental caries is an infectious and multifactorial disease. Caries-forming bacteria (ie, *Streptococcus mutans*, *Lactobacillus*, *Actinomyces*) are commonally present in the oral cavity.[1] Dental caries occur when bacterial by-products, that is, acids, cavitate the hard surfaces of teeth. Without intervention, the bacteria will penetrate the cavitated enamel surface and underlying dentin and encroach onto the pulp tissue. The bacteria convert all foods, especially sugar and starch, into acids. Cariogenic bacteria and by-products are found in dental plaque, a sticky organic matrix of bacteria, food debris, dead mucosal cells, and saliary components, adhering to the tooth surface. Bacteria colonize on tooth surfaces and produce polysaccharides that enhance adherence of the plaque to the enamel. A demineralization process occurs, and the underlying tooth surfaces lose calcium, phosphate, and carbonate. Cycles of demeralization and remineralization continue throughout the lifetime of the tooth.[187] Plaque that is not removed from the teeth mineralizes into calculus. Plaque and calculus irritate the gingival tissues, resulting in gingivitis and, ultimately, periodontitis. Plaque begins to accumulate on teeth within 20 minutes after eating, which is the time when most bacterial activity occurs. If this plaque is not removed thoroughly and routinely, tooth decay will not only begin but flourish.

Clinical Features

Initially, cavities are usually painless until they proliferate inside the tooth and destroy the pulpal tissue (Figure 5). If left untreated, a periapical infection can develop, requiring endodontic therapy. In the early years of the twentieth century, basic dental research led to significant advances in the understanding of the histopathology of caries in enamel and dentin, microbial risk factors, the physiology and pathology of saliva, and the understanding of fluoride mechanisms. As a result, the development of new preventive interventions and restorative materials made a significant impact on the restoration of caries and the retention of dentition Additionally, a second major development in caries prevention was scientific validation of the efficacy and effectiveness of sealants and fluoride therapy.

Management

Treatment strategies must be directed to each component of the caries process. Optimal oral

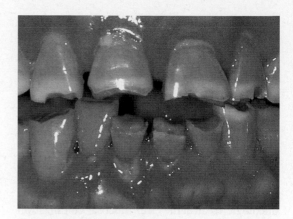

FIGURE 5 A patient on chronic use of analgesia therapy with severe xerostomia and rampant caries.

hygiene must be maintained on a routine basis. Xerostomia should be managed whenever possible by sialogogue therapy or salivary substitutes. Owing to the harmful effect of postradiation caries, patients who have undergone radiation should be treated with a prophylactic regimen, specifically flossing, brushing, and fluoride therapy. Caries resistance can be enhanced with the use of antimicrobial topical fluorides. *Streptococcus mutans*, when exposed to low concentrations of fluoride, produces less acid.[187–190] The combination of oral hygiene, frequent dental follow-up examinations, and appropriate prophylactic treatment procedures is essential to caries prevention, as is fluoride treatment consisting of a daily application of 0.4% stannous fluoride or 1.1% sodium fluoride and applied to the dentition using a brush-on technique or gel-filled trays (ie, fluoride carriers).[1,23,186] The efficacy of topical medication is enhanced with the use of customized carriers that extend the contact time of active drug with tooth structure that leads to increased uptake into the enamel matrices. Fluoride is more readily taken up by demineralized enamel than by sound enamel. Compared with sodium fluoride, stannous fluoride is slightly more acidic, but its uptake into the enamel matrices is four times greater.[1,23] In adults with xerostomia, fluoride leaches out of the enamel within 24 hours; thus, the fluoride regimen must be performed daily for optimal protection. The most efficient method of fluoride application is to use a custom-made polypropylene polypropylene fluoride carrier that completely covers, and extends slightly beyond, the tooth surface.[23] Patients fill the carriers with fluoride gel and place them onto the dentition daily for 10 minutes.[1,23] Patients who receive low doses of radiation and are expected to have a slight degree of xerostomia can use a toothbrush to apply the fluoride gel.[191] Sensitivity and pain are common side effects of fluoride and may necessitate a change in the fluoride concentration or the method of application. A daily fluoride program can decrease postradiation dentinal hypersensitivity, remineralize cavitated enamel matrices, and, more importantly, inhibit caries-forming organisms.[1,23]

Conclusions

The oral cavity should be thoroughly evaluated in all patients diagnosed with cancer, as well as in patients undergoing any immunomyelosuppressive therapy. Preventing and treating the oral complications of cancer are important responsibilities of the oral health care provider, and anticipating primary and secondary mucosal insults and recognizing oral complications promptly in this setting can decrease the incidence of such complications or ameliorate their morbid side effects. By fostering communication and compliance among members of the multidisciplinary team, the dental specialist can ensure quality preventive, therapeutic, and maintenance care to patients with cancer.

References

1. Chambers MS, Toth BB, Martin JW, et al. Oral and dental management of the cancer patient: prevention and treatment of complications. Support Care Cancer 1995;3: 168–75.
2. King GE, Toth BB, Fleming TJ. Oral dental care of the cancer patient. Tex Dent J 1988;105:10–1.
3. National Institutes of Health Consensus Development Conference statement: oral complications of cancer therapies: diagnosis, prevention, and treatment. J Am Dent Assoc 1989;119:179–83.
4. Toth BB, Martin JW, Fleming TJ. Oral and dental care associated with cancer therapy. Cancer Bull 1991;43: 397–402.
5. Hurst PS. Dental considerations in management of head and neck cancer. Otolaryngol Clin North Am 1985;18: 573–603.
6. Lockhart PB, Clark J. Pretherapy dental status of patients with malignant conditions of the head and neck. Oral Surg Oral Med Oral Pathol 1994;77:236–41.
7. Marciani RD, Ownby HE. Treating patients before and after irradiation. J Am Dent Assoc 1992;123:108–12.
8. Niehaus CS, Meiller TF, Peterson DE, Overholser CD. Oral complications in children during cancer therapy. Cancer Nurs 1987;10:15–20.
9. Toth BB, Martin JW, Fleming TJ. Oral complications associated with cancer therapy: an M. D. Anderson Cancer Center experience. J Clin Periodontol 1990;17:508–15.
10. Morton ME, Simpson W. The management of osteoradionecrosis of the jaws. Br J Oral Maxillofac Surg 1986;24: 332–41.
11. Morton M, Roberts H. Oral cancer and precancer: after-care and terminal care. Br Dent J 1990;168:283–7.
12. Poland J. Prevention and treatment of oral complications in the cancer patient. Oncology 1991;5:45–62.
13. Lingeman RE, Singer MJ. Evaluation of the patient with head and neck cancer. In: Suen JY, Myers EN, editors. Cancer of the head and neck. New York: Churchill Livingstone; 1981. p. 15–6.
14. Allard WF, el-Akkad S, Chatmas JC. Obtaining pre-radiation therapy dental clearance. J Am Dent Assoc 1993;124: 88–91.
15. Lowe O. Pretreatment dental assessment and management of patients undergoing head and neck irradiation. Clin Prev Dent 1986;8:24–30.
16. Markitziu A, Zafiropoulos G, Tsalikis L, Cohen L. Gingival health and salivary function in head and neck-irradiated patients. A five year follow up. Oral Surg Oral Med Oral Pathol 1992;73:427–33.
17. Ang KK, Garden AS. General principles of head and neck radiotherapy. In: Ang KK, Garden AS, editors. Radiotherapy for head and neck cancers: indications and techniques. Philadelphia: Lippincott, Williams, and Wilkins; 2002. p. 3–36.

18. Lindquist SF, Hickey AJ, Drane JB. Effects of oral hygiene on stomatitis in patients receiving cancer chemotherapy. J Prosthet Dent 1978;40:312–4.
19. Jackson KC, Chambers MS. Management of oral complications in palliative care. J Pharm Care Pain Symptom Control 2000;8:143–62.
20. Epstein J, Ransier, Lunn R. Enhancing the effect of oral hygiene with the use of a foam brush with chlorhexidine. Oral Surg Oral Med Oral Pathol Oral Radiol Endod 1994; 77:242–7.
21. Toth BB, Chambers MS, Fleming TJ. Prevention and management of oral complications associated with cancer therapies: radiotherapy/chemotherapy. Tex Dent J 1996; 113:23–9.
22. Toth BB, Chambers MS, Fleming TJ, et al. Minimizing oral complications of cancer treatment. Oncology 1995;9: 851–8.
23. Marciani R, Ownby H. Osteoradionecrosis of the jaws. J Oral Maxillofac Surg 1986;4:218–23.
24. National Cancer Institute. Management of oral complications during and after chemotherapy and/or radiation therapy. Available at: www.nci.nih.gov/cancertopics/pdq/supportivecare/oralcomplications/Patient/page5/print.
25. Elting LS, Cooksley C, Chambers MS, et al. The burdens of cancer therapy: clinical and economic outcomes of chemotherapy-induced mucositis. Cancer 2003;98: 1531–9.
26. Kostler WJ, Hejna M, Wenzel C, Zielinski CC. Oral mucositis complicating chemotherapy and/or radiotherapy: options for prevention and treatment. CA Cancer J Clin 2001;51:290–315.
27. Sonis ST, Oster G, Fuchs H, et al. Oral mucositis and the clinical and economic outcomes of blood and bone marrow transplantation. J Clin Oncol 2001;19:2001–5.
28. Rubenstein EB, Peterson DE, Schubert M, et al. Clinical practice guidelines for the prevention and treatment of cancer-induced oral and gastrointestinal mucositis. Cancer 2004;100(9 Suppl):2026–46.
29. Bellm LA, Epstein JB, Rose-Ped A, et al. Patient reports of complications of bone marrow transplantation. Support Care Cancer 2000;8:33–9.
30. Sonis ST. Mucositis as a biological process: a new hypothesis for the development of chemotherapy-induced stomatotoxicity. Oral Oncol 1998;34:39–43.
31. Peterson DE. Oral toxicity of chemotherapeutic agents. Semin Oncol 1992;19:478–91.
32. Fu K, Pajak TF, Trotti A, et al. A Radiation Therapy Oncology Group (RTOG) phase III randomized study to compare hyperfractionation and two variants of accelerated fractionation to standard fractionation radiotherapy for head and neck squamous cell carcinomas: first report of RTOG 9003. Int J Radiat Oncol Biol Phys 2000;48:7–16.
33. Forastiere AA, Goepfert H, Maor M, et al. Concurrent chemotherapy and radiotherapy for organ preservation in advanced laryngeal cancer. N Engl J Med 2003;349: 2091–8.
34. Cooper JS, Pajak TF, Forastiere AA, et al, the Radiation Therapy Oncology Group 9501/Intergro. Postoperative concurrent radiotherapy and chemotherapy for high-risk squamous-cell carcinoma of the head and neck. N Engl J Med 2004;350:1937–44.
35. Sonis S, Clark J. Prevention and management of oral mucositis induced by antineoplastic therapy. Oncology 1991; 5:11–8.
36. Parulekar W, Mackenzie R, Bjarnason G, Jordan RCK. Scoring oral mucositis. Oral Oncol 1998;34:63–71.
37. O'Brien SN, Blijlevens NMA, Mahfouz TH, Anaissie EJ. Infections in patients with hematological cancer: recent developments. Hematology 2003:438–72.
38. Sonis ST, Elting LS, Keefe D, et al. Perspective on cancer therapy-induced mucosal injury: pathogenesis, measurement, epidemiology, and consequences for patients. Cancer 2004;100(9 Suppl):1995–2025.
39. Sonis ST. Transforming growth factor-beta 3 mediated modulation of cell cycling and attenuation of 5-fluorouracil induced mucositis. Oral Oncol 1997;33:47–54.
40. Sonis ST. Defining mechanisms of action of interleukin-11 on the progression of radiation-induced oral mucositis in hamsters. Oral Oncol 2000;36:373–81.
41. Sonis ST, Eilers JP, Epstein JB, et al. Validation of a new scoring system for the assessment of clinical trial research of oral mucositis induced by radiation or chemotherapy. Cancer 1999;85:2103–13.
42. Engelmeier RL. A dental protocol for patients receiving radiation therapy for cancer of the head and neck. Spec Care Dentist 1987;7:54–8.

43. Mahood DJ, Dose AM, Loprinzi CL, et al. Inhibition of fluorouracil-induced stomatitis by oral cryotherapy. J Clin Oncol 1991;9:449–52.
44. Worthington HV, Clarkson JE, Eden OB. Interventions for treating oral mucositis for patients with cancer receiving treatment. Cochrane Database Syst Rev 2002;(1): CD001973.
45. Clarkson JE, Worthington HV, Eden OB. Interventions for preventing oral mucositis for patients with cancer receiving treatment. Cochrane Database of Systematic Reviews 2003;(3).
46. World Health Organization. Cancer pain relief: with a guide to opioid availability. 2nd ed. 1996. Available at: http://whqlibdoc.who.int/publications/9241544821.pdf.
47. Capizzi R. Amifostine: the preclinical basis for broad-spectrum selective cytoprotection of normal tissues from cytotoxic therapies. Semin Oncol 1996;23:2–16.
48. Brizel D, Wasserman TH, Henke M, et al. Phase III randomized trial of amifostine as a radioprotector in head and neck cancer. J Clin Oncol 2000;18:3339–45.
49. Bourhis J, De Crevoisier R, Abdulkarim B, et al. A randomized study of very accelerated radiotherapy with and without amifostine in head and neck squamous cell carcinoma. Int J Radiat Oncol Biol Phys 2000;46:1105–8.
50. Buntzel J, Schuth J, Kuttner K, et al. Radiochemotherapy with amifostine cytoprotection for head and neck cancer. Support Care Cancer 1998;6:155–60.
51. Potten C. Protection of the small intestinal clonogenic stem cells from radiation-induced damage by pretreatment with interleukin 11 also increases murine survival time. Stem Cells 1996;14:452–9.
52. Booth D, Haley J, Bruskin A, et al. Transforming growth factor b3 protects murine small intestinal crypt stem cells and animal survival after irradiation, possibly by reducing stem cell cycling. Int J Cancer 2000;86:53–9.
53. Dorr W, Hamilton CS, Boyd T, et al. Radiation-induced changes in cellularity and proliferation in human oral mucosa. Int J Radiat Oncol Biol Phys 2002;52:911–7.
54. Spielberger R, Stiff P, Bensinger W, et al. Palifermin for oral mucositis after intensive therapy for hematologic cancers. N Engl J Med 2004;351:2590–8.
55. Sonis S. Transforming growth factor-beta 3 mediated modulation of cell cycling and attenuation of 5-fluorouracil induced mucositis. Oral Oncol 1997;33:47–54.
56. Kaplan G, Walsh G, Guido L, et al. Novel responses of human skin to intradermal recombinant granulocyte/macrophage-colony-stimulating factor: Langerhans cell recruitment, keratinocyte growth, and enhanced wound healing. J Exp Med 1992;175:1717–28.
57. Nemunaitis J, Rosenfeld C, Ash R, et al. Phase III randomized, double-blind placebo-controlled trial of rhGM-CSF following allogeneic bone marrow transplantation. Bone Marrow Transplant 1995;15:949–54.
58. Makkonen T. Granulocyte macrophage-colony stimulating factor (GM-CSF) and sucralfate in prevention of radiation-induced mucositis: a prospective randomized study. Int J Radiat Oncol Biol Phys 2000;46:525–34.
59. Rosso M. Effect of granulocyte-macrophage colony-stimulating factor on prevention of mucositis in head and neck cancer patients treated with chemo-radiotherapy. J Chemother 1997;9:382–5.
60. Mantovani G, Massa E, Astara G, et al. Phase II clinical trial of local use of GM-CSF for prevention and treatment of chemotherapy- and concomitant chemoradiotherapy-induced severe oral mucositis in advanced head and neck cancer patients: an evaluation of effectiveness, safety and costs. Oncol Rep 2003;10:197–206.
61. Sprinzl G, Galvan O, De Vries A, et al. Local application of granulocyte-macrophage stimulating factor (GM-CSF) for the treatment of oral mucositis. Eur J Cancer 2001; 37:2003–9.
62. Scherlacher A, Beaufort-Spontin F. Radiotherapy of head-neck neoplasms: prevention of inflammation of the mucosa by sucralfate treatment. HNO 1990;38:24–8.
63. Epstein J, Wong F. The efficacy of sucralfate suspension in the prevention of oral mucositis due to radiation therapy. Int J Radiat Oncol Biol Phys 1994;28:693–8.
64. Etiz D, Erkal H, Serin M, et al. Clinical and histopathological evaluation of sucralfate in prevention of oral mucositis induced by radiation therapy in patients with head and neck malignancies. Oral Oncol 2000;36:116–20.
65. Carter D, Hebert M, Smink K, et al. Double blind randomized trial of sucralfate vs placebo during radiotherapy for head and neck cancers. Head Neck 1999;21:760–6.
66. Cengiz M, Ozyar E, Akol F, et al. Sucralfate in the prevention of radiation-induced oral mucositis. J Clin Gastroenterol 1999;28:40–3.

67. Franzen L, Henriksson R, Littbrand B, et al. Effects of sucralfate on mucositis during and following radiotherapy of malignancies in the head and neck region. Acta Oncol 1995;34:219–23.

68. Lievens Y, Haustermans K, Van der Weyngaert D, et al. Does sucralfate reduce the acute side-effects in head and neck cancer treated with radiotherapy? A double-blind randomized trial. Radiother Oncol 1998;47:149–53.

69. Makkonen T, Bostrom P, Vilja P, et al. Sucralfate mouth washing in the prevention of radiation-induced mucositis: a placebo-controlled double-blind randomized study. Int J Radiat Oncol Biol Phys 1994;30:177–82.

70. Matejka M, Nell A, Kment G, et al. Local benefit of prostaglandin E2 in radiochemotherapy-induced oral mucositis. Br J Oral Maxillofac Surg 1990;28:89–91.

71. Porteder H, Rausch E, Kment G, et al. Local prostaglandin E2 in patients with oral malignancies undergoing chemo- and radiotherapy. J Craniomaxillofac Surg 1988;16:371–4.

72. Sironi M, Pozzi P, Polentarutti N, et al. Inhibition of inflammatory cytokine production and protection against endotoxin toxicity by benzydamine. Cytokine 1996;8:710–6.

73. Epstein JB, Silverman S Jr, Paggiarino DA, et al. Benzydamine HCl for prophylaxis of radiation-induced oral mucositis: results from a multicenter, randomized, double-blind, placebo-controlled clinical trial. Cancer 2001;92:875–85.

74. Ferretti G, Raybould TP, Brown AT, et al. Chlorhexidine prophylaxis for chemotherapy- and radiotherapy-induced stomatitis: a randomized double-blind trial. Oral Surg Oral Med Oral Pathol 1990;69:331–8.

75. Spijkervet F, van Saene HK, Panders AK, et al. Effect of chlorhexidine rinsing on the oropharyngeal ecology in patients with head and neck cancer who have irradiation mucositis. Oral Surg Oral Med Oral Pathol 1989;67:154–61.

76. Foote R, Loprinzi C, Frank A, et al. Randomized trial of a chlorhexidine mouthwash for alleviation of radiation-induced mucositis. J Clin Oncol 1994;12:2630–3.

77. Spijkervet F, van Saene HK, van Saene JJ, et al. Effect of selective elimination of the oral flora on mucositis in irradiated head and neck cancer patients. J Surg Oncol 1991;46:167–73.

78. Okuno S, Foote RL, Loprinzi CL, et al. A randomized trial of a nonabsorbable antibiotic lozenge given to alleviate radiation-induced mucositis. Cancer 1997;79:2193–9.

79. Symonds R, McIlroy P, Khorrami J, et al. The reduction of radiation mucositis by selective decontamination antibiotic pastilles: a placebo-controlled double-blind trial. Br J Cancer 1996;74:312–7.

80. Wijers O, Levendag P, Harms E, et al. Mucositis reduction by selective elimination of oral flora in irradiated cancers of the head and neck: a placebo-controlled double-blind randomized study. Int J Radiat Oncol Biol Phys 2001;50:343–52.

81. El-Sayed S, Nabid A, Shelley W, et al. Prophylaxis of radiation-associated mucositis in conventionally treated patients with head and neck cancer: a double-blind, phase III, randomized, controlled trial evaluating the clinical efficacy of an antimicrobial lozenge using a validated mucositis scoring system. J Clin Oncol 2002;20:3956–63.

82. Trotti A, Garden A, Warde P, et al. A multinational, randomized phase III trial of iseganan HCl oral solution for reducing the severity of oral mucositis in patients receiving radiotherapy for head and neck malignancy. Int J Radiat Oncol Biol Phys 2004;58:674–81.

83. Dodd M, Dibble S, Miaskowski C, et al. Randomized clinical trial of the effectiveness of 3 commonly used mouthwashes to treat chemotherapy-induced mucositis. Oral Surg Oral Med Oral Pathol Oral Radiol Endod 2000;90:39–47.

84. Schubert MM, Jones DL. Management of oral mucositis pain. Tex Dent J 2004;121:507–18.

85. Davies AN, Broadley K, Beighton D. Xerostomia in patients with advanced cancer. J Pain Symptom Manage 2001;22:820–5.

86. Narhi TO. Prevalence of subjective feelings of dry mouth in the elderly. J Dent Res 1994;73:20–5.

87. Liu R, Fleming TJ, Toth BB. Salivary flow rates in patients with head and neck cancer 0.5 to 25 years after radiotherapy. Oral Surg Oral Med Oral Pathol Oral Radiol Endod 1990;70:724–9.

88. Schubert M, Izutsu KT. Iatrogenic causes of salivary gland dysfunction. J Dent Res 1987;66 Suppl:680–8.

89. Chambers MS, Garden AS, Kies MS, Martin JW. Radiation-induced xerostomia in patients with head and neck cancer: pathogenesis, impact on quality of life, and management. Head Neck 2004;26:796–807.

90. Sreebny LM, Schwartz SS. A reference guide to drugs and dry mouth – 2nd edition. Gerodontology 1997;14:33–47.

91. Bergdahl M, Bergdahl J. Low unstimulated salivary flow and subjective oral dryness: association with medication, anxiety, depression, and stress. J Dent Res 2000;79:1652–8.

92. Malone-Lee JG, Walsh JB, Maugourd MF. Tolterodine: a safe and effective treatment for older patients with overactive bladder. J Am Geriatr Soc 2001;49:700–5.

93. California Dental Hygienists Association. Xerostomia: drymouth. Available at: http://www.cdha.org/articles/drymouth.htm (accessed February 7, 2003).

94. Sjogren R, Nordstrom G. Oral health status of psychiatric patients. J Clin Nurs 2000;9:632–8.

95. Nagler RM, Gez E, Rubinov R, et al. The effect of low-dose interleukin-2-based immunotherapy on salivary function and composition in patients with metastatic renal cell carcinoma. Arch Oral Biol 2001;46:487–93.

96. Logemann JA, Smith CH, Pauloski BR, et al. Effects of xerostomia on perception and performance of swallow function. Head Neck 2001;23:317–21.

97. Eisbruch A, Kim HM, Terrell JE, et al. Xerostomia and its predictors following parotid-sparing irradiation of head-and-neck cancer. Int J Radiat Oncol Biol Phys 2001;50:695–704.

98. Webb S. IMRT: general considerations. In: Webb S, editor. Intensity-modulated radiation therapy. Philadelphia: Institute of Physics Publishing; 2001. p. 1–34.

99. Chambers MS, et al. 2005 OOO Article s. mutans

100. Chao KS, Deasy JO, Markman J, et al. A prospective study of salivary function sparing in patients with head-and-neck cancers receiving intensity-modulated or three-dimensional radiation therapy: initial results. Int J Radiat Oncol Biol Phys 2001;49:907–16.

101. Chao KS, Majhail N, Huang CJ, et al. Intensity-modulated radiation therapy reduces late salivary toxicity without compromising tumor control in patients with oropharyngeal carcinoma: a comparison with conventional techniques. Radiother Oncol 2001;61:275–80.

102. Leek H, Albertsson M. Pilocarpine treatment of xerostomia in head and neck patients. Micron 2002;33:153–5.

103. Grotz KA. Prophylaxis of radiogenic sialadenitis and mucositis by coumarin/troxerutine in patients with head and neck cancer—a prospective, randomized, placebo-controlled, double-blind study. Br J Oral Maxillofac Surg 2001;39:34–9.

104. Ripamonti C. A randomized, controlled clinical trial to evaluate the effects of zinc sulfate on cancer patients with taste alterations caused by head and neck irradiation. Cancer 1998;82:1938–45.

105. Cockerham MB, Weinberger BB, Lerchie SB. Oral glutamine for the prevention of oral mucositis associated with high-dose paclitaxel and melphalan for autologous bone marrow transplantation. Ann Pharmacother 2000;34:300–3.

106. Chambers MS. Xerostomia and its role in mucositis: complications and management [abstract]. Support Care Cancer 1997;5:149.

107. Chambers MS, Toth BB, Martin JW, et al. Oral and dental management of the cancer patient: prevention and treatment of complications. Support Care Cancer 1995;3:168–75.

108. Lindegaard JC, Grau C. Has the outlook improved for amifostine as a clinical radioprotector? Radiother Oncol 2000;57:113–8.

109. Hensley ML, Schuchter LM, Lindley C, et al. American Society of Clinical Oncology clinical practice guidelines for the use of chemotherapy and radiotherapy protectants. J Clin Oncol 1999;17:3333–55.

110. Shaha AR, Patel S, Shasha D. Harrison LB. Head and neck cancer. In: Lenhard RE Jr, Osteen RT, Gansler T, editors. Clinical oncology. Atlanta: American Cancer Society; 2001. p. 297–330.

111. Seikaly H, Jha N, McGaw T, et al. Submandibular gland transfer: a new method of preventing radiation-induced xerostomia. Larygoscope 2001;111:347–52.

112. Kaanders JHAM, Fleming TJ, Ang KK, et al. Devices valuable in head and neck radiotherapy. Int J Radiat Oncol Biol Phys 1992;23:639–45.

113. Spiegel JH, Deschler DG, Cheney ML. Microvascular transplantation and replantation of the rabbit submandibular gland. Arch Otolaryngol Head Neck Surg 2001;127:991–6.

114. Spiegel JH, Zhang F, Levin DE, et al. Microvascular transplantation of the rat submandibular gland. Plast Reconstr Surg 2000;106:1326–35.

115. Greer JE, Eltorky M, Robbins KT. A feasibility study of salivary gland autograft transplantation for xerostomia. Head Neck 2000;22:241–6.

116. Nagler RM, Baum BJ. Treatment reduces the severity of xerostomia following radiation therapy for oral cavity cancer. Arch Otolaryngol Head Neck Surg 2003;129:245–51.

117. Delporte C, O'Connell BC, He X, et al. Increased fluid secretion after adenoviral-mediated transfer of the aquaporin-1 cDNA to irradiated rat salivary glands. Proc Natl Acad Sci U S A 1997;94:3268–73.

118. Epperly MW, Gretton JA, DeFilippi SJ, et al. Modulation of radiation-induced cytokine elevation associated with esophagitis and esophageal stricture by manganese superoxide dismutase-plasmid/liposome (SOD2-PL) gene therapy. Radiat Res 2001;155:2–14.

119. Epperly MW, DeFelippi SJ, Sikora CA, et al. Intratracheal injection A manganese superoxide dismutase (MnSOD) plasmid/liposomes protects normal lung but not orthotopic tumors from irradiation. Gene Ther 2000;7:1011–8.

120. Chambers MS. Clinical commentary on prophylactic treatment of radiation-induced xerostomia. Arch Otolaryngol Head Neck Surg 2003;129:251–2.

121. Mercandante S, Calderone L, Villari P, et al. The use of pilocarpine in opioid-induced xerostomia. Palliat Med 2000;14:529–31.

122. LeVeque FG, Montgomery M, Potter D, et al. A multicenter, randomized, double-blind, placebo-controlled, dose-titration study of oral pilocarpine for treatment of radiation-induced xerostomia in head and neck cancer patients. J Clin Oncol 1993;11:1124–31.

123. Fox PC, van der Ven PF, Baum BJ, Mandel ID. Pilocarpine for the treatment of xerostomia associated with salivary gland dysfunction. Oral Surg Oral Med Oral Pathol 1986;61:243–8.

124. Chambers MS, Toth BB, Payne R, et al. Mutans streptococci and salivary flow rates in cancer patients attending a pain clinic [abstract]. J Dent Res 1997;76:358.

125. Chambers M, Martin C, Toth B, et al. Assessment of functional improvement in cancer patients with oral pilocarpine as treatment for analgesia-induced xerostomia [abstract]. Support Care Cancer 1997;5:164.

126. Chambers M, Toth B, Martin C, et al. Assessment of salivary flow improvement in cancer patients with oral pilocarpine as treatment for analgesia-induced xerostomia [abstract]. Proc Am Soc Clin Oncol 1997;16:50a.

127. Wiseman LR, Faulds D. Oral pilocarpine: a review of its pharmacological properties and clinical potential in xerostomia. Drugs 1995;49:143–55.

128. Johnson JT, Ferretti GA, Nethery WJ, et al. Oral pilocarpine for post-irradiation xerostomia in patients with head and neck cancer. N Engl J Med 1993;329:390–5.

129. Atkinson JC, Baum BJ. Salivary enhancement: current status and future therapies. J Dent Educ 2001;65:1096–101.

130. Al-Hashimi I. The management of Sjogren's syndrome in dental practice. J Am Dent Assoc 2001;132:1409–17.

131. Evoxac™ capsules (cevimeline hydrochloride). In: Physician's desk reference. 55th ed. Montvale (NJ): Medical Economics Co; 2001. p. 1110–2.

132. Store G, Boysen M. Mandibular osteoradionecrosis: clinical behaviour and diagnostic aspects. Clin Otolaryngol 2000; 25:378–84.

133. Marx SD. Management of irradiated patients and osteoradionecrosis. In: Marx RE, Stern D, editors. Oral and maxillofacial pathology: a rationale for diagnosis and treatment. Chicago: Quintessence; 2003. p. 375–94.

134. Murray CG, Daly TE, Zimmerman SO. The relationship between dental disease and radiation necrosis of the mandible. Oral Surg Oral Med Oral Pathol 1980;49:99–104.

135. Jereczek-Fossa BA, Orecchia R. Radiotherapy-induced mandibular bone complications. Cancer Treat Rev 2002;28:65–74.

136. Berger RP, Symington JM. Long-term clinical manifestation of osteoradionecrosis of the mandible: report of two cases. J Oral Maxillofac Surg 1990;48:82–4.

137. Marx RE. Osteoradionecrosis: a new concept of its pathophysiology. J Oral Maxillofac Surg 1983;41:283–8.

138. Marx RE, Johnson RP. Studies in the radiobiology of osteoradionecrosis and their clinical significance. Oral Surg Oral Med Oral Pathol 1987;64:379–90.

139. Chong J, Hinckley LK, Ginsberg LE. Masticator space abnormalities associated with mandibular osteoradionecrosis: MR and CT findings in five patients. AJNR Am J Neuroradiol 2000;21:175–80.

140. Bachmann G, Rossler R, Klett R, et al. The role of magnetic resonance imaging and scintigraphy in the diagnosis of pathologic changes of the mandible after radiation therapy. Int J Oral Maxillofac Surg 1996;25:189–95.

141. Chang DW, Oh HK, Robb GL, Miller MJ. Management of advanced mandibular osteoradionecrosis with free flap reconstruction. Head Neck 2001;23:830–5.

142. Feldmeier JJ, Hampson NB. A systematic review of the literature reporting the application of hyperbaric oxygen prevention and treatment of delayed radiation injuries: an evidence based approach. Undersea Hyperb Med 2002; 29:4–30.

143. Feldmeier JJ, Davolt DA, Court WS, et al. Histologic morphometry confirms a prophylactic effect for hyperbaric oxygen in the prevention of delayed radiation enteropathy. Undersea Hyper Med 1998;25:93–7.

144. Feldmeier JJ, Newman R, Davolt DA, et al. Prophylactic hyperbaric oxygen for patients undergoing salvage for recurrent head and neck cancers following full course irradiation [abstract]. Undersea Hyper Med 1998;25 Suppl:10.

145. Marx RE. Radiation injury to tissue. In: Kindwall EP, editor. Hyperbaric medicine practice. Flagstaff: Best Publishing; 1995. p. 464–503.

146. Marx RE, Johnson RP. Problem wounds in oral and maxillofacial surgery: the role of hyperbaric oxygen. In: Davis JC, Hunt TK, editors. Problem wounds: the role of oxygen. New York: Elsevier; 1988. p. 65–123.

147. Blanchaert RH, Bailey J. Osteoradionecrosis of mandible. In: Lydiatt W, Talavera F, editors. eMedicine.com 2001. p. 1–10.

148. Ioannides C, Fossion E, Boeckx W. Surgical management of the osteoradionecrotic mandible with free vascularised composite flaps. J Craniomaxillofac Surg 1994;22:330–4.

149. Lydiatt DD, Lydiatt WM, Hollins RR, et al. Use of free fibula flap in patients with prior failed mandibular reconstruction. J Oral Maxillofac Surg 1998;56:444–6.

150. Shaha AR, Cordeiro PG, Hidalgo DA, et al. Resection and immediate microvascular reconstruction in the management of osteoradionecrosis of the mandible. Head Neck 1997;19:406–11.

151. Beumer J, Silverman S Jr, Benak SB Jr. Hard and soft tissue necrosis following radiation therapy for oral cancer. J Prosthet Dent 1972;27:640–4.

152. Epstein J, Rea G, Wong FL, et al. Osteoradionecrosis: study of the relationship of dental extractions in patients receiving radiotherapy. Head Neck Surg 1987;10:48–54.

153. Marciani RHO. Osteoradionecrosis of the jaws. J Oral Maxillofac Surg 1986;4:218–23.

154. Schweiger J. Oral complications following radiation therapy: a five-year retrospective report. J Prosthet Dent 1987;58: 78–82.

155. Epstein J, Wong, FL, Stevenson-Moore P. Osteoradionecrosis: clinical experience and a proposal for classification. J Oral Maxillofac Surg 1987;45:104–10.

156. Fujita M, Tanimoto K, Wada T. Early radiographic changes in radiation bone injury. Oral Surg Oral Med Oral Pathol 1986;61:641–4.

157. Pappas G. Oral roentgenology. Bone changes in osteoradionecrosis: a review. Oral Surg Oral Med Oral Pathol 1969;27:622–30.

158. Bundgaard T, Tandrup O, Elbrond O. A functional evaluation of patients treated for oral cancer. A prospective study. Int J Oral Maxillofac Surg 1993;22:28–34.

159. Granstrom G, Jacobsson M, Tjellstrom A. Titanium implants in irradiated tissues: benefits from hyperbaric oxygen. Int J Oral Maxillofac Impl 1992;7:15–25.

160. Khan SA, Wingard JR. Infection and mucosal injury in cancer treatment. J Natl Cancer Inst Monogr 2001;29: 31–60.

161. Sonis ST. Oral complications of cancer therapy. In: Bast RC, Kufe DW, Pollack R, editors. Holland-Frei cancer medicine. 5th ed. Hamilton (ON): BC Decker; 2000. p. 2371–9.

162. Scully C, Epstein JB. Oral health care for the cancer patient. Eur J Cancer B Oral Oncol 1996;32B:281–92.

163. Wujcik D. Infection control in oncology patients. Nurs Clin North Am 1993;28:639–50.

164. Cella DF, Tulsky DS, Gray G, et al. The Functional Assessment of Cancer Therapy Scale: development and validation of the general measure. J Clin Oncol 1993; 11:570–9.

165. Cella D, Hahn E, Chang CH. Implementation and application into cross-cultural trials. Qual Life Res 1997; 6:631.

166. Blijlevens NMA, Donnelly JP, De Pauw BE. Mucosal barrier injury: biology, pathology, clinical counterparts and consequences of intensive treatment for haematological malignancy: an overview. Bone Marrow Transplant 2000; 25:1269–78.

167. Redding SW, Zellars RC, Kirkpatrick WR, et al. Epidemiology of oropharyngeal *Candida* colonization and infection in patients receiving radiation for head and neck cancer. J Clin Microbiol 1999;37:3896–900.

168. Fleming ID, Brady LW, Mieszkalski GB, et al. Basis for major current therapies for cancer. In: Murphy GP, Lawrence W, Lenhard RE, editors. American Cancer Society textbook of clinical oncology. 2nd ed. Atlanta: American Cancer Society; 1995. p. 96–134.

169. Lenhard RE, Lawrence W, McKenna RJ. General approach to the patient. In: Murphy GP, Lawrence W, Lenhard RE, editors. American Cancer Society textbook of clinical oncology. 2nd ed. Atlanta: American Cancer Society; 1995. p. 64–74.

170. Tang ITL, Shepp DH. Herpes simplex virus infection in cancer patients: prevention and treatment. Oncology 1992;6:101–9.

171. Greenberg MS. Oral herpes simplex infections in patients with leukemia. J Am Dent Assoc 1987;114:483–6.

172. MacPhail LA, Hilton JF, Heinic GS, Greenspan D. Direct immunofluorescence vs. culture for detecting HSV in oral ulcers: a comparison. J Am Dent Assoc 1995;126:74–8.

173. Montgomery MT, Redding SW, LeMaistre CF. The incidence of oral herpes simplex virus infection in patients undergoing cancer chemotherapy. Oral Surg Oral Med Oral Pathol 1986;61:238–42.

174. Epstein JB, Sherlock CH, Page JL, et al. Clinical study of herpes simplex virus infection in leukemia. Oral Surg Oral Med Oral Pathol 1990;70:38–43.

175. Mealey BL, Semba SE, Hallmon WW. Dentistry and the cancer patient. Part I. Oral manifestations and complications of chemotherapy. Compend Contin Educ Dent 1994;XV:1252–6.

176. Flaitz CM, Hammond HL. The immunoperoxidase method for the rapid diagnosis of intraoral herpes simplex virus infection in patients receiving bone marrow transplants. Spec Care Dent 1988;8:82–5.

177. Rosenberg SW. Oral care of chemotherapy patients. Dent Clin North Am 1990;34:239–50.

178. Cooper B. New concepts in management of acute leukemia. BUMC Proc 1990;3:31–3.

179. O'Sullivan EA, Duggal MS, Bailey CC, et al. Changes in the oral microflora during cytotoxic chemotherapy in children being treated for acute leukemia. Oral Surg Oral Med Oral Pathol 1993;76:161–8.

180. Mattsson T, Arvidson K, Heimdahl A, et al. Alterations in test acuity associated with allogeneic bone marrow transplantation. J Oral Pathol Med 1992;21:33–3.

181. Epstein JB, Vickars L, Spinelli J, Reece D. Efficacy of chlorhexidine and nystatin rinses in prevention of oral complications in leukemia and bone marrow transplantation. Oral Surg Oral Med Oral Pathol 1992; 73:682–9.

182. Ferretti GA, Ash RC, Brown AT, et al. Chlorhexidine for prophylaxis against oral infections and associated complications in patients receiving bone marrow transplants. J Am Dent Assoc 1987;114:461–7.

183. Ferretti GA, Hansen IA, Whittenburg K, et al. Therapeutic use of chlorhexidine in bone marrow transplant patients: case studies. Oral Surg Oral Med Oral Pathol 1987;63: 683–7.

184. Raether D, Walker PO, Bostrum B, Weisdorf D. Effectiveness of oral chlorhexidine for reducing stomatitis in a pediatric bone marrow transplant population. Pediatr Dent 1989;11:37–42.

185. Rutkauskas JS, Davis JW. Effects of chlorhexidine during immunosuppressive chemotherapy. A preliminary report. Oral Surg Oral Med Oral Pathol 1993;76:441–8.

186. Keene HJ, Fleming TJ. Prevalence of caries-associated microflora after radiotherapy in patients with cancer of the head and neck. Oral Surg Oral Med Oral Pathol Oral Radiol Endod 1987;64:421–6.

187. MMWR recommendations and reports: recommendations for using fluoride to prevent and control dental caries in the United States. August 17, 2001/50(RR14);1–42 (CDC).

188. Bowden GHW. Effects of fluoride on the microbial ecology of dental plaque. J Dent Res 1990;69:653–9. [Special issue]

189. Marquis RE. Diminished acid tolerance of plaque bacteria caused by fluoride. J Dent Res 1990;69:672–5. [Special issue]

190. Rosen S, Frea JI, Hsu SM. Effect of fluoride-resistant microorganisms on dental caries. J Dent Res 1978;57: 180.

191. Keene HJ, Fleming TJ, Toth BB. Cariogenic microflora in patients with Hodgkin's disease before and after mantle field radiotherapy. Oral Surg Oral Med Oral Pathol 1994;78:577–81.

Upper Airway Problems

Rex C. Yung, MD, FCCP

The respiratory tract is often involved in cancer, either by primary malignancies or cancers metastatic to the respiratory tract. Bronchogenic carcinoma is the leading cause of cancer mortality, accounting for 30% of cancer-related deaths in both males and females in the United States.[1] Other upper aerodigestive tract malignancies, that is, head and neck and esophageal cancers, are also tobacco related and frequently cause complications in the upper airways. Disease progression, deteriorating patient functional status, and/or the effects of therapies contribute to the overall high morbidity and mortality owing to cancer complications of the respiratory tract.

This chapter focuses on upper airway problems encountered in the care of cancer patients. It reviews the anatomy of the region of interest, that is, the larynx, hypopharynx, and trachea, functional defects of which will lead to the principal problems of upper airway obstruction, vocal cord paralysis (VCP), and aspiration, manifested clinically as respiratory distress and gas-exchange derangements. A myriad of other signs and symptoms can be caused by direct tumor involvement of the upper airway and its adjacent soft tissue and vascular structures or as a result of iatrogenic complications from antineoplastic therapy and adjunctive interventions.

Anatomy of the Upper Airway

The region of the airways under consideration in this chapter is confined to the larynx, hypopharynx, and the central nonconducting airways, including the trachea and main carinal branching into the right and left mainstem bronchi.[2] Malformations and cancer-associated pathologies of the orofacial region and airway segments distal to the zero (trachea) and first-generation (right and left mainstem bronchi) branching can also lead to breathing and gas-exchange abnormalities, but these are addressed in preceding and following chapters.

The larynx is the organ of voice production and consists of the soft tissue structures interposed between the pharynx and the upper trachea. Dysfunction of the vocal cords, cartilage, and muscular and membranous structures of this region may lead to voice dysfunction, airflow obstruction, and increased risk of aspiration.

The pharynx is the upper expanded portion of the digestive tube, with the mouth and nasal cavities above and in front and connected to the esophagus below. The hypopharynx is the longest and most inferior of the three segments of the pharynx and is somewhat funnel shaped, defined superiorly by the level of the epiglottis and anteriorly by the lateral aspects of the thyroid cartilage and narrowing toward the level of the cricopharyngeal muscles. Although it is structurally made up of voluntary smooth muscles arranged in outer circular and inner longitudinal layers, the hypopharynx has a far more complex function than merely serving as a passage for solids and liquids on its way to the digestive tract. The orderly coordination of action with the tongue in propelling a bolus of food, timely relaxation of the cricopharyngeus and subsequent peristaltic action of esophageal musculature, and other dynamic interactions with laryngeal structures allow feeding, swallowing, and avoidance of aspiration. Hypopharyngeal pathology and dysfunction may therefore lead gas-exchange abnormalities and nutritional deficits.

The inferior aspect of the upper airway consists of the trachea, which consists of 16 to 20 hyaline cartilage rings connected by a membranous annular ligament. It extends from the subglottis to the carina, which is superimposed to the level of the fifth to sixth thoracic vertebrae posteriorly and just about inferior to the angle of Louis of the sternum anteriorly. Except for the cricoid cartilage ring, the remaining tracheal cartilage "rings" are C shapes, open in their posterior aspect. This paraesophageal aspect formed by a fibrous and smooth muscular membranous wall allows for deglutition without resistance from a series of firm cartilage. Unfortunately, this functional-anatomic adaptation leaves the posterior portion of the trachea especially vulnerable to direct endotracheal invasion or extrinsic compressive effects by posterior and inferior mediastinal pathology. In addition to airway compromise by upper airway obstruction, fistulae developing in the central tracheobronchial tree from direct tumor invasion or iatrogenic causes from cancer therapies can lead to tracheobronchial-esophageal-pleural fistulae. These pathologic connections clinically manifest themselves as coughing,

aspiration, pneumothorax, and pneumomediastinum. These lead to subsequent mediastinitis and pneumonitis, which can lead to respiratory embarrassment and sepsis. The complex anatomic connections of the trachea and mainstem bronchi to a number of mediastinal, vascular, and bronchial structures, plus the tenuous tracheal blood supply, also limit surgical interventions in relieving obstructions or in repairing an injured trachea. Because of the close anatomic relationship of the thoracic esophagus to the left mainstem bronchus, certain pathology affecting the left and right mainstem bronchi is considered as a continuum of the trachea in this chapter.

Clinical Manifestations of Upper Airway Problems

Clinical manifestations of the upper airway problems associated with cancers are listed in Table 1. Specific signs, symptoms, and physical findings are discussed further in the respective sections on the specified conditions of upper airway obstruction, vocal cord dysfunction, and aspiration.

Upper Airway Problems

Tumor Invasion of the Upper Airways

Cancers affecting the upper airways consist of the following: primary cancers of the upper aerodigestive tract (ie, pharyngeal, laryngeal, and tracheal cancers); cancers that invade this space by direct extension, primarily thyroid, esophageal, bronchogenic carcinomas, mediastinal tumors, including lymphoproliferative disorders; and cancers of almost all origins that may metastasize to the upper airways.

Primary cancers of the upper aerodigestive tract share much that is common in etiology, and they can all present with similar upper airway symptoms. As shown in Table 2, taken together, they still constitute only a minority of all new cases of incident cancers but may have a disproportionately high morbidity and mortality, even acknowledging the overweighing in mortality given to lung cancers by including all bronchogenic cancers.

There are, however, important differences in their cancer biology that lead to different

Table 1 Clinical Signs and Symptoms of Upper Airway Problems

Common Symptoms
  Cough
  Dysphonia: hoarseness, voice change
  Throat, neck, and chest pain
  Dysphagia, including a chronic foreign body sensation
  Dyspnea: from central airway obstruction, parenchymal pneumonia
  Bleeding: oropharyngeal, hematemesis, or hemoptysis
  Fever: from infections (pharyngitis, laryngitis, tracheitis, bronchitis, pneumonitis, mediastinitis, abscess
      formation) or tumor necrosis
  Retained airway secretions, difficulty clearing secretions

Uncommon Symptoms
  Referred otalgia, especially ipsilateral ear pain
  Massive exsanguination from vascular erosion and rupture

Possible findings on physical examination
  Hoarseness
  Fluctuance of the soft tissue of the neck, other signs of inflammation
  External draining sinus tract or skin breakdown
  Crackles and other findings suggesting consolidation owing to pneumonia
  Fever, clinical signs of sepsis
  Stridor and/or wheezing, especially inspiratory and when supine
  Tracheal deviation: compression by extrinsic mass or deviation toward volume loss
  Superior vena cava syndrome: facial plethora and edema, superficial varicosities
  Hamann's crunch and subcutaneous crepitus as a result of pneumomediastinum
  Clubbing and other paraneoplastic syndromes
  Weight loss and generalized cachexia

Table 2

	Estimated New Cancer Cases	Cancer Deaths 2006
All sites	1,399,790	564,830
Pharynx (all oral cavity and pharyngeal)	8,950 (30,990)	2,110 (7,430)
Larynx	9,510	3,740
Lung	174,470	162,460
Esophagus	14,550	13,770
Total of four sites (% of all cancers)	207,480 (14.8)	182,080 (32.2)
Adapted from Jemal A et al.[1]		

prognosis and management goals. Tobacco is a major risk factor for the development of all upper aerodigestive tract malignancies, including tumors of the lung, esophagus, larynx, and hypopharynx.[3] Laryngeal cancer in particular is more likely in heavy smokers; however, unlike hypopharyngeal cancer, it tends to be detected earlier because of clinically obvious and chronic voice changes, as well as the higher diagnostic sensitivity of a direct endoscopic examination. Hypopharyngeal cancer is also due to tobacco use but is also associated with heavy alcohol intake.[4] Patients present with a chronic sore throat, gradual but persistent dysphagia that may be dismissed and adapted to by alterations in diet, and, less commonly, an ipsilateral referred otalgia (ear pain). A foreign body sensation may be felt, but hemoptysis and voice changes are late sequelae of direct tumor extension into the larynx. Diagnosis would most often require detailed esophagoscopy under sedation. Because of the vascular and lymphatic drainage of hypopharyngeal tumors, at the time of diagnosis, many or most of these cancers already have regional or distant spread of disease. Radiologic assessment by computed tomography (CT), magnetic resonance imaging (MRI), and chest radiography to detect synchronous lung primary cancers is needed. Prognostically, laryngeal cancers generally fare better than hypopharyngeal cancers, again because of the latter's late diagnosis and early dissemination, as explained. However, in time, laryngeal tumors can also extend to the hypopharynx and vice versa, and both can extend down into the trachea. Hence, for a discussion of additional etiologic risk factors, these upper airway cancers are considered together.

In addition to tobacco products and alcohol, a number of chemical carcinogens have been linked to laryngeal, hypopharyngeal, and bronchogenic carcinomas. These include arsenic, asbestos, chromates, nickel compounds, cobalt and certain heavy metals, chloromethyl ethers, polycyclic aromatic hydrocarbons, certain mineral oils, and aniline dye compounds.[5] Occupational or environmental radon exposure and previous radiotherapy also increase the risk of the development of upper aerodigestive (UAD) cancers.

Environmental risk factors are admixed with genetic predispositions to greatly increase the risk of the development of UAD cancers. One example is in Fanconi's anemia, a rare autosomal recessive disorder with a high degree of genomic instability in which affected individuals are predisposed to cancers, especially hematologic and squamous cell cancers.[6] Hence, Fanconi's anemia patients in the international registry have been noted to have a 500 times standard incidence ratio for the development of head and neck cancers and a high degree of recurrence approaching 50%, which may be made worse when the patient is given therapeutic external beam radiation.[7] Whether individuals have transmitted germline mutations or acquired losses of tumor suppressor genes, the accumulation of genetic and epigenetic abnormalities leads to the development of precursor lesions and eventually invasive carcinomas, which may be single or multiple primary tumors over time.[8–11]

One nongenetic syndrome complex associated with hypopharyngeal carcinoma is the Plummer-Vinson or Paterson–Brown Kelly syndrome of progressive dysphagia, esophageal and hypopharyngeal webs, vitamin B and iron deficiency anemia, and weight loss identified and characterized between 1914 and 1922.[12–14] The pathophysiologic basis of this association is thought to be due to a chronic inflammation response. It is hoped that improved recognition and management with vitamin B and iron supplementation plus dilation should make this condition an interesting historical vignette.

Acquired immune deficiency syndrome (AIDS)–related malignancies (AIDS-defining cancers) include Kaposi's sarcoma (KS), non-Hodgkin's lymphoma (NHL), and human papillomavirus (HPV)-associated cervical and anal cancers. KS in particular and NHL will involve the aerodigestive tract. In the first decade and a half of AIDS, KS has been listed as the leading cause of AIDS-related malignancy, and pulmonary KS, almost always involving the central airways, has been noted in between a fifth to a third of AIDS-related KS.[15] In fact, pulmonary KS may be the solo or initial site of KS presentation, with between 10 and 20% of patients presenting with pulmonary KS absent cutaneous and oral mucocutaneous lesions.[15,16] Although pulmonary KS lesions can become profuse in the lung parenchyma and lead to significant gas exchange impairment, endobronchial KS lesions may also present in various upper airway locations and lead to significant central airway obstruction or to life-threatening bleeding, especially on biopsy.[17,18] Although KS found in the airways in the AIDS era was most recently associated with human immunodeficiency virus (HIV) infection, it is important to consider KS in other patients in immunocompromised states, such as on transplant-related immunosuppression,[19,20] and episodic spontaneous cases that may present with acute airway obstruction.[21,22] AIDS-related lymphoma may also involve the mediastinum with extrinsic compression or intrinsic involvement of the trachea and mainstem bronchi. In the past decade, perhaps as a result of changes in personal practices limiting exposure to herpes simplex virus 8, the putative causative agent for KS, and/or because of highly active antiretroviral therapy (HAART) reconstituting the immune system, there has been a decline in the number of KS cases.[23,24] Conversely, perhaps because of HAART resulting in longer overall survival, there has been a noted rise in tobacco-related malignancies, including primary bronchogenic and head and neck carcinomas,[25,26] and their consequential upper airway involvement and complications as well.

Another infection-related tumor is squamous papilloma in the larynx and tracheobronchial tree caused by HPV passed by maternal-neonatal transmission during childbirth. Unlike HIV-associated papillomavirus-associated cancers of the female genital and anal tract, this is primarily a benign tumor of childhood that often regresses in adulthood. However, recurrent papillomatosis may be prolific in its polypoid growth, leading to upper airway obstruction and dysphonia. Although uncommon, between 1.6 and 5% of papillomatosis have been reported to undergo malignant transformation into squamous cell and verrucous carcinoma, even in the absence of tobacco products, ionizing radiation, or other carcinogenic exposures.[27] This malignant transformation is most common with HPV type 11 and, as with other cancers, seems especially prone to develop in association with *TP53* and other tumor suppressor gene mutations.[28–30]

Primary tracheal cancers are relatively rare compared with secondary cancers. In the adult patient, most primary cancers are malignant and few are benign (Table 3).[31,32] Although certain primary tracheal tumors, such as adenoid cystic carcinomas, mucoepidermoid carcinomas, and central carcinoid tumors, are clearly tracheal in origin, the most common primary tracheal cancer of the squamous cell type often raises the question as to whether it may be of a metastatic origin from the nearby head and neck, esophageal, or lung origin when these cancers are also present since it is known that metachronous lesions are more common when there is one primary UAD cancer

---

Table 3 Classifications of Laryngeal and Tracheal Tumors

Primary malignancies
  Squamous cell carcinoma (SCC)
  Adenoid cystic carcinoma
  Carcinoid, small cell, undifferentiated
    neuroendocrine cancers
  Mucoepidermoid carcinoma
  Adenocarcinoma
  Leiomyosarcoma
  Chondrosarcoma
  Rhabdomyosarcoma
  Malignant fibrous histiocytoma
  Kaposi's sarcoma
  Primary melanoma
  Recurrent respiratory papillomatosis in
    transformation to SCC

Metastatic malignancies
  Squamous cell carcinoma metastases from
    other primary tumors
  Melanoma
  Renal cell carcinoma
  Colon and gastrointestinal tract malignancies
  Uroepithelial malignancies
  Mesenchymal sarcomas (osteo-, leiomyo-,
    chondro-, rhabdomyosarcoma)
  Lymphomas

---

present, and patients who have had any previous UAD malignancy are at a much increased risk of developing second primary malignancies of the UAD tract.[33–35] Overall, however, most cancers involving the trachea are metastatic in origin, with most by direct extension from tumors arising in the adjacent structures of the thyroid, head and neck, and esophageal sources. Direct tracheal invasion occurs in up to 6.5% of thyroid cancers, and subsequent upper airway obstruction is a leading cause of death.[36] Tracheal involvement by extrinsic compression or by direct extension is a frequent complication of esophageal carcinomas. In this instance, fistulae formation presents as much of a problem as does airway obstruction.

Aside from direct extension from tumors of the UAD tract, cancers of almost any origin may metastasize to the larynx, hypopharynx, and trachea (see Table 3). These are, however, relatively rare, and as documented by Nicolai and colleagues, only 143 cases of cancers metastatic to the larynx were reported by 1996, these being primarily melanoma, renal cell carcinoma, and sporadic cases from the colon and lung.[37] Similarly, sporadic cases of renal cell carcinomas, sarcomas, chondrosarcomas and other mesenchymal cell tumors, and breast, colon, uroepithelial, male genital, and gynecologic tumors have all been reported to have metastasized to the central conducting airways of the trachea and mainstem bronchi.[38] Although melanomas detected in the upper airways are most often metastatic in origin, primary tracheobronchial melanomas have also

---

been diagnosed presumptively when a cutaneous primary source cannot be ascertained.

Prognostically, cancers arriving by distant metastases to the upper airways are rarely, if ever, curable. In fact, only direct thyroid cancer invasion and squamous cell metastases from a lung primary tumor could be considered for curative resection if the metastatic involvement is limited and the patient is a functionally fit candidate. Palliative measures to mechanically reduce or to cytoreduce the tumor bulk and to maintain airway patency are mentioned in the following section.

Vocal Cord Paralysis

VCP is predominantly unilateral in pattern, in which case, symptoms can range from minimal to notable dysphonia, especially progressive hoarseness, and, given the central role of the vocal cords in protecting the airway inlet during swallowing, aspiration symptoms resulting in cough, dyspnea, and pneumonia. At the same time, failure of normal apposition of the cords limits effective coughing and airway clearance. The degree of vocal cord dysfunction ranges from mild paresis with weakened but residual function to complete immobility. The position of the paralyzed cord may be fully lateralized to full medialization. The left vocal cord is much more commonly involved than the right because of the longer path of the recurrent laryngeal nerve looping below the aortic arch and is hence easily entrapped by lung cancers originating in the aortopulmonary window or metastasizing to nodal stations L2, L4, or L5 or by large mediastinal cancers. Bilateral VCP, when present, leads to more severe symptoms, including upper airway obstruction, when both cords are fixed in a medialized position.

The two leading causes of VCP are neoplasia and postsurgical injuries, accounting for between 70 and 80% of adult cases.[39,40] In the cancer patient, iatrogenic causes also include head and neck radiotherapy,[41] but surgical resection of thyroid, head and neck, and mediastinal cancers remains the primary cause. Because of the very different concerns regarding VCP causing airway obstruction and VCP leading to aspiration, the specifics of diagnostic evaluation and therapy of these entities are addressed separately in the respective sections.

Upper Airway Obstruction

Obstruction of the upper airways as a result of cancers of the UAD tract (head and neck, esophagus, and lungs), thyroid, mediastinal structures, and metastatic diseases may present subacutely with progressive symptoms, such as increasing dyspnea, cough, dysphonia, dysphagia, and mild bleeding, or acutely, with life-threatening asphyxiation and massive hemorrhage. The levels of the obstruction may occur anywhere from the soft supraglottic tissues of the hypopharynx to direct involvement of the larynx or the subglottic trachea. The larynx and the trachea together form a semirigid tubular structure in which injuries may irreversibly damage the cartilaginous-membranous network, leading to scarring and fixed stenosis, malacia, or both.

The most common cause of upper airway obstruction in the cancer patient would be direct tumor growth and invasion or extrinsic compression of the tracheobronchial tree by the tumors listed in Table 3. Additional causes are as listed in Table 4, including conditions that may be complications of cancer progression, iatrogenic from cancer therapy, or entirely unrelated.

Critical airway obstruction as a result of vocal cord dysfunction owing to cancer is unusual in that both vocal cords will have to be affected and both vocal cords will have to be paralyzed in a paramedian position to cause critical airflow limitation. In large retrospective series, bilateral (VCP in the adult patient is more commonly secondary to trauma, either owing to external forces or as a result of surgery, especially thyroid resection.[42,43] In the cancer patient, this most commonly results from surgically induced recurrent laryngeal nerve injuries[42,43] or radiation- and other treatment-induced nerve injuries.[44] Rare

cancer-related causes of bilateral VCP included paraneoplastic syndromes, such as bulbar amyotrophic lateral sclerosis secondary to small cell carcinoma.[45] Bilateral VCP may occur in the setting of prolonged endotracheal intubations, especially in patients with conditions of compromised vasculature, including diabetes, stroke, and ischemic heart disease. These individuals have increased risk of developing acute laryngeal injuries from intubations; therefore, cancer patients with these comorbidities who are intubated without immediate prospects of weaning may be candidates for early tracheostomies.[46] Symptomatic or occult gastroesophageal reflux disease is also a predisposing cause of glottic and subglottic stenosis, as well as Barrett's esophagus and esophageal carcinoma.[47] Hence, in cancer patients, especially ones with UAD tract malignancies leading to impaired swallowing function, esophageal cancer patients with resections, and gastric pull-ups or colonic interpositions, reflux as a cause should be considered and evaluated as indicated and preventive measures taken.[48]

Obstruction of the subglottic trachea in the cancer patient may present as a fixed airway narrowing or variable airway collapse. Fixed obstructions are due to extrinsic tracheal

obstruction by upper mediastinal and neck structures, direct tracheal invasion by tumors, or a combination of both processes. Fixed tracheal obstruction may also result from cancer therapies, including external beam radiation, scarring from surgical resection and especially at the anastomotic site, and again as a result of prolonged endotracheal tube intubations. Airway narrowing in the trachea varying with the respiratory cycle, especially during exhalation and cough manuever, is due to tracheomalacia, and in the cancer patient, this may be the result of cancer invasion and destruction of cartilaginous rings, treatment such as thyroidectomy, or a limited tracheal resection or again as a result of tracheal cartilage destruction after prolonged endotracheal intubation or tracheostomy tubes, both of which may cause pressure necrosis of the supportive cartilage.

Hemorrhage may cause upper airway obstruction by direct obstruction of the airway passage or from extrinsic blockage by an enlarging hematoma. Blood clots blocking the trachea and mainstem bronchi leading to potentially life-threatening obstruction have been reported in both pediatric and adult oncology patients.[49,50] In addition to critical narrowing of the airways lumen, the aspirated blood volume, if sufficiently large, may lead to sufficient alveolar filling to impair oxygenation. The source of the blood may originate from anywhere along the oropharynx, larynx, and trachea to oozing or being coughed up from the lung parenchyma itself owing to friable cancer masses or from diffuse alveolar hemorrhage. Retropharyngeal, sublingual, and neck hemorrhages may be spontaneous from a cancer[51] or a malignancy-associated marrow dysfunction[52] and severe enough to cause airway obstruction, or it may be the result of biopsies,[53] postoperative hemorrhage,[54] or anticoagulation therapy.[55–57] Patients with head and neck cancer or lung cancer compounded by severe chronic obstructive pulmonary disease (COPD) may have tracheostomy tubes. Subsequent tracheoinnominate artery fistulae are a rare but potentially devastating cause of bleeding into the airway.[58] Radiation- and chemotherapy-induced mucositis may be severe, leading to diffuse bleeding and oral and esophageal mucosal sloughing. Pain and administered narcotic analgesics and sedatives may further inhibit good airway clearance and cloud the sensorium, and patients may develop frank airway obstruction.[59]

Among the iatrogenic causes of upper airway obstruction, the role of the central lines placed in the jugular or subclavian vessels deserves mention as a large number of cancer patients have long-term indwelling central venous catheters placed for infusion of chemotherapy and nutrition, or they may have temporary lines for hemodynamic monitoring of the administration of fluids, blood products, and medications. Cancer

Table 4 Causes of Upper Airway Obstruction
Physical obstruction by tumor
Intrinsic or by direct extension and invasion
Tumors of tongue
Larynx and hypopharynx
Vocal cords
Trachea and lung
Esophageal
Thyroid
Mediastinal tumors
Metastatic cancers
Extrinsic compression
Thyroid
Esophageal
Mediastinal tumors
Lymphomas
Germ cell tumors
Thymic carcinomas
Malignant adenopathy
Metastatic cancers
Bilateral vocal cord paralysis
Radiation- and chemotherapy-induced mucositis
Tracheobronchial stenosis and post-stenotic segment malacia
Foreign bodies, including food, teeth, and dental appliances that are dislodged or aspirated
Malpositioned artificial airways (endotracheal tubes, tracheostomies, airway stents)
Obstruction of endogenous or artificial airways by secretions, mucus, and/or blood
Airway edema owing to anaphylaxis, angioedema, trauma
Extrinsic compression by hematoma, fluid extravasation
Infections including epiglottitis, pharyngeal and retropharyngeal abscesses
Chemical and heat inhalational airway burn injuries
Congenital anomalies: bronchial and mediastinal cysts in a paratracheal position, piriform sinus cyst, hemangiomas, laryngeal and tracheal webs, tracheolaryngomalacia, vascular anomalies, etc.
Obstructive sleep apnea–related upper airway obstruction
Psychogenic, eg, psychogenic asthma and paradoxic vocal cord dysfunction

patients may have thrombocytopenia and coagulopathy that increase the risk of hemorrhage and impair normal hemostasis. Landmarks used for central venous cannulation may be effaced in the patient with anasarca or the veins collapsed in the dehydrated and debilitated patient. In any case, intravenous fluid extravasation from a malpositioned line,[60] neck hematoma leading to upper airway obstruction,[61] and inadvertent arterial cannulation, with subsequent subcutaneous hemorrhage even leading to death from airway obstruction,[62] have all been reported. Cancer patients may also be hypercoagulable, and even surgically placed tunneled catheters may malfunction when placed into a thrombosed superior vena cava (SVC) and cause a backflow with subsequent upper airway obstruction.[63]

There are many other causes of fixed and variable upper airway obstruction, not specifically related to a malignant condition or antineoplastic therapies, that may predate or develop coincidentally with the cancer diagnosis and subsequent treatment. These are listed in Table 4 as part of the differential diagnosis of upper airway obstruction but are not specifically addressed further in this discussion.

Diagnosis and Evaluation of Upper Airway Obstruction

Patient presentation includes dyspnea, cough, and a variable degree of adventitial breath sounds.[64] Audible stridor and subjective wheezing would occur only with significant compromise of the upper airway lumen, narrowed down to a 4 to 5 mm caliber. The pattern of stridor and wheezing may depend on whether the critical airway narrowing is fixed or variable, as in malacia or edema and hematoma in a location above or below the thoracic inlet.[65] Patients may have difficulty clearing secretions, especially if they also have VCP with incomplete adduction, cancer treatment–related mucositis, neuromuscular weakness, impaired mentation, or any other condition leading to an impaired ability to cough or protect the airways. Exertional dyspnea may also be due to systemic effects of concomitant anemia, advanced COPD, and cardiovascular disease.

Voice change may be due to direct tumor invasion of the larynx and vocal cords or entrapment of one or both of the recurrent laryngeal nerves. The left vocal cord is more likely to be paretic because of the longer path length of the recurrent laryngeal nerve. A patient with known paralysis of one vocal cord and dysphonia who then develops increasing dyspnea while regaining voice quality may be developing fixed bilateral VCP and worsening airway obstruction.

A physical examination should include observation of cutaneous findings of vascular

obstruction leading to SVC syndrome; this would include facial and possibly upper extremity edema, plethora, and prominent skin surface collaterals. Tenderness and swelling, with fluctuance and warmth, may suggest the site of an abscess, hematoma, or fluid extravasation. The trachea should be observed and palpated. Deviation of the trachea may be due to a space-occupying process such as a large parenchymal lung mass or pleural effusion pushing the trachea contralateral, lung volume loss from postoperative changes, or ipsilateral atelectasis. Auscultation and percussion of the chest may detect concomitant pneumonitis and the consolidation and presence of pleural effusion.

For patients who are sufficiently stable as outpatients or who may leave the monitored setting, pulmonary function studies with maximal effort flow-volume loops may clarify whether they have fixed or variable upper airway obstruction and the level of the narrowing by the pattern of flow limitation.[65,66] Baseline lung function studies will also provide a basis for evaluating an objective response to any palliative measures.

Imaging studies of the upper airways are indispensable in the current diagnosis and management of cancer-related upper airway and thoracic problems. Because of the complex anatomy of the UAD tract, planar radiographs of the thorax and neck seldom provide sufficient information about the specific pathology. On the other hand, in the initial evaluation of an unstable patient with upper airway problems who may not tolerate being in a recumbent position, a chest radiograph and posteroanterior and lateral neck films can be easily and rapidly obtained in a monitored setting to provide a global overview of the affected area. The chest radiograph with a properly aligned patient in full inspiratory breath-hold should offer a rapid assessment of gross central airway patency and the presence of any lung masses, infiltrates, pleural effusions, or pneumothoraces that may affect the intrathoracic trachea. Figure 1 illustrates the lateral leftward displacement of the midtrachea by a large right lung tumor. The tracheal air column is narrowed but remains grossly patent. Contrast studies provide additional information by outlining specific structures. Figure 2 illustrates a pharyngeal swallow study of the same patient who complains of dysphagia in addition to dyspnea, hoarseness, cough, and increasing problems with clearing secretions. There is no evidence of a fistula formation, complete esophageal obstruction, or proximal aspiration, but there is impingement and compression of the esophagus. CT has improved significantly such that with multislice detector CT scans, acquisition time is shortened to a single breath-hold and the data can be easily and rapidly manipulated at a workstation to provide three-dimensional imaging information.[67,68]

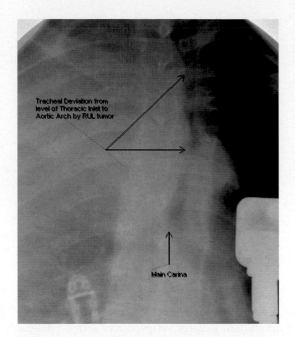

FIGURE 1 Planar anteroposterior upright chest radiograph showing tracheal deviation and narrowing at the level of the thoracic inlet to aortic arch by a large right upper lobe small cell lung cancer.

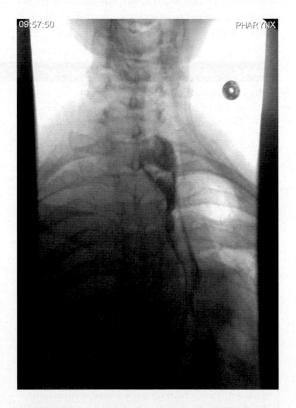

FIGURE 2 A pharyngeal study demonstrates no aspiration but definite esophageal narrowing and is complementary to the planar chest radiograph (see Figure 1).

Unless contraindicated by insufficient renal function or known sensitivity to the intravenous contrast dye, a contrast-enhanced CT scan provides much additional useful information. Given that most, if not all, of the patients in question present with increasing dyspnea and cancers generally increase the risk of thromboembolism, a significant pulmonary embolism may be ruled out at the same time. Contrast enhancement in the chest CT can help distinguish a tumor mass from distal compressive atelectasis. Tumor involvement of the vasculature by direct invasion or extrinsic compression can be assessed and therapeutic decisions regarding the need for vascular stenting or radiotherapy for SVC syndrome taken. Contrast localization of the larger vessels is also important in the planning for surgical or endoscopic interventions to avoid vascular complications. Figure 3 shows the contrast-enhanced CT scan of the same patient in Figures 1 and 2, with greater details of the extent of tumor invasion, including chest wall involvement and developing SVC compression. Another advantage of CT is the ability to view the acquired data in different windows and planar projections. Figure 4 demonstrates even more critical airway narrowing in a patient with concomitant emphysema and radiation fibrosis, all of which contribute to the symptom of dyspnea. MRI and magnetic resonance angiography may more accurately depict vascular anomalies and neural structures, but the length of image acquisition, and with the exception of open magnetic resonance units, may complicate the monitoring of patients with severe upper airway symptoms. These and diagnostic and interventional angiographic studies to detect a significant bleeding source and to direct embolization management of severe bleeding may need to be carried out after elective intubation.

Even with the advent of advanced three-dimensional reconstructions of airways and generation of virtual bronchoscopy "fly-through,"[68,69] direct endoscopic imaging, preferably with anesthetic assistance and emergency surgical standby for tracheostomy, will provide the most direct assessment of the pharyngeal and laryngeal spaces and of the tracheobronchial tree. A variety of rigid and flexible fiberoptic laryngoscopic and bronchoscopic instruments are available.[70] The choice of instrument depends on the purpose of the examination. Initially, a small-caliber instrument with or without a working channel provides visual

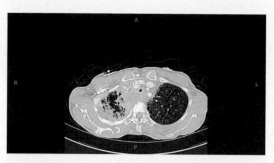

FIGURE 4 A computed tomographic scan demonstrates the extent of critical airways narrowing at the upper trachea caused by concentric tumor encroachment in a patient with progressive non–small cell lung cancer. Note the severe emphysema (*left*) and postradiation scarring (*right*), which is best appreciated in the lung-window setting.

examination and allows passage of a narrowed upper airway segment to assess the integrity of more distal airways.[71] Such small instruments are less likely to induce trauma and further airway edema. Conversely, larger instruments, including rigid bronchoscopes and suspension laryngoscopes with better imaging and suctioning capabilities and the ability to pass accessory instruments, may be needed on follow-up examination to clear secretions, débride obstructing lesions, and deploy stents to maintain the airway patency (Figure 5).[70] These instruments can also be used to secure an airway, whether by passing an endotracheal tube through the rigid instruments or over a flexible endoscope. Hence, endoscopy often encompasses both a diagnostic and a therapeutic component.

In the case of bilateral VCP, provided that the degree of airway obstruction is not critical, a thorough otolaryngology evaluation is performed, including electromyography if direct tumor invasion and involvement of bilateral recurrent laryngeal nerves are not obvious, because in these cases, conservative reconstructive surgery should be

offered rather than destructive procedures, which will leave the patient permanently hoarse, or bypass tracheostomy, with all of its attendant side effects.[72]

Management of Upper Airway Obstruction

The first priority in the management of upper airway obstruction is to preserve the patient's ability to ventilate and to oxygenate. In acute situations, this may require the need for an emergency airway placement, most often by endotracheal intubation but occasionally necessitating emergency tracheostomy or temporizing cricothyroidectomy. Specialized approaches may include the use of jet ventilation to maintain adequate gas exchange when an airway cannot be secured,[73] but the special techniques and technical considerations of surgery are beyond the scope of this discussion. Patients may present with acute airway obstruction anywhere from home to while being monitored in an intensive care unit. In a patient with known cancer, especially one that may involve the upper airways or has progressive symptoms suggestive of upper airway compromise, it is hoped that they will have been assessed and given warning signs for urgent follow-up evaluations to obviate the need for emergency interventions in the field.

For subacute cases of increasing respiratory and gas-exchange compromise, urgent assessment and intervention are still critical, but time and palliative measures may be available to defer immediate invasive airway interventions while the cause for the deterioration is determined. As always, treating the primary cause for the airway compromise is preferable and necessary for a good outcome.

In the hospital setting, especially in institutions in which a number of difficult airways cases are encountered on a regular basis, ideally, there should have been assembled a "difficult airways team" encompassing individuals from disciplines with interest and training in this area. This would include specialists from anesthesia, otolaryngology, pulmonary and critical care, thoracic and foregut surgery, gastroenterology, radiology, and support from respiratory care services. For the general internist or primary care physician triaging the overall care of a cancer patient, the presence of an established team will expedite the evaluation and management of the obstructed airway. Nevertheless, short of an acute deterioration necessitating immediate intubation, some standard orders can be implemented while an urgent assessment proceeds.

Any patients with the potential for a catastrophic airway closure should be placed in a monitored setting, either in the emergency department, a critical care unit, or at least on a

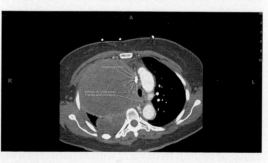

FIGURE 3 Contrast-enhanced computed tomographic scan showing superior vena cava compression, chest-wall involvement, and tracheal compression by tumor.

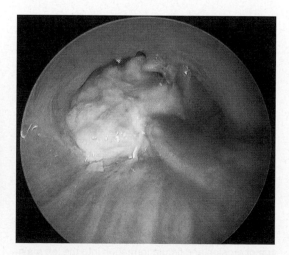

FIGURE 5 Rigid bronchoscopy image of an obstructing central airway non–small cell cancer about to be mechanically débrided.

monitored unit in which cardiac telemetry, circulatory vital signs, and blood oxygen saturations by pulse oximetry are continuously assessed. Unless there is concomitant circulatory arrest, the patient should be encouraged to sit in an upright position and supplemental oxygen as needed provided with adequate humidification since inspissations of tenacious secretions may further compromise a narrowed air passage. Bronchodilators of the β-agonist class and including racemic epinephrine may be given by nebulization, again via a small-volume nebulizer rather than with a metered-dose inhaler (MDI) or by dry powder inhalation (DPI) without humidification. β-Agonists have the advantage of providing airways with smooth muscle relaxation and may assist in mucociliary clearance and in patients with concomitant alveolar edema may assist in alveolar fluid clearance. β-Agonist agents may, however, exacerbate tachyarrhythmias in distressed patients with preexisting cardiac disease who may not tolerate additional adrenergic stimuli. Additional inhalational therapies with quarternary antimuscarinic agents (ipatropium bromide) have proven to have additional benefit in an asthmatic population in the emergency department but may not be extrapolatable to patients with cancer-associated airway narrowing. Corticosteroids are often used to reduce airway edema; however, there would be questionable benefit of giving inhaled steroids, either by standard MDI or DPI preparations in patients with acute airway narrowing. Starting systemic steroids of a stress dosage range between 100 mg of hydrocortisone or 125 mg methylprednisolone (Solu-Medrol) (roughly five times the potency

range) can be given with small risk of severe complications, even in patients with known or suspected glucose intolerance, active infections, or tissue breakdown, such as a mediastinitis or fistulae, as the steroids may be rapidly tapered with the definitive management of airway compromise. Broad-spectrum antibiotic therapy, often empiric, may be started in the cancer patient with upper airway obstruction as these patients are susceptible to infections, may have concomitant neutropenia and impaired mucosal barriers, and are very likely to have follow-up surgical interventions and antineoplastic therapies. The choice of agent should include coverage for oropharyngeal anaerobes and directed therapy against any known pathogen already recovered from the patient.

Although patients with upper airway obstruction and the associated discomforts of dyspnea and other symptoms are understandably anxious, sedative and hypnotic agents should be withheld lest they suppress the respiratory drive and interfere with effective communication. The at-risk patient should be kept fasting and given nothing by mouth to lessen the risk of reflux aspiration during acute intubation and resuscitation if that becomes necessary. As many cancer patients with UAD malignancies have impaired swallowing and are at increased risk of stress gastritis, should they require eventual intubation and mechanical ventilation, empiric therapy with proton pump inhibitors is warranted.[47] Hydration is given intravenously, and these patients should, in fact, always have reliable intravenous access as they may need volume resuscitation and pressor support in the immediate aftermath of intubation and positive pressure ventilation that may precipitously reduce cardiac preload in a malnourished cancer patient who has probably been poorly feeding when he or she has upper airway compromise.

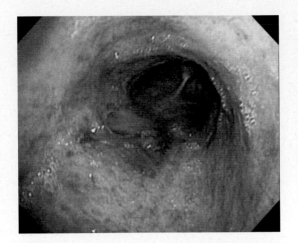

FIGURE 8 Flexible videobronchoscopic image of the tracheal opening of a tracheoesophageal fistula with leakage of methylene Blue dye that had been sipped and swallowed.

The work of breathing may be reduced by several other modes of noninvasive ventilatory assistance. This generally brings to mind noninvasive positive pressure ventilation (NIPPV) in the form of continuous positive airway pressure, bilevel positive airway pressure devices, or a ventilator with pressure support ventilation provided with a tight face mask or nasal mask. However, although there is now ample evidence to support the use of NIPPV in providing temporizing support and thus avoiding the iatrogenic complications of invasive airway ventilation in patients with acute exacerbations of COPD,[74] cardiogenic pulmonary edema,[75] and even with active hematologic malignancies presenting with neutropenia and respiratory insufficiency,[76] in a more recent retrospective analysis of NIPPV, there are insufficient data on this mode of therapy for upper airway obstruction.[77] In fact, in the patient with pure upper airway narrowing without parenchymal lung disease owing to cardiogenic or noncardiogenic edema, COPD exacerbations, or infections, caution must be exercised as the positive pressure may distend the esophagus and abdomen, predisposing the patient to reflux and/or aspirate while the tight mask used will impair communication and the ability to safely vomit. There have been reports of iatrogenic barotraumas leading to pneumomediastinum, especially when anatomic defects, such as esophageotracheal fistulae, may be present.

Another approach at reducing the work of breathing is to reduce airflow turbulence that occurs at the point or length of critical airway stenosis. Helium-oxygen (heliox) gas mixtures at a premixed or blended ratio of 80:20 (percentage ratios of helium to oxygen, with helium replacing nitrogen) or 70:30 are usually available in the respiratory department of most hospitals. Heliox use has a long history of safety in use dating back to 1935[78] in a wide range of patients with airway

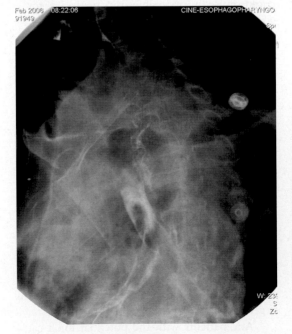

FIGURE 6 Cine-esophagram in an oblique plan showing the leakage of contrast material via an tracheoesophageal fistula into bilateral bronchi.

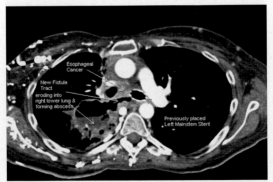

FIGURE 7 Computed tomographic scan of a patient with an esophageal primary cancer with previous tumor erosion and fistula formation into the left mainstem, status stent placement, who now presents with a new fistula connecting into the right lower lung and subsequent abscess formation.

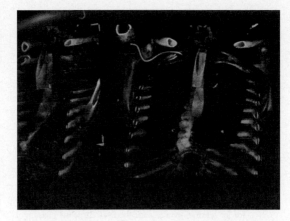

FIGURE 9 Three-dimensional image reconstruction showing the relationship between the tracheal and esophageal stents placed to manage a tracheoesophageal fistula secondary to esophageal primary cancer.

narrowing, from pediatric patients with acute inflammatory epiglottitis to the elderly with multiple comorbidities who have developed upper airway stenosis[79] and specifically in patients with malignancy-associated upper airway obstruction.[64] The limitations of heliox include the limited amount of oxygen that can be mixed in as any percentage of greater than 40% oxygen, or the converse of less than 60% helium, will negate the beneficial effects of reduced airflow turbulence and reduced work of breathing. The choice of whether to select heliox or a higher percentage of oxygen therefore depends largely on the need for supplemetal oxygen.[80] Therefore, for patients with a critical airway narrowing but also with another cause of poor gas exchange, and for patients with neurologic, metabolic, or infectious causes of altered sensorium, endotracheal intubation or elective or emergent tracheostomy may be required for controlled airway management and gas exchange.

When possible, surgical resection of a malignant upper airway obstruction for cure is optimal[31,32]; however, in most instances, palliative treatment measures are more likely. These would include external beam radiotherapy, cytotoxic chemotherapy, and, for the maintenance of airway patency, a variety of interventional endoscopic procedures,[70,81] which are covered in detail in Chapter 44.

Summary

Problems in the upper airways of a cancer patient may present with myriad symptoms and clinical findings. The primary goals, as in the ABCs of life support, are to maintain airway patency and to ensure respiration and adequate gas exchange. Noninvasive supportive maneuvers are preferred; however, given the potential lability of potentially debilitated and unstable patients, careful moni-

toring may be required and preparations made for emergency critical care interventions as the need arises. Upper airway pathology only rarely directly causes circulatory collapse, and iatrogenic causes, such as positive pressure ventilation without adequate volume resuscitation, barotraumas, iatrogenic pneumothoraces, or vascular injuries, should be avoidable. Because the same symptoms may be caused by a variety of pathologies at different levels of the airways and adjacent structures, evaluation should be initially directed by the history. Various imaging modalities often provide the initial and confirmatory diagnostic information, and it is important to retrieve any baseline imaging studies for comparison to determine whether observed findings were actually preexisting and to ascertain the rapidity of any deterioration. Direct physical and endoscopic examination of the oropharynx and laryngeotracheal and esophageal tracts should be performed as indicated. Ideally, an experienced, interested, and cooperative team of specialists, including the otolaryngologist, thoracic and foregut surgeon, pulmonologist, gastroenterologist, anesthesiologist, and diagnostic and interventional radiologist, should be available to lend support to the primary care physician and medical and radiation oncologists. Many patients with cancer-related upper airway problems have curable disease or malignancies that may be put into a period of remission and control. Certain complications, such as paralyzed vocal cords or post-treatment airway stenosis, may not be reversible but can often be remedied. For other, less fortunate patients with progressive and advanced disease, upper airway dysfunction and/or progressive respiratory compromise may herald the inevitable demise. Although supportive and comfort care is always provided, additional palliative procedures may be available, asphyxiation should certainly be avoidable, except in the most challenging cases, and advanced directives should be addressed to avoid further aggressive, often invasive, and, ultimately, futile interventions.

REFERENCES

1. Jemal A, Siegel R, Ward E, et al. Cancer statistics, 2006. CA Cancer J Clin 2006;56:106–30.
2. Cummings otolaryngology-head and neck surgery. 4th ed. St. Louis: Elsevier Mosby; 2005.
3. Rothman KJ, Cann CI, Flanders D, et al. Epidemiology of laryngeal cancer. Epidemiol Rev 1980;2:195–209.
4. Menvielle G, Luce D, Goldberg D, et al. Smoking, alcohol drinking and cancer risk for various sites of the larynx and hypopharynx. A case-control study in France. Eur J Cancer Prev 2004;13:165–72.
5. Alberg AJ, Yung RC, Semet JM. Epidemiology of lung cancer. In: Mason R, editor. Murray & Nadel's textbook of respiratory medicine. 4th ed. Philadelphia: Elsevier Saunders; 2005. p. 1328–48.
6. Rosenberg PS, Socie G, Alter BP, et al. Risk of head and neck squamous cell cancer and death in patients with Fanconi anemia who did and did not receive transplants. Blood 2005;105:67–73.
7. Kutler DI, Auerbach AD, Satagopan J, et al. High incidence of head and neck squamous cell carcinoma in patients

with Fanconi anemia. Arch Otolaryngol Head Neck Surg 2003;129:106–12.
8. Hittelman WN. Genetic instability in epithelial tissues at risk for cancer. Ann N Y Acad Sci 2001;952:1–12.
9. Jang SJ, Chiba I, Hirai A, et al. Multiple oral squamous epithelial lesions: are they genetically related? Oncogene 2001;20:2235–42.
10. Estellar M, Herman JG. Cancer as an epigenetic disease: DNA methylation and chromatin alterations in human tumours. J Pathol 2002;196:1–7.
11. Hung RJ, Hel O, Tartigian SV, et al. Jang SJ, Chiba I, Hirai A, et al. Multiple oral squamous epithelial lesions: are they genetically related? Oncogene 2001;20:2235–42.
12. Vinson PP. Hysterical dysphagia. Minn Med 1922;5:107–8.
13. Paterson DR. A clinical type of dysphagia. J Laryngol Otol.1991;34:289–91.
14. Kelly AB. Spasm at entrance to esophagus. J Laryngol Rhinol Otol 1991;34:285–9.
15. Huang L, Schnapp LM, Gruden JF, et al. Presentation of AIDS-related pulmonary Kaposi's sarcoma diagnosed by bronchoscopy. Am J Respir Crit Care Med 1996;153: 1385–90.
16. Chin R Jr, Jones DF, Pegram PS, et al. Complete endobronchial occlusion by Kaposi's sarcoma in the absence of cutaneous involvement. Chest 1994;105:1581–2.
17. Mochloulis G, Irving RM, Grant HR, et al. Laryngeal Kaposi's sarcoma in patients with AIDS. J Laryngol Otol 1996;110:1034–7.
18. Beitler AJ, Ptaszynski K, Karpel JP. Upper airway obstruction in a woman with AIDS-related laryngeal Kaposi's sarcoma. Chest 1996;109:836–7.
19. Farge D. Kaposi's sarcoma in organ transplant recipients. The Collaborative Transplantation Research Group of Ile de France. Eur J Med 1993;2:339–43.
20. Moray G, Basaran O, Yagmurdur MC, et al. Immunosuppressive therapy and Kaposi's sarcoma after kidney transplantation. Transplant Proc 2004;36:168–70.
21. Rajaratnam K, Desai S. Kaposi's sarcoma of the trachea. J Laryngol Otol 1988;102:951–3.
22. Angouridakis N, Constantinidis J, Karkavelas G, et al. Classic (Mediterranean) Kaposi's sarcoma of the true vocal cord: a case report and review of the literature. Eur Arch Otorhinolaryngol 2006;Feb 23. [E-pub ahead of print]
23. Burgi A, Brodine S, Wegner S, et al. Incidence and risk factors for the occurrence of non-AIDS-defining cancers among human immunodeficiency virus-infected individuals. Cancer 2005;104:1505–11.
24. Bower M, Palmieri C, Dhillon T. AIDS-related malignancies: changing epidemiology and the impact of highly active antiretroviral therapy. Curr Opin Infect Dis 2006;19: 14–9.
25. Frisch M, Biggar RJ, Engels EA, et al. Association of cancer with AIDS-related immunosuppression in adults. JAMA 2001;285:1736–45.
26. Engels EA, Brock MV, Chen J, et al. Elevated incidence of lung cancer among HIV-infected individuals. J Clin Oncol 2006;24:1383–8.
27. Rehberg E, Kleinsasser O. Malignant transformation in non-irradiated juvenile laryngeal papillomatosis. Eur Arch Otorhinolaryngol 1999;256:450–4.
28. Rady PL, Schnadig VJ, Weiss RL, et al. Malignant transformation of recurrent respiratory papillomatosis associated with integrated human papillomavirus type 11 DNA and mutation of p53. Laryngoscope 1998;108:735–40.
29. Cook JR, Hill DA, Humphrey PA, et al. Squamous cell carcinoma arising in recurrent respiratory papillomatosis with pulmonary involvement: emerging common pattern of clinical features and human papillomavirus serotype association. Mod Pathol 2000;13:914–8.
30. Lele SM, Pou AM, Ventura K, et al. Molecular events in the progression of recurrent respiratory papillomatosis to carcinoma. Arch Pathol Lab Med 2002;126:1184–8.
31. McCarthy MJ, Rosado-de-Christenson ML. Tumors of the trachea. J Thorac Imaging 1995;10:180–98.
32. Gaissert HA. Primary tracheal tumors. Chest Surg Clin N Am 2003;13:247–56.
33. Jones AS, Morar P, Phillips DE, et al. Second primary tumors in patients with head and neck squamous cell carcinoma. Cancer 1995;75:1343–53.
34. Yang KY, Chen YM, Huang MH, et al. Revisit of primary malignant neoplasms of the trachea: clinical characteristics and survival analysis. Jpn J Clin Oncol 1997;27: 305–9.
35. Raghavan U, Quraishi S, Bradley PJ. Multiple primary tumors in patients diagnosed with hypopharyngeal cancer. Otolaryngol Head Neck Surg 2003;128:419–25.

36. Muehrcke DD, Surgical treatment of thyroid cancers invading the airway. Surg Rounds 1994;669.

37. Nicolai P, Puxeddu R, Capiello J, et al. Metastatic neoplasms to the larynx: report of three cases. Laryngoscope 1996;106:851–5.

38. Wood DE. Management of malignant tracheobronchial obstruction. Surg Clin North Am 2002;82:621–42.

39. Terris DJ, Arnstein DP, Nguyen HH. Contemporary evaluation of unilateral vocal cord paralysis. Otolaryngol Head Neck Surg 1992;107:84–90.

40. Myssiorek D. Recurrent laryngeal nerve paralysis: anatomy and etiology. Otolaryngol Clin North Am 2004;37:25–44.

41. Lau DP, Yo YL, Wee J, et al. Vocal fold paralysis following radiotherapy for nasopharyngeal carcinoma: laryngeal electromyography findings. J Voice 2003;17:82–7.

42. Holinger LD, Holinger PC, Holinger PH. Etiology of bilateral abductor vocal cord paralysis: a review of 389 cases. Ann Otol 1976;85:428–36.

43. Kearsley J. Vocal cord paralysis (VCP)—an aetiologic review of 100 cases over 20 years. Aust N Z J Med 1981;11:663–6.

44. Khanlou H, Eiger G. Safety and efficacy of heliox as a treatment for upper airway obstruction due to radiation-induced laryngeal dysfunction. Heart Lung 2001;30:146–7.

45. Chang CY, Martinu T, Witsell DL. Bilateral vocal cord paresis as a presenting sign of paraneoplastic syndrome: case report. Otolaryngol Head Neck Surg 2004;130:788–90.

46. Volpi D, Lin PT, Kuriloff DB, et al. Risk factors for intubation injury of the larynx. Ann Otol Rhinol Laryngol 1987;96:684–6.

47. Maronian NC, Azadeh H, Waugh P, et al. Association of laryngopharyngeal reflux disease and subglottic stenosis. Ann Otol Rhinol Laryngol 2001;110:606–12.

48. Jindal JR, Milbrath MM, Shaker R, et al. Gastroesophageal reflux disease as a likely cause of "idiopathic" subglottic stenosis. Ann Otol Rhinol Laryngol 1994;103:186–91.

49. Sanderson PM, Hartsilver E. Acute airway obstruction in a child with acute lymphoblastic leukaemia during central venous catheterization. Paediatr Anaesth 1998;8:516–9.

50. Collins KA, Presnell SE. Asphyxia by tracheobronchial thrombus. Am J Forensic Med Pathol 2005;26:327–9.

51. Draper MR, Sandhu G, Frosh A, et al. Retropharyngeal haematoma causing acute airway obstruction—first presentation of metastatic carcinoma. J Laryngol Otol 1999;113:258–9.

52. Chandrasekara DP, Brennan W. Spontaneous lingual haematoma with airway obstruction in myelodysplastic syndrome: a case report. Aust J Otolaryngol 2004;7:86–9.

53. Roh JL. Intrathyroid hemorrhage and acute upper airway obstruction after fine needle aspiration of the thyroid gland. Laryngoscope 2006;116:154–6.

54. Piper SN, Maleck WH, Kumle B, et al. Massive postoperative swelling of the tongue: manual decompression and tactile intubation as a life-saving measure. Resuscitation 2000;43:217–20.

55. Cohen AF, Warman SP. Upper airway obstruction secondary to warfarin-induced sublingual hematoma. Arch Otolaryngol Head Neck Surg 1989;115:718–20.

56. Duong TC, Burtch GD, Shatney CH. Upper-airway obstruction as a complication of oral anticoagulation therapy. Crit Care Med 1986;14:830–1.

57. Gonzalez-Garcia R, Schoendorff G, Munoz-Guerra MF, et al. Upper airway obstruction by sublingual hematoma: a complication of anticoagulation therapy with acenocoumarol. Am J Otolaryngol 2006;27:129–32.

58. Allan JS, Wright CD. Tracheoinnominate fistula: diagnosis and management. Chest Surg Clin N Am 2003;13:331–41.

59. Chaimberg KH, Cravero JP. Mucositis and airway obstruction in a pediatric patient. Anesth Analg 2004;99:59–61.

60. Clevens RA, Bradford CR. Airway obstruction secondary to central line intravenous fluid extravasation. Arch Otolaryngol Head Neck Surg 1994;120:437–9.

61. Rider MA, Chell J. Iatrogenic haematoma causing airway obstruction in a burned patient. Burns 1994;20:260–1.

62. Lau HP, Lin TY, Lee YW, et al. Delayed airway obstruction secondary to inadvertent arterial puncture during percutaneous central venous cannulation. Acta Anaesthesiol Sin 2001;39:93–6.

63. O'Hara JF Jr, Brand MI, Boutros AR. Acute airway obstruction following placement of a subclavian Hickman catheter. Can J Anaesth 1994;41:241–3.

64. Chen K, Varon J, Wenker OC. Malignant airway obstruction: recognition and management. J Emerg Med 1998;16:83–92.

65. Lunn WW, Sheller JR. Flow volume loops in the evaluation of upper airway obstruction. Otolaryngol Clin North Am 1995;28:721–9.

66. Hyatt RE. Evaluation of major airway lesions using the flow-volume loop. Ann Otol Rhinol Laryngol 1975;84:635–42.

67. Chooi WK, Morcos SK. High resolution volume imaging of airways and lung parenchyma with multislice CT. Br J Radiol 2004;77:S98–105.

68. Hoppe H, Walder B, Sonnenschein M, et al. Multidetector CT virtual bronchoscopy to grade tracheobronchial stenosis. AJR Am J Roentgenol 2002;178:1195–200.

69. Shitrit D, Postinikov V, Grubstein A, et al. Accuracy of virtual bronchoscopy for grading tracheobronchial stenosis: correlation with pulmonary function test and fiberoptic bronchoscopy. Chest 2005;128:3545–50.

70. Yung RC. Endoscopy of the tracheobronchial tree. In: Cummings, Haughey, Thomas, et al, editors. Otolaryngology-head and neck surgery. 4th ed. St. Louis: Elsevier Mosby; 2005. p. 2454–77.

71. Schuurmans MM, Michaud GC, Diacon AH, et al. Use of an ultrathin bronchoscope in the assessment of central airway obstruction. Chest 2003;124:735–9.

72. Hillel AD, Benninger M, Blitzer A, et al. Evaluation and management of bilateral vocal cord immobility. Otolaryngol Head Neck Surg 1999;121:760–5.

73. Standley TD, Smith HL. Emergency tracheal catheterization for jet ventilation: a role for the ENT surgeon? J Laryngol Otol 2005;119:235–6.

74. Bott J, Carroll MP, Conway JH, et al. Randomised controlled trial of nasal ventilation in acute ventilatory failure due to chronic obstructive airways disease. Lancet 1993;341:1555–7.

75. Rusterholtz T, Kempf J, Berton C, et al. Noninvasive pressure support ventilation (NIPSV) with face mask in patients with acute cardiogenic pulmonary edema (ACPE). Intensive Care Med 1999;25:21–8.

76. Hilbert G, Gruson D, Vargas F, et al. Non-invasive continuous positive airway pressure in neutropenic patients with acute respiratory failure requiring intensive care unit admission. Crit Care Med 2000;28:3185–90.

77. Liesching T, Kwok H, Hill NS. Acute applications of noninvasive positive pressure ventilation. Chest 2003;124:699–713

78. Barach AL. The therapeutic use of helium. JAMA 1936;107;1273–80.

79. Berkenbosch JW, Grueber RE, Graff GR. Patterns of helium-oxygen (heliox) usage in the critical care environment. J Intensive Care Med 2004;19:335–44.

80. Ho AM, Dion PW, Karmaker MK, et al. Use of heliox in critical upper airway obstruction. Physical and physiologic considerations in choosing the optimal helium: oxygen mix. Resuscitation 2002;52:297–300.

81. Noppen M, Poppe K, D'Haese J, et al. Interventional bronchoscopy for treatment of tracheal obstruction secondary to benign or malignant thyroid disease. Chest 2004;125:723–30.

Pneumonia in Cancer Patients

Christoph Schmidt-Hieber, MD
Daniel N. Ginn, MPH
John N. Greene, MD

With the increasing number of cancer patients receiving immunomodulating therapy, a growing number of pulmonary infectious complications are developing. These patients are also more likely to develop more severe infections and present in an atypical pattern. Early recognition and timely administration of antimicrobial agents are dependent on the awareness of the clinician of the disease presentation and appropriate imaging and diagnostic testing. Based on the infectious etiology, this chapter reviews common causes of pneumonia in cancer patients.

Bacterial pneumonia is a potentially life-threatening complication in a wide variety of cancer diagnoses and treatments. Many etiologic agents are associated with infections leading to pneumonia, and among the implicated bacteria, five primary organisms and groups are noted: *Streptococcus pneumoniae*, *Legionella* species, gram-negative bacilli, *Staphylococcus aureus*, and *Nocardia* species. Generally, the cancer patients most at risk of bacterial pneumonia are those with chemotherapy-induced neutropenia and patients receiving hematopoietic stem cell transplantation (HSCT). One study reported that during their disease course, approximately 80% of leukemia patients will develop pneumonia and that it is most commonly bacterial in origin.[1]

Bacterial pneumonias generally present atypically as severe sepsis with systemic signs and symptoms in cancer patients with neutropenia.[2,3] Airspace consolidation in the lungs is most commonly caused by bacterial pneumonia. Attributable mortality owing to bacteremic pneumonia in neutropenic patients has been reported at 55%, with 53% for gram-positive cocci and 54.2% for gram-negative bacilli.[2] Pneumonia is the most common cause of acute respiratory failure in cancer patients, which is the most common cause of intensive care unit admission.[3] Mortality rates are generally the highest for patients with ventilator-associated pneumonia and late-stage disease or prolonged neutropenia.[4] Treatment of bacterial pneumonias is typically the same for cancer patients as it is in the general population.[5]

As a consequence of the life-threatening nature of bacterial pneumonia in cancer patients, rapid diagnosis and prompt administration of appropriate antibiotic therapy are essential. The underlying malignancy of a patient can have a significant impact on the etiology of infection, leading to pneumonia, and the patient's immune status is almost always a contributing factor. Keen observation of the immune status of the patient and the antimicrobial resistance patterns in the area are necessary to choose the appropriate treatment for the cancer patient with pneumonia.

S. pneumoniae

S. pneumoniae is an encapsulated gram-positive bacterium and is one of the most common causes of pneumonia in both cancer patients and immunocompetent noncompromised patients.[5] It is typically a community-acquired pathogen and is of increasing concern to the neutropenic patient and as a late infection in HSCT patients with chronic graft-versus-host disease (GVHD).[5,6] Patients with decreased humoral immunity are predisposed to *S. pneumoniae* infection, particularly those with multiple myeloma, chronic lymphocytic leukemia, and Hodgkin's disease who have undergone splenectomy.[5,6–8] The development of neutropenia owing to myeloablative chemotherapy increases the possibility of *S. pneumoniae* infection and the likelihood that previously asymptomatic colonization may become symptomatic.[8] As a cause of 5% of bacteremias in one study, *S. pneumoniae* infection resulted in pneumonia in 71% of those patients.[6] Elsewhere, *S. pneumoniae* has been responsible for 30% of bacteremic pneumonias, including 20% of early-onset pneumonias in neurosurgical patients.[2,9] *S. pneumoniae* has also been implicated as a causative agent of postobstructive pneumonia and aspiration pneumonia, a common complication following laryngectomy.[10,11]

Lung cancer patients are obviously at heightened risk of infection leading to pneumonia. There is an increased risk of respiratory failure and mortality from community-acquired pneumonia (CAP) owing to *S. pneumoniae* in patients with underlying chronic obstructive pulmonary disease (COPD) and malignancy.[10] On a chest radiograph, *S. pneumoniae* infection generally presents as a focal infiltrate that develops in less than 24 hours during the course of pneumonia.[6,12]

Treatment options for community-acquired *S. pneumoniae* pneumonia should be approached syndromically, and efforts to identify the pathogen should be aggressive.[13] Initial treatment for early neutropenic patients with focal infiltrates is the prompt start of empiric broad-spectrum antibiotic therapy.[6] Drug resistance is a paramount concern with *S. pneumoniae*. Approximately 44 to 50% of strains exhibit greatly diminished susceptibility to penicillin, and approximately 16% are fully resistant.[2,6,8] Decreased sensitivity to some β-lactam antibiotics has been reported, with ceftazidime showing poor activity. The recent administration of a β-lactam antibiotic is a risk factor for the appearance of penicillin-resistant strains in adults.[2,8,10] Reported data have also demonstrated in penicillin-resistant *S. pneumoniae* isolates that there is an increase in resistance to erythromycin and cephalosporins, such as ceftriaxone and cefotaxime.[8] Resistance to β-lactam antibiotics has been correlated to increased resistance to macrolides and to trimethoprim-sulfamethoxazole (TMP-SMX). The recommended empiric treatment for *S. pneumoniae* infection is a macrolide, doxycycline, ceftriaxone, or a respiratory fluoroquinolone.[10] Recent studies have also shown all strains to have been susceptible to imipenem and vancomycin.[2] Nevertheless, the likelihood of new resistance remains a cause of concern.

In addition to antibiotics, corticosteroids have been useful in the treatment of severe community-acquired pneumonia[14] and severe viral respiratory infections, such as coronavirus (severe acute respiratory syndrome) and parainfluenza virus (croup in children). A multicenter placebo-controlled study of patients admitted to the intensive care unit with severe CAP demonstrated remarkable results in favor of the use of hydrocortisone. There was a significant improvement in alveolar-arterial oxygen gradient and chest radiograph score, a significant reduction in multiorgan dysfunction syndrome score, C-reactive protein levels, septic shock, length of hospital stay, and mortality in the hydrocortisone treatment arm compared with the placebo arm. Hydrocortisone was infused intravenously as a 200 mg bolus followed by a rate of 10 mg/h for 7 days.

Legionella Species

Of the *Legionella* species that are a threat to the health of cancer patients, *Legionella pneumophila* is responsible for 90% of infections, with serotype 1 responsible for 70% alone.[15] *Legionella* causes an atypical pneumonia (legionnaires' disease) and opportunistically affects patients with malignancies, HSCT patients, and those who are immunosuppressed and/or neutropenic owing to corticosteroid use or chemotherapy; cigarette smoking is also a major risk factor.[7,10,15] A prolonged course of steroid use will put a patient at a 10-fold increased risk of infection.[6] One epidemiologic study has shown that *Legionella* pneumonia is nine times more likely in the immunocompromised host than in the normal population.[16] Unlike *S. pneumoniae*, the primary host defense against *Legionella* is cell-mediated immunity, predisposing both lymphoid leukemia and hairy cell leukemia patients to infection because of their decreased cell-mediated immunity.[15] *Legionella* outbreaks are typically community acquired and are related to some environmental contamination when found nosocomially.[17]

Diagnosis of *Legionella* pneumonia requires a positive urinary antigen, direct fluorescent antibody, or a positive sputum or bronchoalveolar lavage (BAL) culture on charcoal yeast extract.[6,15] Infection is difficult to distinguish based on routine laboratory screenings and chest radiography, but isolation is always indicative of disease.[6,12,15] On a chest radiograph, bilateral or asymmetric infiltrates may be diffuse, cavitary, or nodular and multilobar consolidation is frequently present.[1,5,6,15] Pleural effusion may also been seen on a radiograph.[17] *Legionella* pneumonia follows a subacute progression of symptoms with refractory or late infiltrates that lasts for up to a week or more.[6,12,17] Symptoms include high fever, malaise, myalgia, confusion, multiple rigors, anorexia, and headache.[15] As legionellosis progresses, a slightly productive cough, pleuritic chest pain, hyponatremia, elevated transaminases, gastrointestinal symptoms such as watery diarrhea, and bradycardia may be experienced.[13,15] Left untreated, the pneumonia can progress to stupor, shock, and multiorgan failure and can be fatal. Poor prognostic indicators include acute renal failure, shock, or the need for mechanical ventilation.[18] Although rare, the recurrence of infection is possible in the immunocompromised patient.[15]

In the immunocompromised cancer patient, extrathoracic *Legionella* infection may develop, such as arthritis and encephalitis.[19] Also in those with a compromised immune status, mixed infections are found more commonly than in the immunocompetent. Pathogens found along with *Legionella* include *S. pneumoniae*, *Streptococcus pyogenes*, *Enterococcus faecium*, *Enterobacter*, *Prevotella*, *Listeria*, *Nocardia*, and cytomegalovirus (CMV).[18]

As with other bacterial causes of pneumonia, it is important to begin treatment as soon as possible for *Legionella* pneumonia as it can run a fulminant course in cancer patients. The treatment of any severe CAP should include empiric treatment for *Legionella* as incorrect therapy leads to reported mortality rates approaching 80%. Currently, the best recommended treatment of legionellosis includes new macrolides and fluoroquinolones with or without rifampin. Azithromycin, doxycycline, ofloxacin, ciprofloxacin, and levofloxacin are all preferred to erythromycin.[15]

Gram-Negative Bacteria

There are a number of gram-negative bacteria with the potential to cause pneumonia in the cancer patient. *Pseudomonas aeruginosa*, *Haemophilus influenzae*, *Neisseria meningitidis*, *Klebsiella pneumoniae*, and *Stenotrophomonas maltophilia* are all relevant to the scope of this discussion; however, *P. aeruginosa* and *S. maltophilia* are the most significant. Although there has been an etiologic shift in recent years to gram-positive bacteria as the source of infections in neutropenic patients, 30 to 40% of these infections are due to gram-negative bacteria.[20]

P. aeruginosa is one of the leading causes of bacterial pneumonia in cancer patients.[6,16,20] At the advent of methicillin use, *P. aeruginosa* posed a major threat to persistently neutropenic cancer patients, with a fatality rate of 90%. The β-lactam antibiotics were the first to curb this agent, and the fatality rate has dropped precipitously. One report noted that *P. aeruginosa* and *S. pneumoniae* account for 42 and 30%, respectively, of total pneumonia-causing bacterial infections and that *P. aeruginosa* is responsible for 68% of the gram-negative pneumonias.[20] *P. aeruginosa* infections are primarily nosocomial, and patients with solid tumors and those with acute leukemia are the most affected.[5,20] Also, it is the most frequently isolated bacteria in ventilator-associated pneumonia and is an indicator of poor prognosis.[11,17,21] Patients receiving HSCTs may have coinfection with *P. aeruginosa* and *Aspergillus* species.[16] In neutropenic patients, *P. aeruginosa* may exhibit acute infiltrates with a nodular pattern and cavitation on a chest radiograph.[5,6]

Untreated *Pseudomonas* infections can be rapidly fatal in neutropenic patients. Ever-increasing resistance to available antimicrobial drugs highlights the importance of proper treatment selection. Antipseudomonal penicillins and cephalosporins have declined in efficacy with the emergence of resistance. Multiple studies have measured the resistance of *P. aeruginosa* to meropenem at 6 to 11%; piperacillin, ticarcillin, imipenem, and ceftazidime at 5 to 17%; and cefepime at 17%.[20] Ciprofloxacin resistance has been reported over a range of 21 to 75%, suggesting that corresponding rates are institution specific.[20] After prolonged neutropenia and use of broad-spectrum antibiotics, superinfection with *P. aeruginosa* is possible.[7] Combination therapy recommended for severe *P. aeruginosa* infections includes cefepime, piperacillin-tazobactam, or a carbapenem combined with an aminoglycoside or a fluoroquinolone with antipseudomonal activity. Because of better lung penetration, an antipseudomonal quinolone is preferred over aminoglycosides when used in combination with a β-lactam antibiotic.

S. maltophilia (formerly *Xanthomonas maltophilia*) is an important nosocomial cause of pneumonia in cancer patients. Those infected with *S. maltophilia* tend to have serious underlying conditions, such as lung cancer, acute leukemia, and chronic myelogenous leukemia, resulting in a reported pneumonia mortality rate of 50%.[22] Long-term neutropenia, extended hospitalization (more than 1 week), and the presence of central venous catheters are also risk factors for *S. maltophilia* colonization.[22,23] A reported 42.6% of patients with upper respiratory tract (URT) colonization with *S. maltophilia* developed pneumonia, but for sites other than lung colonization, 14.7% developed pneumonia. The clinical picture of *S. maltophilia* pneumonia is not particularly distinct from other causes of bacterial pneumonia. *S. maltophilia*–induced pneumonia may cause nonspecific alveolar infiltrates and focal areas of necrosis and hemorrhage. In one series, radiographic findings included bilateral infiltration in 50% and pleural effusion in 20%. However, none had cavitation.[22]

The primary challenge presented by *S. maltophilia* is the selection of appropriate therapy as it is especially prone to developing resistance. The agent is universally resistant to imipenem and has shown complete resistance to cefazolin, tobramycin, and amikacin.[22,24] Previous treatment with imipenem is an important risk factor because its ineffectiveness against *S. maltophilia* makes superinfection possible. Other antimicrobials considered to be risk factors include ampicillin, gentamicin, vancomycin, metronidazole, piperacillin, cefotaxime, and ceftazidime.[22,23] Currently effective drugs against *S. maltophilia* strains include ceftazidime, ticarcillin-clavulanate, TMP-SMX, the newer fluoroquinolones and tigecycline of the fluoroquinolones, Moxifloxacin has the highest activity in vitro against *S. maltophilia* (80% susceptibility).[22,23]

S. aureus

S. aureus is also a common cause of life-threatening pneumonia. Infections generally arise in late neutropenia and originate most often from central venous catheters.[9,25,26] In patients receiving HSCTs, matched unrelated and mismatched allogeneic recipients are at risk of more frequent and more severe infection than sibling recipients.[27] Neurosurgical patients may experience early-onset pneumonia and, if there is tracheal colonization, ventilator-associated pneumonia owing to *S. aureus*.[21] Aspiration pneumonia with lung abscess is also a risk of infection.[10,11] The radiographic presentation of *S. aureus* pneumonia includes early focal infiltrates, with cavitary and nodular lesions progressing in less than 24 hours. Abscesses can occur in areas of consolidation where necrosis has developed.[1,5,6,12] A newly discovered virulence factor that produces tissue necrosis has been found in some strains of methicillin-resistant *Staphylococcus aureus* (MRSA), called Panton-Valentine leukocidin (PVL). Severe CAP caused by MRSA carrying the *PVL* gene has been described in healthy adults.[28] In several patients, concomitant influenza A infection contributed to the severity of the illness. Cancer patients could likewise be susceptible to this infection, and MRSA-carrying *PVL* genes should be considered if severe CAP is diagnosed.

This bacterium maintains a genetic plasticity that allows it to continually develop resistance to new antibiotics. MRSA has become a ubiquitous etiology of infection, and resistance to vancomycin, although scarce, is being reported as well.[29] Where resistance has not developed, MRSA frequently demonstrates 100% susceptibility to vancomycin.[25] MRSA susceptibility has been retained by minocycline, TMP-SMX, and a newer agent, linezolid, which has been an effective treatment for nosocomial and ventilator-associated MRSA pneumonia. Recent studies demonstrated the superiority of linezolid over vancomycin for nosocomial MRSA pneumonia and MRSA ventilator-associated pneumonia, with better clinical and microbial response rates and a higher survival rate.[30,31] Another new therapeutic, daptomycin, has shown effectiveness against MRSA but is specifically contraindicated for pneumonia treatment.[2]

Nocardia

Nocardia species are aerobic actinomycetes found universally in soil. *Nocardia* infections are most often due to *Nocardia asteroides* and are pulmonary in nature, affecting patients with lymphomas and lymphocytic leukemias, especially in the terminal stages of disease.[5,32] A review of 1,050 cases of nocardiosis from the 1970s found that 17% of patients had a solid or hematologic malignancy.[33] Prolonged use of corticosteroids (more than 1 month) is a significant risk factor for the development of nocardial infections. Interestingly, neutropenia is not a risk factor for nocardiosis.[32]

Allogeneic HSCT is another risk factor for nocardial infections. One study found that nocardiosis was diagnosed a median of 210 days after transplantation, with an 84% survival rate from the infection.[34] Interestingly, 40% (10 of 25 patients) were receiving oral TMP-SMZ twice-weekly prophylaxis for *Pneumocystis carinii* pneumonia (PCP).

Pulmonary infection presents with fever, night sweats, and cough, but the severity varies with the degree of immunosuppression.[17] Pneumonia caused by *Nocardia* progresses subacutely or chronically with a multifocal pattern, consisting of consolidation and cavitary or nodular lesions that are detectable on a computed tomographic (CT) scan before they can be seen on a chest radiograph.[5,6,12] However, one study indicates that 75% of non–acquired immune deficiency syndrome (AIDS) immunosuppressed patients with pulmonary nocardiosis will exhibit singular nodularity, with only 21% having cavitation.[1] Isolation and identification of *Nocardia* species are diagnostic, and gram staining distinctively shows beaded gram-positive, filamentous rods.[13,16] Distinguishing *Nocardia* from *Actinomyces*, which has a similar Gram stain pattern, requires a modified Kinyoun stain. *Nocardia* is acid-fast positive, whereas *Actinomyces* is acid fast negative.

Nocardia has a propensity to spread to the central nervous system, presenting as a brain abscess, which is frequently asymptomatic. Up to 44% of patients with disseminated nocardiosis will have brain involvement.[33,35] Therefore, all patients with pulmonary nocardiosis should have a CT scan of the brain to rule out central nervous system involvement.

Antibiotics with bactericidal activity are replacing the mainstay of therapy, TMP-SMX, which is bacteriostatic. Treatment for *Nocardia* infections is a combination of a third-generation cephalosporin, such as cefotaxime, or carbapenem and amikacin intravenously followed by oral minocycline or TMP-SMX. Because of the tendency for relapse of *Nocardia* infection, treatment should continue for a prolonged period of time (6–12 months).[32]

Cytomegalovirus

CMV is a member of the Herpesviridae family. More than 50% of adults in the United States and Europe have antibodies against CMV. CMV is a well-known cause of severe infections in HSCT patients, especially following allogeneic HSCT between the first and the third month after transplantation.[36,37] Important risk factors in these patients for developing CMV disease include seropositivity for CMV antibodies of either or both the donor and the recipient, age older than 20 years, GVHD, and failure of reconstitution after HSCT.[38] Prior to the introduction of specific antiviral therapy with ganciclovir and intravenous immunoglobulin (IVIG), CMV pneumonia occurred in 17% of allogeneic SCT patients and had an associated mortality rate of 85%.[37] Since the introduction of preemptive therapy, the overall rate of CMV pneumonia has decreased (6% in one study),[39] but the proportion of patients with late CMV disease (> 100 days after transplantation) has increased,[39,40] and the mortality rate remains high (up to 76%) once pneumonia has developed.[39] Occasionally, *P. carinii* will be found together with CMV in severe pneumonia.

The acute syndrome preceding CMV pneumonia typically consists of flu- or mononucleosis-like symptoms, such as fever and myalgia. Thrombocytopenia, leukopenia, atypical lymphocytosis, and liver function abnormalities may be observed during this time. Once CMV pneumonia has developed, patients present with tachypnea, a nonproductive cough, dyspnea, and unilateral or bilateral rales.[36,41]

On a chest radiograph, pulmonary parenchymal infiltrates will be visible in most patients. The pattern of infiltrates can be consolidation, interstitial, ground-glass, or a combination of all three, and is most often located at the bases of the lungs. More rarely, a nodular pattern or pneumothorax has been described.[42] A CT scan of the lung will most commonly reveals ground-glass opacification, areas of consolidation, and small bilateral nodules.[43]

CMV pneumonia is defined by the presence of symptoms of pulmonary disease combined with the detection of CMV in BAL fluid or lung tissue samples.[44] The preferred diagnostic approaches are deoxyribonucleic acid (DNA) or pp65 antigen detection methods and viral culture. Recently, several real-time polymerase chain reaction (PCR) assays that increase sensitivity and decrease processing time have been described.[45–47]

General prevention strategies in allogeneic SCT patients include matching of seronegative recipients and donors and use of seronegative or leukocyte-reduced blood products. Other than that, two different strategies using antiviral drugs have been studied in recent years: either preemptive or prophylactic treatment. In preemptive therapy, antiviral treatment is started as soon as CMV infection is diagnosed by DNA detection methods or antigenemia assays. By contrast, prophylactic treatment is typically started at engraftment and continued at least during the first 3 months after transplantation. Although several studies have shown prophylactic treatment to decrease early CMV disease, the mortality rate was not changed because of other intercurrent infections and a higher incidence of late CMV disease. Because preemptive treatment seems to reduce mortality, especially when a short-term antigenemia- or DNA-based strategy is used, it has become the strategy favored by most authors for the general situation.[38,40,48] However, prophylactic treatment remains warranted when the risk of severe GVHD is unusually high and when corticosteroids are used for the treatment of GVHD. Usually, no preemptive or prophylactic treatment is required when both donor and recipient are seronegative for CMV. The same holds true for autologous SCT recipients without risk factors.[38,40] Preemptive treatment should be started as soon as CMV is detected in blood by either an antigenemia assay, PCR, or, more rarely, viral culture. Ganciclovir should be used at a dosage of 5 mg/kg twice daily for 1 to 2 weeks, followed by 5 mg/kg daily for 100 days or until no CMV DNA or antigen can be detected on several occasions. Foscarnet at a dosage of 60 mg/kg twice daily can be used instead of ganciclovir when marrow toxicity or ganciclovir resistance is observed.[38,40,48] Prophylactic treatment consists of ganciclovir at a dosage of 5 mg/kg once daily, started at engraftment and continued for 100 days.

Once CMV pneumonia has developed, ganciclovir should be used at a dosage of 5 mg/kg twice a day for 1 or 2 weeks and then at a dosage of 5 mg/kg daily for 3 to 4 weeks. IVIG (500 mg/kg) or CMV immunoglobulin (150 mg/kg) is added every other day for the first 2 weeks and then weekly. Longer treatment may be required in cases of severe immunosuppression. Foscarnet at a dosage of 90 mg/kg twice daily can be used as an alternative to ganciclovir in cases of marrow toxicity or ganciclovir resistance.[40] Other antiviral drugs that have some activity against CMV include valganciclovir and cidofovir. Valganciclovir is an effective oral formulation for treatment of CMV infection with good systemic absorption. Cidofovir is nephrotoxic and is rarely used for the treatment of CMV infection in the setting of HSCT.

Influenza Virus

Influenza virus is one of the most common causes of severe respiratory disease in the world. Most epidemics are caused by influenza A, subtype H3N2, resulting in about 140,000 hospitalizations per year in the United States.[49] Influenza has a typical seasonal distribution, with most cases occurring between November and April.[49,50] Among the cancer population, patients with leukemia and/or undergoing HSCT have an increased risk of developing severe disease from influenza infection. In these patients, the risk of developing influenzal pneumonia has been reported to be between 28 and 80%, with an associated mortality rate of 17 to 33%.[51–55] However, the incidence is relatively low (about 1%), probably owing to prevention measures such as vaccination of both patients and staff. The risk factors for influenza infection include HSCT during the influenza season, female sex, and advanced disease, and the risk factors for progression to pneumonia are lymphocytopenia and steroid use.[54] During the winter of 1993–1994 in Houston, one-third (15 of 45) of adults with leukemia who were hospitalized in a local cancer center with an acute respiratory illness were infected with influenza.[56] Twelve (80%) of the patients infected with influenza virus had pneumonia, and of these, four (33%) died. They expired owing to progressive respiratory failure at a mean of 24 days (range 8–31 days). Patients who died tended to have received chemotherapy more recently and to be more myelosuppressed.

Typical symptoms of respiratory tract infection and pneumonia owing to influenza include fever, productive or nonproductive cough, wheezing, and nasal congestion. More rarely, a sore throat, shortness of breath, myalgia, and chest pain have occurred.[52,57] On a chest radiograph, bilateral or unilateral consolidation and nodular opacities will be seen. A CT scan of the lung will show ground-glass opacities, consolidation, centrilobular nodules, and branching linear opacities.[58]

In the previously mentioned study, the most common presenting symptom in leukemia patients infected with influenza was fever (87%), followed in frequency by cough (73%) and wheezing (67%). Sore throat and nasal congestion were noted, 33% (5 of 15) and 53% (8 of 15) of the time, respectively. Myalgia occurred in only 4 (27%) patients. Five patients had radiographically documented sinusitis (one of whom had concurrent *Aspergillus* sinusitis). Pneumonia was diagnosed at a mean of 8 days (range 0–24 days) after the onset of symptoms in 80% (12 of 15) of the patients. Bilateral infiltrates were noted in 10 patients and unilateral infiltrates in 2. Three (25%) patients with pneumonia were concurrently infected with *Aspergillus* species, respiratory syncytial virus (RSV), and RSV combined with *Candida* species, respectively.

A high frequency of infection occurred in another influenza epidemic recorded in the same city and institution during the winter of 1991–1992.[59,60] Twenty-eight (29%) adult HSCT recipients and 37 (11%) adults with leukemia hospitalized with an acute respiratory illness were infected with influenza virus. The complication rate in those patients was quite high. Seventy-five percent (6 of 8) of the HSCT recipients and 75% (3 of 4) of the leukemia patients with influenza developed pneumonia with a high mortality rate, 17% and 33%, respectively.

Pneumonia complicating influenza is frequently bacterial or mixed bacterial and viral in origin.[56] Cancer patients, especially those with neutropenia, with prolonged corticosteroid therapy, or following HSCT may be particularly vulnerable to coinfection with *Aspergillus* species.

Influenza can be diagnosed by culture or, more rapidly, by antigen assays, neuraminidase activity assays, or reverse transcriptase polymerase chain reaction (RT-PCR). Culturing influenza virus, although time-consuming, may provide important information about the virus subtype and drug resistance[61]; however, RT-PCR has been shown to have a higher sensitivity than viral culture and is therefore now considered the reference standard by some authors.[62] Adequate specimens can be obtained by nasopharyngeal wash, throat swab, or BAL. Using BAL specimens has been reported to increase the diagnostic yield.[63]

Prevention

Although the immune response to immunization with inactive influenza virus vaccine in cancer patients is less than in the general public, its use is highly recommended in this population by the Centers for Disease Control and Prevention.[49,64,65] In addition, chemoprophylaxis is highly recommended in immunosuppressed patients with cancer if they are exposed to the influenza virus. The drug that appears to be the most popular and useful for chemoprophylaxis and treatment for influenza in all populations is the new neuraminadase inhibitor oseltamivir. Its low toxicity, high efficiency, and oral formulation make it favored over the inhaled neuraminadase zanamivir (Relenza). Older drugs that also may be useful for prophylaxis and treatment include amantadine or rimantadine. Of the older drugs, the latter is preferred because of less toxicity. For HSCT patients, vaccination should be begun before transplantation and resumed more than 6 months after transplantation. Chemoprophylaxis with either M2 inhibitors or neuraminidase inhibitors (oseltamivir or zanamivir) should also be considered in times of nosocomial or community outbreaks of influenza.[55,61,66]

Treatment

Both M2 inhibitors and neuraminidase inhibitors are known to be effective in preventing and treating influenza infection in immunocompetent patients. In immunosuppressed HSCT patients, early therapy with oseltamivir or zanamivir has been shown to decrease progression to pneumonia and mortality from influenza infection.[54,67] Since resistance against M2 inhibitors in immunocompromised patients has been reported,[68] it has been suggested that neuraminidase inhibitors should be used either alone or in combination with M2 inhibitors.[54] However, no large-scale clinical studies are available that would justify a general recommendation.

Finally, inhaled ribavirin, used mostly for RSV infections, has also been successfully used in patients with influenza pneumonia. Dosage recommendations are 100 mg twice daily for both rimantadine and amantadine, 10 mg twice daily for zanamivir, and 75 mg twice daily for oseltamivir.[49]

Respiratory Syncytial Virus

RSV, a single-stranded RNA virus of the Paramyxoviridae family, is the most common cause of lower respiratory tract (LRT) disease, such as bronchiolitis and pneumonitis, in infants between 6 weeks and 6 months of age.[69] Among immunocompetent adults, RSV infection usually produces symptoms of the common cold. However, severe respiratory disease is seen in immunocompromised cancer patients with leukemia and those receiving HSCT.[70] RSV infection usually occurs during the winter months, but illness during the summer can occur.[71] RSV can colonize the URT without causing symptoms. However, URT colonization and/or infection frequently lead to LRT infection in HSCT recipients and patients receiving myeloablative chemotherapy. Transmission seems to occur mainly by direct contact with large particulate droplets and/or fomites, with a high risk of nosocomial spread.[72] The mortality rate of RSV pneumonia in immunocompromised patients, especially HSCT recipients, has been reported to approach 100% but can be largely reduced by prompt and adequate therapy.[73–75]

RSV pneumonia in immunocompromised adults typically starts with symptoms of URT infection, such as cough, rhinitis, or sinusitis. Progression to LRT infection is more likely to occur in patients with renal failure, elevated serum lactate dehydrogenase (LDH), or mucositis and recipients of allogeneic HSCT (especially during the immediate post-transplant period) and/or myelosuppressive chemotherapy.[71] RSV has a propensity to cause tracheobronchitis, with resultant necrosis, edema, and increased mucous secretion, resulting in obstruction. Wheezing is a characteristic finding on physical examination. A chest radiograph will show bilateral infiltration in 40%. High-resolution computed tomography (HRCT) of the chest will demonstrate groundglass infiltrates. RSV can be detected by antigen testing (enyzme-linked immunosorbent assay or immunofluorescence) or viral culture. However,

PCR is the most sensitive method for detecting RSV.[76] Although samples can be obtained by nasal wash or throat swab, sensitivity greatly improves when a BAL or an endotracheal aspiration is performed.[77]

In immunocompromised HSCT patients, a combination therapy with aerosolized ribavirin and IVIG has been shown to be effective in RSV URT illnesses and RSV pneumonia.[75,78,79] However, no controlled clinical trials of this regimen have been performed to date, and there is no general consensus on which patients to treat and when to start therapy. Ghosh and colleagues suggested treating patients according to individual risk factors, such as the level of immunosuppression, the age of the patient, the clinical course of the respiratory illness, and the presence of underlying lung disease.[78] A monoclonal antibody against RSV, palivizumab, is 50 to 100 times more active than RSV-specific IVIG and has been approved for prophylactic use in infants at risk of severe RSV infection. Monthly prophylaxis with intramuscular palivizumab has shown a 55% reduction in RSV infection–related hospitalization in premature infants and infants with chronic lung disease (bronchopulmonary dysphasia).[80] It has been reported to be effective in adults following HSCT for prophylaxis and treatment of severe RSV infection as well.[80,81] A short course of therapy with corticosteroids, as shown in several studies of children with RSV tracheobronchitis and croup, may be of benefit.[71,80] The use of aerosolized ribavirin is quickly falling out of favor because of difficulties with administration and a lack of efficacy. Because RSV is transmitted nosocomially at a high frequency, infection control measures, such as contact isolation, gowns, and gloves, are crucial in preventing nosocomial RSV pneumonia outbreaks.[72]

Human Metapneumovirus

Human metapneumovirus (hMPV) was first isolated in 2001 from infants with clinical syndromes closely resembling those caused by RSV infection, including bronchiolitis, croup, asthma exacerbation, and pneumonia.[82] As a member of the Paramyxoviridae family, it belongs to the same subfamily (Pneumovirinae) as RSV. The only other member of its genus (*Metapneumovirus*) identified so far is avian pneumovirus type C, which is known to cause rhinotracheitis in turkeys. Further studies have shown hMPV to be a frequent cause of respiratory tract illness, not only in otherwise healthy infants and children[83] but also in elderly and immunocompromised patients.[84–86] Most cases of hMPV infection have been reported during the winter and early spring months, suggesting a seasonality that is similar to that of RSV infection.[87] Furthermore, some data indicate that hMPV infection might aggravate

respiratory tract disease caused by RSV[88]; however, this finding could not be confirmed in another study.[89] Patients with malignancy are included in a large series of patients with hMPV respiratory infections.[86] However, two patients with cancer and hMPV infection are reported in the literature with significant detail, in a case report fashion.[90,91] Both patients died from severe pneumonia with respiratory failure. One patient was a 17-month-old female with acute lymphoblastic leukemia (ALL),[90] and the other patient was a 33-year-old female also with ALL.[91]

The most common symptoms caused by hMPV include fever, cough, dyspnea, tachypnea, and wheezing. Despite clinical features that are very similar to RSV infection, it has been suggested that hMPV respiratory illness tends to be less severe, with less hypoxemia and dyspnea.[83,86,87] A chest radiograph may show atelectasis, hyperinflation, and infiltrates. HRCT of the chest usually reveals bilateral ground-glass infiltrates. With rapid antigen detection tests being unavailable to date, RT-PCR is currently the method of choice for detecting acute hMPV infection. Adequate primers were recently described by Côté and colleagues.[92] Although samples obtained by nasopharyngeal aspirate have been used in most studies, sensitivity might be increased by BAL as it has been described in the diagnosis of RSV pneumonia.[93]

At the time of writing, no treatment for hMPV infection has been evaluated in any large-scale study. However, a combination of ribavirin and IVIG, as used for RSV infection, has been shown to have some in vitro activity against hMPV and might therefore be considered for severe hMPV respiratory illness in immunocompromised patients.[94]

Rhinovirus

The majority of common cold syndromes are caused by human rhinoviruses (HRVs) and coronaviruses. These are generally considered to replicate principally in the URT. However, severe respiratory infection requiring hospitalization can occur in the elderly and immunosuppressed population. Patients with COPD are particularly at risk of serious infection.[95] In one study, the most common pathogen found as a cause of exacerbation of COPD was the picornaviruses, 75% of which were due to rhinoviruses.[96]

Most patients with common colds present with a self-limited syndrome characterized by nasal obstruction, coryza , sneezing, sore throat, and cough. Fever is uncommon in immunocompetent adults. However, infants, hospitalized elderly patients, and HSCT recipients can develop LRT disease, including viral pneumonia.[97]

One series of myelosuppressed HSCT patients with HRV pneumonia diagnosed by viral culture resulted in a fatal outcome in 32% (7 of 22).[98] All of the patients presented with infection within the first 10 days after transplantation, suggesting nosocomial acquisition.[96] The mean time between the onset of acute respiratory symptoms and respiratory failure was 12 days (range 3–21 days). The duration of viral shedding was 8 days (range 1–18 days). In another study, HSCT recipients with acute pulmonary infiltrates were found to have HRV in 8% (6 of 77 patients) of the cases.[99] All of them were detected by RT-PCR of BAL. Most of the patients presented with HRV infection after the first 100 days after transplantation, which is consistent with a community acquisition of infection. All of the patients had copathogens (three with *Aspergillus* species, three with parainfluenza virus, two with RSV, and one with CMV, *P. aeruginosa*, *S. aureus*, and *S. pneumoniae*). Death occurred in five of six patients, with a mean time of 54 days between illness onset and death. The most sensitive available technique for diagnosing HRV presence is RT-PCR because cell culture is relatively insensitive.[99]

There is no known treatment for severe rhinovirus infection that is readily available. However, a promising agent, pleconaril (a viral capsid function inhibitor), shortens the course of illness but induces the P-450 hepatic enzyme, which could result in drug-to-drug interactions.[95]

Aspergillus

The genus *Aspergillus* consists of more than 600 species, with *A. fumigatus*, *A. flavus*, *A. terreus*, and *A. nidulans* being the most common causes of infection in humans. Because *Aspergillus* species are ubiquitous, infections can occur in the community and in the hospital setting, especially during periods of renovation or construction in the latter case. The respiratory tract is the primary portal of entry, and the pulmonary alveolar macrophage is the first line of defense against infection. Neutrophils and circulating peripheral blood monocytes are the secondary line of defense. Chemotherapy, radiation therapy, and corticosteroids significantly alter these primary and secondary lines of defense to allow for *Aspergillus* infection. The most common risk group that develops invasive pulmonary aspergillosis (IPA) is composed of those with prolonged neutropenia (greater than 7 days) or GVHD and those receiving corticosteroids or another immunosuppressive therapy.

The mortality rates of IPA are 60% or higher in patients with a hematologic malignancy and 80% or higher in patients following allogeneic SCT. The longer the duration of neutropenia, the greater the mortality rate in patients with IPA. A bimodal pattern of IPA has been noted in patients following allogeneic SCT at 16 and 96 days after transplantation, which corresponds to the periods of neutropenia and GVHD, respectively.[100]

The most common clinical finding in patients with IPA includes fever, pleuritic pain, cough (usually nonproductive), and hemoptysis. Decreased breath sounds owing to pulmonary consolidation or a pleural friction rub, which can be evanescent, may be noted on the examination. *Aspergillus* species have a strong predilection to invade blood vessels, resulting in vascular thrombosis, infarction, and tissue necrosis. This, in turn, results in the characteristic radiographic findings, which include bronchopneumonia, lobar consolidation, multiple nodular lesions resembling septic emboli, cavitary lesions, the halo sign, and the air crescent sign. The earliest lesions are best seen by HRCT scans, which can detect infection a week earlier than plain chest radiographs. Peripheral nodular lesions greater than 2 cm are suggestive of *Aspergillus pneumoniae* in high-risk patients. A halo of ground-glass infiltrates can frequently be seen surrounding the dense core of the nodular lesions. In some cases, an air crescent can be visualized within the nodular infiltrates and represents separation of the necrotic center from the hemorrhagic outer rim. After several weeks, cavitation frequently develops from lung necrosis. Although the radiographic findings mentioned above are highly suggestive of IPA in the high-risk patient, definitive diagnosis requires visualization of the pathogen by fungal stains and culture of sputum, BAL, or biopsy of affected tissue. *Aspergillus* species in tissue form angular, dichotomously branching septate hyphae, which are indistinguishable from *Fusarium*, *Scedosporium*, and other pathogenic molds. Culture of *Aspergillus* in the high-risk patient with characteristic radiographic findings is diagnostic of IPA. Serologic testing (galactomannan)[101] and antigen-based testing by PCR are not universally accepted but can be useful for early detection of IPA and for following the response to treatment. Reducing morbidity and mortality from IPA require prophylactic therapy, early detection, effective therapy after diagnosis, and resolution of immunosuppression.

Voriconazole has become the drug of choice for IPA after an improved response, a higher survival rate, and less toxicity were noted when compared with amphotericin B.[102] Combination therapy is considered more effective than monotherapy. Voriconazole combined with caspofungin resulted in a better response rate and a higher survival rate than voriconazole alone in the treatment of IPA.[103] Other drugs that are effective alone or in combination include itraconazole, caspofungin, and lipid formulations of amphotericin B, which are less nephrotoxic than amphotericin B. A newly appoved antifungal, posacongzole, posaconazole, also has excelled activity against Aspergillus as well as other molds, including zygomycosis Granulocyte colony-stimulating factor, granulocyte-macrophage

colony-stimulating factor, or granulocyte transfusions may be used to improve the response to antifungal therapy with IPA.

The duration of therapy ranges from 6 weeks to 6 months depending on resolution of pulmonary lesions by serial CT and the recovery of host immunity. Because the risk of relapse of IPA is over 50% with future episodes of neutropenia, appropriate antifungal therapy is begun with onset.

Fusarium

The *Fusarium* genus belongs to the fungi imperfecti and derives its name from its fusiform spores. It is a ubiquitous fungus and a common soil saprophyte and plant pathogen. In the hospital setting, this mold and other dematiaceous fungi have been shown to be present in water or water-related surfaces and potted plants, which serve as a potential reservoir for infection.[104] In some areas, the rainy season is associated with a two- to sixfold greater incidence of *Fusarium* infections in cancer patients than the drier months.[105] Localized and systemic diseases have been described in the literature in both non-neutropenic and neutropenic hosts. Improved antibiotic treatment, use of prophylactic antibiotics, intensification of antileukemic treatment resulting in profound and prolonged myelosuppression, and HSCT contribute to the emergence of *Fusarium* species as a significant cause of severe, often fatal disease.[104] Almost half of the reported cases of disseminated fusariosis occur in patients with acute leukemia, and prolonged neutropenia is the predominant risk factor.[105] Corticosteroid use has not been identified as a major risk factor for fusariosis and is, therefore, far less frequent than aspergillosis in patients with GVHD receiving corticosteroids.[106] Portals of entry for this fungus include the respiratory tract (nasal passages, sinuses, and lung) and skin, especially between the toes and in the periungal area.

Pulmonary fusariosis resembles aspergillosis with nodular, cavitary, or nonspecific pulmonary infiltrates. The typical course is described as fever, nodular lung lesions or sinusitis, periungal or toe cellulitis, disseminated nodular skin lesions, myalgias, and fungemia. The eventual outcome is resolution with myeloid recovery or death secondary to disseminated infection. Boutati and Anaissie recently reviewed the cases of 43 patients with invasive and/or disseminated fusariosis, all of whom were immunocompromised and most of whom were neutropenic at diagnosis (84%) or undergoing steroid therapy.[107] Skin lesions were present in up to 70% of patients in a review by Richardson and colleagues and in 79% (34 of 43) in the review by Boutati and Anaissie.[107,108] Interestingly, all 18 patients in the latter review who had blood cultures positive for *Fusarium* species had skin lesions. Skin lesions present as multiple painful erythematous subcutaneous nodules approximately 2 to 3 cm in diameter. Occasionally, the lesions form a black necrotic eschar and may ulcerate. Clinical and histopathologic findings of septate branching hyphae, with a propensity for vascular invasion and thrombus formation, are very similar to those for other mold infections. A unique feature of *Fusarium* species, in contrast to other molds, such as *Aspergillus*, is the high rate of positive blood cultures, up to 50% in some reports, and the frequent finding of skin lesions.[104] The frequent finding of fungemia is thought to be due to the propensity for intravascular sporulation of *Fusarium*, which is not a characteristic of *Aspergillus*.

Outcome generally relates to recovery of bone marrow and the overall condition of the host. Susceptibility to antifungal therapy seems to be a significant factor, with *Fusarium* shown to be consistently resistant to 5-fluorocytosine and variably sensitive to amphotericin B and amphotericin B lipid formulations posaconazole, ketoconazole and miconazole.[104] Voriconazole alone or combined with amphotericin B lipid formulations remains the drug of choice. Recurrent infection has been described, generally among patients with repeated episodes of neutropenia.[107] Therefore, prompt reinstitution of antifungal therapy and a search for evidence of recurrence during subsequent neutropenic episodes are essential.[104] HSCT recipients may develop infection before or after engraftment, even when they have adequate neutrophil counts. Overall, the prognosis remains poor with disseminated disease, and early diagnosis and aggressive combination antifungal therapy and surgery or débridement, coupled with leukocyte transfusions or growth factors, remain the best approach.[104]

Scedosporium

Infections owing to *Scedosporium* are primarily caused by *S. apiospermum* and *S. prolificans* (inflatum). *Scedosporium apiospermum* is the asexual form of *Pseudallescheria boydii*, better known as the most common cause of Madura foot in the United States. This phaeohyphomycete, found commonly in soil, standing water, and sewage, has been known to cause locally invasive infections and systemic fungemia in the immunocompromised patient.[110] Locally invasive infections are usually caused by traumatic or penetrating injuries that introduce the fungus into deep tissues, as in Madura foot or mycetoma.[109] Other deep tissue infections have been described, including osteomyelitis, endocarditis, sinusitis, parotitis, pneumonia, and brain abscess.[109] Although *S. apiospermum* infections have been described in immunocompetent patients, disseminated infection is far more common in the immunocompromised host, with prolonged neutropenia or chronic GVHD, or in those receiving corticosteroids or amphotericin B.[110] *Scedosporium* is inherently resistant to amphotericin B.

In one review of the literature, 25 disseminated *Scedosporium* species infections in cancer patients were reported, with a mortality rate of 96%.[110] The time from the onset of symptoms of disseminated infection until death ranged from 1 to 29 days (average 12 days). All patients had a hematologic malignancy in various stages of therapy; 15 patients were receiving amphotericin B therapy when their cultures were positive for *Scedosporium* species.

The triad of fever, nodular skin lesions, and myalgia, once considered to be pathognomonic of disseminated candidiasis (especially *Candida tropicalis*), is common in patients with disseminated *Scedosporium* and *Fusarium*.[105] In addition, positive blood cultures are common with disseminated *Scedosporium* and *Fusarium* but are rare when *Aspergillus* disseminates.[105]

Invasive *Scedosporium* pulmonary disease resembles aspergillosis, with fever, cough, pleuritic pain, and hemoptysis being the most common.[111] In one study, the most common clinical features among the 25 patients with disseminated infection included fever (92%), pulmonary symptoms (48%), central nervous system findings (44%), rash (28%), and arthralgias or myalgias (16%).[110] Findings on chest radiography or CT of the lungs are similar to those of invasive pulmonary aspergillosis with nodular consolidation that may develop cavitation. Multiple brain infarcts can be seen by CT or magnetic resonance imaging of the brain when dissemination to the central nervous system develops. Culture of the organism from involved sites by sputum, BAL, or biopsy sampling is required for diagnosis. The acute angle branching and septation of hyphae seen on histopathology for *Scedosporium* cannot be distinguished from *Aspergillus* and other molds.

Scedosporium is resistant to amphotericin B. Lipid formulations of amphotericin B have been successfully used for *Scedosporium* infections in case reports.[105] However, voriconazole is the drug of choice for *Scedosporium* infections, possibly combined with a lipid formulation of amphotericin B. Posaconazole also has based invitro antivity against Scedosporium. Ultimate recovery from all mold infections is dependent on resolution of neutropenia.

Zygomycosis

Zygomycosis is an opportunistic infection caused by organisms belonging to the class Zygomycetes. The organisms most commonly implicated in clinical disease belong to the genera *Mucor*, *Rhizopus*, *Absidia*, and *Cunninghamella*, with *Rhizopus* being the most common. These organisms are widely disseminated in the environment, and most of the infections are due to the inhalation of spores.

Zygomycosis is an uncommon acute and often fatal opportunistic fungal infection that is classically seen with poorly controlled diabetes mellitus with acidosis, acute leukemia, or other immunosuppressive conditions. Neutrophils and monocytes or macrophages are the essential host defense factors against the Zygomycetes. Patients with acute leukemia are at high risk of developing zygomycosis as a result of prolonged neutropenia. A relatively new association of zygomycosis occurring in patients with iron and aluminum excess who receive deferoxamine therapy has been reported with increasing frequency.[111] Although most commonly noted in patients receiving hemodialysis, zygomycosis develops in patients with various iron overload states such as thalassemia, sideroblastic anemia, and myelodysplasia in which deferoxamine may be used.

The clinical manifestations of zygomycosis consist of rhinocerebral, pulmonary, gastrointestinal, cutaneous, and disseminated infection. The rhinocerebral form is the most common presentation. Rhinocerebral zygomycosis is found most commonly in uncontrolled diabetics with ketoacidosis and then in patients with prolonged neutropenia. It is associated with the development of sinusitis with involvement of the orbit leading to proptosis and ophthalmoplegia. Pulmonary zygomycosis more often occurs in patients with leukemia or lymphoma with prolonged neutropenia.[112] Symptoms of pleuritic chest pain, fever, cough, and hemoptysis with radiographic findings of consolidation and cavity formation are indistinguishable from those of pulmonary aspergillosis.[112]

Hematogenous dissemination can result in brain, spleen, kidney, heart, liver, and omentum metastatic infection. Pulmonary zygomycosis has a predilection to spread to the brain. Cerebral forms of zygomycosis are more like to de?? in patients with a hematologic malignancy and associated neutropenia. Regardless of the anatomic site of the lesion, invasion of blood vessels results in downstream tissue necrosis, and a black necrotic eschar develops if the skin is involved. The diagnosis of zygomycosis is best made by biopsy of involved tissues with histopathology and fungal culture. Microscopy will reveal broad, irregularly shaped, ??? nonseptate hyphae with right-angled branching. The fungi are often seen invading through tissue planes and blood vessels. Thrombosis and resultant infarction of the surrounding tissue ensue. The diagnosis of pulmonary zygomycosis is rarely made antemortem as the yield from sputum fungal smears, culture, and BAL is low.[112]

Without early aggressive therapy, zygomycosis is almost always fatal. Therapy consists of early surgical débridement, administration of amphotericin B or lipid formulations of amphotericin B, and correction of the underlying disease process. Lipid formulations of amphotericin B allow for administration of amphotericin B at higher doses with less nephrotoxicity.[113] Posaconazole with in-vitro antivity against zygomycetes, can be used alone or in combination with lipid formulations of amphotericin B. If surgical débridement or the correction of the underlying conditions is not possible, then the response from medical treatment alone is poor. A better therapeutic response is obtained in patients with diabetic ketoacidosis and zygomycosis than in patients with underlying leukemia and lymphoma because ketoacidosis can be quickly corrected and the sinus, rather than the lung, is usually affected. Therapy with high-dose lipid formulations of amphotericin B, combined with aggressive surgery and immune reconstitution, offers the best chance for survival of cancer patients with zygomycosis.[113] If consolidation chemotherapy is needed in patients with a history of zygomycosis, prophylaxis with amphotericin B or its lipid formulations or posaconazole can prevent a relapse of infection.[114]

P. Carinii Pneumonia

P. carinii is a unicellular eukaryote thought to be a protozoon for more than 80 years. Its taxonomy had remained unclear until 1988, when Edman and colleagues demonstrated it to be a fungus by analyzing its ribosomal ribonucleic acid.[115] *P. carinii* was named after Antonio Carini, who discovered the organism in rats in 1912. A new name for the cause of *Pneumocystis* infection in humans was recently selected: *P. jiroveci*, after Otto Jirovec, who demonstrated the organism in premature newborns who died of interstitial plasma cell pneumonia in l951.[116] We use *P. carinii* in place of *P. jiroveci* in this chapter owing to its familiarity and extensive use in the literature. Most children have acquired antibodies against *P. carinii* by the age of 4 years.[117] Primary infection is usually asymptomatic, and the latency of the organism seems to occur in some cases.[118] However, several studies now suggest that PCP is due to reinfection rather than to reactivation of latent infection.[119] It has been known as a complication in both human immunodeficiency virus (HIV)-positive and HIV-negative immunocompromised patients with T-lymphocyte disorders for a long time.[120,121] In the AIDS population, PCP may develop in more than 75% of persons in the absence of chemoprophylaxis.[122] Because of standard prophylaxis for PCP with TMP-SMX in HIV-infected patients with a CD4 lymphocyte count below 200 cells/mL, PCP has been much less common in this population in recent years. However, in cancer patients, PCP may be increasing because of more intensive and prolonged suppression of cellular immunity with corticosteroids and

monoclonal antibodies. In addition, mortality owing to PCP is higher in cancer patients compared with AIDS patients, partly because of late recognition of the infection.

Several large studies of PCP in HIV-negative patients published recently found that lymphocytic leukemias and lymphomas predominated.[123–126] A few patients had multiple myeloma, acute and chronic myelogenous leukemia, and solid tumors. The primary risk factors were cytotoxic chemotherapy, prolonged corticosteroid therapy, and SCT. Admission to the intensive care unit was required for 45 and 56% of patients in two of the studies, respectively.[124,126] In the same two studies, 30 and 41% required mechanical ventilation, and the mortality rate was 33 and 38%, respectively.[124,126] Poor prognostic indicators were prolonged corticosteroid therapy, a high respiration rate, a high heart rate, an elevated C-reactive protein level, an elevated serum LDH level, and mechanical ventilation.

Antecedent corticosteroid use is cited in 80 to 94% of cases of non-HIV PCP.[126–130] Paradoxically, corticosteroid treatment predisposes patients to PCP and also improves the outcome once PCP occurs. The use of corticosteroid therapy to treat PCP in immunosuppressed patients without HIV was only recently proved to be as effective as in HIV-positive patients.[131] As illustrated in many published series, the high incidence of corticosteroid use as adjuvant therapy may account for the decreased mortality in recent years.[127–129,132]

PCP historically has been noted in children with ALL who are receiving corticosteroids and intensive chemotherapy.[133] It is now relatively uncommon in this age group because of the routine use of TMP-SMX prophylaxis. In adults with ALL, PCP generally occurs during consolidation or early maintenance therapy.[134] However, earlier presentations may occur with more intensive chemotherapy. Because of the association of PCP with the tapering of corticostroids, many ALL treatment protocols institute intermittent TMP-SMX prophylaxis following induction chemotherapy.[135]

Of all of the solid organ tumors, brain cancer metastasis—both primary and secondary—is associated with the highest incidence of risk of PCP. The incidence ranges from 1.7 to 6%.[136,137] The predisposition to PCP stems from long-term use of corticosteroids to reduce cerebral edema in patients with brain tumors.[130,136,137] Two-thirds of cases of PCP become symptomatic during corticosteroid taper. A dose reduction in long-term corticosteroid therapy may unmask an ongoing pulmonary inflammation from PCP that initially developed while the patient was receiving immunosuppressive therapy.

Patients with brain tumors who are receiving corticosteroid treatment for more than 5 weeks are at risk of PCP, especially when the dose is

tapered. Among patients with brain tumors, those with primary central nervous system lymphoma are at the highest risk of PCP, with a mortality of nearly 50%.[138,139] The major risk factors are corticosteroid, high-dose methotrexate, and radiation therapy, all of which reduce CD4 cell counts.

HIV patients with PCP classically present with a gradual onset of fever, nonproductive cough, and dyspnea over a few weeks. However, PCP causes a somewhat different manifestation in HIV-negative immunocompromised patients, in whom symptoms develop more rapidly (few days) and appear to be more fulminant and severe than in AIDS patients.[140] Patients with cancer infected with PCP are hospitalized earlier and present with a more acute disease. The respiration rate is higher (39 breaths per minute vs 22 breaths per minute) and the arterial oxygen partial pressure value (52 mm Hg vs 69 mm Hg) is lower in cancer patients than in patients with HIV infection.[130,140] On physical examination, auscultation of the lungs is often normal, although it may sometimes reveal wheezing, rales, or rhonchi.

Laboratory findings that are helpful in diagnosing PCP include arterial blood gases and serum LDH. Arterial blood gases reflect the severity of pulmonary involvement and typically show hypoxia and an increase in the alveolar-arterial oxygen gradient.[141] LDH is elevated in most cases of PCP, as it is in other diseases causing lung parenchymal damage. Therefore, its increase is nonspecific, but a normal LDH will help rule out PCP with a high negative predictive value.[142]

Classic findings on a chest radiograph show diffuse interstitial infiltration, and, rarely, cystic or cavitary lesions and pneumothorax can be seen.[141] Because the chest radiograph may be normal, HRCT is indicated when the clinical suspicion of PCP is high. The usual finding on an HRCT scan is bilateral ground-glass alveolar infiltration with interstitial pneumonia.[142]

Final diagnosis of PCP can be made only by identification of the organism. Since *P. carinii* cannot be cultured, sputum samples or BAL fluid will have to be obtained for histochemical staining and subsequent microscopic examination. Appropriate staining techniques include the Gomori methenamine silver stain, modified Wright-Giemsa stain, and, more recently, immunofluorescent stain, which increases sensitivity and specificity.[143]

Since the 1970s, multiple clinical trials have clearly shown that TMP-SMX decreases the incidence and mortality of PCP. Currently, TMP-SMX remains the drug of choice for treatment and prevention and is recommended by the Infectious Diseases Society of America for all patients at risk of PCP. Standard treatment starts with intravenous administration at a dose of 15 to 20 mg/kg trimethoprim per day and can be switched to the oral form of the drug when improvement occurs. The duration of treatment is 3 weeks, followed by prophylaxis for 6 months. On rare occasions, mutations in *P. carinii* associated with TMP-SMX failure have been reported, indicating that resistance may be emerging. However, the major limitation of TMP-SMX therapy is side effects. Allergic reactions, primarily rash and myelosuppression, are the most common toxicities that require drug discontinuation.

Alternatives to TMP-SMX include aerosolized pentamidine or dapsone for prophylaxis; intravenous pentamidine, trimetrexate, or combination clindamycin-primaquine for treatment; and the newer agent, atovaquone, which is useful for both treatment and prophylaxis.

In cancer patients, if TMP-SMX prophylaxis is not tolerated, the second drug of choice is atovaquone. One study found that PCP prophylaxis with atovaquone was better tolerated and associated with less toxicity than TMP-SMX following autologous HSCT. In other studies, prophylaxis with dapsone and inhaled pentamidine following HSCT was associated with higher rates of PCP when compared with TMP-SMX.

Adjunctive corticosteroid therapy has been shown to improve survival and decrease the occurrence of respiratory failure in severe cases of PCP both in patients with AIDS[144] and in non-HIV patients.[145] Corticosteroids should be added if the arterial oxygen tension is below 70 mm Hg while on room air.

Mycobacterium tuberculosis

Tuberculosis (TB) is a dramatic problem worldwide, with 2 billion people (one-third of the world's population) infected with *Mycobacterium tuberculosis*. In cancer patients, especially following HSCT, a high incidence of TB might be expected owing to the resultant cellular immunodeficiency from cancer therapy. However, in spite of the worldwide high prevalence, TB has not been described in cancer patients to the extent expected. Nonetheless, the incidence of TB in cancer patients after HSCT has been estimated to be 10 to 40 times higher than in the general population.[146] A similarly high estimated incidence of TB has been found in solid organ transplant patients, in whom TB has been much better studied than in HSCT patients, with more than 270 cases reported.[146] Countries with a high prevalence of TB would be most likely to see significant numbers of cancer patients with active disease. Most of the literature on TB in cancer patients is in the HSCT population.

In Taiwan, where pulmonary TB is endemic, 8 of 350 SCT recipients were found to have pulmonary TB over a 6-year period.[147] The relative risk of having pulmonary TB after HSCT was 13.1-fold higher than in the general population. There was a trend toward an increased risk of having pulmonary TB in allogeneic HSCT patients compared with autologous HSCT patients. All eight patients with pulmonary TB received allogeneic HSCT, and most (seven of eight patients) developed the infection during treatment for GVHD. CT of the chest was normal in one patient, with the rest showing either interstitial (two patients) or alveolar infiltrates (five patients) at the onset of pulmonary TB. The four fatal cases had an obviously shorter duration between HSCT and the onset of infection.

Another study found four patients with *Mycobacterium tuberculosis* infection identified from 641 adult patients who received a HSCT over a 12-year period (prevalence 0.6%).[148] The pretransplantation diagnosis was acute myelogenous leukemia in two patients and chronic myelomonocytic leukemia in the other two. The sites of infection were the lung (two patients), spine (one patient), and central nervous system (one patient). The onset of infection ranged from 120 days to 20 months post-HSCT. Two patients had coexisting CMV infection. One patient had graft failure. The two patients who received anti-TB therapy recovered from the infection.

Of five HSCT series with a total of more than 5,000 patients, only 10 cases of *M. tuberculosis* infection were described, with an overall incidence of 0.19%.[149] The median age of the 10 patients who developed TB was 29 years (range 17–40 years). The median time for onset of symptoms was 150 days (range 23–550 days), with the patients mainly presenting with fever and cough, with infiltrates on a chest radiograph. A respiratory tract specimen, mostly sputum, yielded positive smears for acid-fast bacilli in three patients and positive *M. tuberculosis* culture in eight patients, whereas lung tissue histology was the first diagnostic test in two patients. Treatment with standard anti-TB drugs for a longer duration was highly effective, with no excessive side effects. The risk factors identified for development of TB included allogeneic HSCT, total-body irradiation, and chronic GVHD.[150]

The Infectious Diseases Working Party of the European Blood and Marrow Transplant Group conducted a survey to obtain information about the frequency, presentation, and treatment of mycobacterial infection (MBI) in HSCT recipients.[150] Among 29 centers, MBI was diagnosed in 0.79% of 1,513 allogeneic and 0.23% of 3,012 autologous HSCT recipients during 1994–1998 a median of 160 days after transplantation. The mean interval between first symptoms and diagnosis was 29 days and was still longer for patients with atypical MBI or recipients of corticosteroid therapy. The prevalence of MBI was highest among those who received matched unrelated or mismatched HSTC's from related donors. Of 31 patients, 20 had TB, 8 had atypical MBI, and 3 had diagnoses based on histologic findings only.

Five patients (16%) died, all of whom had received an allogeneic HSCT.

A national survey of TB after HSCT was undertaken to study the incidence, clinical presentation, and outcome.[146] Twenty confirmed cases were found among 8,013 patients (8 in 5,147 autologous and 12 in 2,866 allogeneic HSCT's). The estimated incidence in cases/10 patients/year was 101 (56.5–145) for the whole group, 71.1 (21.8–120) in autologous transplant patients, and 135.6 (58.9–212) in allogeneic transplant patients. Compared with the general population, TB was more frequent after allogeneic (relative risk 2.95) but not after autologous HSCT. TB after HSCT is a late infection (median 324 days posttransplantation), predominantly affects the lungs (80% of the cases), and appears to respond well to treatment but has a high mortality rate (25%) in allogeneic recipients. It can also complicate the post-transplantation management as anti-TB drugs frequently decrease the serum levels of cyclosporine, causing an aggravation of GVHD.[146] GVHD, corticosteroid treatment, and total-body irradiation appear to be associated with TB in allogeneic recipients.[146]

In summary, pulmonary TB is uncommon in cancer patients. Countries and areas with endemic TB will, by nature of frequent exposure, encounter more cancer patients with active disease. As in AIDS patients, those with cancer and profound immunosuppression will have a greater likelihood of developing active infection (the lifetime risk in AIDS patients is 50%) when exposed to TB. In addition, extrapulmonary disease would be expected to be more common in immunosuppressed cancer patients as in AIDS patients (more than 50% of cases). Treatment of TB is the same in the cancer patient as in the noncancer patient, but the potential for drug interactions will be more common. Other than allogeneic HSCT recipients, prognosis with effective therapy is the same in cancer and noncancer patients.

Nontuberculous Mycobacteria

Nontuberculous mycobacteria (NTM) are ubiquitous in the environment and have been recovered from fresh and salt water (including hot water pipes), soil, animals, and milk and food products. Colonization of body surfaces and secretions can occur naturally and without causing disease. As the incidence of TB has declined in the United States and other developed countries, NTM are now the most common isolates detected from clinical specimens. Prior to the AIDS epidemic, most cases of NTM produced an indolent, cavitary pulmonary infection in nonimmunosuppressed patients, mostly male, with COPD or previous TB.[151]

In HIV-infected patients, NTM, mostly *Mycobacterium avium* complex (MAC), usually causes disseminated infection. Pulmonary findings are not as common as fever of unknown origin, with diffuse lymphadenopathy in AIDS patients. Prophylaxis for NTM is a standard recommendation for HIV-infected patients with a CD4 lymphocyte count less than 100 cells/mL.

In cancer patients, NTM can cause catheter-related infections, bacteremia, skin and soft tissue infections, pneumonia, and disseminated infections. Patients with leukemia, lymphoma, or HSCT and those requiring prolonged corticosteroid therapy are at highest risk of NTM infection.

As with TB in cancer patients, NTM infections are more commonly reported in HSCT recipients, who tend to be more profoundly immunosuppressed and thus more likely to develop active disease. An increase in NTM infections in HSCT patients has been observed and may reflect increased numbers of transplants, intensification of immunosuppressive regimens, prolonged survival of transplant recipients, and/or improved diagnostic techniques.[152] The difficulty of diagnosis and the impact associated with infections owing to NTM in HSCT necessitates that, to ensure prompt diagnosis and early initiation of therapy, a high level of suspicion for NTM disease should be maintained.[152] The most common manifestations of NTM infection in HSCT recipients include cutaneous and pleuropulmonary disease and catheter-related infections.[152]

Mycobacterium kansasii is the most virulent of the NTM and usually presents as lung disease that is nearly identical to TB. The major predisposing factor to lung infection is COPD, which is present in over two-thirds of cases. Lung cancer, lymphocytic leukemia, and lymphoma are the most common associated malignancies. The clinical presentation is similar to pulmonary TB, with fever, weight loss, cough, and hemoptysis.[151] Cavitation occurs in 85 to 95% of cases, being bilateral in 20%. In some cases, the cavities tend to have thinner walls and less surrounding parenchymal infiltration than in TB.[153] Treatment is similar to that for *M. tuberculosis*, with rifampin, isoniazid, pyrazinamide, and ethambutol (except without pyrazinamide because of inherent resistance).[151] The duration of treatment, 18 months, is the same for noncancer patients. Radiologic improvement, symptom resolution, and sputum conversion to negative are expected during therapy.

Mycobacterium avium complex

Pulmonary symptoms owing to MAC may be present for months or years before the diagnosis is made. The median interval from onset of symptoms to the correct diagnosis was reported to range from 25 weeks to 10 months.[154] Early cases may be asymptomatic and discovered only by routine screening chest radiographs. Most patients experience chronic cough, usually productive of purulent sputum but usually without hemoptysis. Constitutional symptoms, including fever, night sweats, weight loss, malaise, lethargy, and fatigue, are not common unless patients have extensive lung disease. Symptoms usually improve with successful therapy.

Patients with underlying lung disease and MAC infection often have cavities apparent on the chest radiograph.[154] It has been suggested that MAC-related cavities tend to be thinner, with less surrounding parenchymal opacification and more contiguous but less distal bronchogenic spread of opacification than in TB.[154] In middle-aged and older women without underlying lung disease, MAC primarily involves the lingula and right middle lobe associated with bronchiectasis and subcentimeter peripheral nodules.[154] This entity is known as Lady Windermere syndrome, after the play with the same name.[155] Often reticular changes, a single nodule, or multiple small nodules are present. Pleural effusions are not common in MAC lung infections.

HRCT is more sensitive than chest radiography for detecting the abnormalities associated with MAC lung disease.[156] The presence of bronchiectasis and multiple small nodules is predictive of MAC lung disease, especially when they are adjacent to each other.[156] In a study, one-quarter of patients with typical changes of fibronodular bronchiectasis produced sputum that grew MAC on culture.[156] Other reported abnormalities include atelectasis, consolidation, "tree in bud," and ground-glass opacities.[156] Serial CT in MAC lung disease has shown that bronchiectasis tends to become more severe and nodules spread to other segments over time.[156] The development of consolidation and ground-glass opacities is preceded by the appearance of nodules. Some small nodules will disappear with successful treatment.[156]

The reported rates of treatment success have ranged from 20 to 90% in individual studies, but if patients who were unable or unwilling to complete treatment, those requiring surgery, those who died, and those with relapse during an adequate follow-up period are included, the cure rate is approximately 40%.[156] Serious toxicity limited the number of medications, dose, and duration of therapy in these regimens.[156] Some have suggested that adjusting therapy to sensitivity testing results improves outcome in MAC lung disease, but others have not been able to show a benefit.[156]

The newer macrolides, clarithromycin and azithromycin, are concentrated in alveolar macrophages and have good activity against MAC, an intracellular organism.[156] Clarithromycin and azithromycin, administered alone or in combination with other medications, are effective for pneumonia owing to MAC in cancer patients. Emergence of resistance to the macrolide may be prevented by the addition of ethambutol, rifabutin, or streptomycin. Newer fluoroquinolones (such as moxifloxacin and levofloxacin) and linezolid may also be useful for treatment of MAC and other mycobacteria, such as *Mycobacterium tuberculosis* and rapidly growing mycobacteria (RGM). The recognition that these patients have a failure of the interferon-γ pathways has led to some preliminary studies of cytokine therapy in MAC lung disease, and preliminary results suggest that interferon-γ may have a role in the treatment of MAC.[156]

Rapidly Growing Mycobacteria

RGM will grow on solid media in less than 7 days, unlike other NTM and TB, which grow slowly. *M. fortuitum*, *M. chelonae*, and *M. abscessus* are the most common RGM-causing infections in cancer patients. Other risk factors include underlying lung disease (such as emphysema), achalasia and rheumatologic conditions, HSCT, and cancers that require immunosuppressive therapy. *M. chelonae* primarily causes cutaneous disease, whereas *M. fortuitum* and *M. abscessus* primarily cause lung infection. One report reviewed the epidemiology and clinical manifestations of 154 patients with RGM pulmonary disease and found that 82% was due to *M. abscessus*.[157]

Most patients with pneumonia owing to RGM are white, female nonsmokers who are at least 60 years of age.[158] Forty percent have an underlying medical condition, such as previously treated pulmonary MAC, cystic fibrosis, lipoid pneumonia, achalasia, or lung transplantation.[159] The symptoms, signs, and radiographic findings are indistinguishable from those of MAC pneumonia. Treatment of RGM is very similar to that of MAC infection and is reviewed above and in Daley and Griffith.[158] If limited disease is found, surgical resection of the involved lung may be curative. Patients with pulmonary or disseminated NTM infections can be safely transplanted by receiving effective antimicrobial therapy before, during, and after HSCT.[152]

Mycobacterium bovis

Bacille Calmette-Guérin (BCG) is a live attenuated strain of *Mycobacterium bovis* and when administered intravesicularly is an effective treatment for patients with superficial transitional cell carcinoma of the bladder. By inducing granulomatous inflammation, the host immune system destroys the cancer in the mucosa and submucosa of the bladder.

Although infection owing to dissemination of *M. bovis* outside the bladder is rare, it can be quite debilitating. One report of adverse effects of BCG therapy reported in a study of more than 1,200 patients included a 2.9% incidence of high fever (>39°C), 1.0% major hematuria, 0.9% granulomatous prostatitis, 0.7% granulomatous pneumonitis or hepatitis, 0.5% arthritis or arthralgia, 0.4% epididymo-orchitis, 0.4% life-threatening BCG sepsis, 0.3% urethral obstruction, 0.2% bladder contracture, 0.1% renal abscess, and 0.1% cytopenia.[159]

The mechanism of complications in patients after disseminated BCG infections is that the hematogenous spread of mycobacteria to sites such as the liver, bone, or lung induces direct organ damage, and a hypersensitivity response to *M. bovis* occurs at the same time. For this reason, the recommended treatment for patients with severe *M. bovis* infections in the acute setting is a combination of antimycobacterial therapy and corticosteroids.[160] Symptoms of BCG dissemination with pneumonitis include shortness of breath, nonproductive cough, fever, sweats, weight loss, and malaise.[160] Radiographic findings are best seen with HRCT scans of the chest with a miliary pattern of 2 to 5 mm nodules seen in the lower lobes of the lung.[160] Diagnosis requires open lung biopsy since BAL or biopsy is usually unsuccessful. However, the readily apparent clinical diagnosis and usual response to appropriate therapy preclude the need for a surgical diagnosis. PCR for *M. bovis* of a blood sample may be positive during active dissemination of BCG from the bladder. Treatment of disseminated BCG or pneumonia includes isoniazid and rifampin for 3 to 6 months. Corticosteroids are considered when severe symptoms or a poor response to antimicrobial therapy occurs.

REFERENCES

1. Hiorns MP, Screaton NJ, Müller NL. Acute lung disease in the immunocompromised host. Radiol Clin North Am 2001;39:1137–51.
2. Carratala J, Roson B, Fernandez-Sevilla A, et al. Bacteremic pneumonia in neutropenic patients with cancer: causes, empirical antibiotic therapy, and outcome. Arch Intern Med 1998;158:868–72.
3. Pastores S. Diagnosing acute respiratory failure in patients with cancer, part 1. J Respir Dis 2003;24:492–8.
4. Pastores S. Managing acute respiratory failure in patients with cancer, part 2. J Respir Dis 2003;24:543–7.
5. Cunha BA. Pneumonias in the compromised host. Infect Dis Clin North Am 2001;15:591–612.
6. Collin BA, Ramphal R. Pneumonia in the compromised host including cancer patients and transplant patients. Infect Dis Clin North Am 1998;12:781–805.
7. Rolston KVI. The spectrum of pulmonary infections in cancer patients. Curr Opin Oncol 2001;13:218–23.
8. Gill JK, Field T, Vincent AL, et al. Antibiotic susceptibility among penicillin-resistant pneumococcal isolates in cancer patients. Infect Med 2003;20:439–44.
9. Greene JN. Infectious complications in stem cell transplant recipients. In: Greene JN, editor. Infections in cancer patients. New York: Marcel Dekker; 2004. p. 151–61.
10. Somboonwit C, Craig C, Greene JN. Infections in patients with lung cancer. In: Greene JN, editor. Infections in cancer patients. New York: Marcel Dekker; 2004. p. 187–97.
11. Somboonwit C, Greene JN. Infections in patients with head and neck cancer. In: Greene JN, editor. Infections in cancer patients. New York: Marcel Dekker; 2004. p. 177–85.
12. White P. Evaluation of pulmonary infiltrates in critically ill patients with cancer and marrow transplant. Crit Care Clin 2001;17:647–70.
13. Talbot EA, Hicks CB. Opportunistic thoracic infections: bacteria, viruses, and protozoa. Chest Surg Clin North Am 1999;9:167–92.
14. Confalonieri M, Urbino R, Potena A, et al. Hydrocortisone infusion for severe community-acquired pneumonia. Am J Respir Crit Care Med 2005;171:242–8.
15. Tsambiras PE, Tsambiras BM, Greene JN, et al. Legionella pneumophila pneumonia in cancer patients: case report and review. Infect Dis Clin Pract 2000;9:261–8.
16. Agustí C, Rañó A, Sibila O, Torres A. Nosocomial pneumonia in immunosuppressed patients. Infect Dis Clin N Am 2003;17:785–800.
17. Somboonwit C, Greene JN. Pulmonary infections in cancer patients. In: Greene JN, editor. Infections in cancer patients. New York: Marcel Dekker; 2004. p. 289–306.
18. Pedro-Botet ML, Sabria-Leal M, Sopena N, et al. Role of immunosuppression in the evolution of legionnaires' disease. Clin Infect Dis 1998;26:14–9.
19. Roig J, Sabria M, Pedro-Botet ML. Legionella spp.: community acquired and nosocomial infections. Cur Opin Infect Dis 2003;16:145–51.
20. Bodey GP. Pseudomonas aeruginosa infections in cancer patients: have they gone away? Curr Opin Infect Dis 2001;14:403–7.
21. Stoll CM, Vincent AL. Infections in patients with brain tumors. In: Greene JN, editor. Infections in cancer patients. New York: Marcel Dekker; 2004. p. 163–76.
22. Fujita J, Yamadori I, Xu G, et al. Clinical features of Stenotrophomonas maltophilia pneumonia in immunocompromised patients. Respir Med 1996;90:35–8.
23. Schaumann R, Stein K, Eckhardt C, et al. Infections caused by Stenotrophomonas maltophilia—a prospective study. Infection 2001;29:205–8.
24. Abbas AA, Fryer CJ, Felimban SK, et al. Stenotrophomonas maltophilia infection related mortality during induction in childhood acute lymphoblastic leukemia. Med Pediatr Oncol 2003;41:93–4.
25. Aksu G, Ruhi MZ, Akan H, et al. Aerobic bacterial and fungal infections in peripheral blood stem cell transplants. Bone Marrow Transplant 2001;27:201–5.
26. Kolbe K, Domkin D, Deriga HG, et al. Infectious complications during neutropenia subsequent to peripheral blood stem cell transplantation. Bone Marrow Transplant 1997; 19:143–7.
27. van Kraaij MGJ, Verdonck LF, Rozenberg-Arska M, Dekker AW. Infections post-transplant—early infections in adults undergoing matched related and matched unrelated/mismatched donor stem cell transplantation: a comparison of incidence. Bone Marrow Transplant 2002; 30:303–9.
28. Francis JS, Doherty MC, Lopatin U, et al. Severe community-onset pneumonia in healthy adults caused by methicillin-resistant Staphylococcus aureus carrying the Panton-Valentine leukocidin genes. Clin Infect Dis 2005; 40:100–7.
29. Anstead GM, Owens AD. Recent advances in the treatment of infections due to resistant Staphylococcus aureus. Curr Opin Infect Dis 2004;17:549–55.
30. Wunderink RG, Bello J, Cammarata SK, et al. Linezolid vs. vancomycin, analysis of two double-blind studies of patients with methicillin-resistant Staphylococcus aureus nosocomial pneumonia. Chest 2003;124:1789–97.
31. Kollef MH, Rello J, Cammarata SK, et al. Clinical cure and survival in gram-positive ventilator-associated pneumonia: retrospective analysis of two double-blind studies comparing linezolid with vancomycin. Intensive Care Med 2004;30:388–94.
32. Watkins A, Greene JN, Vincent AL, Sandin RL. Nocardial infections in cancer patients: our experience and a review of the literature. Infect Dis Clin Pract 1999;8:294–300.
33. Beaman BL, Burnside J, Edwards B, et al. Nocardial infections in the United States 1972-1974. J Infect Dis 1976; 134:286.
34. van Burik J, Hackman RC, Nadeem SQ, et al. Nocardiosis after bone marrow transplantation: a retrospective study. Clin Infect Dis 1997;24:1154–60.
35. Lederman ER, Crum NF. A case series and focused review of nocardiosis: clinical and microbiologic aspects. Medicine (Baltimore) 2004;83:300.
36. Fishman JA, Rubin RH. Infection in organ-transplant recipients. N Engl J Med 1998;338:1741–51.
37. Meyers JD, Flournoy N, Thomas ED. Risk factors for cytomegalovirus infection after human marrow transplantation. J Infect Dis 1986;153:478–88.
38. Zaia JA. Prevention and management of CMV-related problems after hematopoietic stem cell transplantation. Bone Marrow Transplant 2002;29:633–8.
39. Nguyen Q, Champlin R, Giralt S, et al. Late cytomegalovirus pneumonia in adult allogeneic blood and marrow transplant recipients. Clin Infect Dis 1999;28:618–23.
40. Boeckh M, Nichols WG, Papanicolaou G, et al. Cytomegalovirus in hematopoietic stem cell transplant recipients: current status, known challenges, and future strategies. Biol Blood Marrow Transplant 2003;9:543–58.
41. Williams DM, Krick JA, Remington JS. Pulmonary infection in the compromised host. Part II. Am Rev Respir Dis 1976;114:593–627.
42. Olliff JFC, Williams MP. Radiological appearances of cytomegalovirus infections. Clin Radiol 1989;40:463–7.
43. Franquet T, Lee KS, Muller NL. Thin-section CT findings in 32 immunocompromised patients with cytomegalovirus pneumonia who do not have AIDS. AJR Am J Roentgenol 2003;181:1059–63.
44. Ljungman P, Griffiths P, Paya C. Definitions of cytomegalovirus infection and disease in transplant recipients. Clin Infect Dis 2002;34:1094–7.
45. Boeckh M, Huang M, Ferrenberg J, et al. Optimization of quantitative detection of cytomegalovirus DNA in plasma by real-time PCR. J Clin Microbiol 2004;42:1142–8.
46. Hong KM, Najjar H, Hawley M, Press RD. Quantitative real-time PCR with automated sample preparation for diagnosis and monitoring of cytomegalovirus infection in bone marrow transplant patients. Clin Chem 2004;50:846–56.
47. Ikewaki J, Ohtsuka E, Satou T, et al. Real-time PCR assays based on distinct genomic regions for cytomegalovirus reactivation following hematopoietic stem cell transplantation. Bone Marrow Transplant 2005;35:403–10.
48. Meijer E, Boland GJ, Verdonck LF. Prevention of cytomegalovirus disease in recipients of allogeneic stem cell transplants. Clin Microbiol Rev 2003;16:647–57.
49. Centers for Disease Control and Prevention. Prevention and control of influenza. Recommendations of the Advisory Committee on Immunization Practices. MMWR Morb Mortal Wkly Rep 2004;53(RR06):1–40.
50. World Health Organization. Influenza in the world. Wkly Epidemiol Rec 2004;79:385–92
51. Whimbey E, Elting LS, Couch RB, et al. Influenza A virus infections among hospitalized adult bone marrow transplant recipients. Bone Marrow Transplant 1994;13: 437–40.
52. Yousuf HM, Englund J, Couch R, et al. Influenza among hospitalized adults with leukemia. Clin Infect Dis 1997;24: 1095–9.
53. Ljungman P, Ward KN, Crooks BN, et al. Respiratory virus infections after stem cell transplantation: a prospective study from the Infectious Diseases Working Party of the European Group for Blood and Marrow Transplantation. Bone Marrow Transplant 2001;28:479–84.
54. Nichols WG, Guthrie KA, Corey L, Boeckh M. Influenza infections after hematopoietic stem cell transplantation: risk factors, mortality, and the effect of antiviral therapy. Clin Infect Dis 2004;39:1300–6.
55. Hayden FG. Prevention and treatment of influenza in immunocompromised patients. Am J Med 1997;102:55–60.
56. Yousuf HM, Englund J, Couch R, et al. Influenzae among hospitalized adults with leukemia. Clin Infect Dis 1997;24: 1095–9.
57. Oliveira EC, Marik PE, Colice G. Influenza pneumonia. A descriptive study. Chest 2001;119:1717–23.
58. Oikonomou A, Müller NL, Nantel S. Radiographic and high-resolution CT findings of influenza virus pneumonia in patients with hematologic malignancies. AJR Am J Roentgenol 2003;181:507–11.
59. Whimbey E, Elting LS, Couch RG, et al. Influenza A virus infection among hospitalized adults bone marrow transplant recipients. Bone Marrow Transplant 1994;13: 437–40.
60. Elting LS, Whimbey E, Lo W, et al. Epidemiology of influenzae A virus infection in patients with acute or chronic leukemia. Support Care Cancer 1995;3:198–202.
61. Salgado C, Farr BM, Hall KK, Hayden FG. Influenza in the acute hospital setting. Lancet Infect Dis 2002;2:145–55.
62. Ruest A, Michaud S, Deslandes S, Frost EH. Comparison of the Directigen A+B test, the QuickVue influenza test, and clinical case definition to viral culture and reverse transcription-PCR for rapid diagnosis of influenza virus infection. J Clin Microbiol 2003;41:3487–93
63. Rañó A, Agustí C, Jimenez P, et al. Pulmonary infiltrates in non-HIV immunocompromised patients: a diagnostic approach using non-invasive and bronchoscopic procedures. Thorax 2001;56:379–87.

64. Centers for Disease Control and Prevention. Guidelines for preventing opportunistic infections among hematopoietic stem cell transplant recipients. Recommendations of CDC, the Infectious Disease Society of America, and the American Society of Blood and Marrow Transplantation. MMWR Morb Mortal Wkly Rep 2000;49(RR10):1–128.
65. Hayden FG. Prevention and treatment of influenza in immunocompromised patients. Am J Med 1997;102:55–60.
66. Cooper NJ, Sutton AJ, Abrams KR, et al. Effectiveness of neuraminidase inhibitors in treatment and prevention of influenza A and B: systematic review and meta-analyses of randomised controlled trials. BMJ 2003;326:1235–41.
67. Johny AA, Clark A, Price N, et al. The use of zanamivir to treat influenza A and B infection after allogeneic stem cell transplantation. Bone Marrow Transplant 2002;29: 113–5.
68. Englund JA, Champlin RE, Wyde PR, et al. Common emergence of amantadine- and rimantadine-resistant influenza A viruses in symptomatic immunocompromised adults. Clin Infect Dis 1998;26:1418–24.
69. Simoes EAF. Respiratory syncytial virus infection. Lancet 1999;354:847–52.
70. Whimbey E, Englund JA, Couch RB. Community respiratory virus infections in immunocompromised patients with cancer. Am J Med 1997;102 Suppl 3A:10–8.
71. Araisse EJ, Mahfouz TH, Aslan T, et al. The natural history of respiratory syncytial virus infection in cancer and transplant patients: implications for management. Blood 2004;103:1611–7.
72. Raad I, Abbas J, Whimbey E. Infection control of nosocomial respiratory viral disease in the immunocompromised host. Am J Med 1997;102 Suppl 3A:48–52.
73. Whimbey E, Champlin RE, Englund JA, et al. Combination therapy with aerosolized ribavirin and intravenous immunoglobulin for respiratory syncytial virus disease in adult bone marrow transplant recipients. Bone Marrow Transplant 1995;16:393–9.
74. Bowden RA. Respiratory virus infections after marrow transplant: the Fred Hutchinson Cancer Research Center experience. Am J Med 1997;102 Suppl 3A:27–30.
75. Machado CM, Vilas Boas LS, Mendes AVA, et al. Low mortality rates related to respiratory virus infections after bone marrow transplantation. Bone Marrow Transplant 2003;31:695–700.
76. van Elden LJR, van Kraaij MGJ, Nijhuis M, et al. Polymerase chain reaction is more sensitive than viral culture and antigen testing for the detection of respiratory viruses in adults with hematological cancer and pneumonia. Clin Infect Dis 2002;34:177–83.
77. Englund JA, Piedra PA, Jewell A, et al. Rapid diagnosis of respiratory syncytial virus infections in immunocompromised adults. J Clin Microbiol 1996;34:1649–53.
78. Ghosh S, Champlin RE, Englund J, et al. Respiratory syncytial virus upper respiratory tract illnesses in adult blood and marrow transplant recipients: combination therapy with aerosolized ribavirin and intravenous immunoglobulin. Bone Marrow Transplant 2000;25:751–5.
79. Whimbey E, Champlin RE, Englund JA, et al. Combination therapy with aerosolized ribavirin and intravenous immunoglobulin for respiratory syncytial virus disease in adult bone marrow transplant recipients. Bone Marrow Transplant 1995;16:393–9.
80. Boeckh M, Berrey MM, Bowden RA, et al. Phase 1 evaluation of the respiratory syncytial virus-specific monoclonal antibody palivizumab in recipients of hematopoietic stem cell transplants. J Infect Dis 2001;184:350–4.
81. El Saleeby CM, Suzich J, Conley ME, DeVincenzo JP. Quantitative effects of palivizumab and donor-derived T cells on chronic respiratory syncytial virus infection, lung disease, and fusion glycoprotein amino acid sequences in a patient before and after bone marrow transplantation. Clin Infect Dis 2004;39:e17–20.
82. van den Hoogen BG, de Jong JC, Groen J, et al. A newly discovered human pneumovirus isolated from young children with respiratory tract disease. Nat Med 2001;7: 719–24.
83. Williams JV, Harris PA, Tollefson SJ, et al. Human metapneumovirus and lower respiratory tract disease in otherwise healthy infants and children. N Engl J Med 2004;350: 443.
84. van den Hoogen BG, van Doornum GJJ, Fockens JC, et al. Prevalence and clinical symptoms of human metapneumovirus infection in hospitalized patients. J Infect Dis 2003;188:1571–7.
85. Cane PA, van den Hoogen BG, Chakrabarti S, et al. Human metapneumovirus in a haematopoietic stem cell transplant recipient with fatal lower respiratory tract disease. Bone Marrow Transplant 2003;31:309–10.
86. Boivin G, Abed Y, Pelletier G, et al. Virological features and clinical manifestations associated with human metapneumovirus: a new paramyxovirus responsible for acute respiratory-tract infections in all age groups. J Infect Dis 2002;186:1330–4.
87. Hamelin ME, Abed Y, Boivin G. Human metapneumovirus: a new player among respiratory viruses. Clin Infect Dis 2004;38:983–90.
88. Greensill J, McNamara PS, Dove W, et al. Human metapneumovirus in severe respiratory syncytial virus bronchiolitis. Emerg Infect Dis 2003;9:372–5.
89. Lazar I, Weibel C, Dziura J, et al. Metapneumovirus and severity of respiratory syncytial virus disease. Emerg Infect Dis 2004;10:1318–20.
90. Palletier G, Dery P, Yacine A, et al. Respiratory tract reinfections by the new human metapneumovirus in an immunocompromised child. Emerg Infect Dis 2002;8:976–8.
91. Cane PA, van den Hoogen BG, Chakrabarti S, et al. Human metapneumovirus in a hematopoietic stem cell transplant recipient with fatal lower respiratory tract disease. Bone Marrow Transplant 2003;31:309–10.
92. Côté S, Abed Y, Boivin G. Comparative evaluation of real-time PCR assays for detection of the human metapneumovirus. J Clin Microbiol 2003;41:3631–5.
93. Englund JA, Piedra PA, Jewell A, et al. Rapid diagnosis of respiratory syncytial virus infections in immunocompromised adults. J Clin Microbiol 1996;34:1649–53.
94. Wyde PR, Chetty SN, Jewell AM, et al. Comparison of the inhibition of human metapneumovirus and respiratory syncytial virus by ribavirin and immune serum globulin in vitro. Antiviral Res 2003;60:51–9.
95. File TM. Viral respiratory tract infections: increasing importance and a new pathogen. Curr Opin Infect Dis 2003;16: 125–7.
96. Greenberg SB, Allen M, Wilson J, et al. Respiratory viral infections in adults with and without chronic obstructive pulmonary disease. Am J Respir Crit Care Med 2000;162: 167–73.
97. Bowden RA. Respiratory virus infections after marrow transplant: the Fred Hutchinson Cancer Research Center experience. Am J Med 1997;102:27–30, 42–3.
98. Ghosh S, Champlin R, Couch R, et al. Rhinovirus infections in myelosuppressed adult blood and marrow transplant recipients. Clin Infect Dis 1999;29:528–32.
99. Ison MG, Hayden FG, Kaiser L, et al. Rhinovirus infections in hematopoietic stem cell transplant recipients with pneumonia. Clin Infect Dis 2003;36:1139–43.
100. Wald A, Leisenring W, van Burik JA, Bowden RA. Epidemiology of Aspergillus infections in a large cohort of patients undergoing bone marrow transplantation. J Infect Dis 1997;175:1459–66.
101. Marr KA, Balajee SA, McLaughlin L, et al. Detection of galactomannan antigenemia by enzyme immunoassay for the diagnosis of invasive aspergillosis: variables that affect performance. J Infect Dis 2004;190:641–9.
102. Herbrecht R, Denning DW, Patterson TF, et al. Voriconazole versus amphotericin B for primary therapy of invasive aspergillosis. N Engl J Med 2002;347:408–15.
103. Marr KA, Boeckh M, Carter RA, et al. Combination antifungal therapy for invasive aspergillosis. Clin Infect Dis 2004; 39:797–802.
104. Poblete SJ, Greene JN, Sandin RL. Disseminated *Fusarium* in the immunocompromised host. Infect Dis Clin Pract 1998;7:339–44.
105. Jahagirdar BN, Morrison VA. Emerging fungal pathogens in patients with hematologic malignancies and marrow/stem-cell transplant recipients. Semin Respir Infect 2002; 17:113–20.
106. Chandrasekar PH. Fungi other than Candida and Aspergillus. In: Wingard JR, Bowden RA, editors. Management of infection in oncology patients. Martin Dunitz; 2003. New York, London, pp. 203–221.
107. Boutati EI, Anaissie EJ. Fusarium, a significant emerging pathogen in patients with hematologic malignancy: ten years' experience at a cancer center and implications for management. Blood 1997;90:999–1008.
108. Richardson SE, Bannatyne RM, Summerbell RC, et al. Disseminated fusarial infection in the immunocompromised host. Rev Infect Dis 1988;10:1171–81.
109. Husain S, Munoz P, Forrest G, et al. Infections due to Scedosporium apiospermum and Scedosporium prolificans in transplant recipients: clinical characteristics and impact of antifungal agent therapy on outcome. Clin Infect Dis 2005;40:89–99.
110. Strickland LB, Greene JN, Sandin RL, et al. *Scedosporium* species infections in cancer patients: three cases and review of the literature. Infect Dis Clin Pract 1998;7: 4–11.
111. Venkattaramanabalaji GV, Foster D, Greene JN, et al. Mucormycosis associated with deferoxamine therapy after allogeneic bone marrow transplantation. Cancer Control 1997;4:168–71.
112. Kontoyiannis DP, Wessel VC, Bodey GP, et al. Zygomycosis in the 1990s in a tertiary-care cancer center. Clin Infect Dis 2000;30:851–6.
113. Larkin JA, Montero JA. Efficacy and safety of amphotericin B lipid complex for zygomycosis. Infect Med 2003;20: 201–6.
114. Nosari A, Oreste P, Montillo M, et al. Mucormycosis in hematologic emergencies and emerging fungal infections. Haematologica 2000;85:1068–71.
115. Edman JC, Kovacs JA, Masur H, et al. Ribosomal RNA sequence shows *Pneumocystis carinii* to be a member of the Fungi. Nature 1988;334:519–22
116. Sajadi MM, Fanthy GT, Fantry LE. A Czech researcher and Pneumocystis. Clin Infect Dis 2004;39:270.
117. Peglow SL, Smulian AG, Linke MJ, et al. Serologic responses to *Pneumocystis carinii* antigens in health and disease. J Infect Dis 1990;161:296–306.
118. Vargas SL, Hughes WT, Wakefield AE, et al. Limited persistence in and subsequent elimination of *Pneumocystis carinii* from the lungs after *P. carinii* pneumonia. J Infect Dis 1995;172:506–10.
119. Wakefield AE. *Pneumocystis carinii*. Br Med Bull 2002;61: 175–88.
120. Rosen P, Armstrong D, Ramos C. *Pneumocystis carinii* pneumonia: a clinicopathologic study of twenty patients with neoplastic diseases. Am J Med 1972;53:428–36.
121. Fauci AS, Macher AM, Longo DL, et al. Acquired immunodeficiency syndrome epidemiologic clinical, immunologic, and therapeutic considerations. Ann Intern Med 1984;100:92–106.
122. Baez-Escudero JL, Greene JN, Sandin RL, et al. *Pneumocystis carinii* pneumonia in cancer patients. Abstr Hematol Oncol 2004;7(1):24–30.
123. Roblot F, Godet C, Le Moal G, et al. Analysis of underlying diseases and prognosis factors associated with *Pneumocystis carinii* pneumonia in immunocompromised HIV-negative patients. Eur J Clin Microbiol Infect Dis 2002;21: 523–31.
124. Pagano L, Fianchi L, Mele L, et al. *Pneumocystis carinii* pneumonia in patients with malignant hematological diseases: 10 years' experience of infection in GIMEMA centres. Br J Haematol 2002;117:379–86.
125. Roblot F, Le Moal G, Godet C, et al. *Pneumocystis carinii* pneumonia in patients with hematologic malignancies: a descriptive study. J Infect 2003;47:19–27.
126. Yale SH, Limper AH. *Pneumocystis carinii* pneumonia in patients without aacquired immunodeficiency syndrome: associated illnesses and prior corticosteroid therapy. Mayo Clin Proc 1996;71:5–13.
127. Varthalitis I, Aoun M, Daneau D, et al. *Pneumocystis carinii* pneumonia in patients with cancer. An increasing incidence. Cancer 1993;71:481–5.
128. Sepkowitz KA, Brown AE, Telzak EE, et al. *Pneumocystis carinii* pneumonia among patients without AIDS at a cancer hospital. JAMA 1992;267:832–7.
129. Schiff D. Pneumocystis pneumonia in brain tumor patients: risk factors and clinical features. J Neurooncol 1996;27: 235–40.
130. Pareja JG, Garland R, Koziel H. Use of adjunctive corticosteroids in severe adult non-HIV *Pneumocystis carinii* pneumonia. Chest 1998;113:1215–24.
131. Mansharamani NG, Garland R, Delaney D, et al. Management and outcome patterns for adult *Pneumocystis carinii* pneumonia, 1985 to 1995; comparison of HIV-associated cases to other immunocompromised states. Chest 2000;118:704–11.
132. Arend SM, Kroon FP, van't Wout JW. *Pneumocystis carinii* pneumonia in patients without AIDs, 1980 through 1993. An analysis of 78 cases. Arch Intern Med 1995;155: 2436–41.
133. Hughes W, Feldman S, Aur R, et al. Intensity of immunosuppressive therapy and the incidence of *Pneumocystis carinii* pneumonia. Cancer 1975;36:2004–9.
134. Chanock S. Evolving risk factors for infectious complications of cancer therapy. Hematol Oncol Clin North Am 1993;7: 771–93.

135. Hughes W, Rivera G, Schnell M, et al. Successful intermittent chemoprophylaxis for *Pneumocystis carinii* pneumonitis. N Engl J Med 1987;316:1627–32.

136. Henoon JW, Jalai JK, Walker RW, et al. *Pneumocystis carinii* pneumonia in patients with primary brain tumors. Arch Neurol 1991;48:406–9.

137. Slivka A, Wen PY, Shea WN, et al. *Pneumocystis carinii* pneumonia during steroid taper in patients with primary brain tumors. Am J Med 1993;94:216–9.

138. Mathew BS, Grossman SA. *Pneumocystis carinii* pneumonia prophylaxis in HIV negative patients with primary CNS lymphoma. Cancer Treat Rev 2003;29:105–19.

139. Mahindra AK, Grossman SA. *Pneumocystis carinii* pneumonia in HIV negative patients with primary brain tumors. J Neurooncol 2003;63:263–70.

140. Kovacs JA, Hiemenz JW, Macher AM, et al. *Pneumocystis carinii* pneumonia: a comparison between patients with acquired immunodeficiency syndrome and patients with other immunodeficiencies. Ann Intern Med 1989; 100:663–71.

141. Hopewell PC. *Pneumocystis carinii* pneumonia: diagnosis. J Infect Dis 1988;157:1115–9.

142. Quist J, Hill AR. Serum lactate dehydrogenase (LDH) in *Pneumocystis carinii* pneumonia, tuberculosis, and bacterial pneumonia. Chest 1995;108:415–8.

143. Ng VL, Yajko DM, McPhaul LW, et al. Evaluation of an indirect fluorescent antibody stain for detection of *Pneumocystis carinii* in respiratory specimens. J Clin Microbiol 1990;28:975–9.

144. Gagnon S, Boota AM, Fischl MA, et al. Corticosteroids as adjunctive therapy for severe *Pneumocystis carinii* pneumonia in the acquired immunodeficiency syndrome. N Engl J Med 1990;323:1444–50.

145. Pareja JG, Garland R, Koziel H. Use of adjunctive corticosteroids in severe adult non-HIV *Pneumocystis carinii* pneumonia. Chest 1998;113:1215–24.

146. de la Camara R, Martino R, Granados E, et al. Tuberculosis after hematopoietic stem cell transplantation: incidence, clinical characteristics and outcome. Bone Marrow Transplant 2000;26:291–8.

147. Ku S-C, Tang J-L, Hsueh P-R, et al. Pulmonary tuberculosis in allogeneic hematopoietic stem cell transplantation. Bone Marrow Transplant 2001;27:1293–7.

148. Aljurf M, Gyger M, Alrajhi A, et al. Mycobacterium tuberculosis infection in allogeneic bone marrow transplantation patients. Bone Marrow Transplant 1999;24:551–4.

149. IP MS, Yuen KY, Woo PC, et al. Risk factors for pulmonary tuberculosis in bone marrow transplant recipients. Am J Respir Crit Care Med 1998;158:1173–7.

150. Cordonnier C, Martino R, Trabasso P, et al. Mycobacterial infection: a difficult and late diagnosis in stem cell transplant recipients. Clin Infect Dis 2004;38:1229–36.

151. Kourbeti IS, Maslow MJ. Nontuberculous mycobacterial infections of the lung. Curr Infect Dis Rep 2000;2:193–200.

152. Doucette K, Fishman JA. Nontuberculous mycobacterial infection in hematopoietic stem cell and solid organ transplant recipients. Clin Infect Dis 2004;38:1428–39.

153. Christiansen EE, Dietz GW, Ahn CH, et al. Radiographic manifestation of pulmonary Mycobacterium kansaii infections. AJR Am J Roentgenol 1978;131:985.

154. Chalermskulrat W, Gilbey JG, Donohue JF. Nontuberculous mycobacteria in women, young and old. Clin Chest Med 2002;23:1–14.

155. Reich JM, Johnson RE. *Mycobacterium avium* complex pulmonary disease presenting as an isolated lingular or middle lobe pattern. The Lady Windermere syndrome. Chest 1992;101:1605–9.

156. Field SK, Fisher D, Cowie RL. Mycobacterium avium complex pulmonary disease in patients without HIV infection. Chest 2004;126:566–81.

157. Griffith DE, Girard WN, Wallace RJ Jr. Clinical features of pulmonary disease caused by rapidly growing mycobacteria. Rev Infect Dis 1993;147:1271–8.

158. Daley CL, Griffith DE. Pulmonary disease caused by rapidly growing mycobacteria. Clin Chest Med 2002 Sep;23(3):423–32, vii.

159. Lamm DL, van der Meijden PM, Morales A, et al. Incidence and treatment of complications of bacillus Calmette-Guerin intravesicular therapy in superficial bladder cancer J Urol 1992;147:596–600.

160. Elkabani M, Greene JN, Vincent AL, et al. Disseminated Mycobacterium bovis after intravesicular bacillus Calmette-Guerin treatments for bladder cancer. Cancer Control 2000;7:476–81.

Noninfectious Pulmonary Problems in the Patient with Cancer

Shirin Shafazand, MD

Jeffrey Rubins, MD

Gene L. Colice, MD

In 2006, about 1,900,000 people in the United States will be diagnosed with cancer.[1] In the United States, the lifetime probability of developing cancer at any site is now one in two (about 50%) for a man and one in three (about 33%) for a woman. Although overall cancer survival rates have improved over the last three decades, death rates in cancer are still substantial. In 2004, slightly more than 560,000 deaths in the United States were caused by cancer. These statistics vividly demonstrate the importance of cancer as a public health concern but actually represent just a portion of the problem. Cancer also causes substantial morbidity. Pulmonary complications are especially common, including those relating to pulmonary spread of the cancer, initiated by systemic procoagulant effects of cancer, and owing to toxicity from the chemotherapy and radiotherapy regimens used to treat the primary cancer. This chapter reviews these major noninfectious pulmonary complications of cancer.

Pleural Effusions in Cancer Patients

In evaluating the cancer patient with a pleural effusion, clinicians should be concerned about pleural metastases. An estimated 50% of all cancer patients develop a malignant pleural effusion at some point during the course of their illness, and approximately 15% of cancer patients die with malignant effusions.[2] Malignant effusions are most common in lung and breast cancer (50–75% of malignant effusions), lymphoma (both Hodgkin's and non-Hodgkin's), mesothelioma, and colon and ovarian cancer.[2,3] Malignant effusions indicate a very poor prognosis, with 30-day mortality rates of 30 to 50% and a median survival of 4 months.[2] Because of the poor prognosis in many cancer patients with pleural effusions, clinicians should make decisions regarding the aggressiveness of the diagnostic and therapeutic procedures based on maximizing the patient's quality of life.

Nonmalignant pleural effusions must also be considered in the cancer patient. Depressed immune defenses predispose these patients to pneumonia, which may be complicated by parapneumonic effusions. Increased levels of tissue factor or activation of the coagulation cascade predispose cancer patients to pulmonary embolism (PE), which can produce pleural effusion. Bronchial obstruction by cancer can produce postobstructive pneumonia or atelectasis, which, in turn, can cause effusions. Mediastinal nodes can obstruct the thoracic duct, producing an exudative effusion or a chylothorax.[2] Pleural effusions may complicate cancer treatments. Chest radiation for lung cancer, mesothelioma, lymphoma, or breast cancer can cause a direct radiation pleuritis, resulting in pleural effusion.[4] Effusions usually appear within 6 months of radiation therapy, although they occasionally pose a diagnostic puzzle when occurring years later. Mediastinal radiation can cause mediastinal fibrosis, which can lead to effusions by obstructing pleural lymphatic drainage. Chemotherapy can produce pleuritis and pleural effusions, most commonly with the use of methotrexate, procarbazine, cyclophosphamide, or bleomycin.[2]

Diagnosis

The etiology of a pleural effusion in cancer patients can often be suspected based on the patient's clinical presentation and history of previous treatments. A definitive diagnosis, however, usually requires diagnostic thoracentesis. Thoracentesis should be considered in any cancer patient with an unexplained pleural effusion. Relative contraindications to thoracentesis include a bleeding diathesis, anticoagulation, mechanical ventilation, and cellulitis at the puncture site. If pleural fluid is not obtained readily or in patients with smaller effusions, ultrasonography is useful in identifying an appropriate puncture site.

The initial diagnostic studies to order on pleural fluid in cancer patients can be remembered as the "5 C's." The first "C" is a reminder to "see" the gross appearance of the fluid and order additional studies accordingly. A bloody pleural fluid suggests malignancy, PE, or parapneumonic causes, although bloody fluid can also be seen in asbestos effusions and in postpericardiotomy syndrome. A purulent effusion is diagnostic of an empyema requiring drainage. A milky effusion indicates either a chylous or pseudochylous effusion, which can be distinguished by testing pleural cholesterol and triglyceride levels.

The second "C" is for chemistries to distinguish transudates from exudates (Table 1). Although transudative effusions may be

Table 1 Causes of Pleural Effusions in Cancer Patients
Transudates
Congestive heart failure
Cirrhosis with ascites
Nephrotic syndrome
Hypoalbuminemia
Peritoneal dialysis
Glomerulonephritis
Atelectasis
Superior vena cava
Constrictive pericarditis
Malignancy (< 5%)
Pulmonary embolism (< 35%)
Urinothorax
Exudates
Metastatic disease
Parapneumonic
Pulmonary embolism
Radiation
Chylothorax
Pancreatitis
Esophageal perforation
Tuberculosis pleuritis obstruction
Post–cardiac injury syndrome
Drug induced
Viral pleuritis

interpreted to indicate that no further evaluation is needed, pleural effusions from PE and malignancy rarely present as transudates. In contrast, exudative effusions indicate inflammatory or malignant diseases that require further diagnostic studies. The criteria identified by Light and colleagues in 1972 have high sensitivity for distinguishing transudates from exudates but require simultaneous measurement of pleural and serum protein and lactate dehydrogenase (LDH).[5] Newer criteria have a sensitivity and a specificity similar to those of Light and colleagues and require only pleural fluid measurements of protein, LDH, and cholesterol.[6] A low pleural fluid glucose and pH in a patient with a parapneumonic effusion indicate the need for drainage. A low pleural fluid glucose and pH suggest a very poor prognosis in patients with malignant effusions.[4,7]

The third "C," cell count differential, may indicate possible etiologies for exudative effusions. Pleural fluid with greater than 50% neutrophils indicates an acute process, such as parapneumonic effusions and those owing to PE or pancreatitis, but tends to exclude malignancy and tuberculosis. A differential with greater than 50% lymphocytes suggests malignancy or tuberculosis.[8] Pleural fluid eosinophilia, defined as greater than 10% eosinophils, is often caused by blood or air in the pleural space but may be seen with malignant effusions or those caused by drug reactions (such as dantrolene, bromocriptine, or nitrofurantoin). Increased numbers of mesothelial cells tend to exclude the diagnosis of tuberculosis,[8] whereas markedly increased numbers of mesothelial cells in bloody or eosinophilic effusions in the absence of trauma suggest PE.[9]

The fourth "C," pleural fluid cultures for bacterial, fungal, and tuberculous pathogens, should be performed routinely in cancer patients with exudative effusions. When tuberculosis is suspected, pleural fluid adenosine deaminase levels >40 U/L strongly suggest tuberculous pleuritis.[8] The fifth "C," cytology, should also be obtained routinely because of the high prevalence of malignant effusions in these patients. The yield of cytology varies from 62 to 90%, depending on the extent of disease and the propensity of the pleural malignancy to shed tumor cells into the pleural fluid.[2] Mesothelioma, squamous cell carcinoma, lymphoma, and sarcoma involving the pleura may be missed in more than 50% of cases by pleural fluid cytology.[8]

In an appreciable proportion of patients, the etiology of an exudative effusion will remain undiagnosed after a single thoracentesis. Repeat thoracentesis will increase the diagnostic yield.[10] Pleural fluid LDH on serial thoracenteses may guide the aggressiveness of the evaluation. A rising LDH suggests an active inflammatory process that should be pursued further, whereas a decreasing LDH supports a less aggressive approach.[8] If more aggressive diagnostic steps are warranted, closed-needle pleural biopsy can increase the diagnostic yield for malignancy by 7 to 12%.[2] However, video-assisted thoracoscopy (VATS) has emerged as the procedure of choice for undiagnosed pleural effusions because it allows visualization of the pleural space and directed biopsies.[10] VATS has diagnostic yields up to 95% compared with 62% for cytology and 44% for closed-needle biopsy.[11] After VATS, fewer than 10% of exudative effusions remain undiagnosed compared with >20% after cytology and needle biopsy.[2] Some patients may not tolerate the general anesthesia and single-lung ventilation required for VATS. In these patients, medical thoracoscopy, performed under conscious sedation and local anesthesia in an endoscopy suite using either rigid or semiflexible instruments, should be considered.

Treatment

Management of pleural effusions in the cancer patient is usually directed at relieving dyspnea, which is the most common presenting symptom. Accumulation of large amounts of pleural fluid may cause dyspnea by decreasing chest wall compliance, shifting the mediastinum to the contralateral hemithorax, decreasing ventilation of the ipsilateral lung, and stimulating reflexes within the lungs and chest wall.[12] However, dyspnea may be unrelated to the pleural effusion, caused instead by underlying heart or lung disease, PE, pericardial effusion, or tumor infiltration of the lung parenchyma. For cancer patients with dyspnea and pleural effusions, the prime considerations are (1) whether removal of the pleural fluid relieves dyspnea, (2) the patient's general health and functional status, and (3) the patient's expected survival.[13] The goals in such patients should be to provide relief of dyspnea, minimize discomfort, and limit hospitalization time.

For patients with effusions owing to small cell lung cancer and for some with effusions from lymphoma and germ cell tumors, chemotherapy may effectively reduce effusions and relieve symptoms.[13] Most cancer patients with symptomatic pleural effusions, however, require therapeutic thoracentesis for palliation. Drainage of pleural fluid by therapeutic thoracentesis or placement of a pleural drainage catheter relieves dyspnea by increasing lung ventilation. Typically, total lung capacity increases by approximately one-third of the volume of fluid removed, and forced vital capacity increases by about one-sixth of the volume removed.[14] However, many cancer patients with pleural effusions do not benefit from removal of pleural fluid either because the underlying lung cannot reexpand or because the dyspnea is caused by other underlying conditions. When considering therapeutic thoracentesis, mediastinal position may predict whether a patient is likely to benefit from this procedure. Mediastinal shift away from the pleural effusion indicates a positive pleural pressure and compression of the underlying lung that likely will be relieved by thoracentesis. In contrast, the absence of mediastinal shift or shift toward the pleural effusion implies lung entrapment by obstruction of the mainstem bronchus or extensive pleural involvement that will prevent reinflation of the lung when the pleural fluid is removed.

At initial therapeutic thoracentesis, removal of even 300 cc of fluid should be sufficient to determine whether relief of dyspnea will occur. Removal of more than 1,500 cc of fluid is not advised because of the risk of causing reexpansion pulmonary edema. In patients with lung entrapment, far less fluid can be safely removed before unduly stretching the underlying lung. If large-volume thoracentesis is planned, using pleural manometry to ensure that pleural pressure does not fall below −20 cm H_2O is the safest approach and may allow removal of much larger volumes than otherwise recommended.[15] Generally, reexpansion pulmonary edema can be avoided by removing <1,500 cc of pleural fluid and stopping the thoracentesis if the patient begins to feel chest pain or shortness of breath.

After therapeutic thoracentesis, relief of dyspnea should be evaluated by objective measures, such as the ability to walk a defined distance without shortness of breath, and documented for future reference. A chest radiograph should be obtained immediately after thoracentesis to determine the extent of lung reexpansion. Hydropneumothorax on the postprocedure radiograph, especially when the apparent volume of airspace within the lung appears to be unchanged, signals lung entrapment. A thickened pleura on chest computed tomography (CT) supports this diagnosis and indicates that further thoracentesis will probably be of little value. If the lung has reexpanded, but the patient reports no relief of dyspnea, the clinician should consider contrast-enhanced chest CT to evaluate for lymphangitic carcinomatosis, thromboembolism, tumor embolism,[2] and other nonmalignant cardiopulmonary diseases that can produce dyspnea.

Patients whose symptoms improve after thoracentesis should be followed for recurrence of symptomatic effusions. Those remaining asymptomatic should simply be observed.[16] For cancer patients with poor performance status (Karnofsky score <70) and limited life expectancy (<3 months), recurring symptomatic pleural effusions can be managed with repeated outpatient thoracentesis, which avoids hospitalization for more invasive and potentially morbid procedures.[13,16] If effusions recur quickly and patients have sufficient support at home, insertion of an indwelling tunneled catheter is a reasonable option to palliate dyspnea.[16,17] The only tunneled catheter approved by the US Food and Drug Administration (the Pleurx catheter, marketed by Denver Biomedical, Golden CO) is a 15.5F silicone catheter. A proximal polyester cuff causes subcutaneous fibrosis, which prevents dislodgement and lessens the risk of infection. The catheter has a valved hub that keeps the system closed, except when a specific dilator attached to a 600 mL vacuum bottle system is inserted. The catheter can be inserted as an outpatient procedure, and the effusion can be drained at home with the disposable vacuum bottles as frequently as necessary to relieve symptoms. The Pleurx catheter has been shown to be equivalent to or better than pleurodesis in relief of dyspnea and improvement in quality of life and induces spontaneous pleurodesis in up to 20 to 45% of patients over a median 29 days after placement.[17-19] However, approximately 20% of patients have complications related to the catheter, most commonly chest pain in the first week after catheter placement (10–14%). Catheter obstruction may necessitate replacement (2–8%). More serious complications, such as local cellulitis (6%), tumor seeding of the catheter track (1–3%), and pleural infection (1–5%), also occur.[17-19]

Cancer patients with better performance status (Karnofsky score of 70 or higher) whose lungs reexpand after the initial thoracentesis should be considered for pleurodesis if they have recurrence of a symptomatic effusion.[2,13,20] After complete drainage of the pleural effusion, sclerosing agents are instilled to produce acute pleural injury and inflammation, causing bridging pleural fibrosis that effectively "glues" the lungs to the chest wall and obliterates the potential pleural space. Systemic corticosteroids should be avoided or reduced to the lowest possible doses prior to pleurodesis to avoid suppressing sclerosant-induced inflammation and thereby causing pleurodesis failures.[21] Pleurodesis through a chest tube using a talc slurry appears to be as effective as that performed using talc powder insufflated (poudrage) during VATS.[22-24] For most patients, pleural effusions can be drained as effectively and with less pain using small-bore (10–14F) intercostal pleural catheters as opposed to large-bore (24–32F) chest tubes.[16,25-27] The main disadvantage to pleurodesis by a pleural catheter or chest tube is that a longer hospitalization may be required to fully drain the effusion prior to instillation of the sclerosing agent, but it avoids general anesthesia and intubation with VATS.

Talc is the most effective agent for pleurodesis and the least expensive. It has been recommended as the agent of choice by the European, American, and British thoracic societies.[2,16] Talc, which prevents recurrent effusions in 90 to 95% of patients, was found to be more effective than bleomycin,

tetracycline, mustine, or tube drainage alone in a systematic review of 10 studies including 308 patients.[23] The talc preparations used for pleurodesis are asbestos-free powders that require sterilization by dry heat, ethylene oxide, or gamma irradiation prior to use in talc slurry or are available in aerosol-propellent bottles for use in poudrage. Although more effective than other sclerosants, talc pleurodesis has a higher incidence of complications, including fever, empyema, and acute lung injury. Fever occurs in up to 65% of patients within 4 to 12 hours of talc pleurodesis and may last up to 72 hours before resolving spontaneously.[2] Empyema has been reported in up to 11% of patients, presumably related to difficulties in preparation of an adequately sterilized product for instillation. The most worrisome complication is acute lung injury and adult respiratory distress syndrome (ARDS), which has been estimated to occur in up to 9% of patients.[2] Because talc particles are known to be absorbed into lymphatic and venous drainage during sclerosis, the incidence of ARDS may be related to the particle size of talc and the dose used. Most cases of talc-induced ARDS have been reported in the United States, where 11 to 20 µ of talc is used, rather than in Europe, where "French talc," with a 34 µ particle size, is used.[28] In addition, doses of talc up to 14 g were used in earlier studies when ARDS was first recognized, in contrast to the 3 to 5 g doses now recommended.

Pleurodesis is unsuccessful in 10 to 40% of patients, depending on the approach, the sclerosant, and, most importantly, whether the underlying lung reinflates fully as the effusion is drained. Treatment options for most cancer patients who fail pleurodesis include a repeat attempt at pleurodesis, serial thoracenteses to remove fluid as necessary, or placement of a Pleurx catheter and drainage at home.[16] The Pleurx catheter was shown to effectively palliate dyspnea in 10 of 11 patients with lung entrapment, even when pleurodesis was not achieved.[29] Some centers place a pleuroperitoneal shunt in such patients to drain the effusion into the abdominal space, but these devices have the same complications as the Pleurx catheter and a higher rate of catheter occlusion.

Pleurectomy is an invasive surgical option that effectively prevents recurrence of effusions by complete resection of the pleural space. However, the procedure is associated with complications of empyema, hemorrhage, and cardiorespiratory failure and carries an operative mortality of 10 to 13%.[16] Thus, it should rarely be used in cancer patients who have an already limited prognosis.

In summary, pleural effusions in cancer patients may herald metastatic malignancy, infection, or thromboembolism or may be related to underlying diseases. When symptomatic,

palliative therapies should be chosen based on maximizing the patient's quality of life. Repeated serial thoracenteses, pleurodesis, or indwelling tunneled catheters are palliative options to consider, depending on prognosis and patient choices.

Approach to Pneumothorax in Cancer Patients

Pneumothorax is classified as iatrogenic, traumatic, or spontaneous in origin (Table 2).[30] Cancer patients are at risk of iatrogenic pneumothoraces because they often undergo such diagnostic procedures as transthoracic needle biopsy of the lung and mediastinal lesions, percutaneous biopsy of the liver and adrenal lesions, and transbronchial biopsy or needle aspirates. Therapeutic procedures performed in cancer patients, such as insertion of central venous catheters for administration of chemotherapy or antibiotics, performing celiac plexus block to relieve abdominal pain from cancer, percutaneous insertion of needles into the chest for brachytherapy, radiofrequency ablation or direct immunotherapy, and laser bronchoscopy also can cause iatrogenic pneumothoraces. Pneumothorax can be a late complication of chemotherapy or radiation therapy.

Patients with bronchogenic cancer or cancer metastatic to the lungs rarely develop spontaneous pneumothorax. Rapid dissolution of a tumor mass during chemotherapy of small cell carcinoma[31] and a "check-valve" bronchial obstruction by bronchoalveolar cell carcinoma[32]

Table 2 Cancer-Related Causes of Pneumothorax
Iatrogenic
Related to diagnostic procedures
Transthoracic needle biopsy of pulmonary lesions
Transthoracic mediastinal biopsy
Percutaneous needle biopsy of adrenal glands and liver
Transbronchial needle aspirate
Related to therapeutic procedures
Central venous catheters
Chemotherapy: upper lobe fibrosis after BCNU
Transthoracic radiation therapy
Laser bronchoscopy
Percutaneous fine-needle brachytherapy
CT-guided radiofrequency ablation of pulmonary lesions
CT-guided immunotherapy of pulmonary metastases
Celiac plexus block
Spontaneous
Associated with primary lung cancer
Associated with cancer metastatic to lungs
BCNU = carmustine; CT = computed tomography.

have been reported to produce large spontaneous pneumothoraces. Bronchogenic carcinoma may cavitate or rupture into the pleural space[33,34]; similar mechanisms may explain spontaneous pneumothoraces seen with osteogenic sarcoma metastatic to the lung.[35,36]

Almost all cancer patients with pneumothorax have acute pleuritic chest pain or shortness of breath. Pneumothorax occurring immediately after a procedure is rarely a diagnostic dilemma. However, delayed iatrogenic pneumothorax or spontaneous pneumothorax may be more difficult to detect as chest pain may be minimal and symptoms may resolve within 24 hours, even without resolution of the pneumothorax. A clinically significant pneumothorax is usually readily detected on a standard chest radiograph; chest CT is usually not necessary.

The management of iatrogenic pneumothorax occurring immediately after a diagnostic or therapeutic procedure is comparable to that recommended for treatment of primary spontaneous pneumothorax.[37] For clinically stable patients with small pneumothoraces (<3 cm from the apex to the cupola on a chest radiograph), observation with monitoring of clinical stability and a repeat chest radiograph in 4 to 6 hours may be sufficient in up to 60% of patients. Patients with a stable pneumothorax on a repeat radiograph can be discharged and followed with repeat chest radiographs every 1 to 2 days until the pneumothorax has resolved. Patients who cannot readily access emergency services or are considered unreliable should be admitted for observation. Supplemental oxygen can accelerate reabsorption of pleural air.[38]

Patients with significant symptoms, large pneumothoraces, or enlarging pneumothoraces on repeat radiographs should be treated by insertion of a small-bore (7–14F) pleural catheter. Simple aspiration of the pneumothorax through the catheter is successful in the majority of patients who are younger than 50 years of age and have less than 2.5 L of air aspirated.[30] If the lung remains reexpanded for 6 hours after aspiration, patients with reliable access to emergency services can be discharged and followed with repeat chest radiographs in 2 to 3 days.[37]

Patients who cannot be managed with simple aspiration should have the pleural catheter attached to a one-way Heimlich valve or a water-seal. The Heimlich valve allows patients to ambulate in the hospital more easily and may even allow carefully selected patients whose lungs have reexpanded to be treated as outpatients. However, Heimlich valves can become occluded by coexisting inflammatory or bloody pleural fluid and do not allow easy determination of the presence of a persistent air leak. In contrast, a water-seal permits prompt detection of a persistent air leak, indicating a bronchopleural

fistula, and allows application of suction to evacuate the pneumothorax. Pleural catheters should be attached to the water-seal if patients fail the Heimlich valve, are expected to have persistent bronchopleural fistula, or have underlying cardiopulmonary disease that decreases their ability to tolerate a recurrent pneumothorax.

A bronchopleural fistula is uncommon with iatrogenic pneumothorax but may occur in those patients who have underlying lung disease. If the bronchopleural fistula persists beyond 4 days, patients should be considered for pleurodesis by thoracoscopy if possible.[37] If surgery is contraindicated or patients refuse the procedure, pleurodesis via the chest tube is an alternative approach.

In contrast to the management of patients with iatrogenic pneumothorax, cancer patients with a spontaneous pneumothorax generally should be hospitalized. Those who are clinically stable and have small pneumothoraces (<3 cm from the apex to the cupola on a chest radiograph) can be observed with serial radiographs and, if the pneumothorax worsens, can be managed by placement of a small-bore pleural catheter as described above. In contrast, unstable patients or those with large pneumothoraces should have 24F to 28F chest tubes inserted and placed to water-seal. Most cancer patients with spontaneous pneumothorax should be considered for pleurodesis to prevent recurrence of pneumothorax, depending on their performance status and prognosis. Pleurodesis by medical or surgical thoracoscopy is the preferred management strategy discussed in consensus guidelines, but instillation of sclerosing agents via a chest tube may be more appropriate for cancer patients with a poorer performance or prognosis.[37]

In summary, cancer patients are at risk of iatrogenic pneumothorax related to diagnostic or therapeutic procedures or spontaneous pneumothorax related to bronchogenic or metastatic lung cancer. Management by observation or evacuation of the pneumothorax is determined by the patient's clinical stability and the size of the pneumothorax. Patients with persistent bronchopleural fistula and those with spontaneous pneumothorax should be considered for pleurodesis to prevent recurrent pneumothoraces.

Cancer and Venous Thromboembolism

Since Armand Trousseau's initial report of migratory thrombophlebitis observed in patients with cancer in 1865,[39] numerous studies have shown an association between cancer and venous thromboembolism (VTE). The incidence of VTE in cancer patients is not clearly known and varies from 4 to 31% depending on the tumor histology, the methods used to diagnose VTE, and patient

characteristics.[40] Although a higher risk of VTE has traditionally been associated with pancreatic adenocarcinoma, recent information suggests that in men, the highest incidence of VTE is observed in patients with lung, prostate, and colorectal cancer and in women with breast, lung, and ovarian cancer.[41]

The strong association between cancer and VTE is further demonstrated by the often observed increased incidence of cancer during the first year after a thromboembolic event (2–4% absolute risk),[42] with the risk being highest among those with idiopathic VTE (on average five times higher than those with secondary causes for thrombosis).[43–45] Two large population-based Scandinavian studies confirmed the increased incidence of cancer during the first year postdiagnosis of VTE and showed a 10 to 30% increased long-term risk (up to 10 years of follow-up) of cancer compared with the general population.[46,47] Despite the strong association demonstrated in these studies, very little information exists on the impact of aggressive screening for cancer following the initial VTE and patient survival. Furthermore, the costs and morbidity associated with screening, coupled with a lack of sufficiently sensitive and specific diagnostic tests for many cancers associated with VTE, make recommendations for extensive screening for malignancy in patients presenting with idiopathic VTE controversial. However, it is reasonable to consider the possibility of occult malignancy in patients with primary VTE and to provide a thorough clinical evaluation, including a history and physical examination, routine laboratory tests, and chest radiography, for such patients. Additional testing should be offered in accordance with findings from the initial evaluation.[48]

Pathogenesis and Risk Factors

The pathogenesis of VTE in cancer is complex, involving all elements of Virchow's triad (Table 3). Vessel wall injury may occur as a result of direct invasion by malignant cells or release of vascular permeability factors by tumor cells. Additionally, extrinsic factors, including surgical procedures and insertion of indwelling venous catheters, contribute to vessel wall injury. Disability from advanced disease and immobilization associated with surgical interventions increase the risk of venous stasis, whereas obstruction of blood flow by an intrinsic or extrinsic tumor mass further compounds the problem. Finally, cancer is a hypercoaguable state. Tumor cells express cell markers and can release soluble factors that have procoagulant activity; the two best described are tissue factor (TF) and cancer procoagulant (CP). TF activates factor VII, forming a complex that activates factors IX and X and increases thrombin formation. The overall effect of TF is production of fibrin and platelet

Table 3 Pathogenesis of Venous Thromboembolism in Malignancy

Vessel wall injury
    Invasion by malignant cells
    Release of vascular permeability factors by
        malignant cells
    Indwelling central venous catheter
    Surgical manipulation
    Chemotherapy

Venous stasis
    Obstruction of blood flow: intrinsic or extrinsic
        compression by tumor mass
    Prolonged immobilization secondary to
        surgical intervention
    Thrombocytosis

Hypercoagulability
    Release of procoagulant factors, including
        tissue factor and cancer procoagulant
    Release of inflammatory mediators: TNF and
        IL-1
        Up-regulation of tissue factor and platelet-
            activating factor, leukocyte and cellular
            adhesion molecules
        Down-regulation of thrombomodulin,
            endothelial cell protein C receptor
    Necrosis of tumor
        Reduced levels of antithrombin III, proteins
            C and S

IL = interleukin; TNF = tumor necrosis factor.

activation.[49,50] CP is a cysteine protease that directly activates factor X in the absence of factor VII and can induce platelet activation.[49,50] Inflammatory cytokines such as tumor necrosis factor (TNF) and interleukin-1 further enhance the procoagulant activity of tumor cells. Unfortunately, many of the cytotoxic and hormonal therapies offered to cancer patients may also increase the risk of thromboembolism by augmenting endothelial cell reactivity and platelet adhesion, directly damaging vessel walls, or decreasing levels of natural coagulation inhibitors (eg, protein C or S).[51] The increased risk of VTE in patients with cancer, combined with the higher probability of death,[52] necessitates a heightened awareness on the part of clinicians and an aggressive approach to the prophylaxis, diagnosis, and treatment of thromboembolic events.

Prophylaxis

VTE prophylaxis is routinely recommended after major surgery owing to the increased risk of postoperative thrombosis.[53] Compared with patients undergoing surgery for benign disease, patients with cancer are estimated to have twice the risk of postoperative deep venous thrombosis (DVT) and more than three times the risk of fatal PE.[54] Internists taking care of postoperative cancer patients play an important role in ensuring that adequate prophylaxis is provided.

Prophylactic options include mechanical measures, for example, compression stockings, low-dose unfractionated heparin (UFH), and low molecular weight heparins (LMWHs). Only a few large trials have compared various anticoagulation regimens for surgical prophylaxis, and most were not designed specifically to evaluate cancer patients. In a meta-analysis, Mismetti and colleagues concluded that once-daily LMWH appears to be as safe and efficacious as multidose UFH in patients with and without malignancy.[55] The ENOXACAN study was the first randomized trial comparing the prophylactic use of enoxaparin, 40 mg once daily with UFH, 5,000 units three times a day, in 631 patients undergoing elective curative abdominal or pelvic surgery for cancer.[56] The study showed no statistically significant difference in efficacy and safety between enoxaparin and UFH in the prevention of venographically detected DVT and symptomatic VTE (14.7 vs 18.2%, respectively; $p > .05$).[57] The ENOXACAN II investigators studied the extended use of enoxaparin prophylaxis versus placebo beyond initial hospitalization in postoperative cancer patients. They concluded that extended (3 months) use of enoxaparin led to a significant absolute risk reduction in VTE of 7%. This absolute risk reduction means that 14 postoperative cancer patients need to be treated for 21 days to prevent one case of VTE. The majority of DVTs in the ENOXACAN II study were asymptomatic and distal. Although extended prophylaxis will likely reduce clinically relevant proximal DVTs, more studies are needed to confirm the results of this trial prior to definitive recommendations for long-term prophylaxis following oncologic surgery.

Neurosurgical patients, many of whom undergo craniotomy for neoplasms, have an elevated risk of developing VTE in the immediate postoperative period, and this risk remains as high as 23% at 1 year.[58,59] Prophylaxis with LMWH, initiated within 24 hours of craniotomy, can reduce the risk of VTE without significantly increasing serious bleeding.[60–62] VTE prophylaxis has not been studied extensively in other surgical oncology settings. In general, medical prophylaxis is recommended after any surgery for cancer owing to the increased risk of thrombosis. If the risk of bleeding is considered to far outweigh the risk of VTE, then mechanical methods of prophylaxis are strongly recommended until the risk of bleeding has decreased.[53]

Treatment

The management of VTE in cancer patients is challenging. In addition to the increased risk of VTE, cancer patients are more likely to have recurrent VTE (annual risk estimated to be 20.7%)[63] and have a three- to sixfold increased risk of hemorrhagic complications compared

with patients without cancer.[63,64] The prognosis of cancer patients with VTE is far worse than that of their thrombosis-free counterparts. In one study, the 1-year survival rate was 12% in patients with cancer and VTE compared with 36% in similar patients without VTE.[52] Finally, any therapeutic recommendation should take into account the patient's quality of life and minimize morbidity as much as possible.

Standard therapy for acute VTE is UFH or LMWH followed by long-term therapy with warfarin for secondary prophylaxis. Several randomized controlled trials and meta-analyses have shown that LMWHs are at least as effective as UFH in decreasing the recurrence of thrombosis[65–67] and may be associated with a lower risk of major bleeding and heparin-induced thrombocytopenia. Although these trials were not designed specifically to assess treatment options in patients with malignancy, extrapolation of the results from a large subgroup of patients with cancer in these studies suggests that LMWHs are as efficacious as UFH for the initial treatment of VTE in patients with malignancy. The convenience of use, without the need for frequent laboratory monitoring, has made LMWHs agents of choice in the inpatient and outpatient management of clinically stable patients with DVT. In many countries, outpatient LMWH is even being used for the treatment of hemodynamically stable PE.[58] The decrease in the length of hospital stay and possibility of outpatient treatment with LMWH will likely have a positive impact on the quality of life of patients with cancer and should be an important consideration in the choice of pharmacologic therapy.

Traditionally, long-term anticoagulation has been achieved with warfarin, started in combination with LMWH or UFH within the first 24 hours of diagnosis and continued for at least 3 months. This approach necessitates frequent laboratory monitoring to maintain an international normalized ratio (INR) of between 2.0 and 3.0.[68] In patients with malignancy, maintenance of therapeutic-range INR can be difficult, and more treatment failures are noted than in the general population. Two recent randomized trials support the use of LMWH instead of warfarin for long-term secondary prophylaxis of VTE. The CANTHANOX trial compared 3 months of warfarin therapy with enoxaparin, 1.5 mg/kg once daily, in patients with cancer and a diagnosis of proximal DVT, PE, or both.[69] There was no statistically significant difference between the two groups in terms of recurrence of symptomatic VTE or major bleeding. However, the warfarin group showed a trend toward more bleeding. In a similar study, the CLOT trial, investigators randomized cancer patients with VTE to receive either dalteparin alone for 6 months or dalteparin followed by warfarin therapy.[70] The 6-month cumulative risk of VTE was significantly reduced from 17% in the warfarin group to 9% in the dalteparin group, with no difference in adverse bleeding complications. The main practical limitation of long-term LMWH use for secondary prophylaxis is the cost of the drug. Although evidence supports its use as superior to warfarin therapy and it is at least as safe, it remains to be determined whether long-term use of LMWH is cost-effective.

Given the increased incidence of recurrence of VTE in patients with cancer, it is prudent to continue secondary prophylaxis for several months following the initial diagnosis. However, the optimal duration of therapy is unknown in cancer patients. Most recommendations are extrapolated from studies in the general population, of whom patients with malignancy are a subset. In patients with idiopathic DVT, 6 months of therapy with oral anticoagulation was better than 6 weeks and 2 years was better than 3 months in preventing recurrent VTE.[71,72] In another study, 1-year prophylaxis was better than 3 months of anticoagulation, but the benefits were not sustained after discontinuation of prophylaxis at 1 year.[73] Some authors have recommended long-term low-intensity warfarin therapy (maintaining an INR of 1.5–1.9) after 3 months of conventional therapy. Two randomized controlled trials investigating this option have conflicting results.[74,75] It is not clear whether low-intensity anticoagulation is as effective and safer than conventional warfarin therapy, and more studies are needed before definitive recommendations can be made. Despite the increased risk of hemorrhage, in the cancer population, it is prudent to continue anticoagulation indefinitely or at least as long as the cancer is active to reduce the risk of recurrent VTE.[76]

Failure of Anticoagulation

The management of cancer patients who develop recurrent VTE despite adequate warfarin therapy is difficult. Several options are currently available, none of which have been compared in clinical trials. After initial treatment with UFH or LMWH, the options are to continue anticoagulation with warfarin, targeting a higher INR (3.0–4.0) and accepting a higher risk of bleeding; switch to twice-daily, adjusted-dose UFH; use once-daily, weight-adjusted LMWH; or insert an inferior vena cava (IVC) filter. IVC filters have also been used for patients in whom anticoagulation is contraindicated. Decousus and colleagues evaluated the role of IVC filters in preventing PE and DVT recurrence. All patients were diagnosed with proximal DVT and received anticoagulation for 3 months after initial management with either LMWH or dose-adjusted UFH. At 12 days, 4.8% of patients without filters developed PE compared with 1.1% with filters ($p = .03$). After 2 years, however, this initial benefit was no longer

sustained, and a statistically significant mortality benefit was not found with the use of an IVC. Ironically, the IVC filter group had a higher risk of DVT recurrence at 2 years.[40,77] Thus, IVC filters should be used cautiously in patients who are anticipated to have long-term survival following cancer therapy. Pharmacologic anticoagulation should be initiated whenever possible to decrease the recurrence of DVT and associated morbidity. Although the evidence is not very strong, long-term therapy with LMWHs may be the best option currently available in the management of patients who develop recurrent VTE while on adequate warfarin therapy.[70]

In summary, the management of patients with malignancy and VTE is challenging. Cancer patients are at increased risk of VTE, they are more likely to develop complications while on anticoagulation, the incidence of recurrence is high, and often the prognosis is worse than in similar patients who do not develop VTE. LMWHs are becoming the agent of choice for prophylaxis, treatment, and extended anticoagulation in patients with cancer. Interestingly, there is some indirect evidence that LMWHs may exert an antineoplastic effect in cancer patients.[78,79] More study is needed to further establish this potential benefit. Antithrombotic agents, such as direct thrombin inhibitors and inhibitors of factor Xa, are being evaluated in clinical trials. Their effectiveness in the cancer population is yet unknown, but they are promising and, it is hoped, will improve our management of patients with malignancy and VTE.

Cancer and Hemoptysis

Hemoptysis is defined as expectoration of blood from the tracheobronchial tree or pulmonary parenchyma. It must be distinguished from bleeding from the gastrointestinal tract and upper airways. Hemoptysis ranges from blood streaking of sputum to gross blood. The term *massive hemoptysis* is reserved for bleeding that is potentially life-threatening but is arbitrarily defined by bleeding ranging from more than 100 mL to more than 600 mL over a 24-hour period. Although only 5% of hemoptysis is massive, it has been associated with a mortality rate as high as 85%.[80]

Etiology

The bronchial arteries are generally the site of bleeding in patients with hemoptysis. In addition to having higher pressures than the pulmonary arteries, they perfuse the airways, and hemoptysis usually originates in airway mucosal lesions (Table 4).[81] Hemoptysis may be the first manifestation of lung cancer in 25 to 50%[82] of patients but is infrequently responsible for massive bleeding in this patient population.[83] In one series, cancer patients with massive hemoptysis typically

Table 4 Etiology of Hemoptysis in Cancer Patients

Neoplasm
   Bronchial carcinoma
   Bronchial adenoma
   Tracheal tumors
   Carcinoid
   Metastatic cancer

Infectious
   Tuberculosis
   Aspergilloma
   Cryptococcosis
   Histoplasmosis
   Atypical *Mycobacteria*
   Bacterial pneumonia
   Lung abscess

Vascular
   Pulmonary embolism
   Ruptured thoracic aneurysm
   Arteriovenous malformation

Cardiac
   Mitral stenosis
   Congestive heart failure

Hematologic
   Thrombocytopenia
   Coagulopathy
   Platelet dysfunction
   Disseminated intravascular coagulation

Pulmonary
   Acute or chronic bronchitis
   Pulmonary infarct
   Bronchiectasis
   Bronchovascular fistula

Miscellaneous
   Iatrogenic
   Autoimmune disorders
   Drugs

had large, centrally located tumors, usually squamous cell carcinoma. More often, hemoptysis is a late manifestation of lung cancer.[83] The etiology of hemoptysis may not be established in more than 40% of patients.[84] In many of these cases, nonmalignant causes were probably the source of hemoptysis. In the cancer patient, particular attention should be paid to the diagnosis and management of other factors that might exacerbate or cause hemoptysis, such as thrombocytopenia and coagulopathy secondary to deficiencies in vitamin K–dependent coagulation factors seen in patients with liver metastases.

Diffuse alveolar hemorrhage (DAH) originates from pulmonary vessels. Patients undergoing chemotherapy for leukemia or those who have received bone marrow transplantation are at risk of DAH and occasionally massive hemoptysis. Although the etiology of DAH is not entirely clear, it probably involves small pulmonary vessel injury secondary to a combination of drugs, thrombocytopenia, coagulopathy, infection, and radiation. Management is supportive, with correction of thrombocytopenia and coagulopathy and prescription of high-dose corticosteroids.

Management

The approach to management of a patient with hemoptysis should be initially directed toward ensuring that the patient's airway is patent and oxygenation is adequate. Volume resuscitation and correction of coagulopathy are important next steps. The urgency of evaluation and therapeutic interventions is determined by the briskness of bleeding and the patient's clinical stability. A history and physical examination, chest radiography, complete blood count, renal function, liver function tests, and prothrombin time and partial thromboplastin time are routinely recommended. Sputum samples should be evaluated for the presence of infection. The chest radiograph may be normal in patients with hemoptysis in almost half of the cases.[85,86] When a parenchymal infiltrate is visualized on the chest radiograph, it may not accurately reflect the site of bleeding because blood can be aspirated into portions of the lung distal from the source of bleeding.[87]

Fiberoptic bronchoscopy and chest CT are complementary diagnostic tests for identifying the bleeding site. Bronchoscopy can detect bleeding sites in the proximal airways, such as bronchitis and central endobronchial lesions. In addition to detection of parenchymal lesions, chest CT is valuable at detecting bronchiectasis, lung abscesses, and many peripheral tumors not accessible to the bronchoscope. The optimal timing for bronchoscopy is controversial.[88] Visualization of the airways is difficult in the setting of massive bleeding. However, the chance of identifying the bleeding site is enhanced if the lesion is actively bleeding at the time of bronchoscopy.

For patients with massive hemoptysis, diagnostic tests and rapid management often occur concurrently to decrease the elevated risk of death secondary to asphyxiation. Early consultation with pulmonary and thoracic surgery specialists is recommended. Protection of the nonbleeding lung is a priority; this will require knowledge of the site of bleeding, which may not be readily available. If the bleeding site is known, the patient should be placed in the lateral decubitus position with the bleeding site dependent to decrease spillage of blood into the unaffected lung. If oxygenation is compromised or bleeding continues at a brisk pace, then oral intubation should be performed. This can be achieved simultaneously with bronchoscopy. A single-lumen endotracheal tube placed into the mainstem bronchus of the nonbleeding lung can be used to selectively ventilate that lung. This is easier to achieve if the left lung is bleeding and the right mainstem bronchus is selectively intubated. However, there is the potential problem of blocking the right upper lobe bronchus and further compromising oxygenation and ventilation. A double-lumen endotracheal tube may be used as an alternative. However, they are difficult to place, even by experienced personnel. Ensuring proper positioning as the patient moves is important and may require paralysis and sedation. The individual lumen size of double-lumen tubes is often too small to permit passage of a bronchoscope and is prone to obstruction by an intraluminal clot. Given these difficulties, double-lumen tubes are not recommended unless other approaches have failed.

In addition to localization of the bleeding site, flexible bronchoscopy may offer therapeutic options. Tamponade of the bleeding site may be achieved with the placement of a 4F, 100 cm Fogarty balloon catheter, alongside the bronchoscope, into the segmental or subsegmental bronchus leading to the bleeding site for 24 to 48 hours. Bleeding may slow or stop with intrabronchial administration of iced saline or topical epinephrine (diluted 1:20,000). Rigid bronchoscopy, performed under general anesthesia, will allow for more effective suctioning, direct cautery, and packing of the bleeding site. However, its range of visualization is limited, and it is often used in conjunction with flexible bronchoscopy if bleeding persists.

Arteriography is an increasingly important addition to available therapeutic options. Because hemoptysis usually originates from the bronchial arteries, bronchial angiography is the first step. Arteriography more commonly hints at the possible bleeding site by the indirect observation of tortuous vessels and hypervascularized regions rather than by direct visualization of extravasation of contrast. Bronchial artery embolization may stop hemoptysis acutely in more than 85% of cases. Unfortunately, in 10 to 20% of cases, rebleeding occurs in the ensuing 6 to 12 months.[89–91] Complications of bronchial artery embolization include bronchial wall necrosis and the risk of paralysis owing to inadvertent embolization of the anterior spinal artery. The anterior spinal artery arises from the bronchial circulation in 5% of the population; fortunately, the risk of paraplegia is less than 1% in experienced hands.[80,91,92]

Surgery is emergently indicated when life-threatening pulmonary hemorrhage persists despite adequate medical therapy. Morbidity and mortality are greater for emergent lung resection compared with elective resection in patients who have been stabilized and are no longer actively bleeding.[80]

In nonmassive cases of hemoptysis, nonspecific treatment with antibiotics, bed rest, and antitussives will usually be effective in decreasing the bleeding. This allows identification of the bleeding site and directed therapy. Local external beam radiation may be effective in controlling hemoptysis in patients with bronchogenic tumors. Endobronchial brachytherapy may be useful in patients with endobronchial tumors not responsive to external radiation. In cancer patients, hemoptysis may be caused by PE.[93] In these cases, the risk of further hemoptysis with anticoagulation needs to be balanced against recurrent thromboembolism and its inherent complications. If the decision is made for anticoagulation, LMWHs have been associated with a lower risk of bleeding than warfarin therapy.[94] IVC filters should be considered in these patients.

In patients with advanced cancer, the treatment of hemoptysis should take into consideration not only the cause and severity of the bleeding but also the patient's life expectancy, quality of life, expectations, and family wishes. It is important to discuss the patient's wishes regarding life-sustaining therapies and resuscitation early in the management of disease. In patients with end-stage cancer, aggressive diagnostic and treatment modalities may not be indicated. Palliation and sedation with benzodiazepines and intravenously administered opioids to allow patient comfort, in addition to emotional support of both the patient and family, may be the best approach.

In summary, hemoptysis can be a difficult management problem. Massive hemoptysis may be life-threatening. Airway protection is the vital first step. Bronchial artery embolization may be useful in controlling bleeding acutely and allowing directed therapy to the source of bleeding. Careful attention must be paid to factors such as thrombocytopenia and coagulopathy, which may contribute to the bleeding. DAH is a less common cause of hemoptysis but may also cause respiratory failure.

Radiation-Induced Pneumonitis

Pathogenesis

Ionizing radiation injures cells and causes cell death in a variety of ways. Cellular injury has generally been attributed to deoxyribonucleic acid (DNA) damage.[95] Extensive single- and double-stranded breaks in DNA can overwhelm cellular repair mechanisms. Disruption of genomic sequences will ultimately impair vital cellular processes and cause cell death. Rapidly dividing cells are most vulnerable to this damage. DNA damage may not be noticeable in resting cells but may become apparent as these cells enter mitosis. The direct effects of radiation on the cell membrane may also induce apoptosis through the effects on cell membrane sphingomyelin.[96] Recent evidence suggests that radiation will cause the enzyme acid sphingomyelinase to convert sphingomyelin to ceramide. Ceramide will ultimately be transported to the mitochondria, where it will activate apoptosis.[97] Initiation of apoptosis through this sequence of events may be most important in endothelial cells because these cells have high levels of acid sphingomyelinase.[98] Radiation may also damage cells by initiating complex inflammatory processes. Reactive oxygen species are generated by ionizing radiation. These reactive oxygen species can up-regulate expression of a variety of proinflammatory mediators, such as TNF and intracellular adhesion molecule 1,[99,100] and stimulate recruitment of inflammatory cells. Inflammation within the lung is characteristically found after radiation therapy. Gene expression profiling indicates that profibrotic and growth factors, such as platelet-derived growth factor and transforming growth factor, are activated shortly after the pulmonary inflammatory process begins.[101] These observations demonstrate that the acute inflammatory response to ionizing radiation is inextricably linked to the development of subsequent pulmonary fibrosis.

Clinical Manifestations

Radiation pneumonitis presents in one of two fundamentally different ways. Acute radiation pneumonitis has been defined as developing within 90 days of radiation therapy. Radiation-induced pulmonary fibrosis is defined as becoming evident 6 months after radiation therapy and may progress over years. However, a clear distinction between these two forms of radiation pneumonitis may be artificial as the pathogenesis of the disease suggests that acute inflammation is the basis for the development of fibrosis. The most widely accepted method for categorizing the severity of acute radiation pneumonitis and radiation-induced pulmonary fibrosis has been developed by the Radiation Therapy Oncology Group (RTOG) (Table 5).[102]

It is difficult to precisely define the incidence of the two forms of radiation pneumonitis. Following radiation therapy, radiographic and pulmonary function testing may show subtle abnormalities in a substantial number of patients, but most will not have symptoms related to these changes. These effects have been clearly documented in a prospective study of patients receiving radiation therapy for management of lung cancer. Standard measures of lung function, the forced expiratory volume in 1 second (FEV_1) and the diffusing capacity for carbon monoxide (DLCO), decreased between 10 and 15% over the 6 months following treatment.[103] Interestingly, the FEV_1 tended to improve by 12 months, but the DLCO remained decreased. The reduction in the DLCO may be the most sensitive indicator of radiation pneumonitis. It can reflect changes in the lung interstitium related to either fibrosis or inflammation. It is also sensitive to a reduction in lung perfusion related to endothelial cell injury, which has also been demonstrated following thoracic radiation.[104] Changes in DLCO, a physiologic test, nicely reflect the pathogenesis of radiation pneumonitis, which involves both endothelial damage and interstitial inflammation.

Symptomatic radiation pneumonitis may affect more than 30% of treated patients, but most will have transient symptoms that resolve without treatment.[105–107] In these patients, the usual presenting complaint is shortness of breath. Dry, nonproductive cough may also be described. Hypoxia, sometimes to a severe degree, will commonly accompany these symptoms. Probably less than 10% of patients receiving radiation therapy will develop more problematic pulmonary involvement (RTOG grades 3 and 4). Fortunately, respiratory failure is unusual.[108]

The diagnosis of radiation pneumonitis is usually established by the chest radiograph. Interstitial changes, typically described as reticulonodular shadows, are found corresponding to the radiation field or portal. In the classic example of the radiographic findings of radiation pneumonitis, the interstitial changes have sharp edges with a geometric shape (Figure 1). The shape does not correspond to lung anatomy, again emphasizing the relationship to the radiation portal. However, in unusual cases, radiographic changes may be found diffusely, or "out of (the radiation) field." ARDS, reflecting diffuse lung disease, has been described in patients following localized lung radiation. In these cases, radiation may have induced a lymphocyte-mediated hypersensitivity reaction against lung antigens.[109]

Radiation pneumonitis occurs primarily in patients with lymphoma, lung cancer, bone marrow transplantation, esophageal cancer, and breast cancer who may receive ionizing radiation to the thorax. The risk of developing radiation pneumonitis is most clearly related to the dose of radiation received, the volume of lung irradiated, and the treatment schedule. The role of these factors is demonstrated by the following clinical observations. Upper hemibody irradiation with a dose of 8 Gy results in a high risk of life-threatening pulmonary complications, and a single-fraction dose of 10 Gy to the entire lungs is nearly always fatal.[110] The threshold dose for causing radiation pneumonitis seems to be 20 to 25 Gy administered in 1.8 to 2 Gy per dose fractions. This threshold dose is well below the usual curative intent dose administered to patients with lung cancer, which is between 63 and 70 Gy.[111] Tangential radiation of the breast after lumpectomy or the chest wall after mastectomy results in very low risk of radiation pneumonitis.[112] Daily treatments of 1.8 to 2 Gy seem to pose minimal risk,[113] whereas daily treatment sizes of greater than 2.67 Gy present greater risk. Continuous hyperfractionated accelerated radiotherapy, which involves using smaller doses of radiation therapy given two to three times per day, may also effectively reduce the risk of radiation pneumonitis.[114,115] Almost certainly genetic factors play a role in determining the susceptibility of patients to developing radiation pneumonits, but future work is needed to more fully understand this interaction.

Understanding the relationship among radiation dose, lung volume irradiated, and treatment schedule was an essential step in developing more sophisticated methods to minimize the risk of radiation pneumonitis. Three-dimensional CT-based conformal treatment planning is currently used to determine the ideal radiation dose and portal. The ideal radiation dose is defined as the maximal dose that can be delivered to the tumor while simultaneously minimizing radiation delivered to surrounding normal tissue. Based on the results of chest CT, a dose-volume histogram is constructed that essentially graphs

Table 5 Severity Categorization of Radiation Pneumonitis and Radiation Fibrosis						
	Grade 0	*Grade 1*	*Grade 2*	*Grade 3*	*Grade 4*	*Grade 5*
Radiation pneumonitis	No adverse effects	Mild symptoms of dry cough or dyspnea	Persistent cough requiring narcotic antitussives/dyspnea with minimal effort	Severe cough refractory to narcotic antitussives or dyspnea at rest, radiographic evidence of pneumonitis, intermittent oxygen needs, or requirement for steroids	Severe respiratory insufficiency with requirement for continuous oxygen or assisted ventilation	Death
Radiation fibrosis	No adverse effects	Asymptomatic or mild symptoms: dry cough, slight radiographic changes	Moderate symptomatic fibrosis	Severe symptomatic fibrosis, dense radiographic changes	Severe respiratory insufficiency, oxygen required or assisted ventilation	Death

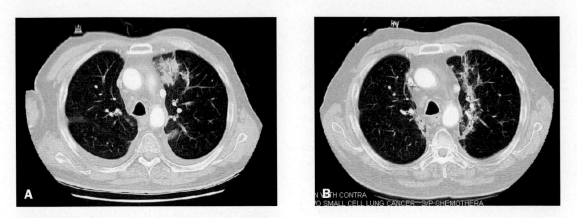

FIGURE 1 A computed tomographic scan of a patient with acute radiation pneumonitis (*left*) with subsequent development of radiation-induced pulmonary fibrosis (*right*). Note the sharp line demarcating the parenchymal infiltrate from the normal-appearing lung and the geometric shape of the infiltrate, both of which are characteristic features of radiation pneumonitis.

the cumulative dose going to the lung versus the tumor. Cases that may benefit most from this approach are those tumors that are situated adjacent to radiosensitive tissue, such as the heart, esophagus, and spinal cord. Limiting this approach in lung cancer is the frequent combination of tumor and atelectasis. Distinguishing between tumor and either atelectatic lung or postobstructive pneumonia may be difficult. This approach does allow the average radiation dose to be calculated for normal lung; this can be a useful guide to the probability of radiation pneumonitis.[116] The risk of radiation pneumonitis increases from 10% in portions of lung receiving less than 10 Gy to 50% in portions of lung receiving, on average, over 30 Gy.[117]

Management

Treatment of acute, symptomatic radiation pneumonitis is based on the use of corticosteroids. Although randomized controlled clinical trials have not demonstrated the value of this approach, nonrandomized clinical studies support the use of corticosteroids in patients with grade 2 or greater severity disease.[118] The dose and duration of therapy vary, with tapering adjusted by individual response. For patients with grade 3 severity, prednisone given at 1 mg/kg is the usual starting dose, which should be tapered by reductions of no more than 10 mg every 2 weeks. Recurrence of symptoms is common during the tapering process and requires dose escalation. Corticosteroids should not be used to prevent acute radiation pneumonitis. Patients with grade 3 severity radiation pneumonitis or fibrosis should be carefully evaluated for use of chronic oxygen supplementation and ventilatory assist devices.

There has been considerable interest in developing pharmacologic approaches to prevent radiation pneumonitis. Amifostine (Ethyol, Medimmune) is a drug approved for use as a radiation protector, but only for patients receiving radiation therapy for cancers of the head and

neck region. It may act as a scavenger of reactive oxygen species. The drug may be preferentially taken up by normal cells, protecting them from reactive oxygen species generated by irradiation. Small clinical trials in patients with advanced non–small cell lung cancer suggest that amifostine may prevent acute radiation pneumonitis, but further long-term trials are needed to clearly demonstrate this benefit.[119,120] Pentoxyfilline (Trental, Aventis) was also found in a small double-blind randomized trial to protect against radiation pneumonitis.[121] The protective effects of pentoxyfilline may occur by interference with TNF signaling. There is active interest in a variety of other classes of drugs as protective agents. Angiotensin-converting enzyme inhibitors have been shown in preclinical studies with rodents to have promise in protecting against radiation pneumonitis, but the mechanism of action is unclear.[122] Future studies will be directed at inhibitors of cytokines and other mediators of the inflammatory and fibrotic response.

In summary, radiation pneumonitis occurs through the effects of ionizing radiation on normal lung and endothelial cells. Factors predisposing patients to radiation pneumonitis relate to the amount of normal tissue being exposed to irradiation, the total dose, and the dosing schedule. Modern radiotherapy techniques have successfully reduced the risk of radiation pneumonitis by carefully adjusting the radiation portal according to three-dimensional visualization of the tumor obtained by CT scans. Radiation pneumonitis can usually be controlled with corticosteroids, but severe toxicity still may occur. There is promise for the development of pharmacologic approaches to prevent radiation pneumonitis.

Chemotherapy-Related Lung Disease

Pathogenesis and Risk Factors

The mechanism by which chemotherapeutic agents cause lung damage is not well understood.

This is in large part because so many different chemotherapeutic drugs, with multiple different modes of action, have been implicated as causes of lung injury. Finding a common mechanism among the various classes of chemotherapeutic agents implicated in causing lung damage has not been possible. Further complicating the relationship between drug and lung injury is the possibility that the drug itself may not be causing the injury; rather, the lung damage may be caused by a metabolite of the drug.

A possible common theme for chemotherapy-induced pneumonitis is that the alveolar epithelial cell seems to be the target cell for injury. One possible mechanism for chemotherapeutic agents to damage this cell is through enhanced apoptosis. Apoptosis pathways can be initiated through interaction of an anticancer drug with the cell surface molecule Fas ligand. Alternatively, chemotherapeutic agents may trigger apoptosis through interactions with cytochrome *c* in the mitochondria. A key intermediate step leading to cell death in both the Fas ligand and the mitochondrial apoptosis pathways is activation of the caspase cascade.[123] Toxic drug metabolites may be an alternative way for chemotherapeutic agents to damage alveolar epithelial cells. Biotransformation of drugs usually occurs through oxidation. This process can produce reactive oxygen species; accumulation of these reactive oxygen species may cause cell death through oxidative stress and lipid peroxidation. This observation may be particularly relevant to the alveolar epithelial cell because of its exposure to ambient air. Hyperoxia has been clinically implicated as being associated with an increased susceptibility to chemotherapeutic drug–induced lung toxicity. Hyperoxia will also increase the production of reactive oxygen species.[123] Toxic drug metabolites may also trigger an immune response.[124] Whatever mechanism is responsible for the initial alveolar epithelial cell injury, the inflammatory response also triggers increased production of growth factors, particularly members of the epidermal growth factor family. Activation of growth factors is probably critical for epithelial cell repair but may also be responsible for initiation of pulmonary fibrosis.[123]

Other important issues in the pathogenesis of chemotherapy-induced lung disease are the relationship of genetic factors with risk and the enhanced risk associated with either combined chemotherapy and radiation therapy or concomitant administration of multiple drugs that have pulmonary toxicity. The importance that genetic factors might play in the susceptibility of population groups to chemotherapy-induced pneumonitis became apparent with the introduction of gefinitib, an epidermal growth factor receptor tyrosine kinase inhibitor, into Japan. The reported incidence of interstitial lung disease following the use of gefinitib in Japan was 1.9%, which is higher than reported rates for the rest of the world. Whether part of this increase in risk was due to unsuspected, preexisting lung disease in patients treated with gefinitib is still unclear.[125] Combined administration of chemotherapy and radiation therapy seems to increase the risk of lung injury.[126] Chemotherapy given prior to the initiation of radiation therapy (neoadjuvant chemotherapy) seems not to increase the risk of radiation pneumonitis, but concomitant administration of chemotherapy and radiation therapy is associated with a substantially higher risk of radiation pneumonitis.[102] Chemotherapeutic agents that seem to be associated with this increased risk include gemcitabine, bleomycin, and anthracyclines.[127–129] Another chemotherapeutic agent that possibly might increase the likelihood of radiation pneumonitis is paclitaxel.[130] There is concern that taxine-containing regimens pose a greater risk of inducing radiation pneumonitis than platin-vinca and platin-etoposide regimens.[102] The simultaneous use of multiple drugs that are associated with pulmonary toxicity may also be a significant hazard. The combination of gemcitabine and bleomycin seems to be associated with an unacceptably high rate of pulmonary toxicity.[131] Interestingly, amiodarone has been associated with enhancing the pulmonary toxicity of cyclophosphamide.[132]

Clinical Manifestations

Chemotherapy-induced lung injury may present in multiple different ways, ranging from acute respiratory failure to the more insidious development of dyspnea and nonproductive cough. Although the symptoms and radiographic manifestations of chemotherapy pneumonitis are often nonspecific, in general, lung injury associated with the use of chemotherapeutic agents will usually fall into one of six different types.[133] These six different categories are differentiated definitively by histologic means, but the diagnosis may often be suspected by the combination of clinical and radiographic findings.

Diffuse alveolar damage has been associated most commonly with bleomycin.[134,135] Clinically, it may present with an acute to subacute course, with symptoms of dyspnea and nonproductive cough developing over weeks. Radiographic changes are most clearly seen on chest CT, which demonstrates diffuse ground-glass opacities. Histologically, it is characterized by hyaline membrane formation in alveolar spaces along with alveolar and interstitial edema. Hypersensitivity pneumonitis has been related to the use of methotrexate and cyclophosphamide.[133,136] In some cases, it may present in a similar way clinically to diffuse alveolar damage, with an acute to subacute onset of symptoms. However, it may also present in a more indolent fashion. Radiographic

abnormalities may consist of ground-glass opacities, especially with the more acute onset of symptoms; with chronic presentation, it is more likely that poorly defined nodular opacities will be found on a chest radiograph or CT scan. The histologic appearance of hypersensitivity pneumonitis shows granulomas, indicating an immunologically mediated disorder. Bronchoalveolar lavage will reveal high numbers of lymphocytes.

Probably the most common form of chemotherapy-induced pneumonitis, confirmed histologically, is nonspecific interstitial pneumonitis.[137] It has most commonly been associated with methotrexate. This form of drug-related lung injury tends to present over a longer time course. Radiographic changes are often described as patchy, but diffuse ground-glass opacities may also be seen in more severe cases. As the disease progresses, chest CT will begin to show such evidence of pulmonary fibrosis as a reticular pattern and peripheral traction bronchiectasis with honeycombing. Lung biopsy will show infiltration of interstitial spaces with fibrosis and a mononuclear inflammatory process. Bronchiolitis obliterans organizing pneumonia, formerly known as BOOP and now referred to as cryptogenic organizing pneumonia, has been described with methotrexate, cyclophosphamide, bleomycin, and busulfan.[135,137] The clinical symptoms usually progress in a more chronic fashion, similar to nonspecific interstitial pneumonits. Radiographically, patchy infiltrates are seen either peripherally or peribronchially. Histologically, nonspecific inflammation and fibrosis are found in the interstitial spaces and plugs of loose connective tissue with immature fibroblasts are seen within respiratory bronchioles.

Unusual forms of chemotherapy-induced pneumonitis include eosinophilic pneumonia and pulmonary edema. Eosinophilic pneumonia has been described in association with the use of methotrexate.[134,135] The clinical presentation may be either acute or subacute, and respiratory failure may occur. Bilateral airspace consolidation, characteristically involving the lung periphery, is the typical radiographic appearance. The alveoli, and often the interstitium, are filled with eosinophils. Peripheral eosinophilia may not be apparent, but bronchoalveolar lavage will show a very high percentage of eosinophils. Diffuse capillary leak syndrome may cause acute pulmonary edema. Capillary leak has been associated with cytosine arabinoside and docetaxel; it has been clearly described in the all-*trans* retinoic acid syndrome.[138] Patients present within days of beginning all-*trans* retinoic acid with respiratory distress, pleural and pericardial effusions, and bilateral, diffuse airspace consolidation on a chest radiograph or CT scan. Lung histology is nonspecific, with alveoli filled with proteinaceous material.

Management

Treatment is based on first establishing the diagnosis. Usually, the onset of symptomatic chemotherapy-induced lung injury and associated radiographic abnormalities and changes in pulmonary function tests coincide temporally with the use of the drug. Unfortunately, serial measurements of the DLCO do not always predict the development of drug-induced lung disease.[131] Disease recognition should prompt discontinuation of the offending agent, which may be sufficient to allow reversal of the disease. The standard approach to treatment of symptomatic chemotherapy pneumonitis is the use of corticosteroids. With severe forms presenting with respiratory failure, high-dose corticosteroids (methylprednisolone at a dose of 250 mg four times per day) is most often advised.[133] In less severe cases, as with radiation-induced pneumonitis, the use of prednisone 1 to 2 mg/kg/d is an accepted approach. Tapering is a slow process, often taking months, and may be complicated by recurrences of symptoms. Immunosuppressive agents, such as azathioprine, have been used as corticosteroid-sparing agents in patients suffering from intolerable side effects, but the value of these agents has never been demonstrated. Interest in developing pharmacologic approaches to either preventing or treating chemotherapy-induced lung disease is high.

In summary, chemotherapeutic agents can damage the lungs in a variety of ways, with the alveolar epithelial cells appearing to be most vulnerable. Chemotherapy-induced lung damage may develop acutely or insidiously. Presenting symptoms are usually dyspnea and nonproductive cough with either ground-glass opacifications or reticulonodular infiltrates found on CT. Histologic abnormalities vary widely, but fibrosis may be an ultimate end point. Early recognition and timely withdrawal of the offending agent, along with corticosteroids, are usually effective in controlling the disease.

Conclusion

Noninfectious pulmonary problems in the patient with cancer range widely in type. This chapter has reviewed the major types that should be considered. These problems are associated with metastatic spread of the cancer (to the pleura, causing effusions and pneumothorax, or to the airways, precipitating hemoptysis), systematic procoagulant effects of the cancer (promoting the risk for VTE), and side effects of the treatments (radiotherapy and/or chemotherapy) used to treat the primary disease. Unfortunately, many of these noninfectious pulmonary problems are associated with an overall poor prognosis. Sensitivity to this issue in cancer patients suffering from noninfectious pulmonary problems should be an important aspect of the management approach.

REFERENCES

1. American Cancer Society. Available at: www.americancancersociety.org (accessed March 12, 2006).

2. Antony VB, Loddenkemper R, Astoul P, et al. Management of malignant pleural effusions. Eur Respir J 2001;18:402–19.

3. Alexandrakis MG, Passam FH, Kyriakou DS, et al. Pleural effusions in hematologic malignancies. Chest 2004;125:1546–55.

4. Heffner JE, Nietert PJ, Barbieri C. Pleural fluid pH as a predictor of survival for patients with malignant pleural effusions. Chest 2000;117:79–86.

5. Light RW, Macgregor MI, Luchsinger PC, et al. Pleural effusions: the diagnostic separation of transudates and exudates. Ann Intern Med 1972;77:507–13.

6. Heffner JE, Brown LK, Barbieri CA. Diagnostic value of tests that discriminate between exudative and transudative pleural effusions. Chest 1997;111:970–80.

7. Sahn SA, Good JT Jr. Pleural fluid pH in malignant effusions. Diagnostic, prognostic, and therapeutic implications. Ann Intern Med 1988;108:345–9.

8. Light RW. Clinical practice. Pleural effusion. N Engl J Med 2002;346:1971–7.

9. Romero Candeira S, Hernandez Blasco L, et al. Biochemical and cytologic characteristics of pleural effusions secondary to pulmonary embolism. Chest 2002;121:465–9.

10. Rivera MP, Detterbeck F, Mehta AC. Diagnosis of lung cancer: the guidelines. Chest 2003;123S:129–36.

11. Loddenkemper R. Thoracoscopy—state of the art. Eur Respir J 1998;11:213–21.

12. Estenne M, Yernault JC, De Troyer A. Mechanism of relief of dyspnea after thoracocentesis in patients with large pleural effusions. Am J Med 1983;74:813–9.

13. Kvale PA, Simoff M, Prakash UB. Lung cancer. Palliative care. Chest 2003;123S:284–311.

14. Light RW, Stansbury DW, Brown SE. The relationship between pleural pressures and changes in pulmonary function after therapeutic thoracentesis. Am Rev Respir Dis 1986;133:658–61.

15. Light RW, Jenkinson SG, Minh VD, et al. Observations on pleural fluid pressures as fluid is withdrawn during thoracentesis. Am Rev Respir Dis 1980;121:799–804.

16. Antunes G, Neville E, Duffy J, et al. BTS guidelines for the management of malignant pleural effusions. Thorax 2003;58 Suppl 2:ii29–38.

17. Pollak JS. Malignant pleural effusions: treatment with tunneled long-term drainage catheters. Curr Opin Pulm Med 2002;8:302–7.

18. Putnam JB Jr, Light RW, Rodriguez RM, et al. A randomized comparison of indwelling pleural catheter and doxycycline pleurodesis in the management of malignant pleural effusions. Cancer 1999;86:1992–9.

19. Putnam JB Jr, Walsh GL, Swisher SG, et al. Outpatient management of malignant pleural effusion by a chronic indwelling pleural catheter. Ann Thorac Surg 2000;69:369–75.

20. Martinez-Moragon E, Aparicio J, Sanchis J, et al. Malignant pleural effusion: prognostic factors for survival and response to chemical pleurodesis in a series of 120 cases. Respiration 1998;65:108–13.

21. Xie C, Teixeira LR, McGovern JP, et al. Systemic corticosteroids decrease the effectiveness of talc pleurodesis. Am J Respir Crit Care Med 1998;157:1441–4.

22. Dressler CM, Olak J, Herndon JE, et al. Phase III intergroup study of talc poudrage vs talc slurry sclerosis for malignant pleural effusion. Chest 2005;127:909–15.

23. Shaw P, Agarwal R. Pleurodesis for malignant pleural effusions. Cochrane Database Syst Rev 2004;CD002916.

24. Yim AP, Chan AT, Lee TW, et al. Thoracoscopic talc insufflation versus talc slurry for symptomatic malignant pleural effusion. Ann Thorac Surg 1996;62:1655–8.

25. Clementsen P, Evald T, Grode G, et al. Treatment of malignant pleural effusion: pleurodesis using a small percutaneous catheter. A prospective randomized study. Respir Med 1998;92:593–6.

26. Patz EF Jr, McAdams HP, Erasmus JJ, et al. Sclerotherapy for malignant pleural effusions: a prospective randomized trial of bleomycin vs doxycycline with small-bore catheter drainage. Chest 1998;113:1305–11.

27. Tattersall DJ, Traill ZC, Gleeson FV. Chest drains: does size matter? Clin Radiol 2000;55:415–21.

28. West SD, Davies RJ, Lee YC. Pleurodesis for malignant pleural effusions: current controversies and variations in practices. Curr Opin Pulm Med 2004;10:305–10.

29. Pien GW, Gant MJ, Washam CL, et al. Use of an implantable pleural catheter for trapped lung syndrome in patients with malignant pleural effusion. Chest 2001;119:1641–6.

30. Sahn SA, Heffner JE. Spontaneous pneumothorax. N Engl J Med 2000;342:868–74.

31. O'Connor BM, Ziegler P, Spaulding MB. Spontaneous pneumothorax in small cell lung cancer. Chest 1992;102:628–9.

32. Minami H, Sakai S, Watanabe A, et al. Check-valve mechanism as a cause of bilateral spontaneous pneumothorax complicating bronchioloalveolar cell carcinoma. Chest 1991;100:853–5.

33. Woodring JH. Unusual radiographic manifestations of lung cancer. Radiol Clin North Am 1990;28:599–618.

34. Steinhauslin CA, Cuttat JF. Spontaneous pneumothorax. A complication of lung cancer? Chest 1985;88:709–13.

35. Seo JB, Im JG, Goo JM, et al. Atypical pulmonary metastases: spectrum of radiologic findings. Radiographics 2001;21:403–17.

36. Smevik B, Klepp O. The risk of spontaneous pneumothorax in patients with osteogenic sarcoma and testicular cancer. Cancer 1982;49:1734–7.

37. Baumann MH, Strange C, Heffner JE, et al. Management of spontaneous pneumothorax: an American College of Chest Physicians Delphi consensus statement. Chest 2001;119:590–602.

38. Northfield TC. Oxygen therapy for spontaneous pneumothorax. Br Med J 1971;4:86–8.

39. Trousseau A. Phlegmasia alba dolens, textbook (Clinique Medicale de l'Hotel-Dieu de Paris). Vol 3. R. Hardiwicke, London, 1865.

40. Deitcher SR. Cancer-related deep venous thrombosis: clinical importance, treatment challenges, and management strategies. Semin Thromb Hemost 2003;29:247–58.

41. Sallah S, Wan JY, Nguyen NP. Venous thrombosis in patients with solid tumors: determination of frequency and characteristics. Thromb Haemost 2002;87:575–9.

42. Sorensen HT, Johnsen SP, Norgard B, et al. Cancer and venous thromboembolism: a multidisciplinary approach. Clin Lab 2003;49:615–23.

43. Hettiarachchi RJ, Lok J, Prins MH, et al. Undiagnosed malignancy in patients with deep vein thrombosis: incidence, risk indicators, and diagnosis. Cancer 1998;83:180–5.

44. Prandoni P, Lensing AW, Buller HR, et al. Deep-vein thrombosis and the incidence of subsequent symptomatic cancer. N Engl J Med 1992;327:1128–33.

45. Prandoni P, Piccioli A. Venous thromboembolism and cancer: a two-way clinical association. Front Biosci 1997;2:e12–20.

46. Baron JA, Gridley G, Weiderpass E, et al. Venous thromboembolism and cancer. Lancet 1998;351:1077–80.

47. Sorensen HT, Mellemkjaer L, Steffensen FH, et al. The risk of a diagnosis of cancer after primary deep venous thrombosis or pulmonary embolism. N Engl J Med 1998;338:1169–73.

48. Mandala M, Ferretti G, Cremonesi M, et al. Venous thromboembolism and cancer: new issues for an old topic. Crit Rev Oncol Hematol 2003;48:65–80.

49. Kwaan HC, Parmar S, Wang J. Pathogenesis of increased risk of thrombosis in cancer. Semin Thromb Hemost 2003;29:283–90.

50. Lee AY. Cancer and thromboembolic disease: pathogenic mechanisms. Cancer Treat Rev 2002;28:137–40.

51. Rickles FR, Falanga A. Molecular basis for the relationship between thrombosis and cancer. Thromb Res 2001;102:V215–24.

52. Sorensen HT, Mellemkjaer L, Olsen JH, et al. Prognosis of cancers associated with venous thromboembolism. N Engl J Med 2000;343:1846–50.

53. Geerts WH, Pineo GF, Heit JA, et al. Prevention of venous thromboembolism: the Seventh ACCP Conference on Antithrombotic and Thrombolytic Therapy. Chest 2004;126S:338–400.

54. Kakkar AK, Williamson RC. Prevention of venous thromboembolism in cancer patients. Semin Thromb Hemost 1999;25:239–43.

55. Mismetti P, Laporte S, Darmon JY, et al. Meta-analysis of low molecular weight heparin in the prevention of venous thromboembolism in general surgery. Br J Surg 2001;88:913–30.

56. Efficacy and safety of enoxaparin versus unfractionated heparin for prevention of deep vein thrombosis in elective cancer surgery: a double-blind randomized multicentre trial with venographic assessment. ENOXACAN Study Group. Br J Surg 1997;84:1099–103.

57. Bergqvist D, Agnelli G, Cohen AT, et al. Duration of prophylaxis against venous thromboembolism with enoxaparin after surgery for cancer. N Engl J Med 2002;346:975–80.

58. Lee AY. Anti-thrombotic therapy in cancer patients. Expert Opin Pharmacother 2003;4:2213–20.

59. Marras LC, Geerts WH, Perry JR. The risk of venous thromboembolism is increased throughout the course of malignant glioma: an evidence-based review. Cancer 2000;89:640–6.

60. Agnelli G, Piovella F, Buoncristiani P, et al. Enoxaparin plus compression stockings compared with compression stockings alone in the prevention of venous thromboembolism after elective neurosurgery. N Engl J Med 1998;339:80–5.

61. Iorio A, Agnelli G. Low-molecular-weight and unfractionated heparin for prevention of venous thromboembolism in neurosurgery: a meta-analysis. Arch Intern Med 2000;160:2327–32.

62. Nurmohamed MT, van Riel AM, Henkens CM, et al. Low molecular weight heparin and compression stockings in the prevention of venous thromboembolism in neurosurgery. Thromb Haemost 1996;75:233–8.

63. Prandoni P, Lensing AW, Piccioli A, et al. Recurrent venous thromboembolism and bleeding complications during anticoagulant treatment in patients with cancer and venous thrombosis. Blood 2002;100:3484–8.

64. Palareti G, Legnani C, Lee A, et al. A comparison of the safety and efficacy of oral anticoagulation for the treatment of venous thromboembolic disease in patients with or without malignancy. Thromb Haemost 2000;84:805–10.

65. Low-molecular-weight heparin in the treatment of patients with venous thromboembolism. The Columbus Investigators. N Engl J Med 1997;337:657–62.

66. Gould MK, Dembitzer AD, Doyle RL, et al. Low-molecular-weight heparins compared with unfractionated heparin for treatment of acute deep venous thrombosis. A meta-analysis of randomized, controlled trials. Ann Intern Med 1999;130:800–9.

67. Koopman MM, Prandoni P, Piovella F, et al. Treatment of venous thrombosis with intravenous unfractionated heparin administered in the hospital as compared with subcutaneous low-molecular-weight heparin administered at home. The Tasman Study Group. N Engl J Med 1996;334:682–7.

68. Ansell J, Hirsh J, Poller L, et al. The pharmacology and management of the vitamin K antagonists: the Seventh ACCP Conference on Antithrombotic and Thrombolytic Therapy. Chest 2004;126S:204–33.

69. Meyer G, Marjanovic Z, Valcke J, et al. Comparison of low-molecular-weight heparin and warfarin for the secondary prevention of venous thromboembolism in patients with cancer: a randomized controlled study. Arch Intern Med 2002;162:1729–35.

70. Lee AY, Levine MN, Baker RI, et al. Low-molecular-weight heparin versus a coumarin for the prevention of recurrent venous thromboembolism in patients with cancer. N Engl J Med 2003;349:146–53.

71. Kearon C, Gent M, Hirsh J, et al. A comparison of three months of anticoagulation with extended anticoagulation for a first episode of idiopathic venous thromboembolism. N Engl J Med 1999;340:901–7.

72. Schulman S, Lindmarker P. Incidence of cancer after prophylaxis with warfarin against recurrent venous thromboembolism. Duration of Anticoagulation Trial. N Engl J Med 2000;342:1953–8.

73. Agnelli G, Prandoni P, Santamaria MG, et al. Three months versus one year of oral anticoagulant therapy for idiopathic deep venous thrombosis. Warfarin Optimal Duration Italian Trial Investigators. N Engl J Med 2001;345:165–9.

74. Kearon C, Ginsberg JS, Kovacs MJ, et al. Comparison of low-intensity warfarin therapy with conventional-intensity warfarin therapy for long-term prevention of recurrent venous thromboembolism. N Engl J Med 2003;349:631–9.

75. Ridker PM, Goldhaber SZ, Danielson E, et al. Long-term, low-intensity warfarin therapy for the prevention of recurrent venous thromboembolism. N Engl J Med 2003;348:1425–34.

76. Levine MN. Managing thromboembolic disease in the cancer patient: efficacy and safety of antithrombotic treatment options in patients with cancer. Cancer Treat Rev 2002;28:145–9.

77. Decousus H, Leizorovicz A, Parent F, et al. A clinical trial of vena caval filters in the prevention of pulmonary embolism in patients with proximal deep-vein thrombosis. Prevention du Risque d'Embolie Pulmonaire par Interruption Cave Study Group. N Engl J Med 1998;338:409–15.

78. Kakkar AK. An expanding role for antithrombotic therapy in cancer patients. Cancer Treat Rev 2003;29 Suppl 2:23–6.

79. Kakkar AK, Levine MN, Kadziola Z, et al. Low molecular weight heparin, therapy with dalteparin, and survival in advanced cancer: the Fragmin Advanced Malignancy Outcome Study (FAMOUS). J Clin Oncol 2004;22: 1944–8.

80. Thompson AB, Teschler H, Rennard SI. Pathogenesis, evaluation, and therapy for massive hemoptysis. Clin Chest Med 1992;13:69–82.

81. Deffebach ME, Charan NB, Lakshminarayan S, et al. The bronchial circulation. Small, but a vital attribute of the lung. Am Rev Respir Dis 1987;135:463–81.

82. Ripamonti C, Fusco F. Respiratory problems in advanced cancer. Support Care Cancer 2002;10:204–16.

83. Miller RR, McGregor DH. Hemorrhage from carcinoma of the lung. Cancer 1980;46:200–5.

84. Millar AB, Boothroyd AE, Edwards D, et al. The role of computed tomography (CT) in the investigation of unexplained haemoptysis. Respir Med 1992;86:39–44.

85. Marshall TJ, Flower CD, Jackson JE. The role of radiology in the investigation and management of patients with haemoptysis. Clin Radiol 1996;51:391–400.

86. Naidich DP, Funt S, Ettenger NA, et al. Hemoptysis: CT-bronchoscopic correlations in 58 cases. Radiology 1990; 177:357–62.

87. Bobrowitz ID, Ramakrishna S, Shim YS. Comparison of medical v surgical treatment of major hemoptysis. Arch Intern Med 1983;143:1343–6.

88. Gong H Jr, Salvatierra C. Clinical efficacy of early and delayed fiberoptic bronchoscopy in patients with hemoptysis. Am Rev Respir Dis 1981;124:221–5.

89. Swanson KL, Johnson CM, Prakash UB, et al. Bronchial artery embolization: experience with 54 patients. Chest 2002;121:789–95.

90. Uflacker R, Kaemmerer A, Picon PD, et al. Bronchial artery embolization in the management of hemoptysis: technical aspects and long-term results. Radiology 1985;157: 637–44.

91. Yu-Tang Goh P, Lin M, Teo N, et al. Embolization for hemoptysis: a six -year review. Cardiovasc Intervent Radiol 2002;25:17–25.

92. Wong ML, Szkup P, Hopley MJ. Percutaneous embolotherapy for life-threatening hemoptysis. Chest 2002;121: 95–102.

93. Carson JL, Kelley MA, Duff A, et al. The clinical course of pulmonary embolism. N Engl J Med 1992;326:1240–5.

94. Levine MN, Lee AY, Kakkar AK. From Trousseau to targeted therapy: new insights and innovations in thrombosis and cancer. J Thromb Haemost 2003;1:1456–63.

95. Ward JF. DNA damage produced by ionizing radiation in mammalian cells: identities, mechanisms of formation, and reparability. Prog Nucleic Acid Res Mol Biol 1988; 35:95–125.

96. Paris F, Fuks Z, Kang A, et al. Endothelial apoptosis as the primary lesion initiating intestinal radiation damage in mice. Science 2001;293:293–7.

97. Santana P, Pena LA, Haimovitz-Friedman A, et al. Acid sphingomyelinase-deficient human lymphoblasts and mice are defective in radiation-induced apoptosis. Cell 1996;86:189–99.

98. Marathe S, Schissel SL, Yellin MJ, et al. Human vascular endothelial cells are a rich and regulatable source of secretory sphingomyelinase. Implications for early atherogenesis and ceramide-mediated cell signaling. J Biol Chem 1998;273:4081–8.

99. Hallahan D, Kuchibhotla J, Wyble C. Cell adhesion molecules mediate radiation-induced leukocyte adhesion to the vascular endothelium. Cancer Res 1996;56:5150–5.

100. Hallahan DE, Spriggs DR, Beckett MA, et al. Increased tumor necrosis factor alpha mRNA after cellular exposure to ionizing radiation. Proc Natl Acad Sci U S A 1989;86: 10104–7.

101. Thornton SC, Walsh BJ, Bennett S, et al. Both in vitro and in vivo irradiation are associated with induction of macrophage-derived fibroblast growth factors. Clin Exp Immunol 1996;103:67–73.

102. Machtay M. Pulmonary complications of anticancer treatment. In: Abeloff M, Armitage J, Niederhuber J, et al, editors. Clinical oncology. Elsevier Press; Philadelphia, PA 2004. p. 1237–50.

103. Miller KL, Zhou SM, Barrier RC Jr, et al. Long-term changes in pulmonary function tests after definitive radiotherapy for lung cancer. Int J Radiat Oncol Biol Phys 2003;56: 611–5.

104. Theuws JC, Kwa SL, Wagenaar AC, et al. Dose-effect relations for early local pulmonary injury after irradiation for malignant lymphoma and breast cancer. Radiother Oncol 1998;48:33–43.

105. Marks LB. The pulmonary effects of thoracic irradiation. Oncology (Huntingt) 1994;8:89–106; discussion 100, 103–4.

106. Marks LB. Dosimetric predictors of radiation-induced lung injury. Int J Radiat Oncol Biol Phys 2002;54:313–6.

107. Marks LB, Fan M, Clough R, et al. Radiation-induced pulmonary injury: symptomatic versus subclinical endpoints. Int J Radiat Biol 2000;76:469–75.

108. Monson JM, Stark P, Reilly JJ, et al. Clinical radiation pneumonitis and radiographic changes after thoracic radiation therapy for lung carcinoma. Cancer 1998;82:842–50.

109. Roberts CM, Foulcher E, Zaunders JJ, et al. Radiation pneumonitis: a possible lymphocyte-mediated hypersensitivity reaction. Ann Intern Med 1993;118:696–700.

110. Fryer CJ, Fitzpatrick PJ, Rider WD, et al. Radiation pneumonitis: experience following a large single dose of radiation. Int J Radiat Oncol Biol Phys 1978;4:931–6.

111. Roach M III, Gandara DR, Yuo HS, et al. Radiation pneumonitis following combined modality therapy for lung cancer: analysis of prognostic factors. J Clin Oncol 1995; 13:2606–12.

112. Lind PA, Marks LB, Hardenbergh PH, et al. Technical factors associated with radiation pneumonitis after local +/– regional radiation therapy for breast cancer. Int J Radiat Oncol Biol Phys 2002;52:137–43.

113. Carruthers SA, Wallington MM. Total body irradiation and pneumonitis risk: a review of outcomes. Br J Cancer 2004; 90:2080–4.

114. Jenkins P, D'Amico K, Benstead K, et al. Radiation pneumonitis following treatment of non-small-cell lung cancer with continuous hyperfractionated accelerated radiotherapy (CHART). Int J Radiat Oncol Biol Phys 2003; 56:360–6.

115. Saunders M, Dische S, Barrett A, et al. Continuous hyperfractionated accelerated radiotherapy (CHART) versus conventional radiotherapy in non-small-cell lung cancer: a randomised multicentre trial. CHART Steering Committee. Lancet 1997;350:161–5.

116. Rodrigues G, Lock M, D'Souza D, et al. Prediction of radiation pneumonitis by dose-volume histogram parameters in lung cancer—a systematic review. Radiother Oncol 2004;71:127–38.

117. Hernando ML, Marks LB, Bentel GC, et al. Radiation-induced pulmonary toxicity: a dose-volume histogram analysis in 201 patients with lung cancer. Int J Radiat Oncol Biol Phys 2001;51:650–9.

118. Moss WT, Haddy FJ, Sweany SK. Some factors altering the severity of acute radiation pneumonitis: variation with cortisone, heparin, and antibiotics. Radiology 1960;75: 50–4.

119. Antonadou D, Coliarakis N, Synodinou M, et al. Randomized phase III trial of radiation treatment +/– amifostine in patients with advanced-stage lung cancer. Int J Radiat Oncol Biol Phys 2001;51:915–22.

120. Komaki R, Lee JS, Kaplan B, et al. Randomized phase III study of chemoradiation with or without amifostine for patients with favorable performance status inoperable stage II-III non-small cell lung cancer: preliminary results. Semin Radiat Oncol 2002;12:46–9.

121. Ozturk B, Egehan I, Atavci S, et al. Pentoxifylline in prevention of radiation-induced lung toxicity in patients with breast and lung cancer: a double-blind randomized trial. Int J Radiat Oncol Biol Phys 2004;58:213–9.

122. Ward WF, Lin PJ, Wong PS, et al. Radiation pneumonitis in rats and its modification by the angiotensin-converting enzyme inhibitor captopril evaluated by high-resolution computed tomography. Radiat Res 1993;135:81–7.

123. Higenbottam T, Kuwano K, Nemery B, et al. Understanding the mechanisms of drug-associated interstitial lung disease. Br J Cancer 2004;91 Suppl 2:S31–7.

124. Kaplowitz N. Biochemical and cellular mechanisms of toxic liver injury. Semin Liver Dis 2002;22:137–44.

125. Camus P, Kudoh S, Ebina M. Interstitial lung disease associated with drug therapy. Br J Cancer 2004;91 Suppl 2:S18–23.

126. Abid SH, Malhotra V, Perry MC. Radiation-induced and chemotherapy-induced pulmonary injury. Curr Opin Oncol 2001;13:242–8.

127. Cassady JR, Richter MP, Piro AJ, et al. Radiation-Adriamycin interactions: preliminary clinical observations. Cancer 1975;36:946–9.

128. Catane R, Schwade JG, Turrisi AT III, et al. Pulmonary toxicity after radiation and bleomycin: a review. Int J Radiat Oncol Biol Phys 1979;5:1513–8.

129. Scalliet P, Goor C, Galdermans D. Gemzar with thoracic radiotherapy [abstract]. Proc Am Soc Clin Oncol 1988; 17:499.

130. Willner J, Schmidt M, Kirschner J, et al. Sequential chemo- and radiochemotherapy with weekly paclitaxel (Taxol) and 3D-conformal radiotherapy of stage III inoperable non-small-cell lung cancer. Results of a dose escalation study. Lung Cancer 2001;32:163–71.

131. Friedberg JW, Neuberg D, Kim H, et al. Gemcitabine added to doxorubicin, bleomycin, and vinblastine for the treatment of de novo Hodgkin disease: unacceptable acute pulmonary toxicity. Cancer 2003;98:978–82.

132. Bhagat R, Sporn TA, Long GD, et al. Amiodarone and cyclophosphamide: potential for enhanced lung toxicity. Bone Marrow Transplant 2001;27:1109–11.

133. Muller NL, White DA, Jiang H, et al. Diagnosis and management of drug-associated interstitial lung disease. Br J Cancer 2004;91 Suppl 2:S24–30.

134. Cleverley JR, Screaton NJ, Hiorns MP, et al. Drug-induced lung disease: high-resolution CT and histological findings. Clin Radiol 2002;57:292–9.

135. Rossi SE, Erasmus JJ, McAdams HP, et al. Pulmonary drug toxicity: radiologic and pathologic manifestations. Radiographics 2000;20:1245–59.

136. Ellis SJ, Cleverley JR, Muller NL. Drug-induced lung disease: high-resolution CT findings. AJR Am J Roentgenol 2000; 175:1019–24.

137. Erasmus JJ, McAdams HP, Rossi SE. Drug-induced lung injury. Semin Roentgenol 2002;37:72–81.

138. Jung JI, Choi JE, Hahn ST, et al. Radiologic features of all-trans-retinoic acid syndrome. AJR Am J Roentgenol 2002;178:475–80.

Cancer-Related Issues in Mechanical Ventilation

Bruce P. Krieger, MD, FCCP

Mark Rumbak, MD, FCCP

Acute respiratory failure (ARF) is the most common diagnosis among adult cancer patients who require admission to the intensive care unit (ICU).[1,2] Recent reports noted that approximately 50[1,3,4] to 87%[5] of oncology patients with ARF will require mechanical ventilatory support (MVS). Advances in our understanding of ARF and MVS, especially in the spectrum of acute lung injury (ALI) and acute respiratory distress syndrome (ARDS),[6] have been applied to patients in the ICU and resulted in significant improvements in their survival. These encouraging techniques have been adopted for use in cancer patients with ALI/ARDS with the expectation of improved survival. The majority of diseases that precipitate ARF in cancer patients are potential causes of ARDS/ALI (Table 1). However, the precise number of cancer patients who develop ARDS is not known.[2] One series of 153 patients who suffered from hematologic and solid neoplasms and developed ARF documented a 30% incidence of ARDS and a 35% incidence of other causes of acute hypoxemic and ventilatory failure.[3] A more recent series documented a 20% incidence of ARDS among 203 cancer patients with ARF.[1]

Until the past decade, most clinicians and experts maintained a very pessimistic attitude toward the outcome of using MVS in oncology patients after the development of ARF. A review of the literature prior to 1999 disclosed mortality rates between 72 and 98% in this group of patients.[3] The mortality for patients with hematologic malignancies who required MVS exceeded 80%, whereas it was slightly lower (70%) in reports of patients with solid malignancies. The requirement for MVS in oncology patients who were admitted to an ICU significantly increased the risk of mortality in recent series ($p < .05$), raising the odds ratio of dying by 3.55 to 13.7 (Table 2).[3–5] However, more recent studies have evoked a less nihilistic opinion because of better survival rates, especially in hematologic patients who required MVS (Table 3).[3,5–7] Some of the proposed reasons for

Table 1 Causes of Acute Respiratory Failure in Oncology Patients
Underlying malignancy
Progression of the original malignancy
Airway obstruction from the malignancy
Lymphangitic carcinomatosis*
Pulmonary leukostasis*
Pulmonary hemorrhage*
Tumor emboli*
Paraneoplastic syndromes
Postoperative respiratory failure
Treatment-related complications
Radiation-induced lung injury*
Chemotherapy-induced pneumonitis*
Transfusion-associated lung injury*
Chemotherapy-induced cardiomyopathy
Chemotherapy-induced tumor lysis syndromes*
Chemotherapy-induced neutropenia and resulting infections*
Acute respiratory distress syndrome/acute lung injury
Pulmonary infections*
Bacterial, fungal, mycobacterial, viral
Nonpulmonary sepsis*
Aspiration*
Any of the above conditions marked with an asterisk
Miscellaneous
Venous thromboembolic disease
Renal failure
Gastrointestinal bleeding with aspiration

the improved outcomes include advances in critical care and invasive MVS,[6] targeted therapy for septic shock,[5] better treatments for malignancies, improved ventilatory strategies for MVS,[3] better support of nonpulmonary organ failures,[5] and noninvasive positive pressure ventilation (NIPPV).[8–13] This chapter explores the etiologies of ARF in oncology patients, problems with airway management in cancer patients, conventional MVS, lung-protective strategies for ventilating patients with ARDS, and how NIPPV has been used in treating cancer patients with ARF. A pragmatic algorithm is also presented that will aid interested clinicians in their approach to the adult oncology patient who requires MVS.

Incidence of and Indications for MVS in Oncology Patients

Various studies have reported the incidence of MVS that was required in adult oncology patients who were admitted to an ICU. However, because of the general nihilistic attitude toward this aggressive modality,[3] the actual need for ventilatory assistance in the cancer patient who develops ARF may be far greater than the reported incidence. Kress and colleagues documented the need for MVS in 46% of 44 lung cancer patients who were admitted to a university hospital ICU.[3] This was similar to the 54% incidence noted by Azoulay and colleagues in a group of 120 patients

Table 2 Effect of Mechanical Ventilatory Support on the Risk of Mortality in Oncology Patients Admitted to the Intensive Care Unit					
Study	Year	No. of Patients	Odds Ratio	95% Confidence Intervals	Population
Kress et al[3]	1999	44	13.7	1.6–120.6*	Bone marrow transplant only
Kress et al[3]	1999	77	10.0	3.4–29.9*	Neutropenic patients
Azoulay et al[4]	2000	120	3.55	1.09–1.44*	Solid tumors
Darmon et al[5]	2005	100	6.36	1.76–22.94*	Hematologic and solid tumors
*$p < .05$.					

Table 3 Survival Rates in Recent Studies of Oncology Patients Who Required Mechanical Ventilatory Support

Study	Year	No. of Patients	Survival (%)	Population
Kress et al.[3]	1999	153	33	Hematologic and solid tumors
Azoulay et al.[4]	2000	65	46	Solid tumors
Lin et al.[7]	2003	81	15	Bronchogenic carcinoma
Depuydt et al.[6]	2004	166	35	Mixed tumors; 16% NIPPV
Darmon et al.[5]	2005	87	45	Hematologic and solid tumors; 34% NIPPV

NIPPV = noninvasive positive pressure ventilation.

with solid tumors who presented with ARF, of whom 27% had lung cancer.[4] Azoulay and colleagues extended their findings in a later study to include hematologic malignancies in addition to solid tumors.[1] They also included patients who were prescribed noninvasive MVS. The requirement for MVS was similar to that in their earlier study (56%), with an additional 17% of patients treated with NIPPV alone.[1] NIPPV was used alone in 33% of 100 patients with hematologic and solid malignancies reported by Darmon and colleagues.[5] An additional 54% of these patients were intubated for MVS. In 80 patients with leukemia who developed ARF, 41% required MVS compared with 53% of 47 patients with lymphoma.[3] As noted earlier in this chapter, the need to institute MVS significantly increased the risk of mortality in all patient groups (see Table 2).

ARF is the most common diagnosis for oncology patients who were admitted into an ICU. Collating the data from three studies that involved 568 patients, the incidence of ARF was 40%.[3–5] The only recent study that provided detailed information concerning the etiology of ARF in cancer patients was Azoulay and colleagues' analysis of 203 cancer patients with ARF.[1] The majority (91%) of these patients had a hematologic malignancy, and 35% were neutropenic when admitted to the ICU. Infectious pneumonia was the cause of ARF in 58% of the patients, and multilobar radiologic involvement was present in 79% of all the subjects. Bacterial pneumonia was the most frequent infection (29.5%) and was associated with a statistically increased risk of mortality ($p = .04$) by univariate analyses but not multivariable analyses. Pneumocystis pneumonia, viral pneumonia, tuberculosis, and invasive aspergillosis were also diagnosed. The odds ratio of dying by multivariable analysis for patients with aspergillosis was significantly increased (3.78; $p < .05$). Twenty percent of their patients met the criteria for the diagnosis of ARDS. Noninfectious etiologies for ARF included congestive heart failure (12.3%), isolated alveolar hemorrhage (6%), toxic pneumonia (4%), pulmonary infiltration by malignant cells (8%), and no definite diagnoses despite an invasive diagnostic workup (21%). Patients with no definite diagnosis also had an increased risk of

dying ($p < .01$ by univariate analysis), whereas those who developed congestive heart failure had a lower risk of mortality by both univariate and multivariable analyses ($p = .01$). Although the authors did not comment on the incidence of ALI (which is a diagnosis that has a less impaired level of oxygenation compared with ARDS), it is likely that this was present in a significant number of their patients. Therefore, the remainder of this chapter focuses on caring for adult oncology patients with ARF who require MVS, especially in the presence of ALI and ARDS.

Airway Management

Upper Airway Obstruction

Upper airway obstruction is a medical emergency in any patient group and must be dealt with as soon as possible.[14] The causes of upper airway obstruction in cancer patients are similar to those in noncancer patients (Table 4), except the prevalence of obstruction in cancer patients is higher. Physicians with experience in these disorders, especially otolaryngologists, should be consulted early. The initial management is important, and a diagnosis should be made if at all possible.

Table 4 Causes of Upper Airway Obstruction

Nasopharyngeal
  Benign masses
  Malignant masses
Oropharyngeal
Infective
  Angioedema
  Stevens-Johnson syndrome
  Toxic epidermolysis
  Trauma
  Obstructive sleep apnea
Laryngeal
  Infectious
Iatrogenic
  Related to intubation
Miscellaneous
  Sarcoid
  Functional
  Neoplastic
  Wegener's granulomatosis
  Angioedema

Early symptoms and signs include shortness of breath, difficulty in breathing, anxiety, increased pulse rate, heart rate, blood pressure, and stridor. Later manifestations include increasing stridor, little movement of air, abnormal mentation including agitation, use of accessory muscles of respiration, and arterial desaturation. The obstruction is now severe, and reestablishing the airway is urgent and vital. The most experienced physician on the team should attempt the reestablishment of the airway as quickly as possible. Finally, if reestablishment of the airway fails, the pulse slows and the blood pressure drops as the patient's heart begins to stop. At this point, even if the patient is finally resuscitated, brain damage can occur if hypoxia is prolonged.[14]

If the cancer itself is the cause of the obstruction, then the airway may be maintained while the cancer is treated. Successful treatment allows the patient to be safely extubated. It is important to explain to patients or their health care surrogate that if treatment fails, withdrawal of life support becomes a possibility. In these patients, it is expected that a cancer is obstructing the airway, but infection and bleeding are also common causes of airway obstruction. A diagnosis should be made as soon as possible as the treatment of cancer, infection, or hemorrhage is different. Major bacterial infections include *Streptococcus* sp, *Staphylococcus aureus* (which often may be methicillin resistant), and *Haemophilius influenzae*. Sometimes fungal infections may occlude the airway, usually when immunity recovers. Antibiotics, antivirals, antifungals, treating the coagulopathy, and, if necessary, drainage are the definitive treatments. Massive bleeding can occlude the airway, and reestablishment of the airway is performed before attention to the primary lesion is given. Laryngeal abnormalities should be diagnosed as soon as possible, especially preextubation.[15,16] If the latter necessitates reintubation, a tracheostomy is performed to allow the edema and other damage to resolve itself. In these cases, decannulation is performed only after inspection of the larynx, usually 2 weeks later. Otolaryngology should be involved in every step. Most patients are intubated, but some can be treated conservatively. However, if they are not intubated immediately, they must be carefully observed in the ICU with a tracheostomy, difficult airway, or cricoidotomy tray at the bedside.

Translaryngeal Intubation

After the patient has failed noninvasive mechanical ventilation or if it is decided to intubate directly, an endotracheal tube (ET tube) is inserted into the trachea. The ET tube can be inserted through the nose or mouth. It is sometimes easier to insert the ET tube through the nose when the patient is awake, obese, or combative. Cancer patients are preferably intubated through the nose because they have low platelet counts. The prevalence of sinusitis and subsequent ventilator-associated pneumonia is increased in the nasally intubated patient.[17,18]

Tracheostomy

The exact timing of tracheostomy is controversial. In patients in whom long-term mechanical ventilation or other reasons for long-term tracheostomy is suspected, tracheostomy is performed as early as possible. In most patients, tracheostomy is performed at some time during the ventilation of patients who fail to wean easily. Prolonged translaryngeal intubation has the disadvantages and complications of injury to the mouth, larynx, and trachea, as well as the dangers of self-extubation and malposition, parasinusitis, extreme physical discomfort, and needing increased sedation.[19–23]

A tracheostomy provides a relatively stable, well-tolerated airway. It makes oral feedings possible, enhances communication, permits earlier ambulation, and facilitates pulmonary toilet and oral hygiene. Unfortunately, tracheostomy is associated with such complications as stomal infection, pneumothorax, subcutaneous emphysema, hemorrhage, tracheal stenosis, tracheomalacia, granulation tissue, and, rarely, death.

Most recent studies support the American College of Chest Physicians recommendations on the timing of tracheostomies.[24] Patients are treated for 5 days or so and assessed for extubation. If they will be extubated in the next day or so, they are left translaryngeally intubated. If they are not expected to be extubated soon, then a tracheostomy is performed.[24] The advantages and disadvantages of early tracheostomy are listed in Table 5, and the disadvantages of translaryngeal intubation are found in Table 6.

Table 5 Advantages and Disadvantages of Tracheostomy

Advantages
  Oral feedings
  Communications
  Earlier ambulation
  Oral hygiene
  Discharge from the intensive care unit
  Stable, well-tolerated airway

Disadvantages
  Stomal infection
  Subcutaneous emphysema
  Pneumothorax
  Hemorrhage
  Tracheal stenosis and tracheomalacia
  Granulation tissue

Table 6 Complications of Translaryngeal Intubation

Injury to mouth, larynx, and trachea
Self-extubation
Malposition
Sinusitis
Physical discomfort

Mechanical Ventilatory Support

Cancer patients are ventilated when they cannot support themselves and develop respiratory failure. In most cases, the patients are ventilated until the disease, which causes the respiratory failure, is treated.[25] Occasionally, the respiratory failure is due to the cancer itself and the patient is ventilated until the cancer is treated sufficiently enough to allow the patient to breathe on his or her own. Patients and their families must be warned that if radiation, chemotherapy, or surgery fails, then withdrawal of life support should be withdrawn. Cancer patients are treated similarly to noncancer patients for the most part. However, there are some differences. Cancer patients are intubated through the mouth rather than the nose. Many of these patients are immunosuppressed, and bacterial and nonbacterial pathogens are diagnosed by protected specimen brush, bronchoalveolar lavage (BAL), or mini-BAL.[24]

Conventional Mechanical Ventilation

Most cancer patients are ventilated using conventional mechanical ventilation. Patients can be ventilated using pressure modes (pressure support or pressure-regulated volume control) or volume modes (volume control or synchronized intermittent mandatory ventilation [SIMV]). The most commonly used mode is volume controlled followed by SIMV and then pressure support ventilation (PSV). Pressure-regulated volume control is used when the peak pressures in the airway are high.[26]

Volume Control Ventilation or Assist Control

The volume control or assist control ventilation is the most commonly used mode. The patient can trigger a preset volume (tidal volume [V_t]) after exerting enough of a negative pressure to overcome the preset trigger sensivity. There is also a preset backup rate (frequency). Positive end-expiratory pressure (PEEP) can be used with this mode. This is a good mode at which to rest the patient during ventilation. The flow rate is also preset. Caution must be exercised in patients with hyperinflated lungs as they need time to exhale fully before the ventilator gives the next breath. Increasing the flow rate to greater than 80 L per minute will help ensure that there is enough time

for adequate exhalation. Assist control is the best mode at which to rest the patient.[26]

Synchronized Intermittent Mandatory Ventilation

If the patient is not breathing spontaneously, then there is no difference between assist control and SIMV. SIMV is also a popular ventilatory mode. It is used mainly with pressure support (see below). There is usually a preset backup rate. The patient can breathe on his or her own but has no extra support unless pressure support is also used. This mode is used to gradually allow the patient to breathe on his or her own as the rate is decreased. Many authors feel that this is a poor mode to ventilate or wean patients unless it is used with pressure support.[26]

Pressure Support Ventilation

PSV is a patient-initiated, pressure-regulated ventilatory mode. The ventilator senses the patient's inspiratory flow and will then give a volume up to a preset pressure. As the patient's flow rate decreases, the ventilator will cease its flow. Nonbreathing the patient does not trigger the ventilator, and the patient will become apneic as there is no backup rate. Here the patient can breathe spontaneously with pressure support. Pressure support can be used as a primary ventilation mode provided that the patient can initiate a spontaneous breath. To ventilate a patient, the PSV_{max} is used. This is giving enough pressure support to return 10 mL/kg ideal body weight from the ventilator. Pressure support can be used with SIMV, the so-called "SIPS" (SIMV with pressure support). Patients are usually ventilated using the assist control mode and weaned using the SIPS mode.[26] Table 7 contrasts the ventilator parameter for normal lungs, hyperinflated lungs, and lungs with ALI or ARDS.

Ventilating the Patient with ALI or ARDS

Any patient who presents with bilateral infiltrates and a ratio of partial pressure of oxygen in arterial blood to fraction of inspired oxygen (FiO_2) of between 300 and 200 (ALI) or less than 200 (ARDS), with no evidence of heart failure, must be ventilated using a lung-protective strategy.[25] Patients with ALI/ARDS will have some of their alveoli filled with fluid, whereas others are normal. If the usual tidal volume is given to these patients, then those normal alveoli will be overdistended, causing a production of cytokines and further damage to the lung. This will further perpetuate the systemic inflammatory response syndrome (SIRS). The ARDS Network published a large study using lower tidal volumes, which decreased the all-cause mortality by 9% and decreased the SIRS response. Low V_t (6 mL/kg ideal body

Table 7 Difference between Ventilation of Common Disease States

Lung Type	Vt (Ideal Body Weight; mL/kg)	pH Goal	Oxygen Saturation Goal (%)
Normal	8–10	7.36–7.45	92–100
Hyperinflated	8–10	7.36–7.45	92–95
ALI/ARDS	4–6	7.15–7.45	88–95
Neuromuscular disease	10	7.36–7.45	92–100

ALI = acute lung injury; ARDS = acute respiratory distress syndrome; Vt = tidal volume.

weight) was used compared with 12 mL/kg ideal body weight. The plateau pressures should be as far below 30 cm/H_2O as possible. Once the ALI/ARDS is diagnosed, then the lower V_t is reached after 1 to 4 hours. If the plateau pressures are still above 30 cm/H_2O, then the V_t can be reduced to 4 mL/kg. Lower tidal volumes allow the arterial carbon dioxide pressure to rise to the so-called "permissive hypercarbia." The respiratory rate may be increased to a maximum of 35 per minute. The pH is allowed to fall to 7 or more. The arterial oxygenation goal using this protocol is an arterial saturation greater than 88%. There is an arbitrary ratio of PEEP to FiO_2. Prone positioning of patients with severe ARDS has fallen out of favor. Ideal body weight calculation for females is 45.5 + 2.5(height in inches −60) and for males is 50 + 2.5(height in inches −60).[25]

Outcomes of Cancer Patients Undergoing Mechanical Ventilation

The expectations and management of cancer patients admitted to an ICU are difficult to predict. Many patients are young and may have undergone chemotherapy and radiation therapy. Physicians may not be receptive to either applying full measures or to cease these same measures when appropriate. Unfortunately, most studies of this patient group are retrospective with heterogeneous populations. Azoulay and colleagues reported on the 30-day mortality of 120 patients with solid malignancies.[4] This was 58.7%, with 92% occurring in the ICU. Not surprisingly, previous surgery, pulmonary edema, and remission were good prognostic factors. Knaus scale D or C, vasopressor use, and late failure from noninvasive ventilation were poor prognostic factors. This is better than previous studies. Lin and colleagues studied lung cancer patients with ARF requiring mechanical ventilation in a tertiary care hospital.[7] The overall mortality rate was 85.2%. The adverse prognostic features were FiO_2 greater than 0.6, more than two organ failures, and an APACHE III (Acute Physiology and Chronic Health Evaluation III) score greater than 70. Kress and colleagues documented 348 consecutive critically ill cancer patients from their ICU.[3] They looked at different common types of patients and found that there was no mortality difference between leukemia, lung cancer, or lymphoma. Neutropenia was not an independent risk factor for death except when combined with mechanical ventilation (53%). Persistent ARF (eg, ARDS) and hepatic and cardiovascular failure predicted mortality (41%). In the bone marrow transplant group, the overall mortality rate was 39%. The mechanical ventilation and allogeneic bone marrow transplant groups had a higher mortality rate. Darmon and colleagues found that the mortality of patients with newly diagnosed malignancies who come to the ICU depends on the number and nature of the organ failure and not on the type of malignancy or extent of the malignancy at presentation.[27] Finally, patients over the age of 60 years have a poorer prognosis. However, selected older patients can have better prognoses.[28] Therefore, cancer patients should be encouraged to be treated as aggressively as possible.

Noninvasive MVS

Noninvasive MVS has only recently been applied to oncology patients with ARF.[1,5,6,8,9] Thoracic societies from America, Britain, and Europe have published consensus guidelines concerning the indications for noninvasive MVS (NIPPV), contraindications, monitoring, establishing teams to provide NIPPV in the hospital setting, training, infection control, and equipment safety.[29,30] NIPPV delivers mechanically assisted breaths via a tight-fitting nasal, oronasal, or full facial mask without requiring intubation. The oronasal mask is the most commonly used interface, and newer designs and safer anxiolytic medications have helped patients tolerate wearing the device for longer periods of time.[9] The tight-fitting system allows high concentrations of oxygen to be delivered. In the machines that have been devoted to delivering NIPPV, the patient's spontaneous V_t is augmented by an operator-set amount of pressure during inspiration. The inspiratory pressure commences when the machine senses a predetermined drop in airway pressure. When the inspiratory flow decelerates to a threshold value, the added inspiratory pressure ceases and the patient is able to exhale passively to an operator-set expiration pressure (PEEP level). Thus, the difference between the preset inspiratory and expiratory pressures is analogous to a pressure-supported breath delivered by a conventional ventilator. Many ventilator manufacturers have modified their standard machines to allow conventional volume and pressure-positive pressure modes to be delivered via a mask interface. NIPPV has been well established as a preferred mode of MVS in patients with exacerbations of chronic obstructive pulmonary disease as a means of avoiding intubation and the associated higher complication and mortality rates.[11,13,29,30] In these patients, NIPPV not only improved hypoxemia and hypercarbia, it also reduced diaphragmatic energy expenditure and dyspnea.[31] NIPPV, especially in the form of continuous positive airway pressure, has also been accepted as a useful adjunct in treating patients with cardiogenic pulmonary edema. Although mortality rates were not significantly reduced, the time to resolution of the acute phase of respiratory failure was significantly shortened, whereas oxygenation improved more rapidly.[11,13,32] Intubation may also be avoided in the subgroup of hypercarbic patients owing to cardiogenic pulmonary edema.[11,32] However, its role in hypoxemic respiratory failure is not as well established.[11,13,30]

Interestingly, one of the first patient populations with hypoxemic respiratory failure in which NIPPV showed statistically significant efficacy was in immunocompromised patients with diffuse radiographic pulmonary infiltrates, fever, and ARF.[8] Greater than 50% of the 52 adult patients who were prospectively studied by Hilbert and colleagues had a hematologic malignancy complicated by neutropenia.[8] The 26 patients who were assigned to the NIPPV modality via a face mask and pressure-supported ventilator mode experienced lower mortality (relative risk reduction of 0.56; $p = .03$) and lower rates of intubation ($p = .03$). They also developed fewer ($p = .03$) fatal ICU complications, such as nosocomial pneumonia, severe sepsis, and sinusitis. These observations were similar to those of another study that randomized 40 immunosuppressed solid organ transplant recipients with ARF to NIPPV or conventional therapy.[33] The allure of these results led Hilbert and colleagues to suggest in a review that NIPPV may be the preferred mode of ventilation in immunocompromised patents with ARF because of the lower rates of fatal infectious complications and lower overall mortality.[9,12] However, in a later study that compared 26 patients with hematologic malignancies who received NIPPV for ARF with 52 case-controlled matched patients who underwent invasive MVS, there was no difference in in-hospital mortality rates (65% in both groups).[6]

An accompanying editorial to the Hilbert and colleagues' article warned that the indiscriminate use of NIPPV in oncology patients with ARF may be harmful.[12] This admonition was actually borne out in another group of patients (postextubation respiratory failure) in whom NIPPV was originally touted to be helpful but proven to be harmful because its use significantly delayed necessary reintubation.[31] The patients in Hilbert and colleagues' study were highly selected.[8] They excluded patients who suffered multiorgan failures, uncorrected bleeding diathesis, poor neurologic status, or hemodynamic instability. In addition, NIPPV was applied early in the patients' treatment. This latter observation may be clinically relevant as evidenced by the results of Azoulay and colleagues' recent study.[1] When NIPPV was the only means of MVS that was required, the mortality rate was significantly less than that of invasive MVS. However, late NIPPV failure (>3 days) and the need to change from NIPPV to invasive MVS both carried a statistically increased risk ($p < .05$) of in-hospital death. Various conditions may preclude the successful application of NIPPV in oncology patients (see Table 7).[13,30] When a noninvasive MVS strategy is instituted, then either physiologic improvement (pH, oxygenation, or ventilation) or favorable changes in the physical examination (less tachypnea, improved thoracoabdominal coordination) should be realized within the first 1 to 3 hours if NIPPV is to be safely continued.[13,b] Continued use without signs of improvement has been shown to place the patient at risk of a worse outcome.[12,13,30–34]

Conclusions

As outlined in this chapter, the prognosis for adult critically ill oncology patients has significantly improved over the past decade. The more favorable outcomes also extend to patients with ARF who require MVS.[1,3,5,6] Although the decision to commence MVS is not always straightforward, it needs to be decided early in the course of a patient's ICU admission since delayed intubation has been associated with significantly increased mortality rates.[1] NIPPV offers an alternative form of MVS that may be more "acceptable" when tackling the question of whether to be "aggressive" in the care of the individual with ARF and an underlying malignancy.

Table 8 Conditions that May Preclude the Use of Noninvasive Positive Pressure Ventilation

Hemodynamic instability
  Hypotension, shock
  Cardiac dysrhythmias, uncontrolled cardiac
    ischemia
Unfavorable patient characteristics
  Inability to clear secretions
  Facial abnormalities (trauma, edentulous
    individuals, surgery)
  Upper gastrointestinal bleeding
  Recent esophageal surgery
  Inability to protect airway, cough, or swallow
  Inability to fit or tolerate mask
  Confusion or impaired consciousness
Institution's lack of experience with NIPPV

NIPPV = noninvasive positive pressure ventilation.

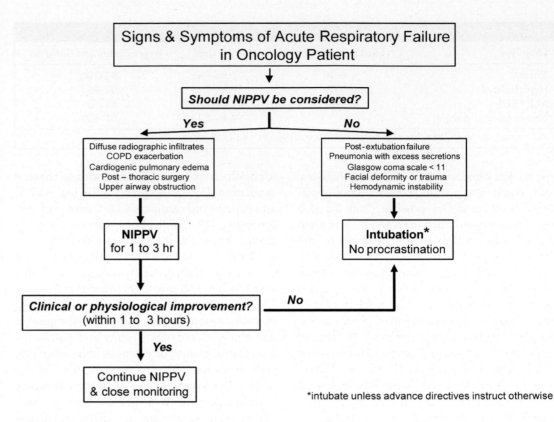

FIGURE 1 Suggested approach to mechanical ventilatory support for the adult oncology patient with acute respiratory failure. COPD = chronic obstructive pulmonary disease; NIPPV = noninvasive positive pressure ventilation.

However, NIPPV is not a panacea.[12,13,34] Indeed, when used in the wrong clinical setting[31] (Table 8) or when its use is continued despite the patient showing no physiologic or clinical improvement within 1 to 3 hours,[11,13,34] then the patient's outcome may be negatively impacted.[1,31] Figure 1 outlines our approach to this vexing decision. Advances in the understanding of ARF and the application of MVS, along with better care of the airway in patients who require prolonged MVS, have contributed to attenuating the pessimism that, until recently, pervaded the clinician's thinking when treating adult oncology patients who developed ARF.

REFERENCES

1. Azoulay E, Thiery G, Chevret S, et al. The prognosis of acute respiratory failure in critically ill cancer patients. Medicine 2004;83:360–70.
2. Pastores SM. Acute respiratory failure in critically ill patients with cancer. Diagnosis and management. Crit Care Clin 2001;17:623–46.
3. Kress JP, Christenson J, Pohlman AS, et al. Outcomes of critically ill cancer patients in a university hospital setting. Am J Respir Crit Care Med 1999;160:1957–61.
4. Azoulay E, Moreau D, Alberti C, et al. Predictors of short-term mortality in critically ill patients with solid malignancies. Intensive Care Med 2000;26:1817–23.
5. Darmon M, Thiery G, Ciroldi M, et al. Intensive care in patients with newly diagnosed malignancies and a need for cancer chemotherapy. Crit Care Med 2005;33:2488–93.
6. Depuydt PO, Benoit DD, Vandewoude KH, et al. Outcome in noninvasively and invasively ventilated hematologic patients with acute respiratory failure. Chest 2004;126:1299–306.
7. Lin Y-C, Tsai Y-H, Huang C-C, et al. Outcome of lung cancer patients with acute respiratory failure requiring mechanical ventilation. Respir Med 2004;98:43–51.
8. Hilbert G, Gruson D, Vargas F, et al. Noninvasive ventilation in immunosuppressed patients with pulmonary infiltrates, fever, and acute respiratory failure. N Engl J Med 2001;344:481–7.
9. Hilbert B, Gruson D, Vargas F. Noninvasive mechanical ventilation in immunocompromised patients. Clin Pulm Med 2004;11:175–82.
10. Keenan SP, Sinuff T, Cook DJ, et al. Does noninvasive positive pressure ventilation improve outcome in acute hypoxemic respiratory failure? A systematic review. Crit Care Med 2004;32:2516–23.
11. Caples SM, Gay PC. Noninvasive positive pressure ventilation in the intensive care unit: a concise review. Crit Care Med 2005;33:2651–8.
12. Hill NS. Noninvasive ventilation for immunocompromised patients. N Engl J Med 2001;344:522–4.
13. Krieger BP. Evidence-based review of noninvasive mechanical ventilation in the ICU. Pulm Perspect 2005;22:6–8.
14. Aboussouan LS, Stoller JK. Diagnosis and management of upper airway obstruction. Clin Chest Med 1999;15:35.
15. Jaber S, Chanques G, Mateck S, et al. Post-extubation stridor in intensive care patients: risk factors evaluation and importance of the cuff-leak test. Intensive Care Med 2003;29:69.
16. Bradley PJ. The treatment of the patient with upper airway obstruction caused by cancer of the larynx. Otolaryngol Head Neck Surg 1999;120:737.
17. Frerk CM. Predicting difficult intubation. Anesthesia 1991;46:1005.
18. Sakles JC, Laurin EG, Rantapaa AA, et al. Airway management in the emergency department: a one year study of 620 tracheal intubations. Ann Emerg Med 1998;31:326.
19. Whited RE. A prospective study of laryngotracheal sequelae in long-term intubation. Laryngoscope 1984;94:367–77.
20. Gaynor EB, Greenberg SB. Untoward sequelae of prolonged intubation. Laryngoscope 1985;95:1461–7.
21. Rodriguez JL, Steinberg SM, Luchetti FA, et al. Early tracheostomy for primary airway management in the surgical critical care setting. Surgery 1990;108:65–9.

22. Heffner JE. Medical indications for tracheostomy. Chest 1989;96:186–90.

23. Marsh HM, Gillespie DJ, Baumgarener AE. Timing of tracheostomy in the critically ill patient. Chest 1989;96: 190–3.

24. Rumbak MJ, Newton M, Truncale, et al. A prospective, randomized study comparing early percutaneous dilatational tracheotomy to prolonged translaryngeal intubation in critically ill medical patients. Crit Care Med 2004;32: 1689–94.

25. Surviving Sepsis Campaign guidelines for the management of severe sepsis and septic shock. Crit Care Med 2004; 32:858–73.

26. Schmidt G, Hall JB. Management of the ventilated patient. In: Hall JB, Schmidt GA, Wood LDH, editors. Principles of critical care medicine. New York: McGraw Hill; 2005.

28. Darmon M, Thiery G, Ciroldi M, et al. Intensive care in patients with newly diagnosed malignancies and the need for cancer chemotherapy. Crit Care Med 2005;33: 2689–93.

28. Soares M, Carvalho MS, Salluh JIF, et al. Effect of age on the survival of critically ill patients with cancer. Crit Care Med 2006;34:715–21.

29. American Thoracic Society, et al. International consensus conferences in intensive care medicine: noninvasive positive pressure ventilation in acute respiratory failure. Am J Respir Crit Care Med 2001;163:283–91.

30. British Thoracic Society Standard of Care Committee. Non-invasive ventilation in acute respiratory failure. Thorax 2002;57:192–211.

31. Esteban A, Frutos-Vivar F, Niall D, et al. Noninvasive positive-pressure ventilation for respiratory failure after extubation. N Engl J Med 2004;350:2452–60.

32. Nava S, Carbone G, DiBattista N, et al. Non-invasive ventilation in cardiogenic pulmonary edema: a multicenter randomized trial. Am J Respir Crit Care Med 2003;168: 1432–7.

33. Vitacca, et al. Am J Respir Crit Care Med 2001;164:638–

34. Truwitt JD, Bernard GR. Noninvasive ventilation—don't push too hard. N Engl J Med 2004;350:2512–5.

Bronchoscopy and Lung Cancer: Diagnostic and Therapeutic Modalities

Michael J. Simoff, MD

Bronchoscopy has evolved tremendously over the past several years. It has become a more developed diagnostic tool and a more effective therapeutic one. This chapter discusses the great variety of forms that bronchoscopy has taken on in the diagnosis and management of lung cancer.

This topic is geared toward those physicians who do not practice bronchoscopy. It is important that those physicians who send patients to have bronchoscopies for diagnosis or rely on the pathologic answer for the management of their patients realize the scope of diagnostic procedures available, their advantages, and their limitations. This further understanding will enhance the capacity for management. The therapeutics section informs the physician managing cancer about interventions, which can be used in the event of an airway obstruction or the sequelae of one (eg, postobstructive pneumonia).

History

The history of bronchoscopy is actually not that of a diagnostic tool; rather, it is a therapeutic technique. In 1897, Gustav Killian, a professor of otorhinolaryngology at the University of Freiburg, Germany, successfully removed a bone splinter from the right mainstem bronchus of a farmer using a rigid bronchoscope. His techniques and methods improved with time and expanded to different physicians and countries. In 1904, Chevalier Jackson, of Philadelphia, Pennsylvania, continued to advance the field of therapeutic bronchoscopy by improving on the equipment first developed by Professor Killian. It was not until the Ninth International Congress of Diseases of the Chest in August 1966 that Professor Dr. Shigeto Ikeda presented his new invention, the bronchofiberscope.[1] In the early 1970s, the fiberoptic bronchoscope went from a novelty to a routine tool in the diagnosis of diseases of the chest. It took about 70 years of use for the bronchoscope to become a diagnostic tool from its therapeutic roots. As this chapter progresses, I discuss how the future of this medically historical tool continues to evolve.

Bronchoscope

Initially, the fiberoptic bronchoscope was just that, a bundle of about 25,000 image- and light-specific guide fibers. As recently as the early 1990s, the fiberoptic bronchoscope was still state of the art. The fibers were smaller and transmitted images and light better than their predecessors, but in many ways, they remained essentially the same scope.

The next evolution to bronchoscopy was the addition of charge-coupled device (CCD) cameras to the tips of scopes, introducing digital technology to the bronchoscopy suite. The CCD cameras permitted the development of video-bronchoscopes, which allowed bronchoscopists and their assistants to view the procedure on a television screen. As video chip technology continues to improve, the optical systems available with modern bronchoscopes also advance significantly. These new developments not only provide improved visualization, they also allow the scopes to have smaller and smaller external diameters with larger working channels through which to perform procedures, creating a more flexible and dexterous tool for working within the airways.

The modern video bronchoscope has a working length of 60 cm (Figure 1). The typical diagnostic bronchoscope (eg, Olympus P160, Olympus Inc., Tokyo, Japan) has an external diameter of 4.2 mm with a working channel of 2.0 mm. The working channel is a conduit through the length of the bronchoscope, which allows the passage of forceps, brushes, and laser fibers, to name a few. The tip of the bronchoscope can flex (bend up) 180° and retroflex (bend down) 130°. The small external diameter makes the scope more comfortable to the patient as it is routinely passed through one of the nares and more agile for the bronchoscopist to use. Larger fiberoptic bronchoscopes can be used as therapeutic and diagnostic tools. As an example, the Olympus XT160 (Olympus America Inc., Melville, NY) has an external diameter of 6.2 mm but provides a working channel of 3.2 mm. Although the additional 1.2 mm may not sound like a

significant amount of additional space, it provides a distinct advantage to the bronchoscopist performing more advanced procedures or in the event of significant bleeding in the airways. Currently, some bronchoscopes are becoming available that use hybrid technology, using fiberoptic bundles from the tip of the scope up to the handle, which is where the CCD camera chip is located to provide excellent digital images, but provide smaller external diameters and larger working channels and maintain improved flexibility.

Diagnostic Bronchoscopy

Diagnostic bronchoscopy would be defined as those procedures and techniques that are used to make the diagnosis of disease, in the case of this chapter, specifically lung cancer. The following is a brief overview of the available techniques, their advantages, and their limitations. This review is meant to provide the nonbronchoscopist with an understanding of the everyday techniques used to diagnose lung cancer. Further discussion will then continue toward the more modern tools and advanced diagnostic techniques available commercially, as well as some that are just becoming available, to fully understand the diagnostic capabilities of bronchoscopy.

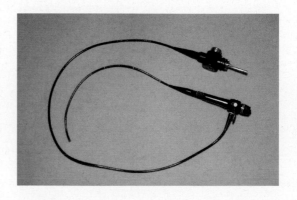

FIGURE 1 Bronchoscope: Olympus flexible videoscope.

Airway Examination

The object from the inception of bronchoscopy was to look into the airways. The modern flexible bronchoscope makes this much easier to do than with the still available but much less common rigid bronchoscope. Typical airway anatomy begins just distal to the cricoid within the trachea and continues branching through multiple generations to the level of the respiratory bronchioles and, finally, the alveoli. There are usually 24 to 26 generations of airways branching from the level of the trachea.[2] With a typical diagnostic flexible bronchoscope, the bronchoscopist can visualize down through three to five generations of airways. This limitation may seem surprising to some, but the diameter of the airways quickly gets smaller with each generation of airway and modern bronchoscopes, with diameters of 4.2 to 6.0 mm are currently limited purely by size. The use of smaller bronchoscopes, termed "thin" or "ultrathin" bronchoscopes, is currently being explored, but at this time, they would not be used in the "usual" bronchoscopic examination of the airway.

Another advantage of modern digital scopes is that as video technology continues to improve, the available CCD camera chips used to create visual images continue to improve, creating images that give detail that far surpasses previous generations of bronchoscopes. The improved optics improve the diagnostic capability of modern bronchoscopes by allowing bronchoscopists the advantage of picking up more subtle changes of the mucosa, which often mask underlying sites of early cancer growth.

What may seem obvious is that in those patients with lesions that are endoscopically visible, the diagnostic yield is greater than in those in whom the airway examination is otherwise normal. A variety of techniques can be used to sample both the visible and the, in essence, endoscopically invisible lesion. There are multiple techniques used by bronchoscopists to diagnose lung cancer. Diagnostic procedures used by the bronchoscopist obtain both cytologic and histologic samples. A significant advantage of cytology is that it often requires very little cellular material to make a diagnosis. Histologic samples, when enough tissue is acquired, can help further refine the cell type of the cancer.

Airway Washes and Bronchoalveolar Lavage

After the airways have been examined, the bronchoscopist next begins collecting samples to make the diagnosis of cancer. The simplest of these sampling methods is merely collecting the secretions, which are always present within the airways. This random collection of secretions is both simple and of little risk to the patient but usually is of very low yield as to making the diagnosis. The bronchoscopist may also choose to instill small amounts (10 to 40 mL) of saline into the airways before suctioning to improve the potential yield of this procedure. Reported cytologic yields of washes vary from 31.6 to 45.1%.[3,4]

Bronchoalveolar lavage (BAL) is another technique that uses a more directed approach to sampling of the airways for cancer cells to make the diagnosis. The tip of the flexible bronchoscope is moved into the lobe, then the segment, and eventually the subsegment that the bronchoscopist suspects as the location of the cancer. The leading edge of the bronchoscope is thus placed into a "wedge" position. This wedging seals off the bronchial tree from that point out to the level of the alveoli. Instead of just collecting the secretions that are then in this location, the bronchoscopist instills 20 to 50 mL aliquots of normal saline into this area and then suctions back the instillate after allowing a short time for the liquid to move into the distal airways. Continuous suction is then used to collect the infused saline. Approximately 120 mL of collected BAL fluid is often the goal of the procedure.[5] Some bronchoscopists will routinely collect only 35 to 50 mL of sample for diagnosis. Typically, returns of 40 to 60% of the infused volume are achieved with this procedure. The yield can be affected by the amount of fluid instilled, the site lavaged (dependent segments having lower yields), and how well the bronchoscope was wedged.[6–8] BAL is only occasionally used in the evaluation of the patient for lung cancer. The few studies available report a diagnostic yield of 33 to 69%.[9–11]

Cytologic Brushing

This technique uses a flexible cytology brush that is passed through the working channel of the bronchoscope and then "brushed" onto a visible lesion, blindly into an area of suspicion, or directed to a peripheral lesion under fluoroscopic guidance (Figure 2). Once the brush is placed at the location of interest, it is vigorously agitated in a back-and-forth manner. This motion assists the bristles in picking up as many cells as may be in the area, actually rubbing cells off the tumor. The brush is then removed through the working channel of the bronchoscope and is used to create slides, which are fixed with spray preservetive or placed in 95% ethyl alcohol to prepare them for interpretation. Often the brush is then placed into a cytologic solution so that any remaining cells can be removed and possibly help improve the cytologic diagnosis of cancer.

As in washes, and soon to be discussed in biopsies, endobronchial tumor (visible tumor in the airway) has a higher yield when using cytologic brushing. In cases of endobronchially

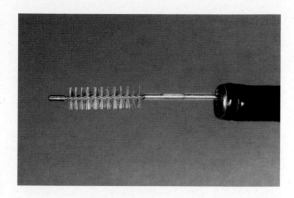

FIGURE 2 A cytology brush exiting the working channel of a bronchoscope.

visible tumor, the reported sensitivities vary from 65.9 to 84%.[3,4,12,13] Cytologic brushings of lesions invisible to the bronchoscopist have lower diagnostic sensitivities, from 22 to 47%.[12,13] Overall, cytologic techniques, including washing and brushings, add a significant amount to the diagnostic yield of bronchoscopy for lung cancer. Both of these techniques are relatively simple to perform and are low-risk procedures.

Endobronchial Biopsy

An endobronchial biopsy is the sampling of a lesion that is endoscopically visible during the bronchoscopy. Biopsies through a bronchoscope are performed with flexible biopsy forceps, which are passed through the working channel of the bronchoscope. The forceps themselves have hinged cups with either a smooth or a serrated cutting edge. When open, the forceps have a diameter of 6 mm, allowing a reasonably sized biopsy specimen to be obtained. Once the forceps exit the distal end of the bronchoscope, there is no way to guide the forceps independent of the bronchoscope. Biopsies must therefore be performed in reasonably close approximation to the end of the bronchoscope (1–3 cm). When the biopsy forceps are passed through the working channel of a bronchoscope, they nearly occlude the working channel (normal working channel 2.0 mm, with an average forceps diameter of 1.8 mm). As the forceps are pushed out of the bronchoscope, secretions, tissue, and/or blood can be pushed out in front of the forceps, obscuring the bronchoscopists' vision of the previously identified lesion that they want to biopsy. Owing to the size of the forceps, there is little to no room for suctioning away these secretions, making the procedure much more difficult (Figure 3).

It is not uncommon for the bronchoscopist to see a lesion in the airway that can be reached using forceps and/or a brush to sample for diagnosis. Although it may seem simple to make a diagnosis at this point, it is not always true. The reported diagnostic yield of endobronchial biopsy for bronchogenic carcinoma ranges from 73 to

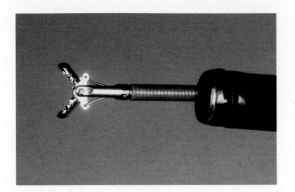

FIGURE 3 Biopsy forceps exiting the working channel of a bronchoscope.

96%.[14–19] Nonbronchoscopists may ask why the yield is not 100% if you can see the lesion. The answer is that although sometimes a lesion can be seen, its position in the airway makes it difficult, if not impossible, to direct biopsy forceps or a brush into the location of the lesion. Second, many rapidly growing cancers have necrotic slough and tissue on their surfaces, and the initial samples, or possibly all of the samples, may be of this material, which will not provide a histologic diagnosis. Lastly, owing to the fact that the "view" of the lesion may change as discussed above, it is recommended that three to five biopsies of an endoscopically visible lesion will give the highest sensitivity (90–100%) for this diagnostic procedure.[19,20] If less than four biopsies are performed, the diagnostic yield for this procedure can be reduced, thereby potentially not yielding a diagnosis.[18]

Transbronchial Biopsy

The solitary pulmonary nodule or, in many cases, the large radiologically evident mass has to be biopsied for diagnosis. This requires performing biopsies on lesions that are not endoscopically visible; instead, using previously performed chest radiographs and computed tomographic (CT) scans, bronchoscopists must identify very specifically where they believe the lesion to be within the lung and, subsequently, which airways will lead to it. This procedure is known as transbronchial lung biopsy. Procedurally, it entails entering the airways with the bronchoscope, identifying the appropriate lobar, segmental, and subsegmental bronchi that will direct the biopsy forceps toward the previously identified lesion. Once the bronchoscope is in place, the tip of the bronchoscope is advanced until it can advance no further. This positioning is known as a wedge position. The advantage of the wedge positioning is that it will leave the bronchoscope in one place for the entirety of the procedure, allowing repeated introduction of biopsy forceps, a cytology brush, or other diagnostic tools the bronchoscopist chooses to use. The added benefit is that if there is

significant bleeding, it is localized and controlled within the airways distal to the tip of the bronchoscope, minimizing the risk to the patient.

Once in position, many bronchoscopists will use fluoroscopy to assist with transbronchial biopsies. Fluoroscopy can be performed in a single plane, or, to improve accuracy, several planes can be used to assist in the three-dimensional assessment of the lesion and the location of the bronchoscope in the chest. The lesion is first localized with fluoroscopy. The bronchoscope tip is then assessed for proper positioning in relation to the lesion. The forceps (or other diagnostic tool) are then watched moving toward and optimally directly into the desired lesion. Once in position, the forceps are drawn backward, opened, and moved into position (Figure 4). Many bronchoscopists like to observe the lesion being tugged by the forceps as the biopsy is taken fluoroscopically.

Many factors influence the diagnostic yield of transbronchial biopsy techniques. The first is the size of the lesion to be biopsied. As might be expected, the smaller the lesion, the lower the diagnostic yield. For those peripheral tumors less than 2 cm in size, the diagnostic yield is 28 to 30%. Tumors greater than 2 cm but less than 4 cm in diameter have a diagnostic yield of 64%, and those greater than 4 cm up to 80%.[21–25] The number of biopsies performed also influences the diagnostic yield of transbronchial biopsies. Diagnostic yields of 21 to 52% are reported when four or fewer biopsies were taken for a peripheral lesion (size indeterminate). This is compared with a diagnostic yield of 70 to 78% when more than four biopsies were taken during the bronchoscopic procedure.[26–28]

As might be expected, blind biopsies into the lung parenchyma, even when fluoroscopically guided, have risks. The two greatest risks with transbronchial biopsies are bleeding and pneumothorax. The reported risk of pneumothorax is 3 to 5%. The use of fluoroscopy reduces the risk of pneumothorax versus blind procedures.[29–32]

Bleeding in excess of 50 mL is considered significant when induced by a bronchoscopic biopsy. There is a less than 3% risk of serious bleeding with transbronchial biopsies. When the procedure is performed by maintaining a good wedge position, the risk to the patient of a poor outcome is significantly reduced.[29,31,32]

Transbronchial Needle Aspiration

Transbronchial needle aspiration (TBNA) is anther technique to assist in the diagnosis of patients with lung cancer. This technique is used when the mass in question lies outside the bronchus. TBNA can be used to sample centrally located masses, lymph nodes, and peripheral tumors. TBNA can be used for cytologic or histologic samples. A number of different types of needles are available for this technique, each with specific characteristics to maximize efficiency when using them. The two most common types of needles are the 22-gauge cytology needle and the 19-gauge histology needle.

Both needles are 1.9 mm in diameter. They are passed through the working channel of the bronchoscope with the needle withdrawn into the needle sheath. Once the hub of the needle has been passed out of the end of the bronchoscope, the needle can be exposed. The cytology needle is 13 mL long. The histology needle actually has a 21-gauge needle inside its core. When projected, this 19- or 21-gauge needle is 18 mm long; once the 21-gauge needle is withdrawn, the 19-gauge needle is 15 mm long (Figure 5). The tip of the TBNA needle (any size) is then placed against the wall of the bronchus (in approximation to the node or tumor that the bronchoscopist wishes to sample) and is pushed through the wall as perpendicular to the mucosa as possible to maximize the depth of penetration of the needle. The initial concern of most newcomers to TBNA is that this procedure must have a high risk of the development of pneumothorax and bleeding. This is actually incorrect; there are only two reported cases of pneumothorax in the literature, with a

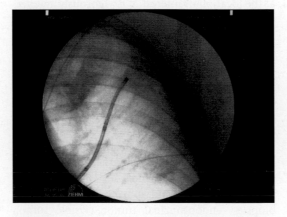

FIGURE 4 Fluoroscopic image of a transbronchial biopsy.

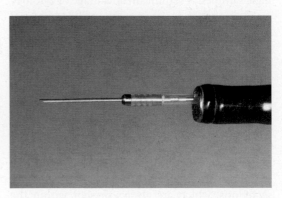

FIGURE 5 A transbronchial needle aspiration needle exiting the working channel of a bronchoscope.

reported risk of pneumothorax of 1.4%.[33,34] The risk of bleeding is also very small. To illustrate this, it is best to look at invasive cardiac and hemodynamic studies performed via the airways in the 1940s and 1950s. Large-bore needles were used to penetrate the bronchial wall and then directed into the pulmonary artery, aorta, and/or the left atrium to perform various imaging and/or hemodynamic measurements.[35,36] With these significantly more invasive studies, there were no reported deaths or major complications of bleeding. There is actually only one reported hemomediastinum as a result of TBNA.[37]

TBNA is an excellent procedure for the diagnosis of lung cancer. The procedure has a degree of operator variability in the potential diagnostic yield. Reported yields in the literature vary from 38 to 73%,[38–40] and when a mucosal abnormality or external compression of the airway was evident, there was a reported positive aspiration yield of 88%.[41] As pulmonologists continue to gain experience with this procedure, the number of mediastinoscopies can be reduced for the mediastinal staging of lung cancer. In experienced hands, the bronchoscopist can clearly stage the mediastinum, minimizing further invasive procedures for our patients with lung cancer.

TBNA can also be used as part of the evaluation of a solitary pulmonary nodule. The use of the smaller, 22-gauge cytology needle for peripheral lesions is the ideal tool. After the bronchoscope is wedged, as above, the needle is passed through the working channel of the bronchoscope and extended toward the lesion. The needle is then extended and pushed into the tumor being assessed. The diagnostic yield of this procedure is up to 35%.[27] Other reports further define the yield as it relates to the size of the lesion. Shure and Fedullo differentiate between lesions less than and greater than 2 cm.[42] The yield for TBNA when tumors were less than 2 cm is 33% and 76% for those greater than 2 cm. Another study uses the cutoff of 3 rather than 2 cm and found the diagnostic yield of tumors less than 3 cm to be 27.5% and 65.5% for lesions greater than 3 cm.[43]

TBNA is a necessary procedure for the evaluation of patients with lung cancer. Overall, this technique is an excellent addition to the evaluation of patients with a lung mass or mediastinal lymphadenopathy, for the diagnosis of primary disease, and the staging necessary for managment.

Bronchoscopy: Putting It All Together

Individually, each of the procedures discussed above is good for the diagnosis of lung cancer. Clinically, however, most or all of these procedures are used at the discretion of the bronchoscopist performing the procedure. Aggressive bronchoscopists will almost always use several techniques to maximize the chance of making a diagnosis at the time of the first bronchoscopy. Several studies demonstrate a much greater opportunity to diagnose lung cancer with the combination of several techniques, some with up to 80% diagnostic yields.[22,24,44–46] A combination of a biopsy (endobronchial or transbronchial), brushing, and washings (or BAL) should be considered the standard bronchoscopic approach in making the diagnosis of lung cancer. If there is lymphadenopathy on the CT scan of the mediastinum or hilum, TBNA should also be performed to maximize the chance of staging and diagnosing the patient with one procedure.

The procedures, which were discussed above, are routine in most medical centers. Those to be discussed below are available at only a few referral centers. These advanced diagnostic procedures are excellent additional techniques for the diagnosis and management of patients with lung cancer. As clinical experience with them continues to grow, they may become part of mainstream diagnostic bronchoscopy.

Autofluorescence Bronchoscopy

Despite advancements in chemotherapeutic agents, radiation, and surgical techniques, the recurrence rate of lung cancer is 3.6 to 4% per year. Second primary tumors occur in 17% of patients within 3 years of treatment of their primary disease.[47,48] With 10 to 20% of patients having a second primary tumor or recurrence, it suggests a more complicated process than a single tumor alone. The pathologic changes of dysplasia, carcinoma in situ, and microinvasive carcinoma are very superficial. These changes develop in the intraepithelial to superficial submucosal layers of the bronchial wall. The diagnostic yield of finding these subtle visible changes with standard white light bronchoscopy is actually quite low. To improve the yield of identifying these changes requires a new diagnostic tool.

Autofluorescence uses a little known and very weak physical property of light: fluorescence. Fluorescence is always present with visible light, but it is 10,000 times dimmer than reflected light and as such is not visible to the naked eye or with standard bronchoscopy. Autofluorescence is a property of the upper submucosa, the same anatomic location of many early cancers.

Autofluorescence bronchoscopy is achieved by stimulating certain cells within the submucosa, called fluorophores. The fluorophores are stimulated by light of 390 to 460 nm (blue light), which excites them to a higher energy level. With a rapid decay from the excited state, light of predominantly 520 nm (green) and to a lesser extent 630 nm (red) is released. When the airway is visualized in autofluorescence, the airways appear green. Owing to a variety of physical characteristics of light and pathologic changes secondary to the development of a cancer, a precancerous lesion, and microinvasive cancer, all appear red (Figure 6).

In reviewing 11 clinical studies including 1,084 patients, the sensitivity of white light bronchoscopy to autofluorescence bronchoscopy was found to be 52.4 to 84%, respectively, for the identification of early endobronchial lesions.[49–58] Autofluorescence is an excellent clinical tool for the detection of early lung cancer. As its popularity continues to grow, we will find more and more applications for its use. Its greatest limitation lies in the fact that only several generations of the airways can currently be examined with a bronchoscope; therefore, we can see only some of the problems that exist.

Endobronchial Ultrasonography and Endobronchial Ultrasonography–Directed Transbronchial Biopsy

Endoluminal ultrasonography has been established as a routine diagnostic procedure in many fields of medicine owing to its diagnostic advantages over traditional radiologic evaluations.[59] This is especially true of gastrointestinal endoscopy. Ultrasound imaging is generated owing to the difference in resistance of various tissues to ultrasound waves (impedance). The different impedance of various soft tissues has made ultrasonography an indispensable diagnostic tool in medicine.

Two techniques exist to perform endobronchial ultrasonography (EBUS) within the airways. The first is the use of a 20 MHz transducer that uses a saline-filled balloon to eliminate an air-transducer interface, allowing delivery of the ultrasound waves to the tissue. This technique allows a 360° image of the parabronchial and paratracheal structures. Under favorable conditions, structures at a distance of up to 4 cm from the probe can be visualized.

The second technique uses a 7.5 MHz linear array transducer, which is built into the tip of a flexible bronchoscope. As the bronchoscopist is inspecting the airways, he or she can put the ultrasound probe up against the wall of the airway and visualize structures (eg, lymph nodes, tumors, blood vessels). This bronchoscope has another advantage in that a specially designed transbronchial needle can be used to sample lesions under direct ultrasound visualization. This bronchoscope is, in essence, the same as the endoscopic ultrasound gastroesophagoscopes used by gastroenterologists. By visualizing the target tissue and watching its sampling, it is hoped that greater and greater yields can be obtained with diagnostic bronchoscopy. Indications for the use of EBUS can be reviewed in Table 1.

EBUS has been used in the evaluation of patients with small radiologically invisible tumors, in which the physicians will use endobronchial therapy alone to manage the disease.[60–62] EBUS is

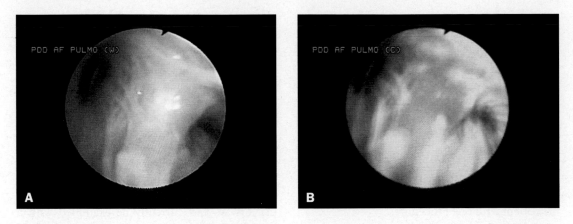

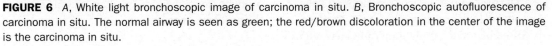

FIGURE 6 *A*, White light bronchoscopic image of carcinoma in situ. *B*, Bronchoscopic autofluorescence of carcinoma in situ. The normal airway is seen as green; the red/brown discoloration in the center of the image is the carcinoma in situ.

Table 1 Indications for Endobronchial Ultrasonography

Endobronchial cancer
  Intraluminal extension
  Invasion/impression
  Early cancer depth of invasion
  Vascular invasion

Mediastinal and hilar nodal staging
Mediastinal mass evaluation
Peripheral lesions

---

also used in the localization of peripheral tumors, which are not endoscopically visible, to improve the yield of transbronchial biopsy procedures.[63,64] The use of the 20 MHz system has been shown to improve identification of mediastinal lymph nodes, also improving yields of TBNA.[65,66] The use of directional ultrasonography has not been studied enough to demonstrate its potential addition to the technique of blind TBNA. Lastly, EBUS has been used to differentiate between tumor approximation and tumor invasion of mediastinal structures. In a prospective study, it was demonstrated that differentiation of external tumor invasion versus impression of the tracheobronchial wall by EBUS was reliable in 90% of patients compared with contrast CT (50%).[67] This may help influence the management of lung cancer patients who were initially thought to be unresectable, allowing them the opportunity to go to the operating room for a more definitive therapy.

Overall, EBUS is not yet a routine tool in most institutions. Its acceptance and popularity continue to grow in face of the advances being made in this tool and the corresponding bronchoscopes. The use of this technology will continue to grow with respect to managing cancer of the chest.

Future Techniques

Despite continued advancement in diagnostic techniques and treatment protocols, lung cancer remains the number 1 cancer killer. With this in mind, we must continue to look forward in our goal of discovering, diagnosing, and treating this disease. A few of the novel diagnostic tools being clinically explored are now discussed. The first tool is electromagnetic navigation. Electromagnetic navigation is a new technology to allow improved manipulation throughout the airways to approach a peripheral lung lesion. This technology incorporates the merging of CT with three-dimensional generation imaging, an electromagnetic field formed around the patient's body, and a directional probe, which is bronchoscopically placed into the airways.

Electromagnetic navigation is currently entering more complete clinical trials. The technology is very exciting for the sampling of not only peripheral lesions but also adding the capacity of potentially using therapeutic modalities at the time of the original biopsy. There is also promise for mediastinal node sampling to be enhanced with concurrent use of this very exciting tool. There is limited clinical experience at this time with external navigation systems, but, in the future, this technology will very likely play an important part in the diagnosis and, it is hoped, management of lung cancer.[68]

Another area of possible future advancement in bronchoscopy is that of "optical biopsies." Optical biopsying is actually a variety of techniques that fall under this very unusual heading. An optical biopsy is actually the use of structural imaging technology, which depends predominantly on the scattering properties of light at a tissue interface. This technology includes optical coherence tomography (OCT), confocal microscopy, and light-scattering spectroscopy.

OCT is discussed here as it has entered the phase of clinical trials. This technology is in many ways analogous to ultrasonography, but instead of sound, it measures the intensity of back-reflected infrared light. As it is light, there OCT does not require direct contact with tissue or a transducing medium and can be performed through air, which is ideal for the lungs. In essence, OCT performs a high-resolution assessment of tissue microstructure. The images produced are equivalent to a low to moderate mechanical-level biopsy obtained during diagnostic procedures at the micron scale of resolution. The goal would be to "look" at a mass in the airways and diagnose it as a cancer to being therapy at the time of the original bronchoscopy, without having to wait for sample processing.[69,70]

Electromagnetic navigation and OCT are two of the potential tools being developed for the bronchoscopic diagnosis of lung cancer. The future would have us looking toward early, more complete diagnosis and staging, with possible nonsurgical approaches to the treatment and cure of the solitary pulmonary nodule.

Therapeutic Bronchoscopy

Setting for Intervention

Most of the estimated 173,770 new cases of lung cancer diagnosed in the United States in 2004, accounting for 13% of all new cancer cases, will be in an advanced stage.[71] Central airways disease can be in the form of bulky endobronchial disease, endobronchial extension of cancer, or extrinsic compression of the airways by the tumor or lymphadenopathy. Shortness of breath, hemoptysis, and cough are frequent complaints of patients with lung cancer. Those patients with an endobronchial component to their disease may benefit from a bronchoscopic intervention as part of the management of their disease.

Not all endobronchial disease causes complete obstruction of the airways. Sometimes patients have partial obstruction, which often has a less severe symptom complex. As these patients enter treatment programs, the endobronchial component of their disease, in response to these treatments, can lead to more complicated concerns. External beam radiotherapy can induce endobronchial inflammation and swelling, further compromising the airways. Radiation or chemotherapy can lead to necrosis of the endobronchial component of the cancer. The inflammation and necrotic tissue can cause further airway compromise by inducing airway obstruction, lung collapse, and possible postobstructive pneumonia. Therefore, endobronchial techniques should be considered throughout the management of lung cancer patients.[72,73] Many studies not only demonstrate improvement in clinical symptoms and quality of life, they also suggest increased overall survival with the use of endobronchial management techniques.[74–87]

Lastly, when all management options have been used, end-stage patients will often develop compromise of their airways as the cancer continues to progress.

Endobronchial management options may help relieve some of their symptoms, allowing them freedom from shortness of breath as they go home in conjunction with hospice or other palliative therapies.[88–90]

Most endobronchial techniques are performed on an outpatient basis. Unless a patient presents with respiratory failure, many of the procedures performed provide immediate relief of symptoms. This rapid symptomatic improvement allows patients to return home with an improved quality of life or better prepares them to continue treatment at their local programs. Although interventional procedures are not definitive therapies, they often provide partial to total relief of the strangling sensation produced by complete airway occlusion.

Interventional pulmonology is the practice of advanced techniques via a bronchoscope and thoracoscope. The direction of this chapter again concentrates on bronchoscopic techniques. Programs that include endobronchial procedures need an armamentarium of therapeutic modalities rather than a single invasive approach to manage patients with complicated lung cancer. As each patient's anatomy differs, the manner in which the patient's cancer leads to symptoms varies. Several procedures used in conjunction (ie, laser and stenting) may be necessary to provide the most efficacious management of the disease. Offering a multitude of modalities allows the best selection of approaches for the patient.[88,89]

The following sections discuss a variety of techniques and tools available to the interventionalist for the endobronchial management of lung cancer. In many cases, no one technique is better than the others; most often, some combination of these techniques offers the greatest benefit to the patient.

Bronchoscopy

Since the inception of flexible fiberoptic bronchoscopy in the late 1960s in Japan and in 1970 in the United States, the flexible bronchoscope has become the most widespread tool for evaluating and diagnosing diseases of the airways and lungs.[1] The rigid bronchoscope, the flexible bronchoscope's predecessor, was in many regards forgotten as a tool until interventional pulmonology evolved in the 1980s. Interventional pulmonologists reevaluated this tool and found its properties advantageous to the procedures that are currently performed. A survey in 1991 by the American College of Chest Physicians reported that only

8% of responding pulmonologists used a rigid bronchoscope.[91]

Overall, concurrent use of the flexible bronchoscope with the rigid bronchoscope is necessary for the practice of interventional pulmonology. The rigid bronchoscope offers many advantages to the interventional pulmonologist, one of which is the superior control of the airway achieved with its use. Ventilation is performed through the scope itself rather than around the flexible bronchoscope. The larger-bore rigid bronchoscopes allow optical systems, large-caliber suction catheters, and the laser to pass through the scope simultaneously. Large rigid biopsy forceps are used through the rigid bronchoscope, which can provide more significant tissue biopsies and assist in mechanical debulking of lesions. However, the rigid bronchoscope is a more difficult tool to use that requires additional training. In addition, rigid bronchoscopy is most commonly performed in the operating room requiring general anesthesia, making the logistics of its use difficult for many. Overall, in difficult airway conditions, rigid bronchoscopy is an excellent technique for the management of endobronchial disease.

The rigid bronchoscope can be used not only as a delivery device of therapeutic tools; the scope itself can be used as a tool in the management of endobronchial disease. The distal end of the bronchoscope has a beveled end. This edge can be used to shear large sections of endobronchial tumor away from the airway wall in a technique often referred to as "applecoring." Mathisen and Grillo described their experience with 56 patients with endobronchial obstruction from the trachea to the distal mainstem bronchi.[92] After an applecoring application of the rigid bronchoscope, they reported an improvement in 90% of their patients. Only 3 of the 56 patients had more than minor bleeding with this procedure. Although this procedure is technically difficult, applecoring combined with the use of larger biopsy forceps allows the tumor to be quickly resected from the obstructed airway.

Ablative Techniques

This includes all of those technologies used in the debulking and/or resection of endobronchial cancer. They include laser, electrocautery, argon plasma coagulation, cryotherapy, and photodynamic therapy. Each is discussed below.

Laser Therapy

Laser is an acronym derived from light amplification by stimulated emission of radiation. Lasers have many medical uses, including the endobronchial management of lung cancer. The most common laser used within the bronchi is the neodymium:yttrium-aluminum-garnet (Nd:YAG) laser. The potassium-titanyl-phosphate

and diode lasers are also occasionally used. As in all lasers, the Nd:YAG laser delivers a very specific wavelength of light, 1,064 nm. This wavelength allows the laser energy to be conducted via a quartz monofilament and thus can be easily used with either the rigid or the flexible bronchoscope. Normally, the Nd:YAG laser is used at 30 to 60 watts, but it has a wide range of power outputs, up to 100 watts. Depending on the energy level used, the laser can affect tissue several millimeters to several centimeters in depth (Figure 7).

The predominant tissue effects of Nd:YAG lasers are thermal necrosis and photocoagulation. Of these, photocoagulation is the most commonly used effect. Using lower energy levels, the surface of the tumor is heated, causing shrinkage of the tumor and diminishing the blood flow to that region. By devascularizing the tumor, more rapid mechanical debulking can be performed, with improved control of bleeding.

Thermal necrosis uses higher energy levels to destroy tissue, causing the formation of eschar. The problem with this approach is that most tumors are significantly vascular, and in destroying tissue with laser energy, large blood vessels can also be destroyed. These blood vessels may then perforate with the tissue destruction, leading to significant hemorrhage and an increase rather than a decrease in morbidity and mortality with this procedure. Despite this, cautious use of the thermal necrosis technique of laser therapy can be safely and efficiently used in the airway.

Ablative therapy with a laser can be performed via flexible or rigid bronchoscopy. The majority of interventionalists use rigid bronchoscopy as the predominant tool for the performance of laser procedures when possible owing to the ease of the debulking part of the procedure. Using the flexible bronchoscope, the Nd:YAG fiber can be passed through the working channel, and thereby energy can be delivered to areas that cannot otherwise be reached with the rigid bronchoscope.[74–87,92]

The reported success rate of symptom palliation using laser energy in the endobronchial management of lung cancer is high. Reports of

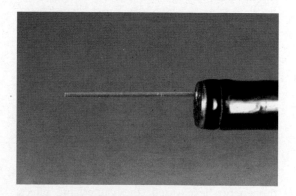

FIGURE 7 A laser fiber exiting the working channel of a bronchoscope.

clinical improvement rates range from 84 to 92% following laser bronchoscopy.[78,81,93–95] Further review of the literature identifies studies that demonstrate improved survival in patients treated with laser bronchoscopy.[80,84,85,96] Brutinel and colleagues compared 25 historical controls (ie, patients who would have been candidates for laser management but did not receive it secondary to the unavailability of the procedure at the time of their management) with 71 patients treated with laser bronchoscopy as part of the treatment program.[80] The authors reported 76 and 100% mortality rates at 4 and 7 months, respectively, in the control population. In the group treated with laser bronchoscopy, survival rates at 7 months and 1 year were 60% and 28%, respectively. Although no definitive randomized studies are available, review of historical studies would suggest improved survival in patients treated with endobronchial techniques.

Electrocautery

Electrocautery is another ablative technique available to the interventional pulmonologist. Similarly to laser, thermal energy is used to cauterize and/or cut through tissue. This thermal effect is secondary to the resistance of tissue to the flow of electrical current. This phenomenon leads to tissue temperatures elevating to 160°F (71°C), with cellular or tissue destruction. Electrocautery delivers electrical energy via one of several introducer devices to cut and/or destroy tumor cells. The various tools of electrocautery can be introduced through a rigid or flexible bronchoscope (the bronchoscope must be grounded to prevent the physician operator from receiving electrical energy). The tools include a blunt probe for delivering higher-level electrical energy and destroying tissue; a "hot" forceps, which can cauterize before debulking or biopsying; a snare that cauterizes as it cuts; and an electrosurgical scalpel for resecting tumor. Electrocautery techniques continue to gain popularity, and its use continues to spread.[97]

Argon Plasma Coagulation

Argon plasma coagulation (APC) is another electrically based technique. Instead of using one of the varieties of contact probes available for electrocautery procedures, the APC is a form of noncontact electrocautery. Argon gas is ionized as it exits the delivery catheter. This ionized argon gas then acts as a conductor for the electrical energy being delivered. The advantages of this system are that the electrical energy can be used to "paint" the surface of the tumor, cauterizing the entire surface quickly (similar to a laser). Depending on the energy level used, the cauterizing effects of APC can penetrate 3 to 5 mm of the tumor surface. The added benefit to this tool is that the

argon, being a gas, flows as any gas and therefore can form eddies around corners. When the proper orientation of flow across an obstruction is used, this eddying allows cautery around corners to maximize the surface area being covered.[98]

Cryotherapy

Cryotherapy differs from the other ablative techniques thus far discussed in its use of cold rather than heat to destroy tissue. A probe is placed through a bronchoscope and then onto or directly into an obstructing tumor mass. The probe tip is cooled by the use of either liquid nitrogen (−196°C) or nitrous oxide (−80°C). Tissue freezing causes destruction of all cells in an area of approximately 1 cm in diameter around the probe tip. Vascular thrombosis occurs with the supercooling of tissue, minimizing bleeding during resection of the tumor.

Overall, cryotherapy is an excellent technique for tumor ablation. One of the limiting factors to the use of cryotherapy is that the tissues destroyed with the freezing take 24 to 36 hours to die and necrose. This therefore requires repeating the bronchoscopy in 36 to 48 hours to remove the necrosed tissue. In many cases, repeat treatments with cryotherapy are performed at the time of the second bronchoscopy, requiring a third debulking. Although cryotherapy is effective at tumor destruction and management, the necessity of repeated procedures makes this a more time-consuming procedure to perform, limiting its usefulness in the management of symptomatic bulky endobronchial disease.[99]

Photodynamic Therapy

Photodynamic therapy (PDT) is an important adjunctive modality to the management of endobronchial lung cancer. PDT can be used with bulky disease, but most interventionalists feel that it is of limited benefit in this role.[100,101] The most suitable lesions for PDT are in situ carcinomas or those limited to 4 to 5 mm of microinvasion.[102]

PDT requires that a photosensitizing drug be intravenously administered to the patient 48 to 72 hours prior to the procedure. Porfimer sodium (Photofrin) is the most common agent currently used for this. This photosensitizer penetrates all cells systemically. Photofrin is not cleared as quickly in cancer cells as in the other cells of the surrounding tissue 48 to 72 hours after injection and is therefore found in higher concentrations in cancer cells as opposed to the endothelium surrounding the tumor.[102,103] An argon dye laser is then used to provide a 630 nm wavelength of light energy to activate the intracellular porfimer sodium. The laser energy is transmitted via a flexible quartz fiber, which can be used through a flexible or rigid bronchoscope. The fiber tip can

be placed in close approximation to the tumor with a directed or cylindrically diffused laser delivery, or it can be imbedded into the tumor to provide the energy needed to start the intracellular activation of the porfimer sodium. This reaction leads to cellular destruction by a variety of mechanisms. Tissue necrosis then ensues as the cancer cells die over the next 24 to 36 hours.[102–104]

As the neoplastic tissue necrotizes, it must be removed by repeated bronchoscopies. Flexible bronchoscopy is commonly performed daily or every other day for up to 1 week to remove the necrotic tissue. The necrosis of bulky tumor can be dangerous to the patient if the necrotic tissue separates from the bronchial wall and occludes the airway. In some programs that use only PDT, patients remain intubated following the procedure for 1 to 2 days secondary to this concern. If necrotic tissue is removed over the first 24 to 48 hours, a second laser application to the cancer can be performed, thus improving the cancer tissue destruction. PDT is an excellent therapeutic modality for patients with early-stage cancers. It destroys neoplastic tissue effectively and is an outstanding therapeutic modality in carcinoma in situ and microinvasive cancers. PDT is a necessary tool in our armamentarium of endobronchial treatments, but the time delays and multiple steps of management make it a more cumbersome therapy for the management of late-stage endobronchial lung cancer.[104]

A great limitation to the use of PDT is that the drug stays not only in tumor cells for an extended period of time but also in the skin and cells of the eyes. This therefore makes patients photosensitive, not only to the argon laser but also to any source of white light, most significantly sunlight, which contains light with wavelengths of 630 nm. Patients must therefore stay out of all forms of white light for at least 6 weeks to prevent damage to their skin and/or eyes. If a patient were to have advanced disease, this limitation to the patient's life seems very cumbersome indeed. Owing to PDT's excellent management of early disease, the inconvenience may well be worth it.

Endobronchial Prosthesis

Endobronchial prostheses are most often referred to as stents, which can be used in several clinical situations: intrinsic, extrinsic, or mixed endobronchial obstruction. Stents work well in conjunction with other modalities, such as laser and mechanical debulking of tumors. Currently, there is no one perfect stent. The stents clinically available are composed of Silastic rubber, metal alloys, and hybrids of materials. The advantages and disadvantages of each stent type are noted in Tables 2 and 3.

Table 2 Advantages and Disadvantages of Silastic Stents

Advantages
   Removable and replaceable
   No growth through stent
   Low cost
   Low likelihood of granulation tissue formation

Disadvantages
   Potential for migration/dislodgment
   Rigid bronchoscopy needed for placement
   Possible secretion adherence

Table 3 Advantages and Disadvantages of Metal Stents

Advantages
   Easy to place
   Good wall–internal diameter relationship
   Powerful radial force
   Excellent conformity for irregular tracheal or
      bronchial walls
   Good epithelialization

Disadvantages
   Permanent
   Tumor regrowth (noncovered)
   Possible migration of covered stents
   Significant granulation tissue stimulation
   Epithelialization affecting wall mechanics and
      secretion clearance
   Radial force causing necrosis of bronchial wall,
      erosion, fistulae, perforation

Silastic Stents

In 1990, Dumon reported the use of what is now referred to as the Dumon stent (Bryan Corp., Woburn, MA).[105] Developed in 1987, it is a Silastic stent with evenly spaced studs along its outside walls (Figure 8). These studs not only assist in maintaining placement of the stent in the airway, they also allow the clearance of secretions around the walls of the stent. Although the use of expandable wire mesh stents is increasing, the Dumon stent remains the most commonly used stent worldwide.

When placed endobronchially, the Dumon stent is effective in maintaining the structural integrity. Its solid walls prevent tumor growth from reobstructing airways. Endobronchial tumors are often debulked, and then a stent is placed to relieve the airways obstruction. This can be performed prior to the initiation of radiotherapy and/or chemotherapy. This may afford the patient a clinical advantage owing to the improved ability to breathe. Patients may be able to tolerate more aggressive treatment programs owing to their improved ability to breath.

Another advantage of the Dumon stent is its ease of removal. This can be significant when endobronchial procedures are used early in the management of cancer patients. After definitive therapies have been used (radiation, chemotherapy), reevaluation of the airway can be performed, and the stent can be left in place, removed (if deemed of no further clinical advantage), or replaced with a larger stent that would further improve the caliber and stability of the airway. The disadvantages of the Dumon stent are the potential for migration and the need for a rigid bronchoscope for placement. The migration issue, although often referred to, occurs less often when an experienced interventional endoscopist places the stent.[105–111] In regard to the need for rigid bronchoscopy, the number of interventional pulmonologists using this technique is small but continues to grow.

Other Silastic stents include the Hood stent (Hood Laboratories, Decatur, GA) and the hybrid Rüsch Y stent (Rüsch Inc, Duluth, GA). The Hood stent is similar to the Dumon stent in design and use. The Hood stent (Figure 9) is placed in the same manner as the Dumon stent.[112]

The Rüsch Y stent (Figure 10) is a Silastic stent with stainless steel C-rings that artificially replicate the cartilage. The posterior wall of the stent is made of a thinner Silastic plastic to make it more functional, similar to the membranous trachea itself. The three available sizes of this stent are designed to traverse the entire length of the trachea with branches into the right and left

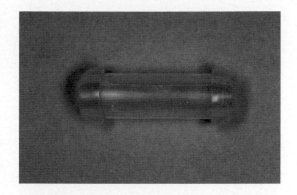

FIGURE 9 Hood bronchial stent.

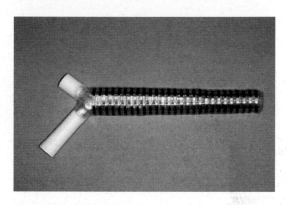

FIGURE 10 Rüsch Y stent.

mainstem bronchi. The Rüsch Y stent requires rigid bronchoscopy and a special delivery device. This stent is difficult to place and remains uncommon in clinical practice.

Metallic Stents

Metal stents, such as the historical Gianturco (Cook Inc, Bloomington, IN), Palmaz (Johnson & Johnson Interventional Systems, Warren, NJ), and Wallstent (Schneider Inc, Minneapolis, MN) stents, as well as the commonly used Ultraflex (Boston Scientific, Natick, MA) stent and soon to be released Alveolus stent (Alveolus Inc., Charleston, SC), have been used in the endobronchial management of lung cancer.

The advantage of metal stents is the relative ease of placement via a flexible bronchoscope with or without fluoroscopic assistance. This ease of placement allows some bronchoscopists to use these stents as their sole modality in the management of endobronchial disease. This practice, however, limits the options to patients that may otherwise be available if all interventional modalities are considered. The wire mesh design of many of the original metal stents did not prevent the tumor from growing through the stent over time. The Ultraflex and Alveolus stents are both available covered. The wrap is applied to the outside of the wire mesh to prevent tumor invasion through the stent.[106,107,113–115]

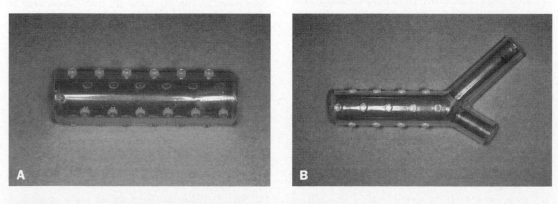

FIGURE 8 *A,* Dumon tracheobronchial stent. *B,* Dumon Y stent.

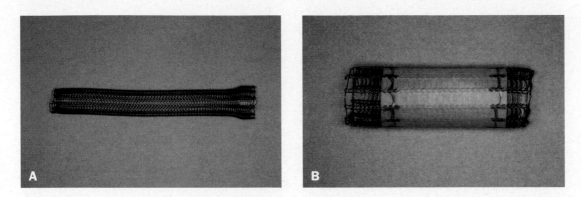

FIGURE 11 *A*, Ultraflex uncovered stent. *B*, Ultraflex covered stent.

The Ultraflex stent is made of nitinol, a titanium and nickel alloy, which has little bioreactivity. This stent has an excellent inner to outer diameter and conforms well to various airway shapes, maintaining an equal pressure along the entire length of the stent. The Ultraflex stent is available in a variety of lengths and diameters. It is available in both covered and noncovered forms. The covered stent uses a polyurethane wrapping around all but the proximal and distal 1 cm of the stents. The covered version of this stent is excellent for use in the palliation of airway obstruction in lung cancer patients (Figure 11).

The Alveolus stent is also a wire mesh stent. At the time of the writing of this chapter, this stent is not commercially available, although it should be in the near future. This stent is also made of nitinol but is completely covered, preventing all tumor ingrowth. This stent's design characteristics make it very promising, but no clinical studies exist to validate its use (Figure 12).

Stents are effective tools for the endobronchial management of lung cancer. The choice of which stent to use should be made carefully, weighing the advantages and disadvantages of each so that the proper tool is used in all situations. Multiple stent types need to be available to the endoscopist to allow the proper choice for the appropriate clinical situation.

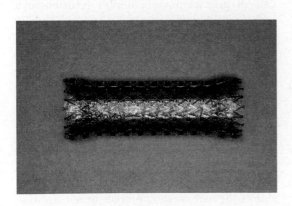

FIGURE 12 Alveolus stent.

Conclusion

Bronchoscopy has expanded the bounds of the innovative thinkers who created this wonderful technique. The goal of this chapter was to introduce the techniques and technologies of both diagnostic and therapeutic bronchoscopy. Both areas continue to evolve, with the goal of new innovative thinkers being the earliest conceivable detection of lung cancer, with the opportunity to treat it more aggressively and, it is hoped, more successfully.

REFERENCES

1. Ikeda S. Flexible bronchofiberscope. Laryngology 1970; 79:916–23.
2. Horsfield K, Cumming G. Morphology of the bronchial tree in man. J Appl Physiol 1968;24:273–383.
3. Karahalli E, Yilmaz A, Turker H, Ozvaran K. Usefulness of various diagnostic techniques during fiberoptic bronchoscopy for endoscopically visible lung cancer; should cytologic examinations be performed routinely? Respiration 2001;68:611–4.
4. Jones AM, Hanson IM, Armstrong GR, O'Driscoll BR. Value and accuracy of cytology in addition to histology in the diagnosis of lung cancer at flexible bronchoscopy. Respir Med 2001;95:374–8.
5. Kelly CA, Kotre CJ, Ward C, et al. Anatomical distribution of bronchoalveolar lavage fluid as assessed by digital subtraction radiography. Thorax 1987;42:624–8.
6. Davis GS, Giancola MS, Constanze MC, Low RB. Analyses of sequential bronchoalveolar lavage samples from healthy human volunteers. Am Rev Respir Dis 1982;126:611–6.
7. Pingleton SK, Harrison GF Stechschulte DJ, et al. Effect of location, pH, and temperature of instillate in bronchoalveolar lavage in normal volunteers. Am Rev Respir Dis 1983;128:1035–7.
8. Ettensohn DB, Jankowski MJ, Duncan PG, Low RB. Bronchoalveolar lavage in the normal volunteer subject. I. Technical aspects and intersubject variability. Chest 1988;94:275–80.
9. De Gracia J, Bravo C, Miravitalles M, et al. Diagnostic value of bronchoalveolar lavage in peripheral lung cancer. Am Rev Respir Dis 1993;147:649–52.
10. Linder J, Radio SJ, Robbins RA, et al. Bronchoalveolar lavage in the cytologic diagnosis of carcinoma of the lung. Acta Cytol 1987;31:796–801.
11. Pirozynski M. Bronchoalveolar lavage in the diagnosis of peripheral, primary lung cancer. Chest 1992;102:372–4.
12. Augusseau S, Mouriquand J, Brambilla C, et al. Cytological survey of bronchial brushings and aspirations performed during fiberoptic bronchoscopy. Arch Geschwulstforsch 1978;48:245–9.
13. Ehya H, Young N. Cytologic approach to tumors of the tracheobronchial tree. Chest Surg Clin N Am 2003;13: 41–62.
14. Dierkesmann R. The diagnostic yield of bronchoscopy. Cardiovasc Intervent Radiol 1991;14:24–8.
15. Mak VH, Johnston ID, Hetzel MR, Grubb C. Value of washings and brushings at fiberoptic bronchoscopy in the diagnosis of lung cancer. Thorax 1990;45:373–6.
16. Zisholtz BM, Eisenberg H. Lung cancer cell type as a determinant of bronchoscopy yield. Chest 1983;84: 428–30.
17. Lam WK, So SY, Hsu C, Yu DY. Fiberoptic bronchoscopy in the diagnosis of bronchial cancer: comparison of washings, brushings and biopsies in central and peripheral tumours. Clin Oncol 1983;9:35–42.
18. Popovich J Jr, Kvale PA, Eichnhorn MS, et al. Diagnostic accuracy of multiple biopsies from flexible fiberoptic bronchoscopy. A comparison of central versus peripheral carcinoma. Am Rev Respir Dis 1982;125:521–23.
19. Gellert AR, Rudd RM, Sinha G, Geddes DM. Fibreoptic bronchoscopy effect of multiple bronchial biopsies on diagnostic yield in bronchial carcinoma. Thorax 1982; 37:684–7.
20. Shure D, Astarita RW. Bronchogenic carcinoma presenting as an endobronchial mass: optimal number of biopsy specimens for diagnosis. Chest 1983;83:865–7.
21. Arroliga AC, Matthay RA. The role of bronchoscopy in lung cancer. Clin Chest Med 1993;14:87–98.
22. Radke JR, Conway WA, Eyler WR, et al. Diagnostic accuracy in peripheral lung lesions. Chest 1979;76:176–9.
23. Wallace JM, Deutsch AL. Flexible fiberoptic bronchoscopy and percutaneous needle lung aspiration for evaluating the solitary pulmonary nodule. Chest 1982;81:665–71.
24. Zavala DC. Diagnostic fiberoptic bronchoscopy: techniques and results of biopsy in 600 patients. Chest 1975;68: 12–9.
25. Savage C, Morrison RJ, Zwischenberger JB. Bronchoscopic diagnosis and staging of lung cancer. Chest Surg Clin N Am 2001;4:701–21.
26. Descombes F, Gardiol D, Leunberger PH. Transbronchial lung biopsy: an analysis of 530 cases with reference to the number of samples. Monaldi Arch Chest Dis 1997;53: 324–9.
27. Milman N, Faurschou P, Munch EP, et al. Transbronchial lung biopsy through the fiberoptic bronchoscope: results and complications in 452 examinations. Respir Med 1994;88:749–53.
28. Mazzone P, Jain P, Arroliga AC, Matthay RA. Bronchoscopy and needle biopsy techniques for diagnosis and staging of lung cancer. Clin Chest Med 2002;23:137–58.
29. Anderson HA, Fontana RS, Harrision EG Jr. Transbronchial lung biopsy in diffuse pulmonary disease. Dis Chest 1965;48:187–92.
30. Anderson HA, Fontana RS. Transbronchoscopic lung biopsy for diffuse pulmonary diseases: technique and results in 450 cases. Chest 1972;62:125–8.
31. Palojoki A, Sutinen S. Transbronchoscopic lung biopsy as aid in pulmonary diagnostics. Scand J Respir Dis 1972;53: 120–4.
32. Andersen HA, Miller WE, Bernatz PE. Lung biopsy: transbronchoscopic, percutaneous, open. Surg Clin North Am 1973;53:785–93.
33. Wang KP, Haponik EF, Britt EF, et al. Transbronchial needle aspiration of peripheral pulmonary nodules. Chest 1984; 86:819–23.
34. Wang KP, Haponik EF, Gupta PK, Erozan YS. Flexible transbronchial needle aspiration: technical considerations. Acta Otol Rhinol Laryngol 1984;93:233–6.
35. Morrow AG, Braunwald E, Haller JA, Sharp EH. Left heart catheterization by the transbronchial route. Circulation 1957;16:1033–9.
36. Crymes TP, Fish RG, Smith ED, et al. Complications of transbronchial left atrial puncture. Am Heart J 1959;58: 46–52.
37. Kucera RF, Wolfe GK, Perry ME. Hemomediastinum after transbronchial needle aspiration. Chest 1986;90:466.
38. Shure D, Fedullo PF. The role of transcarinal needle aspiration in the staging of bronchogenic carcinoma. Chest 1984;86:693–6.
39. Harrow EM, Oldenburg FA, Smith AM. Transbronchial needle aspiration in clinical practice. Thorax 1985;40: 756–9.
40. Wang KP, Terry PB. Transbronchial needle aspiration in the diagnosis and staging of bronchogenic carcinoma. Am Rev Respir Dis 1983;127:344–7.
41. Gay PC, Brutinel WM. Transbronchial needle aspiration in the practice of bronchoscopy. Mayo Clin Proc 1989;64: 158–62.
42. Shure D, Fedullo PF. Transbronchial needle aspiration of peripheral masses. Am Rev Respir Dis 1983;128:1090–2.

43. Reichenberger F, Weber J, Tamm M, et al. The value of transbronchial needle aspiration in the diagnoses of peripheral pulmonary lesions. Chest 1999;116:704–8.

44. Arroliga AC, Matthay RA. The role of bronchoscopy in lung cancer. Clin Chest Med 1993;14:87–98.

45. Cortese DA, McDougall JC. Biopsy and brushing of peripheral lung cancer with fluoroscopic guidance. Chest 1979; 75:141–5.

46. Kvale PA, Bode FR, Kini S. Diagnostic accuracy in lung cancer. Comparison of techniques used in association with flexible fiberoptic bronchoscopy. Chest 1976;69: 752–7.

47. Thomas P, Rubinstein L, Lung Cancer Study Group. Cancer recurrence after resection: T1N0 non-small cell lung cancer. Ann Thorac Surg 1990;49:242–7.

48. Woolner LB, Fontana RS, Cortese DA. Roentgenographically occult lung cancer: pathologic findings and frequency of multicentricity during a 10-year period. Mayo Clin Proc 1984;59:453–66.

49. Lam S, MacAuley C, LeRiche J, et al. Early localization of bronchogenic carcinoma. Diagn Ther Endosc 1994;1: 75–8.

50. Lam S, MacAuley C, Hung J, et al. Detection of dysplasia and carcinoma in situ with a lung imaging fluorescence endoscope device. J Thorac Cardiovasc Surg 1993;105: 1035–40.

51. Lam S., Hung J, Kennedy S, et al. Detection of dysplasia and carcinoma in situ by ratio fluorometry. Am Rev Respir Dis 1992;146:1458–61.

52. Ikeda N, Kim K, Okunaka T, et al. Early localization of bronchogenic cancerous/precancerous lesions with lung imaging fluorescence endoscope. Diagn Ther Endosc 1997;3: 197–201.

53. Yokomise H, Yanagihara K, Fukuse T, et al. Clinical experience with lung-imaging fluorescence endoscope (LIFE) in patients with lung cancer. J Bronchol 1997;4:205–8.

54. Venmans B, Linden H, Van Boxem T, et al. Early detection of preinvasive lesions in high risk patients. J Bronchol 1998;5:280–3.

55. Lam S, Kennedy T, Unger M, et al. Localization of bronchial intraepithelial neoplastic lesions by fluorescence bronchoscopy. Chest 1998;113:696–702.

56. Venmans B, Van Boxem T, Smi, E, et al. Results of two years experience with fluorescence bronchoscopy in detection of preinvasive bronchial neoplasia. Diagn Ther Endosc 1999;5:77–84.

57. Haubinger K, Stanzel F, Huber R, et al. Autofluorescence detection of bronchial tumors with the D-Light/AF. Diagn Ther Endosc 1999;5:105–12.

58. Venmans BJ, Linden van der JC, Elbers JRJ, et al. Observer variability in histopathological reporting of bronchial biopsy specimens: influence on the results of autofluorescence bronchoscopy in detection of bronchial neoplasia. J Bronchol 2000;7:210–4.

59. Kleinau H, Liebeskind U, Zaiaic M, Schlag PM. Endoluminal and intraoperative ultrasound. Onkologie 1993;16: 435–42.

60. Kurimoto N, Murayama M, Morita K, et al. Assessment of usefulness of endobronchial ultrasonography in determination of depth of tracheobronchial tumor invasion. Chest 1999;115:1500–6.

61. Herth F, Becker HD. EBUS for early cancer detection. Eur Respir J 2000;16 Suppl 31:189.

62. Miyazu Y, Miyazawa T, Iwamoto Y, et al. The role of endoscopic techniques, laser-induced fluorescence endoscopy, and endobronchial ultrasonography in choice of appropriate therapy for bronchial cancer. J Bronchol 2001;8: 10–6.

63. Becker HD, Herth F. Computer assisted analysis of endosonographic I,ages in solitary pulmonary nodules. Eur Respir J 2002;20 Suppl 38:462.

64. Herth F, Ernst A, Becker HD. Endobronchial ultrasound-guided transbronchial lung biopsy in solitary pulmonary nodules and peripheral lesions. Eur Respir J 2002;20: 972–4.

65. Shannon JJ, Bude RO, Orens JB, et al. Endobronchial ultrasound-guided needle aspiration of mediastinal adenopathy. Am J Respir Crit Care Med 1996;153: 1424–30.

66. Herth F, Ernst A, Becker HD. Ultrasound-guided transbronchial needle aspiration: an experience in 242 patients. Chest 2003;123:604–7.

67. Herth F, Becker HD. Tumor invasion or impression? Endobronchial ultrasound (EBUS) allows differentation in patients with lung cancer. Eur Respir J 2001;16 Suppl 31:6.

68. Schwarz Y, Mehta AC, Ernst A, et al. Electromagnetic navigation during flexible bronchoscopy. Respiration 2003;70: 516–22.

69. Brezinski ME, Tearney GJ, Bouma BE, et al. Optical coherence tomography for optical biopsy: properties and demonstration of vascular pathology. Circulation 1996;93: 1206–13.

70. Boppart SA, Bouma BE, Pitris C, et al. In vivo subcellular optical coherence tomography imaging in Xenopus laevis: implications for the early diagnosis of neoplasms. Nat Med 1998;4:861–5.

71. Cancer facts and figures, 2004. Atlanta: American Cancer Society; 2004.

72. Edell ES, Cortese DA, McDougall JC. Ancillary therapies in the management of lung cancer: photodynamic therapy, laser therapy, and endobronchial prosthetic devices. Mayo Clin Proc 1993;68:685–90.

73. Cortese DA, Edell ES. Role of phototherapy, laser therapy, brachytherapy, and prosthetic stents in the management of lung cancer. Clin Chest Med 1993;14:149–59.

74. Hetzel MR, Millard FJ, Ayesh R, et al. Laser treatment for carcinoma of the bronchus. Br Med J 1983;286:12–6.

75. Mehta AC, Golish JA, Ahmad M, et al. Palliative treatment of malignant airway obstruction by Nd-YAG laser. Cleve Clin Q 1985;52:513–24.

76. McDougall JC, Corese DA. Neodymium-YAG laser therapy of malignant airway obstruction: a preliminary report. Mayo Clin Proc 1983;58:35–9.

77. Toty L, Personne C, Colchen A, et al. Bronchoscopic management of tracheal lesions using the neodymium yttrium aluminum garnet laser. Thorax 1981;36:175–8.

78. Dumon JF, Reboud E, Garbe L, et al. Treatment of tracheobronchial lesions by laser photoresection. Chest 1982;81: 278–84.

79. Arabian A, Spagnolo SV. Laser therapy in patients with primary lung cancer. Chest 1984;86:519–23.

80. Brutinel WM, Cortese DA, McDougall JC, et al. A two-year experience with the neodymium-YAG laser in endobronchial obstruction. Chest 1987;91:159–65.

81. Beamis JF Jr,Vergos K, Rebeiz EE, et al. Endoscopic laser therapy for obstructing tracheobronchial lesions. Ann Otol Rhinol Laryngol 1991;100:413–9.

82. Sonett JR, Keenan RJ, Ferson PF, et al. Endobronchial management of benign, malignant, and lung transplantation airway stenosis. Ann Thorac Surg 1995;59:1417–22.

83. Macha HN, Becker KO, Kemmer HP. Pattern of failure and survival in endobronchial laser resection: a matched pair study. Chest 1994;105:1668–72.

84. Desai SJ, Mehta AC, Vanderbug Medendorp S, et al. Survival experience following Nd:YAG laser photoresection for primary bronchogenic carcinoma. Chest 1988;94: 939–44.

85. Stanopoulos IT, Beamis JF Jr, Martinez FJ, et al. Laser bronchoscopy in respiratory failure from malignant airway obstruction. Crit Care Med 1993;21:386–91.

86. Cavaliere S, Foccoli P, Toninelli C, et al. Nd:YAG laser therapy in lung cancer: an 11-ear experience with 2,253 applications in 1,585 patients. J Bronchol 1994;1:105–11.

87. Ross DJ, Mohsenifar Z, Koerner SK. Survival characteristics after neodymium:YAG laser photoresection in advanced stage lung cancer. Chest 1990;98:581–5.

88. Edell ES, Cortese DA, McDougall JC. Ancillary therapies in the management of lung cancer: photodynamic therapy, laser therapy, and endobronchial prosthetic devices. Mayo Clin Proc 1993;68:685–90.

89. Cortese DA, Edell ES. Role of phototherapy, laser therapy, brachytherapy, and prosthetic stents in the management of lung cancer. Clin Chest Med 1993;14:149–59.

90. Sutedja G, Schramel F, van Kralingen K, et al. Stent placement is justifiable in end-stage patients with malignant airway tumours. Ann Otol Rhinol Respir 1995;62: 148–50.

91. Prakash UB, Stubbs SE. The bronchoscopy survey: some reflections. Chest 1991;100:1660–7.

92. Mathisen DJ, Grillo HC. Endoscopic relief of malignant airway obstruction. A five-year experience with 1,396 applications in 1,000 patients. Ann Thorac Surg 1989; 48:469–75.

93. Cavaliere S, Foccoli P, Farina PL. Nd:YAG laser bronchoscopy. Chest 1988;94:15–21.

94. Kvale PA, Eichenhorn MS, Radke JR, et al. YAG laser photoresection of lesions obstructing the central airways. Chest 1985;87:283–8.

95. Eichenhorn MS, Kvale PA, Miks VM, et al. Initial combination therapy with YAG laser photoresection and irradiation for inoperable non-small cell carcinoma of the lung: a preliminary report. Chest 1986;89:782–5.

96. Petrovich Z, Stanley K, Cox JD, et al. Radiotherapy in the management of locally advanced lung cancer of all cell types: final report of randomized trial. Cancer 1981; 48:1335–40.

97. Gerasin VA, Safirovsky BB. Endobronchial electrosurgery. Chest 1988;93:270–4.

98. Reichle G, Freitag L, Kullmann H-J, et al. Argon plasma coagulation in bronchology: a new method—alternative or complementary. J Bronchol 2000;7:109–17.

99. Maiwand MO, Homasson JP. Cryotherapy for tracheobronchial disorders. Clin Chest Med 1995;16:427–43.

100. Lam S. Photodynamic therapy of lung cancer. Semin Oncol 1994;21:15–9.

101. Sutedja T, Lam S, LeRiche JC, et al. Response and pattern of failure after photodynamic therapy for intraluminal stage I lung cancer. J Bronchol 1994;1:295–8.

102. Furuse K, Fukuoka M, Kato H, et al. A prospective phase II study on photodynamic therapy with Photofrin II for centrally located early-stage lung cancer: the Japan Lung Cancer Photodynamic Therapy Study Group. J Clin Oncol 1993;11:1852–7.

103. Hayata Y, Kato H, Konaka C, et al. Photodynamic therapy (PDT) in early stage lung cancer. Lung Cancer 1993;9: 287–94.

104. Moghissi K, Dixon K, Stringer M, et al. The place of bronchoscopic photodynamic therapy in advanced unresectable lung cancer: experience of 100 cases. Eur J Cardiothorac Surg 1999;15:1–6.

105. Dumon JF. A dedicated tracheobronchial stent. Chest 1990; 97:328–32.

106. Colt HG, Dumon JF. Tracheobronchial stents: indications and applications. Lung Cancer 1993;9:301–6.

107. Tojo T, Iioka S, Kitamura S, et al. Management of malignant tracheobronchial stenosis with metal stents and Dumon stents. Ann Thorac Surg 1996;61:1074–8.

108. Dumon JF, Cavaliere S, Diaz-Jimenez JP, et al. Seven-year experience with the Dumon prosthesis. J Bronchol 1996; 3:6–10.

109. Diaz-Jimenez JP, Munoz EF, Ballarin JIM, et al. Silicone stents in the management of obstructive tracheobronchial lesions: 2-year experience. J Bronchol 1994;1:15–8.

110. Freitag L, Eicker K, Donovan TJ, et al. Mechanical properties of airway stents. J Bronchol 1995;2:270–8.

111. Clarke CP, Ball DL, Sephton R. Follow-up of patients having Nd:YAG laser resection of bronchostenotic lesions. J Bronchol 1994;1:19–22.

112. Gaer JA, Tsang V, Khaghani A, et al. Use of endotracheal silicone stents for relief of tracheobronchial obstruction. Ann Thorac Surg 1992;54:512–6.

113. Colt HG, Dumon J-F. Airway obstruction in cancer: the pros and cons of stents. J Respir Dis 1991;12:741–4, 746, 748–9.

114. Bolliger CT, Probst R, Tschopp K, et al. Silicone stents in the management of inoperable tracheobronchial stenoses: indications and limitations. Chest 1993;104:1653–9.

115. Gelb AF, Zamel N, Colchen A, et al. Physiologic studies of tracheobronchial stents in airway obstruction. Am Rev Respir Dis 1992;146:1088–90.

Direct Neurologic Complications of Cancer

Robert Cavaliere, MD
David Schiff, MD

Neurologic complications of systemic cancer are common and widely recognized. The entire neuraxis, from the muscle to the cerebral hemispheres, is susceptible to the adverse effects of cancer and its treatments. The consequences of neurologic complications of cancer can be considerable, as the resulting pain and functional and cognitive dysfunction may result in significant degradation of quality of life. As advances in therapies for systemic cancer improve patient survival, an increasing incidence of neurologic complications can be expected. Patients may present to the medical system at any level, from the office of the primary care physician or oncologist to the emergency room. It is essential that all clinicians become familiar with common neurologic complications of cancer. The focus of this chapter is common direct neurologic complications of systemic cancer that affect the peripheral and central nervous systems. Typical presentation, diagnostics, and therapies will be reviewed. Indirect neurologic complications of cancer and its therapies are covered in other chapters in this volume.

Plexopathy

Brachial Plexus

The brachial plexus is an anastomotic collection of nerves formed by the nerve roots of the fifth cervical through first thoracic spinal segments. The malignant involvement of the brachial plexus occurs by two mechanisms, compression by a mass or infiltration by cancer cells. The former arises by metastases to axillary lymph nodes or direct extension of apical lung tumor, both of which lie in close proximity to the lower trunk of the brachial plexus. The most common malignancies to do so are breast and lung cancers, accounting for approximately 70% of cases of malignant plexopathy.[1,2] Both lesions tend preferentially to involve the lower trunk of the plexus derived primarily from C8 and T1 spinal segments. Lymphomas occasionally infiltrate the brachial plexi.[3,4] Pain is the most common and

significant symptom. It commonly involves the shoulder region and radiates down the medial aspect of the arm into the fourth and fifth digits of the hand. Muscle weakness and sensory loss may also be present (Table 1). A Horner's syndrome is present in approximately 50% of patients.[1]

Lumbosacral Plexus

Colorectal tumors, genitourinary tumors and sarcomas are the most common cancers to impact the lumbosacral (LS) plexus.[5,6] Tumors invade the plexus by direct extension from the primary site in a majority of cases although metastases from extra-abdominal malignancies occurred in 27% of cases.[5] Similar to neoplastic brachial plexopathy, the predominant symptom among patients with neoplastic LS plexopathy is pain. Weakness and sensory abnormalities are common, the distribution dependant on the extent of plexus involvement (see Table 1).[7] Symptoms are typically unilateral.[6] Incontinence is rare, and its presence suggests epidural extension of tumor.[5]

Diagnosis

Electrophysiologic evaluation, including nerve conduction studies and electromyography, may help localize the disease as well as help differentiate it from other disease processes such as radiation plexopathy.[8,9] CT scanning of the plexi has been employed in the work-up of patients with suspected neoplastic plexopathies, identifying abnormalities in 89% and 74% of patients with brachial and LS plexopathy respectively[6,10]. There are several limitations of this technique, including beam hardening artifact from surrounding bone, limited separation vascular structures from nerve bundles, and single-plane imaging.[11] Magnetic resonance imaging (MRI) provides much better anatomic detail and has become the imaging modality of choice. The most common finding with both CT and MRI is a mass either in or near the plexus.[10,11] Increased T2 signal adjacent to the brachial plexus is occasionally seen on MRI.[11] Often, imaging is sufficient to

Table 1 Neurologic Deficits Associated with Injuries of the Plexus	
Lower Brachial Plexus	
Muscle Weakness	Finger Flexion
	Wrist Flexion
	Grip and intrinsic muscles of hand
Sensory Loss	Inner border of arm
	Inner border of forearm
	Inner border of hand
Horner's Syndrome	Ipsilateral ptosis
	Ipsilateral miosis
	Anhidrosis
Posture	"Claw hand deformity"
Upper Brachial Plexus	
Muscle Weakness	Shoulder abduction
	Flexion at elbow
	External rotators of the arm
	Supination of forearm
Sensory Loss	Outer surface of upper arm
Reflex	Depressed bicep and brachioradialis
Posture	"Waiter's tip"
Lumbar Segment of Lumbosacral Plexus	
Muscle Weakness	Hip flexion
	Leg extension
	Leg Adduction
Sensory Loss	Inguinal region
	Lateral, anterior and medial thigh
	Medial lower leg
Reflex	Depressed patellar reflex
Sacral Segment of Lumbosacral Plexus	
Muscle Weakness	Dorsiflexors and plantar flexors of ankle
	Inversion and eversion of foot
	Hip abduction
	Hip extension
Sensory loss	Outer leg
	Dorsum and sole of foot
	Posterior thigh
Reflex	Depressed ankle jerk
Adapted from Brazis PW.[7]	

establish the diagnosis. Nine percent of MR scans, however, are normal, and surgical exploration is often necessary.[1,2,11] More recently, positron emission tomography (PET) has been employed and may help confirm metastases in patients with indeterminate MRI.[12–14] Experience with this modality is limited to small case series, and more research is necessary to evaluate its utility. Spine imaging may also be indicated, as coexistent epidural disease is present in approximately 50% of cases.[1,5] Restaging with systemic imaging to evaluate for active disease outside of the plexus should be considered.[1] Hydronephrosis should be ruled out in patients with LS plexopathy; it was detected in 44% of cases in one series.[5]

Treatment

Depending on tumor type, a variety of treatment modalities have been used, including radiation, chemotherapy, and steroids. Response to treatment, however, has been poor. Pain control is improved in only 15% of patients with LS and 46% of patients with brachial lesions. Only rarely do patients improve neurologically.[1,10] Supportive treatment, including pain management with opioids, is essential to ensure patient comfort.

Leptomeningeal Metastases

Once thought to be rare, infiltration of the leptomeninges by tumor is increasing in incidence, estimated to be approximately 4 to 15%, 7 to 15%, and 5 to 15% in patients with solid tumors, lymphoma, and leukemias, respectively.[15] The reported incidence of leptomeningeal metastases (LMM) varies depending on method of case ascertainment (Table 2).

The clinical presentation of LMM is variable and dependant on the area of the nervous system involved. Multifocality is typical (Table 3).[15,16] Headache and back and neck pain arise from meningeal irritation and may be non-localizing. Headaches may also be secondary to hydrocephalus resulting from obstruction of cerebrospinal fluid (CSF) flow or impaired CSF reabsorption.

Table 2 Frequency of LMM by Cancer Type

Cancer Type	Frequency of LMM (%)	Proportion if all cases LMM
Lung		10 to 26%
NSCL	1–5	
SCLC	6	
Breast	1–2	12 to 34%
Melanoma	5	17 to 25%
GI	1	4 to 14%
Unknown Primary	1 to 7%	

Adapted from Hitchins RN et al,[33] Chamberlain MC and Kormanik,[42] Boogerd W et al,[30] Fizazi K et al,[40] and Chamberlain MC.[15]

Table 3 Signs and symptoms of LMM

Symptoms	Signs
Cerebral symptoms	
Headache	Mental change
Mental change	Seizures
Difficulty walking	Papilledema
Nausea/Vomiting	Diabetes Insipidus
Cranial Nerve	
Diplopia	Ocular nerve palsies
Hearing loss	Facial weakness
Vertigo	Diminished hearing
Vision loss	Diminished facial sensation
Facial numbness	Lingual weakness
Dysphagia	Diminished gag
Hoarseness	Optic neuropathy
Spinal symptoms	
Lower motor neuron weakness	Reflex asymmetry
Paresthesias	Weakness
Radicular pain	Sensory loss
Back or neck pain	Positive straight leg raise
Bowel or bladder dysfunction	Decreased rectal tone
	Nuchal rigidity

Adapted from Wasserstrom WR et al.[16]

Nerve root involvement may cause neuropathic type pain in a radicular distribution. Limb weakness may result from involvement of the cerebral hemispheres and spinal cord (upper motor distribution) or cauda equina and nerve roots (lower motor neuron distribution). Often patients have a cauda equina syndrome including paraparesis and bowel or bladder function disturbance. Cerebral hemispheric dysfunction may result from underlying brain irritation, compression, or strokes (secondary to vascular compression or infiltration).

Diagnosis

CSF analysis is an essential component of the evaluation of patients with suspected LMM. Nearly all patients with LMM have CSF abnormalities, the most common finding being elevated protein often with a lymphocytic pleocytosis. Occasionally, opening pressure is elevated, and glucose is low. Although suggestive of LMM in the appropriate clinical setting, these findings are not diagnostic. The identification of malignant cells within the CSF is considered the gold standard. Cytology is positive on the first analysis in approximately 54 to 91% of cases. The yield increases to approximately 76 to 100% by the third analysis.[17] The yield of additional lumbar punctures is small. In about 10% of cases, cytology remains negative. The variability may be accounted for by several factors, including the method by which fluid is collected and processed and case ascertainment. It is not uncommon for

fluid that has been collected at night, on weekends, or even during the workday to be refrigerated prior to processing. Such delays may decrease the yield of cytology relative to immediate processing by a cytopathologist.[17] Variations in CSF composition at different levels of the neuraxis in the absence of a CSF block have been demonstrated.[17–21] The extent of disease may partially account for the variation.[15,20] CSF collected from an Ommaya reservoir or ventricular shunt may be falsely negative in the presence of more caudal disease, such as in the brain stem or spinal cord.[21] Conversely, fluid obtained from the lumbar cistern via a lumbar puncture may be falsely negative in a patient with cerebral or brain stem disease.[22] CSF obtained in the vicinity of a radiographic abnormality or clinically defined lesion may have a greater yield.[17,18] Often, an insufficient volume of CSF is submitted for cytopathologic review. A minimum of 10 cc is recommended for cytology alone.[17] Flow cytology, especially in patients with hematological malignancies, may further increase the yield of CSF analysis. Other testing with potential benefit includes testing for tumor markers and immunohistochemistry.[15,23]

Neuroimaging is a valuable tool in the evaluation of patients with suspected LMM, particularly in those with a coagulopathy or elevated intracranial pressure prohibiting lumbar puncture. In addition, in the appropriate clinical context, typical radiographic findings may be sufficient to establish the diagnosis, even in the absence of positive cytology. Previously, cranial computerized tomography (CT) and spinal myelography were frequently utilized. MRI is now the method of choice as it is readily available, has better sensitivity and is less invasive. Leptomeningeal or subependymal linear or nodular enhancement is the most common finding. This may take the form of enhancement of the sulci within the cerebral hemispheres, or of the folia in the cerebellum. Enhancement may outline the brainstem or spinal cord. Frequently, enlargement of the cranial nerves or roots and matting of the cauda equina is evident. Hydrocephalus is often present. MRI also has the advantage of detection of coexistent parenchymal or spinal epidural disease that may require additional intervention.[22,24,25] MRI demonstrates leptomeningeal seeding in approximately 75% and 36 to 46% of patients with and suspected LMM, positive and negative cytology respectively.[22,26]

CSF flow studies are often performed in patients with LMM, especially when intrathecal (IT) chemotherapy is planned. Flow abnormalities may be detected that were otherwise not predicted based on conventional imaging and clinical evaluation.[27,28] Only 31% to 42% of patients with flow abnormalities had hydrocephalus.[27,28] On occasion, flow studies may detect asymptomatic areas of disease.[27] The presence of flow abnormalities is associated with a worse prognosis and may interfere with the distribution of drugs administered intrathecally.[15,27–29] Once identified, areas of CSF block can be corrected with radiation in about 50% of cases, thus restoring flow and improving survival.[15,27,28]

Treatment

The disseminated nature of LMM is such that the entire neuraxis must be treated. Craniospinal radiation effectively targets not only the leptomeninges, but also the parenchyma of the CNS and vertebral column. As such, coexistent disease in the structures is treated as well. Craniospinal radiation, however, is associated with significant toxicity, including severe myelosuppression, that may limit the delivery treatments to systemic disease. In addition, large areas of the gastrointestinal tract are included in the treatment field, resulting in mucosal damage and notable morbidity. As such, radiation therapy (RT) is generally reserved for the focal treatment of bulky disease, symptomatic regions, or areas of CSF block. Doing so may palliate symptoms, especially pain, or restore normal CSF flow dynamics.[15,27,30–33]

Systemic or IT delivery of chemotherapy is commonly used to treat LMM. A notable advantage of systemic chemotherapy is the treatment of coexistent active systemic disease. In addition, the distribution of the agents is not dependant on the normal flow of CSF. In fact, therapeutic levels of medications have been detected both proximal and distal to known CSF blocks.[34] Systemically delivered chemotherapy may penetrate bulky disease more effectively than agents delivered intrathecally. Intravenous administration of chemotherapy obviates the need for repeated lumbar punctures or placement of an Ommaya reservoir, the latter of which is associated with significant complications.[34,35] A wider array of agents is available for systemic delivery than IT delivery. The blood-brain barrier, however, limits the penetration of most chemotherapies used to treat malignancies that most commonly metastasize to the leptomeninges. The impact of this barrier is debatable, as the blood-brain barrier is known to be disturbed in this setting.

IT chemotherapy, delivered via an Ommaya reservoir or repeated lumbar punctures, is perhaps the most common treatment employed. Cytotoxic agents administered directly into the CSF bypass the blood brain barrier that excludes agents given systemically. Also, systemic toxicity is reduced without compromising effective treatment of leptomeningeal disease. Repeated lumbar punctures, however, are inconvenient and uncomfortable. Placement of an Ommaya reservoir requires a surgical procedure and is associated with short and long-term complications, including infection, hemorrhage, catheter malfunction, and peri-catheter necrosis. Furthermore, CSF dynamics are frequently disturbed in the setting of LMM and homogenous distribution of medication cannot be ensured. Neurotoxicity may occur in areas of trapped chemotherapy.[27,29] Alternatively, insufficient levels of chemotherapy may be achieved at other sites.

Methotrexate (MTX), cytosine arabinoside and thiotepa are the agents available for Intrathecal (IT) administration. Traditionally, they have been given as single-dose injections 2 days per week during an induction phase. Depending on the response, the frequency of administration is tapered during a consolidation phase. The optimal duration of therapy is unknown. The short half-life and rapid clearance of these medications has raised the concern that the exposure of tumor cells to cytotoxic levels of the agents is insufficient, particularly distant from the injection site.[36] Alternative schedules have been developed in which IT chemotherapy is given on several consecutive days, thereby ensuring a steady drug level is maintained for an adequate period of time.[15] However, the frequent injections required may be difficult and inconvenient for the patient. Recently, a lipid-encapsulated version of cytosine arabinoside (DepoCyt, Enzon Pharmaceuticals, Bridgewater, NJ) was developed that effectively increases the half-life such that cytotoxic levels are maintained for 14 days.

Several retrospective and prospective trials have been performed evaluating the effectiveness of IT therapy. Most trials differed in their inclusion criteria, treatment methods and schedules, and criteria for diagnosis and response. Thus, comparisons of the results are difficult. Nonetheless, some conclusions can be drawn. Approximately 20 to 30% of patients die during early phases of treatment.[30,35,37] The agents all appear to have equal efficacy, although there is a trend towards better survival and longer time to disease progression with DepoCyt in the treatment of both solid and hematologic tumors.[38,39] Clinical response rates vary between 9 and 69%. Cytologic response rates are about 25 to 50%. Melanoma and non-small cell lung cancer are relatively more resistant, and breast cancer, small cell lung cancer, and lymphomas are more responsive. Duration of response is short, and median survival remains only 4 to 5 months with aggressive therapy. One study of MTX in breast cancer patients suggested a benefit of IT therapy on a concentration, versus time, schedule.[40] Most studies failed to demonstrate a benefit when multiple agents were administered simultaneously[33,41] although Kim and colleagues, in a small retrospective study, noted improved survival and response rate among those treat with MTX, cytosine arabinoside, and hydrocortisone, compared to MTX alone.[31] Patients with normal CSF flow dynamics have better responses.[28,42] Toxicity is similar among the agents and includes headache and nausea. Arachnoiditis is common and can be minimized with the administration of dexamethasone several days prior to and after IT treatment.[15] As the agents are cleared into systemic circulation, systemic toxicity may occur. IT MTX is occasionally associated with mucositis and myelosuppression. Folinic acid is generally given in conjunction with MTX to minimize this complication.

Systemic chemotherapy, particularly MTX, is occasionally given to treat LMM. MTX penetrates the CNS poorly when given at standard doses. When given at high doses, however, cytotoxic concentrations are obtained within the CSF. In addition, clearance from the CSF is slower relative to IT administration of MTX.[34] Significant hematologic and gastrointestinal toxicity can be prevented with folinic acid rescue. Few studies have been published reviewing the effectiveness of this intervention in the treatment of LMM, although the data available are encouraging.[34]

Although systemic chemotherapy is generally thought to penetrate the CNS poorly, patients with LMM treated with a variety of chemotherapeutic regimens specifically directed at the underlying systemic malignancy have a better response than those who do not receive systemic treatment.[30,40,43] Bokstein and colleagues compared patients treated prospectively in two separate trials differing only in the use of IT chemotherapy.[35] Exclusion of IT chemotherapy did not change the overall response to treatment, the median survival or the proportion of long-term survivors. The rates of early and delayed IT treatment-related complications were decreased significantly.

Survival of patients with LMM is poor. Untreated, patients succumb to their illness within 1 to 2 months. Even with aggressive management, survival is typically less than 6 months. Patients with hematological malignancies are more responsive than those with solid malignancies.[44] Patients with better prognostic features, including little neurologic disability, limited systemic or parenchymal CNS disease, and higher performance status may benefit more from treatment.

Epidural Spinal Cord Compression (ESCC)

ESCC is a common problem among patients with systemic cancer. A recent population-based study reported an incidence of 2.5% of patients preceding death. The cancers with the greatest propensity to cause this problem are multiple myeloma and prostate carcinomas. However, reflecting the higher incidence within the population, breast, prostate, and lung cancer account for most cases, approximately 20% each.[45,46]

ESCC results most commonly from the growth of metastases present within the vertebral body into the spinal canal. Alternatively, the resulting bony destruction results in compression fractures. Less commonly, lesions in the paraspinal region grow into the spinal canal through the neural foramina. Any segment of the spinal column can be involved, although thoracic and lumbar segments are most often involved. Multiple lesions are common, occurring in one-third of patients.[47,48]

Pain is the most common symptom, affecting almost all patients with this condition. It is usually the first symptom and may precede decline in neurologic status by weeks to months. Pain is progressive and severe and occasionally positional, with exacerbation in the supine position. It is often localized to the symptomatic vertebral segment. A coexistent radiculopathy is often associated with neuropathic discomfort in the limbs. As the disease progresses, focal deficits develop, including lower extremity weakness and, ultimately, loss of ambulation. As a result, there is significant decline in performance status and quality of life. As neurologic status at presentation is strongly predictive of functional outcome, it is imperative that a high index of suspicion is present such that the appropriate diagnostic and therapeutic interventions can be instituted in a timely manner.

Diagnosis

The cornerstone of diagnosis is the radiographic detection of a lesion within the spinal canal. The imaging modality of choice is MRI. MRI is a non-invasive means of imaging the entire spinal axis thereby detecting not only the clinically suspected lesion but also other lesions less clinically apparent.[49] It provides superior anatomic detail of the spinal cord and surrounding structures, such as leptomeninges, vertebral body, and bone marrow. Alternative or coexistent non-malignant pathology that may be present can be seen.[49] Certain patients, including those with metallic objects such as artificial heart valves, cannot receive MRIs. A high-quality MR image necessitates that the patient remain still during the study to prevent movement artifact. The pain associated with ESCC, often exacerbated by recumbancy, may limit the ability of the patient to tolerate the exam. This is particularly true given the duration of an MRI study, which is typically longer than myelography. Otherwise, few other contraindications exist, and the procedure is generally well tolerated.

Alternatively, CT myelography, which, prior to MRI, was the imaging modality of choice, may be performed. It requires the injection of a dye directly into the epidural space via a lumbar puncture. The dye is than allowed to diffuse caudal and rostral to the injection site, after which a CT is performed. The dye forms a "cast" of the epidural space that may be deformed by a lesion, malignant or non-malignant, extending into it. Myelography, however, is invasive and, in the presence of a complete block, requires a second cervical injection to visualize the rostral extent of the lesion. Although CT allows visualization of anatomic structures, it is less sensitive and more limited than MRI.[50]

Treatment

ESCC is a true neurologic emergency. Without treatment, it follows a relentless course resulting in significant pain and progressive neurologic deterioration culminating in death. A delay in therapy may result in rapid, irreversible loss of function. Treatment is palliative as most patients succumb to their underlying systemic disease. Median reported survival remains approximately 6 months, although certain patients may survive longer. Prognostic factors have been elucidated and scales established to assist the clinician in identifying appropriate patients for more aggressive surgery.[51,52] Prognostic factors include underlying tumor histology, medical and neurologic status at presentation, extent of systemic disease, and number of vertebral metastases.

Although corticosteroids have long been used to treat patients with ESCC, it was not until recently that their benefit was demonstrated in a prospective, randomized clinical trial.[53] In this study, successful treatment, defined as retained ability to walk in pretreatment ambulatory patients and recovery of ambulation of non-ambulatory patients, was demonstrated in 81% of those who received dexamethasone compared to 63% of those who did not. At 1 year, a significantly greater percentage of treated patients remained ambulatory. The high-dose regimen tested in this study, however, is associated with significant toxicity.[54,55] Subsequently, a second study randomized patients to either a 100 mg or 10 mg bolus of dexamethasone followed by 16 mg daily. No difference was found in pain control, ambulation, or continence.[56] The optimal dose of steroids in ESCC remains unknown. High-dose regimens are typically reserved for patients with notable neurologic deficits or those progressing rapidly, while less symptomatic patients are treated more conservatively.[46] Occasionally, steroids can be avoided entirely.[57]

RT is routinely used in the treatment of patients with ESCC. Besides effectively controlling pain, it preserves ambulation in 90% of ambulatory patients. In addition, 30 to 40% of paraparetic and 10% of paraplegic patients regain ambulation. Several regimens have been evaluated, although none have been found to be superior.[58] Generally, the treatment field includes one uninvolved spinal segment above and below the lesion.

Response to treatment may be dependant on the degree of radio-responsiveness of the underlying tumor. Breast carcinoma, lymphoma, multiple myeloma, and small cell lung cancer are among the tumors responsive to RT. Conversely, melanoma, sarcoma, and renal cancer are considered relatively resistant. A smaller proportion of patients are ambulatory at completion of RT in the latter group, and responses are less durable.[59–61] The effectiveness of radiation therapy may be diminished in patients with structural disease such as vertebral body collapse and compression by bony fragments.[62,63] Such patients are often treated with surgery to stabilize the spine and relieve the compression.

Radiation is generally well tolerated. The presence of hematological precursors sensitive to radiation within the spinal canal increases the risk of bone marrow suppression if sufficient spinal segments are included within the treatment field. Other innocent bystanders include the mucosal lining of the gastrointestinal tract, made up of rapidly dividing cells that, when extensively irradiated, may result in mucositis and diarrhea. In addition, patients are at risk of radiation-induced myelopathy especially those treated with large fractions. This complication is rare, however, even in those retreated with RT for a loco-regional recurrence.[64–66]

Though surgery is frequently employed in the treatment of ESCC, its role is controversial. Laminectomy had long been the procedure of choice. Laminectomy, however, provides only limited exposure to the anterior elements of the spine that are most frequently involved by metastases. In addition, removal of posterior support elements in the setting of vertebral body disease further destabilizes the spine. This results in potential instability and increases the risk of future complications. Not surprisingly, early studies did not demonstrate benefit when laminectomy was performed in conjunction with radiation therapy.[67,68] With the advent of modern instrumentation, surgeons can implant a variety of devices that provide necessary support. Studies of posterior approach surgeries, including laminectomy, that incorporate instrumentation have demonstrated improved results with 60 to 70% of non-ambulatory patients regaining ambulation.[69,70] Other surgical approaches have been attempted as well.[51,71–77] These frequently include an anterior approach through body cavities, which provides a direct route to the vertebral body for decompression and stabilization. Among the advantages relative to the posterior approach, the anterior approach permits minimal removal of uninvolved bone and reconstruction of the often diseased and unstable, weight-bearing, anterior column. With modern imaging, surgeons can now determine the extent of disease within the spine as well as the structures involved.

Hence, the type of surgery employed may now be tailored to the individual case. Modern reports of such techniques have been encouraging, with 60 to 82% of patients having improvement in their neurologic status.[71–73,76,77] Only recently, however, has modern surgery has been compared to RT. Patchell and colleagues reported a randomized control trial of surgery and postoperative RT versus RT alone for patients with a single level of compression.[78] Fifty-six percent of patients in the surgery-plus-radiation group regained the ability to walk, versus 19% of those who received radiation alone. Those who received surgery were ambulatory for 126 days, versus 35 days who were only treated with radiation. Narcotic use was significantly lower in those who were operated on. The authors concluded that surgery plus radiation was more effective then radiation alone.

Surgery, like every invasive procedure, is associated with complications. Most modern surgical series report about a 30% complication rate.[71,73,77,79] Many of the complications are medical, including pneumonia, gastrointestinal bleeding, and pulmonary embolus. About 12 to 20% of patients sustain wound dehiscence or infection or failure of instrumentation.[70,76–78] Frequently, such complications require a second surgery. Nonetheless, surgical mortality remains low, with most series reporting a 30-day mortality of less than 7%.[71,72,75–77,79] Preoperative RT increases the risk of wound and instrumentation failure.[72,76,78,79] Patients with poor performance status may also be at higher risk of complication.[72,79]

Cerebral Metastases

Cerebral metastases represent the most common complication of systemic cancer. Although any malignancy can metastasize to the brain, the most common to do so are melanoma and lung cancer. However, given the relatively higher incidence within the population, non-small cell and breast cancer account for the majority of cases (Table 4).[80,81] Hematological malignancies only rarely metastasize to brain parenchyma.

Table 4 Proportion of Cerebral Metastases by Primary Cancer Type

Cancer Type	Proportion of cases (%)
Lung	40 to 64
Non-small cell	24 to 49
Small Cell	15
Breast	14 to 17
Unknown Primary	5 to 8
Melanoma	4 to 11
Gastrointestinal	3 to 6
Genitourinary	2 to 6

Adapted from Zimm S et al[80] and Nussbaum ES et al.[81]

Any region of brain can be involved by metastases. The most common locations are the cerebral and cerebellar hemispheres. Usually lesions are located at the gray white junction. In the CT era, approximately 50% of patients with metastatic disease had solitary lesions.[81] This undoubtedly is an overestimate as MRI is more sensitive in detecting lesions. In a recent study, 31% of patients with solitary lesions on contrasted head CT had multiple lesions on MRI.[82] Typical symptoms include headache and focal neurologic deficits, the latter dependant on the region of brain involved by the lesion. Patients can also present with seizures, altered mental status, cognitive decline, and behavioral changes. Occasionally, metastases are asymptomatic and detected only on staging imaging. Symptoms may be acute or subacute in onset. Most commonly, cerebral metastases develop over the course of one's illness. Occasionally, cerebral metastases, most commonly from a lung primary, may represent the first symptom of a systemic malignancy.

MRI is the preferred diagnostic imaging modality. Typically, lesions enhance following the administration of gadolinium, either in a ring or homogenous pattern. Usually, surrounding T2 signal abnormality is present, occasionally resulting in significant mass effect and shift. Metastases in the cerebellum may result in compression of the fourth ventricle and secondary hydrocephalus. CT scanning is also used in the evaluation of patients with suspected metastases, although it is less sensitive than MRI. MRI provides better anatomic detail for surgical planning, is less susceptible to bony artifact, is able to visualize smaller lesions, and provides superior visualization of the posterior fossa.[82–84]

Once detected, systemic staging is indicated to establish the extent of disease. Usually, a CT of the chest, abdomen, and pelvis is performed. Occasionally, PET scanning is employed in patients with cerebral metastases of unknown primary. In one study, PET scanning identified the primary tumor in 24% of patients.[85] However, survival was not altered by the discovery of the primary tumors. More research is necessary to define the role of this imaging modality.

Prognostication is important in the treatment planning of patients with cerebral metastases. Several factors have been identified to correlate with outcome, including extent of systemic disease, patient age and performance status, and underlying tumor histology. Recursive partitioning analysis has stratified patients based on prognostic factors into three classes (Table 5).[86]

Treatment

Corticosteroids, usually dexamethasone, may provide rapid although transient, palliation by reducing the surrounding edema.[87] The optimal

Table 5 Recursive Partitioning Analysis (RPA) of Prognostic Factors in Patients with Cerebral Metastases

RPA Class	Prognostic Factors	Median Survival
Class I	KPS[1] > 70; Age < 65; Primary tumor controlled; No additional metastases	7.1 months
Class II	KPS > 70; Age > 65; Primary uncontrolled; Additional metastases	4.2 months
Class III	KPS < 70	2.3 months

KPS = Karnofsky Performance Status. Adapted from Gaspar L et al.[86]

dose is unknown, although lower doses have been shown to be as effective as higher doses.[88] Furthermore, lower doses are associated with fewer side effects. In the event of impending herniation, larger doses may be required. Once patients are symptomatically improved, steroids should be tapered to the lowest effective dose.

Patients with seizures require an antiepileptic medication. Phenytoin is most often used because it is effective and can be rapidly loaded. Phenytoin, however, is highly protein-bound and interacts with the cytochrome P-450 system thereby predisposing to drug interactions. The use of antiseizure medications in patients who have not had a seizure is controversial. Several studies have failed to demonstrate a statistically significant reduction in patients who subsequently develop seizures.[89,90] Thus, patients may unnecessarily be exposed to possible side effects and complications of these medications. As such the prophylactic use of antiseizure medications is not recommended.[91]

More definitive treatment directed at the metastases involves surgery, radiation and sometimes chemotherapy. Which interventions are employed depends on a number of factors, including status of systemic disease, patient performance status, previous treatments, and number and location of metastases.

Radiation Therapy

Radiation therapy has been the mainstay of therapy for patients with metastatic deposits within the CNS. Traditionally, treatment has been delivered to the whole brain. Several treatment schedules and doses have been assessed although none has been found to be superior to the others.[92–94] A commonly utilized treatment plan is 30 gray divided in 10 fractions delivered over 2 weeks. Early studies reported that approximately 40 to 50% of patients had improvement in their neurologic status and that 60 to 90% of specific symptoms improve.[92,94] However, more recent studies failed to show such a significant clinical benefit. In a prospective study of 85 symptomatic patients with metastases from solid tumors, 19% improved and 55% died or progressed 1 month following radiation therapy. Furthermore, there was a statistically significant decline in performance status with a trend toward worse quality of life.[87] Assessment of the response to whole brain radiation therapy (WBRT) is difficult to separate from the effects of dexamethasone given concomitantly.

Surgery

Until recently, the disseminated nature of metastatic malignancies has limited surgery to palliative interventions directed at symptomatic lesions. Early retrospective studies have demonstrated a benefit of resection of solitary metastases, although interpretation was limited by selection bias. Two prospective, randomized trials performed in the CT era, however, demonstrated a survival advantage when resection of a solitary metastasis was performed in conjunction with radiation compared to radiation alone.[95,96] Patients who underwent resection remained independent for a significantly longer period of time and had better local control of the metastatic disease. Patients with active extracranial disease, however, did not benefit from surgery, and overall survival approximated that of those treated with radiation alone in this group.[96] Age was a significant, independent prognostic factor in both studies. A third prospective randomized trial failed to demonstrate an advantage to resection of a solitary metastases, although ten of 43 patients randomized to radiation alone underwent resection. In addition, a greater proportion of patients had active systemic disease.[97] Nonetheless, the weight of the evidence supports resection of solitary cerebral metastases in patients with controlled systemic disease.

The use of surgery in patients with multiple metastases is less clear. Patients with a dominant lesion causing significant mass effect or symptoms are frequently resected. One retrospective study assessed the impact of resection of up to three lesions on survival.[98] Survival of patients who underwent gross total resection of all lesions closely approximated that of patients with solitary lesions. This intervention has yet to be tested in a prospective fashion, and surgery in patients with multiple metastases should be reserved for select cases.

The role of WBRT following the resection of a solitary metastasis remains a matter of debate. The only prospective study published to date found that postoperative WBRT reduced the rate of failure both in the vicinity of, and distant to,

the resected lesion. In addition, patients were less likely to die of neurologic causes. However, there was no difference in overall survival or the time in which patients remained functionally independent.[99] Yet the potential toxicity of WBRT may outweigh the benefit. One study reported an 11% incidence of dementia in one-year survivors with metastatic disease treated with WBRT.[100] Patients reported in this study, however, were treated with unconventional treatment regimens that included high-dose fractions. Furthermore, several patients were treated with methotrexate, a medication with higher CNS toxicity, especially when given in conjunction with radiation therapy. On further analysis, none of the patients treated with conventional treatment schemes developed cognitive disturbances. In addition, it is difficult to separate the effects of treatment from the underlying tumor. Most patients with metastatic disease may not survive long enough to suffer from this delayed complication, although the acute and subacute toxicities of radiation therapy and the inconvenience of daily treatment sessions remain problematic. Alternatively, careful radiographic surveillance for patients who choose to defer radiation therapy may detect recurrences early, prior to development of symptoms and associated performance decline, such that they can then be treated with additional focal therapies or WBRT. This is particularly true since MRI, which is more sensitive than CT and capable of detecting smaller lesions, has become readily available.

Stereotactic Radiosurgery

Stereotactic radiosurgery (SRS, Elekta, Stockholm, Sweden), as delivered by Gamma Knife or a modified linear accelerator, is an emerging technology that accurately delivers high doses of radiation to a target in a single treatment session. As a treatment modality, it has several advantages over both conventional surgery and radiation therapy. Neurosurgeons are often limited by the anatomic constraints of the central nervous system. As such, even patients with solitary lesions may not be candidates for resection. Surgical resection entails a craniotomy that is associated with significant mortality and morbidity and requires a several-day hospitalization. SRS, although not risk-free, is less invasive and, in many facilities, done as an outpatient procedure. Patients with a surgically inaccessible solitary lesion or multiple metastases can be treated in a single session. Unfortunately, SRS does not provide tissue for pathological examination. As many as 11% of cancer patients with a solitary cerebral lesion suspected to be a metastases based on preoperative imaging are found to have an alternative pathological diagnosis.[95] Also, larger lesions, which may be amenable to surgery, are less responsive to SRS, and their treatment is associated with greater toxicity.[101]

Relative to WBRT, SRS has several distinct advantages. The precision with which radiation is delivered with SRS, as well as the steep dose gradient, spares the normal surrounding brain tissue thereby minimizing CNS toxicity. In addition, even radioresistant tumors are sensitive to the high doses of radiation delivered by SRS.[102–104] Fractionation of conventional WBRT requires daily visits to a treatment facility, which may be difficult and inconvenient for both the patients and their caregivers. Recurrent lesions can be retreated without significant toxicity. However, SRS is a focal treatment strategy similar to surgery and does not treat micrometastases not visualized on head CT or MRI. The addition of WBRT to surgical resection reduces failure distant from surgical site to 14% from 37%.[99] The cost of SRS at present is significantly greater than that of WBRT.

Solitary Metastases

Several studies have demonstrated the effectiveness of SRS in the treatment of solitary metastases.[103,105–107] When employed with WBRT, local control rates of 80 to 85% at 1 year and median survival of 56 weeks are similar to that reported in trials of surgical resection followed by WBRT[95,99] and exceed control rates of patients treated either with surgery[99] or WBRT alone.[95,103] Randomized, prospective trials comparing surgery to SRS have not been performed, and retrospective reports have yielded conflicting results. Binda and colleagues demonstrated superior survival among patients treated with conventional surgery[108] whereas others reported similar survival between the two groups.[109,110] Local control appears better with surgery, and patients die less often from neurologic causes.[108,109] Short-term toxicity is minimized with SRS relative to surgery[103,109] although one study found the contrary.[108] Long-term morbidity, however, may be greater in patients treated with SRS.[109]

Multiple Metastases

SRS can be used to treat patients with multiple metastatic deposits, a distinct advantage over conventional surgery. Two prospective, randomized trials of WBRT with or without SRS that included patients with multiple lesions demonstrated significantly improved local control and time to brain failure in patients treated with SRS.[105,111] Although there was no difference in overall survival, patients treated with SRS required lower steroid doses and had a better performance status.[105] Alternatively, retrospective studies of patients with multiple metastases demonstrated similar local control when patients were treated with SRS with or without WBRT. As expected, failure at sites distant from the originally treated lesions was greater in patients treat with SRS alone.[112,113] As such, SRS appears to be an effective intervention in patients with multiple cerebral metastases.

The role of upfront WBRT in patients treated with SRS is a matter of debate. Several retrospective reviews have been undertaken to address this question, although no prospective, randomized studies have been reported to date.[106,112,114] The addition of WBRT does not appear to improve survival relative to SRS alone. Intracranial control, however, is better with upfront WBRT, although a greater proportion of patients initially treated with SRS alone received salvage therapy at recurrence.[112,114] This difference may account for the similar survival between the two groups. The results of an interim analysis of a prospective randomized trial support the findings of the previously reported retrospective series. Although survival and preservation of Karnofsky Performance Score (KPS) was equivalent between the two groups, in- and out-of-field failure was more common when treated with SRS alone.[115]

Chemotherapy

The role of chemotherapy in the treatment of cerebral metastases is the least well studied of all treatment modalities. Like WBRT, chemotherapy would treat the whole brain. Although it is now recognized that chemotherapy is associated with cognitive impairment, presumably it is less toxic than WBRT, thereby serving as an effective alternative. The intact blood-brain barrier (BBB) excludes many chemotherapeutics used to treat systemic disease. In the presence of metastatic lesions, however, the BBB is leaky as indicated by the presence of enhancement on imaging. BBB disruption with mannitol and intra-arterial chemotherapy have been attempted to bypass this barrier, although their role has yet to be definitively established. Occasionally, chemotherapy is given at high doses, such that the concentration gradient across the BBB is sufficient for agents to cross it. The most common agent to be delivered in this manner is methotrexate with folinic acid rescue. More recent, intracavitary chemotherapy in the form of Gliadel wafers has been employed. Novel agents, such as temozolomide, which are capable of penetrating the blood-brain barrier, are also promising.[116–118]

Chemotherapy has most extensively been evaluated in the treatment of small cell lung cancer, a tumor with known chemosensitivity. Most often, it has been used in the setting of recurrence following RT.[119,120] One randomized trial of teniposide versus teniposide with WBRT found patients treated with both modalities to have a higher response rate and longer progression-free survival. Overall survival was identical.[121] Small series have reported the utility of chemotherapy in the treatment of breast cancer, non-small cell lung cancer, and melanoma.[122–127] Thus far, data are limited, and the role of chemotherapy has yet to be defined.

Conclusion

The neurologic complications of cancer are not uncommon. As therapies for systemic disease improve, one can expect an increased incidence of these conditions. Clinicians must be familiar with these conditions so that therapeutic interventions that palliate and cure patients can be instituted.

REFERENCES

1. Kori SH, Foley KM, Posner JB. Brachial plexus lesions in patients with cancer: 100 cases. Neurology 1981;31: 45–50.
2. Wittenberg KH, Adkins MC. MR imaging of nontraumatic brachial plexopathies: frequency and spectrum of findings. Radiographics 2000;20:1023–32.
3. Baehring JM, Damek D, Martin EC, Betensky RA, Hochberg FH. Neurolymphomatosis. Neuro-oncol 2003;5:104–15.
4. Pietrangeli A, Milella M, De Marco S, et al. Brachial plexus neuropathy as unusual onset of diffuse neurolymphomatosis. Neurol Sci 2000;21:241–5.
5. Jaeckle KA, Young DF, Foley KM. The natural history of lumbosacral plexopathy in cancer. Neurology 1985;35: 8–15.
6. Thomas JE, Cascino TL, Earle JD. Differential diagnosis between radiation and tumor plexopathy of the pelvis. Neurology 1985;35:1–7.
7. Brazis PW. The localization of lesions affecting the cervical, brachial and lumbosacral plexuses. In: Brazius PW, Masdeu JC, Biller J, editors. Localization in clinical neurology. 4th ed. Boston: Lippincott Williams & Wilkins; 2001. 107–119.
8. Krarup C, Crone C. Neurophysiological studies in malignant disease with particular reference to involvement of peripheral nerves. J Neurol 2002;249:651–61.
9. Harper CM Jr, Thomas JE, Cascino TL, Litchy WJ. Distinction between neoplastic and radiation-induced brachial plexopathy, with emphasis on the role of EMG. Neurology 1989;39:502–6.
10. Cascino TL, Kori S, Krol G, Foley KM. CT of the brachial plexus in patients with cancer. Neurology 1983;33: 1553–7.
11. Thyagarajan D, Cascino T, Harms G. Magnetic resonance imaging in brachial plexopathy of cancer. Neurology 1995;45(3 Pt 1):421–7.
12. Ahmad A, Barrington S, Maisey M, Rubens RD. Use of positron emission tomography in evaluation of brachial plexopathy in breast cancer patients. Br J Cancer 1999;79:478–82.
13. Hathaway PB, Mankoff DA, Maravilla KR, et al. Value of combined FDG PET and MR imaging in the evaluation of suspected recurrent local-regional breast cancer: preliminary experience. Radiology 1999;210:807–14.
14. Trojan A, Jermann M, Taverna C, Hany TF. Fusion PET-CT imaging of neurolymphomatosis. Ann Oncol 2002;13: 802–5.
15. Chamberlain MC. Leptomeningeal metastases: a review of evaluation and treatment. J Neurooncol 1998;37:271–84.
16. Wasserstrom WR, Glass JP, Posner JB. Diagnosis and treatment of leptomeningeal metastases from solid tumors: experience with 90 patients. Cancer 1982;49:759–72.
17. Glantz MJ, Cole BF, Glantz LK, et al. Cerebrospinal fluid cytology in patients with cancer: minimizing false-negative results. Cancer 1998;82:733–9.
18. Chamberlain MC, Kormanik PA, Glantz MJ. A comparison between ventricular and lumbar cerebrospinal fluid cytology in adult patients with leptomeningeal metastases. Neuro-oncol 2001;3:42–5.
19. Murray JJ, Greco FA, Wolff SN, Hainsworth JD. Neoplastic meningitis. Marked variations of cerebrospinal fluid composition in the absence of extradural block. Am J Med 1983;75:289–94.
20. Glass JP, Melamed M, Chernik NL, Posner JB. Malignant cells in cerebrospinal fluid (CSF): the meaning of a positive CSF cytology. Neurology 1979;29:1369–75.
21. Schiff D, Feske SK, Wen PY. Deceptively normal ventricular fluid in lymphomatous meningitis. Arch Intern Med 1993;153:389–90.
22. Freilich RJ, Krol G, DeAngelis LM. Neuroimaging and cerebrospinal fluid cytology in the diagnosis of leptomeningeal metastasis. Ann Neurol 1995;38:51–7.

23. Thomas JE, Falls E, Velasco ME, Zaher A. Diagnostic value of immunocytochemistry in leptomeningeal tumor dissemination. Arch Pathol Lab Med 2000;124:759–61.
24. Collie DA, Brush JP, Lammie GA, et al. Imaging features of leptomeningeal metastases. Clin Radiol 1999;54:765–71.
25. Gomori JM, Heching N, Siegal T. Leptomeningeal metastases: evaluation by gadolinium enhanced spinal magnetic resonance imaging. J Neurooncol 1998;36:55–60.
26. Straathof CS, de Bruin HG, Dippel DW, Vecht CJ. The diagnostic accuracy of magnetic resonance imaging and cerebrospinal fluid cytology in leptomeningeal metastasis. J Neurol 1999;246:810–4.
27. Glantz MJ, Hall WA, Cole BF, et al. Diagnosis, management, and survival of patients with leptomeningeal cancer based on cerebrospinal fluid-flow status. Cancer 1995;75: 2919–31.
28. Chamberlain MC, Kormanik PA. Prognostic significance of 111indium-DTPA CSF flow studies in leptomeningeal metastases. Neurology 1996;46:1674–7.
29. Mason WP, Yeh SD, DeAngelis LM. 111Indium-diethylene-triamine pentaacetic acid cerebrospinal fluid flow studies predict distribution of intrathecally administered chemotherapy and outcome in patients with leptomeningeal metastases. Neurology 1998;50:438–44.
30. Boogerd W, Hart AA, van der Sande JJ, Engelsman E. Meningeal carcinomatosis in breast cancer. Prognostic factors and influence of treatment. Cancer 1991;67:1685–95.
31. Kim DY, Lee KW, Yun T, et al. Comparison of intrathecal chemotherapy for leptomeningeal carcinomatosis of a solid tumor: methotrexate alone versus methotrexate in combination with cytosine arabinoside and hydrocortisone. Jpn J Clin Oncol 2003;33:608–12.
32. Danjoux CE, Jenkin RD, McLaughlin J, et al. Childhood medulloblastoma in Ontario, 1977–1987: population-based results. Med Pediatr Oncol 1996;26:1–9.
33. Hitchins RN, Bell DR, Woods RL, Levi JA. A prospective randomized trial of single-agent versus combination chemotherapy in meningeal carcinomatosis. J Clin Oncol 1987;5:1655–62.
34. Glantz MJ, Cole BF, Recht L, et al. High-dose intravenous methotrexate for patients with nonleukemic leptomeningeal cancer: is intrathecal chemotherapy necessary? J Clin Oncol 1998;16:1561–7.
35. Bokstein F, Lossos A, Siegal T. Leptomeningeal metastases from solid tumors: a comparison of two prospective series treated with and without intra-cerebrospinal fluid chemotherapy. Cancer 1998;82:1756–63.
36. Fisher PG, Kadan-Lottick NS, Korones DN. Intrathecal thiotepa: reappraisal of an established therapy. J Pediatr Hematol Oncol 2002;24:274–8.
37. Jaeckle KA, Batchelor T, O'Day SJ, et al. An open label trial of sustained-release cytarabine (DepoCyt) for the intrathecal treatment of solid tumor neoplastic meningitis. J Neurooncol 2002;57:231–9.
38. Glantz MJ, Jaeckle KA, Chamberlain MC, et al. A randomized controlled trial comparing intrathecal sustained-release cytarabine (DepoCyt) to intrathecal methotrexate in patients with neoplastic meningitis from solid tumors. Clin Cancer Res 1999;5:3394–402.
39. Glantz MJ, LaFollette S, Jaeckle KA, et al. Randomized trial of a slow-release versus a standard formulation of cytarabine for the intrathecal treatment of lymphomatous meningitis. J Clin Oncol 1999;17:3110–6.
40. Fizazi K, Asselain B, Vincent-Salomon A, et al. Meningeal carcinomatosis in patients with breast carcinoma. Clinical features, prognostic factors, and results of a high-dose intrathecal methotrexate regimen. Cancer 1996;77: 1315–23.
41. Giannone L, Greco FA, Hainsworth JD. Combination intra-ventricular chemotherapy for meningeal neoplasia. J Clin Oncol 1986;4:68–73.
42. Chamberlain MC, Kormanik P. Carcinoma meningitis secondary to non-small cell lung cancer: combined modality therapy. Arch Neurol 1998;55:506–12.
43. Siegal T, Lossos A, Pfeffer MR. Leptomeningeal metastases: analysis of 31 patients with sustained off-therapy response following combined-modality therapy. Neurology 1994; 44:1463–9.
44. Mason WP. Leptomeningeal metastases. In: Schiff D, Wen PY, editors. Cancer neurology in clinical practice. 1st ed. Totowa: Humana Press Inc., NJ 2003. 107–119.
45. Loblaw DA, Laperriere NJ, Mackillop WJ. A population-based study of malignant spinal cord compression in Ontario. Clin Oncol (R Coll Radiol) 2003;15:211–7.
46. Cavaliere R, Schiff D. Epidural spinal cord compression. Curr Treat Options Neurol 2004;6:285–95.

47. Schiff D, O'Neill BP, Wang CH, O'Fallon JR. Neuroimaging and treatment implications of patients with multiple epidural spinal metastases. Cancer 1998;83:1593–601.
48. Heldmann U, Myschetzky PS, Thomsen HS. Frequency of unexpected multifocal metastasis in patients with acute spinal cord compression. Evaluation by low-field MR imaging in cancer patients. Acta Radiol 1997;38:372–5.
49. Husband DJ, Grant KA, Romaniuk CS. MRI in the diagnosis and treatment of suspected malignant spinal cord compression. Br J Radiol 2001;74:15–23.
50. Carmody RF, Yang PJ, Seeley GW, et al. Spinal cord compression due to metastatic disease: diagnosis with MR imaging versus myelography. Radiology 1989;173:225–9.
51. Tomita K, Kawahara N, Kobayashi T, et al. Surgical strategy for spinal metastases. Spine 2001;26:298–306.
52. Tokuhashi Y, Matsuzaki H, Toriyama S, et al. Scoring system for the preoperative evaluation of metastatic spine tumor prognosis. Spine 1990;15:1110–3.
53. Sorensen S, Helweg-Larsen S, Mouridsen H, Hansen HH. Effect of high-dose dexamethasone in carcinomatous metastatic spinal cord compression treated with radiotherapy: a randomised trial. Eur J Cancer 1994;30A: 22–7.
54. Weissman DE, Dufer D, Vogel V, Abeloff MD. Corticosteroid toxicity in neuro-oncology patients. J Neurooncol 1987;5:125–8.
55. Weissman DE. Glucocorticoid treatment for brain metastases and epidural spinal cord compression: a review. J Clin Oncol 1988;6:543–51.
56. Vecht CJ, Haaxma-Reiche H, van Putten WL, et al. Initial bolus of conventional versus high-dose dexamethasone in metastatic spinal cord compression. Neurology 1989;39:1255–7.
57. Maranzano E, Latini P, Beneventi S, et al. Radiotherapy without steroids in selected metastatic spinal cord compression patients. A phase II trial. Am J Clin Oncol 1996;19:179–83.
58. Loblaw DA, Laperriere NJ. Emergency treatment of malignant extradural spinal cord compression: an evidence-based guideline. J Clin Oncol 1998;16:1613–24.
59. Katagiri H, Takahashi M, Inagaki J, et al. Clinical results of nonsurgical treatment for spinal metastases. Int J Radiat Oncol Biol Phys 1998;42:1127–32.
60. Kim RY, Spencer SA, Meredith RF, et al. Extradural spinal cord compression: analysis of factors determining functional prognosis--prospective study. Radiology 1990; 176:279–82.
61. Maranzano E, Latini P. Effectiveness of radiation therapy without surgery in metastatic spinal cord compression: final results from a prospective trial. Int J Radiat Oncol Biol Phys 1995;32:959–67.
62. Tomita T, Galicich JH, Sundaresan N. Radiation therapy for spinal epidural metastases with complete block. Acta Radiol Oncol 1983;22:135–43.
63. Helweg-Larsen S. Clinical outcome in metastatic spinal cord compression. A prospective study of 153 patients. Acta Neurol Scand 1996;94:269–75.
64. Schiff D, Shaw EG, Cascino TL. Outcome after spinal reirradiation for malignant epidural spinal cord compression. Ann Neurol 1995;37:583–9.
65. Maranzano E, Bellavita R, Floridi P, et al. Radiation-induced myelopathy in long-term surviving metastatic spinal cord compression patients after hypofractionated radiotherapy: a clinical and magnetic resonance imaging analysis. Radiother Oncol 2001;60:281–8.
66. Grosu AL, Andratschke N, Nieder C, Molls M. Retreatment of the spinal cord with palliative radiotherapy. Int J Radiat Oncol Biol Phys 2002;52:1288–92.
67. Young RF, Post EM, King GA. Treatment of spinal epidural metastases. Randomized prospective comparison of laminectomy and radiotherapy. J Neurosurg 1980;53: 741–748.
68. Gilbert RW, Kim JH, Posner JB. Epidural spinal cord compression from metastatic tumor: diagnosis and treatment. Ann Neurol 1978;3:40–51.
69. Bauer HC. Posterior decompression and stabilization for spinal metastases. Analysis of sixty-seven consecutive patients. J Bone Joint Surg Am 1997;79:514–22.
70. Rompe JD, Hopf CG, Eysel P. Outcome after palliative posterior surgery for metastatic disease of the spine—evaluation of 106 consecutive patients after decompression and stabilisation with the Cotrel-Dubousset instrumentation. Arch Orthop Trauma Surg 1999;119: 394–400.
71. Fourney DR, Abi-Said D, Rhines LD, et al. Simultaneous anterior-posterior approach to the thoracic and lumbar spine for the radical resection of tumors followed by reconstruction and stabilization. J Neurosurg Spine 2001;94:232–44.
72. Sundaresan N, Steinberger AA, Moore F, et al. Indications and results of combined anterior-posterior approaches for spine tumor surgery. J Neurosurg 1996;85:438–46.
73. Gokaslan ZL, York JE, Walsh GL, et al. Transthoracic vertebrectomy for metastatic spinal tumors. J Neurosurg 1998;89:599–609.
74. Tomita K, Kawahara N, Baba H, et al. Total en bloc spondylectomy for solitary spinal metastases. Int Orthop 1994;18:291–8.
75. Bilsky MH, Boland P, Lis E, et al. Single-stage posterolateral transpedicle approach for spondylectomy, epidural decompression, and circumferential fusion of spinal metastases. Spine 2000;25:2240–50.
76. Sundaresan N, Rothman A, Manhart K, Kelliher K. Surgery for solitary metastases of the spine: rationale and results of treatment. Spine 2002;27:1802–6.
77. Weigel B, Maghsudi M, Neumann C, et al. Surgical management of symptomatic spinal metastases. Postoperative outcome and quality of life. Spine 1999;24:2240–6.
78. Patchell R, Tibbs W, Regine R, et al. Direct decompressive surgical resection in the treatment of spinal cord compression caused by metastatic cancer: a randomized trial. The Lancer 366(9486):643–648.
79. Wise JJ, Fischgrund JS, Herkowitz HN, et al. Complication, survival rates, and risk factors of surgery for metastatic disease of the spine. Spine 1999;24:1943–51.
80. Zimm S, Wampler GL, Stablein D, et al. Intracerebral metastases in solid-tumor patients: natural history and results of treatment. Cancer 1981;48:384–94.
81. Nussbaum ES, Djalilian HR, Cho KH, Hall WA. Brain metastases. Histology, multiplicity, surgery, and survival. Cancer 1996;78:1781–8.
82. Schellinger PD, Meinck HM, Thron A. Diagnostic accuracy of MRI compared to CCT in patients with brain metastases. J Neurooncol 1999;44:275–81.
83. Sze G, Milano E, Johnson C, Heier L. Detection of brain metastases: comparison of contrast-enhanced MR with unenhanced MR and enhanced CT. AJNR Am J Neuroradiol 1990;11:785–91.
84. Davis PC, Hudgins PA, Peterman SB, Hoffman JC Jr. Diagnosis of cerebral metastases: double-dose delayed CT vs contrast-enhanced MR imaging. AJNR Am J Neuroradiol 1991;12:293–300.
85. Kole AC, Nieweg OE, Pruim J, et al. Detection of unknown occult primary tumors using positron emission tomography. Cancer 1998;82:1160–6.
86. Gaspar L, Scott C, Rotman M, et al. Recursive partitioning analysis (RPA) of prognostic factors in three Radiation Therapy Oncology Group (RTOG) brain metastases trials. Int J Radiat Oncol Biol Phys 1997;37:745–51.
87. Bezjak A, Adam J, Barton R, et al. Symptom response after palliative radiotherapy for patients with brain metastases. Eur J Cancer 2002;38:487–96.
88. Vecht CJ, Hovestadt A, Verbiest HB, et al. Dose-effect relationship of dexamethasone on Karnofsky performance in metastatic brain tumors: a randomized study of doses of 4, 8, and 16 mg per day. Neurology 1994;44:675–80.
89. Cohen N, Strauss G, Lew R, et al. Should prophylactic anticonvulsants be administered to patients with newly-diagnosed cerebral metastases? A retrospective analysis. J Clin Oncol 1988;6:1621–4.
90. Glantz MJ, Cole BF, Friedberg MH, et al. A randomized, blinded, placebo-controlled trial of divalproex sodium prophylaxis in adults with newly diagnosed brain tumors. Neurology 1996;46:985–91.
91. Glantz MJ, Cole BF, Forsyth PA, et al. Practice parameter: anticonvulsant prophylaxis in patients with newly diagnosed brain tumors. Report of the Quality Standards Subcommittee of the American Academy of Neurology. Neurology 2000;54:1886–93.
92. Borgelt B, Gelber R, Kramer S, et al. The palliation of brain metastases: final results of the first two studies by the Radiation Therapy Oncology Group. Int J Radiat Oncol Biol Phys 1980;6:1–9.
93. Murray KJ, Scott C, Greenberg HM, et al. A randomized phase III study of accelerated hyperfractionation versus standard in patients with unresected brain metastases: a report of the Radiation Therapy Oncology Group (RTOG) 9104. Int J Radiat Oncol Biol Phys 1997;39:571–4.
94. Haie-Meder C, Pellae-Cosset B, Laplanche A, et al. Results of a randomized clinical trial comparing two radiation schedules in the palliative treatment of brain metastases. Radiother Oncol 1993;26:111–6.
95. Patchell RA, Tibbs PA, Walsh JW, et al. A randomized trial of surgery in the treatment of single metastases to the brain. N Engl J Med 1990;322:494–500.
96. Vecht CJ, Haaxma-Reiche H, Noordijk EM, et al. Treatment of single brain metastasis: radiotherapy alone or combined with neurosurgery? Ann Neurol 1993;33: 583–90.
97. Mintz AH, Kestle J, Rathbone MP, et al. A randomized trial to assess the efficacy of surgery in addition to radiotherapy in patients with a single cerebral metastasis. Cancer 1996;78:1470–6.
98. Bindal RK, Sawaya R, Leavens ME, Lee JJ. Surgical treatment of multiple brain metastases. J Neurosurg 1993;79:210–6.
99. Patchell RA, Tibbs PA, Regine WF, et al. Postoperative radiotherapy in the treatment of single metastases to the brain: a randomized trial. Jama 1998;280:1485–9.
100. DeAngelis LM, Delattre JY, Posner JB. Radiation-induced dementia in patients cured of brain metastases. Neurology 1989;39:789–96.
101. Chang EL, Hassenbusch SJ 3rd, Shiu AS, et al. The role of tumor size in the radiosurgical management of patients with ambiguous brain metastases. Neurosurgery 2003; 53:272–81.
102. Brown PD, Brown CA, Pollock BE, et al. Stereotactic radiosurgery for patients with "radioresistant" brain metastases. Neurosurgery 2002;51:656–67.
103. Auchter RM, Lamond JP, Alexander E, et al. A multiinstitutional outcome and prognostic factor analysis of radiosurgery for resectable single brain metastasis. Int J Radiat Oncol Biol Phys 1996;35:27–35.
104. Manon R, O'Neill A, Knisely J, et al. Phase II Trial of Radiosurgery for One to Three Newly Diagnosed Brain Metastases From Renal Cell Carcinoma, Melanoma, and Sarcoma: An Eastern Cooperative Oncology Group Study (E 6397). *Journal of Clinical Oncology* 2005;23(34):8870–6.
105. Andrews DW, Scott CB, Sperduto PW, et al. Whole brain radiation therapy with or without stereotactic radiosurgery boost for patients with one to three brain metastases: phase III results of the RTOG 9508 randomised trial. Lancet 2004;363:1665–72.
106. Hasegawa T, Kondziolka D, Flickinger JC, et al. Brain metastases treated with radiosurgery alone: an alternative to whole brain radiotherapy? Neurosurgery 2003;52: 1318–26.
107. Flickinger JC, Kondziolka D, Lunsford LD, et al. A multi-institutional experience with stereotactic radiosurgery for solitary brain metastasis. Int J Radiat Oncol Biol Phys 1994;28:797–802.
108. Bindal AK, Bindal RK, Hess KR, et al. Surgery versus radiosurgery in the treatment of brain metastasis. J Neurosurg 1996;84:748–54.
109. O'Neill BP, Iturria NJ, Link MJ, et al. A comparison of surgical resection and stereotactic radiosurgery in the treatment of solitary brain metastases. Int J Radiat Oncol Biol Phys 2003;55:1169–76.
110. Muacevic A, Kreth FW, Horstmann GA, et al. Surgery and radiotherapy compared with gamma knife radiosurgery in the treatment of solitary cerebral metastases of small diameter. J Neurosurg 1999;91:35–43.
111. Kondziolka D, Patel A, Lunsford LD, et al. Stereotactic radiosurgery plus whole brain radiotherapy versus radiotherapy alone for patients with multiple brain metastases. Int J Radiat Oncol Biol Phys 1999;45:427–34.
112. Sneed PK, Lamborn KR, Forstner JM, et al. Radiosurgery for brain metastases: is whole brain radiotherapy necessary? Int J Radiat Oncol Biol Phys 1999;43:549–58.
113. Kihlstrom L, Karlsson B, Lindquist C. Gamma Knife surgery for cerebral metastases. Implications for survival based on 16 years experience. Stereotact Funct Neurosurg 1993;61(Suppl 1):45–50.
114. Sneed PK, Suh JH, Goetsch SJ, et al. A multi-institutional review of radiosurgery alone vs. radiosurgery with whole brain radiotherapy as the initial management of brain metastases. Int J Radiat Oncol Biol Phys 2002;53:519–26.
115. Hidefumi A, Hiroki S, Masao T, et al. Stereotactic Radiosurgery Plus Whole-Brain Radiation Therapy vs Stereotactic Radiosurgery Alone for Treatment of Brain Metastases. A Randomized Controlled Trial. *JAMA* 2006;295:2483–91.
116. Christodoulou C, Bafaloukos D, Kosmidis P, et al. Phase II study of temozolomide in heavily pretreated cancer patients with brain metastases. Ann Oncol 2001;12: 249–54.
117. Abrey LE, Olson JD, Raizer JJ, et al. A phase II trial of temozolomide for patients with recurrent or progressive brain metastases. J Neurooncol 2001;53:259–65.
118. Verger E, Gil M, Yaya R, et al. Temozolomide and concomitant whole brain radiotherapy in patients with brain metastases: A phase II randomized trial. Int J Radiat Oncol Biol Phys 2005;61:185–91.

119. von Pawel J. The role of topotecan in treating small cell lung cancer: second-line treatment. Lung Cancer 2003;41 (Suppl 4):3–8.

120. Korfel A, Oehm C, von Pawel J, et al. Response to topotecan of symptomatic brain metastases of small-cell lung cancer also after whole-brain irradiation. A multicentre phase II study. Eur J Cancer 2002;38:1724–9.

121. Postmus PE, Haaxma-Reiche H, Smit EF, et al. Treatment of brain metastases of small-cell lung cancer: comparing teniposide and teniposide with whole-brain radiotherapy —a phase III study of the European Organization for the Research and Treatment of Cancer Lung Cancer Cooperative Group. J Clin Oncol 2000;18:3400–8.

122. Ebert BL, Niemierko E, Shaffer K, Salgia R. Use of temozolomide with other cytotoxic chemotherapy in the treatment of patients with recurrent brain metastases from lung cancer. Oncologist 2003;8:69–75.

123. Lin NU, Bellon JR, Winer EP. CNS metastases in breast cancer. J Clin Oncol 2004;22:3608–17.

124. Hwu WJ. New approaches in the treatment of metastatic melanoma: thalidomide and temozolomide. Oncology (Huntingt) 2000;14(12 Suppl 13):25–8.

125. Biasco G, Pantaleo MA, Casadei S. Treatment of brain metastases of malignant melanoma with temozolomide. N Engl J Med 2001;345:621–2.

126. Boogerd W, Dalesio O, Bais EM, van der Sande JJ. Response of brain metastases from breast cancer to systemic chemotherapy. Cancer 1992;69:972–80.

127. Franciosi V, Cocconi G, Michiara M, et al. Front-line chemotherapy with cisplatin and etoposide for patients with brain metastases from breast carcinoma, nonsmall cell lung carcinoma, or malignant melanoma: a prospective study. Cancer 1999;85:1599–605.

Neurologic Toxicity of Radiotherapy

Kimberly Keene, MD
James Larner, MD

Radiation therapy is one of the cornerstones of cancer therapy and is often used in combination with surgery and chemotherapy as a multimodality approach to improve tumor control. While high doses of radiation can sterilize cancer cells, normal tissue tolerance to radiation limits the total dose that can safely be administered. The pathophysiology of radiation injury is not fully understood but likely represents a constellation of responses from vascular, stromal and epithelial cells. Experimental and clinical data have been used to establish the clinical limits of prescribed dose. Normal tissue toxicity is directly related to the total dose, the dose per fraction, the number of fractions, and the volume of tissue irradiated as well as the time interval between fractions. As the total dose, volume treated or dose per fraction increases, the likelihood of normal tissue damage increases. Conversely, as the interval between delivered fractions decreases, toxicity will increase. The $TD_{5/5}$ and $TD_{5/50}$, (the tolerance dose at 5 years where 5% and 50% of the population would express injury, respectively); are used to set dose limitations. Most dose response curves for normal tissue toxicity are sigmoidal in shape. As a result, a small increase in prescribed dose can lead to a large (exponential) increase in normal tissue toxicity. Patient factors, such as age and comorbid illnesses, including diabetes and hypertension, predispose patients to normal tissue toxicity. The addition of chemotherapy to radiation treatment lowers the threshold for radiation-induced damage to normal cells. There is also a genetic basis for the heterogeneity of normal tissue toxicity. For example, individuals with diseases such as Fanconi's anemia and ataxia telangiectasia are hypersensitive to radiation. There is little doubt that other unidentified genes also play a significant role in determining which patients manifest normal tissue toxicity at a given dose/volume level.

New techniques, such as three-dimensional-conformal, intensity-modulated, and stereotactic radiation therapy are designed to spare normal tissues while treating the tumor to higher doses, thereby improving local control and cure. Intensity-modulated radiation therapy uses multiple blocking patterns to vary the radiation beam intensity to conform to the target and avoid normal structures, while stereotactic radiation uses many focused slender beams of radiation that intersect within the target to deliver the prescribed dose of therapy. These exciting technologic improvements allow radiation to be sculpted in elegant ways. The use of dose volume histograms allows physicians to graphically visualize the total dose received to various volumes of different tissue and provide quantitative data for planning therapy. Modifications to the plan are then made to provide maximum dose to the target tissues while sparing normal tissues. Radiosensitizers and radioprotectors are also under exploration to improve therapeutic ratios by increasing the cancer cell's susceptibility to radiation while protecting normal tissues.

CNS Toxicity of the Brain

The critical target of radiation, which is responsible for cell death, is thought to be deoxyribonucleic acid (DNA). Irradiation of cells causes single- and double-strand DNA breaks that, if not repaired, result in cell death. Radiation also results in induction of various genes and altered protein expression, which serve to enhance repair or facilitate apoptosis. Multiple cell types, including subependymal cells, oligodendroglial cells and endothelial cells undergo apoptosis following radiation; this forms the basis of many acute effects. After injury, the progenitor cells must repopulate before differentiating into functional cells. While DNA damage occurs instantaneously after exposure, the latency to expression of injury, or of a tumor response, varies with the number and cycling time of surviving clonogens. However, the latency time to injury is not an indicator of the severity of the injury, and there is little correlation between acute and late radiation damage to normal tissue. For example, lymphocyte progenitor cells have a rapid division and turnover rate so the expression of injury is observed within days after irradiation. On the other hand, organs and tissues with a slow proliferation rate, like the kidney, heart, and brain, may take a year or more before damage is clinically apparent.[1]

Normal tissues are made up of many different stem cells, each with their own inherent cell kinetics, leading to different latency periods for expression of injury. Clinical toxicity of the brain has been separated temporally into acute, subacute, and late effects based on the time period to the clinical manifestation of the injury. Acute effects of radiation have been described in a few instances at autopsy, while most pathologic and radiographic changes reported are for late effects. Toxicities are related to treatment techniques, which include partial brain, whole brain and stereotactic radiosurgery.

Acute Effects

The mechanistic basis of acute effects of radiation is unclear although radiation-induced cerebral edema appears to be a major cause. Edema results in increased intracranial pressure, headaches, nausea, fatigue, or an intensification of presenting tumor signs and symptoms. The correlation of imaging studies with the severity of acute effects of radiation (increased edema) is weak. Nonetheless, acute toxicities almost always resolve with corticosteroid administration, supporting edema as the etiology. Compromise of the blood-brain barrier is one hypothesis for the pathogenesis of radiation-induced cerebral edema. Animal studies suggest the blood-brain barrier disruption is caused by radiation–induced apoptosis of endothelial cells.[2,3] Other common, even universal, acute toxicities of whole or partial brain radiation include alopecia, blockage of the eustachian tubes, fatigue, and skin erythema. Serous otitis media frequently resolves spontaneously with time; however, histamine blockers or even a myringotomy may be required. Skin erythema is treated with supportive care, including water-based lotions and aloe.

Partial Brain Toxicity

Both low- and high-grade astrocytomas are frequently treated with portals that not only include the tumor itself but also a margin of 1 to 2 cm (in order to cover microscopic tumor infiltrating into normal brain) to a dose of 54 to 60 gray (Gy) (1.8 to 2.0 Gy per fraction) combined with chemotherapy and/or surgery. Partial brain irradiation is generally well tolerated, with most patients experiencing no severe toxicity; however, mild toxicities occur, including skin erythema (34%), otitis (5%), vomiting (8%), lethargy (7%) and headache (25%).[4,5] The North Central Cancer Treatment Group (NCCTG) and Radiation Therapy Oncology Group (RTOG) prospectively compared two different doses of postoperative radiation therapy, 50.4 Gy versus 64.8 Gy for the treatment of low-grade gliomas. Interestingly, there was no difference in acute toxicities between the treatment arms. However, late toxicity, as discussed subsequently, was significantly higher for the patients receiving the higher dose.[6]

Whole Brain Toxicity

Whole brain radiotherapy (WBRT) using two lateral opposed fields is commonly used as a palliative regimen for patients with brain metastases to alleviate symptoms such as headaches. Since the life expectancy of these patients is short, WBRT is given in larger fractions over a shorter time period than treatment schedules employed for primary central nervous system (CNS) tumors. A standard WBRT schedule is 30 Gy in 10 fractions (ie, each fraction is 300 cGy). In contrast to partial brain irradiation, all patients treated with WBRT experience complete alopecia and skin erythema. Typically, the alopecia resolves over a period of several months, although pretreatment hair density is seldom recovered. Since both eustachian tubes are included in WBRT fields, eustachian tube dysfunction is also common.

When the dose per fraction of WBRT is escalated, severe acute complications can occur. For example, half of the patients treated with a whole brain radiation dose of 15 Gy given in 2 fractions over 3 days experienced symptoms ranging from severe headaches to pyrexia and cerebral herniation.[3,6,7] A single dose of 10 Gy to the whole brain has been reported to cause severe toxicity including death.[8]

Stereotactic radiosurgery uses multiple noncoplanar small beams that intersect within the target to produce highly conformal dose distributions while reducing the dose to normal tissues. Stereotactic radiosurgery can either be given as primary treatment or as a boost in addition to fractionated therapy. Single fraction stereotactic radiosurgery was studied in patients previously treated with external beam radiotherapy for either solitary brain tumors or metastasis. The incidence of severe acute toxicities was related not only to the prescribed dose but also tumor size. Patients with a tumor diameter of 31 to 40 mm had severe acute toxicities in up to 17% of cases at a dose of 18 Gy, while those with smaller tumor diameters, less than 20 mm, had no severe acute toxicities at 24 Gy.[5,8,9] The RTOG randomized 333 patients with 1–3 brain metastases between WBRT alone

or combination with stereotactic radiosurgery. In the group treated with WBRT and stereotactic radiosurgery, most toxicities were mild (43%) or moderate (18%) with only one severe toxicity. Patients receiving WBRT alone had similar toxicities although no severe toxicities were noted.[10] Stereotactic radiosurgery can be used safely in combination with WBRT provided appropriate doses are used.

Subacute Toxicity

Subacute toxicity presents a few weeks to a few months after completion of radiation therapy. Symptoms include fatigue, decreased concentration, and exacerbation of presenting signs and symptoms of the tumor itself. Subacute effects of radiation are indistinguishable from tumor progression on imaging studies; however, the radiation effects resolve on subsequent scans.[11]

Somnolence syndrome is most frequently reported in the pediatric population and represents a constellation of one or more effects, such as fatigue, anorexia, headache, nausea and vomiting, irritability, fever, dysphagia, dysarthria, and ataxia. Up to 60% of children treated with WBRT for acute lymphoblastic leukemia have experienced this syndrome. The syndrome is typically self-limited, lasting anywhere from 2 days to 8 weeks. However, there have been reports of fatality from subacute radiation toxicity. Findings at autopsy revealed gliosis, necrosis, and diminished numbers of oligodendroglial cells. Neurons and axons are preserved.[12] The etiology of somnolence syndrome is thought to be related to either demyelination or vascular damage. Interestingly, the likelihood of patients experiencing somnolence syndrome does not appear to be dose-related.[13] Prophylactic steroids appear to decrease the likelihood of somnolence syndrome. Thirty-two acute lymphoblastic leukemia pediatric patients treated with WBRT (18 Gy in 9 fractions) were randomized between two prophylactic doses of dexamethasone. Patients receiving 2 mg and 4 mg of dexamethasone during radiation therapy had 64% and 17.6% incidences of somnolence syndrome, respectively.[14]

Late Toxicity

Late radiation toxicity manifests several months to years after the completion of treatment. The probability of severe complications increases with dose and the volume of brain irradiated. The $TD_{5/5}$ of normal brain is 50 Gy if two-thirds of the brain is irradiated, and 60 Gy if one-third of the brain is irradiated.[15] Complications also increase if radiation is given concurrently with chemotherapy.[15,16] The principal late effects include radiation necrosis, white matter injury, brain atrophy, and vascular injury.

Most cases of severe radiation necrosis occur when small volumes of brain are taken to high

doses, either with stereotactic or partial brain techniques. Focal radiation necrosis is usually confined to the volume receiving high doses of radiation. Computed tomography reveals low-density white matter changes with irregular enhancement, associated with surrounding edema and various degrees of mass effect. These changes are difficult to differentiate from tumor progression or from tumor-associated necrosis (Figure 1A, 1B).[17] MRI demonstrates increased gadolinium uptake with necrosis with increased perilesional signal abnormality on T2 and FLAIR sequences. The abnormal signal intensity is usually periventricular but it can extend out to the cortex.[18] Positron emission tomography (PET) and single photon emission computed tomography (SPECT) can sometimes distinguish between metastatic brain tumor and glioma recurrences versus radiation necrosis.[19–21]

Pathologically, radiation necrosis may be described as yellow-brown with a waxy appearance on gross examination. Coagulation and fibrinoid necrosis with edema and dystrophic calcium deposits are seen histologically. Plaques of demyelination in the white matter and ischemic infarction are often noted. Radiation-induced infarcts demonstrate irregular reactive astrocytes, glitter cell accumulation, gliosis and vascular granulations. Blood vessel occlusion from medial fibrosis and organized thrombi are causes of cerebral infarction and necrosis. Ganglion cells are generally well preserved. (Figures 1C to 1E).[22]

Clinically, radiation necrosis causes symptoms related to mass effect and increased intracranial pressure, such as headache, ataxia, and nausea. Seizures and focal deficits, such as hemiparesis, hemisensory loss, and aphasia, are also seen. Treatment includes the use of high doses of corticosteroids, and surgery may be necessary to evacuate the necrotic mass. Surgical decompression can shorten the time the patient requires steroids and therefore lessens the side effects associated with long-term corticosteroid use.[23] Radiation necrosis is most commonly seen following stereotactic radiosurgery or when partial brain doses are above 60 Gy. Shaw and colleagues noted an incidence of radionecrosis of 5% and 11% at 6 and 24 months, respectively, in patients treated with radiosurgery following previous external beam radiation.[24] Of the 16 patients with radionecrosis, 15 required operation. In low-grade glioma patients randomized to 50.4 Gy versus 64.8 Gy external beam radiation, the two-year actuarial incidence of severe radiation necrosis was 2.5% and 5%, respectively.[25]

White matter injury is the most common late radiation injury and typically extends beyond the high-dose volume of irradiation. Magnetic resonance imaging (MRI) studies have found that 50% of patients show a significant alteration in

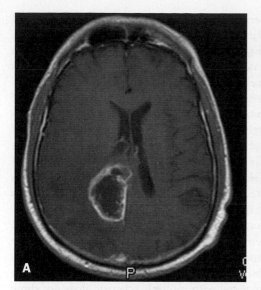

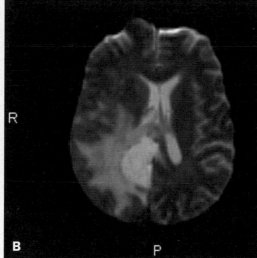

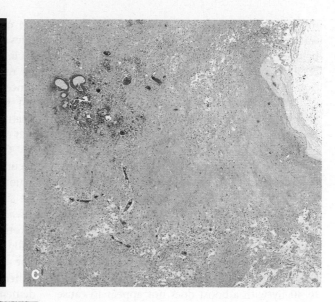

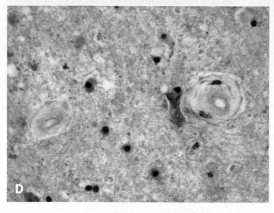

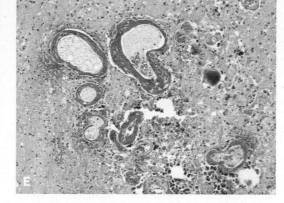

FIGURE 1 Computed tomography reveals low-density white matter changes with irregular enhancement, associated with surrounding edema and various degrees of mass effect (A, B). Blood vessel occlusion from medial fibrosis and organized thrombi are causes of cerebral infarction and necrosis. Ganglion cells are generally well preserved (C, D, E).

white matter signaling. High-grade lesions are associated with radiation to large volumes and higher doses, and, therefore, have a greater likelihood of white matter injury. The frequency of white matter changes is very high. In one series, 100% of 33 patients treated with conventional radiation to a median dose of 54 Gy in 1.8 Gy fractions for primary brain tumors expressed white matter changes on MRI 6 to 25 years after treatment. Patients with confluent white matter changes reported significant physical, cognitive and social impairment. The addition of chemotherapy increased the severity of white matter injury. However, not all severe white matter changes are clinically expressed.[26,27] Pathology reveals white matter pallor and reactive astrocytosis. Clinically, symptoms range from mild fatigue and personality changes, to dementia. Intellectual impairment and learning disabilities are most commonly seen in children.[28]

Leukoencephalopathy is a syndrome characterized by white matter changes associated with the symptoms of lassitude, dysarthria, cognitive dysfunction, and seizures. More severe CNS damage manifests as ataxia, confusion, memory loss, dementia, and death. This syndrome usually appears within 4 years after completion of radiation therapy. It was first described in children with acute lymphatic leukemia (ALL) who were

treated after radiation with intrathecal methotrexate. The syndrome is now also recognized in adults. Imaging reveals white matter injury initially near the ventricles with progression to the entire cerebral white matter. MRI demonstrates an increase in T2 signal throughout the white matter. Calcifications may be scattered or confluent.[29] The clinical course is slowly progressive; however, stabilization has been described.[30]

One of the most widely recognized long-term complication of CNS radiation is a deterioration of cognitive function; however, other therapies, including medication, chemotherapy, surgery, and comorbid illnesses, as well as the tumor itself, contribute to the decline of intellectual ability. Isolating and quantifying the role of radiation therapy in cognitive decline has been extremely difficult.

Many retrospective studies examining the impact of radiation on cognitive dysfunction were methodologically flawed in that no pretreatment baseline cognitive testing was performed. Typically these studies compared neurocognitive function in long-term survivors of brain tumors treated with radiation therapy or surgery alone. Cognitive impairment has been reported in patients receiving high-dose radiation therapy for low- and high-grade gliomas, and from lower-dose radiation therapy such as prophylactic

cranial irradiation for lung cancer, as well as radiation for the pediatric malignancies.[31,32] In a study of surgically treated, low-grade glioma patients, 28 patients who received radiation and 23 treated with surgery alone were alive and eligible for neuropsychological testing. The group receiving postoperative radiation therapy demonstrated significantly decreased neuropsychological performance compared with the cohort treated with surgery alone. However, 19 of the 28 patients treated with radiation therapy received whole brain radiation to a dose of 40 Gy followed by a boost of 20 to 28 Gy. This study strongly suggests that whole brain radiation therapy to a dose of 40 Gy followed by a boost leads to significant neurocognitive impairment.[33] However, in current practice, whole brain irradiation to a dose of 40 Gy is rarely used, and patients are now treated with focal irradiation. Another study compared the neurocognitive outcomes of patients with low-grade glioma, about half of whom were treated with radiation therapy (90% with focal radiation) and half with surgery only, to patients with low-grade non-Hodgkin's lymphoma/chronic lymphocytic leukemia patients and healthy controls. Low-grade glioma patients had a decreased ability in all neurocognitive domains compared to low-grade hematologic patients or healthy controls. The authors concluded that the tumor itself, and not the radiation therapy, was felt to have the most deleterious affects on neurocognitive outcome, although radiotherapy resulted in some long-term memory deterioration.[28,29,34]

Komaki and colleagues prospectively evaluated the cognitive function of patients receiving prophylactic cranial irradiation (PCI) (total dose of 25 Gy in 10 fractions over 2 weeks). Prior to PCI administration, 29 out of the 30 patients had preexisting cognitive dysfunction. Almost all the cognitive dysfunction was due to disease, as opposed to other factors, such as substance abuse or previous history of neurologic disease. Neuropsychological testing 6 to 20 months later showed no significant differences from the pretreatment state.[35] Thus, WBRT at a dose of 25 Gy as opposed to 40 Gy with a boost does not appear to cause any significant decline in cognition. Neurocognitive function was also determined in patients with non-small cell lung carcinoma treated with PCI (30 Gy in 15 fractions over 3 weeks). Impairments of attention and visual memory in both those treated with PCI and in the control group were noted, but there were no significant differences in neurocognitive functioning between the two treatment groups. However, MRI imaging revealed white matter abnormalities of higher grades in those receiving PCI.[36] Although it is extremely difficult to dissect the role of radiation therapy in the production of neurocognitive deterioration, the bulk of the evidence suggests that the whole brain can tolerate between 25 and 30 Gy without significant impairment. However, when the whole brain receives an excess of 30 Gy, the risk of neurocognitive dysfunction increases dramatically. The principal reason for neurologic deterioration in most cases is the tumor itself. When fraction sizes exceed 2 Gy, the risk of radiation-induced neurocognitive deterioration increases.

In addition to dose and fraction size, age is also a predictive factor for neurocognitive dysfunction. Pediatric cases are often treated with lower-dose irradiation in comparison to adults in the hope of reducing long-term sequela, including cognitive effects. Ris and colleagues reported the intellectual outcome in 43 pediatric patients treated with craniospinal radiation therapy with adjuvant chemotherapy for medulloblastoma. Diminished functioning from baseline was found in verbal IQ, nonverbal IQ and full-scale IQ. Young children were more negatively affected, and patients with higher baseline functioning suffered sharper declines than those with lower baseline scores.[37]

Other causes of neurocognitive decline, including paraneoplastic disorders, endocrine dysfunction, nutritional deficits, medication, depression, and cancer, per se, should be addressed. Improved radiation techniques and the use of smaller treatment fields suggest the role of RT in contributing to neurocognitive decline is small. Although there is no treatment for radiation-induced cognitive dysfunction, the concerns of late neurocognitive dysfunction are not a strong reason for omitting RT for the treatment plan in cases in where there is evidence that radiation therapy has been beneficial.[38]

Cerebrovascular effects of radiation therapy occur frequently after treatment to the parasellar region. Pathologic changes after radiation therapy are similar to severe atherosclerosis. Moyamoya disease results from occlusion of the internal carotid artery typically affecting the anterior and middle cerebral branches of the circle of Willis. The disease presents with multiple and diffuse ischemic or hemorrhagic vascular insults causing dementia or death, which can occur years after irradiation. Patient factors such as underlying comorbid disease (including neurofibromatosis), surgery, and tumor encasement of vessels also impact the development of vasculopathy.[39,40] Angiograms show a characteristic "puff of smoke" or blush at the base of the brain from the collateral blood vessel formation.[41]

Spinal Cord

Radiation myelopathy is a dreaded but rare complication following radiation treatment for either primary spinal cord malignancy, spinal cord metastasis, or after definitive treatment for a thoracic, head and neck, or upper abdominal malignancy. Myelopathy may involve the white or grey matter and typically results in a chronic progressive course.[42] Clinically, spinal cord myelopathy occurs in a subacute (early delayed) or late fashion with either sensory or motor symptoms. Fractionated radiation therapy has a $TD_{5/5}$ for spinal myelopathy of 57 to 60 Gy and a $TD_{5/50}$ of 68 to 73 Gy.[43] The spinal cord is rarely treated beyond a conservative dose of 50 Gy to limit the frequency of spinal cord injury. Neurotoxic chemotherapy agents such as methotrexate, cisplatin, cytarabine, taxanes, and vinblastine may reduce the tolerance of the spinal cord to radiation. Intrathecal chemotherapy during radiation therapy is contraindicated because of the overlapping spinal cord toxicity.[44]

Early Spinal Cord Toxicity

Subacute myelopathy is marked by sensory changes, including paresthesias. The latency period for subacute myelopathy is 1 to 6 months and symptoms gradually improve without specific treatment over 2 to 9 months. Lhermitte's sign is described as an electrical shock with flexion of the neck. It is thought that the flexion of the neck elongates the spinal cord, and this tension results in the clinical symptoms. Only with a long latency period does the appearance of Lhermitte's sign foretell of permanent spinal cord injury.[12] From a cohort of 1,112 patients with malignancies of the upper respiratory system treated with radiation therapy, 40 patients (3.6%) developed Lhermitte's sign with a mean time of development of 3 months and duration of 6 months. No patient progressed to transverse myelitis. An increased risk for the development of Lhermitte's sign in patients receiving more than 2 Gy per fraction (one fraction per day) or a total of more than 50 Gy to the spinal cord has been noted.[45] Pathologically, early radiation injury to the spinal cord results in focal areas of demyelination, fibrinoid necrosis of blood vessels, and edema.[22] Positron emission tomography may demonstrate increased activity. MRI, although sensitive enough to diagnose demyelination associated with multiple sclerosis, does not show any pathologic change in patients with transient or chronic Lhermitte's sign. Recovery from spinal injury has been associated with an increase in PET signaling.[42,46]

Late Spinal Cord Toxicity

Late radiation injury to the spinal cord generally occurs months to years after treatment. The median latency period is 20 months with 75% of cases occurring within 30 months of treatment. The latency period is dose-dependent, with shorter periods for patients receiving higher doses. Children have shorter latency periods than adults. Patients undergoing repeat radiation therapy to the same segment of spinal cord are at particularly high risk of damage and have a mean latency period of only 5 months.[12]

Signs and symptoms of myelitis may be insidious or acute onset, with functional deficits ranging from paresthesias to severe sensory and motor changes, urine and bowel incontinence, and paresis. Brown-Séquard syndrome, which consists of motor weakness and pyramidal tract signs on one side with a decrease in temperature and pain sensations on the contralateral side, can precede a complete myelopathy. On the other hand, some patients present with both extremities equally affected. Radiation-induced cord changes are generally irreversible, and many die from secondary complications.[12]

Delayed late radiation myelopathy is a result of demyelination and axonal loss of the sensory and motor tracts. Pathology reveals white matter, tumor-like masses of cord necrosis with spongiform degeneration and vascular lesions leading to telangiectasia, fibrinoid necrosis, edema, focal hemorrhage, and hemorrhagic necrosis. Neurons are usually spared. Calcifications may be present in older lesions, and, with time, the cord may contract. The etiology of radiation injury is multifactorial. Vascular damage with resultant infarction, parenchymal radiation injury (including damage to oligodendrocytes and astrocytes), as well as damage to the spinal cord–blood barrier all contribute to the pathogenesis of spinal cord myelitis.[22]

Radiographic imaging of eight patients, treated to an accidental mean dose of 136 Gy and who developed late spinal myelopathy, revealed a high-intensity signal on T2-weighted MRI images as well as gadolinium enhancement on T1-weighted MRI images.[46] However, some patients with myelopathy have no abnormality on MRI.[47] Myelography is often normal, but there may be expansion or attenuation at the level of irradiation. Cerebral spinal fluid evaluation may reveal a mildly elevated protein, but most often is normal without the presence of abnormal cells.[12] Myelin basic protein levels are increased.[48]

In order to qualify for a diagnosis of radiation myelopathy, several criteria must be met: (1) history of prior radiation treatment at or above the level of deficit; (2) the radiation dose must be high enough to cause the deficit; (3) the latency period must be appropriate; (4) other potential etiologies, such as tumor metastasis and cord compression, or a paraneoplastic syndrome, must be excluded.[12]

There is no effective treatment for radiation-induced myelopathy. Prevention, therefore, is critical. Steroids have been used to slow progression and anticoagulation in those with radionecrosis, in order to reverse radiation-induced small-vessel endothelial injury, and have led to clinical improvement in some patients.[49] If neurologic decline is due to hemorrhage into the spinal cord, the patient may recover slowly and future avoidance of nonsteroidal anti-inflammatory drugs and anticoagulants is prudent.[3]

Cranial Nerves

Cranial neuropathies from radiation therapy are rare since tolerance of the cranial nerves is higher than that of the brain or spinal cord. Injury to cranial nerves is typically expressed 1 to 20 years post-radiation, and recurrent malignancy must be ruled out. Myokymic discharges can be seen on EMG due to hyper-excitability of demyelinated axons.[50,51] Most reported cases have been associated with stereotactic as opposed to external beam radiotherapy. The most common tumor site treated with external beam in which cranial nerve damage has been observed is carcinoma of the nasopharynx, where a 1 to 5% incidence of cranial nerve palsy has been noted.[52] The etiology of cranial neuropathy is thought to be due to either fibrotic encasement, vasculitis, or direct radiation damage.[53]

Radiation-induced olfactory nerve dysfunction is difficult to diagnose because of its close ties to the function of taste, which is often altered during and after radiation therapy. Patients sometimes report a pungent smell which may be due to stimulation of the olfactory receptors by the free radicals and ozone formed in the nasal mucosa during therapy.[54] Patients also report a transient decreased ability to smell when radiation fields include the olfactory nerves.[55,56]

Radiation can affect visual function through multiple mechanisms, including production of dry eye syndrome, cataract formation, glaucoma, retinopathy, or by directly damaging the optic nerve.[57] Damage to the lacrimal gland from doses of 40 to 50 Gy, which are commonly used in treatment of head and neck carcinomas, may result in a dry eye leading to corneal opacification, ulceration, and, ultimately, in loss of vision. Dry eye syndrome has a latency period of 6 to 10 months.[12] Occasionally, enucleation is necessary to alleviate the pain produced by dry eye syndrome. Cataract formation can occur with doses of fractionated radiation as low as 5 Gy and has a latency period of up to 3 years.[58] Retinopathy is seen after 45 to 50 Gy and is expressed 1.5 to 3 years after high-dose radiation therapy. The clinical characteristics are strikingly similar to diabetic retinopathy, with occlusion of small vessels, neovascularization, hemorrhage, retinal ischemia, cotton wool spots, and retinal arterial narrowing.[59] Secondary angle closure glaucoma may result from neovascularization.[12] During radiation therapy some patients complain of seeing visual lights, which is completely benign. Optic neuropathy is thought to be caused by microangiopathy, which may lead to complete visual loss. In order to make a diagnosis of optic neuropathy, the following criteria must be met: (1) irreversible visual loss with visual field defects; (2) absence of visual pathway compression due to recurrence or progression of tumor, radiation-induced neoplasm, arachnoidal adhesions around the chiasm, radiation retinopathy or any other obvious cause; (3) absence of optic disc edema; and (4) optic nerve atrophy must coincide temporally with the onset of visual loss.[60-62] Radiation-induced optic neuropathy is characterized by bilateral or monocular painless blindness and diplopia. MRI reveals enhancement of the optic nerve, and, pathologically, the nerve show demyelination and gliosis.[3,58]

There is no specific treatment for optic neuropathy, although steroids, anti-coagulants and hyperbaric oxygen have been tried.[63] Prevention of radiation damage by decreasing dose to the eye whenever possible can reduce the likelihood of visual loss. However, for tumors such as pituitary adenomas, optic gliomas, and ocular lymphomas, complete shielding of the involved optic structures may not be possible.

Oculomotor, abducens, or trochlear nerve palsies usually present with a prior history of radiation to the sella turcica or parasellar region, and patients complain of intermittent diplopia or blurred vision. Neuromyotonia, characterized by spontaneous spasm of eye muscles secondary to spontaneous discharges of the ocular nerves has been described.[64] Demyelination is thought to be the etiology of radiation neuropathy, and there is no treatment; however, in the case of neuro-myotonia, membrane-stabilizing agents such as carbamazepine have been used with success.[65].

Trigeminal nerve palsy occurs in 15 to 29% of patients treated with radiosurgery for acoustic neuroma, with a median onset of 5 months.[66] Symptoms include facial nerve pain progressing to numbness, which differentiates this syndrome from trigeminal neuralgia. Atrophy of the muscles of mastication may occur. Tumor recurrence involving the trigeminal nerve must be ruled out. Full or partial spontaneous improvement is seen in approximately one-half of patients.[67]

Facial nerve palsy is rarely seen with external beam but it does occur following radiosurgical procedures for acoustic neuroma cases, where incidences vary from 17 to 67%.[68] Facial nerve palsy has a median onset of 6 months, and approximately one-half of patients have spontaneous partial or full recovery.[69].

Taste is also a function of the seventh cranial nerve, through the chorda tympani nerve, and is frequently affected during the treatment of head and neck carcinomas with external beam radiation. Cancer patients often have some alteration in taste before the initiation of treatment, due either to general malnutrition or vitamin deficiency. Patients begin to notice a loss of taste after two weeks of radiation therapy and one-half to two-thirds of patients have partial to complete taste loss 2 months after completion of radiation therapy. At 12 to 24 months, most have partial recovery. Xerostomia and mucositis can contribute to perceived loss of taste. The perception of sweet had the fastest recovery, with sour having the slowest rate of recovery. After 12 to 24 months, bitter and salt were still the qualities most impaired. The $TD_{5/50}$ for loss of taste is in the 50 to 60 Gy range.[70,71]

Radiation-induced acute hearing loss from external beam treatments is usually from a serous effusion which resolves spontaneously. Late acoustic nerve palsy is difficult to diagnose because it can also be due to normal aging, trauma to the eustachian tube, or tympanic membrane perforation.[72] Kwong and colleagues reported on sensorineural hearing loss in 132 patients treated for nasopharyngeal carcinoma with irradiation and cisplatin. Twenty-two percent had evidence of hearing loss, with higher frequencies affected the most; however, it is unclear how much was due to the cisplatin.[73] Late acoustic nerve damage has been reported in 33 patients treated for supratentorial brain tumors. Seventy-seven percent of patients treated for vestibular schwannomas with radiosurgery have hearing preservation. Significantly reduced sensorineural hearing loss was found for all frequencies tested in both air (28 of 33 patients) and bone conduction (15 of 33 patients). Patients treated to less than 54 Gy did not have severe hearing loss. Vestibular function was also reduced in three patients, with two patients having symptoms of balance disturbances.[74]

The remaining cranial nerves (glossopharyngeal, vagus, spinal accessory, and hypoglossal) all course through the neck and are all potentially susceptible to encasement by radiation fibrosis after treatment for head and neck cancer, which can lead to dysfunction.[75] Radiosurgery of acoustic neuromas or vestibular schwannomas can result in damage to the nerves depending on the volume of the lesion and the dose prescribed. Patients with dysfunction of the ninth and tenth cranial nerves complain of dysphagia, dysphonia and, in severe cases, dyspnea due to abnormal glottic closure. Xerostomia can also contribute to dysphagia, and a trial of pilocarpine may prove beneficial.[76] Although xerostomia affects the perception of poor swallowing, it does not alter the physiologic aspects of bolus transport.[77] Axonal degeneration from microvascular damage and direct Schwann cell injury have also been implicated in the damage of nervous tissue from radiation therapy.[78] Treatment includes supportive care and palliative procedures such as gastrostomy tubes for dysphagia, and a laryngoplasty or tracheostomy to relieve hoarseness of voice or dyspnea, and reduce the risk of aspiration.

Peripheral Nerves

When peripheral nerves are damaged by radiation, symptoms include pain, paresthesias, and, rarely, weakness. Of all peripheral nerves the brachial and lumbosacral plexi are the most frequently damaged. The etiology is largely speculative; however, demyelination of axon fibers, fibrosis, and nerve ischemia from radiation-induced vasculature damage have been hypothesized.

Brachial plexopathy is seen in 1.8 to 5% of patients treated for breast, lung, lymphoma, and other tumors involving the upper extremity. Latency periods range from 1 month to 18 years.[79] Radiation doses higher than 50 Gy, the use of chemotherapy, and extensive axillary node dissection are predisposing factors.[80] Before attributing the damage to radiation, other causes must be ruled out, such as tumor recurrence, vasculopathy with subclavian occlusion, or surgical structural damage. EMG studies show abnormal motor and sensory nerve conduction with myokymic discharges, which are helpful in distinguishing radiation-induced plexopathy from paraneoplastic causes.[81] Clinically, radiation neuropathies present as paresthesias but may progress to weakness and sensory loss to full paresis. Although pain may be a prominent

feature; the severity is usually less in radiation plexopathy compared with neoplastic plexopathy. MRI may reveal either increased or decreased T2 signal with a decreased T1 signal.[82] If radiation-induced fibrosis is the basis of nerve damage, enhancement with gadolinium is seen. Therapeutic options for radiation-induced plexopathies are limited. No treatment exists that will restore full function. Surgery with neurolysis, grafting of the latissimus dorsi or omentoplasty may be of some benefit. Hyperbaric oxygen, which has been successful in the treatment of osteoradionecrosis and hemorrhagic cystitis, is not useful.[83]

Lumbosacral plexopathy presents with lower extremity weakness and sensory loss, which may remain stable for years or professes to paralysis. Often, foot drop is the first presenting symptom. EMG reveals myokymic discharges, suggesting radiation damage instead of tumor recurrence. The etiology of lumbosacral plexopathy is thought to be similar to brachial plexopathy. Like brachial plexopathy, the latency period for lumbosacral plexopathy is long.[84,85] Lumbosacral plexopathy is most commonly seen in patients treated for endometrial, bladder, and other pelvic tumors, including rectal carcinoma.[86,87] As with brachial plexopathy, it is essential to exclude tumor recurrence before attributing the damage to radiation. Post-radiation therapy lumbosacral polyradiculopathy can also demonstrate nodular and leptomeningeal enhancement of the cauda equina and conus medullaris on MRI.[88]

Clinically, lumbosacral plexopathy is commonly bilateral, and the pain is milder in comparison to tumor-associated plexopathy. Incontinence is not typically a feature of radiation-induced plexopathy.[89] No effective treatment exists; however, supportive care with pain management and occupational/physical therapy are helpful to improve quality of life.[90].

Second Malignancies

One of the most serious late complications of radiation therapy is the induction of a secondary malignancy. Radiation-induced tumors include benign and malignant processes including meningiomas, schwannomas, sarcomas, and gliomas. Typically radiation-induced lesions are high-grade and have an aggressive natural history.[91]

Criteria to support a diagnosis of a radiation-induced tumor include: (1) the tumor must have a different histology than the original tumor; (2) the tumor must develop within/adjacent to the radiation field; (3) a minimum period of several years must have elapsed since the radiation was received; and (4) the patient must not suffer from underlying genetic disease that favors the development of tumors, such as von Recklinghausen's disease or Li-Fraumeni syndrome. Confirmation of the presumed diagnosis must always be made

by biopsy.[92] Fortunately, radiation-induced CNS neoplasms are rare, with 34 cases of sarcomas and 312 cases of meningiomas reported as of 1995. The overall relative risk of developing a second neoplasm is 1 to 3% with a latency of 15 to 30 years.[93,94] Factors that may increase the risk of a secondary malignancy include the use of chemotherapy, young age, and genetic predisposition. Secondary tumors may arise from both low- and high-dose radiation therapy.[3,77,95,96] Radiation-induced tumors of the peripheral nervous system have also been described.[76,79,97–100]

Endocrine Dysfunction

Loss of endocrine function is common when radiation therapy is delivered to the base of skull, pharynx, or directly to the hypothalamus-pituitary axis. In general, the hypothalamus is more sensitive than the anterior pituitary. Posterior pituitary dysfunction has not been reported.[101] The time to develop an endocrine abnormality can vary from a few months to 10 or more years following radiation therapy.[102]

The different hypothalamic-pituitary axes respond to irradiation with varying degrees of sensitivity. The growth hormone axis is the most sensitive, while the prolactin axis is the least sensitive. Growth hormone deficiency after irradiation has been reported after doses as low as 12 to 24 Gy. Abnormalities of growth can be subtle and may only manifest at puberty. In children, a high index of suspicion is prudent, and it is advisable to test for growth hormone (GH) deficiency every 6 months after therapy. To diagnose GH deficiency in children treated with spinal irradiation, it is necessary to measure growth velocity of long bones such as the femur, which is outside of the radiation field. When a decrease in growth rate is noted, growth hormone deficiency cannot be assumed. Further testing is necessary to rule out competing diagnoses, such as thyroid disease and malnutrition, before more definitive growth hormone testing is pursued.[103][81] Recombinant human growth hormone can restore the normal velocity of growth in children; however, catch-up growth may not occur.[104] Adults do not often have clinical symptoms from growth hormone deficiency, although a decrease in lean muscle mass can be seen.[105] Growth hormone replacement in adults after radiation therapy, therefore, remains controversial.[106,107]

After doses of 50 Gy to the hypothalamic-pituitary axis, 29 to 35% will have gonadotropin deficiency. Gonadotropin dysfunction may lead to precocious puberty in children.[24,108,109] Adults may experience infertility, abnormal menses, and decreased libido. The diagnosis of gonadotropin deficiency is based on elevated serum LH and FSH levels. A gonadotropin releasing hormone test may also be of use. Females with complete gonadotropin deficiency require estrogen and progestin replacement, while those with a partial deficiency need periodic progestin administration to induce menses. Males require androgen replacement.

TSH deficiency leading to hypothyroidism presents with lethargy, weight gain, cold sensitivity and other signs of decreased thyroxin. Children may also demonstrate a decreased growth rate. Data are limited as to a threshold dose. Pediatric series report an incidence of 3 to 6% after doses of 40 to 50 Gy to the hypothalamic-pituitary axis. In adults, the incidence is 60 to 65% after doses of 50 to 57 Gy.[110,111] Treatment consists of thyroxin replacement and monitoring of therapy with serum TSH, T4, and T3 levels.

Symptoms of adrenocorticotropic hormone (ACTH) deficiency include lethargy, fasting hypoglycemia and dilutional hyponatremia. Incidences range from 19 to 35% after a dose of more than 50 Gy to the HPA axis and latency time varies from 5 to 15 years.[112,113] Random cortisol levels below 18 μg/dL suggest the diagnosis and further testing can be pursed with an insulin hypoglycemic challenge and metyrapone. Treatment consists of replacement with hydrocortisone.[114]

Prolactin is controlled by the hypothalamic neurotransmitter dopamine. When the hypothalamus is damaged, the inhibitory effects of dopamine on prolactin are released and hyperprolactinemia results. Prolactin functions to initiate lactation and regulate cyclic ovulation in the female.[115] Hyperprolactinemia is seen after doses of 50 Gy to the HPA axis, with an incidence of 50%, and results in menstrual irregularity, galactorrhea, and infertility in the female. Treatment consists of dopamine agonists such as bromocriptine, which will reduce prolactin levels.[116]

REFERENCES

1. Perez CA, BL,HE, Principles and practice of radiation oncology. Philadelphia: Lippincott Williams and Wilkins; 2004.
2. Li YQ, Chen P, Jain V, et al. Early radiation-induced endothelial cell loss and blood-spinal cord barrier breakdown in the rat spinal cord. Radiat Res 2004;161:143–52.
3. Posner J. Neurologic complications of cancer. Philadelphia: F. A. Davis Co.; 1995.
4. Karim AB, Afra D, Cornu P, et al. Randomized trial on the efficacy of radiotherapy for cerebral low-grade glioma in the adult: European Organization for Research and Treatment of Cancer Study 22845 with the Medical Research Council study BRO4: an interim analysis. Int J Radiat Oncol Biol Phys 2002;52:316–24.
5. Shaw E, Arusell R, Scheithauer B, et al. Prospective randomized trial of low- versus high-dose radiation therapy in adults with supratentorial low-grade glioma: initial report of a North Central Cancer Treatment Group/Radiation Therapy Oncology Group/Eastern Cooperative Oncology Group study. J Clin Oncol 2002;20:2267–76.
6. Shaw E, Arusell R, Scheithauer B, et al. Prospective randomized trial of low- versus high-dose radiation therapy in adults with supratentorial low-grade glioma: initial report of a North Central Cancer Treatment Group/Radiation Therapy Oncology Group/Eastern Cooperative Oncology Group study. J Clin Oncol 2002;20:2267–76.
7. Young DF, Posner JB, Chu F, Nisce L. Rapid-course radiation therapy of cerebral metastases: results and complications. Cancer 1974;34:1069–76.
8. Hindo WA, DeTrana FA III, Lee MS, Hendrickson FR. Large dose increment irradiation in treatment of cerebral metastases. Cancer 1970;26:138–41.
9. Shaw E, Scott C, Souhami L, et al. Single dose radiosurgical treatment of recurrent previously irradiated primary brain tumors and brain metastases: final report of RTOG protocol 90–05. Int J Radiat Oncol Biol Phys 2000;47:291–8.
10. Andrews DW, Scott CB, Sperduto PW, et al. Whole brain radiation therapy with or without stereotactic radiosurgery boost for patients with one to three brain metastases: phase III results of the RTOG 9508 randomised trial. Lancet 2004;363:1665–72.
11. Graeb DA, Steinbok P, Robertson WD. Transient early computed tomographic changes mimicking tumor progression after brain tumor irradiation. Radiology 1982;144:813–7.
12. Gutin PH LSSG. Radiation injury to the nervous system. New York: Raven Press; 1991.
13. Littman P, Rosenstock J, Gale G, et al. The somnolence syndrome in leukemic children following reduced daily dose fractions of cranial radiation. Int J Radiat Oncol Biol Phys 1984;10:1851–3.
14. Uzal D, Ozyar E, Hayran M, et al. Reduced incidence of the somnolence syndrome after prophylactic cranial irradiation in children with acute lymphoblastic leukemia. Radiother Oncol 1998;48:29–32.
15. Emami B, Lyman J, Brown A, et al. Tolerance of normal tissue to therapeutic irradiation. Int J Radiat Oncol Biol Phys 1991;21:109–22.
16. Johannesen TB, Lien HH, Hole KH, Lote K. Radiological and clinical assessment of long-term brain tumour survivors after radiotherapy. Radiother Oncol 2003;69:169–76.
17. Schultheiss TE, Kun LE, Ang KK, Stephens LC. Radiation response of the central nervous system. Int J Radiat Oncol Biol Phys 1995;31:1093–112.
18. Giglio P, Gilbert MR. Cerebral radiation necrosis. Neurologist 2003;9:180–8.
19. Tsuyuguchi N, Sunada I, Iwai Y, et al. Methionine positron emission tomography of recurrent metastatic brain tumor and radiation necrosis after stereotactic radiosurgery: is a differential diagnosis possible? J Neurosurg 2003;98:1056–64.
20. Henze M, Mohammed A, Schlemmer HP, et al. PET and SPECT for detection of tumor progression in irradiated low-grade astrocytoma: a receiver-operating-characteristic analysis. J Nucl Med 2004;45:579–86.
21. Benard F, Romsa J, Hustinx R. Imaging gliomas with positron emission tomography and single-photon emission computed tomography. Semin Nucl Med 2003;33:148–62.
22. Fajardo L BMAR. Radiation pathology. New York; 2001.
23. Schultheiss TE, Kun LE, Ang KK, Stephens LC. Radiation response of the central nervous system. Int J Radiat Oncol Biol Phys 1995;31:1093–112.
24. Shaw E, Scott C, Souhami L, et al. Single dose radiosurgical treatment of recurrent previously irradiated primary brain tumors and brain metastases: final report of RTOG protocol 90–05. Int J Radiat Oncol Biol Phys 2000;47:291–8.
25. Shaw E, Arusell R, Scheithauer B, et al. Prospective randomized trial of low- versus high-dose radiation therapy in adults with supratentorial low-grade glioma: initial report of a North Central Cancer Treatment Group/Radiation Therapy Oncology Group/Eastern Cooperative Oncology Group study. J Clin Oncol 2002;20(9):2267–2276.
26. Johannesen TB, Lien HH, Hole KH, Lote K. Radiological and clinical assessment of long-term brain tumour survivors after radiotherapy. Radiother Oncol 2003;69:169–76.
27. Constine LS, Konski A, Ekholm S, et al. Adverse effects of brain irradiation correlated with MR and CT imaging. Int J Radiat Oncol Biol Phys 1988;15:319–30.
28. Schultheiss TE, Kun LE, Ang KK, Stephens LC. Radiation response of the central nervous system. Int J Radiat Oncol Biol Phys 1995;31:1093–112.
29. Schultheiss TE, Kun LE, Ang KK, Stephens LC. Radiation response of the central nervous system. Int J Radiat Oncol Biol Phys 1995;31:1093–112.
30. Keime-Guibert F, Napolitano M, Delattre JY. Neurological complications of radiotherapy and chemotherapy. J Neurol 1998;245:695–708.
31. Scheibel RS, Meyers CA, Levin VA. Cognitive dysfunction following surgery for intracerebral glioma: influence of histopathology, lesion location, and treatment. J Neurooncol 1996;30:61–9.
32. Surma-aho O, Niemela M, Vilkki J, et al. Adverse long-term effects of brain radiotherapy in adult low-grade glioma patients. Neurology 2001;56:1285–90.
33. Surma-aho O, Niemela M, Vilkki J, et al. Adverse long-term effects of brain radiotherapy in adult low-grade glioma patients. Neurology 2001;56:1285–90.
34. Klein M, Heimans JJ, Aaronson NK, et al. Effect of radiotherapy and other treatment-related factors on mid-term to long-term cognitive sequelae in low-grade gliomas: a comparative study. Lancet 2002;360:1361–68.
35. Komaki R, Meyers CA, Shin DM, et al. Evaluation of cognitive function in patients with limited small cell lung cancer prior to and shortly following prophylactic cranial irradiation. Int J Radiat Oncol Biol Phys 1995;33:179–82.
36. Stuschke M, Pottgen C. Prophylactic cranial irradiation as a component of intensified initial treatment of locally advanced non-small cell lung cancer. Lung Cancer 2003;42 (Suppl 1):53–6.
37. Ris MD, Packer R, Goldwein J, et al. Intellectual outcome after reduced-dose radiation therapy plus adjuvant chemotherapy for medulloblastoma: a Children's Cancer Group study. J Clin Oncol 2001;19:3470–6.
38. Brown PD, Buckner JC, Uhm JH, Shaw EG. The neurocognitive effects of radiation in adult low-grade glioma patients. Neuro-oncol 2003;5:161–7.
39. Rudoltz MS, Regine WF, Langston JW, et al. Multiple causes of cerebrovascular events in children with tumors of the parasellar region. J Neurooncol 1998;37:251–61.
40. Hillemanns A, Kortmann RD, Herrlinger U, et al. Recurrent delayed brain hemorrhage over years after irradiation and chemotherapy for astrocytoma. Eur Radiol 2003;13:1891–4.
41. Schultheiss TE, Kun LE, Ang KK, Stephens LC. Radiation response of the central nervous system. Int J Radiat Oncol Biol Phys 1995;31:1093–112.
42. Esik O, Csere T, Stefanits K, et al. A review on radiogenic Lhermitte's sign. Pathol Oncol Res 2003;9:115–20.
43. Rubin P. Extradural spinal cord compression by tumor. I. Experimental production and treatment trials. Radiology 1969;93:1243–8.
44. Allen JC. Complications of chemotherapy in patients with brain and spinal cord tumors. Pediatr Neurosurg 1991;17:218–24.
45. Fein DA, Marcus RB Jr, Parsons JT, et al. Lhermitte's sign: incidence and treatment variables influencing risk after irradiation of the cervical spinal cord. Int J Radiat Oncol Biol Phys 1993;27:1029–33.
46. Alfonso ER, De Gregorio MA, Mateo P, et al. Radiation myelopathy in over-irradiated patients: MR imaging findings. Eur Radiol 1997;7:400–4.
47. Maranzano E, Bellavita R, Floridi P, et al. Radiation-induced myelopathy in long-term surviving metastatic spinal cord compression patients after hypofractionated radiotherapy: a clinical and magnetic resonance imaging analysis. Radiother Oncol 2001;60:281–8.
48. Rubin P. Extradural spinal cord compression by tumor. I. Experimental production and treatment trials. Radiology 1969;93:1243–48.
49. Glantz MJ, Burger PC, Friedman AH, et al. Treatment of radiation-induced nervous system injury with heparin and warfarin. Neurology 1994;44:2020–7.
50. Mizobuchi K, Kincaid J. Accessory neuropathy after high-dose radiation therapy for tongue-base carcinoma. Muscle Nerve 2003;28:650–1.
51. Lee AW, Law SC, Ng SH, et al. Retrospective analysis of nasopharyngeal carcinoma treated during 1976–1985: late complications following megavoltage irradiation. Br J Radiol 1992;65:918–28.
52. Huang S-C. Nasopharyngeal cancer: Study II. Int J Radiat Oncol Biol Phys 1981;713–6.
53. Lin YS, Jen YM, Lin JC. Radiation-related cranial nerve palsy in patients with nasopharyngeal carcinoma. Cancer 2002;95:404–9.
54. Sagar SM, Thomas RJ, Loverock LT, Spittle MF. Olfactory sensations produced by high-energy photon irradiation of the olfactory receptor mucosa in humans. Int J Radiat Oncol Biol Phys 1991;20:771–6.
55. Ophir D, Guterman A, Gross-Isseroff R. Changes in smell acuity induced by radiation exposure of the olfactory mucosa. Arch Otolaryngol Head Neck Surg 1988;114:853–5.
56. Ho WK, Kwong DL, Wei WI, Sham JS. Change in olfaction after radiotherapy for nasopharyngeal cancer—a prospective study. Am J Otolaryngol 2002;23:209–14.

57. Cackett P, Stebbing J, Dhillon B. Complications of therapy and a diagnostic dilemma case. Case 1. Radiation maculopathy following treatment of nasopharyngeal carcinoma. J Clin Oncol 2003;21:4650–1.

58. Hempel M, Hinkelbein W. Eye sequelae following external irradiation. Recent Results Cancer Res 1993;130:231–6.

59. Cackett P, Stebbing J, Dhillon B. Complications of therapy and a diagnostic dilemma case. Case 1. Radiation maculopathy following treatment of nasopharyngeal carcinoma. J Clin Oncol 2003;21:4650–1.

60. van den Bergh AC, Dullaart RP, Hoving MA, et al. Radiation optic neuropathy after external beam radiation therapy for acromegaly. Radiother Oncol 2003;68:95–100.

61. Parsons JT, Bova FJ, Fitzgerald CR, et al. Radiation optic neuropathy after megavoltage external-beam irradiation: analysis of time-dose factors. Int J Radiat Oncol Biol Phys 1994;30:755–63.

62. Kline LB, Kim JY, Ceballos R. Radiation optic neuropathy. Ophthalmology 1985;92:1118–26.

63. van den Bergh AC, Dullaart RP, Hoving MA, et al. Radiation optic neuropathy after external beam radiation therapy for acromegaly. Radiother Oncol 2003;68:95–100.

64. Lessell S, Lessell IM, Rizzo JF III. Ocular neuromyotonia after radiation therapy. Am J Ophthalmol 1986;102:766–70.

65. Frohman EM, Zee DS. Ocular neuromyotonia: clinical features, physiological mechanisms, and response to therapy. Ann Neurol 1995;37:620–6.

66. Ito K, Shin M, Matsuzaki M, et al. Risk factors for neurological complications after acoustic neurinoma radiosurgery: refinement from further experiences. Int J Radiat Oncol Biol Phys 2000;48:75–80.

67. Miller RC, Foote RL, Coffey RJ, et al. Decrease in cranial nerve complications after radiosurgery for acoustic neuromas: a prospective study of dose and volume. Int J Radiat Oncol Biol Phys 1999;43:305–11.

68. Miller RC, Foote RL, Coffey RJ, et al. Decrease in cranial nerve complications after radiosurgery for acoustic neuromas: a prospective study of dose and volume. Int J Radiat Oncol Biol Phys 1999;43:305–11.

69. Miller RC, Foote RL, Coffey RJ, Sargent DJ, Gorman DA, Schomberg PJ et al. Decrease in cranial nerve complications after radiosurgery for acoustic neuromas: a prospective study of dose and volume. Int J Radiat Oncol Biol Phys 1999;43:305–11.

70. Mossman K, Shatzman A, Chencharick J. Long-term effects of radiotherapy on taste and salivary function in man. Int J Radiat Oncol Biol Phys 1982;8:991–7.

71. Maes A, Huygh I, Weltens C, et al. De Gustibus: time scale of loss and recovery of tastes caused by radiotherapy. Radiother Oncol 2002;63:195–201.

72. Lin YS, Jen YM, Lin JC. Radiation-related cranial nerve palsy in patients with nasopharyngeal carcinoma. Cancer 2002;95:404–9.

73. Kwong DL, Wei WI, Sham JS, Ho WK, Yuen PW, Chua DT et al. Sensorineural hearing loss in patients treated for nasopharyngeal carcinoma: a prospective study of the effect of radiation and cisplatin treatment. Int J Radiat Oncol Biol Phys 1996;36(2):281–289.

74. Johannesen TB, Rasmussen K, Winther FO, Halvorsen U, Lote K. Late radiation effects on hearing, vestibular function, and taste in brain tumor patients. Int J Radiat Oncol Biol Phys 2002;53(1):86–90.

75. Lin YS, Jen YM, Lin JC. Radiation-related cranial nerve palsy in patients with nasopharyngeal carcinoma. Cancer 2002;95(2):404–409.

76. Fisher J, Scott C, Scarantino CW, et al. Phase III quality-of-life study results: impact on patients' quality of life

77. Logemann JA, Smith CH, Pauloski BR, et al. Effects of xerostomia on perception and performance of swallow function. Head Neck 2001;23:317–21.

78. Mizobuchi K, Kincaid J. Accessory neuropathy after high-dose radiation therapy for tongue-base carcinoma. Muscle Nerve 2003;28:650–1.

79. Wadd NJ, Lucraft HH. Brachial plexus neuropathy following mantle radiotherapy. Clin Oncol (R Coll Radiol) 1998; 10:399–400.

80. Rubin DI, Schomberg PJ, Shepherd RF, Panneton JM. Arteritis and brachial plexus neuropathy as delayed complications of radiation therapy. Mayo Clin Proc 2001;76:849–52.

81. Lederman RJ, Wilbourn AJ. Brachial plexopathy: recurrent cancer or radiation? Neurology 1984;34:1331–5.

82. van Es HW. MRI of the brachial plexus. Eur Radiol 2001;11:325–36.

83. Pritchard J, Anand P, Broome J, et al. Double-blind randomized phase II study of hyperbaric oxygen in patients with radiation-induced brachial plexopathy. Radiother Oncol 2001;58:279–86.

84. Abu-Rustum NR, Rajbhandari D, Glusman S, Massad LS. Acute lower extremity paralysis following radiation therapy for cervical cancer. Gynecol Oncol 1999;75:152–4.

85. Georgiou A, Grigsby PW, Perez CA. Radiation induced lumbosacral plexopathy in gynecologic tumors: clinical findings and dosimetric analysis. Int J Radiat Oncol Biol Phys 1993;26:479–82.

86. Frykholm GJ, Sintorn K, Montelius A, et al. Acute lumbosacral plexopathy during and after preoperative radiotherapy of rectal adenocarcinoma. Radiother Oncol 1996;38:121–30.

87. Ashenhurst EM, Quartey GR, Starreveld A. Lumbo-sacral radiculopathy induced by radiation. Can J Neurol Sci 1977;4:259–63.

88. Hsia AW, Katz JS, Hancock SL, Peterson K. Post-irradiation polyradiculopathy mimics leptomeningeal tumor on MRI. Neurology 2003;60:1694–6.

89. Iglicki F, Coffin B, Ille O, et al. Fecal incontinence after pelvic radiotherapy: evidences for a lumbosacral plexopathy. Report of a case. Dis Colon Rectum 1996;39:465–7.

90. Cooper J. Occupational therapy intervention with radiation-induced brachial plexopathy. Eur J Cancer Care (Engl) 1998;7:88–92.

91. Al Mefty O, Topsakal C, Pravdenkova S, et al. Radiation-induced meningiomas: clinical, pathological, cytokinetic, and cytogenetic characteristics. J Neurosurg 2004;100:1002–13.

92. Cahan WG, Woodard HQ, Higinbotham NL, et al. Sarcoma arising in irradiated bone: report of eleven cases. 1948. Cancer 1998;82:8–34.

93. Amirjamshidi A, Abbassioun K. Radiation-induced tumors of the central nervous system occurring in childhood and adolescence. Four unusual lesions in three patients and a review of the literature. Childs Nerv Syst 2000;16:390–397.

94. Salvati M, Frati A, Russo N, et al. Radiation-induced gliomas: report of 10 cases and review of the literature. Surg Neurol 2003;60:60–7.

95. Salvati M, Frati A, Russo N, Caroli E, Polli FM, Minniti G et al. Radiation-induced gliomas: report of 10 cases and review of the literature. Surg Neurol 2003;60:60–7.

96. Stavrou T, Bromley CM, Nicholson HS, et al. Prognostic factors and secondary malignancies in childhood medulloblastoma. J Pediatr Hematol Oncol 2001;23:431–6.

97. Salvati M, Polli FM, Caroli E, et al. Radiation-induced schwannomas of the nervous system. Report of five cases and review of the literature. J Neurosurg Sci 2003;47:113–6.

98. Gorson KC, Musaphir S, Lathi ES, Wolfe G. Radiation-induced malignant fibrous histiocytoma of the brachial plexus. J Neurooncol 1995;26:73–7.

99. Hussussian CJ, Mackinnon SE. Postradiation neural sheath sarcoma of the brachial plexus: a case report. Ann Plast Surg 1999;43:313–7.

100. Salvati M, Frati A, Russo N, et al. Radiation-induced gliomas: report of 10 cases and review of the literature. Surg Neurol 2003;60:60–7.

101. Sklar CA, Constine LS. Chronic neuroendocrinological sequelae of radiation therapy. Int J Radiat Oncol Biol Phys 1995;31:1113–21.

102. Pai HH, Thornton A, Katznelson L, et al. Hypothalamic/pituitary function following high-dose conformal radiotherapy to the base of skull: demonstration of a dose-effect relationship using dose-volume histogram analysis. Int J Radiat Oncol Biol Phys 2001;49:1079–92.

103. Sklar CA, Constine LS. Chronic neuroendocrinological sequelae of radiation therapy. Int J Radiat Oncol Biol Phys 1995;31:1113–21.

104. Meacham L. Endocrine late effects of childhood cancer therapy. Curr Probl Pediatr Adolesc Health Care 2003;33:217–42.

105. Sklar CA, Constine LS. Chronic neuroendocrinological sequelae of radiation therapy. Int J Radiat Oncol Biol Phys 1995;31(5):1113–1121.

106. Sklar CA, Constine LS. Chronic neuroendocrinological sequelae of radiation therapy. Int J Radiat Oncol Biol Phys 1995;31(5):1113–1121.

107. Piersanti M. Growth hormone replacement for patients with adult onset growth hormone deficiency—what have we learned. Neurosurg Focus 2004;16:E12.

108. Pai HH, Thornton A, Katznelson L, et al. Hypothalamic/pituitary function following high-dose conformal radiotherapy to the base of skull: demonstration of a dose-effect relationship using dose-volume histogram analysis. Int J Radiat Oncol Biol Phys 2001;49:1079–92.

109. Constine LS, Woolf PD, Cann D, et al. Hypothalamic-pituitary dysfunction after radiation for brain tumors. N Engl J Med 1993;328:87–94.

110. Samaan NA, Vieto R, Schultz PN, et al. Hypothalamic, pituitary and thyroid dysfunction after radiotherapy to the head and neck. Int J Radiat Oncol Biol Phys 1982;8:1857–67.

111. Constine LS, Woolf PD, Cann D, et al. Hypothalamic-pituitary dysfunction after radiation for brain tumors. N Engl J Med 1993;328:87–94.

112. Constine LS, Woolf PD, Cann D, Mick G, McCormick K, Raubertas RF et al. Hypothalamic-pituitary dysfunction after radiation for brain tumors. N Engl J Med 1993; 328(2):87–94.

113. Pai HH, Thornton A, Katznelson L, Finkelstein DM, Adams JA, Fullerton BC et al. Hypothalamic/pituitary function following high-dose conformal radiotherapy to the base of skull: demonstration of a dose-effect relationship using dose-volume histogram analysis. Int J Radiat Oncol Biol Phys 2001;49(4):1079–1092.

114. Sklar CA, Constine LS. Chronic neuroendocrinological sequelae of radiation therapy. Int J Radiat Oncol Biol Phys 1995;31(5):1113–1121.

115. Sklar CA, Constine LS. Chronic neuroendocrinological sequelae of radiation therapy. Int J Radiat Oncol Biol Phys 1995;31(5):1113–1121.

116. Sklar CA, Constine LS. Chronic neuroendocrinological sequelae of radiation therapy. Int J Radiat Oncol Biol Phys 1995;31(5):1113–1121.

Neurologic Complications of Chemotherapy

Denise M. Damek, MD

Despite differing mechanisms of action and modes of administration, the final common pathway of chemotherapeutic agents is the reduction or cessation of abnormal cancer cell proliferation. Consequently, normal body tissues with rapid cell turnover are the most susceptible to chemotherapy-related toxicity. Neurotoxicity is not commonly seen for several reasons. First of all, in the adult central nervous system, active cell turnover is limited to neuroglial cells, macrophages, and endothelial cells. In addition, the central nervous system is protected by a blood-brain barrier which effectively excludes many large molecules and hydrophilic compounds. The peripheral nervous system is similarly protected by a blood-nerve barrier. The blood-brain barrier can be circumvented by directly administering chemotherapy into the cerebrospinal fluid or brain, providing a drug in large doses systemically or intra-arterially, or utilizing agents to disrupt the blood-brain barrier. Prior or concurrent brain irradiation, or the presence of structural lesions within the brain, may increase drug penetration into the central nervous system. As such, neurotoxicity is variable and depends not only on the drug itself, but also upon the dose provided, the route of administration, and concomitant or prior therapies. In some instances, neurotoxicity is dose-limiting.

Not all neurotoxicity is the result of direct chemotherapy action on the nervous system. Chemotherapy-mediated alteration of electrolytes, fluid balance, the coagulation system, the immune system, and body organ function may cause or exacerbate central and peripheral nervous system dysfunction.

This chapter addresses the neurologic complications of some of the most commonly used chemotherapy agents (Table 1). Central and peripheral nervous system toxicity is discussed (Table 2). Neurologic complications related to radiation are addressed in another chapter in this volume (see Chapter 42, "Neurologic Toxicity of Radiotherapy").

Chemotherapy-Induced Toxicities of the Peripheral Nervous System

Peripheral Neuropathy

Peripheral neuropathies result from altered function and structure of peripheral nerves. Depending on the underlying cause, there may be selective involvement of motor, sensory, or autonomic nerve fibers; or more diffuse involvement of all fibers. Toxins such as chemotherapy cause peripheral neuropathy through axonal degeneration, primary neuronal degeneration, or segmental demyelination.

Axonal degeneration is the most common cause of peripheral neuropathy. Here, a toxin acts at multiple sites along nerve axons, ultimately causing degeneration of the nerve axon and myelin sheath beginning at the most distal part of the nerve and progressing proximally towards the nerve cell body. Descriptively, these neuropathies are often referred to as dying-back neuropathies or length-dependent peripheral neuropathies. The clinical presentation is a symmetrical, distal to proximal graded loss of sensory and motor function. The sensory loss occurs in a stocking-glove distribution. By the time the sensory abnormality reaches the level of the knees, symptoms are often recognized in the hands. If large sensory nerve fiber involvement predominates, symptoms include loss of proprioception and gait ataxia. Small fiber involvement leads to paresthesias, and loss of pin and temperature sensation. Distal muscle weakness and atrophy occur when motor nerves are affected. Likewise, loss of ankle jerks occurs first, followed by other reflexes (depending on the degree of proximal spread). Axonal regeneration can occur, albeit slowly. Recovery may be significantly delayed and is often incomplete.

In primary neuronal degeneration, a toxin damages or destroys the dorsal root ganglion neurons, which are the sensory nerve cell bodies. Degeneration of the entire peripheral and central axonal processes follows. Clinically, there is prominent loss of ability to localize the extremities in space (proprioception), diffuse areflexia, and ataxia. Neuronal regeneration does not occur.

As such, symptom recovery is contingent upon the degree of damage to the dorsal root ganglion cells. Recovery is poor, but incomplete reversal of some symptoms may occur over a long interval.

With segmental demyelination, toxins injure and break down either the myelin sheath or the Schwann cells along the entire length of nerve fibers with relative sparing of the underlying axons. This most commonly occurs in the setting of immune-mediated inflammatory processes, but occasionally can be mediated by toxins. The functional correlate of demyelination is nerve signal conduction block, resulting in motor weakness and mild sensory loss. Sensory modalities relayed via small-diameter myelinated fibers or unmyelinated fibers, such as temperature and light touch, are generally spared. Remyelination of nerve fibers and clinical recovery can occur within days to weeks.

Many neuropathies present towards the end of therapy or after completion of chemotherapy, limiting the clinician's ability to impact symptomatology with drug cessation. For this reason, the early detection of neuropathy prior to the development of symptoms is paramount. Unfortunately, the use of electrophysiologic testing, in particular nerve conduction studies, to identify high risk patients, or for the early detection of peripheral neuropathy, has for the large part been disappointing. However, a decrease in sensory nerve action potentials (SNAPs) may be used to monitor the severity of a neuropathy objectively in some cases.[1]

Platinum Compounds

The main neurologic complication of cisplatin is a cumulative dose-dependent sensory neuropathy. Cisplatin almost exclusively affects the large myelinated sensory nerves, both clinically and by objective measurement of nerve conduction studies.[2] Subclinical signs of cisplatin neuropathy, primarily absent ankle jerks and decreased vibratory function, are seen at cumulative doses > 200 mg/m^2. Some patients perceive sensory symptoms after cumulative doses

Table 1 Chemotherapeutic Agents Causing Neurotoxicity			
Chemotherapeutic Agent and Drug Class	**Mechanism of Action**	**Mode of Administration**	**Use**
Alkylating Agents **Platinum-based**			
Cis-platinum	Inhibits DNA synthesis by the formation of DNA cross-links	IV, IA	Head and neck, breast, testicular, and ovarian CA, sarcomas, bladder, gastric, lung esophageal, cervical, and prostate CA, myeloma, melanoma, small cell lung cancer, osteosarcoma, Hodgkin's and non-Hodgkin's lymphoma, neuroblastoma
Carboplatin	Covalently binds to DNA bases and disrupts DNA function	IV, IA	Ovarian cancer. Lung, head and neck, endometrial, esophageal, bladder, breast, cervical, CNS tumors, germ cell tumors, osteogenic sarcoma, and high-dose therapy with stem cell/bone marrow support
Oxaliplatin	Binds to DNA, RNA, or proteins	IV	Advanced colorectal carcinoma. Head and neck cancer, non-Hodgkin's lymphoma, ovarian cancer
Nitrosoureas			
Carmustine (BCNU)	Interferes with DNA function by alkylation and formation of DNA cross-links	IV, implantable wafer	CNS tumors, multiple myeloma, Hodgkin's and non-Hodgkin's lymphoma, melanoma, lung and colon carcinoma
Lomustine (CCNU)	Inhibits DNA and RNA synthesis via carbamylation of DNA polymerase, alkylation of DNA, and alteration of RNA proteins	PO	CNS tumors, Hodgkin's and non-Hodgkin's lymphoma, melanoma, renal carcinoma, lung and colon carcinoma
Mustards			
Ifosfamide (with mesna)	Inhibits DNA synthesis by the formation of DNA cross-links	IV	Lung cancer, Hodgkin's and non-Hodgkin's lymphoma, breast CA, acute and chronic lymphocytic leukemias, ovarian CA, sarcomas, pancreatic and gastric carcinomas
Cyclophosphamide	Inhibits DNA synthesis by the formation of DNA cross-links	IV	Hodgkin's and non-Hodgkin's lymphoma, Burkitt's lymphoma, leukemia (CLL, CML, AML, ALL), mycoses fungoides, multiple myeloma, neuroblastoma, retinoblastoma, sarcomas, breast, testicular, endometrial, ovarian, and lung CA. Conditioning regimens for bone marrow transplant
Melphalan	Inhibits DNA and RNA synthesis by the formation of carbonium ions and DNA cross-links	PO, IV	Palliative treatment of multiple myeloma, nonresectable epithelial ovarian carcinoma, neuroblastoma, rhabdomyosarcoma, breast CA
Other			
Thiotepa	Inhibits DNA, RNA, and protein synthesis by the cross-linking of DNA	IV, IT, intravesicular	Superficial bladder tumors, breast and ovarian adenocarcinoma, lymphoma, sarcoma, CNS leptomeningeal disease and metastases
Procarbazine	Mechanism of action is unclear; methylates nucleic acids, inhibits DNA, RNA, and protein synthesis, may damage DNA directly and suppress mitoses	PO	Hodgkin's and non-Hodgkin's lymphoma, CNS tumors, melanoma, lung cancer, multiple myeloma
Plant Alkaloids **Vincas**			
Vincristine	Disrupts the formation of the mitotic spindle by binding to tubulin and inhibiting microtubule formation	IV	Leukemia, Hodgkin's and non-Hodgkin's lymphoma, Wilms' tumor, neuroblastoma, rhabdomyosarcoma
Podophyllins			
Etoposide (VP-16)	Delays transit of cells through the S phase and arrests cells in the late S or early G2 phase. Inhibits topoisomerase II and appears to cause DNA strand breaks.	IV	Lymphoma, lung, testicular, bladder, and prostate CA, hepatoma, rhabdomyosarcoma, uterine CA, neuroblastoma, mycosis fungoides, Kaposi's sarcoma, histiocytosis, gestational trophoblastic disease, Ewing's sarcoma, Wilms' tumor, and CNS tumors
Others			
Paclitaxel	Promotes microtubule assembly and distorts mitotic spindles	IV	Breast, lung (small cell and non-small cell), and ovarian cancers
Docetaxel	Inhibits DNA, RNA, and protein synthesis by stabilization of microtubules	IV	Breast and non-small cell lung cancer

Table 1 *Continued*

Chemotherapeutic Agent and Drug Class	Mechanism of Action	Mode of Administration	Use
Antimetabolites			
Antifolates			
Methotrexate	Folate antimetabolite. Inhibits DNA synthesis by inhibiting purine and thymidylic acid synthesis	IV, IT	Trophoblastic neoplasms, leukemias, breast, head and neck, and lung carcinoma, osteosarcoma, soft-tissue sarcomas, GI tract, esophageal, and testicular CA, lymphomas
Cytidine Analogs			
Cytarabine	Inhibits DNA synthesis by incorporating into DNA and inhibiting DNA polymerase	IV, IT	Leukemias, lymphomas
Fluorinated Pyrimidines			
Fluorouracil	Pyrimidine antimetabolite. Interferes with DNA synthesis by blocking the methylation of deoxyuridylic acid	IV, topical	Breast, colon, head and neck, pancreas, rectum, and stomach CA. Used topically to treat skin cancer.
Purine Analogs			
Fludarabine	Inhibits DNA synthesis by inhibition of DNA polymerase and ribonucleotide reductase	IV	Chronic lymphocytic leukemia, non-Hodgkin's lymphoma
Others			
Hydroxyurea	Mechanism is unclear. Thought to inhibit DNA synthesis by inhibition of ribonucleoside diphosphate reductase	PO	CML, acute leukemia, radiosensitizing agent in the treatment of CNS tumors, head and neck tumors, uterine, cervix, and non-small cell lung cancer
Gemcitabine	Pyrimidine antimetabolite. Inhibits DNA synthesis by inhibition of DNA polymerase and ribonucleotide reductase	IV	Adenocarcinoma of the pancreas, non-small cell lung cancer
Antineoplastic Antibiotics			
Anthracyclines			
Doxorubicin	Inhibition of DNA and RNA synthesis by intercalation between DNA base pairs	IV	Leukemias, lymphomas, multiple myeloma, sarcoma, mesotheliomas, germ cell tumors of the ovary and testes, neuroblastoma, head and neck, thyroid, lung, breast, stomach, pancreas, liver, ovary, bladder, prostate, and uterine CA
Antineoplastic Enzymes			
L-Asparaginase	Inhibits protein synthesis through the depletion of asparagine	IV, IM, subcutaneous	Acute lymphocytic leukemia, lymphoma
Antineoplastic Biologics			
Cytokines			
Interleukin-2	Promotes differentiation, and proliferation, and recruitment of T and B cells, natural killer cells, and thymocytes; stimulates lymphokine-activated killer cells and tumor-infiltrating lymphocytes	IV, Subcutaneous	Renal cell CA, melanoma, multiple myeloma, colorectal CA, non-Hodgkin's lymphoma
Interferon	Stimulates the immune system against tumor cells; direct and indirect cytotoxic activity; increases the expression of tumor-associated antigens	Subcutaneous	Chronic myelogenous leukemia, hairy cell leukemia, Kaposi's sarcoma, malignant melanoma, follicular non-Hodgkin's lymphoma
Anti-angiogenesis Agents			
Thalidomide	Inhibits tumor necrosis factor-alpha; inhibits fibroblast growth factor and vascular endothelial growth factor-induced angiogenesis	PO	Multiple myeloma, Waldenström's macroglobulinemia, CNS tumors, Kaposi's sarcoma
Suramin	Inhibits a number of growth factors and enzymes essential to cell proliferation. May also have anti-angiogenic activity	IV	Chemosensitizing agent for various solid tumors; investigational use in prostate cancer and many other cancer types

ALL = acute lymphoblastic leukemia; AML = acute myelogenous leukemia; CA = cancer; CLL = chronic lymphocytic leukemia; CML = chronic myelogenous; CNS = central nervous system; DNA = deoxyribonucleic acid; GI = gastrointestinal; IA = intra-arterially; IM = intramuscularly; IV = intravenously; PO = oral.

>300 mg/m²,[3,4] but almost all patients have evidence of neuropathy at cumulative doses greater than 500 to 600 mg/m².[5] Symptom onset is often delayed and may not manifest until after completion of therapy.[6] In fact, symptoms can worsen in the weeks to months following discontinuance of the drug.[7] The first symptoms are paresthesias and numbness of the feet, progressing to involve the lower and upper extremities. Loss of proprioception results in gait ataxia. Muscle cramps are frequently reported during symptom progression and gradually resolve after symptom stabilization.[7] Lhermitte's sign is occasionally present. Autonomic symptoms, while reported, rarely occur.[3,8,9] Somatosensory-evoked responses (SSER) may facilitate early detection of cisplatin neuropathy by showing a slight impairment of nerve conduction prior to the presence of

Table 2 Neurologic Complications Of Chemotherapy

Chemotherapeutic Agent and Drug Class	Peripheral Neuropathy	Toxic/Metabolic Encephalopathy	Leukoencephalopathy	RPLS	Cognitive Dysfunction	Seizures	Cerebellar Syndrome	Movement Disorder	Visual Symptoms	Aseptic Meningitis	Stroke/Vascular disorder	Spinal cord abnormalities
Alkylating Agents												
Platinum-based												
Cis-platinum	X	X	X	X	X	X			X		X	X
Carboplatin	X	X		X	X	X					X	
Oxaliplatin	X											
Nitrosureas												
Carmustine (BCNU)	X	X	X						X		X	
Lomustine (CCNU)		X							X			
Mustards												
Ifosfamide (with mesna)		X		X								
Cyclophosphamide				X	X				X			
Melphalan												
Other												
Thiotepa			X		X					X		
Procarbazine	X											
Plant Alkaloids												
Vincas												
Vincristine	X	X		X		X		X	X			
Podophyllins												
Etoposide (VP-16)	X	X		X								
Others												
Placlitaxel (Taxol)	X	X			X							
Docetaxel (Taxotere)	X											
Antimetabolites												
Antifolates												
Methotrexate		X	X	X	X	X			X	X		X
Cytidine Analogs												
Cytarabine		X	X	X		X	X	X	X	X		X
Fluorinated Pyrimidines												
Fluorouracil		X	X		X	X	X	X	X		X	
Purine Analogs												
Fludarabine		X	X									
Others												
Hydroxyurea	X											
Gemcitabine	X											
Antineoplastic Antibiotics												
Anthracyclines												
Doxorubicin				X	X							
Antineoplastic enzymes												
L-Asparaginase		X				X					X	
Antineoplastic Hormones												
Anti-estrogens												
Tamoxifen		X							X			
Antineoplastic Biologics												
Cytokines												
Interleukin-2			X									
Interferon			X									
Anti-angiogenesis Agents												
Thalidomide	X					X						
Suramin	X											

abnormal signs or symptoms.[10]; however, clinical applicability has yet to be demonstrated. SSER may be more accurate than conventional electrophysiologic studies in evaluating the progression of cisplatin neuropathy.

Cisplatin preferentially accumulates in the dorsal root ganglia, dorsal roots, and peripheral nerve, and appears to remain there indefinitely in an acutely neurotoxic state.[10,11] Platinum levels in the dorsal root ganglia correlate with cumulative cisplatin doses and possibly symptom severity.[10] However, the mechanism of cisplatin-induced neuropathy remains unknown. Prior exposure to platinum compounds is generally thought to be a major risk factor for the development of peripheral neuropathy. However, no substantial neurotoxicity was reported with re-treatment of cisplatin in one study.[12] Components of the neuropathy, including muscle cramps and Lhermitte's sign, are self-limited symptoms. The remaining neuropathic features, in particular the sensory deficits, are often permanent. However, a small percentage of patients show slow gradual symptom improvement.

The role of neuroprotective agents in preventing or ameliorating cisplatin-induced neurotoxicity is unclear. One randomized, double-blind, placebo-controlled trial of Org-2766, a synthetic corticotropin(4-9) analogue, in patients treated with cisplatin for ovarian cancer found that treated patients showed stable vibratory perception thresholds and less prominent neurologic deficits compared to untreated patients.[13] However, this result was not duplicated in a later study.[14] Less impairment of sensory nerve conduction abnormalities was seen in gastric cancer patients given glutathione with cisplatin chemotherapy.[15] Amifostine, a thiol prodrug, has shown mixed results in three clinical trials.[16–18] Despite some initial promising results, to date, none of these therapies has shown unequivocal benefit.

At standard doses, carboplatin causes paresthesias in approximately 5% of patients. However, high-dose carboplatin can cause a sensory neuropathy similar to that produced by cisplatin.

Oxaliplatin-induced peripheral neuropathy is indistinguishable from that produced by cisplatin. Peripheral neuropathy develops following long-term drug administration, presumptively corresponding to the cumulative dose provided. Oxaliplatin-induced neuropathy symptomatically may respond to temporary cessation of the drug. Forty percent of patients have complete symptom resolution 6 to 8 months following cessation of therapy.[19] Anecdotal evidence suggests some symptomatic benefit with carbamazepine and amifostine.[20,21]

Thalidomide

Peripheral neuropathy usually occurs following prolonged administration of thalidomide. Up to 70% of patients treated for more than 6 months

have signs and symptoms of peripheral neuropathy.[22] Peripheral neuropathy can be dose-limiting. Clinical trials utilizing a variety of daily doses report a frequency of mild neuropathic symptoms of 13 to 41%, and severe neuropathic symptoms of 5 to 20%.[23] The incidence of peripheral neuropathy is higher in elderly patients, patients with preexisting neuropathy, and those treated with additional neurotoxic chemotherapy. The risk is greater when the cumulative dose exceeds 50 g.[24] Genetically determined alterations in drug metabolism (ie, "slow acetylators") may be more susceptible to toxicity due to slower drug excretion.[22]

Clinical symptoms initially relate to small fiber sensory nerve involvement, with paresthesias and numbness of the toes and fingers that extends proximally. Later, large fiber involvement is seen with abnormal vibratory perception, deep pressure sensation, and poor position sense. Eventually ataxia, progressive gait disturbance, and postural tremor are seen. If the neuropathy is severe, pyramidal tract damage, proximal muscle weakness, and muscular atrophy develop. Magnetic resonance imaging (MRI) of the spinal cord of patients with neuropathy show signal abnormalities in the posterior columns, consistent with degeneration of the posterior columns.[25] Symptom improvement typically occurs within 3 weeks of discontinuance of the drug; however, the extent of recovery is variable.[22] Discontinuance of the drug at the onset of neuropathic symptoms increases the probability of recovery. Likewise, better recovery is generally seen in younger patients and those treated with lower cumulative doses of thalidomide.[26]

Vincristine

Vincristine causes significantly more neurotoxicity than the other vinca alkaloids. Peripheral neuropathy is rarely seen with vindesine sulfate and vinblastine treatment; however, it may complicate vinorelbine therapy in 20 to 25% of patients. Approximately 50% of individuals treated with a typical dose of vincristine (2 mg/dose limit) develop paresthesias of the fingers and toes. If single doses in excess of 2 mg are provided, the incidence of symptomatic neuropathy is approximately 90%.[27] In fact, a mixed sensorimotor polyneuropathy is dose-limiting for vincristine.

Muscle cramps affecting the arms and legs may be the first manifestation of neuropathy and may be the last symptom to resolve. Typical progression of signs and symptoms includes the early development of paresthesias in fingers and toes, loss of ankle reflexes, and then symmetrical length-dependent distal sensory and motor deficits. Impairment of fine motor skills often precedes clinically detectable weakness of the hands and feet. Vibratory sensation is generally spared. As symptoms progress, gait ataxia may

occur. Autonomic neuropathy is common, occurring in as many as one-third of patients.[28] Bowel motility dysfunction, manifesting as colicky abdominal pain and constipation, paralytic ileus, or megacolon, may precede the development of sensory or motor symptoms.[27] Orthostatic hypotension, urinary retention from an atonic bladder, impotence, and disturbed heart rate occur infrequently. Cranial nerve involvement occurs in approximately 10% of cases. Laryngeal nerve paresis is the most commonly described. Patients present with hoarseness generally after several courses of vincristine. Symptom resolution occurs 4 to 6 weeks following discontinuance of the drug.[29] In addition, diplopia, facial nerve palsy, ophthalmoplegia,[30] and sensorineural hearing loss[31] have been reported.

Risk factors for developing vincristine neurotoxicity include single doses greater than 2 mg, frequent vincristine administration, poor nutritional state, advanced age, liver dysfunction, and concurrent neurotoxic drugs.[32] Individuals with preexisting abnormalities of peripheral nerve, such as the demyelinating type of Charcot-Marie-Tooth disease (hereditary motor and sensory neuropathy type I) can develop a severe, often irreversible and sometimes fatal neuropathy.[30,33]

There is no clearly effective treatment for vincristine-induced neuropathy other than discontinuance of the drug. Overall, the long-term prognosis for recovery is good. If vincristine is discontinued, when paresthesias first appear, symptoms promptly resolve. Mild symptoms generally resolve within a couple of months after drug cessation.[27] However, when prominent, motor weakness may take months to regress, and sensory symptoms may linger for years.[34]

Paclitaxel

The occurrence and severity of peripheral neuropathy with the taxanes is single-dose and cumulative-dose–related.[35–37] Paclitaxel-induced neuropathy is the best characterized. Symptoms manifest following cumulative doses of 100 to 200 mg/m^2.[36] At a single paclitaxel dose of 135 mg/m^2, approximately 2% of patients develop paresthesias of the hands and feet,[38] but following a dose of 250 mg/m^2, approximately 60% of patients develop neuropathic symptoms.[28] Neuropathy is the dose-limiting toxicity when paclitaxel doses >250 mg/m^2 are administered in combination with granulocyte colony-stimulating factor.[39,40]

Paclitaxel and docetaxel produce a predominantly sensory neuropathy. The pathophysiologic mechanism of paclitaxel-induced neuropathy is thought to be related to microtubule aggregation in neurons, axons, and Schwann cells, which leads to demyelination and abnormal axoplasmic transport.[35] Unlike the sensory neuropathy elicited by cisplatin, all sensory modalities are affected. Within 48 hours of treatment, patients develop paresthesias, numbness, and pain in the feet and hands. Pruritus can be a prominent feature. The rapid onset of symptoms and early presence of hand symptoms suggests preferential involvement of dorsal root ganglia and/or myelin sheath.[41] Fine motor skills are often compromised, but weakness is not generally seen. However, some patients may develop disabling proximal muscle weakness mimicking myopathy.[42] Arthralgia and myalgias, especially in the legs, can often be seen 2 to 7 days after the drug is given.[43] Rare autonomic neuropathy has been reported.[44] In addition, Lhermitte's sign can develop following docetaxel administration.[37] Symptoms are usually reversible after discontinuation of the drug, and may even resolve despite continued therapy.[28] However, there are reports of permanent neuropathy.[45] Predisposing factors include high-dose cycles, high cumulative doses, diabetes mellitus, and preexisting neuropathy.[28]

Suramin

Suramin produces a predominantly motor peripheral neuropathy in up to 40% of patients whose blood levels of the drug exceed 350 µg/ml.[28] Patients commonly describe paresthesias of the face and limbs followed by rapid onset of proximal muscle weakness that can progress to quadriplegia with bulbar and respiratory muscle weakness. The presentation is similar to acute inflammatory demyelinating polyneuropathy (AIDP) or Guillain-Barré syndrome. The underlying pathogenic mechanism is thought to be conduction block in peripheral nerves due to demyelination. Symptoms resolve after the drug is discontinued. Unlike the other neuropathies, this neuropathy can be prevented through careful monitoring of suramin blood levels.

Bortezomib

The clinical spectrum of bortezomib-induced peripheral neuropathy is not yet fully defined. Bortezomib causes a painful peripheral neuropathy in approximately 40% of patients.[46] This symptom may be dose-limiting, and, currently, dose adjustments are recommended for disabling neuropathic symptoms, which occur in approximately 15% of patients.[46] Nerve conduction studies in a small number of patients were consistent with axonal degeneration.[46] Symptom improvement is seen following discontinuance of the drug, but the time course of recovery or extent of recovery remain largely unknown.

Other Chemotherapeutic Agents

Various other chemotherapy drugs can produce peripheral neuropathy. A reversible peripheral neuropathy characterized by distal paresthesias, decreased deep tendon reflexes, and myalgias is fairly common during procarbazine therapy. High-dose cytarabine, particularly when given in combination with other potentially neurotoxic drugs, rarely causes an axonal and/or demyelinating peripheral neuropathy.[28] Fludarabine can cause a mild peripheral neuropathy generally presenting with paresthesias or weakness. In addition, high-dose etoposide rarely causes a reversible axonal sensory neuropathy.[47] Furthermore, peripheral neuropathies rarely occur as a complication of treatment with high-dose ifosfamide, fluorouracil, and gemcitabine hydrochloride.

Muscle Weakness/Arthralgia

Muscle weakness and arthralgia most commonly occurs in the setting of sensorimotor neuropathy, such as that seen with vincristine and paclitaxel. However, a chemotherapeutic-agent–induced primary muscle disorder has been implicated in some cases. A toxic myopathy was implicated in one patient following paclitaxel administration on the basis of clinical signs and symptoms, electrophysiologic studies, and muscle biopsy findings of accumulation of acid phosphatase in lysosomes.[26] Dose dependent weakness and fatigue can occur 1 to 2 months from the onset of thalidomide therapy.[22] Furthermore, steroid-induced myopathy is a common and well-recognized complication of long-term steroid provision. Muscle aching and pseudoarthritis are frequent manifestations of steroid withdrawal.

Peripheral Nerve Hyperexcitability

Acutely, oxaliplatin can produce a unique syndrome that resembles neuromyotonia. Sensory manifestations are the most prominent, and generally develop within hours or days of therapy. Patients report fairly dramatic paresthesias and dysesthesias of the hands, feet, and perioral region. Pharyngo-laryngo-dysesthesias cause a subjective sense of difficulty in breathing. Cold exposure may trigger or exacerbate these symptoms. Motor nerves or muscle may also be affected, presenting as jaw tightness and pain, eye pain, ptosis, leg cramps, visual field abnormalities, and voice changes. Symptoms usually resolve spontaneously over hours to days. However, repeated drug administration may produce more severe and more prolonged symptoms.[21] Electrophysiologic examination findings are identical to those seen in neuromyotonia, which is produced by excessive nerve excitability of peripheral nerve axons.[21] Oxaliplatin may produce a transient channelopathy, acting as a direct toxin against either voltage-gated potassium or sodium channels in axons.[21]

Chemotherapy-Induced Toxicities of the Central Nervous System

Toxic and Metabolic Encephalopathy

Toxic and metabolic encephalopathies are a group of neurologic disorders characterized by altered mental status attributable to the presence of an exogenous or endogenous drug or toxin, or non-brain organ failure. Chemotherapeutic agents or their metabolites may act as direct toxins. Alternatively, they may cause electrolyte or fluid imbalance, renal or liver dysfunction, or other metabolic derangements. Symptoms do not distinguish causative agents in acute encephalopathy. The hallmark of acute encephalopathy is confusion, disorientation, and altered behavior. Symptoms range from simply appearing depressed and withdrawn to an agitated delirium and florid hallucinations. Seizures may represent the only manifestation of acute encephalopathy or may accompany other symptoms. Motor system abnormalities may include increased tone, tremor, multifocal myoclonus, muscle cramps, asterixis, and weakness. Widespread neurologic dysfunction can be seen.

Ifosfamide

The reported incidence of high-dose ifosfamide- and mesna-induced encephalopathy ranges widely from 8 to 14% to greater than 50%.[48–50] A transient confusional state is most commonly seen, but in some patient groups more severe symptoms of confusion, visual hallucinations, cerebellar dysfunction, seizures, cranial nerve palsies, extrapyramidal signs, and, occasionally, coma occur. Symptoms manifest hours to several days post drug administration. Diffuse slow wave activity is frequently seen on electroencephalography (EEG) following treatment, even in asymptomatic patients.[49,51] EEG findings are consistent with a diffuse encephalopathy of toxic or metabolic origin. Symptoms typically resolve spontaneously after several days.[52] However, irreversible deficits and death have been reported.[52–54] Successful rechallenge with ifosfamide has been reported.[51] Accumulation of a metabolite of ifosfamide, Chloracetaldehyde, has been implicated as the responsible toxic agent. Risk factors for encephalopathy include short infusion times (24-hour),[51] renal dysfunction,[49] low serum albumin,[49,48] presence of pelvic tumor,[49] underlying brain disease,[55] phenobarbital use,[56] and previous ifosfamide-induced encephalopathy.

Other Chemotherapeutic Agents

An acute encephalopathy can complicate the treatment course of many other chemotherapeutic agents. The resultant symptoms are indistinguishable from those of a metabolic encephalopathy. Paclitaxel can cause a severe acute encephalopathy at doses in excess of 600 mg/m^2 with stem cell support.[57] Likewise, high-dose therapy with methotrexate, lomustine, and etoposide can produce an acute encephalopathy. In addition, encephalopathy can occur following standard dose treatment with cisplatin, vincristine, asparaginase, procarbazine, 5-fluorouracil, cytarabine, interleukin-2 (IL-2), and tamoxifen.

Toxic Leukoencephalopathy

Neuroimaging and neuropathology have identified cerebral white matter as a target of chemotherapy-induced toxicity. Toxins may affect any component of the white matter, including myelin, nerve axons, oligodendrocytes, astrocytes, and blood vessels; however, myelin often bears the brunt of the damage.[58] This acute or delayed structural change in cerebral white matter is called leukoencephalopathy. White matter injury has been associated with a number of chemotherapeutic agents including methotrexate, carmustine, cisplatin, cytarabine, fluorouracil, levamisole, fludarabine, thiotepa, interleukin-2, and interferon-α.[58] Both the route of administration and the dose administered influence the development of leukoencephalopathy. Less than 10% of patients treated with intravenous methotrexate develop leukoencephalopathy; however, this complication is seen in up to 40% of patients receiving intrathecal methotrexate.[59,60] Likewise, cytarabine and thiotepa may produce a leukoencephalopathy when administered intrathecally. On the other hand, cisplatin and carmustine can cause leukoencephalopathy when injected intra-arterially. Conventional doses of fludarabine, cytarabine, and 5-fluorouracil are rarely associated with cerebral white matter changes on MRI. However, high-dose therapy with these same agents may produce profound white matter changes.[58].

A wide and diverse range of signs and symptoms have been reported.[61] The most prominent clinical manifestation is the presence of neurobehavioral changes, which can range from a mild chronic confusional state with inattention, memory loss, and emotional dysfunction, to a devastating white matter dementia syndrome, abulia, stupor, and coma. Focal neurologic deficits such as hemiparesis, visual loss, and sensory deficits are frequently described. Notably absent are signs of cortical gray matter involvement, such as aphasia and seizures.

The diagnosis of toxic leukoencephalopathy requires clinical symptoms of white matter dysfunction and correlative neuroradiographic white matter abnormalities. Magnetic resonance imaging offers better resolution of white matter than other neuroimaging methods and is the imaging method of choice. Characteristic T2-weighted imaging findings are diffuse, increased signal intensity within the white matter, often extending from the ventricles to the cortical medullary junction. A scalloped lateral margin results from the sparing of the subcortical arcuate fibers and overlying cortex. In patients with intraventricular catheters, radiographic findings are fairly localized to white matter adjacent to the catheter path.[62] In patients with more widespread toxin exposure, the extent of radiographic involvement is variable. In some cases, white matter changes can be seen on MRI in asymptomatic patients. The clinical significance of this is uncertain, but it may be a harbinger for the development of symptomatic leukoencephalopathy if additional treatment is provided.

The spectrum of neuropathologic findings in toxic leukoencephalopathy ranges from patchy intramyelinic edema with preservation of myelin, to widespread edema and demyelination with preservation of axons, and to destruction of oligodendrocytes, axonal loss, and necrosis.[63] However, the most common findings are gliosis, macrophage infiltration, and demyelination. The distribution of lesions and corresponding symptomatology is variable, ranging from isolated optic nerve involvement to multifocal white matter lesions, to confluent symmetrical subcortical white matter involvement.[61]

Drugs delivered directly into the ventricles can flow back along the reservoir catheter path and can accumulate in the white matter.[62] This complication can occur with properly placed catheters or a misplaced catheter tip that is directed into the brain parenchyma. Rarely, this may occur in patients with an indwelling intraventricular catheter who receive only systemic chemotherapy. In addition, factors such as increased intracranial pressure, the presence of widespread leptomeningeal tumor, or obstruction of cerebrospinal fluid outflow may increase drug concentrations within the ventricular system. The provision of intra-arterial drug is particularly conducive to vascular injury. Even though the route of drug delivery may predispose to toxicity, it does not elucidate the mechanism of white matter injury. The pathogenesis largely remains unknown, but most certainly consists of a variety of mechanisms. Proposed mechanisms include a direct toxic effect on myelin, disruption of myelin synthesis via injury to oligodendrocytes, cerebral edema secondary to breakdown of the blood-brain barrier, or reversible axonal swelling secondary to metabolic deterioration.[58,64]

Many patients fully recover; however, others may experience a progressive course with devastating sequelae. The prognosis depends largely on the extent of white matter injury and whether or not that injury is reversible or irreversible. If the nerve axons remain spared, and tissue necrosis has not occurred, the prognosis for recovery is favorable. Discontinuance of the inciting toxin early on in the disease process before irreversible damage has occurred remains critical. Often, however, chemotherapeutic-induced toxic leukoencephalopathy symptoms do not manifest until after the completion of therapy. This limits the value of early detection and cessation or alteration of drug therapy. Several therapeutic interventions have been tried with variable success. These include corticosteroids, anticoagulation therapy, and ventriculoperitoneal shunting, and leucovorin for methotrexate-induced toxicity.[58]

Methotrexate-Induced Mild Leukoencephalopathy

Methotrexate (MTX) can cause acute or subacute neurotoxicity that is characterized by somnolence, confusion, and focal neurologic deficits. Focal symptoms present with a stroke-like onset and include hemiparesis, aphasia, and hemisensory loss. Even though this syndrome is more commonly associated with high-dose MTX treatment, intrathecal and low-dose methotrexate therapy can also produce transient neurologic symptoms.[65] Prior to the routine use of leucovorin rescue in conjunction with methotrexate therapy, reported incidences of this syndrome approached 15%.[66] Since then, however, the incidence is approximately 3%.[67]

Symptoms commonly occur within 24 hours of drug administration, but can manifest up to 2 weeks following therapy. Evaluation usually reveals normal head CT, either normal MRI or diffuse periventricular high signal on T2-weighted images, normal cerebrospinal fluid (CSF), and generalized slowing on EEG. Restricted diffusion (high-intensity signal on diffusion-weighted imaging with decreased apparent diffusion coefficient) in the periventricular deep white matter bilaterally was reported in one case.[64] Abnormal signal on T2-weighted MR images can be found in asymptomatic patients or patients with minimal symptoms following MTX treatment.[68–71] The severity of the white matter insult on MRI does not correlate with clinical symptomatology.[70] Most patients fully recover within 72 hours; however, a chronic leukoencephalopathy has been reported.[72] Even though additional cycles have been provided without symptom recurrence,[67,73] the syndrome may recur with drug rechallenge.

The mechanism remains unknown, but an underlying vascular etiology induced or worsened by metabolic disturbance has been proposed. Proposed mechanisms include MTX-induced altered neurotransmitter levels secondary to inhibition of tetrahydrobiopterin synthesis,[66] increased adenosine,[74] or increased homocysteine levels.[65]

Methotrexate-Induced Disseminated Necrotizing Leukoencephalopathy

In some cases, rapid severe neurologic deterioration occurs following MTX treatment characterized by personality changes, confusion, somnolence, ataxia, spasticity, seizures, dementia, and even coma and death. CT and MRI demonstrate extensive white matter damage.[71,75] This imaging abnormality in conjunction with rapid clinical deterioration represents disseminated necrotizing leukoencephalopathy (DNL), a rare complication of MTX. DNL is associated with both intravenous and intrathecal methotrexate and cranial irradiation. Characteristic histopathologic findings include discrete or confluent foci of demyelination, scattered areas of coagulative necrosis, astrocytosis, and, occasionally, dystrophic calcification.[75]

Chronic Methotrexate-Induced Leukoencephalopathy

Leukoencephalopathy is the most common delayed central nervous system (CNS) effect of MTX. It is associated with multiple prior doses of intra-CSF or high-dose intravenous MTX, prior or concurrent provision of whole brain irradiation, and age greater than 60 years at the time of methotrexate treatment. The most significant risk factor is the provision of cranial irradiation before or during MTX therapy. The risk for leukoencephalopathy is less than 2% in patients receiving intravenous MTX alone, compared to approximately 45% in patients receiving intrathecal and intravenous MTX and brain irradiation.[76] Combined chemoradiotherapy for the treatment of primary central nervous system lymphoma demonstrates an overwhelming risk of dementia in patients more than 60 years of age.[77,78] However, treatment approaches without the use of radiation have not reported this complication.[79,80] Symptoms manifest months to years following methotrexate provision and include personality or behavioral change and global cognitive impairment, often progressing to severe dementia, quadriplegia, gait apraxia, and incontinence. Coma and death can eventually occur. Brain imaging studies show diffuse white matter hyperintensities most prominent in the corona radiate, cortical atrophy, and ex-vacuo ventriculomegaly. The histopathologic spectrum seen in chemotherapy/radiation-induced leukoencephalopathy ranges from myelin pallor with foamy macrophages and gliosis to severe vasculitis and necrosis.[81,82] The prognosis of patients developing late neurotoxicity is poor, with a 50% risk of death at 12 months despite continued remission of cerebral lymphoma.

Carmustine

Carmustine (BCNU)-mediated encephalopathy has been observed months following intravenous doses greater than 1,200 mg/m^2.[83,84] More significant, however, is the neurotoxicity associated with intra-arterial BCNU. Once quite popular, intracarotid infusion of BCNU has been largely abandoned due to unacceptable toxicity. Patients frequently reported ipsilateral eye, neck, and head pain following the procedure. Infraophthalmic carotid artery infusion is associated with the formation of retinal and choroidal emboli and thrombosis, producing optic neuropathy and

retinopathy.[85] Subclinical retinal rod and cone dysfunction was also documented in the majority of patients in one series.[86] More significant, however, was the fairly common development of a potentially life-threatening necrotizing leukoencephalopathy.[87–89] In one series, delayed cerebral necrosis occurred in 80% of patients receiving supraophthalmic intra-arterial carotid BCNU infusions.[85] Generally 1 to 6 months following intra-arterial BCNU therapy, patients presented with seizures, altered mental status, and focal neurologic deficits. Unrelenting symptom progression leading to coma and death was often seen. Imaging revealed predominantly nonenhancing white matter edema and mass effect within the vascular territory of the injected artery. Pathological examination of brain tissue in patients succumbing to the disorder revealed either miliary foci of necrosis and mineralizing axonopathy or more diffuse confluent necrotizing leukoencephalopathy changes within the white matter of the treated vascular distribution.

Cisplatin

Encephalopathy as a complication of cisplatin therapy is more common with intra-arterial drug administration than intravenous drug administration. Cisplatin-induced encephalopathy is often characterized by focal brain dysfunction, in particular cortical blindness, and seizures. Imaging findings resemble reversible posterior leukoencephalopathy syndrome.[90] Symptoms occur during, immediately after, or as long as 10 days following cisplatin infusion. Drug-induced encephalopathy must be differentiated from that precipitated by the hydration preceding cisplatin treatment, electrolyte imbalance (hypomagnesemia and hypocalcemia), nephropathy, or hyponatremia secondary to syndrome of inappropriate anti-diuretic hormone secretion (SIADH). In almost all reported cases, spontaneous symptom resolution occurs. Limited information exists on recurrence with subsequent doses, but at least one report details readministration of drug without syndrome recurrence.[91]

Cytarabine

Encephalopathy is a well-recognized complication of high-dose intravenous cytarabine (ara-C). In contrast, intrathecal cytarabine-mediated encephalopathy is uncommon.[92] Symptoms ranging from an altered level of consciousness to coma have been reported.[93–95] Focal neurologic deficits may accompany diffuse cerebral symptomatology, including visual loss, anosmia, hemiparesis, and myelopathy. Some have suggested that the appearance of focal neurologic deficits early on in the treatment course may be predictive of those at risk for severe neurotoxicity.[95] Persistent dementia may follow concomitant radiation therapy and high-dose cytarabine.[96]

Fludarabine

A delayed progressive encephalopathy may occur at fludarabine doses greater than 40 mg/m^2 per day.[28] Cortical blindness, dementia, coma, and death can develop. Autopsy shows a diffuse necrotizing leukoencephalopathy. Toxicity may increase when fludarabine is combined with cytarabine.

Multifocal Inflammatory Leukoencephalopathy Associated with 5-Fluorouracil and Levamisole

5-Fluorouracil (5-FU) given in combination with levamisole rarely produces a multifocal inflammatory leukoencephalopathy. Symptom onset generally begins 6 weeks to 5 months after initiation of therapy.[97] Over a period of several weeks, patients develop encephalopathy and focal neurologic deficits such as hemiparesis, ataxia, aphasia, and sensory loss. Acutely, neurologic signs and symptoms correlate with multiple contrast-enhancing periventricular white matter lesions.[98–102] Even though these lesions appear similar radiographically to the acute demyelinating lesions of multiple sclerosis, in the cancer population, they may be mistaken for brain metastases or infectious etiologies. In some cases, [201]thallium chloride single photon emission computed tomography may provide a noninvasive method of distinguishing between a malignant and nonmalignant process. In other cases, stereotactic brain biopsy may be necessary to establish a definitive diagnosis. The histopathologic findings are indistinguishable from multiple sclerosis and include areas of demyelination, perivascular lymphocytic infiltration, and relative axonal sparing.[99] Discontinuance of chemotherapy and the provision of corticosteroids results in gradual symptom resolution over weeks to months. Likewise, sequential imaging studies show loss of enhancement followed by a decrease in lesion size.[98,99,103] Continued radiographic improvement was seen for at least 18 months in one reported case.[98] It remains unclear whether or not the combination of 5-FU and levamisole, 5-FU alone, or levamisole alone is causative. Patients rechallenged with 5-FU alone did not experience syndrome recurrence.[104,105] Likewise, there are reports of patients tolerating continued levamisole therapy without 5-FU or with reduced doses of 5-FU.[99] One reported patient deteriorated with continued levamisole therapy.[106] The pathogenesis of this multifocal inflammatory demyelinating syndrome is unknown. Proposed mechanisms include an immune-mediated process, as well as a levamisole-induced cell-mediated reaction to 5-FU-induced direct myelin damage.

Encephalopathy can occur with 5-FU alone, manifesting weeks to months following initiation of 5-FU therapy and quickly resolving after discontinuance of the drug.[107] In addition, there is one report of an acute onset, severe encephalopathy progressing to coma within 72 hours in a patient treated with a 5-FU-based chemotherapy regimen who was later found to have a severe dihydropyrimidine dehydrogenase (DPD) deficiency.[108] Brain MRI was normal. Prompt symptom resolution coincided temporally with the provision of infusional thymidine. DPD is the rate-limiting enzyme responsible for 5-FU catabolism. DPD-deficient patients are often asymptomatic and remain undiagnosed until they present with unusually severe 5-FU mediated toxicities. It is estimated that severe DPD deficiency may occur in as many as 3% of cancer patients.[109,110] As such, patients should be appropriately evaluated for DPD if any untoward side effects of 5-FU manifest.

Interferons

Most CNS toxicities are seen with Interferon-α (IFN-α) and IFN-γ. Neurobehavioral symptoms are the most common. Typically within the first week of therapy, patients manifest somnolence, personality changes, cognitive slowing, and headache.[111] Symptoms appear to be dose-related, although age may also be a predisposing factor.[112,113] Imaging studies are often normal, but may demonstrate periventricular white matter changes or non-specific white matter changes.[111] Electroencephalography demonstrates diffuse slow wave activity.[114] Typically symptoms resolve without any specific intervention; however, some patients demonstrate persistent or progressive neurobehavioral symptoms.[115,116]

Interleukins

High doses of IL-2 and IL-1 have been associated with a mild diffuse encephalopathy characterized by headache, depressed mood, delusions, hallucinations, and mild cognitive dysfunction. Symptoms completely resolve within several weeks of the discontinuance of therapy. More significant, however, is the rare recognition of a severe leukoencephalopathy following intraventricular or intravenous IL-2 treatment. The pathogenesis is unknown, but IL-2–stimulated release of neuroendocrine hormones and cytokines has been implicated.[117]

Reversible Posterior Leukoencephalopathy Syndrome

Reversible posterior leukoencephalopathy syndrome (RPLS) is a reversible encephalopathy with distinct clinico-radiographic features. It is characterized by subacute onset of headache, cortical blindness, altered mental status, and seizures associated with symmetrical parieto-occipital region white matter edema. Hypertension inconsistently heralds symptom onset. There is increasing recognition of RPLS as a complication of hematopoietic stem cell transplantation in both childhood and adult cancers. In addition, there are case reports of RPLS in adults during cytotoxic chemotherapy with single-agent[90,118] and multiple-agent chemotherapeutic regimens [119–121] utilizing cisplatin, cytarabine, doxorubicin, cyclophosphamide, vincristine, ifosfamide, and etoposide. RPLS has not been linked with a particular drug or mode of drug administration. This entity is also recognized with non-oncologic diagnoses such as renal failure, acute hypertension, fluid overload, eclampsia, and immunosuppressive drug therapy.[122,123] The primary mechanism is thought to be loss of cerebral autoregulatory vascular control with subsequent microvascular infarction, petechial hemorrhage, and fluid transudation. Control of hypertension, cerebral edema, and other inciting factors leads to complete or near complete symptom resolution within days to weeks.

Cognitive Dysfunction

A growing body of literature supports the hypothesis that adult cancer patients experience cognitive deficits associated with cancer treatments including cranial irradiation, conventional chemotherapy, high-dose chemotherapy and hematopoietic transplantation, and biologic response modifiers. Patients often use the term "chemobrain" to describe their symptoms. The majority of published studies focus on the cognitive effects of adjuvant chemotherapy or high-dose chemotherapy with stem cell transplantation for the treatment of breast cancer. These retrospective, post-chemotherapy reports identify a subgroup of patients in which cognitive decline could be attributable to chemotherapy. The reported incidence of chemotherapy-related cognitive dysfunction in these studies ranges from 16 to 75%. Cognitive deficits may be seen during or shortly after treatment [124–126], approximately 2 years following treatment [127–129], and 10 years following completion of therapy.[130] The development of cognitive deficits has not been linked to a particular drug. Cisplatin may have a long-term effect on cognitive function.[131] In addition, implicated breast cancer regimens consist of numerous chemotherapeutic agents, including 5-fluorouracil, epirubicin, cyclophosphamide, thiotepa, carboplatin, methotrexate, doxorubicin, paclitaxel, and vinblastine.

In four small studies of women receiving chemotherapy for breast cancer utilizing the High Sensitivity Cognitive Screen, the incidence of moderate or severe cognitive dysfunction ranged from 16 to 50%.[126–129] Memory and concentration appear to be especially vulnerable to the effects of cancer therapy; however, subtle dysfunction has been reported in several cognitive domains, including verbal and nonverbal memory, information processing speed, and visuospatial processing. Patients receiving chemotherapy consistently score lower on performance tests compared to patients treated with local therapy. However, even so, they generally score within the normal range when compared with published norms. As such, while meaningful to an individual patient, the cognitive effects of chemotherapy are relatively subtle.

Few prospective studies have been reported. No differences in Mini Mental Status Examination (MMSE) scores were seen in one heterogeneous cancer patient group comparing pretreatment and approximately 4 months into treatment.[132] However, the MMSE is a screening measure designed to capture fairly gross cognitive dysfunction, such as dementia, and is not sensitive to subtle cognitive abnormalities. One prospective, randomized, longitudinal trial evaluated formal neuropsychometric testing prechemotherapy, and at 1- and 2-year intervals following chemotherapy. Overall, the reported results were consistent with previously reported conclusions that a subgroup of patients do experience subtle, but meaningful cognitive decline following chemotherapy.

The mechanism by which chemotherapy causes subtle cognitive deficits is unknown, and may differ from one chemotherapeutic agent to another. Likewise, it is uncertain if a particular chemotherapy drug or specific combinations of drugs are causative. Cognitive deficits might be attributable to a direct toxic effect on cerebral gray and white matter, microvascular injury, or secondary injury as a consequence an immunologic-mediated inflammatory response stimulated by the chemotherapy agent(s).

Drowsiness

Numerous chemotherapy drugs are associated with drowsiness and fatigue. However, it is often unclear whether or not these symptoms reflect inherent drug effect, or the side effects from a multitude of confounding factors. In some cases, the drug is clearly causative. Thalidomide is the prototypic example. Somnolence is the most common acute side effect of thalidomide, noted in approximately 50% of patients. This dose-dependent symptom is generally mild and may be ameliorated by timing drug administration near bedtime. Many patients develop tachyphylaxis to this side effect after 2 to 3 weeks of therapy. Rebound insomnia after cessation of thalidomide has been reported.[133]

Seizures

Chemotherapy-related seizures may occur as an isolated symptom or as part of a generalized encephalopathy. They may represent a direct effect of the drug, or result from a drug-induced metabolic derangement or a chemotherapy drug-anticonvulsant medication interaction. Seizures may accompany chemotherapy-induced aseptic meningitis. In addition, they have been reported in association with intra-arterial chemotherapy injection. Structural brain lesions and a preexisting history of seizures are risk factors. However, in this setting, the contribution of the chemotherapeutic agent(s) is often unclear. Seizures have been reported with cisplatin, vincristine,[134] 5-FU,[135] L-asparaginase,[136] cytarabine,[28] and thalidomide.[22]

Most often, seizures are related to metabolic abnormalities. Cisplatin is a notorious cause of metabolic derangements. Approximately 60% of patients receiving cisplatin develop hypomagnesemia and secondary hypocalcemia from impaired magnesium reabsorption in the proximal renal tubule.[137] Hyponatremia secondary to SIADH may occur.[138] In addition, seizures can also result from water intoxication/cerebral edema due to the hydration before and after cisplatin infusion.

Chemotherapeutic agents can also alter the pharmacokinetics of enzyme-inducing anticonvulsant medications. Cisplatin can decrease phenytoin levels, and doxorubicin and cisplatin can reduce carbamazepine and valproic acid levels.[139] Furthermore, 5-FU and high-dose tamoxifen can cause elevations in phenytoin levels and subsequent drug toxicity.[139]

Cerebellar Syndromes

Acute cerebellar syndromes are caused by only a few drugs, mainly cytarabine and 5-fluorouracil. Cerebellar syndromes caused by high dose ara-C and 5-fluorouracil have in common a dose-related incidence, symptom resolution with discontinuance of the drug, and the occasional presence of a transient ocular palsy.

Cytosine Arabinoside (Cytarabine, Ara-C)

High-dose ara-C is associated with an irreversible cerebellar syndrome as well as reversible cerebellar abnormalities. Dose-limiting cerebellar toxicity occurs at cumulative doses exceeding 48 g/m²; however, individual doses > 3g/m² may be more significant than the cumulative dose. Regimens providing 3 g/m² every 12 hours for 8 to 12 doses produce an acute or subacute cerebellar syndrome in 10 to 25% of patients.[93,140,141] Additional risk factors include renal insufficiency,[142] abnormal liver function (elevated transaminase, total bilirubin, or alkaline phophastase),[93] age over 50 years,[93,94] and underlying neurologic dysfunction. Of these, renal insufficiency seems to be the most significant.[142]

Several days after initiating therapy, patients may develop subtle signs of cerebellar dysfunction, including a mildly unsteady gait, nystagmus, or other oculomotor abnormalities. Extracerebellar symptoms including somnolence, confusion, and, rarely, seizures may precede or coincide with the initial cerebellar dysfunction. If treatment is continued, progressive and potentially disabling gait ataxia, appendicular ataxia, and dysarthria may develop. Following cessation of ara-C, maximal symptom recovery occurs within two weeks. The degree of recovery is inversely proportional to the severity and extent of cerebellar symptoms seen. Patients with a full cerebellar syndrome or significant disability, generally have irreversible symptoms. Conversely, if only some features of a full cerebellar syndrome develop and symptoms are mild, complete symptom recovery is often seen. If no significant cerebellar toxicity is seen, a second course can be safely administered.[93] Imaging studies may initially show white matter abnormalities within the cerebellum, and later demonstrate cerebellar atrophy. Pathologically, Purkinje cell dropout, loss of neurons in the dentate nucleus, and proliferation of Bergmann cells is seen.[140]

5-Fluorouracil

5-Fluorouracil–induced neurotoxicity is rare with conventional drug dosing. However, with high-dose therapy (> 15 mg/kg/week), an acute cerebellar syndrome indistinguishable from that produced by ara-C is seen in approximately 2% of patients.[143] The concomitant provision of allopurinol, N-phosphonoacetyl-L-aspartate (PALA), thymidine, and levamisole may enhance 5-FU neurotoxicity.[28] Symptoms generally manifest weeks to months following initiation of chemotherapy and are reversible with discontinuation of the drug or a reduction in the dosage. If additional 5-FU is provided, symptoms may recur.[144,145]

Movement Disorders

Movement disorders are rarely reported in conjunction with chemotherapeutic agents. 5-Fluorouracil may cause focal dystonia and parkinsonian symptoms, likely due to basal ganglia dysfunction.[146,147] Reversible athetosis, ataxia, and parkinsonian symptoms have been reported following vincristine administration.[148,149] Additionally, one patient who received high doses of cytarabine developed a parkinsonian syndrome that resolved within 12 weeks of drug discontinuance.[150] Cytarabine is also associated with painful leg, moving toes syndrome.[28]

Visual Symptoms

There is increasing recognition of eye and visual pathway toxicity from chemotherapeutic agents. Of the orbital structures, the retina seems particularly vulnerable; but chemotherapy-related toxicity can involve any component of the eye. Visual toxicity often accompanies more widespread cerebral dysfunction, manifesting as visual field deficits or cortical blindness. Intrathecal drug administration is associated with optic neuropathy. In addition, retinopathy is a prominent complication of intracarotid drug administration. Visual complications range from transient eye irritation to irreversible blindness. When studied prospectively, subclinical abnormalities are often reported. This underscores the need for surveillance ophthalmologic examinations in patients receiving drugs with known ocular toxicity. Overall, the majority of ocular symptoms are mild, and, often, visual function is maintained following treatment.

Cisplatin

Intravenous cisplatin rarely causes papilledema, retrobulbar neuritis, or retinal cone dysfunction.[151,152] In addition, the focal neurologic symptoms seen with cisplatin-induced encephalopathy may include homonymous hemianopia and cortical blindness. More commonly, visual symptoms complicate intra-arterial cisplatin infusion.

Intra-arterial infusion of cisplatin into the common carotid artery produces cranial neuropathies in approximately 6% of patients.[153] Any cranial nerve may be affected by itself or in combination. Ocular toxicity is in part contingent upon placement of the intra-arterial catheter. If drug is delivered proximal to the origin of the ophthalmic artery (infraophthalmic), clinically significant ipsilateral visual loss occurs in up to 60% of cases.[86] Ipsilateral and, sometimes, bilateral retinal infarcts and frank retinal necrosis may occur.[86]. There is one report of a patient developing a cavernous sinus syndrome following intra-arterial cisplatin infusion.[85] Supraophthalmic intra-arterial carotid drug delivery spares ocular complications, but is associated with cerebral toxicity. Visual symptoms are particularly common and include cortical blindness and visual field deficits. Additional complications include headache (HA), confusion, and seizures.[154] Many patients will recover within a few weeks; however, some patients remain blind or have permanent visual field deficits.

Nitrosureas

Oral lomustine (CCNU) when used in conjunction with low-dose cranial irradiation and/or possibly multi-agent chemotherapeutic regimens, may cause damage to ocular structures. Patients generally present with sudden-onset total blindness followed in a few weeks by optic atrophy. Pathology from one reported case showed severe demyelination, axonal loss, and hyalinized vessels. Ocular structure damage due to low-dose cranial irradiation is exceedingly rare, further implicating CCNU as contributing factor.[68]

Retinal infarcts can occur following high-dose intravenous or intracarotid carmustine (BCNU). The mechanism is likely fibrinoid necrosis of vessels and necrotizing vasculitis.[84,88,155]

5-Fluorouracil

5-FU can cause oculomotor abnormalities, in particular vergence disturbances, and optic neuropathy.[111,156] Symptoms generally precede the development of typical features of 5-FU cerebellar neurotoxicity. Patients present with diplopia attributable to poor fusional capacity as a consequence of convergence and divergence weakness. Extraocular muscle paresis may occur later in the clinical course. Discontinuance of drug facilitates complete or near complete recovery in most patients. Recurrent oculomotor abnormalities may occur if additional 5-FU is provided.[156] Generally, each subsequent episode increases in severity and duration. Symptoms likely represent 5-FU–mediated neurotoxicity at the level of the brainstem.[156] Additional ocular toxicities include a presumed toxic optic neuropathy. Fluorocitrate, a breakdown product of 5-FU metabolism and potent inhibitor of Krebs cycle, has been implicated in the pathogenesis of this syndrome.[157]

Cyclophosphamide

Blurring of vision, interfering with a patient's ability to read, can occur minutes to hours following the provision of high-dose cyclophosphamide therapy.[158] Recovery generally mirrors time to onset, and complete symptom resolution is seen hours to days. Continuation of cyclophosphamide therapy does not result in symptom recurrence. No abnormalities have been detected on ophthalmologic examination, but often symptoms have resolved prior to evaluation.

Cytarabine

Cytarabine rarely produces reversible ocular toxicity, including blurred vision, photophobia, burning eye pain, blindness, Horner syndrome, and reversible bilateral lateral rectus palsies. Optic nerve damage from intrathecally administered cytarabine, when severe, can result in blindness.

Vincristine

Visual loss is occasionally reported when vincristine is used in conjunction with multiple chemotherapeutic agents.[159–162] In addition, vincristine may cause cortical blindness.[163] Spontaneous recovery was seen in all of the reported cases. However, one patient developed recurrent symptoms with repeated vincristine administration.

Methotrexate

High-dose, intrathecal methotrexate therapy, often in conjunction with cranial irradiation and/or multiple chemotherapeutic agents, may produce visual loss.[164–166] No cases have been reported with intravenous methotrexate.

Tamoxifen

Infrequently, tamoxifen produces ocular toxicity involving the cornea, retina, or optic nerve. Ocular symptoms are more common in patients treated with high daily doses or high cumulative tamoxifen doses, but have been reported with standard doses as well.[167] Symptoms may be reversible if recognized early on in the disease process.

High-dose Multidrug Chemotherapy

High-dose multidrug chemotherapy regimens provided with hematopoietic stem cell support, in particular in breast cancer patients, have been associated with cognitive dysfunction and ophthalmologic disorders, including retinopathy, optic neuritis, and, rarely, cortical blindness.[81] Patients report decreased visual acuity, visual field abnormalities, or frank visual loss. Ocular symptoms can involve one or both eyes simultaneously or sequentially.[81]

Hearing Loss

Cisplatin

Cisplatin commonly produces dose-dependent ototoxicity due to peripheral receptor (hair cell) loss in the organ of Corti. Transient tinnitus is often the first symptom to appear, but persistent tinnitus is uncommon, affecting only about 7% of patients.[168] Subclinical high-frequency hearing loss (4,000 to 8,000 hertz[Hz]) is detected by audiometry in approximately 70% of patients. However, symptomatic hearing loss within frequencies important for speech discrimination (500 to 3,000 Hz) is less frequent, occurring in roughly 10% of patients.[168].

Prior cranial irradiation,[169] concurrent provision of ototoxic drugs,[168,170] young age, and the presence of a CNS neoplasm potentiate cisplatin-induced hearing loss. The risk of substantial hearing loss is proportional to the cumulative cisplatin dose, and is nominal at cumulative doses < 540 mg/m². [169,171] Furthermore, the presence of high-frequency hearing loss is fairly predictive of the risk of hearing loss within speech frequencies. If high-frequency hearing loss is present, a patient is at substantial risk of developing symptomatic hearing loss with the provision of two to four additional courses of cisplatin if no cranial irradiation has been provided, or with the provision of one additional course of cisplatin if the patient was previously treated with cranial irradiation.[169] As such, routine hearing screening is recommended at doses exceeding 360 mg/m².[171] Recovery of hearing loss is unlikely[169,171]; however,

acceptable hearing thresholds can often be achieved with hearing aids. Thus, the development of ototoxicity does not necessarily mandate discontinuance of cisplatin therapy in those patients with clear anti-tumor benefit from the drug.

Cisplatin may also cause a vestibulopathy, which may or may not be associated with hearing loss. Symptoms include vertigo and ataxia. Patients frequently complain of difficulty walking in the dark and on uneven surfaces. Patients with abnormal or asymmetric vestibular function prior to initiating chemotherapy may be particularly at risk.[172] Vestibulopathy seems to be cumulative-dose–dependent with the greatest risk occurring at cumulative doses > 400 mg/m².[172] Prior use of aminoglycosides may exacerbate the vestibulopathy.[168,172]

Aseptic Meningitis

Aseptic meningitis is a well-recognized and usually transient complication of intra-cerebrospinal fluid (intra-CSF) chemotherapy. It has also been reported following intravenous cytarabine.[28] This side effect occurs in 5 to 40% of patients after intra-CSF methotrexate administration, and in approximately 10% of patients following intra-CSF cytarabine administration. Symptoms are more frequent following lumbar injection compared to intrathecal injection. Symptoms of headache, nuchal rigidity, back pain, nausea or emesis, fever, and lethargy generally manifest 2 to 4 hours after intra-CSF drug administration and last 12 to 72 hours. Seizures and subacute encephalopathy are rarely seen.[92,173] Aseptic meningitis may follow the first, or any subsequent, intra-CSF drug injection, although, once it occurs, patients usually do not experience difficulty with continued injections. CSF evaluation reveals a lymphocytic pleocytosis and elevated protein. This syndrome differentiates itself from bacterial meningitis by time of onset relative to injection. Once symptoms occur, only supportive care is indicated. However, the concurrent provision of corticosteroids, either injected intrathecally with the chemotherapeutic agent or orally is preventative.

Stroke and Other Vascular Complications

Cerebrovascular complications of chemotherapy may be the result of a direct toxic insult to blood vessels, or represent an indirect effect of chemotherapy on the vascular system. For instance, doxorubicin-induced cardiomyopathy and subsequent thrombus formation can lead to stroke. Stroke is most commonly seen in the setting of multidrug regimens, making it difficult to determine the primary culprit. The pathogenic mechanisms appear quite diverse, and in many cases unknown.

Cisplatin

Cisplatin has been associated with vascular toxicity including myocardial infarction, cerebrovascular ischemic events, hypertension, and Raynaud's phenomenon. Vascular complications are most common when cisplatin is administered in combination with other agents, but they have also been reported following cisplatin monotherapy.[174–178] Some patients present during the course of chemotherapy. However, in others, strokes occur months following completion of therapy.[178] Angiograms may be normal or show focal vessel occlusion. It is unclear whether vascular toxicity results from cisplatin-induced endothelial injury, hypomagnesemia-induced vasospasm, or coagulopathy. Other agents provided concomitantly with cisplatin as part of multidrug regimens may also contribute to vascular toxicity.

Carmustine

Intra-arterial infusion of BCNU is associated with a vasculopathy of the carotid, ophthalmic, retinal, and choroidal arteries, with arterial emboli or thrombosis, or both, in up to 80% of patients.[85]

L-Asparaginase

Cerebral venous and dural sinus thrombosis, cerebral venous infarction, and/or cerebral hemorrhage occur in 1 to 2% of patients treated with L-asparaginase.[179] Arterial infarcts are notably absent.[179,180] These vascular complications are more frequent at higher drug doses; however, a clear dose-dependency has not been established. L-asparaginase hydrolyzes asparagine to aspartic acid, depleting asparagine and inhibiting protein synthesis. This leads to the depletion of plasma proteins, including those involved in coagulation (anti-thrombin III, protein C and S, fibrinogen, and factors IX and XI) and fibrinolysis (plasminogen).[181] Elevation of serum prothrombin time (PT), partial thrombin time (PTT), and thrombin time is routinely seen during treatment in most patients but is not thought to have clinical significance.[180] Hemorrhagic events generally occur early on in the course of therapy, and thrombotic events are typically seen after 5 days to several weeks of therapy.[179] On occasion, thrombotic complications do not manifest until treatment is completed. Presenting signs and symptoms of cerebral venous and dural sinus thrombosis include severe headaches, seizures, altered mental status, focal neurologic deficits, and papilledema. Routine imaging studies may implicate venous sinus thrombosis or demonstrate secondary complications, such as venous infarcts or cerebral hemorrhage. However, definitive diagnosis is typically established by CT venogram or MR venogram demonstrating clot in cerebral sinuses.

Treatment is controversial. In the absence of hemorrhage, most recommend heparin anticoagulation, but others provide fresh frozen plasma to prevent clot extension.[179,181] Most patients, even those with cerebral hemorrhage, fully recover.[179] No patient has ever been reported to have a second cerebrovascular event with continued L-asparaginase therapy, either with or without prophylactic pretreatment, but many propose prophylactic pretreatment with fresh frozen plasma or heparin.

Bleomycin

Bleomycin, especially when used as part of a cisplatin-based chemotherapy regimen, has been rarely associated with delayed cerebral and myocardial infarcts. It is unclear which drug is specifically at fault, although bleomycin is thought to be the main culprit. The specific mechanism is unknown, although hypomagnesemia may be a risk factor.[28]

Other Chemotherapy Agents

Other chemotherapeutic agents have been rarely associated with cerebrovascular disorders. Cerebral infarcts are rarely reported with 5-fluorouracil.[182] Likewise, there is one reported case of carboplatin-induced thrombotic microangiopathy that resulted in numerous small cortical infarcts, coma, and death.[28] Necrosis and hemorrhagic cerebral infarcts occasionally follow intracarotid doxorubicin injection when provided in conjunction with osmotic blood-brain-barrier opening.[28]

Spinal Cord Syndromes

Lhermitte's Sign

Lhermitte's sign, characterized by paresthesias or electrical shock–like sensations in the back and extremities precipitated by neck flexion, is seen in 20 to 40% of patients receiving cisplatin. In some cases, arm abduction precipitates distal paresthesias, suggesting traction on a demyelinated brachial plexus.[28] Symptoms typically develop during or after several weeks of treatment.[183] A sensory neuropathy often precedes the development of Lhermitte's sign. Rare reports of myelopathy exist.[184] Proposed mechanisms include transient demyelination of the posterior columns[170] or toxic insult to the central processes of the dorsal root ganglion cells, which travel in the dorsal columns.[181] Lhermitte's phenomenon is generally not associated with chemotherapeutic agents other than cisplatin, although two patients did develop Lhermitte's sign following docetaxel administration.[37]

Myelopathy

One of the most emphasized complications of intrathecal chemotherapy is myelopathy, which is reported for both methotrexate and ara-C, either alone or in combination. Even though this complication is rare, it has the potential for severe and persistent neurologic disability and even death. In fact, the provision of intrathecal vincristine is contraindicated due to the occurrence of fatal myeloencephalopathy.[185]

Methotrexate   Methotrexate-induced myelopathy is generally seen following several intrathecal treatments. Symptoms typically manifest half an hour to 48 hours following intrathecal drug, but can be delayed for 2 weeks.[186] Clinically, patients present with back or leg pain, followed by progressive weakness of the legs, ascending sensory loss, and sphincter dysfunction. In severe cases, progressive quadriplegia, brainstem dysfunction, and death can occur. Concurrent provision of radiation, presence of active CNS leukemia, or frequent MTX treatments appear to increase risk. Gadolinium enhancement of the anterior nerve roots of the cauda equina has been reported in three patients presenting with progressive, flaccid weakness of the lower extremities.[187] Elevated CSF IgG synthesis and myelin basic protein has been reported.[187,188] Symptoms are often transient, but variable clinical improvement is seen.[189,190] The pathologic changes are maximal in the outer one-third of the spinal cord, similar to the expected penetration of intrathecal drug. Vacuolar myelin loss, axonal swelling, and necrosis in the absence of inflammation is reported.[191] The pathogenesis is unknown, but may be an idiosyncratic drug reaction.[28]

Cytarabine   Rarely, intrathecal cytarabine administration causes a transverse myelopathy identical to that seen with intrathecal methotrexate. Symptoms present acutely generally weeks to months following initiation of intrathecal cytarabine.[192] In two reported cases, clinical symptoms and pathologic changes extended beyond the spinal cord into the brainstem producing a locked-in syndrome in one patient[193] and edema, cerebrospinal fluid outflow obstruction, and a herniation syndrome in another patient.[188] Risk factors for the development of myelopathy include concurrent intravenous ara-C, prior or concurrent intrathecal (IT) MTX, or prior or concurrent radiation therapy to the spinal cord, and daily drug administration.[92] Most patients recover spontaneously, but symptoms may be irreversible and fatalities have been reported.[92,192–195] Histopathologically, widespread spinal cord and nerve root demyelination, white matter microvascuolization, and axonal swelling are seen.[192,196,197]

REFERENCES

1. Molloy FM, Floeter MK, Syed NA, et al. Thalidomide neuropathy in patients treated for metastatic prostate cancer. Muscle Nerve 2001;24:1050–7.
2. Riggs JE, Ashraf M, Snyder RD, et al. Prospective nerve conduction studies in cisplatin therapy. Ann Neurol 1988;23: 92–4.

3. Boogerd W, Ten Bokkel Huinink WW, Dalesio O, et al. Cisplatin-induced neuropathy: central, peripheral, and autonomic nerve involvement. J Neurooncol 1990;9: 255–63.

4. Gregg RW, Molepo JM, Monpetit VJA, et al. Cisplatin neurotoxicity: the relationship between dosage, time and platinum concentration in neurologic tissues and morphologic evidence of toxicity. J Clin Oncol 1992;10: 795–803.

5. Roelofs RI, Hruskesky W, Rogin J, Rosenberg L. Peripheral sensory neuropathy and cisplatin chemotherapy. Neurology 1984;34:934–8.

6. Lomonaco M, Milone M, Batocchli AP, et al. Cisplatin neuropathy: clinical course and neurophysiological findings. J Neurol 1992;239:199–204.

7. Siegal T, Haim N. Cisplatin-induced peripheral neuropathy: frequent off-therapy deterioration, demyelinating syndromes, and muscle cramps. Cancer 1990;15: 1117–23.

8. Rosenfeld CS, Broder LE. Cisplatin-induced autonomic neuropathy. Cancer Treat Rep 1984;68:659–60.

9. Cohen SC, Mollman JE. Cisplatin-induced gastric paresis. J Neurol Oncol 1987;5:237–40.

10. Gregg RW, Molepo JM, Monpetit VJ, et al. Cisplatin neurotoxicity: the relationship between dosage, time, and platinum concentration in neurologic tissues, and morphologic evidence of toxicity. J Clin Oncol 1992;10: 795–803.

11. Gormley PE, Gangji D, Wood JH, et al. Pharmacokinetic study of cerebrospinal fluid penetration of cis-diamminedichloroplatinum II. Cancer Chemother Pharmacol 1981;5:257–60.

12. van den Bent MJ, van Putten WL, Hilkens PH, et al. Retreatment with dose-dense weekly cisplatin after previous cisplatin chemotherapy is not complicated by significant neurotoxicity. Eur J Cancer 2002;38:387–91.

13. Gerritsen van der Hoop R, Vecht CJ, van der Burg ME, et al. Prevention of cisplatin neurotoxicity with an ACTH(4-9) analogue in patients with ovarian cancer. N Engl J Med 1990;322:89–94.

14. Neijt J, van der Burg M, Vecht C, et al. A double-blind randomized study with Org 2766, an ACTH(4-9) analog, to prevent cisplatin neuropathy [abstract A827]. Proc ASCO 1994:13:261.

15. Cascinu S, Cordella L, Del Ferro E, et al. Neuroprotective effect of reduced glutathione on cisplatin-based chemotherapy in advanced gastric cancer: a randomized double-blind placebo-controlled trial. J Clin Oncol 1995;13: 26–32.

16. Kemp G, Rose P, Lurain J, et al. Amifostine pretreatment for protection against cyclophosphamide-induced and cisplatin-induced toxicities: results of a randomized control trial in patients with advanced ovarian cancer. J Clin Oncol 1996;14:2101–12

17. Rick O, Beyer J, Schwella N, et al. Assessment of amifostine as protection from chemotherapy-induced toxicities after conventional-dose and high-dose chemotherapy in patients with germ cell tumor. Ann Oncol 2001;12: 1151–1155.

18. Gradishar WJ, Stephenson P, Glover DJ, et al. A phase II trial of cisplatin plus WR-2721 (Amifostine) for metastatic breast carcinoma: an Eastern Coooperative Oncology Group Study (E8188). Cancer 2001;92:2517–22.

19. Brienza S, Vignoud J, Itzhaki M, et al. Oxaliplatin (L-OHP): Global safety in 682 patients. Proc Am Soc Clin Oncol 1995;14:209 (abstr 513) Eckel F, Schmelz R, Adelsberger H, et al. Prevention of oxaliplatin-induced neuropathy by carbamazepine: a pilot study. Dtsch Med Wochenschr 2002;127:78–82.

20. Schmelz R, Adelsberger H, et al. Prevention of oxaliplatin-induced neuropathy by carbamazepine: a pilot study. Dtsch Med Wochenschr 2002;127:78–82.

21. Wilson RH, Lehky T, Thomas RR, et al. Acute oxaliplatin-induced peripheral nerve hyperexcitability. J Clin Oncol 2002;20:1767–74.

22. Dimopoulos MA, Eleutherakis-Papaiakovou V. Adverse effectse of thalidomide administration in patients with neoplastic disease. Am J Med 2004;117:508–15.

23. Offidani M, Corvatta L, Marconi M, et al. Common and rare side-effects of low-dose thalidomide in multiple myeloma: focus on the dose-minimizing peripheral neuropathy. Eur J Haematol 2004;72:403–409.

24. Bastuji-Garin S, Ochonisky S, Bouche P, et al. Incidence and risk factors for thalidomide neuropathy: a prospective study of 135 dermatologic patients. J Invest Dermatol 2002;119:1020–6.

25. Giannini F, Volpi N, Rossi S, et al. Thalidomide-induced neuropathy: a gangliopathy? Neurology 2003;60:877–8.

26. Chaudhry V, Cornblath DR, Corse A, et al. Thalidomide-induced neuropathy. Neurology 2002;59:1872–5.

27. Haim N, Epelbaum R, Ben-Shahar M, et al. Full dose vincristine (without 2-mg dose limit) in the treatment of lymphomas. Cancer 1994;15:2515–9.

28. Posner JB. Side effects of chemotherapy. In: Neurologic Complications of Cancer. Philadelphia: FA Davis; 1995. p. 282–310.

29. Delaney P. Vincristine-induced laryngeal nerve paralysis. Neurology 1982;32:1285–8.

30. Sandler SG, Tobin W, Henderson ES. Vincristine-induced neuropathy: a clinical study of fifty leukemic patients. Neurology 1969;19:367–74.

31. Lugassy G, Shapira A. Sensorineural hearing loss associated with vincristine treatment. Blut 1990;61:320–1.

32. Legha SS. Vincristine neurotoxicity. Pathophysiology and management. Med Toxicol 1986;1:421–7.

33. Naumann R, Mohm J, Reuner U, et al. Early recognition of hereditary motor and sensory neuropathy type I can avoid life-threatening vincristine neurotoxicity. Br J Haematol 2001;115:323–5.

34. Postma TJ, Benard BA, Huijgens PC, et al. Long term effects of vincristine on the peripheral nervous system. J Neurooncol 1993;15:23–7.

35. Lipton RB, Apfel SC, Dutcher JP, et al. Taxol produces a predominantly sensory neuropathy. Neurology 1989;39: 368–73.

36. van Gerven JM, Moll JW, van den Bent MJ, et al. Paclitaxel (taxol) induces cumulative mild neurotoxicity. Eur J Cancer 1994;30A:1074–7.

37. Hilkens PHE, Verweij J, Stoter G, et al. Peripheral neurotoxicity induced by docetaxel. Neurology 1996;46: 104–8.

38. Trimble EL, Adams JD, Vena D, et al. Paclitaxel for platinum-refractory ovarian cancer; results from the first 100 patients registered to National Cancer Institute Treatment Referral Center 9103. J Clin Oncol 1993;11: 2405–10.

39. Sarosy G, Kohn E, Stone DA, et al. Phase I study of Taxol and granulocyte colony-stimulating factor in patients with refractory ovarian cancer. J Clin Oncol 1992;10:1165–70.

40. Schiller JH, Storer B, Tutsch K, et al. Phase I trial of 3-hour infusion of paclitaxel with or without granulocyte colony-stimulating factor in patients with advanced cancer. J Clin Oncol 1994;12:241–8.

41. Schaumburg HH, Spencer PS. Toxic neuropathies. Neurology 1979;29:429–31.

42. Freilich R, Balmaceda C, Seidman A, et al. Motor neuropathy due to docetaxel and paclitaxel. Neurology 1996;47: 115–8.

43. Lorenz E, Hagen B, Himmelmann A, et al. A phase II study of biweekly administration of paclitaxel with recurrent epithelial ovarian cancer. Int J Gynecol Cancer 1999;9: 373–6.

44. Jerian SM, Sarosy GA, Link CJ, et al. Incapacitating autonomic neuropathy precipitated by taxol. Gynecol Oncol 1993:51:277–80.

45. Kaplan JG, Einzig AI, Schaumburg HH. Taxol causes permanent large fiber peripheral nerve dysfunction: a lesson for preventative strategies. J Neurooncol 1993;16:105–107.

46. Kane RC, Bross PF, Farrell AT, Pazdur R. Velcade: U.S. FDA approval for the treatment of multiple myeloma progressing on prior therapy. Oncologist 2003;8:508–13.

47. Imrie KR, Couture F, Turner CC, et al. Peripheral neuropathy following high-dose etoposide and autologous bone marrow transplantation. Bone Marrow Transplant 1994;13:77–9.

48. Curtin JP, Koonings PP, Gutierrez M, et al. Ifosfamide-induced neurotoxicity. Gynecol Oncol 1991; 42:193–6.

49. Meanwell CA, Blake AE, Kelly KA, et al. Prediction of ifosfamide/mesna associated encephalopathy. Eur J Cancer Clin Oncol 1986;22:815–9.

50. Zalupski M, Baker LH. Ifosfamide. J Natl Cancer Inst 1988; 80:556–66.

51. Pratt CB, Goren MP, Horowitz ME, et al. Central nervous system toxicity following treatment of pediatric patients with ifosfamide/mesna. J Clin Oncol 1986;4:1253–61.

52. Watkin SW, Husband DJ, Green JA, et al. Ifosfamide encephalopathy: a reappraisal. Eur J Cancer 1989;25: 1303–10.

53. Verdeguer A, Castel V, Esquembre C, et al. Fatal encephalopathy with ifosfamide/mesna. Pediatr Hematol Oncol 1989;6:383–5.

54. Shuper A, Stein J, Goshen J, et al. Subacute central nervous system degeneration in a child: an unusual manifestation of ifosfamide intoxication. J Child Neurol 2000;15: 481–3.

55. Chastagner P, Sommelet-Olive D, Kalifa C, et al. Phase II study of ifosfamide in childhood brain tumors: a report by the French Society of Pediatric Oncology (SFOP). Med Pediatr Oncol 1993;21:49–53.

56. Ghosn M, Carde P, Leclerq B, et al. Ifosfamide/mesna related encephalopathy: a case report with a possible role of Phenobarbital in enhancing neurotoxicity. Bull Cancer 1988;75:391–2.

57. Nieto Y, Cagnoni PJ, Bearman SI, et al. Acute encephalopathy: a new toxicity associated with high dose paclitaxel. Clin Cancer Res 1999;5:501–6.

58. Filley CM. Toxic leukoencephalopathy. Clin Neuropharmacol 1999;22:249–60.

59. Asato R, Akiyama Y, Ito M, et al. Nuclear magnetic resonance abnormalities of the cerebral white matter in children with acute lymphoblastic leukemia and malignant lymphoma during and after central nervous system prophylactic treatment with intrathecal methotrexate. Cancer 1992;70:1997–2004.

60. Mahoney DH, Shuster JJ, Nitschke R, et al. Acute neurotoxicity in children with B-precursor acute lymphoid leukemia: an association with intermediate-dose intravenous methotrexate and intrathecal triple therapy – a Pediatric Oncology Group study. J Clin Oncol 1998;16:1712–22.

61. Moore-Maxwell CA, Datto MB, Hulette CH. Chemotherapy-induced toxic leukoencephalopathy causes a wide range of symptoms: a series of four autopsies. Modern Pathology 2004;17:241–7.

62. Lemann W, Wiley RG, Posner JB. Leukoencephalopathy complicating intraventricular catheters: clinical, radiographic and pathologic study of 10 cases. J Neurooncol 1988;6:67–74.

63. Filley CM, Kleinschmidt-DeMasters BK. Toxic leukoencephalopaty. N Engl J Med 2001;345:425–32.

64. Lee S, Kim M. Diffusion-weighted MRIs in an acute leuko-encephalpathy following intrathecal chemotherapy. Meurology 2004;62:832–3.

65. Winick NJ, Bowman WP, Kamen BA, et al. Unexpected acute neurologic toxicity in the treatment of children with acute lymphoblastic leukemia. J Natl Cancer Inst 1992;84: 252–6.

66. Jaffe N, Takaue Y, Anzai T, Robertson R. Transient neurologic disturbances induced by high-dose methotrexate treatment. Cancer 1985;56:1356–60.

67. Rubnitz JE, Relling MV, Harrison PL, et al. Transient encephalopathy following high-dose methotrexate treatment in childhood acute lymphoblastic leukemia. Leukemia 1998;12:1176–81.

68. Wilson DA, Nitschke R, Bowman ME, et al. Transient white matter changes on MR images in children undergoing chemotherapy for acute lymphocytic leukemia. Radiology 1991;180:205–9.

69. Lien HH, Blomlie V, Saeter G, et al. Osteogenic sarcoma: MR signal abnormalities of the brain in asymptomatic patients treated with high-dose methotrexate. Radiology 1991;179: 547–50.

70. Pääkko E, Vainionpää L, Lanning M, et al. White matter changes in children treated for acute lymphoblastic leukemia. Cancer 1992;70:2728–33.

71. Ebner F, Ranner G, Slavic I, et al. MR findings in methotrexate-induced CNS abnormalities. AJR Am J Roentgenol 1989;153:1283–8.

72. Allen JC, Rosen G, Mehta BM, Horten B. Leukoencephalopathy following high-dose IV methotrexate chemotherapy with leucovorin resuce. Cancer Treatm Rep 1980; 64:1261–73.

73. Phillips PC. Methotrexate toxicity. In: Neurological complications of cancer treatment. Rottenberg DA, editor. Boston: Butterworth-Heinemann; 1991. p. 115–34.

74. Bernini JC, Fort DW, Griener JC, et al. Aminophylline for methotrexate-induced neurotoxicity. Lancet 1995;345: 544–7.

75. Oka M, Terae S, Kobayashi R, et al. MRI in methotrexate-related leukoencephalopathy: disseminated necrotizing leukoencephalopathy in comparison with mild leukoencephalopathy. Neurorad 2003;45:493–7.

76. Glass JP, Lee YY, Bruner J, Fields WS. Treatment-related leukoencephalopathy: a study of three cases and literature review. Medicine 1986;65:154–62.

77. Abrey LE, DeAngelis LM, Yahalom J. Long-term survival in primary CNS lymphoma. J Clin Oncol 1998;16:859–63.

78. Blay JY, Conroy T, Chevreau C, et al. High-dose methotrexate for the treatment of primary cerebral lymphomas: analysis of survival and late neurologic toxicity in a retrospective series. J Clin Oncol 1998;16:864–71.
79. McAllister LD, Doolitte ND, Guastadisegni PE, et al. Cognitive outcomes and long-term follow-up results after enhanced chemotherapy delivery for primary central nervous system lymphoma. Neurosurg 2000;46:21–61.
80. Guha-Thakurta N, Damek D, Pollack C, Hochberg FH. Intravenous methotrexate as initial treatment for primary central nervous system lymphoma: response to therapy and quality of life of patients. J Neurooncol 1999;43: 259–68.
81. Cossaart N, SantaCruz KS, Preston D, et al. Fatal chemotherapy-induced encephalopathy following high-dose therapy for metastatic breast cancer: a case report and review of the literature. Bone Marrow Transplant 2003:31: 57–60.
82. Lai R, Abrey LE, Rosenblum MK, DeAngelis LM. Treatment-induced leukoencephalopathy in primary CNS lymphoma: a clinical and autopsy study. Neurology 2004;62: 451–6.
83. Phillips GL, Fay JW, Herzig GP, et al. Intensive 1,3-bis(2-chloroethyl)-1-nitrosourea (BCNU), NSC #4366650 and cryopreserved autologous marrow transplantation for refractory cancer. A phase I-II study. Cancer 1983;52: 1792–1802.
84. Burger PC, Kamenar E, Schold SC, et al. Encephalomyelopathy following high-dose BCNU therapy. Cancer 1981;48:1318–27.
85. Miller DF, Bay JW, Lederman RJ, et al. Ocular and orbital toxicity following intracarotid injection of BCNU (carmustine) and cisplatinum for malignant gliomas. Ophthalmology 1985;92: 402–6.
86. Kupersmith MJ, Frohman LP, Choi IS, et al. Visual system toxicity following intra-arterial chemotherapy. Neurology 1988;38:284–9.
87. Foo SH, Choi IS, Berenstein A, et al. Supraophthalmic intracarotid infusion of BCNU for malignant glioma. Neurology 1986;36:1437–44.
88. Kleinschmidt-DeMasters BK. Intracarotid BCNU leukoencephalopathy. Cancer 1986;57:1276–80.
89. Rosenblum MK, Delattre J-Y, Walker RW, Shapiro WR. Fatal necrotizing encephalopathy complicating treatment of malignant gliomas with intra-arterial BCNU and irradiation: a pathological study. J Neurooncol 1989;7: 269–81.
90. Ito Y, Arahata Y, Goto Y, et al. Cisplatin neurotoxicity presenting as reversible posterior leukoencephalopathy syndrome. Am J Neuroradiol 1998;19:415–7.
91. Berman IJ, Mann MP. Seizures and transient cortical blindness associated with cis-platinum (II) diamminedichloride (PDD) therapy in a thirty-year-old man. Cancer 1980; Feb 15;45:764–66.
92. Resar LM, Phillips PC, Kastan MB, et al. Acute neurotoxicity after intrathecal cytosine arabinoside in two adolescents with acute lymphoblastic leukemia of B-cell type. Cancer 1993;71:117–23.
93. Herzig RH, Hines JD, Herzig GP, et al. Cerebellar toxicity with high dose cytosine arabinoside. J Clin Oncol 1987;5: 927–32.
94. Gottlieb D, Bradstock K, Koutts J, et al. The neurotoxicity of high-dose cytosine arabinoside is age-related. Cancer 1987;60:1439–41.
95. Hoffman DL, Howard JR, Sarma R, et al. Encephalopathy, myelopathy, optic neuropathy, and anosmia associated with intravenous cytosine arabinoside. Clin Neuropharmacol 1993;16:258–62.
96. Maher EA, Fine HA. Primary CNS lymphoma. Semin Oncol 1999;26:346–56.
97. Franco DA, Greenberg HS. 5-FU multifocal inflammatory leukoencephalopathy and dihydropyrimidine dehydrogenase deficiency. Neurology 2001;56:110–2.
98. Israel ZH, Lossos A, Barak V, et al. Multifocal demyelinative leukoencephalopathy associated with 5-fluorouracil and levamisole. Acta Oncologica 2000;39:117–20.
99. Hook CC, Kimmel DW, Kvoois LK, et al. Multifocal inflammatory leukoencephalopathy with 5-fluorouracil and levamisole. Ann Neurol 1992;31:262–7.
100. Savarese DM, Gordon J, Smith TW, et al. Cerebral demyelination syndrome in a patient treated with 5-fluorouracil and levamisole. Cancer 1996;77:387–94.
101. Lynch HT, Droszcz CP, Albano WA, Lynch JF. "Organic brain syndrome" secondary to 5-fluorouracil toxicity. Dis Colon Rectum 1981;24:130–1.
102. Fassas AB, Gattani AM, Morgello S. Cerebral demyelination with 5-fluorouracil and lavamisole. Cancer Invest 1994;12: 379–83.
103. Mak W, Cheng PW, Cheung RTF. Leukoencephalopathy following chemotherapy for colonic carcinoma. Clin Radiol 2001;56:333–5.
104. Leichman L, Brown T, Poplin B. Symptomatic radiologic and pathologic changes in the central nervous system (CNS) associated with 5-fluorouracil (5-FU) and levamisole (LV) [abstract 582]. Proc ASCO 1993;12:198.
105. Chen TC, Hinton DR, Leichman L, et al. Multifocal inflammatory leukoencephalopathy associated with levamisole and 5-fluorouracil:case report. Neurosurgery 1994;35: 1138–43.
106. Kimmel DW, Schutt AJ. Multifocal leukoencephalopathy: occurrence during 5-fluorouracil and levamisole therapy and resolution after discontinuance of chemotherapy. Mayo Clin Proc 1993;68:363–5.
107. Greenwald ES. Organic mental changes with fluorouracil therapy. JAMA 1976;235:248–9.
108. Takimoto CH, Long Z, Zhang R, et al. Severe neurotoxicity following 5-fluorouracil-based chemotherapy in a patient with dihydropyrimidine dehydrogenase deficiency. Clin Cancer Res 1996;2:477–81.
109. Diasio RB, Lu Z. Dihydropyrimidine dehydrogenase activity and fluorouracil chemotherapy. J Clin Oncol 1994;12: 2239–42.
110. Etienne MC, Lagrange JL, Dassonville O, et al. Population study of dihydropyrimidine dehydrogenase in cancer patients. J Clin Oncol 1994;12:2248–53.
111. Adams F, Quesada JR, Gutterman JU. Neuropsychiatric manifestations of human leukocyte interferon therapy in patients with cancer. JAMA 1984;252:938–41.
112. Kirkwood JM, Ernstoff MS, Davis CA, et al. Comparison of intramuscular and intravenous recombinant alpha-2 interferon in melanoma and other cancers. Ann Intern Med 1985;103:32–6.
113. Spiegel RJ. The alpha interferons: clinical overview. Sem Oncol 1987;14:1–12.
114. Smedley H, Katrak M, Sikora K, Wheeler T. Neurological effects of recombinant human interferon. Br Med J Clin Res 1983;286:262–4.
115. Merimsky O, Reider-Groswasser I, Inbar M, Chaitchik S. Interferon-related mental deterioration and behavioral changes in patients with renal cell carcinoma. Eur J Cancer 1990;26-596–600.
116. Meyers CA, Scheibel FS, Forman AD. Persistent neurotoxicity of systemically administered interferon-alpha. Neurology 1991;41:672–6.
117. Denicoff KD, Durkin TM, Lotze MT, et al. The neuroendocrine effects of interleukin-2 treatment. J Clin Endocrinol Metab 1989;69:402–10.
118. Vaughn DJ, Jarvik JG, Hackney D, et al. High-dose cytarabine neurotoxicity: MR findings during the acute phase. AJNR 1993;14:1014–6.
119. Honkaniema J, Kahara V, Dastidar P, et al. Reversible posterior leukoencephalopathy after combination chemotherapy. Neuroradiology 2000;42:895–9.
120. Shin RK, Stern JW, Janss AJ, et al. Reversible posterior leukoencephalopathy during the treatment of acute lymphocytic leukemia. Neurology 2001;56:388–91.
121. Edwards MJ, Walker R, Vinnicombe S, et al. Reversible posterior leukoencephalopathy syndrome following CHOP chemotherapy for diffuse large B-cell lymphoma. Ann Oncol 2001;12:1327–9.
122. Hinchey J, Chaves C, Appignani B, et al. A reversible posterior leukoencephalopathy syndrome. N Engl J Med 1996; 334:494–500.
123. Fisher NC, Ruban E, Carey M, et al. Late onset fatal acute leucoencephalopathy in liver transplant recipient. Lancet 1997;349:1884–5.
124. Komaki R, Meyers CA, Shin DM, et al. Evaluation of cognitive function in patients with limited small cell lung cancer prior to and shortly following prophylactic cranial irradiation. Int J Radiat Oncol Biol Phys 1995;33:179–82.
125. Wieneke MH, Dienst ER. Neuropsychological assessment of cognitive functioning following chemotherapy for breast cancer. Psychooncology 1995;4:61–6.
126. Tchen N, Juffs HG, Downie FP, et al. Cognitive function, fatigue, and menopausal symptoms in women receiving adjuvant chemotherapy for breast cancer. J Clin Oncol 2003;21:4175–83.
127. van Dam FS, Schagen SB, Muller MJ, et al. Impairment of cognitive function in women receiving adjuvant treatment for high risk breast cancer: high dose versus standard dose chemotherapy. J Natl Cancer Inst 1998;90: 210–8.
128. Schagen SB, van Dam FS, Muller MJ, et al. Cognitive deficits after postoperative adjuvant chemotherapy for breast carcinoma. Cancer 1999;85:640–50.
129. Brezden CB, Philips KA, Abdolell M, et al. Cognitive function in breast cancer patients receiving adjuvant chemotherapy. J Clin Oncol 2000;18:2695–701.
130. Ahles TA, Saykin AJ, Furstenberg CT, et al. Neuropsychologic impact of standard-dose systemic chemotherapy in long-term survivors of breast cancer and lymphoma. J Clin Oncol 2002;20:485–93.
131. Troy L, McFarland K, Littman-Power S, et al. Cisplatin-based therapy: a neurological and neuropsychological review. Psychooncology 2000;9:29–39.
132. Iconomou G, Mega V, Koutras A, et al. Prospective assessment of emotional distress, cognitive function, and quality of life in patients with cancer treated with chemotherapy. Cancer 2004;101:404–11.
133. Escudier B, Lassau N, Couanet D, et al. Phase II trial of thalidomide in renal cell carcinoma. Ann Oncol 2002;13: 1029–35.
134. Dallera F, Gamoletti R, Costa P. Unilateral seizures following vincristine intravenous injection. Tumori 1984;70:243–4.
135. Pirzada NA, Ali II, Dafer RM. Fluorouracil-induces neurotoxicity. Ann Pharmacol 2000;34:25–38.
136. Hamdan MY, Frenkel EP, Bick R. L-asparaginase-provoked seizures as singular expression of central nervous toxicity. Clin Appl Thromb Hemostasis 2000;6:234–8.
137. Shilsky RL, Anderson T. Hypomagnesemia and renal magnesium wasting in patients receiving cisplatin. Ann Intern Med 1979;90:929–31.
138. Ritch PS. Cis-dichlorodiammineplatinum II-induced syndrome of inappropriate secretion of antidiuretic hormone. Cancer 1988;61:448–50.
139. Vecht CJ, Wagner GL, Wilms EB. Treating seizures in patients with brain tumors: drug interactions between antiepileptic and chemotherapeutic agents. Semin Oncol 2003;30:49–52.
140. Winkleman MD, Hines JD. Cerebellar degeneration caused by high dose cytosine arabinoside: a clinicopathological study. Ann Neurol 1983;14:520–7
141. Hwang Tl, Yung A, Estey EH, et al. Central nervous system toxicity with high dose cytosine arabinoside. J Clin Oncol 1987;60:1439–41.
142. Smith GA, Damon LE, Rugo HS, et al. High-dose cytarabine dose modification reduces the incidence of neurotoxicity in patients with renal insufficiency. J Clin Oncol 1997;15: 833–9.
143. Riehl J, Brown WJ. Acute cerebellar syndrome secondary to 5-fluorouracil therapy. Neurology 1964;14:961–7.
144. Gottlieb JA, Luce JK. Cerebellar ataxia with weekly 5-fluorouracil administration. Lancet 1971;1:138–9.
145. Boileau G, Piro AJ, Lahiri SR, et al. Cerebellar ataxia during 5-fluorouracil therapy (NSC-19893). Cancer Chemother Rep 1971;55:595–8.
146. Brashear A, Siemers E. Focal dystonia after chemotherapy: a case series. J Neurooncol 1997;34:163–7.
147. Bergevin PR, Patwardhan VC, Weissman J, Lee SM. Neurotoxicity of 5-fluorouracil [letter]. Lancet 1975;1: 410.
148. Verstappen CC, Heimans JJ, Hoekman K, et al. Neurotoxic complications of chemotherapy in patients with cancer. Drugs 2003;63:1549–63.
149. Carpentiere U, Lockhart LH. Ataxia and athetosis as side effects of chemotherapy with vincristine in non-Hodgkin's lymphoma. Cancer Treatm Rep 1978;62: 561–2.
150. Luque FA, Selhorst JB, Petruska P. Parkinsonism induced by high-dose cytosine arabinoside. Movem Disorders 1987;2: 219–22.
151. Ostrow S, Hahn D, Wiernik PH, Richards RD. Ophthalmologic toxicity after cisdichlorodiammineplatinum (II) therapy. Cancer Treatm Rep 1978;62:1591–4.
152. Wilding G, Caruso R, Lawrence TS, et al. Retinal toxicity after high-dose cisplatin therapy. J Clin Oncol 1985;3: 1683–9.
153. Frustaci S, Barzan L, Comoretto R, et al. Local neurotoxicity after intra-arterial cisplatin in head and neck cancer. Cancer Treat Rep 1987;71:257–9.
154. Tfayli A, Hentschel P, Madajewicz S, et al. Toxicities related to intraarterial cisplatin and etoposide in patients with brain tumors. J Neurooncol 1999;42:73–7.
155. Shingleton BJ, Bienfang DC, Albert DM, et al. Ocular toxicity associated with high-dose carmustine. Arch Ophthalmol 1982;100:1766–72.
156. Bixenman WW, Nicholls JV, Warwick OH. Oculomotor disturbances associated with 5-flourouracil chemotherapy. Am J Ophthalmol 1977;83:789–93.
157. Koenig H, Patel A. Acute cerebellar syndrome in 5-fluorouracil chemotherapy: a manifestation of fluorocitrate intoxication. Neurology 1970;20: 416.

158. Kende G, Sirkin SR, Thomas PRM, Freeman AI. Blurring of vision: a previously undescribed complication of cycloophosphamide therapy. Cancer 1979;44:69–71.

159. Sanderson PA, Kuwabara T, Cogan D. Optic neuropathy presumably caused by vincristine therapy. Am J Ophthalmol 1976;81:146–50.

160. Norton SW, Stockman JA. Unilateral optic neuropathy following vincristine chemotherapy. J Pediatr Ophthalmol Strabismus 1979;16:190–3.

161. Awidi AS. Blindness and vincristine. Ann Intern Med 1980; 93:781.

162. Shurin SB, Rekate HL, Annable W. Optic atrophy induced by vincristine. Pediatrics 1982;70:288–91.

163. Byrd RL, Rohrbaugh TM, Raney RB, Norris DG. Transient cortical blindness secondary to vincristine therapy in childhood malignancies. Cancer 1981;47:37–40.

164. Bleyer WA, Drake JC, Chabner BA. Neurotoxicity and elevated cerebrospinal fluid methotrexate concentration in meningeal leukemia. N Engl J Med 1973;289:770–3.

165. Price RA, Jamieson PA. The central nervous system in childhood leukemia: II. Subacute encephalopathy. Cancer 1975;35:306–18.

166. Haghbin M, Tan CT, Clarkson BD, et al. Treatment of acute lymphoblastic leukemia in children with "prophylactic" intrathecal methotrexate and intensive systemic chemotherapy. Cancer Res 1975;35:807–11.

167. Ah-Song R, Sasco AJ. Tamoxifen and ocular toxicity. Cancer Detect Prev 1997;21:522–31.

168. Moroso MJ, Blair RL. A review of cis-platinum ototoxicity. J Otolaryngol 1983;12:365–9.

169. Schell MJ, McHaney VA, Green AA, et al. Hearing loss in children and young adults receiving cisplatin with or without prior cranial irradiation. J Clin Oncol 1989;7: 754–60.

170. Walsh TJ, Clark AW, Paarhad IM, et al. Neurotoxic effects of cisplatin therapy. Arch Neurol 1982;39:719–20.

171. Schaefer SD, Post JD, Close LG, Wright CG. Ototoxicity of low- and moderate-dose cisplatin. Cancer 1985;56: 1934–9.

172. Black FO, Myers EN, Schramm VL, et al. Cisplatin vestibular ototoxicity: preliminary report. Laryngoscope 1982;92: 1363–8.

173. Eden OB, Goldie W, Wood T, et al. Seizures following intrathecal cytosine arabinoside in young children with acute lymphoblastic leukemia. Cancer 1978;42:53–8.

174. Licciardello JTW, Moade JL, Rudy CK, et al. Elevated plasma von Willebrand factor levels and arterial occlusive complications associated with cisplatin-based chemotherapy. Oncology 1985;42:296–300.

175. Doll DC, List AF, Greco FA, et al. Acute vascular ischemic events after cisplatin-based combination chemotherapy for germ-cell tumors of the testis. Ann Intern Med 1986; 105:48–51.

176. Samuels BL, Vogelzang NJ, Kennedy BH. Severe vascular toxicity associated with vinblastine, bleomycin, and cisplatin chemotherapy. Cancer Chemother Pharmacol 1987;19:253–6.

177. Icli F, Karaoguz H, Dincol D, et al. Severe vascular toxicity associated with cisplatin-based chemotherapy. Cancer 1993;72:587–93.

178. Apiyasawat S, Wongpraparut N, Jacobson L, et al. Cisplatin induced localized aortic thrombus. Echocardiography 2003;20:199–200.

179. Feinberg WM, Swenson MR. Cerebrovascular complications of L-asparaginase therapy. Neurology 1988;38:127–33.

180. Priest JR, Ramsay NK, Steinherz PR, et al. A syndrome of thrombosis and hemorrhage complicating L-asparaginase therapy for childhood acute lymphoblastic leukemia. J Pediatr 1982;100:984–9.

181. Hammack JE, Cascino TL. Chemotherapy and other common drug-induced toxicities of the central nervous system in patients with cancer. In: Handbook of clinical neurology. Vecht CJ, editor. Amsterdam: Elsevier Science; 1998. p. 481–514.

182. Gradishar WJ, Vokees EE, Schilsky RI, et al. Catastrophic vascular events in patients receiving 5-fluorouracil (5-FU) based chemotherapy. Proc Am Assoc Cancer Res 1990;31:A1128.

183. Dewar J, Lunt H, Abernethy DA, et al. Cisplatin neuropathy with Lhermitte's sign. J Neurol Neurosurg Psychiatry 1986;49:96–9.

184. List AF, Kummet TD. Spinal cord toxicity complicating treatment with cisplatin and etoposide. Am J Clin Oncol 1990;13:256–8.

185. Bain PG, Lantos PL, Djurovic V, et al. Intrathecal vincristine: a fatal chemotherapeutic error with devastating central nervous system effects. J Neurol 1991;238:230–4.

186. McLean DR, Clink HM, Enst P, et al. Myelopathy after intrathecal chemotherapy. A case report with unique magnetic resonance imaging changes. Cancer 1994;73:3037–40.

187. Koh S, Nelson MD Jr, Kovanlikaya A, Chen LS. Anterior lumbosacral radiculopathy after intrathecal methotrexate treatment. Pediatr Neurol 1999;21:576–8.

188. Bates S, McKeever P, Masur H, et al. Myelopathy following intrathecal chemotherapy in a patient with extensive Burkitt's lymphoma and altered immune status. Am J Med 1985;78:697–702.

189. Gagliano RG, Costanzi JJ. Paraplegia following intrathecal methotrexate. Cancer 1976;37:1663–8.

190. Back EH. Death after intrathecal methotrexate. Lancet 1969; 2:1005.

191. Clark AW, Cohen SR, Nissenblatt MJ, Wilson SK. Paraplegia following intrathecal chemotherapy. Cancer 1982;50: 42–7.

192. Dunton SF, Nitschke R, Spruce WE, et al. Progressive ascending paralysis following administration of intrathecal and intravenous cytosine arabinoside. Cancer 1986; 57:1083–8.

193. Kleinschmidt-Demasters BK, Yeh M. 'Locked-in syndrome' after intrathecal cytosine arabinoside for malignant immunoblastic lymphoma. Cancer 1992;70:2504–7.

194. Saiki JH, Thompson S, Smith F, Atkison R. Paraplegia following intrathecal chemotherapy. Cancer 1972;29: 370–4.

195. Breuer AC, Pitman SW, Dawson DM, Schoene WC. Paraparesis following intrathecal cytosine arabinoside: a case report with neuropathologic findings. Cancer 1977;40: 2817–22.

196. Boogerd W, van der Sande JJ, Moffie D. Acute fever and delayed leukoencephalopathy following low dose intraventricular methotrexate. J Neurol Neurosurg Psychiatry 1988;51:1277–83.

197. Mena H, Garcia JH, Velandia F. Central and peripheral myelinopathy associated with systemic neoplasia and chemotherapy. Cancer 1981;48:1724–37.

Paraneoplastic Neurologic Disorders

Steven Vernino, MD, PhD

The term paraneoplastic literally means "around or near cancer." Paraneoplastic syndromes are remote medical complications of cancer that cannot be attributed to direct effects of the neoplasm or its metastases. Paraneoplastic syndromes can affect almost any organ system. In a broad sense, common problems like fatigue, opportunistic infections, and side effects of chemotherapy and radiation could be considered paraneoplastic syndromes. Other paraneoplastic disorders are related to inappropriate production of secreted compounds by the tumor, leading to hypercalcemia, hyponatremia, hyperadrenalism, or cancer-associated coagulopathy. Organs distant from the tumor can also be affected when a malignancy stimulates tissue-specific autoimmunity. The most dramatic example of cancer-related autoimmunity is the paraneoplastic neurologic disorder (PND).

Patients can spontaneously mount an effective anti-cancer immune response, particularly when malignancy cells spread early to regional lymph nodes. The immune response to cancer is certainly important, and there is great interest in developing treatments that stimulate anti-tumor immunity. In several clinicopathologic studies, tumors that are heavily infiltrated with lymphocytes have a better prognosis.[1,2] However, in rare cases, a vigorous anti-tumor immune response may become misdirected and cause damage in remote tissues, including the nervous system.

Paraneoplastic neurologic disorders have been recognized for over 50 years, since the first descriptions of sensory neuronopathy and limbic encephalitis.[3,4] Recent evidence indicates that most of the recognized PNDs are a consequence of an autoimmune response to cancer. A prevailing theory is that this occurs when tumor cells inappropriately express onconeural proteins that are usually restricted to the nervous system. Tumors of neuroendocrine lineage, small-cell lung carcinoma for instance, often express neuronal nuclear, cytoplasmic or membrane proteins.[5–7] These neuronal antigens expressed in an abnormal environment may stimulate paraneoplastic neurologic autoimmunity through a variety of mechanisms. In addition to tumor factors, many patients with PND have a personal or family history of other autoimmune conditions. Cytotoxic T-cells are thought to be the principal effectors,[8] presumably by recognizing autoantigens in the context of MHC Class I on both tumor cells and neurons. Antibodies against the same or similar antigens may be produced as well, but these autoantibodies are usually not directly pathogenic. The autoimmune attack on the nervous system, although misdirected, is characteristically highly specific for one or more cell types or regions of the nervous system. In other words, these syndromes are not associated with systemic or widespread neurologic inflammation. When reported, the neuropathologic findings in PND are often rather non-specific (Figure 1).[9,10]

General Principles

PND can affect any part of the nervous system and often affects multiple levels of the nervous system simultaneously (Table 1). Some PNDs have unique clinical characteristics and should be easily recognized (eg, paraneoplastic cerebellar degeneration, sensory neuronopathy, and limbic encephalitis). However, similar or identical syndromes may also occur, in the absence of cancer, as idiopathic autoimmune disorders or due to other causes.[11,12] Furthermore, the presentation of PND may be indistinguishable from common neurologic disorders (eg, peripheral neuropathy, myasthenia gravis, motor neuron disease, and myelitis). In these cases, the association with cancer may be under-recognized because of the absence of clinical suspicion.

Because PND can affect any part of the nervous system, the symptoms and signs of the disease can be quite varied. However, certain features are typical. Most PNDs have a subacute and progressive course. The neurologic symptoms typically develop over weeks or months, but can progress more rapidly (over a few days) in some cases. The median age of onset is around 65 years, but with a wide range. There is a strong female predominance (about 2:1) even when cases of gender-specific tumors (breast, ovary, and testes) are not considered.[13,14] In the majority of cases, there is no prior history of cancer, and the neurologic illness precedes the diagnosis of cancer. Misdiagnosis or delay in diagnosis of PND is common. The initial intensive search for malignancy may be unrevealing, which may put the diagnosis of PND in question. In some cases, non-specific symptoms (fever, fatigue, anorexia,

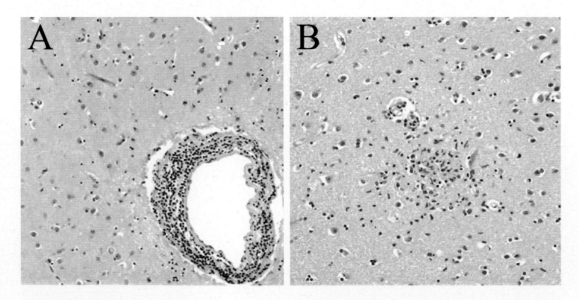

FIGURE 1 Neuropathologic findings in paraneoplastic limbic encephalitis. The pathological changes in paraneoplastic disorders of the central nervous system are non-specific. Common findings regardless of the site of pathology include (A) perivascular lymphocytic infiltration, gliosis and (B) microglial nodules. The lymphocytic infiltrate is composed predominantly of T-cells. Similar findings can be seen in viral encephalitis. Adapted from Vernino et al.[10]

Table 1 Paraneoplastic Neurological Syndromes
Brain
Cerebellar degeneration[19,20]
Limbic encephalitis[3,29]
Brainstem encephalitis[32]
Opsoclonus-myoclonus[11,48]
Chorea[10]
Eye and Cranial nerve
Optic neuritis[33]
Retinal degeneration[49]
Ageusia/anosmia[10,42]
Subacute hearing loss[23]
Spinal cord
Myelopathy[50]
Myelitis with rigidity and spasms ("stiff-person" and "stiff-limb" syndromes)[51,52]
Motor neuronopathy[53,54]
Nerve
Sensory neuronopathy (Pure Sensory Neuropathy)[4,13]
Sensorimotor peripheral neuropathy (subacute or chronic)[36]
Painful or pruritic sensory neuropathy[37]
Pure motor neuropathy
Polyradiculoneuropathy (Guillain-Barré Syndrome)[55]
Mononeuritis multiplex
Brachial plexitis
Autonomic neuropathy, gastrointestinal dysmotility[13,56]
Neuromuscular junction / muscle
Lambert-Eaton myasthenic syndrome[57]
Myasthenia Gravis[23]
Dermatomyositis[58]
Neuromyotonia[59]
Multifocal Disorders (Encephalomyeloneuropathies)

and weight loss) and findings (such as hyponatremia, anemia, or elevated sedimentation rate) may support the suspicion of occult malignancy. In patients with a previous history of cancer, the neurologic illness may herald cancer recurrence. When found, the tumors tend to be limited in stage and respond well to treatment.[15] In fact, several reports suggest that patients with PND have a favorable cancer survival compared to those with identical tumors without PND.[16–19] On the other hand, the neurologic response to treatment tends to be poor (with some exceptions for specific syndromes) and patients are often left with significant neurologic disability.[16,20,21]

Overall, paraneoplastic neurologic disorders are quite rare (estimated at 0.01% of cancer patients).[22] Certain malignancies are more likely to be associated with PND. About 30% of patients with thymoma have some form of neurologic autoimmunity, mostly myasthenia gravis.[23] Small-cell carcinoma, most commonly arising in the lung, is associated with one or more PNDs in up to 3% of cases.[24,25] Other malignancies with

definite PND associations include gynecologic malignancies, arising from the breast, ovary, fallopian tube, and peritoneum, Hodgkin's and non-Hodgkin's lymphoma, testicular cancer, and neuroblastoma. PND occurs at a much lower frequency in patients with non-small cell lung, renal cell, uterine, and melanotic skin cancers. Many of the most common malignancies (adenocarcinoma of the colon or prostate, transitional cell bladder carcinoma, and skin carcinomas) are highly unlikely to be associated with PND. Case report associations of these cancers with neurologic disease could be coincidental due to the high frequency of these malignancies. When one of these tumors is found in a patient with suspected PND, the search for a second malignancy should continue. Alternatively, the pathology of the tumor should be carefully examined for the possibility of mixed pathology with small-cell neuroendocrine features. Common primary tumors of the adult nervous system (glioma or meningioma) are essentially never associated with PND—it would also be very difficult to dissociate paraneoplastic phenomena from direct effects of the tumor. All PND are rare, but several syndromes are distinctive enough to warrant specific attention.

Paraneoplastic Cerebellar Degeneration

Paraneoplastic cerebellar degeneration (PCD) begins as mild unsteadiness of walking, which progresses to a severe cerebellar ataxia over a few weeks or months. In some cases, a more acute onset may be misdiagnosed as brainstem or cerebellar stroke. More insidious onset may lead to a diagnosis of an inherited and degenerative cause. The typical presenting features are disabling incoordination of gait, trunk and limbs and an ataxic dysarthria. Often, severe vertigo and motion sickness with nausea, diplopia, nystagmus and oscillopsia are early complaints. As a result, within a few months, most patients will lose the ability to walk or even sit independently, lose the ability to write, or feed themselves, and lose the ability to communicate effectively.[19,20] Dramatic tremors of the limbs and head (titubation) are typical. However, the syndrome usually remains restricted to the cerebellum. Strength, sensation, and cognition are not affected. Symptoms often stabilize spontaneously, but unfortunately, the usual outcome is irreversible severe ataxia and loss of independence. Severe depression is a commonly associated comorbidity.

It is estimated that 50% of patients with subacute, severe, adult-onset ataxia have an underlying malignancy. Many of the non-paraneoplastic cases are probably idiopathic autoimmune disorders.[26,27] PCD is more common in women since the classical association is with ovarian or

breast carcinoma. Usually, the onset of symptoms precedes the diagnosis of cancer or heralds a cancer recurrence. Autoantibodies reactive against the cytoplasm of cerebellar Purkinje cells (Purkinje cell antibody-type I [PCA-1] or "anti-Yo") may be found in the serum or cerebrospinal fluid (CSF) as markers of these tumors. Imaging of the breast and pelvis and measurement of tumor biomarkers should be performed but may be normal. Thus, when PCA-1 antibodies are found, exploratory laparotomy is usually warranted, even if imaging is negative.[28] A poorly differentiated adenocarcinoma may be identified involving the fallopian tube or peritoneal wall even if the ovaries are pathologically normal or surgically absent. PCD may also occur in the context of other malignancies (small-cell lung carcinoma or Hodgkin's lymphoma) with different antibody markers (Table 2). The pathological outcome of PCD is a near complete loss of cerebellar Purkinje cells. Early in the disease course, imaging of the cerebellum is usually unremarkable. Later, cranial MRI and CT show diffuse cerebellar atrophy which corresponds to permanent neuronal loss.

Limbic Encephalitis

Paraneoplastic limbic encephalitis (PLE) is characterized by the triad of short-term memory impairment, temporal lobe seizures and psychiatric symptoms (commonly depression, psychosis or a change in personality). Two-thirds of patients have overt seizures (usually complex partial temporal lobe seizures) that may be difficult to control, and all patients show abnormalities on electroencephalography.[29] The differential diagnosis includes primary psychiatric illness, viral encephalitis, Creutzfeldt-Jacob disease, vasculitis, and non-paraneoplastic autoimmune encephalopathies.[30] PLE may stabilize or partially improve following treatment of the cancer or treatment with immunomodulatory therapies, but most patients are left with residual memory impairment and seizures.

The pathology of PLE is focused in the anteromedial temporal cortex, hippocampus, and amygdala, although adjacent limbic structures (eg, the hypothalamus and insular cortex) may be involved, and the process may be quite asymettrical.[29] MRI typically shows non-enhancing signal changes in the mesial temporal lobes (Figure 2). Later in the disease course, marked hippocampal atrophy is associated with permanent cognitive impairment and epilepsy.

The most common tumors associated with PLE are small-cell lung carcinoma (SCLC), testicular cancer, breast cancer, and thymoma. Again, the syndrome usually occurs when the cancer is occult and limited in stage. A variety of

Table 2 Neuronal Paraneoplastic Autoantibodies

Antibody	Antigen(s)	Tumor	Associated syndromes
Neuronal nuclear and cytoplasmic antibodies*			
ANNA-1 (anti-Hu)[13,21]	HuD, HuC, Hel-N1	SCLC	Encephalomyelitis, sensory neuronopathy, autonomic and sensorimotor neuropathies, ataxia
CRMP-5 (anti-CV2)[42]	CRMP-5 (66kD)	SCLC or thymoma	Encephalomyelitis, chorea, neuropathy, optic neuritis
PCA-1 (anti-Yo)[19]	CDR34 and CDR62	Ovarian or breast cancer	Paraneoplastic cerebellar degeneration
Anti-Ma [32]	Ma1 and Ma2	Lung, breast or testicular	Limbic and brainstem encephalitis
Amphiphysin [60]	Amphiphysin	Lung or breast cancer	Encephalomyelitis, neuropathy, stiff-person syndrome
PCA-2 [61]	Unknown (280kD)	SCLC	Encephalomyelitis
ANNA-2 (anti-Ri)[31]	Nova	Lung or breast cancer	Ataxia, opsoclonus-myoclonus, neuropathy
PCA-Tr (anti-Tr)[62]	Unknown	Hodgkin lymphoma	Paraneoplastic cerebellar degeneration
ANNA-3 [63]	Unknown (170kD)	SCLC	Encephalomyelitis
Recoverin	Recoverin	SCLC	Cancer-associated retinopathy
Ion channel antibodies			
P/Q-type VGCC [43]	Neuronal Ca⁺⁺ channels	SCLC (60%)	Lambert-Eaton syndrome
N-type VGCC [43]	Neuronal Ca⁺⁺ channels	Lung or breast cancer	Encephalomyelitis, neuropathy
Muscle AChR [23]	Muscle acetylcholine receptor	Thymoma (15%)	Myasthenia gravis
Ganglionic AChR [64]	Neuronal acetylcholine receptor	SCLC (15%)	Autonomic neuropathy
VGKC [65]	Neuronal K⁺ channels	Thymoma or SCLC	Neuromyotonia; limbic encephalitis
mGluR1 [66]	Metabotropic glutamate receptor	Hodgkin lymphoma	Paraneoplastic cerebellar degeneration

* Alternate nomenclature is indicated in parentheses

AChR = acetylcholine receptor; ANNA = antineuronal nuclear antibody; CDR = cerebellar degeneration related protein; CRMP-5 = collapsing response mediator protein antibody; mGluR1 = metabotropic glutamate receptor, type 1; PCA = Purkinje cell antibody; SCLC = small-cell lung carcinoma; VGCC = voltage-gated calcium channel; VGKC = voltage-gated potassium channel.

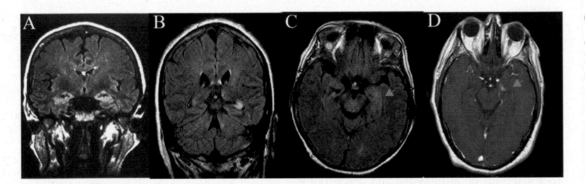

FIGURE 2 Radiographic features of paraneoplastic limbic encephalitis. (A) Bilateral signal abnormality in the medial temporal/hippocampal cortex is the most typical finding. (B) The changes can be subtle, restricted and unilateral in some cases. The characteristic abnormalities are best appreciated on coronal fluid-attenuated inversion recovery (FLAIR) magnetic resonance imaging.[29] (C) Findings on axial FLAIR findings can be easily missed, as in this case, which shows swelling and mild signal change in the left mesial temporal lobe (arrowhead). (D) Gadolinium contrast enhancement is usually not conspicuous. When seen, the contrast-enhancing region (arrowhead) reflects only a small portion of the affected limbic cortex.[29]

autoantibody markers are associated with PLE, including antineuronal nuclear antibody-type 1 (ANNA-1) and anti-Ma (see Table 2). The autoantibody findings are very useful in directing the search for occult malignancy, but up to 30% of patients with PLE and cancer have negative antibody studies.[29] In those cases, a search for malignancy must be conducted according to the patient's individual cancer risk factors.

Brainstem Encephalitis

This syndrome is characterized by prominent eye movement abnormalities (vertical gaze palsy, ophthalmoplegia, double vision, complex nystagmus or other involuntary eye movements) often associated with disorders of sleep and wakefulness (including excessive somnolence or central sleep apnea). Other cranial nerve findings include ptosis, facial weakness, flaccid dysarthria, dysphagia, subacute hearing loss, and jaw or eyelid dystonia.[31,32] Symptoms of brainstem encephalitis may also occur in combination with those of PLE, PCD, or opsoclonus-myoclonus. Brain MRI may be normal or may show brainstem abnormalities involving the medulla, pons, midbrain, or even rostrally into the hypothalamus and medial thalamus. Several different cancers have been associated with this syndrome, including SCLC, testicular, and breast cancer.

Opsoclonus-Myoclonus

Opsoclonus describes involuntary, random, high-amplitude, conjugate eye movements often associated with diffuse or focal myoclonus (involuntary brief muscle contraction causing jerks of the trunk or limbs). This syndrome was initially described in children with neuroblastoma (also known as "dancing eyes, dancing feet" syndrome). However, less than half of patients with opsoclonus-myoclonus have cancer. Other causes include viral encephalitis, drug intoxication and idiopathic autoimmune cause. Patients without cancer often make a good recovery and respond to treatment. Children with opsoclonus-myoclonus may also respond to well to adrenocorticotropic hormone, prednisone and other immunomodulatory treatments. In children with neuroblastoma, the neurologic symptoms often improve following treatment of the tumor, and the cancer survival rate is excellent. However, many children are left with some degree of incoordination or other neurologic deficits. In adults, this syndrome may coexist with features of PCD, PLE or brainstem encephalitis. In this situation, the presence of underlying malignancy (lung or breast cancer) is much more likely.

Paraneoplastic Chorea

Common movement disorders, such as essential tremor and parkinsonism, are very unlikely to occur as paraneoplastic neurologic manifestations of occult malignancy. However, the subacute onset of generalized or focal chorea may represent a paraneoplastic neurologic disorder.

Chorea (or choreoathetosis) refers to involuntary, random, and coordinated but purposeless movements of one or more parts of the body. The patient may be unconcerned by or even unaware of the movements, and observers may attribute the movements to simple restlessness. Choreic movements of the body and limbs are often described as writhing and are much slower than myoclonic jerks. Chorea of the face (orofacial dyskinesia) can consist of excessive pursing of the lips or blinking and may be associated with a strained voice. Chorea in adults can have many causes, but subacute onset in a patient over 60 years old and association with other neurologic symptoms (vision loss, limbic encephalitis or neuropathy) should strongly raise the possibility of a paraneoplastic disorder.[10] Additionally, unlike other causes, paraneoplastic chorea may present asymmetrically.

Paraneoplastic chorea appears to be the result of a "striatal" encephalitis. Cranial magnetic resonance imaging (MRI) may show characteristic transient non-enhancing signal abnormalities in the striatum, which consists of the caudate and putamen (Figure 3).[10] The most commonly associated malignancy is SCLC often associated with collapsing response mediator protein (CRMP-5) autoantibodies in serum and CSF.

Paraneoplastic Vision Loss

Progressive vision loss can occur as a paraneoplastic phenomenon although the exact incidence is unknown since non-specific visual complaints

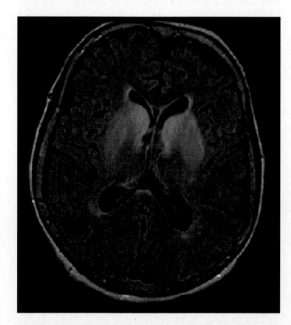

FIGURE 3 Radiographic features of paraneoplastic chorea. In many cases of paraneoplastic chorea, cranial T2-weighted and fluid-attenuated inversion recovery magnetic resonance imaging demonstrates signal abnormalities in the striatum (caudate and putamen). These areas do not enhance with gadolinium and show no changes on diffusion-weighted imaging.[10]

in cancer patients are fairly common. Subacute unilateral vision loss in the elderly must raise the possibility of ischemic, infectious or non-paraneoplastic inflammatory optic neuropathy. Paraneoplastic vision loss can present in a similar way with painless generalized or scotomatous loss of acuity, abnormalities of color vision or photosensitivity. Most cases start as monocular vision loss that becomes bilateral within weeks or months. Two forms of paraneoplastic vision loss are recognized. Cancer-associated retinopathy (CAR) is associated with an abnormal electroretinogram and positive visual symptoms (sparkling lights, shimmering scotomata or color distortion). Classically, CAR is associated with SCLC and with antibodies against any of several retinal antigens (most commonly the photoreceptor protein recoverin). Paraneoplastic optic neuritis, on the other hand, is often associated with a swollen, leaky optic disc, SCLC, and CRMP-5 antibodies.[33]

Encephalomyelitis with Rigidity

Stiff-person syndrome, first described in 1956,[34] is a rare disorder characterized by muscle rigidity and spasms characteristically affecting the axial muscles. Patients have an inability to relax their muscles, hyperlordotic posture due to involuntary back extension, and exaggerated muscle responses to cutaneous and auditory stimuli. This classic form of stiff-person syndrome is more common in women and often associated with antibodies against glutamic acid decarboxylase (GAD)[35] and with autoimmune diabetes. These patients usually do not have cancer and do not have any other paraneoplastic autoantibodies. They have a chronic disorder that may respond to immunosuppression or to treatment with high doses of benzodiazepines.

A similar disorder may occur in a paraneoplastic context. Various terms, including paraneoplastic stiff-person syndrome or encephalomyelitis with rigidity, have been used to differentiate this entity from the classic syndrome. The best described association is with breast cancer and autoantibodies against amphiphysin, although the syndrome can occur with other cancers, and antibody tests may be negative despite a paraneoplastic cause. Clinical features that should increase the suspicion of a paraneoplastic disorder include stiffness and spasms that affect one limb much more than the axial muscles (sometimes referred to as "stiff-limb" syndrome), presence of diffuse rigidity coexisting with brain or spinal cord signs (encephalomyelitis with rigidity), the absence of GAD antibodies, and the lack of a response to benzodiazepines.

Sensorimotor Peripheral Neuropathy

Autonomic neuropathy and pure sensory neuropathy represent recognized paraneoplastic

syndromes of the peripheral nerves and ganglia and are discussed separately below. Signs and symptoms of a peripheral sensorimotor neuropathy (numbness in the feet and fingers or distal weakness) are very common in cancer patients. The incidence of paraneoplastic peripheral neuropathy, however, is unknown since cancer patients often have several plausible reasons to develop neuropathy including nutritional deficiencies and exposure to chemotherapeutic agents. Nevertheless, neuropathy may present well in advance of the cancer diagnosis and is arguably the most common paraneoplastic neurologic syndrome. In many cases, the characteristics of a paraneoplastic peripheral neuropathy are those of a mixed sensory and motor length-dependent axonal neuropathy indistinguishable from those of non-paraneoplastic causes that are commonly encountered in the neurology clinic. One study estimated that 4.5% of patients with unexplained adult onset axonal sensorimotor neuropathy have a malignancy.[36] A few clinical features should increase the suspicion of PND. The onset of paraneoplastic neuropathy tends to be more rapid, with progression of symptoms, signs, and electrophysiologic changes over weeks or months. Pain is typical, and there may be unusual manifestations (such as intense itching reported in association with breast cancer).[37] On electrophysiological studies, there may be evidence of more widespread nerve involvement affecting nerve roots as well as peripheral nerves. Analysis of CSF may show mild abnormalities.

Paraneoplastic peripheral neuropathy has been associated with a number of cancers (small-cell and non–small-cell lung cancer, breast cancer and thymoma) and with several autoantibody markers (see Table 2), notably ANNA-1, CRMP-5 and N-type calcium channel antibodies. However, antibody studies can be negative in many patients with paraneoplastic peripheral neuropathy.[36]

A demyelinating polyneuropathy occurs commonly in patients with the rare osteosclerotic form of plasmacytoma as part of the polyneuropathy, organomegaly, endocrinopathy, M protein, and skin changes (POEMS) syndrome.[38] There are no specific antibody tests, although serum protein electrophoresis can detect the monoclonal protein, and a radiographic bone survey may reveal an osteosclerotic focus. Treatment of the tumor in these cases can lead to improvement in the neuropathy.

Paraneoplastic Sensory Neuronopathy

Progressive neuropathy that exclusively affects the sensory nerves has been termed pure sensory neuropathy, sensory ganglionopathy, or sensory neuronopathy. About 20% of cases of sensory neuronopathy are paraneoplastic; the remainder are associated with systemic autoimmune disease (notably Sjögren syndrome) or toxin exposure or remain idiopathic. Initial symptoms may commence in the upper or lower extremity and consist of distal pain, numbness, and paresthesias, which can be asymmetric. Clumsiness and gait unsteadiness develops because of marked loss of joint position sense. This sensory ataxia is distinct from ataxia due to a cerebellar disorder; speech and eye movements are normal. When the patient closes the eyes, the loss of balance and coordination becomes much worse, and slow wandering movements of the digits or limbs (pseudoathetosis) may be seen. Muscle stretch reflexes are usually absent. Often, the disorder progresses relentlessly over weeks or months and leads to significant disability—inability to walk or attend to basic needs. Because of marked insensitivity, the patient may be unaware of serious injuries to the extremities.

The pathological correlate of paraneoplastic sensory neuronopathy is destruction of neurons and inflammation in the dorsal root ganglia. Any of several paraneoplastic antibodies may be found, but the typical correlation is with ANNA-1 (anti-Hu) antibody. SCLC is the most commonly associated tumor. Typically, the neurologic syndrome precedes the diagnosis of cancer, and the detection of cancer is often delayed by over a year despite close surveillance.

Paraneoplastic Autonomic Neuropathy

In other cases, paraneoplastic autoimmunity can specifically target the neurons and nerves of the autonomic nervous system and spare the motor and sensory nerves. The autonomic nervous system has myriad functions, including regulation of body temperature, blood pressure, heart rate, urination, digestion, and sexual function. Complete or partial autonomic failure can be a troublesome or even life-threatening problem. Autonomic dysfunction has many causes, but many cases of subacute autonomic failure have an autoimmune basis, and some of these patients have an underlying malignancy. Common symptoms are syncope (due to orthostatic hypotension), heat intolerance (due to anhidrosis), dry mouth, severe constipation, and vomiting. The latter symptoms are due to abnormalities of gastrointestinal motility. A common presentation of paraneoplastic autonomic neuropathy is unexplained gastroparesis or intestinal pseudo-obstruction. This presentation of PND may be unrecognized as the patient undergoes extensive and unrevealing gastrointestinal evaluations. When autonomic symptoms occur in concert with another neurologic syndrome (like PLE or sensory neuronopathy), a paraneoplastic cause should be strongly suspected.

The most common association is with SCLC and ANNA-1 (anti-Hu) antibodies. Many patients with SCLC and autonomic failure who do not have ANNA-1 have antibodies against the neuronal ganglionic acetylcholine receptor.[39] Mild abnormalities of autonomic function (dry mouth and impotence) are also present in a majority of patients with the Lambert-Eaton syndrome.

Myasthenia Gravis and Lambert-Eaton Syndrome

These two disorders differ from the disorders described above in two important respects. First, these diseases are directly caused by antibodies that are also a specific diagnostic marker, and second, patients often respond well to treatment. Myasthenia gravis (MG) is the prototypical autoimmune neurologic disorder. Patients present with fatiguable weakness that usually affects the eyes (causing ptosis and diplopia). Antibodies against acetylcholine receptors (AChR) at the neuromuscular junction cause the disease and can be detected in the serum in about 85% of MG patients. MG is generally not thought of as a paraneoplastic disorder, yet up to 15% of patients with MG have thymoma. MG has also been rarely associated with SCLC. The possibility of thymoma should be considered in any patient with a new diagnosis of MG, and certain antibody results should increase the suspicion of thymoma.[23] The incidence of thymoma is highest when the onset of MG is at an older age. When present, thymoma can usually be detected with routine computed tomography of the chest. Although histologically benign, thymoma should be resected if possible since untreated thymoma can be invasive and locally metastatic. Unlike other PND, MG will usually respond to immunosuppressive drugs (such as steroids and azathioprine) and to symptomatic treatment with acetylcholinesterase inhibitor (pyridostigmine) to improve neuromuscular transmission. Most MG patients will need some form of long-term treatment for MG even after thymectomy. Paraneoplastic MG is very difficult to control unless the thymoma is removed.

Like MG, Lambert-Eaton syndrome (LES) is an antibody-mediated disorder. Antibodies against P/Q-type voltage-gated calcium channels on the motor nerve terminal lead to inefficiency of neuromuscular transmission. LES is a paraneoplastic disorder associated with SCLC in about 60% of adult patients. Patients with paraneoplastic LES usually present after age 40 with complaints of generalized weakness and fatigue. Back and proximal leg pain may be a prominent feature leading to a misdiagnosis of lumbar spinal stenosis. On examination, muscle weakness may be minimal and out of proportion to the patient's complaints. A consistent finding is decreased or

absent tendon reflexes. Many patients also have mild autonomic symptoms, consisting of dry mouth, constipation and impotence (in men). When LES is associated with SCLC, features of other neurologic syndromes may coexist, and other paraneoplastic antibodies may be detected in addition to calcium channel antibodies. If the cancer is found and treated, the symptoms of LES generally improve although rarely remit completely. Immunosuppression and other drugs (pyridostigmine and 3,4-diaminopyridine) are usually effective in improving strength.

Laboratory Findings

Since PND usually predates the diagnosis of cancer, and routine laboratory tests in patients with these disorders are usually normal, diagnosis of PND depends on clinical suspicion. In some cases, mild elevation of erythrocyte sedimentation rate, C-reactive protein or antinuclear antibody may provide a non-specific indicator of ongoing inflammation and autoimmunity. Analysis of CSF may be normal or show only mild lymphocytic pleocytosis and elevated protein. Oligoclonal bands and increased CSF immunoglobulin γ synthesis rate are seen in a minority of cases. The advent and expansion of paraneoplastic serological testing in neurology has been a great help in diagnosing PND.

Paraneoplastic Autoantibodies

The use and interpretation of antibody testing in suspected PND is an area of much confusion and intellectual debate. Furthermore, the number of antibodies associated with autoimmune neurologic disorders has been growing steadily. Many small laboratories offer testing for individual paraneoplastic antibodies, but the major reference laboratories have moved toward offering comprehensive testing panels to improve sensitivity and to relieve the clinician from the burden of having to keep up with this evolving field. Conceptually, it is useful to consider paraneoplastic antibodies in two distinct groups because the implications of testing differ.

Antibodies against Neuronal Nuclear and Cytoplasmic Antigens

The first group consists of antibodies directed against intracellular antigens in the nucleus or cytoplasm of neurons (see Table 2). In some cases, the protein antigen has been definitively identified, and testing using Western blot against recombinant protein is available. In other cases, the antibody is defined descriptively based on the pattern of immunohistochemical staining of brain sections. In most cases, the antibodies have been shown to recognize antigens both in neurons and in the appropriate tumor cells. It is unlikely that these antibodies are directly pathogenic since their specific antigens are intracellular and not readily accessible in living neurons. Furthermore, the antibodies often bind to a wide variety of neurons (ANNA-1, for example, binds to the nuclei of all neurons) even though the associated clinical syndromes are usually restricted to a specific region or cell type of the nervous system. These antibodies are important as surrogate markers of a specific immune response to cancer. Because of these characteristics, neuronal nuclear and cytoplasmic antibodies are highly specific for the presence of cancer and also predictive of the cancer type. Nearly 90% of patients with ANNA-1 antibodies have SCLC,[13] and over 90% of patients with PCA-1 have cancer (76% ovarian or related peritoneal tumors and 13% breast cancer).[40] Thus, finding a neuronal nuclear or cytoplasmic antibody in a patient with a neurologic syndrome should mandate a thorough evaluation for occult malignancy and close oncologic follow-up if cancer is not detected on the initial search. The antibody specificity helps direct the search for cancer by predicting the most likely cancer.

On the other hand, individual neuronal nuclear and cytoplasmic paraneoplastic antibodies are not very specific for a particular neurologic syndrome. These antibodies also may be found in a small but significant proportion of cancer patients who have no neurologic symptoms.[41] Each antibody can be associated with several distinct syndromes or with unique presentations in individual patients. For example, PCA-1 antibodies are usually associated with PCD, but can also be associated with motor neuropathy. ANNA-1 and CRMP-5 antibodies have been associated with nearly every recognized paraneoplastic neurologic syndrome.[21,42] Additionally, individual neuronal and nuclear cytoplasmic antibodies are not sensitive diagnostic tools. The most common paraneoplastic antibody, ANNA-1, is found in only 25% of patients with PLE and proven SCLC.[29] Even when the most complete battery of paraneoplastic antibodies is obtained, as many as 30% of patients with a subacute neurologic syndrome and cancer have no paraneoplastic antibody detected.[14,29] Thus, negative antibody tests cannot exclude a PND.

Ion Channel Antibodies

The other group of antibodies that may be associated with PND are antibodies against neuronal ion channels (see Table 2). The implications of ion channel antibody results are very different than the nuclear and cytoplasmic antibodies described above. Ion channel antibodies are usually very sensitive and quite specific for a particular neurologic disorder, but not specific for paraneoplastic disease. For example, antibodies against neuronal P/Q-type voltage-gated calcium channels are found in nearly all patients with the Lambert-Eaton myasthenic syndrome, but only about 60% of adult patients with LES have cancer.[43] Hence, the antibody is a marker of the disease but not a marker of cancer. Likewise, myasthenia gravis is highly associated with muscle AChR antibodies, but MG is a paraneoplastic disorder associated with thymoma in only 15% of patients.

Voltage- and ligand-gated ion channels are integral to the proper functioning of all neurons, but they are relatively low in abundance in the cell membrane. Thus, ion channel antibodies are generally not detectable using tissue immunohistochemistry. These antibodies are detected using more sensitive and quantitative methods. Ion channel antibodies are also unique in that they may be directly pathogenic. Muscle AChR antibodies are the cause of MG, and P/Q-type calcium channel antibodies cause LES.

Evaluation and Treatment

The evaluation of a PND requires an initial clinical suspicion. These disorders usually precede a diagnosis of cancer, and the cancers are typically very limited in stage and usually asymptomatic. Some of the clinical syndromes should immediately raise the possibility of PND in the clinician's mind. However, many patients with PND have atypical, unusual, or multifocal neurologic complaints that are impossible to localize neuroanatomically. Thus, it is appropriate to consider a paraneoplastic cause in nearly every unexplained subacute neurologic syndrome. The presence of cancer risk factors or constitutional symptoms, such as unexplained weight loss, should increase the suspicion further.

Testing for paraneoplastic antibodies can help confirm the diagnosis of PND and help direct the search for occult malignancy. Negative paraneoplastic serology, however, cannot be used to "rule-out" a PND. If there is a prior history of cancer, specific cancer risk factors, or high suspicion based on the neurologic syndrome, one should proceed with cancer screening even without serological confirmation.

The cancer work-up starts with a detailed medical history and a complete medical examination, including palpation of lymph nodes, breasts, and testes, plus rectal and pelvic examination. The search for suspected lung cancer would start with computed tomography (CT) of the chest. If the chest CT is indeterminate or normal, positron emission tomography (PET) has been shown to be more sensitive for detecting small foci of malignancy (Figure 4).[14,44] If initial imaging studies are normal, repeat examination and chest CT should be performed at 3-month intervals. For suspected pelvic gynecologic malignancies, evaluation starts with bimanual pelvic examination, CT, or ultrasonography of the abdomen and pelvis, and measurement of the serum CA-125 tumor marker. In some situations, it is necessary to proceed with exploratory laparotomy even if screening studies are normal. Breast cancer evaluation requires physical examination and mammography (supplemented by ultrasonography or MRI). Evaluation for testicular cancer includes physical and ultrasound examination of the testes, tumor markers (α-fetoprotein and β-hCG) and CT of the abdomen and pelvis. Suspicious findings on the imaging studies should be subjected to biopsy to confirm the cancer diagnosis and guide treatment.

Tumor therapy is the standard approach to treating PND. A complete oncologic remission can be associated with stabilization or improvement in the neurologic syndrome.[14] Hence, early tumor diagnosis and prompt institution of therapy is critical. Even though these patients may have a poor performance score due to their neurologic deficits, aggressive tumor treatment offers the best chance of a favorable neurologic outcome. In addition to eliminating the tumor as the stimulus for the autoimmune syndrome, many chemotherapy regimens also provide direct immunosuppressive effects. These cancers are often found at a limited stage and are held in check by a vigorous anti-tumor immune response. Hence, the oncologic outcome in patients with PND is better than in patients with similar tumors.[16–19] Once a tumor remission is achieved, the serum titers of paraneoplastic antibodies tend to decline slowly over time but may never normalize. A relapse of neurologic symptoms or onset of a new unexplained neurologic syndrome may herald tumor recurrence. A rise in the paraneoplastic antibody titer can also signal the return of cancer, but monitoring of paraneoplastic serology over time is not efficient or reliable for this purpose. Standard oncologic follow-up and imaging studies according to the type of malignancy is important, especially if immunosuppression is used to treat the PND. Theoretically, treatments that impair cytotoxic T-cell function would facilitate tumor growth. However, immunosuppression has thus far not been associated with increased risk of cancer recurrence in small treatment studies for PND.[16,45]

In cases of PND where cancer cannot be identified, despite an exhaustive search, or where the neurologic symptoms progress despite cancer remission, immunomodulatory therapies can be applied.[16] These might include corticosteroids, immunosuppressants, intravenous immunoglobulin, or plasma exchange.[45] The role of these immunomodulatory therapies in combination with standard cancer treatment is not known.

Some PND syndromes typically respond to treatment better than others. Paraneoplastic disorders of the neuromuscular junction

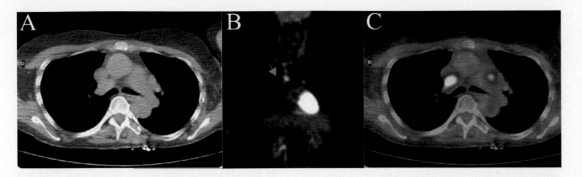

FIGURE 4 Positron-emission tomography detection of occult cancer. A patient with paraneoplastic encephalitis, PCA-2 and CRMP-5 antibodies, and a long smoking history was evaluated. (A) Computed tomography (CT) of the chest was unremarkable, but (B) ^{18}F-fluorodeoxyglucose positron emission tomography (PET) revealed hypermetabolic foci in the right mediastinum lymph node chain (arrowhead). (C) With current technology, the PET abnormalities can be identified anatomically and coregistered with CT. In this case, directed mediastinoscopic biopsy revealed small-cell lung carcinoma.

(myasthenia gravis and LES) are antibody mediated disorders and respond well to plasma exchange, intravenous immunoglobulin or long-term immunosuppression (eg, prednisone, azathioprine). In general, other disorders of the peripheral nervous system (paraneoplastic neuropathies) are more likely to improve than those of the central nervous system.[46] Paraneoplastic sensory and sensorimotor neuropathies may stabilize or improve modestly after cancer treatment, but residual deficits are the rule. Paraneoplastic autonomic disorders can sometimes improve dramatically after treatment.[39]

Among common central nervous system paraneoplastic disorders, limbic encephalitis and opsoclonus-myoclonus are most amenable to treatment.[11,46] In combination with cancer treatment, high-dose steroid treatment may be useful in promoting recovery in these disorders. Typical paraneoplastic cerebellar degeneration, on the other hand, rarely responds to treatment.[16] Even with effective cancer treatment and adjunctive immunosuppression, the best outcome of PCD is an arrest of neurologic progression. Patients and their families need to understand the inherent difficulties in treating these disorders and set reasonable expectations. Median survival for PND of the central nervous system is 2 to 4 years from the onset of neurologic symptoms.[14]

Because PND is so devastating and because an autoimmune etiology is likely, immunomodulatory therapies are often utilized. However, very few prospective studies have been performed to establish the efficacy or futility of such treatments. Based on retrospective data, it is generally thought that immunomodulatory treatment is ineffective, and that treatment of the underlying malignancy is the only available treatment for these disorders.[11,13,21,46,47] Yet, there have been individual case reports of neurologic improvement using corticosteroids, intravenous immunoglobulin, plasma exchange, protein A immunoabsorption, rituximab, tacrolimus, mycophenolate mofetil, or cyclophosphamide. Based on a few systematic prospective case series,[16,45] immunomodulatory treatments may lead to a stabilization or mild improvement of disability in patients who are still ambulatory, but offer little benefit to those with severe disability. Syndromes limited to the peripheral nervous system seem to be more likely to respond than those affecting the CNS.

Symptomatic therapies are also important for the management of patients with PND. Patients with PLE need anticonvulsants to control their seizures. Patients with myoclonus or chorea can benefit from clonazepam or neuroleptics.[10] Paraneoplastic neuropathies are often associated with significant pain that might benefit from analgesics, tricyclic antidepressants, or anticonvulsants (gabapentin or carbamazepine). Neuromuscular junction disorders can respond to acetylcholinesterase inhibitors (pyridostigmine) or 3,4-diaminopyridine (for LES). Most importantly, PND is psychologically devastating to patients and their families. Patients are faced not only with a progressive and disabling neurologic syndrome but also with a new diagnosis of cancer and an uncertain future. Severe depression is a common factor, which may interfere with the patient's treatment. This must be recognized and addressed. Finally, rehabilitation services are important. If the neurologic syndrome can be stabilized, physical and occupational therapies can help these patients reestablish some degree of independence.

Summary

Paraneoplastic neurologic syndromes represent a rare, but severe immunologic complication of certain malignancies (most notably small-cell lung carcinoma, ovarian cancer, and thymoma). Clinical manifestations can be quite varied and multifocal in the nervous system. Several distinct clinical syndromes are recognized including sensory neuronopathy, cerebellar degeneration, limbic encephalitis, and Lambert-Eaton myasthenic syndrome. These disorders are usually associated with a subacute onset and significant disability. Typically, the neurologic presentation antedates the diagnosis of malignancy, and the cancer, when found, tends to be localized and responsive to treatment. Diagnosis depends on clinical suspicion, serology for paraneoplastic antibodies, and a focused search for cancer. Current treatments for the neurologic symptoms are effective in only a minority of cases. Optimum management includes early diagnosis, treatment of cancer to remission, immunosuppression, symptomatic therapies, and compassionate support.

References

1. Zhang L, Conejo-Garcia JR, Katsaros D, et al. Intratumoral T cells, recurrence, and survival in epithelial ovarian cancer. N Engl J Med 2003;348:203–13.
2. Eerola AK, Soini Y, Paakko P. A high number of tumor-infiltrating lymphocytes are associated with a small tumor size, low tumor stage, and a favorable prognosis in operated small cell lung carcinoma. Clin Cancer Res 2000;6:1875–81.
3. Corsellis J, Goldberg G, Norton A. Limbic encephalitis and its association with carcinoma. Brain 1968;91:481–96.
4. Denny-Brown D. Primary sensory neuropathy with muscular changes associated with carcinoma. J Neurol Neurosurg Psychiatry 1948;11:73–87.
5. Cunningham JM, Lennon VA, Lambert EH, Scheithauer B. Acetylcholine receptors in small cell carcinomas. J Neurochem 1985;45:159–67.
6. Kiers L, Altermatt HJ, Lennon VA. Paraneoplastic anti-neuronal nuclear IgG autoantibodies (type I) localize antigen in small cell lung carcinoma. Mayo Clin Proc 1991;66:1209–16.
7. Oguro-Okano M, Griesmann GE, Wieben ED, et al. Molecular diversity of neuronal-type calcium channels identified in small cell lung carcinoma. Mayo Clin Proc 1992;67:1150–9.
8. Albert ML, Darnell JC, Bender A, et al. Tumor-specific killer cells in paraneoplastic cerebellar degeneration. Nature Medicine. 1998;4:1321–4.
9. Bakheit A, Kennedy P, Behan P. Paraneoplastic limbic encephalitis: clinico-pathological correlations. J Neurol Neurosurg Psychiatry 1990;53:1084–8.
10. Vernino S, Tuite P, Adler CH, et al. Paraneoplastic chorea associated with CRMP-5 neuronal antibody and lung carcinoma. Ann Neurol 2002;51:625–30.
11. Bataller L, Graus F, Saiz A, et al. Clinical outcome in adult onset idiopathic or paraneoplastic opsoclonus-myoclonus. Brain 2001;124(Pt 2):437–43.
12. Font J, Ramos-Casals M, de la Red G, et al. Pure sensory neuropathy in primary Sjogren's syndrome. Longterm prospective followup and review of the literature. J Rheumatol 2003;30:1552–7.
13. Lucchinetti CF, Kimmel DW, Lennon VA. Paraneoplastic and oncologic profiles of patients seropositive for type I antineuronal nuclear autoantibodies. Neurology 1998;50:652–7.
14. Candler PM, Hart PE, Barnett M, et al. A follow up study of patients with paraneoplastic neurological disease in the United Kingdom. J Neurol Neurosurg Psychiatry 2004;75:1411–5.
15. Graus F, Dalmou J, Rene R, et al. Anti-Hu antibodies in patients with small-cell lung cancer: association with complete response to therapy and improved survival. J Clin Oncol 1997;15:2866–72.
16. Vernino S, O'Neill BP, Marks RS, et al. Immunomodulatory treatment trial for paraneoplastic neurological disorders. Neuro-oncol 2004;6:55–62.
17. Maddison P, Newsom-Davis J, Mills KR, Souhami RL. Favourable prognosis in Lambert-Eaton myasthenic syndrome and small-cell lung carcinoma. Lancet 1999;353(9147):117–8.
18. Altman AJ, Baehner RL. Favorable prognosis for survival in children with coincident opso-myoclonus and neuroblastoma. Cancer 1976;37:846–52.

19. Hammack JE, Kimmel DW, O'Neill BP, Lennon VA. Paraneoplastic cerebellar degeneration: a clinical comparison of patients with and without Purkinje cell cytoplasmic antibodies. Mayo Clin Proc 1990;65:1423–31.

20. Rojas I, Graus F, Keime-Guibert F, et al. Long-term clinical outcome of paraneoplastic cerebellar degeneration and anti-Yo antibodies. Neurology 2000;55:713–5.

21. Dalmau J, Graus F, Rosenblum M, Posner J. Anti-Hu associated paraneoplastic encephalomyelitis/sensory neuronopathy. A clinical study of 71 patients. Medicine 1992;71:59–72.

22. Darnell RB, Posner JB. Paraneoplastic syndromes involving the nervous system. N Engl J Med 2003;349:1543–54.

23. Vernino S, Lennon VA. Autoantibody profiles and neurological correlations of thymoma. Clin Cancer Res 2004;10:7270–7275.

24. Elrington GM, Murray NM, Spiro SG, Newsom-Davis J. Neurological paraneoplastic syndromes in patients with small cell lung cancer. A prospective survey of 150 patients. J Neurol Neurosurg Psychiatry 1991;54:764–7.

25. Sculier JP, Feld R, Evans WK, et al. Neurologic disorders in patients with small cell lung cancer. Cancer 1987;60:2275–83.

26. Honnorat J, Saiz A, Giometto B, et al. Cerebellar ataxia with anti-glutamic acid decarboxylase antibodies: study of 14 patients. Arch Neurol 2001;58:225–30.

27. Hadjivassiliou M, Grunewald RA, Chattopadhyay AK, et al. Clinical, radiological, neurophysiological, and neuropathological characteristics of gluten ataxia. Lancet 1998;352(9140):1582–5.

28. Hetzel DJ, Stanhope CR, O'Neill BP, Lennon VA. Gynecologic cancer in patients with subacute cerebellar degeneration predicted by anti-Purkinje cell antibodies and limited in metastatic volume. Mayo Clin Proc 1990;65:1558–63.

29. Lawn ND, Westmoreland BF, Kiely MJ, et al. Clinical, magnetic resonance imaging, and electroencephalographic findings in paraneoplastic limbic encephalitis. Mayo Clin Proc 2003;78:1363–8.

30. Thieben MJ, Lennon VA, Boeve BF, et al. Potentially reversible autoimmune limbic encephalitis with neuronal potassium channel antibody. Neurology 2004;62:1177–82.

31. Pittock SJ, Lucchinetti CF, Lennon VA. Anti-neuronal nuclear autoantibody type 2: paraneoplastic accompaniments. Ann Neurol 2003;53:580–7.

32. Voltz R, Gultekin SH, Rosenfeld MR, et al. A serologic marker of paraneoplastic limbic and brain-stem encephalitis in patients with testicular cancer. N Engl J Med 1999;340:1788–95.

33. Cross SA, Salomao DR, Parisi JE, et al. Paraneoplastic autoimmune optic neuritis with retinitis defined by CRMP-5-IgG. Ann Neurol 2003;54:38–50.

34. Moersch F, Woltman H. Progressive fluctuating muscular rigidity and spasm ("stiff-man" syndrome): report of a case and some observations in 13 other cases. Proc Staff Meet Mayo Clin 1956;31:421–7.

35. Walikonis JE, Lennon VA. Radioimmunoassay for glutamic acid decarboxylase (GAD65) autoantibodies as a diagnostic aid for stiff-man syndrome and a correlate of susceptibility to type 1 diabetes mellitus. Mayo Clin Proc 1998;73:1161–6.

36. Antoine JC, Mosnier JF, Absi L, et al. Carcinoma associated paraneoplastic peripheral neuropathies in patients with and without anti-onconeural antibodies [see comment]. J Neurol Neurosurg Psychiatry 1999;67:7–14.

37. Peterson K, Forsyth PA, Posner JB. Paraneoplastic sensorimotor neuropathy associated with breast cancer. J Neurooncol 1994;21:159–170.

38. Dispenzieri A, Gertz MA. Treatment of POEMS syndrome. Curr Treat Options Oncol 2004;5:249–57.

39. Vernino S, Low PA, Fealey RD, et al. Autoantibodies to ganglionic acetylcholine receptors in autoimmune autonomic neuropathies. N Engl J Med 2000;343:847–55.

40. Pittock SJ, Kryzer TJ, Lennon VA. Paraneoplastic antibodies coexist and predict cancer, not neurological syndrome. Ann Neurol 2004;56:715–719.

41. Galanis E, Frytak S, Rowland KM, Jr, et al. Neuronal autoantibody titers in the course of small-cell lung carcinoma and platinum-associated neuropathy. Cancer Immunol Immunother 1999;48(2-3):85–90.

42. Yu Z, Kryzer T, Griesmann G, et al. CRMP-5 neuronal autoantibody: marker of lung cancer and thymoma-related autoimmunity. Ann Neurol 2001;49:146–54.

43. Lennon VA, Kryzer TJ, Griesmann GE, et al. Calcium-channel antibodies in the Lambert-Eaton syndrome and other paraneoplastic syndromes. N Engl J Med 1995;332:1467–74.

44. Antoine JC, Cinotti L, Tilikete C, et al. [18F]fluorodeoxyglucose positron emission tomography in the diagnosis of cancer in patients with paraneoplastic neurological syndrome and anti-Hu antibodies. Ann Neurol 2000;48:105–8.

45. Keime-Guibert F, Graus F, Fleury A, et al. Treatment of paraneoplastic neurological syndromes with antineuronal antibodies (Anti-Hu, anti-Yo) with a combination of immunoglobulins, cyclophosphamide, and methylprednisolone. J Neurol Neurosurg Psychiatry 2000;68:479–82.

46. Graus F, Keime-Guibert F, Rene R, et al. Anti-Hu-associated paraneoplastic encephalomyelitis: analysis of 200 patients. Brain 2001;124(Pt 6):1138–48.

47. Grisold W, Drlicek M, Liszka-Setinek U, Wondrusch E. Anti-tumour therapy in paraneoplastic neurological disease. Clin Neurol Neurosurg 1995;97:106–11.

48. Dale RC. Childhood opsoclonus myoclonus. Lancet Neurol 2003;2:270.

49. Adamus G, Ren G, Weleber RG. Autoantibodies against retinal proteins in paraneoplastic and autoimmune retinopathy. BMC ophthalmol 2004;4:5.

50. Babikian VL, Stefansson K, Dieperink ME, et al. Paraneoplastic myelopathy: antibodies against protein in normal spinal cord and underlying neoplasm. Lancet 1985;2(8445):49–50.

51. Brown P, Marsden CD. The stiff man and stiff man plus syndromes. J Neurol 1999;246:648–52.

52. Barker RA, Revesz T, Thom M, et al. Review of 23 patients affected by the stiff man syndrome: clinical subdivision into stiff trunk (man) syndrome, stiff limb syndrome, and progressive encephalomyelitis with rigidity. J Neurol Neurosurg Psychiatry 1998;65:633–40.

53. Younger DS. Motor neuron disease and malignancy. Muscle Nerve 2000;23:658–60.

54. Forsyth PA, Dalmau J, Graus F, et al. Motor neuron syndromes in cancer patients. Ann Neurol 1997;41:722–30.

55. Lisak RP, Mitchell M, Zweiman B, et al. Guillain-Barre syndrome and Hodgkin's disease: three cases with immunologic studies. Trans Am Neurol Assoc 1975;100:140–4.

56. Pardi DS, Miller SM, Miller DL, et al. Paraneoplastic dysmotility: loss of interstitial cells of Cajal Am J Gastroenterol 2002;97:1828–33.

57. Greene JG, Divertie MB, Brown AL, Lambert EH. Small cell carcinoma of lung. Observations on four patients including one with a myasthenic syndrome. Arch Intern Med 1968;122:333–9.

58. Stockton D, Doherty VR, Brewster DH. Risk of cancer in patients with dermatomyositis or polymyositis, and follow-up implications: a Scottish population-based cohort study. Br J Cancer 2001;85:41–5.

59. Newsom-Davis J, Mills KR. Immunological associations of acquired neuromyotonia (Isaacs' syndrome) Report of five cases and literature review. Brain 1993;116:453–69.

60. Antoine JC, Absi L, Honnorat J, et al. Antiamphiphysin antibodies are associated with various paraneoplastic neurological syndromes and tumors. Arch Neurol 1999;56:172–7.

61. Vernino S, Lennon VA. New Purkinje cell antibody (PCA-2): marker of lung cancer-related neurological autoimmunity. Ann Neurol 2000;47:297–305.

62. Bernal F, Shams'ili S, Rojas I, et al. Anti-Tr antibodies as markers of paraneoplastic cerebellar degeneration and Hodgkin's disease. Neurology 2003;60:230–4.

63. Chan K, Vernino S, Lennon V. ANNA-3 Anti-neuronal nuclear antibody marker of lung cancer-related autoimmunity. Ann Neurol 2001;50:301–11.

64. Vernino S, Adamski J, Kryzer TJ, et al. Neuronal nicotinic ACh receptor antibody in subacute autonomic neuropathy and cancer-related syndromes. Neurology 1998;50:1806–11.

65. Vernino S, Lennon VA. Ion channel and striational antibodies define a continuum of autoimmune neuromuscular hyperexcitability. Muscle Nerve 2002;26:702–7.

66. Sillevis Smitt P, Kinoshita A, De Leeuw B, et al. Paraneoplastic cerebellar ataxia due to autoantibodies against a glutamate receptor. N Engl J Med 2000;342:21–7.

Neuropathic Pain

Leslie J. Blackhall MD, MTS

Neuropathic pain is defined as pain due to an injury to, or dysfunction of, the nervous system. In patients with cancer, neuropathic pain can occur from the tumor itself, infiltrating or compressing neural structures, or as a consequence of cancer treatment. The pathophysiology of neuropathic pain is complex, and may involve both peripheral and central mechanisms. For example, patients with peripheral nerve damage from chemotherapy may manifest hyperesthia (hypersensitivity to noxious stimuli), allodynia (pain to stimuli that normally do not cause pain), and spontaneous pain (pain occurring in the absence of any stimulation). In these cases, damage to the sensory neurons may cause spontaneous ectopic activity, due to focal demyelination producing exposure of sodium channels[1] and accumulation of inflammatory mediators and cytokines that sensitize nociceptor terminals so that they respond to normally innocuous stimli.[2] Neuroma formation in regenerating afferent nerves can cause an accumulation of sodium channels and an increase in ectopic activity. Peripheral nerve injury may cause disinhibition in the dorsal root ganglia through multiple mechanisms, including a reduction in GABA (down-regulated on injured nerves) and an up-regulation of cholecystokinin receptors. This disinhibition can lead to exaggerated or even spontaneous firing of dorsal horn neurons. Central neurons can become sensitized as well, as in the phenomenon known as "wind up" where repetitive C-fiber input causes increased central response to subsequent stimuli (mediated through the NMDA receptors). Finally, patients with phantom limb pain may have cortical reorganization as well.

The diagnosis of neuropathic pain in cancer may be obvious, or more subtle as part of a mixed pain complex in which nociceptive and neuropathic components are both present. In the latter case, neuropathic pain may be identified by the quality of the pain. Patients with this type of pain complain of burning, shooting, or radiating pain. Paroxysms of pain, often described as having an "electric shock" quality, may be present. Allodynia, hyperesthesia and paresthesias are characteristic of neuropathic pain, and patients may report a paradoxical feeling of numbness and pain in the same area.

Treatment of Neuropathic Pain in Cancer

Cancer-related neuropathic pain is common, and may be more severe and difficult to treat than other types of cancer-related pain. Epidural spinal cord compression, leptomeningeal disease, brachial plexus infiltration and lumbosacral plexopathies are examples of neuropathic syndromes that will often require aggressive pain management. While treatment of the underlying disease with radiation, surgical decompression or chemotherapy may provide relief of pain, not all patients will respond to these treatments, and even those who respond may have a prolonged lag time before their pain improves. Radiation, surgery, and chemotherapy may themselves cause neuropathic pain (see "Treatment-Related Neuropathic Pain Syndromes" below for a discussion of treatment related pain). Finally, at the end of life, patients with these syndromes may not be candidates for further treatment of their primary disease. For these reasons, the symptomatic treatment of neuropathic pain is an important issue in cancer care. In the following section, we will discuss the pharmacologic management of neuropathic pain, with emphasis on medications specific for treatment of neuropathic pain. It is important to remember, however, that opioids, even those without specific efficacy for neuropathic pain, have an important place in the management of neuropathic pain, and will almost always be required in treating moderate to severe pain.[3,4] This is especially true because patients with cancer-related neuropathic pain will often have other types of cancer pain syndromes. Treatment-related pain syndromes may be a special case, and these are discussed in a later section (see "Treatment-Related Neuropathic Pain Syndromes" below).

As we discuss the medications commonly used for neuropathic pain, it should be noted that most of the evidence for the efficacy of these agents has been for nonmalignant conditions. In general, this section has been organized by class of drug (eg, antidepressant, anticonvulsant). However, another and potentially more useful way of thinking about medications for neuropathic pain is by mechanism of action.[5,6] Thus, mode of action, where known, has been discussed in each section and is also shown in Table 1.

Although it is beyond the scope of this chapter to discuss neurosurgical and anesthetic techniques for the treatment of cancer-related pain, patients who do not respond to pharmacologic treatment, or who are unable to tolerate the side effects of treatment, may benefit from nerve blocks, epidural or intrathecal medications,[7] or even to neurosurgical approaches such as cordotomy.[8] Referral to a specialist in cancer-related pain syndromes is recommended in difficult cases like these.

Tricyclic Antidepressants.

Mechanism of Action

A tricyclic antidepressant (TCA) acts as a modulator of descending inhibitory pathways via inhibition of reuptake of norepinephrine and serotonin (imipramine, amitriptyline, clomipramine), or, in some cases, norepinephrine alone (desipramine and maprotiline).[5,6] Successful treatment of pain is independent of improvement of depression, and usually occurs at dosages below those prescribed for antidepressant effects.

Efficacy in Specific Conditions

In studies of painful polyneuropathies (usually diabetic), TCAs have been shown to be effective, with a number needed to treat (NNT) (ie, the number of patients needed to treat to obtain at least 50% pain relief for one patient) of 3.0 across 13 separate studies.[6,9] Balanced reuptake inhibitors have generally been more effective for this condition than those inhibiting the reuptake of NE alone, with a NNT of 2.0 for the balanced reuptake inhibitors, versus 3.4 for the selective NE reuptake inhibitors. This situation may be reversed in postherpetic neuralgia, where data for effectiveness is fairly strong and the NNT overall is about 2.3. These agents, amitriptyline in particular, may be effective for both lancinating and steady pain, and may also be effective in neuropathic pain caused by peripheral nerve injury. Some caution is needed in generalizing the results of studies done mainly on benign peripheral neuropathy (primarily of diabetic origin) to cancer-related peripheral neuropathies (usually

Table 1 Medications to Combat Neuropathic Pain NMDA = N-methyl-D-aspartic acid

Location of Action	Mechanism of Action	Medication
Peripheral nervous system	Sodium channel blocker	Lidocaine (patch and systemic), mexiletine, lamotrigine, carbamazepine, oxcarbazepine, topiramate
Peripheral nervous system	Depletion of substance P	Topical capsaicin
Central nervous system (spinal cord)	Calcium channel blocker	Gabapentin, levetiracetam
Central nervous system (spinal cord)	NMDA receptor blocker	Ketamine, methadone
Central nervous system (brain, modulating descending inhibitory pathways)	Norepinephrine and/or serotonin reuptake inhibition	TCAs, venlafaxine, duloxetine, paroxetine, citalopram, bupropion, tramadol
Central nervous system (brain, modulating descending inhibitory pathways)	Opioid receptors	Opioids (including methadone), tramadol

Adapted from Beydoun A, Backonja M.[5]

caused by chemotherapeutic agents). Several studies on TCAs in the treatment of HIV-related peripheral neuropathy, for example, have failed to show benefit.[10,11]

Several studies have looked specifically at TCAs in cancer-related neuropathic pain. In a study of radiation-induced mucositis pain in head and neck cancer, the TCA nortriptyline hydrochloride provided effective relief in 8 of 19 patients; 11 of 19 required the addition of morphine to provide effective relief.[12] In a study of postmastectomy pain, 8 of 15 patients had more than 50% reduction in pain intensity with amitriptyline (average dose 50 mg). Unfortunately, most of the good responders did not wish to continue the medication because of side effects, especially sedation.[13] These authors suggested using a less sedating TCA.

Side Effects

Side effects of TCAs are generally related to their anticholinergic effects and include sedation, dizziness, weight gain, orthostatic hypotension, dry mouth, urinary retention, constipation, arrhythmias and confusion. (Some of these side effects, in particular, weight gain and sedation, can be useful in cancer patients; and amitriptyline, in particular, may be prescribed at night for patients with neuropathic pain and difficulty sleeping). TCAs can lower the seizure threshold and should be used with caution in liver disease. Overdose can be fatal, usually secondary to cardiac complications. Drug interactions are common and include imidazoles such as Diflucan (increased blood levels of TCAs), carbamazepine (decreased blood levels of TCA and carbamazepine). The risk of dose-limiting side effect may be reduced in TCAs by choice of agent. Desipramine has fewer anticholinergic side effects but, as an NE inhibitor, it may be less effective than amitriptyline. If avoidance of sedation is desired,

then nortriptyline is a good choice. It is a major metabolite of amitriptyline and has fewer sedating side effects.[14]

Other Antidepressants

Since the use of TCAs for pain control has been limited by the high incidence of side effects, the newer, better-tolerated antidepressants have been studied as treatments for neuropathic pain. Although there are far fewer data for SSRIs than for TCAs, it appears that they are relatively ineffective compared to TCAs for this indication,[4,15] although there is some evidence for paroxetine[16] and citalopram.[17] Bupropion has also shown some efficacy in the treatment of neuropathic pain syndromes.[18,19]

Two newer antidepressants that have shown particular promise in treating neuropathic pain are venlafaxine and duloxetine. Both of these agents inhibit reuptake of serotonin and norepinephrine, although venlafaxine affects the NE system more weakly and mainly at higher doses.[20] These agents presumably work through the same mechanisms as the TCAs, but have a better side effect profile. Several articles have presented evidence for the use of venlafaxine for diabetic neuropathy.[20-23] One article looked at the use of perioperative venlafaxine for the prevention of postmastectomy pain syndrome and found it to be effective in preventing postoperative chest wall, arm and axilla pain[24]; otherwise, reports have mainly focused on nonmalignant pain syndromes.

Duloxetine is an antidepressant related to venlafaxine, but with more robust NE inhibition and has been studied for the treatment of painful physical symptoms associated with depression.[25,26] Data on cancer-related neuropathic pain are lacking, but in theory, this agent is promising.

In summary, antidepressants, especially the TCAs have been the mainstay of treatment for

neuropathic pain for many years. More recently, however, TCAs have fallen out of favor because of their many adverse side effects. Judicious choice of TCA may allow them to be used effectively, however. Newer antidepressants, such as venlafaxine and duloxetine, show promise in treating neuropathic pain, with an improved side effect profile. More data are needed on their use in cancer-related pain.

Gabapentin

Mechanism of Action

The mechanism of action is still unclear for this agent, although evidence points to central mechanisms, perhaps at the level of the spinal cord, where it acts to inhibit the calcium channel current.[5,6]

Efficacy in Specific Conditions

Early evidence for the effectiveness of gabapentin for neuropathic pain, in the form of case studies, led to randomized controlled trials of this agent for specific conditions. Well-designed studies have found gabapentin to be effective for diabetic peripheral neuropathy,[27] postherpetic neuralgia,[28,29] and other neuropathic pain syndromes.[30] Improvement has also been seen in phantom limb pain.[31] Doses used in one study, which showed a positive effect for gabapentin, were much higher than those used for the management of seizures, with patients requiring up to 3,600 mg/day.[32]

Because of the success of gabapentin in treating nonmalignant neuropathic pain, and its relatively favorable side-effect profile (see "Side Effects" below) it has become widely used in treating cancer patients with a variety of neuropathic pain syndromes.[33] One study looked at the efficacy of gabapentin as an adjuvant to opioid therapy in cancer patients with a variety of neuropathic pain syndromes, including brachial plexopathy, sciatic neuropathy, and radiculopathy from meningeal disease. In this uncontrolled trial, 20 of 22 patients experienced significant improvement following addition of gabapentin.[34]

Side Effects

Gabapentin is generally well tolerated. The most common side effects of this medication are sedation, ataxia, and dizziness. Peripheral edema, abdominal cramping, and nausea are less common. The central nervous system (CNS) side effects of gabapentin mainly occur during the titration phase and may be ameliorated by starting with lower doses and titrating slowly.

In summary, gabapentin is increasingly used as a first line agent for cancer-related neuropathic pain, either alone or in combination with opioids. Because patients with advanced cancer are frequently debilitated and already suffering from fatigue for a variety of reasons, it is our clinical experience that the aggressive titration schedules used in studies on nonmalignant neuropathic pain syndromes are not appropriate in this population. For these patients, tolerance to gabapentin-related sedation may be improved by starting at doses as low as 100 mg three times a day and titrating up each dose by 100 mg every day or two until pain is improved or intolerable side effects occur.

Lamotrigine is a newer antiepileptic agent that has been studied for its use in nonmalignant neuropathic pain syndromes. Its mechanisms of action are unknown although it probably acts as both a sodium channel modulator in the peripheral nervous system (PNS) and a calcium channel inhibitor at the level of the spinal cord.[5] Specific data on its use in cancer patients are lacking; however, it has been shown to benefit patients with trigeminal neuralgia,[35] HIV-associated neuropathy,[36,37] diabetic neuropathy,[38] and post-stroke pain.[39] Adverse effects are similar to those seen in gabapentin, including somnolence, dizziness, and ataxia, but are more common with this agent than with gabapentin. Rarely, severe rash—and even Stevens-Johnson syndrome—may occur. Slow titration is required to avoid the more severe CNS side effects.

Carbamazepine and oxcarbazepine have also been used for neuropathic pain. The mechanism of action is probably the same as that of lamotrigine. Carbamazepine is an agent that has long been used to treat trigeminal neuralgia and has been the drug of choice for that condition.[40,41] The use of this medication has been limited, however, by its side effects which commonly include sedation, dizziness, ataxia, and nausea, as well as rare, but potentially fatal, hematological effects. Oxcarbazepine is a metabolite of carbamazepine, which appears to have similar benefits, with an improved side effect profile.[42] As with many agents, data from patients with cancer-related pain are not yet available.

Other anticonvulsants, including pregabalin,[43] topiramate,[44] and levetiracetam[45,46] have also been used for neuropathic pain, and are likely to find increasing use for this indication. Clonazepam is probably not effective for neuropathic pain.[47]

NMDA Receptor Antagonists

Ketamine is an anesthetic agent whose mode of action in the treatment of neuropathic pain is NMDA receptor antagonism, acting at the level of the spinal cord. The NMDA receptor is involved in central sensitization and in opioid tolerance, so NMDA receptor antagonists have been used as single agents for the treatment of pain and also to improve efficacy of opioid medications.

Efficacy in specific conditions

Although ketamine has been studied for peripheral neuropathy,[48] post-amputation pain[49] and postherpetic neuralgia,[50] its utility for these conditions has been limited by the severe and near-universal side effects, including sedation and even hallucinations. However, this agent has found a niche in the treatment of intractable, opioid-resistant cancer-related pain. Most of the evidence for the use of ketamine in this setting is anecdotal, including case reports,[51-54] open-label audits,[55] and other uncontrolled trials,[56] with relatively few randomized controlled trials.[57-59] Like the case reports, those trials showed the efficacy of ketamine in cancer patients with neuropathic pain. Hallucinations and sedation, however, were frequently reported in all studies.

The importance of ketamine in cancer pain management becomes clear when one looks at the patients treated in the case reports. These patients were suffering from very advanced cancer nearing the end of life, with serious complications of their disease, such as spinal cord compression, which caused severe neuropathic pain. They were generally on very high-dose opioids and multiple adjuvant medications without significant relief, and their pain greatly improved, albeit at the frequent cost of sedation, with ketamine. One such report, for example, describes a patient with neuropathic pain from cervical cancer.[52] Despite 1,000 mg/day of oral morphine and 200 mcg/hr of transdermal fentanyl and numerous adjuvant analgesics, she was experiencing severe pain, reported as 8 to 9 out of 10 on a numeric rating scale. This patient responded to IV ketamine in conjunction with IV morphine. This patient is characteristic of many of the case reports concerning intravenous ketamine for patients near the end of their lives. Oral ketamine has also been used for cancer-related neuropathic pain, in the outpatient setting.[56] Seven of nine patients improved on oral ketamine in this study, although three withdrew because of side effects, including sedation and feelings of unreality.

Side Effects

As discussed above, side effects include sedation, hallucinations, dizziness, and feelings of unreality. These side effects are frequent and may be severe. They appear to be dose-related. Several of these studies reported the concomitant use of haloperidol, diazepam, or midazolam to prevent or treat hallucinations or dissociative symptoms.[52,58] Dose reduction also generally results in improvement or elimination of these side effects.[55]

In summary, ketamine is an effective treatment for severe neuropathic cancer pain. For selected patients, it can be extremely beneficial, providing relief in desperate situations. Because of the potential for severe side effects, however,

IV ketamine should be reserved for those patients whose symptoms are refractory to other medications and should generally be given under the supervision of a clinician experienced in cancer pain management. The starting dose should be low: 0.1 to 0.15 mg/kg/hour continuously, with gradually increasing doses while monitoring for CNS side effects and using haloperidol, diazepam, or midazolam if necessary. For patients close to the end of their lives, especially those who are not expected to survive the hospitalization, a continuous infusion can be maintained intravenously or subcutaneously. Other patients may benefit from the transition to oral ketamine,[53,54] and there is evidence that, for some patients, a "burst" of IV ketamine may provide continued pain relief even after it has been discontinued.[55]

Methadone

Mechanism of Action

Methadone is an opioid finding increasing use for the treatment of neuropathic pain in cancer. It acts at both the μ-opioid and δ-opioid receptors. It also is an NMDA receptor antagonist, which has led to interest in its use in neuropathic pain. The methadone marketed in this country is a racemic mixture of the d and l isomer; it is the d isomer that blocks the NMDA receptor.[60] It may also inhibit the reuptake of norepinephrine and serotonin.[61]

Efficacy in Specific Conditions

Because of its long, and highly variable half-life, methadone has been considered a second-line agent for the treatment of cancer-related pain. Recently, however, there has been increasing interest in this agent, especially for neuropathic pain. Methadone has the advantage of being inexpensive, well-absorbed orally, and dosed two or three times a day. Since it lacks neuroactive metabolites, it can be used in renal failure. Its mechanism of action has led to interest in its use for neuropathic pain; however, there is little evidence to support the idea that methadone is superior to morphine or other opioids for this indication, and scant data to suggest that methadone is more effective for neuropathic pain than for other types of pain.

Several studies on methadone have showed efficacy for cancer pain treatment comparable to morphine.[62-65] Other studies have shown methadone to be efficacious in patients with cancer pain who are poorly responsive to morphine.[66,67]

None of the studies cited above focused specifically on methadone's effect on neuropathic pain. One study, which attempted to examine this issue by looking retrospectively at the ratio of morphine and hydromorphone to methadone during opioid rotation for the treatment of cancer-related neuropathic and non-neuropathic pain, did not find a difference in the equianalgesic ratios for these two indications, suggesting no greater efficacy for methadone in neuropathic cancer pain than in non-neuropathic pain.[68]

Side Effects

Side effects are similar to those of other narcotics, including confusion, sedation, constipation, diplopia, dizziness, dry mouth, nausea, and respiratory depression with overdose.

In summary, methadone is increasingly used in the management of cancer pain, especially in patients with neuropathic pain, and is used by some clinicians as a first-line agent for that indication. There is currently a paucity of data to support its specific use for neuropathic pain as compared to other types of cancer-related pain. That said, it is an effective agent for cancer-related pain of all types, and may have particular utility in patients who are poorly responsive to morphine. It can be used safely as long as attention is paid to its unique characteristic, in particular its long and variable half-life, which makes equianalgesic conversion difficult.[69,70]

Topical Agents

Lidocaine 5% Patch

Mechanism of Action

Lidocaine is a sodium channel antagonist. Such antagonists have been shown to bind to abnormal sodium channels with high affinity, and reduce the frequency of ectopic discharges. The rationale for the use of the lidocaine patch is to deliver this drug locally to an area of nerve damage, while reducing or eliminating systemic side effects.

Efficacy in Specific Conditions

The lidocaine 5% patch has been mostly studied as an agent for postherpetic neuralgia. Several well-designed trials have found it to be safe and effective for this indication.[71–73] Other focal peripheral neuropathic pain syndromes can be treated by the lidocaine patch as well.[74] The NNT for this study was 4.4, which is comparable to other treatments for this condition. The major indication for this agent is a focal peripheral neuropathy, especially with a component of allodynia. In terms of cancer-related pain, it seems reasonable to consider this agent for postmastectomy pain and post-thoracotomy pain, as they fit this definition, despite a lack of specific studies for these indications.

Side Effects

Side effects are mild and mainly consist of local reactions to the patch, including rash, pruritus, and sweating.

In summary, the lidocaine 5% patch is an easy-to-use agent with few side effects. It is a first-line agent for the treatment of postherpetic neuralgia, and may be combined with other agents for more severe pain syndromes. It effectively relieves allodynia, and should be considered for patients with postmastectomy, post-thoracotomy, and other postsurgical pain syndromes where focal peripheral neuropathic pain is present.

Topical Capsaicin

Mechanism of Action

Topical capsaicin is an agent derived from red peppers whose mode of action is felt to be depletion of substance P from sensory fibers.

Efficacy in Specific Conditions

Capsaicin applied topically has been studied for postherpetic neuralgia in a 0.025% concentration.[75] In this open-label uncontrolled trial, 56% of 23 patients reported good or excellent pain relief after 4 weeks. A burning sensation after application of the drug was common, however, and led to a 1/3 drop-out rate. A randomized controlled trial of 0.075% capsaicin for this indication also showed significant improvement.[76] Studies on the efficacy of this agent for diabetic and other peripheral neuropathies have been mixed, with some reporting improvement[77,78] and others no improvement compared to placebo.[79,80] Several articles have specifically addressed the use of topical capsaicin for postmastectomy pain syndrome. Two open-label studies showed improvement with this agent.[81,82] A randomized controlled trial of 0.075% capsaicin had somewhat more mixed results, with no improvement in "steady pain," but significant improvement in stabbing and overall pain, compared to vehicle cream.[83]

Side Effects

Side effects are mainly local in nature. The most common is a burning sensation, and it may be severe enough to cause discontinuation of the agent. Rash has been reported as well. Rarely, coughing and sneezing may occur.

In summary, capsaicin is a topical agent that may be effective in some types of cancer-related neuropathic pain syndromes. It is less useful as a topical agent than lidocaine only because of the burning sensation it frequently causes.

Antiarrhythmics

Systemic Lidocaine

Mechanism of Action

Lidocaine acts as a sodium channel blocker, suppressing ectopic discharges from injured nerve endings.

Efficacy in Specific Conditions

Intravenous lidocaine has been described for the treatment of neuropathic pain for many years. Acute postoperative pain,[84] phantom limb pain,[85] and peripheral nerve injury[86] are conditions in which there is some evidence of efficacy for lidocaine. One randomized, double-blind study comparing a 30-minute infusion of intravenous (IV) lidocaine to saline for diabetic peripheral neuropathy showed a reduction in symptoms (such as pain and sleep disturbance) lasting from days to several weeks.[87] A similar trial comparing IV lidocaine to saline for postherpetic neuralgia showed reduction in pain as measured by visual analog scores in the lidocaine group, with efficacy similar to morphine.[88]

Case reports have documented efficacy of lidocaine in neuropathic cancer pain.[89,90] One recent paper reviewed the use of intravenous lidocaine in an inpatient hospice unit. Sixty-one patients who had pain characterized as opioid refractory (ineffective pain relief despite the equivalent of 200 mg/d of oral morphine or more) were studied. Most of these patients were diagnosed with neuropathic pain (78%). The underlying diagnoses of these patients are not discussed, although, nationwide, cancer patients make up the majority of those enrolled in hospice care. Of these patient, 80% were deemed to have a "major" response to lidocaine, usually delivered as a bolus, followed by continuous IV infusion if response to the bolus was noted. Major response was defined as a decrease of at least 3 points on an 11-point pain scale. In this group of terminally ill patients (78% of whom died prior to discharge), the major side effect was sedation. One patient died suddenly, although sudden in this context is a relative term, and the cause of death was not clear.[91]

Side Effects

Side effects may be severe, which is why this drug is not a first-line agent. They include confusion, sedation, disorientation, lightheadedness, and cardiac arrhythmias. CNS side effects are not uncommon, especially in older patients. These are less concerning if the medication is given as a "burst" and not continued indefinitely.

Mexiletine Hydrochloride

The success of lidocaine in treating some types of neuropathic pain led to interest in other agents in this class. Mexiletine hydrochloride, a structural analog of lidocaine, which can be given orally, has received attention as a treatment for neuropathic pain.

The mechanism of action is the same as that for lidocaine.

Efficacy in Specific Conditions

Several studies found mexiletine hydrochloride to be beneficial for the treatment of diabetic peripheral neuropathy.[92–94] In at least one study, patients with stabbing and burning pain sensations were most likely to experience benefit from treatment with this agent.[94] Other studies have not found mexiletine hydrochloride to be effective in the treatment of diabetic peripheral neuropathy,[95] and its use for the treatment of other peripheral neuropathies, such as those associated with HIV disease, has been disappointing.[96,97] Adverse effects were not uncommon in all studies, although serious cardiac side effects were quite rare, perhaps because they tended to exclude patients with cardiac histories, or even abnormal EKGs.

Aside from its general use in the treatment of peripheral neuropathies, mexiletine hydrochloride has been studied for cancer-related pain syndromes. One randomized, placebo-controlled study examined the use of intraoperative regional block and 6 days of oral mexiletine hydrochloride postoperatively, given alone or in combination, on immediate and chronic pain in patients undergoing surgery for breast cancer. While both regional block and oral mexiletine hydrochloride seemed to provide some immediate benefit in reducing postoperative pain, development of chronic postmastectomy pain syndrome was not affected by mexiletine hydrochloride or regional block given in this manner.[98] Open-label studies[99] and case reports[100] have had mixed results in the treatment of neuropathic pain in patients with advanced cancer.

Side Effects

As mentioned above, serious arrhythmias are a known side effect of drugs in this class, and, for this reason, they should generally not be used in patients with serious cardiac disease, including heart failure and known arrhythmias. Confusion, sedation, and dizziness are also side effects of this and similar medications. Gastrointestinal side effects, including nausea, diarrhea, vomiting, and abdominal pain, are common. Side effects tend to increase as dose increases. This is unfortunate, as at least some studies have shown dose-dependent improvement in pain.

In summary, lidocaine and its oral analog mexiletine hydrochloride are drugs that have shown some benefit in the treatment of neuropathic pain, including cancer-related neuropathic pain. Because of their potentially serious side effects, they are considered second- or third-line agents. Some would recommend a trial of intravenous lidocaine, and, if benefit is seen, continue ongoing treatment with mexiletine hydrochloride.[101]

Tramadol

Mechanism of Action

Tramadol is a unique agent that is a relatively weak (compared to opioids) agonist at μ-opioid receptors. It is also a relatively weak inhibitor of the norepinephrine and serotonin reuptake (compared to antidepressants). Because of the latter property, this agent has attracted interest as a treatment for neuropathic pain.

Efficacy in Specific Conditions

Tramadol has shown benefit in the treatment of diabetic neuropathy,[102,103] postherpetic neuralgia[104] and other painful polyneuropathies.[105] The latter study is of particular interest because it showed not just generalized relief of pain but also specific relief of allodynia, a symptom that has been thought to be relatively opioid-resistant, perhaps indicating specific efficacy of this agent for neuropathic pain. With respect to cancer-related pain, one open-label, non-placebo controlled study on the use of a slow-release preparation of tramadol on cancer-related pain found that 71% of patients reported good to complete pain relief at 6 weeks.[106] Although this study looked at all types of cancer-related pain, more than 40% of these patients had a neuropathic cause of their pain. Two other studies compared morphine to tramadol for cancer-related pain.[107,108] Both studies found morphine to be more efficacious for this indication; however, neither looked specifically at neuropathic pain and therefore could not answer the question of whether tramadol might have specific action on cancer pain of neuropathic origin.

Side Effects

Side effects are similar to those of other μ-receptor agonists, but less severe[107,108] including dizziness, sedation, confusion, constipation, nausea and vomiting, dry mouth, and urinary retention. Sweating is also common.

In summary, tramadol is an agent with a unique mode of action, with both opioid effects and effects related to NE and SE reuptake inhibition. It is a relatively weak opioid and, for this reason, is less likely to be effective for very severe cancer-related pain; however, there is some evidence it may have specific efficacy for neuropathic pain. Its side effect profile is relatively favorable, and it has a lower abuse potential than other opioids. Some of the studies cited above have used doses greater than the 400 mg/day generally recommended for this drug.[106]

Treatment-Related Neuropathic Pain Syndromes

The following section will discuss neuropathic pain syndromes that are caused by treatments for cancer. Emphasis will be on mechanism of action, diagnosis and prevention, as well as general guidelines for treatment.

Post-thoracotomy Chest Pain

Cause and Incidence

Persistent pain following thoracic surgery for lung cancer (and other conditions) is probably related to injury to the intercostal nerves, which produces a neurogenic pain syndrome, often including radiating pain, allodynia, and other sensory disturbances. Post-thoracotomy pain, defined as postoperative pain of at least 2 months duration where other causes of pain have been excluded,[109] is a common occurrence, with most studies finding an incidence of > 50% at 6 months[110–112] (although some studies have found lower rates).[113,114] Patients undergoing surgery for malignancy may be more likely to develop chronic pain than those have surgery for other reasons.[115] For most patients, the pain will be mild; however, a subset will have severe and difficult-to-control pain.[114]

Prevention

Several factors have been shown to correlate with an increased likelihood of chronic pain following thoracotomy, including increasing age and female gender. Intensity of acute postoperative pain has been shown to correlate with the presence of chronic pain in most studies.[112,116] This observation has led to studies on preemptive analgesia: attempts to improve or eliminate acute postoperative pain and to prevent the development of chronic pain. One study found that preoperative thoracic epidural analgesia (TEA) (using bupivacaine and morphine), combined with epidural patient-controlled anesthesia (PCA) postoperatively reduced perioperative and chronic pain, compared to postoperative pain control only using IV PCA.[110] Other studies have supported the clinical utility of preemptive analgesia to prevent post-thoracotomy pain,[117] while some have not.[113] Other aspects of the surgical procedure have been studied as well. Preemptive analgesia of the skin,[118] muscle-sparing surgery,[119] and video-assisted thoracic surgery (VATS)[120,121] have not been shown to reduce the incidence of chronic postoperative pain. One study reported that the use of intracostal sutures led to a decreased pain experience at up to three months postoperatively compared to the usual pericostal sutures.[122]

Treatment

Treatment of established chronic post-thoracotomy pain should be individualized; however, many would start with the lidocaine 5% patch[74]. Capsaicin cream is another possibility, as this agent has almost no systemic side effects; however, the local reactions to this agent are more severe than with lidocaine. If local agents are ineffective or incompletely effective, TCAs have been a first-line treatment (see "Tricyclic Antidepressants" above). However, because of the relatively unfavorable side-effect profile, many would now institute a trial of gabapentin. If the pain is severe or refractory enough to warrant a narcotic, tramadol is a reasonable first choice. It is important to note that post-thoracotomy pain usually begins days to, at most, weeks following surgery, and pain that starts after this time frame, or that worsens after initially improving, should raise suspicion for recurrent disease.

Postmastectomy Pain

Cause and Incidence

The breast, axilla, and upper arm are innervated by a variety of nerves: the lateral cutaneous branch of the T2 (the intercostobrachial nerve), T3, and T4 provide innervation to the anterior chest wall and upper back, the torso, and nipple. Sympathetic innervation for the cutaneous structures of the breast is provided by the medial and lateral branches of the ventral ramus of the 3rd to 6th intercostal nerves.

Because of the number of different types of procedures performed on breast cancer patients (mastectomy, lumpectomy, sentinel node biopsy, axillary node dissection, reconstructive procedures etc.), as well as the frequent association of these procedures with chemotherapy and/or radiation, classifying the causes and incidence of pain following surgery for breast cancer is complex. While both nociceptive pain (due to damaged muscles or ligaments) and neuropathic pain can result in pain following surgery for breast cancer, neuropathic pain is more likely to persist long after wound healing has occurred. By all accounts, this type of pain is common following surgery for breast cancer.

One article distinguishes four pain syndromes: phantom breast pain, intercostobrachial neuralgia, neuroma pain, and other nerve injury pain.[123] Phantom breast pain is the painful sensation that a removed breast is still present (nonpainful breast phantoms occur as well). One prospective study interviewed patients 3 weeks and 1 year after mastectomy with a prevalence of 13.3% for painful breast phantoms (PBP) at 3 weeks, and 12.7% at one year.[124] Other studies have found higher rates, up to 44%.[123,125] PBP is often described as knife-like, or shooting.

Intercostobrachial neuralgia, usually known as postmastectomy pain syndrome (PMP) consists of pain in the axilla, medial upper arm, and anterior chest wall, and is often caused by nerve damage during axillary node dissection.[126,127] Lumpectomy as well as mastectomy can result in damage to the intercostobrachial nerve. PMP is usually described as a continuous aching or burning, with intermittent shooting or shock-like sensations. Allodynia and hyperesthesia are common. It is often worsened by movement. Estimates of the prevalence of this syndrome vary widely. In one study, 20% of patients undergoing treatment of breast cancer at outpatient oncology centers had symptoms whose history and characteristics were consistent with postmastectomy syndrome.[128] Of those reporting pain, half reported that the pain interfered with daily chores,

and half reported sleep disturbances. A retrospective questionnaire found that 43% of responders reported a intercostobrachial-type (postmastectomy) pain syndrome.[129] Pain was severe enough to affect sleep in a third of these women. Younger women were more likely than older women to experience pain following breast surgery in this study.

Neuroma pain can occur in the scars from either mastectomy or lumpectomy, but may be more common in patients undergoing mastectomy and radiation than those who have had a modified radical mastectomy.[130] Estimates of the prevalence of neuroma pain range from 23 to 49%.[123]

Other nerve-injury pain can occur during surgery even when the intercostobrachial nerve has been spared; estimates of these types of injuries are not available. Breast reconstruction, especially procedures involving implants, seems to increase the risk of chronic pain following mastectomy for breast cancer.[131]

Prevention

As with the post-thoracotomy syndrome and other postoperative pain syndromes, preemptive analgesia to prevent or diminish perioperative pain has been proposed as a means of decreasing the incidence of chronic pain following surgery for breast cancer. One study evaluated the use of a single 1,200 mg dose of gabapentin given preoperatively. Acute movement-related pain, and morphine consumption were reduced in the study group, but chronic postmastectomy pain was not evaluated.[132] One well-designed study found that venlafaxine given for two weeks perioperatively significantly reduced the incidence of PMP at 6 months. Interestingly, this effect occurred despite the fact that acute pain was not reduced in the study group.[133]

Treatment of Established Postmastectomy Pain

Amitriptyline is effective in the treatment of PMP; however, as mentioned above, many women will not tolerate this medication because of its adverse effects.[13] If a trial of a TCA is desired, nortriptyline should probably be tried first because it is less sedating.[14] Venlafaxine has also been shown to be somewhat effective in the treatment of PMP.[134] As mentioned above, topical agents, such as lidocaine 5% patch[74] and capsaicin,[81,82] can be effective, usually with minimal side effects, especially in patients with allodynia. The use of other medications, including gabapentin and opioids, will need to be individualized, depending on severity of pain and the patient's tolerance of various side effects.

Phantom Limb Pain

Cause and Incidence

Phantom limb pain (PLP) is the sensation of pain in a limb that has been amputated. As compared

to stump pain, which is experienced at the site of the stump, the patient with phantom limb pain actually feels that the toe, or foot or other portion of the amputated limb is hurting. (This should also be distinguished from non-painful phantom sensations.) Incidence of this puzzling condition is from 50 to 80% in various studies.[135–139] The pain is usually intermittent and described in terms common in neuropathic pain, such as shooting, stabbing, and burning. It is usually perceived as being localized in distal parts of the amputated limb. Almost all patients with this syndrome develop pain within days of surgery.[140] It tends to decrease or disappear over time, and patients often experience a process known as "telescoping" where the phantom limb initially experienced as the full size of the missing part becomes smaller, with the most distal part (the foot or hand) shrinking back towards the stump. A minority, however, will have long-lasting, severe pain.[141]

The pathophysiology of phantom limb pain is complex and includes both peripheral and central factors. Because manipulation of the stump often causes pain in the phantom limb, some have theorized that neuromas formed at the site of severed nerve endings generate abnormal impulses in the CNS, leading to phantom pain. This theory is bolstered by the observation that phantom limb pain more often occurs in patients with observable stump pathology,[142] and may be improved by local injection of lidocaine into the stump.[143] Unfortunately, however, stump revision, including removal of neuromas, has had limited success in improving phantom limb pain, which suggests other mechanisms of action as well, including sensitization of dorsal horn neurons in the spine, mediated through NMDA receptors,[144] and cortical reorganization.[145]

Few consistent risk factors for the development of phantom limb pain have been found. Cause of amputation does not seem to correlate with development of painful phantoms; however, several studies have shown that pain in the limb prior to amputation is a risk factor for phantom limb pain after amputation.[144,146]

Prevention

Preemptive epidural analgesia may reduce phantom limb pain,[147,148] underlining the need for patients undergoing amputation to have their pre- and perioperative pain control maximized. Ongoing tissue damage (such as that caused by residual or recurrent tumor) near the stump also seems to predispose to, and increase the severity of, PLP. Patients with increasing PLP syndromes should be evaluated for tumor recurrence.[149]

Treatment

Treatment of established phantom limb pain may be difficult; however, several studies have been published with positive results. Morphine and other narcotics have been used for this indication. One small but well-designed study comparing extended-release morphine to placebo for PLP showed that morphine reduced the intensity of PLP, and that this reduction was associated with a decrease in cortical reorganization, at least in some of the patients tested.[150] Ketamine was effective in one study, presumably through its effect on the NMDA receptor.[144] Calcitonin, given by infusion, was effective in one double-blind trial in reducing both the intensity and frequency of PLP, an effect which lasted for up to months after the infusion. Mechanism for this improvement is unclear, although it may be related to effects on serotonin receptors.[151] Nonpharmacologic methods, including TENS[152] and sensory discrimination training,[153] have shown promise in treating this condition as well.

Post Radical Neck Dissection

Cause and Incidence

Neuropathic pain following neck dissection for head and neck cancer is a well-known syndrome, occurring in perhaps 23 to 28% of patients.[154–156] One prospective study found that 25% of cancer-free patients had pain at 12 and 24 months postoperatively, although only 3 to 4% had severe pain.[156] Others have found lower levels of postoperative pain.[157] This pain is usually described as continuous, burning with hyperesthesia, allodynia, and intermittent paroxysms of "shock-like" pain. A myofascial component to this pain is often present as well. The neuropathic pain is apparently caused by damage to the superficial cervical plexus (C2-4),[158] and may be improved, at least temporarily, with nerve blocks to that area. Incidence of pain is not necessarily correlated with aggressiveness of the surgery or use of radiation.[156,158]

Treatment

Specific treatment protocols for this syndrome have not been reported in the literature. One study reported effective relief with nonspecific combinations of narcotic and adjuvant medications (including gabapentin, TCAs and mexiletine hydrochloride) as is generally recommended for neuropathic pain, supplemented in some cases by nerve blocks.[158] Botulinum toxin injection into trigger points may improve pain in some patients as well.[159]

Postradiation Pain Syndromes

Several well-described pain syndromes occur as a result of radiation. As with the postsurgical pain syndromes mentioned above, one of the main challenges is to differentiate pain caused by the treatment (radiation or surgery) from pain caused by residual or recurrent tumor. Brachial plexopathy is the best described of these syndromes. It is more likely to occur with higher doses of radiation (greater than 6,000 cGy), and may appear months to years following completing of radiation. Clinical features of the pain syndrome, such as distribution and intensity, cannot reliably distinguish between malignant and postradiation plexopathy,[160] although plexopathies caused by recurrent cancer are more likely to be painful. Magnetic resonance imaging is probably the best modality for distinguishing brachial plexopathy due to tumor infiltration from radiation effects, especially in the classic delayed-onset injury,[161] with the finding of a discrete mass adjacent to the brachial plexus highly predictive of tumor infiltration. Less common causes of brachial plexopathy include chemotherapy, nerve entrapment from lymphedema, and occlusion of the subclavian artery.[161]

Radiation damage may cause other painful neurologic syndromes, including lumbosacral plexopathy[162] and radiation myelopathy.[163] Once again, patients with these syndromes need careful evaluation for recurrent tumor.

Treatment

While specific treatment protocols have not been described, it is our experience that severe postradiation pain requires a narcotic, often in combination with adjuvant medications such as gabapentin. Symptomatic treatment will need to be individualized using the agents discussed above.

Chemotherapy-Induced Peripheral Neuropathy

Many chemotherapeutic agents are neurotoxic. In particular, the taxanes, the vinca alkaloids and cisplatin are known to cause peripheral neuropathy, which may be very painful. In general, the neuropathy caused by these agents is dose-related (either to cumulative dose or dose intensity). Although peripheral neuropathy can occur in any patient, those with preexisting neuropathy due to diabetes mellitus or other causes may be at higher risk for the development of severe peripheral neuropathic complications of chemotherapy. Below we will briefly discuss the data regarding risk factors for, and prevention of, chemotherapy-related peripheral neuropathy. Research into neuroprotective agents will be discussed, although the use of these agents is, for the most part, still investigational.

Cisplatin and Other Platinum Compounds

Peripheral neuropathy is common with cisplatin, starting with exposure to doses as low as 200 mg/m^2, and is almost universal at doses >400 mg/m^2. Deterioration may start within a month after initiation of treatment and continue for up to 6 months after completion of treatment (a phenomenon known as "coasting").[164–166] This is primarily a sensory neuropathy, with both negative (numbness, loss of vibration sensation, loss of tendon reflexes) and positive symptoms (paresthesias of varying intensities). The exact mechanism of this neuropathy is not completely clear; however, the drug appears to accumulate in the dorsal root ganglia. Oxaliplatin can cause both acute and chronic neurotoxic reactions. The acute reactions occur 30 to 60 minutes after infusion and resolve within days of treatment. They consist of paresthesias, allodynia, jaw and leg cramps, and, occasionally, visual changes,[167] and are related to infusion time and dose, and reappear with each infusion. Chronically, oxaliplatin causes a peripheral neuropathy similar to that caused by cisplatin. Carboplatin appears to be less neurotoxic than cisplatin; however, it can cause peripheral neuropathy as well.[168]

Prevention of Platinum-Related Neuropathy

Because neurotoxicity is related to dose intensity and cumulative dose, reduction of dose and longer intervals between infusions may reduce the severity of neuropathic complications of cisplatin. Several neuroprotective agents have been studied for use with cisplatin, including a synthetic ACTH analog, which has had mixed results.[169,170] Amifostine, a thiol prodrug, showed benefit in preventing cisplatin neuropathy in one study[171]; however, subsequent studies have not been positive.[172,173] Glutathione showed some benefit in one study of patients with advanced gastric cancer.[174] Finally, nerve growth factors show some promise in both prevention and treatment of cisplatin peripheral neuropathy.[175]

Cumulative neurotoxicity from oxaliplatin is usually reversible after discontinuation of therapy, and may be managed by temporary cessation of treatment. One pilot study showed reduction of chronic neuropathy with administration of carbemazepine.[176] Some success has been seen with amifostine as well.[177]

Taxanes

Paclitaxel causes peripheral neuropathy by promoting the rigid microtubules that act to inhibit axonal transport. Patients may develop neuropathy after even a single dose of paclitaxel, especially if used in combination with cisplatin, but the neuropathy is most common in doses >250 mg/m^2 and usually begins 48 hours after infusion.[178,179] Symptoms include paresthesias, numbness and pain in feet and hands, ataxia, and muscle weakness. Neuropathy may be the dose-limiting side effect, interfering with the ability to perform activities of daily living.[180] Docetaxel can cause peripheral neuropathy, as well, in a dose-dependent way.[181,182] Both paclitaxel and docetaxel neuropathies may reverse after discontinuation of treatment, although permanent neuropathy can occur.[183]

Prevention of Taxane-Induced Neuropathy

Because neuropathy is dose-dependent, changes in dosing schedule may reduce or prevent this complication, especially in patients with diabetes mellitus.[184,185] Various agents, including glutamine[186] and an ACTH analog[187] have shown some promise as neuroprotective agents. Corticosteroids are probably not effective in preventing taxane-related neuropathy.[188] Amifostine has had mixed results but is probably not useful.[189,190] Nerve growth factors are under investigation.[191]

Vinca Alkaloids

Peripheral sensory neuropathies are very common in patients treated with vinca alkaloids, and are felt to be due to alterations in cellular microtubule structure causing edema of fast- and slow-conducting axons.[192] Toxicity is dose-dependent, and risk is increased with hepatic insufficiency.[193] Paresthesias and pain of the hands and feet are the initial symptoms of neurotoxicity; some patients will go on to develop muscle cramps and weakness. Autonomic insufficiency, including constipation (to the point of megacolon), bladder insufficiency, orthostatic hypotension, and impotence, may occur.[194] Most of the neuropathic side effects of these agents are reversible within a few months after discontinuing treatment.[195]

Prevention of Vinca Alkaloid-Related Neuropathy

Manipulation of dosing schedule by giving smaller doses per interval or longer intervals between doses may reduce the neuropathic symptoms of vincristine and related agents. Treatment is usually interrupted if patients experience more severe symptoms, such as muscle weakness.[196] Glutamic acid may reduce vincristine peripheral neuropathy.[197]

Treatment of Established Neuropathies

Treatment of established peripheral neuropathies has been extensively covered above in the section on medications for neuropathic pain. As noted in that section, however, much of the research on treatment of peripheral neuropathy has been done on patients with diabetic neuropathy. For patients with mild to moderate peripheral neuropathy, TCAs have generally been used as first-line agents; however, many would now use gabapentin first because of its more favorable side-effect profile. Carbamazepine may be effective, especially for oxaliplatin-related neuropathies. Tramadol or opioids may be needed alone or in combination with adjuvant medications for more severe pain, and many would consider methadone when an opioid is needed because of its theoretical benefit for neuropathic pain. Specific treatments for chemotherapy-induced peripheral neuropathy that are still investigational include decompression of peripheral nerves[198] and ethosuximide.[199]

Postherpetic Neuralgia

Cause and Incidence

Although postherpetic neuralgia (PHN) is not a direct complication of cancer, it has been included here because herpes zoster infection, including disseminated disease, is a not an uncommon result of the immunosuppression that accompanies cancer and/or its treatment. Herpes zoster infection causes neuropathic pain during the acute infection (as a prodrome and for ≈ 30 days after the onset of the rash), subacutely (for 1 to 4 months after onset of the rash) and as a chronic painful condition known as postherpetic neuralgia.[200] Pathologic evaluation of patients with PHN reveals scarring of peripheral nerves, ganglion, and sensory roots, with damage (including inflammation and atrophy) at the level of the dorsal horn of the spinal cord, as well.[201,202]

Risk factors for the development of persistent pain include age ≥ 50, prodromal symptoms, rash severity, and moderate to severe pain during the acute phase of illness.[203] This means that patients with cancer, who are often elderly and are more likely have disseminated (and more acutely painful) disease, are at higher risk of chronic pain following acute infection.

Prevention of PHN

Prevention of PHN has been extensively studied. Most studies agree that treatment with antiviral agents (acyclovir, famciclovir, and valacyclovir), especially when initiated early, reduces the duration and likelihood of postherpetic neuralgia.[204–208] Because acute pain during zoster infection predicts the development of chronic postherpetic neuralgia, some have tried preemptive analgesia to prevent PHN. One study suggested that acute treatment with low-dose amitriptyline reduces the incidence of postherpetic neuralgia.[209] Anesthetic techniques, including sympathetic blocks[210] and epidural blocks,[211] have also been tried; while these techniques reduce acute pain, problems with study design make it difficult to say definitively that they reduce PHN.[212] Corticosteroids have also been advocated to prevent PHN, but results of clinical trials have not shown this to be effective.[213,214]

Treatment of Established PHN

TCAs have traditionally been the first-line agents for PHN.[6,9,215] Unfortunately, the side effects of these medications make them poorly tolerated, especially in elderly patients (although, as stated above, nortriptyline is better than amitriptyline in this respect[14]). For this reason, gabapentin (as discussed above) would be a first-line agent, used prior to TCAs, by most clinicians.[28,29] Lidocaine 5% patch is also a first-line agent once the open lesions are gone. It is easy to apply, works quickly and without a long titration schedule, and works especially well for the treatment of allodynia.[71,72,73]

For patients whose pain is not controlled with non-narcotic medications alone, opioids can be an effective treatment. Both morphine and oxycodone have been proven to be effective for this indication.[88,216,217] Tramadol is another reasonable choice for PHN.[104]

Combinations of several of the above medications may be necessary to achieve an acceptable level of pain control in many patients.[218] In particular, the lidocaine 5% patch is easy to combine with oral agents because of its lack of systemic side effects and its special efficacy for allodynia. Patients who do not respond to these agents may benefit from referral to a pain specialist for more aggressive therapy.

Conclusion

As patients with cancer survive longer, with a greater disease burden, helping them maintain an adequate quality of life becomes ever more crucial. In this setting, treatment of cancer-related neuropathic pain is an essential part of the overall palliative care plan. Careful assessment and individualized treatment are the keys to successful management of neuropathic pain in cancer. Patience and persistence are required, as trials of multiple different agents may be needed before a satisfactory regimen is determined. Because much of the work on neuropathic pain syndromes has been done on nonmalignant conditions, more research on cancer-related neuropathic pain is needed.

REFERENCES.

1. Elliott KJ. Taxonomy and mechanisms of neuropathic pain. Semin Neurol 1994;14:195–205.
2. Woolf CJ, Mannion RJ. Neuropathic pain: aetiology, symptoms, mechanism, and management. Lancet 1999; 353:1959–64.
3. Raja SN, Haythornthwaite JA, Pappagallo M et al. Opioids versus antidepressants in postherpetic neuralgia. Neurology 2002;59:1015–21.
4. Ehrnrooth E, Grau C, Zachariae R, Anderson J. Randomized trial of opioids versus tricyclic antidepressants for radiation-induced mucositis pain in head and neck cancer. Acta Onc 2001;40:745–50.
5. Beydoun A, Backonja M. Mechanistic stratification of antineuralgic agents. J Pain Sympt Manage 2003;25 (Suppl 1):18–30.
6. Sindrup SH, Jensen TS. Efficacy of pharmacological treatments of neuropathic pain: an update and effect related to mechanism of drug action. Pain 1999;83:389–400.

7. Mercadante S. Intrathecal morphine and bupivicaine in advanced cancer patients implanted at home. J Pain Symptom Manage 1994; 15:166–172.

8. Sanders M, Zuurmond W. Safety of unilateral and bilateral percutaneous cervical cordotomy in 80 terminally ill cancer patients. J Clin Oncol 1995;13:1509–12.

9. McQuay HJ, Tramer M, Nye BA, et al. A systemic review of antidepressants in neuropathic pain. Pain 1996;68: 217–27.

10. Kieburtz K, Simpson D, Yiannoutos C, et al. A randomized trial of amitriptyline and mexiletene for painful neuropathy in HIV infection. Neurology 1998;51: 1682–8.

11. Shlay, Chaloner K, Max M, et al. A randomized, placebo-controlled trial of a standardized acupuncture regimen or amitriptyline for pain caused by HIV-associated peripheral neuropathy. JAMA 1998;280:1590–5.

12. Ehrnrooth E, Grau C, Zachariae R, Anderson J. Randomized trial of opioids versus tricyclic antidepressants for radiation-induced mucositis pain in head and neck cancer. Acta Onc 2001;40:745–50.

13. Kalso E, Tasmuth T, Pertti J. Amitriptyline effectively relieves neuropathic pain following treatment of breast cancer. Pain 1995;64:293–302.

14. Watson C, Vernich L, Chipman M, Reed K. Nortriptyline versus amitriptyline in postherpetic neuralgia: a randomized trial. Neurology 1998;51:1166–71.

15. Max MB, Lynch SA, Muir J, et al. Effects of desipramine, amitriptyline, and fluoxetine on pain in diabetic neuropathy. N Eng J Med 1992:326:1250–6.

16. Sindrup SH, Gram LF, Brosen K, et al. The selective serotonin reuptake inhibitor paroxetine is effective in the treatment of diabetic neuropathy symptoms. Pain 1990;42:135–144.

17. Sindrup SH, Bjerre U, Dejgaard A et al. The selective serotonin reuptake inhibitor citalopram relieves the symptoms of diabetic neuropathy. Clin Pharmacol Ther 1992;52: 547–52.

18. Semenchuk MR, Davis B. Efficacy of sustained-release bupropion in neuropathic pain: an open-label study. Clin J Pain 2000;16:6–11.

19. Semenchuk MR, Sherman S, Davis B. Double-blind, randomized trial of bupropion SR for the treatment of neuropathic pain. Neurology 2001;57:1583–8.

20. Sindrup SH, Bach FW, Madsen C, et al. Venflaxine versus imipramine in painful polyneuropathy. Neurology 2003;60:1284–1284.

21. Davis JL, Smith RL. Painful peripheral diabetic neuropathy treated with venflaxine extended release capsules. Diabetes Care 1999;22:1909–10.

22. Kiayias JA, Vlachou ED, Lakka-Papadodima E. Venflaxine HCl in the treatment of painful peripheral diabetic neuropathy. Diabetes Care 2000;23:699.

23. Simpson DA. Gabapentin and venflaxine for the treatment of painful diabetic neuropathy. J Clin Neromusc Dis 2001;3:53–62.

24. Reuben SS, Makari-Judson G, Lurie SD. Evaluation of efficacy of the perioperative administration of venflaxine XR in the prevention of postmastectomy pain syndrome. J Pain Symp Manage 2004;27:133–9.

25. Mallinckrody CH, Goldstein DJ, Detke MJ, et al. Duloxitene: a new treatment for the emotional and physical symptoms of depression. Primary Care Companion J Clin Psychiatry 2003;5:19–28.

26. Goldstein DJ, Lu Y, Detke MJ, et al. Effects of duloxitene on painful symptoms associated with depression. Psychosomatics 2004. 45:17–28.

27. Backonja M, Beydoun A, Edwards KR, et al. Gabapentin for the symptomatic treatment of painful neuropathy in patients with diabetes mellitus. JAMA 1998.

28. Rowbotham M, Harden N, Stacey B, et al. Gabapentin for the treatment of postherpetic neuralgia. JAMA 1998;280: 1837–42.

29. Rice AS, Maton S, Postherpetic Neuralgia Study Group. Gabapentin in postherpetic neuralgia. Pain 2001;94: 215–24.

30. Serpell MG, Neuropathic Pain Study Group. Gabapentin in neuropathic pain syndromes. Pain 2002;99:557–66.

31. Bone M, Critchley P, Buggy DJ. Gabapentin in postamputation phantom limb pain. Reg Anesth Pain Med. 2002;27:481–6.

32. Backjona M, Glanzman P.L. Gabapentin dosing for neuropathic pain. Clin Ther 2003;25:81–104.

33. Oneschuk D, al-Shahri MZ. The pattern of gabapentin use in a tertiary palliative care unit. J Palliat Care 2003;19: 185–7.

34. Caraceni A, Zecca E, Martini C, et al. Gabapentin as an adjuvant to opioid analgesia for neuropathic cancer pain. J Pain Symptom Manage 1999;17:441–5.

35. Zakrzewska JM, Chaudhry Z, Nurmikko TJ, et al. Lamotrigine (lamictal) in refractory trigeminal neuralgia: results from a double-blind placebo controlled crossover trial. Pain 1997;73:223–30.

36. Simpson DM, Olney R, McArthur JC, et al. A placebo-controlled trial of lamotrigine for painful HIV-associated neuropathy. Neurology 2000;54:2115–9.

37. Simpson DM, McArthur JC, Olney D, et al. Lamotrigine for HIV-associated painful sensory neuropathies: a placebo-controlled trial. Neurology 2003;60:1508–14.

38. Eisenberg E, Alon N, Yarnitsky D. Lamotrigene in the treatment of painful diabetic neuropathy. Eur J Neurol 1998;5:167–73.

39. Vestergaard K, Andersen G, Gottrup H, et al. Lamotrigine for central poststroke pain: a randomized controlled trial. Neurology 2001;56:184–90.

40. Campbell FG, Graham JG, Zilkha KJ. Clinical trial of carbamazepine (Tegretol) in trigeminal neuralgia. J Neurol Neurosurg Psychiat 1966;29:265–7.

41. Killian M, Fromm GH. Carbamazepine in the treatment of neuralgia: use and side effects. Arch Neurol 1968;19: 129–36.

42. Carrazana E, Mikoshiba I. Rationale and evidence for the use of oxcarbazepine in neuropathic pain. J Pain Symptom Manage 2003;25(Suppl 5):31–35.

43. Dworkin RH, Corbin AE, Young JP Jr et al. Pregabalin for the treatment of postherpetic neuralgia: a randomized, placebo-controlled trial. Neurology 2003;60:1274–83.

44. Backonja MM. Anticonvulsants (antineuropathics) for neuropathic pain syndromes. Clin J Pain 2000;16 (Suppl 2):67–72.

45. Price MJ. Levetiracetam in the treatment of neuropathic pain: three case studies. Clin J Pain 2004;20:33–6.

46. Ward S, Jenson M, Royal M, et al. Gabapentin and levetiracetam in combination for the treatment of neuropathic pain. J Pain 2002;3(2 Suppl 1):38.

47. Reddy S, Patt RB. The benzodiazepines as adjuvant analgesics. J Pain Symptom Manage 1994;9:510–4.

48. Felsby S, Nielsen J, Arendt-Nielsen L, Jensen TS. NMDA receptor blockade in chronic neuropathic pain: a comparison of ketamine and magnesium chloride. Pain 1996;64:283–91.

49. Nickolajsen L, Hansen PO, Jensen TS. Oral ketamine therapy in the treatment of post amputation stump pain. Acta Anaesthesiol Scand 1997;41:329–31.

50. Eide PK, Jorum E, Strubhaug A, et al. Relief of post herpetic neuralgia with the NMDA receptor antagonist ketamine. Pain 1994;58:347–54.

51. Tarumi Y, Watanabe S, Bruera E, et al. High-dose ketamine in the management of cancer-related neuropathic pain. J Pain Symptom Manage 2000;19:405–7.

52. Kotilnska-Lemieszek A, Luczak J. Subanesthetic ketamine: an essential adjuvant for intractable cancer pain. J Pain Symptom Manage 2004; 28:100–2.

53. Fitzgibbon EJ, Hall P, Schroder C, et al. Low dose ketamine as an analgesic adjuvant in difficult pain syndromes: a strategy for conversion from parenteral to oral ketamine. J Pain Symptom Manage 2002;23:165–70.

54. Benitez-Rosario MA, Feria M, Salinas-Martin A, et al. A retrospective comparison of the dose ratio between subcutaneous and oral ketamine. J Pain Symptom Manage 2003;25:400–2.

55. Jackson K, Ashby M, Martin P, et al. "Burst" ketamine for refractory cancer pain: an open-label audit of 39 patients. J Pain Symptom Manage 2001;22:834–42.

56. Kannan TR, Saxena A, Bhatnagar S, et al. Oral ketamine as an adjuvant to oral morphine for neuropathic pain in cancer patients. J Pain Symptom Manage 2002;23:60–5.

57. Bell RF, Eccleston C, Kalso E. Ketamine as an adjuvant to opioids for cancer pain: a qualitative systemic review. J Pain Symptom Manage 2003;26:867–75.

58. Mercadante S, Arcuri E, Tirelli W, et al. Analgesic effect of intravenous ketamine in cancer patients on morphine therapy: a randomized, controlled, double-blind, crossover, double-dose study. J Pain Symptom Manage 2000;20:246–52.

59. Lauretti GR, Lima IC, Reis MP, et al. Oral ketamine and transdermal nitroglycerin as analgesic adjuvants to oral morphine therapy for cancer pain management. Anesthesiology 1999;90:1528–33.

60. Davis AM, Inturrisi CE. d-methadone blocks morphine tolerance and N-methyl-D-aspartate-induced hyperalgesia. J Pharmacol Exp Ther 1999;289:1048–53.

61. Foley K. Opioids and chronic neuropathic pain. N Eng J Med 2003;348:1279–81.

62. Mercadante S, Casuccio A, Agnello A, et al. Morphine versus methadone in the pain treatment of advanced cancer patients followed up at home. J Clin Oncol 1998;16: 3656–61.

63. Ventafridda V, Ripamonti C, Bianchi M, et al. A randomized study on oral morphine and methadone in the treatment of cancer pain. J Pain Symptom Manage 1986;1:203–7.

64. Gourlay GK, Cherry DA, Cousins MJ. A comparative study of the efficacy and pharmacokinetics of oral methadone and morphine in the treatment of severe pain in patients with cancer. Pain 1986;25:297–312.

65. Bruera E, Palmer JL, Bosnjak S, et al. Methadone versus morphine as a first-line strong opioid for cancer pain: a randomized,double-blind study. J Clin OC 2004;22: 185–92.

66. Mercadante S, Casuccio A, Fulfaro F, et al. Switching from morphine to methadone to improve analgesia and tolerability in cancer patients: a prospective study. J Clin Oncol 2001;19:2898–904.

67. Mercadante S, Casuccio A, Calderone L. Rapid switching from morphine to methadone in cancer patients with poor response to morphine. J Clin Oncol 1999;17: 3307–12.

68. Gagnon B, Bruera E. Differences in the ratios of morphine to methadone in patients with neuropathic versus non-neuropathic pain. J Pain Symptom Manage 1999;18 120–5.

69. Davis MP, Walsh D. Methadone for relief of caner pain: a review of pharmacokinetics, pharmacodynamic, drug interactions and protocols of administration. Support Care Cancer 2001;9:73–83.

70. Nicholson, AB Methadone for cancer pain. Cochrane Database of Systematic Reviews 2004;3.

71. Rowbotham MC, Davies PS, Verkempinck C, Galer BS. Lidocaine patch: double-blind controlled study of a new treatment method for postherpetic neuralgia. Pain 1996;65:39–444.

72. Galer BS, Rowbotham MC, Perander, Friedman E. Topical lidocaine patch relieves postherpetic neuralgia more effectively than a vehicle topical patch. Pain 1999;80: 533–8.

73. Galer BS, Jensen MP, Ma T, et al. The lidocaine patch 5% effectively treats all neuropathic pain qualities. Clin J Pain 2002;18:297–301.

74. Meier T, Wasner G, Faust M, et al. Efficacy of lidocaine patch 5% in the treatment of focal peripheral neuropathic pain syndromes. Pain 2003;106:151–8.

75. Watson CP, Evans RJ, Watt VR. Postherpetic neuralgia and topical capsaicin. Pain 1988;33:333–40.

76. Watson CP, Tyler KL, Bickers DR, et al. A randomized vehicle-controlled trial of topical capsaicin in the treatment of postherpetic neuralgia. Clin Theraputics 1993;15: 510–26.

77. Capsaicin Study Group. Treatment of painful diabetic peripheral neuropathy with topical capsaicin. Arch Intern Med 1991;15:2225–9.

78. Capsaicin Study Group. Effect of treatment with capsaicin on daily activities of patients with painful diabetic neuropathy. Diabetes Care 1992;15:159–65.

79. Chad DA, Aron N, Lundstrom R, et al. Does capsaicin relieve the pain of diabetic neuropathy? Pain 1990;42:387–8.

80. Low PA, Opfer-Gehrking TL, Dyck PJ, et al. Double-blind, placebo controlled study of the application of capsaicin cream in chronic distal painful polyneuropathy. Pain 1995;62:163–8.

81. Dini D, Bertelli G, Gozza A, Forno GG. Treatment of the postmastectomy pain syndrome with topical capsaicin. Pain 1993;54:223–6.

82. Watson CP, Evans RJ, Watt VR. The post mastectomy pain syndrome and the effect of topical capsaicin. Pain 1989;38:177–86.

83. Watson CP, Evans RJ. The post mastectomy syndrome and topical capsaicin. Pain 1992;51:375–9.

84. Cassuto J Wallin G, Hogstrom S, et al. Inhibition of postoperative pain by continuous low dose intravenous infusion of lidocaine. Anesth Analg 1985;64:971–4.

85. Boas RA, Covino BG, Shahnarian A. Analgesic responses to IV lidocaine. Br J Anesth 1982;54:501–5.

86. Edwards WT, Habib F, Burney RG, et al. Intravenous lidocaine in the management of various chronic pain states. Reg Anesth 1982;10:1–6.

87. Bath FW, Jensen TS, Kastrup J. The effect of intravenous lidocaine on nociceptive processing in diabetic neuropathy. Pain 1990;40:29–34.

88. Rowbotham M, Reisner-Keller, LA, Fields HL. Both intravenous lidocaine and morphine reduced the pain of postherpetic neuralgia. Neurology 1991;41:1024–8.

89. Brose WG, Cousins MJ. Subcutaneous lidocaine for the treatment of neuropathic cancer pain. Pain 1991;45:145–8.

90. Devulder JE, Ghys L, Dhondt W, et al. Neuropathic pain in a cancer patient responding to subcutaneously administered lignocaine. Clin JPain 1993;9:220–3.

91. Thomas J, Kronenberg R, Cox MC, et al. Intravenous lidocaine relieves severe pain. J Pall Med 2004;7:660–7.

92. Oskarsson P, Ljunggren JG, Lins PE. Efficacy and safety of mexilitene in the treatment of painful diabetic neuropathy. Diabetes Care 1997;20:1594–7.

93. Dejgard A, Peterson P, Kastrup J. Mexilitene for the treatment of chronic painful diabetic neuropathy. Lancet 1988;2:9–11.

94. Stracke H, Meyer UE, Schumacher HE, Federlin K. Mexilitene in the treatment of diabetic neuropathy. Diabetes Care 1992;15:1550–5.

95. Wright JM, Oki JC, Graves L. Mexilitene in the symptomatic treatment of diabetic peripheral neuropathy. Annal Pharmacotherapy 1997;31:29–34.

96. Kieburtz K, Simpson D, Yiannoutsous, et al. A randomized trial of amitriptyline and mexilitene for painful neuropathy in HIV infection. Neurology 1998;51:1682–8.

97. Kemper C, Kent G, Burton S, Derensinski C. Mexilitene for HIV-infected patients with painful peripheral neuropathy. J Acquir Immune Defic Syndr 1998;19:367–72.

98. Fassoulaki A, Sarantopoulos C, Melemeni A, Hogan Q. Regional block and mexilitene: the effect on pain after cancer breast surgery. Reg Anesth Pain Med 2001;26:223–8.

99. Chong SF, Bretscher ME, Mailliard JA, et al. Pilot study evaluating local anesthetics administered systemically for the treatment of pain in patients with advanced cancer. J Pain Sympt Manag 1997;13:112–7.

100. Sloan P, Basta M, Storey P, von Gunten C. Mexilitene as an adjuvant analgesic for the management of neuropathic cancer pain. Anesth Analges 1999;89:760–4.

101. Mao J, Chen LL. Systemic lidocaine for neuropathic pain relief. Pain 2000;87:7–17.

102. Harati Y, Gooch C, Swenson M, et al. Double-blind randomized trial of tramadol for the treatment of the pain of diabetic neuropathy. Neurology 1998;50:1842–6.

103. Erdine S. Efficacy of tramadol hydrochloride in chronic painful diabetic neuropathy. Proceedings of the 8th World Congress on Pain; 1997; Seattle: IASP Press. p. 271.

104. Gobel H, Stradler TH. Treatment of pain due to postherpetic neuralgia with tramadol. Clin Drug Invest 1995;10:208–14.

105. Sindrup SH, Anderson G, Madsen C, et al. Tramadol relieves pain and allodynia in polyneuropathy. Pain 1999;83:85–90.

106. Petzke F, Radbruch L, Sabatowski R, et al. Slow-release tramadol for the treatment of chronic malignant pain—an open multicenter trial. Support Care Cancer 2000:9:48–54.

107. Wilder-Smith CH, Schimke J, Osterwalder B, et al. Oral tramadol, a mu-opioid agonist and monoamine reuptakeblocker, and morphine for strong cancer-related pain. Ann Oncol 1994;5:141–6.

108. Leppart W. Analgesic efficacy and side effects of oral tramadol and morphine administered orally in the treatment of cancer pain. Nowotwory 2001;51:257–66.

109. Macrae WA. Chronic pain after surgery. Br J Anaesth 2001;87:88–98.

110. Senturk M, Ozcan P, Perihan E, et al. The effects of three different analgesia techniques on long-term postthoracotomy pain. Anesth Anal 2002;94:11–5.

111. Dajczman E, Gordon A, Kreisman H, Wolkove N. Long-term postthoracotomy pain. Chest 1991;99:270–4.

112. Katz J, Jackson M, Kavanagh B, Sandler AN. Acute pain after thoracic surgery predicts long-term postthoracotomy pain. Clin J Pain 1996;12:50–5.

113. Ochroch EA, Gottschalk A, Augostides J, et al. Long-term pain and activity during recovery from major thoracotomy using thoracic epidural analgesia. Anesthesiology 2002;97:1234–44.

114. Richardson J, Sabanthan S, Mearns AJ, et al. Postthoracotomy neuralgia. Pain Clin 1994;7:87–97.

115. Matsunaga M, Dan K, Manabe FY, et al. Residual pain of thoracotomy patients with malignancy and non-malignancy. Pain 1990;Suppl 1:148.

116. Kalso E, Perttunnen K, Kaasinen S. Pain after thoracic surgery. Acta Anaesthesiol Scand 1992;36:96–100.

117. Obata H, Saito S, Fujita N, et al. Epidural block with mepivicaine before surgery reduces long-term postthoracotomy chest pain. Can J Anaesth 1999;46:1127–32.

118. Cerfolio RJ, Bryant AS, Bass CS, Bartolucci AA. A prospective double-blinded, randomized trial evaluating the use of preemptive analgesia of the skin before thoracotomy. Ann Thorac Surg 2003;76:407–12.

119. Landreneau RJ, Pigula F, Luketich JD, et al. Acute and chronic morbidity differences between muscle sparing versus standard postlateral thoracotomy on pulmonary function, muscle strength and postoperative pain. J Thoracic Cardiovasc Surg 1996;112:1346–51.

120. Kirby TJ, Mack MJ, Landrenau RJ, et al. Video-assisted thoracic surgery versus muscle-sparing thoracotomy. J Thorac Cardiovasc Surg 1995;109:997–1002.

121. Furrer M, Rechsteiner R, Eigenmann V, et al. Thoracotomy and thorascopy: postoperative pulmonary chest wall complaints. Eur J Cardio-thorac Surg 1997;12:82–7.

122. Cerfolio RJ, Price TN, Bryant AS, et al. Intracostal sutures decrease the pain of thoracotomy. Ann Thorac Surg 2003;76:407–12.

123. Jung BF, Ahrendy GM, Oaklaner, Dworkin RH. Neuropathic pain following breast cancer surgery: proposed classification and research update. Pain 2003;104:1–13.

124. Kroner K, Krebs B, Skov J, Jorgensen HS. Immediate and long term phantom breast syndrome after mastectomy. Pain 1989;36:327–34.

125. Jamison K, Wellisch DK, Katz RL, Pasnau RO. Phantom breast syndrome. Arch Surg 1979;114:93–5.

126. Granek I, Ashikai R, Foley K. The postmastectomy pain syndrome: clinical and anatomical correlates. Proc Am Soc Clin Oncol 1984;3:122.

127. Foley KM. Pain syndromes in patients with cancer. Med Clin North Am 1987;71:169–84.

128. Stevens PE, Dribble SL, Miakowski C. Prevalence, characteristics and impact of postmastectomy pain syndrome. Pain 1995;61:61–8.

129. Smith WCS, Bourne D Squair J, et al. A retrospective cohort study of postmastectomy pain syndrome. Pain;1999;83:91–5.

130. Tasmuth T, von Smitten K, Hietamem P, et al. Pain and other symptoms after different treatment modalities of breast cancer. Ann Oncol 1995;6:453–9.

131. Wallace MS, Wallace AM, Lee J, et al. Pain after breast surgery: a survey of 282 women. Pain 1996;66:195–205.

132. Dirks J, Fredsborg BB, Christensen D, et al. A randomized study of the effects of single-dose gabapentin versus placebo on postoperative pain and morphine consumption after mastectomy. Anesthesiology 2002;97:560–4.

133. Reuben SS, Makari-Judson G, Lurie SD. Evaluation of efficacy of the perioperative administration of venflaxine XR in the prevention of poatmastectomy pain syndrome. J Pain Symptom Manage 2004;24:133–9.

134. Tasmuth T, Hartel B, Kalso E. Venflaxine in neuropathic pain following treatment of breast cancer. Eur J Pain 2002;6:17–24.

135. Jensen TS, Krebs B, Nielsen J, Rasmussen P. Immediate and long-term phantom limb pain in amputees. Pain 1985:21:267–78.

136. Nickolajsen L, Ilkjaer S, Kroner K, et al. The influence of preamputation pain on post amputation stump and phantom pain. Pain 1997: 393–405.

137. Parkes CM. Factors determining the persistence of phantom pain in the amputee. J Psychosom Res 1973;17:97–108.

138. Sherman RA, Sherman CJ, Parker L. Chronic phantom and stump pain among American veterans. Pain 1984;18:83–95.

139. Nikolajsen L, Jensen TS. Phantom limb pain. Br J Anaesth 2001;87:107–16.

140. Jensen TS, Krebs B, Nielsen J, et al. Phantom limb, phantom pain and stump pain in amputees during the first 6 months following limb amputation. Pain 1983;17:243–56.

141. Wartan SW, Harmann W, Wedley JR, McColl I. Phantom pain and sensation among British veteran amputees. Br J Anaesth 1997;78:652–9.

142. Sherman RA. Stump and phantom limb pain. Neurol Clin 1989;7:249–64.

143. Chabal C, Jacobson L, Russel L, Burchiel KJ. Pain responses to perineuromal injection of normal saline gallamine and lidocaine in humans. Pain 1989;36:321–5.

144. Nikolassen L, Hansen CL, Nielsen J, et al. The effect of ketamine on phantom pain: a central neuropathic disorder maintained by peripheral input. Pain 1996;67:69–77.

145. Flor H, Elbert T, Muhlnickel, et al. Cortical reorganization and phantom phenomena in congential and traumatic upper extremity amputees. Exp Brain Res 1998;119:205–12.

146. Houghton AD, Nicholls G, Houghton AL, et al. Phantom pain: natural history and association with rehabilitation. Ann R Coll Surg Engl 1994;76:22–5.

147. Bach S, Noreng MF, Tjelden NU. Phantom limb pain in amputees during the first 12 months following limb amputation, after preoperative lumbar epidural blockade. Pain 1988;33:297–301.

148. Katz J. Prevention of phantom limb pain by regional anaesthesia. Lancet 1997;349:519–20.

149. Sugarbaker PH, Weiss CM, Davidson DD, et al. Increasing phantom limb pain as a symptom of cancer recurrence. Cancer 1984;54:373–5.

150. Huse E, Larbig W, Flor H, Birbaumer N. The effect of opioids on phantom limb pain and cortical reorganization. Pain 2001;90:47–55.

151. Jaeger H, Maier C. Calcitonin in phantom limb pain: a double blind study. Pain 1992:48:21–7.

152. Katz J, Melzk R. Auricular transcutaneous electrical nerve stimulation (TENS) reduces phantom limb pain. J Pain Sympt Manage 1991;6:73–83.

153. Flor H, Denke C, Shaefer M, Grusser S. Effects of sensory discrimination training on cortical reorganization and phantom limb pain. Lancet 2001;357:1763–4.

154. Vecht CJ, Hoff AM Kansen PJ, et al. Types and causes of pain in cancer of the head and neck. Cancer 1992;70:178–84.

155. Grond S, Zech D, Lynch J, et al. Validation of World Health Organization guidelines for pain relief in head and neck cancer. Ann Otol Rhino Laryngol 1993;102:342–8.

156. Chaplin JM, Morton RP. A prospective longitudinal study of pain in neck and neck cancer patients. Head and Neck 1999;21:531–7.

157. Talmi YP, Horowitz Z, Pefeffer R, et al. Pain in the neck after neck dissection. Otolaryn Head Neck 2003;123:302–6.

158. Sist T, Miner M, Lema M. Characteristics of postradical neck pain syndrome: a report of 25 cases. J Pain Sympt Manage 1999;18:95–102.

159. Wittekindt C, Liu W, Klussman J, Guntinas-Linchius O. Botulinum toxin type A for the treatment of chronic neck pain after neck dissection. Head Neck 2004;26:39–45.

160. Lederman RJ, Wilbourne AJ. Brachial plexopathy: recurrence cancer or radiation? Neurology 1984:34:1331–5.

161. Thyagarajan D, Cascino T, Harms G. Magnetic resonance imaging in brachial plexopathy of cancer. Neurology 1995;45:421–7.

162. Thomas JE, Cascino Tl, Earle JD. Differential diagnosis between radiation and tumor plexopathy of the pelvis. Neurology 1985;35:1–7.

163. Watling CJ, Moulin DE. Neuropathic pain. In: Bruera ED, Portenoy RK, editors. Cancer pain: assessment and management. New York: Cambridge University Press; 2003. p. 400.

164. Boogerd W, Ten Bokkel Huinink WW, Dalesio O, et al. Cisplatin-induced neuropathy: central, peripheral and autonomic involvement. J Neurooncol 1990;255–63.

165. Lomonasco M, Milone M, Batocchli AP, et al. Cisplatin neuropathy: clinical course and neurophysiological findings. J Neurolo 1992;239:199–204.

166. Siegal T, Haim N. Cisplatin induced peripheral neuropathy: frequent off-therapy deterioration, demyelinatin syndromes and muscle cramps. Cancer 1990;15:117–1123.

167. Extra JM, Marty M, Brienza S, Misset JL. Pharmacokinetics and safety profile of oxaliplatin. Semin Oncol 1998;25:13–22.

168. Markman M, Kennedy A, Webster K, et al. Neurotoxicity associated with a regimen of carboplatin and paclitaxel employed in the treatment of gynecological malignancies. J Cancer Res Clin Oncol 2001;127:55–8.

169. Gerritsen van der Hoop R, Vecht CJ, van der Burg ME, et al. Prevention of cisplatin neurotoxicity with an ACTH (4–9) analogue in patients with ovarian cancer. N Engl J Med 1990.

170. Neijt J, van der Burg M Vecht C, et al. A double-blind randomized study with Org 2766, an ACTH (4-9) analog, to prevent cisplatin neuropathy [abstract]. Proc ASCO 1994;13:261.

171. Kemp G, Rose P, Lurain J, et al. Amifostine pretreatment for protection against cyclophosphamide-induced and cisplatin-induced toxicities: results of a randomized control trial in patients with advanced ovarian cancer. J Clin Oncol 1996;14:2101–12.

172. Rick O, Beyer J, Schwella N, et al. Assessment of amifostine as protection from chemotherapy-induced toxicities after conventional-dose and high-dose chemotherapy

in patients with germ cell tumor. Ann Oncol 2001;12:1151–5.

173. Gradishar WJ, Stephenson P, Glover DJ, et al. A phase II trial of cisplatin plus WR-2721 (amifostine) for metastatic breast carcinoma: an Eastern Cooperative Oncology Group Study (E8188). Cancer 2001;92:2517–22.

174. Cascinu S, Cordella L, Del Ferro E, et al. Neuroprotective effect of reduced glutathione on cisplatin-based chemotherapy in advanced gastric cancer. J Clin Oncol 1995;13:26–332.

175. Apfel SC, Arezzo JC, Lipson L, Kessler JA. Nerve growth factor prevents experimental cisplatin neuropathy. Ann Neurol 1992;31:76–80.

176. Eckel F, Schmelz R, Adelsberger H, et al. Prevention of oxaliplatin-induced neuropathy by carbamazepine: a pilot study. Dtsch Med Wochenschr 2002;127:78–82.

177. Wilson RH, Lehky T, Thomas RR, et al. Acute oxaliplatin-induced peripheral nerve hyperexcitability. J Clin Oncol 2002;20:1767–74.

178. van Gerven JM, Moll JW, van den Bent MJ, et al. Paclitaxel (taxol) induces cumulative mild neurotoxicity. Eur J Cancer 1994;30:1074–7.

179. Postma TJ, Vermorken JB, Liefting AJ, et al. Paclitaxel-induced neuropathy. Ann Oncol 1995;6:489–94.

180. Schiller JH, Storer B, Tutsch K, et al. Phase I trial of 3-hour infusion of paclitaxel with or without granulocyte colony-stimulating factor in patients with advanced cancer. J Clin Oncol 1994;12:241–8.

181. New PZ, Jackson CE, Rinaldi D, et al. Peripheral neuropathy secondary to docetaxel (Taxotere). Neurology 1996;46:108–11.

182. Hilkens PH, Verweij J, Stoter G, et al. Peripheral neurotoxicity induced by docetaxel. Neurology 1996;46:104–8.

183. Kaplan JG, Einzig AI, Schaumburg HH. Taxol causes permanent large fiber peripheral nerve dysfunction: a lesson for preventative strategies. J Neurooncol 1993;16:105–7.

184. Trimble EL, Adams JD, Vena D, et al. Paclitaxel for platinum-refractory ovarian cancer: results from the first 1000 patients registered to National Cancer Institute Treatment Referral Center 9103. J Clin Oncol 1993;11:2405–10.

185. Lipton RB, Apfel SC, Dutcher JP, et al. Taxol produces a predominantly sensory neuropathy. Neurology 1989;39:368–73.

186. Vahdat L, Papadopoulos K, Lange D, et al. Reduction of paclitaxel-induced peripheral neuropathy with glutamine. Clin Cancer Res 2001;7:1192–7.

187. Hamers FP, Pette C, Neijt JP, et al. The ACTH(4-9) analog, Org2766 prevents Taxol-induced neuropathy in rats. Eur J Pharmacol 1993b;233:177–8.

188. Pronk LC, Hilkens PH, van der Bent MJ, et al. Corticosteroid co-medication does not reduce the incidence and severity of neurotoxicity induced by docetaxel. Anticancer Drugs 1998;9:759–64.

189. Vahdat L, Papadopoulos K, Lange D, et al. Reduction of paclitaxel-induced peripheral neuropathy with glutamine. Clin Cancer Res 2001;7:1192–7.

190. DiPaola RS, Rodriguez R, Goodin S, et al. Amifostine and dose intense paclitaxel in patients with advanced malignancies. Cancer Ther 1998;1:11–7.

191. Hayakawa K, Itoh T, Niwah H, et al. NGF prevention of neurotoxicity induced by cisplatin, vincristine and taxol depends on toxicity of each drug and NGF treatment schedule. Brain Res 1998;794:313–9.

192. Quasthoff S, Hartung HP. Chemotherapy-induced peripheral neuropathy. J Neurol 2002;249:9–17.

193. Sandler SG, Tobin W, Henderson ES. Vincristine-induced neuropathy: a clinical study of fifty leukemic patients. Neurology 1969;19:367–74.

194. Haim N, Epelbaum R, Ben-Sahar M, et al. Full dose vincristine (without 2-mg dose limit) in the treatment of lymphomas. Cancer 1994;15:2515–9.

195. Postma TJ, Benard BA, Huijgens PC, et al. Long term effects of vincristine on the peripheral nervous system. J Neurooncol 1993;15:23–7.

196. Legha SS. Vincristine neurotoxicity, pathophysiology and management. Med Toxicol 1986;1:421–7.

197. Jackson DV, Wells HB, Atkins JN, et al. Amelioration of vincristine neurotoxicity by glutamic acid. Am J Med 1988;84:1016–22.

198. Dellon AL, Swier P, Maloney CT, et al. Chemotherapy-induced neuropathy: treatment by decompression of peripheral nerves. Plastic Reconstruct Surg 2004;114:478–83.

199. Flatters SJL, Bennett GJ. Ethosuximide reverses paclitaxel and vincristine-induced painful peripheral neuropathy. Pain 2004;109:150–61.

200. Dworkin RH, Schmader KE. Treatment and prevention of postherpetic neuralgia. Clin Infect Disease 2003;36:877–82.

201. Watson CPN, Deck JH, Morshead C, et al. Postherpetic neuralgia: postmortem examination of a case. Pain 1988;34:129–38.

202. Watson CPN, Deck JH, Morshead C, et al. Postherpetic neuralgia: further postmortem studies of cases with and without pain. Pain 1991;44:105–17.

203. Whitley RJ, Shukla S, Crooks RJ. The identification of risk factors associated with persistent pain following herpes zoster. J Infect Disease 1998;178 (Suppl 1):71–5.

204. Tyring S, Barbarash RA, Nahlik JE, et al. Famciclovir for the treatment of acute herpes zoster: effects on acute disease and postherpetic neuralgia. Ann Intern Med 1995;123:89–96.

205. Dworkin RH, Boon RJ, Griffithe DRG, Phung D. Postherpetic neuralgia: impact of famciclovir, age rash severity and acute pain in herpes zoster patients. J Infect Disease 1998;178(Suppl 1):76–80.

206. Wood MJ, Shukla S, Fiddian AP, Crooks RJ. Treatment of acute herpes zoster: effect of early (48h) versus late (48–72h) therapy with acyclovir and valciclovir on prolonged pain. J Infect Disease 1998;178(Suppl 1):81–4.

207. Wood MJ, Kay R, Dworkin RH, et al. Oral acyclovir therapy accelerates pain resolution in patients with herpes zoster: a meta-analysis of placebo-controlled trials. Clin Infect Dis 1996;22:341–7.

208. Jackson JL, Gibbons R, Meyer G, Inouye L. The effect of treating herpes zoster with oral acyclovir in preventing postherpetic neuralgia: a meta-analysis. Arch Intern Med 1997;157:909–12.

209. Bowsher D. The effects of pre-emptive treatment of postherpetic neuralgia with amitriptyline. J Pain Symptom Manage 1997;13:327–31.

210. Wu CL, Marsh A, Dworkin RH. The role of sympathetic nerve blocks in herpes zoster and postherpetic neuralgia. Pain 2000;87:121–9.

211. Pasqualucci A, Pasqualucci V, Galla F, et al. Prevention of postherpetic neuralgia: acyclovir and prednisilone versus epidural local anesthetic and methyprednisilone. Acta Anaesthesiol Scand 2000;44:910–8.

212. Opstelten W, van Wijck AJM, Stolker RJ. Interventions to prevent postherpetic neuralgia: cutaneous and percutaneous techniques. Pain 2004;107:202–6.

213. Whitley RJ, Weiss H, Gnann JW, et al. Acyclovir with and without prednisone for the treatment of herpes zoster: a randomized placebo-controlled trial. Ann Intern Med 1996;125:376–83.

214. Wood MJ, Johnson RW, McKendrick MW, et al. A randomized trial of acyclovir for 7 or 21 days with or without prednisilone for treatment of acute herpes zoster. N Engl J Med 1994;330:896–900.

215. Max MB. Thirteen consecutive well-designed randomized trials show that antidepressants reduce pain in diabetic neuropathy and postherpetic neuralgia. Pain Forum 1995;4:248–53.

216. Watson CPN, Babul N. Efficacy of oxycodone in neuropathic pain: a randomized trial in postherpetic neuralgia. Neurology 1998;50:1837–184141.

217. Raja SN, Haythornthwaite JA, Pappagallo M, et al. Opioids versus antidepressants in postherpetic neuralgia: a randomized, placebo-controlled trial. Neurology 2002;59:1015–21.

218. Dworkin RH, Schmader KE. Treatment and prevention of postherpetic neuralgia. Clin Infect Disease 2003;36:877–82.

Psychiatric Issues in Oncology

Gabrielle Marzani-Nissen, MD
Lora D. Baum, PhD

As the array of therapeutic options for oncologic patients increases, more individuals now live with, or have undergone treatment for, cancer. As such, more patients and clinicians are experiencing cancer as a chronic process. In 2003, it was estimated that 9.6 million people were living after a cancer diagnosis.[1] For these and others, issues related to quality of life and sustained health have taken on prominence. The impact of stress and mood has been shown to have direct effects on disease outcome. This is elucidated by the now 20-year-old field of psychoneuroimmunology.[2–6]

The most common psychiatric diagnoses seen by the internist are delirium, adjustment disorders, and depression. A classic study by Derogatis and colleagues found a 44% prevalence of psychiatric disorders in cancer patients.[7] Although the most quoted study, it is based on criteria from an older Diagnostic and Statistical Manual of Psychiatry, the DSM-III. It is now thought that clinically significant levels of depression and/or anxiety develop in 15 to 40% of cancer patients, and depend on the site of cancer and the stage of disease.[8,9] The incidence of delirium also depends on the stage of illness for cancer patients and ranges from 15 to 85%.

Throughout this chapter, emphasis is placed upon a combined approach using both pharmacologic management of mood or anxiety disorders with adjunctive psychotherapy. Although some cancer patients are initially too distressed to participate fully in psychotherapy as they contend with a life-threatening illness, once a medication or treatment begins to take effect, this experience changes. Patients often want to examine the way they look at the world, and many readily grasp the connection between their thoughts, emotions, and behaviors, and how changing one can impact another.

The goal of this chapter is to provide clinicians with practical information and strategies for the cancer patients they care for. It is also designed to assist practitioners with populations who may have special needs, such as those with schizophrenia and bipolar illness. It will cover delirium, frontal lobe syndromes, anxiety disorders, mania and bipolar illnesses, personality disorders, schizophrenia, and, finally, depression and the assessment of suicide risk.

Delirium and Cognitive Impairment Disorders

Delirium

Clinical Manifestations

Delirium, characterized by a fluctuating disturbance in consciousness, is reported to affect 8 to 40% of inpatients at any given time.[10] Symptoms, which can be subtle, often occur abruptly, with an average onset of 3.3 days in the oncologic population (see DSM-IV criteria for delirium).[11] The incidence of delirium in the cancer population is cited at 13 to 25%, although up to 85% of terminally ill cancer patients are delirious.[12] Vulnerable populations include the elderly, brain injured, demented or cognitively impaired, those recovering from procedures or surgeries, and those who are very ill. The 3-month mortality is 23 to 33%.[13,14] In cancer populations, associated risk factors include advanced age, cognitive impairment, low albumin level, bone metastasis, hematologic malignancy, use of opioids, and alcoholism.[11,15] Family or nursing staff are often the first to notice delirium manifesting itself as restlessness, anxiety, change in attention, and easy distractibility. It can unmask old cerebrovascular events and cause memory impairment, disorganized speech, disorientation, misperceptions, illusions, change in sleep, aphasia, tremor, asterixis, myoclonus, and reflex and tone changes.[13]

Psychiatric symptoms and mimickers include mania, depression, tearfulness, personality changes, irritability, delusions, hallucinations, and psychosis. Subtypes include the hyperalert (agitated type), the hypoalert (lethargic type), and a mixed or alternating type.[10,12] The latter is often mistaken for depression—part of the reason that the most common consult for psychiatrist is "Evaluate for depression" while the most common diagnosis given is "Delirium."

Pathophysiologic Manifestations

The earliest sign of delirium is a disruption of the sleep-wake cycle, which is controlled by the suprachiasmatic nuclei of the anterior hypothalamus. As the sleep-wake cycle is normally synchronized with external environmental cues, a loss of light and unfamiliar hospital environments will promote delirium in vulnerable populations. The term "sundowning" is a misnomer; it is not related to light, but rather, the time of day (late afternoon). The neurotransmitter glutamate in the ascending reticular activating system (ARAS) in the brainstem, is involved in levels of consciousness and in maintaining wakefulness.[16,17] Dysregulation of other transmitters, such as acetylcholine, norepinephrine, and histamine have been implicated, with acetylcholine likely a major contributor.[17,18]

Etiology

The causes of delirium in the cancer patient are often different than in the general population. This is due to the nature of the disease and the modality of treatments. For example, intentional alkalinization of urine is produced to minimize the risk of tumor lysis syndromes. Table 1 reviews some of these features.[10,12,18–20] Even when mild, combinations of states such as anemia, and slight hypercalcemia may produce delirium in a vulnerable individual.

Diagnosis

The electroencephalograms (EEG) is often very sensitive and shows diffuse background slowing, although certain events such as delirium tremens and hyperthermia have a normal or increased amount of activity.[18,21] An EEG can rule out nonconvulsive status epilepticus, a mimicker of delirium. Although a Folstein Mini-Mental State score is often low, a normal result can occur in individuals with high premorbid functioning. Delirium can take up to 3 months to clear[22] in certain vulnerable populations; thus, internists will often care for those with resolving delirium. The evaluation for delirium involves the identification of an underlying medical cause and the removal of offending agents.

Pharmacologic Treatments

There are no medications approved by the United States Food and Drug Administration (FDA)

Table 1 Special Causes of Delirium in the Cancer Patient

Medical Illnesses

CNS: primary CNS cancer, secondary metastasis, stroke, post-operative state, whole brain radiation, non-convulsive status epilepticus

Hepatic: hepatic failure or dysfunction; hyperammonemia,

Hematologic: anemia

Metabolic: prophylactic alkalinization in patients vulnerable for tumor lysis syndrome or other hypercarbia; metabolic disarray

Renal: renal disease or failure

GI: constipation, ileus

Endocrine: hypercalcemia from bone metastasis or paraneoplastic syndromes; hyper- and hypoglycemia, adrenal pathology or crisis, hypomagnesemia, thyrotoxicosis; SIADH, hyper- and hyponatremia

Deficiencies: B_1, B_{12} and niacin deficiency

Pulmonary: hypoxia from primary lung disease, infection, or pulmonary embolus

Infections: sepsis; infections in immunosuppressed or elderly individuals, meningitis, encephalitis, or opportunistic infections

Vascular: thromboembolic events such as deep venous thrombosis, disseminated intravascular coagulation

Withdrawal: alcohol, benzodiazepines, barbiturates, narcotics

Medications that can cause Delirium in the Cancer Patient

Antibiotics (particularly quinolones, penicillins, cephalosporins)

Antifungals

Anesthesia

Anticholinergic/antihistaminergic medications (including benztropine mesylate, diphenhydramine, Phenergan, and tricyclic antidepressants)

Antihypertensives (especially β-blockers and clonidine),

Chemotherapeutic agents: L-asparaginase, bleomycin, cisplatin, cytosine arabinoside (ara-C), fludarabine, 5-fluorouracil, interferon, interleukin, ifosfamide, methotrexate (with high dose or intrathecal administration), prednisone, procarbazine, vinblastine, vinca alkaloids (vincristine)

Dopaminergic agents

Sedatives, such as benzodiazepines and other hypnotics such as zolpidem

Corticosteroids and other immunosuppressants such as azathioprine

Muscle relaxants

Opioid medications

Stimulants

Salicylates

Toxic levels of valproate, lithium, carbamazepine, digitalis

for the treatment of delirium except for alcohol withdrawal. However, the literature provides recommendations for agitated delirium. These consist of low-dose antipsychotics. Antipsychotics are divided into typical agents and atypical agents (see "Schizophrenia"). There are new warnings by the manufacturers on all atypical agents. Therefore, risks, benefits, and alternatives need to be discussed with the patients primary dellsion maker prior to giving these medicatives, for the demented elderly.[23,24] These are due to four randomized controlled trials that found an association with increased cerebrovascular events and an increase in all-cause mortality with these agents. Low-dose quetiapine beginning at 25 mg/d and increasing by 25 mg/d up to 25 mg tid has been asked. Quetiapine is very sedating, so it is useful at night. Typical agents such as haloperidol at 0.5 mg to 1 mg bid can also be started and titrated slowly.[12] Haloperidol is not particularly sedating. In the elderly, some typical agents such as chlorpromazine are avoided because of their anticholinergic activity. The partial dopamine agonist aripiprazole, and the atypical agent ziprasidone have little data to support their use in delirium. Akathisia is a common side effect of all antipsychotics, although it is seen more frequently in older agents. Higher doses have been recommended in some textbooks, but that brings the possibility of extrapyramidal side effects, such as dystonia and parkinsonism. Prolonged Q–Tc intervals, torsades de pointes, and neuroleptic malignant syndromes (discussed elsewhere), are also major concerns.[25] Vital signs should be monitored, an electrocardiogram (EKG) ordered, and Q–Tc intervals monitored for moderate to high doses.

If a person is severely agitated, some recommend a higher dose of haldol, such as 5 to 10 mg. Checking for acute hypoxia and other vital-sign abnormalities is important before doing so. As the delirium is resolving, plan to taper because there is a risk of tardive dyskinesia. Tardive dyskinesia is thought to be related to extrapyramidal side effects. Typical neuroleptics have a 25% incidence of tardive dyskinesia in the elderly at 1 year, which is often irreversible. The incidence of tardive dyskinesia is thought to be much lower in the newer agents, but quetiapine, which is thought

to have the least EPS of all the agents, is still reported to have 4 to 6% at low doses and 6 to 8% at high doses.[26]

Benzodiazepines should not be used for delirium unless it is due to alcohol or benzodiazepine withdrawal. It is critical to determine if this is delirium is due to alcohol or benzodiazepine withdrawal because all antipsychotic agents can lower the seizure threshold.

Recommendations for the treatment of agitated delirium are as follows.

- Check vital signs, rule out an acute medical process
- Rule out offending medications
- Rule out alcohol withdrawal
- Obtain a baseline EKG and Q–Tc (with a monitored bed if high doses of medication required)
- Begin with haloperidol 0.5-1 mg bid, or quetiapine 25mg at night, and titrate slowly
- Consider giving two-thirds of the total dose in the evening and one-third in morning, or morning and noon
- Consider the possibility that increased agitation is due to akathisia

Psychological interventions

Establishing a routine and providing visual cues wtih clocks, calendars, exposure to daytime sunlight, and the closing of curtains at night can help the confused patient reestablish a sleep-wake cycle.[27] Decreasing stimulation and activities at night will minimize and help prevent delirium. Providing familiar objects from home, such as a favorite pillow case or piece of music can assist with the reorienting process. Individuals with poor eyesight and hearing need their hearing aid and glasses to prevent misinterpretation of shadows and noises, which fosters delusions.[18,28] If a patient is in the hospital, a single room without undue distractions is helpful. Having consistent caregivers, who provide confident, consistent care will help reassure the frightened patient and help from feel safe. The family should be briefed on ways to help the patient, such as the calm repetition of information. Limiting the number of caregivers and restricting visitors to a few familiar people can be very helpful.

Frontal Lobe Syndromes

Frontal lobe syndromes occur with bilateral lesions. This may be due to a variety of insults including ischemia, mass effect such as tumor, and degenerative or demyelinating processes.[29] Individuals manifest these syndromes with a delay in processing information and retrieving information, poor judgment, and a decrease in curiosity. This social withdrawal or apathy can quickly shift to irritability, abrupt behavioral aggression, and disinhibition. An intact unilateral lobe does not generally produce this behavior. Lesions of the frontal lobes have three presentations: changes in motor activities, personality changes, and cognitive dysfunction.[30] There are predictable responses to specific lesions. For example, damage to orbitofrontal regions is associated with behavioral disinhibition, lack of guilt, and poor insight. Dorsolateral regions affect higher functioning behaviors and produce mood disorders. Injury in the medial region causes lethargy, amotivation, and less spontaneous movements and use of language.[29]

For patients who have had primary brain tumors or secondary metastasis, personality changes may be evident. It is important to rule out offending medications, which can potentially worsen or cause other effects. For example, benzodiazepines may contribute to behavioral disinhibition. Although antipsychotic medications are often recommended and used for behavioral dyscontrol, parkinsonism often occurs. Seizures are not uncommon in this population. Levetiracetam (Keppra), which is often successfully used as an antiepileptic drug (AED), may worsen behavior in some individuals. In this case, other AEDs such as valproate (VPA), carbamazepine (CBZ), lamotrigine, and oxcarbazepine may be more appropriate. It is best to use an AED that has some mood-stabilizing properties, rather than phenytoin in this population. Additionally, delirium may also be very subtle in this population.

Families often need to be educated to understand that behaviors that appear to be laziness, depression, or antisocial behavior are due to frontal lobe injury. Depending on the needs and limitations of the individual, referrals to occupational therapy and physical therapy can be helpful.

Anxiety Disorders

Anxiety per se is often a healthy and adaptive response to the diagnosis of cancer and its treatments.[31] In cancer patients, stressful periods occur at points of transition. These include a new cancer diagnosis, beginning any new treatment, waiting for test results, and preparing for medical procedures. In advanced cancer patients, the failure of treatment or a recurrence can produce anxiety.[32] Shock and disbelief commonly follow the diagnosis of cancer. Anxiety, intrusive thoughts, impaired attention, irritability, dysphoric mood, and vegetative symptoms such as loss of appetite and difficulty sleeping, will often occur but should slowly resolve over 7 to 10 days.[32] However, significant anxiety and depressive disorders can persist in between 25 to 48% of individuals.[7,10,32–34] About 4 to 5% of patients with cancer have preexisting anxiety disorders, which is the most prevalent psychiatric disorder in the general adult population. Adjustment disorders (see

DSM-IV chart on adjustment disorders), an exaggerated form of normal anxious response, are the mos t common type of disorder in cancer patients.[35] Anticipatory anxiety can occur before appointments or treatments and can become a conditioned response to the treatment setting.[36]

Diagnosis

Standard screening instruments and criterion, including the DSM, may overdiagnose anxiety (see TWS is a charts?? for Generalized Anxiety disorder) and mood disorders in medically ill individuals because they include neurovegetative criteria that can artificially elevate the score of an individual who may have difficulty with sleep or appetite due to the cancer or the cancer treatment.[32,34] The Hospital Anxiety and Depression Scale (HADS) has been validated to assess patients with medical illnesses.[32,37]

Cancer is now considered a risk factor for the development of Acute Stress Disorder (ASD) and Post-traumatic Stress Disorder (PTSD) (see chart).[38] Acute stress disorder begins within 2 days of the event, such as the cancer diagnosis, and lasts up to 4 weeks (see TWS is a charts??).

If at that point symptoms continue, the criterion for post-traumatic stress disorder is met. Symptoms include the reexperiencing of the event, avoidance, a sense of numbing, detachment or lack of emotional responsiveness, reduced awareness of surroundings, derealization and impaired recall. PTSD includes nightmares and flashbacks (see DSM-IV criteria for PTSD). In this context, the individual may not hear critically important information. As a practical matter, a physician should write down important information, and ideally have a friend or family member in the room to assist with later recall. Many factors, including biologic vulnerability, prior trauma, and poor social supports play a role in the development of ASD and PTSD.[38] In the cancer population, other factors include youth, previous health, and dissatisfaction with the manner in which they were told about cancer.[38] The stage of illness affects the content of anxiety. For example, anticipated alopecia has been shown to be "the most disturbing factor" in 47 to 58% of women with cancer, while other body-image issues predominate in metastatic disease.[39,40] There is debate as to whether anxiety disorders predominate among different sites of cancer.[32,41]

The diagnosis or treatment of cancer can exacerbate generalized anxiety disorders, which are present in 1.5 to 3% of the population.[42] However, some cancers, such as pancreatic cancer, can produce anxiety, panic attacks and depression, and precede the diagnosis in up to 50% of patients.[43] Symptoms must cause "clinically significant" distress or impairment in an important area of functioning, last at least six months,

and not be due to a substance, medicine, or medical problem (see the chart from DSM-IV).

The Diagnostic and Statistical Manual of Psychiatry, Fourth Edition, text revision (DSM-IV-TR) requires that a primary anxiety disorder be excluded if the etiology is due to a substance, medication or medical illness that can cause the symptoms.[44] Therefore, any patient who has a sudden increase in distress should be evaluated for an acute medical or metabolic process. It is not unusual for a patient to who was on steroids, or given benzodiazepines for nausea or narcotics in the hospital to develop withdrawal that unwittingly occurred in the transition into or from the hospital. Clarifying which medications were given in the hospital, not just the discharge medications, can be very important. Patients may have been started on medications that produced anxiety as a side effect. These may include steroids or beta agonists. Acute anxiety in populations who have a statistically high association with alcohol, such as head and neck, esophageal, gastric, and pancreatic cancers should be thought to be possibly from alcohol withdrawal. Additionally, patients who are heavy smokers may have nicotine withdrawal.

In cancer patients, symptoms of anxiety should also prompt the clinician to consider brain metastases, pulmonary embolus, thyroid disease, rapid withdrawal from steroids, hypoglycemia, and adrenal disease as appropriate. Anxiety due to a medication should be considered. Akathisia, a subjective sense of motor restlessness that manifests as pacing, and inability to sit still, or skin crawling, is often associated with typical and atypical neuroleptics, Phenergan, Compazine, and selective serotonin reuptake inhibitors (SSRIs).[18,45]

Medical Illnesses That Can Present as Anxiety

- Cardiac: ischemia, arrhythmias, systolic and diastolic failure and diastolic dysfunction, valvular disease
- Endocrine: carcinoid, adrenal crisis or disease, disorders of calcium, thyroid disease, pheochromocytoma
- Metabolic: potassium disorders, hypoglycemia, hyponatremia, uremia, hypercarbia from pain, and prophylactic alkalinization of urine
- Respiratory/Pulmonary: hypoxia, asthma/reactive airways, COPD, pneumothorax, pulmonary edema, pulmonary embolism
- Heme: porphyrias (anxiety and panic attacks), anemia
- Neurologic: delirium, brain tumor, infarcts (particularly left frontal lobe infarcts), traumatic brain injury, mass effects, epilepsy / seizures (particularly temporal lobe epilepsy), vertigo

- Gastrointestinal: acute or chronic bleeding (hypovolemia)
- Immunologic: anaphylaxis, transfusion reaction
- Substances: alcohol, barbiturate, or benzodiazepine withdrawal; amphetamines and sympathomimetic agents, caffeine and caffeine withdrawal, nicotine withdrawal, opioid withdrawal, akathisia from Phenergan, Compazine, typical or atypical antipsychotic agents, corticosteroids

Pharmacologic Treatments

Medications FDA-approved and traditionally used for anxiety disorders include SSRIs, selective serotonin/noradrenergic reuptake inhibitors (SNRIs) such as venlafaxine hydrochloride, mirtazapine, tricyclic agents, monoamine oxidase inhibitors (MAO-I) and benzodiazepines. Tricyclic medications and MAO-Is are avoided as first-line agents due to their side effects and danger or lethality in overdose.

Generalized anxiety disorders have also been treated successfully with azapirone agents such as buspirone hydrochloride (Buspar).[46–48] Gabapentin and lamotrigine have some reported efficacy. SSRIs and SNRIs may induce nausea, but controlled release forms may avoid the stimulation of upper gastrointestinal serotonin receptors that mediate nausea. Although generally regarded as safe and first-line agents, SSRIs (and possibly SNRIs) may increase the risk of intraoperative bleeding.[49] For cancer patients, the clinician should be aware that these medications cause an SIADH-like hyponatremia, and lower the seizure threshold by about 0.1%.

The anxiety seen in cancer patients is associated with more autonomic hyperactivity than in other patients with anxiety disorders.[32] These patients may be more sensitive to the side effects of some medications such as the SSRIs, venlafaxine and buspirone. A clinical pearl in treating anxiety with SSRIs and venlafaxine is the recognition that there is often an initial burst of anxiety in the first days of use with this medications; this anxiety usually dissipates within a few days. Clinical effects take 2 to 4 weeks. Telling the patient to anticipate a small increase in anxiety is therapeutically reassuring and often allows them to better tolerate the initial days. Working patients may prefer to start the medication on a weekend to minimize stress. Slow titration at half the recommended starting dose, with a dose increase in a week can often minimize side effects. Although the dose required to treat anxiety is lower than that for depression, complete resolution of panic symptoms will often not occur until higher doses are used. All SSRIs and medications in the antidepressant family have now been given warnings about the increased risk of suicidal ideation. This is likely multifactorial, and will now likely require

a routine follow-up sooner than the usual 1-month follow-up as (recommendations are being formalized by consensus guidelines). So long as patients understand that they need to contact someone immediately if they feel suicidal, or proceed to the nearest emergency room, it is reasonable to prescribe these medications for anxiety, especially since depression and panic themselves carry a risk of suicidal ideation. Although many practitioners prescribe benzodiazepines for the initial days, this can promote dependence on these agents. If prescribing a benzodiazepine, a longer acting one, such as clonazepam (Klonopin) is preferred, as there is less of an initial "rush" and less tendency to become dependent on the instant relief of anxiety. Although not FDA-approved, psychiatrists will often use low doses of quetiapine 25 to 50 mg instead of benzodiazepines for sleep and anxiety.[50]

Classes of Medications used for Anxiety Disorders

The following medications are for GAD, ASDs, and PTSDs. All SSRIs and SNRIs cause hyponatremia, and all can lower seizure threshold, as can Wellbutrin.

SSRIs are the most prevalent medications used for their safety profile and efficacy. The oldest agents have the most P-450 interactions, which is important for patients on complex medication regimens. They are fluoxetine (Prozac), paroxetine (Paxil), sertraline (Zoloft), citalopram (Celexa), and escitalopram (Lexapro). The longer acting forms generally have less initial anxiety and gastrointestinal distress, but the medications with the long-acting (sustained release (SR), XR, XL forms (paroxetine, fluoxetine, venlafaxine) also have the most P-450 interactions. All of these medications cause sexual dysfunction and weight gain. Start at half of the recommended dose.

Bupropion (Wellbutrin) is generally avoided for panic disorder as it can worsen panic attacks. Although most notorious for lowering the seizure threshold, the long-acting forms have the same incidence as SSRIs and SNRIs. It has no sexual dysfunction associated with it. It may be activating, but also may have better effect on sleep architecture. The SR form may reduce fatigue in cancer patients [51]

Mirtazepine (Remeron) is good for cancer patients with nausea (it may stimulate appetite), and insomnia (lower doses are more sedating than higher doses), anorexia (causes weight gain), and it has a sol tab. It has P-450 interaction. Start at 15 mg and increase if the patient is too sedated.

Duloxetine: (Cymbalta) uses NE and serotonin simultaneously, and has efficacy for pain. It has more than 1,000 inactive metabolites,

and should not be used with renal or hepatic dysfunction. Start at 30 mg.

Venlafaxine, (Effexor XR form) at low doses acts like an SSRI, and at higher doses has NE effects (BP). It appears to have efficacy for pain. It has mild effects on blood pressure at higher doses (about 10 mm). Start at 37.5 mg, and titrate slowly by 37.5 mg increments.

Tricyclics are generally avoided because of anticholinergic and muscarinic side effects, and high lethality in overdose.

MAO-Is (eg, phenelzine) are generally avoided because of lethality in overdose and strict dietary requirements.

Buspirone (Buspar) is recommended for generalized anxiety disorders, and usually is not effective for patients who have a history of using benzodiazepines. Start at 5 mg at night and increase slowly in a bid or tid fashion. When taken with food, there is less of a side effect of dizziness.

Gabapentin (Neurontin, Micromedex, Inc.) is sedating, has no antidepressant properties, but may have efficacy for social phobia. Start at 100 mg at night and increase by 100 mg in a bid or tid fashion.

Atypical Antipsychotics such as quetiapine, olanzapine, risperidone are used at times for severe anxiety as an augmentation strategy, and are sedation. Quetiapine has the least extrapyramidal side effects, and can be started at 25 mg a night titrating rapidly by 25 mg doses.

Benzodiazepines are used with caution by many psychiatrists because of their risk of dependence. Longer acting medications, such as clonazepam are useful because there is less of an initial "rush" with the medication. Clonazepam additionally has few active metabolites, although it is long-acting so should be used with caution for patients with hepatic dysfunction. If used, Clonazepam should be initiated at 0.25 mg twice a day before beginning the SSRI or SNRI, and then removed within weeks.[52] Alprazolam is avoided by psychiatrists because of the "rush" associated with it and the risk of addiction with this short-acting agent.

There are open labeled studies with valproate, carbamazepine, and topiramate. Clonidine hydrochloride and propranolol have both been cited as helpful for anxiety, but both can cause depression in some individuals. Trazodone hydrochloride (Desyrel), a very weak antidepressant, is good for sleep architecture, and can be used for sleep augmentation. Early studies in Europe found that it compared well against diazepam; using 25 mg tid found the anxiolytic effect to be equivalent to diazepam (Valium) 5 mg tid for anxiety.[52–54] Trazodone has been associated with priapism. Other sedative hypnotics such as zolpidem tartrate (Ambien) can be helpful for short periods, as efficacy decreases with long-term use.

An elixir is available for fluoxetine, and a soluble tablet is available for mirtazapine.

For acute stress disorders and post-traumatic stress, SSRIs have been shown to be effective. Tricyclics and MAO-Is (phenelzine) have been shown to be efficacious, but for the reasons above, are generally avoided. Open label studies with valproate, carbamazepine, and topiramate have shown mixed or limited efficacy. There is one controlled trial with lamotrigine showing efficacy (note, however, the risk of rash). Additionally, there is preliminary evidence that olanzapine, quetiapine, and risperidone may be helpful. Propranolol may reduce the onset of post-traumatic symptoms, and clonidine hydrochloride may have effects, but both can cause depression. Benzodiazepines are anxiolytic, but, again, raise a concern for tolerance and addiction, as they act on the GABA receptor complex that is shared with alcohol.[55]

Drug Interactions

The cytochrome P-450 system is a hepatic enzyme system that has clinically significant interactions with psychotropic agents and chemotherapy. Medications that are metabolized by this system will often interact with one another. In a healthy general population on no other medications P-450 interactions are rarely an issue. However, in cancer populations, certain chemotherapeutic agents and other medications used for nausea and side effects will interact with this system. Medication catabolism can be increased or decreased. There are helpful resources that are free and available on the Internet (eg, <http://medicine.iupui.edu/flockhart/table.htm>) as well as books that can guide the practitioner. Additionally, pharmacists are a helpful resource. Many antidepressants and antipsychotic agents use the P-450 systems. A helpful rule of thumb for SSRIs is that the newer ones often have the least P-450 interaction. Even with interactions, these medications can be used. The key is to go slow. Some common substrates include antidepressants (eg, amitriptyline, imipramine, bupropion, all SSRIs, mirtazapine, venlafaxine), antipsychotics (typical and atypical agents including clozapine, haloperidol, olanzapine, perphenazine, risperidone, thioridazine) chemotherapeutic agents, (eg, cyclophosphamide, ifosfamide, paclitaxel, tamoxifen), antinausea agents (eg, ondansetron, metoclopramide) and pain medications, such as celecoxib and methadone.

The P-450 interaction can increase levels of these agents substantially and cause adverse events. For example, excess stimulation of central serotonin receptors are thought to cause serotonin syndrome. This causes autonomic dysfunction, similar to neuroleptic malignant syndrome, and includes tachycardia, fever, diaphoresis, hypertension, diarrhea and myoclonus. When extreme, it can lead to shock and death. Of note,

the chemotherapeutic agent procarbazine, a weak MAO-I, should be used cautiously with any medication that has tricyclic, serotonergic, or noradrenergic components because of the risk of hypertensive crisis and serotonin syndromes.[56] This would include many psychiatric medications.

Psychological Interventions

Many anxious cancer patients are reluctant to take more medication, especially if they are also taking chemotherapy. Cognitive and behavioral techniques are often quite effective and have the added benefit of the patient's active participation in their care, a factor that adds to feelings of self-efficacy (the confidence of a person in their ability to successfully complete a task) and increased control. This idea forms the basis for many of the cognitive-behavioral interventions that will be helpful to cancer patients. Recently, a meta-analysis of many studies found that psychological interventions for anxiety were effective even when offered preventively to cancer patients on the basis of their medical diagnosis, and not psychological distress.[57] Initial treatment involves education about the nature of anxiety, and then the teaching of relaxation techniques, guided imagery, self-hypnosis, or distraction. These techniques are useful for many of the treatment-related side effects of chemotherapy, such as nausea, vomiting, and fatigue, as well as for anxiety.[58] For instance, many patients can be taught to modify pain or nausea sensations through self-hypnosis, which can decrease their intake of medication, thus allowing them choices in how symptoms are managed.[59] Biofeedback may be used to help monitor training in these techniques, but is usually not necessary, since patients often experience subjective improvement rather quickly.

The experience of anxiety is often both cognitive and physical. Patients describe racing thoughts; obsessive, repetitive thoughts; and a future-oriented sensation of dread or impending doom. In addition, the physiologic sensations include a subjective feeling of tension (often in the stomach and chest) and muscle tension (usually in the neck and shoulders). Hand and jaw clenching can occur, even in sleep, which can leave muscles feeling fatigued. Cognitive-behavioral interventions for anxiety thus must be targeted to an individual's experience to achieve optimum symptom relief.

Interventions for anxiety can take many different forms. Most produce what Herbert Benson has termed a "relaxation response," which is characterized by a decreased sympathetic arousal.[60] Meditation, yoga, and exercise are examples of techniques that patients can pursue independently through community-based courses.[61,62] Many psychologists trained in behavioral

medicine techniques can teach patients diaphragmatic breathing, autogenics (a technique used to induce vasodilation or constriction through increasing or decreasing peripheral blood flow), progressive muscle relaxation, and self-hypnosis, all of which have been found helpful in reducing anxiety.[63]

Most patients with anxiety are aware of a mind-body connection, because they notice the somatic effects of anxiety. To take advantage of an anxious patient's propensity to imagine the worst, a statement such as, "I already know you have a good imagination because you're a great worrier" can be used. This comment provides a positive use for what can be perceived as a negative trait, and does so with compassion and humor. Here are two examples of easy-to-teach cognitive techniques, which can be taught to a patient in a few moments during an office visit.

Thought Stopping   This technique serves as both a distraction and a focal point, which allows a cycle of obsessive thoughts to be broken and then redirected. The patient is asked to picture a big, red, stop sign and to focus on the octagonal shape, the red background with white letters. The stop sign's powerful influence in everyday culture is emphasized: everybody obeys stop signs. As the stop sign is envisioned, the thought process is interrupted, and the patient is directed to then focus on something pleasant and positive, such as a pleasant memory, or a place that recalls good feelings. Redirecting activity, such as moving to a different room, or taking a brief walk outside, can also serve to break the chain of obsessive thoughts.

Worry Time   Worry can be framed as an inefficient use of free time, which does not change the outcome of a feared event, but does negatively impact quality of life. Therefore, the patient is directed to continue to worry (since they have undoubtedly failed at not worrying), but to do it at a prescribed time only. For instance, worrying for the first five minutes of each hour would be allowed, but worrying outside of this time is prohibited. Through this technique, patients will often realize that nothing bad happens if they miss their "worry time" and they might even enjoy life in the meantime.

One component of anxiety in cancer patients that is not addressed by some of the cognitive-behavioral interventions discussed here is the anxiety that is a part of having a life-threatening illness. For many, cancer is the first time that mortality has become a clear possibility. This existential anxiety is best addressed through the exploration of beliefs and fears about the dying process and what lies beyond. For instance, many patients fear a painful, lonely death. Allowing a person to discuss what would constitute an optimal death experience can relieve some of the anxiety and fear associated with dying. Encouraging a patient to open a discussion with relatives about end-of-life planning can deepen relationships with significant others and lead to healing on many levels.

Adjustment Disorders

Cancer patients who have clinically significant symptoms of anxiety or depression and do not meet criteria for other disorders often have adjustment disorders. In a study of patients referred to a psycho-oncology service, 40% had an adjustment disorder.[64] These individuals usually had good functioning before their diagnosis, and the stress of the cancer diagnosis or treatment engenders subjective feelings of distress, and difficulty coping or functioning at work or at home. Patients may or may not report these to their primary medical provider or oncologist, but because psychological distress is so common in cancer patients, it is important to inquire about overall coping when seeing them. In most cases, the level of psychological distress in adjustment disorders does not warrant psychotropic medication. Psychological interventions that are effective for adjustment disorders include supportive psychotherapy, group peer support, and group psycho-educational therapy.

Supportive psychotherapy targets specific symptoms, such as depression, anxiety or insomnia, and places the symptoms into a context that normalizes the reaction, given the extreme circumstances of a cancer diagnosis. Often, patients have never consulted a mental health professional and are now more open to it because having cancer is universally understood as a stressor. This can be an opportunity for a patient to gain support in a confidential, professional setting, and not to burden relatives with fears and concerns. Patients often look forward to leaving their troubles at the therapist or doctor's office so they can feel emotionally stronger around family. Small interventions, such as ways to improve sleep[65] and nutrition, can often improve physical and emotional functioning in tandem.

Peer group support is a good choice for those who prefer a community-based intervention, and fellow patients can provide a sense of authenticity missing from a purely professional encounter. The informal support that occurs as a result of exchanging tips for thriving through treatment help not only in the short term, but also in the relationships that often grow out of these groups. Social support has been found to be a key variable in successful adjustment to cancer,[66] and support groups provide this in many ways.

In 1989, David Spiegel and colleagues published a surprising analysis of data that showed that weekly supportive group therapy with self-hypnosis for pain in women with metastatic breast cancer improved survival when compared to a randomized control group.[67] This article was based upon an intervention that was designed to test the effectiveness of their model to decrease pain and increase quality of life, which it also did. However, upon a retrospective analysis of the survival of the groups, Spiegel was surprised to notice that the women in the intervention group lived about twice as long as those in the control group. This finding swept through the cancer community, and soon patients were calling for support groups with the belief that, if they participated, they would live longer. Subsequently, other researchers, including those mentored by Spiegel[68] have provided a mixed outcome with regards to increased longevity. In an editorial,[69] Spiegel states that 5 of 10 published trials report that psychotherapy prolongs survival. He explains the trials that do not show this effect by the large changes in both medical care and the widespread demand for psychosocial support that have occurred since his original study was begun in the late 1970s. Regardless of whether longevity is increased, almost all trials demonstrate improvement in psychological functioning, with the more distressed patients benefiting the most.[68]

When recommending support groups for patients, it is important to distinguish between those that are completely peer-led and those that are professionally led. While peer-led groups can be helpful for those who are exhibiting mild symptoms, professionally led groups have the benefit of being able to provide specific skills training in coping techniques, relaxation therapy, and credible information. More distressed or more isolated patients can usually benefit from this increased level of monitoring and mentoring.

Lastly, exercise is an intervention that is often overlooked, yet can be very effective in preventing cancer related-fatigue, and improving mood.[70] In both breast cancer[71] and prostate cancer[72] patients, randomized trials of exercise in patients receiving radiotherapy found that patients who engaged in a moderate, home-based exercise program had no increase in fatigue from baseline, while patients who did not exercise had significant increases in fatigue. The exercise programs also improved overall physical functioning, which added to self-efficacy and self-esteem during a time when many patients feel discouraged. Pinto and Turnzo[73] found that, among breast cancer patients, those who exercised reported higher satisfaction with body image and better mood than sedentary patients. Overall, for patients with mild to moderate symptoms characteristic of adjustment disorders, significant improvements in quality of life can be made by addressing symptoms such as mood, insomnia, and fatigue.

Mood Disorders

Major Depression

Rates of depression in cancer patients vary from 1 to 50%, depending on the type of malignancy and study.[74–76] Major depression likely affects about 25% of the cancer population.[74,75,77,78] In a study at Memorial Sloan-Kettering Cancer Center, 31% of patients seen by the consult psychiatry service had a major depressive disorder or an adjustment disorder with depressed mood.[75] Factors, including interferon, appear to be involved in certain types of depression. Thus, individuals treated with interferon therapy may be vulnerable.[79–83] The site of cancer has been associated with various levels of psychological distress.[9] The assessment of depression in the cancer patient is discussed in another chapter (see Chapter 9, "Cancer and Depression"). Before prescribing an antidepressant in any patient, a screen to rule out hidden bipolar illness, alcohol abuse, and suicidal ideation is warranted. This includes an assessment for hypomania, with questions such as: "Have you ever seemed to need less sleep than usual, felt rested or energized, with clarity of thought or racing thoughts?" All SSRIs and medications in the antidepressant family have now been given warnings about the increased risk of suicidal ideation. As discussed in the section on anxiety, this is likely multifactorial, and will now likely require a routine follow-up sooner than the usual 1-month follow-up as recommendations are being formalized by consensus guidelines. So long as patients understand that they need to contact someone immediately if they feel suicidal, or proceed to the nearest emergency room, it is reasonable to prescribe these medications, especially since depression carries its own risk of suicidal ideation and suicide. In using these medications, it should be noted that many interact through the P-450 pathway (see "Anxiety Disorders").

The pharmacologic treatment of depression depends on whether or not the patient is undergoing treatment with chemotherapy, radiation, or surgery. If none of those, the treatment of depression should be the same as for the general population. Traditional first-line agents for depression include SSRIs, venlafaxine, mirtazapine, and bupropion. Gender and age differences have been noted with these agents in the treatment of depression. This is thought to be related to the presence or absence of estrogen. In some studies, premenopausal women have better responses to SSRIs than men or postmenopausal women. There is some suggestion that venlafaxine may have more efficacy than SSRIs in men and postmenopausal women. For example, there was a 2.5 times greater trend in improvement for women over 50 years old on venlafaxine compared with younger women on SSRIs.[84,85] A new agent, duloxetine (Cymbalta) appears to be very good for some pain syndromes. Optimizing side effects can be helpful in choosing an agent. For example, mirtazapine is helpful for nausea, weight gain, and sedation, and causes no sexual dysfunction. Bupropion is activating, weight-neutral, causes no sexual dysfunction, but has a risk of seizures in its warning label. The longest acting versions have the equivalent risk of seizure as SSRIs. Both of these agents interact with the P-450 system (see "Anxiety Disorders"). The newest SSRIs have the least P-450 interaction. SSRIs and venlafaxine appear to have efficacy for women for hot flashes, which can be useful for women who cannot be on estrogen replacement.[86,87] However, venlafaxine can also cause sweating. SSRIs and venlafaxine are associated with headache. Duloxetine tends not to cause headache. Second-line agents such as tricyclics and MAO-Is carry more side effects and can be lethal in overdose. For more details on the agents discussed above, the reader is referred to the section on anxiety and Table 2.

Psychological Interventions

The treatment of depression using cognitive therapy has long been a mainstay in psychotherapy.[88] Beck described the "cognitive triad" as (1) a negative view of the self (as unworthy, inadequate, and bad); (2) a negative view of the environment (as unsatisfying, demanding, and difficult); and (3) a negative view of the future (as unchangeable, unfulfilling, and hopeless). The thoughts related to this triad are the key cognitions in depression. Cognitive therapy serves to correct

misconceptions and errors in judgment and generate an array of possibilities for the future through demonstrating that choices are available even in difficult situations. This approach was recently found to be effective in decreasing depression and increasing optimism in women with early-stage breast cancer treated with a 10-week, group cognitive-behavioral stress management intervention.[89]

When providing primary medical care to a depressed patient, practitioners can sometimes begin to feel hopeless. The faulty logic that characterizes some patients' thoughts, as well as the subjectively difficult circumstances they have, can at times be hard to counter. However, maintaining professional distance while showing empathy, and continuous positive reframing of negative or irrational thoughts serves to model optimism.

Here are a few interventions that can be used to help remind patients that they do have some control over what can feel like a hopeless situation:

Identifying Automatic Thoughts

Ask patients if they have thoughts that seem to repeat over and over, like a broken record. Many depressed patients will readily describe them when prompted. Some examples might be "I'm not going to survive this," "I'm a terrible burden to my family," or "Why should I bother with all this?" A short examination of the usually skewed perceptions, by refuting with logical information, can be helpful. Examples based on your knowledge of the patient's situation can be helpful here, such as: "Just as you cared for your husband after his surgery, he now wants to help you through

this." Patients can be surprised how unrealistic—yet pervasive—these thinking patterns can be when they identify and discard their negative automatic thoughts.

Positive Reframing

Pessimism often only allows a glass to seem half empty, when in fact it is also half full. Language is an important framer of possibility. Illness can be seen to be an impediment or an opportunity for change with regard to interpersonal relationships, work, and recreation. If a patient continually verbalizes what they can't do, ask, "What can you do now that you couldn't before?" A pause in life, even a forced one, is still a break in routine, and allows for thinking and doing things differently.

Identifying Dichotomous Thinking

Many depressed patients see only black-and-white outcomes. They are blind to the myriad possibilities that exist in the gray area in between. When you hear patients being very rigid in their dichotomous thinking, you can challenge them to generate more possibilities. ("Are the only two choices available to stay in bed or to jog your usual mile? What other activities could you pursue at this time?")

The role of a primary medical doctor for the cancer patient with depression can seem daunting. However, what patients value as much as medical expertise is the human ability to understand. By providing a depressed patient with the correct 'prescription' to see clearly, they can take back control of a situation that can, at times, feel overwhelming.

Suicide

In the general population, individuals with mood disorders have a 15% lifetime risk of suicide and account for 50 to 70% of successful suicides. There is a higher risk with anxiety or panic symptoms and alcohol abuse. Fifteen to 25% of suicides are due to alcohol dependence and other substance abuse. However, these individuals often have a comorbid depression and have experienced an "interpersonal loss."[90] There is a correlation between low serotonin levels and suicidal behavior.[91–93]

In general, the risk factors for suicide are listed in Table 3.[88,92]

Suicide in the Cancer Patient

Suicide should not be considered a "rational act" in the cancer patient.[75] It should be attributed to an underlying state, such as depression, delirium or pain.[95] Cancer patients have twice the risk of suicide than that of the general population.[95,96] The same risk factors, such as male gender, older age, marital status, and social isolation apply as

SSRIs	starting dose in mgs	dose range in mgs	metabolized by	inhibitor	stimulator
Fluoxetine (Prozac)	10–20	20–80	2D6		
Paroxetine (Paxil)			2D6	+ + +2D6	-for both
Immediate Release	10	10–50			
Controlled Release	12.5	12.5–62.5			
Sertraline (Zoloft)	25–50	50–200	No for both	-for both	-for both
Citalopram (Celexa)	10	20–60	No for both	-for both	-for both
Escitalopram (Lexapro)	5	10–20	No for both	+2D	-for both
Bupropion (Wellbutrin)			No for both	+ +2D6	-for both
Immediate Release	100	100–150 TI0			
Sustained Release	150	150–300			
Extended Release	150	300–450			
Venlafaxine XR (Effexor XR)	37.5	75–225	2D6	-for both	-for both
Mirtazapinee (Remeron)	15	15–45	No for both	-for both	-for both
Duloxetine (Cymbalta)	30	30–60	2D6	+ +2D6	-for both

Table 2 Selective Medications Used for the Treatment of Depression in Cancer Patients

+ = least interaction; + + = moderate interaction; + + + = most interaction

Table 3 Risk Factors for Suicide in the General Population

Male gender

Social isolation

Social status (being divorced, widowed or single)

Unemployment, change in social or economic status, legal problems, moving

Psychiatric illness (particularly, major depression or bipolar illness), co morbid psychiatric illness, psychological turmoil, previous attempts, alcohol use, anxiety

Physical illness

Family history

Presence of firearms

Recent loss

Hopelessness

Psychosis (particularly with command hallucinations)

Older age

Presence of a specific plan, means available to carry out the plan, and rehearsal of the plan.

in the general population. For example, men with cancer who are in their 60s and 70s have a 1.55 to 2.3 times greater risk for suicide than that of the general population.[97] As with the general population, poor social support, personal or family history of mood disorders, or prior attempts at suicide increase the risk, as do drug and alcohol abuse. For patients, risk is highest in the first few months after diagnosis.[97]

Psychological distress and "existential suffering" are also related to suicide.[98] Greater physical impairment or dependency, transition states (treatment decisions, undergoing treatment), emotional stress related to the diagnosis of cancer, plus social and cultural attitudes have been found to increase the risk of suicide. Additionally, pain, change in physical appearance, terminal illness or anxiety due to a poor prognosis, and issues related to death and dying are risk factors for suicide.[74,75,90,99] Hopelessness is more significant than the diagnosis of depression in determining risk of suicide.[75]

Confounding variables such as metabolic abnormalities (eg, hypercalcemia) and medications, including steroids and β-blockers, should be identified to rule out medication-induced depression. Certain medications, such as levetiracetam (Keppra) have been associated with suicidal ideation in small numbers of individuals.[100] A diagnosis of cancer, particularly brain cancer, has been associated with a higher risk of suicide.[101] Others report the highest risk in head and neck,[102] gastrointestinal (GI),[96] genitourinary, lung, and other respiratory cancers.[97] Additionally, breast cancer has been associated with a higher risk of suicide compared to other types of cancer.

As noted above, comorbid substance abuse with alcohol in general increases the risk for

suicide. This may be one reason why suicide risk in head, neck, and GI cancers may be higher than with other cancers.

Assessment of depression and suicidality should include asking the patient if there have been periods of hypomania (bipolar II symptoms), as these individuals may be more likely to enter a "mixed state," where they are energized and dysphoric, a highly dangerous combination. The most likely time to commit suicide is when the person has the energy to do it. Individuals naturally may go though a mixed state as the energy returns and they may look better, but still report severe depression. SSRIs have been associated with a risk of suicidal ideation, and this may be, in part, due to the temporary phenomenon of a mixed state. However, the risk of suicide in an unmedicated, depressed population is higher than that for a medicated one. Delirium, by producing a depressed affect, may induce suicidal behavior.[75] It is noted that, before committing suicide, 8 of 10 patients who were suicidal had asked for better pain control.[78] Medications such as interferon, steroids, and other agents that are contributing to the symptoms should be halted and reassessed.

Assessment of suicidal ideation in the cancer patient entails the following.[75]

- Be empathic
- Establish a relationship
- Identify depression, anxiety, or other psychiatric illness
- Evaluate for delirium
- Identify risk factors in the patient (demographics, family history of psychiatric illness and suicides, past depressions or anxiety, substance abuse, suicide history)
- Identify risk factors related to the cancer (prognosis, stage, pain)
- Identify social and other support systems (who they live with; where they live)
- Identify hopelessness
- Identify suicidal ideation
- If suicidal or hopeless, identify if there is plan
- Identify if it is possible to implement the plan (access to guns in the home, for example)

When in doubt, the patient should be evaluated immediately by a mental health professional to determine need for admission to a hospital. If admitted, a sitter with a psychiatric consult-service following should be assigned to the individual, or admission to a psychiatric service should be instituted as appropriate.

Bipolar Disorder and Secondary Mania

Traditionally, when the term mania is used, it refers to the manic pole of a bipolar (or

manic-depressive) illness. Unipolar depression, also known as Major Depressive Disorder is described elsewhere. Bipolar disorders have two subtypes. Bipolar type I is associated with mania, mixed states, and depression, whereas bipolar type II has hypomania and depression. Hypomania by definition does not require hospitalization (see DSM-IV criteria for mania and hypomania).

Etiology and Diagnosis

In cancer patients, mania can be a manifestation of a primary bipolar illness, a side effect of a medication, or a manifestation of an underlying condition, such as a brain tumor or delirium. Although it is debated as to whether one has to have a bipolar diathesis to become manic on medications, in vulnerable patients, mania can be induced with antidepressants, stimulants, steroids, INH, L-dopa, and caffeine.[103–105]

Cerebrovascular events and neuro-oncologic events can also precipitate mania or exacerbate a stable condition.[104,106–109] The role of the right side of the brain in secondary mania is well established,[110] although there are instances documented of left hemispheric injury.[111] A high index of suspicion should be used to assign a diagnosis of a new bipolar illness in a cancer patient. Substance abuse (including alcohol, amphetamines, cocaine), thyroid or other endocrine dysfunction, cerebrovascular events, partial complex seizures, and personality disorders can mimic bipolar illness.

Pharmacologic Treatments

There is solid literature and expert consensus guidelines for the treatment of mania due to a bipolar I disorder. Drugs that are FDA-approved for bipolar mania include: lithium, valproate, olanzapine, risperidone, quetiapine, and anpipir ziprasidone.[112] There is solid literature for carbamazepine and lamotrigine FDA-approved for maintenance in bipolar depression). Other off-label medications include oxcarbamazepine[113] and topiramate. Electroconvulsive therapy (ECT) is also recognized as a valid treatment for bipolar mania.

However, these guidelines neither automatically apply, nor should be reflexively used for secondary mania. Secondary mania does not appear to respond as well to lithium and may respond better to divalproex sodium or olanzapine.[114] In secondary mania, the first task, if possible, is to remove the offending agent.

For cancer patients, there are specific concerns with mood stabilizers, as some depress bone marrow functioning (VPA and CBZ) and have other important effects. For example, valproate (Depakote, Depakene) is bound to albumin. Any process that affects albumin alters the levels of valproate. It is important, then, to check a free and total level of valproate, particularly in low-albumin states. Valproate interacts with many medications used in cancer patients, including antiemetics of the phenothiazine class (promethazine hydrochloride and prochlorperazine) and antipsychotic agents.

The choice of mood stabilizer varies for the type of bipolar disorder (eg,, euphoric vs. mixed) (see DSM-IV criteria for mixed state) and is still actively debated in the literature. For euphoric mood or "classic" mania: lithium is considered to be the gold standard, although valproate is a first-line agent. For mixed episodes, dysphoric mood, or rapid cycling, the treatment of choice is VPA or CBZ, although some think that lithium is still a first-line agent (Table 4). When rapid loading is required, oral VPA at 10 to 15 mg/kg is recommended in a divided dose. When psychotic, antipsychotic medications are utilized, the FDA has approved antipsychotic agents for the treatment of mania. There are no consensus guidelines for the treatment of substance-induced mania.

Due to the complexity of these medication interactions, providers are strongly encouraged to check for them before prescribing these medications.

Personality Disorders

In clinical practice, patients who have a diagnosis of a personality disorder, or traits of such, are deemed difficult, challenging, or even hateful.[116] One of the hallmarks in recognizing patients with personality disorders is the ability to evoke intense negative feelings in their caregivers. When this occurs in patients who have a medical illness, and especially a life-threatening disease such as cancer, the clinician is placed in a difficult bind: how to help with compassion while setting limits with a patient who demands attention.

According to the DSM–IV, a personality disorder is "an enduring pattern of inner experience and behavior that deviates markedly from the expectations of the individual's culture, is pervasive and inflexible, has an onset in adolescence or early adulthood, is stable over time, and leads to distress or impairment."[44] A review of the 10 specific personality disorders is beyond the scope of this text, but instead, certain traits of patients with borderline personality disorder (BPD) will be used to identify ways in which treatment by the primary care provider can contribute to an overall positive outcome.

About 2% of the general population carries a diagnosis of BPD,[44] and therefore these patients interact frequently with the medical system, where they often present with chronic pain, hypochondriasis, multiple somatic complaints, medication

sensitivity, and drug-seeking behavior.[117] Even though many have occasional, extreme episodes of psychiatric symptoms (such as brief psychotic episodes, dissociative episodes, impulsivity, and rage), often the diagnosis is missed because of a superficially intact ability to function in society. It is only under stress that intense feelings of abandonment can resurface, an issue in which the medical system can play an unwitting part. Characteristic office behaviors include boundary violations (premature familiarity, requesting

special treatment), medical neediness, atypical presentation (self-inflicted wounds), mediation-seeking behavior, and a lack of cooperation with medical treatment (nothing works, or there are reasons for why interventions can't be tried, leading to an escalating and complex treatment plan). Often, the clinician is left with the sense that "I'm trying too hard and nothing is helping." This is one of the classic binds of the BPD patient: "You must help me/You can't help me." Another, more complicated bind is when the clinician

Table 4 Guidelines for use of Mood Stabilizers*

Lithium
Used for classic euphoric mania
As a salt, is affected by sodium and medications that affect sodium (see below):
Has Effects on renal, thyroid, cardiac, neurologic (tremor, cognitive impairment) skin (acne), GI), metabolic (weight gain) systems
Lowers seizure threshold
Increases white blood cell count (demarginates white cells)
Toxicity and overdose: narrow therapeutic window) Has risk of check level at 12 hours after last dose
Increased by: Thiazides, spironolactone, triamterene, ACE inhibitors, indomethacin (as much as 60%), NSAIDs, calcium channel blockers, tetracycline
Note: aspirin does not increase lithium levels
Decreased by: NaCl and sodium bicarbonate, acetazolamide, psyllium, theophylline

Valproate (VPA):
Used for mixed/rapid cycling
Is an Anticonvulsant
Can cause sedation, nausea, vomiting, diarrhea, tremor weight gain, LFT elevation and pancreatitis
Needs free and total levels 12 hours after last dose
Can be loaded
Has sprinkles that can be used
Is Protein bound, affected by low albumin states and competing medications
Affects bone marrow, often platelets more than other lines
Increased by: Phenobarbital, magnesium and aluminum hydroxide, aspirin, fluoxetine
Decreased by; CBZ

Carbamazepine (CBZ):
Used for mixed/rapid cycling mania
Is an Anticonvulsant
Needs level at 12 hours after last dose
Structurally similar to TCAs, so consider when on other SSRIs or TCAs
Can affect bone marrow, cause transient leukopenia, mild thrombocytopenia, both idiopathic and dose related, elevated liver function tests including a cholestatic picture, and can cause a rash
SIADH
Multiple drug-drug interactions:
Increases levels of erythromycin, antiarrhythmics, diltiazem, cimetidine, verapamil, VPA (lowers VPA level)
Lowers levels of acetaminophen, alprazolam, amitriptyline, bupropion, clonazepam, cyclosporine, desipramine, fentanyl, fluphenazine, haloperidol, hormonal contraceptives, imipramine, neuroleptics, lamotrigine, methylprednisolone, phenytoin, theophylline, valproate, warfarin.
CBZ levels increased by allopurinol, cimetidine, clarithromycin, diltiazem, erythromycin, fluoxetine, and fluoxamine, gemfibrozil, levetiracetam, itraconazole, ketoconazole, lamotrigine, loratadine, macrolides, nefazodone, Valproate, verapamil.
CBZ levels decreased by: doxorubicin, cisplatin, CBZ (induces own metabolism), phenytoin, valproate.
Interactions where no level was elevated: Levetiracetam/Carbamazepine, led to CBZ toxicity in 4 patients, no elevations of CBZ.[115]
CBZ/Quetiapine. Active metabolite of CBZ increased with addition of Quetiapine[115]

*In general, recommendations for mood stabilizers include: check levels at trough 12 hours after last dose; check free levels of VPA and CBZ. All patients need to be aware that these medications have effects on fetal development, and that hormonal contraceptive levels are decreased by CBZ.
ACE = angiotensin converting enzyme; NaCl = sodium chloride; LFT = liver function test; NSAID = nonsteroidal anti-inflammatory drug; SIADH = syndrome of inappropriate antidiuretic hormone; SSRI = selective serotonin reuptake inhibitors.

becomes unwittingly enmeshed in the problems of the BPD patient, and ultimately becomes irritated with the demands, communicating a sense of frustration. The patient, exquisitely sensitive to rejection, becomes rageful, yet dependent: "I hate you/Don't leave me."

The first element in setting up a successful patient interaction between a medical professional and a patient with BPD is recognizing the disorder by using your own reactions as a guide. The following treatment guidelines will help.

- Structure the office environment to model consistency and clear communication;
- set limits and remain neutral emotionally;
- outline the limits of treatment and when referral might be necessary;
- incorporate mental health treatment into overall medical care;
- prescribe psychotropic medications for symptom relief.[117]

There is no defined medication regimen, but treating target symptoms of depressive effect, anxiety, impulsive behavior, or distorted thinking will often provide some relief.

In addition to the difficulty with interpersonal relationships by patients with BPD, the stress of cancer can reactivate some maladaptive coping strategies, the so-called "lower-level defenses" such as splitting or denial.[116] Splitting consists of unconsciously dividing caregivers into "the good ones" and "the bad ones." These categories can shift around, and the staff can be lured into taking sides for or against a patient. Denial, in its most rigid form, can lead patients to avoid knowledge of their disease and of their treatment options, and to flee from the medical system. These defenses may seem unreasonable, but are merely attempts to manage an overwhelming reality. In summary, treatment of patients with personality disorders and cancer is a difficult task, requiring recognition by staff of a patient's limitations, and a coordinated plan involving consistency, consultation, and caring.

Schizophrenia

The incidence of cancer in the schizophrenic population is debated but appears to be the same as in the general population which is 1 to 1.5%.[119] Internists are caring for more and more patients with both illnesses. Important in caring for schizophrenic individuals with cancer is assessment of capacity. Assessing for capacity involves only the patient understanding the nature of the medical illness; the risks, benefits, and alternatives to procedures; and the ability to manipulate this information, not their psychiatric illness. Often, these individuals have family or case managers to aid in decision making. An individual may have limited capacity for one aspect of

care, but not be able to fully manipulate information. In the state of Virginia, two physicians must deem a patient to not have such a capacity, and then, a legally authorized representative is appointed. Other jurisdictions have other requirements. Assessment for capacity is a dynamic and fluid event. If an individual with schizophrenia, who previously had the capacity, has an acute change in behavior, one should consider the onset of delirium. For individuals with schizophrenia, familiar environments are important. It is best to have consistency of caregivers such as the same doctor and nurse.[119]

Medications used in schizophrenia, such as olanzapine, are often metabolized through the P-450 pathway (see "Anxiety Disorders") and are affected by smoking. There may be a 40% decrease increase in metabolism if the patient suddenly stops smoking. Thus, a previously therapeutic dose may be excessive in the inpatient setting. It is very reasonable to have a psychiatric consult for these individuals to help guide their care, and aid in enhancing services such as case management during these periods of stress.

The type of schizophrenia an individual has is important. Those with paranoid schizophrenia are often highly functional. In fact, 15 to 25% of schizophrenics were found to have IQs in the normal to above average range.[120] This disease process manifests with delusions and paranoia more than with hallucinations. Men manifest the illness earlier so tend to be unmarried; women manifest later and tend to be divorced. Up to 55% of schizophrenics attempt suicide once in their lives.[121] The risk of suicide is high: 10 to 15% die by suicide.

Pathophysiology

Schizophrenia is felt to be due to a disturbance in the level of dopamine (and serotonin) in the brain. There are four main regions of the brain that are of pharmacologic interest. These include the mesocortical (frontal lobes), mesotemporal (temporal lobes), nigrostriatal (basal ganglia) and tuberinfundibular region (involved in prolactin). The mesotemporal region is involved in the production of hallucinations and delusions, which are historically called positive symptoms. The mesocortical regions are involved in executive processing and motivation. PET scans demonstrate decreased frontal metabolism in individuals with schizophrenia. The oldest medications used for schizophrenia are called the typical antipsychotics (or neuroleptics). Examples of typical antipsychotics include chlorpromazine (Thorazine) which is also used for hiccups, fluphenazine (Prolixin), haloperidol (Haldol), and perphenazine (Trilafon)

Typical antipsychotics decrease the levels of dopamine across all four regions. Although there

is a decrease in hallucinations and delusions, there is also a further depletion in the already decreased frontal regions and a decrease in areas that require it for normal functioning. These include the basal ganglia, and the tuberinfundibular pathway. The classic profile of an individual on this medication is a "treated" schizophrenic with parkinsonism, amotivation, decreased cognitive functioning, with possible lactation (loss of tonic inhibition of prolactin). The atypical antipsychotics tend to maintain or increase the level of dopamine in the frontal cortices, thus allowing individuals to function at a higher level. However, for unclear reasons, some individuals do not respond as well to the atypical medications compared to the typical medications.

Pharmacologic Treatment

Table 5 provides dosing recommendations and outlines side effect profiles of these agents drawn from affinity information.[122,123]

If an individual cannot take an oral tablet, olanzapine sol tabs (Zydis), the elixir, intravenous (IV) or intramuscular forms can be used. Elixirs are available for fluphenazine (Prolixin), haloperidol (Haldol), and risperidone (Risperdal). By report, there are fewer extrapyramidal effects with IV medications than oral medications. Side effects that must be recognized include akathisia, dystonic reactions, and neuroleptic malignant syndrome (NMS). Dystonic reactions are more common in young, muscular men. NMS is felt to be a spectrum illness that is associated with muscular rigidity and cogwheeling, manifested by elevated creatine kinase (CK), autonomic instability (fever, diaphoresis, tachycardia, hypertension), leukocytosis, and change in mental status including delirium. It can be subtle initially and, if unrecognized, can lead to coma and death. It usually begins within the first weeks of treatment, and is precipitated by dehydration, medical illness, high doses of neuroleptics, and in conjunction with other agents that act on dopamine blockade. Treatment is supportive, although dantrolene (a skeletal muscle relaxant) and bromocriptine are sometimes used.[18,45] In the cancer patient, it is important to note that clozapine, an atypical antipsychotic, has been associated with agranulocytosis and severe leukopenia and thus is monitored weekly when first begun. A psychiatrist should be involved in decision-making to determine how best to monitor this medication.

Summary

Across the entire spectrum of patients with cancer, the most common psychiatric co-morbidities include delirium, anxiety disorders, adjustment disorders, and mood disorders. The prevalence of

Table 5 Dosing and Comparison of Typical and Atypical Antipsychotics

Atypical (year) *FDA for mania	Trade name Geriatric Dosing	Geriatric Dosing (mg)	Psychois in adult population	Schizophrenia (refractory)	D2 (EPS)	Severse H1 (Sedation)	M1 (Anticholinergic)	Alpha 1 (hypotension)
Clozapine (1974, 1989)	Clozaril	*not recommendes	N/A	(400–600) weekly CBCs at first for agranulocytosis	0/+	+++	+++	+++
Risperidone (1994)*	Risperdal	*Warning for dementia 0.25–0.5 (5–1.5)	2–4	2–4 (4–8)	+++	++	0/+	+++
Olanzapine (1996)*	Zyprexa/Zydis	*Warning for dementia 2.5–5 (5.7.5)	10–15	10–15 (15–40)	+++	+++	+++	++
Quetiapine (1997)*	Seroquel	*12.5–25 (50–200)	25–600	400–600 (400–900+)	0/+	++	0/+	++
Ziprasodone hydrochloride (2001)*	Geodon	*QTC warning		40–120 (120–200)	+++	+/++	0/+	++
Aripiprazole* (2004)	Abilify	*Not yet fully studied 2–5 (8–12)	2.5–15	10–15 (10–15)	+++	+/++	0/+	+
Typical Comparison	**AKA**				**D2**	**H1**	**M2**	**Alpha1**
Haloperidol (high potency)	Haldol	0.5–20 mg	0.5–20 mg	max 20 mg daily**	+++	+	0/+	+++
Fluphenazine (high potency)	Prolixen	1–10 mg	2–20 mg	max 40 mg daily	+++	+	+	+
Perphenazine, (Medium potency)	Trilafon	2–12 mg	12–24 mg	max 64 mg daily	++	++	++	++
Chlorpromazine, thioridazine (Low potency)	Thorazine	not recommendes	100–1000 mg	max 2,000	+	+++	+++	+++

High potency = SE EPS, safer IM (less orthostasis)
Low potency = SE drowsiness, dizziness, dry mouth
*Warning for dementia (all atypicals now have warnings)
**Newer data supports lower dosing with haldol based on receptor occupancy
CBC = complete blood count; EPS = extra pyramidal signs ; FDA = Food and Drug Administration; M1 = muscarinic receptor; M2 = histaminic receptor; 0 = none; + = least; ++ = moderate; +++ = most

these conditions varies, depending upon the medical status of the patient population. Common issues that span these diagnoses are disturbances in body image, relationship problems, occupational concerns, issues of loss, and anticipatory grief. Treatments range from the purely medical to the essentially psychological, with a blend of therapies usually being most effective. Many cancer centers have developed multidisciplinary psycho-oncology services to help address these needs. These professionals are often helpful in providing individual assessment, therapy and referral for patients and their family members with cancer.

REFERENCES

1. Croyle RT, Rowland JH. Mood disorders and cancer: a national cancer institute perspective. Bio Psych 2003;54:191–194.
2. Adler R, Madden K, Felten DL, et al. Psychoneuroimmunology: interactions between the brain and the immune system. In: Fogel BS, Shiffer RB, Rao SM, editors. Neuropsychiatry. Baltimore (MD): Williams & Wilkins; 1996. p. 193–221.
3. Deakin W, Graeff F. 5-HT and mechanisms of defense. J Psychopharmacol 1991;(5):305–15.
4. Kiecolt-Glaser JK, Glaser R. Psychosomatics 1986;27:621–4.
5. McEwen BS. Stress and neuroendocrine function. In: Psychoneuroendocrinology Editors. p. 513–46.
6. Mohl PC, Huang L, Bowden C, et al. Natural killer cell activity in major depression. American J Psych 144:1619a.
7. Derogatis LR, Morrow GR, Fetting J, et al. The prevalence of psychiatric disorders among cancer patients. JAMA 1983;249:751–7.
8. Sheard T, Maguire P. The effect of psychological interventions on anxiety and depression in cancer patients: results of two meta-analyses. Br J Cancer 1999;80:1770–80.
9. Zabora J, Brintzenhofeszoc K, Curbow B, et al. The prevalence of psychological distress by cancer site. Psychooncology 2001;10:19–28.
10. Mazzocato C, Stiefel F, Buclin T, Berney A. Psychopharmacology in supportive care of cancer: a review for the clinician. Support Care Cancer 2000;8:89–97.
11. Gagnon P, Habel M, Hervouet S, et al. [Prevalence of psychiatric disorders and factors associated with delirium in patients referred to a psycho-oncology service] Fr. Bulletin du Cancer 2002;89:1093–8.
12. Breitbart W, Cohen KR. Delirium. In: Holland C, editor. Psychooncology. New York: Oxford University Press; 1998. p. 564–75.
13. Bourgeois JA, Seaman JS, Servis ME. Delirium, dementia, and amnestic disorders. In: Hales RE, Yudofsky SC, editors. Textbook of clinical psychiatry. 4th ed. Washington (DC): American Psychiatric Publishing, Inc.; 1999. p. 259–308.
14. Lipowski ZJ. Update on delirium. Psychiatr Clin North Am 1992;15:335–46.
15. Ljubisavljevic V, Kelly B. Risk factors for development of delirium among oncology patients. Gen Hosp Psychiatry 2003;25:345–52.
16. Seigel, J. Brain mechanisms that control sleep and waking. Naturwissenschaften 2004;91:355–65.
17. Qureshi A, Lee-Chiong T Jr. Medications and their effects on sleep. Med Clin North Am 2004;8:751–66.
18. Cohen B. Theory and practice of psychiatry. New York: Oxford University Press 2003.
19. Morrison, C. Identification and management of delirium in the critically ill patient with cancer. AACN Clin Issues Adv Practice Acute Critical Care 2003;14:92–111.
20. Plotkin, SR, Wen, PY. Neurologic complications of cancer therapy. Neurol Clin 2003;21:279–318.
21. Bostwick JM, Philbrick KL. The use of electroencephalopathy in psychiatry of the medically ill. Psychiatr Clin North Am 2002;(25)1:1725.
22. Gleason, OC. Delirium. Am Fam Physician 2003;67:1027–34.
23. Duff G. Atypical antipsychotic drugs and stroke. Available at: http://medicines.mhra.gov.uk.
24. Olanzapine, risperidone. New safety information regarding use in elderly patients with dementia. WHO Pharmaceuticals Newsletter No. 2; 2004; p. 1.
25. Sadock BJ, Sadock VA, editors. Kaplan and Sadock's comprehensive textbook of psychiatry. 7th ed. Lippincott Williams & Williams; 2000.
26. Physicians Desk Reference.
27. Clary, Greg L;Krishnan, K. Ranga. Delirium: diagnosis, neuropathogenesis and treatment. J Psychiatr Pract 2001;7:310–23.
28. Finkel SI. Behavioral and psychologic symptoms of dementia. Clin Geriatr Med 2003;19:799–824.

29. Sadock B, Sadock V, editors. Kaplan and Sadock's synopsis of psychiatry, 9th ed. Philadelphia: Lippincott Williams & Wilkins; 2003.
30. Skuster DZ, Digre KB, Corbett JJ. Neurologic conditions presenting as psychiatric disorders. Psychiatr Clin North Am 1992;15:311–33.
31. Fawzy FI, Servis MC, Greenberg DB. Oncology and psychooncology. In: The American Psychiatric Publishing textbook of consultation liaison psychiatry. 2nd ed. Washington (DC):American Psychiatric Publishing, Inc.; 2002. p. 657–78.
32. Noyes R, Holt CS, Massie MJ. Anxiety disorders. In: Holland JC, editor. Psycho-oncology. New York: Oxford University Press; 1998. p. 548–63.
33. Smith EM, Gomm SA, Dickens CM. Assessing the independent contribution to quality of life from anxiety and depression in patients with advanced cancer. Palliat Med 2003;17:509–13.
34. Stark D, Kiely M, Smith A, et al. Anxiety disorders in cancer patients: their nature, associations, and relation to quality of life. J Clin Oncol 2002;20:3137–48.
35. Massie MJ, Holland JC. Consultation and liaison issues in cancer care. Psychiatr Med 1987;5:343–59.
36. Matteson S, Roscoe J, Hickok J, et al. The role of behavioral conditioning in the development of nausea. Am J Obstet Gynecol 2002;186(5 Suppl):239–43.
37. Smith AB, Selby PJ, Velikova G, et al. Factor analysis of the hospital anxiety and depression scale from a large cancer population. Psychology & Psychotherapy: Theory, Research & Practice 2002;75(Pt 2):165–75.
38. McGarvey EL, Canterbury RJ, Cohen RB. Evidence of acute stress disorder alter diagnosis of cancer. South Med J 1998;91:864–6.
39. McGarvey EL, Baum LD, Pinkerton RC, et al. Psychological sequelae and alopecia among women with cancer. Cancer Pract. 2001;9:283–9.
40. Kissane DW, Grabsch B, Love A, et al. Psychiatric disorder in women with early stage and advanced breast cancer: a comparative analysis. Aust N Z J Psychiatry 2004;38: 320–6.
41. Chen EI, Kunkel. Oncology. In: Kornstein SG, Clayton AH, editors. Women's mental health. New York: Guilford; 2002. p. 369–89.
42. Kessler RC, Keller MB, Wittchen H. The epidemiology of generalized anxiety disorder. Psychiatr Clin North Am 2001;24:19–39.
43. Passik SD, Roth AJ. Anxiety symptoms and panic attacks preceding pancreatic cancer diagnosis. Psychooncology 1999;8:268–72.
44. Diagnostic and Statistical Manual of Mental Disorders. 4th ed. Text Revision DSM-IV-TR. American Psychiatric Association; 2000.
45. Stahl SM. Essential pharmacology: neuroscientific basis and practical applications. 2nd ed. Cambridge: Cambridge University Press; 2000.
46. Brawman-Mintzner O. The pharmacologic treatment of generalized anxiety disorder. Psychiatr Clin North Am 2001:24:119–37.
47. Golden RN. Making advances where it matters: improving outcomes in mood and anxiety disorders. CNS Spectrums 2004;9(6 Suppl 4):14–22.
48. Solvason HB, Ernst H, Roth W. Predictors of response in anxiety disorders. Psychiatr Clin North Am 2003; 26:411–33.
49. Psychiatry Drug Alerts, Jan 2004.
50. Sajatovic M. Treatment for mood and anxiety disorders: quetiapine and aripiprazole. 2003;5(4):320–6.
51. Cullum JL, Wojciechowski AE, Pelletier G, Simpson JS. Bupropion sustained release treatment reduces fatigue in cancer patients. Can J Psychiatry 2004;49:139–44.
52. Liebowitz MD. Anxiety disorders. In: Rakel RE, Bope ET, editors. Conn's current therapy 2004. 56th ed. Saunders (Elsevier); 2004. p. 1151–5.
53. Bertoletti P. [Evaluation of the effectiveness of and tolerance to a new psychopharmalogical agent in the anxiety-depression syndrome (comparison in a double blind study with diazepam)] Ital. G Clin Med 1977;58 (9–10):393–400.
54. Brogden RN, Heel RC, Speight TM et al. Trazodone: a review of it's pharmacologic properties and therapeutic use in depression and anxiety. Drugs 1981;21:401–29.
55. Practice guidelines for the treatment of patients with acute stress disorder and posttraumatic stress disorder. Am J Psych 2004;161(11 Suppl).
56. Micromedex, University of Virginia, 1974 – 2004. Thomson MICROMEDEX(R) Healthcare Series Vol. 122.
57. Sheard T, Maguire P. The effect of psychological interventions on anxiety and depression in cancer patients: results of two meta-analyses. Br J Cancer 1999;80:1770–80.
58. Baider L, Uziely B, De-Nour AK. Progressive muscle relaxation and guided imagery in cancer patients. Gen Hosp Psychiatry 1994;16:340–7.
59. Lyles JN, Burish TG, Krozely MG, Oldham RK. Efficacy of relaxation training and guided imagery in reducing the aversiveness of cancer chemotherapy. J Consult Clin Psychol 1982;50:509–24.
60. Benson H. The relaxation response. New York: Morrow; 1975.
61. Kabat-Zinn J, Massion AO, Kristeller J, et al. Effectiveness of a meditation-based stress reduction program in the treatment of anxiety disorders. *Am J Psychiatry* 1992; 149:936–43.
62. Speca M, Carlson LE, Goodey E, Angen M. A randomized, wait-list controlled clinical trial: the effect of a mindfulness meditation-based stress reduction program on mood and symptoms of stress in cancer outpatients. *Psychosom Med* 2000;62:613–22.
63. Lehrer PM, Woolfolk RL, editors. Principles and practice of stress management. 2nd ed. New York: Guilford Press; 1993.
64. ullivan R, Crown J, Walsh N. The use of psychotropic medication in patients referred to a psycho-oncology service. Psychooncology 1998;7:301–6.
65. Savard J, Morin CM. Insomnia in the context of cancer: a review of a neglected problem. J Clin Oncol 2001;19: 895–908.
66. Trunzo JJ, Pinto BM. Social support as a mediator of optimism and distress in breast cancer survivors. J Consul Clin Psychol 2003;71:805–11.
67. Spiegel D, Bloom JR, Kraemer HC, Gottheil E. Effect of psychosocial treatment on survival of patients with metastatic breast cancer. Lancet 1989;2(8668):888–91.
68. Goodwin PJ, Leszcz M, Ennis M, et al. The effect of group psychosocial support on survival in metastatic breast cancer. New Eng J Med 2001;345:1719–26.
69. Spiegel D. Mind matters—group therapy and survival in breast cancer. New Eng J Med 2001;345:1767–8.
70. Watson T, Mock V. Exercise as an intervention for cancer-related fatigue. Phys Ther 2004;84:736–43.
71. Mock V, Dow KH, Meares CJ, et al. Effects of exercise on fatigue, physical functioning, and emotional distress during radiation therapy for breast cancer. Oncol Nurs Forum 1997;24:991–1000.
72. Windsor PM, Nicol KF, Potter J. A randomized, controlled trial of aerobic exercise for treatment-related fatigue in men receiving radical external beam radiotherapy for localized prostate carcinoma. Cancer 2004;101:550–7.
73. Pinto BM, Trunzo JJ. Body esteem and mood among sedentary and active breast cancer survivors. Mayo Clin Proc 2004;79:181–6.
74. Chochinov HM. Depression in cancer patients. Lancet Oncol 2001;2:499–505.
75. Brietbart W, Krivo S. Suicide. In: Holland, JC, editor. Psycho-oncology. New York: Oxford University Press; 1998. p. 541–7.
76. Spiegel D, Sands S, Koopman C. Pain and depression in patients with cancer. Cancer 1994;74:2570–8.
77. Bottomley A. Depression in cancer patients: a literature review. Eur J Cancer Care (Engl) 1998:73:181–91.
78. Valente SM, Saunders JM, Cohen MZ. Evaluating depression among patients with cancer. Cancer Pract 1994;2:65–71.
79. Passik SD, Brietbart, WS. Depression in patients with pancreatic carcinoma; diagnostic and treatment issues. Cancer 1996;78:615–23.
80. Dusheiko G. Side effects of alpha interferon in chronic hepatitis C. Hepatology 1997 26(3 Suppl 1):112–21.
81. Malaguarnera M, et al. Interferon alpha-induced depression in chronic hip c patients: comparison between different types of interferon alpha. Neuropsychobiolog 1998;37: 93–7.
82. Mohr D, et al. Treatment of depression improves adherence to interferon beta-1b therapy for multiple sclerosis. Arch Neurol 1997;54:531–3.
83. Morikawa O, Sakai N, Obara H, et al. Effects of interferon-alpha, interferon-gamma, and cAMP on the transcriptional regulation of the serotonin receptor. Eur J Pharmacol 1998;349(2-3):317–24.
84. Thase ME, Bhargava M, Sachs GS. Treatment of bipolar depression: current status, continued challenges, and the STEP-BD approach. Psychiatr Clin North Am 2003; 26:495–518.
85. Sloan D, Kornstein S. Gender differences in depression and response to antidepressant treatment. Psychiatr Clin North Am 2003;26:581–94.
86. Loprinzi CL, Kugler JW, Sloan JA, et al. Venlafaxine in management of hot flashes in survivors of breast cancer: a randomised controlled trial. Lancet 2000;356(9247): 2059–63.
87. Barton DL, Loprinzi CL, Novotny P, et al. Pilot evaluation of citalopram for the relief of hot flashes. J Support Oncol 2003;1:47–51.
88. Beck AT, Rush AJ, Shaw BF, Emery G. Cognitive therapy of depression. New York: Guilford; 1979.
89. Antoni MH, Lehman JM, Kilbourn KM, et al. Cognitive-behavioral stress management intervention decreases the prevalence of depression and enhances benefit finding among women under treatment for early-stage breast cancer. Health Psychol 2001;20:20–32.
90. Jacobs DG, Brewer M, Klein-Benheim M. Suicide assessment. An overview and recommended protocol. In: Jacobs D, editor. Harvard Medical School guide to suicide assessment and intervention. San Francisco: Jossey-Bass; 1999.
91. Alvarez JC, Cremniter D, Lesieur P, et al. Low blood cholesterol and low platelet serotonin levels in violent suicide attempters. Biol Psychiatry 1999;45:1066–9.
92. Brown GL, Goodwin FK. Cerebrospinal fluid correlates of suicide attempts and aggression. Ann N Y Acad Sci 1986;487:175–88.
93. Mann JJ, Arango V, Underwood MD. Serotonin and suicidal behavior. Ann N Y Acad Sci 1990;600:476–84.
94. Klerman GL. Clinical epidemiology of suicide. J Clin Psychiatry 1987;48(Suppl):33–8.
95. Roth AJ, Breitbart W. Psychiatric emergencies in terminally ill cancer patients. Hematol Oncol Clin North Am 1996;10:235–59.
96. Louhivuori KA, Hakama M. Risk of suicide among cancer patients. Am J Epidemiol 1979;109:59–65.
97. Hem E, Loge JH, Haldorson T, et al. Suicide risk in cancer patients from 1960-1999. J Clin Onc 2004;22:4209–16.
98. Filiberti A, Ripamonti C. Suicide and suicidal thoughts in cancer patients. Tumori 2002;88:193–9.
99. Noor-Mahmood SB, Schlebusch L, Bosch BA. Suicidal behavior in patients diagnosed with cancer of the cervix. Crisis: The Journal of Crisis Intervention and Suicide Prevention 2003;24:168–72.
100. White J, Walczak T, Leppik I, et al. Discontinuation of levetiracetam because of behavioral side effects: a case control study. Neurology 2003;61:1218–21.
101. Hughes D, Kleepsies P. Suicide in the medically ill. Suicide Life Threat Behav 2001;31(1 Suppl):48–59.
102. Harris EC, Barraclough BM. Suicide as an outcome for medical disorders. Medicine 1994;73:281–96.
103. Arnaldi G. J Clin Endocrinol Metab 2003;88:5593–602.
104. Burke WJ, Wengel S. Late life mood disorders. Clin Geriatr Med 2003;19:777–97.
105. Gerner R. Treatment of acute mania. Psychiatric Cl of N. America 1993;16 (3):443–460.
106. Benke T, Kurzthaler I, Schmidauer CH et al. Mania caused by a diencephalic lesion. Neuropsychologia. 2002;40 (3):245–52.
107. Gafoor R, O'Keane V. Three case reports of secondary mania: evidence supporting a right frontotemporal locus. Eur Psychiatry 2003;18:32–3.
108. Mendez MF. Mania in neurologic disorders. Curr Psychiatry Rep 2000;2:440–5.
109. Sokolski KN. Exacerbation of mania secondary to right temporal lobe astrocytoma in a bipolar patient previously stabilized on valproate. Cogn Behav Neurol 2003;16: 234–8.
110. Ghika-Schmid F, Bogousslavsky J. Affective disorders following stroke. Eur Neurol 1997;38:75–81.
111. Lim LC. Mania following left hemisphere injury. Singapore Med J 1996;37:448–50.
112. Bauer MS, Mitchner L. What is a "mood stabilizer"? An evidence-based response. Am J Psychiatry;161:3–18.
113. Suppes, T, Dennehy EB. Texas Medication Algorithm Project: TIMA Procedural Manual: Bipolar Disorder Algorithm [PDF]. Available at: http://www.dshs.state.tx.us/mhprograms/TIMABDman.pdf.
114. Bowden CL. Clinical correlates of therapeutic response in bipolar disorder. J Affect Disord 2001;67(1–3):257–65.
115. Drug interactions: carbamazepine/quetiapine. Psychiatry Drug Alerts. January 2004, (18) 1.

116. Groves JE. Taking care of the hateful patient. New Eng J Med 1978;298:883–7.
117. Sansone RA, Sansone LA. Borderline personality disorder. Interpersonal and behavioral problems that sabotage treatment success. Postgrad Med 1995;97:169–79.
118. Hay JL, Passik SD. The cancer patient with borderline personality disorder: suggestions for symptom-focused management in the medical setting. Psychooncology 2000;9:91–100.

119. Shuster, JL. Schizophrenia. In: Holland, JC, editor. Psychooncology. New York: Oxford University Press; 1998. p. 614–8.
120. Flashman LA, Green MF. Review of cognition and brain structure in schizophrenia: profiles, longitudinal course and effects of treatment. Psychiatr Clin North Am 2004;27:1–18.
121. Risk management foundation of the Harvard Medical Institutions Incorporated. Guidelines for identification, assessment and treatment planning for suicidality

[appendix]. In: Jacobs D, editor. Harvard Medical School guide to suicide assessment and intervention. San Francisco: Jossey-Bass; 1999. p. 579–91.
122. Nasrallah, HA, Smeltzer DJ. Contemporary diagnosis and management of the schizophrenia. Newton (PA): Handbook in Healthcare Company; 2002.
123. Ryan, JM. Antipsychotic therapies in geriatric patients: the important of safety and tolerability. Presented at the American Psychiatric Association meeting, New York, 2004.

Renal Failure and Renal Tubular Defects

John R. Foringer, MD

Kevin W. Finkel, MD

Renal disease is a common and complex problem in patients being treated for malignancy. Cancer patients are often hospitalized for treatment of their disease or the complications that arise from such treatment and are therefore vulnerable to the same renal risks seen in the general hospitalized population. In addition, unique injuries may occur from the use of chemotherapy, immunosuppressant agents, hematopoietic stem cell transplantation, release of toxic intracellular constituents, or malignancy itself. The presence of preexisting renal disease in cancer patients is another complicating factor. The detection of an elevated serum creatinine may exclude participation in a chemotherapeutic trial or lead to its early termination. Furthermore, there is little data on the effects of dialysis on serum concentrations and therapeutic benefit of numerous chemotherapy agents. Finally, as survival rates of patients with cancer improve, an increasing number will develop end stage renal disease (ESRD) requiring chronic dialysis or renal transplantation. These patients will require additional expertise in care.

Acute Renal Failure

Background

Acute renal failure (ARF) is characterized by an abrupt decrease in glomerular filtration rate (GFR) over hours to days. It occurs in approximately 5% of all hospitalized patients and 30% of those in the intensive care unit (ICU).[1] The morbidity and mortality associated with ARF are well described. In ICU patients with ARF mortality rates approaching 60 to 80%.[2–4] Over the last 30 years, there has been little change in the mortality associated with hospital-acquired ARF. In 1979, the incidence of ARF was reported to be 4.9%, with an overall mortality of 29%. If the rise in creatinine was greater than 3 mg/dL, then mortality increased to 64%.[1] A more recent report in 1996 also looked at incidence and outcomes of ARF. Using the same definition for ARF as the previous study, the incidence of ARF was 7.4%.[5] The overall mortality rate was 19.4%, while the mortality in patients with sepsis and ARF it was 76%.[5] Acute renal failure significantly increases hospital length

of stay and cost of care.[6,7] Additional morbidity and cost result from chronic dialysis therapy needed by 5% to 30% of surviving patients.[8]

Equally important is the need to recognize that small changes in serum creatinine levels are associated with significant increases in mortality rates. In one study of over 4,000 patients who underwent cardiothoracic surgery with cardiopulmonary bypass, 21-day mortality was 30% in patients whose creatinine increased more than 0.5 mg/dL within 48 hours compared to 9% or less for patients with smaller or no increase in postoperative creatinine.[9] In a large cohort study of 5,000 patients who received intravenous radiocontrast, a 50% increase in serum creatinine within 48 hours was associated with a sixfold increase in 30-day mortality rates.[10] Therefore, early recognition and treatment of ARF may improve patient outcome.

Defining Acute Renal Failure

To date, there is no standard definition for ARF. Acute renal failure is detected by a change in the serum creatinine concentration that serves as a surrogate for a change in GFR. However, no consensus exists on what degree of change in the creatinine level constitutes ARF. This variability in the definition makes it difficult to compare individual treatment or intervention trials. It also delays the recognition of ARF in the clinical setting. Typically, ARF is defined as a 50% increase in serum creatinine if the baseline is ≤ 1.5 mg/dL. A small increase in the serum creatinine level is clinically significant because it is an insensitive and delayed marker of decreased GFR. The discordance between changes in creatinine levels and GFR exist because creatinine excretion occurs through both glomerular filtration and proximal tubular secretion. As filtration of creatinine declines, tubular secretion will increase; thus, no measurable change in the serum creatinine develops until there is a profound decrease in the GFR. In addition, the nonsteady state of creatinine levels in ARF makes it impossible to accurately determine GFR with the use of 24-hour urine collections or the Cockcroft-Gault formula. The Cockcroft-Gault formula is accepted as a

standard method for estimating GFR only when the serum creatinine level is stable.[11,12]

$$GFR = (140-age) \times Pt\ weight\ (0.85)\ if\ female/(72 \times SCr)$$

where Pt weight = patient's weight in kg and SCr = serum creatinine

The insensitivity in serum creatinine change as a marker for declines in GFR makes it difficult to identify early ARF and initiate timely intervention. A lack of sensitivity for identifying small declines in the GFR have led to attempts to develop biomarkers of tubular injury that are both sensitive and specific for early ARF. Recently described, kidney injury molecule-1 (KIM-1) is a novel protein that is expressed during tubular injury and acute tubular necrosis (ATN).[13] Urinary KIM-1 is being evaluated as a possible biomarker for the early diagnosis of ATN. Thus far, other urinary markers for the early detection of ATN have not been proven useful for clinical use.

Evaluation of Acute Renal Failure

In the evaluation of ARF, the most useful clinical indices include the history, physical examination, and urinary output. Useful laboratory data are urinalysis, urinary specific gravity, examination of urinary sediment, and measurement of urine electrolytes. Under certain circumstances, evaluation of urine osmolality and staining for urine eosinophils are helpful. Measurements of the serum blood urea nitrogen (BUN) and creatinine are routine for following the progression of ARF. When assessing the hemodynamic changes in patients and evaluating the adequacy of renal perfusion, central hemodynamic monitoring is often required.

Although the first indication of renal hypoperfusion or tubular injury may be changes in urine output, urine output is an insensitive measure of renal perfusion pressure. Prerenal azotemia with intact tubular function results in increased tubular sodium reabsorption and decreased water excretion. The renal hypoperfusion can result in a fall in the urine output to less than 20 mL/hour. Oliguria, defined as a urine output <400 mL/d, may ensue. Oliguria is present in approximately 50% of ARF cases, regardless of cause. In the evaluation of suspected prerenal azotemia, urine indices are predictable based on the effect of norepinephrine, angiotensin II, aldosterone, and antidiuretic hormone (ADH) on renal blood flow and sodium and water reabsorption. Typical urine indices are illustrated in Table 1. During low urine flow states, tubular reabsorption of BUN increases and the serum BUN-to-creatinine ratio is often elevated to >20:1. An increased BUN-to-creatinine ratio also develops with gastrointestinal bleeding, obstructive uropathy, and hypercatabolic states common in critically ill patients. With the increased avidity of the proximal and distal tubule for sodium, the urine sodium typically is <20 milliequivalent/L (mEq/L). An alternative measure to evaluate the kidneys' ability to conserve sodium during oliguric ARF is the fractional excretion of sodium (FENa). The FENa has been adopted to distinguish intact tubular function (prerenal) from compromised tubular function (acute tubular necrosis) in the oliguric patient. With simultaneous measurements of the plasma sodium and creatinine (PCr mg/dL) and the urinary sodium and creatinine (UCr mg/dL) the FENa is calculated as follows:

$$FENa\ (\%) = (UNa \times PCr \times 100)/CPNa \times UCr$$

where UNa is urinary sodium and PNa is plasma sodium.

The FENa is <1% (see Table 1) in healthy people, demonstrating that less than 1% of the daily sodium load filtered by the kidneys is normally excreted in the urine. In the face of suppressed atrial natriuretic peptide release and high serum levels of aldosterone during prerenal azotemia, the FENa is also <1%, indicating intact tubular function. In contrast, in ATN the FENa is usually >1%.[14,15] Although the FENa can be a useful tool in differentiating prerenal azotemia from ATN, there are many pitfalls to its use when confounding factors are present. In chronic renal disease, impaired sodium and water reabsorption can increase the FENa despite the presence of prerenal azotemia. Similarly, administration of diuretics, bicarbonate, and saline can also raise the urine sodium content. In contrast, there are

numerous reports of patients with ATN from radiocontrast, rhabdomyolysis, sepsis, transplant rejection, urinary obstruction, acute glomerulonephritis, and hepatorenal syndrome in which the FENa is <1%.[16] Therefore the utility of calculating the FENa to differentiate prerenal azotemia from ATN is dependent on the patient's clinical disease and the use of ancillary urine and serum tests.

Urinalysis and examination of the urinary sediment can help differentiate the underlying etiology of ARF. Prerenal azotemia is typically associated with a normal urinalysis or occasional fine granular and hyaline casts. In ATN, tubular epithelial cells, epithelial cell casts, and coarse granular casts are seen. Pyuria and white blood cell casts are indicative of glomerulonephritis, infection, or acute tubulo-interstitial nephritis (TIN). Staining for the presence of urine eosinophils can help identify TIN, although, their detection is not a finding exclusive to TIN. Eosinophils have been seen in patients with rapidly progressive glomerulonephritis, bacterial prostatitis, acute cystitis, and post-infectious glomerulonephritis.[17] Red blood cell casts indicate acute or rapidly progressive glomerulonephritis. Nephrotic range proteinuria suggests intrinsic glomerular disease. In hemoglobinuria and myoglobinuria, the urine dipstick is positive for large blood in the absence of red blood cells on microscopic analysis. The classification of ARF and the typical urine findings are listed in Table 2.

Prerenal Azotemia

Prerenal azotemia accounts for approximately 50 to 60% of hospital acquired ARF.[1,18] It is a normal physiologic response to decreased renal perfusion pressure resulting in a hemodynamically mediated reduction in the GFR. No immediate injury occurs to the renal parenchyma, and the GFR rapidly returns to normal with reversal of the hemodynamic insult. Overt pathologic changes can occur if the renal hypoperfusion is sustained. The decrease in glomerular ultrafiltration pressure can be secondary to a true decrease in the arterial blood volume or a decrease in the effective arterial blood volume as in congestive heart failure, cirrhosis, capillary leak syndromes, and

sepsis. When the mean arterial pressure falls below 80 to 90 mm Hg there is a reduction in renal blood flow. Progression of the prerenal state can lead to ATN. Prerenal azotemia and ischemic ATN are manifestations of renal hypoperfusion. The severity and duration of the insult will dictate the likelihood of progression from prerenal azotemia to ischemic tubular damage.

In renal hypoperfusion states, GFR is maintained by the interplay of several neurohumoral systems. The renin-angiotensin axis increases the vasomotor tone of the efferent arteriole, while afferent arteriolar vasomotor tone decreases under the influence of nitric oxide, vasodilatory prostaglandins, and the kallikrein-kinin system. The sympathetic nervous system reacts to hypoperfusion with release of norepinephrine and ADH. With sustained reductions in renal blood flow, the ability of the kidney to maintain glomerular perfusion pressure is overwhelmed; the GFR declines, resulting in azotemia and cellular hypoxia with ischemic tubular damage.

Common causes of prerenal azotemia are listed in Table 3. In patients with cancer, prerenal azotemia is often the result of loss of extracellular fluid volume from vomiting, diarrhea, and poor oral intake during the treatment of cancer or as a complication of the malignancy itself. Capillary leak syndrome with an increase in third-space volume loss is a complication in cancer patients associated with bone marrow transplant and, in particular, interleukin-2 therapy as discussed later in this chapter (see "Chemotherapeutic Agents").[19,20] Other common causes of third-space fluid losses leading to intravascular volume depletion include ascites, sepsis, and peripheral edema secondary to lymphatic obstruction.

Specific Causes of Prerenal Azotemia

Non-steroidal Anti-inflammatory Drugs

Non-steroidal anti-inflammatory drugs (NSAIDs) can be divided into nonselective inhibitors of both cyclooxygenase-1 (COX-1) and cylcooxygenase-2 (COX-2) or selective inhibitors of COX-2. Patients at greatest risk for NSAID-induced ARF include the elderly and patients with congestive heart failure, advanced liver disease, atherosclerotic vascular disease, or chronic kidney disease.[21,22] Special attention should be given to elderly patients treated with NSAIDs of any type. In a population-based study, the risk of ARF in the elderly increased by 58% with prescription NSAID use.[23] The nonselective NSAIDs are inhibitors of the prostaglandins responsible for vasodilatation in the kidney and can promote prerenal azotemia in susceptible patients. The selective COX-2 inhibitors also cause a similar renal vasoconstriction. The renal safety profile of celecoxib (a COX-2 inhibitor) is similar to ibuprofen. One selective COX-2 inhibitor, rofecoxib, was found

Table 1 Urinary Indices in the Differential Diagnosis of ARF				
Index	*Normal Value*	*Prerenal Azotemia*	*Acute Tubular Necrosis*	*Obstruction*
Urinary volume	≥0.5 mL/kg/hr	≤0.5 mL/kg/hr	Variable	Variable
Urine specific gravity	1.003–1.025	≥1.020	1.010	Variable
Urinary sodium	Variable	<20 mEq/L	>40 mEq/L	<40 mEq/L early >40 mEq/L late
FENa	<1%	<1%	>3%	<1% early >3% late
BUN/creatinine ratio	10:1	>20:1	Variable	Variable
BUN = blood urea nitrogen; FENa = fractional excretion of sodium; mEq = milliequivalent				

Table 2 Urinary Findings and Confirmatory Test in the Common Causes of AKF

Prenatal Azotemia

Common Scenarios in Cancer Patients	Suggestive Clinical Findings	Typical Urine Analysis	Confirmation
Emesis	Volume depletion	FeNa < 1%	Rapid resolution of ARF
Poor oral intake	Decreased EABV	UNa < 20	with correction of
Ascites		SG > 1.020	renal hypoperfusion
Heart failure			Invasive monitoring—
Hemorrhage			CVP or PCWP
Capillary leak syndrome			
Diuretics			
NSAID			
ACE-I or ARB			

Postrenal Azotemia

Obstruction from pelvic	Abdominal or flank pain	Hematuria without	Abdominal X-ray
or ureteral cancer,	Palpable bladder	dysmorphic red blood	Renal ultrasound
metastasis, lymphoma, etc.	Enlarged prostate	cells, RBC casts,	CT or MRI
Retroperitoneal fibrosis	Urinary frequency,	or proteinuria	IVP
Hemorrhagic cystitis	oliguria, or anuria	Variable FeNa and UNa	Retrograde pyelography
Nephrolithiasis			

Intrinsic Renal Azotemia

Common Scenarios in Cancer Patients	Cause of ARF	Typical Urine Analysis	Confirmation
Initiation of a new medication with onset of ARF	Acute tubulointerstitial nephritis	Positive urine WBC Urine eosinophils White cell casts	Peripheral eosinophilia Renal biopsy Biopsy of skin rash
Recent NSAID use		Red blood cells	
Recent blood transfusion	Hemolysis	Rarely red blood cell casts	Elevated K⁺, PO₄, and uric acid, LDH
		Urine supernatant is pink and heme + Hemoglobinuria	Hypocalcemia Peripheral smear with fragmented red blood cells
Six months to a year post BMT	Hemolytic uremic syndrome and	Urine red blood cells Heme +	Renal biopsy Peripheral smear with
Use of tacrolimus or cyclosporine	thrombotic thrombocytopenic		schistocytes and fragmented red cells
Radiation nephritis	purpura		Thrombocytopenia
24 to 48 hours after radiocontrast	Radiocontrast	Early FeNa < 1%, UNa < 20	Temporal relationship to the contrast
		Progression to FeNa > 1% and UNa > 20	infusion
Severe hypophosphatemia after chemotherapy induced renal tubular injury	Rhabdomyolysis	Urine supernatant Heme + without red blood cells Myoglobinuria	Elevated creatine kinase, PO₄, uric acid, K⁺ Hypocalcemia Elevated serum myoglobin
Initiation of chemotherapy in any malignancy with a large tumor burden	Tumor lysis syndrome	Urate crystals	Elevated K⁺, PO₄, uric acid Decreased Ca²⁺
Autolysis of cells with an aggressive leukemia or lymphoma			
Progression of prerenal azotemia	Ischemia	FeNa > 1%, UNa > 20 SG = 1.010	Clinical assessment and urine findings usually
Sepsis		Muddy brown, granular,	sufficient
Hemorrhage		or tubule epithelial cell cast	

ARF = acute renal failure; ACE-I = angiotensin converting enzyme inhibitor; ARB = angiotensin receptor blocker; BMT = bone marrow transplantation; Ca²⁺ = serum calcium; CT = computed tomography; CVP = ; EABV = effective arterial blood volume; FeNa = fractional excretion of sodium; IVP = intravenous pyelography; K⁺ = serum potassium; MRI = magnetic resonance imaging; NSAID = non-steroidal anti-inflammatory drugs; LDH = ; lactate dehydrogenase; PCWP = ; PO₄ = serum phosphorous; RBC = red blood (cell) count; SG = urine specific gravity; UNa = urine sodium concentration; WBC = white blood (cell) count;

Table 3 Causes of Prerenal Azotemia

Intravascular volume depletion
Cutaneous losses
  Burns
  Hyperthermia
    Cutaneous graft vs. host disease
    Cutaneous T-cell lymphoma
Gastrointestinal fluid loss
  Vomiting
  Diarrhea
  Enterocutaneous fistula
  Nasogastric suction
    Ileus or bowel obstruction
Renal losses
  Drug-induced or osmotic diuresis
  Diabetes insipidus
  Adrenal insufficiency
"Third-space" losses
  Capillary leak syndrome (Graft vs. host disease, interferon therapy, SIRS)
  Pancreatitis
  Hypoalbuminemia
Blood losses
  Gastrointestinal bleeding
  Hemorrhagic cystitis
  Surgical blood loss
  Intra-abdominal or retroperitoneal bleeding

Decreased effective arterial blood volume
Decreased cardiac output
  Myocardial, valvular, pericardial disease
  Pulmonary embolism
  Pulmonary hypertension
  Positive pressure ventilation
Cirrhosis
Nephrotic syndrome
Sepsis
Anesthesia

Impaired renal vascular autoregulation
Angiotensin-converting enzyme inhibitors
Angiotensin-receptor blockers
Non-steroidal anti-inflammatory drugs
Cyclooxygenase 2 inhibitors
Cyclosporine A
Tacrolimus
Hypercalcemia
Hepatorenal syndrome

to have a higher incidence of renal toxicity than the nonselective inhibitors or celecoxib.[24] The renal toxicity of NSAIDs is increased when they are used in combination with other medications, with the potential to alter the kidneys' ability to autoregulate glomerular filtration pressure such as angiotensin-converting enzyme (ACE) inhibitors and angiotensin receptor blockers (ARBs). The renal vascular changes associated with NSAID use are typically reversible, although prolonged use can lead to permanent renal injury. Non-steroidal anti-inflammatory drugs are also known to cause acute TIN, in which case, there is often a sudden change in GFR that may persist for days to weeks.

ACE Inhibitors and ARBs

The renin-angiotensin system contributes to the autoregulation of glomerular perfusion pressure, and inhibition of this system has the potential to induce prerenal azotemia. Angiotensin-converting enzyme inhibitors reduce blood pressure by inhibiting the proteolytic cleavage of angiotensin I to angiotensin II. Angiotensin receptor blockers occupy the angiotensin receptor. Much like the prostaglandin inhibitors, ACE inhibitors and ARBs increase the risk of ARF in the elderly, in patients using diuretics, and in patients with volume depletion, congestive heart failure, or diabetes.[25,26] Their use in conjunction with NSAIDs, cyclosporine, and tacrolimus puts patients at an even greater risk for ARF.[25,27] The incidence of ARF is also higher in patients with chronic kidney disease of any etiology. Patients with chronic kidney disease may depend on local angiotensin II production to maintain GFR in the face of decreased functional renal mass. Therefore, a decline in GFR when these patients receive ACE-inhibitors is not unexpected. The rise in serum creatinine is typically less then 30% and does not constitute ARF. More dramatic increases in serum creatinine suggest the presence of underlying renal vascular disease.

Calcineurin Inhibitors

The calcineurin inhibitors cyclosporine A (CSA) and tacrolimus are widely used as immunosuppressants in bone marrow transplantation to prevent graft-versus-host disease (GVHD). Both CSA and tacrolimus cause ARF. Nephrotoxicity is the result of direct afferent arteriolar vasoconstriction leading to a decrease in the glomerular filtration pressure and GFR. The vascular effect associated with CSA and tacrolimus is reversible with discontinuation of the drug. A dose reduction is sometimes enough to reverse the prerenal affect. Chronic nephrotoxicity is a potential complication with more prolonged use of the calcineurin inhibitors. Proteinuria, tubular dysfunction, arterial hypertension, and rising creatinine are clinical findings consistent with chronic CSA or tacrolimus nephrotoxicity. It typically takes more than 6 months of therapy for the chronic changes to occur. Arteriolar damage, interstitial fibrosis, tubular atrophy, and glomerulosclerosis are found on renal biopsy specimens. The pathologic changes of the chronic nephrotoxicity are irreversible.[28-30] A rare complication of CSA and tacrolimus therapy is hemolytic uremic syndrome (HUS). The mechanism of CSA or tacrolimus-induced HUS is direct damage to the vascular endothelium in a dose-dependent fashion. With discontinuation of the drug, patients may have partial recovery.[31-33] Calcineurin inhibitors have also been associated with hyperkalemia, thought to be secondary to tubular resistance to aldosterone.[34]

Hepatorenal Syndrome

Hepatorenal syndrome (HRS) is a unique cause of renal vasoconstriction with a decline in GFR in the face of normal renal histology that occurs in the setting of liver failure. The clinical picture associated with HRS is that of a prerenal azotemia. In true HRS without confounding renal injuries, the renal failure will resolve with liver transplantation. The pathogenesis of HRS is not completely understood. Systemic and splanchnic vascular resistance is decreased, leading to a decrease in the effective arterial volume and hypoperfusion of the renal vasculature. The compensatory response is an increase in the mediators of renal vasoconstriction, including increased renin-angiotensin-aldosterone activity, ADH levels, sympathetic tone, and endothelin levels. The renal response is an increase in salt and water avidity leading to worsening ascites and edema.[35,36] Clinically, HRS is characterized by oliguric ARF with very low urine sodium and bland urine sediment. The diagnosis of HRS is a diagnosis of exclusion. Other causes for the ARF should be ruled out, including causes of prerenal azotemia, intrinsic renal disease, and obstructive nephropathy. Major and minor criteria have been established for the diagnosis of HRS (Table 4). Liver transplant is the definitive therapy for HRS. However, patients who develop HRS prior to transplant have worse graft and patient survival.[37] Newer pharmacologic therapy with vasopressin analogs (eg, ornipressin and terlipressin), which are splanchnic vasoconstrictors, has shown some benefit. However, the major complication associated with these medications is mesenteric

---

Table 4 Diagnostic Criteria for Hepatorenal Syndrome

Major Criteria

Acute or chronic liver disease with advanced hepatic failure and portal hypertension

Depressed GFR with a serum creatinine > 1.5 mg/dL or a creatinine clearance < 40 mL/min

Absence of shock, ongoing bacterial infection, fluid loss, and treatment with nephrotoxic medications

No sustained improvement in renal function after withdrawal of diuretics and fluid resuscitation with 1.5L of isotonic saline

Proteinuria < 500 mg/d and no evidence of obstructive nephropathy on ultrasonography

Minor Criteria

Oliguria

Urine sodium < 10 mEq/L

Urine osmolality > plasma osmolality

Urine red blood cells < 50 per high-power field

Serum sodium concentration < 130 mEq/L

Adapted from Arroyo V, et al.[45]
mEq = milliequivalent.

---

ischemia.[38-40] Oral midodrine hydrochloride (a selective α_1-adrenergic agonist) in combination with octreotide showed benefit in renal function in a small series of patients.[41] N-acetylcysteine was shown to increase renal blood flow without changing the hemodynamic derangements associated with HRS.[42] Several small studies have shown that transjugular intrahepatic portosystemic shunting (TIPS) has prolonged survival and improved renal function in patients with HRS.[43,44] Given the poor prognosis of HRS, in a patient with rapid onset of renal failure, dialysis is usually not instituted unless the patient is a candidate for liver transplant or has a chance of hepatic recovery.[35,36,45]

Abdominal Compartment Syndrome

Abdominal compartment syndrome (ACS) may develop in patients with massive ascites or in the postoperative state. It was first reported in 1876 in a paper describing the reduction in urine flow associated with elevated intra-abdominal pressure (IAP).[46] Acute increases in IAP are deleterious for both intra-abdominal and distant organ function including the kidneys.[47] Acutely, the abdomen functions as a closed space; thus, any increase in the volume of its contents leads to a rise in compartmental pressure. Abdominal compartment syndrome is characterized by an acute rise in IAP coupled with evidence of organ dysfunction, usually reduced urine output. The pathogenesis of this reduction in urine formation is complex and attributed to three major factors: (1) compression of the great veins reduces venous return to the right heart, which manifests as relative volume depletion that is coupled with increased renal venous back pressure from high central venous pressures, as well as renal vein compression; (2) direct pressure on the renal cortex shunts blood away from the corticomedullary junction by altering renal vascular resistance and induces an ischemic injury; and (3) direct pressure on the ureters causing obstructive nephropathy. Regardless of the underlying cause, a reduction in urine output and azotemia in the presence of a measured IAP over 15 cm H_2O is certainly cause for concern and should prompt intervention.

The causes of an increased IAP are listed in Table 5. Abdominal compartment syndrome should be managed with attention to preservation of underlying organ function, and is usually treated with urgent surgical decompression. This is a highly complex condition and skilled surgical intervention is required.

Obstructive (Postrenal) Nephropathy

Urinary tract obstruction is a relatively common cause of renal failure in patients with malignancy

Table 5 Causes of Increased Intra-abdominal Pressure

Peritoneal tissue edema (trauma, peritonitis)
Fluid overload in shock
Retroperitoneal hematoma
Surgical trauma
Reperfusion injury after bowel ischemia
Pancreatitis
Ileus or obstruction
Abdominal packing to control hemorrhage
Abdominal closure under tension
Severe ascites

and is discussed in detail in a later chapter (see Chapter 48, "Urinary Tract Infections").

Intrinsic Acute Renal Failure

Intrinsic ARF (Table 6) is associated with renal parenchymal injury. The most common cause of intrinsic renal failure is ATN. It accounts for approximately 85% of intrinsic ARF episodes in hospitalized patients.[48] The etiology of the tubular injury may be nephrotoxic (35%) or ischemic (50%) in origin. However, ATN is often a multifactorial process, developing in the setting of a critical illness with nephrotoxic medications, renal hypoperfusion, and sepsis all playing a role. With prolonged episodes of renal hypoperfusion, cortical necrosis can occur and lead to irreversible renal failure. The pathophysiologic abnormalities that result in a fall in GFR include intrarenal vasoconstriction, decreased glomerular filtration pressure, intra-tubular obstruction, transtubular back-leak of filtrate, and interstitial inflammation. The clinical course of ATN is divided into three components: initiation, maintenance, and recovery. The period in which a patient first experiences a renal injury is the initiation phase of ATN. The renal injury is potentially reversible if the precipitating insult is corrected. With progression of the injury, parenchymal damage ensues and abrupt changes in the GFR occur. The maintenance phase can last several days to weeks, during which the GFR remains depressed and the patient can have variable urine output. In the recovery phase, the GFR returns to normal as cellular regeneration and tubular repair occurs.

Specific Causes of Intrinsic Renal Failure

Radiocontrast Nephropathy (RCN)

Ten percent of hospital-acquired ARF is the result of contrast-induced nephrotoxicity, making it one of the most common causes of ATN.[5] Patients at particular risk for RCN are the elderly, diabetics, and patients with chronic kidney disease, congestive heart failure or volume depletion. Contrast nephropathy often occurs in the cancer

Table 6 Causes of Intrinsic Renal Failure in Cancer Patients

Acute tubular necrosis
Ischemic
  Hypotension
  Sepsis
  Cardiopulmonary arrest
Exogenous nephrotoxins
  Acyclovir
  Aminoglycosides
  Amphotericin B
  Cisplatin
  Cyclosporine
  Foscarnet
  Ifosfamide
  Pentamidine
  Radiocontrast
Intrinsic nephrotoxins
  Myoglobinuria
  Hemoglobinuria
  Hyperuricosuria

Acute glomerulonephritis
Post-infectious
Endocarditis-associated
Systemic vasculitis

Vascular syndromes
Renal artery thromboembolism
Renal vein thrombosis
Atheroembolic disease
HUS/TTP

Acute tubulointerstitial nephritis
Drug-induced
  Penicillins
  Cephalosporins
Bactrim
  Fluoroquinolones
  NSAID
Furosemide
Thiazides
  Interferon-α
Infectious causes
  Bacterial
  Viral
  Cytomegalovirus
  Fungal
  Tuberculosis
Malignancy
  Lymphoma
  Leukemia
  Myeloma

patient with an early prerenal azotemia from volume depletion when the serum creatinine is still normal. Cancer-induced hypercalcemia is a particular risk factor for contrast-induced renal failure, and the calcium should be lowered to normal levels prior to contrast administration. Patients receiving NSAIDs, ACE inhibitors, ARBs, CSA, or tacrolimus are also at increased risk for RCN. In patients with multiple myeloma, a potential interaction between contrast agents and light chains has been found.[49] Contrast nephropathy causes ARF by renal

vasoconstriction and direct tubular injury.[50,51] The vasoconstriction associated with RCN has been linked to increased levels of vasoconstrictors, such as calcium, endothelin, and adenosine, and inhibition of the vasodilator nitric oxide. Oxidant injury through free radical oxygen species has also been implicated and has been a target of preventative measures.[52] Clinically, patients usually have an elevation in the serum creatinine 24 to 48 hours after the exposure to the contrast. The creatinine typically peaks at 3 to 5 days and returns to baseline in 7 to 10 days. The diagnosis of RCN is often based on the temporal relationship. It is common to see a FENa < 1% with RCN secondary to the renal vasoconstriction and a prerenal-like picture. Although RCN is typically a transient event, it is associated with a hospital mortality rate five times greater than in matched controls who receive radiocontrast but do not develop ARF.[10] Many trials have been done to evaluate the use of n-acetyl-cysteine, low-dose dopamine, and fenoldopam mesylate for prophylaxis against RCN and are discussed later in this chapter (see "Specific Measures"). The administration of intravenous fluid has become commonplace for the prevention of RCN. It has been shown that 0.45% sodium chloride significantly decreased the incidence of ARF when compared to the administration of intravenous fluid with either mannitol or furosemide.[53] Although radiocontrast is a renal tubular toxin, it also causes intense renal vasoconstriction, which may explain the salutatory effects of fluid administration. Another study suggests that a solution containing 0.9% sodium chloride is more efficacious in preventing ARF than one containing 0.45% sodium chloride.[54]

Aminoglycosides

Aminoglycosides cause intrinsic ARF in approximately 10% of patients who are treated with them for more than 2 to 3 days. The serum creatinine typically rises 7 to 10 days after the drug is initiated. Aminoglycosides concentrate in the proximal tubular cells causing cellular damage. Once overt nephropathy develops, the urinalysis shows tubular epithelial cells and tubular cell casts. Proximal tubular injury is evident by wasting of electrolytes such as potassium, magnesium, and calcium in the urine.[55] The FENa is typically >2%. Aminoglycosides can also cause nephrogenic diabetes insipidus because the tubulointerstitial injury inhibits adenylate cyclase activity leading to ADH resistance.[56] Risk factors for aminoglycoside-induced ARF are advanced age, chronic kidney disease, volume depletion, liver disease, and prolonged use of the drug. Monitoring of aminoglycoside blood levels is important in preventing renal toxicity. Studies suggest that once-daily dosing of aminoglycosides decreases the risk of ARF without altering the antimicrobial efficacy.[57,58]

Amphotericin B

Amphotericin B and its liposomal derivatives are a common cause of ATN, particularly in patients who have undergone bone marrow transplant. Eighty percent of patients who receive amphotericin B will develop some degree of renal impairment. The initial nephrotoxic injury from amphotericin B results from renal vasoconstriction of the preglomerular arterioles and predisposes the patient to an ischemic insult.[59,60] Direct tubular toxicity follows. As with many tubular toxins, amphotericin B results in tubular wasting of potassium and magnesium. A renal tubular acidosis (RTA) causing a hyperchloremic metabolic acidosis, as well as a nephrogenic diabetes insipidus from ADH resistance, are common findings.[26,60,61] The newer liposomal forms of amphotericin B lack the solubilizing agent deoxycholate that contributes to tubular toxicity. Such preparations reduce, but do not eliminate, the development of ATN.[62] Although the renal failure associated with amphotericin B is usually temporary and improves with discontinuation of the drug, reinstitution often results in recurrence of the ARF.[63] In the prevention of amphotericin-B–induced ARF, clinical studies have shown that hydration with normal saline prior to the amphotericin infusion provides some protection.[64,65]

Pigmented Nephropathy

The principal cause of the pigmented nephropathies is rhabdomyolysis and hemoglobinuria from transfusion reactions or post–bone-marrow transplant. The majority of rhabdomyolysis cases are subclinical with mild elevations in the creatine kinase (CK), lactic dehydrogenase, or aspartate transaminase. In severe cases, ARF may ensue from myoglobinuria. Hemoglobinuria can be induced by the infusion of hemolyzed red blood cells.[66] Preservation of bone marrow with dimethyl sulfoxide (DMSO) will cause hemolysis of red blood cells present in the stored specimen, and subsequent infusion will result in hemoglobinuria. Mismatched blood products and transfusion reactions produce hemoglobinuria. Myoglobinuria as well as hemoglobinuria have been thought to cause ARF through three mechanisms: renal vasoconstriction, intratubular cast formation, and heme-mediated proximal tubular injury. It is also known that oxidant stress is increased with the release of heme proteins. Free heme proteins are suspected to reduce the formation of nitric oxide and increase endothelin levels leading to vasoconstriction and the decline in GFR. Intratubular obstruction occurs with the interaction of myoglobin and Tamm-Horsfall mucoprotein in an aciduric environment.[67] The diagnosis of myoglobin-induced nephrotoxicity is suspected on history and by a CK level greater than 10 times

the normal range. The urine dipstick is commonly positive for blood, with no red blood cells on microscopic examination. The FENa may be <1% despite tubular injury. Evaluation of the urine sediment typically reveals heme-pigmented casts. Serum electrolyte derangements are common, including hyperkalemia, hyperphosphatemia, hyperuricemia, and hypocalcemia. The majority of patients will experience recovery of renal function with resolution of the hemoglobinuria or myoglobinuria. In the recovery phase of rhabdomyolysis, hypercalcemia develops in 30% of patients secondary to increased levels of vitamin D and parathyroid hormone. Replacement of serum calcium should be withheld in asymptomatic patients to prevent severe hypercalcemia after recovery. To prevent and treat the ARF of rhabdomyolysis, aggressive hydration is effective. Alkalinization of the urine has also been advocated to increase the solubility of the heme proteins in the urine. Alkalinization may also reduce the production of reactive oxygen species, thus reducing the oxidant stress.[68]

Chemotherapeutic Agents

Cisplatin

Nephrotoxicity is the most common dose-limiting side effect of cisplatin administration. The primary site for clearance of cisplatin is the kidney. The most common clinical scenario is the gradual onset of nonoliguric ARF; electrolyte wasting is seen, however, especially with high doses of cisplatin.[69] Apoptosis of renal proximal tubular cells is induced, resulting in wasting of electrolytes such as potassium, magnesium, calcium, and bicarbonate.[69] A common electrolyte abnormality is hypomagnesemia, which often occurs with prolonged exposure to the drug.[70] The direct tubular toxicity associated with cisplatin is exacerbated in a low-chloride environment. In the intracellular compartment, chloride molecules are replaced with water molecules in the cis position of cisplatin, forming hydroxyl radicals that injure the neutrophilic binding sites on DNA.[71,72] The decline in GFR associated with cisplatin toxicity usually occurs 3 to 5 days after the exposure.[69] Doses of cisplatin >50 mg/m² are sufficient to cause renal failure. The renal injury is typically reversible, but repeated doses of cisplatin in excess of 100 mg/m² may cause irreversible renal damage.[72] Hydration with isotonic saline and avoidance of concomitant nephrotoxins is the most effective way to prevent cisplatin-induced nephrotoxicity. Amifostine has been shown to reduce cisplatin nephrotoxicity through promotion of better DNA repair and elimination of free radicals.[73,74] With the cessation of cisplatin therapy, the majority of patients will recover renal function. However, it has been reported that the GFR is reduced on average 15% in patients followed long-term for resolved ARF from cisplatin nephrotoxicity.[75]

Ifosfamide

Ifosfamide is an alkylating drug that causes renal toxicity either directly or through a metabolite. The metabolite of ifosfamide, chloroacetaldehyde, causes direct tubular epithelial cell damage.[76] The renal injury occurs throughout the kidney, including the glomerulus, proximal and distal tubule, and interstitium. The proximal tubule is most seriously affected, causing wasting of electrolytes similar to cisplatin. The degree of hypokalemia, hypophosphatemia, hypomagnesemia, and hyperchloremic acidosis experienced with ifosfamide toxicity can be severe. Patients can develop Fanconi syndrome with hypophosphatemic rickets and osteomalacia, as well as nephrogenic diabetes insipidus.[77] A potential marker for ifosfamide nephrotoxicity is increased urinary β_2-microglobulin excretion.[78] Risk factors for ifosfamide nephrotoxicity include previous exposure to cisplatin, chronic kidney disease, and a cumulative dose > 84 g/m².[79,80] Recent data suggest that amifostine may have a protective role against ifosfamide, as well as cisplatin nephrotoxicity.[81] The majority of patients will recover from ifosfamide-induced tubular injury; however, there are reports of long-term complications. Ifosfamide has been attributed to chronic renal fibrosis with a decline in the GFR over time and, in one case, leading to end-stage renal disease.[82,83] In pediatric literature, the chronic and progressive nature of ifosfamide-induced renal toxicity is well documented.[84]

Methotrexate

Methotrexate (MTX)-induced ARF is caused by the precipitation of the drug and its more insoluble metabolite, 7-hydroxymethotrexate, in the tubular lumen.[72,85] At a pH of <5.5, the drug and its metabolite precipitate when their concentration exceeds 2×10^{-3} molar, whereas solubility increases with a urine pH of 7.[86] Acute renal failure occurs from intrarenal obstruction, direct tubule toxicity, and prerenal azotemia from afferent arteriolar vasoconstriction. Acute renal failure is reported in 30 to 50% of patients treated with high-dose MTX (>1 g/m²).[86] For the prevention of renal toxicity, hydration and high urine output is essential. Isotonic saline infusion and furosemide may be necessary to keep the urine output >100 mL/h. An increase in the clearance rate of MTX is seen when the urine pH is increased from 5.5 to 8.4, which can be accomplished with an isotonic solution containing bicarbonate.[87] Once ARF develops, the excretion of MTX is reduced, the systemic toxicity of MTX is increased, and treatment is mainly supportive. It may be necessary to remove the drug with dialysis. Hemodialysis, using high blood flow rates with a high-flux dialyzer is an effective method of removing methotrexate.[88] High-dose leucovorin therapy can reduce the systemic toxicity associated with MTX and ARF.[89,90] In the majority of cases, MTX-induced ARF will resolve. Often the plasma creatinine will peak within one week and return to baseline at 3 weeks.[91]

Biologic Agents
Acute renal failure is well described with the administration of α-interferon and interleukin-2.[92,93] Acute renal failure secondary to interferon-α (IFN-α) therapy is uncommon and has been associated with and without massive proteinuria.[94] Renal biopsy in IFN-α–associated ARF has revealed glomerular lesions, including focal segmental glomerulosclerosis and minimal change disease.[94-96] Other renal lesions include acute tubular interstitial nephritis and acute tubular necrosis.[97,98] The ARF can be reversible with cessation of the drug; however, some patients may have CKD or require long-term dialysis. After recovery of the ARF, proteinuria may persist, and these patients should be monitored for progression of renal disease.[94] With interleukin-2–induced renal dysfunction, a systemic capillary leak syndrome occurs resulting in volume depletion, hypotension, and prerenal azotemia.[19,20] Unlike IFN-α, interleukin-2 produces a decreased GFR in the majority of patients who receive the drug, and the incidence of ARF is high.[99]

Imatinib mesylate is a protein-tyrosine kinase inhibitor that inhibits the BCR-ABL tyrosine kinase as well as the receptor tyrosine kinase for platelet-derived growth factor and stem cell factor c-kit.[100] Two reports in the literature described acute renal failure associated with Gleevec. One case reported renal failure requiring temporary hemodialysis with ATN found on renal biopsy.[101] Both cases reported recovery of renal function with the cessation of imatinib mesylate. It is now recommended that renal function be monitored closely during therapy with Gleevec.

Bisphosphonates

Bisphosphonates are commonly used to manage hypercalcemia of malignancy and to reduce skeletal complications in patients with bone metastases and multiple myeloma. All three generations of bisphosphonates have been shown to cause renal failure. The most common pathologic finding on renal biopsy is acute tubular necrosis. A recent study reports biopsy-proven toxic ATN in six patients treated with zoledronic acid, a potent bisphosphonate. Renal function recovered with cessation of the drug but did not return to baseline levels.[102] Pamidronate has been shown to cause ATN as well as the nephrotic syndrome from a collapsing variant of focal segmental glomerular sclerosis.[103,104] The exact mechanism of bisphosphonate-induced renal failure is not known; however, direct toxicity to the tubular epithelial cells is suspect.

Renal Diseases Associated with Malignancy

Multiple Myeloma

Fifty percent of patients with multiple myeloma (MM) will develop some degree of renal functional impairment, and 10% will require dialysis. The pathogenesis of MM-induced renal failure includes myeloma kidney, renal tubular dysfunction, light-chain deposition disease, amyloidosis, and plasma cell infiltration. Hypercalcemia can also complicate MM and induce renal failure. Patients with MM are at increased risk for other causes of renal failure, in particular contrast nephropathy. The overproduction of monoclonal immunoglobulin light chains is the primary factor associated with the renal disease of MM. The recommended diagnostic tool for identifying the presence of urinary light chains is urine protein electrophoresis with immunofixation. Light chains can combine with Tamm-Horsfall mucoproteins to form casts that cause intratubular obstruction. Factors that influence tubular cast formation include low tubular flow rate, acidity of the urine, radiocontrast infusion, and distal nephron sodium, chloride, and calcium concentration. The therapy of MM-induced renal disease is limited to treating the MM. In patients with high tumor burdens, acute renal failure may ensue. Partial recovery of the GFR may occur in up to 50% of patients who undergo treatment of the MM.[105] Small case series suggest that plasmapheresis improves renal survival in patients who require dialysis for ARF from myeloma kidney.[106,107] However, renal biopsy may be necessary to identify those patients likely to respond to plasmapheresis therapy. Given the limited clinical experience and need for biopsy, plasmapheresis for myeloma kidney has not gained wide acceptance.

Patients with MM are at increased risk for developing ARF from nephrotoxic injury, particularly radiocontrast. The incidence of contrast nephropathy in MM patients is 0.6% to 1.25%.[108] It is postulated that iodinated contrast enhances the precipitation of intratubular proteins leading to obstruction. Adequate hydration and avoiding low urine flow states is the best protection against ARF in MM patients.

Hypercalcemia Associated with Multiple Myeloma

Hypercalcemia complicates MM in 15% of patients at presentation. Hypercalcemia induces prerenal azotemia by causing nephrogenic diabetes insipidus, renal vasoconstriction, and intratubular calcium deposition.[109] When the serum calcium level is >13 mg/dL, most patients will have some degree of volume depletion. Volume repletion and a saline diuresis are essential to the therapy. Isotonic saline should be infused intravenously in large volumes to increase calcium excretion. Furosemide may be used to increase the calciuresis once volume depletion is corrected. Thiazide diuretics should be avoided because they decrease urinary calcium excretion. Bisphosphonates, pyrophosphate analogs with a high affinity for hydroxyapatite, may be necessary to control the serum calcium in severe cases.[110,111] Pamidronate and clodronate, two second-generation bisphosphonates, are commonly used preparations. Both drugs are potent inhibitors of osteoclast bone resorption without significant bone demineralization.[112] Pamidronate can be given as a single intravenous dose of 30 to 90 mg and may normalize the calcium for several weeks.[111] Calcitonin, derived from the thyroid C-cell, inhibits osteoclast activity. The onset of calcitonin is rapid but with a short half-life and is usually not given as a sole therapy.[113] Plicamycin (mithramycin) is an inhibitor of RNA synthesis and impairs osteoclast activity. It is an effective means to acutely lower serum calcium. However, the multiple toxicities associated with plicamycin have made its use uncommon. Glucocorticoids are also effective in the therapy of hypercalcemia in patients with hematologic malignancies. Hemodialysis with a low calcium bath is the preferred method of reducing serum calcium levels in patients with a severely depressed GFR.

Tumor Lysis Syndrome

Tumor lysis syndrome is often a dramatic presentation of ARF in patients with malignancy. It is characterized by the development of hyperphosphatemia, hypocalcemia, hyperuricemia, and hyperkalemia. Tumor lysis syndrome can occur spontaneously during the rapid growth phase of malignancies such as bulky lymphoblastomas and Burkitt's and non-Burkitt's lymphomas that have extremely rapid cell turnover rates.[114] More commonly, it is seen when cytotoxic chemotherapy induces lysis of malignant cells in patients with large tumor burdens. Tumor lysis syndrome has developed in patients with non-Hodgkin's lymphoma, acute lymphoblastic leukemia, chronic myelogenous leukemia in blast crises, small cell lung cancer, and metastatic breast cancer.[115] In most patients, the ARF is reversible after aggressive supportive therapy including dialysis.

The pathophysiology of ARF associated with tumor lysis syndrome is related to two main factors, preexisting volume depletion prior to the onset of renal failure and the precipitation of uric acid and calcium phosphate complexes in the renal tubules and tissue.[116] Patients may be volume-depleted from anorexia or nausea and vomiting associated with the malignancy, or from increased insensible losses from fever or tachypnea. Therefore, it is important to establish brisk flow of hypotonic urine to prevent or ameliorate ARF associated with tumor lysis syndrome.

Hyperuricemia is either present before treatment with chemotherapy or develops after therapy despite prophylaxis with allopurinol.[117] Uric acid is nearly completely ionized at physiologic pH, but becomes progressively insoluble in the acidic environment of the renal tubules. Precipitation of uric acid causes intratubular obstruction leading to increased renal vascular resistance and decreased GFR.[118] Moreover, a granulomatous reaction to intraluminal uric acid crystals and necrosis of tubular epithelium can be found on biopsy specimens.

Hyperphosphatemia and hypocalcemia also occur in tumor lysis syndrome. In patients who do not develop hyperuricemia in tumor lysis syndrome, ARF has been attributed to metastatic intra-renal calcification or acute nephrocalcinosis.[119] Tumor lysis with release of inorganic phosphate results in acute hypocalcemia and metastatic calcification resulting in ARF.

Therefore, ARF associated with tumor lysis syndrome is the result of the combination of volume depletion in the face of urinary precipitation of uric acid in the renal tubules and parenchyma, and acute nephrocalcinosis from severe hyperphosphatemia. Since patients at risk for tumor lysis often have intra-abdominal lymphoma, urinary tract obstruction can be a contributing factor in the development of ARF. Given the aforementioned pathogenetic factors for ARF, patients who are undergoing treatment with malignancies likely to experience rapid cell lysis should receive vigorous intravenous hydration to maintain good urinary flow and urinary dilution. In addition, because uric acid is very soluble at physiologic pH, sodium bicarbonate should be added to the intravenous fluid to achieve a pH greater than 6.5 in the urine. Alkalinization can be achieved by the administration of 100 mEq/L of sodium bicarbonate in 1 liter of D_5W (5% dextrose in water) at a rate of 200 mL/h. Since metabolic alkalosis can aggravate hypocalcemia, caution should be exercised when using alkali in patients with low serum calcium levels. It is advisable to stop the infusion if the serum bicarbonate level is greater than 30 mEq/L. Allopurinol is administered to inhibit uric acid formation. Through its metabolite oxypurinol, allopurinol inhibits xanthine oxidase and thereby blocks the conversion of hypoxanthine and xanthine to uric acid. During massive tumor lysis, uric acid excretion can still increase, despite the administration of allopurinol, so that intravenous hydration is still necessary to prevent ARF. Since allopurinol and its metabolites are excreted in the urine, the dose should be reduced in the face of impaired renal function. Urate oxidase has been recently approved for use in the United States. It converts uric acid to water-soluble allantoin, thereby decreasing serum uric acid levels and urinary uric acid excretion.[120] The use of urate oxidase may obviate the need for urinary alkalinization, but good urine flow with hydration should be maintained given the probability of preexisting volume depletion.

Dialysis for ARF associated with tumor lysis syndrome may be required for the traditional indications of fluid overload, hyperkalemia, hyperphosphatemia or hyperuricemia unresponsive to medical management. There is some interest in using dialysis in patients at high risk of tumor lysis syndrome to prevent the development of renal failure. In a small trial in five children, continuous hemofiltration was started prior to administration of chemotherapy and appeared to prevent renal failure in 80% of the patients.[121] However, given that continuous dialysis is complicated, expensive, and not without risk, its routine use as prophylaxis cannot be recommended.

Thrombotic Microangiopathy

Thrombotic microangiopathy (TMA) in the form of hemolytic-uremic syndrome (HUS) and thrombocytopenic purpura (TTP) is a disease of multiple etiologies manifesting as non-immune hemolytic anemia, thrombocytopenia, varying degrees of encephalopathy, and renal failure due to platelet thrombi in the microcirculation of the kidneys. Laboratory findings include elevated indirect bilirubin and lactate dehydrogenase (LDH) levels, depressed serum haptoglobin values, and schistocytes on peripheral blood smear. The characteristic renal lesion consists of vessel wall thickening in capillaries and arterioles, with swelling and detachment of endothelial cells from the basement membranes and accumulation of subendothelial fluffy material.[122] These vascular lesions are indistinguishable from those seen in malignant hypertension or scleroderma renal crisis.

Typically, HUS develops in children with hemorrhagic colitis from verotoxin-producing *Escherichia coli* infection associated with ingestion of undercooked meat.[123] Renal failure is pronounced, and altered sensorium is not consistently present. In contrast, idiopathic TTP is usually seen in adult women where encephalopathy is the predominant clinical feature whereas renal involvement is less severe. However, because of similar laboratory findings and the great overlap in clinical features, these syndromes likely share the same pathogenesis—endothelial cell dysfunction.[124]

In cancer patients, malignancy, chemotherapy, radiation, immunosuppressive agents, and bone marrow transplantation can induce endothelial dysfunction leading to TMA and renal failure (Table 7).

Treatment of renal failure and TMA in cancer patients is mainly supportive, with initiation of dialysis as necessary. Stopping any causative medications is advised. However, the role of

Table 7 Thrombotic Microangiopathy in Cancer Patients

Chemotherapy
Mitomycin C
Platinum
Bleomycin
Holmium

Immunosuppressive agents
Cyclosporine
Tacrolimus

Malignancy
Gastric carcinoma

Bone Marrow Transplantation
BMT nephropathy

Radiation
Acute radiation nephritis
Malignant hypertension

plasmapheresis remains controversial. Although all forms of TMA share the same underlying pathogenesis of endothelial cell injury and dysfunction, the actual inciting event may be different in each case and not amenable to plasmapheresis. As an example, plasmapheresis has not been found to be an effective therapy for HUS in children, despite its clear benefit in the treatment of idiopathic TTP.[125] In TTP, an autoantibody to the von Willebrand's factor-cleaving protease has been described.[126] Inhibition of the cleaving enzyme leads to unusually large von Willebrand multimers that may agglutinate circulating platelets at sites with high levels of intravascular shear stress and trigger TMA. Plasma infusion may provide an exogenous source of cleaving protease to compete with the autoantibody while plasmapheresis will remove the pathogenic antibody. In HUS, no autoantibody has been found and may explain the ineffectiveness of plasmapheresis in this disorder.[127] Reports on the use of plasmapheresis in cancer patients are confined to those with bone marrow transplantation (BMT) nephropathy. Most studies are small case series that are unable to clearly demonstrate true benefit. Nevertheless, when faced with a patient with the clinical characteristics of severe TTP after BMT, a trial of plasmapheresis is probably warranted.

Bone Marrow Transplantation

Acute renal failure, defined as doubling of the baseline serum creatinine level, may occur in up to 50% of patients who undergo BMT, of which half will undergo hemodialysis.[128] Initially, it was assumed that the cause of ARF was multifactorial in nature, given the severity of illness and the amount of nephrotoxin exposure. Instead, three distinctive renal syndromes associated with BMT were described and are categorized according to the time of onset.[129] Renal complications are more prevalent in patients who undergo allogeneic transplants. When autologous stem cell transplants became the predominant method of BMT, the incidence of these disorders decreased.[130]

Within the first few days after transplantation, ARF may develop from hemoglobinuria caused by infusion of hemolyzed red blood cells.[66] Preservation of bone marrow with DMSO will cause hemolysis of red blood cells present in the stored specimen, and subsequent infusion will result in hemoglobinuria. Three mechanisms are involved in the pathogenesis of hemoglobinuric ARF: renal vasoconstriction, direct cytotoxicity of hemoglobin, and intratubular cast formation. By scavenging nitric oxide and stimulating the release of endothelin and thromboxane, hemoglobin causes renal vasoconstriction. Hemoglobin is also toxic to renal tubular epithelial cells either directly or through release of iron, and by generation of reactive oxygen species.[131] Intratubular cast formation occludes urinary flow, thereby decreasing GFR, and prolongs cellular exposure to the harmful effects of hemoglobin. Another renal syndrome usually occurs 10 to 21 days after transplantation and is associated with the development of veno-occlusive disease (VOD) of the liver.[129] VOD of the liver is characterized by tender hepatomegaly, fluid retention with ascites formation, and jaundice. It is the result of fibrous narrowing of small hepatic venules and sinusoids triggered by the pre-transplant cytoreductive regimen, and is more common after allogeneic than autologous BMT. The ARF is similar in appearance to hepatorenal syndrome. Patients have hyperdynamic vital signs, along with hyponatremia, oliguria, and low urinary sodium concentration. The urinalysis shows minimal proteinuria and muddy brown granular casts as a result of bile salts and bilirubin in the urine. The patients are usually resistant to diuretics, and spontaneous recovery is rare. Risk factors for the development of ARF include weight gain, hyperbilirubinemia, use of amphotericin B, and a baseline serum creatinine level greater than 0.7 mg/dL. The development of ARF adversely affects survival. In patients who require dialysis, the mortality rate approaches 80%. Although VOD can be diagnosed by either direct measurement of sinusoidal pressures or liver biopsy, these procedures are difficult or hazardous in BMT patients. Therefore the diagnosis of VOD is usually made on clinical criteria. However, studies have shown that clinical criteria alone may not be sufficient to recognize or exclude a diagnosis of VOD.[132] Small trials using infusions of prostaglandin E, pentoxifylline, or low-dose heparin to prevent the development of VOD have been promising .[133–135] However, their use is not commonplace because of the associated risks of bleeding.

A late-stage renal manifestation of transplantation referred to as "BMT nephropathy" usually occurs more than 6 months after the procedure. It is characterized by the development of ARF with microangiopathic hemolytic anemia, worsening thrombocytopenia, hypertension, and fluid retention. Hence, BMT nephropathy is a form of HUS.[136] Patients may also have varying degrees of encephalopathy resembling TTP. It occurs in patients who receive cyclosporine for prevention of graft-versus-host disease, as well as those who do not. Radiation may play a role because its incidence appears higher after allogeneic compared with autologous BMT.[130] Although plasmapheresis therapy is often successful in treating idiopathic TTP, the results in BMT nephropathy have been disappointing.[137] Prognosis of BMT nephropathy is variable. Those patients who present with a modest rise in creatinine concentration and normal level of consciousness may have either spontaneous resolution or slow progression to chronic hemodialysis. Those patients who present with a fulminant course of TTP uniformly do poorly, despite aggressive dialysis and plasmapheresis, and often succumb to the disease.

GVHD is a complication of BMT not typically associated with renal disease. Renal lesions associated with GVHD have been described, and the primary manifestation is proteinuria. Immune-complex–mediated glomerular disease is the predominant finding on biopsy, with membranous nephropathy the pathologic lesion most commonly found.[138–140] In the majority of cases, the proteinuria improved or resolved with treatment of the GVHD with steroids or cyclosporin A.[139]

ARF associated with Lymphoma and Leukemia

Lymphoma

Infiltration of the kidneys by lymphoma cells may be detected in up to 90% of cases at autopsy. However, clinical renal disease as a result of infiltration is rare, most commonly seen in highly malignant and disseminated disease.[141–144] The diagnosis of renal failure resulting from lymphomatous infiltration is necessarily one of exclusion because more common explanations for renal failure usually exist. The diagnosis may be suspected from clinical features and imaging studies. Patients may present with flank pain and hematuria. Renal ultrasonography reveals diffusely enlarged kidneys, sometimes with multiple focal lesions. Although definitive diagnosis depends on renal biopsy, this procedure is often impossible because of the presence of contraindications. In such cases the following criteria support the diagnosis of renal failure as a result of lymphomatous infiltration: (1) renal enlargement without obstruction; (2) absence of other causes of renal failure; and (3) rapid improvement of renal failure after radiotherapy or systemic chemotherapy.

Cytotoxic Nephropathy/Hemophagocytic Syndrome

Hemophagocytic syndrome (HPS) is a reactive disorder that results from intense macrophage activation and cytokine release.[145] It has developed in patients with malignant lymphoma, severe bacterial and viral infections, and in patients receiving prolonged parenteral nutrition with soluble lipids. Patients present with fever, rash, respiratory failure, lymphadenopathy and hepatosplenomegaly. There have been recent reports of HPS in association with occult peripheral T-cell lymphomas causing severe ARF.[146] Renal biopsy specimens are characterized by an unusually severe degree of interstitial edema with limited interstitial cellular infiltrate. A number of cytokines, including interferon-α, tumor necrosis factor (TNF), interleukin-6, macrophage colony-stimulating factor, and CD-8 are up-regulated in HPS and may explain the marked macrophage activation and cytokine release. In patients with lymphadenopathy who develop unexplained multiple organ dysfunction, markedly elevated cytokine levels support the diagnosis.

Leukemia

Leukemic infiltration of the kidneys is present in 60 to 90% of patients with chronic lymphocytic leukemia (CLL). Although uncommon, many cases of renal failure attributable to leukemic infiltration are known.[147–149] Ultrasonography usually reveals bilateral renal enlargement. Chemotherapy often produces a dramatic improvement in renal function.

There are reports of patients with CLL who develop ARF from leukemic infiltration and are infected with polyomavirus.[150] Urine from patients demonstrates viral inclusions in tubular cells ("decoy" cells), and blood is positive for polyomavirus (BK type) DNA. Therefore, in leukemia patients with ARF considered due to leukemic infiltration, evidence for coexisting BK virus infection should be sought.

Patients with significantly elevated white cell counts can develop ARF from leukostasis. Leukemic cells occlude the peritubular and glomerular capillaries, thereby decreasing GFR. Patients may be oliguric but their renal function often improves with therapeutic leukopheresis or chemotherapy. Leukostasis has been described in both acute and chronic leukemia.

Radiation Nephritis

Renal failure and hypertension develop when the kidneys are exposed to more than 2,300 rads of radiation in fractionated doses over a period of 3 to 5 weeks.[151] A characteristic of radiation injury is the long latent period between radiation and overt nephrotoxicity. The effects of DNA damage from radiation are not evident until cell division occurs. The latency period depends on the proliferation rate of a particular tissue. The recognition of radiation injury has led to treatment protocols that have significantly minimized exposure and the incidence of radiation nephropathy. In the past, abdominal radiation and total body irradiation for bone marrow transplantation were leading causes of radiation nephritis. Today, sequential radiosensitizing chemotherapy with radiation is a more prevalent mode.[152]

Five clinical syndromes of radiation injury to the kidney are described: (1) acute radiation nephropathy; (2) chronic radiation nephropathy; (3) asymptomatic proteinuria; (4) benign hypertension; and (5) malignant hypertension.

Acute Radiation Nephropathy

Acute radiation nephropathy usually occurs after a latent period of 6 to 12 months.[153,154] Patients present with ARF accompanied by microangiopathic hemolytic anemia with schistocytes, thrombocytopenia, hypertension, and fluid overload with edema. Renal biopsy findings are not specific to radiation injury and are typical of HUS. The onset of ARF can be abrupt, and the degree of anemia and hypertension is severe. Although progression to chronic renal failure is the rule, there are reports of response to ACE inhibitor therapy in stabilizing the renal function.[155] The development of end stage renal disease (ESRD) is a poor prognostic event in these patients because survival on chronic dialysis is poor compared to that of age-matched, non-diabetic and diabetic patients.

Malignant hypertension as a complication of radiation to the kidney has been reported as a feature of acute radiation nephropathy, but also occasionally as an isolated late manifestation presenting 18 months to 11 years after irradiation. The incidence of this complication is much less with the availability of the new classes of antihypertensive agents, in particular, the ACE inhibitors.

Tubulointerstitial Nephritis

Acute tubulointerstitial nephritis (TIN) is a common cause of ARF accounting for 10% of cases in hospitalized patients.[156] On renal biopsy, an interstitial cellular infiltrate is the hallmark of TIN. The infiltrate is predominantly mononuclear with T- and B- lymphocytes, macrophages, and natural killer cells.[157] Scattered neutrophils, eosinophils, basophils, and plasma cells are also present. The infiltrate results in interstitial edema, disruption of tubular basement membrane, and destruction of the interstitial architecture. Similar to glomerulonephritis, most forms of acute TIN are immune-mediated.[158] Although earlier investigations concentrated on humeral

mechanisms with deposition of antibody or antigen-antibody immune complexes in the tubular basement membrane, there is abundant evidence now to suggest that cell-mediated immune responses account for most cases of acute TIN.[159–162] Experimental studies demonstrate that renal tubular epithelial cells can process and present target antigens to T-cells, as well as strongly express Class II major histocompatibility complex (MHC) determinants when stimulated by pro-inflammatory cytokines such as interferon-γ and tumor necrosis factor-α.

The clinical features of TIN are variable and in part depend on the inciting process.[163] In general, besides renal failure, disruption of the normal tubulointerstitial compartment will produce findings consistent with renal tubular dysfunction, including urinary concentrating defect, hyperchloremic metabolic acidosis, hypo- or hyperkalemia, and hypomagnesemia. Modest proteinuria can be present, but nephrotic range proteinuria is distinctly unusual and associated with use of only a few medications: NSAIDs, interferon-α, and methicillin.

Drug-Induced Acute Tubulointerstitial Nephritis

Drug reactions are a major cause of acute TIN in patients with cancer because they are exposed to a large number of medications of different classes. The most commonly implicated agents are the penicillins, cephalosporins, and NSAIDs. It can be difficult to establish a direct link between a particular drug and ARF because patients typically receive a variety of potentially nephrotoxic medications, making it uncertain which is the responsible agent. Also, comorbid conditions that could cause renal dysfunction are usually present. Since renal biopsy to determine the etiology of ARF is not routine, the diagnosis of acute TIN is presumptive. Acute TIN occurs within days to a few weeks of exposure to a drug, and there is no relationship between its development and the cumulative dose. Most patients present with symptoms of edema, hypertension, diminished urine output, and renal failure. The classical manifestations of allergic phenomena such as skin rash, arthralgias, fever, and eosinophilia are present in only a minority of patients.[164] Occasionally, flank pain is a prominent feature of the presentation. The presence of urinary eosinophils is of limited utility in the evaluation of ARF.[165] The finding of eosinophils in the urine has a positive predictive value for diagnosing acute TIN of only 40%. Absence of urinary eosinophils is more helpful in excluding the diagnosis although the negative predictive value is still only 70%. Hansel (rather than Wright's) stain is the preferred method of detecting eosinophiluria.[17] Pyuria in the absence of an infectious organism (sterile pyuria) can be seen with acute TIN; however,

leukopenia can limit the appearance of white blood cells in the urine. Therefore, the diagnosis of acute TIN requires a high index of suspicion and knowledge of the potential causes. Clues to the presence of acute TIN are listed in Table 8.

Treatment of drug-induced acute TIN is cessation of the causative agent. Small case series have reported significant clinical response to corticosteroid administration.[163,166,167] There are no large, randomized, placebo-controlled trials to guide treatment. Given the potential side effects of corticosteroids, their use should be restricted to patients with progressive renal failure despite stopping the offending drug. Consideration of renal biopsy in these cases is strongly recommended because the clinical diagnosis of TIN is presumptive and the risks from corticosteroid use in critically ill patients are high. Drug-induced acute TIN has been associated with a wide spectrum of medications, as listed in Table 9.

Fluoroquinolones

All members of this class have been reported to cause acute TIN.[164] Typically, there is fever, rash, and eosinophilia, but no other systemic features of an allergic reaction. Granulomatous TIN has been reported, as well as necrotizing vasculitis of the skin, lung, bladder, and kidney.[168]

Vancomycin

Although the nephrotoxicity of vancomycin has been attributed to impurities in the older

Table 8 Medications Causing Acute Tubulointerstitial Nephritis

Antibiotics
Cephalosporins
Fluoroquinolones
Penicillins
Rifampin
Sulfonamides
Vancomycin

Biologic agents
Interleukin 2
α-interferon

Anti-inflammatory agents
NSAIDs
COX-2 inhibitors

Diuretics
Furosemide
Thiazide diuretics

Immunosuppressive agents
Azathioprine
OKT3

Miscellaneous
Allopurinol
Cimetidine/ ranitidine/famotidine
Omeprazole
Pamidronate

COX-2 = cylcooxygenase-2; OKT = .

Table 9 Clinical Features of Acute Tubulointerstitial Nephritis
Absence of other major causes to explain renal failure
Prior implication of drug as a cause of acute TIN
Non-oliguric acute renal failure
Microscopic or gross hematuria
Sterile pyuria
White blood cell casts
Eosinophilia
Eosinophiluria
Fever
Skin rash
Arthralgias
Hyperchloremic metabolic acidosis (RTA)
Urinary concentrating defect
Hypo- or hyperkalemia
Hypomagnesemia
RTA = renal tubular acidosis; TIN = tubulointerstitial nephritis.

preparations of the drug, there remains a small incidence of ARF associated with its use.[169] Vancomycin nephrotoxicity typically develops when administered in combination with other drugs, particularly aminoglycosides, and when given at higher-than-recommended doses. There may be some signs of a hypersensitivity reaction, such as skin rash and eosinophilia.

Rifampin

There are several reports of hypersensitivity reactions to rifampin associated with its intermittent use, manifesting as fever, nausea, diarrhea, and oliguric ARF.[170] Rifampin is associated with several immune-mediated phenomena. The drug acts as a hapten and results in antibody and immune-complex formation, and the subsequent development of interstitial nephritis with renal failure.[171]

Penicillins

Acute tubulointerstitial nephritis has been reported with all the penicillins.[164] Renal manifestations include hematuria, proteinuria, and oliguric ARF. Fever, rash, arthralgias, eosinophilia, pyuria, and eosinophiluria may also be present, particularly associated with the use of methacillin.

Cephalosporins

All generations of cephalosporins produce nephrotoxicity. Most cases involve direct toxicity to the renal tubular cells, resulting in ATN. In addition, cephalosporins can produce hypersensitivity reactions with skin rash, fever, eosinophilia, hematuria, and TIN.[163,164] In some reports, renal failure was the only finding. Cephalosporins are structurally similar to the penicillins, and cross-reactivity has been reported in 1 to 20% of patients.

Infective Tubulointerstitial Nephritis

Bacterial Infection

Bacterial pyelonephritis may result in ARF.[172] This occurs most commonly in the setting of an ascending urinary tract infection superimposed on obstructive nephropathy. In patients with urinary tract infection or pyelonephritis who develop ARF, urgent imaging of the kidneys and urinary tract is necessary to exclude the presence of obstruction. Acute renal failure as a result of pyelonephritis can also occur in the absence of urinary tract obstruction. Occasionally, renal involvement results from hematogenous spread. In such cases, blood cultures are frequently positive, and there may be evidence of overt sepsis. Clinical distinction from ATN secondary to septicemia and septic shock may therefore be difficult. Renal histopathologic findings reveal an acute polymorphonuclear infiltrate in the interstitium with microabscess formation.

The prognosis in acute bacterial TIN is significantly worse than for ATN. Whereas patients with ATN are expected to make full recovery, bacterial TIN often progresses to severe interstitial scarring and progressive chronic renal failure. Patients require prolonged antibiotic treatment to eradicate the infection and close monitoring to minimize chronic progressive renal damage.

Renal Candidiasis

Mucosal ulceration and long-dwelling intravascular catheters are major risk factors for invasion of the blood stream by Candida species. Other important risk factors include prolonged hospitalization, prior exposure to antimicrobial agents, corticosteroid therapy, the postoperative state, surgical wounds, chronic indwelling urinary catheters, and underlying malignancy. The kidneys are particularly vulnerable to candidal invasion. The presence of hyphae in the urine does not have diagnostic significance, while the absence of pyuria does not rule out a diagnosis of renal candidiasis especially in the severely neutropenic patient. Therefore, a positive culture of Candida from urine in the septicemic patient is considered as proof of renal candidiasis.[173] The Candida organisms progressively penetrate the renal parenchyma, forming hyphae and microabcesses, especially in the cortical regions. Involvement of renal vasculature may result in renal infarction and papillary necrosis. Penetration of the organisms into the renal tubules may result in multiple sites of tubular obstruction, or the formation of large aggregates of fungi within the collecting system in the form of fungal balls or bezoars.[174] This complication should be suspected in the presence of flank pain and microscopic hematuria. Candida species differ in virulence capacity to involve the kidneys. *Candida albicans* and

C. tropicalis have the greatest propensity to cause widespread metastatic disease and renal invasion.

The patient with renal candidiasis usually presents with fever, candiduria, and unexplained progressive renal failure.[175] There usually are no symptoms referable to the kidneys, while there may be symptoms arising from involvement of other organs, including skin, mucosa, muscle, and eyes. Contrary to the case with bacterial urinary tract infections, there is no consensus as to the critical concentrations of candiduria required for a diagnosis of renal candidiasis. High colony counts may be a reflection of colonization rather than infection in patients with indwelling bladder catheters or nephrostomy tubes. Diagnosis is further complicated by the lack of any tests to localize infection to the kidneys. Candida casts are highly suggestive of renal infection but are an unusual finding. The presence of fungal bezoars in the upper urinary tract can be excluded with renal ultrasonography or other suitable imaging procedures. A useful diagnostic test in the catheterized patient with candiduria, bladder washings with amphotericin B will clear the urine of colonization but not renal candidosis.[176]

Zygomycosis

Invasive zygomycosis (mucormycosis) occurs predominantly in immunocompromised patients. Patients present with bilateral flank pain, fever, hematuria, pyuria, and renal failure, with radiographic evidence of enlarged non-functioning kidneys.[177] Mortality is high, and nephrectomy is usually required along with systemic anti-fungal therapy.

Adenovirus Infections

Opportunistic infections secondary to systemic adenovirus infection occur in immunocompromised patients. Adenovirus type II appears to have a predilection for urothelial membrane surfaces, and infections of the urothelium are frequent. As a result, adenovirus type II has been associated with urinary tract obstruction and hemorrhagic cystitis in this patient population. There are several reports of acute TIN with oliguric ARF in the setting of a severe of pneumonitis, hepatitis, meningoencephalitis, myocarditis, and hemorrhagic cystitis.[178,179]

Polyomavirus (BK Type) Infection

Polyomaviruses are ubiquitous, usually acquired in childhood, and have a predilection for the urothelial surfaces. They have been associated with renal dysfunction and urinary tract obstruction from ureteral ulcerations and strictures. An acute TIN (BK nephropathy) has been reported in patients who received renal or bone marrow transplants.[180] The diagnosis of BK nephropathy is suggested by the presence of inclusion-bearing cells in the urine ("decoy" cells) and the detection by polymerase chain reaction of BK virus DNA in the serum.

Epstein-Barr Virus Infection

Epstein-Barr virus (EBV) is associated with acute TIN and renal failure in both immunocompetent and immunocompromised patients.[181] Other renal lesions associated with EBV and infectious mononucleosis includes acute glomerulonephritis, hemolytic-uremic syndrome, and rhabdomyolysis-induced ARF.[182]

Disseminated Histoplasmosis

Immunocompromised patients can develop multiple organ failure from disseminated histoplasmosis. The disease usually follows a rapidly progressive course with a high mortality rate. Although uncommon, ARF does occur.[183,184] Biopsy specimens show aggregates of phagocytosed macrophages in the glomerular capillaries and the tubular interstitium.

Prevention of Acute Tubular Necrosis

There currently exist no known therapeutic options to ameliorate ARF or hasten its recovery. Dialysis remains only a supportive measure to treat or prevent the metabolic and hypervolemic complications of renal failure. Therefore, prevention of ARF remains a keystone in the treatment of the critically ill patient.

Volume Resuscitation

Most cases of ARF are the result of multiple factors, including exposure to nephrotoxic agents and relative or frank renal hypoperfusion. Avoidance of potential nephrotoxins such as intravenous radiocontrast, aminoglycoside antibiotics, and anti-fungal agents, when possible, is prudent. Maintenance of adequate intravascular volume to preserve renal perfusion pressure is essential. Many cancer patients have capillary leak associated with the systemic inflammatory response syndrome (SIRS) resulting in severe interstitial edema and renal hypoperfusion. Often, these patients also are receiving intravenous vasopressor agents and positive pressure ventilation that further impair renal blood flow. How exactly to maintain effective arterial blood volume in such circumstances remains a contentious issue. Aggressive hydration with crystalloid solutions such as 0.9% sodium chloride can worsen interstitial edema and pulmonary function. Colloidal solutions, such as various starches and human albumin, might appear to be attractive alternatives, but there is little solid evidence that establishes their superiority in clinical trials.[185–187] Systematic reviews of randomized controlled

trials comparing crystalloids with colloids have yielded conflicting results. Some trials have found an increased mortality rate associated with the administration of human albumin and hydroxyethylstarch while others have not.[188,189] So despite the importance of fluid therapy in the prevention of ARF, the nature of the optimum fluid resuscitation regimen remains a disputed topic. For the time being, it appears that treatment of the underlying diagnosis, usually sepsis, and general supportive efforts, including ultrafiltration if necessary, are the mainstays of therapy.

In the critically ill patient, it is often difficult to predict when a potential insult to the kidneys will occur, making true prophylaxis difficult.

Specific Measures

N-acetylcysteine

N-acetylcysteine (NAC) is an antioxidant and causes renal vasodilatation by generating increased levels of nitric oxide (NO). Based on these effects, NAC was used in several small human trials for the prevention of ARF from radiocontrast agents in high-risk individuals. The trials have shown that its administration results in a significantly smaller change in baseline serum creatinine values compared to changes in the placebo group.[190,191] However, whether or not NAC prevents severe ARF and the need for dialysis has not been determined. At this point, it is probably reasonable to provide NAC prior to radiocontrast administration in patients at risk for the development of ARF. However, no convincing data exist to support the routine administration of NAC in other clinical circumstances to prevent the development of ARF.

Low-Dose Dopamine

Low-dose dopamine administration (1-3 µg/kg/min) to normal individuals causes renal vasodilatation and increased glomerular filtration rate (GRF), and acts as a proximal tubule diuretic. Due to these effects, numerous studies have used low-dose dopamine to either prevent or treat ARF in a variety of clinical settings. It has been given as prophylaxis for ARF associated with radiocontrast administration, repair of aortic aneurysms, orthotopic liver transplantation, unilateral nephrectomy, renal transplantation, and chemotherapy with interferon.[192,193] Yet despite more than 20 years of clinical experience, prevention trials with low-dose dopamine all have been small, inadequately randomized, of limited statistical power, and with end-points of questionable clinical significance. Furthermore, there is concern for the potential harmful effects of dopamine, even at low doses. It can trigger tachyarrhythmias and myocardial ischemia, decrease intestinal blood flow, and suppress T-cell function.[192–194] It has also been shown to

increase the risk of radiocontrast nephropathy when given as prophylaxis to patients with diabetic nephropathy.[195] Therefore, the use of low-dose dopamine for renal protection should be abandoned.

Low-Dose Fenoldopam Mesylate

Fenoldopam mesylate is a pure dopamine type-1 receptor agonist that has similar hemodynamic effects to dopamine in the kidney without α- and β-adrenergic stimulation. Limited trials suggest administration of fenoldopam mesylate reduces the occurrence of ARF from radiocontrast agents and from the repair of aortic aneurysms.[196,197] However, as in the case of low-dose dopamine, no randomized controlled trials exist to support its indiscriminate use and it should be restricted to well-designed clinical studies.

Diuretics

Furosemide is a loop diuretic and vasodilator that may decrease oxygen consumption in Henle's loop by inhibiting sodium transport, thus lessening ischemic injury. By increasing urinary flow, it may also reduce intratubular obstruction and backleak of filtrate. Based on these properties, furosemide might be expected to prevent ARF. However, few data support its use. Furosemide was found to be ineffective when used to prevent ARF after cardiac surgery, and was found to increase the risk of ARF when given to prevent contrast nephropathy.[53,198]

Mannitol is an osmotic diuretic that can also scavenge free-radicals. It may be beneficial when added to organ preservation solutions during renal transplantation and protect against ARF caused by rhabdomyolysis if given extremely early.[199,200] Otherwise, mannitol has not been shown to be useful in the prevention of ARF. In fact, mannitol may aggravate ARF from radiocontrast agents.[195]

Atrial Natriuretic Peptide

Atrial natriuretic peptide (ANP) causes vasodilatation of the afferent arteriole and constriction of the efferent arteriole resulting in an increased GFR. It also inhibits renal tubular sodium reabsorption. Most studies with ANP concern the treatment of established ARF. However, in two studies that administered ANP in renal transplant recipients to prevent primary renal dysfunction, no benefit was found.[201,202] As with low-dose dopamine and mannitol, one study suggested that ANP prophylaxis might worsen renal function in diabetic patients receiving radiocontrast material.[195]

Insulin-like Growth Factor-1

Insulin-like growth factor-1 (IGF-1) increases renal blood flow and induces cell proliferation and differentiation. In addition, it reverses apoptosis. In animal models, it ameliorates renal injury associated with ischemia and may prevent injury following renal transplantation.[203,204] IGF-1 was given to a small group of patients in a single trial for prophylaxis of ARF following aortic aneurysm repair.[205] IGF-1 was started postoperatively in a randomized placebo-controlled fashion. It was well tolerated, and produced a modest increase in the creatinine clearance in the treated group compared to the placebo group. However, no patient developed ARF necessitating dialysis. Hence, the role, if any, for IGF-1 in the prevention of ARF remains unknown.

Clinical Trials in the Treatment of Acute Tubular Necrosis

Effective treatment of ARF in critically ill patients is lacking despite substantial advances in the understanding of its pathogenesis at a cellular and molecular level. This lack of efficacy results from numerous factors: the multifactorial nature of ARF in the intensive care unit (ICU), reliance on changes in serum creatinine levels to detect changes in GFR, varying definitions of ARF, the high mortality rate of ICU patients in general, and the lack of consensus on the timing and appropriate form of acute dialysis. Although a wide variety of agents, including loop diuretics, low-dose dopamine, ANP, thyroid hormone, and IGF-1, are effective in animal models, they have not been effective in the treatment of ARF in the clinical setting.[48,206]

The reasons that these therapies have been highly effective only in animals remain speculative. Most human trials involve moderately or severely ill patients in the ICU with multiple organ failure, whereas animal models of ARF rely on a single mechanism of injury in otherwise healthy animals.[207] In addition, the time of the renal insult is known precisely in the models, allowing for early administration of the intervention. In clinical trials, on the other hand, therapy is delayed because of reliance on a change of the serum creatinine level to indicate ARF. By the time the serum creatinine concentration has increased, there has been a significant decline in the GFR and the renal injury has been present for a prolonged period. Timing of the intervention may be critical to its success. Very early in ARF, hemodynamic factors and oxidant injury may predominate, while, later, inflammation may play a more prominent role. Unfortunately, there still exists no easily available reliable marker of early ARF. Therefore, therapy of ARF remains primarily supportive.

Low-Dose Dopamine

Numerous trials using low-dose dopamine to treat ARF suggest that its use is beneficial.[192,193,208]

However, most studies were either uncontrolled case series or small randomized trials with limited statistical power. More recently, a large randomized placebo-controlled trial in 328 critically ill patients with early ARF sufficiently powered to detect a small benefit was reported.[209] There was no effect of low-dose dopamine on renal function, need for dialysis, ICU or hospital length-of-stay, or mortality. These findings combined with the aforementioned potential deleterious effects of low-dose dopamine are strong arguments for abandoning its use entirely in ARF.

Diuretics

In patients with ARF, several studies have found no benefit from loop diuretics.[210–214] Their use did not accelerate renal recovery, decrease the need for dialysis, or reduce mortality. It was shown that the mortality rate of oliguric patients who responded to furosemide with a diuresis was lower than those who did not.[18,214] However, the clinical characteristics, severity of renal failure, and mortality rates were similar in patients with either spontaneous non-oliguric ARF or patients who became non-oliguric after furosemide. This implies that those patients able to respond to furosemide are less sick and have intrinsically less severe renal damage than non-responders, rather than there existing any true therapeutic benefit to furosemide administration. Although administration of furosemide might improve fluid management if it induces a diuresis, a retrospective review of a recent trial in critically ill patients with ARF found diuretic use to be associated with an increased risk of death and non-recovery of renal function.[215] Most of the increased risk, however, was seen in those patients unresponsive to high doses of diuretics, implying they had more severe disease. Therefore, diuretics should be used with caution in critically ill patients. Diuretics should be withdrawn if there is no response. In patients who experience an increase in urine output, volume status must be closely monitored because the injured kidneys are susceptible to further damage from mild changes in perfusion pressure. To maintain the diuresis, a continuous infusion of drug is probably preferable to intermittent bolus administration.[216] Although there are no large randomized controlled trials, the overall evidence suggests that continuous infusion of diuretics as opposed to bolus administration is more effective and associated with less toxicity and delayed development of diuretic resistance.

Atrial Natriuretic Peptide

ANP improved renal blood flow and GRF in an uncontrolled trial of 11 patients who developed ARF after cardiac surgery.[217] In an open-labeled trial, infusion of ANP to patients with ARF increased GFR and decreased the need for dialysis by nearly 50%.[218] Based on these results, a

randomized placebo-controlled trial of 504 critically ill patients with ARF was conducted.[219] Despite the large size of the trial, ANP administration had no effect on 21-day dialysis-free survival, mortality, or change in plasma creatinine concentration. Although a subgroup analysis of the study suggested that ANP might be beneficial in those patients with oliguric renal failure, a subsequent similar trial in patients with oliguric renal failure failed to demonstrate any benefit of ANP.[220] Hence, there is no convincing evidence to support the use of ANP in the treatment of ARF.

Insulin-Like Growth Factor-1

Based on the positive effects of IGF-1 in animal models of ARF, a randomized placebo-controlled trial was conducted in 72 critically ill patients with ARF.[221] The results showed there was no difference in the two groups in post-treatment GFR, need for dialysis, or mortality. In anuric patients, IGF-1 administration was associated with a slower rate of improvement in urine output and GFR. So despite the ample evidence that IGF-1 accelerates renal recovery in animal models of ARF, there is no support for its use in humans.

Thyroxine

The administration of thyroid hormone following the initiation of ARF in a variety of ischemic and nephrotoxic animal models was found to be effective in promoting recovery of renal function.[222–225] Based on these results, thyroxine was administered to 59 patients with ARF in a randomized placebo-controlled trial.[226] Patients were well matched in baseline characteristics. Administration of thyroxine had no effect on any renal parameter. However, the trial was terminated early because of a significantly higher mortality rate in the patients who received thyroxine.

Renal Replacement Therapy

Dialysis initially entered clinical practice more than 50 years ago, yet there is no consensus on the appropriate timing for initiation of dialysis, the dose or intensity of dialysis, or the mode of dialysis (intermittent versus continuous) in patients with ARF. By tradition, clinical parameters such as severe electrolyte imbalance, pulmonary edema, intractable metabolic acidosis, azotemia (BUN > 100 mg/dL), and uremia are used as indications for starting dialysis, but these parameters may be inappropriate in the critically ill patient. No studies have clearly defined the optimal time to initiate dialysis. Retrospective trials done more than 30 years ago suggested that maintaining a BUN level below 150 mg/dL conferred a survival benefit.[227,228] In a later prospective trial, more intensive dialysis (maintaining the BUN level below 60 mg/dL compared to 100 mg/dL) did not improve mortality.[229] Part of the problem is that the dialysis procedure itself may be harmful. Bleeding and infection from vascular access, and hypotension and arrhythmias from changes in volume, may complicate dialysis. Studies also show that the dialysis procedure may prolong the course of ARF.[230] Delayed recovery may result from hypotension or activation of an inflammatory cascade by the interaction of blood components with the dialyzer membrane.[231]

Intensity of Dialysis

Once dialysis has been initiated, it has not been established how often and how long it should be prescribed. In other words, what is the optimal intensity of dialysis that provides the patient the benefits of the procedure without exposure to undue risk? Equally germane to the issue is identifying appropriate end-points to define "adequate" dialysis in an ICU patient. Survival rate appears most relevant. However, given the severity of the patients' comorbid diseases, it may be unrealistic to expect that various intensities of dialysis will impact mortality, or at the very least, to expect clinical trials to be powered sufficiently to prove any effect. Currently there is interest in applying some form of measuring urea removal in patients with ARF to define dialysis adequacy analogous to the circumstance in chronic outpatient dialysis. The National Cooperative Dialysis Study demonstrated that morbidity and hospitalization rates were inversely related to the amount of urea removal per treatment in chronic, stable hemodialysis patients.[232] Whether such a relationship exists in acutely ill patients with higher urea generation rates because of hypercatabolism is unknown. Recent trials have begun to address this issue. A study from the Cleveland Clinic showed a link between dialysis intensity and outcome in ICU patients when underlying comorbidity was accounted for using the Cleveland Clinic Severity of Illness Score.[233] Dialysis had no effect on the outcome of patients with low or high severity scores, but a beneficial effect in those with intermittent scores. Higher delivery of dialysis as measured by the reduction of urea concentration was associated with a significant decrease in morbidity when compared to low dose delivery in patients with an intermediate severity score. A more recent study in 72 critically ill patients with ARF randomized to daily or alternate day dialysis reported improved survival with the more intense regimen.[234] However, in this study, the dose of dialysis per session was significantly lower than what would be considered adequate for a stable patient on chronic hemodialysis. It thereby proves that under-dosing dialysis in a critically ill patient is detrimental, but failed to define what should be considered adequate for such patients. Although one could take the position that more dialysis is better, given the aforementioned risks associated with dialysis, that attitude may be cavalier. In fact, in a trial of chronic renal-failure patients, increasing the dose of dialysis beyond what is currently considered adequate conferred no additional benefit to patients.[235] Therefore, "excessive" dialysis in critically ill patients may only increase the exposure to risk without imparting any additional benefit. Until these issues are resolved by ongoing clinical trials, it seems prudent to rely on clinical parameters such as electrolyte and acid-base balance, control of volume overload, and avoidance of azotemia (maintaining the BUN below 60 mg/dL) to guide dialytic therapy.

Mode of Dialysis

In the past, intermittent hemodialysis (IHD) was the treatment of choice for ARF. However, as a result of the rapid solute removal and large volume shifts associated with its use, patients with hemodynamic instability poorly tolerate it. Because of the risk of hypotension and the possibility of prolonging ARF, newer modes of dialysis to minimize hypotension have been devised. Continuous renal replacement therapy (CRRT) removes solute and fluid at a much slower rate than IHD, thus minimizing hypotension.[236,237] Use of CRRT was originally reserved for patients with hemodynamic instability or massive fluid overload who could not otherwise tolerate IHD. Although dialysis was usually successful in such patients, the mortality rate remained high due to the underlying severity of illness. Given the better hemodynamic profile of CRRT, as well as potentially better solute clearance and removal of inflammatory cytokines, it was thought that CRRT would lead to better outcomes in critically ill patients who could otherwise tolerate IHD.

CRRT and IHD have been compared in a number of non-randomized or retrospective trials that have championed CRRT as the modality of choice in critically ill patients. However, prospective or randomized trials comparing IHD and CRRT have not found CRRT to confer a better outcome.[238,239] This somewhat surprising finding may be the result of studying critically ill patients where multiple factors play a role in the ultimate outcome. For now, it appears that IHD and CRRT are equivalent methods of treatment for ARF in the ICU.

There is also interest in using CRRT for non-renal indications, including sepsis and acute respiratory distress syndrome (ARDS).[240] It is based on the assumption that dialytic removal of inflammatory cytokines such as TNF-α and interleukins improves survival.[241] Small trials suggesting CRRT is beneficial all have serious methodological flaws. In addition, although cytokines can be removed by filtration and/or absorption to the filter, the actual quantity is low compared to endogenous clearance.[242] Clearance is also indiscriminant and can remove cytokines that may be beneficial in the face of critical illness. Until adequate clinical trials are completed, the use of CRRT for non-renal indications cannot be recommended.

Summary

In cancer patients, renal failure has become a difficult problem to prevent, diagnose early, and ultimately treat. The number of cancer survivors is rising and chronic kidney disease is too often the result of ARF, especially from nephrotoxic injury sustained during chemotherapy. To date, there is little data supporting prophylactic measures against ARF except volume expansion to prevent toxic nephropathy from contrast and chemotherapy. Even less clinical data is available in the treatment of established ARF. It is important to understand dialysis is not a therapy for ARF but simply a therapy to control the metabolic and volume complications associated with ARF. Unfortunately, to date, there are no large randomized trials to help define when dialysis should be started, what type of dialysis should be used, or for how long dialysis should be done in this patient population. With this in mind, the prevention of ARF becomes the best hope of a successful renal outcome in the treatment of cancer patients. To this end, it is important to recognize the potential risk factors for ARF, to diagnose ARF quickly, and work towards a rapid resolution of the renal insult.

REFERENCES

1. Hou S, Bushinsky D, Wish J, et al. Hospital-acquired renal insufficiency: a prospective study. Am J Med 1983;74: 243–8.
2. Albright RC Jr. Acute renal failure: a practical update. Mayo Clin Proc 2001;76:67–74.
3. Brivet FG, et al. Acute renal failure in intensive care units—causes, outcome, and prognostic factors of hospital mortality; a prospective, multicenter study. French Study Group on Acute Renal Failure. Crit Care Med 1996; 24:192–8.
4. van Bommel EF, Leunissen KM, Weimar W. Continuous renal replacement therapy for critically ill patients: an update. J Intensive Care Med 1994;9:265–80.
5. Nash K, Hafeez A, Hou S. Hospital-acquired renal insufficiency. Am J Kidney Dis 2002;39:930–6.
6. Huynh TT, et al. Determinants of hospital length of stay after thoracoabdominal aortic aneurysm repair. J Vasc Surg 2002;35:648–53.
7. Dimick JB, et al. Complications and costs after high-risk surgery: where should we focus quality improvement initiatives? J Am Coll Surg 2003;196:671–8.
8. Silvester W. Outcome studies of continuous renal replacement therapy in the intensive care unit. Kidney Int 1998; 66(Suppl):138–41.
9. Lassnigg A, et al. Minimal changes of serum creatinine predict prognosis in patients after cardiothoracic surgery: a prospective cohort study. J Am Soc Nephrol 2004;15: 1597–605.
10. Levy EM, Viscoli CM, Horwitz RI. The effect of acute renal failure on mortality. A cohort analysis. Jama 1996;275: 1489–94.
11. Robertshaw M, Lai KN, Swaminathan R. Prediction of creatinine clearance from plasma creatinine: comparison of five formulae. Br J Clin Pharmacol 1989;28:275–80.
12. Vervoort G, Willems HL, Wetzels JF. Assessment of glomerular filtration rate in healthy subjects and normoalbuminuric diabetic patients: validity of a new (MDRD) prediction equation. Nephrol Dial Transplant 2002;17: 1909–13.

13. Han WK, et al. Kidney Injury Molecule-1 (KIM-1): a novel biomarker for human renal proximal tubule injury. Kidney Int 2002;62:237–44.

14. Espinel CH, Gregory AW. Differential diagnosis of acute renal failure. Clin Nephrol 1980;13:73–7.

15. Miller TR, et al. Urinary diagnostic indices in acute renal failure: a prospective study. Ann Intern Med 1978;89:47–50.

16. Zarich S, Fang LS, Diamond JR. Fractional excretion of sodium. Exceptions to its diagnostic value. Arch Intern Med 1985;145:108–12.

17. Nolan CR 3rd, Anger MS, Kelleher SP. Eosinophiluria—a new method of detection and definition of the clinical spectrum. N Engl J Med 1986;315:1516–9.

18. Anderson RJ, et al. Nonoliguric acute renal failure. N Engl J Med 1977;296:1134–8.

19. Memoli B, et al. Interleukin-2-induced renal dysfunction in cancer patients is reversed by low-dose dopamine infusion. Am J Kidney Dis 1995;26:27–33.

20. Mercatello A, et al. Acute renal failure with preserved renal plasma flow induced by cancer immunotherapy. Kidney Int 1991;40:309–14.

21. Whelton A. Nephrotoxicity of nonsteroidal anti-inflammatory drugs: physiologic foundations and clinical implications. Am J Kidney Dis 1999;28(1) (suppl 1):13–24.

22. Bennett WM, Henrich WL, Stoff JS. The renal effects of nonsteroidal anti-inflammatory drugs: summary and recommendations. Am J Kidney Dis 1996;28(1 Suppl 1): 56–62.

23. Griffin MR, Yared A, Ray WA. Nonsteroidal antiinflammatory drugs and acute renal failure in elderly persons. Am J Epidemiol 2000;151:488–96.

24. Zhao SZ, et al. A comparison of renal-related adverse drug reactions between rofecoxib and celecoxib, based on the World Health Organization/Uppsala Monitoring Centre safety database. Clin Ther 2001;23:1478–91.

25. Knight EL, et al. Predictors of decreased renal function in patients with heart failure during angiotensin-converting enzyme inhibitor therapy: results from the studies of left ventricular dysfunction (SOLVD). Am Heart J 1999; 138(5 Pt 1):849–55.

26. Schoolwerth AC, et al. Renal considerations in angiotensin converting enzyme inhibitor therapy: a statement for healthcare professionals from the Council on the Kidney in Cardiovascular Disease and the Council for High Blood Pressure Research of the American Heart Association. Circulation 2001;104:1985–91.

27. Adhiyaman V, et al. Nephrotoxicity in the elderly due to co-prescription of angiotensin converting enzyme inhibitors and nonsteroidal anti-inflammatory drugs. J R Soc Med 2001;94:512–4.

28. Myers BD, L Newton. Cyclosporine-induced chronic nephropathy: an obliterative microvascular renal injury. J Am Soc Nephrol 1991;2(2 Suppl 1):45–52.

29. Myers BD, et al. The long-term course of cyclosporine-associated chronic nephropathy. Kidney Int 1988;33: 590–600.

30. Lopau K, et al. Tacrolimus in acute renal failure: does L-arginine-infusion prevent changes in renal hemodynamics? Transpl Int 2000;13:436–42.

31. Medina PJ, Sipols JM, George JN. Drug-associated thrombotic thrombocytopenic purpura-hemolytic uremic syndrome. Curr Opin Hematol 2001;8:286–93.

32. Busca A, Uderzo C. BMT: bone marrow transplant associated thrombotic microangiopathy. Hematol 2000;5: 53–67.

33. Gharpure VS, et al. Thrombotic thrombocytopenic purpura associated with FK506 following bone marrow transplantation. Bone Marrow Transplant 1995;16:715–6.

34. Kamel KS, et al. Studies to determine the basis for hyperkalemia in recipients of a renal transplant who are treated with cyclosporine. J Am Soc Nephrol 1992;2:1279–84.

35. Kramer L, Horl WH. Hepatorenal syndrome. Semin Nephrol 2002;22:290–301.

36. Gines P, Arroyo V. Hepatorenal syndrome. J Am Soc Nephrol 1999;10:1833–9.

37. Gonwa TA, et al. Impact of pretransplant renal function on survival after liver transplantation. Transplantation 1995;59:361–5.

38. Guevara M, et al. Reversibility of hepatorenal syndrome by prolonged administration of ornipressin and plasma volume expansion. Hepatology 1998;27:35–41.

39. Uriz J, et al. Terlipressin plus albumin infusion: an effective and safe therapy of hepatorenal syndrome. J Hepatol 2000;33:43–8.

40. Mulkay JP, et al. Long-term terlipressin administration improves renal function in cirrhotic patients with type 1 hepatorenal syndrome: a pilot study. Acta Gastroenterol Belg 2001;64:15–9.

41. Angeli P, et al. Reversal of type 1 hepatorenal syndrome with the administration of midodrine and octreotide. Hepatology 1999;29:1690–7.

42. Holt S, et al. Improvement in renal function in hepatorenal syndrome with N-acetylcysteine. Lancet 1999;353(9149): 294–5.

43. Guevara M, et al. Transjugular intrahepatic portosystemic shunt in hepatorenal syndrome: effects on renal function and vasoactive systems. Hepatology 1998;28:416–22.

44. Brensing KA, et al. Long term outcome after transjugular intrahepatic portosystemic stent-shunt in non-transplant cirrhotics with hepatorenal syndrome: a phase II study. Gut 2000;47:288–95.

45. Arroyo V, et al. Definition and diagnostic criteria of refractory ascites and hepatorenal syndrome in cirrhosis. International Ascites Club. Hepatology 1996;23:164–76.

46. Wendt EC. Uber den Einflus des intra-abdominellen Drukkes auf dies Absonderungsgeschwindigkeit des Hames. Arch Heilkunde 1876;17:527.

47. McNelis J, Marini CP, Simms HH. Abdominal compartment syndrome: clinical manifestations and predictive factors. Curr Opin Crit Care 2003;9:133–6.

48. Star RA. Treatment of acute renal failure. Kidney Int 1998;54:1817–31.

49. Holland MD, et al. Effect of urinary pH and diatrizoate on Bence Jones protein nephrotoxicity in the rat. Kidney Int 1985;27:46–50.

50. Murphy SW, Barrett BJ, Parfrey PS. Contrast nephropathy. J Am Soc Nephrol 2000;11:177–82.

51. Solomon R. Contrast-medium-induced acute renal failure. Kidney Int 1998;53:230–42.

52. Bakris GL, et al. Radiocontrast medium-induced declines in renal function: a role for oxygen free radicals. Am J Physiol 1990;258(1 Pt 2):115–20.

53. Solomon R, et al. Effects of saline, mannitol, and furosemide to prevent acute decreases in renal function induced by radiocontrast agents. N Engl J Med 1994;331:1416–20.

54. Mueller C, et al. Prevention of contrast media-associated nephropathy: randomized comparison of 2 hydration regimens in 1620 patients undergoing coronary angioplasty. Arch Intern Med 2002;162:329–36.

55. Swan SK. Aminoglycoside nephrotoxicity. Semin Nephrol 1997;17:27–33.

56. Humes HD, Weinberg JM. The effect of gentamicin on antidiuretic hormone-stimulated osmotic water flow in the toad urinary bladder. J Lab Clin Med 1983;101: 472–8.

57. Barza M, et al. Single or multiple daily doses of aminoglycosides: a meta-analysis. BMJ 1996;312(7027):338–45.

58. Hatala R, Dinh TT, Cook DJ. Single daily dosing of aminoglycosides in immunocompromised adults: a systematic review. Clin Infect Dis 1997;24:810–5.

59. Sawaya BP, et al. Direct vasoconstriction as a possible cause for amphotericin B-induced nephrotoxicity in rats. J Clin Invest 1991;87:2097–107.

60. Sawaya BP, Briggs JP, Schnermann J. Amphotericin B nephrotoxicity: the adverse consequences of altered membrane properties. J Am Soc Nephrol 1995;6:154–64.

61. Barton CH, et al. Renal magnesium wasting associated with amphotericin B therapy. Am J Med 1984;77:471–4.

62. Sorkine P, et al. Administration of amphotericin B in lipid emulsion decreases nephrotoxicity: results of a prospective, randomized, controlled study in critically ill patients. Crit Care Med 1996;24:1311–5.

63. Sacks P, Fellner SK. Recurrent reversible acute renal failure from amphotericin. Arch Intern Med 1987;147:593–5.

64. Branch RA. Prevention of amphotericin B-induced renal impairment. A review on the use of sodium supplementation. Arch Intern Med 1988;148:2389–94.

65. Llanos A, et al. Effect of salt supplementation on amphotericin B nephrotoxicity. Kidney Int 1991;40:302–8.

66. Smith DM, et al. Acute renal failure associated with autologous bone marrow transplantation. Bone Marrow Transplant 1987;2:195–201.

67. Holt SG, Moore KP. Pathogenesis and treatment of renal dysfunction in rhabdomyolysis. Intensive Care Med 2001;27:803–11.

68. Moore KP, et al. A causative role for redox cycling of myoglobin and its inhibition by alkalinization in the pathogenesis and treatment of rhabdomyolysis-induced renal failure. J Biol Chem 1998;273:31731–7.

69. Arany I, Safirstein RL. Cisplatin nephrotoxicity. Semin Nephrol 2003;23:460–4.

70. Vogelzang NJ, Torkelson JL, Kennedy BJ. Hypomagnesemia, renal dysfunction, and Raynaud's phenomenon in patients treated with cisplatin, vinblastine, and bleomycin. Cancer 1985;56:2765–70.

71. Leibbrandt ME, et al. Critical subcellular targets of cisplatin and related platinum analogs in rat renal proximal tubule cells. Kidney Int 1995;48:761–70.

72. Ries F, Klastersky J. Nephrotoxicity induced by cancer chemotherapy with special emphasis on cisplatin toxicity. Am J Kidney Dis 1986;8:368–79.

73. Hensley ML, et al. American Society of Clinical Oncology clinical practice guidelines for the use of chemotherapy and radiotherapy protectants. J Clin Oncol 1999;17: 3333–55.

74. Santini V, Giles FJ. The potential of amifostine: from cyto-protectant to therapeutic agent. Haematologica 1999;84: 1035–42.

75. Osanto S, et al. Long-term effects of chemotherapy in patients with testicular cancer. J Clin Oncol 1992;10: 574–9.

76. Skinner R. Strategies to prevent nephrotoxicity of anticancer drugs. Curr Opin Oncol 1995;7:310–5.

77. Skinner R, et al. Nephrotoxicity after ifosfamide. Arch Dis Child 1990;65:732–8.

78. Lee BS, et al. Ifosfamide nephrotoxicity in pediatric cancer patients. Pediatr Nephrol 2001;16:796–9.

79. Skinner R, Cotterill SJ, Stevens MC. Risk factors for nephrotoxicity after ifosfamide treatment in children: a UKCCSG Late Effects Group study. United Kingdom Children's Cancer Study Group. Br J Cancer 2000;82:1636–45.

80. Aleksa K, Woodland C, Koren G. Young age and the risk for ifosfamide-induced nephrotoxicity: a critical review of two opposing studies. Pediatr Nephrol 2001;16:1153–8.

81. Hartmann JT, et al. The use of reduced doses of amifostine to ameliorate nephrotoxicity of cisplatin/ ifosfamide-based chemotherapy in patients with solid tumors. Anticancer Drugs 2000;11:1–6.

82. Friedlaender MM, et al. End-stage renal interstitial fibrosis in an adult ten years after ifosfamide therapy. Am J Nephrol 1998;18:131–3.

83. Berns JS, et al. Severe, irreversible renal failure after ifosfamide treatment. A clinicopathologic report of two patients. Cancer 1995;76:497–500.

84. Prasad VK, et al. Progressive glomerular toxicity of ifosfamide in children. Med Pediatr Oncol 1996;27: 149–55.

85. Condit PT, Chanes RE, Joel W. Renal toxicity of methotrexate. Cancer 1969;23:126–31.

86. Perazella MA. Crystal-induced acute renal failure. Am J Med 1999;106:459–65.

87. Sand TE, Jacobsen S. Effect of urine pH and flow on renal clearance of methotrexate. Eur J Clin Pharmacol 1981;19:453–6.

88. Wall SM, et al. Effective clearance of methotrexate using high-flux hemodialysis membranes. Am J Kidney Dis 1996;28:846–54.

89. Kepka L, et al. Successful rescue in a patient with high dose methotrexate-induced nephrotoxicity and acute renal failure. Leuk Lymphoma 1998;29(1–2):205–9.

90. Ackland SP, Schilsky RL. High-dose methotrexate: a critical reappraisal. J Clin Oncol 1987;5:2017–31.

91. Abelson HT, et al. Methotrexate-induced renal impairment: clinical studies and rescue from systemic toxicity with high-dose leucovorin and thymidine. J Clin Oncol 1983;1:208–16.

92. Webb DE, et al. Metabolic and renal effects of interleukin-2 immunotherapy for metastatic cancer. Clin Nephrol 1988;30:141–5.

93. Ault BH, et al. Acute renal failure during therapy with recombinant human gamma interferon. N Engl J Med 1988;319:1397–400.

94. Shah M, et al. Interferon-alpha-associated focal segmental glomerulosclerosis with massive proteinuria in patients with chronic myeloid leukemia following high dose chemotherapy. Cancer 1998;83:1938–46.

95. Coroneos E, et al. Focal segmental glomerulosclerosis with acute renal failure associated with alpha-interferon therapy. Am J Kidney Dis 1996;28:888–92.

96. Horowitz R, et al. Interferon-induced acute renal failure: a case report and literature review. Med Oncol 1995;12: 55–7.

97. Fahal IH, et al. Acute renal failure during interferon treatment. BMJ 1993;306(6883):973.

98. Averbuch SD, et al. Acute interstitial nephritis with the nephrotic syndrome following recombinant leukocyte a interferon therapy for mycosis fungoides. N Engl J Med 1984;310:32–5.

99. Ponce P, et al. Renal toxicity mediated by continuous infusion of recombinant interleukin-2. Nephron 1993;64:114–8.

100. Druker BJ, et al. Efficacy and safety of a specific inhibitor of the BCR-ABL tyrosine kinase in chronic myeloid leukemia. N Engl J Med 2001;344:1031–7.

101. Pou M, et al. Acute renal failure secondary to imatinib mesylate treatment in chronic myeloid leukemia. Leuk Lymphoma 2003;44:1239–41.

102. Markowitz GS, et al. Toxic acute tubular necrosis following treatment with zoledronate (Zometa). Kidney Int 2003;64:281–9.

103. Markowitz GS, et al. Collapsing focal segmental glomerulosclerosis following treatment with high-dose pamidronate. J Am Soc Nephrol 2001;12:1164–72.

104. Banerjee D, et al. Short-term, high-dose pamidronate-induced acute tubular necrosis: the postulated mechanisms of bisphosphonate nephrotoxicity. Am J Kidney Dis 2003;41:E18.

105. Winearls CG. Acute myeloma kidney. Kidney Int 1995;48:1347–61.

106. Zucchelli P, et al. Controlled plasma exchange trial in acute renal failure due to multiple myeloma. Kidney Int 1988;33:1175–80.

107. Johnson WJ, et al. Treatment of renal failure associated with multiple myeloma. Plasmapheresis, hemodialysis, and chemotherapy. Arch Intern Med 1990;150:863–9.

108. McCarthy CS, Becker JA. Multiple myeloma and contrast media. Radiology 1992;183:519–21.

109. Smolens P, Barnes JL, Kreisberg R. Hypercalcemia can potentiate the nephrotoxicity of Bence Jones proteins. J Lab Clin Med 1987;110:460–5.

110. Lin JH. Bisphosphonates: a review of their pharmacokinetic properties. Bone 1996;18:75–85.

111. Fleisch H. Bisphosphonates. Pharmacology and use in the treatment of tumour-induced hypercalcaemic and metastatic bone disease. Drugs 1991;42:919–44.

112. Singer FR, Minoofar PN. Bisphosphonates in the treatment of disorders of mineral metabolism. Adv Endocrinol Metab 1995;6:259–88.

113. Hosking DJ, Gilson D. Comparison of the renal and skeletal actions of calcitonin in the treatment of severe hypercalcaemia of malignancy. Q J Med 1984;53(211):359–68.

114. Cohen L, Balow J, Magrath I, et al. Acute tumor lysis syndrome. A review of 37 patients with Burkitt lymphoma. Am J Med 1980;68:486–491.

115. Silverman P, Distelhorst CW. Metabolic emergencies in clinical oncology. Semin Oncol 1989;16:504–15.

116. Arrambide K, Toto RD. Tumor lysis syndrome. Semin Nephrol 1993;13:273–80.

117. Kjellstrand CM, Campbell D, von Hartitzsch B, Buselmeier TJ. Hyperuricemic acute renal failure. Arch Intern Med 1974;133:349–59.

118. Conger J. Acute uric acid nephropathy. Semin Nephrol 1981;1:69–74.

119. Boles JM, et al. Acute renal failure caused by extreme hyperphosphatemia after chemotherapy of an acute lymphoblastic leukemia. Cancer 1984;53:2425–9.

120. Masera G, et al. Urate-oxidase prophylaxis of uric acid-induced renal damage in childhood leukemia. J Pediatr 1982;100:152–5.

121. Saccente SL, Kohaut EC, Berkow RL. Prevention of tumor lysis syndrome using continuous veno-venous hemofiltration. Pediatr Nephrol 1995;9:569–73.

122. Symmers W. Thrombotic microangiopathic haemolytic anaemia (thrombotic microangiopathy). Br Med J 1952;2:897–903.

123. Riley LW, et al. Hemorrhagic colitis associated with a rare Escherichia coli serotype. N Engl J Med 1983;308:681–5.

124. Remuzzi G, Ruggenenti P. The hemolytic uremic syndrome. Kidney Int 1995;48:2–19.

125. Rizzoni G, et al. Plasma infusion for hemolytic-uremic syndrome in children: results of a multicenter controlled trial. J Pediatr 1988;112:284–90.

126. Tsai H, Lian C. Antibodies to von Willebrand factor-cleaving protease in acute thrombotic thrombocytopenic purpura. N Engl J Med 1998;339:1585–1594.

127. Furlan M, et al. von Willebrand factor-cleaving protease in thrombotic thrombocytopenic purpura and the hemolytic-uremic syndrome. N Engl J Med 1998;339:1578–84.

128. Zager RA, et al. Acute renal failure following bone marrow transplantation: a retrospective study of 272 patients. Am J Kidney Dis 1989;13:210–6.

129. Zager RA. Acute renal failure in the setting of bone marrow transplantation. Kidney Int 1994;46:1443–58.

130. Gruss E, et al. Acute renal failure in patients following bone marrow transplantation: prevalence, risk factors and outcome. Am J Nephrol 1995;15:473–9.

131. Zager RA. Rhabdomyolysis and myohemoglobinuric acute renal failure. Kidney Int 1996;49:314–26.

132. Carreras E, et al. On the reliability of clinical criteria for the diagnosis of hepatic veno-occlusive disease. Ann Hematol 1993;66:77–80.

133. Attal M, et al. Prevention of hepatic veno-occlusive disease after bone marrow transplantation by continuous infusion of low-dose heparin: a prospective, randomized trial. Blood 1992;79:2834–40.

134. Gluckman E, et al. Use of prostaglandin E1 for prevention of liver veno-occlusive disease in leukaemic patients treated by allogeneic bone marrow transplantation. Br J Haematol 1990;74:277–81.

135. Bianco JA, et al. Phase I-II trial of pentoxifylline for the prevention of transplant-related toxicities following bone marrow transplantation. Blood 1991;78:1205–11.

136. Loomis LJ, et al. Hemolytic uremic syndrome following bone marrow transplantation: a case report and review of the literature. Am J Kidney Dis 1989;14:324–8.

137. Silva VA, et al. Plasma exchange and vincristine in the treatment of hemolytic uremic syndrome/thrombotic thrombocytopenic purpura associated with bone marrow transplantation. J Clin Apheresis 1991;6:16–20.

138. Lee GW, et al. Membranous glomerulopathy as a manifestation of chronic graft-versus-host-disease after non-myeloablative stem cell transplantation in a patient with paroxysmal nocturnal hemoglobinuria. J Korean Med Sci 2003;18:901–4.

139. Lin J, et al. Membranous glomerulopathy associated with graft-versus-host disease following allogeneic stem cell transplantation. Report of 2 cases and review of the literature. Am J Nephrol 2001;21:351–6.

140. Sato N, et al. Nephrotic syndrome in a bone marrow transplant recipient with chronic graft-versus-host disease. Bone Marrow Transplant 1995;16:303–5.

141. Kanfer A, et al. Acute renal insufficiency due to lymphomatous infiltration of the kidneys: report of six cases. Cancer 1976;38:2588–92.

142. Koolen MI, et al. Non-Hodgkin lymphoma with unique localization in the kidneys presenting with acute renal failure. Clin Nephrol 1988;29:41–6.

143. Malbrain ML, et al. Acute renal failure due to bilateral lymphomatous infiltrates. Primary extranodal non-Hodgkin's lymphoma (p-EN-NHL) of the kidneys: does it really exist? Clin Nephrol 1994;42:163–9.

144. Miyake JS, Fitterer S, Houghton DC. Diagnosis and characterization of non-Hodgkin's lymphoma in a patient with acute renal failure. Am J Kidney Dis 1990;16:262–3.

145. Gauvin F, et al. Reactive hemophagocytic syndrome presenting as a component of multiple organ dysfunction syndrome. Crit Care Med 2000;28:3341–5.

146. Holt S, et al. Cytokine nephropathy and multi-organ dysfunction in lymphoma. Nephrol Dial Transplant 1998;13:1853–7.

147. Comerma-Coma MI, et al. Reversible renal failure due to specific infiltration of the kidney in chronic lymphocytic leukaemia. Nephrol Dial Transplant 1998;13:1550–2.

148. Pagniez DC, et al. Reversible renal failure due to specific infiltration in chronic lymphocytic leukemia. Am J Med 1988;85:579–80.

149. Phillips JK, et al. Renal failure caused by leukaemic infiltration in chronic lymphocytic leukaemia. J Clin Pathol 1993;46:1131–3.

150. Boudville N, et al. Renal failure in a patient with leukaemic infiltration of the kidney and polyomavirus infection. Nephrol Dial Transplant 2001;16:1059–61.

151. Krochak RJ, Baker DG. Radiation nephritis. Clinical manifestations and pathophysiologic mechanisms. Urology 1986;27:389–93.

152. Cassady JR. Clinical radiation nephropathy. Int J Radiat Oncol Biol Phys 1995;31:1249–56.

153. Cohen EP. Radiation nephropathy after bone marrow transplantation. Kidney Int 2000;58:903–18.

154. Moulder JE, Fish BL, Abrams RA. Renal toxicity following total-body irradiation and syngeneic bone marrow transplantation. Transplantation 1987;43:589–92.

155. Cohen EP, et al. Captopril preserves function and ultrastructure in experimental radiation nephropathy. Lab Invest 1996;75:349–60.

156. Michel DM, Kelly CJ. Acute interstitial nephritis. J Am Soc Nephrol 1998;9:506–15.

157. Rastegar A, Kashgarian M. The clinical spectrum of tubulointerstitial nephritis. Kidney Int 1998;54:313–27.

158. Kelly CJ. T cell regulation of autoimmune interstitial nephritis. J Am Soc Nephrol 1990;1:140–9.

159. Eddy AA, et al. A relationship between proteinuria and acute tubulointerstitial disease in rats with experimental nephrotic syndrome. Am J Pathol 1991;138:1111–23.

160. Neilson EG. Pathogenesis and therapy of interstitial nephritis. Kidney Int 1989;35:1257–70.

161. Neilson EG, et al. Molecular characterization of a major nephritogenic domain in the autoantigen of anti-tubular basement membrane disease. Proc Natl Acad Sci U S A 1991;88:2006–10.

162. Wilson CB. Nephritogenic tubulointerstitial antigens. Kidney Int 1991;39:501–17.

163. Linton AL, et al. Acute interstitial nephritis due to drugs: review of the literature with a report of nine cases. Ann Intern Med 1980;93:735–41.

164. Rossert J. Drug-induced acute interstitial nephritis. Kidney Int 2001;60:804–17.

165. Ruffing KA, et al. Eosinophils in urine revisited. Clin Nephrol 1994;41:163–6.

166. Galpin JE, et al. Acute interstitial nephritis due to methicillin. Am J Med 1978;65:756–65.

167. Pusey CD, et al. Drug associated acute interstitial nephritis: clinical and pathological features and the response to high dose steroid therapy. Q J Med 1983;52(206):194–211.

168. Lien YH, et al. Ciprofloxacin-induced granulomatous interstitial nephritis and localized elastolysis. Am J Kidney Dis 1993;22:598–602.

169. Downs NJ, et al. Mild nephrotoxicity associated with vancomycin use. Arch Intern Med 1989;149:1777–81.

170. Gabow PA, Lacher JW, Neff TA. Tubulointerstitial and glomerular nephritis associated with rifampin. Report of a case. JAMA 1976;235(23k0):2517–8.

171. Quinn BP, Wall BM. Nephrogenic diabetes insipidus and tubulointerstitial nephritis during continuous therapy with rifampin. Am J Kidney Dis 1989;14:217–20.

172. Huang JJ, et al. Acute bacterial nephritis: a clinicoradiologic correlation based on computed tomography. Am J Med 1992;93:289–98.

173. Ramsay AG, Olesnicky L, Pirani CL. Acute tubulo-interstitial nephritis from Candida albicans with oliguric renal failure. Clin Nephrol 1985;24:310–4.

174. Bhattacharya S, Bryk D, Wise GJ. Clinicopathological conference: renal pelvic filling defect in a diabetic woman. J Urol 1982;127:751–3.

175. Wise GJ, Silver DA. Fungal infections of the genitourinary system. J Urol 1993;149:1377–88.

176. Wise GJ, Kozinn PJ, Goldberg P. Amphotericin B as a urologic irrigant in the management of noninvasive candiduria. J Urol 1982;128:82–4.

177. Levy E, Bia MJ. Isolated renal mucormycosis: case report and review. J Am Soc Nephrol 1995;5:2014–9.

178. Myerowitz RL, et al. Fatal disseminated adenovirus infection in a renal transplant recipient. Am J Med 1975;59:591–8.

179. Erdogan O, et al. Acute necrotizing tubulointerstitial nephritis due to systemic adenoviral infection. Pediatr Nephrol 2001;16:265–8.

180. Rosen S, et al. Tubulo-interstitial nephritis associated with polyomavirus (BK type) infection. N Engl J Med 1983;308:1192–6.

181. Frazao JM, et al. Epstein-Barr-virus-induced interstitial nephritis in an HIV-positive patient with progressive renal failure. Nephrol Dial Transplant 1998;13:1849–52.

182. Mayer HB, et al. Epstein-Barr virus-induced infectious mononucleosis complicated by acute renal failure: case report and review. Clin Infect Dis 1996;22:1009–18.

183. Nasr SH, et al. Granulomatous interstitial nephritis. Am J Kidney Dis 2003;41:714–9.

184. Walker JV, et al. Histoplasmosis with hypercalcemia, renal failure, and papillary necrosis. Confusion with sarcoidosis. JAMA 1977;237:1350–2.

185. Klahr S. Obstructive nephropathy. Kidney Int 1998;54:286–300.

186. Schierhout G, Roberts I. Fluid resuscitation with colloid or crystalloid solutions in critically ill patients: a systematic review of randomised trials. BMJ 1998;316(7136):961–4.

187. Choi PT, et al. Crystalloids vs. colloids in fluid resuscitation: a systematic review. Crit Care Med 1999;27:200–10.

188. Schortgen F, et al. Effects of hydroxyethylstarch and gelatin on renal function in severe sepsis: a multicentre randomised study. Lancet 2001;357(9260):911–6.

189. Boldt J, et al. Volume therapy in the critically ill: is there a difference? Intensive Care Med 1998;24:28–36.

190. Durham JD, et al. A randomized controlled trial of N-acetylcysteine to prevent contrast nephropathy in cardiac angiography. Kidney Int 2002;62:2202–7.

191. Kay J, et al. Acetylcysteine for prevention of acute deterioration of renal function following elective

coronary angiography and intervention: a randomized controlled trial. JAMA 2003;289:553–8.

192. Burton CJ, Tomson CR. Can the use of low-dose dopamine for treatment of acute renal failure be justified? Postgrad Med J 1999;75(883):269–74.

193. Denton MD, Chertow GM, Brady HR. "Renal-dose" dopamine for the treatment of acute renal failure: scientific rationale, experimental studies and clinical trials. Kidney Int 1996;50:4–14.

194. Segal JM, Phang PT, Walley KR. Low-dose dopamine hastens onset of gut ischemia in a porcine model of hemorrhagic shock. J Appl Physiol 1992;73:1159–64.

195. Weisberg LS, Kurnik PB, Kurnik BR. Risk of radiocontrast nephropathy in patients with and without diabetes mellitus. Kidney Int 1994;45:259–65.

196. Tumlin JA, et al. Fenoldopam mesylate blocks reductions in renal plasma flow after radiocontrast dye infusion: a pilot trial in the prevention of contrast nephropathy. Am Heart J 2002;143:894–903.

197. Sheinbaum R, et al. Contemporary strategies to preserve renal function during cardiac and vascular surgery. Rev Cardiovasc Med 2003;4(Suppl 1):21–8.

198. Lassnigg A, et al. Lack of renoprotective effects of dopamine and furosemide during cardiac surgery. J Am Soc Nephrol 2000;11:97–104.

199. Better OS, et al. Mannitol therapy revisited (1940–1997). Kidney Int 1997;52:886–94.

200. Bonventre JV, Weinberg JM. Kidney preservation ex vivo for transplantation. Annu Rev Med 1992;43:523–53.

201. Ratcliffe PJ, et al. Effect of intravenous infusion of atriopeptin 3 on immediate renal allograft function. Kidney Int 1991;39:164–8.

202. Sands JM, et al. Atrial natriuretic factor does not improve the outcome of cadaveric renal transplantation. J Am Soc Nephrol 1991;1:1081–6.

203. Petrinec D, et al. Insulin-like growth factor-I attenuates delayed graft function in a canine renal autotransplantation model. Surgery 1996;120:221–6.

204. Miller SB, et al. Insulin-like growth factor I accelerates recovery from ischemic acute tubular necrosis in the rat. Proc Natl Acad Sci U S A 1992;89:11876–80.

205. Franklin SC, et al. Insulin-like growth factor I preserves renal function postoperatively. Am J Physiol 1997;272(2 Pt 2):257–9.

206. Thadhani R, Pascual M, Bonventre JV. Acute renal failure. N Engl J Med 1996;334:1448–60.

207. Miller SB, et al. Rat models for clinical use of insulin-like growth factor in acute renal failure. Am J Physiol 1994;266(6 Pt 2):949–56.

208. Graziani G, Casati S., Cantaluppi A. Dopamine-furosemide therapy in acute renal failure. Proc EDTA 1982;19:319–324.

209. Bellomo R, et al. Low-dose dopamine in patients with early renal dysfunction: a placebo-controlled randomised trial. Australian and New Zealand Intensive Care Society (ANZICS) Clinical Trials Group. Lancet 2000;356(9248):2139–43.

210. Cantarovich F, et al. High dose furosemide in established acute renal failure. Br Med J 1973;4(5890):449–50.

211. Minuth AN, Terrell JB Jr, Suki WN. Acute renal failure: a study of the course and prognosis of 104 patients and of the role of furosemide. Am J Med Sci 1976;271:317–24.

212. Kleinknecht D, et al. Furosemide in acute oliguric renal failure. A controlled trial. Nephron 1976;17:51–8.

213. Brown CB, Ogg CS, Cameron JS. High dose furosemide in acute renal failure: a controlled trial. Clin Nephrol 1981;15:90–6.

214. Shilliday IR, Quinn KJ, Allison ME. Loop diuretics in the management of acute renal failure: a prospective, double-blind, placebo-controlled, randomized study. Nephrol Dial Transplant 1997;12:2592–6.

215. Mehta RL, et al. Diuretics, mortality, and nonrecovery of renal function in acute renal failure. JAMA 2002;288:2547–53.

216. Martin SJ, Danziger LH. Continuous infusion of loop diuretics in the critically ill: a review of the literature. Crit Care Med 1994;22:1323–9.

217. Sward K, Valson F, Ricksten SE. Long-term infusion of atrial natriuretic peptide (ANP) improves renal blood flow and glomerular filtration rate in clinical acute renal failure. Acta Anaesthesiol Scand 2001;45:536–42.

218. Rahman SN, et al. Effects of atrial natriuretic peptide in clinical acute renal failure. Kidney Int 1994;45:1731–8.

219. Allgren RL, et al. Anaritide in acute tubular necrosis. Auriculin Anaritide Acute Renal Failure Study Group. N Engl J Med 1997;336:828–34.

220. Lewis J, et al. Atrial natriuretic factor in oliguric acute renal failure. Anaritide Acute Renal Failure Study Group. Am J Kidney Dis 2000;36:767–74.

221. Hirschberg R, et al. Multicenter clinical trial of recombinant human insulin-like growth factor I in patients with acute renal failure. Kidney Int 1999;55:2423–32.

222. Siegel NJ, et al. Beneficial effect of thyroxin on recovery from toxic acute renal failure. Kidney Int 1984;25:906–11.

223. Cronin RE, Newman JA. Protective effect of thyroxine but not parathyroidectomy on gentamicin nephrotoxicity. Am J Physiol 1985;248(3 Pt 2):F332–9.

224. Cronin RE, Brown DM, Simonsen R. Protection by thyroxine in nephrotoxic acute renal failure. Am J Physiol 1986;251(3 Pt 2):408–16.

225. Sutter PM, et al. Beneficial effect of thyroxin in the treatment of ischemic acute renal failure. Pediatr Nephrol 1988;2:1–7.

226. Acker CG, et al. A trial of thyroxine in acute renal failure. Kidney Int 2000;57:293–8.

227. Parsons FM, Hobson F, Blagg CR, McCracken BH. Optimal time for dialysis in acute reversible renal failure. Lancet 1961;1:129–134.

228. Kleinknecht D, et al. Uremic and non-uremic complications in acute renal failure: evaluation of early and frequent dialysis on prognosis. Kidney Int 1972;1:190–6.

229. Gillum DM, et al. The role of intensive dialysis in acute renal failure. Clin Nephrol 1986;25:249–55.

230. Conger J. Dialysis and related therapies. Semin Nephrol 1998;18:533–40.

231. Hakim RM, Wingard RL, Parker RA. Effect of the dialysis membrane in the treatment of patients with acute renal failure. N Engl J Med 1994;331:1338–42.

232. Lowrie EG, et al. Effect of the hemodialysis prescription of patient morbidity: report from the National Cooperative Dialysis Study. N Engl J Med 1981;305:1176–81.

233. Paganini EP, T.M., Goormastic M, Halstenberg W, et al. Establishing a dialysis therapy patient outcome link in intensive care unit acute dialysis for patient with acute renal failure. Am J Kidney Dis 1996;28(Suppl 3):81–89.

234. Schiffl H, Lang SM, Fischer R. Daily hemodialysis and the outcome of acute renal failure. N Engl J Med 2002;346:305–10.

235. Eknoyan G, Beck G, Cheung A, et al. Effect of dialysis dose and membrane flux in maintenance hemodialysis. N Engl J Med 2002;347:2010–9.

236. Ronco C. Continuous renal replacement therapies in the treatment of acute renal failure in intensive care patients. Part 1. Theoretical aspects and techniques. Nephrol Dial Transplant 1994;9(Suppl 4):191–200.

237. Ronco C. Continuous renal replacement therapies in the treatment of acute renal failure in intensive care patients. Part 2. Clinical indications and prescription. Nephrol Dial Transplant 1994;9(Suppl 4):201–9.

238. Rialp G, et al. Prognostic indexes and mortality in critically ill patients with acute renal failure treated with different dialytic techniques. Ren Fail 1996;18:667–75.

239. Mehta RL, et al. A randomized clinical trial of continuous versus intermittent dialysis for acute renal failure. Kidney Int 2001;60:1154–63.

240. van Bommel EF. Should continuous renal replacement therapy be used for 'non-renal' indications in critically ill patients with shock? Resuscitation 1997;33:257–70.

241. Bellomo R, et al. Preliminary experience with high-volume hemofiltration in human septic shock. Kidney Int Suppl 1998;66:S182–5.

242. Schetz M, et al. Removal of pro-inflammatory cytokines with renal replacement therapy: sense or nonsense? Intensive Care Med 1995;21:169–76.

Urinary Tract Infections

Diana I. Jalal, MD

B.V.R. Bhamidipati Murthy, MD

Urinary tract infection (UTI) is the most common bacterial infection in the general population and is also a common clinical problem in cancer patients. While UTI affects all ages, significant differences are seen in age prevalence between the two sexes. While it is common at all ages in females, it occurs mostly at extremes of life in males. Patients with structural or functional abnormalities of the urinary tract, patients who are immunosuppressed, such as transplant recipients and cancer patients on chemotherapy, are particularly susceptible to UTI. UTIs are classified either according to the anatomic site—bladder (cystitis) or kidney (pyelonephritis)—or into uncomplicated or complicated (Table 1). Although the definitions of uncomplicated and complicated UTIs vary depending on the source of the definition, most agree that an acute uncomplicated UTI is typically an episode of acute cystitis or pyelonephritis that occurs in a young, healthy, non-pregnant woman with no functional or anatomic abnormalities of the urinary tract. It is also reasonable to consider UTIs that occur in healthy, ambulatory, postmenopausal women as uncomplicated. Similarly, episodes of acute cystitis that affect healthy young men are classified as uncomplicated by some, although this is more controversial.[1] A complicated infection is associated with an underlying condition that increases the risk for acquiring a UTI or that is likely to be associated with failing antimicrobial therapy.[2] Considering this definition, UTI in cancer patients should be considered complicated when it occurs as a result of suppressed immunity. The epidemiology and prevalence of UTI in cancer patients are not established; it is believed that the pathogenesis and treatment issues of UTI in cancer patients are no different from those in the general population. Hence, this review will primarily discuss UTI as it occurs in the general population. In addition, unique urinary tract infections that occur in certain specific situations in cancer patients such as patients on intensive chemotherapy and bone marrow transplantation (BMT) recipients will be discussed in more detail.

Traditionally, infection of the upper urinary tract has been termed "pyelonephritis," which indicates that there is inflammation of renal parenchyma as well as pelvis of the kidney in this condition. However, from a clinical standpoint, this term refers to a disorder of the kidney resulting from bacterial invasion. While this simple characterization amply describes acute pyelonephritis, the role of bacterial infection in chronic pyelonephritis is more complex. It is unusual for bacterial infection alone to cause chronic damage to the kidney, and in almost all of these patients, there is either a demonstrable urinary tract abnormality such as vesicoureteral reflux (VUR) or an anatomic obstruction to the flow of urine. Since chronic pyelonephritis is not a common problem in cancer patients, this review will restrict the discussion of upper urinary tract infection to acute pyelonephritis. Similarly, the long-term effects of UTI, such as chronic renal disease, hypertension, or both, and its effects on longevity and survival will not be discussed. Urinary tract obstruction and its management as it relates to cancer patients are discussed in another chapter (see Chapter 49, "Urologic Disorders").

Epidemiology of UTI

Surveys of office practice and general hospital admissions in the United States estimate that approximately 7 million episodes of acute cystitis, and at least 250,000 episodes of acute pyelonephritis, occur per year.[2,3] After infancy, and until age 55, UTI is predominantly a female disease occurring most often in sexually active women.[4] The frequency of UTI after infancy and until 10 years of age is about 1.2%. Approximately 1 to 3% of women between the ages of 15 and 24 years have bacteriuria; the incidence increases by 1 to 2% for each decade thereafter, up to a level of about 10 to 15% by the 6th or the 7th decades. Approximately 40 to 50% of women will have at least one UTI in their lifetime.[5]

The incidence of UTI in men under the age of 50 years is much lower than in women, ranging from 5 to 8 in 10,000 men annually.[6,7] As the aging process progresses and prostatic disease becomes more common, the frequency of UTI in men rises dramatically.[5] The frequency of bacteriuria in the elderly non-catheterized patient lies somewhere between 11 and 15%. Despite the fact that most of these resolve spontaneously, genitourinary infections are the second most common cause of infections in this patient population.[4] With the onset of chronic debilitating illness and long-term institutionalization, bacteriuria rates in both sexes reach 15 to 50%, the incidence in women here being only slightly higher than in men.[5]

Unfortunately, little data exist that can shed light on the epidemiology of complicated UTIs. UTIs are the most common nosocomially acquired infections, accounting for 42% of all nosocomial infections.[8] A recent European study reported a general incidence of nosocomially acquired UTI of 3.55 per 1,000 patient hospital days.[9] The most important identified risk factor for developing a nosocomial UTI is the presence of an indwelling urinary catheter. Catheter-related infections account for more than one million cases in hospitals and nursing homes.[10]

Other populations at increased risk include pregnant women, patients with paraplegia or quadriplegia as a result of spinal cord injuries, and recipients of kidney transplants. The reported incidence of a urinary tract infection in kidney transplant patients ranges between 35% and 79% if antimicrobial prophylaxis is not administered.[11,12]

Pathogenesis of Urinary Tract Infections

Microbial Virulence Factors and Host Defenses

Normally, the urinary tract is sterile and well protected against microbial infection. In the past, host susceptibility to UTIs has been studied in

Table 1 Classification of Urinary Tract Infections (UTI) in Adults
Young women with acute uncomplicated cystitis
Young women with recurrent cystitis
Young women with acute uncomplicated pyelonephritis
All adults with complicated UTI
All adults with asymptomatic bacteriuria

patients with structural or functional abnormalities; however, most patients with UTIs have no such abnormalities. Recent research has focused on the host behavioral factors, in addition to genetically determined cellular mechanisms that predispose to sporadic and recurrent UTI.[13]

Most of the urinary pathogens enter the urinary tract by ascending through the urethra into the bladder. They typically originate from the fecal flora, although the importance of the vagina as a bacterial reservoir and a source of pathogens in women has recently become appreciated.[13] *Escherichia coli* is the most common pathogen, and hence, the best characterized. Not all strains of fecal *E. coli* are capable of infecting the urinary tract; certain distinctive properties are needed to enable these microorganisms to overcome the local host defenses and invade the urinary tract.

Pathogen Factors

As mentioned above, few clones of *E. coli* that colonize the gastrointestinal tract possess the ability to spread to the urinary tract and to produce clinically notable disease, these clones are termed uropathogenic *E. coli* (UPEC).[14] They possess genes encoding a diverse array of specialized properties that are thought to contribute to virulence, the so-called "virulence factors." Clinical isolates from patients with cystitis and pyelonephritis are commonly derived from *E. coli* groups that express a limited range of distinctive O, K, and H antigens.[15] O antigens (surface cell wall antigens) O1, O2, O4, O6, O7, 016, O18, and O75 are expressed in 80% of UPEC. The capsular polysaccharide (K antigens) particularly K1, K2, K5, K12, K13, and K51 are antiphagocytic.[14]

Gram-negative bacteria carry adhesins, most commonly fimbriae with lectin-like domains that recognize oligosaccharide epitopes on cell surface glycolipids or glycoproteins. The resulting specific adherence not only promotes colonization but has also been identified as the most important virulence factor these bacteria possess.[16] There is strong epidemiologic evidence linking the adhesins with disease severity.[17,18] Adherence to the uroepithelium allows bacteria to resist the flushing action of the urine flow and bladder emptying, as well as facilitates tissue attack and invasion.[16] It is also felt to be the primary enhancer of cytokine responses by the host cells.[13] Most *E. coli* adhesins are fimbrial, but some are amorphous fibers, or capsule-like. Irrespective of morphology, adhesins contain defined molecular regions that interact with specific host receptor epitopes. In most cases, the bulk of each fiber is composed of nonadhesive structural subunits, whereas the adhesin is attached to the tip of the fiber.

These adhesins are categorized according to receptor specificity to mannose-sensitive and mannose-resistant. The mannose-resistant adhesins are more diverse and further subdivided into various families. Mannose-sensitive adhesins

in *E. coli* consist of type 1 fimbriae, also known as common pili, since they are present in almost all *E. coli* and broadly among other Enterobacteriaceae.[15] Type-I pili are composite fibers consisting of a long thick cylindrical rod joined at the distal end to a short thin tip fibrillum (FimH).[19] Type-I pili bind to the mannose-containing glycoproteins present on the bladder epithelial surface and are critical to the establishment of cystitis.[20] Immunization against the type I fimbrial adhesin molecule FimH has been shown to be protective against experimental UTI in mice and monkeys.[21,22] Of the mannose-resistant adhesins, the best-known group is the P fimbriae family. They are named as such due to their ability to bind specifically to Gal(1-4)Gal B disaccharide galabiose, which is present within the antigens of the human P blood system.[15] These receptors predominate in the kidney. Consequently, P pili have been shown to be critical in the ability of *E. coli* to cause pyelonephritis. They also are associated with sepsis as well as the development of prostatitis.

Other virulence factors include siderophores (which allow for iron acquisition), toxins produced by the bacteria (such as alpha hemolysin), and protectin, a polysaccharide coating that interferes with phagocytosis and protects against complement-mediated opsonization or lysis.[15]

In addition to the different virulence factors, certain *E. coli* enzymes may contribute to bacterial virulence in nutrient-limited environments by allowing the biosynthesis of essential metabolites. Two examples are guaA and argC, which participate in the synthesis of guanine and arginine, respectively.[23] Due to its toxic effect, lipopolysaccharide (LPS) should be considered when discussing virulence factors. LPS, which is a structural component of *E. coli*, interacts with Toll-like and other receptors in the host cell initiating signal transduction cascades that stimulate cytokine and chemokine synthesis.[15]

Local Defenses

In women, estrogen stimulates the vaginal mucosa to grow and proliferate, thereby providing a sloughing mechanism for the removal of the bacteria. It also results in conditions that aid the cultivation of lactobacilli in the vaginal vestibule. These organisms create an environment with an acidic pH, which is particularly hostile for the Enterobacteriaceae, and which inhibits bacterial proliferation.

Other vaginal factors include the presence of certain types of cell surface antigens, such as the Lewis blood group. This exists at two genetic loci: Lea, and Leb. Patients who are Le(a+b+) and Le(a-b+) are referred to as secretors and have a lower incidence of UTIs compared to the nonsecretors, who are Le(a+b-) and Le(a-b-).

Local defenses in the male are different and appear to be more effective. The most notable is

length of the urethra and the mechanical action of urine flow.[24] In males who are circumcised, this mechanical clearing appears to be enough to prevent the occurrence of UTI.[25] In addition, the prostate gland elaborates several proteins that have significant antibacterial effects, such as prostate antibacterial factor (PAF), spermine and spermidine. When an inflammatory process overwhelms host defenses, these substances are reduced, and the risk of infection may be increased.

The urine itself possesses several characteristics that render it inhibitory to bacterial growth. Low osmolality inhibits bacterial proliferation, as does high osmolality coupled with a low pH.[24] Furthermore, certain substances in the urine, such as urea, inhibit bacterial growth and proliferation.[13] In addition, urine contains a variety of oligosaccharides and glycoproteins with receptor affinity. For example, Tamm-Horsfall glycoprotein is produced by the tubular cells in the ascending loop of Henle and the convoluted tubule and is secreted into the urine. It helps combat bacterial infections in the urinary tract via several mechanisms. It has a receptor for type I pili of *E. coli*, thus functioning as a mechanical barrier to bacterial binding and facilitating removal of the organism from the urogenital tract.[26,27] Additionally, Tamm-Horsfall protein binds to polymorphonuclear leukocytes (PMNs) enhancing their phagocytic function and complement expression.

The ureter also plays a role in protecting the urogenital tract from infection, namely through its peristaltic activity. The significance of this activity is evident when ureteral peristalsis is impaired, such as in pregnancy or obstruction. There are factors within the kidney itself that help protect the host against UTI; for example, 10,000 times the bacterial load needed to initiate infection in the renal medulla would be needed to initiate infection in the renal cortex when bacteria are directly injected into the kidney. This is thought to be due to the relatively reduced blood supply to the medulla and concomitant hypoxia, both of which reduce the immune response.[24]

The role of the immune system in protection against UTI is not well-characterized. Patients who are known to have an ineffective immune system, such as diabetics, transplant recipients, and patients receiving corticosteroids, have an increased number of UTIs.[14] The local immune response is primarily mediated by PMNs. Despite the fact that these cells play no role in the prevention of the initial phase of the infection, they do appear to limit tissue invasion. The adherence of the bacteria to the uroepithelium is followed by PMN activation and their immediate appearance in the urine. They are recruited by certain cytokines and other chemoattractants, after which they undergo transepithelial migration to the site of bacterial colonization. Through the mannose residues on the surface of the PMNs, they are able to bind the bacteria leading to phagocytosis and removal.[24]

The protective role of the humoral immune response and that of acquired resistance is more controversial, despite the reported specific antibody response that accompanies UTI. This response is typically noted 7 to 10 days after the onset of the infection, with the magnitude of antibody appearance being greater in pyelonephritis than in cystitis. The main protective function of the antibodies applies to deep parenchymal bacterial infection in pyelonephritis, thus serving to reduce local tissue damage and prevent the spread of the bacteria.[13]

Although T cells are locally and systemically activated as a consequence of UTI, the role cell-mediated immunity plays in protecting against infection remains to be determined.[14]

A Dynamic Interaction

The early phase of any bacterial infection is a battle between the innate defenses of the host and the virulence factors elaborated by the infecting pathogen.[19] The initial phase of cystitis involves UPEC adhering to the bladder surface epithelium. This incites a variety of events within the host uroepithelial cells. The first event involves the invasion process, which results from the direct interaction between FimH and host cell signaling cascades, leading to host cell cytoskeleton rearrangements and the internalization of the adherent E. coli.[19,28] The second event triggered by this interaction is exfoliation of the superficial bladder epithelial cells, which occurs via an apoptotic-like mechanism that involves activation of caspases and cysteine proteases and DNA fragmentation.

The bacterial cells, however, do not wait for their impending clearance by exfoliation; instead, they have been noted to replicate yielding disorganized bacterial clusters termed "bacterial factories." UPEC can then flux out of the dying cell before the completion of exfoliation, thereby allowing bacteria to escape this innate host defense mechanism. This allows for persistence of the bacteria in the bladder for several months, without being shed in the urine.[29] In fact, these bacteria have been shown to form intracellular biofilms, creating pod-like protrusions on the bladder surface. These pods contain the bacteria encased in a polysaccharide-rich matrix surrounded by a protective shell of uroplakin. Thus, in addition to the intestine and the vagina, the bladder itself may serve as a reservoir for UPEC and a source of recurrent cystitis seen in a large portion of young women after the first episode of cystitis.[30]

The third series of events, which appears to be induced directly by the interaction between the bacterial adhesins and their specific cell-surface epitopes, is cytokine and chemokine production.

For example, the interaction between the P-fimbriae and their specific motif on the uroepithelial cell surface leads to activation of several signaling pathways, such as the ceramide signaling pathway, which is involved in the induction of cytokine responses. They also recruit Toll-like receptor-4 (TLR-4) and activate the accompanying signaling pathway. Whether LPS participates in triggering host response mechanisms remains unclear. There are studies supporting a role for LPS in epithelial cell activation, and others suggesting direct activation of these cells via the fimbriae independent of LPS. Among the evidence for P-pili–dependant activation of the host response, individuals were subjected to intravesicular inoculation with either a nonfimbriated asymptomatic bacteriuria strain or transformed asymptomatic bacteriuria strains expressing P-fimbriae. The latter group were found to have invariably higher Inter-Leukin (IL)-8 and IL-6 levels and greater neutrophil responses in the urinary tract as compared to the non-transformant group.[31]

On the other hand, type-I fimbriae E. coli are capable of activating the host cell responses, and have been shown more consistently to incite these responses through an LPS and TLR-4-dependant activation signal.[16,32] Of note, this was thought to occur despite the fact that epithelial cells are CD-14 negative and thus have a poor response to LPS.[31] Recently, however, there is evidence that CD-14 (which is part of the receptor complex for LPS) is expressed on the bladder epithelial cell surface, and is required in association with a TLR for these cells to respond to LPS and type-I fimbriated E. coli. This response appears to be mediated by the activation of nuclear factor kappa B (NF-κB) and p38 mitogen-activated protein kinase (MAPK) signaling pathways.[20] Regardless of the exact mechanism by which bacteria trigger the cascade of innate responses, once the intruder is recognized, proinflammatory cytokines and chemokines such IL-1, IL-6, and IL-8 are produced and lead to the recruitment and the activation of inflammatory cells.[19]

As indicated in the prior section, neutrophils are crucial for bacterial clearance from the kidneys and the bladder.[33] In response to the chemotactic gradient, neutrophils leave the circulation, traverse the submucosa, and reach the epithelial barrier. The last step of exit to the lumen, transepithelial migration is aided partially by epithelial intercellular adhesion molecule 1 (ICAM-1), as well as by IL-8. A role for IL-8 in neutrophil recruitment was suggested by the strong correlation between the urinary IL-8 levels and the urinary neutrophils numbers in individual patients.[34] It is now appreciated that IL-8 is the main chemokine involved in neutrophils migrating across infected epithelial cells in vitro. In vivo studies in the murine UTI model have identified macrophage-inflammatory protein-2 as an epithelial IL-8 equivalent in the mouse urinary tract.

In the IL-8 receptor knockout mouse, neutrophils fail to cross the epithelial barrier and accumulate in the tissue in massive numbers resulting in abscess formation and extensive fibrosis.[35,36] Use of anti-IL-8 antibody reduces neutrophil migration across the epithelial cell layers indicating its central role in this process.[34,37] These interactions explain the emergence of leukocytes in the urine, known as pyuria, which is a clinically utilized sign in the diagnosis of UTI.

Host Risk Factors Predisposing To UTI

The host factors predisposing to UTI are shown in Table 2. Each of these will be discussed in more detail here.

Obstruction

Obstruction to the urinary tract, whether acute or chronic, leads to an increased risk of UTI.[38] A noted increase in the incidence of UTI is associated with obstruction in male infants, female children, pregnancy, as well as with calculi, bladder neck obstruction, and extrinsic compression of the ureters (tumors or retroperitoneal fibrosis). All these conditions are accompanied by a high incidence of pyelonephritis.[13] Several proposed mechanisms may account for this, including that obstruction results in decreased urinary flow and reduced efficiency of micturition, impairing clearance of the bacteria from the genitourinary tract.[38] Bladder over-distention may interfere with local mucosal defense mechanisms. Increased residual volume also predisposes to, and maintains, bladder infection by providing a continuous pool of media suitable for bacterial growth, and thus may enhance multiplication of the bacteria in the urine, as well as increase the capacity of the bacteria to multiply in the renal parenchyma, allowing the infection to be transmitted from one part of the kidney to another. Proof for the importance of obstruction in the pathogenesis of UTI is derived from the animal model of experimental hematogenous pyelonephritis, in which the kidney appears relatively resistant to infection, unless the ureter is ligated.[13]

Diabetes Mellitus

Although it has been shown that bacterial growth is enhanced by high glucose content in the urine, patients with diabetes who have no neurologic complications affecting bladder function and

Table 2 Host Factors Predisposing to Urinary Tract Infections
Urinary tract obstruction
Diabetes mellitus
Advanced age
Immune compromised state
Urologic interventions

who have not undergone instrumentation are not at greater risk for developing UTI. Following instrumentation, however, or in the presence of autonomic neuropathy, ascending infection is more common and usually more severe.[13]

Advanced Age

Aging is associated with an increased prevalence of bacteriuria, occurring in 10% of men, and 20% of women over the age of 65. Possible reasons for the higher incidence of UTI include poor bladder emptying, loss of bactericidal effect of the prostate in elderly men, uterine prolapse and cystocele in elderly women, neuromuscular disease, and the risk of increased instrumentation in both genders.[13]

Immunocompromised Host

When considering the susceptibility of different populations of immune-suppressed patients to a particular form of infection, it is important to realize that such susceptibility is not caused by one factor, but is likely due to several factors interacting in an individual patient. It is determined by the underlying disease, the dose and duration of the immunosuppressive therapy, and the presence or absence of granulocytopenia.[39] These factors may play an important role in the increased susceptibility, and hence increased incidence of severity, of UTI in cancer patients. The interaction of certain therapies with any pre-existing immune abnormality makes it extremely difficult to establish a pathophysiology underlying the types of infections encountered in these patients. However, some disease processes are felt to be associated with increased infection susceptibility due to immune defects associated with the disease itself rather than the therapy. One potential example of this is multiple myeloma, since almost all the episodes of gram-negative bacteremia in these patients seem to occur in non-granulocytopenic individuals.[40] Most infections occurring in such patients involve the urinary, as well as the respiratory, tracts. Globally, up to 55% of the nosocomial infections affecting this group of patients are urinary tract infections, with *E. coli* being the most frequently isolated microorganism.[40]

Although neutropenia in and of itself does not appear to predispose the individual patient to acquiring a urinary tract infection, it blunts the clinical manifestations of an acquired infection, and predisposes the patient to bacteremia.[41] In one report, out of 56 patients with underlying malignancy and vancomycin-resistant enterococcus (VRE) infection (90% of whom had hematologic malignancies), 71% had bacteremia, whereas only 14% had a urinary infection.[42]

Broad-spectrum antibiotics play an important role in the compromised host, since they can alter the normal bacterial flora in the periurethral area suppressing the growth of the lactobacilli leading to a greater incidence of colonization with resistant pathogenic microorganisms. They also predispose to fungemia with hematogenous seeding of the urinary tract.[41]

Surgical trauma, drainage catheters, chemicals, and certain diseases can breach the integrity of the mucopolysaccharide lining of the bladder mucosa, providing a nidus for infection and a conduit for bacterial invasion.

Other factors, such as malnutrition, have been independently associated with an increased risk of nosocomially acquired infections.[43] In addition to uremia, hyperglycemia and the potential immunomodulating effect of certain viral infections (such as cytomegalovirus [CMV], Epstein-Barr virus, and human immunodeficiency virus [HIV]) may contribute to weakening the host defenses. Thus, it is not surprising that infection by low virulence microorganisms becomes much more common once the immune system and/or the integrity of the urinary tract is compromised.[39] In fact, most of the *E. coli* isolated from compromised patients with a urinary infection are negative for P-fimbriae.[44] Further, most *E. coli* strains isolated from patients with a catheter-related urinary infection do not carry the virulence genes that *E. coli* from patients with community-acquired UTIs carry.[45]

Urologic Procedures

Patients subjected to urologic procedures pose a special risk for developing UTIs. Any drain from the urinary tract to the external surface will increase the risk—the longer the catheter has been in place, the greater the risk.[46] The risk of infection varies further with the type of surgery; when the surgery in carried out on infected tissue or in a patient with an infected stone, then infection is almost inevitable. Deposition of implants such as stents and other foreign bodies also increases the risk.[46] Not surprisingly, the most commonly reported complication of urinary diversion procedures is urinary tract infection, occurring in 35 to 40% of patients undergoing such procedures.[39,47,48] This high rate is not surprising when taking into account the high likelihood of other complications associated with these procedures, such as ureteral strictures (11%), incontinence (9%), and urinary stone formation (7%).[47] The renal calculi that accompany such diversion procedures are usually composed of calcium and struvite, and the concomitant infection is classically due to *Proteus* spp.[38] Of note, urine cultures from these patients are difficult to interpret because of the interference from residual bowel flora.[49]

Microbiology

The spectrum of etiologic agents is similar in uncomplicated upper and lower UTI, with *E. coli* being the causative pathogen in 80 to 85% and *Staphylococcus saprophyticus* in 5 to 20% of cases.[50] Occasionally, other Enterobacteriaceae, such as *Proteus mirabilis* and *Klebsiella* spp or enterococci are isolated. However, the spectrum of pathogens causing a complicated UTI is much broader than that causing an uncomplicated infection. While *S. saprophyticus* is rarely seen in patients with a complicated UTI, several microorganisms are relatively more common in this group of patients, including *Proteus, Klebsiella, Pseudomonas,* and *Serratia,* in addition to the *Enterococci, Staphylococcus, Citrobacter,* and certain fungi.[1] One report from Germany on nosocomially acquired UTIs found *E. coli* to be the most common pathogen accounting for 32% of these infections in 2001, followed by *Enterococcus* spp in 22% of patients, and coagulase-negative staphylococcus in 10%.[51] It has been noted that other microorganisms have become more common over the past two decades, such as yeast and *K. pneumonia.*[52]

These uropathogens, including *E. coli,* are more likely to be resistant to the commonly used antibacterial agents in the immunocompromised host, where bacterial pathogens remain the most common cause of infection.[8] For example, with the advent of antimicrobials and the increasing use of cephalosporins, increasing rates of colonization and infections with *Enterococci,* particularly VRE, are occurring. These microorganisms typically colonize the intestinal tract, the respiratory tract, and vagina of otherwise healthy individuals. *Enterococcus faecalis* and *Enterococcus faecium* are responsible for 85 to 90% and 5 to 10% of infections in humans, respectively. UTI is the most common nosocomial infection caused by these microorganisms. VRE, especially *Enterococcus faecium,* is prevalent in hospitalized individuals across the United States. The reported prevalence of VRE colonization in the urine varies according to the center, ranging from 1 to 26% in one study, with *Enterococcus faecium* accounting for about 88% of all VREs isolated.[53]

Clinical Syndromes and Diagnosis

Asymptomatic Bacteriuria

Asymptomatic bacteriuria is defined as the isolation of bacteria from the urine in significant quantities consistent with infection (greater than or equal to 10^5 colony forming units (CFU)/mL) preferably on two occasions, but without the local or systemic symptoms and signs.[4,54] Although asymptomatic bacteriuria commonly precedes a UTI, with an estimated prevalence of 3.5% in the general population, it does not always lead to symptomatic infection. Certain factors increase the risk for asymptomatic bacteriuria, such as parity, diabetes in women, a history of UTI, and a lower education level. An estimated 4 to 10%

of pregnant women are diagnosed with asymptomatic bacteriuria.[4] During pregnancy, asymptomatic bacteriuria has been associated with progression to pyelonephritis as well as with preterm labor and cerebral palsy.[55] In most other populations, however, including the elderly, spinal cord injury patients, and patients with diabetes, asymptomatic bacteriuria does not denote increased risk of disease; hence screening and treatment are not recommended.[4,10]

Acute Uncomplicated Cystitis

Acute cystitis is generally considered uncomplicated unless it is associated with a predisposing factor, such as instrumentation with a catheter, the presence of a bladder stone, bladder outlet obstruction by benign prostate hypertrophy, or an underlying malignancy.[2] At the time of presentation with symptoms of an acute UTI, it is usually difficult to classify patients as having a complicated or an uncomplicated infection. It is, however, generally safe to assume that a premenopausal, sexually active, non-pregnant woman with recent onset of dysuria, frequency, or urgency, who has not been recently instrumented or treated with antibiotics, has an uncomplicated UTI.[2]

In young, sexually active women presenting with acute dysuria, three possible causes would need to be considered: acute cystitis, acute urethritis (caused by *Chlamydia trachomatis*, *Neisseria gonorrhea*, or *Herpes simplex*), and vaginitis. A distinction among these three entities can usually be made with a high degree of certainty after performing a good history and physical examination, and by reviewing the urinalysis findings.[54] The typical symptoms of acute cystitis are urgency, frequency, dysuria, and suprapubic pain. Vaginitis is more likely if patients have an associated vaginal discharge or odor, pruritus, or dyspareunia. Nearly all young women with acute cystitis have been shown to have pyuria, defined as 10 or more leukocytes per mm³ on an unspun voided midstream urine specimen.[2] The leukocyte esterase test has a widely reported sensitivity of 75 to 96% for detecting pyuria associated with acute UTI.[56] Thus, for patients with symptoms suggestive of a urinary infection, a negative leukocyte esterase test does not exclude the presence of an infection, and should prompt a microscopic urinary examination as well as urinary culture. UTI appears to be more likely with the presence of hematuria, since about 40% of women with an acute urinary infection are noted to have hematuria.[2] Gram stain is usually not performed since pathogens with low counts ($< 10^4$ CFU/mL) are difficult to visualize.[2] In symptomatic young women with suspected acute cystitis, a urine culture demonstrating 100 or more CFU/mL of uropathogenic species is indicative of infection.[54,56,57] However, from a practical point of view,

obtaining urine culture is not necessary in young women with acute uncomplicated cystitis, since the causative microorganisms and their antimicrobial susceptibilities are predictable.[2]

Recurrent Cystitis in Women

About 20% of young women with an initial episode of cystitis have recurrent infections. Occasionally, such recurrences are due to persistent infections, but most cases of recurrences are due to episodes of exogenous reinfection, typically months apart.[58] Most of these patients have no underlying anatomic abnormalities.[54] This increased susceptibility in certain individuals is of unclear etiology. In some patients, certain habits, such as the use of diaphragms and spermicides may account for some of the recurrences.[59] In others, there may be a genetic predisposition.[54] In postmenopausal women, the risk of recurrent UTI appears related to presence of factors that impair bladder emptying, such as cystocele and increased postvoid residual.[60] Recurrence should be documented by urine culture at least once, and then managed either by continuous or postcoital prophylaxis, or by therapy initiated by the patients at onset of symptoms. Topical estradiol may be of benefit in postmenopausal women.[54]

Acute Uncomplicated Pyelonephritis

Acute pyelonephritis should be considered uncomplicated, as well, in an otherwise healthy host infected with a virulent uropathogen unless it is associated with an underlying predisposing condition similar to those mentioned above, even though the infection does involve the upper urinary tract. The presentation of pyelonephritis can vary, from mild to moderate illness, to a life-threatening illness with gram-negative septicemia.[57] The severity of an infection seems to be related to cytokine expression, especially IL-6 and IL-8 responses, both locally and systemically. These cytokine responses are influenced, as indicated earlier, by host and bacterial variables.[61] Acute pyelonephritis is suggested by flank pain, nausea and vomiting, fever > 38°C, or by costovertebral angle tenderness.[2] Urinary frequency occurs in up to 98% of the women with acute pyelonephritis, suggesting a concomitant cystitis.[62] As in acute uncomplicated cystitis, pyuria occurs in the vast majority of the patients with acute pyelonephritis, and hematuria can be similarly evident. Urine culture reveals $> 10^5$ CFU/mL of uropathogens in > 80% of the cases, although some patients may have colony counts as low as 10^3 CFU/mL. Contrary to acute uncomplicated cystitis, a urine culture and sensitivity should always be performed in patients with acute pyelonephritis, since there are potentially serious sequelae to the use of inappropriate antimicrobial therapy.[1,63] Blood culture obtained in patients with acute pyelonephritis who are admitted to the

hospital reveal that up to 20% of these patients may have a positive result; however, the presence of bacteremia is not likely to affect the choice of antimicrobial therapy in this particular group of patients.[64–69]

Urologic Evaluation of Women with UTI

Most women with an episode of acute UTI, and recurrent uncomplicated cystitis have no underlying anatomic or functional abnormality, and, therefore, routine urologic evaluation would not be indicated in such patients.[1] For patients with two or more episodes of pyelonephritis, further evaluation is indicated. Typically, such an evaluation includes renal ultrasonography and/or computed tomography scan to rule out nephrolithiasis or obstructive uropathy. A complete evaluation, including cystoscopy and excretory urography, should be reserved for patients with persistent hematuria after eradicating the infection.[2]

Acute Uncomplicated UTI in Young Healthy Men

Due to the infrequency of UTIs in men, it has been traditional to consider all such infections in men complicated.[70] However, it is now clear that a small number of men between the ages 15 and 50 years old may suffer from an acute uncomplicated UTI without associated urologic abnormalities. Risk factors associated with these infections include homosexuality, intercourse with an infected female partner, and the lack of circumcision.[71,72] The etiologic agents are similar to those in women, and the causative microorganisms seem to have the same susceptibility patterns.[1] As in women, dysuria, frequency, urgency, and suprapubic pain or hematuria are the typical symptoms in a patient presenting with cystitis; fever and flank pain would suggest pyelonephritis. The absence of pyuria suggests a noninfectious etiology. Urethritis must be considered in sexually active men; examination for penile ulcerations and evaluation of a urethral swab with gram stain to exclude *N. gonorrhea* or *C. trachomatis* infections is important. A midstream urine culture using colony count criteria similar to that recommended for women is recommended to confirm the diagnosis.[1] Young healthy men presenting with an acute cystitis syndrome with no discernable complicating factors, who respond promptly to therapy, usually demonstrate no abnormalities on urologic evaluation; thus, routine urologic evaluation is not necessary in this clinical setting.[54] Urologic evaluation should probably be done routinely in adolescents, men with pyelonephritis, recurrent infections, or in the presence of a complicating factor.[1]

Complicated Urinary Tract Infections

Complicated UTIs are those that occur in patients with functional, metabolic, or anatomic abnormalities of the urinary tract; they also include infections caused by pathogens that are resistant to antibiotics (Table 3). The clinical spectrum is wide and includes asymptomatic bacteriuria, mild cystitis, pyelonephritis, and life-threatening urosepsis. As mentioned earlier, there are a vast number of diverse microorganisms that might be responsible for a complicated UTI.[54] It is important to take this into consideration when contemplating the different therapeutic options.

Urine and blood cultures must be obtained from individuals suspected of having a complicated UTI in order to identify the infecting pathogen and its potential susceptibility pattern. Correction of the underlying predisposing condition is necessary, when feasible, to prevent recurrence of the infection.

Antimicrobial Treatment of Urinary Tract Infections

Acute Uncomplicated Cystitis

Despite the fact that little change has occurred in the epidemiology of the causative microorganisms of acute uncomplicated cystitis, the management of these infections has become more complicated by the trend towards increased

---

Table 3 Causes of Complicated Urinary Tract Infections

Structural abnormalities
Obstruction
Prostatic infection
Nephrolithiasis
Urinary diversion procedures
Infected cysts
External drainage urinary catheters, and
    nephrostomy tubes
Stents
Vesicoureteral reflux
Neurogenic bladder
Bladder or renal abscesses
Fistula

Metabolic/Hormonal Abnormalities
Diabetes mellitus
Pregnancy
Chronic kidney disease
Xanthogranulomatous pyelonephritis

Impaired Host Responses*
Transplant recipients
Neutropenia
Congenital or acquired immunodeficiency

Unusual Pathogens
Yeast and fungi
Mycoplasma spp
Resistant bacteria including *pseudomonas
    aeruginosa*

Reproduced with permission from Elsevier Inc.[30]
* Includes patients with malignancy because of their immune compromised state either from disease or from therapy.

---

antimicrobial resistance. In the United States, the prevalence of resistance to trimethoprim-sulfamethoxazole (TMP-SMX) among *Escherichia coli* strains causing cystitis varies by region, and is higher than 20% in some regions.[73] Nitrofurantoin and fluoroquinolones remain highly active against almost all strains of *Escherichia coli*, although resistant strains to the fluoroquinolones are being reported in the US and in other countries[1]. The prevalence of resistance among uropathogens to β-lactams is high, ranging from 26 to 38%; hence, they are not recommended for first-line empiric therapy.[73] TMP-SMX is the most studied therapeutic agent, effective at eradicating initial bacteriuria in up to 93% of cases. It is, according to the clinical practice guidelines for management of acute uncomplicated cystitis published by the Infectious Diseases Society of America (IDSA), the recommended current standard of therapy.[74] Based on multiple studies revealing that 3 days therapy of an antimicrobial is generally as effective as the same antimicrobial agent given for longer durations, 3-day regimens are advocated. Single-dose therapy, in general, is less effective and associated with higher recurrence rates; accordingly, it is not recommended. Ofloxacin is as effective as TMP-SMX, as are probably the newer fluoroquinolones, but they are recommended as initial empirical therapy only in communities with higher than 20% resistance rates to TMP-SMX. β-lactams in 3-day regimens are less effective than TMP-SMX or fluoroquinolones in eradicating the infections and should not be used as first-line therapy. The role of nitrofurantoin may become more prominent in the treatment of acute uncomplicated cystitis, especially with the increasing resistance to TMP and TMP-SMX.[74]

Acute Uncomplicated Pyelonephritis

For decades, the traditional therapy for pyelonephritis has been hospitalization and treatment with intravenous antimicrobials for 6 weeks. This has recently changed, however, with the recent studies suggesting that, for most patients with an episode of acute uncomplicated pyelonephritis, an adequate outcome can be achieved with 2 weeks of therapy. Shorter durations (7 days) are likely feasible in patients with mild pyelonephritis. Due to the seriousness of an acute uncomplicated pyelonephritis, the high prevalence of resistance of the causative pathogens to TMP-SMX, and the high risk of failure when TMP-SMX is used for resistant bacteria, the recommended empirical antibiotic choice is an oral fluoroquinolone. TMP-SMX and β-lactams should not be used alone unless the organism is known to be susceptible to the particular agent being used. If the patient is suspected of having a gram-positive infection based on gram stain, amoxicillin or amoxicillin-clavulanic acid is recommended.

Nitrofurantoin should not be used to treat pyelonephritis since it does not achieve reliable tissue or serum levels.

If the patient requires hospitalization due to high fever, dehydration, vomiting, and/or sepsis, then he/she should be treated with parenteral antibacterial therapy. Several agents are considered effective in this setting. The IDSA recommends the use of an intravenous fluoroquinolone as first-line therapy here as well, but intravenous ceftriaxone or an aminoglycoside, with or without ampicillin, are also acceptable choices.[74] If Enterococcus is suspected, then ampicillin with gentamicin is a reasonable option.[1,74]

Acute Cystitis in Postmenopausal Women

There are few studies of the treatment of acute cystitis in postmenopausal women. Three-day therapy with ofloxacin was shown to be superior to cephalexin for 7 days in one study.[75] Unfortunately, there are no studies comparing the same antibacterial agent for different durations in older healthy ambulatory women. It is likely that the 3-day regimen as described for younger females is effective in this group of patients as well.[1]

Acute Uncomplicated UTI in Men

Data on the treatment of young healthy males with a UTI are lacking due to the low frequency of such infections in the group of individuals. Due to the potential of an accompanying prostatitis in this setting, most sources recommend the use of a fluoroquinolone for 7 days as first-line of empiric therapy since it provides the best antimicrobial spectrum and prostatic penetration. A 7-day course of TMP-SMX can also be used. Nitrofurantoin and β-lactams should not be used in young males with an acute UTI since they would not reach adequate tissue levels.[1]

Complicated UTI

In order to ensure effective eradication of an infection, the antibacterial agent has to be directed against the causative pathogen. Identification of the microorganisms and their susceptibility patterns by conventional laboratory methods takes 2 to 3 days in most cases. Unfortunately, in the situation of a complicating UTI, therapy cannot be delayed for long, and is typically initiated empirically. The ideal agent would need to offer coverage to the broad spectrum of pathogens that might be responsible for such an infection depending on the clinical setting. Due to their broad antibacterial spectrum and their favorable pharmacokinetics, the fluoroquinolones (eg, ciprofloxacin, levofloxacin, gatifloxacin), which achieve high bioavailability in the urine, can be considered the agents of choice in patients with mild to moderate illness. For initial empiric therapy in the more seriously ill hospitalized patients, the choice of antibiotic must offer good activity against pathogens such as *Pseudomonas aeruginosa* as well as most of the enterococci. Combination of agents such as ampicillin and gentamicin, piperacillin and tazobactam, imipenem and cilastatin sodium would be appropriate.[8,54] Once the infecting strain and the antimicrobial susceptibilities are known, therapy can be modified accordingly. Usually 2 weeks of treatment are recommended, and patients who are receiving parenteral antibiotics can be switched to oral therapy when they improve clinically. Naturally, eliminating the underlying complicating factor, if plausible, is of great importance in preventing recurrence of the infectious disease.

Types of UTI More Common in Cancer Patients:

As mentioned earlier, very little information is available with regard to the epidemiology of UTI in patients with malignancy. However, certain types of UTI appear to be more frequently observed in cancer patients: for example, fungal UTI and viral hemorrhagic cystitis secondary to an immunocompromised state. It is reasonable to discuss catheter-related UTI in this context, although it is not specific to cancer patients, because of the high morbidity of these patients and the frequency with which it is observed in these patients. For these reasons, these three types of UTI will be discussed in more detail.

Catheter-Related Infections

Between 15% and 25% of patients in general hospitals may have a catheter inserted at some point during the course of their stay.[76] Up to half the patients requiring an indwelling urethral catheter for 5 days or longer will develop bacteriuria or candiduria.[77] The urinary tract of the catheterized patient appears to be highly susceptible to infection, once a small number of microorganisms gain access. Low-level bacteriuria or candiduria has been shown to progress to > 10[5] CFU/ml 96% of the time.[78] Catheter-related UTIs are the most common nosocomial infections in hospitals and nursing homes, constituting > 40% of all institutionally-acquired infections.[76] The risk of bacteriuria with short-term catheterization is 5% per day.[79] Furthermore, Platt and colleagues observed that acquiring a urinary tract infection (defined as bacteriuria > 10[5] CFU/mL in the study) during indwelling bladder catheterization is associated with nearly a threefold increase in mortality among hospitalized patients.[80] Less than 5% of catheter-associated bacteriuria will be complicated by bacteremia; however, due to the large number of catheterized patients, nosocomial UTIs are the source of up to 15% of nosocomial blood stream infections.[81]

Risk Factors for Catheter-Associated UTI

The most important risk factor for acquiring a UTI in the setting of an indwelling bladder catheter is the duration of catheterization, particularly past 6 days. Other risk factors include female gender, lack of administration of systemic antibiotics during the period of catheterization, catheter insertion outside the operating room, being on a urology service, other active sites of infection, diabetes, and malnutrition.[77] The presence of azotemia (creatinine > 2 mg/dL), ureteral stent, or use of the catheter to monitor urine output further increase the risk.[77,79,82]

Definition of Catheter-Related UTIs

Most sources advocate considering the new appearance of > 10[3] CFU/mL of bacteria or fungi to represent a catheter-acquired UTI.[77–79] Most of these infections are unimicrobial, although they have been reported to be polymicrobial in up to 15% of the cases.[81] The most commonly isolated microorganism is *Escherichia coli*. Other gram-negative pathogens such as *Klebsiella*, *Enterobacter*, *Citrobacter*, and *P. aeruginosa* are common, as well. In one report, up to 27% of catheter-acquired UTIs were caused by enterococci or staphylococci, and up to one-third of the isolates were *Candida* species.[83] Yeast UTIs are particularly common when antibiotics are in use, and are increasing in incidence.[52]

Pathogenesis

Most catheter-associated UTIs are endogenous—that is, from the patient's own colonic flora. The indwelling catheter offers conduits for bacterial entry along its external and internal surfaces.[81] Organisms can gain access into the urinary tract in one of two ways. Extraluminal contamination may occur early, by direct inoculation when the catheter is inserted, or later by organisms ascending from the perineum by capillary action in the thin mucous film contiguous to the external catheter surface. Intraluminal contamination may occur by reflux of microorganisms gaining access into the lumen from failure of closed drainage or contamination of urine in the collecting bag.[79] Although these infections have been shown to occur by both extraluminal and intraluminal routes, they seem to derive preponderantly from organisms that gain access extraluminally.[84] Some suggest that the latter is of even greater importance in women, perhaps because of the shorter urethra and its closer proximity to the anus.[85]

Urinary catheters are tubular latex or silicone devices which, when inserted, may acquire biofilms on the inner or the outer surface.[86] The initial adherence occurs to the irregular surfaces surrounding the catheter eyeholes. Microcolonies form in the depressions on these surfaces and spread to cover the entire surface around the eyeholes.[87] A distinguishing characteristic of biofilms is the presence of an extracellular polymeric matrix, containing open water channels and primarily composed of polysaccharides, surrounding and encasing the cells.[88] Most of the biofilm volume is actually composed of this layer rather than of pathogenic cells. Organisms contained within the biofilms seem to be well protected against antimicrobials and the urine flow.[86] Urinary catheter biofilms may initially be composed of a single microorganism, but longer exposure inevitably leads to the presence of multiple species.[89] Organisms commonly present in biofilms of bladder catheters are *S. epidermidis*, *Enterococcus faecalis*, *Escherichia coli*, *Proteus mirabilis*, and *Pseudomonas*, among others.[86] Other than biofilm formation, the catheter, as a foreign body, may lead to a complex defect in PMN function, which may be partially responsible for these patients' higher susceptibility to infection.[81,86]

Clinical Features

Most patients with a catheter-acquired UTI are asymptomatic, with less than 10% of those with a microbiologically documented UTI reporting any symptoms. Placement of an indwelling urethral catheter can, in and by itself, cause dysuria or urgency; however, these complaints do not appear to denote an underlying infection. Neither fever nor peripheral leukocytosis has been shown to be predictive of a urinary infection in this setting. Continuous drainage by the catheter with the resultant decompression of the infected bladder may prevent the urgency and frequency that would be expected in the setting of cystitis.[77] Similarly, most patients do not demonstrate pyuria, even with a microbiologically documented, catheter-associated UTI when the catheterization was short-term.[83] The sensitivity of pyuria was calculated at merely 37% in this prospective study, and based on this study, pyuria should not be used as the sole criteria for obtaining a urine culture if UTI is suspected in catheterized individuals.[83] In any event, the importance of such infections stems from the fact that they comprise the largest institutional reservoir for antibiotic resistant pathogens such as *Enterococci*, *Klebsiella*, *Citrobacter*, *Pseudomonas*, and others.[77]

Prevention

Several catheter-care practices are universally recommended to prevent, or at least delay, the onset of catheter-associated UTIs: avoid unnecessary catheterizations; consider other methods of bladder drainage, such as condom catheters or suprapubic catheters; and ensure a trained professional inserts the catheter under aseptic conditions. Maintenance of closed drainage with as little manipulation as possible, and maintenance of dependant drainage by keeping the collecting tubing and bag below the bladder level, are important. However, it is of greater importance to limit the duration of catheterization by prompt removal of the indwelling catheter once deemed unnecessary. Other techniques, such as anti-infective lubricant, antireflux valves, and instillation of an antibiotic into the collection bag remain of unproven efficacy.[79]

Use of systemic antimicrobials, such as TMP-SMX or ciprofloxacin, appears to be effective in the prevention of catheter-related UTIs[90]; however, infections that occur despite prophylaxis are far more likely to be caused by antibiotic-resistant bacteria. Furthermore, since most of these infections are asymptomatic and rarely lead to bacteremia, it is difficult to justify the use of systemic antibiotics in every patient subjected to an indwelling urethral catheter.[79] An exception to this would be renal transplant recipients, where prophylaxis has been shown to be cost-effective in the prevention of UTI.[11]

Treatment

Treatment of asymptomatic bacteriuria in the setting of an indwelling bladder catheter is not generally recommended. There are, however, specific groups of patients in whom it appears necessary, for example, patients with granulocytopenia or other immune compromising conditions or those undergoing urologic procedures.[79] Removal of the catheter results in eradication of infection unless predisposing factors for UTI persist. Treatment should be directed at the specific microorganism isolated.

Fungal UTI

There appears to be a steady increase in the rate of nosocomial fungal infections, from 2.0 to 3.8 per 1,000 discharges in the United States, as reported to the Centers for Disease Control and Prevention (CDC) National Nosocomial Infections Surveillance (NNIS) system. High rates of infection are not limited to oncology wards and high-risk nurseries; they also occur on cardiac surgery, burn, and trauma wards.[91] In patients with an indwelling catheter, up to 27% of UTIs have been reported to be caused by fungi.[82] Table 4 shows the CDC criteria for diagnosis of nosocomially-acquired UTI. Since the majority of the renal fungal infections result from *Candida* sp, the remainder of this discussion will be focused on the clinical findings and the treatment of *Candida* infections of the urinary tract.

Candiduria is a rare finding in healthy, non-hospitalized individuals. In hospitalized patients, the prevalence of candiduria is variable, but seems to be most common in the intensive care unit. *Candida* UTIs represent 10 to 15% of all nosocomial UTIs.[92,93] Analysis of reports from the NNIS system showed that *Candida albicans* ranked

Table 4 CDC Criteria for Diagnosis of Nosocomially-Acquired Urinary Tract Infections

One of the following: fever (> 38°C), urgency, frequency, dysuria, or suprapubic tenderness **AND** a urine culture $\geq 10^5$ CFUs/mL urine with no more than two species of organisms.

Two of the following: fever (> 38°C), urgency, frequency, dysuria, or suprapubic tenderness **AND** any of the following:

Dipstick test positive for leukocyte esterase and/or nitrite

Pyuria (≥ 10 WBCs/μL or ≥ 3 WBC/high-power field of unspun urine

Organisms seen on Gram stain of unspun urine

Two urine cultures with repeated isolation of the same uropathogen (gram-negative bacteria or *Staphylococcus saprophyticus*) with $\geq 10^2$ CFUs/mL urine in non-voided specimen

Urine culture with $\leq 10^5$ CFUs/mL urine of single uropathogen in a patient being treated with appropriate antimicrobial therapy

Physician's diagnosis

Physician institutes appropriate antimicrobial therapy

CDC = Centers for Disease Control and Prevention; WBC = white blood (cell) count.

seventh among all hospital pathogens isolated from a major infections site in 1996.[91] More recently, it was reported as the fourth most common cause of blood stream infection in the United States.[94] Over the past decade, there has been a definite increase in the incidence of non-*albicans Candida* species causing serious disease in humans.[95–97] In one retrospective series by Abbas and colleagues that evaluated patients with underlying malignancies, *Candida krusei* accounted for 5% of fungemias during 1989 through 1992; the incidence increased to 10% during the period 1993 to 1996.[97] The major risk factor for of non-*albicans* infections, including *Candida krusei* and *Candida glabrata*, was fluconazole prophylaxis given to patients undergoing treatment for leukemia.[95,97]

Most nosocomial *Candida* infections are thought to be endogenous, arising from colonization of the mouth, colon, vagina, or skin. *Candida* typically gains access to the urinary tract by the ascending route; thus, it occurs more frequently in women.[98] Other risk factors associated with *Candida* infections are summarized in Table 5.

According to a prospective multicenter study by Kauffman and colleagues, *Candida albicans* is the most common agent isolated in the urine (52%), followed by *Candida glabrata* in 16% of the patients. Ten percent of the patients had more than one species of *Candida* present.[99] A common problem is determining whether the presence of *Candida* in the urine is indicative of infection or merely colonization. Although pyuria usually supports the presence of an underlying infection, it might also be the result of concomitant

Table 5 Risk Factors for Candida Urinary Tract Infections

Diabetes Mellitus

Extremes of age

Female gender

Use of antimicrobial agents

Use of indwelling bladder catheters

Urinary tract disease: neurogenic bladder, prostatic disease, renal failure

Malignancy

Malnutrition

Use of immunosuppressive therapy, and/or radiation therapy

Adapted from Kauffman CA et al,[99] Vazquez JA et al,[93] and Rivett AG et al.[100]

bacteriuria. In any event, the presence of colony counts $\geq 10^3$ CFU/mL would need to be interpreted according to the clinical situation and to the patient's symptoms.

Most patients with funguria are asymptomatic, with less than 5% reporting dysuria, frequency, urgency, or flank pain. Hematuria also appears to be uncommon. Fever occurs more frequently (up to 22%); however, in most cases, it is not clear whether it is due to the candidal infection itself or the underlying disease.[99] Asymptomatic candiduria is usually viewed as a benign condition that rarely leads to invasive disease.[100] When invasion of the upper urinary tract does occur, however, the clinical signs and symptoms are indistinguishable from those associated with bacterial infection. The formation of perinephric abscesses and fungal balls (bezoars) that commonly include sloughed renal papillae (papillary necrosis) can occur in the compromised host, especially in the presence of obstruction, and in diabetics.

In a prospective multi-center study, Sobel and colleagues randomized 316 patients with asymptomatic candiduria $\geq 10^3$ CFU/mL to either fluconazole or placebo. In the untreated group, they demonstrated that candiduria resolved in 41% of patients merely upon removal of the indwelling bladder catheter. Higher eradication rates were noted in the treated group as compared to the placebo group, initially (63% vs. 35%). However, patients who had received either fluconazole or placebo had similar rates of candiduria two weeks after the completion of therapy.[101] Accordingly, treatment of asymptomatic candiduria is not recommended by the IDSA except in specific circumstances. Candiduria should be treated if the patient is symptomatic, neutropenic, a renal allograft recipient, or about to undergo urologic manipulation. Removal of the urinary instrument should be undertaken if feasible. Choices for therapy include fluconazole at 200 mg/d for 7 to 14 days, amphotericin B at 0.3 to 1.0 mg/kg/d for 1 to 7 days, or, in the absence of renal insufficiency, flucytosine at 25 mg/kg qid.

The latter may be especially effective in patients with non-*albicans Candida* species.[102] The management of perinephric abscesses, bezoars, and papillary necrosis requires invasive urologic procedures to ensure adequate drainage in addition to the systemic therapy.[103]

Candiduria may be a source of subsequent dissemination, as in patients with urinary tract obstruction, or a marker of acute hematogenous dissemination as in neutropenic patients.[103] Renal involvement was present in one study in 90% of patients who died of disseminated candidiasis, on autopsy.[98] Among the NNIS hospitals, there has been a dramatic increase in the rate of all nosocomial bloodstream infections caused by fungi—from 5.4% in 1980 to 9.9% in 1990, the most common fungus being *Candida* spp.[91] Increased susceptibility to invasive candidiasis is typically attributed to host factors such as a severe illness, immunocompromised status, or malnutrition. Unlike candiduria, disseminated candidiasis carries a grave prognosis, with an estimated crude mortality of 50 to 60%.[91]

In patients with known disseminated candidiasis, renal involvement has no specific treatment implications unless renal function deteriorates or the patient develops flank pain. In these settings, imaging studies of the kidney such as ultrasonography or computed tomography are needed to exclude obstruction, perinephric abscess, and papillary necrosis.[102]

Prophylaxis reduces the incidence of both superficial and deep candidiasis in high-risk populations. The best data on prophylaxis of fungal infections include two randomized controlled trials that compared fluconazole with placebo in bone marrow transplantation recipients.[104,105] Both studies observed that fluconazole was both safe and effective in preventing *Candida* infections caused by all species except *Candida krusei*, and both studies demonstrated improvement in morbidity. In the trial by Slavin and colleagues, the probability of survival was greater in the group receiving the prophylaxis.[104] In the guidelines for the treatment of candidiasis, the IDSA advocates prophylaxis for neutropenic patients in limited situations: standard chemotherapy for acute myelogenous leukemia, allogeneic bone marrow transplantation, and high-risk autologous bone marrow transplantation.

Hemorrhagic Cystitis

Hemorrhagic cystitis (HC) is one of the frequent complications in bone marrow transplant (BMT) recipients.[106] The incidence of HC is reported to vary widely, from 6 to 38% of patients after bone marrow transplantation.[107–111] Two distinct clinical types of HC have been described in these patients: an early and a late type. The early type is principally from chemotherapeutic agents—busulfan, cyclophosphamide, and ifosfamide—which are used during the conditioning regimen

in these patients. This is usually mild, and can often be prevented by modifying the conditioning regimen[107]; occasionally, it can be severe. On the other hand, the late onset type is related to either graft-versus-host disease (GVHD) or viral infections.[107] This review will discuss HC as it relates to viral infections in bone marrow transplantation recipients.

Viruses that have been incriminated in causing HC include the adenovirus and polyomaviruses. HC caused by human polyomavirus is from two types, BK virus (BKV) and JC virus (JCV). BKV causes cystitis and nephropathy in immunosuppressed and renal transplant recipients, while JCV is uncommonly associated with renal disorders. A polyomavirus of simian origin, SV40, has been associated recently with HC after bone marrow transplantation.[112]

The clinical features of HC with either adenovirus or BKV infections appear to be similar. Based on clinical features, Bedi and classified HC into four grades as shown in Table 6.[108] Grades 0 to 2 are considered mild disease, while grades 3 and 4 are considered severe disease. Apart from hematuria and clot retention or obstruction, other clinical features include pain, dysuria, renal failure, and problems associated with disseminated disease, such as pneumonia, enteritis, and neurologic complications. In a study on children who underwent allogeneic bone marrow transplantation, Hale and colleagues observed that the prevalence of severe HC was 11%, the mean duration of symptoms was 73 days, and in a multivariate analysis, male sex and unrelated donor grafts were significantly associated with HC.[113] In a study from the M. D. Anderson Cancer Center in Houston, TX, where the study was also limited to allogeneic BMT patients, of the 105 patients with acute lymphocytic leukemia, 32 patients developed HC within the first year after transplantation with a cumulative incidence of 30%.[114] The median time of onset of HC was 23 days with only one patient developing HC after 100 days. The mean duration of symptoms of HC was 30 days. Grade 2 HC occurred in 56%, grade 3 in 31%, and grade 4 in 13%; 59% were attributed to polyomavirus, with 17% attributed to adenovirus. An interesting feature in this study was a high CMV reactivation rate (63%) among patients with HC. While polyomavirus infection was

similar in both younger and older patients, adenovirus infection was exclusive to patients younger than 25 years. The two main factors that were associated with HC included transplantation from a matched, unrelated donor, and age <26 years. Interestingly, the use of cyclophosphamide in the preparative regimen was not associated with HC.[114]

The published studies that have looked at HC in BMT recipients can be summarized as those associated with adenovirus infections or with BKV infections.

Adenovirus-Associated HC

In another study from M. D. Anderson Cancer Center, 85 out of 2,889 (3%) of adult patients who received BMT were diagnosed with adenovirus infection.[115] Of the 85, 13% were diagnosed with HC. There was no significant difference in the incidence of HC between patients who received allogeneic versus autologous BMT. The mean duration of symptoms of patients with HC was 26 days, compared with 21 days for pneumonia and 60 days for disseminated disease. Overall mortality was 26%, but none of the patients with isolated HC died; 85% of patients with disseminated disease had GVHD. The predictors for disseminated disease in a multivariate analysis were GVHD (odds ratio [OR] 6.23) and treatment with ≥ 2 immunosuppressive drugs (OR 74.0).[115]

In a study from Japan, Akiyama and colleagues observed that HC was more common after allogeneic BMT, rather than after autologous or syngeneic BMT.[116] In addition, the preparative regime, GVHD prophylaxis, grade of GVHD, and use of mesna were significantly associated with HC. Adenovirus was responsible for HC in 60% of patients, and 85% of the adenovirus-associated HC were due to infection by type II.[116] The serological status of adenovirus was not a risk factor for subsequent development of HC among these patients. In most studies, asymptomatic shedding of adenovirus was not common in BMT recipients. In the study by Akiyama and colleagues, the prevalence of adenovirus in urine samples in patients without HC was 3%, compared with 60% among patients with HC.[116]

BKV/JCV Infections

BKV and JCV, named after the initials of the patients from whom the viruses were first discovered, are common problems in BMT recipients. In the general population, infection with these viruses occurs early in childhood, and seroconversion occurs throughout childhood such that, by 10 years of age, 60% of children would have acquired the antibodies.[117] The prevalence of a prior infection among adults is 60 to 80%.[118] Asymptomatic viruria occurs in 0.3% of non-immunosuppressed patients, 3% of pregnant women, 10 to 45% of renal transplant recipients

Table 6	Grading of Hemorrhagic Cystitis
Grade 0	No hematuria
Grade 1	> 50 erythrocytes per high-power microscopic field
Grade 2	Macroscopic hematuria
Grade 3	Macroscopic hematuria with clots
Grade 4	Macroscopic hematuria with clots and obstruction with elevated creatinine

Adapted from Bedi et al.[108]

and 50% of BMT recipients.[119–121] BKV is probably transmitted through the respiratory secretions, although isolation of the virus from respiratory secretions has not been easy. After replication and dissemination, BKV invades the renal and urothelial cells where it establishes a latent infection. Infection can also be carried to the recipient through the organ, particularly in solid organ transplant patients. In renal transplant recipients, BKV infection is identified with graft dysfunction and is often associated with rejection.[122] The degree of viremia was higher in patients with rejection and graft dysfunction than in those without.[122]

HC in association with BKV infection in BMT recipients has been shown in a number of studies.[106–108,123–126] While BKV infection does not always lead to HC in these patients, HC is four times more common among patients with BKV infection than among those without the infection.[121] HC and renal infections in association with BKV infection are also seen in severely immunosuppressed patients, such as patients with HIV or /acquired immunodeficiency syndrome.[127–129] BKV infection causing nephropathy or HC is likely to be a secondary infection or reactivation of a previous primary infection.[122]

Diagnosis of BKV infection is principally made by urine examination. Presence of decoy cells in the urine is a morphologic marker for viral replication. Decoy cells are caused by infection of urinary epithelial cells by BKV and can be identified by light microscopy.[121] The nuclei of these cells are enlarged, and nuclear chromatin is completely homogenized by viral cytopathic effect. Urine BKV deoxyribonucleic acid (DNA) polymerase chain reaction (PCR) is highly sensitive and specific for diagnosing the infection. BKV DNA PCR in the plasma is also highly sensitive and specific for diagnosing BKV nephropathy, but may also be useful in diagnosis of HC. The predictive value of BKV DNA PCR is limited in children because an incidental primary BKV infection that is common in childhood may not be differentiated from a secondary infection or reactivation of a prior primary infection in these immunosuppressed patients.

Treatment

In most cases, the clinical course of HC is mild and requires only volume expansion (also termed hyperhydration). When the hematuria is severe, analgesics may be required to relieve the pain from passing clots. An indwelling catheter is useful to prevent clot retention and urinary obstruction, but this is likely to be more successful in adults than in children because of the small catheter lumen required in children.[111] Evacuation of blood clots can also be carried out with transurethral catheterization, particularly in adults. Suprapubic catheter insertion and/or

surgical removal of clots may have to be performed if clot retention cannot be relieved through transurethral catheterization. Many urologists prefer an open surgical procedure for suprapubic catheter insertion, rather than a blind procedure because of better hemostasis with the former, as many of these patients are thrombocytopenic.

Several other local treatments have been tried with varied success in controlling hematuria in HC. These include prostaglandin E2 and F2α, alum irrigation, instillation of formalin, intravesical hydrostatic pressure, hyperbaric oxygen, and laser vaporization of the bleeding areas.[110,130,131]

Specific treatment of viral diseases causing HC are still evolving. Cidofovir has been tried for adenovirus infections, as well as in an occasional patient with BKV infection, with varying success.[121,132–135] Two studies showed promising results: one showed that all patients prospectively treated with cidofovir for adenovirus infections responded.[134] All adenovirus infections, pneumonia, enteritis, HC and disseminated disease, were included in this study. None of these patients had nephrotoxicity from the drug at the dosage of 1mg/kg/d given three times weekly, and continued until virologic remission is achieved. In the other study that included only BMT patients with HC, 10 of the 14 (71%) patients showed clinical improvement with cidofovir.[135] Seven patients had nephrotoxicity from the drug, despite the dosage being the same as in the above study, and in four of them, the drug had to be discontinued. No prospective randomized trials are yet available with cidofovir. Breakthrough infections with CMV and herpes simplex virus (HSV) have been observed while on treatment with cidofovir in these immunosuppressed patients.[135] Cidofovir for adenovirus-associated HC has generally been reserved for grade 3 and 4 HC, and the preliminary results are certainly promising.

Intravenous ribavirin has also been tried in adenovirus infections in BMT patients, including HC. However, the results have been disappointing. In a study from M. D. Anderson Cancer Center, intravenous ribavirin was tried in 12 of 85 BMT patients with adenovirus infection, with only one of them responding to the treatment.[115] Among these 12 patients, only one patient had HC, and that patient did not respond to ribavirin. So, at the current time, for adenovirus-associated high-grade HC, cidofovir may be the treatment of choice, despite its significant nephrotoxic potential.

There is no consensus on optimum antiviral therapy to date for BKV/JCV infections. It is not certain whether asymptomatic viruria needs treatment, and no trials exist that show prevention of symptomatic infections by preempted treatment of asymptomatic patients. Cidofovir

has not met with the same degree of success in BKV infections. One complicating feature is that BKV can cause nephropathy, particularly in renal transplant recipients, and cidofovir also is nephrotoxic. It has also not been established that treatment of BKV nephropathy improves the graft survival in these patients. The experience of treating BKV-associated HC with cidofovir is limited to two case reports. In one report, a successful clearance of viruria after treatment with cidofovir in a BMT recipient with HC was observed; the patient also had a simultaneous reactivation of CMV infection.[133] In another report, no response was observed with cidofovir in a patient with HIV infection and HC.[127] In an extreme case of HC with hematuria, intravenous vidarabine was used in a BMT patient with BKV-associated HC with improvement of symptoms, although viruria persisted.[136]

Thus, more prospective studies are needed to establish the optimum therapy in both adenovirus and BKV-associated urinary infections in these immunocompromised patients.

Conclusions

Urinary tract infections remain among the most common medical problems encountered, both in the general population and in hospitalized individuals, including patients with an underlying diagnosis of cancer. There are multiple local and systemic factors that predispose this latter group of patients to such infections. Patients with malignancies of the abdomen and the pelvis are at high risk of developing obstruction by virtue of the mass itself, or as a result of radiation therapy. UTIs are the most commonly reported complication among patients undergoing diversion procedures.

Systemic immune deficiency may be secondary to the disease itself or, more commonly, a consequence of the introduced therapies. Neutropenic patients are more susceptible to infection with resistant microorganisms such VRE. Although they typically do not develop dysuria or pyuria, they are at increased risk of septicemia once a UTI has occurred. Thus, the presence of bacteriuria and candiduria needs to be taken seriously and should warrant antimicrobial therapy in these immunocompromised patients.

Certain subsets of patients, such as those undergoing BMT, are at higher risk of viral hemorrhagic cystitis. They are particularly prone to adenoviral and BKV infections. Despite the advent of newer antiviral agents, their treatment continues to pose a clinical challenge.

Unfortunately, little effort has been made to define the incidence and the microorganism patterns of UTIs in this group of patients. Further, the potential impact of UTIs on morbidity and mortality of cancer patients remains to be explored.

REFERENCES

1. Hooton TM. The current management strategies for community-acquired urinary tract infection. Infect Dis Clin North Am 2003;17:303–32.

2. Hooton TM, Stamm WE. Diagnosis and treatment of uncomplicated urinary tract infection. Infect Dis Clin North Am 1997;11:551–81.

3. Schappert SM. Ambulatory care visits to physician offices, hospital outpatient departments, and emergency departments: United States, 1997. Vital Health Stat 13 1999:i–iv, 1–39.

4. Foxman B. Epidemiology of urinary tract infections: incidence, morbidity, and economic costs. Dis Mon 2003;49:53–70.

5. Tolkoff-Rubin N.E. CRS, Rubin, R.H. Urinary Tract Infections, Pyelonephritis, and Reflux Nephropathy. In: Brenner BM, ed. The Kidney. Philadelphia, PA: Saunders W.B.; 2000:1449-508.

6. Krieger JN, Ross SO, Simonsen JM. Urinary tract infections in healthy university men. J Urol 1993;149:1046–8.

7. Vorland LH, Carlson K, Aalen O. An epidemiological survey of urinary tract infections among outpatients in Northern Norway. Scand J Infect Dis 1985;17:277–83.

8. Wagenlehner FM, Naber KG. Emergence of antibiotic resistance and prudent use of antibiotic therapy in nosocomially acquired urinary tract infections. Int J Antimicrob Agents 2004;23(Suppl 1):24–9.

9. Bouza E, San Juan R, Munoz P, et al. A European perspective on nosocomial urinary tract infections II. Report on incidence, clinical characteristics and outcome (ESGNI-004 study). European Study Group on Nosocomial Infection. Clin Microbiol Infect 2001;7:532–42.

10. Foxman B, Brown P. Epidemiology of urinary tract infections: transmission and risk factors, incidence, and costs. Infect Dis Clin North Am 2003;17:227–41.

11. Tolkoff-Rubin NE, Cosimi AB, Russell PS, Rubin RH. A controlled study of trimethoprim-sulfamethoxazole prophylaxis of urinary tract infection in renal transplant recipients. Rev Infect Dis 1982;4:614–8.

12. Prat V, Horcickova M, Matousovic K, et al. Urinary tract infection in renal transplant patients. Infection 1985;13:207–10.

13. Sobel JD. Pathogenesis of urinary tract infection. Role of host defenses. Infect Dis Clin North Am 1997;11:531–49.

14. Tolkoff-Rubin NE, Rubin RH. Urinary tract infection in the immunocompromised host. Lessons from kidney transplantation and the AIDS epidemic. Infect Dis Clin North Am 1997;11:707–17.

15. Johnson JR. Microbial virulence determinants and the pathogenesis of urinary tract infection. Infect Dis Clin North Am 2003;17:261–78, viii.

16. Hedlund M, Frendeus B, Wachtler C, et al. Type 1 fimbriae deliver an LPS- and TLR4-dependent activation signal to CD14-negative cells. Mol Microbiol 2001;39:542–52.

17. Sandberg T, Kaijser B, Lidin-Janson G, et al. Virulence of Escherichia coli in relation to host factors in women with symptomatic urinary tract infection. J Clin Microbiol 1988;26:1471–6.

18. Vranes J, Kruzic V, Sterk-Kuzmanovic N, Schonwald S. Virulence characteristics of Escherichia coli strains causing asymptomatic bacteriuria. Infection 2003;31:216–20.

19. Schilling JD, Mulvey MA, Hultgren SJ. Dynamic interactions between host and pathogen during acute urinary tract infections. Urology 2001;57:56–61.

20. Schilling JD, Martin SM, Hunstad DA, et al. CD14- and toll-like receptor-dependent activation of bladder epithelial cells by lipopolysaccharide and type 1 piliated Escherichia coli. Infect Immun 2003;71:1470–80.

21. Langermann S, Palaszynski S, Barnhart M, et al. Prevention of mucosal Escherichia coli infection by FimH-adhesin-based systemic vaccination. Science 1997;276:607–11.

22. Langermann S, Mollby R, Burlein JE, et al. Vaccination with FimH adhesin protects cynomolgus monkeys from colonization and infection by uropathogenic Escherichia coli. J Infect Dis 2000;181:774–8.

23. Russo TA, Jodush ST, Brown JJ, Johnson JR. Identification of two previously unrecognized genes (GUAA and ARGC) important for uropathogenesis. Mol Microbiol 1996;22:217–29.

24. Neal DE Jr. Host defense mechanisms in urinary tract infections. Urol Clin North Am 1999;26:677–86, vii.

25. To T, Agha M, Dick PT, Feldman W. Cohort study on circumcision of newborn boys and subsequent risk of urinary-tract infection. Lancet 1998;352:1813–6.

26. Orskov I, Ferencz A, Orskov F. Tamm-Horsfall protein or uromucoid is the normal urinary slime that traps type 1 fimbriated Escherichia coli. Lancet 1980;315:887.

27. Parkkinen J, Virkola R, Korhonen TK. Identification of factors in human urine that inhibit the binding of Escherichia coli adhesins. Infect Immun 1988;56:2623–30.

28. Martinez JJ, Mulvey MA, Schilling JD, et al. Type 1 pilus-mediated bacterial invasion of bladder epithelial cells. Embo J 2000;19:2803–12.

29. Mulvey MA, Schilling JD, Hultgren SJ. Establishment of a persistent Escherichia coli reservoir during the acute phase of a bladder infection. Infect Immun 2001;69:4572–9.

30. Anderson GG, Palermo JJ, Schilling JD, et al. Intracellular bacterial biofilm-like pods in urinary tract infections. Science 2003;301:105–7.

31. Wullt B, Bergsten G, Connell H, et al. P-fimbriae trigger mucosal responses to Escherichia coli in the human urinary tract. Cell Microbiol 2001;3:255–64.

32. Wullt B, Bergsten G, Fischer H, et al. The host response to urinary tract infection. Infect Dis Clin North Am 2003;17:279–301.

33. Haraoka M, Hang L, Frendeus B, et al. Neutrophil recruitment and resistance to urinary tract infection. J Infect Dis 1999;180:1220–9.

34. Godaly G, Proudfoot AE, Offord RE, et al. Role of epithelial interleukin-8 (IL-8) and neutrophil IL-8 receptor A in Escherichia coli-induced transuroepithelial neutrophil migration. Infect Immun 1997;65:3451–6.

35. Frendeus B, Godaly G, Hang L, et al. Interleukin 8 receptor deficiency confers susceptibility to acute experimental pyelonephritis and may have a human counterpart. J Exp Med 2000;192:881–90.

36. Hang L, Frendeus B, Godaly G, Svanborg C. Interleukin-8 receptor knockout mice have subepithelial neutrophil entrapment and renal scarring following acute pyelonephritis. J Infect Dis 2000;182:1738–48.

37. Godaly G, Hang L, Frendeus B, Svanborg C. Transepithelial neutrophil migration is CXCR1 dependent in vitro and is defective in IL-8 receptor knockout mice. J Immunol 2000;165:5287–94.

38. Ronald AR, Harding GK. Complicated urinary tract infections. Infect Dis Clin North Am 1997;11:583–92.

39. Mohamed Mohamed-Abdallah Z, Esteban Fuertes M, Hermida Gutierrez J, et al. [Diversions of the upper urinary tract in oncologic patients]. Actas Urol Esp 1994;18 Suppl:465–7.

40. Paradisi F, Corti G, Cinelli R. Infections in multiple myeloma. Infect Dis Clin North Am 2001;15:373–84, vii–viii.

41. Korzeniowski OM. Urinary tract infection in the impaired host. Med Clin North Am 1991;75:391–404.

42. Raad I, Hachem R, Hanna H, et al. Treatment of vancomycin-resistant enterococcal infections in the immunocompromised host: quinupristin-dalfopristin in combination with minocycline. Antimicrob Agents Chemother 2001;45:3202–4.

43. Schneider SM, Veyres P, Pivot X, et al. Malnutrition is an independent factor associated with nosocomial infections. Br J Nutr 2004;92:105–11.

44. Dowling KJ, Roberts JA, Kaack MB. P-fimbriated Escherichia coli urinary tract infection: a clinical correlation. South Med J 1987;80:1533–6.

45. Guyer DM, Kao JS, Mobley HL. Genomic analysis of a pathogenicity island in uropathogenic Escherichia coli CFT073: distribution of homologous sequences among isolates from patients with pyelonephritis, cystitis, and catheter-associated bacteriuria and from fecal samples. Infect Immun 1998;66:4411–7.

46. Johansen TE. Nosocomially acquired urinary tract infections in urology departments. Why an international prevalence study is needed in urology. Int J Antimicrob Agents 2004;23 Suppl 1:30–4.

47. Salom EM, Mendez LE, Schey D, et al. Continent ileocolonic urinary reservoir (Miami pouch): the University of Miami experience over 15 years. Am J Obstet Gynecol 2004; 190:994–1003.

48. Ramirez PT, Modesitt SC, Morris M, et al. Functional outcomes and complications of continent urinary diversions in patients with gynecologic malignancies. Gynecol Oncol 2002;85:285–91.

49. Rubenstein JN, Schaeffer AJ. Managing complicated urinary tract infections: the urologic view. Infect Dis Clin North Am 2003;17:333–51.

50. Hooton TM, Besser R, Foxman B, et al. Acute uncomplicated cystitis in an era of increasing antibiotic resistance: a proposed approach to empirical therapy. Clin Infect Dis 2004;39:75–80.

51. Hofstetter A, Schilling A. [Urinary tract infections caused by hospital infections (nosocomial infections). A long-term study]. Urologe A 1984;23(3):134–40.

52. Bronsema DA, Adams JR, Pallares R, Wenzel RP. Secular trends in rates and etiology of nosocomial urinary tract infections at a university hospital. J Urol 1993;150:414–6.

53. Zhanel GG, Laing NM, Nichol KA, et al. Antibiotic activity against urinary tract infection (UTI) isolates of vancomycin-resistant enterococci (VRE): results from the 2002 North American Vancomycin Resistant Enterococci Susceptibility Study (NAVRESS). J Antimicrob Chemother 2003;52:382–8.

54. Stamm WE, Hooton TM. Management of urinary tract infections in adults. N Engl J Med 1993;329:1328–34.

55. Naeye RL. Causes of the excessive rates of perinatal mortality and prematurity in pregnancies complicated by maternal urinary-tract infections. N Engl J Med 1979;300(15):819–23.

56. Pappas PG. Laboratory in the diagnosis and management of urinary tract infections. Med Clin North Am 1991;75:313–25.

57. Stamm WE, Counts GW, Running KR, et al. Diagnosis of coliform infection in acutely dysuric women. N Engl J Med 1982;307:463–8.

58. Nicolle LE, Ronald AR. Recurrent urinary tract infection in adult women: diagnosis and treatment. Infect Dis Clin North Am 1987;1:793–806.

59. Foxman B, Gillespie B, Koopman J, et al. Risk factors for second urinary tract infection among college women. Am J Epidemiol 2000;151:1194–205.

60. Raz R, Gennesin Y, Wasser J, et al. Recurrent urinary tract infections in postmenopausal women. Clin Infect Dis 2000;30:152–6.

61. Benson M, Jodal U, Agace W, et al. Interleukin (IL)-6 and IL-8 in children with febrile urinary tract infection and asymptomatic bacteriuria. J Infect Dis 1996;174:1080–4.

62. Fairley KF, Carson NE, Gutch RC, et al. Site of infection in acute urinary-tract infection in general practice. Lancet 1971;2:615–8.

63. Hooton, TM, Stamm WE. Acute Pyelonephritis: Symptoms; diagnosis; and treatment. UpToDate 2007. (Accessed March 21st, 2007, at http://www.utdol.com/utd/content/topic.do?topicKey=uti_infe/6922&type=-A&selectedTitle=6~119.)

64. Velasco M, Martinez JA, Moreno-Martinez A, et al. Blood cultures for women with uncomplicated acute pyelonephritis: are they necessary? Clin Infect Dis 2003;37:1127–30.

65. Pasternak ELI, Topinka MA. Blood cultures in pyelonephritis: Do results change therapy? (Abs). Acad Emerg Med 2000;7(10):1170

66. Wing DA, Park AS, Debuque L, Millar LK. Limited clinical utility of blood and urine cultures in the treatment of acute pyelonephritis during pregnancy. Am J Obstet Gynecol 2000;182:1437–40.

67. Thanassi M. Utility of urine and blood cultures in pyelonephritis. Acad Emerg Med 1997;4:797–800.

68. McMurray BR, Wrenn KD, Wright SW. Usefulness of blood cultures in pyelonephritis. Am J Emerg Med 1997;15:137–40.

69. MacMillan MC, Grimes DA. The limited usefulness of urine and blood cultures in treating pyelonephritis in pregnancy. Obstet Gynecol 1991;78:745–8.

70. Lipsky BA. Urinary tract infections in men. Epidemiology, pathophysiology, diagnosis, and treatment. Ann Intern Med 1989;110:138–50.

71. Barnes RC, Daifuku R, Roddy RE, Stamm WE. Urinary-tract infection in sexually active homosexual men. Lancet 1986;1:171–3.

72. Spach DH, Stapleton AE, Stamm WE. Lack of circumcision increases the risk of urinary tract infection in young men. JAMA 1992;267:679–81.

73. Gupta K, Sahm DF, Mayfield D, Stamm WE. Antimicrobial resistance among uropathogens that cause community-acquired urinary tract infections in women: a nationwide analysis. Clin Infect Dis 2001;33:89–94.

74. Warren JW, Abrutyn E, Hebel JR, et al. Guidelines for antimicrobial treatment of uncomplicated acute bacterial cystitis and acute pyelonephritis in women. Infectious Diseases Society of America (IDSA). Clin Infect Dis 1999;29:745–58.

75. Raz P. Urinary tract infection in elderly women. Int J Antimicrob Agents 1998;10:177–9.

76. Warren JW. Catheter-associated urinary tract infections. Int J Antimicrob Agents 2001;17:299–303.

77. Tambyah PA, Maki DG. Catheter-associated urinary tract infection is rarely symptomatic: a prospective study of 1,497 catheterized patients. Arch Intern Med 2000; 160:678–82.

78. Stark RP, Maki DG. Bacteriuria in the catheterized patient. What quantitative level of bacteriuria is relevant? N Engl J Med 1984;311:560–4.

79. Maki DG, Tambyah PA. Engineering out the risk for infection with urinary catheters. Emerg Infect Dis 2001; 7:342–7.

80. Platt R, Polk BF, Murdock B, Rosner B. Mortality associated with nosocomial urinary-tract infection. N Engl J Med 1982;307:637–42.

81. Warren JW. Catheter-associated urinary tract infections. Infect Dis Clin North Am 1997;11:609–22.

82. Platt R, Polk BF, Murdock B, Rosner B. Risk factors for nosocomial urinary tract infection. Am J Epidemiol 1986;124:977–85.

83. Tambyah PA, Maki DG. The relationship between pyuria and infection in patients with indwelling urinary catheters: a prospective study of 761 patients. Arch Intern Med 2000;160:673–7.

84. Tambyah PA, Halvorson KT, Maki DG. A prospective study of pathogenesis of catheter-associated urinary tract infections. Mayo Clin Proc 1999;74:131–6.

85. Daifuku R, Stamm WE. Association of rectal and urethral colonization with urinary tract infection in patients with indwelling catheters. JAMA 1984;252:2028–30.

86. Donlan RM. Biofilms and device-associated infections. Emerg Infect Dis 2001;7:277–81.

87. Stickler D, Young R, Jones G, et al. Why are Foley catheters so vulnerable to encrustation and blockage by crystalline bacterial biofilm? Urol Res 2003;31:306–11.

88. Donlan RM. Biofilms: microbial life on surfaces. Emerg Infect Dis 2002;8:881–90.

89. Stickler DJ, King JB, Winters C, Morris SL. Blockage of urethral catheters by bacterial biofilms. J Infect 1993;27: 133–5.

90. van der Wall E, Verkooyen RP, Mintjes-de Groot J, et al. Prophylactic ciprofloxacin for catheter-associated urinary-tract infection. Lancet 1992;339:946–51.

91. Fridkin SK, Jarvis WR. Epidemiology of nosocomial fungal infections. Clin Microbiol Rev 1996;9:499–511.

92. Febre N, Silva V, Medeiros EA, et al. Microbiological characteristics of yeasts isolated from urinary tracts of intensive care unit patients undergoing urinary catheterization. J Clin Microbiol 1999;37:1584–6.

93. Vazquez JA, Sobel JD. Mucosal candidiasis. Infect Dis Clin North Am 2002;16:793–820, v.

94. Kao AS, Brandt ME, Pruitt WR, et al. The epidemiology of candidemia in two United States cities: results of a population-based active surveillance. Clin Infect Dis 1999;29:1164–70.

95. Abi-Said D, Anaissie E, Uzun O, et al. The epidemiology of hematogenous candidiasis caused by different *Candida* species. Clin Infect Dis 1997;24:1122–8.

96. Pfaller MA. Epidemiology of candidiasis. J Hosp Infect 1995;30 Suppl:329–38.

97. Abbas J, Bodey GP, Hanna HA, et al. *Candida krusei* fungemia. An escalating serious infection in immunocompromised patients. Arch Intern Med 2000;160: 2659–64.

98. Lehner T. Systemic candidiasis and renal involvement. Lancet 1964;41:1414–6.

99. Kauffman CA, Vazquez JA, Sobel JD, et al. Prospective multicenter surveillance study of funguria in hospitalized patients. The National Institute for Allergy and Infectious Diseases (NIAID) Mycoses Study Group. Clin Infect Dis 2000;30:14–8.

100. Rivett AG, Perry JA, Cohen J. Urinary candidiasis: a prospective study in hospital patients. Urol Res 1986;14: 183–6.

101. Sobel JD, Kauffman CA, McKinsey D, et al. Candiduria: a randomized, double-blind study of treatment with fluconazole and placebo. The National Institute of Allergy and Infectious Diseases (NIAID) Mycoses Study Group. Clin Infect Dis 2000;30:19–24.

102. Rex JH, Walsh TJ, Sobel JD, et al. Practice guidelines for the treatment of candidiasis. Infectious Diseases Society of America. Clin Infect Dis 2000;30:662–78.

103. Ostrosky-Zeichner L, Rex JH, Bennett J, Kullberg BJ. Deeply invasive candidiasis. Infect Dis Clin North Am 2002; 16:821–35.

104. Slavin MA, Osborne B, Adams R, et al. Efficacy and safety of fluconazole prophylaxis for fungal infections after marrow transplantation—a prospective, randomized, double-blind study. J Infect Dis 1995;171:1545–52.

105. Goodman JL, Winston DJ, Greenfield RA, et al. A controlled trial of fluconazole to prevent fungal infections in patients undergoing bone marrow transplantation. N Engl J Med 1992;326:845–51.

106. Leung AY, Mak R, Lie AK, et al. Clinicopathological features and risk factors of clinically overt haemorrhagic cystitis complicating bone marrow transplantation. Bone Marrow Transplant 2002;29:509–13.

107. Seber A, Shu XO, Defor T, et al. Risk factors for severe hemorrhagic cystitis following BMT. Bone Marrow Transplant 1999;23:35–40.

108. Bedi A, Miller CB, Hanson JL, et al. Association of BK virus with failure of prophylaxis against hemorrhagic cystitis following bone marrow transplantation. J Clin Oncol 1995;13(5):1103–9.

109. Miyamura K, Takeyama K, Kojima S, et al. Hemorrhagic cystitis associated with urinary excretion of adenovirus type 11 following allogeneic bone marrow transplantation. Bone Marrow Transplant 1989;4:533–5.

110. Vogeli TA, Peinemann F, Burdach S, Ackermann R. Urological treatment and clinical course of BK polyomavirus-associated hemorrhagic cystitis in children after bone marrow transplantation. Eur Urol 1999;36:252–7.

111. Brugieres L, Hartmann O, Travagli JP, et al. Hemorrhagic cystitis following high-dose chemotherapy and bone marrow transplantation in children with malignancies: incidence, clinical course, and outcome. J Clin Oncol 1989;7:194–9.

112. Comar M, D'Agaro P, Andolina M, et al. Hemorrhagic cystitis in children undergoing bone marrow transplantation: a putative role for simian virus 40. Transplantation 2004;78:544–8.

113. Hale GA, Rochester RJ, Heslop HE, et al. Hemorrhagic cystitis after allogeneic bone marrow transplantation in children: clinical characteristics and outcome. Biol Blood Marrow Transplant 2003;9:698–705.

114. El-Zimaity M, Saliba R, Chan K, et al. Hemorrhagic cystitis after allogeneic hematopoietic stem cell transplantation: donor type matters. Blood 2004;103:4674–80.

115. La Rosa AM, Champlin RE, Mirza N, et al. Adenovirus infections in adult recipients of blood and marrow transplants. Clin Infect Dis 2001;32:871–6.

116. Akiyama H, Kurosu T, Sakashita C, et al. Adenovirus is a key pathogen in hemorrhagic cystitis associated with bone marrow transplantation. Clin Infect Dis 2001;32: 1325–30.

117. Brown P, Tsai T, Gajdusek DC. Seroepidemiology of human papovaviruses. Discovery of virgin populations and some unusual patterns of antibody prevalence among remote peoples of the world. Am J Epidemiol 1975;102:331–40.

118. Shah KV, Daniel RW, Warszawski RM. High prevalence of antibodies to BK virus, an SV40-related papovavirus, in residents of Maryland. J Infect Dis 1973;128:784–7.

119. Coleman DV, Gardner SD, Field AM. Human polyomavirus infection in renal allograft recipients. Br Med J 1973;3: 371–5.

120. Coleman DV, Daniel RA, Gardner SD, et al. Polyoma virus in urine during pregnancy. Lancet 1977;2:709–10.

121. Pahari A, Rees L. BK virus-associated renal problems—clinical implications. Pediatr Nephrol 2003;18:743–8.

122. Hirsch HH, Knowles W, Dickenmann M, et al. Prospective study of polyomavirus type BK replication and nephropathy in renal-transplant recipients. N Engl J Med 2002; 347:488–96.

123. Peinemann F, de Villiers EM, Dorries K, et al. Clinical course and treatment of haemorrhagic cystitis associated with BK type of human polyomavirus in nine paediatric recipients of allogeneic bone marrow transplants. Eur J Pediatr 2000;159:182–8.

124. Apperley JF, Rice SJ, Bishop JA, et al. Late-onset hemorrhagic cystitis associated with urinary excretion of polyomaviruses after bone marrow transplantation. Transplantation 1987;43:108–12.

125. Azzi A, Fanci R, Bosi A, et al. Monitoring of polyomavirus BK viruria in bone marrow transplantation patients by DNA hybridization assay and by polymerase chain reaction: an approach to assess the relationship between BK viruria and hemorrhagic cystitis. Bone Marrow Transplant 1994;14:235–40.

126. Leung AY, Suen CK, Lie AK, et al. Quantification of polyoma BK viruria in hemorrhagic cystitis complicating bone marrow transplantation. Blood 2001;98:1971–8.

127. Barouch DH, Faquin WC, Chen Y, et al. BK virus-associated hemorrhagic cystitis in a human immunodeficiency virus-infected patient. Clin Infect Dis 2002;35:326–9.

128. Behzad-Behbahani A, Klapper PE, Vallely PJ, et al. Detection of BK virus and JC virus DNA in urine samples from immunocompromised (HIV-infected) and immunocompetent (HIV-non-infected) patients using polymerase chain reaction and microplate hybridisation. J Clin Virol 2004;29:224–9.

129. Nebuloni M, Tosoni A, Boldorini R, et al. BK virus renal infection in a patient with the acquired immunodeficiency syndrome. Arch Pathol Lab Med 1999;123: 807–11.

130. Ravi R. Endoscopic neodymium:YAG laser treatment of radiation-induced hemorrhagic cystitis. Lasers Surg Med 1994;14:83–7.

131. Gweon P, Shanberg A. Treatment of cyclophosphamide induced hemorrhagic cystitis with neodymium:YAG laser in pediatric patients. J Urol 1997;157:2301–2.

132. Hatakeyama N, Suzuki N, Kudoh T, et al. Successful cidofovir treatment of adenovirus-associated hemorrhagic cystitis and renal dysfunction after allogeneic bone marrow transplant. Pediatr Infect Dis J 2003;22:928–9.

133. Held TK, Biel SS, Nitsche A, et al. Treatment of BK virus-associated hemorrhagic cystitis and simultaneous CMV reactivation with cidofovir. Bone Marrow Transplant 2000;26:347–50.

134. Hoffman JA, Shah AJ, Ross LA, Kapoor N. Adenoviral infections and a prospective trial of cidofovir in pediatric hematopoietic stem cell transplantation. Biol Blood Marrow Transplant 2001;7:388–94.

135. Nagafuji K, Aoki K, Henzan H, et al. Cidofovir for treating adenoviral hemorrhagic cystitis in hematopoietic stem cell transplant recipients. Bone Marrow Transplant 2004;34:909–14.

136. Vianelli N, Renga M, Azzi A, et al. Sequential vidarabine infusion in the treatment of polyoma virus-associated acute haemorrhagic cystitis late after allogeneic bone marrow transplantation. Bone Marrow Transplant 2000; 25:319–20.

49

Urologic Disorders

Glenn A. McDonald, MD
John R. Foringer, MD

Urologic Complications in Cancer

Optimal care of patients with neoplastic disorders requires not only proper therapy but also the anticipation of complications from both primary disease and associated therapeutic interventions. Abnormalities of the urinary tract commonly herald the presence of a neoplastic process or result from its therapy. Common urologic complications associated with neoplastic disorders include hematuria, hemorrhagic cystitis, and urinary obstruction. The presence of these abnormalities is associated with significant prognostic implications as well as management challenges. This chapter will review the salient features of these disorders and their therapy.

Hematuria

Hematuria is the presence of abnormal numbers of red blood cells (RBCs) in the urine. It may present with obvious discoloration of the urine, as in macroscopic (gross hematuria), or with visibly normal urine, as with microscopic hematuria. The pattern of hematuria may be intermittent or persistent. Clinically, hematuria can be divided into two distinct categories, asymptomatic isolated hematuria and symptomatic hematuria. Asymptomatic isolated hematuria presents in the absence of any evidence suggesting the cause or site of the hematuria. Symptomatic hematuria occurs in the presence of associated historical clues, physical signs and symptoms, or abnormal laboratory values. Distinguishing between asymptomatic isolated and symptomatic hematuria can help guide the diagnostic work-up.

Gross hematuria is always associated with urinary tract pathology and commonly presents as red-colored urine. However, red-colored urine is not always caused by hematuria. The ingestion of several foods (rhubarb, beets), drugs (phenolphthalein, phenothiazines, phenindione, phenazopyridine), or in the presence of porphyrins (as in porphyria) may lead to red-colored urine.[1] Thus, in gross hematuria it is necessary to confirm the presence of hematuria by urine dipstick and microscopic evaluation. The urine

dipstick is a colorimetric test to detect free heme. In addition to RBCs, the presence of free hemoglobin (intravascular hemolysis) and myoglobin (rhabdomyolysis) will result in a positive dipstick test.[2] Contamination with iodine-containing products (Betadine) or other oxidizing agents can result in false positive urine results. Ascorbic acid excretion and old (air-exposed) dipsticks have been associated with false negative results.[3] The limitations of the urine dipstick test demonstrate the necessity for microscopic evaluation of urine in the evaluation of hematuria.

Under normal circumstances, people excrete up to 1.2×10^6 red blood cells per day. Hematuria is defined as the presence of RBCs in the urinary tract that exceeds the amount normally found in a fresh urine sample. Since it is impractical to quantitate the number of RBCs over 24 hours, clinically significant hematuria is defined as ≥ 3 RBCs per high-powered field in 2 of 3 properly collected urine specimens.[4] Once the presence of RBCs in the urine has been confirmed, the objective is to identify the site and cause of bleeding. The site of bleeding may originate from any location in the urinary tract, which can be divided into three broad categories: extra renal diseases, non-glomerular renal disease, and glomerular renal disease. The predominant causes of hematuria in cancer patients are most commonly attributed to extra-renal disease and non-glomerular renal disease.

Hematuria Associated with Extra-Renal Disease

In the general population, extra-renal causes of hematuria account for approximately 65% of the cases of hematuria. This percentage is markedly increased in cancer patients. Extra-renal causes of hematuria include uroepithelial neoplasm, benign prostatic hypertrophy, urinary tract infections, and nephrolithiasis (Table 1).

Extra-Renal Neoplasms

Uroepithelial neoplasms include transitional cell carcinoma and squamous cell carcinoma. The incidence of transitional cell carcinoma progressively increases above the age of 35. It is

Table 1 Extrarenal Causes of Hematuria

Neoplasms
Transitional cell carcinoma
Squamous carcinoma
Adenocarcinoma and benign hypertrophy

Infections
Acute cystitis, prostatitis, and urethritis
Tuberculosis
Schistosoma haematobium

Drugs
Anticoagulation (heparin, warfarin)
Cyclophosphamide (hemorrhagic cystitis)

Nephrolithiasis/Crystalluria
Drugs
Uric Acid

Adapted from Lieberthal W, Mesler DM. Hematuria and the acute nephritic syndrome. In: Jacobson HR, Striker GE, Klahr S, editors. The principles and practice of nephrology. 2nd ed. St Louis: Mosby; 1995. p. 102–110.

the fourth leading cause of cancer in men aged 60 to 79 (behind prostate, lung, and colon cancer).[5] The risk factors that are associated with the development of transitional cell carcinoma include age, sex, race, amount of hematuria, tobacco use, toxic exposures, and parasitic infection (Table 2).[6] These tumors occur approximately four times more frequently in men than women and twice as likely in white versus black males. They account for approximately 15 to 20% of the cases of hematuria in adult white men.[7] These tumors are 10 times more likely to occur in the bladder than the renal pelvis. Involvement of the renal pelvis is suggested by the presence of hydronephrosis on renal ultrasonography. The diagnosis of transitional cell carcinoma should be considered in patients with hematuria and a history of heavy tobacco use or exposure to occupational toxins.[8] While transitional cell carcinomas account for the majority of tumors of the bladder, squamous cell carcinoma has been associated with chronic shistosomiasis.[8] Abnormal urine cytology is present in approximately 70 to 80% of the cases of bladder cancer, but is approximately 95% specific. The low sensitivity of urine cytology makes flexible cystoscopy the preferred test to evaluate for neoplasms of the bladder.

Table 2 Factors Associated with an Increased Incidence of Uroepithelial Malignancy

Age
Progressive increase in risk as age rises above 35 yr

Sex
Male > female

Race
Whites > blacks

Hematuria
Gross > microscopic

Exposure to carcinogens
Phenacetin abuse
Pelvic irradiation
Occupational exposures
Aniline dyes
Benezidine (rubber)
Plastic industry

Parasitic infection
Schistosoma haematobium

Adapted from Lieberthal W, Mesler DM. Hematuria and the acute nephritic syndrome. In: Jacobson HR, Striker GE, Klahr S, editors. The principles and practice of nephrology. 2nd ed. St Louis: Mosby; 1995. p. 102–110.

Adenocarcinoma of the prostate is a common cause of hematuria. In contrast to transitional cell carcinoma, the incidence adenocarcinoma of the prostate increases above the age of 45 and is the most common malignancy of the urinary tract in men above the age of 55 (National Cancer Institute (U.S.). Division of Cancer Prevention and Control., 1987 #23). Benign prostatic hypertrophy (BPH) is also associated hematuria.[9] BPH is so prevalent in elderly men that the presence of hematuria merits formal evaluation.

Urinary Tract Infections

Infections of the urinary tract such as urethritis, cystitis, or prostatitis account for approximately 20 to 25% of all cases of hematuria in the general population. Cancer patients are at an increased risk for these infections from both the primary disease and the associated therapy. Three factors that predispose cancer patients to infections of the urinary tract include an obstructive process related to the primary tumor, immunosuppression from chemotherapeutic agents, and the presence of a foreign body (such as a Foley catheter or nephrostomy tube). These infections may present as microscopic or macroscopic hematuria and are associated with pyuria. The presence of hematuria and pyuria should raise suspicion for infection and necessitates obtaining a urine culture. Two infectious organisms that are commonly associated with negative urine cultures are *Chlamydia trachomatis* and *Mycobacterium tuberculosis*.[10,11] It is important to note that other diseases can present with hematuria and pyuria. Three disorders that should be considered are inflammatory glomerulonephritis, interstitial nephritis, and multiple myeloma (myeloma kidney). Unlike infections of the urinary tract, these disorders are commonly associated with renal insufficiency.

Nephrolithiasis/Crystalluria

Nephrolithiasis accounts for 20% of the cases of hematuria in the general population. The classic presentation consists of flank pain, associated with either microscopic or macroscopic hematuria and the presence of crystals in the urine. Cancer patients may develop hematuria associated with crystalluria as a toxic effect from a therapeutic agent. Medications that are associated with crystalluria include sulphadiazine, triamterene, acyclovir, and indivir.[12] Additionally, a sudden rise in the serum uric acid from conditions such as tumor lysis syndrome has been associated with hematuria and uric acid crystaluria.[13]

Non-glomerular Renal Causes of Hematuria

Hematuria in cancer patient may also result from non-glomerular renal disorders. These disorders most commonly arise from the primary neoplasm, such as renal cell carcinoma or a therapeutic intervention (Table 3). The most common causes of hematuria in this category include: renal cell carcinoma, metabolic abnormalities, such as hypercalcemia or hyperuricemia, and coagulopathies.

Table 3 Non-Glomerular Renal Parenchymal Causes of Hematuria

Neoplasms
Renal cell carcinoma
Wilms' tumor
Benign cysts

Vascular
Renal infarct renal vein thrombosis malignant hypertension
Arteriovenous malformation
Papillary necrosis
Loin pain hematuria syndrome

Metabolic
Hypercalciuria
Hyperuricosuria

Familial
Polycystic kidney disease
Medullary sponge kidney

Papillary necrosis
Analgesic abuse
Sickle cell disease and triat
Renal tuberculosis
Diabetes obstructive uropathy

Drugs
Anticoagulants (heparin, warfarin)
Drug induced acute interstitial nephritis

Renal Cell Carcinoma

Renal cell carcinoma (RCC) represents approximately 20% of all urinary tract neoplasms. The incidence of RCC is about half that of transitional cell carcinoma, but has a poorer prognosis, with a 5-year survival of only 60%.[5] The classic triad of hematuria, an abdominal mass, and flank pain are found in less than 5% of cases. The most common presentation of RCC is as asymptomatic hematuria or an incidental finding on an imaging study. Risk factors for RCC include heavy metal, asbestos, and hydrocarbon exposures; tobacco use; and acquired cystic disease in patients with end stage kidney disease.[14] The majority of RCC cases may be part of an autosomal dominant disorder, the von Hippel-Lindau disease resulting from biallelic mutation of the VHL gene.[15] Other clinical features that are commonly associated with RCC include fever, hypertension, erythrocytosis, and hypercalcemia. Renal cell carcinomas are most commonly identified by renal ultrasonography as a solid mass or complex cyst. Computed tomography and magnetic resonance imaging are useful in determining local spread plus renal vein and inferior vena cava involvement, respectively.[16,17]

Hypercalciuria and Hyperuricosuria

Hypercalcemia and hyperuricemia have been demonstrated in cancer patients associated with the neoplasm or related therapeutic interventions.[18] If these conditions lead to hypercalciuria or hyperuricosuria, this may manifest as hematuria.[19] Both conditions would predispose the patient to either calcium or uric acid nephrolithiasis. Treatment for the elevated urine uric acid or calcium (with allopurinol or hydrochlorothiazide, respectively) resolved the hematuria.[19]

Other Causes of Hematuria

Disorders of Coagulation

Hematuria may present, associated with bleeding diathesis. Cancer patients commonly develop bleeding diathesis from abnormalities of the coagulation system related to the neoplastic disease or therapy, and for hypercoagulable states or thrombosis. Hematuria associated with coagulopathic states always requires further evaluation.[20]

Evaluation of Hematuria

Hematuria commonly presents with signs, symptoms, or abnormalities on urinalysis, or with laboratory values that provide clues to the etiology. Thus, the first step in the evaluation of hematuria is a complete history and physical examination. The pattern of hematuria can give insight into the site of bleeding. Prominent hematuria associated with the initiation of the stream suggests a urethral lesion, whereas hematuria at termination is consistent with a bladder bleeding. Hematuria that is present continuously throughout urination is consistent with bladder, ureteral, or renal bleeding. The pattern of hematuria can be confirmed by obtaining a split urine specimen. Features associated with hematuria can often provide clues to the site and/or cause of hematuria. Bleeding from the upper urinary tract may be associated with ureteral casts, which form long serpentine clots compared to broad clots associated with lower urinary tract bleeding. Lower urinary tract bleeding may also present as bright red blood that clears with urination.

Other constellations of symptoms can suggest specific causes of hematuria. The presence of urgency, urinary frequency, and dysuria are commonly present with urinary tract infections. The presence of hematuria with associated unilateral flank pain is suggestive of urinary tract obstruction from renal stone disease. People over the age of 50 who present with hematuria and flank pain should be evaluated for renal cell carcinoma. All men above the age of 50 who present with hematuria should be asked about hesitancy, inability to empty the bladder, and the quality of the urinary stream to investigate for prostatic disease. Finally, in women who menstruate, it is important to rule out the possibility of contamination with RBCs from menstrual blood.

A patient's family history can often provide important clues to the etiology of hematuria. Both polycystic kidney disease and glomerular basement membrane diseases are inherited renal diseases that may present as hematuria. Careful attention to the medication history can be important. Drug-induced interstitial nephritis, cyclophosphamide associated hemorrhagic cystitis, or the presence of anticoagulation may present as hematuria. On physical examination, the presence of a renal mass or evidence of prostate disease on rectal examination, are critical in the evaluation of hematuria. The combination of hypertension, edema, and hematuria are consistent with glomerulonephritis. Hereditary disorders of the glomerular basement membrane are associated with sensory-neural hearing loss and anterior lenticonus. Careful examination of the urine can aid in the evaluation of hematuria. The presence of dysmorphic RBCs (fragmented or distorted), RBC casts, and proteinuria is suggestive of a glomerular disease.

Clinical Approach to Hematuria

Because of the arbitrary nature of the definition of hematuria, it is important to consider the clinical presentation and demographic data of the patient with established hematuria. In the absence of associated symptoms (asymptomatic isolated hematuria) the evaluation is directed by the patient's age (Table 4). Hematuria in asymptomatic patients under the age of 35 years old is very different from those over the age of 35. Glomerular and metabolic disease account for the majority of asymptomatic, isolated hematuria in adults under the age of 35. The evaluation of all patients with isolated hematuria should include renal ultrasonography as an initial imaging study. In patients under the age of 35, a 24-hour urine collection should be obtained to evaluate for metabolic disorders such as hypercalciuria or hyperuricosuria. In the absence of a metabolic cause, the focus of the evaluation turns to glomerular diseases. Specific attention should be paid to the family history for any first-degree relatives with familial glomerular disease. Prior to obtaining a renal biopsy, intravenous pyelography (IVP) should be performed to exclude the rare case of medullary sponge kidney. The incidence of a neoplasm presenting as asymptomatic, isolated hematuria markedly increases above the age of 35. If the initial renal ultrasonography is normal, IVP with nephrotomography should be performed with attention to visualization of the renal pelvis and ureters. Radiolucent filling defects would indicate the presence of a tumor. In the event of an inadequate visualization of the collecting system, retrograde pyelography should be performed. In addition to visualizing the collecting system, cystoscopy is indicated to rule out bladder involvement. If the above imaging studies are normal, urine cytology should be obtained. Urine cytology is abnormal in only 75 to 80% of patients with bladder. If the above evaluation is normal, a work-up for metabolic and glomerular etiologies should be performed.

Hemorrhagic Cystitis

Hemorrhagic cystitis is defined as acute or insidious diffuse vesicular inflammation with hemorrhage.[21] The presence of associated bleeding diathesis due to the cancer or its treatment may exacerbate vesicular bleeding. Gross hematuria commonly requires emergency therapy and palliation. The majority of cases of hemorrhagic cystitis in cancer patients are due to metabolites of chemotherapeutic agents such as cyclophosphamide, bladder injury from radiation therapy, and viral infections in an immunocompromised host (Table 5). Other important causes of bladder hemorrhage that occur in cancer patients (but that will not be discussed) include hemorrhage due to the primary neoplasm; or bacterial, fungal, or parasitic infection associated with an immunosuppressed state.

Drug-Induced Hemorrhagic Cystitis

The urinary tract is exposed to the toxic effects of many therapeutic agents and their metabolites. Many of these agents are concentrated in the urine and have prolonged exposure to the mucosa of the bladder. A prominent example is the oxazaphosphorine alkylating agents that include cyclophosphamide and ifosfamide. Initial experience with these agents was associated with bladder damage manifesting as dysuria, increased urinary frequency, urgency, and microscopic and macroscopic hematuria.[22] Similar effects were subsequently noted with ifosfamide.[23] The incidence of hemorrhagic cystitis in patients receiving high-dose cyclophosphamide therapy has been reported to be as high as 20%—and as high as 8% of those receiving ifosfamide. Hemorrhagic cystitis is associated with a high morbidity and may result in life-threatening vesicular hemorrhage, with reported mortality rates in bone marrow transplantation patients of up to 75%.[24] The toxic effects of these agents commonly occur at the time of, or shortly after, the administration of these agents. Bladder hemorrhage may present later in the course of therapy in patients who are on chronic oral therapy. Other complications with chronic therapy include the development of fibrosis and transitional cell carcinoma of the bladder.[25,26]

It was initially thought that these agents were directly toxic to the vesical mucosa. Work by

Table 4 Major Causes of Asymptomatic Isolated Hematuria

Patients < 35 years old	
Glomerular	IgA nephropathy
	Thin basement membrane disease
	Benign familial hematuria
	Presymptomatic Alport syndrome
Other renal parynchymal disease	Medullary sponge kidney
	Polycystic kidney disease
Metabolic	Hypercalciuria
Hyperuricosuria	
Patients > 35 years old	
Bladder cancer	
Transitional cell carcinoma of the urothelium	
Renal cell carcinoma	

Adapted from Salant DJ. Approach to the patient with asymptomatic isolated hematuria. In Nethrology Rounds. Snell; 2004: 2(5).

Table 5 Causes of Hemorrhagic Cystitis

Major Causes	
Cyclophosphamide	
Radiation	
Viral	
Other Causes	
Drug Toxicity	Busulfan, Thiotepa, Gentian, Contraceptive suppository, Penicillin and Methenamine
Systemic Disease	Amyloidosis
Hemorrhage—primary tumor	

Philips and colleagues, demonstrated that there were no toxic effects with direct exposure of the bladder to these agents.[27] Systemic administration resulted in bladder toxicity within 24 hours of receiving the first dose. Furthermore, untreated animals developed cystitis when urine from treated animals was instilled into their bladder, suggesting the presence of a toxic metabolite. The animals developed transmural edema, mucosal ulceration, and necrosis within 24 hours of administration of cyclophosphamide. The toxicity was dose-dependent and abrogated by inducing a diuresis. Subsequently, the hepatic metabolite of cyclophosphamide, acrolein, has been implicated as the toxic agent.[28,29] In other studies characterizing histologic and cytology features of cyclophosphamide toxicity, edema and hyperemia was noted within 4 hours of administration of a single dose and persisted for up to 36 hours.[25,26] Both increased dosage and repeated exposure are associated with progressive fibrosis.

Patients commonly present with signs of bladder irritation that include dysuria, increased frequency, urgency, and microscopic or gross hematuria. In one study of 100 patients who developed cyclophosphamide-induced hemorrhagic cystitis, microhematuria was present in 93% of the cases; 78% presented with gross hematuria; and 45% had symptoms associated with voiding.[30] Hemorrhage severe enough to require transfusion occurred in 20% of the patients. Bladder hemorrhage occurred after a mean cumulative intravenous dose of 18 g or an oral dose of 90 g. Hemorrhagic cystitis occurred after one dose in three patients. Cystectomy was required in 9 patients, and 10 patients died from uncontrolled bleeding or a complication thereof.[30] The primary clinical risk factor for developing hemorrhagic cystitis is the presence of thrombocytopenia at the time of treatment.[31] It is clear that bladder toxicity is a major limiting factor with the use of these agents. Therefore, effort to prevent or limit this toxicity is of paramount importance.

As mentioned above, initial studies indicated that prehydration with associated diuresis decreased the incidence of bladder hemorrhage.[24,32] Prehydration decreases bladder toxicity by diluting and washing out acrolein, the toxic metabolite of cyclophosphamide. Subsequent studies evaluating the effects of hydration on cyclophosphamide toxicity have been mixed, specifically, in the setting of high-dose therapy and chronic oral therapy.[24,33] A different strategy to limit the toxicity of acrolein is to bind and neutralize its toxic effects. Mesna (2-mercaptoehane sulfonate) is an agent that binds acrolein, limiting its toxicity and thereby allowing maximum therapeutic efficacy of oxazaphosphorine alkylating agents.[34,35] An added benefit of preventing bladder injury will also prevent the subsequent development of transitional cell carcinoma associated with this therapy.[36] In addition to aggressive oral hydration, mesna is given intravenously in doses of 800 mg/m^2 or 20 mg/kg at time of cyclophosphamide administration and every 4 hours for 2 to 3 subsequent doses. To protect against ifosfamide toxicity, patients should receive intravenous hyperhydration and an intravenous bolus of mesna 15 minutes prior to treatment that equals 20% of the ifosfamide dose, and every 4 hours for 2 doses. The total mesna dose should equal 60% of the ifosfamide dose. Mesna can be administered as a continuous infusion at 100% of the ifosfamide dose. Mesna should be continued 4 to 8 hours after the infusion of ifosfamide is complete. In the case of high-dose cyclophosphamide as used in bone marrow transplantation, mesna is given in doses ranging from 60 to 160% of the cyclophosphamide dose by continuous infusion or in 3 to 5 divided doses.[36–39]

Radiation Cystitis

Radiation is a common therapeutic modality employed in the treatment of gynecologic, genitourinary, and rectal cancer. Approximately 20% of the patients who receive pelvic irradiation of these tumors experience some form of bladder toxicity.[40,41] Bladder toxicity most commonly manifests as dysuria, urgency, and increased frequency due to reduced bladder compliance and capacity. Unlike cyclophosphamide toxicity, hematuria may occur months to years after therapy, presenting as microscopic hematuria or life-threatening hemorrhagic cystitis.[42] Hemorrhagic cystitis has been reported in up to 9% of the patients who received full-dose irradiation for genitourinary cancer.[43]

The initial toxic effect of radiation on the bladder is on the vesical mucosa with the development of diffuse mucosal edema. This is followed by the development of vascular telangiectasia, submucosal hemorrhage, and interstitial fibrosis.[21] The long-term consequence of this process is a small fibrotic bladder that is noncompliant. As this process resolves, the greatest danger is the development of obliterative endarteritis leading to ischemia of the vessel wall and hemorrhage.[44] In addition to hemorrhagic cystitis, one study demonstrated that 85% of macroscopic hematuria post-radiation therapy was attributed to recurrent disease.[40] This observation underscores the importance of cystoscopy with any episode of hematuria post-radiation therapy.

Viral Hemorrhagic Cystitis

Hemorrhagic cystitis in cancer patients associated with viral infection has been predominantly seen in the bone marrow transplantation population. Viral-induced hemorrhagic cystitis was initially noted in the mid-1970s, when an outbreak of adenovirus type II was associated with urinary symptoms and gross hematuria in immunocompetent children.[45,46] Adenovirus II has been recovered from the urine of patients who developed hemorrhagic cystitis after marrow transplantation.[47] Additionally, the BK type of human polyomavirus has been implicated in the development of hemorrhagic cystitis in the bone marrow transplantation population.[48] BK virus is indigenous in the general population and persists in a latent form in the kidney following a primary infection.[49] Subsequent immunosuppression (bone marrow transplantation) activates the latent virus resulting in viruria.[50] In a prospective study of patients undergoing marrow transplantation, BK virus was found in the urine in 55% of patient with hemorrhagic cystitis, compared to 11% who had no cystitis.[51] Furthermore, Priftakis and colleagues demonstrated that greater than 1×10^4 copies/µL by real time polymerase chain reaction was associated with an increased risk of hemorrhagic cystitis.[52] The use of cyclophosphamide in the preparation for transplantation has been associated with persistent BK viruria and hemorrhagic cystitis.[53] In light of the role of the BK virus in hemorrhagic cystitis in this patient population, DNA gyrase inhibitors such as vidarabine are being incorporated in the uroprotective regimen.[54]

Treatment

The best treatment for any disorder is prevention. Appropriate uroprotective regimens, as outlined for cyclophosphamide-induced hemorrhagic cystitis above, are critical for optimal therapy. The two clinical issues in the treatment of acute hemorrhagic cystitis are urinary obstruction due to clot formation and ongoing bladder hemorrhage. Dissolution of formed clots is accomplished by intermittent or constant bladder irrigation with water, or antibiotic-containing saline or endoscopic clot evacuation. Ongoing diffuse hemorrhage after clot removal is an indication for either systemic or intravesical administration of various hemostatic agents. These agents include aminocaproic acid, silver nitrate, alum, prostaglandins, and formalin (Table 6). In extreme cases, vascular

Table 6 Therapeutic Agents for Hemorrhagic Cystitis
Bladder Irrigation/Clot Evacuation—simple vs continuous
Aminocaproic Acid
Silver Nitrate
Alum
Hyperbaric Oxygen
Formalin
Hypogastric artery embolization
Open cystotomy with bladder packing
Cystectomy with urinary diversion

embolization and emergency cystectomy are utilized to avoid exsanguination.

The initial therapeutic approach to hemorrhagic cystitis consists of clot evacuation with bladder irrigation. Commonly removing clots and decompressing the bladder will decrease or resolve bladder hemorrhage.[55] This process is usually carried out with a multichannel catheter with intermittent or constant irrigation with water or antibiotic-containing saline. Continuous bedside irrigation for recalcitrant clots can result in increased intravesical pressure and bladder rupture.[55] Clots that have been present for many hours may require mechanical disruption under direct visualization with an endoscope. Direct visualization offers the additional advantage of cauterizing any focal site of bleeding.

ε-Aminocaproic acid, an inhibitor of plasminogen activator substances, promotes hemostasis in hemorrhagic cystitis by inhibiting fibrinolysis.[56] Aminocaproic acid has the untoward effect of increasing the density of existing clots, further complicating their disolution.[57] Thus, it is important to make every effort to remove any existing clots prior to treatment with this agent. It is administered either intravenously or orally, with a maximal effect seen at 8 to 12 hours. The use of this agent is contraindicated in patients with upper tract bleeding in the presence of ureteral reflux.[58] It has also been associated with severe hypotension.[58]

The intravesical instillation of silver nitrate has been used to treat diffuse bladder hemorrhage.[59] This agent is instilled for 10 to 20 minutes and may require several treatments. In one study, silver nitrate was associated with a 68% success rates in stopping bladder hemorrhage.[60] Unfortunately, follow-up studies have been associated with short-term efficacy with recurrent bleeding rates of up to 80% at 2 years. Additionally, precipitation of silver salts in the urinary tract has resulted in functional obstruction and renal failure.[61]

Alum is an ammonium or potassium salt of aluminum which can be administered without anesthesia for hemorrhagic cystitis.[62,63] Continuous irrigation of a 1% solution is used to chemically cauterize the bladder. Continuous infusion for an average of 21 hours is required to achieve optimal outcomes. Allergic reactions have been reported, requiring termination of therapy. Alum is reportedly not absorbed by the bladder mucosa but has been associated with increased serum aluminum levels with encephalopathy.[63–65] Prostaglandin E_2 and $F_{2\alpha}$ are normally present in the bladder and have been reported to improve healing of the microvasculature and epithelium, inhibit edema, and have a protective effect on mucosal ulceration.[66,67] When instilled in the bladder, both have been demonstrated to control intractable bladder hemorrhage.[66,68] Severe

bladder spasms have limited the therapeutic efficacy of these agents.

Hyperbaric oxygen is a noninvasive form of therapy for hemorrhagic cystitis. Successful treatment of radiation-induced bone necrosis initiated the evaluation of hyperbaric oxygen in radiation-induced hemorrhagic cystitis. In multiple studies, hyperbaric oxygen therapy has resulted in the reversal of hematuria in patients with radiation-induced cystitis.[44,69] In subsequent studies, this therapy has proven effective in cyclophosphamide-induced hemorrhagic cystitis.[70] Hyperbaric oxygen is thought to promote wound healing in areas of the bladder where perfusion is limited due to scar tissue.

Formalin, the aqueous solution of formaldehyde, is the most effective local treatment for intractable bladder hemorrhage.[71] It is used in tissue preparation for its ability to rapidly crosslink proteins and fix tissues. Intravesical administration of formalin rapidly crosslinks proteins on the bladder mucosa, preventing further tissue necrosis, breakdown, and bleeding. It has been reported to be effective in alleviating bladder hemorrhage in up to 80% of the cases.[71] Unlike alum and the prostaglandins, the administration of formalin requires general or regional anesthesia due to the pain associated with instillation. Adverse effects of formalin administration are related to its ability to fix tissue. Formalin is administered in the reverse Trendelenburg's position to decrease the chance of reflux of formalin in the ureters resulting in fibrosis and hydronephrosis.[72]

Selective vascular embolization has been utilized to control massive bleeding from the bladder. Bleeding from virtually any site involving the bladder or prostate can be addressed by

selective embolization of the hypogastric artery.[73,74] This approach is commonly used in patients with refractory bladder hemorrhage and in patients who are not operative candidates and are medically unstable. Occluding the hypogastric artery may result in transient ischemia of the gluteal muscles, transient unilateral lower limb paralysis, and bladder necrosis.[75,76]

In cases where the above modalities have failed to control the bleeding, open cystotomy with bladder packing or cystectomy with urinary diversion may be required to avoid exsanguinations.[77,78] Surgical intervention under these circumstances is associated with high morbidity and mortality rates due to hemodynamic instability at the time of the procedure. The primary goal of these procedures is to gain hemodynamic instability. While most patients who undergo surgical intervention for bladder hemorrhage require urinary diversion, every effort should be made to avoid cystectomy in favor of bladder reconstruction.

Clinical Approach to Hemorrhagic Cystitis

The therapeutic strategy in hemorrhagic cystitis is predicated on the severity of the bleeding. Devries and Freiha suggested dividing hemorrhage in three categories: mild, moderate, and severe (Table 7).[21] Mild hemorrhage is controlled by simple measures, such as bladder irrigation with water or saline, silver nitrate, alum, and aminocaproic acid. Moderate bladder hemorrhage results in a decrease in hemoglobin requiring 6 units or less of packed red blood cells over several days. Urinary obstruction due to clot formation is a common complication of this level of bleeding.

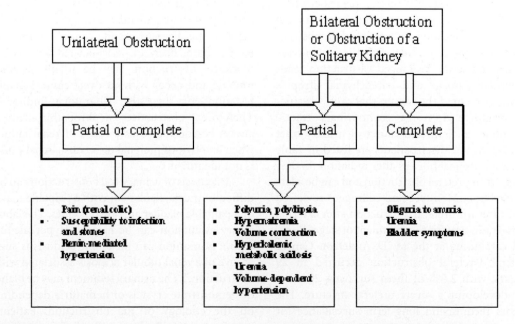

FIGURE 1 Adapted from Schrier R. Atlas of diseases of the kidney. Current Medicine, Inc.; 1999.

Table 7	Therapeutic Approach to Hemorrhagic Cystitis

Mild Hemorrhage
Bladder irrigation/clot removal
Silver nitrate
Alum
Aminocaproic acid

Moderate hemorrhage
Bladder irrigation/clot removal
Silver nitrate
Alum
Aminocaproic acid
Formalin

Severe hemorrhage
Bladder irrigation/clot removal
Aminocaproic acid
Formalin
Hypogastric artery embolization
Surgical intervention

Table 8	Causes of Obstruction in Cancer Patients

Intratubular obstruction
Uric acid crystals from tumor lysis syndrome
Methotrexate
Light chains from multiple myeloma
Acyclovir crystals

Ureteral obstruction
Stones
Blood clot
Sloughed renal papillae
Uric acid
Iatrogenic ligation
Extrinsic compression
  Abscess
  Hemorrhage
  Tumor (lymphoma)
Radiation induced strictures
Transitional cell cancer

Bladder Neck Obstruction
Stones
Hemorrhagic cystitis (cyclophosphamide, holmium)
Prostatic hypertrophy
Bladder carcinoma
Neurogenic bladder (spinal cord compression)

Urethral Obstruction
Stricture
Tumor

Evacuation and prevention of clot formation is the first goal of therapy. Intravesical instillation of aminocaproic acid, alum, or silver nitrate should be considered first-line agents to control this level of bleeding. In resistant cases, the instillation of a diluted formaldehyde solution or an open surgical procedure. Severe hematuria is defined as continued hemorrhage that does not resolve with simple irrigation, instillations, or aminocaproic acid, and requiring greater than 6 units of packed red blood cells. In this clinical setting, formalin appears to have the best chance of controlling intractable hemorrhage.

Obstructive (Postrenal) Nephropathy

Urinary tract obstruction is a relatively common cause of renal failure in patients with malignancy. Regardless of cause, obstruction of urinary flow leads to renal impairment, which, early in the course of the condition, is reversible if the obstruction is alleviated. Tubular function is initially affected; however, prolonged obstruction leads to tubular damage and parenchymal atrophy. Seventy percent of the cancers that cause obstruction originate from the genitourinary tract.[55] Commonly encountered causes of urinary tract obstruction in cancer patients are listed in Table 8. Retroperitoneal fibrosis after radiation therapy can result in ureteral obstruction and can be a late complication. McIntyre and colleagues reviewed 1,784 cases for ureteral obstruction after external beam irradiation for the treatment of stage IB cervical carcinoma at the M. D. Anderson Cancer Center.[79] Ureteral obstruction occurred in 29 patients, with 2.5% of them surviving 20 years after developing a severe ureteral stricture. The authors recommend long-term surveillance for late onset ureteral obstruction.

Clinical manifestations of urinary tract obstruction vary, depending on the location, duration, and degree of obstruction. In patients with complete bilateral obstruction or with an obstructed solitary kidney, anuria (<50 mL of urine output in 24 hours) can be the presenting feature, whereas, in patients with partial obstruction, the urinary output can vary from oliguria to polyuria. In a review of 50 patients with acute renal failure secondary to bilateral ureteral obstruction, 76% had a malignancy as the cause, and half of these patients presented with uremia prior to the diagnosis of the cancer.[80] Although pain is more likely to be associated with acute blockage, obstruction may be totally asymptomatic and occur without overt clinical manifestations or suggestive laboratory findings.[81] Therefore, obstructive nephropathy should always be considered as a cause of renal failure when an obvious prerenal or intrinsic renal cause is not identified.

Diagnosis of urinary tract obstruction can be difficult. Anuria, flank pain with a palpable mass, or a palpable bladder are obvious clues. The laboratory evaluation can be helpful. Hyperkalemia with a non-anion gap metabolic acidosis is suggestive of a renal tubular acidosis associated with obstruction.[82] The urinary sediment may be bland or demonstrate crystals or hematuria depending on the etiology of the obstruction. Patients may have very dilute urine due to the presence of an acquired form of nephrogenic diabetes insipidus.[83]

Ultrasonography is the most useful test to evaluate for the presence of obstruction. Although hydronephrosis is usually demonstrated, there are circumstances when hydronephrosis is not seen, despite urinary tract obstruction: (1) early in the course of obstruction (12 to 24 hours), when the collecting system is relatively noncompliant; (2) in the face of severe volume depletion, when glomerular filtration is severely depressed; and (3) when the collecting system is encased by retroperitoneal lymphadenopathy or fibrosis. Conversely, the finding of hydronephrosis on ultrasonography does not prove the presence of obstruction since it is also seen in high urinary flow states, such as diuretic use and diabetes insipidus, pregnancy, previous obstruction, and congenital megaureter. The lack of functional obstruction can be verified in these cases by a normal renal scan with furosemide-washout. In this test an intravenously injected radioisotope will collect in the dilated collecting system but be promptly excreted by the increased urinary flow induced by the diuretic.

Once obstruction is identified, it should be corrected with either percutaneous nephrostomy tubes or ureteral stenting, depending on local expertise and availability. The duration and severity of obstruction are the major determinants for the recovery of renal function after its correction. The longer the duration of obstruction, the less likely are the chances for complete renal recovery. In the past, open surgical procedures carried a high major complication rate, and now, both percutaneous and cystoscopic techniques are used to decompress obstructed kidneys with greater safety. Relative indications to proceed with percutaneous nephrostomy tube placement include large intravesicular tumors, large prostate tumors, tortuous ureters, more than one site of obstruction, or long occlusions.[84] An internal Double-J stent should be placed after decompression of the collecting system. Antegrade placement of the stent can be done using the nephrostomy tube. Metallic, self-expanding stents are now being used, often in conjunction with Double-J stents to avoid percutaneous nephrostomy tubes.[85–87] If the stent fails rapidly or cystoscopic management of the stent cannot be done, nephrostomy tubes may be permanent or an internal-external stent may be used.

Although renal function can be rapidly regained with percutaneous nephrostomy tubes or ureteral stents, the long-term prognosis for patients who develop obstructive uropathy from metastatic or locally advanced tumors is poor. Donat and Russo from the Memorial Sloan Kettering Cancer Center reported the outcomes of 78 patients treated for ureteral obstruction from locally advanced or metastatic non-urologic tumors.[88] From the time of the first ureteral decompression, the median survival for all patients was 6.8 months. Fifty percent of the patients had a complication related to the placement of the percutaneous nephrostomy tubes or stents. In a report of 103 patients with advanced malignancies undergoing palliative urinary diversion, the average survival was 5 months with a complication rate of 63%.[89] It has been recommended that decompression procedures not be performed in patients with metastatic gastric and pancreatic cancer because the median survival is only 1.4 months after the procedure.[55,88]

Post-Obstructive Diuresis

Post-obstructive diuresis occurs when there is correction of complete bilateral obstruction or complete obstruction of a solitary kidney. It involves the production of a large volume of urine that results from a defect in urinary concentrating ability, impaired reabsorption of urinary sodium, and solute diuresis from retained urea and intravenous administration of sodium-containing solutions. Patients with relief of complete obstruction who are at risk for developing post-obstructive diuresis should be carefully monitored. It has been recommended, for patients without pulmonary edema, congestive heart failure, or altered consciousness from uremia, that urine losses be replaced by oral intake.[90] Replacement fluids are given only if the patients develop orthostatic hypotension, tachycardia, hyponatremia, or a urine output more than 200 mL/hr. On the other hand, in high-risk patients with altered sensorium, congestive heart failure, or pulmonary edema, replacement of half the hourly urine output with half-normal saline has been recommended. If the patient is hyponatremic, normal saline should be used instead.[55,90]

REFERENCES

1. Paola AS. Hematuria: essentials of diagnosis. Hosp Pract (Off Ed) 1990;25:144–52.
2. Sutton JM. Evaluation of hematuria in adults. JAMA 1990;263:2475–80.
3. Tomson C, Porter T. Asymptomatic microscopic or dipstick haematuria in adults: which investigations for which patients? A review of the evidence. BJU Int 2002;90:185–98.
4. Massry SG, Glassock RJ. Massry & Glassock's textbook of nephrology. Philadelphia: Lippincott Williams & Wilkins; 2001. pp. xl, 2072.
5. Jemal A, Murray T, Samuels A, et al. Cancer statistics, 2003. CA Cancer J Clin 2003;53:5–26.
6. Pashos CL, Botteman MF, Laskin BL, Redaelli A. Bladder cancer: epidemiology, diagnosis, and management. Cancer Pract 2002;10:311–22.
7. Cohen SM, Shirai T, Steineck G. Epidemiology and etiology of premalignant and malignant urothelial changes. Scand J Urol Nephrol Suppl 2000;105–15.
8. Marcus PM, Hayes RB, Vineis P, et al. Cigarette smoking, N-acetyltransferase 2 acetylation status, and bladder cancer risk: a case-series meta-analysis of a gene-environment interaction. Cancer Epidemiol Biomarkers Prev 2000;9:461–7.
9. Kearney MC, Bingham JB, Bergland R, et al. Clinical predictors in the use of finasteride for control of gross hematuria due to benign prostatic hyperplasia. J Urol 2002;167:2489–91.
10. Wathne B, Hovelius B, Mardh PA. Causes of frequency and dysuria in women. Scand J Infect Dis 1987;19:223–9.
11. Christensen WI. Genitourinary tuberculosis: review of 102 cases. Medicine (Baltimore) 1974;53:377–90.
12. Fogazzi GB. Crystalluria: a neglected aspect of urinary sediment analysis. Nephrol Dial Transplant 1996;11:379–87.
13. Davidson MB, Thakkar S, Hix JK, et al. Pathophysiology, clinical consequences, and treatment of tumor lysis syndrome. Am J Med 2004;116:546–54.
14. Jonasch E. GDJ, Atkins MB. Renal neoplasia. In: Brenner BM, editor. Brenner and Rector's the kidney. Philadelphia: Saunders; 2004. p. 1895–923.
15. Maher ER, Yates JR, Harries R, et al. Clinical features and natural history of von Hippel-Lindau disease. Q J Med 1990;77:1151–63.
16. Ergen FB, Hussain HK, Caoili EM, et al. MRI for preoperative staging of renal cell carcinoma using the 1997 TNM classification: comparison with surgical and pathologic staging. AJR Am J Roentgenol 2004;182:217–25.
17. Wehle MJ, Thiel DD, Petrou SP, et al. Conservative management of incidental contrast-enhancing renal masses as safe alternative to invasive therapy. Urology 2004;64:49–52.
18. Flombaum CD. Metabolic emergencies in the cancer patient. Semin Oncol 2000;27:322–34.
19. Andres A, Praga M, Bello I, et al. Hematuria due to hypercalciuria and hyperuricosuria in adult patients. Kidney Int 1989;36:96–9.
20. Brigden ML. When bleeding complicates oral anticoagulant therapy. How to anticipate, investigate, and treat. Postgrad Med 1995;98:153–65.
21. deVries CR, Freiha FS. Hemorrhagic cystitis: a review. J Urol 1990;143:1–9.
22. Rubin JS, Rubin RT. Cyclophosphamide hemorrhagic cystitis. J Urol 1966;96:313–6.
23. Cohen MH, Creaven PJ, Tejada F, et al. Phase I clinical trial of isophosphamide (NSC-109724). Cancer Chemother Rep 1975;59:751–5.
24. Droller MJ, Saral R, Santos G. Prevention of cyclophosphamide-induced hemorrhagic cystitis. Urology 1982;20:256–8.
25. Forni AM, Koss LG, Geller W. Cytological study of the effect of cyclophosphamide on the epithelium of the urinary bladder in man. Cancer 1964;17:1348–55.
26. Koss LG. A light and electron microscopic study of the effects of a single dose of cyclophosphamide on various organs in the rat. I. The urinary bladder. Lab Invest 1967;16:44–65.
27. Philips FS, Sternberg SS, Cronin AP, Vidal, PM. Cyclophosphamide and urinary bladder toxicity. Cancer Res 1961;21:1577.
28. Cox PJ. Cyclophosphamide cystitis—identification of acrolein as the causative agent. Biochem Pharmacol 1979;28:2045–9.
29. Brade WP, Herdrich K, Varini M. Ifosfamide—pharmacology, safety and therapeutic potential. Cancer Treat Rev 1985;12:1–47.
30. Stillwell TJ, Benson RC Jr. Cyclophosphamide-induced hemorrhagic cystitis. A review of 100 patients. Cancer 1988;61:451–7.
31. Brugieres L, Hartmann O, Travagli JP, et al. Hemorrhagic cystitis following high-dose chemotherapy and bone marrow transplantation in children with malignancies: incidence, clinical course, and outcome. J Clin Oncol 1989;7:194–9.
32. Shepherd JD, Pringle LE, Barnett MJ, et al. Mesna versus hyperhydration for the prevention of cyclophosphamide-induced hemorrhagic cystitis in bone marrow transplantation. J Clin Oncol 1991;9:2016–20.
33. Hows JM, Mehta A, Ward L, et al. Comparison of mesna with forced diuresis to prevent cyclophosphamide induced haemorrhagic cystitis in marrow transplantation: a prospective randomised study. Br J Cancer 1984;50:753–6.
34. Skinner R, Sharkey IM, Pearson AD, Craft AW. Ifosfamide, mesna, and nephrotoxicity in children. J Clin Oncol 1993;11:173–90.
35. Freedman A, Ehrlich RM, Ljung BM. Prevention of cyclophosphamide cystitis with 2-mercaptoethane sulfonate: a histologic study. J Urol 1984;132:580–2.
36. Schmahl D, Habs MR. Prevention of cyclophosphamide-induced carcinogenesis in the urinary bladder of rats by administration of mesna. Cancer Treat Rev 1983;10 Suppl A:57–61.
37. Burkert H. Clinical overview of mesna. Cancer Treat Rev 1983;10 Suppl A:175–81.
38. Brock N, Pohl J, Stekar J. Detoxification of urotoxic oxazaphosphorines by sulfhydryl compounds. J Cancer Res Clin Oncol 1981;100:311–20.
39. Ehrlich RM, Freedman A, Goldsobel AB, Stiehm ER. The use of sodium 2-mercaptoethane sulfonate to prevent cyclophosphamide cystitis. J Urol 1984;131:960–2.
40. Dean RJ, Lytton B. Urologic complications of pelvic irradiation. J Urol 1978;119:64–7.
41. Schellhammer PF, Jordan GH, el-Mahdi AM. Pelvic complications after interstitial and external beam irradiation of urologic and gynecologic malignancy. World J Surg 1986;10:259–68.
42. McGuire EJ, Weiss RM, Schiff M Jr, Lytton B. Hemorrhagic radiation cystitis. Treatment. Urology 1974;3:204–8.
43. Ram MD. Complications of radiotherapy for carcinoma of the bladder. Proc R Soc Med 1970;63:93–5.
44. Schoenrock GJ, Cianci P. Treatment of radiation cystitis with hyperbaric oxygen. Urology 1986;27:271–2.
45. Mufson MA, Belshe RB. A review of adenoviruses in the etiology of acute hemorrhagic cystitis. J Urol 1976;115:191–4.
46. Numazaki Y, Kumasaka T, Yano N, et al. Further study on acute hemorrhagic cystitis due to adenovirus type II. N Engl J Med 1973;289:344–7.
47. Ambinder RF, Burns W, Forman M, et al. Hemorrhagic cystitis associated with adenovirus infection in bone marrow transplantation. Arch Intern Med 1986;146:1400–1.
48. Rice SJ, Bishop JA, Apperley J, Gardner SD. BK virus as cause of haemorrhagic cystitis after bone marrow transplantation. Lancet 1985;2:844–5.
49. Shah KV, Daniel RW, Warszawski RM. High prevalence of antibodies to BK virus, an SV40-related papovavirus, in residents of Maryland. J Infect Dis 1973;128:784–7.
50. Heritage J, Chesters PM, McCance DJ. The persistence of papovavirus BK DNA sequences in normal human renal tissue. J Med Virol 1981;8:143–50.
51. Arthur RR, Shah KV, Baust SJ, et al. Association of BK viruria with hemorrhagic cystitis in recipients of bone marrow transplants. N Engl J Med 1986;315:230–4.
52. Priftakis P, Bogdanovic G, Kokhaei P, et al. BK virus (BKV) quantification in urine samples of bone marrow transplanted patients is helpful for diagnosis of hemorrhagic cystitis, although wide individual variations exist. J Clin Virol 2003;26:71–7.
53. Bedi A, Miller CB, Hanson JL, et al. Association of BK virus with failure of prophylaxis against hemorrhagic cystitis following bone marrow transplantation. J Clin Oncol 1995;13:1103–9.
54. Chapman C, Flower AJ, Durrant ST. The use of vidarabine in the treatment of human polyomavirus associated acute haemorrhagic cystitis. Bone Marrow Transplant 1991;7:481–3.
55. Russo P. Urologic emergencies in the cancer patient. Semin Oncol 2000;27:284–98.
56. Aroney RS, Dalley DN, Levi JA. Haemorrhagic cystitis treated with epsilon-aminocaproic acid. Med J Aust 1980;2:92.
57. Covey WG. Epsilon-aminocaproic acid therapy in cyclophosphamide-induced bladder hemorrhage. A case report. Conn Med 1971;35:160–3.
58. Pitts TO, Spero JA, Bontempo FA, Greenberg A. Acute renal failure due to high-grade obstruction following therapy with epsilon-aminocaproic acid. Am J Kidney Dis 1986;8:441–4.
59. Kumar AP, Wrenn EL Jr, Jayalakshmamma B, et al. Silver nitrate irrigation to control bladder hemorrhage in children receiving cancer therapy. J Urol 1976;116:85–6.
60. Jerkins GR, Noe HN, Hill DE. An unusual complication of silver nitrate treatment of hemorrhagic cystitis: case report. J Urol 1986;136:456–8.
61. Raghavaiah NV, Soloway MS. Anuria following silver nitrate irrigation for intractable bladder hemorrhage. J Urol 1977;118:681–2.
62. Kennedy C, Snell ME, Witherow RO. Use of alum to control intractable vesical haemorrhage. Br J Urol 1984;56:673–5.
63. Goel AK, Rao MS, Bhagwat AG, et al. Intravesical irrigation with alum for the control of massive bladder hemorrhage. J Urol 1985;133:956–7.
64. Ostroff EB, Chenault OW Jr. Alum irrigation for the control of massive bladder hemorrhage. J Urol 1982;128:929–30.
65. Kavoussi LR, Gelstein LD, Andriole GL. Encephalopathy and an elevated serum aluminum level in a patient receiving

intravesical alum irrigation for severe urinary hemorrhage. J Urol 1986;136:665–7.

66. Mohiuddin J, Prentice HG, Schey S, et al. Treatment of cyclophosphamide-induced cystitis with prostaglandin E2. Ann Intern Med 1984;101:142.

67. Jeremy JY, Tsang V, Mikhailidis DP, et al. Eicosanoid synthesis by human urinary bladder mucosa: pathological implications. Br J Urol 1987;59:36–9.

68. Shurafa M, Shumaker E, Cronin S. Prostaglandin F2-alpha bladder irrigation for control of intractable cyclophosphamide-induced hemorrhagic cystitis. J Urol 1987;137:1230–1.

69. Weiss JP, Boland FP, Mori H, et al. Treatment of radiation-induced cystitis with hyperbaric oxygen. J Urol 1985;134:352–4.

70. Yazawa H, Nakada T, Sasagawa I, et al. Hyperbaric oxygenation therapy for cyclophosphamide-induced haemorrhagic cystitis. Int Urol Nephrol 1995;27:381–5.

71. Kumar S, Rosen P, Grabstald H. Intravesical formalin for the control of intractable bladder hemorrhage secondary to cystitis or cancer. J Urol 1975;114:540–3.

72. Bright JF, Tosi SE, Crichlow RW, Selikowitz SM. Prevention of vesicoureteral reflux with Fogarty catheters during formalin therapy. J Urol 1977;118:950–2.

73. Schuhrke TD, Barr JW. Intractable bladder hemorrhage: therapeutic angiographic embolization of the hypogastric arteries. J Urol 1976;116:523–5.

74. Lang EK, Deutsch JS, Goodman JR, et al. Transcatheter embolization of hypogastric branch arteries in the management of intractable bladder hemorrhage. J Urol 1979;121:30–6.

75. Braf ZF, Koontz WW Jr. Gangrene of bladder. Complication of hypogastric artery embolization. Urology 1977;9:670–1.

76. Carmignani G, Belgrano E, Puppo P, et al. Transcatheter embolization of the hypogastric arteries in cases of bladder hemorrhage from advanced pelvic cancers: followup in 9 cases. J Urol 1980;124:196–200.

77. Golin AL, Benson RC Jr. Cyclophosphamide hemorrhagic cystitis requiring urinary diversion. J Urol 1977;118:110–1.

78. Pomer S, Karcher G, Simon W. Cutaneous ureterostomy as last resort treatment of intractable haemorrhagic cystitis following radiation. Br J Urol 1983;55:392–4.

79. McIntyre JF, Eifel PJ, Levenback C, Oswald MJ. Ureteral stricture as a late complication of radiotherapy for stage IB carcinoma of the uterine cervix. Cancer 1995;75:836–43.

80. Norman RW, Mack FG, Awad SA, et al. Acute renal failure secondary to bilateral ureteric obstruction: review of 50 cases. Can Med Assoc J 1982;127:601–4.

81. Klahr S. Obstructive nephropathy. Kidney Int 1998;54:286–300.

82. Batlle DC, Arruda JA, Kurtzman NA. Hyperkalemic distal renal tubular acidosis associated with obstructive uropathy. N Engl J Med 1981;304:373–80.

83. Schlueter W, Batlle DC. Chronic obstructive nephropathy. Semin Nephrol 1988;8:17–28.

84. Dyer RB, Assimos DG, Regan JD. Update on interventional uroradiology. Urol Clin North Am 1997;24:623–52.

85. vanSonnenberg E, D'Agostino HB, O'Laoide R, et al. Malignant ureteral obstruction: treatment with metal stents—technique, results, and observations with percutaneous intraluminal US. Radiology 1994;191:765–8.

86. Wakui M, Takeuchi S, Isioka J, et al. Metallic stents for malignant and benign ureteric obstruction. BJU Int 2000;85:227–32.

87. Tekin MI, Aytekin C, Aygun C, et al. Covered metallic ureteral stent in the management of malignant ureteral obstruction: preliminary results. Urology 2001;58:919–23.

88. Donat SM, Russo P. Ureteral decompression in advanced nonurologic malignancies. Ann Surg Oncol 1996;3:393–9.

89. Shekarriz B, Shekarriz H, Upadhyay J, et al. Outcome of palliative urinary diversion in the treatment of advanced malignancies. Cancer 1999;85:998–1003.

90. Vaughan ED Jr, Gillenwater JY. Diagnosis, characterization and management of post-obstructive diuresis. J Urol 1973;109:286–92.

Ischemic Heart Disease in Cancer Patients

Atiar M. Rahman, MD, PhD

Table 1 Definitions

Acute coronary syndromes	A spectrum of clinical conditions encompassing ST segment elevation and non-ST segment elevation (unstable angina and non-Q wave myocardial infarction) myocardial infarction
Unstable angina	Ischaemic-type chest pain which is of recent origin; is more frequent, severe, or prolonged than the patient's usual angina; is more difficult to control with drugs; or is occurring at rest or minimal exertion; cardiac enzyme concentrations are not raised
Non-Q wave myocardial infarction	Myocardial infarction (increase in cardiac enzyme concentrations to greater than twice the upper limit of normal) occurring without the subsequent development of new Q waves on the 12 lead electrocardiogram
ST elevation myocardial infarction	Myocardial infarction with ST segment elevation on the presenting electrocardiogram

Epidemiology

Collectively, cardiovascular disease, and cancer account for approximately two-thirds of all deaths in the United States.[1] Coronary artery disease (CAD) is the leading cause of death in the Western world, being responsible for about 1,400,000 annual deaths in the United States alone.[2] Similarly, cancer is second only to cardiovascular diseases as a cause of mortality and accounts for about one-quarter of all deaths in developed countries. In the United States, more than 563,700 people died from cancer in 2004.[3] About 1.37 million new cases of cancer would have been diagnosed in 2004 alone not including in situ (pre-invasive) cancer or the more than one million cases of non-melanomatous skin cancer. Cancer and CAD are true global health problems, although both disease states have often been regarded as a problem belonging principally to the developed world. In reality, more than half of all cancers occur in developing countries; and more than 80% of the global burden of cardiovascular disease occurs in low-income and middle-income countries.[4] The lifelong probability of developing cancer is 45% for men and 38% for women,[5] while the lifelong probability of developing CAD is 49% for men and 32% for women.[6] Indeed, cancer will become the leading cause of death in many countries early in this century. Worldwide there will be more than 30 million people living with cancer by 2015. The increasingly long survival of cancer patients raises a question as to whether there might be an associa-

tion between coronary disease and different types of cancer, since, as with many cancers, the prevalence of CAD is age-dependent, and these different diseases share some of the same risk factors (such as smoking). The attributable risk of age to coronary heart disease and cancer is significant and increases with age: the annual rate of first cardiovascular events in men aged 35 to 44 years of 7 in 1,000 increases almost tenfold to 68 in 1,000 for those aged greater than 85 years (for women, comparable rates occur 10 years later in life).[6] Although no definitive relationship is known to exist between cancer and CAD, in one retrospective autopsy study of 1,642 cancer patients, the incidence of MI was noted to be 6.5%, with significantly higher rates noted in patients with squamous cell cancers.[7] An emerging concept is that cancer is a manageable disease, similar to hypertension or diabetes, and requires early detection, periodic surveillance, and coordinated therapeutic decision-making. It is therefore critical for cancer survivors to limit comorbid illnesses. Many cancer survivors will actually be at as great a risk from cardiac disease as from recurrent cancer.[8]

Economic Impact of Cancer and Heart Disease

According to the American Heart Association (AHA) and the National Center for Chronic Disease Prevention and Health Promotion, the cost of cardiovascular disease in the United States in 2005 was $393.5 billion (US), of which CAD

contributes $142 billion (US) equally split between direct medical costs and indirect costs, such as lost productivity. The National Institutes of Health (NIH) estimated that the overall costs for cancer in 2004 were at $190 billion (US), including $69 billion (US) for direct medical costs and $121 billion (US) for indirect costs, such as lost productivity.[6] However, Americans' risk of dying from cancer continues to decline, and survival rates for many cancers continue to improve. Overall observed rates from all cancers dropped 1.1% per year from 1993 to 2001. The age-adjusted death rates for heart disease (ie, coronary heart disease) have decreased from 307.4 in 1950 to 134.6 per 100,000 persons (standardized to the 1940 population) in 1996. These data reflect progress in prevention, early detection, and treatment of both cancer and CAD. Paradoxically, however, this decline in mortality and resultant increased survival from both disease states combined with graying of the population would more likely translate into more patients with concurrent disease.

CAD and cancer are among the most significant contributors of health care spending in the US. Average monthly health care costs for cancer ranges from $2,187 (US) for each patient with prostate cancer to $7,616 (US) for those with pancreatic cancer, compared to the average health care costs for individuals without cancer of $329 (US) per month.[9] This calculation excludes the average monthly indirect costs for cancer patients estimated at $954 (US), attributed to an average loss of two working days and five days with short-term disability each month. Eisenstein and colleagues calculated that mean 10-year discounted inpatient medical costs of an acute coronary syndrome (ACS) patient were $45,253 (US) ($23,510 [US] acute phase and $21,819 [US] post-acute phase) with similar figures for unstable angina and myocardial infarction patients.[10]

Risk Stratification in Suspected CAD

Extensive clinical and statistical studies have identified several risk factors for coronary artery disease. Most of our knowledge about prevalence of coronary artery disease and its risk factors are mainly derived from studies done in populations of European origin,[11] and data from studies in populations of non-European descent suggest that there may be variations in risk factors between different ethnic populations for coronary heart disease. Hypertension and hyperlipidemia do not represent a similar risk in south Asian[12] and Chinese populations.[13] Although commonly known risk factors (smoking, hypertension, hyperlipidemia, and diabetes) have been claimed to account for only half the risk of a myocardial infarction,[14] evidence from a recent large global case-control study (15,152 cases and 14,820 controls, undertaken in 52 countries in five continents) showed that easily measurable risk factors (including smoking, abnormal lipids, psychosocial factors, hypertension, diabetes, and abdominal obesity) are associated with more than 80% of the risk of an acute myocardial infarction (AMI).[4] The role of these attributes is verified by the fact that a strategy to reduce traditional cardiovascular risk factors through public awareness against smoking, by lowering low-density lipoprotein cholesterol and blood pressure, and by promoting a healthy lifestyle has contributed significantly to the decline in CAD-related deaths in the developed countries. In large cohorts from the United States, those without abnormal electrocardiogram (ECG) results, diabetes, a smoking habit, high cholesterol, and high blood pressure had an 80 to 90% lower risk of coronary heart disease compared with the rest of the population.[14] Similarly, in European studies, non-smokers with low blood pressure and low cholesterol had an age-adjusted relative risk of 0·09, which was much lower that for than the average population (relative risk 1·0).[4,15] The latest data show smoking—a common risk factor for many cancers—as one of the most important risk factors, accounting for about 36% of the worldwide attributable risks of acute myocardial infarction. Additional factors including apolipoprotein ratios (ApoB/A1—marker of the balance of atherogenic and antiatherogenic particles),[16] and psychosocial factors,[17] may add substantially to traditional risk factors.

Risk Stratification in ACS patient

Once a patient presents with ACS, a different approach of risk stratification becomes an integral component in the decision-making for such patient. Several such risk stratification tools are available; however, one that is frequently used is the Thrombolysis in Myocardial Infarction (TIMI) risk score (Table 2).[18,19] This tool combines seven variables (age ≥ 65 years; ≥ three risk factors for CAD; prior coronary stenosis of ≥ 50%; ST-segment deviation on ECG at presentation; at least two anginal events in prior 24 hours; use of aspirin in prior 7 days; and elevated serum cardiac markers) in an evenly weighted scale that can predict short- and long-term risk based on the calculated score[20,21] and identify

Table 2 TIMI* Risk Score for Unstable Angina and Non-ST-Segment Elevation

Age > 65 yr
Three or more risk factors for coronary artery disease
Prior coronary stenosis of 50%
ST-segment deviation on presenting ECG
Use of aspirin in prior 7 days
Elevated serum cardiac markers
Two or more anginal events in previous 24 hr

*One point per risk factor: 5 to 7 points—high risk; 3 to 4 points—intermediate risk; 0 to 2 points—low risk
TIMI = thrombolysis in myocardial infarction

patients that would benefit most from an early invasive strategy.[22,23] Other important predictors in stratifying the early delivery of appropriate treatments in Non ST elevation acute coronary syndrome (NSTE-ACS) patients include hemodynamic instability, signs and symptoms of heart failure, renal insufficiency, elevated levels of C-reactive protein and natriuretic peptides.[24–27]

Coronary Complications of Cancer Therapy

There has been dramatic progress in cancer therapy in recent years, and the therapeutic options now include increasingly complex combinations of medications, radiation therapy, and surgical intervention. While a clear-cut link between cancer and CAD has not been established, many of the cancer treatments have important ischemic cardiac effects and are likely to have significant effects on patient outcomes. Several patient-related factors, including advanced age, preexisting coronary disease, concomitant radiation therapy, and metabolic abnormalities, increase the risk for chemotherapy-induced ischemic cardiac events in these patients. Additionally, each chemotherapeutic agent has the ability to potentiate the adverse effects of other agents. In one prospective study, cancer alone was associated with a fourfold risk of thrombosis, whereas chemotherapy increased the risk by 6.5 times.[28] Radiation therapy also plays an important role in magnifying cardiac toxicity (see below). It is, however, important to bear in mind that cancer patients undergoing intensive therapy are often severely ill, and cause-and-effect relationships of cardiac ischemia and therapies are often not very clear.

Coronary ischemia associated with chemotherapy agents are listed below according to drug class (Table 3).

Anthracyclines/Anthraquinolones

Anthracycline is the most studied of the anticancer drugs related to drug-induced cardiotoxicity, which is probably related to its ability to cause direct myocardial injury via formation of free

Table 3 Adverse Cardiovascular Events Associated With Chemotherapeutic Agents

Agents Associated with Left Ventricular Dysfunction
Anthracyclines
Mitoxantrone
High-dose Cyclophosphamide
Trastuzumab
Ifosfamide
All-*trans* retinoic acid

Agents associated with arterial thromboembolic events
Bevacizumab
Bleomycin
Etoposide
Granulocyte colony-stimulating factor

Agents associated with myocardial ischemia
5- Fluorouracil
Cisplatin
Capecitabine
Interleukin-2
Bleomycin
Etoposide
Tamoxifen
Bevacizumab

Agents associated with hypertension
Bevacizumab
Cisplatin

Agents associated with hypotension
Etoposide
Paclitaxel
Alemtuzumab
Cetuximab
Rituximab
IL-2
Denileukin
Interferon-μ
All-*trans* retinoic acid
Homoharringtonine

Agents Associated with Bradyarrhythmias
Thalidomide
Paclitaxel

Agents Associated with QT Prolongation or Torsades de Pointes
Arsenic trioxide

Agents Associated with Other Toxic Effects
Cardiac tamponade: busulfan
Hemorrhagic myocarditis: cyclophosphamide
Raynaud phenomenon: vinblastine
Autonomic neuropathy: vincristine
Pulmonary fibrosis: bleomycin
Endomyocardial fibrosis: busulfan

radicals.[29] Acute cardiotoxicity may manifest as nonspecific ST-segment and T-wave abnormalities, a common feature with chronic CAD. Anthracycline-induced cardiac toxicity has a dismal prognosis, but it can be greatly altered by early recognition and treatment.

Alkylating Agents

These may cause endothelial and myocyte injury mediated through a toxic metabolite[30] resulting in hemorrhagic myocardial necrosis.[31] The toxic effects can last up to 6 days, but long-term effects are not usually seen in those who survive.[32] Ifosfamide may cause a dose-related incidence of arrhythmia.[33] Cisplatin infusion may be associated with chest pain, palpitations, and, occasionally, elevated cardiac enzymes indicative of myocardial infarction (MI).[34] Cisplatin is unique in that it can cause late cardiovascular complications such as hypertension, myocardial ischemia, and MI as long as 10 to 20 years after the remission of metastatic testicular cancer.[35] Mitomycin may adversely affect the heart via formation of superoxide radicals under aerobic conditions.[36]

Antimetabolites

5-fluorouracil (5-FU), widely used in the treatment of many solid tumor treatment protocols, has been well described to induce cardiac ischemic syndrome,[37] which varies clinically from angina pectoris to acute MI. A "rechallenge" with 5-FU frequently reproduces the cardiac events. The ischemia is usually reversible on cessation of the 5-FU and implementation of anti-ischemic medical therapy. Although ischemic events can occur in patients without underlying CAD (incidence, 1.1%), the incidence is higher in patients with known CAD (4.5%).[38] Capecitabine, currently used in the treatment of breast and gastrointestinal cancers, has been associated with inducible angina or MI,[39] arrhythmias, and ischemic ECG changes.

Antimicrotubule Agents

Paclitaxel is used extensively in the treatment of many solid tumors and is increasingly being used in coated stents for coronary interventions. Post-intervention intracoronary thrombosis is a known complication of coated stents, and require extended antiplatelet therapy in patients with CAD.[40] Paclitaxel is also known to cause sinus bradycardia, heart block, premature ventricular contractions, and ventricular tachycardia.[41] In a large study of approximately 1,000 patients, the incidence of cardiac toxicity was 14%, and most incidents (76%) were grade I asymptomatic bradycardia.[42]

Vinca alkaloids are used primarily in the treatment of leukemia and lymphoma. Vinorelbine-related ischemic cardiac events, including angina with ECG changes,[43] and myocardial ischemia and MI[44] are more likely to occur in women than in men.[45] The occasional clinical presentation of Prinzmetal's angina and reversible ECG changes has led to the hypothesis of ischemia induced by coronary spasm.[43]

Monoclonal Antibodies

Monoclonal antibodies are being increasingly used to manage many hematologic malignancies and solid tumors.[46-49] Infusion of these agents may result in massive release of cytokines leading to hypotension, dyspnea, hypoxia, or even death.[49,50]

Cytokines

Interleukins

High-dose interleukin-2 (IL-2), a T-cell growth factor, used for the treatment of metastatic renal cell carcinoma and melanoma may result in vascular leak syndrome,[51] cardiac arrhythmias, MI, and myocarditis.[52] Improvements in patient selection and treatment protocols may substantially reduce IL-2–treatment–related cardiac ischemic events.[53] Denileukin diftitox (Ontak), an IL-2/diphtheria toxin fusion protein used in the treatment of T-cell lymphoma, may predispose to arterial thrombosis in cancer patients,[54] which may also translate into ischemic symptoms.

Interferon

Interferon, produced by macrophages and lymphocytes and approved for the treatment of many types of cancer, may cause hypotension or hypertension, tachycardia,[55] and, in severe cases, angina and MI.

Miscellaneous Agents

All-*trans* Retinoic Acid

This is a vitamin A derivative and is used in the treatment of acute promyelocytic leukemia. Fatal MI and thrombosis are known complications following use of all-*trans* retinoic acid[56] and may result in substantial decline in the LV ejection fraction[57].

Arsenic Trioxide

Arsenic Trioxide is used in the treatment of refractory or relapsed acute promyelocytic leukemia. Arsenic is commonly known to cause ECG abnormalities. Soignet observed significant prolongation of the QT segment in ≈50% of patients with acute promyelocytic leukemia.[58] They also noted sinus tachycardia, nonspecific ST-T changes, and torsades de pointes. Other reported cardiac complications include complete heart block[59,60] and sudden cardiac death.[61] In all these situations, the infusion of arsenic trioxide had been completed 7 to 22 hours before the events.[61]

Pentostatin

Pentostatin, a purine analogue used in the treatment of hairy cell leukemia and other hematologic malignancies, may induce myocardial infarction and arrhythmias,[62] especially when given with high doses of cyclophosphamide in preparation for bone marrow transplantation.[63]

Thalidomide

Thalidomide is currently used to treat a variety of hematologic and solid malignancies,[64] is relatively safe with regard to coronary complications, and is generally well tolerated. Cardiotoxic effects of thalidomide include sinus bradycardia and deep venous thrombosis.[64]

Etoposide

Etoposide used in the treatment of refractory testicular tumors and small-cell lung carcinoma has been reported to cause myocardial ischemic symptoms and MI.[65] The risk of myocardial ischemic events is significantly increased in patients who have previously undergone chemotherapy or mediastinal radiation.[66] Concomitant chemotherapy with other agents may also increase the risk for MI.[65]

Homoharringtonine

Most often used in the treatment of leukemia, homoharringtonine can be associated with severe hypotension. This dose-related effect is probably related to its calcium-channel–blocking activity.[67] Although not directly linked to coronary artery related complications, ventricular tachycardia and atrial fibrillation have been reported after administration of homoharringtonine,[68] which may complicate management in a known CAD patient.

Radiation Therapy

Radiation therapy is commonly used in the treatment of many types of cancer, particularly breast cancer and Hodgkin's lymphoma. Meta-analysis of randomized clinical trials confirmed increased cardiovascular mortality among patients treated for early breast cancer[69] and Hodgkin's lymphoma.[70] The precise incidence of radiation-induced accelerated atherosclerosis is difficult to confirm, but it has been reported in patients who did not have the traditional risk factors for CAD.[71] Radiation to the thorax can damage coronary arteries in addition to its toxic effect on the pericardium, myocardium, and cardiac valves. Despite its promise to reduce in-stent restenosis, intracoronary irradiation therapy has been almost abandoned because of a high incidence of late thrombosis and an increased risk of myocardial infarction.[72] The morphologic changes observed in radiation-induced coronary artery disease are similar to those observed in spontaneous atherosclerosis.[73] The exact mechanisms by which radiation produces atherosclerosis are not known, but endothelial injury from radiation has been suggested as the initiating factor. Ionizing energy accelerates the deposition of cholesterol in the arterial wall, contributes to intimal and adventitial proliferation, as well as plaque ulceration, all of which may lead to acute coronary thrombosis.[74] Ionizing radiation also produces reactive oxygen species, including superoxide anion, hydrogen peroxide, and hydroxyl radicals that increase oxidative stress to the endothelium and to circulating lipoproteins. The oxidized lipoproteins, in turn, recruit inflammatory monocytes and macrophages into the arterial wall[75] starting the cascade of inflammatory process that leads to ACS Endothelial damage from radiation reduces the bioavailability of nitric oxide resulting in impaired arterial vasodilatation, increased platelet aggregation, and leukocyte adherence. The smaller baseline size of radiated coronary arteries may be a result of increased apoptosis, which in turn, is a result of decreased availability of nitric oxide.[76] The higher the doses of radiation therapy, the higher the incidence of radiation-induced heart disease. The incidence of cardiac toxicity is also higher in patients who undergo concurrent therapy with doxorubicin.[77] Patients with preexisting CAD are especially vulnerable. The mean interval for developing CAD after radiation therapy is approximately 82 months.[78] However, vascular injury from radiation therapy can be silent, with as high as 50% of asymptomatic patients demonstrating new myocardial perfusion defects.[79] Sudden cardiac death has also been reported in patients treated with radiation therapy,[80] which may be attributed to diffuse intimal hyperplasia of coronary arteries or from discrete left main stenosis.[71] Endothelial cell involvement is an early sign of radiation-induced vascular damage.[81] Radiation-induced vascular injury often involves long segments of an artery.[82]

Management of radiation-induced CAD is difficult but not different than that of non–radiation–induced CAD. Both percutaneous coronary intervention and coronary artery bypass grafting have been used for revascularization.[71] However, concomitant radiation-induced mediastinal fibrosis may render surgical bypass grafting more difficult in these patients.[71]

Cancer Prevention, Cylcooxygenase-2 and Cardiovascular Complications

The identification of cylcooxygenase-2 (COX-2) as a promoter of intestinal tumorigenesis led to the concept that COX-2 inhibitors would prevent premalignant colorectal adenomas.[83-87] This looked especially attractive since neither prior clinical trials nor observational studies had reported a clearly increased risk of cardiovascular events with celecoxib use.[88-93] However, in a large prospective, randomized, double-blind, multicenter trial, celecoxib use was associated with a significant dose-related increase in serious cardiovascular events, including myocardial infarction and death.[94] In addition, the number of venous thromboembolic events also increased. Similar observation of an increased incidence of death from cardiovascular causes, myocardial infarction, or stroke among patients receiving rofecoxib in the Adenomatous Polyp Prevention on Vioxx trial resulted in early termination[95,96] and voluntary withdrawal of the drug from the market. Use of other selective COX-2 inhibitors, including valdecoxib, and parecoxib, has also been associated with an increased rate of cardiovascular events.[97,98] The reason for increase in cardiovascular risk associated with the use of COX-2 inhibitors is uncertain. One possible mechanism involves the effects of COX-2 inhibitors on blocking the production of prostacyclin without affecting the synthesis of thromboxane A$_2$,[95] thereby potentially creating a prothrombotic state. Significant increase in cardiovascular thromboembolic events were also noted when parecoxib and valdecoxib were used for pain control in the immediate postoperative period after coronary artery bypass surgery.[99,100]

Cancer and the Prothrombotic State

Cancer appears to cause a prothrombotic or hypercoagulable state through an altered balance between the coagulation and fibrinolytic system. However, for reasons presently unclear, arterial thromboembolism is much less common than venous thrombosis in cancer. This dichotomy may be partly explained by the large amount of fibrin, which is excessively formed in the large venous thrombi, compared to the relatively small amount of fibrin in arterial clots. The pathogenic mechanisms of thrombosis in cancer patients are multifactorial. A major mechanism involves activation of factor VII at the extrinsic coagulation system by tissue factor, which is expressed by most tumor cells.[101] Another important mechanism is triggered by cancer procoagulant, a cysteine protease which directly activates factor X and is expressed by certain human tumor cells.[102] An association between arterial disease and disturbances in hemostasis, thrombosis, and vascular function, have also been reported to be present in cancer.[103] Tumor cells may be directly prothrombotic by generation of excess thrombin and procoagulant proteins, such as tissue factor, fibrinogen, and plasminogen activator inhibitor. Cancer cells can also activate the coagulation system through interactions with platelets, thus shifting the balance to induce a prothrombotic state. In cancer, monocytes may also be activated by immune complexes or cytokines, such as tumor necrosis factor[104,105] and certain malignant cells,[106,107] whereas other cells, including those of sarcoma, melanoma, neuroblastoma, lymphoma, and acute promyelocytic leukemia, can express tissue factor per se.[108] Concentrations of several other proteins within the coagulation cascade are also abnormally raised in cancer, and this is often associated with a fall in the activity of anticoagulant factors[109,110] leading to a prothrombotic or hypercoagulable state. Although these mechanisms play major roles in venous thromboembolism, their exact roles in ACS are unknown; they might contribute to a rapid transition of a vulnerable plaque from a subintimal lesion to a thrombotic occlusion.

Clinical manifestations of arterial thromboembolic phenomenon in cancer may include localized arterial occlusion, nonbacterial thrombotic endocarditis (NBTE), disseminated intravascular coagulation, and thrombotic thrombocytopenic purpura. This variety of clinical syndromes may appear prior to diagnosis of cancer, in the course of overt malignant disease, or following initiation of chemotherapeutic agents. Although certain tumors (such as mucous carcinoma of the pancreas, lung, and gastrointestinal tract) have been traditionally associated with thromboembolism,[111] other solid neoplasms as well as hematologic malignancies are often associated with thrombosis. Notably, NBTE (which is not uncommon in patients with solid tumors[112]) is particularly prevalent in patients with myeloproliferative disorders in whom it may be associated with systemic thrombosis.[113]

Pathogenesis of ACS

ACS encompasses unstable angina (UA), non–ST-segment elevation myocardial infarction (NSTEMI) and ST-segment elevation myocardial infarction (STEMI). STEMI is a distinct clinical entity, which results from an occlusive thrombus. UA/NSTEMI, on the other hand, is the combination of two closely related clinical entities (ie, a syndrome), characterized by decreased myocardial perfusion resulting from nonocclusive thrombus formation subsequent to disruption of an atherosclerotic plaque.

Views of the pathophysiology of atherothrombosis have evolved substantially over the last two decades. Insights into the pathophysiology have advanced beyond the notion of progressive chronic occlusion of the coronary artery, to the recognition that plaque disruption and superimposed thrombus formation are the leading causes of acute coronary syndromes (ACS). The term ACS was used, instead of acute myocardial infarction, in the 1996 guideline publication of the American College of Cardiology/American Heart Association (ACC/AHA) to emphasize this emerging concept of disruption of a vulnerable or high-risk plaque during myocardial ischemia.[114]

Plaque composition rather than luminal stenosis, has become the major focus of the pathophysiologic process of ACS. Plaques consist of inflammatory and smooth muscle cells, cellular debris, and fatty deposits trapped within the vessel wall. Depending on the composition, they are classified into either "stable" (with little risk of acute rupture) or unstable (or "vulnerable"—ie, likely to spontaneously rupture and trigger clot formation initiating ACS). There are two aspects to the transition from vulnerable plaque to acute coronary event: one is associated with characteristics of the atheromatous subintimal lesion, and the other involves factors that make it likely that an obstructive thrombus will form at the site of the atheroma (the "vulnerable patient").

Histologically, stable coronary plaques are rich in collagen and have thick fibrous caps. In contrast, vulnerable or rupture-prone lesions consist of a large number of inflammatory cells, including macrophages, foam cells, monocytes, granulocytes, and lymphocytes, reduced numbers of vascular smooth muscle cells (SMCs), and a thin fibrous cap (<65 μm) of collagen type I, with an underlying necrotic lipid-filled core occupying approximately 35% of the lesion.[115] Therefore, they are less stable and have a higher propensity to rupture. Typically, the underlying cross-sectional luminal narrowing is less than 50%. Plaque disruption usually occurs at the weakest point (the "shoulder"), frequently where the cap is thinnest and most heavily infiltrated with inflammatory cells.[116]

Characteristics of the patient that increase vulnerability include evidence of systemic inflammation (eg, increased levels of C-reactive protein, intercellular adhesion molecule 1, or vascular cell adhesion molecule 1) and hypercoagulability (elevated levels of fibrinogen, D-dimer, and factor V Leiden) as well as decreased anticoagulation factors such as protein S and C, thrombomodulin, and antithrombin III.[117]

Once the cap covering a vulnerable plaque erodes or is disrupted, the highly thrombogenic lipid-rich core, abundant in tissue factor, is exposed to the bloodstream, activating the clotting cascade. This triggers the formation of a superimposed thrombus that leads to vessel occlusion and subsequent ischemic symptoms distal to the occlusion.[118,119] These changes in the plaque are a result of a combination of internal and external influences. Overall plaque burden is greater in the symptomatic than in the asymptomatic patients.

Endothelial Dysfunction

Endothelial dysfunction is a reversible systemic disorder characterized by a reduction of the bioavailability of vasodilators, in particular nitric oxide (NO), and an increase in endothelium-derived vasoconstrictor factors.[120,121] A dysfunctional endothelium promotes lipid and cell permeability, lipoprotein oxidation, inflammation, SMC proliferation, extracellular matrix deposition or lysis, platelet activation, and thrombus formation[122] and generates a proatherogenic environment by creating a proinflammatory, proliferative, and prothrombotic milieu that favors atherogenesis.[123] Endothelial dysfunction is also involved in the recruitment of inflammatory cells into the vessel wall and in the initiation of atherosclerosis. Monocytes migrate into the subendothelium, where they transform into macrophages and modulate inflammatory reactions and the secretion of chemoattractants. Activated macrophages and smooth muscle cells in the atheroma then release lytic enzymes that can degrade the fibrous cap,[124,125] resulting in rupture of the lesion.

Many of the cardiovascular risk factors, as well as cancers, are associated with increased oxidative stress, and it is considered to be a major mechanism involved in the pathogenesis of endothelial dysfunction and may serve as a common pathogenic mechanism of the effect of risk factors on the endothelium.[126,127]

Inflammation and Atherothrombosis

There is a strong link between inflammation and atherothrombosis.[128] Early in atherogenesis, patches of arterial endothelial cells, in particular vascular cell adhesion molecule-1 (VCAM-1), begin to express on their surface selective adhesion molecules that bind to various classes of leukocytes. Once they are in the arterial wall, the blood-derived inflammatory cells participate in and perpetuate a local inflammatory response which not only promote initiation and evolution of atherosclerosis, but also contributes decisively to acute thrombotic complications of atheroma. The activated macrophages produce proteolytic enzymes (eg, matrix metalloproteinases [MMP]) which degrade the collagen in the plaque's protective fibrous cap, rendering it thin, weak, and vulnerable to rupture.[129,130] Indeed, the predictive value for coronary events of high levels of C-reactive protein may be a manifestation of such systemic phenomenon.[131]

Tissue Factor

Tissue factor (TF) is a potent initiator of coagulation cascade, and is a key determinant of the vulnerability of the atherosclerotic plaque. The presence of abundant tissue factor[132] and apoptotic microparticles[133] in the shoulder region and in the acellular, lipid-rich core of the plaque suggests that they're the thrombogenic potential in disrupted atherosclerotic plaque. Circulating tissue factor is strikingly increased in patients with cancer[134]; hence, it may also play a role in the formation of the thrombus upon atherosclerotic plaque disruption. Infective intracellular organisms have also been proposed as major contributors to plaque inflammation, activation, and vulnerability.[135] Overall plaque burden is greater in symptomatic than in asymptomatic patients, and rupture of the plaques is associated with a sudden increase in the intralesional pressure. This increase can occur if there is a loss of integrity of vessels in the vasa vasorum resulting in intraplaque hemorrhage.[136]

Microembolization and Microvascular Obstruction

In the setting of acute MI, the presence of distal microembolization is evident clinically by "no-reflow" phenomenon following reperfusion. Microvascular obstruction, however, is demonstrated very early in the course of ACS, and is most likely caused by embolization rather than by edema or reperfusion injury.[137] One of the postulated mechanisms suggests that plaque rupture results in the release of prothrombotic materials into the coronary circulation, which embolize the microvascular bed. Evidence for the role of distal embolization in the pathogenesis of ACS is found in autopsy studies demonstrating the presence of platelet/fibrin microemboli in the cardiac tissue of up to 50 to 80% of patients with fatal MI.[138] These platelet aggregates contain thrombus overlying a ruptured atheromatous plaque and are located distal to epicardial coronary arteries, making it highly likely to represent emboli rather than mere platelet hyperactivity.[138] A prothrombotic milieu in cancer will likely exacerbate this phenomenon.

Role of Risk Factors and Cancer

In about one-third of the cases of sudden coronary death, there is no significant disruption of atheromatous plaque except for some superficial erosion of markedly stenotic and fibrotic plaque.[139] In such cases, thrombus formation may depend on a hyperthrombogenic state triggered by systemic factors including elevated LDL cholesterol, cigarette smoking, hyperglycemia, and altered hemostasis[140]. Poorly controlled diabetics[141] as well as cancer[142] patients are known to have hyperthrombogenicity.

Role of Platelets in Acute Coronary Syndrome

The role of the platelet and the endothelium in the pathogenesis of atherosclerosis and subsequent ischemic events has been the subject of extensive investigation.[140] The role of platelets is especially important in the context of ACS in cancer patients since patients with malignancy often have thrombocytopenia and are denied antiplatelet therapy, which forms the cornerstone of management in ACS patients (Table 4).

Platelets play a key role in thrombotic vascular occlusion at the ruptured coronary atherosclerotic plaque; and also interact with both

Table 4 Predisposing Factors of ACS in Cancer Patients
Coronary atherosclerosis
Coronary embolization from tumor
Non-bacterial endocarditis
Coronary thrombosis from disseminated intravascular coagulation
Cardiac metastasis
External compression of coronary artery
Coronary ostial lesion from radiotherapy
Tumor-related coagulopathy (especially in patients with leukemia)
Radiation- and chemotherapy-related vasculopathy

the coagulation and fibrinolytic systems in the pathogenesis of thrombosis. Multiple synergistic stimulations of platelet receptors by the corresponding ligands are involved in the process of platelet activation. Following plaque disruption or endothelial injury, platelets attach to the exposed subendothelium, releasing thromboxane A$_2$, serotonin, adenosine diphosphate, platelet activating factor, oxygen-derived free radicals, activated thrombin, and tissue factor, which promotes further platelet aggregation and dynamic vasoconstriction that in turn lead to transient or permanent coronary artery thrombosis.[143] The von Willebrand factor-GP Iba interaction and the collagen-GP VI interaction are the two most important receptor-ligand interactions in the process of platelet thrombus formation on the surface of collagen.[144] In addition, both embolization of platelet aggregates and direct, receptor-mediated platelet adhesion to the post-ischemic microvascular surface result in obstruction and impairment of coronary microcirculation. Such microvascular disturbance may lead to significant additional tissue injury and aggravate myocardial contractile dysfunction. Platelets play another important role in conversion of chronic stable coronary disease to acute unstable process. Platelets inhibit the production of endogenous inhibitors of platelet aggregation and vasoconstriction including prostacyclin, endothelium-derived relaxing factor (nitric oxide). Tissue plasminogen activator is reduced at the sites of endothelial injury, resulting in a vasoconstrictive and prothrombotic environment with conversion from chronic to acute coronary syndromes.[145] Furthermore, new investigations have demonstrated that platelets not only contribute to acute thrombotic vascular occlusion but also participate in the inflammatory and matrix-degrading processes of coronary atherosclerosis itself.[143] Platelet–endothelial-cell interactions at lesion-prone sites might trigger an inflammatory response in the vessel wall early in the genesis of atherosclerosis and contribute to destabilization of advanced atherosclerotic lesions.[146]

ACS in Cancer Patients

Patients with cancer have a prothrombotic milieu: endothelial damage from radiotherapy and chemotherapy.[147] The possible mechanisms responsible for radiation-induced CAD have been described above. Although not clearly defined, it is thought to have a synergistic role with other traditional risk factors.[148] High-dose radiation may damage the vascular endothelium, resulting in fibrosis or medial degeneration in the coronary arteries.[149] Case studies have been reported linking coronary spasm, acute vascular toxicity, and thromboembolism to various chemotherapeutic agents, notably 5-flurouracil (and its analogue capecitabine), cisplatin, vinblastine, bleomycin, and cyclophosphamide.[150-154] Insulin resistance and metabolic disturbance in patients with bone marrow transplantation[155] and chemotherapy-induced early menopause may predispose them to premature coronary atherosclerosis.[156] The exact mechanism behind these vascular events is unknown, but activation of clotting factors following disturbances of microcirculation caused by the release of toxic substance from necrotic tissue and/or malignant cells has been thought to play a leading role. Details of various cardiotoxic events have been described above.

In cancer patients, gross mismatch in myocardial supply and demand may also contribute to initiating coronary syndromes. Increased myocardial oxygen demand in the prolonged perioperative setting, fever, and tachycardia, combined with reduced coronary perfusion in hypotension, anemia, and hypoxemia are common in cancer patients.

Patients undergoing radiation therapy of mediastinal tumors such as lymphoma[157] and seminoma[158,159] may experience accelerated CAD. This is especially true for patients who are also treated with chemotherapy.[160] Other mechanisms involved in accelerated CAD include chemotherapy-induced premature menopause, which is a recognized risk factor for coronary artery disease.[161] Meta-analyses of randomized clinical trials[162,163] and studies of population-based cancer registry data[164-166] show an increased risk of cardiac death in breast cancer patients exposed to radiation therapy, more so among those who received treatment to the left side. The risk of radiation-induced heart disease correlates with radiation-dose volume[163] and fractionation.[167] This risk is further compounded because hormone replacement therapy is not generally recommended for patients with breast cancer. Better prognosis and increased survival these days from better management of cancer patients make them more vulnerable to this radiation-induced heart disease over the long term. However, recently published data from our institution, which comprised improved radiation techniques and dosage,

failed to replicate these earlier claims of increased risk of myocardial infarction among breast cancer patients treated with radiation therapy.[168]

Other causes of tumor-related ACS are listed in Table 4 and include coronary embolization due to papillary fibroelastomas[169] and atrial myxomas,[170-172] and leukemic infiltration into the myocardium or pericardium.[173]

Presentation of ACS in Cancer Patients

The classic or typical symptoms of acute coronary syndromes are substernal or left-sided chest pain, or discomfort that the patient often describes as pressure or heaviness, which may radiate to the left arm, neck, jaw, or shoulder. The discomfort associated with acute MI usually lasts at least 20 minutes, but may be shorter in duration. The discomfort is not positional in nature, nor is it affected by deep inspiration or movement. Unexplained nausea and vomiting, persistent shortness of breath secondary to left ventricular failure, and unexplained weakness, dizziness, lightheadedness, or syncope (or a combination of these) should arouse suspicion. This is more important in light of recent studies evaluating people presenting with AMI symptoms, which show that up to 43% of patients had atypical elements in the description of their chest pain or pressure,[174] and as many as 33 to 47% of all patients having an AMI will present without chest pain.[175,176] In a recently published, large study of 20,881 patients with ACS, more than 8% presented without any chest pain, of whom one in four were not initially recognized as having an acute coronary syndrome.[177]

Because symptoms like dyspnea, pleuritic chest pain, fatigue, weakness, discomfort in the upper abdomen and between the shoulder blades, palpitations, and confusion, are so common in cancer patients, it could easily be confused with symptoms of thoraco-abdominal involvement in preexisting malignancies. The differential diagnosis of chest pain is listed in Table 5. Consequently, these complaints may go unrecognized or may be erroneously labeled as those related to the cancer. Additionally, many cancer patients may not consider them serious enough to seek immediate assistance, therefore delaying prompt recognition and leading to delay in treatment—or misdiagnosis and inappropriate treatment. Therefore, it is imperative to be aware of patients who are at high risk for ACS in order to facilitate diagnosis and treatment. Often, more cases are identified from the "routine" blood test that follows complaints of any of these "atypical" symptoms. However, these "infarclets" allow appropriate secondary prevention leading to reduced costs for subsequent cardiac care. In contrast to these small MI/"infarclets" (identifiable by elevation of cardiac troponin alone), the patient with

Table 5 Differential Diagnostic Considerations in Severe or Prolonged Chest Pain in Cancer Patient

Myocardial infarction
Unstable angina
Pericarditis
Aortic dissection
Chest-wall pain (musculoskeletal or neurologic)
Pulmonary disease (pulmonary embolism, pneumonia, pleurisy, pneumothorax)
Gastrointestinal disease (esophagitis, esophageal spasm, peptic ulcer disease, biliary colic, pancreatitis)
Psychogenic hyperventilation syndrome

Table 6 ECG Changes Mimicking Myocardial Ischemia in Cancer

Pericarditis
Early repolarization
Intracranial pathology including metastasis
Pneumothorax
Hypocalcemia
Hyperkalemia
Pulmonary embolism
Tumor involvement of heart

classic "large myocardial infarction" may often present with heart failure, cardiogenic shock, or life-threatening arrhythmia. Finally, myocardial necrosis may also occur without any symptoms and might be detected only by an ECG or cardiac imaging.

Diagnosis

Today, ACS is detected by several different modalities, including ECG changes, measurement of biochemical markers, and imaging studies such as echocardiography and myocardial perfusion imaging.[178,179] Each of these techniques is able to quantify the extent of damage, from minimal to small to large myocardial infarction. However, the sensitivity and specificity of each of these techniques to quantitate the extent of necrosis accurately differ significantly. Pathologically, infarcts are usually classified as focal/microscopic necrosis, small (< 10% of the left ventricle [LV]), medium (10 to 30% of the LV) or large (> 30% of the LV).

Electrocardiography

ECG remains the time-honored and single most important tool in the diagnosis of ischemic heart disease. ECG criteria have emerged as one of the most powerful tools for the diagnosis and treatment of ACS. By using data from clinical and pathoanatomical correlative studies, significant accuracies and complex algorithms have been developed for standard 12-lead ECG to diagnose evolving MI. In the absence of QRS confounders

like bundle branch block, left ventricular hypertrophy, Wolff-Parkinson-White syndrome, ST segment elevation signifies acute myocardial injury in the right clinical setting. Tall and peaked "hyperacute" T waves may precede these changes during early phases of acute MI. Similarly, ST segment depression and/or T wave abnormalities, noted in two or more contiguous leads on two consecutive ECGs several hours apart, indicates ongoing ischemia. However, in cancer patients, ST segment elevation is more often indicative of pericarditis or myopericarditis (Table 5). In pericarditis, there is absence of reciprocal changes and depression of the PR segment. However, since biochemical markers enable detection of myocardial necrosis too small to be associated with QRS abnormalities, many patients will have a normal or unchanged ECG during microinfarcts. Newer ECG techniques with higher sensitivity and specificity may also be useful for the noninvasive detection of coronary artery disease.[180]

Biochemical Markers of Myocardial Necrosis

Myocardial infarction is diagnosed when specific biomarkers are increased in the setting of acute ischemia.[181] Different myocardial proteins are released into the circulation due to the damaged myocytes: myoglobin, cardiac troponins T and I, creatine kinase, lactate dehydrogenase, as well as many others. These biomarkers merely reflect myocardial damage and not the mechanism of injury. As mentioned above, myopericarditis is relatively common in cancer patients. Therefore, an elevated value in the absence of clinical evidence of ischemia in a patient with cancer should prompt a search for causes, such as myocarditis, or myopericarditis.

Because total creatine kinase (CK) has wide tissue distribution, its measurement is not commonly used for the routine diagnosis of acute MI except when combined with a more sensitive fraction, such as creatine kinase myocardial band (CK-MB) or troponins. The latter is the most preferred biomarker for detection of myocardial injury because of its high tissue specificity and sensitivity. CK-MB is more tissue-specific than total CK but less tissue-specific than cardiac troponin. However, the data documenting its clinical specificity for myocardial necrosis are more abundant. A trend from two or more successive blood samples of CK-MB or troponin is used to diagnose MI. For most patients, these serial enzymes are obtained every 4 to 6 hours but may need to be extended beyond 12 hours if, despite high clinical index of suspicion, the earlier samples are negative. For patients with low suspicion and in need of an early diagnosis, a rapidly appearing biomarker, such as myoglobin, may help to rule out myocardial injury. Although no formal grading system of infarct size exists, the

level of biomarker elevation is often used to quantify extent of myocardial damage (small, medium, or large). In the past, markers like Serum glutamic oxaloacetic transaminase, Alaninc Amino transferase, Aspartate Aminotransferase and Lactate Dehydrogenase (Glutamic-oxaloacetic transaminase, aspartate amino transferase, lactate dehydrogenase and lactate dehydrogenase isoenzymes) were used to diagnose ACS. However, these have been substituted by the newer biomarkers (CK-MB, troponin) and are no longer used in the diagnosis of MI.

It is important to remember that cardiac troponin values may remain elevated for 7 to 10 days or longer after myocardial necrosis, especially in cancer patients with renal insufficiency. This may make it difficult to time the initial event accurately and influence subsequent management decisions. In such cases, a high cardiac troponin value on presentation or on first sample should be correlated to CK-MB or myoglobin and to very recent clinical events.

Imaging

Echocardiographic and myocardial single-photon emission computed tomographic (SPECT) perfusion imaging techniques have revolutionized identifying ischemic from nonischemic causes in cancer patients. Although commonly used in the cardiology outpatient setting for evaluation of inducible ischemia, both may be helpful to rule out or confirm the presence of myocardial ischemia in the acute setting, specially when ECGs are nondiagnostic or uninterpretable. Furthermore echocardiography allows assessment of frequent nonischemic causes of acute chest pain in patients with cancer (eg, perimyocarditis, pulmonary embolism, valvular heart disease like aortic stenosis, and aortic dissection. Echocardiography is also the diagnostic procedure of choice for identification of mechanical complications of MI, namely coexisting valvular dysfunction, infarct expansion, mural thrombus and decrement in left ventricular ejection fraction. While both techniques can determine the localization and extent of infarction, it should be emphasized that a normal echocardiographic exam does not exclude myocardial infarction, since injury involving > 20% of myocardial wall thickness is required before a segmental wall motion abnormality can be detected. Similarly > 10 g of myocardial tissue must be injured before perfusion defect is obvious on a radionuclide perfusion image. Advances in contrast echocardiography hold promise for the routine assessment of myocardial perfusion. Vasodilator stress in conjunction with contrast echocardiography will likely play an important role in the noninvasive evaluation of myocardial perfusion and coronary blood flow reserve.[182]

Several new techniques in cardiovascular (CV) imaging like computed tomography (CT) angiography and magnetic resonance (MR) are extensively used in the diagnosis and follow-up of cancer patients. Newer techniques to image high risk/vulnerable atherosclerotic plaques are appearing on the horizon.[183] CT imaging of the coronary arteries, using either electron beam tomography or multidetector row CT, offer possibilities to assess coronary atherosclerosis and visualization of noncalcified plaque. Coronary calcium imaging may be clinically useful in young cancer patients at intermediate risk for coronary artery disease.[184]

CT pulmonary angiogram (CTPA) is increasingly used for the detection of pulmonary embolism (PE) in cancer patients. Most patients investigated have pathology other than PE as a cause of their symptoms. Careful analysis of CTPA allows assessment of not only the pulmonary arteries for embolism, but the heart as well. Potentially life-threatening, coexistent, underlying or incidental cardiac disease in a patient with chest symptoms can be reliably identified. Pathologies of the myocardium, including hypertrophic cardiomyopathy, pericardial disease, valvular disease, coronary artery disease, and intracardiac abnormalities, are demonstrated. It is important to have a clear understanding of the features of cardiac disease that may be seen on a CTPA.[185] Cardiac MR is also emerging as a powerful imaging technique in Ischemic Heart disease.[186] It is extremely capable of showing infracted myocardium even in the presence of normal coronaries.[187]

Treatments

Non–ST-Segment Elevation Acute Coronary Syndrome (NSTE-ACS)

Acute coronary syndrome in a cancer patient presents a difficult challenge. There is no evidence-based guideline addressing specifically the management of cancer patients with ACS although there is no reason why general guidelines (Table 4) should not be applicable in the majority of cancer patients.

Aspirin

An optimal antiplatelet regimen for patients with NSTE-ACS remains to be defined. Aspirin irreversibly inhibits platelet activation and aggregation by inhibiting cyclooxygenase-1 (prostaglandin H synthase) in platelets and megakaryocytes, which is a key enzyme in the pathway of synthesis of thromboxane A_2, a potent vasoconstrictor and platelet aggregant.[188] Only the parent form of aspirin (acetylsalicylic acid) has any significant effect on platelet function. The inhibited platelets are unable to regenerate cyclooxygenase, therefore, the immediate antithrombotic effect of aspirin remains for the lifespan of the platelet. Following discontinuation of aspirin therapy, normal hemostasis is restored when approximately 20% of platelets regain normal cyclooxygenase activity,[189] making daily intake of aspirin necessary for useful platelet inhibition.

Aspirin reduces the incidence of death and nonfatal MI in patients with unstable angina[190,191] or acute MI,[192] with only a minor increase in the risk of major bleeding (0.2%). Since higher doses of aspirin do not provide greater benefit,[192,193] dosages >75 mg daily may be less desirable in cancer patients due to increased susceptibility to bleeding, especially when combined with clopidogrel. It is important to remember that non-aspirin non-steroidal anti-inflammatory drugs, which are often used by many cancer patients, may attenuate the antiplatelet effects of aspirin.[194–196]

Adenosine Diphosphate Receptor Antagonists

The thienopyridine derivatives (clopidogrel and ticlopidine hydrochloride) are metabolized in the liver to active compounds that covalently bind to the adenosine phosphate (ADP) receptors on platelets and dramatically reduce platelet activation. Clopidogrel is as safe as aspirin, but is more expensive. It is an appropriate alternative to aspirin for long-term secondary prevention in patients who cannot tolerate aspirin, have experienced a recurrent vascular event while taking aspirin, or are at very high risk of a vascular event (>20% per year). An oral loading dose of 300 mg clopidogrel produces detectable inhibition of ADP-induced platelet aggregation after 2 hours, which becomes maximal after 6 hours.[197,198] If a loading dose of clopidogrel is not used, repeated daily oral doses of 75 mg clopidogrel are required to achieve a steady-state maximal platelet inhibition, which is comparable with that produced by 250 mg ticlopidine hydrochloride orally, twice daily.[199] In the Clopidogrel vs Aspirin in Patients at Risk of Ischemic Events trial,[196] there was a modest relative risk reduction in adverse CV events (5.3% vs 5.8%, $p = .04$) with clopidogrel in known atherosclerotic vascular disease patients compared to aspirin. However, addition of clopidogrel to aspirin reduces the risk of serious vascular events among patients with non-ST-segment elevation acute coronary syndromes by 20%, and patients undergoing percutaneous coronary intervention by 30%, compared with aspirin alone. Therefore, cancer patients with NSTE-ACS who are considered to be at low bleeding risk may be started on dual antiplatelet therapy and continued for up to 12 months[200,201] for additional benefit in all-cause mortality, cardiovascular death, MI, and/or stroke. Cancer patients on clopidogrel undergoing surgery may be at increased risk of bleeding if the drug is administered within 5 days of surgery.[202,203] Accordingly, clopidogrel should be withheld 5 days before planned surgery.

Glycoprotein IIb/IIIa Inhibitors

Short-term addition of an intravenous infusion of a glycoprotein (Gp) IIb/IIIa antagonist to aspirin prevents vascular events in high-risk patients having a percutaneous coronary intervention (PCI), and those with NSTE-ACS, but causes increased bleeding. For patients undergoing an early conservative strategy, the benefit of Gp IIb/IIIa inhibitors is less pronounced. However, based on their ability to prevent ischemic complications following PCI, Gp IIb/IIIa inhibitors may be used in NSTE-ACS patients managed with an early invasive strategy.[114] There may even be a paradoxical worse outcome with longer infusions of abciximab in patients for whom PCI is not planned.[204]

Anticoagulation

Unfractionated heparin reduces ischemia in NSTE-ACS through its potentiation of circulating antithrombins and its ability to inhibit clot propagation.[205] However, heparin requires frequent monitoring and can be associated with delays in achieving therapeutic anticoagulation.[206] Low molecular weight heparin (LMWH) provides better bioavailability, more predictable pharmacokinetics, a longer half-life, and is associated with less platelet activation and heparin-induced thrombocytopenia. Regardless, many oncologists have been hesitant to use LMWH because of concerns of reduced efficacy, increased bleeding, and an inability to easily monitor anticoagulation. In two recent large trials in patients with NSTE-ACS, major bleeding episodes were more common with LMWH compared to heparin.[207,208]

Thrombolytics

Despite the role of thrombosis in UA/NSTEMI, thrombolytic agents have not been shown to provide benefit in patients with UA/NSTEMI; in fact, the outcome may be worse with thrombolytics.[209–211] Consequently, thrombolytic agents are contraindicated for use in the treatment of patients who have UA/NSTEMI.

Angiotensin Converting Enzyme Inhibitors

Angiotensin converting enzyme (ACE) inhibitors have emerged as standard care for most patients with atherosclerosis, diabetes mellitus, and left ventricular systolic dysfunction. However, they have not been evaluated in placebo-controlled trials of patients with NSTE-ACS. Nonetheless, support for their long-term outpatient use has come from the Heart Outcomes Prevention Evaluation trial[212] and the European Trial on Reduction of Cardiac Events with Perindopril in Stable Coronary Artery Disease,[213] which showed approximately 20% relative risk reduction in the combined end point of cardiovascular death, MI, and stroke or cardiac arrest ($p < .001$ for all) for the ACE inhibitor arm. In low-risk patients, however, ACE inhibitors do not provide the same benefit.[214]

Angiotensin Receptor Blockade

There is no reason to change the current practice of choosing ACE inhibitors as first-line treatment for these conditions. If ACE inhibitors cannot be used, AngiotensinII receptor blockers represent an acceptable alternative.[215]

β-Blockers

β-blockers reduce cardiac workload and myocardial oxygen demand, and their use in the acute setting may yield a 13% relative risk reduction in the rate of progression to an acute MI[216] and a 29% relative risk reduction in death among high-risk individuals with a threatened or evolving MI.[217] When used in patients following an MI, β-blockers also produce significant reductions in adverse CV events.[218-220] For low- to intermediate-risk patients with angina and for all high-risk patients, intravenous β-blockers should be given in the setting of chest pain, followed by long-term use.

Blood Pressure Control

Because high blood pressure (BP) increases myocardial oxygen demand, its treatment remains an important goal in the management of patients with NSTE-ACS. Although current guidelines recommend a BP of less than 130/85 mm Hg (reserving < 130/80 mm Hg for patients with diabetes or chronic kidney disease,[221] recent evidence suggests that the optimal level may be even lower (ie, 125/75 mm Hg) in patients with stable CAD.[222,223] Either ACE inhibitors and β-blockers or amlodipine may be used for BP reduction in those with stable CAD.

Cholesterol Treatment

The 3-hydroxy-3-methylglutaryl coenzyme-A reductase inhibitors (statins) inhibiting the rate-limiting step in cholesterol synthesis, and have become standard care for most patients with NSTE-ACS. Their sustained use results in a significant reduction in the level of low-density lipoprotein cholesterol (LDL-C), along with more modest but favorable effects on levels of other serum lipids. Based on a recommended LDL-C goal of less than 70 mg/dL (1.8 mmol/L),[224] nearly all patients with NSTE-ACS should begin treatment with a high-dose, potent statin during their hospitalization. The benefits of statins are seen as early as 30 days after treatment.[225] Because of comorbid conditions in cancer patients, including hepatic metastasis, all patients treated with a high-dose, potent statin should have creatine

kinase and transaminase levels closely monitored, with dose adjustment or discontinuation of medication as needed.

Smoking Cessation

All smokers with ACS should be encouraged to quit smoking since abstinence has been found to greatly lower the risk of future coronary events.[226,227] Behavioral support,[228,229] as well as bupropion with or without nicotine replacement,[230] have been shown to have the greatest efficacy in helping patients quit, and thus should be offered to all cancer patients to improve long-term smoking cessation.

Diabetes Management, Diet, and Exercise

All patients with diabetes should maintain strict glycemic control with a glycosylated hemoglobin level of less than 7.0%[231].

STE-ACS

Treatment strategies for STE-ACS in cancer patients remains suboptimal due to the perceived complexity, and a lack of guideline and agreement on the aggressiveness of therapy. There is no evidence-based guideline addressing specifically the management of cancer patients with STE-ACS, although there is no reason why general guidelines should not be applicable in the majority of cancer patients. This lack of consensus for the optimal reperfusion strategy in cancer patients with STE-ACS stems from the exclusion or nonrepresentation of cancer patients in large clinical trials.

In the clinical setting, two key concepts are of profound importance when considering optimal treatment for STE-ACS. The Reimer and Jennings wavefront hypothesis of evolving infarction has driven the entire field of reperfusion therapy for almost last 3 decades[23]; and there is a very strong relationship between time to treatment and extent of myocardial salvage. Whether the therapy given is primary PCI or fibrinolytics depends on the policy of an individual institution, but speed is of the essence. Emphasis should be on restoring arterial patency as soon as possible, especially in high-risk cardiac patients (Table 7). The main concern for use of either strategy in cancer patients is the risk of major bleeding. Whether benefit outweighs risk depends largely on the duration of symptoms or ischemia and the nature of adjunctive therapy (ie, full- or reduced-dose fibrinolytics, platelet inhibitors, or heparin alone). As in elderly persons, patients with hypertension, and those with low body weight,[232] the risk of intracranial bleeding must be considered in cancer patients in the context of multiple preexisting comorbidities (eg, low platelets, presence of metastasis and associated hepatorenal

dysfunction). However, in the elderly who are also at a high risk of bleeding, multiple clinical trials and observational studies indicate improved survival and low risk of stroke with primary PCI compared with thrombolysis with STEMI. Since many cancer patients are managed at facilities without advanced cardiac interventional capability, thrombolytics are viable alternatives if transfer to a tertiary care center is delayed. Survival is greatest when reperfusion by thrombolytics is obtained within the first 3 hours of the onset of symptoms, and incremental delays thereafter do not yield significant additional mortality effect.[233] Moreover, the benefits of thrombolytics late after symptom onset are decreased and the risk of myocardial rupture may be increased.[234,235] However, because thrombolytic therapy requires, on average, 45 to 60 minutes before reperfusion occurs,[236] a case can be made for transfer for PCI without preceding fibrinolytic therapy in patients presenting relatively late (ie, ≥ 3 hours after symptom onset).[237] Moreover, given the altered hemostatic milieu in cancer patients, the efficacy of thrombolytic agents may be unpredictable. Access-site hemorrhage following PCI may be a major issue in cancer patients. It is not clear whether data from studies in patients > 75 years showing an increased risk of intracerebral bleeding with combination of a fibrin-specific agent and a glycoprotein IIb/IIIa receptor antagonist may be extrapolated to the cancer population. Clearly, different approaches to reperfusion therapies need to be placed within the context of the presence of other comorbid conditions in cancer patient presenting with of STE-ACS.

Large-scale targeted clinical trials are needed to evaluate the relative merits of available reperfusion strategies as well as newer antithrombotic adjunctive therapies in cancer patients presenting with STEMI.

Summary

Acute coronary syndrome in a cancer patient presents a difficult challenge. The pathogenic mechanisms of ACS in cancer patients are multifactorial. A major mechanism involves activation of the coagulation system by components expressed by most tumor cells. Another important mechanism is triggered by changes in platelet volume and functions in cancer. There is no evidence-based guideline specifically addressing the management of cancer patients with ACS, although there is no reason why general guidelines should not be applicable in the majority of cancer patients. The main concern for use of primary PCI or fibrinolytics, platelet inhibitors, or heparin in cancer patients is the risk of major bleeding. Nevertheless, many cancer patients with ACS would qualify for the same management as others without cancer. However, a significant

Table 7 The ABCDE Mnemonic for Treatment of ACS

A = Antiplatelet agents—aspirin
 Adenosine diphosphate receptor inhibitor Clopidogrel—in patients who cannot tolerate aspirin
B = β-blocker in patients without contraindications
 Blood pressure control
C = Converting enzyme inhibition in patients with congestive heart failure, left ventricular dysfunction
 (ejection fraction below 40%), hypertension, or diabetes
 Cholesterol lowering agent—statin
 Cessation of smoking
D = Diabetes control
 Diet (heart-healthy)
E = Early invasive approach (cardiac catheterization) in high risk patients and those in whom conservative
 management fails

Table 8 Determinants of short-term high risk of fatal or nonfatal myocardial infarction

Prolonged (>20 min) ongoing pain at rest
Pulmonary edema, most likely related to ischemia
Angina at rest, with dynamic ST-segment changes >1 mm
Angina with new or worsening mitral regurgitant murmur
Angina with S3 or new or worsening rales
Angina with hypotension

number of patients pose a challenge in their management because of several comorbid conditions (specifically, profound thrombocytopenia and metastatic lesions). A subset of high-risk patients may not be candidates for any of the conventional treatments; potential alternatives and a conservative therapeutic modality of treatments may have to be taken into consideration in this setting. An approach of intensive observation and aggressive pain control may of paramount importance in such cancer patients.

With increased complexity of effective cancer therapy, it is important to identify the subset of cancer patients at high risk for cardiovascular events, particularly those with no clinical history of coronary disease. Using novel and improved diagnostic techniques, it is possible to detect coronary artery disease at a much earlier stage, which can be managed with optimized medical therapy. Additionally, an increasing population of older, more deconditioned cancer patients with many comorbidities are under consideration for major surgery. Many such major surgeries are performed before or after chemotherapy and/or radiation, which increases the risk of cardiac ischemic events. Many chemotherapeutic agents have important ischemic cardiac effects, while others have the ability to potentiate the adverse effects of other agents and are likely to have significant effects on patient outcome. It is therefore very important to take into account several patient-related factors, including advanced age, preexisting coronary disease, concomitant radiation

therapy, and metabolic abnormalities in these patients.

REFERENCES

1. Eyre H, Kahn R, Robertson RM, et al. Preventing cancer, cardiovascular disease, and diabetes: a common agenda for the American Cancer Society, the American Diabetes Association, and the American Heart Association. Stroke 2004;35:1999–2010.
2. Miller DD, Shaw LJ. Screening for coronary heart disease: cardiology through the oncology looking glass. J Nucl Cardiol 2005;12:158–65.
3. www.cancer.org. Estimated new cancer cases and deaths by sex for all sites, 2004.
4. Yusuf S, Hawken S, Ounpuu S, et al. Effect of potentially modifiable risk factors associated with myocardial infarction in 52 countries (the INTERHEART study): case-control study. Lancet 2004;364(9438):937–52.
5. Jemal A, Tiwari RC, Murray T, et al. Cancer statistics, 2004. CA Cancer J Clin 2004;54:8–29.
6. http://www.americanheart.org. Heart disease and stroke statistics-2005 update, 2005.
7. Ogawa A, Kanda T, Sugihara S, et al. Risk factors for myocardial infarction in cancer patients. J Med 1995;26 (5-6):221–33.
8. Schultz PN, Beck ML, Stava C, Vassilopoulou-Sellin R. Health profiles in 5836 long-term cancer survivors. Int J Cancer 2003;104:488–95.
9. Chang S, Long SR, Kutikova L, et al. Estimating the cost of cancer: results on the basis of claims data analyses for cancer patients diagnosed with seven types of cancer during 1999 to 2000. J Clin Oncol 2004;22:3524–30.
10. Eisenstein EL, Shaw LK, Anstrom KJ, et al. Assessing the clinical and economic burden of coronary artery disease: 1986-1998. Med Care 2001;39:824–35.
11. Yusuf S, Reddy S, Ounpuu S, Anand S. Global burden of cardiovascular diseases: part I: general considerations, the epidemiologic transition, risk factors, and impact of urbanization. Circulation 2001;104:2746–53.
12. Pais P, Pogue J, Gerstein H, et al. Risk factors for acute myocardial infarction in Indians: a case-control study. Lancet 1996;348(9024):358–63.
13. Yusuf S, Reddy S, Ounpuu S, Anand S. Global burden of cardiovascular diseases: Part II: variations in cardiovascular disease by specific ethnic groups and geographic regions and prevention strategies. Circulation 2001;104:2855–64.
14. Stamler J, Stamler R, Neaton JD, et al. Low risk-factor profile and long-term cardiovascular and noncardiovascular mortality and life expectancy: findings for 5 large cohorts of young adult and middle-aged men and women. JAMA 1999;282:2012–8.
15. Rosengren A, Dotevall A, Eriksson H, Wilhelmsen L. Optimal risk factors in the population: prognosis, prevalence, and secular trends; data from Goteborg population studies. Eur Heart J 2001;22:136–44.
16. Walldius G, Jungner I, Holme I, et al. High apolipoprotein B, low apolipoprotein A-I, and improvement in the prediction of fatal myocardial infarction (AMORIS study): a prospective study. Lancet 2001;358(9298):2026–33.
17. Rosengren A, Hawken S, Ounpuu S, et al. Association of psychosocial risk factors with risk of acute myocardial infarction in 11119 cases and 13648 controls from 52 countries (the INTERHEART study): case-control study. Lancet 2004;364(9438):953–62.
18. Antman EM, Cohen M, Bernink PJ, et al. The TIMI risk score for unstable angina/non-ST elevation MI: a method for prognostication and therapeutic decision making. JAMA 2000;284(7):835–42.
19. Giugliano RP, Braunwald E. Selecting the best reperfusion strategy in ST-elevation myocardial infarction: it's all a matter of time. Circulation 2003;108:2828–30.
20. Gersh BJ, Anderson JL. Thrombolysis and myocardial salvage. Results of clinical trials and the animal paradigm—paradoxic or predictable? Circulation 1993;88:296–306.
21. Singh M, Ting HH, Berger PB, et al. Rationale for on-site cardiac surgery for primary angioplasty: a time for reappraisal. J Am Coll Cardiol 2002;39:1881–9.
22. Wennberg DE, Lucas FL, Siewers AE, et al. Outcomes of percutaneous coronary interventions performed at centers without and with onsite coronary artery bypass graft surgery. JAMA 2004;292:1961–8.
23. Reimer KA, Jennings RB. The "wavefront phenomenon" of myocardial ischemic cell death. II. Transmural progression of necrosis within the framework of ischemic bed size (myocardium at risk) and collateral flow. Lab Invest 1979;40:633–44.
24. Braunwald E. Myocardial reperfusion, limitation of infarct size, reduction of left ventricular dysfunction, and improved survival. Should the paradigm be expanded? Circulation 1989;79:441–4.
25. Califf RM, Topol EJ, Gersh BJ. From myocardial salvage to patient salvage in acute myocardial infarction: the role of reperfusion therapy. J Am Coll Cardiol 1989;14:1382–8.
26. Sadanandan S, Buller C, Menon V, et al. The late open artery hypothesis—a decade later. Am Heart J 2001;142:411–21.
27. Topol EJ, Califf RM, George BS, et al. A randomized trial of immediate versus delayed elective angioplasty after intravenous tissue plasminogen activator in acute myocardial infarction. N Engl J Med 1987;317:581–8.
28. Heit JA, Silverstein MD, Mohr DN, et al. Risk factors for deep vein thrombosis and pulmonary embolism: a population-based case-control study. Arch Intern Med 2000;160:809–15.
29. Myers C. Role of iron in anthracycline action. In: Hacker M, Lazo J, Tritton T, editors. Organ directed toxicities of anticancer drugs. Boston: Martinus Nijhoff; 1988. p. 17–30.
30. Kupari M, Volin L, Suokas A, et al. Cardiac involvement in bone marrow transplantation: electrocardiographic changes, arrhythmias, heart failure and autopsy findings. Bone Marrow Transplant 1990;5:91–8.
31. Dow E, Schulman H, Agura E. Cyclophosphamide cardiac injury mimicking acute myocardial infarction. Bone Marrow Transplant 1993;12:169–72.
32. Gottdiener JS, Appelbaum FR, Ferrans VJ, et al. Cardiotoxicity associated with high-dose cyclophosphamide therapy. Arch Intern Med 1981;141:758–63.
33. Quezado ZM, Wilson WH, Cunnion RE, et al. High-dose ifosfamide is associated with severe, reversible cardiac dysfunction. Ann Intern Med 1993;118:31–6.
34. Berliner S, Rahima M, Sidi Y, et al. Acute coronary events following cisplatin-based chemotherapy. Cancer Invest 1990;8:583–6.
35. Meinardi MT, Gietema JA, van der Graaf WT, et al. Cardiovascular morbidity in long-term survivors of metastatic testicular cancer. J Clin Oncol 2000;18:1725–32.
36. Tomasz M, Mercado CM, Olson J, Chatterjie N. The mode of interaction of mitomycin C with deoxyribonucleic acid and other polynucleotides in vitro. Biochemistry 1974;13:4878–87.
37. Gradishar WJ, Vokes EE. 5-Fluorouracil cardiotoxicity: a critical review. Ann Oncol 1990;1:409–14.
38. Labianca R, Beretta G, Clerici M, et al. Cardiac toxicity of 5-fluorouracil: a study on 1083 patients. Tumori 1982;68:505–10.
39. Frickhofen N, Beck FJ, Jung B, et al. Capecitabine can induce acute coronary syndrome similar to 5-fluorouracil. Ann Oncol 2002;13:797–801.
40. Sevelda P, Mayerhofer K, Obermair A, et al. Thrombosis with paclitaxel. Lancet 1994;343(8899):727.
41. Rowinsky EK, McGuire WP, Guarnieri T, et al. Cardiac disturbances during the administration of taxol. J Clin Oncol 1991;9:1704–12.
42. Trimble EL, Adams JD, Vena D, et al. Paclitaxel for platinum-refractory ovarian cancer: results from the first

1,000 patients registered to National Cancer Institute Treatment Referral Center 9103. J Clin Oncol 1993;11:2405–10.

43. Yancey RS, Talpaz M. Vindesine-associated angina and ECG changes. Cancer Treat Rep 1982;66:587–9.

44. Lejonc JL, Vernant JP, Macquin J, Castaigne A. Myocardial infarction following vinblastine treatment. Lancet 1980;2(8196):692.

45. Lapeyre-Mestre M, Gregoire N, Bugat R, Montastruc JL. Vinorelbine-related cardiac events: a meta-analysis of randomized clinical trials. Fundam Clin Pharmacol 2004;18:97–105.

46. Dillman RO. Monoclonal antibodies in the treatment of malignancy: basic concepts and recent developments. Cancer Invest 2001;19:833–41.

47. Baselga J. Herceptin alone or in combination with chemotherapy in the treatment of HER2-positive metastatic breast cancer: pivotal trials. Oncology 2001;61 Suppl 2:14–21.

48. Jurcic J. Antibody based treatments for leukemia and lymphoma. ASCO Annual Meeting Summaries 2002, Alexandria, Va. p. 180–186.

49. Mellstedt H. Monoclonal antibodies in human cancer. Drugs Today (Barc) 2003;39 (Suppl C):1–16.

50. Albanell J, Baselga J. Systemic therapy emergencies. Semin Oncol 2000;27:347–61.

51. White RL Jr, Schwartzentruber DJ, Guleria A, et al. Cardiopulmonary toxicity of treatment with high dose interleukin-2 in 199 consecutive patients with metastatic melanoma or renal cell carcinoma. Cancer 1994;74:3212–22.

52. Nora R, Abrams JS, Tait NS, et al. Myocardial toxic effects during recombinant interleukin-2 therapy. J Natl Cancer Inst 1989;81:59–63.

53. Kammula US, White DE, Rosenberg SA. Trends in the safety of high dose bolus interleukin-2 administration in patients with metastatic cancer. Cancer 1998;83:797–805.

54. Olsen E, Duvic M, Frankel A, et al. Pivotal phase III trial of two dose levels of denileukin diftitox for the treatment of cutaneous T-cell lymphoma. J Clin Oncol 2001;19:376–88.

55. Vial T, Descotes J. Immune-mediated side-effects of cytokines in humans. Toxicology 1995;105:31–57.

56. Tallman MS, Andersen JW, Schiffer CA, et al. All-trans-retinoic acid in acute promyelocytic leukemia. N Engl J Med 1997;337:1021–8.

57. Tallman MS, Andersen JW, Schiffer CA, et al. Clinical description of 44 patients with acute promyelocytic leukemia who developed the retinoic acid syndrome. Blood 2000;95:90–5.

58. Soignet SL. Clinical experience of arsenic trioxide in relapsed acute promyelocytic leukemia. Oncologist 2001;6 Suppl 2:11–6.

59. Huang SY, Chang CS, Tang JL, et al. Acute and chronic arsenic poisoning associated with treatment of acute promyelocytic leukaemia. Br J Haematol 1998;103:1092–5.

60. Huang CH, Chen WJ, Wu CC, et al. Complete atrioventricular block after arsenic trioxide treatment in an acute promyelocytic leukemic patient. Pacing Clin Electrophysiol 1999;22(6 Pt 1):965–7.

61. Westervelt P, Brown RA, Adkins DR, et al. Sudden death among patients with acute promyelocytic leukemia treated with arsenic trioxide. Blood 2001;98:266–71.

62. Grem JL, King SA, Chun HG, Grever MR. Cardiac complications observed in elderly patients following 2'-deoxycoformycin therapy. Am J Hematol 1991;38:245–7.

63. Gryn J, Gordon R, Bapat A, et al. Pentostatin increases the acute toxicity of high dose cyclophosphamide. Bone Marrow Transplant 1993;12:217–20.

64. Rajkumar SV, Gertz MA, Lacy MQ, et al. Thalidomide as initial therapy for early-stage myeloma. Leukemia 2003;17:775–9.

65. Airey CL, Dodwell DJ, Joffe JK, Jones WG. Etoposide-related myocardial infarction. Clin Oncol (R Coll Radiol) 1995;7:135.

66. Schecter JP, Jones SE, Jackson RA. Myocardial infarction in a 27-year-old woman: possible complication of treatment with VP-16-213 (NSC-141540), mediastinal irradiation, or both. Cancer Chemother Rep 1975;59:887–8.

67. Zhou DC, Zittoun R, Marie JP. Homoharringtonine: an effective new natural product in cancer chemotherapy. Bull Cancer 1995;82:987–95.

68. Ajani JA, Dimery I, Chawla SP, et al. Phase II studies of homoharringtonine in patients with advanced malignant melanoma; sarcoma; and head and neck, breast, and colorectal carcinomas. Cancer Treat Rep 1986;70:375–9.

69. Effects of radiotherapy and surgery in early breast cancer. An overview of the randomized trials. Early Breast Cancer Trialists' Collaborative Group. N Engl J Med 1995;333:1444–55.

70. Hull MC, Morris CG, Pepine CJ, Mendenhall NP. Valvular dysfunction and carotid, subclavian, and coronary artery disease in survivors of Hodgkin lymphoma treated with radiation therapy. JAMA 2003;290:2831–7.

71. Orzan F, Brusca A, Conte MR, et al. Severe coronary artery disease after radiation therapy of the chest and mediastinum: clinical presentation and treatment. Br Heart J 1993;69:496–500.

72. Leon MB, Teirstein PS, Moses JW, et al. Localized intracoronary gamma-radiation therapy to inhibit the recurrence of restenosis after stenting. N Engl J Med 2001;344:250–6.

73. Stewart JR, Fajardo LF, Gillette SM, Constine LS. Radiation injury to the heart. Int J Radiat Oncol Biol Phys 1995;31:1205–11.

74. Theodoulou M, Seidman AD. Cardiac effects of adjuvant therapy for early breast cancer. Semin Oncol 2003;30:730–9.

75. Tribble DL, Barcellos-Hoff MH, Chu BM, Gong EL. Ionizing radiation accelerates aortic lesion formation in fat-fed mice via SOD-inhibitable processes. Arterioscler Thromb Vasc Biol 1999;19:1387–92.

76. Beckman JA, Thakore A, Kalinowski BH, et al. Radiation therapy impairs endothelium-dependent vasodilation in humans. J Am Coll Cardiol 2001;37:761–5.

77. Basavaraju SR, Easterly CE. Pathophysiological effects of radiation on atherosclerosis development and progression, and the incidence of cardiovascular complications. Med Phys 2002;29:2391–403.

78. Veinot JP, Edwards WD. Pathology of radiation-induced heart disease: a surgical and autopsy study of 27 cases. Hum Pathol 1996;27:766–73.

79. Gyenes G, Fornander T, Carlens P, et al. Detection of radiation-induced myocardial damage by technetium-99m sestamibi scintigraphy. Eur J Nucl Med 1997;24:286–92.

80. Brosius FC 3rd, Waller BF, Roberts WC. Radiation heart disease. Analysis of 16 young (aged 15 to 33 years) necropsy patients who received over 3,500 rads to the heart. Am J Med 1981;70:519–30.

81. Paris F, Fuks Z, Kang A, et al. Endothelial apoptosis as the primary lesion initiating intestinal radiation damage in mice. Science 2001;293(5528):293–7.

82. Cheng SW, Ting AC, Lam LK, Wei WI. Carotid stenosis after radiotherapy for nasopharyngeal carcinoma. Arch Otolaryngol Head Neck Surg 2000;126:517–21.

83. Marnett LJ, Kalgutkar AS. Cyclooxygenase 2 inhibitors: discovery, selectivity and the future. Trends Pharmacol Sci 1999;20:465–9.

84. Steinbach G, Lynch PM, Phillips RK, et al. The effect of celecoxib, a cyclooxygenase-2 inhibitor, in familial adenomatous polyposis. N Engl J Med 2000;342:1946–52.

85. Giardiello FM, Yang VW, Hylind LM, et al. Primary chemoprevention of familial adenomatous polyposis with sulindac. N Engl J Med 2002;346:1054–9.

86. Baron JA. Epidemiology of non-steroidal anti-inflammatory drugs and cancer. Prog Exp Tumor Res 2003;37:1–24.

87. Hawk ET, Viner J, Richmond E, Umar A. Non-steroidal anti-inflammatory drugs (NSAIDs) for colorectal cancer prevention. Cancer Chemother Biol Response Modif 2003;21:759–89.

88. Silverstein FE, Faich G, Goldstein JL, et al. Gastrointestinal toxicity with celecoxib vs nonsteroidal anti-inflammatory drugs for osteoarthritis and rheumatoid arthritis: the CLASS study: a randomized controlled trial. Celecoxib Long-term Arthritis Safety Study. JAMA 2000;284:1247–55.

89. Mamdani M, Juurlink DN, Lee DS, et al. Cyclo-oxygenase-2 inhibitors versus non-selective non-steroidal anti-inflammatory drugs and congestive heart failure outcomes in elderly patients: a population-based cohort study. Lancet 2004;363(9423):1751–6.

90. Solomon DH, Schneeweiss S, Glynn RJ, et al. Relationship between selective cyclooxygenase-2 inhibitors and acute myocardial infarction in older adults. Circulation 2004;109:2068–73.

91. Ray S, Stacey R, Imrie M, Filshie J. A review of 560 Hickman catheter insertions. Anaesthesia 1996;51:981–5.

92. Ray WA, Stein CM, Daugherty JR, et al. COX-2 selective non-steroidal anti-inflammatory drugs and risk of serious coronary heart disease. Lancet 2002;360(9339):1071–3.

93. Mamdani M, Rochon P, Juurlink DN, et al. Effect of selective cyclooxygenase 2 inhibitors and naproxen on short-term risk of acute myocardial infarction in the elderly. Arch Intern Med 2003;163:481–6.

94. Solomon SD, McMurray J Jr, Pfeffer MA, et al. Cardiovascular Risk Associated with Celecoxib in a Clinical Trial for Colorectal Adenoma Prevention. N Engl J Med 2005;352:1071–80.

95. Fitzgerald GA. Coxibs and cardiovascular disease. N Engl J Med 2004;351:1709–11.

96. Bresalier RS, Sandler RS, Quan H, et al. Cardiovascular events associated with rofecoxib in a colorectal adenoma chemoprevention trial. N Engl J Med 2005;352:1092–102.

97. Furberg CD, Psaty BM, FitzGerald GA. Parecoxib, valdecoxib, and cardiovascular risk. Circulation 2005;111:249.

98. Juni P, Nartey L, Reichenbach S, et al. Risk of cardiovascular events and rofecoxib: cumulative meta-analysis. Lancet 2004;364(9450):2021–9.

99. Ott E, Nussmeier NA, Duke PC, et al. Efficacy and safety of the cyclooxygenase 2 inhibitors parecoxib and valdecoxib in patients undergoing coronary artery bypass surgery. J Thorac Cardiovasc Surg 2003;125:1481–92.

100. Nussmeier NA, Whelton AA, Brown MT, et al. Complications of the COX-2 inhibitors parecoxib and valdecoxib after cardiac surgery. N Engl J Med 2005;352:1081–91.

101. Donati MB, Semeraro N. Cancer cell procoagulants and their pharmacological modulation. Haemostasis 1984;14:422–9.

102. Falanga A, Iacoviello L, Evangelista V, et al. Loss of blast cell procoagulant activity and improvement of hemostatic variables in patients with acute promyelocytic leukemia administered all-trans-retinoic acid. Blood 1995;86:1072–81.

103. Blann AD, Lip GY. Virchow's triad revisited: the importance of soluble coagulation factors, the endothelium, and platelets. Thromb Res 2001;101:321–7.

104. Lwaleed BA, Chisholm M, Francis JL. The significance of measuring monocyte tissue factor activity in patients with breast and colorectal cancer. Br J Cancer 1999;80(1-2):279–85.

105. Conkling PR, Greenberg CS, Weinberg JB. Tumor necrosis factor induces tissue factor-like activity in human leukemia cell line U937 and peripheral blood monocytes. Blood 1988;72:128–33.

106. Kakkar AK, Lemoine NR, Scully MF, et al. Tissue factor expression correlates with histological grade in human pancreatic cancer. Br J Surg 1995;82:1101–4.

107. Shigemori C, Wada H, Matsumoto K, et al. Tissue factor expression and metastatic potential of colorectal cancer. Thromb Haemost 1998;80:894–8.

108. Rickles FR, Hair GA, Zeff RA, et al. Tissue factor expression in human leukocytes and tumor cells. Thromb Haemost 1995;74:391–5.

109. De Lucia D, De Vita F, Orditura M, et al. Hypercoagulable state in patients with advanced gastrointestinal cancer: evidence for an acquired resistance to activated protein C. Tumori 1997;83:948–52.

110. Nand S, Fisher SG, Salgia R, Fisher RI. Hemostatic abnormalities in untreated cancer: incidence and correlation with thrombotic and hemorrhagic complications. J Clin Oncol 1987;5:1998–2003.

111. Donati MB, Poggi A. Malignancy and haemostasis. Br J Haematol 1980;44:173–82.

112. Edoute Y, Haim N, Rinkevich D, et al. Cardiac valvular vegetations in cancer patients: a prospective echocardiographic study of 200 patients. Am J Med 1997;102:252–8.

113. Reisner SA, Rinkevich D, Markiewicz W, et al. Cardiac involvement in patients with myeloproliferative disorders. Am J Med 1992;93:498–504.

114. Braunwald E, Antman EM, Beasley JW, et al. ACC/AHA guideline update for the management of patients with unstable angina and non-ST-segment elevation myocardial infarction—2002: summary article: a report of the American College of Cardiology/American Heart Association Task Force on Practice Guidelines (Committee on the Management of Patients With Unstable Angina). Circulation 2002;106:1893–900.

115. Kolodgie FD, Virmani R, Burke AP, et al. Pathologic assessment of the vulnerable human coronary plaque. Heart 2004;90:1385–91.

116. van der Wal AC, Becker AE, van der Loos CM, Das PK. Site of intimal rupture or erosion of thrombosed coronary atherosclerotic plaques is characterized by an inflammatory process irrespective of the dominant plaque morphology. Circulation 1994;89:36–44.

117. Naghavi M, Libby P, Falk E, et al. From vulnerable plaque to vulnerable patient: a call for new definitions and risk assessment strategies: Part II. Circulation 2003;108: 1772–8.

118. Farb A, Burke AP, Tang AL, et al. Coronary plaque erosion without rupture into a lipid core. A frequent cause of coronary thrombosis in sudden coronary death. Circulation 1996;93:1354–63.

119. Fuster V, Fayad ZA, Badimon JJ. Acute coronary syndromes: biology. Lancet 1999;353 Suppl 2:SII5–9.

120. Behrendt D, Ganz P. Endothelial function. From vascular biology to clinical applications. Am J Cardiol 2002; 90(10C):40L–48L.

121. Weiss N, Keller C, Hoffmann U, Loscalzo J. Endothelial dysfunction and atherothrombosis in mild hyperhomocysteinemia. Vasc Med 2002;7:227–39.

122. Callow AD. Endothelial dysfunction in atherosclerosis. Vascul Pharmacol 2002;38:257–8.

123. Malek AM, Alper SL, Izumo S. Hemodynamic shear stress and its role in atherosclerosis. JAMA 1999;282:2035–42.

124. Orbe J, Fernandez L, Rodriguez JA, et al. Different expression of MMPs/TIMP-1 in human atherosclerotic lesions. Relation to plaque features and vascular bed. Atherosclerosis 2003;170:269–76.

125. Kong YZ, Huang XR, Ouyang X, et al. Evidence for vascular macrophage migration inhibitory factor in destabilization of human atherosclerotic plaques. Cardiovasc Res 2005;65:272–82.

126. Tomasian D, Keaney JF, Vita JA. Antioxidants and the bioactivity of endothelium-derived nitric oxide. Cardiovasc Res 2000;47:426–35.

127. Cai H, Harrison DG. Endothelial dysfunction in cardiovascular diseases: the role of oxidant stress. Circ Res 2000; 87:840–4.

128. Ballantyne CM, Nambi V. Markers of inflammation and their clinical significance. Atheroscler Suppl 2005;6:21–9.

129. Herman MP, Sukhova GK, Libby P, et al. Expression of neutrophil collagenase (matrix metalloproteinase-8) in human atheroma: a novel collagenolytic pathway suggested by transcriptional profiling. Circulation 2001;104: 1899–904.

130. Libby P, Geng YJ, Aikawa M, et al. Macrophages and atherosclerotic plaque stability. Curr Opin Lipidol 1996;7: 330–5.

131. Ridker PM, Hennekens CH, Buring JE, Rifai N. C-reactive protein and other markers of inflammation in the prediction of cardiovascular disease in women. N Engl J Med 2000;342:836–43.

132. Moons AH, Levi M, Peters RJ. Tissue factor and coronary artery disease. Cardiovasc Res 2002;53:313–25.

133. Mallat Z, Tedgui A. Current perspective on the role of apoptosis in atherothrombotic disease. Circ Res 2001;88: 998–1003.

134. Rauch U, Antoniak S, Boots M, et al. Association of tissue-factor upregulation in squamous-cell carcinoma of the lung with increased tissue factor in circulating blood. Lancet Oncol 2005;6:254.

135. Momiyama Y, Ohmori R, Taniguchi H, et al. Association of Mycoplasma pneumoniae infection with coronary artery disease and its interaction with chlamydial infection. Atherosclerosis 2004;176:139–44.

136. Kolodgie FD, Gold HK, Burke AP, et al. Intraplaque hemorrhage and progression of coronary atheroma. N Engl J Med 2003;349:2316–25.

137. Topol EJ, Yadav JS. Recognition of the importance of embolization in atherosclerotic vascular disease. Circulation 2000;101:570–80.

138. Davies MJ, Thomas AC, Knapman PA, Hangartner JR. Intramyocardial platelet aggregation in patients with unstable angina suffering sudden ischemic cardiac death. Circulation 1986;73:418–27.

139. Virmani R, Kolodgie FD, Burke AP, et al. Lessons from sudden coronary death: a comprehensive morphological classification scheme for atherosclerotic lesions. Arterioscler Thromb Vasc Biol 2000;20:1262–75.

140. Rauch U, Osende JI, Fuster V, et al. Thrombus formation on atherosclerotic plaques: pathogenesis and clinical consequences. Ann Intern Med 2001;134:224–38.

141. Osende JI, Badimon JJ, Fuster V, et al. Blood thrombogenicity in type 2 diabetes mellitus patients is associated with glycemic control. J Am Coll Cardiol 2001;38:1307–12.

142. Caine GJ, Stonelake PS, Lip GY, Kehoe ST. The hypercoagulable state of malignancy: pathogenesis and current debate. Neoplasia 2002;4:465–73.

143. Massberg S, Schulz C, Gawaz M. Role of platelets in the pathophysiology of acute coronary syndrome. Semin Vasc Med 2003;3:147–62.

144. Goto S. Role of von Willebrand factor for the onset of arterial thrombosis. Clin Lab 2001;47(7-8):327–34.

145. Willerson JT. Conversion from chronic to acute coronary heart disease syndromes. Role of platelets and platelet products. Tex Heart Inst J 1995;22:13–9.

146. Massberg S, Brand K, Gruner S, et al. A critical role of platelet adhesion in the initiation of atherosclerotic lesion formation. J Exp Med 2002;196:887–96.

147. Fajardo LF. The pathology of ionizing radiation as defined by morphologic patterns. Acta Oncol 2005;44:13–22.

148. Howe GR, Zablotska LB, Fix JJ, et al. Analysis of the mortality experience amongst U.S. nuclear power industry workers after chronic low-dose exposure to ionizing radiation. Radiat Res 2004;162:517–26.

149. Virmani R, Farb A, Carter AJ, Jones RM. Comparative pathology: radiation-induced coronary artery disease in man and animals. Semin Interv Cardiol 1998; 3(3-4):163–72.

150. Lestuzzi C, Viel E, Picano E, Meneguzzo N. Coronary vasospasm as a cause of effort-related myocardial ischemia during low-dose chronic continuous infusion of 5-fluorouracil. Am J Med 2001;111:316–8.

151. Schwarzer S, Eber B, Greinix H, Lind P. Non-Q-wave myocardial infarction associated with bleomycin and etoposide chemotherapy. Eur Heart J 1991;12:748–50.

152. Stefenelli T, Kuzmits R, Ulrich W, Glogar D. Acute vascular toxicity after combination chemotherapy with cisplatin, vinblastine, and bleomycin for testicular cancer. Eur Heart J 1988;9:552–6.

153. Stefenelli T, Zielinski CC, Mayr H, Scoheithauer W. Prinzmetal's angina during cyclophosphamide therapy. Eur Heart J 1988;9:1155–7.

154. Cheriparambil KM, Vasireddy H, Kuruvilla A, et al. Acute reversible cardiomyopathy and thromboembolism after cisplatin and 5-fluorouracil chemotherapy—a case report. Angiology 2000;51:873–8.

155. Taskinen M, Saarinen-Pihkala UM, Hovi L, Lipsanen-Nyman M. Impaired glucose tolerance and dyslipidaemia as late effects after bone-marrow transplantation in childhood. Lancet 2000;356(9234):993–7.

156. Thompson SG, Greenberg G, Meade TW. Risk factors for stroke and myocardial infarction in women in the United Kingdom as assessed in general practice: a case-control study. Br Heart J 1989;61:403–9.

157. Miltenyi Z, Keresztes K, Garai I, et al. Radiation-induced coronary artery disease in Hodgkin's disease. Cardiovasc Radiat Med 2004;5:38–43.

158. Vallebona A. Cardiac damage following therapeutic chest irradiation. Importance, evaluation and treatment. Minerva Cardioangiol 2000;48:79–87.

159. Whipple GL, Sagerman RH, van Rooy EM. Long-term evaluation of postorchiectomy radiotherapy for stage II seminoma. Am J Clin Oncol 1997;20:196–201.

160. Lederman GS, Sheldon TA, Chaffey JT, et al. Cardiac disease after mediastinal irradiation for seminoma. Cancer 1987; 60:772–6.

161. Muscari Lin E, Aikin JL, Good BC. Premature menopause after cancer treatment. Cancer Pract 1999;7:114–21.

162. Cuzick J, Stewart H, Rutqvist L, et al. Cause-specific mortality in long-term survivors of breast cancer who participated in trials of radiotherapy. J Clin Oncol 1994;12: 447–53.

163. Giordano SH, Kuo YF, Freeman JL, et al. Risk of cardiac death after adjuvant radiotherapy for breast cancer. J Natl Cancer Inst 2005;97:419–24.

164. Favourable and unfavourable effects on long-term survival of radiotherapy for early breast cancer: an overview of the randomised trials. Early Breast Cancer Trialists' Collaborative Group. Lancet 2000;355(9217):1757–70.

165. Rutqvist LE, Johansson H. Mortality by laterality of the primary tumour among 55,000 breast cancer patients from the Swedish Cancer Registry. Br J Cancer 1990;61:866–8.

166. Stracci F, La Rosa F, Falsettini E, et al. A population survival model for breast cancer. Breast 2005;14:94–102.

167. Whelan TJ, MacKenzie RG, Levine M. A randomized trial comparing two fractionation schedules for breast irradiation postlumpectomy in node-negative breast cancer. Proc Am Soc Clin Oncol 2000;19:2a.

168. Vallis KA, Pintilie M, Chong N, et al. Assessment of coronary heart disease morbidity and mortality after radiation therapy for early breast cancer. J Clin Oncol 2002;20: 1036–42.

169. Takada A, Saito K, Ro A, et al. Papillary fibroelastoma of the aortic valve: a sudden death case of coronary embolism with myocardial infarction. Forensic Sci Int 2000;113 (1-3):209–14.

170. Abascal VM, Kasznica J, Aldea G, Davidoff R. Left atrial myxoma and acute myocardial infarction. A dangerous duo in the thrombolytic agent era. Chest 1996;109: 1106–8.

171. Panos A, Kalangos A, Sztajzel J. Left atrial myxoma presenting with myocardial infarction. Case report and review of the literature. Int J Cardiol 1997;62:73–5.

172. Denniston AK, Beattie JM. An unusual case of multiple infarcts. Postgrad Med J 2002;78(921):431–5.

173. Jachmann-Jahn U, Cornely OA, Laufs U, et al. Acute anterior myocardial infarction as first manifestation of acute myeloid leukemia. Ann Hematol 2001;80:677–81.

174. Summers RL, Cooper GJ, Carlton FB, et al. Prevalence of atypical chest pain descriptions in a population from the southern United States. Am J Med Sci 1999;318:142–5.

175. Canto JG, Shlipak MG, Rogers WJ, et al. Prevalence, clinical characteristics, and mortality among patients with myocardial infarction presenting without chest pain. JAMA 2000;283:3223–9.

176. Horne R, James D, Petrie K, et al. Patients' interpretation of symptoms as a cause of delay in reaching hospital during acute myocardial infarction. Heart 2000;83:388–93.

177. Brieger D, Eagle KA, Goodman SG, et al. Acute coronary syndromes without chest pain, an underdiagnosed and undertreated high-risk group: insights from the Global Registry of Acute Coronary Events. Chest 2004;126: 461–9.

178. Antman EM, Anbe DT, Armstrong PW, et al. ACC/AHA guidelines for the management of patients with ST-elevation myocardial infarction—executive summary. A report of the American College of Cardiology/American Heart Association Task Force on Practice Guidelines (Writing Committee to revise the 1999 guidelines for the management of patients with acute myocardial infarction). J Am Coll Cardiol 2004;44:671–719.

179. Klocke FJ, Baird MG, Lorell BH, et al. ACC/AHA/ASNC guidelines for the clinical use of cardiac radionuclide imaging—executive summary: a report of the American College of Cardiology/American Heart Association Task Force on Practice Guidelines (ACC/AHA/ASNC Committee to Revise the 1995 Guidelines for the Clinical Use of Cardiac Radionuclide Imaging). J Am Coll Cardiol 2003;42:1318–33.

180. Rahman AM, Gedevanishvili A, Bungo MW, et al. Non-invasive detection of coronary artery disease by a newly developed high-frequency QRS electrocardiogram. Physiol Meas 2004;25:957–65.

181. Alpert JS, Thygesen K, Antman E, Bassand JP. Myocardial infarction redefined—a consensus document of The Joint European Society of Cardiology/American College of Cardiology Committee for the redefinition of myocardial infarction. J Am Coll Cardiol 2000;36:959–69.

182. Mulvagh SL. Advances in myocardial contrast echocardiography and the role of adenosine stress. Am J Cardiol 2004;94(2A):12D–18D.

183. Mollet NR, Cademartiri F, de Feyter PJ. Non-invasive multislice CT coronary imaging. Heart 2005;91:401–7.

184. Achenbach S, Daniel WG. Imaging of coronary atherosclerosis using computed tomography: current status and future directions. Curr Atheroscler Rep 2004;6:213–8.

185. McKie SJ, Hardwick DJ, Reid JH, Murchison JT. Features of cardiac disease demonstrated on CT pulmonary angiography. Clin Radiol 2005;60:31–8.

186. Constantine G, Shan K, Flamm SD, Sivananthan MU. Role of MRI in clinical cardiology. Lancet 2004;363 (9427):2162–71.

187. Rahman AM, Ahmad N. Recurrent myocardial infarction with near-normal coronary angiogram and myocardial ischemia detected by Tc-99m SPECT and magnetic resonance perfusion imaging. J Nucl Cardiol 2003;10: 439–41.

188. Patrono C. Aspirin as an antiplatelet drug. N Engl J Med 1994;330:1287–94.

189. Awtry EH, Loscalzo J. Aspirin. Circulation 2000;101: 1206–18.

190. Lewis HD Jr, Davis JW, Archibald DG, et al. Protective effects of aspirin against acute myocardial infarction and death in men with unstable angina. Results of a Veterans Administration Cooperative Study. N Engl J Med 1983; 309:396–403.

191. Cairns JA, Gent M, Singer J, et al. Aspirin, sulfinpyrazone, or both in unstable angina. Results of a Canadian multicenter trial. N Engl J Med 1985;313:1369–75.

192. Collaborative meta-analysis of randomised trials of antiplatelet therapy for prevention of death, myocardial infarction, and stroke in high risk patients. Br Med J 2002;324(7329):71–86.

193. Peters RJ, Mehta SR, Fox KA, et al. Effects of aspirin dose when used alone or in combination with clopidogrel in patients with acute coronary syndromes: observations from the Clopidogrel in Unstable angina to prevent Recurrent Events (CURE) study. Circulation 2003;108: 1682–7.

194. Moyad MA. An introduction to aspirin, NSAIDs, and COX-2 inhibitors for the primary prevention of cardiovascular events and cancer and their potential preventive role in bladder carcinogenesis: part I. Semin Urol Oncol 2001; 19:294–305.

195. Tanasescu S, Levesque H, Thuillez C. [Pharmacology of aspirin]. Rev Med Interne 2000;21 Suppl 1:18–26.

196. A randomised, blinded, trial of clopidogrel versus aspirin in patients at risk of ischaemic events (CAPRIE). CAPRIE Steering Committee. Lancet 1996;348(9038):1329–39.

197. Savcic M, Hauert J, Bachmann F, et al. Clopidogrel loading dose regimens: kinetic profile of pharmacodynamic response in healthy subjects. Semin Thromb Hemost 1999;25 Suppl 2:15–9.

198. Helft G, Osende JI, Worthley SG, et al. Acute antithrombotic effect of a front-loaded regimen of clopidogrel in patients with atherosclerosis on aspirin. Arterioscler Thromb Vasc Biol 2000;20:2316–21.

199. Patrono C, Coller B, Dalen JE, et al. Platelet-active drugs : the relationships among dose, effectiveness, and side effects. Chest 2001;119(1 Suppl):39–63.

200. Yusuf S, Mehta SR, Zhao F, et al. Early and late effects of clopidogrel in patients with acute coronary syndromes. Circulation 2003;107:966–72.

201. Yusuf S, Zhao F, Mehta SR, et al. Effects of clopidogrel in addition to aspirin in patients with acute coronary syndromes without ST-segment elevation. N Engl J Med 2001;345:494–502.

202. Yende S, Wunderink RG. Effect of clopidogrel on bleeding after coronary artery bypass surgery. Crit Care Med 2001; 29:2271–5.

203. Hongo RH, Ley J, Dick SE, Yee RR. The effect of clopidogrel in combination with aspirin when given before coronary artery bypass grafting. J Am Coll Cardiol 2002;40:231–7.

204. Quinn MJ, Plow EF, Topol EJ. Platelet glycoprotein IIb/IIIa inhibitors: recognition of a two-edged sword? Circulation 2002;106:379–85.

205. Oler A, Whooley MA, Oler J, Grady D. Adding heparin to aspirin reduces the incidence of myocardial infarction and death in patients with unstable angina. A meta-analysis. JAMA 1996;276:811–5.

206. Cohen M, Demers C, Gurfinkel EP, et al. A comparison of low-molecular-weight heparin with unfractionated heparin for unstable coronary artery disease. Efficacy and Safety of Subcutaneous Enoxaparin in Non-Q-Wave Coronary Events Study Group. N Engl J Med 1997;337: 447–52.

207. Blazing MA, de Lemos JA, White HD, et al. Safety and efficacy of enoxaparin vs unfractionated heparin in patients with non-ST-segment elevation acute coronary syndromes who receive tirofiban and aspirin: a randomized controlled trial. JAMA 2004;292:55–64.

208. Ferguson JJ, Califf RM, Antman EM, et al. Enoxaparin vs unfractionated heparin in high-risk patients with non-ST-segment elevation acute coronary syndromes managed with an intended early invasive strategy: primary results of the SYNERGY randomized trial. JAMA 2004;292:45–54.

209. Bar FW, Verheugt FW, Col J, et al. Thrombolysis in patients with unstable angina improves the angiographic but not the clinical outcome. Results of UNASEM, a multicenter, randomized, placebo-controlled, clinical trial with anistreplase. Circulation 1992;86:131–7.

210. Schreiber TL, Rizik D, White C, et al. Randomized trial of thrombolysis versus heparin in unstable angina. Circulation 1992;86:1407–14.

211. Effects of tissue plasminogen activator and a comparison of early invasive and conservative strategies in unstable angina and non-Q-wave myocardial infarction. Results of the TIMI IIIB Trial. Thrombolysis in myocardial ischemia. Circulation 1994;89:1545–56.

212. Yusuf S, Sleight P, Pogue J, et al. Effects of an angiotensin-converting-enzyme inhibitor, ramipril, on cardiovascular events in high-risk patients. The Heart Outcomes Prevention Evaluation Study Investigators. N Engl J Med 2000;342:145–53.

213. Fox KM. Efficacy of perindopril in reduction of cardiovascular events among patients with stable coronary artery disease: randomised, double-blind, placebo-controlled, multicentre trial (the EUROPA study). Lancet 2003; 362(9386):782–8.

214. Braunwald E, Domanski MJ, Fowler SE, et al. Angiotensin-converting-enzyme inhibition in stable coronary artery disease. N Engl J Med 2004;351:2058–68.

215. Pfeffer MA, McMurray JJ, Velazquez EJ, et al. Valsartan, captopril, or both in myocardial infarction complicated by heart failure, left ventricular dysfunction, or both. N Engl J Med 2003;349:1893–906.

216. Yusuf S, Wittes J, Friedman L. Overview of results of randomized clinical trials in heart disease. II. Unstable angina, heart failure, primary prevention with aspirin, and risk factor modification. JAMA 1988;260:2259–63.

217. Metoprolol in acute myocardial infarction. Mortality. The MIAMI Trial Research Group. Am J Cardiol 1985;56(14):15–22.

218. Timolol-induced reduction in mortality and reinfarction in patients surviving acute myocardial infarction. N Engl J Med 1981;304:801–7.

219. A randomized trial of propranolol in patients with acute myocardial infarction. II. Morbidity results. JAMA 1983; 250:2814–9.

220. Gottlieb SS, McCarter RJ, Vogel RA. Effect of beta-blockade on mortality among high-risk and low-risk patients after myocardial infarction. N Engl J Med 1998;339:489–97.

221. Chobanian AV, Bakris GL, Black HR, et al. The seventh report of the joint national committee on prevention, detection, evaluation, and treatment of high blood pressure: the JNC 7 report. JAMA 2003;289:2560–72.

222. Nissen SE, Tuzcu EM, Libby P, et al. Effect of antihypertensive agents on cardiovascular events in patients with coronary disease and normal blood pressure: the CAMELOT study: a randomized controlled trial. JAMA 2004;292: 2217–25.

223. Pepine CJ. What is the optimal blood pressure and drug therapy for patients with coronary artery disease? JAMA 2004;292:2271–3.

224. Grundy SM, Cleeman JI, Merz CN, et al. Implications of recent clinical trials for the National Cholesterol Education Program Adult Treatment Panel III Guidelines. J Am Coll Cardiol 2004;44:720–32.

225. Schwartz GG, Olsson AG, Ezekowitz MD, et al. Effects of atorvastatin on early recurrent ischemic events in acute coronary syndromes: the MIRACL study: a randomized controlled trial. JAMA 2001;285:1711–8.

226. Mora S, Kershner DW, Vigilante CP, Blumenthal RS. Coronary artery disease in postmenopausal women. Curr Treat Options Cardiovasc Med 2001;3:67–79.

227. Stampfer MJ, Hu FB, Manson JE, et al. Primary prevention of coronary heart disease in women through diet and lifestyle. N Engl J Med 2000;343:16–22.

228. Fiore MC. US public health service clinical practice guideline: treating tobacco use and dependence. Respir Care 2000;45:1200–62.

229. Lancaster T, Stead LF. Individual behavioural counselling for smoking cessation. Cochrane Database Syst Rev 2002: CD001292.

230. Woolacott NF, Jones L, Forbes CA, et al. The clinical effectiveness and cost-effectiveness of bupropion and nicotine replacement therapy for smoking cessation: a systematic review and economic evaluation. Health Technol Assess 2002;6:1–245.

231. Standards of medical care for patients with diabetes mellitus. Diabetes Care 2003;26 Suppl 1:33–50.

232. Van de Werf F, Barron HV, Armstrong PW, et al. Incidence and predictors of bleeding events after fibrinolytic therapy with fibrin-specific agents: a comparison of TNK-tPA and rt-PA. Eur Heart J 2001;22:2253–61.

233. Brodie B, Cox D, Stuckey T. How important is time to treatment with primary percutaneous coronary intervention for acute myocardial infarction? results from the CADILLAC trial. J Am Coll Cardiol 2003;41(Suppl A):368.

234. Becker RC, Charlesworth A, Wilcox RG, et al. Cardiac rupture associated with thrombolytic therapy: impact of time to treatment in the Late Assessment of Thrombolytic Efficacy (LATE) study. J Am Coll Cardiol 1995;25: 1063–8.

235. Honan MB, Harrell FE Jr, Reimer KA, et al. Cardiac rupture, mortality and the timing of thrombolytic therapy: a meta-analysis. J Am Coll Cardiol 1990;16:359–67.

236. Lew AS, Laramee P, Cercek B, et al. The effects of the rate of intravenous infusion of streptokinase and the duration of symptoms on the time interval to reperfusion in patients with acute myocardial infarction. Circulation 1985;72: 1053–8.

237. Dalby M, Bouzamondo A, Lechat P, Montalescot G. Transfer for primary angioplasty versus immediate thrombolysis in acute myocardial infarction: a meta-analysis. Circulation 2003;108:1809–14.

Cardiac Manifestations of Malignancy

Joseph Swafford, MD, FACC

S. Wamique Yusuf, MD, FACC

The cardiac manifestations of cancer are actually quite rare. Many times these clinical entities are found on routine surveillance; sometimes they are found as a result of clinical symptomatology; and most of the times, the malignant manifestations of these disorders cancer involvement of the heart carry a poor prognosis. We will review metastatic malignancies of the heart, and then briefly, primary tumors of the heart. Sometimes these tumors have a higher prevalence for different cardiac chambers and entrance points to the heart (Figure 1). This chapter will conclude with a discussion of amyloidosis, which can be found in multiple myeloma patients. We will initiate our discussion with the clinical presentation and diagnostic techniques for patients with cardiac tumors.

Clinical Presentation of Cardiac Tumors

Cancer patients may very well have constitutional symptoms consisting of fever, weight loss, fatigue, and malaise. These are not very helpful symptoms in focusing to suggest cardiac involvement. There are several categories of clinical presentation for cardiac tumors: (1) arrhythmias, (2) valvular and chamber obstructive symptoms, (3) congestive heart failure, (4) cardioembolic presentation events, and (5) cardiac tamponade.

Arrhythmias

Depending on the size of the cardiac tumor and its location, there may be various arrhythmias that are manifested.[1] Most patients will complain of palpitations, or ectopiay is found on routine electrocardiogram. Patients can have either tachyarrhythmia or bradyarrhythmia. The important thing to remember, particularly in the cancer patient, is that these arrhythmias should warrant some workup, further investigation, keeping cardiac tumors as part of the differential diagnosis of the underlying cause. Cancer patients with arrhythmias routinely should have echocardiography. That, which serves as one of the best screening tests to determine if there is cardiac involvement from cancer.[2,3]

Tachyarrhythmias may include atrial fibrillation, atrial flutter,[4] and ventricular tachycardia. On rare occasions, patients can present with sudden cardiac death from ventricular fibrillation.[5] Patients can also have bradyarrhythmias that may manifest as syncope, near syncope, or extreme dizziness with palpitation. These bradyarrhythmias may result from invasion of the conduction system, such as the atrioventricular (AV) node resulting in the heart block[6] or the bundle branches causing right and left bundle branch block, or can result in sinoatrial node destruction with sinus arrest.

Obstructive Symptoms

Obstructive symptoms can be either the result of impaired filling or outflow obstruction.

The size of some intracardiac masses and tumors can cause obstructions of the valve orifice or major blood vessels, resulting in sudden cessation of cardiac output and resulting syncope. If cardiac tumors are particularly large, limiting cardiac filling, sudden decreases in intravascular volume in these cancer patients, such as with severe hemorrhage or dehydration, can also precipitate syncope more readily. Some cardiac tumors are on a pedunculated stalk and, therefore, can prolapse across different valvular structures. It is with this clinical scenario that you can find the classic tumor plop on auscultation.[7,8] When patients lie in different positions, they may facilitate obstructing one of the cardiac valves, resulting in positional syncope. An example of this is a patient with a left atrial tumor, such as a myxoma,[9] who can have their tumor prolapse across the mitral valve orifice. When lying on the left side, there is a greater tendency to occlude

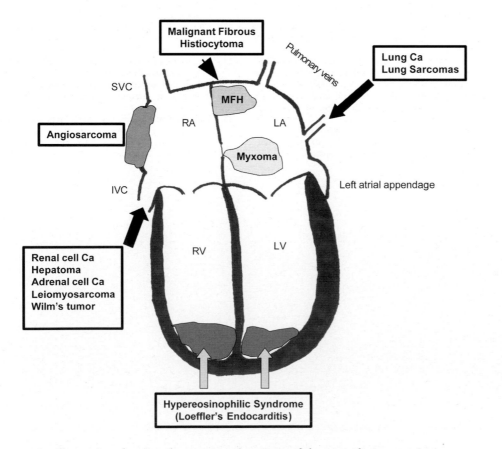

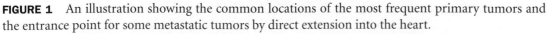

FIGURE 1 An illustration showing the common locations of the most frequent primary tumors and the entrance point for some metastatic tumors by direct extension into the heart.

that mitral valve orifice, resulting in positional syncope.

Congestive Heart Failure

Patients also can have congestive heart failure as a result of chamber or valvular obstruction. With large masses, there is a decrease in the ability to empty cardiac chambers, resulting in elevation of intracardiac pressures and resulting in classic congestive heart failure. This would be very similar to stenotic valvular lesions.[10] Depending on if the tumors are in the left cardiac chambers, you may get symptoms of left heart failure with pulmonary vascular congestion and pulmonary edema. If the tumors involve the right heart chambers, you can get hepatic congestion, ascites, and peripheral edema.

In addition to the obstructive mechanism for the development of congestive heart failure, there may be enough myocardial infiltration by tumors to cause actual pump failure in the form of a restrictive cardiomyopathy.[11]

Cardioembolic Symptoms

Tumors can very frequently be friable[12,13] and can result in the presence of changes in flow pattern within the cardiac chambers, can result in thrombus development. There can be some surface clot that develops over the tumor surface. Any of these factors can result in thromboembolic phenomena lead to thromboembolism. When cardiac tumors in left heart chambers are involved, they can result in stroke,[14] coronary embolization with acute myocardial infarction, renal embolization with renal failure, peripheral arterial embolization[15] with gangrene, or mesentery embolization with an acute abdomen. There has even be a report of cutaneous embolization from a cardiac myxoma.[16] The right-sided embolic phenomena usually manifest a pulmonary embolus.[17]

Cardiac Tamponade

Cardiac tamponade is a frequent clinical presentation for patients with cardiac tumors. Patients will complain of constriction feelings within the chest; they may be restless or have a depressed sensorium because of decreased cardiac output. On physical exam, they may be hypotensive with a pulsus paradoxus, tachycardic, or tachypneic with a respiratory alkalosis. On cardiac auscultation, you can frequently hear a pericardial friction rub. This clinical scenario is often the initial presentation for patients with primary cardiac tumors.[18–20] The great majority of these presentations are the result of associated pericardial involvement; however, there can be cardiac rupture of tumors through the myocardium into the pericardial sac.[21]

Diagnostic Work-Up

Chest X-rays are nonspecific for the diagnosis of cardiac tumors. You may see the enlarged globular cardiac silhouette for those patients that develop cardiac tamponade. Many tumors are intracavitary and therefore won't be picked up by this technique. A higher index of suspicion for cardiac tumors should be maintained for the patient who has primary lung tumors or metastatic tumors to the lung.

Echocardiography can be one of the best screening and most portable imaging techniques for identifying intracardiac masses. The discovery of an intracardiac echodensity on echocardiography can also create a significant diagnostic dilemma, as these densities can represent a primary cardiac tumor, a metastatic tumor, a portion of a thrombus, large vegetation, or an ultrasound artifact. Often, localizing the source or defining the tissue character of the image can be difficult, since echocardiographic images are generated from reflected or refracted ultrasound waves. The probable diagnosis of an intracardiac density can depend upon the clinical situation under which the echocardiogram was performed (Figure 2 and 3). In the cancer patient, echocardiography is ordered to evaluate coexisting cardiac disease, baseline assessment, follow-up of cardiotoxic chemotherapy, or for evaluation of a cardioembolic event such as a pulmonary embolus or stroke. In this clinical decision tree, the type of cancer must be considered, as certain cancers are more likely to metastasize to the heart or produce thrombus. Predisposing factors to development of thrombus, such as the presence of a central venous catheter or recurrent atrial fibrillation, is also important clinical information. The recent development of gas-filled microbubbles allows opacification of left-sided chambers. These bubbles are very small (4 to 10 microns) and can traverse the pulmonary

capillary bed. The main use for this new technique is left ventricular opacification to enhance endocardial definition. Contrast perfusion echocardiography[22] might be indicated, as many cardiac tumors are vascular and will be enhanced by microbubbles, just like the myocardium in myocardial contrast echocardiography.[23,24] Often, a mass found on transthoracic echocardiography (TTE) needs further evaluation by transesophageal echocardiography (TEE) to help exclude the presence of artifact and determine the attachment site of the intracardiac tumor. It is important to remember that this technique is contraindicated for patients with esophageal cancer or head and neck irradiation.

Additional imaging techniques include computerized tomography (CT), magnetic resonance imaging (MRI), and positron emission tomography (PET).

The use of CT and MRI can be most helpful in looking at the relationship of mediastinal or lung masses and how they relate to an intracardiac tumor. These techniques may help delineate invasion through a myocardial wall or an extension from one of the great vessels into the heart. MRI has the additional properties of soft tissue characterization, and that often gives the needed information to decide whether a mass is tumor versus thrombus. Contrast enhancement with gadolinium provides assessment of tumor vascularity. PET imaging has proven useful for tumors in the right atrium, right ventricle, and the left atrium. Tumors are usually hypermetabolic and can be demonstrated with a metabolic tracer. It may be more difficult to image smaller tumors in the left ventricle because the myocardium is thicker and shows metabolic properties of its own.

Endomyocardial biopsy by a transvenous catheter-based bioptome has rarely been performed.[25,26] There are a few cases of percutaneous needle biopsy.[27,28] In the cancer patient, it is most

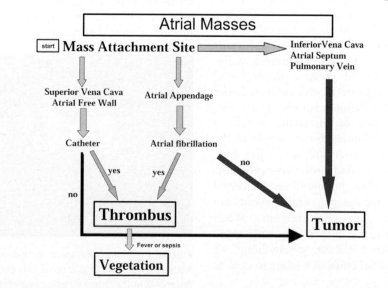

FIGURE 2 A decision tree to help facilitate whether an atrial mass could be tumor versus thrombus. Begin by determining the attachment site of the mass.

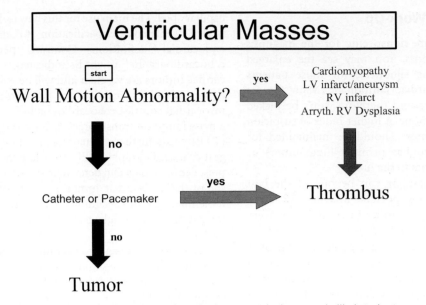

Ventricular Masses

start

Wall Motion Abnormality? — yes → Cardiomyopathy
LV infarct/aneurysm
RV infarct
Arryth. RV Dysplasia

no

Catheter or Pacemaker — yes → Thrombus

no

Tumor

FIGURE 3 A decision tree to help determine whether a ventricular mass is likely to be tumor vs. thrombus. Begin by determing whether there is an right ventricular or left ventricular wall motion abnormality.

probably related to their primary malignancy. If the patient has a reasonable prognosis, then resection not only provides diagnostic pathology, but helps to avoid the clinical consequences mentioned earlier, such as embolism, congestive heart failure, and obstruction. Coronary angiography may be helpful if this will change the surgical approach or identify additional disease that need to be addressed.

Metastatic Cardiac Tumors

Although autopsy studies have shown that metastatic disease to the heart and pericardium can be found in 10 to 20% of patients who died of malignancy; many cases of malignant tumors in the heart remain clinically silent. Metastasis to the heart occurs nearly 100 times more frequently than do primary cardiac tumors.[29] Metastasis may result from direct extension, lymphatic spread, or hematogenous spread into the heart. In absolute numbers, metastasis from lung cancer,[30,31] lymphoma,[32] and breast cancer[33–35] are the most common metastatic tumors. Of all tumors, malignant melanoma has the greatest propensity to metastasize to the heart.[36,37] Such lesions are found in nearly 71% of melanoma patients at autopsy. The most likely site of metastatic disease is the pericardium, although disease spread to the myocardium and/or endocardium is not rare. Because they are so frequently asymptomatic, the tumors can often be found as incidental finding on echocardiography while patients are being evaluated for other reasons. When symptoms do occur, they are frequently those of congestive heart failure, dysrhythmia, or increasing pericardial effusion leading to cardiac tamponade.

Tumor progression through the inferior vena cava may also involve the heart. In adults, this

phenomenon is seen in 4 to 10% of patients with renal cell carcinoma(Figure 4).[38] Other tumors that may spread to the heart through the inferior vena cava included hepatocellular carcinoma[39] and leiomyosarcoma[40] and, in children, Wilms' tumor. Such spread is usually diagnosed with a combination of echocardiography, computed tomography, and magnetic resonance imaging.[41] Most patients with these tumors do not have cardiac symptoms, but they may demonstrate an onset of hypertension or lower extremity edema without other finding of congestive heart failure.

Although these next two examples are not classic metastatic malignancies to the heart, these entities occur in the clinical setting of hematogenous malignancy.

Leukemia

There have been descriptions of cardiac masses inside the cardiac chambers in association with different leukemias and were thought to be do due to leukemic infiltration.[42–44]

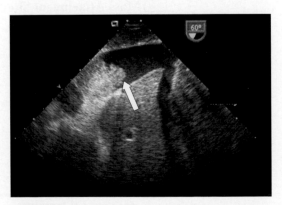

FIGURE 4 Transesophageal echocardiogram done intraperatively showing a renal cell carcinoma tumor thrombus in the inferior vena cava(white arrow). Borrowed from the case files of Dilip Thakar, MD. IVC = inferior vena cava.

Hypereosinophilic Syndrome (Löffler's Endocarditis)

Elevated eosinophil levels from any cause, including leukemia and other neoplastic disorders, can result in myocarditis, cardiac infiltration, or cardiac mass development.[45,46] The pathologic cardiac involvement consists of biventricular apical endocardial thickening, frequently with laminar mural thrombosis that contains eosinophils as part of the thrombus. The clinical scenario is congestive heart failure with hemodynamics similar to other restrictive cardiomyopathies (see Chapter 53, "Pericardium in the Cancer Patient"). Patients can develop embolism from the bilateral mural thrombi. Treatment include routine therapy for CHF, chemotherapy with hydroxyurea and imatinib,[47] and, late in the clinical course, surgical extraction of the fibrotic thrombusi can ameliorate symptoms.

Primary Cardiac Tumors

Malignant and benign primary cardiac tumors are extremely rare, with an incidence in autopsy series reported to be between 0.001% and 0.03%.[48] The occurrences of primary benign and malignant tumors of the heart are unique entities to diagnose and manage.

Benign Primary Cardiac Tumors

Seventy-five percent of primary cardiac tumors are benign; myxomas comprise about one half of this group. Most myxomas are found in the left atrium (75%) and in decreasing frequencies in the right atrium, right ventricle, and left ventricle. The incidence of myxomas peaks at 40 to 60 years of age; they are more common in women, with a female-to-male ratio of 3:1.[49] They are generally friable and tend to fragment, which gives them the potential of embolizing.[50] Most myxomas occur sporadically. Some are familial, and, occasionally, have been described in relation to a particular syndrome called Carney's complex, an autosomal-dominant condition associated with cardiac myxomas, myxomas in other regions (cutaneous or mammary), hyperpigmented skin lesions, hyperactivity of the adrenal or testicular glands, and pituitary tumors.[51–53] Carney's complex occurs at a younger age, and should be considered when cardiac myxomas are discovered in atypical locations in the heart.[54]

In children, the most common benign cardiac tumors are the rhabdomyomas, usually found in the ventricles. One-third of patients with these tumors also have tuberous sclerosis and a much poorer prognosis; death is frequently the result of unstable dysrhythmias. Rhabdomyomas that occur as an isolated finding have a much better prognosis.

Other benign primary tumors of the heart include fibromas (also located in the ventricles), which may be intramural and may become calcified. Lipomas, also seen in the heart, are histologically the same as those in other locations in the body. They usually occur in the left ventricle or the right atrium but may be found anywhere in the heart as well as the pericardium. Although frequently asymptomatic, they may grow large enough to cause obstructive symptoms.

Papillary fibroelastomas, which usually occur on cardiac valves, are often found incidentally (Figure 5). They may result in embolic phenomena,[14] and, when situated on the aortic valve, can cause coronary ostial occlusion.[55] Mesotheliomas[20] of the atrioventricular node, which is now called the cystic tumor of the AV node have the distinction of being the smallest tumor that may cause sudden cardiac death, death resulting from complete heart block, or, occasionally, ventricular fibrillation.

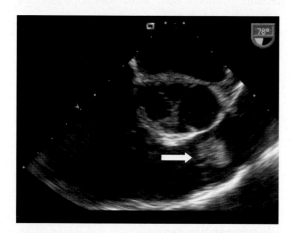

FIGURE 5 Transesophageal echocardiogram showing a pulmonic valve papillary fibroelastoma (arrow) which was found incidentally during thoracic surgery. Borrowed from the case files of Dilip Thakar, MD. AoV = aortic valve, RVOT = right ventricular outflow tract, MPA = main pulmonary artery.

Paragangliomas (pheochromocytomas)[20] may be found as intrapericardial tumors. The very rare hemangiomas are usually found postmortem; they are identified sometimes in vivo during coronary angiography where they may cause a characteristic "tumor blush".

Malignant primary cardiac tumors

Primary cardiac malignancies are of connective tissue origin and are classified as sarcomas.[56,57] There is no gender predilection, and the mean age of presentation is approximately 40 years. Angiosarcomas, the most common type of malignant cardiac tumors, usually occur in the right atrium (Figure 6) and present clinically as hemopericardium or with right-sided congestive heart failure. Eighty percent of these tumors have metastasized at the time of diagnosis, often to the lungs, liver, bone, or lymph nodes.

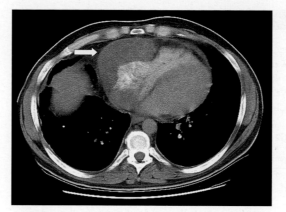

FIGURE 6 Computed axial tomography scan of the heart demonstrating an angiosarcoma in the right atrium. White arrow demonstrates the tumor actually infiltrating the right atrial wall.

Malignant fibrous histiocytomas[58] and fibrosarcomas are most frequently found in the left atrium, and both have a poor prognosis (Figure 7). Occasionally, these tumors are confused with left atrial myxomas.

Treatment of Cardiac Tumors

The optimal treatment for cardiac tumors is resection of the tumor. This obviously has a much better prognosis if the tumor is a benign cardiac tumor. Primary malignancies of the heart can recur, and chemotherapy or radiation therapy may be helpful in controlling them, depending on the histology of the tumor.[40] Metastatic tumors of the heart can be resected, but chemotherapy and bioimmunotherapy may help to control disease. Surgical resection will help avoid obstructive symptoms or cardioembolic events. Cases that involve extensive myocardial infiltration may require explantation of the heart with resection of the tumor, reconstruction of the chambers and valves, and subsequent autotransplantation of the heart.[59–61]

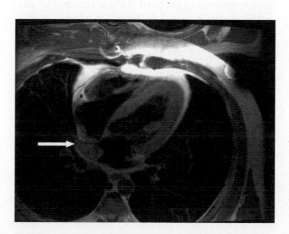

FIGURE 7 A magnetic resonance imaging scan showing a malignant fibrous histiocytoma in the left atrium (white arrow). LV = left ventricle, LA = left atrium.

Cardiac Amyloidosis

The term amyloid was introduced in 1984 by German physician scientist Rudolph Virchow.[62] Amyloid is the term used for the predominantly extracellular deposition of a group of chemically diverse, abnormal proteins that are arranged to a greater or lesser extent in specific beta-pleated fibrils. Amyloidosis is a systemic disorder characterized by tissue deposition of amyloid protein in a wide variety of clinical settings. The conclusive diagnosis of organ involvement with amyloid is with biopsy specimens which, under light microcopy and standard tissue stains, appear as an amorphous, eosinophilic, hyaline-like extracellular substance.[63] To differentiate amyloid deposition from other hyaline deposits like collagen and fibrin, Congo red stain is commonly used which, under ordinary light, imparts a pink or red color to the tissue, and under polarizing microscopy, gives a green birefringence of the stained amyloid.[63] When stained with Congo red, all forms of amyloid appear the same, but biochemically, the fibrils are different. The electron microscopy shows non-branching fibrils of indefinite length and a diameter of approximately 7.5 to 10 nm, and electron microscopy features are identical in all types of amyloidosis.[63]

Classification of Amyloidosis

The classification of amyloidosis is based on the nature of the precursor plasma protein that forms the fibril deposits (Table 1).[64] According to this classification, the amyloid protein is designated A, followed by the protein designation in abbreviated form without any space after first letter A. Thus, the former primary amyloidosis is now AL amyloidosis. The distinction between systemic and localized (organ or tissue limited) is avoided. This is because some amyloid deposits, which may appear to be localized, may represent a predilection site of systemic amyloidosis.

In clinical practice, amyloid deposition may be systemic (generalized) or localized to an organ like the heart or kidney. For clinical practice, the systemic type can be classified as primary (AL type), which is commonly associated with immunocyte dyscrasia, or secondary (AA type), which occurs as a complication of chronic inflammatory process.[63,65,66]

In AL amyloidosis, the κ or λ immunoglobulin light chain is the precursor protein. In AA type, the AA protein (which forms the AA amyloid protein) is derived from circulating acute phase reactant serum amyloid A (SAA), which in itself is synthesized in hepatocytes under the influence of cytokines such as IL-6 and IL-1.

SAA is common in most inflammatory conditions, but an increase in SAA in itself is not sufficient for deposition of amyloid.

Table 1   Characteristics of Common Types of Systemic Amyloidosis

TYPE	Fibril Composition	Precursor Protein	Underlying Disorders
AL(primary)	Monoclonal immunogloulin light chain	λ or κ light chain (ratio of λ to κ,3:1)	Plasma cell dyscrasia
ATTR (familial)	Transthyretin	Variant form of transthyretin	Inheritance
AA(reactive)	Serum amyloid A protein(SAA)	Chronic inflammatory disorders	
Aβ2M	β2 microglobulin	β2 microglobulin	Long term dialysis

Adapted from Ikeda S. Cardiac amyloidosis: heterogenous pathogenic backgrounds. Intern Med 2004;43:1107–14.

The hereditary or familial group includes a heterogeneous group with a variety of clinical manifestation.[65] The most common form in this group is ATTR amyloidosis (previously called pre-albumin), in which the precursor protein is a mutated transthyretin (TTR) and is a normal protein that binds thyroxine and retinol. Hence the name Trans Thy-Retin.

Senile systemic amyloidosis refers to systemic deposition of amyloid in elderly patients. Because of the dominant involvement of the heart, it was previously called "senile cardiac amyloidosis". The amyloid in this form is composed of normal transthyretin molecule.

Cardiac Manifestations:

The amyloid deposits in the extracellular space eventually cause pressure atrophy of the myocardial fibers.[63] The degree of cardiac compromise and subsequent clinical manifestations depend on the extent and location of amyloid deposition. Involvement of conduction system leads to ECG abnormalities, whereas involvement of a large area of myocardium will lead to heart failure.

The cardiac conduction system can be involved in all areas of the conduction system. Particularly, there can be involvement of the sinus node.[67]

Cardiac involvement is a prominent feature of AL amyloidosis,[68] whereas in secondary (AA) amyloidosis, involvement of the heart is found only rarely.[66]

The clinical manifestation of cardiac amyloidosis may be nonspecific, like fatigue, or the patient may present with a wide range of symptoms, from congestive heart failure, coronary insufficiency, heart block, valvular dysfunction, or pericardial effusion.[68] In patients with AL amyloidosis, fatigue and weakness are the most common systemic symptoms noted in more than 56% of patients, followed by weight loss, ecchymosis, and petechiae.[68,69] In these patients, multiorgan involvement should raise the suspicion of cardiac involvement. In one study of AL amyloidosis, heart involvement in the absence of clinical evidence of other system involvement (except the underlying plasma cell dyscrasia) was present in less than 4% of the patients.[68] In these patients, symptoms of left heart failure are predominant followed by fatigue and weakness. Despite predominant symptoms of left heart failure, clinical signs of right heart failure predominate, with jugular venous distention and ankle edema(> 80% of cases).

In some patients, angina pectoris may be the first cardiac manifestation of systemic amyloidosis, and months later, they will develop the full scenario of systemic amyloidosis. These patients have normal coronary angiograms but abnormality of coronary flow reserve.[70] Chest pain is present in about 25% of patients with cardiac amyloidosis, and of those who underwent catheterization, greater than 80% had a normal cardiac catheterization.[68] Chest pain in these patients may be due to small vessel disease. Amyloidosis is known to infiltrate the intramyocardial vessels.

Similarly, another group of patients with angina and amyloidosis had normal epicardial coronary vessels.[71] In one study of primary systemic amyloidosis, the majority of patients did not have severe coexisting coronary atherosclerosis but had amyloid involvement of the epicardial coronary vessels which was nonobstructive.[72] The majority of these patients had intramural coronary amyloidosis. Even of these patients, more than 50% had microscopic changes of myocardial ischemia.[72] In patients with amyloidosis, histologic sections of coronary artery have shown various degrees of diffuse stenosis of the small coronary arteries by amyloid deposition that occurs mainly in the media of the vessels with maintenance of normal intramural epicardial coronary vessels.[71]

Postural hypotension is a predominant feature of cardiac amyloidosis, found in about 40% of patients.[68] In a minority of the patients, chest pain may be preceded by episodes of orthostatic hypotension.[71] Other nonspecific features of cardiac amyloidosis include: syncope (20%), palpitations(17%),hypotension(14%) and hypertension(2.6%).[68] Syncope in these patients may be related to postural hypotension, ventricular arrhythmias or heart block. Patients may also have stress-induced syncope. The prognosis of patients with stress-precipitated syncope is worse when compared to those who do not have stress-induced syncope.[69]

There are no distinguishing clinical features that may differentiate patients with systemic senile amyloidosis (senile cardiac amyloidosis) from those with immunoglobulin-derived amyloid (AL).[73]

Heart failure due to amyloidosis is commonly due to the result of restrictive cardiomyopathy. Progressive deposition of amyloid within the heart leads to thickening of the walls, resulting in small ventricular chambers, noncompliant myocardium, and reduced stroke volume. Eventually, it leads to a diminished cardiac output, which is exacerbated by any increase in the heart rate. Initially, the main problem is diastolic dysfunction rather than systolic dysfunction. In the presence of coexisting hypertension, when clinical suspicion of amyloidosis is low, amyloid cardiac disease can be misdiagnosed as hypertrophy due to hypertension. Amyloid heart disease can mimic hypertrophic cardiomyopathy and remain undiagnosed until development of systolic heart failure.[74]

Investigations

On noninvasive evaluation, cardiac amyloidosis may be confused with hypertrophic cardiomyopathy and other causes of left ventricular hypertrophy. Electrocardiogram (ECG) and echocardiogram findings may be helpful to differentiate a combination of symptoms from other causes of left ventricular hypertrophy. A list of investigations are detailed below and summarized in Table 2.

Electrocardiogram

ECG abnormalities are found in the majority of patients with cardiac amyloidosis. In a study of AL cardiac amyloidosis, about 96% of patients had some ECG abnormality, with low voltage and pseudo-infarct pattern being the most common abnormalities found in > 70% of patients (Figure 8).[68] Conduction abnormalities are found in about 36% of patients. The ECG and echocardiographic features of heart involvement in AA amyloidosis resemble those of AL amyloidosis.[66] In another study in which low voltage (56% of cases) and pseudo-infarct pattern (60%) were the most common ECG findings in biopsy-proven cardiac amyloidosis, it was found that, if an ECG finding of low voltage was present and the echocardiogram showed an intraventricular septum thickness > 1.98 cm, the diagnosis of cardiac amyloidosis can be made with a sensitivity of 72% and a specificity of 91%.[75] In another study, ST depression was found in 70% and T wave changes in 85% of patients with AL Amyloidosis.[71]

Echocardiogram

The most common echocardiogram findings in cardiac amyloidosis are normal LV end diastolic

Table 2 Clinical Evaluation Of A Patient With Suspected Amyloidosis

Clinical Evaluation	Heart (Heart failure, fatigue, syncope, chest pain, murmur, postural hypotension, palpitations)
	Other Systemic Features (macroglosssia, neuropathy, hepatomegaly, malabsorption, diarrhea, proteinuria or frank nephrosis, skin papules or plaques, periorbital ecchymosis, arthritis, carpal tunnel syndrome, pleural effusion due to amyloid heart disease or pleural amyloid deposition)
ECG	Low voltage, pseudoinfarct pattern, heart block
CXR	Heart: Usually normal cardiac silhouette. In later stage Cardiomegaly.
	Lungs: Pulmonary edema, pleural effusion
Echocardiogram	Normal Left ventricular end diastolic dimension, thickening of septum and posterior wall, distinctive sparkling/granular appearance of the myocardium, restrictive physiology.
Holter	Conduction abnormality, Heart rate variability
Blood	Albumin, LFT's Creatinine, electrolyte, Coagulation, Thyroid function.
	BNP and Troponin (in cardiac involment)
Urine	Proteinuria, Creatinine clearance

BNP = brain natriuretic peptide; CXR = chest x ray; ECG = electrocardiogram; LFT = liver function tests.

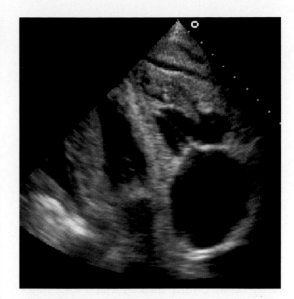

FIGURE 10 A transthoracic two dimensional echocardiogram showing increased echodensity and thickening of the myocardial walls and valves. This also demonstrates the sparkling and granular appearance of the walls.
LV = left ventricle, RV = right ventricle, RA = right ventricle.

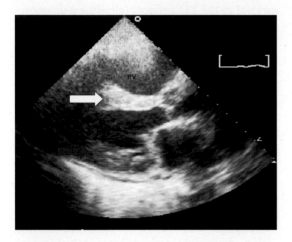

FIGURE 8 A two dimensional echocardiogram showing the parasternal long axis view. The white arrow shows the increased echodensity of the interventricular septum correlating with amyloid deposition compared to normal echocardiographic appearance of the posterior wall of the left ventricle shown by the red arrow.
RV = right ventricle, LV = left ventricle, Ao = aorta, LA = left atrium.

dimension, thickening of both right and left ventricular myocardial walls, restrictive physiology on Doppler, and sparkling/granular appearance of the myocardium (Figure 9 and 10).[75] In cardiac amyloidosis, there is infiltration by amyloid protein, which initially leads to a restrictive diastolic dysfunction, and the left ventricular ejection fraction starts to fall only late in the course of the disease, unless the patient has concomitant coronary artery disease or other etiology for dilated cardiomyopathy.

Chest Roentenograms

The cardiomyopathy in amyloidosis is restrictive in nature, hence the cardiac silhouette may not be enlarged. In senile systemic amyloidosis, cardiomegaly is noted in a majority of patients with associate pleural effusions in >35% of cases.[73]

Nuclear Scintigraphy

Abnormal cardiac uptake of 99mTc-3, 3-disphosphono-1, 2-propodicarboxylic acid (99mTc-DPD) may help differentiate TTR-related cardiac amyloidosis from the AL type of cardiac amyloidosis.[76]

Serology

Serum N-terminal pro-brain natriuretic peptide (BNP) has been found to be a sensitive marker of myocardial dysfunction in patients with AL amyloidosis.[77] In asymptomatic patients with cardiac amyloidosis, BNP levels may be elevated and may help to distinguish between those with or without heart failure.[78] This raises the possibility that elevation of BNP levels in cardiac amyloidosis could be direct myocyte damage due in addition to a rise in left ventricular end diastolic pressure.

In a small study, troponin levels were elevated in all patients with amyloid cardiomyopathy, of which 70% had values above the threshold used for the diagnosis of cardiac ischemia. In this study only 15% of patients had severe coronary artery disease. Amyloid deposition within the intramural epicardial coronary artery was found in all patients, and 38% had obstructive findings with greater than 60% obstruction. Interestingly,

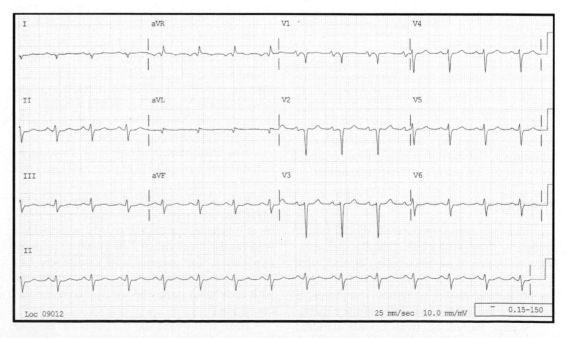

FIGURE 9 A 12 lead EKG demonstrating a pseudo-infarct pattern with Q waves in leads I, AVL, V1 and V2.

troponin I elevation was higher in patients with no or mild coronary artery disease. In this study, no statistical correlation was noted between troponin elevation and left ventricular ejection fraction, left ventricular wall thickness, pulmonary artery wedge pressure, or pulmonary artery pressure. This suggests that, in amyloid cardiomyopathy, elevation in troponins may be due to amyloid infiltration of the heart.[79]

Diagnosis

The diagnosis of cardiac amyloidosis should be considered in any patient who has unexplained cardiomyopathy, in particular in the setting of conditions known to be associated with amyloidosis. Although secondary (AA) amyloidosis rarely causes cardiac involvement, a high index of suspicion is needed in these cases as well. Patients who have amyloid involvement elsewhere, (eg, those with proteinuria or GI involvement with amyloidosis), should have an ECG and an echocardiogram as baseline investigations. In those with a high clinical suspicion of cardiac amyloidosis, the next step would be to establish a diagnosis by cardiac biopsy. When a cardiac biopsy is not possible, then a biopsy of the subcutaneous abdominal fat can be obtained.[80] Once a positive tissue diagnosis is obtained, the next step is to find out the type of amyloidosis. AL amyloidosis is the most common type, and the next step is to search for plasma cell dyscrasia by immunofixation electrophoresis of the serum and urine or by a bone marrow biopsy with immunohistochemical staining of plasma cells for kappa or lambda light chains.[65] The bone marrow biopsy will also help exclude myeloma or other conditions like Waldenström's macroglobulinemia as a cause of amyloidosis. If these are negative, then the next step, even in the absence of a family history of amyloidosis, is to look for a mutant TTR protein in serum, a mutant TTR gene in genomic DNA or both.[65]

Although there may be no clinical features to differentiate senile cardiac amyloidosis from the AL type, the absence of abnormal M protein in serum and urine plus the presence of cardiac amyloidosis in patients greater than 60 years of age with no extracardiac manifestation of primary amyloidosis, raises the possibility of systemic senile amyloidosis (senile cardiac amyloidosis).

Treatment

Treatment of cardiac amyloidosis should not be limited to those with clinical cardiac presentations, as treatment of concomitant disease (such as myeloma, nephrotic syndrome, and neuropathy or Gastrointestinal symptoms symptoms) is essential to the general well-being of the patient.

Angina should be treated with standard anti-anginal medications, albeit with cautious use of β-blockers and calcium channel blockers. In a small group of patients with AL amyloidosis, chest pain on exertion was promptly relieved by nitrates, but recurred frequently despite long-term use of these drugs.[71,81] Due to the recurrence of chest pain despite long-term nitrates, some have advocated the use of anti-anginal medications like nicorandil (not available in the US) which, in a study of normal population, was found to cause a dose-dependent increase in coronary flow velocity and a decrease in coronary vascular resistance, following intracoronary injection.[82] In one case report, despite use of diltiazem and nicorandil, the patient developed recurrent angina with ECG changes.[83]

There is not enough data available to make any firm recommendations on ideal medication for patients with angina and amyloid, but nitrates seem to be the logical and most prevalent choice made in these patients.

Treatment of congestive heart failure is with standard heart-failure medications, which include diuretics, angiotensin-converting enzyme inhibitors (ACE inhibitors) and β-blockers, although these medications have not been systematically studied in any large group of patients with amyloid cardiomyopathy.

ACE inhibitors should be used cautiously because of the potential for causing or exacerbating postural hypotension. This category of drug should be started in small doses, and increments made gradually and cautiously. Calcium channel blockers theoretically have been beneficial in diastolic heart failure,[84] and along with β-blockers and ACE inhibitors have a class 2b indication for treatment of patients with heart failure and normal left ventricular ejection fraction.[85] Calcium channel blockers should also be used cautiously in patients with amyloidosis because they have been reported to precipitate and worsen heart failure even in the presence of normal left ventricular ejection fraction.[86] Discontinuation of verapamil in this case was followed by clinical and echocardiographic improvement with normalization of left ventricular systolic function.[86] Digoxin should be avoided, as it avidly binds to amyloid fibrils,[87] which may lead to toxicity.

Indications for pacemakers are the same as in the general population.[88] However, when there is extensive involvement of the heart by amyloid tissue, successful insertion of pacemaker may still not be life-saving.

Clinical and echocardiographic improvement has been reported with thalidomide treatment in a patient with primary (AL) amyloidosis with cardiac involvement.[89] In a study of primary amyloidosis, for patients with cardiac involvement (21% of the study population), treatment with melphalan improved survival compared to colchicine.[90]

Heart transplantation is a last resort because there is a recurrence of amyloid deposition in transplanted hearts, and, therefore, only provides short-term benefit because it does not influence the underlying disease process.[91] It may have a role in a selective group of patients who are considered to be cured of the primary disease with high-dose chemotherapy and stem cell transplant.

Prognosis

In patients with primary amyloidosis, the presence of cardiac involvement is associated with a worse outcome, and the majority of deaths are cardiac-related.[90] Cardiac amyloidosis is associated with variable prognoses, depending upon the presence of other disease and concomitant involvement of other organs. In patients with primary amyloidosis (AL), the most common cause of death is due to either sudden cardiac death or congestive heart failure.[68] The median survival in the 232 patients following a diagnosis of AL amyloidosis was 1.08 years (range 0.83 to 1.25), and from the date of the index echocardiogram, median survival was 0.50 years (range 0.42 to 0.66).[68] In this study, patients with congestive heart failure median survival from diagnosis was 0.75 years (range 0.59 to 1.00), which was significantly shorter when compared to patients with heart involvement but no congestive heart failure, where median survival was 2.34 years (range 1.58 to 2.92).[68] In patients with systemic amyloidosis, elevated troponin and BNP levels also provide important prognostic information and are predictors of mortality in these patients.[92]

Patients with senile systemic amyloidosis with cardiac amyloidosis, despite being older and exhibiting greater left ventricular wall thickness, appear to have a survival advantage and better prognosis when compared to patients with AL amyloidosis involving the heart.[93]

Amyloid infiltration may affect the geometry of the ventricles in a discordant fashion, and when right ventricular dilation occurs greater than the left ventricle, it is associated with a poor prognosis with a median survival of only 4 months.[94] Right ventricular dilatation in these patients may be due to elevated left ventricular end diastolic pressure or elevated pulmonary vascular resistance and pulmonary hypertension from amyloid involvement of pulmonary arterioles.

REFERENCES

1. Kusano KF, Ohe T. Cardiac tumors that cause arrhythmias. Card Electrophysiol Rev 2002;6:174–7.
2. Meng Q, Lai H, Lima J, et al. Echocardiographic and pathologic characteristics of primary cardiac tumors: a study of 149 cases. Int J Cardiol 2002;84:69–75.
3. Landelius J. Echocardiography and cardiac tumors. Ann Radiol (Paris) 1978;21:324.
4. Hayes D Jr, Liles DK, Sorrell VL. An unusual cause of new-onset atrial flutter: primary cardiac lymphoma. South Med J 2003;96:799–802.
5. Fukuda A, Saito T, Imai M, et al. Metastatic cardiac papillary carcinoma originating from the thyroid in both ventricles with a mobile right ventricular pedunculated tumor. Jpn Circ J 2000;64:890–2.

6. Vinter S, Isaksen C, Vesterby A. Sudden cardiac death in a young woman: tumor of the atrioventricular (AV) node or citalopram intoxication? Am J Forensic Med Pathol 2005;26:349–51.

7. Buksa M, Haracic A. Late diastolic tumor "plop" in an asymptomatic case of right atrial myxoma. Med Arh 1999;53:77–9.

8. Cox WR, Damore S, Rubal BJ, et al. Left atrial myxoma: phonocardiographic, echocardiographic, and micromanometric hemodynamic correlations. South Med J 1984;77:237–41.

9. Vanleeuw P, Calozet Y, Eucher P, et al. Cardiac myxoma. Cardiovasc Surg 1993;1:654–6.

10. Villasenor HR, Fuentes F, Walker WE. Left atrial rhabdomyosarcoma mimicking mitral valve stenosis. Tex Heart Inst J 1985;12:107–10.

11. Christiansen S. Partial left ventriculectomy in patients with neoplasms and severe heart failure who are not candidates for cardiac transplantation. J Thorac Cardiovasc Surg 2004;127:302–3.

12. Smith JA, Davis BB, Stirling GR, et al. Clinicopathological correlates of cardiac myxomas: a 30-year experience. Cardiovasc Surg 1993;1:399–402.

13. Negishi M, Sakamoto H, Sakamaki T, et al. Disaccharide analysis of glycosaminoglycans synthesized by cardiac myxoma cells in tumor tissues and in cell culture. Life Sci 2003;73:849–56.

14. Saw W, Nicholls S, Trim G, et al. Papillary fibroelastoma, a rare but potentially treatable cause of embolic stroke: report of three cases. Heart Lung Circ 2001;10:105–7.

15. Kao CL, Chang JP. Abdominal aortic occlusion: a rare complication of cardiac myxoma. Tex Heart Inst J 2001; 28:324–5.

16. Reed RJ, Utz MP, Terezakis N. Embolic and metastatic cardiac myxoma. Am J Dermatopathol 1989;11:157–65.

17. Skalidis EI, Parthenakis FI, Zacharis EA, et al. Pulmonary tumor embolism from primary cardiac B-cell lymphoma. Chest 1999;116:1489–90.

18. Wilhite DB, Quigley RL. Occult cardiac lymphoma presenting with cardiac tamponade. Tex Heart Inst J 2003;30: 62–4.

19. Aboulafia DM, Bush R, Picozzi VJ. Cardiac tamponade due to primary pericardial lymphoma in a patient with AIDS. Chest 1994;106:1295–9.

20. Vander Salm TJ. Unusual primary tumors of the heart. Semin Thorac Cardiovasc Surg 2000;12:89–100.

21 Corso RB, Kraychete N, Nardeli S, et al. Spontaneous rupture of a right atrial angiosarcoma and cardiac tamponade. Arq Bras Cardiol 2003;81:608–13.

22. Kaul S. Myocardial contrast echocardiography: basic principles. Prog Cardiovasc Dis 2001;44:1–11.

23. Kirkpatrick JN, Wong T, Bednarz JE, et al. Differential diagnosis of cardiac masses using contrast echocardiographic perfusion imaging. J Am Coll Cardiol 2004; 43:1412–9.

24. Tousek P, Orban M, Schomig A, et al. Images in cardiovascular medicine. Real-time perfusion echocardiography of an intracardiac mass. Circulation 2003;107:2390.

25. Scholte AJ, Frissen PH, van der Wouw PA. Transesophageal echocardiography-guided transvenous biopsy of an intracardiac tumor. Echocardiography 2004;21:721–3.

26. Kang SM, Rim SJ, Chang HJ, et al. Primary cardiac lymphoma diagnosed by transvenous biopsy under transesophageal echocardiographic guidance and treated with systemic chemotherapy. Echocardiography 2003; 20:101–3.

27. Yamagami T, Kato T, Tanaka O, et al. Percutaneous needle biopsy under CT fluoroscopic guidance for cardiac tumor during continuous intravenous injection of contrast material. J Vasc Interv Radiol 2005;16:559–61.

28. Khalbuss WE, Gherson J, Zaman M. Pancreatic metastasis of cardiac rhabdomyosarcoma diagnosed by fine needle aspiration. A case report. Acta Cytol 1999;43:447–51.

29. Burke AP, Virmani R; Chap.19, Tumors and Tumor-Like Conditions of the Heart pg583-601. In Silver MD, Gotlieb AI,Schoen FJ. Cardiovascular Pathology, 3rd ed. New York: Churchill Livingstone; 2001.

30. Tamura A, Matsubara O, Yoshimura N, et al. Cardiac metastasis of lung cancer. A study of metastatic pathways and clinical manifestations. Cancer 1992;70:437–42.

31. Weg IL, Mehra S, Azueta V, et al. Cardiac metastasis from adenocarcinoma of the lung. Echocardiographic-pathologic correlation. Am J Med 1986;80:108–12.

32. Koehler F, Borges AC, Fotuhi PC. Large B cell lymphoma with cardiac infiltration. Heart 2003;89:1282.

33. Pavithran K, Doval DC, Ravi S, et al. Cardiac metastasis from carcinoma breast—a case report. Indian J Med Sci 1997;51:15–7.

34. Lieberman EB, Arthur J, Steenbergen C, et al. Antemortem diagnosis of an endomyocardial breast cancer metastasis by transvenous endomyocardial biopsy. Chest 1993;103: 1280–1.

35. Volk MJ, Carbone PP, Pozniak MA, et al. Cardiac involvement in metastatic breast cancer. Wis Med J 1990;89: 56–60.

36. Savoia P, Fierro MT, Zaccagna A, et al. Metastatic melanoma of the heart. J Surg Oncol 2000;75:203–7.

37. Sheldon R, Isaac D. Metastatic melanoma to the heart presenting with ventricular tachycardia. Chest 1991; 99:1296–8.

38. Cheng AS. Cardiac metastasis from a renal cell carcinoma. Int J Clin Pract 2003;57:437–8.

39. Longo R, Mocini D, Santini M, et al. Unusual sites of metastatic malignancy: case 1. Cardiac metastasis in hepatocellular carcinoma. J Clin Oncol 2004;22:5012–4.

40. Raaf HN, Raaf JH. Sarcomas related to the heart and vasculature. Semin Surg Oncol 1994;10:374–82.

41. Gindea AJ, Gentin B, Naidich DP, et al. Unusual cardiac metastasis in hypernephroma: the complementary role of echocardiography and magnetic resonance imaging Am Heart J 1988;116(5 Pt 1):1359–61.

42. Hunkeler N, Canter CE. Antemortem diagnosis of gross cardiac metastasis in childhood leukemia: echocardiographic demonstration. Pediatr Cardiol 1990;11:225–6.

43. Baspinar O, Ucar C, Baysal T, et al. Echocardiographic recognition of cardiac leukemic tumors in a child successfully treated with chemotherapy. Anadolu Kardiyol Derg 2003;3:286.

44. Goncalves Pde A, Almeida MA, Andrade MJ, et al. Cardiac mass in a patient with chronic lymphocytic leukemia. Rev Port Cardiol 2002;21:1371–3.

45. Donahue TP. Images in cardiology: Loeffler's endocarditis resulting from acute lymphoblastic leukemia. Clin Cardiol 2002;25:345.

46. Corssmit EP, Trip MD, JD Durrer. Loffler's endomyocarditis in the idiopathic hypereosinophilic syndrome. Cardiology 1999;91:272–6.

47. Anghel G, De Rosa L, Ruscio C, et al. Efficacy of imatinib mesylate in a patient with idiopathic hypereosinophilic syndrome and severe heart involvement. Tumori 2005; 91:67–70.

48. Virmani R, Burke A,Farb A. Atlas of Cardiovascular Pathology. Philadelphia; Saunders; 1996. Chap 12; Malignant Cardiac Tumors pg 93-100.

49. Pinede L, Duhaut P, Loire R. Clinical presentation of left atrial cardiac myxoma. A series of 112 consecutive cases. Medicine (Baltimore) 2001;80:159–72.

50. Mattle HP, Maurer D, Sturzenegger M, et al. Cardiac myxomas: a long term study. J Neurol 1995;242:689–94.

51. Edwards A, Bermudez C, Piwonka G, et al. Carney's syndrome: complex myxomas. Report of four cases and review of the literature. Cardiovasc Surg 2002;10:264–75.

52. Grossniklaus HE, McLean IW, Gillespie JJ. Bilateral eyelid myxomas in Carney's complex. Br J Ophthalmol 1991; 75:251–2.

53. Ohara N, Komiya I, Yamauchi K, et al. Carney's complex with primary pigmented nodular adrenocortical disease and spotty pigmentations. Intern Med 1993;32:60–2.

54. Tatebe S, Ohzeki H, Miyamura H, et al. Carney's complex in association with right atrial myxoma. Ann Thorac Surg 1994;58:561–2.

55. Granger EK, Rankin J, Larbalestier RI, et al. Obstruction of the right coronary artery ostium by an aortic valve papillary fibroelastoma. Heart Lung Circ 2005;14:266–8.

56. Burke AP, Cowan D, Virmani R. Primary sarcomas of the heart. Cancer 1992;69:387–95.

57. Bear PA, Moodie DS. Malignant primary cardiac tumors. The Cleveland Clinic experience, 1956 to 1986. Chest 1987;92:860–2.

58. Novelli L, Anichini C, Pedemonte E, et al. Malignant fibrous histiocytoma as a primary cardiac tumor. Cardiovasc Pathol 2005;14:276–9.

59. Burjonroppa SC, Reardon MJ, Swafford J. Images in cardiology: right atrial mass: primary angiosarcoma. Heart 2005;91:1271.

60. Reardon MJ, DeFelice CA, Sheinbaum R, et al. Cardiac autotransplant for surgical treatment of a malignant neoplasm. Ann Thorac Surg 1999;67:1793–5.

61. Cooley DA, Reardon MJ, Frazier OH, et al. Human cardiac explantation and autotransplantation: application in a patient with a large cardiac pheochromocytoma. Tex Heart Inst J 1985;12:171–6.

62. Sipe JD, Cohen AS. Review: history of the amyloid fibril. J Struct Biol 2000;130:88–98.

63. Cotran RS, Kumar V, Collins T. Chap 7 Disease of Immunity. pg188-259. In Robbins Pathologic Basis of Disease 6th ed. Eds. Cotran RS, Kumar V, Collins T. Philadelphia: W. B. Saunders 1999.

64. Nomenclature of amyloid and amyloidosis. WHO-IUIS Nomenclature Sub-Committee. Bull World Health Organ 1993;71:105–12.

65. Falk RH, Comenzo RL, Skinner M. The systemic amyloidoses. N Engl J Med 1997;337:898–909.

66. Dubrey SW, Cha K, Simms RW, et al. Electrocardiography and Doppler echocardiography in secondary (AA) amyloidosis. Am J Cardiol 1996;77:313–5.

67. James TN. Pathology of the cardiac conduction system in amyloidosis. Ann Intern Med 1966;65:28–36.

68. Dubrey SW, Cha K, Anderson J, et al. The clinical features of immunoglobulin light-chain (AL) amyloidosis with heart involvement. QJM 1998;91:141–57.

69. Chamarthi B, Dubrey SW, Cha K, et al. Features and prognosis of exertional syncope in light-chain associated AL cardiac amyloidosis. Am J Cardiol 1997;80:1242–5.

70. Al Suwaidi J, Velianou JL, Gertz MA, et al. Systemic amyloidosis presenting with angina pectoris. Ann Intern Med 1999;131:838–41.

71. Hongo M, Yamamoto H, Kohda T, et al. Comparison of electrocardiographic findings in patients with AL (primary) amyloidosis and in familial amyloid polyneuropathy and anginal pain and their relation to histopathologic findings. Am J Cardiol 2000;85:849–53.

72. Neben-Wittich MA, Wittich CM, Mueller PS, et al. Obstructive intramural coronary amyloidosis and myocardial ischemia are common in primary amyloidosis. Am J Med 2005;118:1287.

73. Kyle RA, Spittell PC, Gertz MA, et al. The premortem recognition of systemic senile amyloidosis with cardiac involvement. Am J Med 1996;101:395–400.

74. Morner S, Hellman U, Suhr OB, et al. Amyloid heart disease mimicking hypertrophic cardiomyopathy. J Intern Med 2005;258:225–30.

75. Rahman JE, Helou EF, Gelzer-Bell R, et al. Noninvasive diagnosis of biopsy-proven cardiac amyloidosis. J Am Coll Cardiol 2004;43:410–5.

76. Perugini E, Guidalotti PL, Salvi F, et al. Noninvasive etiologic diagnosis of cardiac amyloidosis using 99mTc-3,3-diphosphono-1,2-propanodicarboxylic acid scintigraphy. J Am Coll Cardiol 2005;46:1076–84.

77. Palladini G, Campana C, Klersy C, et al. Serum N-terminal pro-brain natriuretic peptide is a sensitive marker of myocardial dysfunction in AL amyloidosis. Circulation 2003;107:2440–5.

78. Nordlinger M, Magnani B, Skinner M, et al. Is elevated plasma B-natriuretic peptide in amyloidosis simply a function of the presence of heart failure? Am J Cardiol 2005;96:982–4.

79. Miller WL, Wright RS, McGregor CG, et al. Troponin levels in patients with amyloid cardiomyopathy undergoing cardiac transplantation. Am J Cardiol 2001;88:813–5.

80. Libbey CA, Skinner M, Cohen AS. Use of abdominal fat tissue aspirate in the diagnosis of systemic amyloidosis. Arch Intern Med 1983;143:1549–52.

81. Mueller PS, Edwards WD, GertzMA. Symptomatic ischemic heart disease resulting from obstructive intramural coronary amyloidosis. Am J Med 2000;109:181–8.

82. Hongo M, Takenaka H, Uchikawa S, et al. Coronary microvascular response to intracoronary administration of nicorandil. Am J Cardiol 1995;75:246–50.

83. Yamano S, Motomiya K, Akai Y, et al. Primary systemic amyloidosis presenting as angina pectoris due to intramyocardial coronary artery involvement: a case report. Heart Vessels 2002;16:157–60.

84. Setaro JF, Zaret BL, Schulman DS, et al. Usefulness of verapamil for congestive heart failure associated with abnormal left ventricular diastolic filling and normal left ventricular systolic performance. Am J Cardiol 1990;66: 981–6.

85. Hunt SA, Abraham WT, Chin MH, et al. ACC/AHA 2005 Guideline Update for the Diagnosis and Management of Chronic Heart Failure in the Adult: a report of the American College of Cardiology/American Heart Association Task Force on Practice Guidelines (Writing Committee to Update the 2001 Guidelines for the

Evaluation and Management of Heart Failure): developed in collaboration with the American College of Chest Physicians and the International Society for Heart and Lung Transplantation: endorsed by the Heart Rhythm Society. Circulation 2005;112:154–235.

86. Pollak A, Falk RH. Left ventricular systolic dysfunction precipitated by verapamil in cardiac amyloidosis. Chest 1993;104:618–20.

87. Rubinow A, Skinner M, Cohen AS. Digoxin sensitivity in amyloid cardiomyopathy. Circulation 1981;63:1285–8.

88. Gregoratos G, Abrams J, Epstein AE, et al. ACC/AHA/NASPE 2002 Guideline Update for Implantation of Cardiac Pacemakers and Antiarrhythmia Devices—summary article: a report of the American College of Cardiology/ American Heart Association Task Force on Practice Guidelines (ACC/AHA/NASPE Committee to Update the 1998 Pacemaker Guidelines). J Am Coll Cardiol 2002;40: 1703–19.

89. Oh IY, Kim HK, Kim YJ, et al. An intriguing case of primary amyloidosis with cardiac involvement: Symptomatic and echocardiographic improvement with thalidomide treatment. Int J Cardiol. 2006;113:141-3. Epub 2005 Dec 2.

90. Kyle RA, Gertz MA, Greipp PR, et al. A trial of three regimens for primary amyloidosis: colchicine alone, melphalan and prednisone, and melphalan, prednisone, and colchicine. N Engl J Med 1997;336:1202–7.

91. Dubrey SW, Burke MM, Khaghani A, et al. Long term results of heart transplantation in patients with amyloid heart disease. Heart 2001;85:202–7.

92. Dispenzieri A, Gertz MA, Kyle RA, et al. Serum cardiac troponins and N-terminal pro-brain natriuretic peptide: a staging system for primary systemic amyloidosis. J Clin Oncol 2004;22:3751–7.

93. Ng B, Connors LH, Davidoff R, et al. Senile systemic amyloidosis presenting with heart failure: a comparison with light chain-associated amyloidosis. Arch Intern Med 2005;165:1425–9.

94. Patel AR, Dubrey SW, Mendes LA, et al. Right ventricular dilation in primary amyloidosis: an independent predictor of survival. Am J Cardiol 1997;80:486–92.

The Pericardium in the Cancer Patient

Steven M. Ewer, MD
Michael S. Ewer, MD, JD

Heart disease and cancer are the two most common causes of death in developed countries. While primary cardiac malignancy is relative rare, involvement of the heart either by malignant spread of the tumor, or as a sequel to the various treatment strategies, occurs much more frequently. The pericardium is of especial interest to those treating patients with cancer, as it is the cardiac structure most frequently affected by tumor spread, and it is the cardiac structure most sensitive to the effects of ionizing radiation. Pericardial disease and cancer are therefore two closely related fields of interest.

Approximately 9% of patients who eventually succumb to malignancy have direct cancerous involvement of the pericardium, and for 80% of these patients, their pericardial involvement will contribute to their demise.[1] An even greater number develop pericardial disease via other mechanisms that are related to their malignancy. Likewise, 7% of patients presenting with acute pericardial disease have a neoplastic etiology,[2] and 35% of procedures performed for pericardial disease are done on cancer patients.[3] Usually, pericardial disease in the cancer patient presents well after the diagnosis of cancer has been established. Typical questions that arise include: (1) what aspect of malignancy or its treatment are the cause; (2) what are the implications for prognosis and further cancer treatment; and (3) what is the best way to manage the pericardial disease. In rare cases, however, a patient with no history of cancer may present with malignant pericardial disease as the first manifestation. Sometimes, pericardial involvement during life remains unsuspected and is an incidental finding at autopsy.

Historically, malignant pericardial disease was relegated to a medical curiosity and was diagnosed almost exclusively on autopsy. With the advent of imaging technology in the 20th century, ante mortem diagnosis became possible, but prognosis remained grim and little could be offered to patients besides occasional brief palliation. Currently, even earlier diagnosis of malignant pericardial disease is possible, and a much greater number of treatments are available for the systemic and local management of their malignancy, as well as management of treatment-related pericardial disease. These advances have rendered pericardial disease in the cancer patient increasingly relevant in modern medicine. Despite these accomplishments, however, quality evidence for optimizing diagnostic and therapeutic strategies for these conditions has lagged, and we are left with a considerable degree of uncertainty as to the ideal management of an exceedingly complex group of patients.

Malignant disease and its treatment affect the pericardium in a variety of ways. While primary pericardial tumors are very rare, metastases are quite common. Nearly all cancers (with perhaps the exception of primary brain tumors) are capable of metastasizing to the pericardium through either direct extension (ie, lung, esophageal), retrograde lymphatic spread (ie, lung, breast), or hematogenous seeding (ie, melanoma, lymphoma, leukemia). Other causes of pericardial abnormalities in the cancer patient that do not involve direct invasion include adjacent inflammation, interruption of lymphatic or venous drainage, infection, hypoalbuminemia, congestive heart failure, renal failure, toxicities of chemotherapeutics, and chest irradiation. Many cases of pericardial disease in the cancer patient are idiopathic, and it should be recognized that the pericardial disease is often unrelated to the underlying malignancy. The etiology of a pericardial abnormality in a cancer patient is thus critical to his or her management, having important implications for prognosis and treatment. The possibility that the etiology of a sanguineous pericardial effusion in a lung cancer patient may be caused by tuberculosis, for example, cannot be overemphasized.

Symptoms of pericardial disease are often vague and nonspecific, and can mimic disease in many other organ systems, which are often also affected by the malignancy. Diagnosis can be very challenging, and even after diagnosis, treating existing pericardial disease does not ensure relief of an individual's symptoms. The clinician must approach these patients with a broad view of clinical medicine in order to minimize the possibility of incorrect diagnoses and inappropriate interventions.

Despite the fact that the diagnosis of pericardial problems may be difficult, the management of such problems may be tremendously gratifying. The improvement experienced by a patient following drainage of pericardial fluid in the setting of cardiac tamponade is one of the most dramatic and rewarding interventions that we as internists or cardiologists can undertake. As cancer treatments continue to improve, we will have increasing opportunity to offer our patients both quantity and quality of life through management of their pericardial disease.

After a brief discussion of normal pericardial structure and function, this chapter will examine the spectrum of primary and metastatic tumors of the pericardium, pericardial sequelae of chest radiation, and other aspects of malignancy and its treatment that affect the pericardium. We will then review the more common manifestations of pericardial disease as it pertains to the patient with diagnosed or undiagnosed malignancy. Mechanisms, diagnosis, and treatment of these entities, including acute pericarditis, pericardial effusion, tamponade, and pericardial constriction will be discussed.

Normal Pericardial Structure and Function

The pericardium consists of a fibrous sac that contains the heart. There are two pericardial layers: the inner visceral pericardium, attached directly to the surface of the heart, and the outer parietal pericardium, separated from the visceral pericardium by the pericardial space. The pericardial space contains a small amount of serous fluid. The two layers meet at or near the origin of the great vessels (the superior vena cava, aorta, pulmonary artery, and pulmonary veins), and these attachments serve to anchor the pericardium and heart within the mediastinum. The two layers thus completely enclose the pericardial space, which is often considered a "potential space" because, while usually containing a minimal amount of fluid between the two adjacent surfaces, this space can greatly expand in pathologic states, holding more than two liters of pericardial fluid in some cases.

From an embryologic perspective, the visceral pericardium is a monolayer of mesothelial cells on the surface of the epicardium, which also consists of some connective tissue, adipose tissue, the coronary blood vessels, nerves, and lymphatic vessels. The parietal pericardium consists of a monolayer of mesothelial cells along with a thicker serosa, which is made of fibrous connective tissue including collagen and elastin. The normal thickness of the parietal pericardium is 1 to 3.5 mm, depending on variations in the serosa.[4] The thickness of the parietal pericardium increases with most pericardial disease states, including those related to malignancy, and, indeed, is the primary abnormality in the case of constriction.

Most references to "the pericardium" as a tissue structure are understood to imply the parietal pericardium; the visceral pericardium usually is included as part of the epicardium. While this convention has the potential for confusion, the meaning is usually clear from the context. Metastases to the pericardium, however, may involve both the parietal and visceral layers.

Innervation of the pericardium is derived from the phrenic nerve anteriorly and the esophageal plexus posteriorly, both carrying fibers derived from the vagus nerve. These fibers are the source of chest pain in acute pericarditis. Myocardial innervation is supplied by the same nerves, which helps explain the similarities of anginal pain and pericardial pain when prominent pleuritic features are absent. Lymphatic drainage is to the anterior and posterior mediastinal lymph nodes, and retrograde spread through these vessels is an important source of metastatic tumor spread, especially for cases of breast and lung cancers that involve mediastinal lymph nodes. Obstruction of lymphatics by tumor is also a mechanism for pathologic accumulation of pericardial fluid that does not require invasion of the pericardium per se.

The pericardial space normally contains 15 to 50 mL of fluid, which is continuously secreted by the mesothelial cells of the visceral pericardium. This fluid is essentially a plasma ultrafiltrate and serves to lubricate the movements of the heart. Pericardial fluid is resorbed via lymphatics and veins. When secretion is increased (eg with inflammation) and/or resorption is decreased (eg tumor obstruction), fluid can accumulate abnormally in the pericardial space and is then referred to as an effusion. Three major sinuses, as well as several minor ones within the pericardial space, serve to store accumulated fluid without affecting cardiac function or causing symptoms: the transverse sinus lies between the superior pulmonary veins and the main pulmonary artery; the oblique sinus lies between the right and left pulmonary veins behind the left atrium; and the superior sinus surrounds the base of the

ascending aorta. When preclinical (but nevertheless pathologic) pericardial effusions are present, these sinuses can be seen to be enlarged with various imaging modalities, including computed tomography (CT), magnetic resonance imaging (MRI), and transesophageal echocardiography. Because of their location, the pericardial sinuses are not typically seen on transthoracic echocardiography.

In addition to lubricating the movements of the heart, the pericardium serves many other physiologic functions. The relatively fixed volume and inherent elasticity combine to keep the pericardial sac under tension, which contributes to diastolic pressures within the heart and helps maintain the classic pressure-volume relationships of cardiac physiology. For instance, under conditions that increase left ventricular volume, a condition commonly encountered in the cancer patient (eg, anthracycline cardiomyopathy, renal dysfunction), the structural integrity of the pericardium helps take on some of the burden of increased wall stress. Within the pericardial space, there is a small negative pressure (≈ 3 mmHg) that serves to augment diastolic filling.[4] Other functions include a physical tethering of the heart within the mediastinum, a barrier against infection and inflammation, participation in the cardiac autonomic reflexes, and paracrine functions (releasing mediators such as endothelin and prostacyclins). When cancer results in a diseased pericardium, any of these functions can be altered or disrupted, often leading to complex pathophysiology with subtle, multi-faceted contributions to morbidity.

Primary Tumors of the Pericardium

Primary pericardial tumors are extraordinarily rare. The reported incidence of all cardiac tumors ranges from 0.001% to 0.28% in autopsy series,[5] and pericardial tumors make up only a fraction of these cases. (By comparison, the incidence of pericardial metastases is approximately 2.5% in a similar general autopsy series.) Both benign and malignant pericardial tumors will be addressed. A list of primary tumors of the pericardium is shown in Table 1. Relative incidence as a percentage of all primary pericardial tumors is shown where possible.

Five tumor types make up the vast majority of primary pericardial tumors, accompanied by a longer list of very rare entities (see Table 1). Approximately 25% of primary pericardial tumors are malignant. In general, the benign lesions present more commonly in infancy or childhood, and malignant tumors are seen more frequently after the third decade. The exceptions are slow-growing benign tumors such as lipomas, which may also present later in life. We will briefly discuss some of the more common pericardial tumors below, including pericardial cysts,

Table 1 Primary Tumors of the Pericardium
Benign
Pericardial Cyst (62%)
Teratoma (11%)
Bronchogenic Cyst
Dermoid
Lipoma
Fibroma
Solitary Fibrous Tumor
Neuroma
Lymphangioma
Lymphangioepithelioma
Hemangioma
Neurofibroma
Leiomyoma
Hamartoma
Malignant
Mesothelioma (15%)
Angiosarcoma (7%)
Malignant Teratoma (3%)
Kaposi's Sarcoma
Rhabdomyosarcoma
Fibrosarcoma
Synovial Sarcoma
Spindle Cell Sarcoma
Thymoma
Primary Cardiac Lymphoma
Hodgkin's Lymphoma
Malignant Nerve-Sheath Tumors
Hemangioepithelioma
Liposarcoma
Pheochromocytoma

teratomas, mesotheliomas, and angiosarcomas. Other tumors are found in the literature only as isolated case reports and very small series and will be mentioned briefly. The bulk of epidemiologic data regarding primary cardiac tumors comes from a series of 533 such cases by the Armed Forces Institute of Pathology,[6] and was summarized and updated more recently.[5]

Pericardial Cysts

Pericardial cysts are the most common primary pericardial tumor.[21] They consist of a lining of mesothelial cells surrounded by a layer of fibrous connective tissue, much like the structure of the pericardium itself. Occasionally, hyperplasia of the mesothelium is found, and rarely, inflammatory cells may also be present. The interior of the cyst contains a clear, straw-colored fluid, and may communicate with the pericardial space. Pericardial cysts usually contain only small amounts of fluid (less than 10 cc) and are usually less than 3 cm in their widest dimension. They can, however expand considerably, and may achieve maximal dimensions of up to 15 cm.[5] The most common location is along the right heart border.[5] Pericardial cysts can present at any age, but the majority are diagnosed before the age of 30. They have also been noted as incidental findings at autopsy. Only one-third of patients present with symptoms, which consist primarily of chest pain, but can also include dyspnea and arrhythmias.[4] More typically, an abnormality is seen on chest X-ray obtained for other reasons, which then leads to the diagnosis of a cardiac tumor. More detailed imaging can be obtained with echocardiography, computed tomography, or magnetic resonance imaging. Treatment consists of surgical excision, percutaneous drainage, or thoracoscopic drainage. Pericardial cysts do not have malignant potential, and the prognosis is excellent.

Teratoma

Teratomas are composed of tissue derived from all three germ layers. They are usually, but not always, benign. Pericardial teratomas arise from the base of the pulmonary artery or aorta, which often complicates their surgical removal. Approximately 80% occur in the pediatric population,[5] typically in infancy or in utero.[7,8] There is a remarkable female-to-male preponderance. Clinical presentation is far more dramatic than for pericardial cysts. Because of their location and size, compression of the right atrium is the rule, and right ventricular compression is not uncommon. Furthermore, pericardial teratomas are frequently accompanied by a large pericardial effusion, which exacerbates tamponade physiology. Presentation includes hydrops fetalis, fetal pericardial effusion, and dyspnea, cyanosis, cardiomegaly, cardiac murmurs, and sudden cardiac death in the neonatal or pediatric patient. Treatment includes surgical excision, and a non-trivial operative mortality exists for these patients. Occasionally, fetal pericardiocentesis is also necessary.[9] After recovery from surgery, the prognosis is excellent and recurrences are uncommon. Rarely, teratomas can undergo malignant transformation, invading adjacent structures, including the myocardium. In these unfortunate cases, surgical excision is not feasible and the prognosis is poor; death usually occurs within weeks of the diagnosis.

Mesothelioma

Mesothelioma is the most common primary malignancy of the pericardium. It usually presents in middle age, with males affected twice as often as females.[10] It is unclear from the scant literature available if exposure to inhaled asbestos is a significant risk factor for pericardial mesothelioma as it is for its pleural counterpart, but several cases without any apparent asbestos exposure have been documented.[4,11] Another series, however, found no difference in asbestos exposure in patients with pleural versus pericardial mesothelioma,[12] implying an association. Additionally, the issue is confused by the fact that some mesotheliomas thought to be of pericardial origin are actually derived from the pleura with local

invasion into the pericardium. Some evidence implicates simian virus 40 as well as asbestos in the pathogenesis of mesothelioma; this virus has been found in up to 80% of patients with mesothelioma, and has been found to cause mesothelioma in animal models.[13]

Although localized nodules can exist, mesothelioma usually spreads uniformly throughout the pericardial space. Invasion occurs locally and includes spread to the pleura, mediastinum, mediastinal lymph nodes, and occasionally, through the diaphragm to the peritoneum. Invasion to the deep myocardium or endocardium is rare, in contrast with other pericardial malignancies. Distant metastases are also notably uncommon, but have been found in the brain.[14] Clinical presentation spans the spectrum of pericardial disease, including acute pericarditis, chronic or recurrent pericardial effusions, and constriction. Constitutional symptoms are also common.

Diagnosis of mesothelioma is confirmed by cytologic evaluation of the fluid or pericardial biopsy along with suggestive clinical features. Pathologic distinction between mesothelioma and reactive mesothelial hyperplasia (seen in response to inflammation) can be challenging.[5] Treatment is mainly palliative, and consists of radiation, chemotherapy, and local measures to control pericardial symptoms. Given the behavior patterns of this malignancy, surgical resection is generally impossible. The very high operative mortality makes surgical intervention prohibitively risky, including treatment of pericardial constrictive disease due to mesothelioma. Prognosis is poor with or without surgery, with one series reporting a 60% 6-month mortality.[5]

Angiosarcoma

Angiosarcoma is the second most common primary pericardial malignancy after mesothelioma, and is the most common cardiac sarcoma overall. Angiosarcomas originate in either the right atrium or pericardium in 80% of cases.[5] Patients usually present as young or middle-aged adults, and as is the case with mesothelioma, men are more susceptible than women. Unlike mesothelioma, however, angiosarcoma commonly invades the myocardium and endocardium, and can present with intracardiac masses or valvular obstruction. Distant metastases are possible and occur in approximately one-quarter of all cases,[5] with a predilection for the central nervous system. Symptoms and clinical findings include those of acute pericarditis, pericardial effusion, congestive heart failure (especially right-sided failure resulting from obstruction of the superior or inferior vena cava, or the tricuspid valve), arrhythmias, and constitutional symptoms. Pericardial effusions are typically hemorrhagic. Surgical resection may be possible in selected patients, but treatment is generally palliative, and includes

chemotherapy and radiation. The prognosis is generally poor.

Other Primary Pericardial Tumors

Pericardial lipomas resemble lipomas found elsewhere in the body. They are slow-growing benign tumors that are asymptomatic until they begin to compress adjacent structures. Unlike teratomas, there is no significant inflammatory reaction, and effusion is usually absent. If not compressing critical structures, they can grow to giant proportions—nearly 5 kg in one case report.[15] They are often confused with the more common pericardial cysts, in part because of their homogenous, low-density signal on various imaging modalities. Surgery is curative, and offered only when symptoms warrant intervention or diagnostic uncertainty remains. As with lipomas elsewhere, there is an exceedingly low rate of malignant transformation to liposarcoma. Liposarcomas can recur after surgical resection, and repeat surgery can be an effective way to manage such cases.[16,17]

Occasionally, thymomas can arise from the parietal pericardium without evidence of anterior mediastinal involvement. Tumors can be benign or malignant, and do not appear to be associated with myasthenia gravis. Hemangiomas and lymphangiomas can occur in the pericardium, often mimicking pericardial cysts. Intrapericardial pheochromocytoma is a rare but well-documented phenomenon. Diagnosis includes measurement of active metabolites in the blood and urine, and imaging with MRI or targeted nuclear scanning. Pericardial neurofibromas have been described in the context of von Recklinghausen's disease. Primary cardiac lymphoma is usually of B-cell origin and tends to involve both the myocardium and pericardium simultaneously. Treatment is similar to extracardiac lymphoma.

Metastatic Disease of the Pericardium

In several large autopsy series, 10% of all patients who die because of cancer have metastases to the heart. Of these, approximately 85% have pericardial involvement.[18] Not only is malignant pericardial disease fairly common, it contributes to death in the majority of cases.[1] Pericardial metastases outnumber primary pericardial tumors by about two orders of magnitude, and thus are by far the more important clinical entities. Nearly all cancers have been found to metastasize to the pericardium, but only a handful of these are seen with any meaningful frequency. Table 2 shows a list of these more common pericardial metastases with their relative frequencies.[19–21] Lung cancer, breast cancer, and hematologic malignancies together account for approximately two-thirds of

Table 2 Metastatic Cancers to the Pericardium
Lung Cancer 33% (includes roughly equal numbers of squamous cell, adenocarcinoma, and small cell carcinoma)
Breast Cancer 19%
Hematologic Malignancies 13%
Gastrointestinal Carcinomas 7.7% (includes adenocarcinoma and squamous cell carcinoma)
Malignant Melanoma 4.6%
Prostate Cancer 3.5%
Thyroid Cancer 3.5%
Pancreatic Cancer 3.5%
Gynecologic Malignancies 3.5%

pericardial metastases. In some series, this group accounts for 80%.[18]

Of equal relevance is the likelihood of a given malignancy to metastasize to the pericardium. Melanoma is the most likely to do so, with up to 70% of metastatic cases involving the pericardium.[18] Leukemia and lymphoma are found to involve the pericardium in approximately 33% of cases. Breast cancer metastasizes to the pericardium in approximately 21% of cases, and lung cancer in 19%.[1]

Cancer can metastasize to the pericardium in one of three ways: direct extension, lymphatic spread, and hematogenous spread. All three mechanisms are fairly common and clinically relevant. Direct extension to the pericardium is facilitated by aggressive tumor behavior and proximity to the heart. Malignancies in this category include lung cancer, esophageal cancer, and, to a lesser degree, breast cancer. (The midesophagus is separated from the left atrial cavity by as little as 3 mm of tissue in some locations!) Often overlooked members of this category are primary cardiac tumors that originate elsewhere in the heart and invade the pericardium, such as rhabdomyosarcoma and fibrosarcoma. Angiosarcoma is a unique, albeit confusing, example, in that it can originate in either the myocardium or pericardium and then proceed to invade adjacent structures.

Lymphatic spread is probably the most common mechanism of metastatic spread to the pericardium. As noted above, lymph node groups that receive drainage from the heart are the anterior and posterior mediastinal nodes, and cancers that metastasize to these nodes, most notably breast and lung cancer, can reach the pericardium via retrograde lymphatic spread. Careful histologic study has confirmed this mechanism in the majority of cases involving pericardial metastases.[22–24] Note that invasion and obstruction of these lymphatics is also likely to be the main contributor to malignant and non-malignant pericardial effusions in this group.

Leukemia, lymphoma, and melanoma most commonly seed the heart, including the pericardium, through the blood vessels. Hemorrhage

often accompanies metastases in this category, contributing to the pericardial effusion. It is interesting that these malignancies are precisely the ones most likely to involve the pericardium, implying perhaps that this route of metastasis is more efficient than lymphatic spread or direct extension.

Presentation of metastatic pericardial disease is highly variable. Some cases are asymptomatic and are diagnosed incidentally on autopsy, while others present as life-threatening catastrophic events such as pericardial tamponade. Most patients with pericardial metastases are symptomatic however, and as noted above, pericardial involvement very often leads to their demise.[1] The most common presentations, namely acute pericarditis, chronic effusion, tamponade, and constrictive disease, all occur in cancer patients and will be discussed in detail below. In general, malignant pericardial disease presents more often as chronic pericardial effusions or tamponade, and less often as acute pericarditis. Pericardial constriction can be seen following chest irradiation. However, it is worth mentioning that patients rarely present in classical textbook fashion. Sorting out pericardial disease in the setting of malignancy can be extremely challenging.

Case series have been collected that specifically look at symptoms and signs of metastatic pericardial disease. One study reports dyspnea in 91%, cough in 67%, pleural effusion in 53%, and venous distension in 30%.[25] Another reports tachycardia in 46%, pleural effusion in 44%, dyspnea at rest in 40%, and abnormal chest X-ray in 32%.[19] Other findings include rales, pulsus paradoxus, distant heart sounds, and abdominal symptoms related to congestion. Many of these are nonspecific and can mimic other diseases, especially lung disease, which is frequently coexistent as the primary site of malignancy, another site of metastasis, or pneumonia. Arrhythmias are a common manifestation of malignant pericardial disease,[26] and a new arrhythmia in a cancer patient should raise suspicion for cardiac metastases if this has not previously been diagnosed. Congestive heart failure can present similarly, but symptoms include orthopnea and paroxysmal nocturnal dyspnea, which are usually not present with symptomatic pericardial effusions. Because symptoms are relatively nonspecific, or even misleading, and the differential diagnosis in these patients is always broad, the clinician must have a high index of suspicion to detect clinically relevant pericardial involvement. The adage that pericardial disease can act as a masquerader is especially true in the cancer patient.

Once pericardial disease is suspected based on history and physical examination, the most useful initial test is the transthoracic echocardiogram because of its high diagnostic yield, ready availability, and noninvasive nature. Echocardiographic findings for specific entities

will be discussed below. Chest X-ray may reveal cardiomegaly, pleural effusions, and mediastinal lymphadenopathy, but is not definitive. Electrocardiography may reveal several aspects of pericardial disease, and these will also be considered below. CT and MRI can be helpful adjuncts, especially useful because of their expanded field of view (including lungs, pleura, mediastinum, and great vessels), which helps put malignant pericardial disease in a broader perspective. Indeed, pericardial effusions are often discovered incidentally on chest CT scans done for other indications, such as to rule out pulmonary metastases or thromboembolic disease. Additionally, MRI is especially able to visualize cardiac masses due to its excellent contrast resolution.[27] Melanoma has unique features on MRI because of the ability of melanin to bind paramagnetic metals. This gives melanoma a bright appearance on T1-weighted images, in contrast to other tumors.[27] Both MRI and CT can help determine pericardial thickness if constriction is being considered.

Pathology, including cytology of pericardial fluid and tissue from surgical specimens, is an important aspect of diagnosis. The finding of malignant cells in pericardial fluid or in tissue samples of parietal or visceral pericardium help make the diagnosis of malignant pericardial effusion, which may be defined as an effusion associated with any evidence for malignant invasion of the pericardium. Not all pericardial effusions in a patient with cancer are necessarily malignant. Other mechanisms for effusion in these patients include adjacent inflammation, interruption of lymphatic or venous drainage, infection, hypoalbuminemia, congestive heart failure, renal failure, toxicities of chemotherapeutics, and chest irradiation. The pericardial space has even been found to be a site of extramedullary hematopoiesis in cases of chronic myeloid leukemia,[28,29] and amyloid accumulation in multiple myeloma.[30] Effusions can also be idiopathic, seemingly unrelated to malignancy. In addition to cell morphology, fluid and tissue analysis with chemistry and microbiology may help to diagnose some of these other entities, and will be discussed in more detail below.

Treatment of malignant pericardial disease involves two parallel strategies—local control of the pericardial disease and, where feasible, systemic treatment for the underlying malignancy. Since the overall prognosis of patients with pericardial metastases from any cancer is generally poor, palliation is usually the goal. Tumor type and aggressiveness influence treatment. As with any treatment in oncology, quality and quantity of life must both be considered when choosing a therapeutic strategy. In general, the more definitive procedures carry a higher risk of morbidity and mortality, and less burdensome strategies may sometimes be more prudent. Good communication between the cardiologist, oncologist, primary care physician, patient, and family is essential to arriving at a medically reasonable and appropriate treatment strategy that can be accepted by the patient and his decision-makers.

Malignancy-Related Pericardial Disease

It has been estimated that nearly two-thirds of patients with malignancy who present with pericardial disease do not have direct pathologic invasion of the pericardium by the tumor.[3] In many cases, pericardial disease is related indirectly to the malignancy or its treatment; radiation pericarditis and opportunistic infections are examples of this phenomenon. In some instances, pericardial disease is entirely unrelated to the malignancy. We will discuss some of the non-malignant but malignancy-related conditions here.

Radiation-Induced Pericardial Disease

It has been well established that external radiation to the thorax is associated with cardiac sequelae. All three cardiac layers can be involved, but the pericardium is the most radiosensitive; the myocardium and endocardium are post-mitotic tissues, and thus are less susceptible.[5] Radiation-related cardiac disease depends mostly on radiation dose, volume of the heart exposed, and specific techniques used, but other factors play a role, including age at the time of exposure (younger patients are at higher risk) and even genetic susceptibility, as discovered by examination of certain single nucleotide polymorphisms.[31]

The most common malignancies treated with chest radiation, and thus associated with cardiac disease, are lung cancer, breast cancer, and lymphoma. Other relevant malignancies are esophageal and thyroid cancers. Radiation doses typically associated with cardiac disease start around 25 gray (Gy) (or 2,500 Rads), with disease quite common at doses above 40 Gy. One study found acute pericarditis in over 30% of patients who received greater than 40 Gy to the heart.[5] The incidence of cardiac sequelae also increases when more than 50% of the volume of the heart is contained in the radiation field.[32]

The mechanism of cardiac damage from radiation is not well understood, but is thought to consist of microvascular destruction, including lymphatics, and apoptosis from direct cellular injury.[33] Inflammation from necrosis of tumor cells and hypersensitivity reactions may also play a role.[5] Over time, fibrosis and/or pericardial effusion can form, and pericardial thickening is usually a late manifestation. One theory explaining late development of pericardial disease (over 20 years after exposure in some cases) involves an increased susceptibility or an exaggerated response to infection conferred upon an irradiated pericardium,[4] but little evidence is yet available to support this hypothesis. Although pathologic changes can be found in many patients exposed to radiation, symptoms occur in only a small number of cases.

The exact incidence of radiation-related pericardial disease is difficult to discern because of the potentially long delay between radiation exposure and the development of late pericardial disease. Furthermore, improvement in radiation techniques over the last 30 years have led to remarkable reductions in the incidence of disease, making older epidemiologic studies obsolete. One study examined the burden of cardiac irradiation in all patients with pericardial disease and found radiation to be the cause in 7.3%. This was further broken down, and radiation was implicated in 11% of cases of constriction, 7.5% of pericardial effusion, and 9.1% of acute pericarditis.[20]

Hodgkin's and non-Hodgkin's lymphoma have the highest incidence of radiation-related cardiac disease, attributable to disease prevalence, a younger patient population, and to anatomic considerations. The relative risk of fatal cardiac events has been reported as high as 7.2 after treatment for Hodgkin's lymphoma.[34,35] A typical regimen includes 30 to 39 Gy at 1.5 to 1.8 Gy/fraction over 4 to 5 weeks. Mantle radiation (parallel opposed A-P and P-A fields) is given to the mediastinum, although the heart is usually shielded for part of the treatment. Total radiation dose to the heart depends on the location of the malignancy within the mediastinum. Mantle radiation is associated with a higher incidence of pericarditis than radiation for lung or breast cancer because the total dose to the heart is higher. In one study of 48 long-term Hodgkin's survivors with an average 14-year follow-up and a median dose of 40 Gy, all patients studied were found to have pericardial thickening, and one was found to have constriction.[36] An autopsy study of young patients who received over 35 Gy to the heart found pericardial thickening in 15 of 16 cases, and clinical evidence of tamponade was present in 5 cases prior to death.[37] In the largest cohort to date of patients with mediastinal radiation for Hodgkin's lymphoma, 2.2% of 590 patients developed clinical pericarditis.[38]

Breast cancer is typically treated with 50 Gy at 2 Gy/fraction over 5 to 6 weeks. The radiation field is tangential, such that no more than 2 cm of lung or chest wall tissue is involved. External beam radiation is also sometimes applied to the internal mammary chain of lymph nodes, which is focused at a prescribed depth. The heart is nearly completely shielded during radiation of right-sided breast cancer, and is minimized with the above techniques during left-sided radiation. One study found the mean radiation dose to the heart for left-sided disease to be 3.8 Gy for tangential field alone, and 6.4 Gy when external beam to the internal mammary chain was included.[39] Respiratory gating with breath-holding techniques can further reduce cardiac irradiation.[40] Significant cardiac toxicities of radiation for breast cancer are fairly uncommon, including pericardial disease. One study found no increase in cardiac mortality when comparing patients with left and right-sided breast cancer treated with radiation and followed for 12 years.[41]

Radiation therapy for lung cancer is usually palliative. Regimens consist of 60 Gy to the hilum or mediastinum at 1.8 to 2 Gy/fraction over 7 to 8 weeks. Radiation is usually administered only to active macroscopic lesions, rather than comprehensive inclusion of all potentially involved tissues. Extent of heart involvement thus is highly dependent on location of mediastinal disease. The heart can be fairly effectively shielded during left hilar radiation. Prognosis is generally very poor in this group of patients, so manifestations of late pericardial disease are decidedly rare. Acute pericarditis is possible, but infrequent.

Clinical manifestations of radiation-induced pericardial disease are highly variable. Patients can present acutely during their treatment, subacutely weeks or months later, or as late as decades after radiation exposure. Presentations include acute pericarditis, chronic pericardial effusion, cardiac tamponade, and pericardial constriction. The peak incidence of pericardial sequelae occurs 5 to 9 months after radiation exposure,[32] but all patients are indefinitely susceptible, with incidence increasing with the duration of follow-up.[4] Interestingly, acute disease does not seem to predispose a higher risk of late chronic disease.[32]

Acute pericarditis is an early manifestation and presents with chest pain, fever, a pericardial rub, and electrocardiographic changes. Effusion may or may not be present. The differential diagnosis includes other causes of chest pain, especially pulmonary embolism, which can cause pleuritic chest pain similar to pericarditis, and myocardial infarction, which is also found with increased prevalence after radiation. Malignant pericardial disease is much less likely to present with classic acute pericarditis. Treatment consists of nonsteroidal anti-inflammatory drugs, and corticosteroids are sometimes necessary for refractory cases. Radiation can usually be continued once anti-inflammatory treatment has been initiated. Prognosis is excellent for this form of pericardial disease, but late sequelae may be more frequent in those who experience a significant initial inflammatory reaction.

Subacute or chronic pericardial effusion is the most common manifestation of radiation-induced pericardial disease. Symptoms are similar to other causes of pericardial effusion. Although tamponade is possible with radiation, this entity should raise suspicion for malignant pericardial disease, which is a much more likely cause for tamponade. Effusions range from serous to hemorrhagic, and over time become more fibrinous with evidence of adhesions. Increased protein and lymphocyte count are seen on fluid analysis, and are similar to other inflammatory conditions. The diagnosis is one of exclusion, and diagnostic pericardiocentesis may be required to rule out malignant effusion. Another helpful clinical finding is the absence of metastatic disease elsewhere; if no other metastases are found with appropriate testing, radiation is much more likely to be the cause.[11] Treatment includes anti-inflammatory drugs, with drainage as needed. Definitive surgical procedures are rarely needed, as the condition generally responds well to conservative management. Prognosis is generally good, although some patients do go on to develop constrictive disease.

Pericardial constriction is the feared outcome of chronic radiation-induced pericardial disease. Although its incidence is uncommon, the prognosis is grave. Clinical manifestations of constriction will be discussed below, but a few points specific to radiation disease will be considered here. Although other causes of pericardial constriction (eg, tuberculosis, post-cardiac surgery) typically involve diffuse pericardial calcification, radiation disease tends to be non-calcific.[3] A diagnostic dilemma with this entity is in distinguishing it from myocardial fibrosis, which may also result from cardiac irradiation. Myocardial radiation damage presents as a restrictive cardiomyopathy, which is difficult to distinguish from constriction. In fact, both entities can be present in patients with chest radiation. The distinction is critical, because performing pericardiectomy on patients with predominantly restrictive disease leads to increased operative mortality. Some authors advocate endomyocardial biopsy at the time of catheterization for any patient suspected of having radiation-induced cardiac disease to rule out restriction preoperatively.[4] Even with predominant constriction, operative mortality is very high—21% in one study, with a 5-year survival of only 1%.[3]

A variation of pericardial constriction in the setting of radiation is effusive-constrictive disease, which involves substantial pericardial effusion in addition to the presence of constrictive physiology. This is typically discovered at the time of pericardiocentesis for tamponade, after which constriction becomes evident.

Lastly, a known complication of chest irradiation is the development of secondary malignancies. These can arise from virtually any tissue exposed to the radiation, including the pericardium in very rare instances. Cases involving "primary" pericardial lymphoma,[42] pericardial angiosarcoma,[43] and pericardial mesothelioma[44] have been described, occurring years after radiation therapy to the chest for the initial malignancy.

Chemotherapy-Related Pericardial Disease

Several antineoplastic or related agents have been implicated in pericardial disease,[45] and are summarized in Table 3. The incidence of chemotherapy-related pericardial disease is rare, and the mechanisms are generally poorly understood. They are important, however, in the context of the differential diagnosis of pericardial conditions in the cancer patient. Chemotherapy-related pericardial disease is usually self-limited, and may be treated with anti-inflammatory drugs and removal of the offending agent when practical. In very rare cases, pericardiocentesis may be necessary to treat tamponade or as a diagnostic intervention to help rule out malignant effusion or infection.

Anthracyclines can cause pericarditis (more specifically myopericarditis) as a manifestation of their early cardiotoxicity. These effects are not related to cumulative dose, although the relationship with later cardiac dysfunction has been suggested. The recognition of pericarditis alone, however, should not be considered sufficient grounds for altering the anthracycline-containing chemotherapeutic regimen in patients who are otherwise stable.[46]

All-*trans* retinoic acid is used for induction and maintenance of remission in patients with acute promyelocytic leukemia. The main toxicity of this agent is retinoic acid syndrome, which consists of fever, weight gain, interstitial pulmonary infiltrates, pleural and pericardial effusions, hypotension, and acute renal failure. It is seen during induction in approximately 25% of cases, but has not been observed with maintenance therapy. Pleural and pericardial manifestations occur in about one-third of patients with the syndrome.[47] The mechanism involves the differentiation and extravasation of leukemic cells into affected organs, which causes a brisk inflammatory response and capillary leak. Mortality ranges from 5 to 30%, but cause of death is not usually related directly to the pericardial effusion.[47] Treatment involves early recognition and administration of dexamethasone 10 mg intravenously twice daily. Development of retinoic acid syndrome does not preclude further treatment with this agent, but prophylactic steroids and close monitoring are required.

Infectious Pericardial Disease

Of all pericardial disease with a recognized cause, infections make up the largest category. A long list of potential pathogens exist, including viruses, bacteria, rickettsia, fungi, and parasites.[4] Cancer patients are a uniquely susceptible group as their disease or its treatment routinely causes immunosuppression, leukopenia, multisystem organ disease, and loss of tissue integrity (and hence loss of normal barriers to infection). Frequent hospitalizations and long-term intravascular access catheters add to the infectious burden. Thus, infections should routinely be included in the differential diagnosis of malignant pericardial disease. During any pericardial drainage procedure, samples should always be collected for cell count, Gram stain, and culture, with additional microbiologic studies obtained if indicated. Because treatment is usually curative, correct diagnosis is essential.

Cancer or complications of its treatment can lead to suppurative infections of the pericardium via fistula formation. Given the close proximity of the esophagus to the heart, esophageal cancers can invade locally and create esophagopericardial fistulas with resulting purulent pericarditis.[48–50] Gastric cancer has likewise created fistulas to the pericardium in rare cases.[51] Metallic stents placed into the esophagus for an obstructing tumor can also lead to fistula formation.[52]

Tuberculous pericarditis is especially important in the cancer patient because of this organism's predilection for immunocompromised hosts and the elderly, and because clinical features can often mimic malignant disease. Although *Mycobacterium tuberculosis* can present with the entire spectrum of pericardial syndromes, the most common presentation is an insidious chronic effusive pericarditis, which has a tendency to progress to calcific constrictive disease. Chronic fevers and cachexia are frequent. Interestingly, most patients do not have coexistent pulmonary infection.[4] Diagnosis is challenging because many tests, including acid-fast staining, culture, and tuberculin skin testing all have relatively low sensitivity. Polymerase chain reaction (PCR) to test for mycobacterial DNA is

Table 3 Antineoplastic Agents Associated with Pericardial Toxicity	
Medication	*Comment*
Cytarabine (Ara-C)	Pericarditis, effusion
Cyclophosphamide	Pericarditis
Ifosamide	Pericarditis
Anthracyclines	Myopericarditis, early toxicity, not dose-related
Sargramostim	Effusion, constriction
Busulfan	Tamponade, pericardial fibrosis
Cisplatin	Pericarditis at high doses
Methotrexate	Pericarditis, effusion, possibly immune-mediated
Imatinib	Effusion
All-*trans* Retinoic Acid	Effusion (Retinoic Acid Syndrome)

increasingly being used. Treatment includes multidrug regimens based on local susceptibility patterns as well as pericardiocentesis or surgery as needed. If pericardiectomy is necessary for constriction, earlier intervention leads to better outcomes.[4]

Since human immunodeficiency virus (HIV) is classically associated with certain malignancies and also causes pericardial disease, it is of special interest; HIV can lead to pericardial disease via direct effects, secondary infections, and malignancies. Other cardiovascular sequelae include myocarditis, heart failure, pulmonary hypertension, and premature coronary artery disease.[53] Before the era of highly active antiretroviral therapy (HAART), the incidence of pericardial effusion was found to be 11% per year and was associated with a poor prognosis.[54] Typically, pericardial effusions are small, asymptomatic, and sterile, and do not lead directly to death. Tamponade and constrictive disease are possible, however. Notable secondary pericardial infections include typical and atypical mycobacteria and fungi. HIV-related malignancies such as primary cardiac lymphoma, metastatic lymphoma, and Kaposi's sarcoma have all been known to involve the pericardium.

Pericardial Syndromes in the Cancer Patient

Pericardial disease in the cancer patient can present with a diverse group of clinical syndromes. This spectrum includes acute pericarditis, pericardial effusion, cardiac tamponade, and pericardial constriction. The boundaries between these syndromes are somewhat arbitrary, however, and much overlap is seen in actual practice. Despite its limitations, it is helpful to organize one's approach to pericardial disease within this framework.

Acute Pericarditis

Acute pericarditis is a syndrome of chest pain caused by inflammation of the pericardium and surrounding structures. At least some component of myocarditis is almost universally present and accounts for many of the clinical findings; some authors prefer the term "myopericarditis" for this reason. A clinically apparent pericardial effusion may or may not be present. Of the many possible etiologies, viral infections make up a large segment, and indeterminate etiologies grouped as "idiopathic" constitute a major portion, as well. Many of the less common causes are associated with previously well-established diagnoses or obvious clinical scenarios. The causes of acute pericarditis are summarized in Table 4.

In the general population (ie, without previous diagnosis of malignancy), acute pericarditis is very rarely the first presentation of a malignancy.

Table 4 Causes of Acute Pericarditis

Idiopathic
Viral (Coxsackie viruses, echoviruses, influenza, HIV, etc.)
Tuberculous
Lyme Disease
Other Infections (includes bacterial, fungal, parasitic)
Collagen Vascular Diseases (systemic lupus erythematosus and others)
Drug Reactions
Hypothyroidism
Myocardial Infarction (coexistent or up to months later)
Post-pericardiotomy
Uremia and Renal Dialysis
Neoplastic Pericarditis
Radiation
Trauma

In one series, of 387 patients with acute pericarditis without tamponade, 9 (2.3%) were ultimately found to have occult malignancy as the cause.[2] In this series, features that increased the likelihood of malignancy included the presence of a large effusion and the lack of response to NSAIDs. Of the malignancies that presented with acute pericarditis as the first manifestation, almost all cases were primary lung cancers.

Even in the patient with known malignancy, idiopathic and viral etiologies are still the most likely. Malignant pericarditis moves higher in the differential diagnosis, however, and serious consideration must be given to this entity. In addition to the clinical clues mentioned above, a reasonable search for other metastatic disease is helpful, as the pericardium is very seldom the only site of metastatic spread. Radiation, chemotherapy, renal failure, and post-pericardiotomy, for example, are possible etiologies in the appropriate setting. Infections are also more likely in the cancer patient, given the relative immunosuppression sometimes imposed by malignancy or its treatment.

Acute inflammation of the pericardium presents primarily with chest pain. Other symptoms include fever, dyspnea, and cough. The chest pain is classically located over the left precordium, is sharp in quality and demonstrates pleuritic features. The pain is also positional, worsened by lying supine, and relieved with sitting up. Alternately, the pain can mimic myocardial ischemia with a dull or pressure-like quality and radiation to the jaw, left shoulder, and left arm, a feature probably attributable to the myocarditic component. Onset can be abrupt. Rapid, shallow breathing or splinting are commonly present with pleuritic pain, and can be confused with true dyspnea.

Physical examination findings of acute pericarditis can include low-grade fever, tachycardia, and a pericardial rub. The classic three-component rub is derived from audible movements of the heart within the pericardium. Its phases are timed with systole, early diastole, and atrial contraction, but not all three components of a pericardial rub may be audible. Rubs are characteristically transient and are often positional, and may not be heard at all. Thus, while the presence of a pericardial rub is generally specific for pericarditis, it is not a very sensitive finding. While rubs are more common in cases of pericarditis without significant effusions, they may still be present with large or even hemodynamically significant fluid collections.

Electrocardiographic findings of acute pericarditis are generated by the superficial myocarditis that is almost always present. A current of injury similar to acute ischemia is seen, but it is more generalized as to location and does not correspond anatomically to the distribution of a single coronary artery. A progression of stereotypical electrocardiogram (ECG) changes over the hours and days following the onset of symptoms has been carefully described,[4] but patients can also present with atypical electrocardiographic features or an entirely normal ECG. Initially, ST elevation and PR depression are present in the inferior, anterior, and lateral leads (Figure 1). These changes are the most characteristic of acute pericarditis when they occur. Over hours or days, the ST and PR segments return to baseline, and the T waves flatten and then become inverted. Given more time, the T waves return to normal. Both the ST and T wave changes can mimic acute myocardial ischemia; a helpful feature is the presence of similar ECG changes in leads I and II in pericarditis, which does not correspond to a typical coronary distribution. Diffuse T wave inversions are nonspecific; other features must be used to support the diagnosis.

Echocardiography is useful, especially in the emergency setting, where myocardial infarction is often in the differential diagnosis of acute pericarditis. Echocardiography can rule out significant segmental wall motion abnormalities, and it also detects the presence or absence of pericardial effusions. Even in the hemodynamically stable patient with acute pericarditis, impending cardiac tamponade is occasionally discovered. Earlier diagnosis and prompt treatment of this entity in a controlled setting is far more preferable than waiting until hemodynamic compromise is overt. Echocardiography is also useful for imaging pericardial masses, which are sometimes seen in cases of malignant pericarditis (Figure 2). Fibrinous exudates are sometimes seen, as well, with or without malignant involvement.

Other findings include leukocytosis and other evidence of acute systemic inflammation,

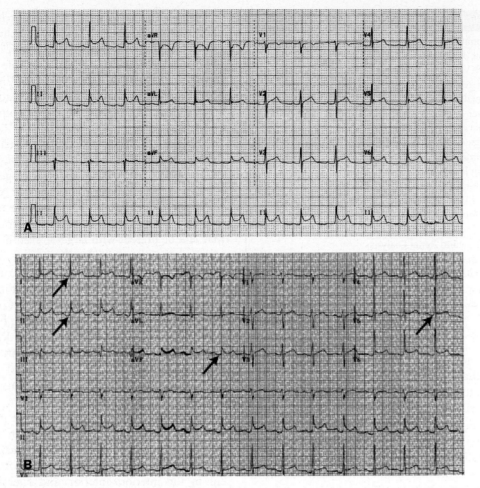

FIGURE 1   A, Electrocardiogram of a patient with multiple myeloma presenting with acute pericarditis. Diffuse ST elevation in a non-coronary distribution is evident. B, Two hours later, the same patient showed diffuse PR depression (arrows) and partial resolution of the ST elevation.

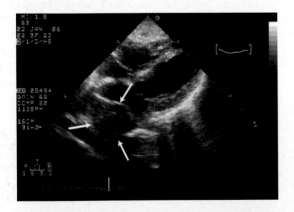

FIGURE 2   Parasternal long axis echocardiographic view showing a large pericardial tumor (arrows) in a patient with metastatic lung cancer compressing the left atrium.

such as C-reactive protein, erythrocyte sedimentation rate, and platelet count. Serum cardiac markers such as troponin can be mildly elevated, reflecting some degree of associated myocarditis.

Differential diagnosis of acute pericarditis includes, most importantly, acute myocardial ischemia. Cancer patients often have multiple risk factors for coronary artery disease, such as advanced age, smoking history, chronic systemic inflammation, chest radiation, etc. Symptom characteristics, ECG abnormalities, and elevated cardiac markers can all mimic an acute myocardial infarction and lead to this misdiagnosis. Distinguishing ischemia from pericarditis in some cases can thus be difficult, especially in the acute setting. Correct diagnosis is crucial, however, as administration of thrombolytics to a cancer patient with pericarditis can have disastrous consequences, such as hemorrhagic tamponade or intracranial bleed. Features that favor the diagnosis of acute pericarditis include pleuritic chest pain, PR depression, generalized distribution of ECG changes, presence of pericardial effusion, and absence of wall motion abnormalities on echocardiography.

Pulmonary embolism is also an important consideration when a cancer patient presents with acute pleuritic chest pain. Given the obvious risk of thromboembolic disease in this population and its high overall incidence, a search for pulmonary embolism is mandatory unless specific findings of pericarditis (such as a pericardial rub) are present. Hypoxemia and obvious lower-extremity, deep venous thrombosis are helpful when present, but pulmonary emboli often present without these features. Pneumonia, other lung diseases, and metastases to the ribs are also in the differential diagnosis of acute pericarditis, but are usually easily excluded after preliminary evaluation.

Management of nonmalignant acute pericarditis consists of a short course of a nonsteroidal anti-inflammatory drug such as aspirin, ibuprofen, or naproxen. Recent evidence suggests that colchicine may also be beneficial, especially in recurrent disease.[55,56] Corticosteroids may be needed for refractory cases but are generally avoided given their substantial side-effect profile and possible increased likelihood of recurrence. A follow-up echocardiogram is often obtained 1 to 2 weeks after symptoms resolve to rule out a late-forming pericardial effusion, even if effusion is absent initially.

Even in the cancer patient, acute pericarditis without effusion that responds rapidly and completely to therapy is unlikely to represent malignant disease, and an exhaustive search for pathologic evidence of pericardial invasion is not warranted. Features that make malignant pericarditis more likely include recurrent or refractory symptoms, large pericardial effusions, and evidence of widespread metastatic disease. Pericardial masses on echocardiography are highly suggestive of malignant involvement. As noted above, when radiation or chemotherapy are the likely causes of pericarditis, the physician can usually continue these treatments after initial symptoms have resolved with the administration of anti-inflammatory drugs; prophylaxis against recurrence with anti-inflammatory drugs has also been successfully employed. When infectious agents are identified as the etiology, appropriate antimicrobial therapy is indicated.

Pericardial Effusion

Pathologic accumulation of fluid in the pericardial space is the most common manifestation of pericardial disease in cancer patients. Clinical presentation is widely variable, and possible etiologies are numerous. Unlike acute "dry" pericarditis, which is typically not related directly to malignancy, a pericardial effusion in a patient with cancer is always of concern, and often a poor prognostic sign. Because malignant invasion of the pericardium occurs frequently, all patients with pericardial effusion need to be carefully evaluated. It should be noted, however, that up to two-thirds of cancer patients who develop pericardial effusions do so through mechanisms other than malignant invasion of the pericardium.[3]

In the general population without preceding diagnosis of malignancy, large pericardial effusions are usually associated with an obvious non-malignant etiology. When a significant effusion is discovered unexpectedly, however, and especially when clinical features of inflammation are absent, the likelihood of finding malignancy is greatly increased. In one series, positive cytology was found in 2 of 63 samples of pericardial fluids from patients without prior diagnosis of malignancy,[57] but true incidence in this group is probably much lower.

Mechanistically, pericardial effusions result from increased production or decreased resorption of pericardial fluid. Alternatively, "foreign" material such as blood, lymph, pus, or tumor can fill the pericardial space. Thus, the nature of the pericardial fluid provides clues as to its origin. Any cause of acute pericarditis (see Table 4), including malignant invasion, radiation, and anti-neoplastic medications, can also lead to an effusion due to increased production of an inflammatory exudate. Diseases that alter the oncotic and hydrostatic balance between serum and tissue, such as heart failure, renal failure, or hypoalbuminemia, can result in effusions as well. Obstruction of pericardial lymphatics or veins by tumor or fibrinous inflammatory debris results in decreased resorption. When malignancy invades and disrupts the normal tissue integrity, hemorrhage can result, and the possibility of infection is increased.

Pericardial effusions of all sizes are frequently asymptomatic and are discovered as incidental findings on chest radiographs or CT scans. Other presentations include acute and chronic pericarditis, gradually worsening dyspnea or functional capacity, and cardiac tamponade with impending hemodynamic collapse. Occasionally, cough or dysphagia is among the presenting symptoms. Symptoms that arise from hemodynamic effects are not predicted by the size of the effusion, but rather are more closely related to intrapericardial pressure, a feature that depends on rapidity of fluid accumulation and distensibility of the pericardium. In the absence of acute pericarditis or frank tamponade, physical examination findings may be absent. Decreased intensity of heart sounds is neither sensitive nor specific. The ECG may show nonspecific findings; decreased QRS voltage can sometimes help to raise suspicion of pericardial effusion, but is also seen with other conditions, such as a left-sided pleural effusion.

If pericardial effusion is suspected or discovered on cardiac imaging, echocardiography is the test of choice for confirmation of the diagnosis and assessment of its hemodynamic significance. First and foremost, it shows the size and location of the effusion. Pericardial effusions appear as echo-free spaces that separate the parietal from the visceral pericardium. When effusions are small (< 100 cc), they tend to appear only posterior to the left ventricle and are < 10 mm in depth when measured in diastole.

Because of the pericardial reflection at the base of the right and left inferior pulmonary veins, small effusions tend not to involve the space posterior to the left atrium (the oblique sinus), and appear to stop at the atrioventricular groove (Figure 3). The oblique sinus can, however, be involved when larger effusions are present. With moderate effusions (100 to 500 cc), a more evenly distributed echo-free space is visualized, including the anterior, lateral, and apical areas. Posteriorly, a moderate effusion measures 10 to 20 mm in diastole. Large effusions (> 500 cc) are obvious in multiple views and > 20 mm thick posteriorly; independent motion of the heart compared with the parietal pericardium may be evident. At the extreme (ie, tamponade), this independent motion manifests as a swinging of the heart within the pericardial space.[58]

In addition to size and location of pericardial effusions, echocardiography can detect multiple other aspects of pericardial pathology seen in cancer patients. A fibrinous exudate can often be seen on the epicardial surface in cases of inflammatory origin and is sometimes confused with tumor. Later manifestations of chronic pericarditis, such as fibrinous bands, loculations, and adhesions, may also be evident. Tumors from metastatic malignancies can be seen on both the parietal and visceral pericardial surfaces. Pericardial calcification and intrapericardial thrombi can also be visualized.

To help determine the cause of a pericardial effusion, and often as a therapeutic maneuver, as well, pericardial fluid can be drained and the fluid analyzed. In the non-emergent setting, this is best done in a controlled fashion by experienced physicians in order to reduce potentially serious complications. Most commonly, pericardiocentesis is performed by a cardiologist with the aid of ultrasonography and/or x-ray fluoroscopy. Alternately, a minimally invasive surgical pericardiotomy under local anesthesia is an option that may allow for additional diagnostic information

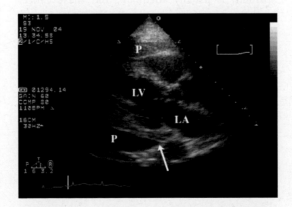

FIGURE 3 Parasternal long axis echocardiographic view showing an anterior and posterior pericardial effusion (P). Although this effusion is large, it is seen extending to the AV groove posteriorly (arrow) between the left ventricle (LV) and left atrium (LA).

through pericardioscopy and pericardial biopsy without a substantially increased risk. Differences between various pericardial drainage procedures will be discussed further under the heading of cardiac tamponade.

The European Society of Cardiology has issued evidence-based guidelines regarding indications for pericardiocentesis.[3] Class I indications include clinical tamponade or a high suspicion for neoplastic or purulent pericarditis. Diagnostic pericardiocentesis for large effusions (as defined above) in asymptomatic patients is a class IIa indication if further diagnostic information may be obtained that would affect management decisions. Level of evidence for these recommendations is *B*, indicating data from non-randomized studies or a single randomized trial. Thus, in a patient with known malignancy, a relatively low threshold exists for drainage as long as it is safe to do so, considering the likelihood of diagnosing malignant pericardial effusion. Findings that favor malignant effusion are larger size, recurrent or persistent effusions despite medical treatment, unclear etiology, widespread metastatic disease elsewhere, and lack of inflammatory features, such as chest pain and fever.

Gross features of pericardial fluid, such as color and consistency at the time of pericardial drainage, can provide useful information. Pus, chylous effusion, and frank hemorrhage are easily recognized. Congestive heart failure and related conditions usually produce a clear, straw-colored fluid (hydropericardium). Increasing levels of inflammation will render the fluid turbid with cells and fibrinous debris, which also increase the viscosity.

Analysis of pericardial fluid should include cell count, leukocyte differential, Gram-stain, culture, and cytology to rule out infection and malignancy; additional studies may also be indicated. Chemistries such as lactate dehydrogenase, glucose, and protein levels are also routinely measured, but are unlikely to add much diagnostic information. Some authors suggest that a bloody effusion with a protein level > 3 mg/dL is highly suggestive of malignancy.[18] One series looking at mean values of various parameters from malignant pericardial effusion found glucose to be 54 mg/dL, protein 5.3 mg/dL, hematocrit 12.9%, leukocyte count 6×10^3/mL, and roughly equal numbers of neutrophils and lymphocytes.[1] Other tests appropriate for pericardial fluid include staining and culture for acid-fast bacilli, lipid levels, and immunologic factors (antinuclear antibody, rheumatoid factor) as indicated by the clinical scenario.

Malignant pericardial effusion, as defined by pathologic evidence for tumor invasion of the pericardium with associated effusion, is the main diagnostic consideration when cancer patients present with pericardial effusion. Among such patients, between one-third and one half will have malignant pericardial disease.[18] Once diagnosed, the prognosis for patients with a malignant effusion is typically measured in months, and aggressive local and systemic cancer treatment is needed to provide palliation and prevent rapid demise. Since up to two-thirds of such patients will have a nonmalignant and easily treatable etiology, the correct diagnosis is of utmost importance.

The mainstay of pathologic diagnosis of malignant pericardial disease is cytology from pericardial fluid. The reported sensitivity ranges generally from 80 to 90% in the literature,[1,11] and the specificity is virtually 100%. The false-negatives that do occur have been attributed to either very low cell counts or large amounts of obscuring blood. Sensitivity of cytology is also lower for certain malignancies, namely leukemia and lymphoma.[11] One problem encountered in sensitivity analysis is that some studies used autopsy findings as the gold standard. Since there is usually a significant time delay between a diagnostic pericardiocentesis and death, there is the possibility that pathologic invasion of the pericardium occurred in the interim, and the presenting effusion may well have been nonmalignant at the time of pericardiocentesis.

In cases of malignant pericardial disease, diagnostic yield can be enhanced with biopsy. Percutaneous biopsy of the parietal pericardium or intrapericardial tumors has been shown to be feasible,[59,60] but surgery is the more usual route of obtaining tissue samples. Through a surgical approach, biopsy specimens from both the visceral and parietal pericardium can be obtained. These are often facilitated by pericardioscopy, which can directly visualize tumors protruding into the pericardial space and thus help direct biopsy. Without direct visualization, pericardial biopsy alone is less sensitive than cytology because of sampling errors.[61] When both cytology and pericardioscopy-guided biopsy are used, sensitivity is maximized. This approach, however, may not be feasible for certain patients or may not be available at certain institutions. Fluid analysis is usually adequate to make the diagnosis, but if the clinical suspicion for malignant effusion is high and cytology findings are benign, a more rigorous investigation is warranted.

Carcinoembryonic antigen (CEA) has been found to be elevated in the pericardial fluid of patients with malignant effusions due to most cancers.[62,63] Although series have been small, results have been promising. Sensitivity and specificity are high, but both false-positive and false-negative results have been reported. One study found the sensitivity of CEA to be 86% for malignant effusion, and, when combined with cytology, the sensitivity was 100%.[63] Another more recent study derived an optimal cutoff for CEA

of 5 ng/mL and found that 14 of 15 patients with a malignant effusion but negative cytology had elevated CEA levels.[62] Given the ease of measurement once pericardial fluid has been obtained, CEA level should probably be routinely included in fluid analysis if malignancy is suspected. With cytology, it promises to increase sensitivity to nearly 100% if it is validated by larger studies.

Analysis of DNA ploidy by flow cytometry has been investigated as an additional means of diagnosing malignant pericardial effusion. In one small series, diploid DNA was associated with benign pathology, and aneuploid and tetraploid with positive cytology. In this series, findings other than diploidy had a sensitivity of 80% and a specificity of 100% for diagnosing malignant effusions.[64] Other studies have found similar results with DNA cytology on various different effusions, including from the pericardium.[65,66] Although not routinely performed in practice, DNA ploidy analysis has the potential to help detect malignancy when cytology is inconclusive. Immunocytochemistry has shown promise, not only in diagnosing malignancy, but also helping to distinguish among various forms. For example, staining with the monoclonal antibody Ber-EP4 was 95.4% sensitive for detecting metastatic carcinoma in effusions, but was not seen in any cases of mesothelioma or in benign effusions.[67] In the future, tumor-specific markers may be available for use in evaluating pericardial effusions of unclear origin in the cancer patient with very high sensitivity and specificity for detecting malignant disease.

Treatment of pericardial effusions in the cancer patient is aimed at the underlying cause. Acute inflammation, infection, hypothyroidism, heart failure, renal failure, etc., can all be managed appropriately, and favorable outcomes with regards to the pericardial disease can be expected. When chemotherapeutic medications or acute chest radiation are the culprit, conservative management is usually adequate, and these cancer treatments need not usually be interrupted. Malignant effusions are managed with a combination of local measures and systemic anti-tumor therapy if indicated. Chest radiation for pericardial metastases can help control aggressive disease as well. Pericardiocentesis, followed by several days of drainage, can often be adequate to prevent recurrences, as well as making the diagnosis. When this fails, a variety of percutaneous and minor surgical approaches can provide more definitive treatment.

Pericardiocentesis is the easiest and least risky of the drainage procedures. It can be done in a catheterization laboratory or at the bedside with echocardiographic guidance. The procedure is described in detail under the section on the emergent management of cardiac tamponade

below (see "Cardiac Tamponade"). Advantages include use of local anesthesia, percutaneous approach, and low complication rate with experienced operators. Fluid is available for analysis, and the catheter can be left in place for several days to allow continued drainage and prevent early recurrence of the effusion. Disadvantages include later recurrence of the effusion and lack of tissue for biopsy.

In some centers, intrapericardial administration of sclerosing agents or anti-tumor agents through the drainage catheter are used to help prevent reaccumulation of pericardial fluid. These interventions have not been the subject of controlled trials, but several small series have been published with encouraging results. Sclerosis with tetracycline analogues provides control of malignant pericardial disease in 90% of patients,[68–70] preventing recurrent effusion and alleviating symptoms. Significant side effects, including pain with administration, fever, and atrial arrhythmias, were more common with tetracycline than with newer agents such as minocycline. Intrapericardial chemotherapy has also shown promise for local control of malignant disease, regardless of primary tumor site. Pharmacokinetic study of intrapericardial cisplatin and 5-fluorouracil has shown much higher drug concentrations and greatly increased half-lives than can be obtained with systemic therapy.[71] Series with cisplatin have shown response rate of virtually 100% with minimal toxicity.[61,72–74] Results with mitoxantrone have been similarly encouraging,[75,76] but 5-fluorouracil appears to be less effective in controlling local pericardial disease.[77] Thiotepa, which has both sclerosing and antineoplastic properties, has recently been studied and showed excellent control of malignant pericardial disease with minimal toxicity.[78]

Subxiphoid pericardiotomy is a minimally-invasive surgical procedure that can be performed under local anesthesia at the bedside. It allows for direct visualization as well as thoracoscopic examination. A pleuropericardial window can also be created via the subxiphoid approach. Fluid and tissue specimens can be obtained for diagnostic purposes. Recurrences of the malignant effusion are possible, but less likely than with pericardiocentesis alone. Complication rates are low, making this the preferred treatment strategy for recurrent malignant effusions at many centers. Pericardioperitoneal shunt is an alternative drainage procedure that is likewise minimally invasive and can be done under local anesthesia. It is technically simpler than subxiphoid pericardiotomy and has been associated with shorter recovery times.[79] Catheter-based pericardiotomy, using a balloon across the pericardium that can be inflated to disrupt the pericardium and allow drainage, has been explored but is seldom undertaken, especially in view of the newer surgical techniques for subxiphoid pericardiotomy. The procedure is especially uncomfortable for the patient, and has only been used in a number of centers.

More definitive surgical management of malignant pericardial disease requires partial or complete pericardiectomy. This requires general anesthesia for anterior thoracotomy or sternotomy, and is associated with significant morbidity and mortality. In most patients with malignant pericardial effusions, prognosis is limited, and less invasive strategies are preferred, but pericardiectomy can be considered in those with a relatively good prognosis in whom more definitive therapy is desired.

Patients who have undergone needle or catheter drainage should have a follow-up cardiac ultrasound examination one month following the procedure, or sooner in the event symptoms of recurrent pericardial tamponade appear. Patients who undergo pericardiotomy or creation of a pleuropericardial window should have a follow-up ultrasonography two months following the procedure; these guidelines are based on personal preference and prudence. There is no clear evidence, however, that discovering a recurrence by ultrasonography prior to the development of symptoms alters the course or improves the quality of life in these patients.

Cardiac Tamponade

Cardiac tamponade is a condition that exists when the pericardial space contains fluid under sufficient pressure to interfere with cardiac filling, resulting in decreased cardiac output and the inability to sustain vital functions. Tamponade is not created merely by a certain quantity of fluid, but by the pressure created by that fluid in the pericardial sac. Life-threatening increases may be seen with relatively small quantities of fluid, as may occur following traumatic injury to the heart with hemorrhage into the pericardium. In the cancer patient, the fluid is more likely to accumulate at a slower rate allowing the pericardial space to expand gradually, and the quantity of fluid required to raise pressure sufficiently to impede cardiac filling is usually much larger. In some instances, the quantity of fluid is greater than two liters.

Malignant pericardial disease is the most frequent cause of cardiac tamponade in the general inpatient population. Furthermore, among the various pericardial syndromes, tamponade is the most likely to be associated with malignancy.[1] It is not rare that cardiac tamponade is the first indication of malignancy; in one clinical series of consecutive patients with tamponade and no prior diagnosis of cancer, 9 of 52 patients (17%) were ultimately diagnosed with malignant effusions.[2] It is more common, however, that a patient with known malignancy who is unaware of malignant spread to the heart experiences cardiac decompensation with cardiac tamponade as the mechanism. Any malignancy that spreads to the pericardium is capable of causing pericardial tamponade, and the phenomenon is seen with some regularity in the face of metastatic breast cancer. Despite the close association between tamponade and malignant pericardial disease, any non-malignant etiology of pericardial disease is capable of causing tamponade—even in a patient with known malignancy. It is thus best to keep open a broad differential for pericardial disease, even in a patient with known malignancy.

Patients with tamponade may not experience the typical chest discomfort of acute pericarditis, and the first clinical manifestation may be increasing shortness of breath. Anxiety, cough, and severe weakness are other common symptoms. Overt tamponade can present as cardiogenic shock or pulseless electrical activity requiring immediate intervention. Physical examination characteristically demonstrates hypotension, tachycardia, and jugular venous distention that may be very pronounced; right atrial activity may be transmitted to the jugular veins with a prominent x descent. Cardiac auscultation may demonstrate distant heart sounds because the fluid separating the heart from the stethoscope may diminish the amplitude. Pericardial friction rubs and pericardial knocks are usually absent or distant on auscultation. The pulse is characteristically weak, and may show an exaggerated decrease during inspiration, known as the phenomenon of pulsus paradoxus. This finding is a manifestation of the interdependence of the right and left cardiac chambers; a preferential filling of the right ventricle during inspiration must be at the cost of left ventricular filling due to the external volume limitation imposed by the pressurized effusion. A paradoxical pulse is defined as a > 10 mm Hg drop in systolic blood pressure with inspiration, and should be measured quantitatively in any patient suspected of having cardiac tamponade. It may also be appreciated by palpating the radial pulse, which can disappear during inspiration in frank tamponade.

Laboratory studies confirm the diagnosis of tamponade. The chest roentgenogram shows an enlarged cardiac silhouette with a sac-like configuration—a helpful, although nonspecific, finding. The electrocardiogram may show electrical alternans, a cyclical variation in QRS voltage occurring with a two-cycle period. Electrical alternans is caused by the heart moving towards and away from the exploring electrode as the heart rocks back and forth within the sac of fluid. Electrical alternans may be seen in some (but not all) electrocardiographic leads; its clear presence in any single lead is sufficient to establish electrical alternans, a very specific (although not especially sensitive) finding in patients with pericardial tamponade.

The most useful noninvasive test is cardiac ultrasonography. A complete transthoracic echocardiogram not only demonstrates the size and location of the pericardial effusion, but several hemodynamic findings suggestive of tamponade as well. One of the earliest findings is compression of the right atrium during systole (Figure 4A), as this chamber typically has the lowest pressures. As tamponade progresses, right ventricular compression during diastole may be evident (Figure 4B). In all patients with frank tamponade, the inferior vena cava is dilated and fails to collapse with inspiration. Doppler echocardiography reveals respiratory variation in ventricular filling velocities that corresponds to the pulsus paradoxus; > 25% decrease in mitral inflow velocities or > 50% decrease in tricuspid inflow velocities with respiration are suggestive of tamponade (Figure 4C). Real-time two-dimensional as well as M-mode echocardiograms may demonstrate the to-and-fro rocking motion of the heart that is responsible for electrical alternans. It should be noted that cardiac tamponade progresses along a continuum, and not all of the above echocardiographic findings may be present in individual patients. Furthermore, care must be taken not to attempt to predict the pace of progression based on echocardiography alone; it is impossible to tell the rate of fluid accumulation and the distensibility of the pericardium. Cardiac tamponade is ultimately a clinical diagnosis, and echocardiography serves a basically confirmatory role.

Advanced pericardial tamponade with hemodynamic collapse constitutes a medical emergency of the first order, and any temporizing in establishing the diagnosis or delay in drainage may prove fatal. Prompt drainage often provides very dramatic symptomatic improvement. When tamponade is hemodynamically compromising, emergent needle drainage is the most expedient.

The most direct technique for needle drainage for patients with pericardial tamponade involves inserting the exploring needle just to the left of the xiphoid process in the angle formed by the xiphoid and the ribs. With the patient lying as flat as can be tolerated, the 18-gauge needle attached to a syringe containing 1% lidocaine is advanced in the direction of the acromial process of the left shoulder until fluid is aspirated. A small aliquot of agitated saline may be injected and visualized under echocardiographic guidance to confirm entry into the pericardial space (Figure 5); echocardiographic visualization has made obsolete the use of the electrocardiographic confirmation of an electrical current of injury as the exploring needle serving as an electrode touches the myocardium.

Once the pericardial space has been entered and the location confirmed, a guide wire is

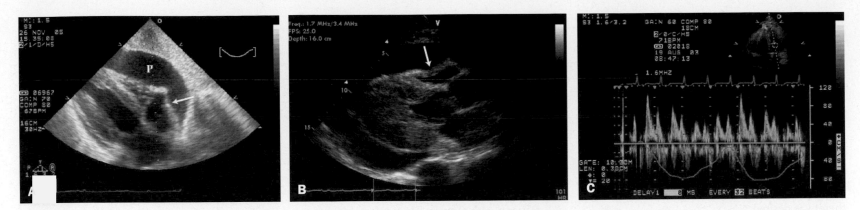

FIGURE 4 Echocardiographic features of pericardial tamponade. A, Non-traditional four-chamber view showing a large pericardial effusion and notching of the right atrium during systole (arrow), one of the early hemodynamic alterations of pericardial tamponade. B, Further hemodynamic embarrassment results in compression of the right ventricle (arrow), seen in this parasternal long axis view. C, Pulse-wave Doppler of the mitral valve showing marked respiratory variation of the mitral inflow velocities consistent with tamponade.

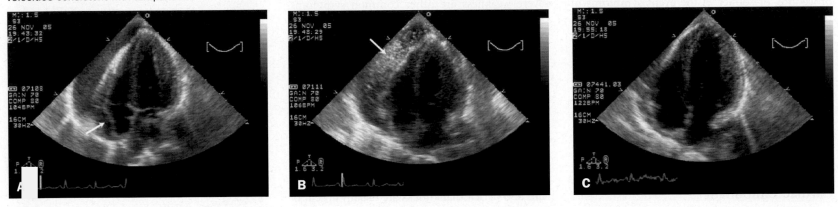

FIGURE 5 Echocardiography-guided pericardiocentesis (apical four-chamber views). A, Large effusion is present with systolic notching of the right atrium (arrow). B, Agitated saline (arrow) has been injected into the pericardial space to confirm proper location of the pericardiocentesis needle. C, After drainage, the effusion is no longer evident and all four cardiac chambers have re-expanded.

advanced through the needle, a dilator is advanced over the wire, and a catheter introducer is inserted into the pericardial space. A catheter may then be inserted and fluid drained through the catheter. In most instances, the fluid is drained in a single sitting using a vacuum bottle. The catheter may remain in place for several days so that additional drainage can be undertaken without reinserting a new catheter. We usually drain each day until the daily aliquot fluid that can be removed is less than 50 mL, the catheter has been in place for five days, or the amount of fluid remains constant at greater than 50 mL for more than two days; while these guidelines have not been scrutinized by clinical trials, they represent a reasonable compromise in that the risk of infection is maintained at safe levels, and the return of fluid is less than would be the case if the catheter were removed immediately following initial drainage.

In cases of cardiac tamponade where hemodynamic collapse does not appear imminent, consideration can be given to some of the other methods of pericardial drainage discussed above. Recurrent pericardial effusion and tamponade may warrant a more definitive procedure, for example. Any therapeutic strategy for tamponade must be instituted without delay, however, as small increases in pericardial fluid volume are associated with large increases in intrapericardial pressure; rapid progression can occur without warning and may be fatal.

Pericardial Constriction

Pericardial constriction occurs when a thick and inflexible shell of pericardium compresses the heart and interferes with normal chamber filling. It causes a syndrome seemingly similar to congestive heart failure, but systolic function of the right and left ventricles are preserved, and important differences exist in the pathophysiology. Constriction is usually seen as a fibrous or calcific response to chronic pericardial inflammation, but can also be caused by direct tumor infiltration.[80] Carcinoid syndrome has also been found to lead to constrictive pericarditis without evidence of pericardial invasion by tumor.[81] In the general population, most causes of pericardial constriction are unknown or follow cases of pericarditis, which are themselves idiopathic.[20] Of the known causes, infection, post-cardiac surgery, and chest radiation are the most commonly implicated. Tuberculous pericarditis was formerly the most common etiology of constriction, but its incidence has decreased in industrialized nations. Any cause of acute or chronic pericardial disease, however, can lead to subsequent constriction.

One surgical pathology series from the Mayo Clinic looked at specimens from 143 consecutive cases of constrictive pericarditis.[20] Etiology was idiopathic in 49%, post-pericardiotomy in 30%, and post-irradiation in 11%. Interestingly, although malignant pericardial disease is a well-established, if uncommon, cause for constrictive pericarditis, no cases were reported, which is likely a reflection of the fact that surgical resection is not feasible in this group.

In the cancer patient exposed to previous chest radiation, this is by far the most likely etiology of constrictive disease. Other possible causes include any pericardial disease that results in a hemorrhagic effusion, as blood typically produces a brisk inflammatory response. Malignant pericardial disease (especially from breast or lung cancer) can lead to constriction, but this is not a common entity, likely because malignant effusions are not especially inflammatory and because the prognosis is so poor in these patients that constriction has not yet had the chance to develop. Complete encasement of the heart by solid tumor in the pericardium can also be clinically indistinguishable from constriction. Mesothelioma has rarely presented as pericardial constriction.[4]

Pericardial constriction can result from pathologic changes to the parietal pericardium, visceral pericardium, or both. These changes primarily include fibrotic thickening and chronic lymphocytic inflammation, with gross calcification present in less than one-third of cases.[20] Pericardial thickening is usually symmetric and completely encases the heart, but other patterns are possible, including loculated or band-like pathology. At its maximum thickness, the parietal pericardium ranged from 1 to 17 mm, with a mean of 4 mm in the Mayo Clinic series of patients with constriction.[20] Interestingly, 4% of cases were categorized as having normal pericardial thickness.

Effusive-constrictive disease is a variation on this theme, which includes features of constriction as well as a significant effusion. It can be seen with malignant pericardial invasion or post-irradiation. Most typically, presentation is consistent with tamponade, and the features of constriction become apparent after pericardiocentesis. Not surprisingly, these cases usually involve constriction by the visceral pericardium.

The pathophysiology of pericardial constriction involves impaired right and left ventricular filling and ventricular interdependence, which is caused by the externally imposed volume limit. Any increased filling in the right heart must be at the expense of left-sided filling, and vice versa. Diastolic pressures in all four cardiac chambers are nearly equalized as well as significantly elevated. Hemodynamic findings with respiratory variation are a key diagnostic feature of constriction; both the right and left atria become insulated from the normal intrathoracic pressure changes, which leads to characteristic patterns during catheterization and echocardiography that are unique to constriction.

Symptoms of constriction arise from elevation of either left- or right-sided filling pressures. Gradually worsening weakness, fatigue, and dyspnea on exertion are prominent, but highly non-specific in the cancer patient. Lower extremity edema, abdominal congestion, and ascites are common, and are often confused with heart failure or tamponade.

Physical examination can be helpful in pericardial constriction. Tachycardia or an irregular heart rate from atrial fibrillation may be present. Pulsus paradoxus may be present, but is less of a phenomenon than it is in the presence of tamponade; it is nearly always under 15 mm Hg. Jugular venous pressure is elevated, and pulsations reveal prominent x and y descents. Kussmaul's sign is a failure of the central venous pressure to decrease with inspiration, owing to high right atrial pressure and the physiologic isolation of the right atrium from changes in intrathoracic pressure. If the central venous pressure is high enough, pulsations of the jugular

vein may be absent and erroneously suggest normal or low pressures. A loud S3, also referred to as a pericardial knock, is due to rapid ventricular filling. Hepatomegaly (sometimes pulsatile), ascites, and lower extremity edema can be present.

Chest radiographs may reveal cardiomegaly, pericardial calcification, an enlarged azygous vein, and pleural effusions. MRI and CT can define pericardial anatomy fairly well and are both more accurate at determining pericardial thickness than echocardiography. They can also show dilation of the superior and inferior vena cavae. ECG findings in constriction are nonspecific. Diagnosis of constriction, however, really requires the hemodynamic data available from echocardiography and catheterization.

Echocardiography can reveal several aspects of pericardial constriction, but the findings can be subtle, and the interpreting cardiologist must have a reasonable index of suspicion to make the diagnosis. Pericardial anatomy can be visible, but image quality is often limited by the high echogenicity of the pericardium, especially when calcification is present. Increased pericardial thickness can sometimes be measured (Figure 6), but this is not a consistent finding and is better evaluated by CT or MRI. The inferior vena cava is dilated and fails to compress with respiration. The interventricular septum can show a characteristic "bounce" corresponding to the rapid ventricular filling in early diastole. An M-mode through the posterior wall of the left ventricle sometimes shows separate densities corresponding to parietal and visceral pericardium that are adherent to the posterior wall and move with the myocardium, a phenomenon known as "tram-tracking" (Figure 7).

Doppler examination of mitral inflow reveals a restrictive filling pattern of severe diastolic dysfunction, including E wave >> A wave velocities and very rapid deceleration time. Unlike restrictive cardiomyopathy, however, tissue Doppler measurements of the mitral annulus can remain

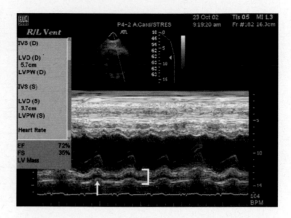

FIGURE 7 M-mode echocardiogram with slice taken through the left ventricle in a patient with constrictive pericarditis. The pericardium is thickened (bracket) and echogenic, and the adherent parietal pericardium (arrow) moves in concert with the contracting ventricle, a finding known as "tram-tracking."

normal. Ventricular interdependence is probably the most specific finding, and is demonstrated by mitral inflow velocities that decrease with inspiration and increase with expiration, and tricuspid velocities that conversely increase with inspiration and decrease with expiration.

Hemodynamic measurements during cardiac catheterization play a confirmatory role. Elevation and equalization of diastolic pressures is seen. Left and right ventricles both show a characteristic diastolic pressure tracing—"dip and plateau"—which reflects rapid early filling followed by abrupt cessation of filling due to a rigid unexpandable heart. This is also affectionately known as the "square-root sign" for obvious reasons (Figure 8). Right atrial pressure tracings demonstrate the prominent x and y descents (Figure 9) and Kussmaul's sign. Simultaneous right atrial and pulmonary capillary wedge tracings can demonstrate the equivalent of ventricular interdependence, with one rising while the other falls.

In practice, diagnosis of pericardial constriction is not straightforward, as many of the above findings can also be seen with tamponade, restrictive cardiomyopathy, or right ventricular failure. The findings that are most specific for constriction are often the hardest to measure. Furthermore, combinations of these entities exist, such as in effusive-constrictive disease or the combined restriction and constriction that frequently occurs after chest irradiation. Sometimes endomyocardial biopsy is used to help rule out a myopathic process if surgical intervention for constriction is being considered. Diagnosis requires a high index of suspicion, an appropriate clinical setting, and radiology, catheterization, and echocardiography findings that help support the diagnosis of pericardial constriction.

Treatment of pericardial constriction is surgical, and complete pericardiectomy is required, usually through a median sternotomy approach.

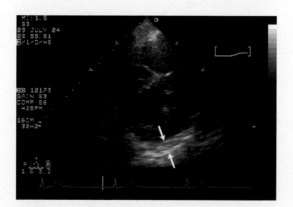

FIGURE 6 Parasternal short axis echocardiographic view through the left ventricle in a patient with constrictive pericarditis. The posterior pericardium (arrows) is markedly thickened and echogenic.

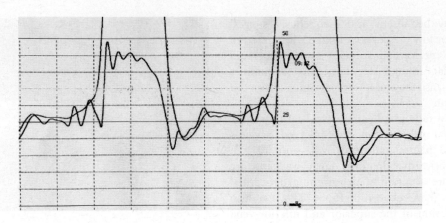

FIGURE 8 Simultaneous pressure tracings from the right and left ventricles demonstrating elevation and equalization of the diastolic pressures as well as the characteristic dip-and-plateau, or "square-root sign", consistent with pericardial constriction.

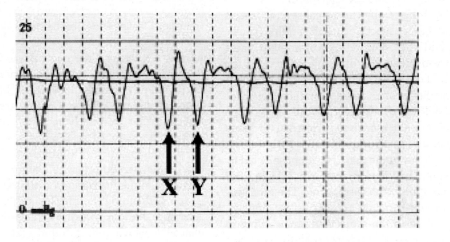

FIGURE 9 Right atrial pressure tracing in constrictive pericarditis, showing elevated mean right atrial pressure (19mmHg) and prominent X and Y descents (labeled).

The surgery is long and technically challenging due to adherent fibrotic debris, and can be complicated by severe bleeding, myocardial damage, arrhythmias, and hypotension. Overall operative mortality is 6 to 12%, and is even higher (21%) in the case of radiation disease.[3] If myocardial fibrosis or atrophy is present, the results after pericardiectomy are dismal. Good outcomes rely on careful patient selection, and it is the rare patient with metastatic cancer who is able to tolerate such a procedure.

REFERENCES

1. Wilding G, Green HL, Longo DL, et al. Tumors of the heart and pericardium. Cancer Treat Rev 1988;15:165–81.
2. Imazio M, Demichelis B, Parrini I, et al. Relation of acute pericardial disease to malignancy. Am J Cardiol 2005; 95:1393–4.
3. Maisch B, Seferovic PM, Ristic AD, et al. Guidelines on the diagnosis and management of pericardial diseases executive summary; the task force on the diagnosis and management of pericardial diseases of the European society of cardiology. Eur Heart J 2004;25:587–610.
4. Spodick DH. The pericardium: a comprehensive textbook. New York: Marcel Dekker, Inc.; 1997.
5. McAllister HA, Jr, Hall RJ, Cooley DA. Tumors of the heart and pericardium. Curr Probl Cardiol 1999;24:57–116.
6. McAllister HA Jr, Fenoglio JJ Jr. Tumors of the cardiovascular system, Fascicle 15. Atlas of tumor pathology. Washington, DC: Armed Forces Institute of Pathology; 1978.
7. Roy N, Blurton DJ, Azakie A, et al. Immature intrapericardial teratoma in a newborn with elevated alpha-fetoprotein. Ann Thorac Surg 2004;78:e6–8.
8. Ragupathy R, Nemeth L, Kumaran V, et al. Successful surgical management of a prenatally diagnosed intrapericardial teratoma. Pediatr Surg Int 2003;19:737–9.
9. Tollens M, Grab D, Lang D, et al. Pericardial teratoma: prenatal diagnosis and course. Fetal Diagn Ther 2003;18:432–6.
10. Thomason R, Schlegel W, Lucca M, et al. Primary malignant mesothelioma of the pericardium. Case report and literature review. Tex Heart Inst J 1994;21:170–4.
11. Hancock EW. Neoplastic pericardial disease. Cardiol Clin 1990;8:673–82.
12. Murai Y. Malignant mesothelioma in Japan: analysis of registered autopsy cases. Arch Environ Health 2001;56:84–8.
13. Carbone M, Rizzo P, Pass H. Simian virus 40: the link with human malignant mesothelioma is well established. Anticancer Res 2000;20(2A):875–7.
14. Bohn U, Gonzalez JL, Martin LM, et al. Meningeal and brain metastases in primary malignant pericardial mesothelioma. Ann Oncol 1994;5:660–1.
15. Lang-Lazdunski L, Oroudji M, Pansard Y, et al. Successful resection of giant intrapericardial lipoma. Ann Thorac Surg 1994;58:238–241.
16. Noji T, Morikawa T, Kaji M, et al. Successful resection of a recurrent mediastinal liposarcoma invading the pericardium: report of a case. Surg Today 2004;34:450–2.
17. Kendall SW, Williams EA, Hunt JB, et al. Recurrent primary liposarcoma of the pericardium: management by repeated resections. Ann Thorac Surg 1993;56:560–2.
18. Kralstein J, Frishman W. Malignant pericardial diseases: diagnosis and treatment. Am Heart J 1987;113:785–90.
19. MacGee W. Metastatic and invasive tumours involving the heart in a geriatric population: a necropsy study.

Virchows Arch A Pathol Anat Histopathol 1991;419:183–9.
20. Oh KY, Shimizu M, Edwards WD, et al. Surgical pathology of the parietal pericardium: a study of 344 cases (1993–1999). Cardiovasc Pathol 2001;10:157–68.
21. Abraham KP, Reddy V, Gattuso P. Neoplasms metastatic to the heart: review of 3314 consecutive autopsies. Am J Cardiovasc Pathol 1990;3:195–8.
22. Kline IK. Cardiac lymphatic involvement by metastatic tumor. Cancer 1972;29:799–808.
23. Williams PL, Warwick, R. Gray's anatomy. Edinburgh: Churchill Livingstone; 1980.
24. Rouviere H. Anatomie des lymphatiques de l'homme. Paris: Mason; 1981.
25. Thurber DL, Edwards JE, Achor RW. Secondary malignant tumors of the pericardium. Circulation 1962;26:228–41.
26. Ewer SM, Yusuf SW. Dysrhythmia in the cancer patient. In: Ewer MS, Yeh E, editors. Cancer and the heart. Hamilton (ON): BC Decker Inc; 2006. p. 139–58.
27. Chiles C, Woodard PK, Gutierrez FR, et al. Metastatic involvement of the heart and pericardium: CT and MR imaging. Radiographics 2001;21:439–49.
28. Bradford CR, Smith SR, Wallis JP. Pericardial extramedullary haemopoiesis in chronic myelomonocytic leukaemia. J Clin Pathol 1993;46:674–5.
29. Shih LY, Lin FC, Kuo TT. Cutaneous and pericardial extramedullary hematopoiesis with cardiac tamponade in chronic myeloid leukemia. Am J Clin Pathol 1988;89:693–7.
30. Kornberg A, Rapoport M, Yona R, et al. Amyloidosis of the pericardium in multiple myeloma: an unusual cause of bloody pericardial effusion. Isr J Med Sci 1993;29:794–7.
31. Janjan NA, Strom E, Perkins G, et al. Effects of radiation on the heart. In: Ewer MS, Yeh E, editors. Cancer and the heart. Hamilton (ON): BC Decker Inc; 2006. p. 75–114.
32. Spodick DH. Pericardial diseases. In: Braunwald E, Zipes DP, Libby P, editors. Heart disease: a textbook of cardiovascular medicine. 6th ed. Philadelphia: W.B. Saunders Company; 2001;1823–1876.
33. Stone RM, Bridges KR, Libby P. Hematological-oncological disorders and the cardiovascular system. In: Braunwald E, Zipes DP, Libby P, editors. Heart disease: a textbook of cardiovascular medicine. 6th ed. Philadelphia: W.B. Saunders Company; 2001;2223–2243.
34. Ewer MS, Benjamin RS, Yeh ETH. Cardiac complications. In: Kufe DW, Pollock RE, Weichselbaum RR, et al, editors. Holland-Frei cancer medicine. 6th ed. Hamilton (ON): BC Decker Inc; 2003;2525–2541.
35. Adams MJ, Hardenbergh PH, Constine LS, et al. Radiation-associated cardiovascular disease. Crit Rev Oncol Hematol 2003;45:55–75.
36. Adams MJ, Lipsitz SR, Colan SD, et al. Cardiovascular status in long-term survivors of Hodgkin's disease treated with chest radiotherapy. J Clin Oncol 2004;22:3139–48.
37. Brosius FC 3rd, Waller BF, Roberts WC. Radiation heart disease. Analysis of 16 young (aged 15 to 33 years) necropsy patients who received over 3,500 rads to the heart. Am J Med 1981;70:519–30.
38. Tarbell NJ, Thompson L, Mauch P. Thoracic irradiation in Hodgkin's disease: disease control and long-term complications. Int J Radiat Oncol Biol Phys 1990;18:275–81.
39. Sautter-Bihl ML, Hultenschmidt B, Melcher U, et al. Radiotherapy of internal mammary lymph nodes in breast cancer. Principle considerations on the basis of dosimetric data. Strahlenther Onkol 2002;178:18–24.
40. Pedersen AN, Korreman S, Nystrom H, et al. Breathing adapted radiotherapy of breast cancer: reduction of cardiac and pulmonary doses using voluntary inspiration breath-hold. Radiother Oncol 2004;72:53–60.
41. Nixon AJ, Manola J, Gelman R, et al. No long-term increase in cardiac-related mortality after breast-conserving surgery and radiation therapy using modern techniques. J Clin Oncol 1998;16:1374–9.
42. Yukiiri K, Mizushige K, Ueda T, et al. Second primary cardiac B-cell lymphoma after radiation therapy and chemotherapy—a case report. Angiology 2001;52:563–5.
43. Killion MJ, Brodovsky HS, Schwarting R. Pericardial angiosarcoma after mediastinal irradiation for seminoma. A case report and a review of the literature. Cancer 1996;78:912–7.
44. Velissaris TJ, Tang AT, Millward-Sadler GH, et al. Pericardial mesothelioma following mantle field radiotherapy. J Cardiovasc Surg (Torino) 2001;42:425–7.
45. Yeh ET, Tong AT, Lenihan DJ, et al. Cardiovascular complications of cancer therapy: diagnosis, pathogenesis, and management. Circulation 2004;109:3122–31.

46. Ewer MS, Benjamin RS. Doxorubicin cardiotoxicity: clinical aspects, recognition, monitoring, treatment, and prevention. In: Ewer MS, Yeh E, editors. Cancer and the heart. Hamilton (ON): BC Decker Inc; 2006. p. 9–32.

47. Tallman MS, Andersen JW, Schiffer CA, et al. Clinical description of 44 patients with acute promyelocytic leukemia who developed the retinoic acid syndrome. Blood 2000;95:90–5.

48. Touati GD, Carmi D, Nzomvuama A, et al. Purulent pericarditis caused by malignant oesophago-pericardial fistula. Eur J Cardiothorac Surg 2003;24:847–9.

49. Kaufman J, Thongsuwan N, Stern E, et al. Esophageal-pericardial fistula with purulent pericarditis secondary to esophageal carcinoma presenting with tamponade. Ann Thorac Surg 2003;75:288–9.

50. Luthi F, Groebli Y, Newton A, et al. Cardiac and pericardial fistulae associated with esophageal or gastric neoplasms: a literature review. Int Surg 2003;88:188–93.

51. Chinnaiyan KM, Ali MI, Gunaratnam NT. Gastric cancer presenting as gastropericardial fistula in a patient with familial adenomatous polyposis syndrome. J Clin Gastroenterol 2004;38:298.

52. Dennert B, Ramirez FC, Sanowski RA. Pericardioesophageal fistula associated with metallic stent placement. Gastrointest Endosc 1997;45:82–4.

53. Hsue PY, Waters DD. What a cardiologist needs to know about patients with human immunodeficiency virus infection. Circulation 2005;112:3947–57.

54. Heidenreich PA, Eisenberg MJ, Kee LL, et al. Pericardial effusion in AIDS. Incidence and survival. Circulation 1995;92:3229–34.

55. Imazio M, Bobbio M, Cecchi E, et al. Colchicine in addition to conventional therapy for acute pericarditis: results of the COlchicine for acute PEricarditis (COPE) trial. Circulation 2005;112:2012–6.

56. Imazio M, Bobbio M, Cecchi E, et al. Colchicine as first-choice therapy for recurrent pericarditis: results of the CORE (COlchicine for REcurrent pericarditis) trial. Arch Intern Med 2005;165:1987–91.

57. Wiener HG, Kristensen IB, Haubek A, et al. The diagnostic value of pericardial cytology. An analysis of 95 cases. Acta Cytol 1991;35:149–53.

58. Sanfilippo AJ, Weyman AE. Pericardial disease. In: Weyman AE, editor. Principles and practice of echocardiography. 2nd ed. Philadelphia: Lea & Febiger; 1994;1102–1134.

59. Ziskind AA, Rodriguez S, Lemmon C, et al. Percutaneous pericardial biopsy as an adjunctive technique for the diagnosis of pericardial disease. Am J Cardiol 1994;74:288–91.

60. Gupta K, Mathur VS. Diagnosis of pericardial disease using percutaneous biopsy: case report and literature review. Tex Heart Inst J 2003;30:130–3.

61. Maisch B, Pankuweit S, Brilla C, et al. Intrapericardial treatment of inflammatory and neoplastic pericarditis guided by pericardioscopy and epicardial biopsy—results from a pilot study. Clin Cardiol 1999;22(1 Suppl 1):17–22.

62. Szturmowicz M, Tomkowski W, Fijalkowska A, et al. Diagnostic utility of CYFRA 21-1 and CEA assays in pericardial fluid for the recognition of neoplastic pericarditis. Int J Biol Markers 2005;20:43–9.

63. Tatsuta M, Yamamura H, Yamamoto R, et al. Carcinoembryonic antigens in the pericardial fluid of patients with malignant pericarditis. Oncology 1984;41:328–30.

64. Bardales RH, Stanley MW, Schaefer RF, et al. Secondary pericardial malignancies: a critical appraisal of the role of cytology, pericardial biopsy, and DNA ploidy analysis. Am J Clin Pathol 1996;106:29–34.

65. Decker D, Stratmann H, Springer W, et al. Benign and malignant cells in effusions: diagnostic value of image DNA cytometry in comparison to cytological analysis. Pathol Res Pract;194:791–5.

66. Fischler DF, Wongbunnate S, Johnston DA, et al. DNA content by image analysis. An accurate discriminator of malignancy in pericardial effusions. Anal Quant Cytol Histol 1994;16:167–73.

67. Motherby H, Kube M, Friedrichs N, et al. Immunocytochemistry and DNA-image cytometry in diagnostic effusion cytology I. Prevalence of markers in tumour cell positive and negative smears. Anal Cell Pathol 1999;19:7–20.

68. Celermajer DS, Boyer MJ, Bailey BP, et al. Pericardiocentesis for symptomatic malignant pericardial effusion: a study of 36 patients. Med J Aust 1991;154:19–22.

69. Grau JJ, Estape J, Palombo H, et al. Intracavitary oxytetracycline in malignant pericardial tamponade. Oncology 1992;49:489–91.

70. Maher EA, Shepherd FA, Todd TJ. Pericardial sclerosis as the primary management of malignant pericardial effusion and cardiac tamponade. J Thorac Cardiovasc Surg 1996;112:637–43.

71. Lerner-Tung MB, Chang AY, Ong LS, et al. Pharmacokinetics of intrapericardial administration of 5-fluorouracil. Cancer Chemother Pharmacol 1997;40:318–20.

72. Fiorentino MV, Daniele O, Morandi P, et al. Intrapericardial instillation of platin in malignant pericardial effusion. Cancer 1988;62:1904–6.

73. Tomkowski W, Szturmowicz M, Fijalkowska A, et al. Intrapericardial cisplatin for the management of patients with large malignant pericardial effusion. J Cancer Res Clin Oncol 1994;120:434–6.

74. Tondini M, Rocco G, Bianchi C, et al. Intracavitary cisplatin (CDDP) in the treatment of metastatic pericardial involvement from breast and lung cancer. Monaldi Arch Chest Dis 1995;50:86–8.

75. Kuhn K, Purea H, Selbach J, et al. Treatment with locally applied mitoxantrone. Acta Med Austriaca 1989;16 (3–4):87–90.

76. Musch E, Gremmler B, Nitsch J, et al. Intrapericardial instillation of mitoxantrone in palliative therapy of malignant pericardial effusion. Onkologie 2003;26:135–9.

77. Morere JF, Delanian S, Boaziz C, et al. Intracavitary 5-fluoro-uracil (5-FU) in combination with systemic chemotherapy. Acta Med Austriaca 1989;16(3-4):74–5.

78. Martinoni A, Cipolla CM, Cardinale D, et al. Long-term results of intrapericardial chemotherapeutic treatment of malignant pericardial effusions with thiotepa. Chest 2004;126:1412–6.

79. Wang N, Feikes JR, Mogensen T, et al. Pericardioperitoneal shunt: an alternative treatment for malignant pericardial effusion. Ann Thorac Surg 1994;57:289–92.

80. Ako J, Eto M, Kim S, et al. Pericardial constriction due to malignant lymphoma. Jpn Heart J 2000;41:673–9.

81. Johnston SD, Johnston PW, O'Rourke D. Carcinoid constrictive pericarditis. Heart 1999;82:641–3.

Treatment-Induced Arrhythmia, Pacemakers, and Automatic Implantable Cardioverter Defibrillators

S. Wamique Yusuf, MD, FACC

Arrhythmias in cancer patients may be due to a condition related to the primary malignancy (eg, pericarditis and pericardial effusion) or related to the treatment of the disease. Various chemotherapeutic agents can lead to a wide variety of cardiovascular problems, including ischemia, prolongation of QT interval and arrhythmias[1]. Atrial fibrillation (AF) and supraventricular tachycardia are probably the most common arrhythmias encountered in the cancer population and have been reported with the use of chemotherapeutic agents,[1–4] following lung surgery[5,6] and bone marrow transplant.[7,8]

Atrial Fibrillation

This is the most common sustained arrhythmia in both the general population and the cancer population.[4–8] The prevalence of atrial fibrillation increases with age and is about 0.5% for patients aged 50 to 59 years and 8.8% for those aged 80 to 89 years.[9] It may become a major drain on health care resources as it is estimated that the lifetime risks for development of atrial fibrillation are 1 in 4 for men and women 40 years of age.[10] It is associated with increased mortality and, in subjects from the original cohort of the Framingham Heart Study, atrial fibrillation was associated with a mortality risk 1.5 to 1.9 times higher after adjustment for the preexisting cardiovascular conditions with which atrial fibrillation was related.[11]

Mechanism of Atrial Fibrillation

Two theories for mechanism of atrial fibrillation have been advanced; enhanced automaticity involving one or more foci firing rapidly or reentry involving one or more circuits.[12,13] The most widely accepted is the multiple wavelet reentry theory.[12] This hypothesis envisions multiple reentrant impulses of variable sizes wandering through the atria creating continuous electrical activity that creates daughter wavelets. The number of wavelets present at any time depends on the refractory period, mass, and the conduction velocity in different parts of the atria.

Risk Factors

The clinical risk factors for atrial fibrillation include advancing age, diabetes, hypertension, congestive heart failure, rheumatic and non-rheumatic valve disease, and myocardial infarction.[14] The echocardiographic risk factors for non-rheumatic atrial fibrillation include left atrial enlargement, increased left ventricular wall thickness, and reduced left ventricular fractional shortening.[15]

Causes and Associated Conditions

Atrial fibrillation is usually precipitated by underlying cardiac or noncardiac disease. The resultant atrial abnormality (frequently inflammation or fibrosis) acts as a substrate for the development of the arrhythmia.[16] In addition, the onset of atrial fibrillation usually requires a trigger. Triggers that may initiate the arrhythmia include alterations in autonomic tone[17] and acute or chronic changes in atrial wall tension.[18] Lung surgery is a potent trigger of atrial fibrillation.[6]

Atrial fibrillation is also the most common arrhythmia after hematopoietic stem cell transplantation, affecting about 4% of patients after transplant, with a relapse rate of 49%.[8] In the vast majority of these patients, multiple antiarrhythmics are needed for rate control.[8]

Various chemotherapeutic agents cause heart failure,[1] and a history of heart failure is significantly more common in patients with chronic atrial fibrillation compared to other forms of atrial fibrillation.[19] Patients with chronic atrial fibrillation also have significantly lower left ventricular ejection fraction compared to patients with paroxysmal or recent atrial fibrillation.[19] The increased propensity for atrial arrhythmias in patients with heart failure results from structural heart disease secondary to congenital, valvular, or ischemic etiologies. These patients have underlying substrate that predisposes them to develop electrically irritable foci, functional or fixed conduction block, and consequently, recurrent tachyarrhythmias. For example, atrial enlargement and hypertrophy predisposes to atrial arrhythmias by decreasing conduction velocity and myocardial refractoriness, while low cardiac output increases sympathetic tone, thereby accelerating the frequency and prolonging the duration of such arrhythmias.

Recently inflammation has been linked to atrial fibrillation,[20] with an elevated C-reactive protein (CRP) level in patients with atrial fibrillation. In the same study, cancer was significantly associated with atrial arrhythmias, with 18.3% of patients with atrial arrhythmias having a history of cancer.[21] Cancer was also significantly associated with elevated CRP levels,[21] although multivariate analysis did not identify cancer as an independent predictor of atrial arrhythmias, leading the authors to suggest that inflammation may be the casual intermediary link between cancer and atrial fibrillation. In another study,[22] patients with colorectal cancer were twice as likely to have atrial fibrillation. At our institution, atrial fibrillation is a common postoperative arrhythmia after lung surgery, with an incidence of about 12%,[6] although others have reported a higher rate of postoperative atrial fibrillation affecting about 26% patients after non-cardiac chest surgery.[23] Male sex, history of arrhythmia, peripheral vascular disease, congestive heart failure, type of procedure performed, and the use of intraoperative transfusion are predictors of postoperative atrial fibrillation.[6] Postoperative atrial fibrillation is usually self-limiting, but in most instances, it is associated with increased duration of hospitalization and higher mortality.[6,23]

Atrial fibrillation may be paroxysmal, persistent, or permanent [24,25]:

- Paroxysmal—self-terminating episodes of atrial fibrillation
- Persistent—atrial fibrillation does not terminate spontaneously, but reverts to sinus rhythm with electrical or pharmacological cardioversion
- Permanent—return of sinus rhythm is not feasible

The term "lone atrial fibrillation" describes atrial fibrillation in the absence of demonstrable underlying cardiac disease or a history of hypertension. Although by definition there is an absence of any demonstrable cardiac disease, it has been found that localized atrial myocarditis frequently (up to 66 %) exists in these patients.[26] It has been estimated that lone atrial fibrillation occurs in approximately 30% of patients with atrial fibrillation.[19]

Conditions associated with atrial fibrillation include:

- Ischemic heart disease/myocardial infarction
- Hypertensive heart disease
- Rheumatic heart disease
- Cardiomyopathy (dilated or hypertrophic)
- Thyrotoxicosis
- Alcohol
- Chronic pulmonary disease
- Post cardiac or other surgery
- Idiopathic
- Sick sinus syndrome.
- Congenital heart disease (eg ASD and Ebstein anomaly)
- Pericarditis
- Tumor
- Catheter in the right atrium

Compared to pre-infarct atrial fibrillation or sinus rhythm, atrial fibrillation that develops in the setting of an acute myocardial infarction is associated with an adverse prognosis.[27]

Clinical Manifestations

Clinical symptoms depends upon the ventricular rate, underlying functional status, presence of any coronary artery disease, obstructive valvular disease, or heart failure.

In an individual, the symptoms vary from the patient being asymptomatic to syncope and congestive heart failure. The dysrhythmia may present for the first time with an embolic complication or exacerbation of heart failure, but most patients with atrial fibrillation complain of palpitations, chest pain, dyspnea, fatigue, lightheadedness, or syncope.[19] Atrial fibrillation associated with a fast ventricular response, may lead to tachycardia-mediated cardiomyopathy,[25] and dilated cardiomyopathy may be the initial presentation, especially in patients who are unaware of the tachycardia. Syncope is an uncommon but serious complication that is usually associated with sinus node dysfunction or hemodynamic obstruction, such as valvular aortic stenosis, obstructive cardiomyopathy, or an accessory atrio-ventricular (AV) pathway.

Clinical History and Physical Examination

The initial evaluation of a patient with suspected or proven atrial fibrillation includes characterizing the pattern of the arrhythmia as paroxysmal or persistent, determining its cause, and defining associated cardiac and extracardiac factors.

Precipitating factors should be specifically enquired for; commonly mentioned triggers include alcohol, sleep deprivation, caffeine, exercise, and emotional stress, but vagally mediated AF episodes may occur during sleep or after a large meal and are more likely to arise during a period of rest after a period of stress. Vagally mediated atrial fibrillation is also suggested when a β-blocker or digitalis has increased the tendency towards atrial fibrillation.[28]

The clinician should determine whether the onset and termination of palpitations is abrupt or gradual; the former favors atrial fibrillation or another supraventricular tachyarrhythmia, whereas the latter suggests a mechanism other than atrial fibrillation, including sinus tachycardia. Are there associated symptoms? Dyspnea may indicate underlying heart disease, whereas angina pectoris points toward coronary artery disease (CAD).

The physical examination may suggest atrial fibrillation on the basis of irregular pulse, irregular jugular venous pulsations, and variation in the loudness of the first heart sound. Examination may also disclose associated valvular heart disease like mitral stenosis or heart failure.

The findings on examination are similar in patients with atrial flutter, except that the rhythm may be regular, and rapid venous oscillations may occasionally be visible in the jugular pulse.

Investigations

Hemoglobin, electrolytes, and thyroid function should be checked. Thyrotoxicosis is important to consider if the heart rate remains uncontrolled, despite therapy.

Electrocardiogram

Normally during atrial fibrillation, the underlying atrial rate is greater than 300 per minute,[25] resulting in small (or "fine"), irregular f (fibrillation) waves. The amplitude of these waves varies and may be especially prominent (or "coarse") in lead V1. As only occasional impulses penetrate the atrioventricular node, a totally irregular ventricular rhythm results, which is the characteristic of this arrhythmia.

In most cases, this is a narrow complex tachycardia, but occasionally, a broad complex tachycardia can be seen in atrial fibrillation. Broad complex tachycardia with atrial fibrillation can occur in the following settings:

- Atrial fibrillation with conduction over an accessory pathway
- Atrial fibrillation with underlying bundle-branch block
- Atrial fibrillation with aberrant ventricular conduction

A review of a previous electrocardiogram (ECG) may show pre-excitation or bundle branch block.

A rapid, irregular, wide-QRS-complex tachycardia strongly suggests atrial fibrillation with conduction over an accessory pathway or atrial fibrillation with underlying bundle-branch block. Extremely rapid rates (over 200 beats per minute [bpm]) suggest the presence of an accessory pathway.

Aberrant ventricular conduction results in wide QRS complexes. In these circumstances, it is important to differentiate atrial fibrillation with aberrant ventricular conduction tachycardia from ventricular tachycardia. This can be done by careful analysis of the rhythm strip.

Factors favoring aberrant ventricular conduction includes long–short cycle length sequence, typical right bundle branch block, relatively rapid ventricular rate, lack of compensatory pause, absence of bundle branch block with shorter cycle length without preceding pause, and normalization of QRS complexes with minimal change in cycle length.[25]

Holter and Event Recorder

If episodes are frequent, then a 24-hour Holter monitor can be used. If episodes are infrequent, then an event recorder, which allows the patient to transmit the ECG to a recording facility when the arrhythmia occurs, may be more useful.

Imaging

A chest radiograph may detect enlargement of the cardiac chambers and heart failure.

Two-dimensional transthoracic echocardiography should be acquired to determine chamber dimensions, function, and to exclude occult valvular, pericardial disease, cardiomyopathy, and pulmonary hypertension. Thrombus should be sought in the left atrium but is seldom detected without a transesophageal echocardiogram (TEE), which is the most sensitive and specific technique to detect sources and potential mechanisms for cardiogenic embolism.[29]

Electrophysiologic Study

An electrophysiologic study is rarely needed to establish the diagnosis of atrial fibrillation but may be useful for other reasons. In patients with paroxysmal atrial fibrillation, an electrophysiologic study may help define the mechanism of atrial fibrillation, which is especially important when curative catheter ablation is considered for selected patients.

Treatment

The major issues in management of patients with atrial fibrillation are related to the arrhythmia itself and to prevention of thromboembolism.

In patients with recurrent, persistent, atrial fibrillation, rate control is an acceptable alternative to rhythm control, and two strategies are associated with a similar number of major cardiovascular events.[30]

General Approach to Antiarrhythmic Drug Therapy

Before any antiarrhythmic agent is administered, reversible cardiovascular and non-cardiovascular precipitants of atrial fibrillation should be addressed. Most of these relate to CAD, valvular heart disease, hypertension, pericardial disease, and heart failure. Those who develop atrial fibrillation in association with alcohol intake should practice abstinence. Prophylactic drug treatment is not usually indicated in case of a first-detected episode of atrial fibrillation. Antiarrhythmic drugs may also be avoided in patients with infrequent and well-tolerated paroxysmal atrial fibrillation. In patients who develop atrial fibrillation only during exercise, administration of a β-blocker may be effective. Selection of an appropriate agent is based first on safety and is tailored to any underlying heart disease that may be present, as well as the number and pattern of previous episodes of atrial fibrillation.[31]

Combination Therapy

When treatment with a single agent fails, combinations of antiarrhythmic drugs may be tried, keeping in mind that combination therapy may cause bradycardia and side effects, some of which may be related to the proarrhythmic effects and prolongation of QT interval. Extra care should be taken in older populations who already have an element of degenerative conduction system disease. Drug interaction should be kept in mind; concurrent administration of amiodarone and propafenone with digoxin may result in a rise in serum digoxin level. Careful follow-up is needed,

as a drug that is initially safe may become proarrhythmic when the patient develops CAD or heart failure or starts other medication that, in combination, may be arrhythmogenic. Thus, the patient should be alerted to the potential significance of such symptoms as syncope, angina pectoris, or dyspnea, and warned about the use of noncardiac drugs that can prolong the QT interval.

Plasma, potassium, and magnesium levels, and renal function should be checked periodically during follow-up because renal insufficiency leads to drug accumulation and predisposes to proarrhythmia.

Drugs for Pharmacologic Cardioversion

Drugs that have proven efficacy for pharmacologic conversion include amiodarone, dofetilide, flecainide, ibutilide fumarate, propafenone, and quinidine.[24]

Digoxin and sotalol are not recommended for pharmacologic conversion and, in fact, has been labeled as class 111 (conditions in which there is evidence and/or general agreement that the procedure or treatment is not useful/effective and, in some cases, may be harmful) in recent ACC guidelines.[24]

Drugs used to maintain sinus rhythm in patients with atrial fibrillation include amiodarone, disopyramide, dofetilide, flecainide, propafenone, quinidine, sotalol.[24]

Like other type IC drugs, propafenone should not be used in patients with ischemic heart disease or LV dysfunction.

There is no evidence to support the antiarrhythmic efficacy of calcium channel antagonist drugs in patients with paroxysmal atrial fibrillation, but they reduce heart rate during an attack.[24]

Medications Used in Special Subgroup of Patients

Heart Failure

Patients with congestive heart failure are particularly prone to the ventricular proarrhythmic effects of antiarrhythmic drugs related to underlying myocardial dysfunction and electrolyte disturbances. Randomized trials have demonstrated the safety of amiodarone and dofetilide (given separately) in patients with heart failure[32,33] and these are the recommended drugs for maintenance of sinus rhythm.

Coronary Artery Disease

In stable patients with CAD, β-blockers may be considered first, as in one study in which more than 50% of patients had hypertension, 26% had CAD, and 26% had CHF, and in which use of metoprolol XL was effective in preventing relapse into atrial flutter or fibrillation.[34] Other β-blockers that reduce the duration and episodes of

paroxysmal atrial fibrillation are sotalol and atenolol.[35] In this study, about 32% of patients had ischemic heart disease.[35] Sotalol has substantial β-blocking activity and may therefore be chosen as the initial antiarrhythmic agent in atrial fibrillation patients with ischemic heart disease because it is associated with less long-term toxicity than amiodarone.

Hypertensive Heart Disease

Patients with left ventricular hypertrophy (LVH) may be at increased risk of developing torsades de pointes related to early ventricular afterdepolarization.[31] Thus, a drug that does not prolong the QT interval is preferable as first-line therapy, and in the absence of CAD or marked LVH (LV wall thickness ≥ 1.4 cm), propafenone and flecainide are reasonable choices.[24] Proarrhythmia with one agent does not predict this type of response to another type of drug. For example, patients with LVH who develop torsades de pointes during treatment with a type III agent may tolerate a type IC agent uneventfully.[24] Amiodarone prolongs the QT interval but carries a very low risk of ventricular proarrhythmia; its extracardiac toxicity profile relegates it to second-line therapy in these individuals, but amiodarone becomes first-line therapy when marked LVH is present. When amiodarone and sotalol either fail or are inappropriate, disopyramide, quinidine, or procainamide may be used as alternatives.[24]

Nonpharmacologic Correction of Atrial Fibrillation

In a selected group of patients, surgical ablation (Maze operation) or catheter ablation can be carried out. In one small study, 64% of patients who were in atrial fibrillation at the beginning of the procedure converted into sinus rhythm during ablation.[36]

Although these procedures have produced promising results, they have not yet been widely applied. Potential complications of catheter ablation for atrial fibrillation include systemic embolism, pulmonary vein stenosis, pericardial effusion, cardiac tamponade, and phrenic nerve paralysis.

Drugs for Heart Rate Control during Atrial Fibrillation

The adequacy of rate control during atrial fibrillation may be judged from clinical symptoms and ECG recordings. The rate is generally considered controlled when the ventricular response ranges between 60 and 80 beats per minute at rest and between 90 and 115 beats per minute during moderate exercise.[37,38] Achieving a target ventricular rate of 90 beats per minute in patients with atrial fibrillation at rest would result in control with the least compromise of cardiac output.[37]

The following agents may be administered to achieve control of the ventricular response to atrial fibrillation in an emergency setting.

Digoxin

Although intravenous digoxin may effectively slow the ventricular rate at rest, there is a delay of at least 60 minutes before onset of a therapeutic effect in most patients, and a peak effect does not develop for up to 6 hours. Digoxin is no more effective than placebo in converting atrial fibrillation to sinus rhythm.[39] Intravenous digoxin offers no substantial advantage over placebo for conversion to sinus rhythm and also provides weak rate control.[40] Given the availability of more effective agents, digoxin is no longer first-line therapy for management of acute atrial fibrillation, except in patients with heart failure or left ventricular dysfunction.

Non-dihydropyridine Calcium Antagonists

The most commonly used calcium channel antagonist agents for treatment of atrial fibrillation are verapamil and diltiazem. Intravenously, each drug is effective in emergency settings, but the response is transient, and repeated doses or a continuous intravenous infusion may be required to maintain heart rate control. These agents, particularly verapamil, generally should not be used in patients with heart failure due to systolic dysfunction.

β-Blockers

Intravenous β-blockade with propranolol, atenolol, metoprolol, or esmolol hydrochloride may help to control the rate of ventricular response to AF in specific settings. β-blockers may be particularly useful in states of high adrenergic tone (eg, postoperative atrial fibrillation). In the immediate postoperative period, β-blockers appear to provide a more rapid conversion to sinus rhythm compared to calcium channel blockers [41].

Amiodarone

Amiodarone has both sympatholytic and calcium antagonistic properties, depresses AV conduction, and is effective in controlling the ventricular rate in patients with atrial fibrillation. Intravenous amiodarone is effective and well tolerated in critically ill patients, and amiodarone is considered a suitable alternative agent for heart rate control when conventional measures are ineffective.[42] It not only decreases heart rate but also significantly improves blood pressure and lowers pulmonary artery wedge pressure in this group of patients.[42] Unlike oral amiodarone, short-term dosing with intravenous amiodarone is not associated with any significant prolongation of action potential duration (QT interval) or use dependent sodium channel blockade,[43] and hence

may be particular useful in the intensive care patients in cancer population, a lot of whom are on antifungals and other medications that prolong QT interval.

In the acute setting, in the absence of conduction over an accessory pathway, the current recommendation[24] is to administer intravenous β-blockers or calcium channel antagonists (verapamil, diltiazem) to slow the ventricular response to atrial fibrillation, exercising caution in patients with hypotension or heart failure. Immediate electrical cardioversion should be performed in patients with acute paroxysmal atrial fibrillation and a rapid ventricular response associated with acute myocardial infarction, symptomatic hypotension, angina, or cardiac failure that does not respond promptly to pharmacological measures.[24]

In patients with accessory pathway (Wolff-Parkinson-White [WPW] syndrome) and symptomatic atrial fibrillation, catheter ablation of the accessory pathway is the treatment of choice.[24]

In hemodynamically stable patients with atrial fibrillation and accessory pathway (WPW syndrome), intravenous quinidine, procainamide, disopyramide, ibutilide fumarate, or amiodarone can be used.[24] In such patients, it is critically important to avoid agents with the potential to increase the refractoriness of the AV node, which could encourage preferential conduction over the accessory pathway. Hence, administration of AV nodal blocking agents such as digoxin, diltiazem, or verapamil is contraindicated in patients with atrial fibrillation in association with WPW syndrome.[24]

Control of heart rate is important not only for prevention of tachycardia-induced cardiomyopathy, but it may also lead to improvement in left ventricular (LV) systolic function and ejection fraction.[25]

Anti-Coagulation in Atrial Fibrillation

In patients with persistent (also known as sustained, and including patients categorized as permanent in certain classification schemes) or paroxysmal (intermittent) atrial fibrillation at high risk of stroke (ie, having any of the following features: prior ischemic stroke, Transient Ischemic Attack (TIA) or systemic embolization, age >75 years, moderately or severely impaired left ventricular systolic function and/or congestive heart failure, history of hypertension or diabetes mellitus) the recommendation is for oral anticoagulation with warfarin (target International Normalized Ratio (INR) 2.5; range 2.0 to 3.0).[44]

In patients with persistent or paroxysmal atrial fibrillation at age 65 to 75 years, in the absence of other risk factors, anti-thrombotic therapy with either warfarin (target INR 2.5; range 2.0 to 3.0) or aspirin 325 mg daily are acceptable alternatives in this group of patients

who are at intermediate risk of stroke.[44] In patients with persistent or paroxysmal atrial fibrillation, who are < 65 years of age and with no additional risk factors, aspirin 325 mg daily is recommended.[44]

Atrial Flutter

Atrial flutter is due to a re-entry circuit in the atrium.[45] This produces atrial contractions at a rate of about 300 beats/min seen on the ECG as flutter (F) waves. These are broad and appear saw-toothed and are best seen in the inferior leads and in lead V1 without an isoelectric baseline between deflections. Atrial flutter may degenerate into atrial fibrillation, or vice versa, which may be reflected on the ECG. The ventricular rate depends on conduction through the atrioventricular node. Typically 2:1 block (atrial rate to ventricular rate) occurs, giving a ventricular rate of 150 beats/min. Identification of a regular tachycardia with this rate should prompt the diagnosis of atrial flutter. The non-conducting flutter waves are often mistaken for, or merged with, T waves and become apparent only if the block is increased. Maneuvers that induce transient atrioventricular block (such as carotid sinus massage or use of adenosine) will slow the conduction and help in identification of flutter waves.

Not all atrial contractions are propagated through to the ventricles due to a variable block within the junctional area (this is due to the refractory nature of the conduction pathway at the higher rate). When conduction through the ventricles does occur, the morphology is normal but the RR interval is irregular.

Cause

The causes of atrial flutter are similar to those of atrial fibrillation, although idiopathic atrial flutter is uncommon. It may convert into atrial fibrillation over time or, after administration of drugs such as digoxin.

The findings on examination are similar to those in patients with atrial fibrillation, except that the rhythm may be regular, and rapid venous oscillations may occasionally be visible in the jugular pulse.

Treatment

The treatment of atrial flutter is almost similar to atrial fibrillation, as these two conditions are frequently present together in the same patient. When rapid control of ventricular response rate to atrial flutter is desired, intravenous administration of a calcium channel blocker (eg, verapamil or diltiazem) or of a β-blocker is usually effective.[45] Sometimes, combination therapy using a calcium channel blocker and a β-blocker is needed for rate control. For ventricular rate control during atrial flutter, drugs should be prescribed that prolong the refractory period of the AV node, such as β-blocking agents, calcium antagonists, digitalis, and amiodarone.[45] With Ibulitide, there is a 60% likelihood of converting atrial flutter to sinus rhythm,[46] and hence, this provides a valuable tool for treatment of atrial flutter.

For prevention of recurrence, class I drugs (flecainide, procainamide, quinidine), β-blockers, class III drugs, and amiodarone can be used.[45] When deciding on pharmacologic therapy, side effects and the possible dangers of drug administration (including arrhythmias and torsades de pointes) should be considered.[47]

Nonpharmacologic Therapy

Electrical Cardioversion and Overdrive Pacing

External electrical cardioversion is safe and effective, terminating atrial flutter in > 90% of episodes.[45] Because external electrical cardioversion requires sedation and anesthesia, some doctors and patients prefer atrial overdrive pacing to terminate atrial flutter. This also has the advantage of being able to pace in the case of sick sinus syndrome after termination of atrial flutter. Implantable devices have become available, allowing both anti-tachycardia and burst pacing, as well as (when needed) internal cardioversion of atrial flutter.

Catheter Ablation   Nowadays, catheter ablation of atrial flutter has become a safe, curative, and highly successful procedure.[45] In a selected group of patients with atrial flutter, the patients treated with catheter ablation reported a significant improvement in their quality of life and symptoms scores.[48] The indications for long-term anticoagulation and anti-thrombotic therapy is the same as for atrial fibrillation.[44]

Anticoagulation for Elective Cardioversion of Atrial Fibrillation or Atrial Flutter   Patients For patients with atrial fibrillation of >48 h or of unknown duration for whom pharmacologic or electrical cardioversion is planned, anticoagulation with warfarin (target INR, 2.5; range 2.0 to 3.0) is recommended for 3 weeks before elective cardioversion and for at least 4 weeks after successful cardioversion.[44]

For patients with atrial fibrillation of >48 h or of unknown duration undergoing pharmacologic or electrical cardioversion, an alternative to the strategy outlined above is anticoagulation (immediate unfractionated intravenous (IV) heparin with target PTT of 60 seconds [range, 50 to 70 seconds], or at least 5 days of warfarin with a target INR of 2.5 [range, 2.0 to 3.0] at the time of cardioversion), and a screening multiplane TEE should be performed. If no thrombus is seen and cardioversion is successful, then anticoagulation (target INR, 2.5; range 2.0 to 3.0) is recommended for at least 4 weeks. If a thrombus

is seen on TEE, then cardioversion should be postponed and anticoagulation should be continued indefinitely. A TEE should be repeated before attempting later cardioversion.[44]

For patients with atrial fibrillation of known duration <48 h, cardioversion can be performed without anticoagulation.[44] However, in patients without contraindications to anticoagulation, anticoagulation with IV heparin (target Activated Partial Thromboriatin Time (APTT), 60 seconds; range 50 to 70 seconds) or Low Mokeular Weight Heparin (LMWH) (at full Deep Veiw Thrombosis (DVT) treatment doses) should be started at presentation.[44]

For patients with risk factors for stroke, it is particularly important to be confident that the duration of AF is <48 h. In such patients with risk factors, a TEE-guided approach is a reasonable alternative strategy. According to ACC/AHA guidelines,[24] cardioversion without TEE guidance during the first 48 hours after the onset of atrial fibrillation is a class 11 b indication.

For emergency cardioversion where a TEE-guided approach is not possible, IV unfractionated heparin (target PTT, 60 seconds; range 50 to 70 seconds) be started as soon as possible, followed by 4 weeks of anticoagulation with warfarin (target INR, 2.5; range 2.0 to 3.0).[44] Following cardioversion, the continuation of anticoagulation beyond 4 weeks is based on whether the patient has experienced more than one episode of atrial fibrillation and on risk factor status. Patients experiencing more than one episode of atrial fibrillation should be considered as having paroxysmal atrial fibrillation.[44]

Anticoagulation increases the frequency and severity of major extracranial and intracranial hemorrhage and the issue of anticoagulation in the cancer population is complex, for most patients in clinical trials are carefully selected, and exclude those with a high risk of bleeding. Presence of thrombocytopenia prevents the use of warfarin in a number of patients with cancer and atrial fibrillation. There are no guidelines in existence regarding how to best manage these patients. Clinical judgment is needed and a decision about initiating anticoagulation, or even aspirin, should be made on an individual basis.

Broad Complex Tacycardia

Broad complex tachycardias occur by various mechanisms and may be ventricular or supraventricular in origin.

Varieties of broad complex tachycardia include ventricular (regular, monomorphic ventricular tachycardia, irregular, torsades de pointes tachycardia, and polymorphic ventricular tachycardia), and supraventricular (bundle branch block with aberrant conduction, and atrial tachycardia with pre-excitation).

Ventricular Tachycardia

Ventricular tachycardia (VT) is defined as three or more ventricular extrasystoles in succession at a rate of more than 100 beats/min. The tachycardia may be self-terminating but is described as "sustained" if it lasts longer than 30 seconds or results in hemodynamic collapse. Ventricular tachycardia is described as "monomorphic" when the QRS complexes have the same general appearance, and "polymorphic" if there is wide beat-to-beat variation in QRS morphology. Monomorphic ventricular tachycardia is the most common form of sustained ventricular tachycardia

Mechanism of Ventricular Tachycardia

The mechanisms responsible for ventricular tachycardia include reentry or increased myocardial automaticity. Ventricular tachycardia in a patient with chronic ischemic heart disease and in post-myocardial infarction patients is caused by reentrant mechanism.[49] The reentry circuits that support ventricular tachycardia can be micro or macro in scale and often occur in the zone of ischemia or fibrosis surrounding damaged myocardium.

Triggered automaticity of a group of cells can result from congenital or acquired heart disease. Once initiated, these tachycardias tend to accelerate, but slow markedly before stopping. The mechanism of ventricular tachycardia in dilated cardiomyopathy is less well understood, but even in patients with nonischemic cardiomyopathy, reentry appears to play a role in the initiation of sustained monomorphic VT.[50]

Ventricular tachycardia may result from direct damage to the myocardium secondary to ischemia or cardiomyopathy, or from the effects of myocarditis or drugs—for example, class 1 antiarrhythmics (such as flecainide, quinidine, and disopyramide).

Broad Complex Tachycardia of Supraventricular Origin

In the presence of aberrant conduction or ventricular pre-excitation, any supraventricular tachycardia may present as a broad complex tachycardia and mimic ventricular tachycardia.

Atrial Tachycardia with Aberrant Conduction

Aberrant conduction is defined as conduction through the atrioventricular node with delay or block, resulting in a broader QRS complex. Aberrant conduction usually manifests as left or right bundle branch block, both of which have characteristic features. The bundle branch block may predate the tachycardia, or it may be a rate-related functional block, occurring when atrial impulses arrive too rapidly for a bundle branch to conduct normally. When atrial fibrillation occurs with aberrant conduction and a rapid ventricular response, a totally irregular broad complex tachycardia is produced.

Wolff-Parkinson-White Syndrome

Broad complex tachycardias may also occur in the Wolff-Parkinson-White syndrome, either as an antidromic atrioventricular reentrant tachycardia or in association with atrial flutter or fibrillation.

Antidromic Atrioventricular Reentrant Tachycardia

In this relatively uncommon tachycardia, the impulse is conducted from the atria to the ventricles via the accessory pathway. The resulting tachycardia has broad, bizarre QRS complexes.

Atrial Fibrillation

In patients without an accessory pathway, the atrioventricular node protects the ventricles from the rapid atrial activity that occurs during atrial fibrillation. In the Wolff-Parkinson-White syndrome, the atrial impulses are conducted down the accessory pathway, which may allow rapid conduction, and consequently, very fast ventricular rates.

Drugs that block the atrioventricular node—such as digoxin, verapamil, and adenosine—should be avoided as they can produce an extremely rapid ventricular response.

The impulses conducted via the accessory pathway produce broad QRS complexes. Occasionally, an impulse will be conducted via the atrioventricular node and produce a normal QRS complex or a fusion beat. The result is a completely irregular, and often rapid, broad complex tachycardia with a fairly constant QRS pattern, except for occasional normal complexes and fusion beats.

Differentiating Between Ventricular and Supraventricular Origin

Clinical Features

The presentation and symptoms related to broad complex tachycardia are similar to other tachycardia and are largely dependent upon heart rate, underlying cardiac function, and hemodynamic consequences of the arrhythmia. Symptoms relate to the heart rate and the underlying cardiac reserve rather than to the origin of the arrhythmia. Rapid tachycardia in the presence of heart disease can lead to syncope and sudden death, whereas those with slower heart rate and normal heart may remain asymptomatic.

It is wrong to assume that a patient with ventricular tachycardia will inevitably be in a state of collapse; some patients look well but present with dizziness, palpitations, syncope, chest pain, or heart failure. In contrast, a supraventricular tachycardia may cause collapse in a patient with underlying poor ventricular function.

A history of coronary artery disease, congestive heart failure, or age >35 years are 90% specific for ventricular tachycardia, but their absence does not establish the diagnosis of supraventricular tachycardia.[51]

Physical Examination

Physical examination of a patient with ventricular tachycardia may reveal the clinical evidence of atrioventricular dissociation—that is, "cannon" waves in the jugular venous pulse or variable intensity of the first heart sound. However, these signs will be absent if there is 1:1 retrograde conduction, and absence of these findings does not exclude the diagnosis.

ECG

Electrocardiographic diagnosis of monomorphic ventricular tachycardia is based on the following features:[52,53]

Duration and Morphology of QRS Complex

In ventricular tachycardia, the sequence of cardiac activation is altered, and the impulse no longer follows the normal intraventricular conduction pathway. As a consequence, the morphology of the QRS complex is bizarre, and the duration of the complex is prolonged (usually to 0.12 seconds or longer). The exception is fascicular ventricular tachycardia, which can have relatively narrow QRS complexes.[52]

As a general rule, the broader the QRS complex, the more likely the rhythm is to be ventricular in origin, especially if the complexes are greater than 0.16 seconds. Duration of the QRS complex may exceed 0.2 seconds, particularly if the patient has electrolyte abnormalities or severe myocardial disease or is taking antiarrhythmic drugs, such as flecainide.

The QRS complex in ventricular tachycardia often has right or left bundle branch morphology. In general, a tachycardia originating in the left ventricle produces a right bundle branch block pattern, whereas a tachycardia originating in the right ventricle results in a left bundle branch block pattern. The intraventricular septum is the focus of the arrhythmia in some patients with ischemic heart disease, and the resulting complexes have left bundle branch block morphology.

Rate and Rhythm

In ventricular tachycardia, the rate is normally 120 to 300 bpm. The rhythm is regular or almost regular (<0.04 seconds beat-to-beat variation), unless disturbed by the presence of capture or fusion beats. If a monomorphic broad complex tachycardia has an obviously irregular rhythm, the most likely diagnosis is atrial fibrillation with either aberrant conduction or pre-excitation.

Frontal Plane Axis

In a normal electrocardiogram, the QRS axis in the mean frontal plane is between $-30°$ and $+90°$, with the axis most commonly lying at around 60°. With the onset of ventricular tachycardia, the mean frontal plane axis changes from that seen in sinus rhythm and is often bizarre. A change in axis of more than 40° to the left or right is suggestive of ventricular tachycardia.

Direct Evidence of Independent Atrial Activity

In ventricular tachycardia, the sinus node continues to initiate atrial contraction. Since this atrial contraction is completely independent of ventricular activity, the resulting P waves are dissociated from the QRS complexes and are positive in leads I and II. The atrial rate is usually slower than the ventricular rate, though occasionally 1:1 conduction occurs. It is important to scrutinize the tracings from all 12 leads of the electrocardiogram, as P waves may be evident in some leads but not in others.

Although evidence of atrioventricular dissociation is diagnostic for ventricular tachycardia, a lack of direct evidence of independent P wave activity does not exclude the diagnosis. Artifacts that simulate P wave activity may complicate the situation.

However, beat to beat differences, especially of the ST segment, suggest the possibility of independent P wave activity, even though it may be impossible to pinpoint the independent P wave accurately.

Indirect Evidence of Independent Atrial Activity

Capture Beat
Occasionally an atrial impulse may cause ventricular depolarization via the normal conduction system. The resulting QRS complex occurs earlier than expected and is narrow. Such a beat shows that, even at rapid rates, the conduction system is able to conduct normally, thus making a diagnosis of supraventricular tachycardia with aberrancy unlikely.

Capture beats are uncommon, and although they confirm a diagnosis of ventricular tachycardia, their absence does not exclude the diagnosis.

Fusion Beats
A fusion beat occurs when a sinus beat conducts to the ventricles via the atrioventricular node and fuses with a beat arising in the ventricles. As the ventricles are depolarized, partly by the impulse conducted through the His-Purkinje system and partly by the impulse arising in the ventricle, the resulting QRS complex has an appearance intermediate between a normal beat and a tachycardia beat.

Like capture beats, fusion beats are uncommon, and although they support a diagnosis of ventricular tachycardia, their absence does not exclude the diagnosis.

QRS Concordance throughout the Chest Leads

Concordance exists when all the QRS complexes in the chest leads are either predominantly positive or predominantly negative. Concordance can be either positive or negative. The presence of concordance suggests that the tachycardia has a ventricular origin.

A previous electrocardiogram may give valuable information. Evidence of a myocardial infarction increases the likelihood of ventricular tachycardia, and a change in mean frontal plane axis during the tachycardia (especially if the change is >40° to the left or right), points to a ventricular origin. Ventricular tachycardia and supraventricular tachycardia with bundle branch block may produce similar electrocardiograms. If a previous electrocardiogram shows a bundle branch block pattern during sinus rhythm that is similar to or identical with that during the tachycardia, the origin of the tachycardia is likely to be supraventricular. But if the QRS morphology or axis changes during the tachycardia, then a ventricular origin is suspected.

Maneuvers to Elicit the Underlying Rhythm

Vagal stimulation—for example, carotid sinus massage or Valsalva's maneuver—does not usually affect a ventricular tachycardia but may affect arrhythmias of supraventricular origin. Transiently slowing or blocking conduction through the atrioventricular node may terminate an atrioventricular nodal reentrant tachycardia or atrioventricular reentrant tachycardia. In atrial flutter transient block may reveal the underlying flutter waves

Adenosine can also be used to block conduction temporarily through the atrioventricular node to ascertain the origin of a broad complex tachycardia, but failure to stop the tachycardia does not necessarily indicate a ventricular origin. In one study of adenosine in broad complex tachycardia, adenosine terminated the arrhythmia or induced diagnostic atrioventricular block in 8 of 9 patients with broad complex Supraventricular tachycardia and all nine patients with narrow complex Supraventricular tachycardia.[54] However, adenosine terminated VT in only 1 of 17 patients.[54]

Danger of Misdiagnosis

The safest option is to regard a broad complex tachycardia of uncertain origin as ventricular tachycardia unless good evidence suggests a supraventricular origin.

If a ventricular tachycardia is wrongly treated as supraventricular tachycardia, the consequences may be extremely serious. Misdiagnosis of broad complex tachycardia and use of verapamil in patients who actually have VT, results in worsening of clinical condition in most of these patients, with poor outcome.[55]

Treatment of Ventricular Tachycardia

In any patient with ventricular tachycardia it is important to exclude coronary ischemia and structural heart disease, including dilated cardiomyopathy, hypertrophic cardiomyopathy, and arrhythmogenic right ventricular dysplasia. Therapy for patients who present with ventricular tachycardia should be determined by the hemodynamic status, symptoms, and history. In unstable patients, electrical cardioversion should be carried out promptly.[56] Treatment of hemodynamically stable ventricular tachycardia depends on whether the VT is monomorphic or polymorphic and whether left ventricular systolic function is normal or impaired. Treatment of polymorphic VT depends on whether QT intervals are normal or prolonged (as in torsades de pointes, when QT is prolonged during sinus rhythm). When polymorphic VT develops in patients who have prolonged QT during sinus rhythm, treatment with magnesium is recommended.[56] Polymorphic VT in the absence of prolong QT is treated the same as monomorphic VT. For stable monomorphic VT in patients with normal LV function, intravenous procainamide, lidocaine, or amiodarone can be used.[56] In patients with stable monomorphic VT and impaired LV function, use of amiodarone or lidocaine is preferred.[56] Ideally, clinicians should attempt to identify whether a broad complex tachycardia is supraventricular or ventricular and treat accordingly. However this is not always possible diagnostically, hence the wise thing is to assume that wide complex tachycardia is VT until proven otherwise. From a statistical point of view, such an assumption sounds like safe practice, since about 90% of wide complex tachycardia are VT.[56] Also, use of medications like verapamil can have disastrous consequences in such cases.[55] Unstable wide complex tachycardia should be treated with immediate cardioversion. For stable wide complex tachycardia of uncertain origin, amiodarone and procainamide are good choices since they are effective for treating both supraventricular tachycardia and ventricular tachycardia.[56] As a general rule, it is better to use just one antiarrhythmic agent in a given patient to avoid proarrhythmic effects. If one agent has not converted a tachycardia after an appropriate dose, then the next step should usually be DC cardioversion.[56] The long-term therapy for patients with sudden cardiac death is largely determined by the

presence of concomitant disease, each of which has specific risk stratification and treatment.[57] Ventricular tachycardia can degenerate into ventricular fibrillation, which should be treated with an unsynchronized electric shock using an initial energy of 200 joules (J). If this is unsuccessful, a second shock using 200 to 300 J and, if necessary, a third shock using 360 J is indicated.[56]

Ventricular fibrillation that is not easily converted by defibrillation may be treated with additional adjunctive measures. Epinephrine (1 mg intravenously) should be given and repeated every 3 to 5 minutes, or Vasopressin (40 units intravenously) as a single dose should be given.[56] For persistent and recurrent VF and ventricular tachycardia (VT), amiodarone in a dose of 300 mg intravenously can be given.[56]

Pacemakers

Pacemakers are increasingly being used in the United States. At our institution, we implanted 22 permanent pacemakers in the 19 months prior to this writing. Cancer patients, particularly in the elderly population who have underlying degenerative conduction system disease, are prone to the side effects of chemotherapeutic agents, a wide variety of which can cause bradycardia and heart block.[1] The treatment of asymptomatic and symptomatic bradycardia in cancer patients is generally the same as in other populations. Where a clear offending agent is considered to be the cause, the approach is to discontinue the medication and observe. In most cases, the bradycardia and heart block resolves over time. In patients who have persistent sinus symptomatic bradycardia and heart block, the indications for pacemakers are the same as those for the general population.[58] In some cancer populations, a particular group of patients (ie, those with ongoing infection) poses a dilemma: any permanent pacemaker implantation in the face of infection creates a potential for infection of the pacemaker pocket site. In these cases, a temporary pacemaker is left in place for few days until the infection is controlled. Although the indication for a pacemaker involves clinical judgment, in the cancer population, this is an overwhelming necessity, as the main objective in some cases is only comfort care.

Pacing Modes

The generic pacemaker code of the North American Society of Pacing and Electrophysiology and the British Pacing and Electrophysiology Group is used to describe various pacing modes. The first letter denotes the chamber or chambers that are paced (A = atrial, V = ventricular, D = dual [atrial and ventricular]). The second letter describes which chambers detect (sense) electrical signals. The third letter represents the response to sensed events (I=inhibition, T=triggering, D=dual [inhibition and triggering]). A fourth letter, R, denotes activation of rate-response features. The most commonly used pacing modes are: AAI(R) single-chamber atrial pacing without (or with) rate response, VVI(R) single-chamber ventricular pacing without (or with) rate response, and DDD(R) dual-chamber pacing without (or with) rate response. In the latest version of the code, a fifth position denotes the chamber or chambers in which multisite pacing is delivered.[59]

Indications

The decision to implant a permanent pacemaker should involve the cardiologist, the primary physician, the patient and the family. Before embarking on a pacemaker insertion, the need for pacing should be clearly documented. To evaluate patients more uniformly, the Joint American College of Cardiology–American Heart Association Task Force established a classification system for the indications for pacemaker implantation.[58] Class I includes all conditions for which it is generally agreed that a permanent pacemaker should be implanted; class II, all conditions for which such pacemakers are frequently used but for which there is disagreement about the need for their use; and class III, all conditions for which it is generally agreed that permanent pacing is not required.

Atrioventricular Block

Atrioventricular heart block can be classified as first-degree, second-degree, or third-degree (ie, complete) heart block. Generally, first-degree atrioventricular block is not considered an indication for pacing, but in some patients with severe first-degree block and who are symptomatic, a pacemaker may be helpful.

Second-degree atrioventricular block is divided into type I (in which there is progressive prolongation of the PR interval before a blocked beat), type II (in which there is no such progressive prolongation), or advanced (in which two or more consecutive P waves are blocked). Second-degree type I atrioventricular block usually occurs in the atrioventricular node, whereas type II and the advanced type usually occur in tissues below the node.[58] When every other beat is conducted (in what is known as 2:1 block), the distinction between types I and II often cannot be made with certainty, and the site of the block may be either at or below the atrioventricular node.[58] Type I second-degree AV block is usually due to delay in the AV node, irrespective of QRS width, and progression to advanced AV block in this situation is uncommon, hence pacing is usually not indicated unless the patient is symptomatic.[58]

Type II second-degree AV block and a wide QRS indicate diffuse conduction system disease and constitute an indication for pacing even in the absence of symptoms[58] as progression to third-degree AV block is common in this condition. However, it is not always possible to determine the site of AV block without electrophysiologic evaluation; hence, if type I second-degree AV block with a narrow or wide QRS is found to be intra- or infra-His upon electrophysiologic study, pacing should be considered.[58] Any form of second-degree atrioventricular block, regardless of the site or type of block that is associated with symptomatic bradycardia, is a class I indication for pacing.[58]

Asymptomatic second-degree type II and advanced atrioventricular blocks are class II indications for pacing.[58] An asymptomatic patient with a second-degree type I atrioventricular block should not receive a permanent pacemaker. Asymptomatic patients who have second-degree atrioventricular block with 2:1 conduction and evidence of infranodal block (based on the results of electrophysiologic study or the presence of a bundle-branch block) are considered to have a class II indication for pacing.[58]

In third-degree atrioventricular block or advanced second degree AV block, class I indication for pacing is present if (1) bradycardia with symptoms are present, (2) arrhythmias or other medical conditions that require drugs result in symptomatic bradycardia, (3) if pauses in the QRS rhythm exceed three seconds in length, or if there are escape rates <40 beats per minute in awake, symptom-free patients.[58]

In general, the decision regarding implantation of a pacemaker must be considered with respect to whether or not AV block will be permanent. In conditions such as electrolyte abnormalities, medications, and conditions causing excessive vagal tone (where a clear precipitating factor is present), correction usually resolves the block. Similarly peri- and postoperative AV block, in which inflammation near the AV conduction system after surgery in this region plays a part, usually resolves over time. In systemic conditions like neuromuscular diseases, sarcoidosis, and amyloidosis, a pacemaker should be considered even if significant heart block is transient, since this may recur.

In patients with chronic bifascicular or trifascicular block, the presence of intermittent third-degree AV block, type II second degree AV block, and alternating bundle branch block is a class I indication for permanent pacing.[58]

In patients with sinus node dysfunction, symptomatic bradycardia (including frequent sinus pauses) that produces symptoms or symptomatic chronotropic incompetence is a class I indication for permanent pacing.[58]

In patients with tachyarrhythmias, like supraventricular tachycardia, in cases in which ablation and/or drugs fail to control arrhythmias, an anti-tachycardia pacing is considered.[58] Other conditions in which prevention of arrhythmias by pacing is a reasonable choice is the Long QT syndrome (LQTS), in which pacing may be especially beneficial for patients with pause-dependent arrhythmias, and use of a pause prevention pacing algorithm for arrhythmia prevention in a young patient with congenital LQTS and documented pause-dependent torsades de pointes has been reported.[60]

Syncope

Syncope in the absence of a clear cardiac cause like marked bradycardia or significant pause with carotid sinus hypersensitivity is, in general, not an indication for a pacemaker. Recurrent syncope caused by carotid-sinus hypersensitivity associated with pauses of more than three seconds in symptomatic patients is a class I indication for pacing.[58] For symptomatic and recurrent neurocardiogenic syncope associated with bradycardia documented spontaneously (or at the time of tilt table test) is a class II indication for pacing.[58] The two conditions where a pacemaker may be may be useful in cardiomyopathy are in patients with hypertrophic or dilated cardiomyopathy. In patients with moderate-to-severe heart failure, cardiac resynchronization therapy (CRT) produced significant improvement in Left Ventricle size and function, improved New York Heart Association functional class, exercise capacity, and quality of life.[61] In patients with hypertrophic obstructive cardiomyopathy (HOCM), those with significant LV outflow tract gradient may obtain symptomatic benefit from pacing,[58] although this may not result in improved survival.[58]

Complications of Pacemakers

Complications related to venous access include hemothorax, air embolism, and pneumothorax. Lead-related complications include perforation, dislodgment, diaphragmatic stimulation, and malposition. Perforation can involve the great vessels, right atrium, or right ventricle. Cardiac tamponade, usually as a result of chamber perforation, is the most ominous implant complication and should be suspected whenever hypotension occurs. Any suspicion of tamponade can be confirmed by hemodynamics or an emergent echocardiogram and definitive treatment via emergent pericardiocentesis should not be delayed. Electrocorticogram during pacing normally should show a Left Bundle Branch Block pattern and any Right Bundle Branch Block pattern raises the questions of pacing lead being in the left ventricle, which is possible in cases of an atrial or ventricular septal defect. However, this configuration (RBBB pattern) is sometimes seen with properly placed right ventricular leads. In clinical practice, a chest radiograph and echocardiogram would usually resolve the issue, although following an algorithm to distinguish right versus left ventricular lead positions when pacing produces a right bundle-branch block configuration by simple ECG is also possible.[62] Pocket-related complications include hematoma, wound pain, pocket erosion, and infection. In cancer patients, some of whom are severely immunosuppressed, every precaution should be taken to avoid pacemaker infection, because when any infection is strongly suspected, the entire system should be regarded as contaminated and the treatment of choice is complete system removal (pulse generator explant plus transvenous lead extraction), and antimicrobial therapy.[63]

Delayed complications of permanent pacing include venous thrombosis, exit block, insulation failure, and conductor fracture. Exit block manifests as increased pacing thresholds. Insulation failure results in decreased lead impedance. Conduction fracture manifests as increased lead impedance. Definitive treatment for these complications is lead replacement.

Implantable Cardioverter Defibrillators

The modern implantable cardioverter defibrillator (ICD) is a transvenous system. The device is implanted either subcutaneously, as for a pacemaker, in the left or right deltopectoral area, or subpectorally in thin patients to prevent the device eroding the skin. The ventricular lead tip is positioned in the right ventricular apex, and a second lead can be positioned in the right atrial appendage to allow dual chamber pacing if required and discrimination between atrial and ventricular tachycardias. The ventricular defibrillator lead has either one or two shocking coils. Most new defibrillators have the ability to record intracardiac electrograms. This allows monitoring of each episode of anti-tachycardia pacing or defibrillation. If treatment has been inappropriate, then programming changes can be made with a programming unit placed over the defibrillator site. Current devices use anti-tachycardia pacing. Should anti-tachycardia pacing fail, then energy shocks are given to terminate the ventricular tachycardia.

Complications

Complications include infection, perforation, displacement, fracture, or insulation breakdown of the leads; over-sensing or under-sensing of the arrhythmia; and inappropriate shocks for sinus tachycardia or supraventricular tachycardia. Psychological problems are common, and counseling plays an important role.

Indications For ICD Implantation

Recommendations for ICD Therapy

The 2002 ACC guidelines[58] indicate that the following are class I indications (ie, conditions for which there is evidence and/or general agreement that a given procedure or treatment is beneficial, useful, and effective) for insertion of ICD:

- Cardiac arrest due to VF or VT not due to a transient or reversible cause
- Spontaneous sustained VT in association with structural heart disease
- Syncope of undetermined origin with clinically relevant, hemodynamically significant sustained VT or VF induced at electrophysiologic study when drug therapy is ineffective, not tolerated, or not preferred
- Non-sustained VT in patients with coronary disease, prior MI, LV dysfunction, and inducible VF or sustained VT at electrophysiologic study that is not suppressible by a class I antiarrhythmic drug
- Spontaneous sustained VT in patients without structural heart disease not amenable to other treatments

Implantation is also appropriate for cardiac conditions with a high risk of sudden death—long QT syndrome, hypertrophic cardiomyopathy, Brugada syndrome, arrhythmogenic right ventricular dysplasia, and after repair of tetralogy of Fallot.[64]

A number of studies of primary and secondary prevention have shown benefit of ICD in patients with cardiomyopathy and depressed left ventricular ejection fraction.[65] In these trials compared with usual care (most commonly amiodarone), ICD significantly reduced mortality.[65] In most of these studies, the EF was < 30%. In the Multicenter Automatic Defibrillator Implantation Trial 2 study,[66] patients with prior myocardial infarction and advanced left ventricular function (LVEF of 30% or less) benefited from prophylactic insertion of automatic implantable cardioverter defibrillators (AICD). In this study, compared with conventional medical therapy, defibrillation therapy was associated with a 31% reduction in the risk of death.[66] This has generated a lot of questions as to which patients with coronary artery disease and depressed LV function should receive a defibrillator and at what time in the course of their disease. Studies have included a heterogeneous group of patients, and, in MADIT 2, almost 88% of patients were enrolled at > 6 months intervals after their myocardial infarction; patients with NYHA class 4 were also excluded.[66] In further analysis of this study,[67] it was shown that ICD provided a substantial reduction in mortality for patients with remote MI, but almost no survival benefit was found in patients with recent MI (< 18 months).[67] In another recent study in which the average time from MI to randomization was 18 days,[68] use of prophylactic ICD implants in high risk patients who recently had an MI and who had low EF (35% or less), prophylactic insertion of ICD did not reduce overall mortality.

In all these studies, the LVEF was taken at one point in time, and in clinical practice, its application post-MI is somewhat difficult for it's known that, by day 90 post-MI, a substantial number of patients who have abnormal baseline ejection fraction and wall motion abnormalities recover their systolic function, with nearly 22% of these patients having complete recovery of function.[69]

Special Considerations for Pacemakers And ICDs in Cancer Patients

Potential life-threatening malfunction of ICDs and pacemakers has been reported in cancer in patients undergoing radiation therapy.[70,71] The three different manufacturers (Medtronic, Guidant, and St Jude Medical) offer widely different guidelines during radiotherapy.[71] Previous recommendations regarding pacemaker and radiation therapy do not include guidelines for ICD.[71] After completion of radiotherapy full interrogation of pacemakers and ICDs should be carried out.[71]

The defibrillator affects the lives of patient and families[72] and, in terminally ill cancer patients, inappropriate triggering of a defibrillator can be an extremely distressing event for all concerned.[73] A deactivation of the ICD may be appropriate in such cases, but a recent review has suggested that clinicians rarely discuss deactivating ICDs, even in those who are perceived to be near death or those who have expressed a desire to limit life prolonging therapy.[74] For a family to see a loved one shocked from an ICD at the end of life can be very distressing.[74] In this survey of 100 patients who died with an ICD in place, the discussion about deactivation occurred in only 27 patients, of which three-quarters of these conversations occurred within the last few days of the patient's life.[74]

REFERENCES

1. Yeh ET, Tong AT, Lenihan DJ, et al. Cardiovascular complications of cancer therapy: diagnosis, pathogenesis, and management. Circulation 2004;109:3122–31.
2. Hashimim LA, Khalyl MF, Salem PA. Supraventricular tachycardia. A probable complication of platinum treatment. Oncology 1984;41:174–5.
3. Jeremic B, Jevremovic S, Djuric L, Mijatovic L. Cardiotoxicity during chemotherapy treatment with 5-fluouracil and cisplatin. J Chemother 1990;2:264–7.
4. Martino S, Ratanatharathorn V, Karanes C, et al. Reversible arrhythmias observed in patients treated with recombinant α₂-interferon. J Cancer Res Clic Oncol 1987;113:376–8.
5. Gibbs HR, Swafford J, Nguyen HD, et al. Postoperative atrial fibrillation in cancer surgery: preoperative risks and clinical outcome. J Surg Oncol 1992;50:224–7.
6. Vaporciyan AA, Correa AM, Rice DC, et al, Risk factors associated with atrial fibrillation after non-cardiac surgery: analysis of 2588 patients. J Thorac Cardiovasc Surg 2004;127:779–86.
7. Murdych T, Weisdorf DJ. Serious cardiac complications during bone marrow transplantation at the University of Minnesota, 1977–1997. Bone Marrow Transplant 2001;28:283–7.

8. Hidalgo JD, Krone R, Rich MW, et al. Supraventricular tachyarrhythmias after hematopoietic stem cell transplantation: incidence, risk factors and outcomes. Bone Marrow Transplant 2004;34:615–9.

9. Wolf PA, Abbot RD, Kennel WB. Atrial fibrillation as independent risk factor for stroke. The Framingham study. Stroke 1991;22:983–8.

10. Lloyd-Jones DM, Wang TJ, Leip EP, et al. Lifetime risk for development of atrial fibrillation. The Framingham Heart Study. *Circulation* 2004;110:1042–6.

11. Benjamin EJ, Wolf PA, D'Agostino RB, et al. Impact of atrial fibrillation on the risk of death. The Framingham study. Circulation 1998;98:946–52.

12. Moe GK, Abildskov JZ. Atrial fibrillation as a self sustaining arrhythmia independent of focal discharge. Am Heart J 1959;58:59–70.

13. Rensma PL, Allessie MA, Lammers WJ. Length of excitation wave and susceptibility to reentrant atrial arrhythmias in normal conscious dogs. Cir Res 1988;62:395–410.

14. Benjamin EJ, Levy D, Vaziri SM, et al. Independent risk factors for atrial fibrillation in a population-based cohort: the Framingham Heart Study. JAMA 1994;271:840–4.

15. Vaziri SM, Larson MG, Benjamin EJ, Levy D. Echocardiographic predictors of nonrheumatic atrial fibrillation: the Framingham Heart Study. Circulation 1994;89:724–30.

16. Falk RH. Etiology and complications of atrial fibrillation: insights from pathology studies. Am J Cardiol 1998; 82(8A):10N–17N.

17. Coumel P. Autonomic influences in atrial tachyarrhythmias. J Cardiovasc Electrophysiol 1996;7:999–1007.

18. Satoh T, Zipes DP. Unequal atrial stretch in dogs increases dispersion of refractoriness conducive to developing atrial fibrillation. J Cardiovasc Electrophysiol 1996;7:833–42.

19. Levy S, Maarek M, Coumel P, Guize L. On behalf of the French Cardiologists. Characterization of different subsets of atrial fibrillation in general practice in France. The ALFA study. Circulation 1999;99:3028–35.

20. Chung MK, Martin DO, Sprecher D, et al. C-reactive protein elevation in patients with atrial arrhythmia's. Inflammation mechanisms and persistence of atrial fibrillation. Circulation 2001;104:2886–91.

21. Chung MK, Martin DO, Sprecher D, et al. Systemic inflammation, atrial fibrillation and cancer. Circulation 2002; 106:e40.

22. Guzzetti S, Costantino G, Sada S, et al. Colorectal cancer and atrial fibrillation: a case control study. Am J Med 2002;112:587–8.

23. Amar D, Roistacher N, Burt M, et al. Clinical and echocardiographic correlates of symptomatic tachyarrhythmias after non-cardiac surgery. Chest 1995;108:374–54.

24. Fuster V, Ryden LE, Asinger RW, et al. ACC/AHA/ESC guidelines for the management of patients with atrial fibrillation: a report of the American College of Cardiology/American Heart Association Task Force on Practice Guidelines and the European Society of Cardiology Committee for Practice Guidelines and Policy Conferences (Committee to Develop Guidelines for the Management of Patients With Atrial Fibrillation). J Am Coll Cardiol 2001;38:1–70.

25. Prystowsky EN, Katz A. Atrial fibrillation. In: Topol E, editor. Textbook of cardiovascular medicine. Philadelphia PA: Lippincott-Raven; 1998. p. 1661–93.

26. Frustaci A, Chimenti C, Bellocci F, et al. Histological substrate of atrial biopsies in patients with lone atrial fibrillation. Circulation 1997;96:1180–4.

27. Rathore SS, Berger AK, Weinfurt KP, et al. Acute myocardial infarction complicated by atrial fibrillation in the elderly: prevalence and outcomes. Circulation 2000;101:969–74.

28. Coumel P. Neural aspects of paroxysmal atrial fibrillation. In: Falk RH, Podrid PJ, editors. Atrial fibrillation: mechanisms and management. New York: Raven Press; 1992. p. 109–25.

29. Pearson AC, Labovitz AJ, Tatineni S, Gomez CR. Superiority of transesophageal echocardiography in detecting cardiac source of embolism in patients with cerebral ischemia of uncertain etiology. J Am Coll Cardiol 1991;17:66–72.

30. Van Gelder IC, Hagens VE, Bosker HA, et al. Rate control versus electrical cardioversion for Persistent Atrial Fibrillation Study Group. N Engl J Med 2002;347: 1834–40.

31. Prystowsky EN. Management of atrial fibrillation: therapeutic options and clinical decisions. Am J Cardiol 2000;85: 3–11.

32. Torp-Pedersen C, Moller M, Bloch-Thomsen PE, et al, for the Danish Investigations of Arrhythmia and Mortality on Dofetilide Study Group. Dofetilide in patients with congestive heart failure and left ventricular dysfunction. N Engl J Med 1999;341:857–65.

33. Singh SN, Fletcher RD, Fisher SG, et al. Amiodarone in patients with congestive heart failure and asymptomatic ventricular arrhythmia: survival trial of antiarrhythmic therapy in congestive heart failure. N Engl J Med 1995;333:77–82.

34. Kuhlkamp V, Schirdewan A, Stangl K, et al. Use of metoprolol CR/XL to maintain sinus rhythm after conversion from persistent atrial fibrillation: a randomized, double-blind, placebo-controlled study. J Am Coll Cardiol 2000; 36:139–46.

35. Steeds RP, Birchall AS, Smith M, Channer KS. An open label, randomised, crossover study comparing sotalol and atenolol in the treatment of symptomatic paroxysmal atrial fibrillation. Heart 1999;82:170–5.

36. Pappone C, Rosanio S, Oreto G, et al. Circumferential radiofrequency ablation of pulmonary vein ostia a new anatomic approach for curing atrial fibrillation. *Circulation* 2000;102:2619–28.

37. Rawles JM. What is meant by a "controlled" ventricular rate in atrial fibrillation? Br Heart J 1990;63:157–61.

38. Resnekov L, McDonald L. Electroversion of lone atrial fibrillation and flutter including haemodynamic studies at rest and on exercise. Br Heart J 1971;33:339–50.

39. Falk RH, Knowlton AA, Bernard SA, et al. Digoxin for converting recent-onset atrial fibrillation to sinus rhythm: a randomized, double-blinded trial. Ann Intern Med 1987;106:503–6.

40. Jordaens L. Conversion of atrial fibrillation to sinus rhythm and rate control by digoxin in comparison to placebo. Eur Heart J 1997;18:643–8.

41. Balser JR, Martinez EA, Winters BD, et al. Beta-adrenergic blockade accelerates conversion of postoperative supraventricular tachyarrhythmias. Anesthesiology 1998;89: 1052–9.

42. Clemo HF, Wood MA, Gilligan DM, Ellenbogen KA. Intravenous amiodarone for acute heart rate control in the critically ill patient with atrial tachyarrhythmias. Am J Cardiol 1998;81:594–8.

43. Naccarelli GV, Jalal S. Intravenous amiodarone. Another option in the acute management of sustained ventricular tachyarrhythmias. Circulation 1995;92:3154–5.

44. Singer DE, Albers GW, Dalen JE, et al. Antithrombotic therapy in atrial fibrillation: the Seventh ACCP Conference on Antithrombotic and Thrombolytic Therapy. Chest 2004;126(3 Suppl):429–56.

45. Wellens HJJ. Contemporary management of atrial flutter. *Circulation* 2002;106:649–52.

46. Ellenbogen KA, Clemo HF, Stambler BS, et al. Efficacy of ibutilide for conversion of atrial fibrillation and flutter. Am J Cardiol 1996;78(Suppl 8A):42–5.

47. Roden RM. Risks and benefits of antiarrhythmic therapy. N Engl J Med 1994;331:785–91.

48. Andrea N, Newby KH, Pisanó E, et al. Prospective randomized comparison of antiarrhythmic therapy versus first-line radiofrequency ablation in patients with atrial flutter. J Am Coll Cardiol 2000;35:1898–904.

49. Richardson AW, Callans DJ, Josephson ME. Electrophysiology of post infarction ventricular tachycardia: a paradigm of stable reentry. J Cardiovasc Electrophysiol 1999;10: 1288–92.

50. Hsia HH, Callans DJ, Marchlinski FE. Characterization of endocardial electrophysiological substrate in patients with nonischemic cardiomyopathy and monomorphic ventricular tachycardia. Circulation 2003;108:704–10.

51. MBaerman JM, Morady F, DiCarlo LA Jr, de Buitleir M. Differentiation of ventricular tachycardia from supraventricular tachycardia with aberration: value of the clinical history. Ann Emerg Med 1987;16:40–3.

52. Griffith MJ, Camm J. Broad complex tachycardia. Hospital Update 1989;531–41.

53. Edhouse J, Morris F. Broad complex tachycardia. Br Med J 2002;324:719–22.

54. Griffith MJ, Ward DE, Linker NJ, Camm AJ. Adenosine in the diagnosis of broad complex tachycardia. Lancet 1988;1(8587):672–5.

55. Stewart RB, Bardy GH, Greene HL. Wide complex tachycardia: misdiagnosis and outcome after emergent therapy. Ann Intern Med 1986;104:766–71.

56. ACLS Provider Manual. American Heart Association 2001. Dallas, Texas Editor Cummins Ro.

57. Priori SG, Aliot E, Blomstrom-Lundqvist C, et al. Task force on sudden cardiac death of the European Society of Cardiology. Eur Heart J 2001;22:1374–450.

58. Gregoratos G, Abrams J, Epstein AE, et al. ACC/AHA/NASPE 2002 guideline update for implantation of cardiac pacemakers and antiarrhythmia devices: a report of the American College of Cardiology/American Heart Association Task Force on Practice Guidelines (ACC/AHA/NASPE Committee on Pacemaker Implantation 2002. J Am Coll Cardiol 2002;40 1703–14.

59. AD Bernstein, JC Daubert, RD Fletcher et al. The revised NASPE/BPEG generic code for antibradycardia, adaptive-rate, and multisite pacing. North American Society of Pacing and Electrophysiology/British Pacing and Electrophysiology Group. Pacing Clin Electrophysiol 2002;25:260–4.

60. Viskin S, Fish R, Roth A, Copperman Y. Prevention of torsades de pointes in the congenital long QT syndrome: use of a pause prevention pacing algorithm. Heart 1998; 79:417–9.

61. St John Sutton MG, Plappert T, Abraham WT, et al. Effect of cardiac resynchronization therapy on left ventricular size and function in chronic heart failure. Circulation 2003;107:1985–90.

62. Coman JA, Trohman RG. Incidence and electrocardiographic localization of safe right bundle branch block configurations during permanent ventricular pacing. Am J Cardiol 1995;76:781–4.

63. Trohman RG, Kim MH, Pinski SL. Cardiac pacing: the state of the art. Lancet 2004;364:1701–19.

64. Houghton T, Kaye GC. Implantable devises for treating arrhythmias. Br Med J 2003;327–336.

65. Ezekwitz JA, Armstrong PW, McAlister FA. Implantable cardiovert defibrillator in primary and secondary prevention; a systemic review of randomized controlled trials. Ann Intern Med 2003;138:445–52.

66. Moss AJ, Zareba W, Hall JW, et al. For the Multicenter Automatic Defibrillator Implantation trial 11 Investigators. Prophylactic implantation of a defibrillator in patients with myocardial infarction and reduced ejection fraction, N Engl J Med 2002;346; 877–83.

67. Wilber DJ, Zareba W, Hall J, et al. Time dependence of mortality risk and defibrillator benefit after myocardial infarction. Circulation. 2004;109:1082–4.

68. Hohnloser SH, Kuck KH, Dorian P, et al, for the DINAMIT Investigators. Prophylactic use of an implantable cardioverter defibrillator after acute myocardial infarction. N Engl J Med 2004;351:2481–8.

69. Solomon SD, Glynn RJ, Greaves S, et al. Recovery of ventricular function after myocardial infarction in the reperfusion era: The Healing and Early Afterload Reducing Therapy Study. Ann Intern Med;134:451–8.

70. Last A. Radiotherapy in patients with cardiac pacemakers. Br J Radiol 1998;71:4–10.

71. Solan AN, Solan MJ, Bednarz G, Goodkin MB. Treatment of patients with cardiac pacemakers and implantable cardioverter-defibrillators during radiotherapy. Int J Radiat Oncol Biol Phys 2004;59:897–904.

72. Eckert M, Jones T. How does an implantable cardioverter defibrillator (ICD) affect the lives of patients and their families? Int J Nurs Pract. 2002;8:152–7.

73. Nambisan V, Chao D. Dying and defibrillation: a shocking experience. Palliat Med 2004;18:482–3.

74. Goldstein NE, Lampert R, Bradley E, et al. Management of implantable cardioverter defibrillators in end-of-life care. Ann Intern Med 2004;141:835–8.

Congestive Heart Failure

J. Christopher Champion, MD

To promote community awareness of the social impact of heart failure (HF), some have utilized a comparison with cancer outcomes (Table 1) to underscore the gravity of this public epidemic as noted in a recent article by Stewart.[1] He keenly observes that cancer, despite tremendous advances in treatment, persists as one of the most recognized but feared disease states. Recent statistics suggest that, in people younger than 85 years of age, cancer exceeds heart disease as the leading cause of death (Figure 1).[2] This approach to raising cancer awareness has energized the subsequent demand for aggressive screening, research, and treatment programs that have established the necessary support for earlier detection of cancer, as well as the development of more effective therapies. This process would appear to be an exemplary model for other disease states and raises an intriguing contrast to heart failure. Though a complex array of medical and device therapies are available for the management of cardiac disease, the prevalence of heart failure continues to rise as the direct and indirect costs of this disease swell at an alarming rate.[3] Yet, the comparisons between cancer and the heart do not end at the socioeconomic level.

The biologic principles underlying cell survival and apoptosis appear to be just as central to the onset of heart failure as in tumor progression, and pathways for cell proliferation and cardiac myocyte hypertrophy are highly conserved.[4] However, the burgeoning field of biologically targeted therapy seen with cancer has not been paralleled in heart failure research.[5] This is, in

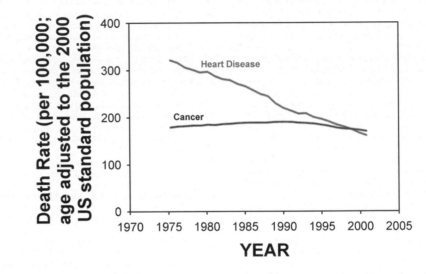

Death Rates from Cancer & Heart Disease in People <85.

FIGURE 1 Death rates from cancer and heart disease in people younger than 85. Redrawn based on data from Jemal A et al.

part, due to the potentially exorbitant cost of randomized, multicenter trials, but there has also been a lack of effective, molecular surrogate end points in cardiovascular research that would make these trials meaningful. In the new era of heart failure research, lessons can be learned from the field of cancer biology whereby future drug development can be tailored to specific molecular targets in order to customize medical care for patients in order to maximize benefits and minimize side effects.

Treatment-Related Cardiomyopathy

Anthracycline Treatment

Background

Anthracyclines are well established as highly efficacious antineoplastic agents for various hemopoietic[6] and solid tumors.[7] However, the cardiotoxicity of these agents has been documented for more than 30 years[8] and remains a potential limitation for many patients with cancer.

Clinical Manifestation

Doxorubicin produces a cardiomyopathy clinically indistinguishable from other forms of congestive heart failure. Patients may be asymptomatic in the early stages and may exhibit only minimal signs of cardiac dysfunction. Among the first signs of cardiac abnormality are new-onset resting tachycardia and loss of normal heart variability due to impaired autonomic function.[9] Without intervention, the cardiac impairment may progress, thus leading to advanced symptomatology with rest dyspnea generally being a poor prognostic sign. Cardiac examination of a patient with decompensated cardiomyopathy often reveals jugular venous distension, an S3 gallop, lower extremity edema, and pulmonary rales. Not all of these physical signs may be present in every patient, but the constellation of findings is generally quite suggestive of acute heart failure.

Three discrete types of anthracycline-induced cardiotoxicity have been described in the literature. First, acute or subacute injury can occur soon after anthracycline exposure. This

Table 1 Comparison of Heart Failure and Cancer Mortality

	Men	Women
Heart failure (Framingham data)	59	45
Breast cancer	—	14
Ovarian cancer	—	45
Colorectal cancer	40*	
Lung Cancer	84*	

Adapted from Stewart S.[1]
*Gender-specific data is not available.

infrequent form of cardiotoxicity may manifest as transient arrhythmias,[10] a pericarditis-myocarditis syndrome, or acute failure of the left ventricle.[11] Second, anthracyclines can induce a chronic form of injury over the course of cumulative exposure that may eventually result in overt cardiomyopathy. This represents the most common type of damage and warrants careful long-term observation for appropriate diagnosis and treatment.[12] Finally, a delayed (or late-onset) anthracycline cardiotoxicity has been well described as a precipitator of left ventricular dysfunction[13] that may manifest years to decades after anthracycline treatment has been completed.[14] Further confounding this presentation is the observation that many individuals may actually have asymptomatic left ventricular dysfunction, thus representing a dormant, subclinical form of toxicity.[15]

Chronic anthracycline-induced cardiomyopathy characteristically presents within 1 year of treatment. Von Hoff describes a large series of patients who developed congestive heart failure secondary to anthracycline-induced chronic cardiomyopathy usually within 231 days after the completion of anthracycline therapy.[16] On the other hand, delayed anthracycline cardiotoxicity may not be apparent for many years. Unfortunately, the concurrent presence of other heart failure risk factors, such as occult hypertension and subclinical coronary artery disease, makes it difficult to precisely ascertain the singular contribution for anthracycline-mediated injury. Nevertheless, anthracyclines are clearly an important independent risk factor leading to both early and delayed congestive heart failure in survivors of cancer.

Pathophysiology

The use of doxorubicin, a highly effective antineoplastic agent of the anthracycline family, has been extensively studied and is associated with various types of cardiotoxicity. Doxorubicin intercalates into the deoxyribonucleic acid (DNA) and thus interferes with both DNA and ribonucleic acid polymerase activity. The exact mechanism of cardiac toxicity is not known; however, it may be related to the generation of highly reactive oxygen species.[17] These free radicals may lead to the production of superoxide anions and highly reactive metabolites, such as hydroxyl radicals and hydrogen peroxide, resulting in membrane lipid peroxidation and direct damage to the cardiac myocytes (Figure 2). This toxic effect may be amplified by the relatively poor antioxidant defense system of the heart.[18] Thus, there is evidence that free-radical scavengers, such as the bispiperazine dexrazoxane, might provide protection from this toxicity.[15] Doxorubicin may interfere with the sarcolemmic sodium-potassium pump, and may also hinder the mitochondrial electron-transport chain. This

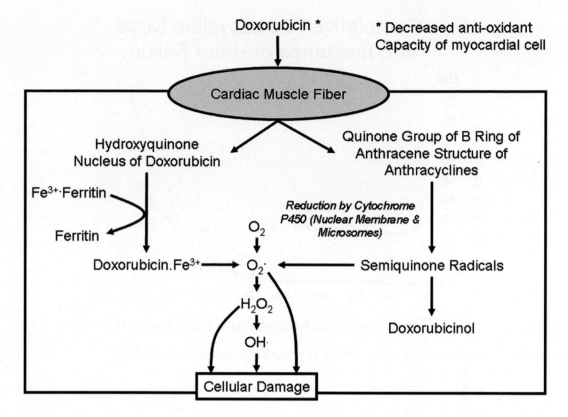

FIGURE 2 Proposed pathways for formation of reactive oxygen species in anthracycline-induced cardiac injury.

may explain the propensity for toxicity in the mitochondrial-rich myocardium. Doxorubicin might stimulate certain immune responses, and induce myocardial apoptosis.[19] Future research will be necessary to elucidate these mechanisms and clarify the underlying pathology that leads to long-term disease sequelae.

Cardiac function is generally preserved until a critical point of myocardial damage is achieved, at which time ventricular impairment progresses rapidly. This is clearly related to the total cumulative dose.[20] Clinically perceptible doxorubicin-induced cardiotoxicity is rarely observed below cumulative doses of 400 mg/m^2, but becomes increasingly common with higher dosages (Figure 3).[16] However, subclinical toxicity is much more frequent and occurs at much lower cumulative dosages. This is demonstrated in the study by Bristow and colleagues of patients who had received doxorubicin and underwent evaluation with serial echocardiography, cardiac catheterization, and endomyocardial biopsy.[21] Twenty-seven of 29 patients who received greater than 272 mg/m^2 had endomyocardial biopsy evidence of myocyte damage, and one patient had histologic changes after only 45 mg/m^2.

Evaluation

Noninvasive cardiac imaging cannot distinguish anthracycline-related cardiomyopathy from other causes of left ventricular dysfunction. Indeed,

the same studies used in the routine evaluation of congestive heart failure are generally employed for surveillance during and after anthracycline exposure to identify functional changes from baseline.

The experience with anthracycline chemotherapy has demonstrated that the early detection of cardiotoxicity in preclinical stages can reduce the development of symptomatic cardiac manifestations through modification of the dosing schedule. There is little consensus on which technique is best when monitoring for evidence of anthracycline-induced cardiotoxicity. Endomyocardial biopsy is considered to be the most sensitive and specific test for the detection of cellular injury; studies have shown the characteristic ultrastructural changes are present before cardiac imaging reveals any evidence of left ventricular dysfunction.[21] Unfortunately, the procedure is limited, not only by its invasive nature but by the expertise required in biopsy interpretation, making it less desirable in the routine evaluation of patients.

Cardiac imaging for the assessment of ventricular structure and function has long been the standard of care for routine follow-up of cancer patients receiving cardiotoxic chemotherapy, despite the lack of clearly established guidelines concerning type, frequency, and duration of testing. The most common method of monitoring for myocardial toxicity with anthracyclines has

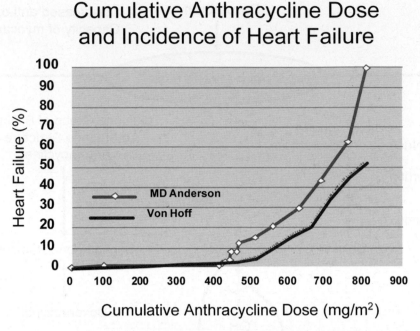

Cumulative Anthracycline Dose and Incidence of Heart Failure

FIGURE 3 Effect of cumulative anthracycline dose on the development of heart failure.

been the assessment of left ventricular systolic function, either with radionuclide ventriculography or echocardiography. The measurement of fractional shortening and the calculation of left ventricular ejection fraction (LVEF) have been the most frequent measurements. These measurements, however, are preload- and afterload-dependent, thereby affecting their reliability as hallmarks of cardiotoxicity. Previous studies have suggested that diastolic dysfunction may actually be the earliest pathology detected by echocardiography in cardiac dysfunction associated with anthracycline toxicity, suggesting a role for diastolic assessment in the preclinical identification of cardiovascular disease.[9]

The echocardiographic evaluation of left ventricular (LV) diastolic filling patterns by Doppler has become widely available and better characterized in recent years, thereby yielding a reliable and noninvasive measure of diastolic performance. Newer methods involve the measurement of transmitral flow, pulmonary venous flow, and, more recently, tissue Doppler imaging.[22] Tissue Doppler imaging (TDI) is a newer ultrasound modality that records systolic and diastolic velocities within the myocardium at the corners of the mitral annulus. It provides information concerning intramyocardial velocity and, thus, LV mechanics during isovolumic contraction and relaxation.[23] Thus, TDI has been proposed as a reliable marker for early identification of myocardial disease before the overt development of LV systolic dysfunction.

Recently, interest has grown in the utilization of circulating markers that may allude to covert myocardial injury or impending decompensation. In the past decade, several studies have confirmed the usefulness of the measurement of the B-type natriuretic peptide (BNP), a cardiac neurohormone, in the diagnosis and management of heart failure. Not only is BNP inversely correlated with ejection fraction, but it is also directly proportional to the degree of heart failure decompensation and left ventricular end diastolic pressure elevation.[24] Notably, elevated secretion of natriuretic peptides has been associated with both left ventricular systolic dysfunction[25] and diastolic filling abnormalities[26] in doxorubicin-treated patients. Transient increases in BNP are seen after administration of a single dose of anthracycline, but the patients with sustained elevation appear to have the greatest risk for developing cardiotoxicity.[27] BNP has also been shown to be elevated prior to the development of LV dysfunction in patients undergoing high-dose therapy and hematopoietic stem cell transplantation.[28] Other biomarkers for early doxorubicin cardiotoxicity, such as cardiac troponins I and T, have recently been shown to be elevated prior to changes in LVEF and before the appearance of cardiac symptoms.[29,30] Such testing is minimally invasive and inexpensive, yielding an excellent means for longitudinal monitoring if further research clearly establishes the utility.

Treatment

Patients who develop congestive heart failure are given standard treatment according to the guidelines of the American College of Cardiology/American Heart Association and the Heart Failure Society of America.[31,32] Our practice and formal recommendation is the use of angiotensin converting enzyme (ACE) inhibitors and β-blockers to treat most anthracycline-associated congestive heart failure. Specific drug regimens are dictated by disease severity, renal function,

and level of symptoms, but they may include a variety of oral and intravenous agents, including vasodilators, nesiritide, inotropes, and pressors as indicated. In patients with heart failure who are black or who have significant renal insufficiency, the combination of nitrates and hydralazine may be employed. Depending upon the prognosis from the patient's cancer, device therapy such as biventricular pacemakers and/or defibrillators may be appropriate. Consideration of cardiac transplantation is generally not warranted unless disease-free survival from cancer is at least five years.

Observational data from our institution supports the long-term continuation of ACE inhibitors and β-blockers is necessary for maintenance of cardiac compensation. Withdrawal of heart failure therapy for chemotherapy-induced cardiac dysfunction at our institution has been shown to commonly result in relapse of heart failure symptoms (New York Heart Association classification) as well as a recurrent decline in left ventricular ejection fraction (Figure 4).[33]

Cardioprotective agents have been developed; however, clinical practice guidelines do not recommend their routine use.[34] Dexrazoxane can be considered for use in breast cancer patients who are receiving more than 300 mg/m^2 of doxorubicin, but this has not been a habitual practice at our institution. Theoretically, if the cardiac complications resulting from anthracycline exposure could be reduced or prevented, higher and potentially more effective doses could be considered. Furthermore, avoidance of cardiotoxicity may preserve alternative therapeutic options should cancer recur in a patient. On a broader scale, such preventative strategies may have favorable economic implications given the annual cost of treating patients with chemotherapy-induced congestive heart failure.[35]

Summary

Certainly, the management of patients with anthracycline-induced cardiomyopathy can pose various dilemmas to oncologists and cardiologists alike. Nevertheless, irrespective of the stage at which it is recognized, the therapeutic tactic remains consistent; that is, to employ appropriate medical therapy that may stabilize the cardiac disease as soon as possible. By accomplishing this task effectively, patients may go on to receive further cancer treatment before disease progression negatively impacts their options and outcomes.

Trastuzumab

Background

Herceptin (Genentech, South San Francisco, CA) (trastuzumab) is a monoclonal antibody effective against breast cancers that overexpress the receptor Her-2/neu (*erb-B2*), a characteristic

Mean LVEF/NYHA in Response to Chemotherapy and ACE-I/Beta Blocker Therapy

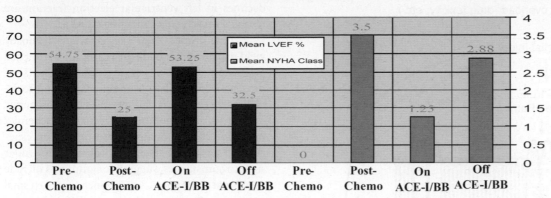

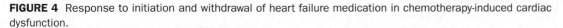

FIGURE 4 Response to initiation and withdrawal of heart failure medication in chemotherapy-induced cardiac dysfunction.

present in about 27% of all breast cancers, through its inhibition of tyrosine kinase. Herceptin used in combination with first-line chemotherapy, including doxorubicin, has been associated with significantly longer time to disease progression, higher response rate, and overall significantly improved survival rates, representing a major advance in therapy for metastatic breast cancer. Importantly, this efficacy has been coupled with a good tolerability profile.

Herceptin alone is infrequently associated with significant cardiomyopathy. However, the incidence of cardiomyopathy has been reported to be as high as 28% in the Herceptin Pivotal Trial (Table 2) among patients who received the combination of Herceptin and anthracyclines.[36]

Clinical Manifestation

As with other cardiac complications of cancer therapy, the precise incidence of trastuzumab-related events is limited by the retrospective nature of their collection and the fact that there is a diminished tendency to report milder, non-specific symptoms. Furthermore, to be able to understand the true significance of trastuzumab-related events, it is important to determine the baseline incidence of systolic dysfunction as well as the influence of other clinical syndromes unrelated to trastuzumab cardiotoxicity, such as sepsis or pulmonary embolism.

Most reported trastuzumab-related cardiac events appear to be asymptomatic decreases in left ventricular ejection fraction. However, when symptoms do occur, they initially tend to be milder in severity and include nonspecific dyspnea, tachycardia, and, occasionally, chest pain. Without appropriate recognition and intervention, symptoms may progress to more advanced stages of heart failure. The clinical findings are identical to those for other causes of cardiomyopathy and are detailed in the prior section for anthracycline-induced cardiomyopathy.

Pathophysiology

As with anthracyclines, the underlying mechanism for this observed cardiomyopathy has not been fully explained, but several hypotheses have been offered. One such theory proposes a "sequential stress" phenomenon that is produced by Herceptin exposure superimposed on the previous or concurrent damage of doxorubicin or other preexisting cardiac disease.[37] Such explanations offer a framework for understanding the concept of this process, but it is laboratory research that has yielded greater insight into a potential cellular basis for this theory. For instance, Chien and colleagues have shown that *ERBB2* knockout mice can develop a dilated cardiomyopathy with impaired systolic and diastolic function in response to hemodynamic stress.[38] Conversely, overexpression of BcL-xL can lead to rescue through the salvage pathway, suggesting that the *erb-B2* myocyte survival pathway may lead to a modifiable predisposition to heart failure.

Such research into the pathophysiology has yielded important findings that may also allude to the regulation of cardiac myocytes. The epidermal growth factor (EGF) signaling system appears to have a vital role in cardiac growth and development. EGF ligands, such as the neuregulins (NRG) seem to mediate interactions between the endothelial cell and the myocyte. The neuregulins promote stabilization of structural proteins and can lead to attenuation of myocyte death.[39] Furthermore, NRG-*erb*-B2 signaling is important not only for cardiac function under normal conditions but also for attenuation of stress-induced myocyte apoptosis.[40] Therefore, trastuzumab, through its effect on *erb-B2*, may down-regulate this essential pathway and impair the counter-regulatory mechanism for preserving cardiac function (Figure 5).

Evaluation

The identification of trastuzumab -induced cardiotoxicity is similar to that used for the monitoring of anthracycline treatment by noninvasive cardiac imaging. Please see "Evaluation" above for further information.

Treatment

Herceptin has an FDA warning for cardiomyopathy and, historically, has not been administered to patients with preexisting LV systolic dysfunction. Traditionally, patients without prior cardiac dysfunction who developed overt heart failure or asymptomatic declines in LV systolic function were denied further trastuzumab treatment. Although congestive heart failure occurring in patients treated with trastuzumab may be moderate or severe, the majority of patients at our center who develop congestive heart failure tend to improve with standard treatment. In fact, the use of angiotensin converting enzyme-inhibitors and β-blockers appears to be quite important in reversing symptomatic and asymptomatic LV dysfunction related to trastuzumab therapy. Our experience has shown that withdrawal of such therapy may lead to recurrent left ventricular dysfunction and relapse of symptoms. Based on observational data from the M. D. Anderson Cancer Center, certain patients with metastatic breast cancer may be safely rechallenged with Herceptin after heart failure has been stabilized with the use of standard HF therapy, especially angiotensin converting enzyme-inhibitors and β-blockers. If clinical benefit from treatment with trastuzumab has been observed then reinitiation must be seriously considered after the risks and benefits of continued use of trastuzumab are thoroughly discussed with the patient. If trastuzumab has been discontinued because of cardiac dysfunction yet symptoms respond to treatment, then resumption of trastuzumab is acceptable with close observation for signs and

Table 2 Incidence of Cardiac Dysfunction according to Background Chemotherapy

	Herceptin Cardiac Dysfunction Results from Pivotal Trials				
	H N = 213	*H+P* N = 91	*P* N = 95	*H+AC* N = 143	*AC* N = 135
Any Cardiac Dysfunction	7%	11%	1%	28%	7%
Class III–IV	5%	4%	1%	19%	3%
AC = anthracycline + cyclophosphamide; H = Herceptin; P = paclitaxel.					

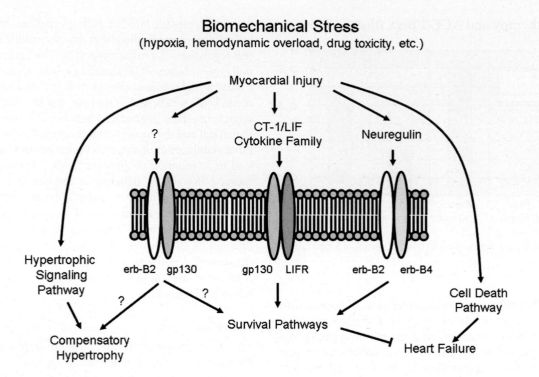

Biomechanical Stress
(hypoxia, hemodynamic overload, drug toxicity, etc.)

FIGURE 5 Proposed pathways involved in trastuzumab-mediated susceptibility to cardiac dysfunction through inhibition of *erb-B2*.

symptoms of heart failure. Routine cardiac imaging and regular clinical assessment should also be performed.

Ischemic Cardiomyopathy

Background

Despite the proliferation of therapeutic interventions for numerous cardiovascular conditions, coronary heart disease continues to be the most common cause of death in the United States and remains the principal reason for heart failure. Ischemic heart disease is identified as the primary etiology for approximately two-thirds of the 5 million heart failure patients in this country. While cancer is observed in a much smaller subset of this group, coronary disease continues to be an exceedingly common comorbid condition that not only complicates therapy, but also often leads to death during the course of treatment for malignancy.

Thus, the effective management of the cancer patient requires careful attention to the signs and symptoms that may signal cardiac decompensation related to myocardial ischemia. The specific issues surrounding the diagnosis and treatment of chronic or acute ischemic syndromes are addressed in another chapter of this book. However, it is worth reiterating that there is a significantly elevated risk for coronary heart disease in cancer patients due to the preponderance of risk factors in this population and to the concurrent existence of conditions that can potentiate ischemia (such as anemia, hypoxia,

and increased myocardial demand). Additionally, several chemotherapeutic agents can actually induce coronary events through vasospasm, thrombosis or other less understood mechanisms. As in non-cancer patients, single or multiple ischemic insults can lead to left ventricular dysfunction requiring medical therapy and/or revascularization to restore compensation. However, many issues unique to cancer patients can complicate the clinical management decisions. These will be discussed in detail in this chapter.

Clinical Manifestation

There is no set pattern for the presenting clinical syndrome of ischemic cardiomyopathy, and this appears to be particularly true of those patients who also have active neoplastic disease. Typical anginal symptoms may not necessarily be noticed prior to presentation with overt heart failure decompensation. Furthermore, misdiagnosis of heart disease may be promoted by the vague presenting complaints that are often attributed to coexisting medical conditions. For instance, general fatigue is a common symptom related to both the presence of cancer and to its treatment with chemotherapy. Similarly, dyspnea may be attributed to the anemia often seen with hematologic malignancies or with myelosuppression from cancer treatment. And many other comorbid conditions such as obstructive lung disease or severe cachexia can confound both the history and physical examination. It is not surprising that the earliest stages of heart failure may go unnoticed, even in experienced hands, and

diagnosis may be made "incidentally" when declines in left ventricular ejection fraction are revealed on screening imaging studies.

These things said, the greatest diagnostic yield may be obtained from a carefully performed evaluation that collects multiple elements of the classic constellation of signs and symptoms. Hallmarks of heart failure caused by ischemic myocardial dysfunction and recurrent ischemia/infarction can dominate the clinical picture, especially at advanced stages of presentation. Under such circumstances, suggestive symptoms include exertional dyspnea, orthopnea, paroxysmal nocturnal dyspnea, fatigue, weight gain, lower extremity edema, and activity tolerance, as well as typical anginal chest pain with radiation and associated symptoms that are relieved with rest or nitroglycerin.

The differentiation of heart disease from other diseases is often made difficult by the frequency with which concurrent illnesses appear in cancer patients. Pulmonary embolism, pericardial disease and pneumonia can all present with varying degrees of dyspnea and chest pain, and each has a dramatically different therapeutic course compared to ischemic cardiomyopathy. Additionally, esophageal disease is not uncommonly observed and may be indistinguishable upon initial presentation.

Pathophysiology

A detailed discussion of the progression of atherosclerotic disease to eventual cardiac dysfunction is beyond the scope of this chapter. Suffice it to say that the process has been well described in a number of animal and human studies. Nevertheless, there are several important points to be made about the coronary pathophysiology as it pertains to the cancer patient:

The underlying mechanism of disease is frequently identical to that seen in other patients with ischemic cardiomyopathy. That is, the disease may be initiated/propagated by a localized infarct with subsequent diffuse fibrosis, areas of dysfunctional ischemic myocardium, or a combination of these.

Several chemotherapeutic agents, such as the antimetabolite 5-fluorouracil, may elicit ischemic symptoms.[41] Usually, the ischemia is reversible with cessation of the agent and initiation of antianginal medical therapy. Underlying coronary artery disease (CAD) is not necessarily a prerequisite to the development of symptoms, but the incidence is higher in those with preexisting coronary disease (1.1% in those without CAD and 4.5% in patients with CAD).[42] Several mechanistic theories have suggested a metabolite that is directly toxic to the myocardium, an autoimmune process, thrombogenesis or inducible vasospastic coronary ischemia.

Radiation has a unique potential for the initiation of coronary vascular disease with an increased risk of death due to ischemic events in patients treated for Hodgkin's disease and breast cancer (see "Effects of Radiation Therapy" below).[43]

Cancer patients commonly exhibit a variety of triggers that may precipitate an acute coronary syndrome, such as anemia, hypoxia, hypotension, infection, up-regulated markers of inflammation, and the need for transfusion of blood products. If these factors are not addressed, recurrent ischemic insult and cardiac decompensation may result.

Evaluation

The evaluation for ischemic disease in the cancer patient is performed using the same methods for non-cancer patients. The history and physical examination may help to identify the presence of suggestive features; however, as noted previously, atypical presentations with non-specific symptoms are quite common. Assessment of global function and regional wall motion by echocardiography or radionuclide ventriculography can allude to areas of anatomic coronary involvement. The decision to pursue further ischemic assessment by invasive or noninvasive imaging should be tempered by the clinical features of comorbid conditions, such as cancer prognosis or general state of illness. At our institution, the needs of the individual patient are taken into consideration and appropriate treatment options such as revascularization are discussed in the context of expected risk/benefit ratio. Factors, such as bleeding risk due to thrombocytopenia or to metastatic brain lesions, for example, are carefully weighed beforehand. A multidisciplinary discussion amongst healthcare providers is often performed to clarify such issues before proceeding with extensive evaluations. Under these circumstances, appropriate candidates will enter a workup that may ultimately culminate in coronary revascularization through percutaneous or surgical means. On occasion, myocardial perfusion imaging or stress echocardiography may be used as a risk assessment tool in the preoperative setting with deferment of cardiac catheterization unless large areas of ischemia are identified.

Treatment

When possible, identification and treatment of a reversible etiology is important for the acute and long-term survival of these patients, as demand ischemia is a common problem throughout the course of cancer treatment. Importantly, the medical management of patients with large areas of hibernating myocardium remains suboptimal compared to revascularization strategies.[44] As with other cardiomyopathies treated at our institution, patients are given standard therapy according to the guidelines of the American College of Cardiology/American Heart Association and the Heart Failure Society of America.[31,32] This generally includes not only angiotensin converting enzyme inhibitors and β-blockers, but also 3-hydroxy-3-methyl-glutaryl-Coenzyme A reductase (HMG-CoA) inhibitors, nitrates and diuretics as indicated. When permissible by bleeding risk and platelet count, aspirin and/or clopidogrel are used. Provided that longevity is expected beyond six months, device therapy with defibrillators or pacemakers is also considered.

Valvular Heart Disease

Specific Disease Entities

While there are several diseases listed below that may lead to valvular heart disease, these entities also may lead to heart failure through other mechanisms. These various syndromes are described in detail separately.

Carcinoid Heart Disease

Pathophysiology Carcinoid tumors are generally rare (1.2 to 2.1 per 100,000).[45] Cardiac involvement may occur in more than 50% of patients diagnosed with carcinoid syndrome, a constellation of symptoms that may include flushing, bronchospasm, and secretory diarrhea. Carcinoid tumors can lead to cardiac valvular disease through the action of peptides that induce the formation of fibromuscular plaques, thereby disrupting valvular integrity. The precise mechanism for plaque creation is somewhat uncertain but may involve several potential mediators of injury including serotonin, 5-hydroxytryptophan, histamine, prostaglandins, bradykinins and tachykinins. Observational data indicates that serotonin levels are higher among carcinoid patients who demonstrate cardiac involvement, compared to patients without cardiac involvement. Such an association implies causality, but does not exclude the role of other cytokines in the pathogenesis.[46]

Mediator release into the hepatic vein from metastatic liver disease predisposes patients to right-sided cardiac lesions. The margins and distal portions of the tricuspid leaflets are often thickened, and involvement of the chordae tendineae may also be seen. Similarly, the pulmonic valve shows thickening and retraction. However, when the primary or metastatic tumor is in the lung, mediators are then released directly into the pulmonary venous bed, thereby bypassing inactivation within the lung tissue and predisposing to left-sided valvular lesions.[47] While left-sided lesions are encountered less frequently than those on the right side, when they are present, they are more likely to result in hemodynamic compromise.

The ultrastructure of cardiac plaques has been studied extensively. These lesions are formed of smooth muscle cells embedded in a stroma of acid mucopolysaccharide and collagen, and they lack elastic fibers.[48] The most important consequence of carcinoid plaques is fibrosis of the valves with resultant distortion of the valvular apparatus and ring. Tricuspid regurgitation and pulmonic stenosis are typically seen, but in the case of progressive destruction, a rigid tricuspid valve may be encountered with characteristic hemodynamic abnormalities. Significant pulmonic regurgitation is rare. Stiffening of the right atrium may be noted and contributes to the neck-vein distention commonly seen with the carcinoid syndrome.

The diagnosis of carcinoid syndrome is usually suggested by the clinical features and established by elevation of 5-hydroxy indole acetic acid (5-HIAA), a product of serotonin metabolism. Urinary 5-HIAA provides a dependable biologic marker, not only for the activity of the tumor but also the response to treatment.[49]

Evaluation Echocardiography is the most useful noninvasive diagnostic tool for evaluating patients with carcinoid heart disease (Figure 6). Echocardiography not only identifies the valvular abnormality but, when coupled with Doppler ultrasonography studies, can also provide hemodynamic data for estimating the degree of valvular involvement.[50]

Concomitant with the thickening and loss of mobility of the tricuspid leaflets, there is increased flow velocity across the tricuspid valve during diastole. Likewise, a regurgitant jet can be seen in the right atrium during systole.[51] Furthermore, chamber enlargement may also be quantified, where both right atrial and right ventricular enlargement are characteristic.

Treatment During the past decade, progress in the management of malignant carcinoid tumors and carcinoid syndrome has resulted in better patient survival. Octreotide acetate (Sandostatin) (Novartis Incorp., New York, NY), the somatostatin analog, is a synthetic octapeptide that binds to subtypes of the somatostatin receptors and inhibits the secretion of bioactive substances that cause the carcinoid syndrome. Treatment with the somatostatin analog relieves symptoms in more than 70% of patients.[52]

Cardiac surgery is the only effective treatment for carcinoid heart disease and should be considered for symptomatic patients whose metastatic carcinoid disease and symptoms of carcinoid syndrome are well controlled. The timing of cardiac operation for carcinoid heart disease remains difficult. No definitive guidelines can be established from the published series to date. Cardiac surgery has been successful in

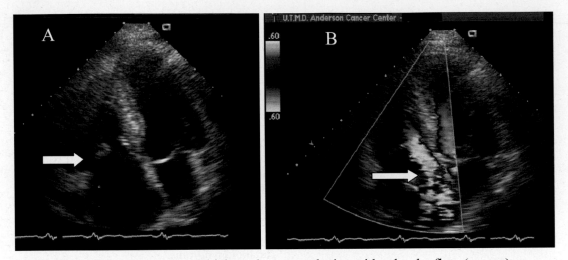

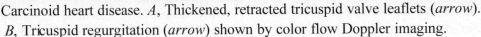

Carcinoid heart disease. *A*, Thickened, retracted tricuspid valve leaflets (*arrow*).
B, Tricuspid regurgitation (*arrow*) shown by color flow Doppler imaging.

FIGURE 6 Echocardiographic feature of carcinoid heart disease.

reducing or relieving the cardiac symptoms of many patients with carcinoid heart disease. However, review of a small surgical series from the Mayo Clinic suggests a high surgical mortality and incomplete symptom resolution among surgical survivors.[53] Despite the high surgical mortality, the survival among surgically treated patients was better than the survival among patients with similar symptoms related to carcinoid heart disease who were treated medically.

Effects of Radiation Therapy   Radiation therapy is frequently utilized as an adjunct to chemotherapy or surgery in the treatment of various cancers. Radiation to the thorax can cause damage to the pericardium, myocardium, valves, and coronary vessels, with pericardium being most frequently involved.[54] The risk of radiation-induced cardiac disease is greater in patients who receive high doses of radiation or concurrent treatment with doxorubicin[43,55] as well as in those patients with cardiac risk factors or preexisting coronary artery disease.[56] Preemptive treatment strategies to minimize the effects of cardiac irradiation include subcarinal shielding techniques, lower total radiation doses, and avoidance of concurrent cardiotoxic agents.

The precise incidence of radiation-induced atherosclerosis is difficult to determine due to the high prevalence of preexisting coronary artery disease in the United States, but it has certainly been observed in a number of patients without the traditional risk factors for coronary heart disease,[57] including young adults. The exact mechanism responsible for vascular injury is not clearly delineated but is possibly related to triggered endothelial damage that leads to accelerated vascular fibrosis.[58]

Vascular injury due to radiotherapy may be silent, considering that half of asymptomatic patients develop new myocardial perfusion defects, possibly due to damage at the microvascular level.[59] Clinically, most symptomatic patients present with angina, dyspnea, or heart failure,[57] though reports of sudden cardiac death have been noted. The mean time interval from radiation treatment to development of coronary heart disease is approximately 82 months according to one study.[54] The management of radiation-induced atherosclerosis is identical to that for atherosclerotic disease due to traditional causes. Both percutaneous intervention and coronary artery bypass graft have been used, though thoracic surgery may pose a particular challenge in these patients due to mediastinal fibrosis and a concomitantly elevated incidence of complications.[57]

Radiation-induced myocardial fibrosis resulting from deposition of fibrous tissues in all three layers of the ventricular wall has also been observed.[54] There is marked alteration in collagen synthesis with increases in collagen as well as increases in the ratio of type I versus type III production.[60]

Similarly, valvular heart disease is commonly seen following radiation treatment due fibrous thickening of cardiac valves with a predilection for left-sided valvular involvement being noted.[58] Only rarely do these patients with radiation-induced valvular disease have clinically moderate or severe dysfunction, with the mean time from radiation to onset of symptoms being approximately 98 months in one observational study.[54] The treatment of valvular disease related to radiotherapy is the same as in the general population.

Radiotherapy may cause fibrous thickening of the pericardium,[58] pericardial effusion, or pericarditis with or without constriction.[54] Pericardial disease is described in greater detail in another chapter of this book (see Chapter 52, "The Pericardium in the Cancer Patient").

REFERENCES

1. Stewart S. Prognosis of patients with heart failure compared with common types of cancer. Heart Fail Monit 2003;3: 87–94.
2. Jemal A, et al. Cancer statistics, 2005. CA Cancer J Clin 2005;55:10–30.
3. Stewart S, et al. Heart failure and the aging population: an increasing burden in the 21st century? Heart 2003;89: 49–53.
4. Hoshijima M, Chien KR. Mixed signals in heart failure: cancer rules. J Clin Invest 2002;109:849–55.
5. Ross JS, et al. Targeted therapies for cancer 2004. Am J Clin Pathol 2004;122:598–609.
6. Hitchcock-Bryan S, et al. The impact of induction anthracycline on long-term failure-free survival in childhood acute lymphoblastic leukemia. Med Pediatr Oncol 1986;14: 211–5.
7. Fisher B, et al. Doxorubicin-containing regimens for the treatment of stage II breast cancer: The National Surgical Adjuvant Breast and Bowel Project experience. J Clin Oncol 1989;7:572–82.
8. Lefrak EA, et al. A clinicopathologic analysis of adriamycin cardiotoxicity. Cancer 1973;32:302–14.
9. Tjeerdsma G, et al. Early detection of anthracycline induced cardiotoxicity in asymptomatic patients with normal left ventricular systolic function: autonomic versus echocardiographic variables. Heart 1999;81:419–23.
10. Steinberg JS, et al. Acute arrhythmogenicity of doxorubicin administration. Cancer 1987;60:1213–8.
11. Ferrans VJ. Overview of cardiac pathology in relation to anthracycline cardiotoxicity. Cancer Treat Rep 1978;62: 955–61.
12. Bristow MR, et al. Clinical spectrum of anthracycline antibiotic cardiotoxicity. Cancer Treat Rep 1978;62: 873–9.
13. Haq MM, et al. Doxorubicin-induced congestive heart failure in adults. Cancer 1985;56:1361–5.
14. Lipshultz SE, et al. Chronic progressive cardiac dysfunction years after doxorubicin therapy for childhood acute lymphoblastic leukemia. J Clin Oncol 2005;23:2629–36.
15. Dorr RT. Cytoprotective agents for anthracyclines. Semin Oncol 1996;23(4 Suppl 8):23–34.
16. Von Hoff DD, et al. Risk factors for doxorubicin-induced congestive heart failure. Ann Intern Med 1979;91:710–7.
17. Horenstein MS, Vander Heide RS, L'Ecuyer TJ. Molecular basis of anthracycline-induced cardiotoxicity and its prevention. Mol Genet Metab 2000;71(1–2):436–44.
18. Pritsos CA, Ma J. Basal and drug-induced antioxidant enzyme activities correlate with age-dependent doxorubicin oxidative toxicity. Chem Biol Interact 2000;127: 1–11.
19. Arola OJ, et al. Acute doxorubicin cardiotoxicity involves cardiomyocyte apoptosis. Cancer Res 2000;60:1789–92.
20. Lipshultz SE, et al. Late cardiac effects of doxorubicin therapy for acute lymphoblastic leukemia in childhood. N Engl J Med 1991;324:808–15.
21. Bristow MR, et al. Doxorubicin cardiomyopathy: evaluation by phonocardiography, endomyocardial biopsy, and cardiac catheterization. Ann Intern Med 1978;88:168–75.
22. Rakowski H, et al. Canadian consensus recommendations for the measurement and reporting of diastolic dysfunction by echocardiography: from the Investigators of Consensus on Diastolic Dysfunction by Echocardiography. J Am Soc Echocardiogr 1996;9:736–60.
23. Miyatake K, et al. New method for evaluating left ventricular wall motion by color-coded tissue Doppler imaging: in vitro and in vivo studies. J Am Coll Cardiol 1995;25: 717–24.
24. Maisel AS, et al. Utility of B-natriuretic peptide as a rapid, point-of-care test for screening patients undergoing echocardiography to determine left ventricular dysfunction. Am Heart J 2001;141:367–74.
25. Hayakawa H, et al. Plasma levels of natriuretic peptides in relation to doxorubicin-induced cardiotoxicity and cardiac function in children with cancer. Med Pediatr Oncol 2001;37:4–9.
26. Nousiainen T, et al. Natriuretic peptides during the development of doxorubicin-induced left ventricular diastolic dysfunction. J Intern Med 2002;251:228–34.

27. Suzuki T, et al. Elevated B-type natriuretic peptide levels after anthracycline administration. Am Heart J 1998;136: 362–3.

28. Snowden JA, et al. Assessment of cardiotoxicity during haemopoietic stem cell transplantation with plasma brain natriuretic peptide. Bone Marrow Transplant 2000;26: 309–13.

29. Cardinale D, et al. Prognostic value of troponin I in cardiac risk stratification of cancer patients undergoing high-dose chemotherapy. Circulation 2004;109:2749–54.

30. Lipshultz SE, et al. Predictive value of cardiac troponin T in pediatric patients at risk for myocardial injury. Circulation 1997;96:2641–8.

31. Hunt SA. ACC/AHA 2005 guideline update for the diagnosis and management of chronic heart failure in the adult: a report of the American College of Cardiology/American Heart Association Task Force on Practice Guidelines (Writing Committee to Update the 2001 Guidelines for the Evaluation and Management of Heart Failure). J Am Coll Cardiol 2005;46:e1–82, 1116–43.

32. Heart Failure Society of America (HFSA) practice guidelines. HFSA guidelines for management of patients with heart failure caused by left ventricular systolic dysfunction—pharmacological approaches. J Card Fail 1999;5:357–82.

33. Abstracts of the 7th Annual Meeting of the Heart Failure Society of America, 21–24 September 2003. J Card Fail 2003;9(5 Abstr Suppl):1–124.

34. Hensley ML, et al. American Society of Clinical Oncology clinical practice guidelines for the use of chemotherapy and radiotherapy protectants. J Clin Oncol 1999;17: 3333–55.

35. Bates M, et al. A pharmacoeconomic evaluation of the use of dexrazoxane in preventing anthracycline-induced cardiotoxicity in patients with stage IIIB or IV metastatic breast cancer. Clin Ther 1997;19:167–84.

36. Seidman A, et al. Cardiac dysfunction in the trastuzumab clinical trials experience. J Clin Oncol 2002;20:1215–21.

37. Ewer MS, et al. Cardiotoxicity in patients receiving trastuzumab (Herceptin): primary toxicity, synergistic or sequential stress, or surveillance artifact? Semin Oncol 1999;26(4 Suppl 12):96–101.

38. Chien KR. Myocyte survival pathways and cardiomyopathy: implications for trastuzumab cardiotoxicity. Semin Oncol 2000;27(6 Suppl 11):9–14, 92–100.

39. Zhao YY, et al. Neuregulins promote survival and growth of cardiac myocytes. Persistence of ErbB2 and ErbB4 expression in neonatal and adult ventricular myocytes. J Biol Chem 1998;273:10261–9.

40. Crone SA, et al. ErbB2 is essential in the prevention of dilated cardiomyopathy. Nat Med 2002;8:459–65.

41. Gradishar WJ, Vokes EE. 5-Fluorouracil cardiotoxicity: a critical review. Ann Oncol 1990;1:409–14.

42. Labianca R, et al. Cardiac toxicity of 5-fluorouracil: a study on 1083 patients. Tumori 1982;68:505–10.

43. Basavaraju SR, Easterly CE. Pathophysiological effects of radiation on atherosclerosis development and progression, and the incidence of cardiovascular complications. Med Phys 2002;29:2391–403.

44. Alderman EL, et al. Results of coronary artery surgery in patients with poor left ventricular function (CASS). Circulation 1983;68:785–95.

45. Modlin IM, Sandor A. An analysis of 8305 cases of carcinoid tumors. Cancer 1997;79:813–29.

46. Robiolio PA, et al. Carcinoid heart disease. Correlation of high serotonin levels with valvular abnormalities detected by cardiac catheterization and echocardiography. Circulation 1995;92:790–5.

47. Millward MJ, et al. Left heart involvement with cardiac shunt complicating carcinoid heart disease. Aust N Z J Med 1989;19:716–7.

48. Lundin L, et al. Histochemical and immunohistochemical morphology of carcinoid heart disease. Pathol Res Pract 1991;187:73–7.

49. Moertel CG. Karnofsky memorial lecture. An odyssey in the land of small tumors. J Clin Oncol 1987;5:1502–22.

50. Tribouilloy C, et al. [Demonstration by Doppler echocardiography of multiple valvular involvement in carcinoid cardiopathy]. Arch Mal Coeur Vaiss 1989;82: 109–14.

51. Callahan JA, et al. Echocardiographic features of carcinoid heart disease. Am J Cardiol 1982;50:762–8.

52. Kvols LK, et al. Treatment of the malignant carcinoid syndrome. Evaluation of a long-acting somatostatin analogue. N Engl J Med 1986;315:663–6.

53. Connolly HM, et al. Outcome of cardiac surgery for carcinoid heart disease. J Am Coll Cardiol 1995;25: 410–6.

54. Veinot JP, Edwards WD. Pathology of radiation-induced heart disease: a surgical and autopsy study of 27 cases. Hum Pathol 1996;27:766–73.

55. Shapiro CL, et al. Cardiac effects of adjuvant doxorubicin and radiation therapy in breast cancer patients. J Clin Oncol 1998;16:3493–501.

56. Glanzmann C, et al. Cardiac risk after mediastinal irradiation for Hodgkin's disease. Radiother Oncol 1998;46:51–62.

57. Orzan F, et al. Severe coronary artery disease after radiation therapy of the chest and mediastinum: clinical presentation and treatment. Br Heart J 1993;69:496–500.

58. Brosius FC 3rd, Waller BF, Roberts WC. Radiation heart disease. Analysis of 16 young (aged 15 to 33 years) necropsy patients who received over 3,500 rads to the heart. Am J Med 1981;70:519–30.

59. Gyenes G, et al. Detection of radiation-induced myocardial damage by technetium-99m sestamibi scintigraphy. Eur J Nucl Med 1997;24:286–92.

60. Chello M, et al. Changes in the proportion of types I and III collagen in the left ventricular wall of patients with post-irradiative pericarditis. Cardiovasc Surg 1996;4(2): 222–6.

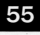

Vascular Disease

Daniel J. Lenihan, MD
Atiar M. Rahman, MD, PhD

The manifestations of vascular disease in patients with cancer can affect any organ and may have a profound influence on overall outcomes. In the general population, arterial and venous thromboembolic disease portends a worse prognosis and is associated with important morbidity, but these complications are even more important in a patient with cancer.[1] Frequently, these patients already have other comorbidities,[2] including immunosuppression and hematologic manifestations, placing them at higher risk of major complications. Thus, optimal therapy for thromboembolic disease, including prevention, is of paramount importance in this particular group of patients. This chapter focuses on a discussion of vascular disease manifested by aortic aneurysms, arterial thromboembolism, and venous thrombosis. The emphasis is on the clinical manifestations, pathophysiologic mechanisms (if known), diagnostic approaches, and optimal treatment in the cancer patient. Additionally, anticipated developments that may further improve the care of these patients are highlighted. The goal of this chapter is to provide a basis for improved understanding of vascular disease in the patient with cancer, which, it is hoped, will lead to development of improved evidence-based treatment and subsequent outcomes.

Aortic Aneurysm

The development of aneurysmal vascular diseases is intimately associated with atherosclerosis, which is typically of a diffuse nature. The common feature involves weakened elastin or collagen that leads to poor arterial tensile strength that results in aneurysmal dilatation.[3] In special populations, such as patients with Ehler-Danlos or Marfan syndrome, the defect may be specifically with elastin or collagen. However, in the cancer patient, there is likely a combination of atherosclerosis, owing to the aging population, and other complications of cancer or cancer therapy that predisposes a patient to the development of aortic aneurysms. Radiation therapy, a known contributor to atherosclerosis,[4–7] and disseminated fungal infections leading to mycotic aneurysms are examples of such conditions.

Clinical Manifestations

The large majority of aneurysms, particularly abdominal aortic aneurysms (AAAs), are asymptomatic and frequently detected at physical examination or during radiologic or ultrasound evaluation. This may occur in up to 75% of patients.[8] The minority of patients will develop abdominal, flank, or back pain if an AAA is present and may have early satiety, occasionally nausea and vomiting, or, uncommonly, ureteral obstruction owing to local compression. However, since these are also manifestations of intra-abdominal malignancy, an unwary physician might miss them. Acute rupture, an immediate life-threatening condition, may occur in up to 20% of cases and results in death more than 50% of the time.[9,10] This may initially manifest clinically with retroperitoneal bleeding and resultant physical findings (psoas sign), which demand immediate recognition. Additionally, thrombus or atheromatous material may embolize distally and patients may develop livido reticularis, renal insufficiency, or blue toe syndrome as a result. Because cancer patients may have mycotic aneurysms in a variety of locations, other manifestations of embolic phenomenon may be evident in the tissues subtended by the aneurysmal segment. Thus, a high degree of suspicion is necessary to detect these serious conditions by both physical examination and radiologic examination (Table 1).

Pathophysiologic Mechanisms

The etiology of aneurysmal disease in general is multifactorial, with genetic predisposition and atherosclerosis, as well as other vascular risk factors (such as hypertension or hyperlipidemia) being most commonly associated. In the patient with cancer, other factors may predominate. Radiation therapy enhances the atherosclerotic process in cancer patients, and this is an important risk factor.[5] For instance, in patients with lymphoma who receive mantle radiation to great vessels, the incidence of significant vascular disease appears to be increased.[4] Additionally, patients with breast cancer have an increased incidence of atherosclerosis and a higher than

Table 1 Risk Factors for and Clinical Manifestations of Aortic Aneurysmal Disease in Cancer Patients
Risk factors
Atherosclerosis
Radiation therapy
Hypertension
Diabetes
Hyperlipidemia
Genetic predisposition (family history)
Disseminated fungal infections (aspergillosis or mucormycosis)
Clinical presentation
Asymptomatic; detected on imaging studies (>50%)
Abdominal or flank pain
Early satiety
Retroperitoneal bleeding
Distal embolism/blue toe syndrome
Livido reticularis
Renal insufficiency

expected mortality.[11] Likewise, immunosuppression from chemotherapy increases the risk of disseminated fungal infections in cancer patients. Certain fungal infections, such as aspergillosis and mucormycosis, are angioinvasive and can result in aneurysmal changes in any vessel in the body (Figures 1 and 2).[12] The final common pathway for development of aneurysmal disease is insufficient elastin, collagen, or both that results in a weakened vessel wall. Once this process produces dilatation and resultant increased wall tension it will continue to progress. Ultimately, rupture is the end result if uncontrolled.

Diagnostic Approaches and Optimal Treatment

The increasing age of the population in general and specifically those being diagnosed with cancer has led to the more common occurrence of multiorgan disease. AAAs are more common in the elderly, and the concomitant occurrence of these two potentially lethal diseases always presents a therapeutic dilemma regarding the priority

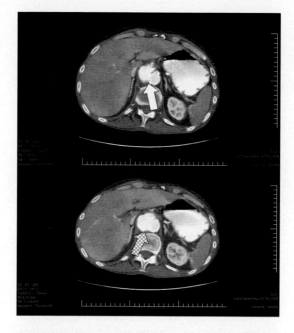

FIGURE 1 Two computed tomographic images of a ruptured mycotic aortic aneurysm in a patient with underlying atherosclerosis and hematologic malignancy. The *top image* indicates the area of rupture (*white arrow*), and the *bottom image* indicates the resultant pseudoaneurysm (*hatched white arrow*).

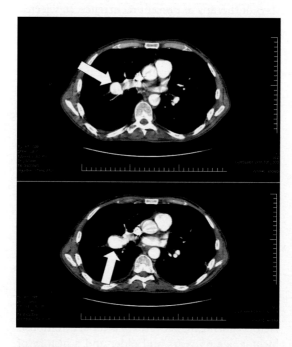

FIGURE 2 Two computed tomographipc images indicating a right pulmonary artery mycotic aneurysm that developed in a patient with a prolonged fungal illness. The *arrows* indicate the aneurysm.

of treatment. Intra-abdominal or thoracic malignancy may be discovered unexpectedly at laparotomy for elective treatment of an AAA and vice versa. The incidence of coexistence ranges from as low as 0.5% to as high as 22% depending on the patient population. Of note, in one study, 22% of patients were found to have abdominal malignancy at the time of AAA repair.[13,14]

Although it is generally agreed that both lesions should be treated to achieve optimal life expectancy, significant uncertainty revolves around whether to treat them simultaneously or as staged procedures. A risk of postoperative rupture of the aneurysm exists when the malignancy is resected first. On the other hand, contamination by gastrointestinal or urinary tract contents may infect the prosthetic graft during simultaneous surgery. Additionally, delaying necessary cancer surgery for approximately 2 months to allow recovery after aneurysmectomy may result in a poorer cancer outcome.

The general principles of surgical approaches for concomitant AAA and intra-abdominal cancer depend on (1) the urgency of the operation, (2) the site and staging of the malignant lesion, (3) the size and location of the aortic aneurysm, and (4) the projected long-term survival of the patient. Aneurysms over 6 cm in diameter pose a greater threat for rupture to the patient and should be treated, initially or simultaneously, in view of the high risk of rupture. This may include a percutaneous repair with a stent graft placement (Figure 3). In many situations, this may be an ideal choice owing to comorbidities.[15] On the other hand, aneurysms of less than 5 cm are usually not life-threatening, and unnecessary reparative surgery may significantly delay the treatment of cancer. For AAAs between 5 and 6 cm in diameter, a multidisciplinary approach to address relative risks would be recommended to determine a strategy. Simultaneous resection, by way of segregated approaches, is useful in some patients with early intra-abdominal cancer. However, eventually both lesions must be resected for improvement of the long-term survival.[16] When both lesions are complicated, a case for simultaneous treatment may be appropriate.[17] Many authors

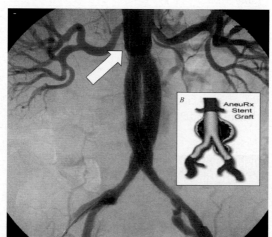

FIGURE 3 *A*, An abdominal aortogram showing the AneuRx (Medtronic Vascular, Santa Rosa, CA) stent graft with the cephalic portion deployed just below renal arteries (*white arrow*) and the caudal end anchored in the common iliac arteries. Proximal stenosis of the left internal iliac artery is noted. *B*, A cartoon depiction of the AneuRx stent graft.

believe that simultaneous AAA repair and resection of an associated, unexpected abdominal neoplasm can be safely performed in most of the patients, sparing the need for a second procedure, except for malignancies requiring major surgical resections.[18]

In patients who are considered too ill for an open AAA repair, endovascular grafting may be a valuable tool in simplifying simultaneous treatment or in staging the procedures with a very short delay.[19] Since the approval of endoluminal grafts for treatment of AAA, endoluminal aortic repair has gained increasing popularity as an alternative to traditional open surgery in the setting of associated malignancy and multiple comorbid conditions. However, despite well-documented, good, early results and the benefits of endoluminal stent graft repair of AAA,[20] the role of endovascular stent grafting in patients with challenging medical and anatomic problems remains a developing area. Some concern has been expressed regarding technical failure and the durability of endovascular grafts, although, overall, the reports are promising.

Many patients with AAA may also have aneurysms at multiple sites within the aorta, for example, thoracoabdominal (TAA) and aortoiliac aneurysms.[3,21] Repair of TAA presents additional challenges secondary to obligate intraoperative visceral, renal, and spinal cord ischemia. Various novel operative techniques for sequential visceral revascularization and reconstruction have been attempted.[22] Others have reported success with endovascular treatment of TAA combined with a simultaneous open AAA repair. In general, patients with at least one of the following categories are considered to be at high risk: age more than 80 years, renal insufficiency (creatinine > 2.0 mg/dl), multivessel coronary artery disease, poor left ventricular function, poor pulmonary reserve, reoperative aortic procedure, a "hostile" abdomen, or an emergent operation.[23] In the case of patients with an aortoiliac aneurysm and a concurrent gastrointestinal tumor, not an infrequent occurrence, there is less of a therapeutic challenge; these patients can be managed as discussed previously, and a multidisciplinary approach is encouraged. With appropriate care to identify high-risk patients, it is feasible to do synchronous conventional resection or use endoluminal techniques.

In summary, the concurrent presence of aortic aneurysmal disease and cancer is a not infrequent occurrence and presents a therapeutic challenge. The open repair of AAA continues to evolve with incorporation of less invasive methods for surgical exposure. Endovascular treatment presents an appealing alternative and will likely continue to develop as a preferred treatment for this condition. In cancer patients, as in the general population, the therapeutic decision remains an individualized approach with a multi-disciplinary input recommended to explore the best therapy for the patient.

Arterial Thromboembolism

The incidence of de novo arterial thromboembolic phenomenon is much lower than that of thrombotic events in the venous system; however, the risk is several-fold higher in cancer patients compared with the general population.[24] This high incidence may be attributable to the general inflammatory condition associated with cancer[25,26] or may be the result of cancer therapy. Atherosclerosis is again the principal culprit when arterial insufficiency is noted; however, in the present and future of cancer therapy, in which antiangiogenesis is a focus, the risk of arterial insufficiency or thrombosis is likely to be increased.[27] An increased awareness and attention to arterial thrombotic events are therefore necessary. There is no better example to illustrate this point than the issues related to rofecoxib and celecoxib, which revealed increased serious arterial thrombotic events in cancer prevention trials.[28–30]

Clinical Manifestations

The complications related to arterial thromboembolism differ significantly from those related to venous thrombosis, mostly owing to the organs supplied by the respective tissues. This could include unstable angina, acute myocardial infarction, stroke, arterial insufficiency, ischemic colitis, and progressive renal insufficiency in specific clinical situations (Table 2). Disseminated intravascular coagulation and marantic endocarditis (Figure 4) are late-stage manifestations of these processes in cancer patients.[31]

Pathophysiologic Mechanisms

In contrast to altered blood flow that may result in venous stasis, arterial thrombosis typically stems from endothelial injury and platelet activation, especially in the presence of atherosclerosis.[32] Platelet activation, rather than inherited hypercoagulability, plays a dominant role in arterial thromboembolism. This may explain the increase in arterial thrombosis in patients with cancer since disorders of platelet number and function

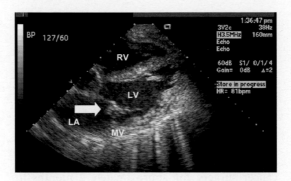

FIGURE 4 Echocardiography indicating marantic endocarditis (*white arrow*), with the left ventricle (LV), mitral valve (MV), right ventricle (RV), and left atrium (LA) indicated in a patient with multiple embolic phenomena or events.

are common in these patients. Arterial thrombosis tends to occur more commonly in hypertensive patients at sites of turbulent blood flow, primarily owing to endothelial injury associated with shearing forces at points of narrowing and branching in the arterial tree. Other pathogenetic mechanisms for arterial thrombosis and thromboembolism include nonbacterial endocarditis,[33] autoimmune vasculitis, aortic aneurysms, the presence of mechanical prosthetic valves, sustained spasm of arteries, precipitation of cryoglobulins or other abnormal proteins in small arteries, direct tumor invasion of arteries, fragmentation and embolization of intracardiac or intra-arterial metastases, and spontaneous arterial thrombosis owing to hypercoagulability.[34,35] Growth factor administration may stimulate atherosclerosis[36] or a hypercoagulable state.[37] It should be noted that hyperhomocysteinemia and the antiphospholipid syndromes are risk factors for both arterial and venous thrombosis (Table 3).

Diagnostic Approaches and Optimal Treatment

Diagnostic approaches to arterial embolic phenomenon in the cancer patient require a high level of suspicion. At times, the ischemic tissue is plainly evident and diagnostic strategies are

obvious. Common locations for arterial thrombi include the cerebral vasculature (stroke), coronary arteries (myocardial infarction or unstable angina), mesenteric arteries (ischemic bowel), and renal arteries (renal insufficiency with casts). These conditions are discussed in greater detail in other sections of this text. In many other clinical situations, the diagnosis of arterial embolism may not be as obvious and frequently eludes diagnosis until there is marked deterioration. For instance, worsening hypertension or proteinuria may be an early indicator of arterial embolic disease to the renal arteries. Livido reticularis, a characteristic rash usually apparent on the lower extremities, may be a harbinger of ischemic vascular injury. Typical risk factors for vascular disease, which are commonly present in those who develop embolic phenomenon, likely contribute in a significant manner.

Various methods of diagnosis and treatment of these conditions have been discussed elsewhere in this text (see Chapter 5). Therapeutic approaches should therefore include aggressive vascular risk factor modification with lipid reduction therapy (particularly statins), control of diabetes and hypertension, and an exercise program. Acetylsalicylic acid and clopidogrel are the mainstays of therapy to prevent recurrence. In selected patients, warfarin-based therapy may be chosen; however, there is an associated increased bleeding risk to consider. In patients with critical limb ischemia, revascularization may be necessary by the usual surgical or percutaneous techniques, and, in general, these approaches are effective. The key for success in management involves prevention of these end-organ manifestations.

It is being recognized that cancer therapy–induced arterial thrombosis may be a separate entity to consider. For example, the results from randomized controlled studies show that patients with colorectal cancer receiving bevacizumab (Avastin) in addition to 5-fluorouracil infusional therapy had a twofold higher risk of serious arterial thromboembolic events, including cerebrovascular accident (stroke), myocardial infarction, transient ischemic attack, and angina, with an estimated overall risk of 5%. Risk factors causing higher rates of arterial thrombosis include age 65 years and older and a history of arterial thromboembolism prior to bevacizumab therapy.[38] The overall effect of this medication is beneficial in selected cancer patients,[39,40] understanding that the increased risk of thrombosis and developing a strategy for minimizing these complications may lead to an even greater beneficial outcome for patients.

Venous Thromboembolism in Cancer Patients

Cancer is inextricably intertwined with thromboembolic phenomenon. Thrombi are solid masses

Table 2 Manifestations of Arterial Thromboembolism in Cancer Patients
Unstable angina
Acute myocardial infarction
Cerebrovascular accident (stroke)
Arterial insufficiency
Progressive renal insufficiency
Ischemic colitis
Disseminated intravascular coagulation
Marantic endocarditis

Table 3 Pathophysiologic Mechanisms for Arterial Thromboembolism in Cancer Patients
Platelet activation
Inherited or acquired hypercoagulability
Vasculitis
Arterial spasm
Cryoglobulinemia
Tumor invasion
Antiphospholipid syndrome
Hyperhomocysteinemia
Atherosclerosis
Compression of vascular bed by tumors

composed of platelets, insoluble fibrin, and entrapped red blood cells that form on flow disturbed endovascular surfaces. By definition, a thrombus is attached to vascular endothelium or to endocardium and a thromboembolus is a detached fragment of a thrombus that is carried forward to occlude a smaller vessel. This association of cancer and thromboembolism was noted 140 years ago by Armand Trousseau. He described phlegmasia alba dolens or migratory thrombophlebitis as a sign of internal malignancy.[41] Recurrent thromboembolism in cancer patients frequently interferes with the management of cancer and the patients' quality of life and may be massive, resulting in death despite early and aggressive treatment. Cancer is usually associated with other known risk factors for thromboembolism, such as old age, extensive surgery, and decreased mobility, all of which increase the risk of thromboembolic disease in these patients. It has been noted, for example, that the incidence of thromboembolism is up to 5 to 7% in breast cancer patients compared with approximately 0.1% in the general population.[42] Furthermore, patients with cancer represent 15 to 20% of all patients with thrombosis; additionally, 10% of patients with venous thromboembolism (VTE) are diagnosed with malignancy in a 2-year period.[43,44] Hence, approximately one-quarter of all VTE are related to malignancy.

Clinical Manifestations

The symptoms and signs of VTE are caused by obstruction to venous flow, vascular inflammation, or embolization. The most common presentation of venous thromboembolic disease in cancer patients is unilateral leg edema. This is usually associated with redness and warmth in the affected extremity. Many patients with cancer, however, do not complain of pain and calf tenderness. A confounding, or perhaps coexistent, condition is cellulitis, and cancer patients with profound immunosuppression are certainly at higher risk of developing this condition. It is not uncommon that patients may develop bilateral lower extremity edema as a manifestation of VTE, but other conditions, such as congestive heart failure, should be considered in that instance. Additionally, thrombosis may be evident in unusual locations, such as the upper extremity,[45] right atrium (Figure 5), or even the internal jugular veins (Figure 6). The most common clinical manifestation of a pulmonary embolus is sudden onset of shortness of breathing and tachypnea. This may be accompanied by pleuritic chest pain, cough, and possibly hemoptysis. Occlusion of small pulmonary arterioles leading to segmental pulmonary infarction may go unnoticed. On the other hand, obstruction of the main pulmonary

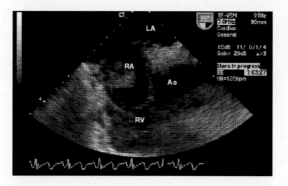

FIGURE 5 A transesophageal echocardiogram with a thrombus evident (*white arrow*) attached to the right atrium (RA). Ao = aorta; LA = left atrium. , RV = right ventricle.

artery by a large thromboembolus can cause acute right ventricular failure, cardiogenic shock, and death (Figure 7). Other clinical consequences of venous thrombosis and thromboembolism include pulmonary hypertension, postphlebitic syndrome, and peripheral venous insufficiency (Table 4).

Pathophysiology of the Coagulation Abnormalities in Cancer

The pathophysiology of thromboembolism in cancer is not clearly understood. It is known that several changes in the coagulation cascade may contribute to this complex phenomenon, resulting in hypercoagulability. In general, the mechanisms involved in thrombus formation include endothelial injury, alterations in blood flow, or hypercoagulability. Normal hemostasis is a balance between opposing coagulative and fibrinolytic mechanisms within intact blood vessels. Intact vascular endothelium produces coagulation inhibitors such as prostacyclin and endothelium-derived nitric oxide, which inhibit intravascular platelet aggregation. Heparin-like molecules on the endothelial surface combine with the plasma antithrombin III to inactivate thrombin, factors Xa and IXa, and most other

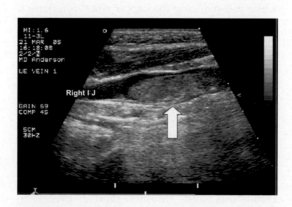

FIGURE 6 A carotid sonogram showing the right internal jugular vein (Right I J) with a thrombus present (*white arrow*).

Table 4 Clinical Manifestations of Venous Thromboembolic Disease in Cancer Patients

Unilateral/bilateral extremity swelling, pain, or numbness
Sudden onset of shortness of breath
Hemoptysis
Pulmonary hypertension
Facial edema
Chronic venous stasis
Sinus tachycardia
Right heart failure
Ascites
Shock
Death

coagulation factors. Another cell surface molecule, thrombomodulin, binds to thrombin. This complex prevents the conversion of fibrinogen to fibrin and activates two other naturally occurring anticoagulants, protein C and protein S, which degrade activated factors V and VIII. Additionally, laminar blood flow without turbulence maintains the platelets in the center and away from the vessel wall, which prevents activation on contact with the endothelium.

Once formed, a thrombus may progress in a variety of stages: (1) the fibrinolytic system may completely degrade the clot, allowing normal blood flow to return, that is, resolution; (2) the thrombus may accumulate more fibrin and platelets and grow along the course of the vessel, that is, propagation (an example is a calf vein thrombus that propagates into the thigh and pelvis becoming high risk of embolism); (3) the thrombus may become incorporated into the vessel wall by the process of fibrosis, that is, organization (an example of this process is postphlebitic syndrome or chronic venous insufficiency); and (4) the thrombus may be partially resorbed despite occlusion of the vessel, resulting in restoration of blood flow, that is, recanalization.[46]

In the specific instance of cancer, neoplastic cells may activate platelets and coagulation proteases by secreting adenosine diphosphate–like activating substances and expressing tissue factor on exposed membrane surfaces.[47] Many cancers generate procoagulants such as tissue factor or enzymes that activate plasma coagulation factors. Levels of protein C and antithrombin III, which are natural anticoagulants, are decreased in malignancy.[48] Tumor necrosis factor and other substances secreted by malignancies induce the release of intracellular tissue thromboplastin into the bloodstream,[42] which promotes thrombin formation. There may be increased turnover of clotting factors such as fibrinogen and factors V, VIII, IX, and XI in patients with malignancy.[49,50] Mucin and the proteases secreted by malignant cells may activate factor X.[51] Thrombocytosis and megakaryocyte hyperplasia are known to be associated with lung, breast, gastric, and ovarian cancers and in Hodgkin's disease.[52] Furthermore, some substances secreted by various human tumors can directly stimulate the aggregation of platelets.[53] The treatment of cancer may also induce abnormalities in the levels of endogenous anticoagulant factors. Levels of protein C and S may be decreased in breast cancer patients treated with cyclophosphamide, methotrexate, and 5-fluorouracil.[54] Similarly, tamoxifen decreases antithrombin III.[55] Corticosteroids are not only known to decrease the platelet count and the levels of clotting factor VIII–von Willebrand factor complex; they may also inhibit blood fibrinolytic activity[56] and decrease the clearance rate of activated clotting factors by reticuloendothelial blockade.[57] The use of estrogen and progesterone agents promotes thrombosis in patients by decreasing coagulation inhibitors antithrombin III, protein C, and protein S. Furthermore, advanced metastatic disease may induce disseminated intravascular coagulation by unknown causes (Table 5).

As a result of these complex interactions, it is clear that thrombus formation is a multifactorial process, but its predisposition is clinically identifiable. In general, well-known risk factors for the development of VTE include prolonged immobilization (bed rest, stroke, prolonged travel), surgical and nonsurgical traumas (including burns), congestive heart failure, pregnancy, estrogen therapy, age over 50 years, malignancy, a history of previous deep venous thrombosis (DVT), acute infectious disease, and immunologic or inherited disorders, such as protein S, protein C, and antithrombin III deficiency.[58,59]

Increased Risk of Venous Thrombosis Unique to Cancer Patients

The presence of cancer itself increases the risk of recurrent thromboembolic disease threefold,[60] more so with metastasis.[61] For example, patients with liver and massive retroperitoneal metastases have more thromboembolic events than those without them. In patients with metastatic liver disease, a predisposing factor for the development of thromboembolism may be the impaired

Table 5 Altered Factors in Malignancy Promoting Thrombosis

Reduced Anticoagulants	Increased Thrombotic Factors
Protein C	Activated platelets
Antithrombin III	Tissue factor
Protein S	Thromboplastin
	Activated factor X
	Thrombocytosis
	Reduced reticuloendothelial system
	Thrombin production
	Factor VIII and fibrinogen

clearance of activated coagulation factors and the decreased synthesis of anticoagulants in the liver.[62] Large retroperitoneal metastases, on the other hand, may increase the risk of thrombosis by mechanical obstruction of the femoral and abdominal vessels.

Similarly, the treatment of cancer may increase the risk of both arterial and venous thromboembolism through a variety of mechanisms,[24] including administration of prothrombotic medications, the placement of long-term venous catheters, and residual mechanical effects resulting from the underlying cancer, as well as the treatment or complications therein.[35]

Prothrombotic Medications in Cancer Patients

In terms of medications with prothrombotic effects, several are known from clinical experience, although there are likely to be many others in which the association is either not established or not suspected at present. Tamoxifen, for example, widely used in the treatment of estrogen receptor–positive breast cancer, is known to be associated with a several-fold increase in thromboembolism.[63–67] The risk of venous and arterial thromboembolism is even higher in patients receiving tamoxifen in combination with chemotherapy compared with those receiving tamoxifen or chemotherapy alone.[64] This increased incidence of venous and arterial thromboembolic complications is more prevalent in premenopausal patients receiving combination therapy. In addition, postmenopausal women also have a higher incidence of venous thromboembolic complications when receiving tamoxifen and chemotherapy compared with those receiving tamoxifen alone.[64] These data, taken together, may suggest that tamoxifen may be dangerous; however, the recurrence rate of breast cancer is markedly reduced with tamoxifen, and, when taken in context, the benefit from cancer reduction outweighs the risk of thrombosis.[68] Furthermore, newer agents, such as raloxifene, may be superior to tamoxifen regarding thrombosis while still reducing the cancer risk.[69] Similarly, a higher incidence of arterial thrombosis has also been reported with multiagent chemotherapy in patients with breast cancer,[63] but it is still unclear if this is due to the medication or the disease itself. Other medications associated with a higher than expected rate of thrombosis include the use of cytokines and hematopoietic growth factors.[36,37,48,70] Furthermore, the use of high-dose corticosteroids and administration of intravenous contrast medium are recognized risk factors for the development of both arterial and venous thrombosis and thromboembolic events in cancer patients.[71–73] Corticosteroids, especially dexamethasone at a dosage of 80 mg or higher per cycle of chemotherapy, increase thromboembolic

complications.[71–74] Thalidomide, a medication used to treat multiple myeloma, is known to significantly increase the rate of venous thrombosis, and current practice includes prophylactic anticoagulation to prevent this complication.[75–77] A burgeoning area of cancer therapy includes antiangiogenic medications intended to decrease the blood supply to specific tumors. It stands to reason that this therapeutic aim will likely have an important impact on vasculature throughout the body. In fact, early studies have confirmed this suspicion. Bevacizumab has been associated with increased thrombotic events and substantial hypertension, although it appears to be effective in reducing cancer recurrence.[78,79] New chemotherapy agents or combinations of established medications should continue to be monitored for an increased risk of thromboembolism.

Catheter-Related Venous Thrombosis

The placement of indwelling long-term central venous catheters is common in cancer patients to aid in administration of chemotherapy, antibiotics, or other drugs. However, an indwelling central venous catheter substantially increases the risk of thromboembolism. The reported incidence of symptomatic catheter-related DVT in adult patients varies from 0.3 to 28.3%.[80,81] These patients are prone to two kinds of catheter-related thromboembolism: sleeve thrombi that build around the indwelling catheters[82] and intraluminal thrombi that build inside the lumen of the catheter.[83] Potential risk factors include the size of the catheter, the position of the catheter, and the site of insertion.[84] The type of chemotherapy appears to influence the rate of catheter-associated thrombosis. Infusion of sclerosing chemotherapy through the catheter increases the risk of thrombosis compared with those patients treated with nonsclerosing chemotherapy.[85] Catheter-associated venous thrombi may partially or completely occlude the blood vessel. In symptomatic patients, swelling or pain of the arm or neck, erythema and numbness of the extremity, jaw pain, and headache may be the presenting symptoms. The prevalence of pulmonary embolism in patients with an upper extremity venous thrombosis is high, and it is close to that observed in cohorts of patients with lower extremity DVT.[86]

Mechanical Effects of Cancer Resulting in Thrombosis

There are many potential examples of how mechanical impingement or obstruction may result in venous thrombosis. Certainly, a large pelvic tumor can physically compress the iliac veins, resulting in lower extremity DVT. Any other location in which a tumor results in compression has the potential for a similar thrombotic complication. These include splenic or hepatic vein thrombosis. An extraordinary example of this concept is a superior vena cava (SVC) thrombosis or SVC syndrome, which is an emergent condition. It is caused by direct invasion and/or compression of the SVC, typically from an intrathoracic malignancy (> 90% of cases). Although any cancer involving the intrathoracic lymph nodes may result in compression of the SVC, the most common cause (67%) is related to advanced lung cancer (particularly right upper lobe tumors or those with paratracheal adenopathy), lymphomas (20%), and metastatic solid malignancy (5%).[87] Some patients may present with an SVC syndrome as their first indication of cancer. Rarely, thrombosis related to a central venous catheter may contribute to an SVC syndrome.

The clinical features of SVC syndrome include swelling of the face, neck, and upper arm; cyanosis; and papilledema and may be associated with shortness of breath and cough. It may very rapidly progress to obstruct the airway, necessitating assisted ventilation. Typically, a complete history and physical examination often reveals the diagnosis of SVC syndrome in a patient with known intrathoracic malignancy; however, additional confirmatory tests are performed, including radiography (a widened mediastinum or a mass in the right side of the chest), computed tomography (CT), or magnetic resonance imaging (MRI) of the chest. CT has replaced invasive contrast venography and may guide attempts at biopsy by mediastinoscopy, bronchoscopy, or percutaneous fine-needle aspiration. It should be kept in mind that biopsy presents an increased risk of bleeding in patients with SVC syndrome secondary to elevated central venous pressure. Sputum cytology and biopsy of a palpable supraclavicular node may give diagnostic information in more than two-thirds of patients.

SVC syndrome may progress rapidly in cancer patients and requires prompt workup and treatment.[88,89] Intravenous steroids and local external beam radiation therapy may give rapid relief by reducing the obstructing mass. Chemotherapy and surgery may also be used in appropriate situations as primary management of SVC syndrome.[90–92] Palliative bypasses may be considered for symptoms that do not respond to medical therapy.[93] Survival in patients with SVC syndrome is related to the course of the underlying malignancy, and patients with untreated malignant SVC syndrome survive, on average, less than 30 days.[94]

Inferior vena cava (IVC) syndrome is a poorly characterized complication of intra-abdominal cancer. It has neither been commonly recognized nor adequately described. This syndrome results from occlusion of the IVC, either by external tumor compression (malignant hepatic enlargement, either secondary or primary), intraluminal tumor invasion (hypernephroma, hepatoma, and adrenal carcinoma), or propagation of thrombotic tumorous material in cancer patients.[95] Clinically, IVC syndrome is characterized by abrupt onset of ascites, bilateral lower extremity edema, and unusual patterns of dilated abdominal wall collateral veins. Up to one-third of patients have thromboembolic complications, but fatal pulmonary embolism is rarely reported. A high index of suspicion must accompany the evaluation of a patient at risk of IVC syndrome. Duplex ultrasonography, CT, or MRI usually yields the diagnosis, and venocavography is rarely needed. Patients with primary or secondary tumoral occlusion of the IVC are difficult to manage with safety and success. When IVC syndrome is identified, prophylactic anticoagulation is recommended. Although patient survival is generally short, life expectancy and treatment depend on the type of accompanying tumor. Nevertheless, their survival may be prolonged by an aggressive surgical approach, chemotherapy, or radiation. Intravascular stenting[96–98] is a rapidly expanding and useful palliative procedural option and will, at least partially, relieve the IVC pressure gradient in these unfortunate patients and provide symptomatic relief by improving lower extremity edema and ascites.

Diagnostic Approaches and Optimal Treatment

VTE is a common disorder associated with significant morbidity and mortality. In the case of patients with cancer, the concurrent mortality associated with DVT or pulmonary embolism is substantially higher than in those without cancer.[1,99] As a result, accurate diagnosis and treatment are crucial. Physical examination is often inadequate for establishing the diagnosis of VTE,[100] and, in most cases, noninvasive testing is needed as an adjunct to clinical assessment.[101] Venography is the diagnostic reference standard[102]; however, because of its invasive nature and technical difficulty, venography is rarely used for routine clinical evaluation of suspected DVT owing to sophisticated and reliable ultrasound techniques. Color flow venous duplex scanning of the proximal and distal veins performed by skilled operators provides the most practical and cost-effective method for assessing DVT of the proximal and distal lower extremity veins. Current ultrasound technology is able to image calf veins in the large majority of patients. Overall, venous duplex scanning has a very high sensitivity and specificity for the diagnosis of symptomatic proximal DVT (above 90%). This allows initiation or withholding anticoagulation treatment without further confirmatory tests. However, a normal bilateral proximal venous sonogram may not exclude a pelvic source of thrombosis. Even in the presence of objective evidence of pulmonary embolism, compression ultrasonography may detect DVT of the proximal lower extremity veins only in approximately 50% of patients.[46] Other less commonly used procedures to diagnose DVT include impedance plethysmography (IPG), CT, and MRI. IPG has a sensitivity for proximal DVT of approximately 65%[103] and was used as the initial noninvasive test for patients with suspected lower extremity DVT before the widespread use of venous duplex scanning.[104] The limitations of IPG include its failure to detect nonocclusive proximal DVT and those isolated to the calf veins or occlusive proximal DVT present in parallel venous systems.[105] Less commonly, a thrombus is noted in the cardiac chambers on echocardiography either related to a catheter or other pathology. Ventilation-perfusion scanning is still being used but is certainly being supplanted by CT angiography. Ultrasonography for extremity swelling has excellent sensitivity and specificity, whereas CT for pulmonary emboli and other organ thromboses is well established as the diagnostic procedure of choice.[68,101] The use of magnetic resonance angiography is also increasing but is limited to tertiary care centers.[106–108] Serologic testing with the measurement of D-dimer is very useful in the general population as a screen for thrombus, but the lack of specificity of the D-dimer assay for VTE in cancer patients warrants interpreting positive assay results with caution.[109]

The diagnostic approaches to venous thrombosis in cancer patients are no different from those for patients without cancer. The level of suspicion must be higher, but the techniques are similar. The diagnosis of catheter-associated DVT may be difficult, and Doppler ultrasonography has a lower accuracy in this setting than it does in symptomatic lower extremity venous thrombosis.[110] Therefore, when the suspicion for catheter-associated thrombosis is high, it should be objectively followed by venography or be treated empirically on clinical suspicion. Catheter-associated DVT (intraluminal) can be lysed in most situations (80–95%) with fibrinolytic agents such as urokinase, streptokinase, and tissue plasminogen activator,[111–114] but if there is a complicating line infection, this catheter will likely have to be removed.

Initiating antithrombotic therapy in cancer patients frequently presents a clinical dilemma. A variety of factors may contribute. These include: difficult venous access, increased risk of bleeding associated with warfarin, hepatic and renal dysfunction, thrombocytopenia, and other comorbid conditions are only a portion of the considerations that often complicate therapeutic decisions in patients with cancer. In general, antithrombotic therapy involves the use of thrombolytics, anticoagulants, and antiplatelet medications. Thrombolytic therapy removes an established thrombus, whereas anticoagulants and antiplatelet drugs are mostly used to prevent or limit the propagation of a thrombus. The treatment of thromboembolism varies significantly depending on which portion of the circulatory system (venous or arterial) is involved; the size and location of the thrombus; the risks of extension, embolization, or recurrence; and the benefits of therapy while balancing the risks of hemorrhage.

Guidelines for antithrombotic therapy for VTE have been published by the Seventh American College of Chest Physicians.[115] Standard treatment for acute VTE traditionally uses low-molecular-weight heparin, unfractionated intravenous heparin, or adjusted-dose subcutaneous heparin, followed by long-term therapy with an oral anticoagulant.[116] The use of unfractionated heparin has been replaced by low-molecular-weight heparin as the first-line treatment in the majority of cancer patients with VTE and cancer, in the hospital or as an outpatient. Long-term oral anticoagulation with warfarin may be complicated by several factors, including drug-drug interactions, malnutrition, nausea and vomiting during chemotherapy, and thrombocytopenia. Additionally, hepatic dysfunction coexisting in cancer patients either from a primary tumor or secondary to chemotherapy may lead to unpredictable levels of anticoagulation, resulting in increased bleeding complications. Recent studies suggest that low-molecular-weight heparin may be more efficient when compared with oral anticoagulant therapy with coumarin for the prevention of recurrent

VTE in patients with cancer who had acute, symptomatic, proximal DVT, pulmonary embolism, or both.[44] Furthermore, low-molecular-weight heparin allows easy dose adjustment, has predictable pharmacokinetic properties, does not require routine laboratory monitoring, and has fewer drug interactions compared with oral anticoagulants. There have also been reports that heparins have antiproliferative, antiangiogenic, antimetastatic effects and that low-molecular-weight heparin may increase the response to chemotherapy and prolong the survival of cancer patients.[117] Thus, secondary prophylaxis with low-molecular-weight heparin may be a more effective and feasible alternative to oral anticoagulant therapy,[44] although the risk of bleeding is not different between the two groups. Very recently, in patients with polycythemia vera, low-dose acetylsalicylic acid has been safely used to prevent thrombotic complications[118] and has been suggested as an alternative option in patients with cancer presenting with paraneoplastic thrombocytosis, who have no contraindications to such treatment.

Recent data suggest that certain anticoagulants might also improve cancer survival rates independently of their effect on thromboembolism.[119,120] New antithrombotic agents, such as oral direct thrombin or long-acting synthetic factor Xa inhibitor, may be useful in cancer patients.[121,122] Furthermore, mechanical treatments, such as compression stockings, used to prevent post-thrombotic syndrome,[123] have value, as well as selected surgical techniques to treat venous ulceration to improve outcomes.[124] In patients with recurrent DVT or in whom the risk of serious bleeding is high, vena cava filters may be employed instead of anticoagulation.[125] It is known that vena cava filters have inherent risks[126] and should be limited to patients with specific contraindications to anticoagulation. Other factors to consider include the life expectancy and quality of life of a cancer patient and the patient's preferences for therapy.

Conclusion

Vascular disease in a cancer patient represents a unique and special entity. Pathogenesis of various vascular and thromboembolic mechanisms may be a feature of the primary malignancy, related to the growth and metastasis of cancer. Patients undergoing chemotherapy or radiation therapy for cancer also mandate a high index of suspicion for thromboembolic complications, and therapy may need to be carefully considered when compared with the general population.

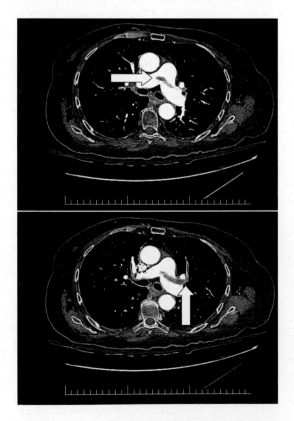

FIGURE 7 Computed tomographic angiographic images of a massive (saddle) pulmonary embolus, indicated by the *white arrows*.

REFERENCES

1. Levitan N, Dowlati A, Remick SC, et al. Rates of initial and recurrent thromboembolic disease among patients with malignancy versus those without malignancy. Risk analysis using Medicare claims data. Medicine (Baltimore) 1999;78:285–91.

2. Piccirillo JF, Tierney RM, Costas I, et al. Prognostic importance of comorbidity in a hospital-based cancer registry. JAMA 2004;291:2441–7.

3. Isselbacher EM. Thoracic and abdominal aortic aneurysms. Circulation 2005;111:816–28.

4. Hull MC, Morris CG, Pepine CJ, Mendenhall NP. Valvular dysfunction and carotid, subclavian, and coronary artery disease in survivors of Hodgkin lymphoma treated with radiation therapy. JAMA 2003;290:2831–7.

5. Giordano SH, Kuo YF, Freeman JL, et al. Risk of cardiac death after adjuvant radiotherapy for breast cancer. J Natl Cancer Inst 2005;97:419–24.

6. Ernemann U, Herrmann C, Plontke S, et al. Pseudoaneurysm of the superior thyroid artery following radiotherapy for hypopharyngeal cancer. Ann Otol Rhinol Laryngol 2003;112:188–90.

7. Auyeung KM, Lui WM, Chow LC, Chan FL. Massive epistaxis related to petrous carotid artery pseudoaneurysm after radiation therapy: emergency treatment with covered stent in two cases. AJNR Am J Neuroradiol 2003; 24:1449–52.

8. Ernst CB. Abdominal aortic aneurysm. N Engl J Med 1993; 328:1167–72.

9. Johansson G, Nydahl S, Olofsson P, Swedenborg J. Survival in patients with abdominal aortic aneurysms. Comparison between operative and nonoperative management. Eur J Vasc Surg 1990;4:497–502.

10. Ouriel K, Green RM, Donayre C, et al. An evaluation of new methods of expressing aortic aneurysm size: relationship to rupture. J Vasc Surg 1992;15:12–8; discussion 19–20.

11. Markopoulos C, Mantas D, Revenas K, et al. Breast arterial calcifications as an indicator of systemic vascular disease. Acta Radiol 2004;45:726–9.

12. Ishikawa T, Kazumata K, Ni-iya Y, et al. Subarachnoid hemorrhage as a result of fungal aneurysm at the posterior communicating artery associated with occlusion of the internal carotid artery: case report. Surg Neurol 2002;58: 261–5.

13. Kurata S, Nawata K, Nawata S, et al. Surgery for abdominal aortic aneurysms associated with malignancy. Surg Today 1998;28:895–9.

14. Carro C, Camilleri L, Garcier JM, De Riberolles C. Periaortic lymphoma mimicking aortic aneurysm. Eur J Cardiothorac Surg 2004;25:1126.

15. Murtagh BM, Lenihan DJ, Smalling R. Endovascular repair of abdominal aortic aneurysms: is this the method of choice? Am J Med Sci 2005;330(4):184-91.

16. Komori K, Okadome K, Funahashi S, et al. Surgical strategy of concomitant abdominal aortic aneurysm and gastric cancer. J Vasc Surg 1994;19:573–6.

17. Morris HL, da Silva AF. Co-existing abdominal aortic aneurysm and intra-abdominal malignancy: reflections on the order of treatment. Br J Surg 1998;85:1185–90.

18. Illuminati G, Calio FG, D'Urso A, et al. Simultaneous repair of abdominal aortic aneurysm and resection of unexpected, associated abdominal malignancies. J Surg Oncol 2004;88:234–9.

19. Jordan WD, Alcocer F, Wirthlin DJ, et al. Abdominal aortic aneurysms in "high-risk" surgical patients: comparison of open and endovascular repair. Ann Surg 2003;237:623–9; discussion 629–30.

20. Dattilo JB, Brewster DC, Fan CM, et al. Clinical failures of endovascular abdominal aortic aneurysm repair: incidence, causes, and management. J Vasc Surg 2002;35: 1137–44.

21. Williamson AE, Annunziata G, Cone LA, Smith J. Endovascular repair of a ruptured abdominal aortic and iliac artery aneurysm with an acute iliocaval fistula secondary to lymphoma. Ann Vasc Surg 2002;16:145–9.

22. Ballard JL, Abou-Zamzam AM Jr, Teruya TH. Type III and IV thoracoabdominal aortic aneurysm repair: results of a trifurcated/two-graft technique. J Vasc Surg 2002;36: 211–6; discussion 216.

23. Szmidt J, Rowinski O, Galazka Z, et al. Simultaneous endovascular exclusion of thoracic aortic aneurysm with open abdominal aortic aneurysm repair. Eur J Vasc Endovasc Surg 2004;28:442–8.

24. Lip GY, Chin BS, Blann AD. Cancer and the prothrombotic state. Lancet Oncol 2002;3:27–34.

25. Naschitz JE, Yeshurun D, Abrahamson J, et al. Ischemic heart disease precipitated by occult cancer. Cancer 1992; 69:2712–20.

26. Mathews J, Goel R, Evans WK, et al. Arterial occlusion in patients with peripheral vascular disease treated with platinum-based regimens for lung cancer. Cancer Chemother Pharmacol 1997;40:19–22.

27. Hamilton DP. Genentech issues Avastin warning. Wall Street Journal 2004 August 16;4.

28. Solomon SD, McMurray JJ, Pfeffer MA, et al. Cardiovascular risk associated with celecoxib in a clinical trial for colorectal adenoma prevention. N Engl J Med 2005;352:1071–80.

29. Bresalier RS, Sandler RS, Quan H, et al. Cardiovascular events associated with rofecoxib in a colorectal adenoma chemoprevention trial. N Engl J Med 2005;352:1092–102.

30. Senior K. COX-2 inhibitors: cancer prevention or cardiovascular risk? Lancet Oncol 2005;6:68.

31. Colman RW, Rubin RN. Disseminated intravascular coagulation due to malignancy. Semin Oncol 1990;17:172–86.

32. Massberg S, Schulz C, Gawaz M. Role of platelets in the pathophysiology of acute coronary syndrome. Semin Vasc Med 2003;3:147–62.

33. Ondrias F, Slugen I, Valach A. Malignant tumors and embolizing paraneoplastic endocarditis. Neoplasma 1985;32:135–40.

34. Pathanjali Sharma PV, Babu SC, Shah PM, et al. Arterial thrombosis and embolism in malignancy. J Cardiovasc Surg (Torino) 1985;26:479–83.

35. Caine GJ, Stonelake PS, Rea D, Lip GY. Coagulopathic complications in breast cancer. Cancer 2003;98:1578–86.

36. Kang HJ, Kim HS, Zhang SY, et al. Effects of intracoronary infusion of peripheral blood stem-cells mobilised with granulocyte-colony stimulating factor on left ventricular systolic function and restenosis after coronary stenting in myocardial infarction: the MAGIC cell randomised clinical trial. Lancet 2004;363:751–6.

37. Fukumoto Y, Miyamoto T, Okamura T, et al. Angina pectoris occurring during granulocyte colony-stimulating factor-combined preparatory regimen for autologous peripheral blood stem cell transplantation in a patient with acute myelogenous leukaemia. Br J Haematol 1997;97:666–8.

38. Ratner M. Genentech discloses safety concerns over Avastin. Nat Biotechnol 2004;22:1198.

39. Bevacizumab combined with chemotherapy improves progression-free survival for patients with advanced breast cancer. Natl Cancer Inst News 2005 www.cancer.gov/newscenter/pressreleases/AvastinBreast.

40. Kabbinavar FF, Hambleton J, Mass RD, et al. Combined analysis of efficacy: the addition of bevacizumab to fluorouracil/leucovorin improves survival for patients with metastatic colorectal cancer. J Clin Oncol 2005.

41. Trousseau A. Clinique medicale de l'hotel-dieu de Paris. Paris: JB, Bailliére et fils; 1868.

42. Goodnough LT, Saito H, Manni A, et al. Increased incidence of thromboembolism in stage IV breast cancer patients treated with a five-drug chemotherapy regimen. A study of 159 patients. Cancer 1984;54:1264–8.

43. Prandoni P, Lensing AW, Buller HR, et al. Deep-vein thrombosis and the incidence of subsequent symptomatic cancer. N Engl J Med 1992;327:1128–33.

44. Lee AY, Levine MN, Baker RI, et al. Low-molecular-weight heparin versus a coumarin for the prevention of recurrent venous thromboembolism in patients with cancer. N Engl J Med 2003;349:146–53.

45. Elting LS, Escalante CP, Cooksley C, et al. Outcomes and cost of deep venous thrombosis among patients with cancer. Arch Intern Med 2004;164:1653–61.

46. Kearon C. Natural history of venous thromboembolism. Circulation 2003;107(23 Suppl 1):I22–30.

47. Uchiyama T, Matsumoto M, Kobayashi N. Studies on the pathogenesis of coagulopathy in patients with arterial thromboembolism and malignancy. Thromb Res 1990;59:955–65.

48. Nand S, Fisher SG, Salgia R, Fisher RI. Hemostatic abnormalities in untreated cancer: incidence and correlation with thrombotic and hemorrhagic complications. J Clin Oncol 1987;5:1998–2003.

49. Rickles FR, Levine M, Edwards RL. Hemostatic alterations in cancer patients. Cancer Metastasis Rev 1992;11:237–48.

50. Bell WR. The fibrinolytic system in neoplasia. Semin Thromb Hemost 1996;22:459–78.

51. Falanga A, Gordon SG. Isolation and characterization of cancer procoagulant: a cysteine proteinase from malignant tissue. Biochemistry 1985;24:5558–67.

52. Eichinger S, Bauer K. Coagulapathic complication of cancer. In: Bast RC, Gansler TS, Holland JF, Frei E, American Cancer Society, editors. Cancer medicine. 5th ed. Hamilton (ON): BC Decker; 2000. p. 2309–16.

53. Hara Y, Steiner M, Baldini MG. Characterization of the platelet-aggregating activity of tumor cells. Cancer Res 1980;40:1217–22.

54. Rogers JS II, Murgo AJ, Fontana JA, Raich PC. Chemotherapy for breast cancer decreases plasma protein C and protein S. J Clin Oncol 1988;6:276–81.

55. Enck RE, Rios CN. Tamoxifen treatment of metastatic breast cancer and antithrombin III levels. Cancer 1984;53:2607–9.

56. van Giezen JJ, Brakkee JG, Dreteler GH, et al. Dexamethasone affects platelet aggregation and fibrinolytic activity in rats at different doses which is reflected by their effect on arterial thrombosis. Blood Coagul Fibrinolysis 1994;5:249–55.

57. Gerrits WB, Prakke EM, van der Meer J, et al. Corticosteroids and experimental intravascular coagulation. Scand J Haematol 1974;13:5–10.

58. Heit JA, Silverstein MD, Mohr DN, et al. Risk factors for deep vein thrombosis and pulmonary embolism: a population-based case-control study. Arch Intern Med 2000;160:809–15.

59. Alikhan R, Cohen AT, Combe S, et al. Risk factors for venous thromboembolism in hospitalized patients with acute medical illness: analysis of the MEDENOX Study. Arch Intern Med 2004;164:963–8.

60. Hassan B, Tung K, Weeks R, Mead GM. The management of inferior vena cava obstruction complicating metastatic germ cell tumors. Cancer 1999;85:912–8.

61. Weijl NI, Rutten MF, Zwinderman AH, et al. Thromboembolic events during chemotherapy for germ cell cancer: a cohort study and review of the literature. J Clin Oncol 2000;18:2169–78.

62. Patrassi GM, Dal Bo Zanon R, Boscaro M, et al. Further studies on the hypercoagulable state of patients with Cushing's syndrome. Thromb Haemost 1985;54:518–20.

63. Wall JG, Weiss RB, Norton L, et al. Arterial thrombosis associated with adjuvant chemotherapy for breast carcinoma: a Cancer and Leukemia Group B study. Am J Med 1989;87:501–4.

64. Saphner T, Tormey DC, Gray R. Venous and arterial thrombosis in patients who received adjuvant therapy for breast cancer. J Clin Oncol 1991;9:286–94.

65. Fisher B, Redmond C, Wickerham DL, et al. Doxorubicin-containing regimens for the treatment of stage II breast cancer: the National Surgical Adjuvant Breast and Bowel Project experience. J Clin Oncol 1989;7:572–82.

66. Fisher B, Costantino JP, Wickerham DL, et al. Tamoxifen for prevention of breast cancer: report of the National Surgical Adjuvant Breast and Bowel Project P-1 Study. J Natl Cancer Inst 1998;90:1371–88.

67. Decensi A, Maisonneuve P, Rotmensz N, et al. Effect of tamoxifen on venous thromboembolic events in a breast cancer prevention trial. Circulation 2005;111:650–6.

68. Goldhaber SZ. Tamoxifen: preventing breast cancer and placing the risk of deep vein thrombosis in perspective. Circulation 2005;111:539–41.

69. Martino S, Cauley JA, Barrett-Connor E, et al. Continuing outcomes relevant to Evista: breast cancer incidence in postmenopausal osteoporotic women in a randomized trial of raloxifene. J Natl Cancer Inst 2004;96:1751–61.

70. Honegger H, Anderson N, Hewitt LA, Tullis JL. Antithrombin III profiles in malignancy, relationship primary tumors and metastatic sites. Thromb Haemost 1981;46:500–3.

71. Cosgriff SW. Thromboembolic complications associated with ACTH and cortisone therapy. J Am Med Assoc 1951;147:924–6.

72. Dawson P. Nonionic contrast agents and coagulation. Invest Radiol 1988;23 Suppl 2:S310–7.

73. Theodossiou C, Kroog G, Ettinghausen S, et al. Acute arterial thrombosis in a patient with breast cancer after chemotherapy with 5-fluorouracil, doxorubicin, leucovorin, cyclophosphamide, and interleukin-3. Cancer 1994;74:2808–10.

74. Kawachi Y, Watanabe A, Uchida T, et al. Acute arterial thrombosis due to platelet aggregation in a patient receiving granulocyte colony-stimulating factor. Br J Haematol 1996;94:413–6.

75. Yeh ET, Tong AT, Lenihan DJ, et al. Cardiovascular complications of cancer therapy: diagnosis, pathogenesis, and management. Circulation 2004;109:3122–31.

76. Rajkumar SV, Gertz MA, Lacy MQ, et al. Thalidomide as initial therapy for early-stage myeloma. Leukemia 2003;17:775–9.

77. Singhal S, Mehta J. Thalidomide in cancer. Biomed Pharmacother 2002;56:4–12.

78. Yang JC, Haworth L, Sherry RM, et al. A randomized trial of bevacizumab, an anti-vascular endothelial growth factor antibody, for metastatic renal cancer. N Engl J Med 2003;349:427–34.

79. Willett CG, Boucher Y, di Tomaso E, et al. Direct evidence that the VEGF-specific antibody bevacizumab has anti-vascular effects in human rectal cancer. Nat Med 2004;10:145–7.

80. Wesenberg F, Flaatten H, Janssen CW Jr. Central venous catheter with subcutaneous injection port (Port-A-Cath): 8 years clinical follow up with children. Pediatr Hematol Oncol 1993;10:233–9.

81. Lokich JJ, Becker B. Subclavian vein thrombosis in patients treated with infusion chemotherapy for advanced malignancy. Cancer 1983;52:1586–9.

82. Hoshal VL Jr, Ause RG, Hoskins PA. Fibrin sleeve formation on indwelling subclavian central venous catheters. Arch Surg 1971;102:253–8.

83. Balestreri L, De Cicco M, Matovic M, et al. Central venous catheter-related thrombosis in clinically asymptomatic oncologic patients: a phlebographic study. Eur J Radiol 1995;20:108–11.

84. Ray S, Stacey R, Imrie M, Filshie J. A review of 560 Hickman catheter insertions. Anaesthesia 1996;51:981–5.

85. Bern MM, Lokich JJ, Wallach SR, et al. Very low doses of warfarin can prevent thrombosis in central venous catheters. A randomized prospective trial. Ann Intern Med 1990;112:423–8.

86. Monreal M, Davant E. Thrombotic complications of central venous catheters in cancer patients. Acta Haematol 2001;106:69–72.

87. Chen JC, Bongard F, Klein SR. A contemporary perspective on superior vena cava syndrome. Am J Surg 1990;160:207–11.

88. Inoue H, Shohtsu A, Koide S, Ogawa J. Resection of the superior vena cava for primary lung cancer: 5 years' survival. Ann Thorac Surg 1990;50:661–2.

89. Dartevelle PG, Chapelier AR, Pastorino U, et al. Long-term follow-up after prosthetic replacement of the superior vena cava combined with resection of mediastinal-pulmonary malignant tumors. J Thorac Cardiovasc Surg 1991;102:259–65.

90. Pass HI, Pogrebniak HW, Steinberg SM, et al. Randomized trial of neoadjuvant therapy for lung cancer: interim analysis. Ann Thorac Surg 1992;53:992–8.

91. Rosell R, Gomez-Codina J, Camps C, et al. A randomized trial comparing preoperative chemotherapy plus surgery with surgery alone in patients with non-small-cell lung cancer. N Engl J Med 1994;330:153–8.

92. Roth JA, Fossella F, Komaki R, et al. A randomized trial comparing perioperative chemotherapy and surgery with surgery alone in resectable stage IIIA non-small-cell lung cancer. J Natl Cancer Inst 1994;86:673–80.

93. Moore WM Jr, Hollier LH, Pickett TK. Superior vena cava and central venous reconstruction. Surgery 1991;110:35–41.

94. Abner A. Approach to the patient who presents with superior vena cava obstruction. Chest 1993;103(4 Suppl):394S–7S.

95. Hartley JW, Awrich AE, Wong J, et al. Diagnosis and treatment of the inferior vena cava syndrome in advanced malignant disease. Am J Surg 1986;152:70–4.

96. Furui S, Sawada S, Kuramoto K, et al. Gianturco stent placement in malignant caval obstruction: analysis of factors for predicting the outcome. Radiology 1995;195:147–52.

97. Kim JK, Park SJ, Kim YH, et al. Experimental study of self-expandable metallic inferior vena caval stent crossing the renal vein in rabbits. Radiologic-pathologic correlation. Invest Radiol 1996;31:311–5.

98. Dondelinger RF, Goffette P, Kurdziel JC, Roche A. Expandable metal stents for stenoses of the vena cava and large veins. Semin Interv Radiol 1991;8:252-263.

99. Sorensen HT, Mellemkjaer L, Olsen JH, Baron JA. Prognosis of cancers associated with venous thromboembolism. N Engl J Med 2000;343:1846–50.

100. Hirsh J, Hoak J. Management of deep vein thrombosis and pulmonary embolism. A statement for healthcare professionals. Council on Thrombosis (in consultation with the Council on Cardiovascular Radiology), American Heart Association. Circulation 1996;93:2212–45.

101. Perrier A, Roy PM, Aujesky D, et al. Diagnosing pulmonary embolism in outpatients with clinical assessment, D-dimer measurement, venous ultrasound, and helical computed tomography: a multicenter management study. Am J Med 2004;116:291–9.

102. Hull R, Hirsh J, Sackett DL, et al. Clinical validity of a negative venogram in patients with clinically suspected venous thrombosis. Circulation 1981;64:622–5.

103. Ginsberg JS, Wells PS, Hirsh J, et al. Reevaluation of the sensitivity of impedance plethysmography for the detection of proximal deep vein thrombosis. Arch Intern Med 1994;154:1930–3.

104. Anderson DR, Lensing AW, Wells PS, et al. Limitations of impedance plethysmography in the diagnosis of clinically suspected deep-vein thrombosis. Ann Intern Med 1993; 118:25–30.

105. Kearon C, Julian JA, Newman TE, Ginsberg JS. Noninvasive diagnosis of deep venous thrombosis. McMaster Diagnostic Imaging Practice Guidelines Initiative. Ann Intern Med 1998;128:663–77.

106. Spritzer CE, Norconk JJ Jr, Sostman HD, Coleman RE. Detection of deep venous thrombosis by magnetic resonance imaging. Chest 1993;104:54–60.

107. Polak JF, Fox LA. MR assessment of the extremity veins. Semin Ultrasound CT MR 1999;20:36–46.

108. Evans AJ, Sostman HD, Witty LA, et al. Detection of deep venous thrombosis: prospective comparison of MR imaging and sonography. J Magn Reson Imaging 1996;6: 44–51.

109. Gaffney PJ, Perry MJ. Unreliability of current serum fibrin degradation product (FDP) assays. Thromb Haemost 1985;53:301–2.

110. Bona RD. Central line thrombosis in patients with cancer. Curr Opin Pulm Med 2003;9:362–6.

111. Hurtubise MR, Bottino JC, Lawson M, McCredie KB. Restoring patency of occluded central venous catheters. Arch Surg 1980;115:212–3.

112. Lawson M, Bottino J, Hurtubise M. The use of urokinase to restore patency of occluded central venous catheters. Am J Intraven Ther Clin Nutr 1982;9:29–32.

113. Frank DA, Meuse J, Hirsch D, et al. The treatment and outcome of cancer patients with thromboses on central venous catheters. J Thromb Thrombolysis 2000;10: 271–5.

114. Kellam B, Fraze D, Kanarek KS. Clot lysis for thrombosed central venous catheters in pediatric patients. J Perinatol 1987;7:242–4.

115. Hirsh J, Guyatt G, Albers GW, Schunemann HJ. The Seventh ACCP Conference on Antithrombotic and Thrombolytic Therapy: evidence-based guidelines. Chest 2004;126 (3 Suppl):172S–3S.

116. Hyers TM, Agnelli G, Hull RD, et al. Antithrombotic therapy for venous thromboembolic disease. Chest 2001;119 (1 Suppl):176S–93S.

117. Smorenburg SM, van Noorden CJ. The complex effects of heparins on cancer progression and metastasis in experimental studies. Pharmacol Rev 2001;53:93–105.

118. Landolfi R, Marchioli R, Kutti J, et al. Efficacy and safety of low-dose aspirin in polycythemia vera. N Engl J Med 2004;350:114–24.

119. Falanga A. Biological and clinical aspects of anticancer effects of antithrombotics. Pathophysiol Haemost Thromb 2003; 33:389–92.

120. Lee AY, Rickles FR, Julian JA, et al. Randomized comparison of low molecular weight heparin and coumarin derivatives on the survival of patients with cancer and venous thromboembolism. J Clin Oncol 2005;23:2123–9.

121. Hoppensteadt D, Walenga JM, Fareed J, Bick RL. Heparin, low-molecular-weight heparins, and heparin pentasaccharide: basic and clinical differentiation. Hematol Oncol Clin North Am 2003;17:313–41.

122. Fiessinger JN, Huisman MV, Davidson BL, et al. Ximelagatran vs low-molecular-weight heparin and warfarin for the treatment of deep vein thrombosis: a randomized trial. JAMA 2005;293:681–9.

123. Prandoni P, Lensing AW, Prins MH, et al. Below-knee elastic compression stockings to prevent the post-thrombotic syndrome: a randomized, controlled trial. Ann Intern Med 2004;141:249–56.

124. Barwell JR, Davies CE, Deacon J, et al. Comparison of surgery and compression with compression alone in chronic venous ulceration (ESCHAR study): randomised controlled trial. Lancet 2004;363:1854–9.

125. Levine M, Rickles FR. Treatment of venous thromboembolism in cancer patients. Haemostasis 1998;28 Suppl 3: 66–70.

126. Decousus H, Leizorovicz A, Parent F, et al. A clinical trial of vena caval filters in the prevention of pulmonary embolism in patients with proximal deep-vein thrombosis. Prevention du Risque d'Embolie Pulmonaire par Interruption Cave Study Group. N Engl J Med 1998;338: 409–15.

Hematologic Complications in Patients with Malignancy

Graeme A.M. Fraser, MD, MSc, FRCPC
Donald M. Arnold, MD, MSc, FRCPC
Agnes Y.Y. Lee, MD, MSc, FRCPC

Hematologic complications are common in patients with cancer and can also complicate and potentially compromise cancer treatment. Furthermore, the morbidity of febrile neutropenic episodes, the risk of hemorrhagic and thrombotic events, and the potential hazards associated with blood product transfusions can further compromise the patients' quality of life. Although some of these clinical problems are due to the malignancy, many are iatrogenic and secondary to treatments for the cancer. Over the past decade, significant advances and technologies have emerged to help guide clinical practice in some of these areas. This chapter provides physicians who care for these patients with a broad overview of the management of secondary hematologic problems in patients with cancer. The topics are organized according to clinical problems that are encountered in daily practice.

Anemia

Anemia is the most common hematologic problem complicating the management of patients diagnosed with cancer. It is associated with increased morbidity, decreased quality of life, and reduced survival compared with similar patients without anemia. A systematic approach to the evaluation of anemia in this patient population is critical because the differential diagnosis is broad and because multiple causes may be occurring simultaneously. Only after an accurate diagnosis is made can appropriate therapies be administered.

The World Health Organization has defined anemia as a hemoglobin concentration below 130 g/L for men and 120 g/L for women.[1] The prevalence of anemia in cancer patients varies across individual studies, depending on the definition used and the patient population evaluated. Data from a recent meta-analysis found that moderate anemia (hemoglobin 80–110 g/L) occurred in 30 to 90% of patients, most frequently in those with an underlying hematologic malignancy or a solid tumor at an advanced stage.[2] In addition, anemic patients had poorer overall survival compared with nonanemic patients in 18 of 19 studies included in this analysis. Whether this represents a causal relationship or simply reflects differences in the population studied is not clear. To date, definitive evidence that correcting anemia improves disease-free or overall survival is lacking.

A comprehensive clinical assessment is important when evaluating a patient with anemia. However, laboratory parameters are often more useful when formulating a diagnostic approach. Historically, the two most common approaches have classified anemia according to either the underlying pathophysiologic mechanism (decreased erythropoiesis, increased red blood cell [RBC] destruction, blood loss) or changes in the RBC mean cell volume (MCV) and reticulocyte count (Table 1).[3] Although the differential diagnosis for anemia is broad, the etiology in cancer patients is usually due to one or more of a few common causes that are associated with the underlying malignancy or its treatment. Cancer-related anemia is a general term used to describe anemia that is due to the underlying malignancy (malignant bone marrow infiltration and anemia of chronic inflammation) and the myelosuppressive effects of cancer therapy (chemotherapy-associated anemia).

Anemia of Chronic Inflammation

Anemia of chronic inflammation (ACI), also called anemia of chronic disease, is one of the most common causes of anemia in cancer patients.[4] It is characterized by normocytic or slightly microcytic anemia (80–110 g/L), low serum iron, normal or elevated serum ferritin, and preserved bone marrow iron stores; however, about 20% of patients may present with severe anemia (< 80 g/L).[5] Clinically, it is often difficult

Table 1 Common Causes of Anemia			
Microcytic Anemia (MCV < 80 FL)	**Normocytic Anemia (MCV 80–100 fl)**		**Macrocytic Anemia (MCV > 100 fl)**
	Increased Reticulocyte Count	*Decreased Reticulocyte Count*	
Iron deficiency*	Blood loss	ACD*	Vitamin B_{12} deficiency*
Thalassemia	Hemolysis	Renal insufficiency	Folate deficiency*
ACD*	Immune hemolysis†	Bone marrow failure*	Clonal bone marrow disorders
Sideroblastic anemia	Nonimmune	Malignant infiltration	MDS*
	Intrinsic RBC abnormalities	Aplastic anemia	Hypothryoidism
	Membranopathies	Pure red cell aplasia	Liver disease
	Enzymopathies	MDS	Reticulocytosis
	Hemoglobinopathies	Drugs/toxins (including	Alcohol
	Microangiopathy*	chemotherapy-associated	Drugs (hydroxyurea,
	HUS-TTP	anemia)	methotrexate, AZT)

ACD = anemia of chronic disease; AZT = azathioprine; HUS = hemolytic-uremic syndrome; MCV = mean cell volume; MDS = myelodysplasia; RBC = red blood cell; TTP = thrombotic thrombocytopenic purpura.
*Diseases associated with an underlying malignancy or its treatment.
†See Table 4 for classification of immune hemolysis.

to differentiate ACI from iron deficiency anemia. Furthermore, concomitant ACI and iron deficiency are not uncommon in cancer patients, particularly those with gastrointestinal malignancies. The diagnostic approach should emphasize the use of serum ferritin and bone marrow aspirate because serum iron, transferrin, and iron saturation may be reduced in both ACI and iron deficiency and, thus, are generally not helpful. A reduced serum ferritin level confirms iron deficiency and should prompt a search for its cause. In the setting of a normal or increased ferritin, bone marrow aspirate may be required to establish a diagnosis of ACI and/or iron deficiency. In ACI, iron staining is classically normal or increased in bone marrow macrophages and absent in erythroid precursors.

The reduction in bone marrow erythropoiesis in ACI is due to impaired iron regulation, trapping of iron in tissue macrophages, decreased erythropoietin production, and poor erythropoietin responsiveness.[6,7] Although the precise mechanisms have not been fully elucidated, recent evidence suggests a central role for the iron regulatory hormone called hepcidin.[8–10] This 25–amino acid protein is a key regulator of intestinal iron absorption and iron release from tissue macrophages. It is synthesized by hepatocytes and induced by infection or inflammation primarily via cytokine-mediated up-regulation (interleukin-6).[8,11]

Treatment

The management of patients with ACI or cancer-related anemia is directed at treating associated diseases, excluding other causes of anemia (see Table 1), and maintaining an adequate hemoglobin in patients with symptomatic anemia. Historically, the administration of allogeneic RBC transfusions was the only option for cancer patients with symptomatic anemia; indeed, they remain an important treatment modality today. Newer strategies include administration of recombinant human erythropoietin (rhEPO) and, possibly in the future, infusion of synthetic oxygen-carrying products.

RBC Transfusions   The indications for RBC transfusion depend on the presence of bleeding or anemia-related symptoms in addition to the absolute hemoglobin concentration prior to transfusion. Since the therapeutic goals are to maintain hemodynamic stability, limit anemia-related symptoms, and prevent ischemic events, the need for transfusion will vary from patient to patient. Setting absolute hemoglobin concentration triggers below which RBC transfusions are indicated are appealing; however, a patient-specific transfusion strategy may be more appropriate than universal RBC transfusion triggers.[12,13] In the absence of randomized clinical trials in

cancer patients, a hemoglobin concentration of 80 g/L is often used as a trigger for RBC transfusions for clinically stable, nonbleeding patients with anemia owing to myelotoxic chemotherapy.[14–16] A review of published clinical practice guidelines for RBC transfusions found that only 1 of 13 guidelines recommended a specific hemoglobin trigger for RBC transfusions and that most others advocated either a range of hemoglobin values based on clinical judgment or clinical judgment alone.[17] One randomized controlled trial in critically ill adult patients admitted to the intensive care unit showed that a restrictive RBC transfusion strategy (transfusion trigger of 70 g/L) was as safe as a liberal transfusion strategy (trigger of 100 g/L).[18] Further studies are needed to determine whether these results can be applied to patients with cancer-associated anemia.

Erythropoiesis-Stimulating Agents (ESAs)   More recently, recombinant erythropoiesis-stimulating agents (ESAs) have been accepted as a standard alternative to RBC transfusion for the treatment of chemotherapy-associated anemia; the best studied of these agents are epoetin alpha and darbepoietin alpha. Tested in large randomized controlled trials that have been summarized in several meta-analyses, the use of ESAs have been outlined in practice guideline recommendations in both North America and Europe.[19–22] Overall, the administration of an ESA has consistently demonstrated a significant reduction in the need for RBC transfusion (approximately 20–55%) and an increase in the hemoglobin concentration from baseline. Evidence for a positive impact on quality of life is more difficult to demonstrate because studies are generally of poorer quality and show conflicting results.[20–22] No clear benefit has been observed in terms of overall survival, tumor response rate, and response duration. Erythropoiesis-stimulating agents are generally well tolerated; however, an increased incidence of thromboembolic events (both venous and arterial) and hypertension has been reported in some clinical trials (Singh AK, Szczch L, Tang KL, Barnhart H, Sapp S et al. Correction of Anemia with Epoetin Alfa in Chronic Kidney Disease. N Engl J Med 2007;355:2085–2098). In a recent meta-analysis of 12 randomized controlled trials evaluating 1,738 cancer patients, treatment with an ESA, increased the relative risk of thromboembolic events (1.58, 95% confidence interval 0.94–2.66), and hypertension (1.19, 95% confidence interval 0.96–1.49) compared with placebo.[23] A recently completed randomized, double-blind, placebo controlled trial evaluated whether the use of epoetin alpha titrated to maintain a hemoglobin level between 120-140 g/L improved quality of life in non-small cell lung cancer patients not receiving chemotherapy (unpublished data). Overall survival was significantly reduced (median 68 days vs. 131 days, p=0.040) in patients

randomized to receive epoetin alpha compared with placebo; in addition, no beneficial effect was observed on quality of life in patients treated with epoetin alpha. These findings have resulted in a black box warning issued by the FDA. Until additional data become available, it remains prudent to inform patients of these potential risks prior to initiating therapy. Acquired pure red cell aplasia (PRCA) owing to antierythropoietin antibodies has not been reported in patients treated for cancer-associated anemia.

The use of ESAs in cancer patients should be limited to patients that are receiving chemotherapy. The smallest dose required to achieve a hemoglobin level sufficient to maintain transfusion independence (approximately 100–120 g/L) should be administered as per manufacturer instructions.

RBC Substitutes   RBC substitutes are an attractive alternative to allogeneic RBC transfusions because they avoid alloimmunity and minimize the risk of transfusion-transmissible disease. Three types of RBC substitutes have been tested in human clinical trials: perfluorocarbons, hemoglobin-based oxygen carriers, and liposomes containing hemoglobin.[24] Perfluorocarbons are chemically and biologically inert substances prepared as emulsions for intravenous administration that are capable of dissolving large volumes of oxygen. In clinical studies, these agents have shown promise in the treatment of perioperative anemia but were associated with toxicities attributed to the emulsifying agent.[25,26] Hemoglobin solutions, derived from outdated human RBCs, bovine RBCs, or recombinant technology, have oxygen-carrying capacity and oxygen delivery properties that are similar to those of endogenous hemoglobin. So far, clinical benefit derived from hemoglobin solutions has been offset by safety concerns.[27,28] Liposomes of bilamellar spheres of phosphatidylcholine loaded with hemoglobin solution can also act as oxygen transporters and may have a role as substitutes for RBC transfusions. These agents have a long half-life in circulation, but they are technically difficult to prepare and currently remain in preclinical stages of investigation only.[29]

Therapy-Related Acute Myeloid Leukemia–Myelodysplastic Syndrome

In rare instances, anemia in patients with a history of cancer may be caused by a secondary hematologic malignancy. Patients treated with radiation therapy or certain chemotherapeutic agents subsequently have an increased risk of developing clonal bone marrow cytogenetic abnormalities, myelodysplasia (MDS), and acute myeloid leukemia (AML). Therapy-related AML-MDS is a devastating late complication of cancer therapy and is associated with specific cytogenetic abnormalities that portend a poor prognosis. Two distinct syndromes have been identified: one is characterized by a prolonged latency period (5–7 years) and an antecedent period of MDS following treatment with alkylating agents; the other has a shorter latency period (1–3 years) and often transforms to AML without an antecedent myelodysplastic phase following treatment with topoisomerase II inhibitors (Table 2).[30] The cumulative incidence of therapy-related AML-MDS varies between 1.5 and 10% and peaks approximately 5 to 9 years after treatment exposure.[31–33] Combined-modality therapy with radio- and chemotherapy results in a synergistic increase in the frequency of therapy-related AML-MDS, thus creating a treatment paradox that can complicate management decisions: improved disease control with combined-modality therapy may be offset by increased morbidity and mortality from delayed therapy-related cancers. Host factors that predispose patients to the development of therapy-related AML-MDS have not been clearly identified; therefore, prevention has focused on reducing the exposure to offending agents where possible.

Treatment

In general, the treatment of therapy-related AML-MDS has been disappointing.[30] Treatment decisions must be individualized. Younger patients with adequate organ function may be candidates for aggressive induction chemotherapy and allogeneic hematopoietic stem cell transplantation (HSCT) with curative intent.[34–36] In contrast, elderly patients may be candidates only for low-dose chemotherapy and palliative, supportive measures.

Acquired PRCA   Acquired PRCA is a rare condition characterized by profound anemia, marked reticulocytopenia, and absent bone marrow erythroid precursors in the setting of normal white blood cell and platelet lineages. Malignancy, thymoma, and lymphoproliferative disorders in particular are well-known causes of PRCA (Table 3).[37–39] Several unique mechanisms, occurring alone or in combination, have been implicated in the pathophysiology of acquired PRCA, including (1) T cell–mediated inhibition of erythropoiesis (thymoma, T-cell lymphoproliferative diseases); (2) development of antibodies with selective cytotoxicity for bone marrow erythroid progenitors; (3) direct infection and lysis of erythroid progenitor cells (parvovirus B19); (4) intrinsic stem cell defects (MDS); and (5) antierythropoietin antibodies (rhEPOs, connective tissue diseases).[37] Diagnostic hallmarks of PRCA include peripheral blood reticulocytopenia (usually < 1%) and absent erythroblasts in a normocellular bone marrow. The presence of giant proerythroblasts in the bone marrow is virtually pathognomonic for parvovirus B19 infection.

The incidence of antibody-associated PRCA in patients treated with rhEPO increased dramatically after 1998, peaked by approximately 2002, and has now sharply declined. This observation was limited almost exclusively to patients treated for anemia owing to end-stage renal disease. This association has been linked to a variety of factors that appear to influence the immunogenicity of the recombinant product, including the route of administration (subcutaneous injection may be more immunogenic compared with intravenous administration) and differences in manufacturing, processing, and storage (formulations stabilized in human serum albumin appear to be less immunogenic than products using polysorbate-based vehicles).[40,41] To date, no cases of rhEPO-induced PRCA have been reported in cancer patients treated for chemotherapy-associated anemia.

Treatment   Management of PRCA should focus on transfusional support in patients with symptomatic anemia and on treatment of any associated conditions, including removal of offending medications. Patients with PRCA owing to infection with parvovirus B19 often respond to therapy with intravenous immunoglobulin (IVIG).[42] Otherwise, first-line therapy for patients with idiopathic PRCA usually consists of immunosuppression based on the assumption that immune mechanisms play an important role in the pathophysiology of PRCA. Owing to a lack of well-designed clinical trials to determine the optimal immunosuppressive regimen, treatment decisions are often empiric. Prednisone, administered at a dose of 1 mg/kg, is a standard first-line agent. In refractory cases, cyclophosphamide, cyclosporine, rituximab (anti-CD20 monoclonal antibody), alemtuzumab (anti-CD52 monoclonal antibody), antithymocyte globulin, and IVIG have been used, with variable success.[43–52]

Autoimmune Hemolytic Anemia

Autoimmune hemolytic anemia (AIHA) represents a group of diseases characterized by the development of autoantibodies with specificity to one or more RBC antigens (Table 4). Subsequent RBC destruction follows owing to (1) intravascular hemolysis if the autoantibody can sufficiently activate complement on RBC membranes and/or (2) extravascular hemolysis owing to Fc and/or complement receptor-mediated destruction by phagocytic cells of the reticuloendothelial system. Among patients with secondary immune hemolysis owing to an underlying malignancy, warm AIHA accounts for greater than 80% of cases and is associated most often with lymphoproliferative diseases or their treatment (fludarabine therapy) and less frequently with solid tumors. Cold agglutinin disease (CAD) accounts for most of the remaining cases of immune-mediated hemolysis and is associated with a similar spectrum of malignancies.

Table 3 Causes of Acquired Pure Red Cell Aplasia

Lymphoid Malignancies
  B- and T-cell chronic lymphocytic leukemia
  Multiple myeloma
  Non-Hodgkin's lymphoma
  Large granular lymphocytic leukemia
Other Malignancies
  Thymoma
  Other solid tumors (rare)
Medications
  Phenytoin
  Sodium valproate
  Recombinant human erythropoietin products
  Mycophenolate mofetil
  Azathioprine
  Isoniazid
Infection
  Parvovirus B19
  Viral hepatitis
  HIV
Immune disorders
  Systemic lupus erythematosus
  Rheumatoid arthritis
  ABO-incompatible hematopoietic stem cell
    transplantation

HIV = human immunodeficiency virus.

Table 2 Clinical Characteristics of Therapy-Related Acute Myeloid Leukemia–Myelodysplastic Syndrome

Therapy	Latency Period (yr)	Clinical Presentation	Cytogenetic Abnormalities	Median Survival (mo)
Alkylating agents or radiation (cyclophosphamide, procarbazine, nitrogen mustard, vinblastine)	5–7	Insidious onset Preceding myelodysplastic phase	Deletions involving chromosomes 5 and 7 Complex (≥ 3) cytogenetic abnormalities	6–8
Topoisomerase II inhibitors (etoposide, tenoposide, doxorubicin)	2–3	AML without a preceding myelodysplastic phase	Translocations involving the *MLL* gene (chromosome 11q23)	6–8

AML = acute myeloid leukemia.

Table 4 Classification of Autoimmune Hemolytic Anemias

	Warm Autoantibodies		Cold Autoantibodies		
	Primary AIHA	Secondary AIHA	Primary CAD	Secondary CAD	PCH
Etiology	Idiopathic	Lymphoproliferative disorders (CLL, LGL, NHL, MM) Drugs (fludarabine, penicillin, methyldopa, quinidine) Autoimmune disorders (SLE) Infections (viral)	Idiopathic	Lymphoproliferative disorders (NHL, CLL, MM, LGL) Infections (EBV, *Mycoplasma pneumonia*)	Syphilis Viral infections
Immunoglobulin Clonality	Polyclonal	Polyclonal	Monoclonal	Monoclonal (malignancy) Polyclonal (infection)	Polyclonal
DAT	IgG	IgG	C3	C3	C3
RBC antigen specificity	Panagglutinin	Panagglutinin	I	I/i	P

AIHA = autoimmune hemolytic anemia; CAD = cold agglutinin disease; DAT = direct antiglobulin test; EBV = Epstein-Barr virus; Ig = immunoglobulin; PCH= paroxysmal cold hemoglobinuria; MM=multiple myeloma; NHL = non-Hodgkin's lymphoma; RBC = red blood cell; SLE = systemic lupus erythematosus.

Warm AIHA

Warm AIHA is usually due to polyclonal immunoglobulin (Ig)G autoantibodies that react more strongly with RBC antigens at core body temperature than at lower temperatures—hence the term "warm." Warm autoantibodies are usually panagglutinins, that is, they react will all cells in a panel of RBC antigens, but occasionally will show specificity, most often to Rh blood group antigens. Definitive diagnosis relies on demonstrating the presence of autoantibody (IgG) or complement (C3) on the RBC surface (positive direct antiglobulin test [DAT]) and laboratory evidence of extravascular hemolysis (reticulocytosis, elevated unconjugated bilirubin and lactate dehydrogenase, decreased or absent haptoglobin, and peripheral blood spherocytosis and polychromasia). Greater than 95% of patients will have a positive DAT owing to IgG and/or C3 coating the RBC surface; the small percentage of DAT-negative patients likely represents IgG autoantibodies below the detectable threshold of the DAT, IgA autoantibodies, or IgM autoantibodies that do not fix and activate complement.[53,54] Delayed hemolytic transfusion reaction, characterized by a positive DAT, the detection of a new alloantibody, and laboratory evidence of extravascular hemolysis 2 to 14 days following transfusion, should be excluded in those patients who have been recently transfused.

Treatment of malignancy-associated warm AIHA should focus on limiting hemolysis by treating the underlying malignancy and the use of immunosuppressive therapy, generally prednisone 1 mg/kg/d. Splenectomy and additional immunosuppressive agents, such as cyclophosphamide, rituximab, cyclosporine, and IVIG, may be beneficial in refractory cases.[55–57] The indications for RBC transfusion are the same as for anemic patients without warm AIHA; however, the presence of panagglutinating autoantibodies usually renders all RBC units cross-match "incompatible." Nevertheless, in the absence of an occult alloantibody, the life span of the transfused RBCs should be similar to that of the patient's own RBCs. Consultation with the transfusion medicine laboratory is often required to exclude occult hemolytic alloantibodies.[58]

Cold Agglutinin Disease

CAD is usually caused by IgM autoantibodies that react optimally between 0 and 4°C, often with specificity to I/i and Pr blood group antigens. The thermal range of the antibody and the titer are important determinants in the degree of hemolysis. Clinically, symptoms relate to the presence of anemia and/or agglutination of RBCs in the distal extremities (acral discoloration, pain, skin ulceration, and necrosis, especially on exposure to a cold environment). A marked spurious increase in the MCV, the presence of RBC agglutination on examination of a peripheral blood smear, and laboratory evidence of hemolysis are clues to the presence of a clinically significant cold agglutinin. IgM antibodies can efficiently fix and activate complement; therefore, the DAT is usually positive with anti-C3 but negative with anti-IgG antibodies.

Treatment of CAD should focus on three issues: (1) keeping patients warm (avoidance of cold environments to reduce hemolytic exacerbations); (2) reducing the antibody titer with systemic chemotherapy for underlying malignancies, additional immunosuppressive therapies, and plasmapheresis, when necessary; and (3) RBC transfusions in symptomatic patients using warmed blood products administered slowly. In contrast to warm AIHA, glucocorticoid therapy and splenectomy are generally not effective therapies for CAD. Cyclophosphamide, rituximab, and plasmapheresis used alone or in combination may be able to reduce autoantibody titer and control hemolysis more effectively.[59–61]

Thrombocytopenia

Thrombocytopenia is defined as a platelet count of less than 150×10^9/L. Clinically significant bleeding rarely develops until the platelet count falls below 50×10^9/L unless there is an accompanying platelet function defect or coagulopathy. Once the platelet count drops below 10 to 20×10^9/L, patients have a higher risk of spontaneous bleeding, ecchymoses, mucosal bleeding (gums, epistaxis, gastrointestinal tract), and intracranial hemorrhage.

A common diagnostic approach divides the causes of thrombocytopenia into disorders associated with increased peripheral platelet destruction, impaired bone marrow platelet production, or splenic sequestration (hypersplenism) (Table 5). Careful examination of the peripheral blood smear is critically important when evaluating thrombocytopenia and should be performed for several reasons: (1) to exclude "pseudothrombocytopenia" owing to ethylenediaminetetraacetic acid–induced platelet clumping; (2) to look for

Table 5 Common Causes of Thrombocytopenia in Cancer Patients

Decreased platelet production
  Myelosuppressive chemotherapy/radiation
  Bone marrow infiltration by malignancy
  Myelodysplastic syndrome
  Vitamin B_{12} or folate deficiency
Increased platelet destruction
  Immune mechanisms:
    Immune thrombocytopenic purpura (often associated with lymphoproliferative diseases)
    Post-transfusion purpura
    Heparin-induced thrombocytopenia
  Nonimmune mechanisms:
    DIC
    HUS-TTP
Hypersplenism
  Splenomegaly (lymphoproliferative diseases, other)

DIC = disseminated intravascular coagulation; HUS = hemolytic-uremic syndrome; TTP = thrombotic thrombocytopenic purpura.

RBC fragments suggestive of a microangiopathic process, such as disseminated intravascular coagulation (DIC), hemolytic-uremic syndrome (HUS), or thrombotic thrombocytopenic purpura (TTP); and (3) to examine for evidence of decreased platelet production (eg, circulating blast cells suggestive of acute leukemia, macrocytosis and hypersegmented neutrophils suggestive of vitamin B_{12} or folate deficiency). Drug-induced causes of thrombocytopenia are common and should always be considered. In particular, physicians should have a high index of suspicion for heparin-induced thrombocytopenia (HIT) in hospitalized patients because of its paradoxical and potentially life-threatening thrombotic complications, and commonly used antibiotics such as Vancomycin must be considered as a cause of severe thrombocytopenia and bleeding (REF Annette Von Drygalski, NEJM 2007). A bone marrow aspirate and biopsy may be required to determine the cause of thrombocytopenia in selected patients, especially when a malignant infiltrate or myelodysplastic syndrome is suspected. Peripheral consumption of platelets is suggested when increased numbers of morphologically normal megakaryocytes are observed in the bone marrow concurrently with peripheral blood thrombocytopenia and megathrombocytes.

Cancer-Related Thrombocytopenia

Thrombocytopenia is common in cancer patients and is most often due to reduced thrombopoiesis from the myelosuppressive effects of radiation or chemotherapy or from bone marrow infiltration by tumor cells. Chemotherapy-induced thrombocytopenia is temporally and predictably related to cancer treatment; bone marrow examination is generally required to diagnose a myelophthisic syndrome.

Treatment

Recombinant Thrombopoietin The discovery of thrombopoietin (TPO), the principal megakaryopoietic growth factor, garnered initial enthusiasm as a potential therapeutic alternative to platelet transfusions for the treatment of chemotherapy-associated thrombocytopenia. Two forms of recombinant human thrombopoietin (rhTPO) have undergone clinical drug development: (1) a full-length molecule (rhTPO) and (2) a truncated molecule called pegylated recombinant human megakaryocyte growth and development factor (PEG-rHuMGDF). Production of PEG-rHuMGDF has now been suspended owing to the development of neutralizing anti-TPO antibodies and clinically significant thrombocytopenia in some patients. rhTPOs have been evaluated in patients with chemotherapy-associated thrombocytopenia, but the results have generally been disappointing thus far. In a series

of randomized controlled trials evaluating patients being treated for acute leukemia, the concomitant administration of rhTPO did not reduce the duration of severe thrombocytopenia or platelet transfusion requirements.[62–64] It is now recognized that the effects of rhTPO are delayed compared with those of other cytokines (ie, granulocyte colony-stimulating factor [G-CSF]). Therefore, ongoing clinical trials have been developed to test alternative dosing regimens in a variety of disease states.

TPO agonists

A new class of molecules that is currently undergoing clinical trials are TPO agonists. These are small molecules that activate the TPO receptor and stimulate platelet production, but are sufficiently different from endogenous TPO that they do not induce anti-TPO antibodies. Results of phase II trials in immune mediate thrombocytopenia have been encouraging (REF Bussel J, Kuter D, George J, NEJM 2006); testing in cancer related thrombocytopenia is ongoing.

Indications for Platelet Transfusions Platelet transfusions are generally indicated for the treatment or prevention of bleeding in patients with thrombocytopenia. Given that the risk of bleeding increases as the platelet count decreases,[65] the absolute platelet count often dictates when platelet transfusions are administered. However, the decision to transfuse platelets should not be influenced only by the platelet count but also by the presence of bleeding or bleeding risk factors, including concurrent coagulopathies or the presence of underlying comorbid illness.[66] Platelet transfusions should generally be avoided in thrombocytopenic patients with TTP[67,68] or HIT[69,70] as platelet transfusions can worsen the outcome of these disease processes.

In clinically stable, nonbleeding thrombocytopenic patients with hematologic malignancies, prophylactic platelet transfusions are recommended for patients with platelet counts below 10×10^9/L. A recent meta-analysis, which included three randomized controlled trials enrolling 492 patients, concluded that bleeding complications were not different using a platelet transfusion trigger of 10×10^9/L or 20×10^9/L. The studies were insufficiently powered to claim that a trigger of 10×109/L is as safe as (or not inferior to) 20×10^9/L. However, platelet transfusion triggers even lower than 10×10^9/L appear to be safe in certain circumstances.[72] Although there is less evidence to guide platelet transfusion practice for patients with solid tumors, a platelet trigger of 10×10^9/L is generally recommended, with the exceptions of patients receiving aggressive therapy for bladder tumors and patients with necrotic tumors (of any type), who may benefit from a more liberal platelet transfusion strategy (trigger of 20×10^9/L) owing to the increased risk of

bleeding from these sites.[73] Additional randomized trials are needed to determine safe triggers for prophylactic platelet transfusions in anticipation of invasive procedures and in thrombocytopenic disorders other than myelotoxic chemotherapy that commonly affect patients with cancer, such as DIC and sepsis. Recommended platelet transfusion triggers for various clinical indications are summarized in Table 6.[73–76]

Platelet Transfusion Alternatives Novel platelet products are being developed to improve on the safety and quality of allogeneic platelet transfusions.[77] Frozen platelets, lyophilized platelets, and hemostatically intact platelet membrane microparticles are currently under investigation. Red cells with surface-bound fibrinogen or RGD (Arg-Gly-Asp) ligand, the fibrinogen peptide that binds to platelet integrin on glycoprotein GpIIb/IIIa, fibrinogen-coated albumin microcapsules or microspheres, and liposome-based hemostatic agents also hold promise as substitutes to platelet transfusions. In addition, recombinant activated factor VII and adequate correction of concomitant anemia may be important adjuncts in the treatment of bleeding owing to thrombocytopenia.[78,79]

Leukopenia

Leukopenia refers to a decrease in the peripheral blood white blood cell count and can be due to lymphopenia, granulocytopenia, or both. Although numerous causes for leukopenia exist, when it occurs in patients with an underlying malignancy, it is usually due to either malignant infiltration of the bone marrow or the myelosuppressive effects of chemo- or radiotherapy. The term *neutropenia* is generally used interchangeably with *granulocytopenia*. Neutropenic fever is one of the most serious complications of cancer therapy and a harbinger of potentially life-threatening infection.

Neutropenia

Neutropenia is defined by an absolute neutrophil count (ANC) of less than 1.5×10^9/L and is further classified as mild (ANC $1.0–1.5 \times 10^9$/L), moderate (ANC $0.5–1.0 \times 10^9$/L), or severe (defined as ANC 0.5×10^9/L or less or 0.1×10^9/L or less). The risk of infection is determined by both the degree and duration of neutropenia. This relationship was demonstrated in a study that evaluated the frequency of infections in 52 patients with acute leukemia and neutropenia of variable duration and severity; 80% of patients with severe neutropenia lasting 2 weeks (ANC $<0.1 \times 10^9$/L) developed an identifiable infection, and 100% of patients with severe neutropenia lasting 3 weeks or more developed an infection.[80] Clinically, the risk of infection begins to increase once the ANC falls below 1.0×10^9/L. Most infections that occur in the setting of

Table 6 Recommended Platelet Transfusion Triggers according to Indications

Indication for Platelet Transfusion	Platelet Count Trigger
Patients with acute leukemia or HSCT and bone marrow failure owing to disease or its therapy, in the absence of additional risk factors such as bleeding, sepsis, or the concomitant use of drugs	10×10^9/L
Chemotherapy-induced thrombocytopenia for the treatment of solid tumors	10×10^9/L
	20×10^9/L for bladder tumors or necrotic tumors
Chronic, stable, severe thrombocytopenia in the absence of bleeding	Observation only
Bone marrow aspiration and biopsy	Generally not recommended
Lumbar puncture and epidural anesthesia	50×10^9/L
Gastroscopy and biopsy	50×10^9/L
Insertion of indwelling endovascular catheters	50×10^9/L
Transbronchial biopsy	50×10^9/L
Liver biopsy	50×10^9/L
Laparotomy	50×10^9/L
Operation in critical sites including brain and eyes	100×10^9/L
Massive transfusion (transfusion of a volume of red cell concentrates equivalent to two blood volumes)	50×10^9/L
Multiple trauma or CNS injury	100×10^9/L
Acute disseminated intravascular coagulation	50×10^9/L
Autoimmune thrombocytopenia	Platelet transfusion should be reserved for life-threatening bleeding

CNS = central nervous system; HSCT = hematopoietic stem cell transplantation.

moderate to severe neutropenia are due to endogenous pyogenic bacteria (both gram positive and gram negative) and certain fungal pathogens. Prolonged neutropenia, therapy with broad-spectrum antibiotics, and treatment with corticosteroids predispose patients to systemic fungal infections.

Patients receiving systemic chemotherapy who become neutropenic are consequently at risk of infection-related morbidity and mortality, cancer treatment delays, and chemotherapy dose reductions. The degree and duration of neutropenia are determined predominantly by the specific chemotherapeutic regimen, but host-related factors are also important. Predictors for the development of chemotherapy-induced neutropenia include advanced patient age, poor functional status, and the presence of underlying comorbid illnesses (eg, renal disease, cardiovascular disease).[81,82] Attempts to limit the degree and duration of neutropenia are accomplished by either chemotherapy dose reduction or myeloid growth factor support. Granulocyte transfusions are no longer routinely used.

Treatment

The prophylactic administration of myeloid growth factors (G-CSF, granulocyte-macrophage colony-stimulating factor) following chemotherapy has been evaluated in randomized controlled trials.[83–86] In general, prophylactic administration of myeloid growth factors results

in a higher ANC nadir, shortened duration of severe neutropenia, and fewer episodes of febrile neutropenia compared with placebo. However, no improvement in overall survival, tumor response rates, or progression-free survival has been shown. Furthermore, economic analyses suggest that the incidence of febrile neutropenia associated with a specific chemotherapeutic regimen must be 40% or higher before prophylaxis with myeloid growth factors is cost-effective.[87,88] With the exception of treatments for advanced germ cell tumors and small cell lung cancer, chemotherapeutic regimens for most common malignant diseases are associated with rates of febrile neutropenia that are substantially below 40%.

Based on the most recent update of the practice guidelines developed by the American Society of Clinical Oncology in 2000, primary prophylaxis with myeloid growth factors is not recommended for most patients because there is no evidence of improved overall or progression-free survival and therapy is not cost-effective. In patients with an expected risk of febrile neutropenia of at least 40%, primary growth factor support is recommended. Therapy in these patients reduces the risk of febrile neutropenia by approximately 50% but does not change response rates or progression-free or overall survival. Also, there may be special circumstances, such as advanced patient age, poor functional status, and poor bone marrow reserve owing to previous chemotherapy

or cytopenias prior to therapy, that may influence the decision to administer primary prophylaxis, but the evidence for a positive impact on clinical outcomes is not strong. Recommendations are similar for secondary prevention of infections in patients with a previous episode of febrile neutropenia. Chemotherapy dose reduction rather than growth factor administration is recommended for most patients. Secondary prophylaxis may be appropriate for a subset of patients undergoing chemotherapy for potentially curable malignancies (eg, germ cell tumors, non-Hodgkin's lymphoma) to maintain dose intensity. There is little evidence to support the routine use of myeloid growth factors for patients with severe neutropenia.

Hemorrhagic Complications

Bleeding is one of the most common hematologic problems encountered in patients with cancer. This is usually directly related to the malignancy, but it may also be due to thrombocytopenia, invasive procedures, and other acquired hemorrhagic syndromes. The two most serious coagulopathies are DIC and acquired inhibition of coagulation factors.

Disseminated Intravascular Coagulation

DIC is common in malignancy. It is a syndrome characterized by widespread fibrin deposition in the vasculature owing to systemic intravascular activation of coagulation. It can be chronic and clinically silent or present acutely with symptomatic thrombosis, mild to catastrophic hemorrhage, or end-organ damage.[89,90] Diagnosis of DIC requires laboratory evidence of microangiopathy, thrombin generation, fibrinolytic activation, and consumption of platelets and pro- and anticoagulant factors in a clinical setting associated with a hypercoagulable state, such as malignancy and sepsis.[91,92] The exact pathogenesis of DIC is not understood, but excessive activation of coagulation via the tissue factor-factor VIIa pathway is considered to be the initiating event. Propagation of this process occurs because there is concomitant suppression of the natural inhibitory pathways, impairment of fibrinolysis, and an inflammatory cytokine response to the initial insult.[93] The most common malignancies that are associated with DIC are acute myelogenous leukemias, particularly M3 and M5, and cancer of the prostate, ovary, or lung.[89,90] Tumor expression of procoagulant molecules is likely involved in the activation of coagulation.

Management

Clinical studies are lacking to guide therapy in patients with DIC. Treatment is usually directed at supporting the patient with blood products if bleeding is the major manifestation and with heparin therapy if symptomatic thromboembolism is present. Intervention is not recommended if the patient is asymptomatic and only laboratory parameters are abnormal. Treatment of the underlying disease is necessary to terminate the ongoing stimulus for activation of coagulation. The role of restoring acquired deficiencies in physiologic anticoagulants such as antithrombin and tissue factor pathway inhibitor has not been evaluated in patients with DIC related to cancer, but these products have had disappointing results in patients with DIC and sepsis.[94,95] Recently, infusion of activated protein C concentrate was shown to improve survival in patients with sepsis; however, patients treated with this product had a higher incidence of bleeding.[96] Whether activated protein C will be beneficial to patients with fulminant DIC and malignancy has not been tested.

Acquired Inhibitors of Coagulation Factors

The development of an acquired inhibitor of a coagulation factor protein represents a rare but potentially life-threatening cause of bleeding in cancer patients.[97] Although the pathophysiology resulting in their formation is not clearly understood, inhibitors are usually IgG autoantibodies that bind to specific epitopes on coagulation factors and interfere with their normal function. Most cases are idiopathic, but approximately 10% are associated with an underlying solid tumor or hematologic malignancy, the presence of which imparts an adverse prognosis.[98] Patients typically present with a bleeding diathesis that can range from mild bruising to catastrophic, life-threatening hemorrhage. The most frequent sites of bleeding include soft tissues, retroperitoneal structures, skin, mucosal surfaces, and the gastrointestinal tract; in contrast to patients with congenital hemophilia A, hemarthroses occur infrequently. An acquired inhibitor should be suspected when a prolonged activated partial thromboplastin time (aPTT), international normalized ratio (INR), or both either fail to correct when patient plasma is mixed in a 1:1 ratio with normal plasma or correct with excess phospholipid, suggesting the presence of an antiphospholipid antibody. Specific coagulation factor assays (guided by whether the aPTT, INR, or both are prolonged) allow subsequent inhibitor identification. The vast majority of acquired inhibitors are directed against factor VIII. The inhibitor titer can be estimated using the Bethesda assay, which measures residual coagulation factor activity after incubation of patient plasma with normal plasma for 2 hours at 37°C.

Treatment

The management of patients with an acquired inhibitor is difficult owing to potentially life-threatening bleeding episodes and a lack of well-designed, prospective clinical trials to help guide treatment decisions. Specific therapeutic recommendations are beyond the scope of this chapter, and referral to a specialist with expertise in disorders of hemostasis and coagulation is recommended. Two main therapeutic goals exist for the treatment of acquired inhibitors: termination of active bleeding and eradication of the inhibitor to prevent future episodes of bleeding. Strategies to control active bleeding include intravenous infusions of specific factor concentrates or factor-bypassing agents such as activated prothrombin complex concentrates, factor VIII inhibitor bypassing activity, or activated factor VII (niastase).[98,99] Initial treatment decisions should be dictated by the severity of the bleeding symptoms and the inhibitor titer. The mainstay of inhibitor eradication has focused on immunosuppressive therapies, most commonly prednisone alone or in combination with cyclophosphamide. Treatment directed toward the underlying malignancy may contribute to inhibitor regression, particularly in patients with hematologic cancers[100]; the relationship in patients with solid tumors is less certain.

Thrombotic Complications

Thrombotic complications in cancer patients may occur spontaneously or secondary to additional risk factors, such as surgery and central venous catheterization. Although the vast majority of the events are venous, arterial thrombosis can also develop. Paradoxically, the two most fulminant thrombotic complications are HIT and TTP, both of which are characterized by an acute onset of severe thrombocytopenia.

Venous Thromboembolism

Active malignancy, with or without chemotherapy, increases the risk of venous thromboembolism (VTE) by four- to sixfold.[101] Cancer is also an independent risk factor for death within 7 days after a thrombotic event, with up to an eightfold increased risk of death in patients receiving chemotherapy.[102] Moreover, cancer patients with VTE have worse survival than cancer patients free of this complication. In a population-based study, the 1-year survival rate of patients diagnosed with cancer and VTE at the same time was 12%, compared with 36% in cancer patients without VTE, who were matched for gender, age at the time of the diagnosis of cancer, and year of cancer diagnosis.[103] The poor prognosis may indicate that patients are dying prematurely of VTE, that VTE is a harbinger of aggressive malignancies, or that activation of coagulation promotes tumor progression. VTE often presents late in the course of malignancy, but it can also be the first manifestation of occult cancer. Approximately 10% of patients with unprovoked or idiopathic VTE are diagnosed with cancer within the first year after their diagnosis of VTE.[104] Although extensive screening for underlying cancer in such patients allows earlier detection of the malignancy, a positive impact on survival has not been demonstrated.[105]

Although the risk of VTE by tumor type remains uncertain for the majority of cancers, the risk appears to be highest for patients with malignant brain tumors and cancer of the ovary, pancreas, and lung.[106] On the other hand, the most common tumor types found in patients with VTE are cancers of the lung, colon, breast, and prostate, which largely reflect the prevalence of these cancers in the general population. The risk of thrombosis is increased with the use of chemotherapy, hormonal therapy, and indwelling central venous catheters.[104] Recent clinical trials also report a high incidence of VTE associated with the use of antiangiogenic agents, such as thalidomide and inhibitors of the vascular endothelial growth factor/receptor pathway.

Venous thrombotic complications in cancer patients can occur in any venous bed, although the most common manifestations are deep venous thrombosis (DVT) of the legs and pulmonary embolism (PE). Most of the clinical studies to date have focused on the prevention and treatment of VTE at these two sites.

Prophylaxis of VTE in Surgical Patients

Anticoagulant prophylaxis is recommended for patients undergoing major surgery because the risk of postoperative thrombosis is substantial.[107] After surgery, cancer patients have twice the risk of DVT and over three times the risk of fatal PE compared with patients free of cancer.[107] Low-molecular-weight heparin (LMWH) or unfractionated heparin (UFH) can reduce the risk by approximately 70%, and these agents are comparable in efficacy and safety for the prevention of postoperative thromboembolism.[108,109] The major advantages of LMWH over UFH are the lower risk of HIT and the requirement for only once-daily injection. Newer and more selective anticoagulants, such as fondaparinux, are also effective for prophylaxis but do not appear to be better than the heparins.[110] More recently, it was shown that extending prophylaxis with LMWH for 3 weeks after hospital discharge in cancer patients can reduce the risk of venographic and proximal VTE by 60%.[111,112] This benefit was achieved without an increase in bleeding. Therefore, cancer patients undergoing surgery should receive pharmacologic prophylaxis with either LMWH or UFH while in hospital. Continuing prophylaxis after hospitalization is reasonable and should be considered in those patients with additional risk factors.

Prophylaxis of VTE in Medical Oncology Patients

The indications for primary prophylaxis in medical oncology patients remain undefined. To date, only one publication has addressed the efficacy and safety of thromboprophylaxis in medical oncology outpatients. In a placebo-controlled trial, it was demonstrated that low-dose warfarin is effective and safe in reducing the incidence of symptomatic thromboembolic events during chemotherapy.[113] However, standard practice does not include routine prophylaxis of ambulatory medical oncology patients because of concerns for anticoagulant-related bleeding and the need for laboratory monitoring. Recent reports of a relatively low incidence of symptomatic VTE (3%) in ambulatory patients with advanced or metastatic malignancies also argue against routine prophylaxis.[114] For hospitalized patients, there is indirect evidence that cancer patients would benefit from thromboprophylaxis with LMWH.[115,116] The risk of bleeding is likely low, but, currently, there are no reliable data about bleeding associated with anticoagulant prophylaxis specifically in cancer patients.[117] In summary, it is reasonable to use LMWH for primary prophylaxis in cancer patients when they are admitted to hospital with an acute illness, but evidence is lacking to support routine prophylaxis in patients in an outpatient setting.

Treatment of VTE

To date, multiple randomized trials and meta-analyses of these trials have confirmed that for initial therapy, LMWHs are at least as efficacious as UFH in reducing recurrent thrombosis and are associated with a lower risk of major bleeding.[118–121] Furthermore, LMWH can be given safely in an outpatient setting without the need for laboratory monitoring and has a lower risk of HIT.[122,123] However, whether LMWHs and UFH perform comparably in patients with cancer and acute VTE has not been formally investigated.

Although vitamin K antagonists are the mainstay of long-term anticoagulant treatment for VTE because they are highly effective in reducing recurrent thrombosis in the general population, treatment failures, serious bleeding, and difficulties with maintaining the INR within the therapeutic range are common problems in patients with cancer. A prospective cohort study reported that the 12-month cumulative incidence of recurrent VTE in cancer patients was 20.7%, versus 6.8% in patients without cancer, whereas the corresponding estimate for major bleeding was 12.4% versus 4.9%, respectively.[124] Patients with cancer also experience recurrent VTE despite having therapeutic INR levels and suffer serious bleeding complications without receiving excessive anticoagulation.[125] Cases of warfarin-induced limb gangrene owing to protein C depletion have also been reported in patients with cancer.[126,127]

Recent evidence from randomized trials shows that LMWH should be the first-line treatment for long-term anticoagulation in cancer patients with VTE.[128,129] In the CLOT trial, LMWH dalteparin was found to reduce the risk of recurrent VTE by 52% (p = .002), from 17 to 9% at 6 months, compared with warfarin therapy.[128] Patients in the dalteparin group received therapeutic doses at 200 U/kg once daily for the first month and then 75 to 80% of the full dose for the next 5 months. Overall, there were no differences in bleeding between the groups. Other trials have suggested that LMWHs may be safer than warfarin therapy for long-term treatment of VTE in cancer patients.[129,130] In addition, LMWHs have few drug interactions, do not require laboratory monitoring, and can readily accommodate thrombocytopenia and invasive procedures. Improvement in overall survival may also be associated with LMWH use in patients with a better prognosis, but further studies are needed to confirm this observation.[114,131,132]

Thrombosis Associated with Central Venous Catheters

Recent studies show that the incidence of catheter-related thrombosis (CRT) is much lower than what was previously reported in historical studies. According to randomized trials and prospective cohort studies, approximately 15% of patients develop CRT that is detectable with venography, but only 4% of patients have symptomatic CRT.[133–135] Furthermore, recent placebo-controlled trials showed that prophylaxis with low-dose warfarin or low-dose LMWH is not effective in reducing symptomatic thrombotic events.[133,134] In addition, low-dose warfarin can produce supratherapeutic anticoagulant levels in one-third of patients receiving fluorouracil-based chemotherapy and therefore should not be given without laboratory monitoring.[136] Therefore, contradictory to previous guideline recommendations, routine prophylaxis for CRT is not warranted.[107]

Treatment The lack of prospective data on the natural history and treatment of CRT precludes any evidence-based recommendation for therapy. In general, patients with symptomatic CRT are treated with anticoagulant therapy, using the same regimens as those for VTE. Some clinicians advocate removal of the involved central line, but this has not been proven to improve short-term morbidity or reduce long-term sequelae. Anticoagulant therapy should be continued for a minimum of 3 months and perhaps until the catheter is no longer needed and is removed.

Arterial Thrombotic Events

Patients with cancer receiving active cancer treatment have an increased risk of arterial thrombotic events. The true incidence is not well defined, but approximately 20% of all thrombotic complications in cancer patients are arterial thrombotic events.[90] These include myocardial infarction, cerebrovascular accidents, nonbacterial thrombotic endocarditis, and peripheral arterial thromboembolism.[90,137–140] The pathogenic mechanisms are unknown, but these events may due to treatment-related injury to the endothelium.[141–143] In reviews of studies evaluating adjuvant therapy for breast cancer, the risk of arterial thrombosis was approximately 1%.[144,145] Estimates in other types of cancer are not available. In general, standard antithrombotic therapies appropriate for the clinical situation are recommended.

Heparin-Induced Thrombocytopenia

HIT is an immune-mediated drug reaction to heparin caused by the development of antibodies directed against an antigenic target formed by heparin bound to platelet factor 4. Binding of the resultant immune complex to the FcγRII receptors on circulating platelets induces platelet activation and aggregation and ultimately leads to thrombin generation.[146] A definitive diagnosis of HIT requires confirmation of the presence of functional HIT antibodies, but treatment should not be withheld until the laboratory result is available. Currently, commercially available assays for HIT antibodies are not completely satisfactory and are not standardized. Enzyme-linked immunosorbent assays are designed to detect the presence of HIT antibodies, whereas functional ^{14}C-serotonin release assays detect antibodies with the ability to induce platelet activation.[147,148] The most common presentation of HIT is new or extension of existing venous or arterial thrombosis in a patient who has received heparin as recently as 5 days previously (or longer) and who has a platelet count of less than 150×10^9/L or a platelet count that has dropped by more than 50% below baseline values. HIT should also be considered in cases of rapid onset thrombocytopenia (less than 5 days after heparin exposure) in patients who have previously received heparin in the past 120 days.[147,149]

Generally, HIT with thrombosis is most commonly described in patients who have inflammatory processes that lower the threshold for platelet activation, for example, surgery. Theoretically, the incidence of HIT may be lower in patients with cancer because of their immunosuppression, but a small retrospective study suggested that cancer patients with HIT are more likely to develop thrombosis than noncancer patients with HIT.[150] In addition, HIT is more difficult to diagnose in this population because thrombocytopenic disorders are relatively common. Therefore, it is important to maintain a high index of suspicion and investigate for HIT in patients presenting with unexplained thrombocytopenia following exposure to heparin.

Treatment

In patients with a confirmed diagnosis of HIT or in whom there is a high clinical suspicion for HIT, alternative anticoagulants are now available for prophylaxis and treatment.[147,149,151] Argatroban and lepirudin are direct thrombin inhibitors that are given intravenously and must be monitored according to the aPTT.[152,153] Argatroban is preferred in patients with renal insufficiency because it is primarily metabolized by the liver, whereas lepirudin is cleared by the kidneys. Danaparoid sodium is a low-molecular-weight heparinoid that can be given as fixed-dose subcutaneous injections, and its anticoagulant effect can be monitored by antifactor Xa activity.[154] In patients with acute thrombosis with HIT, all heparins should be stopped immediately and treatment with one of these alternative anticoagulants should be instituted and continued for a minimum of 5 days. Warfarin should be avoided until thrombocytopenia has resolved. Heparin should also be discontinued in patients with HIT who have isolated thrombocytopenia even without evidence of thrombosis. These patients may benefit from the prophylaxis using an alternate anticoagulant because they have a higher risk of developing thrombosis.[155]

Thrombotic Thrombocytopenic Purpura

TTP is a microangiopathic hemolytic anemia characterized by platelet-rich microvascular thrombosis. The clinical syndrome is characterized by the pentad of thrombocytopenia, microangiopathic hemolytic anemia (schistocytic anemia), neurologic complications, renal impairment, and fever; however, it is uncommon for all five elements to occur concomitantly. A large prospective study of TTP patients found that 100% of patients had schistocytic anemia and thrombocytopenia, 71% had neurologic complications, 59% had renal impairment, and 24% had fever.[156] Significant overlap exists between TTP and HUS, another thrombotic microangiopathy. However, HUS generally affects children, is marked by renal impairment, and, in its classic form, follows a diarrheal illness triggered by an infection with *Escherichia coli* O157:H7.

Excess ultralarge-molecular-weight multimers of von Willebrand's factor (vWF) have been demonstrated in the plasma of patients with TTP and facilitate the formation of microvascular thrombosis, the hallmark of this disease.[157] Recently, using a genome-wide linkage analysis in four pedigrees of affected patients, mutations in the *ADAMTS13* gene (a disintegrin metalloproteinase and thrombospondin-like domain) have been identified as the cause of congenital

TTP.[158] Mutations in this gene result in decreased vWF protease activity and high levels of plasma ultralarge-molecular-weight VWF. The underlying mechanism of acquired TTP, the more common form of the disease, may also be a mutation of *ADAMTS13*; however, vWF protease activity has been shown to be reduced not only in TTP but also in other thrombocytopenic disorders.[159,160]

TTP is a recognized complication of cancer and occurs most commonly in one of three clinical settings: metastatic disease, treatment with chemotherapy, and HSCT. The tumors most commonly associated with TTP are metastatic adenocarcinomas of the stomach, breast, and lung.[161,162] Certain chemotherapeutic agents have been implicated in TTP, in particular, mitomycin C. Up to 10% of patients who receive a cumulative dose of 60 mg or more of mitomycin C have been reported to develop this complication.[163] Chemotherapy-induced TTP portends a poor prognosis with a mortality rate of over 50% within 2 months despite adequate therapeutic plasma exchange (TPE), the mainstay of treatment.[163] For HPCT-associated TTP, a recent systematic review reported that the frequency of diagnosis of TTP-HUS following allogeneic HSCT varied from 0.5 to 63.6%.[164] TTP may mimic other HSCT-related complications, such as sepsis and graft-versus-host disease, which should be excluded prior to initiating therapy with TPE.[165] Risk factors for the development of TTP in the setting of HSCT include total-body irradiation,[166] the use of cyclosporine,[167,168] and graft-versus-host disease.[167] Cyclosporine, a common medication used in the post-HSCT setting, is the most common cause of drug-associated TTP.[169] In general, the prognosis of cancer-associated TTP is worse than sporadic or hereditary TTP and responds poorly to TPE.[170]

Management

The mainstay of treatment for TTP is TPE. Prior to the use of plasma exchange, 90% of patients with TTP died[171]; with current therapies, the mortality from TTP is close to 20%. Patients who respond poorly to once-daily plasma exchange (generally defined as patients with persistence or recurrence of severe thrombocytopenia and hemolysis or patients with new neurologic abnormalities while on TPE) may benefit from increased frequency or increased volume of TPE or the addition of corticosteroids.[172] Other ancillary treatments include vincristine, splenectomy, IVIG, immunosuppressive therapy, or antiplatelet agents.

Transfusion Medicine Issues in Cancer Patients

Blood transfusion is an important component of the care of cancer patients. Roughly half of all RBC transfusions are administered to medical

patients, and patients with hematologic disorders account for approximately 15% of overall RBC use on medical wards.[173–175] In the mid-1980s, blood transfusion was plagued by a high rate of viral disease transmission; however, since then, refined donor testing and better methods of virus inactivation have rendered the current risk of transfusion transmission of known viruses extremely low. Currently, bacterial contamination has become recognized as the most important infectious disease threat to the safety of the blood supply. New and emerging pathogens are a constant threat, and thus, general methods of pathogen inactivation, including the addition of alkylating agents or photosensitive agents such as riboflavin or psoralens, are currently being developed.[176]

Apart from infectious risks, blood transfusion can be associated with important clinical complications that require prompt recognition and treatment. Knowledge of infectious and noninfectious transfusion-associated complications is essential so that these complications can be managed appropriately and prevented when possible and patient requiring blood transfusions can be adequately informed.[177]

Infectious Complications of Blood Transfusion

Virus and Prion Transmission

The risks of transfusion transmission of known viruses are summarized in Table 7. With current nucleic acid-amplification testing (NAT) of blood donors, the residual risk of human immunodeficiency virus (HIV) and hepatitis C virus transmission is approximately 1 in 2 million blood units.[178] The rate of transmission of cytomegalovirus and human T-lymphotrophic virus I and II is effectively reduced by the removal of white blood cells from the donor unit,[179,180] a

Table 7 Infectious risks of blood Transfusion

Infection	Risk per unit transfused
HIV	1: 2–1:4 million
Hepatitis C	1: 2–1:3 million
Hepatitis B	1:30,000–1:500,000
Hepatitis A	Extremely low risk
HTLV I/II	1:2 million; lower rate with leukoreduction
Cytomegalovirus	Up to 1–2% in high-risk patients
Syphilis	Extremely low risk
West Nile virus	Risk unknown
Variant Creutzfeld-Jacob disease	2 cases reported in the United Kingdom

Adapted from Dodd RY et al, Kleinman S et al, and Chiavetta JA et al.[233–235]

HIV = human immunodeficiency virus; HTLV = human T-lymphotrophic virus.

practice that has become routine in many centers. Screening of blood donors for West Nile virus by minipool (six sample) NAT testing was implemented in the United States in June 2003, ever since transfusion-transmission of West Nile virus infection became recognized following the 2002 US epidemic. Seven cases of transfusion transmitted West Nile virus disease have been reported in the United States since testing was implemented, prompting the implementation of more sensitive, single-donor NAT testing.[181,182]

Two cases of transfusion transmission of the prion protein associated with variant Creutzfeldt-Jacob disease have been reported in the recent literature.[183,184] Currently, no effective donor screening test is available; however, many blood collection agencies defer donors who resided in areas where bovine spongiform encephalopathy was prevalent.[185]

Bacterial Contamination

Bacteria are currently the greatest infectious disease risk of blood transfusion[186] and the second most common cause of transfusion-related deaths reported to the US Food and Drug Administration (FDA) after transfusion-related acute lung injury.[187] Platelet products are especially prone to bacterial contamination as they are stored for up to 5 days at room temperature, thus providing an ideal growth medium for bacteria. It is estimated that 1 in 1,000 to 1 in 3,000 platelet concentrates is contaminated with bacteria.[188,189] The incidence is approximately fivefold higher for a typical transfusion of random donor platelets (transfused as a pool of five whole blood–derived platelet concentrates).[190] The prevalence of transfusion-associated sepsis is estimated to occur following one-sixth of contaminated transfusions,[191] and one study estimated a fatality rate of 1 in 500,000 platelet units transfused.[192] The organisms most commonly implicated in bacteria-contaminated platelets are *Staphylococcus aureus*, coagulase-negative staphylococci, *Corynebacterium*, *Propionibacterium*, and *Streptococcus* species. These organisms form part of the normal skin flora that can contaminate the blood unit at the time of donation.

Bacterial contamination of RBCs is much less common; however, RBC-associated sepsis is more often fatal.[193] The most common organisms implicated in septic RBC transfusion reactions are *Yersinia enterocolitica*, *Serratia*, and *Pseudomonas* species. These gram-negative organisms can cause endotoxic shock and are not inactivated during cold storage.

The clinical presentation of septic reactions to platelet transfusions varies from fever and chills to hypotension and shock. Generally, these reactions occur shortly after the transfusion. A body temperature elevation of at least 2°C is invariably present. RBC-associated sepsis tends to be more severe, with shock and DIC often occurring

even before the transfusion is completed. Blood products are often overlooked as the source of sepsis, especially in patients with malignancy, who may acquire infections from multiple other sources. However, vigilance in recognizing and preventing septic transfusion reactions is especially important in cancer patients, who may be at increased risk of infection owing to underlying immunosuppression.

Treatment In cases of new fever and/or hypotension associated with a blood transfusion, the transfusion should be immediately stopped, blood cultures should be drawn from the recipient and from all implicated blood components, and the transfusion medicine service should be notified so that co-components can be recalled if necessary. Hemolytic transfusion reactions should be excluded. Empiric therapy with antibiotics and hemodynamic support are often required even before an organism can be isolated.

To prevent septic reactions owing to bacterial contamination, the American Association of Blood Banks implemented a new safety standard in March 2004 requiring blood banks to implement strategies to limit and detect bacterial contamination of all platelet products.[194] Such strategies may include ensuring proper donor skin antisepsis and initial aliquot diversion from blood collections, bacterial detection of platelets by culture or indirect methods (ie, measurement of oxygen tension or pH), and the use of apheresis platelets instead of pooled random donor platelets.[190] Ensuring the appropriate use of blood products for all patients is another important principle that should be upheld.

Non-infectious Transfusion Complications

Noninfectious complications of blood transfusion are common (Table 8). Discussed in the following section are the clinical emergencies: transfusion-related acute lung injury (TRALI), hemolytic transfusion reactions, anaphylactic transfusion reactions, and post-transfusion

Table 8 Non-infectious risks of blood transfusion

Transfusion Reaction	Risk per unit transfused
Transfusion-related acute lung injury	1:5,000–1:100,000
Acute hemolytic	1:20,000
Anaphylactic	1:1,500–1:23,000
Allergic	1:33–1:300
Delayed hemolytic	1:10,000
Febrile nonhemolytic	1:500 RBC transfusions 1:14 platelet transfusions
Transfusion-associated circulatory overload	1:100

Adapted from Kleinman S et al.[234]
RBC = red blood cell.

purpura (PTP); and the most common transfusion reaction, febrile nonhemolytic transfusion reaction (FNHTR).

Transfusion-Related Acute Lung Injury

TRALI is a rare complication of blood transfusion characterized by the rapid development of acute lung injury occurring within 6 hours of the transfusion. The clinical presentation is indistinguishable from adult respiratory distress syndrome, with hypoxemia, bilateral pulmonary infiltrates on chest radiograph, and preservation of cardiac function (noncardiogenic pulmonary edema). Other features include fever and hypotension that is generally refractory to fluid resuscitation, the need for intubation and mechanical ventilation, and, in most cases, a rapid recovery within 48 to 96 hours.[195] However, TRALI is fatal in approximately 5 to 10% of cases and was the most common cause of transfusion-related deaths reported to the FDA from 2001 to 2003.[187]

Both immune and nonimmune mechanisms have been proposed in the pathophysiology of TRALI. Antileukocyte antibodies, usually with specificity for human leukocyte, granulocyte, or monocyte antigens, have been detected in patients with TRALI or in implicated donors.[187,196,197] These antibodies are thought to react with recipient leukocytes, causing leukosequestration and activation of monocytes and complement, endothelial damage, and a capillary leak syndrome in the lungs.[197] Antileukocyte antibodies may also form immune complexes, causing neutrophil activation.[198] Some authors report a low rate of antibody detection, suggesting that other, nonimmune mechanisms may be important in the pathophysiology of TRALI,[199] such as the accumulation of neutrophil-priming lipids in stored blood products that cause neutrophil activation and lung injury.[200,201] Patients with hematologic malignancy and cardiac disease seem to be at greatest risk of TRALI.[199] It has been hypothesized that two events are required for TRALI to occur: the first is a predisposing clinical condition such as surgery, trauma, or severe infection that results in activation of the pulmonary endothelium and the second is the transfusion of cytokines, biologically active lipids, or leukoagglutinating antibodies that results in neutrophil activation and acute lung injury.[202]

Treatment for TRALI is largerly supportive, and patients often require a brief period of inutbation and mechanical ventilation. Diuretics are generally ineffective, and the benefit of corticosteroids, prostaglandins, nonsteroidal anti-inflammatory medications, and antibody-based therapies remains unproven.[195,203]

Hemolytic Transfusion Reactions

Acute hemolytic transfusion reaction (AHTR) is the accelerated destruction of donor and/or recipient RBCs immediately following or within 24 hours of a transfusion.[204] These reactions most often occur when preexisting antibodies in the recipient's circulation react with RBC antigens on donor cells (ie, group A or red cells transfused to a group O recipient); however, AHTRs may also occur as a result of the passive transfer of hemolytic antibodies in plasma-containing blood products.[205–208] Clerical errors (ie, inadvertently transfusing the wrong units of blood) accounted for 86% of fatal AHTRs reported to the FDA between 1976 and 1985.[209] The consequence is intravascular hemolysis, and the clinical presentation includes fever, pain, hemoglobinemia, and hemoglobinuria. In severe cases, hypotension, DIC, and acute renal failure ensue as a result of cytokine release,[210–212] endothelial tissue factor overexpression,[213] and the nephrotoxic effects of free hemoglobin.[214,215]

The severity of AHTR is directly related to the volume of incompatible blood transfused. Therefore, the transfusion must be stopped as soon as hemolysis is suspected. Vigorous fluid resuscitation and vasopressor agents are often required in cases of hemodynamic compromise. Exchange transfusion with antigen-negative blood should be considered in patients who respond poorly to supportive measures and who have been exposed to large volumes of incompatible blood.

Delayed hemolytic transfusion reaction occurs when the transfusion of RBCs induces an anamnestic antibody response and hemolysis of the transfused cells 2 days to 3 weeks following the transfusion. Patients generally have an alloantibody to RBC antigens that is of sufficiently low titer to elude detection at pretransfusion testing; however, on secondary exposure to the offending antigen, the alloantibody titer rapidly rises and causes hemolysis. Extravascular hemolysis is the main feature of a delayed hemolytic transfusion reaction, which is characterized clinically by an unexplained post-transfusion drop in hematocrit, a positive DAT with IgG or complement coating the cells, and laboratory evidence of hemolysis. Treatment is supportive and, if required, additional transfusions must be antigen negative.[216]

Anaphylactic Transfusion Reactions

Anaphylactic transfusion reactions are characterized by skin rash, respiratory compromise, upper airway obstruction, bronchospasm, cardiovascular collapse, nausea, vomiting, and abdominal pain occurring rapidly within 1 to 45 minutes following the start of the transfusion. The absence of fever and the presence of cutaneous signs distinguished anaphylactic reactions from septic or severe hemolytic reactions. Less severe allergic reactions, generally manifested by cutaneous reactions only, are far more common,

complicating up to 2 to 3% of transfusions.[217] The mechanisms of anaphylactic transfusion reactions include IgE-mediated mast cell activation from allergens in the transfused product; the passive transfer of exogenous anaphylatoxins such as IgE, C3a, C5a, and histamine; and IgG antigen-antibody interactions resulting in endogenous anaphylatoxins. Preformed (IgG) anti-IgA antibodies causing anaphylactic transfusion reactions was first described in 1968 by Vyas and colleagues.[218] However, most anaphylactic reactions are likely not due to anti-IgA[219] but to other mechanisms or perhaps other preformed IgG antibodies in the recipient (eg, antihaptoglobin antibodies).[220]

Anaphylaxis following blood transfusion is a medical emergency and should be managed in the same manner as anaphylaxis to other allergens. The offending agent must be removed immediately by stopping the transfusion, epinephrine should be administered subcutaneously or intravenously depending on the severity of the reaction, and cardiovascular support must be initiated with fluids, inotropes, oxygen therapy, and endotracheal intubation when necessary. Antihistamines may be given for the treatment of urticaria. For mild allergic reactions (itching and hives), administration of antihistamines alone may suffice and the transfusion may be slowly restarted once the reaction abates. Washed RBCs and platelets should be used for patients with repeated anaphylactic or anaphylactoid reactions who required additional transfusions and who do not have anti-IgA antibodies. Patients with undetectable IgA levels in whom anti-IgA antibodies are detected following an anaphylactic transfusion reaction should receive subsequent transfusions from IgA-deficient donors only.[221]

Post-Transfusion Purpura

PTP is characterized by the sudden onset of severe thrombocytopenia 5 to 10 days following blood transfusion in a patient sensitized by previous pregnancies or transfusions.[222] Platelet counts usually fall below 10×10^9/L, and mucocutaneous bleeding, including wet purpura, epistaxis, and gastrointestinal or urinary tract hemorrhage, is common. In fact, PTP is associated with a 7% risk of death owing to intracranial hemorrhage.[223,224] Although other platelet antigens have been implicated in this syndrome, most patients with PTP are homozygous for the human platelet antigen 1b (HPA-1b, formerly PL^A2) and have formed alloantibodies against HPA-1a in response to previous exposure. Blood transfusions containing platelet antigens, including whole blood, RBCs, platelets, and plasma transfusions, invoke a brisk antibody response, which destroys not only transfused antigen-positive platelets but also autologous antigen-negative platelets. The proposed mechanisms for autologous platelet destruction include immune complex formation

and platelet Fc receptor binding,[225] platelet autoantibody formation in response to exogenous platelet antigen,[226] and adsorption of soluble platelet antigen onto autologous platelets.[227] Platelets from patients with PTP should be phenotyped for common platelet antigens using serologic or deoxyribonucleic acid (DNA)-based assays.

PTP is a rare syndrome; only 3% of Caucasians in North America do not express HPA-1a in their platelets, and less than one-third of them would be expected to mount the required immune response.[228] In addition, patients invariably have a history of pregnancies or transfusions. With these figures, 8,000 to 9,000 cases of HPA-1a-negative PTP would be expected per year in the United States; however, approximately 300 cases have been reported in the literature.[223]

IVIG (0.5 g/kg on each of 2 consecutive days) is considered first-line therapy for PTP.[229] Other therapies that have been used include high-dose corticosteroids and therapeutic plasma exchange. Platelet transfusions are generally ineffective; however, in patients with severe bleeding complications, a trial of antigen-negative platelet transfusions should be attempted.[230]

Febrile Nonhemolytic Transfusion Reactions

FNHTRs are characterized by a rise in temperature of at least 1°C that cannot be explained by the patient's clinical condition, often accompanied by chills, rigors, and a feeling of discomfort. The frequency of FNHTR following RBC transfusion ranges from 1 to 12% and following platelet transfusion from 11.4 to 37.5%.[231] Product storage time, leukocyte content, and cytokines present in the transfusion have been associated with FNHTR; thus, leukocyte depletion of platelets, especially prior to storage, use of fresh platelets, and plasma removal of platelets are effective methods of preventing FNHTRs.[232]

FNHTR should be managed according to the severity of the reaction; mild reactions can usually be managed with antipyretics and a brief interruption of the transfusion; for moderate and severe reactions that include hypotension and dyspnea, the transfusion should be stopped and hemolytic or septic reactions should be excluded.[232]

REFERENCES

1. Nutritional anaemias: report of a WHO scientific group. World Health Organ Tech Rep Ser 1968;405:5–37.
2. Knight K, Wade S, Balducci L. Prevalence and outcomes of anemia in cancer: a systematic review of the literature. Am J Med 2004;116 Suppl 7A:11S–26S.
3. Tefferi A. Anemia in adults: a contemporary approach to diagnosis. Mayo Clin Proc 2003;78:1274–80.
4. Spivak JL. Cancer-related anemia: its causes and characteristics. Semin Oncol 1994;21(2 Suppl 3):3–8.
5. Cartwright GE. The anemia of chronic disorders. Semin Hematol 1966;3:351–75.
6. Means RT Jr, Krantz SB. Progress in understanding the pathogenesis of the anemia of chronic disease. Blood 1992;80:1639–47.

7. Means RT Jr. Advances in the anemia of chronic disease. Int J Hematol 1999;70:7–12.

8. Ganz T. Hepcidin, a key regulator of iron metabolism and mediator of anemia of inflammation. Blood 2003; 102:783–8.

9. Nemeth E, Valore EV, Territo M, et al. Hepcidin, a putative mediator of anemia of inflammation, is a type II acute-phase protein. Blood 2003;101:2461–3.

10. Rivera S, Liu L, Nemeth E, et al. Hepcidin excess induces the sequestration of iron and exacerbates tumor-associated anemia. Blood 2005;105(4):1797–802.

11. Nemeth E, Rivera S, Gabayan V, et al. IL-6 mediates hypoferremia of inflammation by inducing the synthesis of the iron regulatory hormone hepcidin. J Clin Invest 2004; 113:1271–6.

12. Blajchman MA, Hebert PC. Red blood cell transfusion strategies. Transfus Clin Biol 2001;8:207–10.

13. Hardy JF. Current status of transfusion triggers for red blood cell concentrates. Transfus Apheresis Sci 2004;31:55–66.

14. Heddens D, Alberts DS, Hannigan EV, et al. Prediction of the need for red cell transfusion in newly diagnosed ovarian cancer patients undergoing platinum-based treatment. Gynecol Oncol 2002;86:239–43.

15. Henry DH. Changing patterns of care in the management of anemia. Semin Oncol 1992;19(3 Suppl 8):3–7.

16. Pavel JN. Red blood cell transfusions for anemia. Semin Oncol Nurs 1990;6:117–22.

17. Calder L, Hebert PC, Carter AO, Graham ID. Review of published recommendations and guidelines for the transfusion of allogenic red blood cells and plasma. CMAJ 1997;156(11 Suppl):S1–8.

18. Hebert PC, Wells G, Blajchman MA, et al. A multicenter, randomized, controlled clinical trial of transfusion requirements in critical care. Transfusion Requirements in Critical Care Investigators, Canadian Critical Care Trials Group. N Engl J Med 1999;340:409–17.

19. Seidenfeld J, Piper M, Flamm C, et al. Epoetin treatment of anemia associated with cancer therapy: a systematic review and meta-analysis of controlled clinical trials. J Natl Cancer Inst 2001;93:1204–14.

20. Bohlius J, Langensiepen S, Schwarzer G, et al. Erythropoietin for patients with malignant disease. Cochrane Database Syst Rev 2004;(3):CD003407.

21. Rizzo JD, Lichtin AE, Woolf SH, et al. Use of epoetin in patients with cancer: evidence-based clinical practice guidelines of the American Society of Clinical Oncology and the American Society of Hematology. Blood 2002; 100:2303–20.

22. Bokemeyer C, Aapro MS, Courdi A, et al. EORTC guidelines for the use of erythropoietic proteins in anaemic patients with cancer. Eur J Cancer 2004;40:2201–16.

23. Bohlius J, Langensiepen S, Schwarzer G, et al. Erythropoietin for patients with malignant disease. Cochrane Database Syst Rev 2004;(3):CD003407.

24. Stowell CP, Levin J, Spiess BD, Winslow RM. Progress in the development of RBC substitutes. Transfusion 2001;41: 287–99.

25. Wahr JA, Trouwborst A, Spence RK, et al. A pilot study of the effects of a perflubron emulsion, AF 0104, on mixed venous oxygen tension in anesthetized surgical patients. Anesth Analg 1996;82:103–7.

26. Stern SA, Dronen SC, McGoron AJ, et al. Effect of supplemental perfluorocarbon administration on hypotensive resuscitation of severe uncontrolled hemorrhage. Am J Emerg Med 1995;13:269–75.

27. Saxena R, Wijnhoud AD, Carton H, et al. Controlled safety study of a hemoglobin-based oxygen carrier, DCLHb, in acute ischemic stroke. Stroke 1999;30:993–6.

28. Sloan EP, Koenigsberg M, Gens D, et al. Diaspirin cross-linked hemoglobin (DCLHb) in the treatment of severe traumatic hemorrhagic shock: a randomized controlled efficacy trial. JAMA 1999;282:1857–64.

29. Phillips WT, Klipper RW, Awasthi VD, et al. Polyethylene glycol-modified liposome-encapsulated hemoglobin: a long circulating red cell substitute. J Pharmacol Exp Ther 1999;288:665–70.

30. Rund D, Ben Yehuda D. Therapy-related leukemia and myelodysplasia: evolving concepts of pathogenesis and treatment. Hematology 2004;9:179–87.

31. Leone G, Mele L, Pulsoni A, et al. The incidence of secondary leukemias. Haematologica 1999;84:937–45.

32. Boivin JF, Hutchison GB, Zauber AG, et al. Incidence of second cancers in patients treated for Hodgkin's disease. J Natl Cancer Inst 1995;87:732–41.

33. Armitage JO, Carbone PP, Connors JM, et al. Treatment-related myelodysplasia and acute leukemia in non-Hodgkin's lymphoma patients. J Clin Oncol 2003;21: 897–906.

34. Taussig DC, Davies AJ, Cavenagh JD, et al. Durable remissions of myelodysplastic syndrome and acute myeloid leukemia after reduced-intensity allografting. J Clin Oncol 2003;21:3060–5.

35. Yakoub-Agha I, de La SP, Ribaud P, et al. Allogeneic bone marrow transplantation for therapy-related myelodysplastic syndrome and acute myeloid leukemia: a long-term study of 70 patients-report of the French Society of Bone Marrow Transplantation. J Clin Oncol 2000;18:963–71.

36. Garrido SM, Bryant E, Appelbaum FR. Allogeneic stem cell transplantation for relapsed and refractory acute myeloid leukemia patients with 11q23 abnormalities. Leuk Res 2000;24:481–6.

37. Charles RJ, Sabo KM, Kidd PG, Abkowitz JL. The pathophysiology of pure red cell aplasia: implications for therapy. Blood 1996;87:4831–8.

38. Chikkappa G, Zarrabi MH, Tsan MF. Pure red-cell aplasia in patients with chronic lymphocytic leukemia. Medicine (Baltimore) 1986;65:339–51.

39. Lacy MQ, Kurtin PJ, Tefferi A. Pure red cell aplasia: association with large granular lymphocyte leukemia and the prognostic value of cytogenetic abnormalities. Blood 1996;87:3000–6.

40. Bennett CL, Luminari S, Nissenson AR, et al. Pure red-cell aplasia and epoetin therapy. N Engl J Med 2004;351: 1403–8.

41. Cournoyer D, Toffelmire EB, Wells GA, et al. Anti-erythropoietin antibody-mediated pure red cell aplasia after treatment with recombinant erythropoietin products: recommendations for minimization of risk. J Am Soc Nephrol 2004;15:2728–34.

42. Young NS. Parvovirus infection and its treatment. Clin Exp Immunol 1996;104 Suppl 1:26–30.

43. Go RS, Li CY, Tefferi A, Phyliky RL. Acquired pure red cell aplasia associated with lymphoproliferative disease of granular T lymphocytes. Blood 2001;98:483–5.

44. Yamada O, Mizoguchi H, Oshimi K. Cyclophosphamide therapy for pure red cell aplasia associated with granular lymphocyte-proliferative disorders. Br J Haematol 1997; 97:392–9.

45. Grigg AP, O'Flaherty E. Cyclosporin A for the treatment of pure red cell aplasia associated with myelodysplasia. Leuk Lymphoma 2001;42:1339–42.

46. Kondo H, Narita K, Iwasaki H, Watanabe J. Effectiveness of cyclosporin A in a patient with pure red cell aplasia associated with T cell-lineage granular lymphocyte proliferative disorders resistant to cyclophosphamide therapy. Eur J Haematol 2000;64:206–7.

47. Yamada O, Motoji T, Mizoguchi H. Selective effect of cyclosporine monotherapy for pure red cell aplasia not associated with granular lymphocyte-proliferative disorders. Br J Haematol 1999;106:371–6.

48. Auner HW, Wolfler A, Beham-Schmid C, et al. Restoration of erythropoiesis by rituximab in an adult patient with primary acquired pure red cell aplasia refractory to conventional treatment. Br J Haematol 2002;116:727–8.

49. Ru X, Liebman HA. Successful treatment of refractory pure red cell aplasia associated with lymphoproliferative disorders with the anti-CD52 monoclonal antibody alemtuzumab (Campath-1H). Br J Haematol 2003;123: 278–81.

50. Dincol G, Aktan M, Nalcaci M, et al. Clonality of acquired primary pure red cell aplasia: effectiveness of antithymocyte globulin. Leuk Lymphoma 2001;42: 1413–7.

51. Larroche C, Mouthon L, Casadevall N, et al. Successful treatment of thymoma-associated pure red cell aplasia with intravenous immunoglobulins. Eur J Haematol 2000;65: 74–6.

52. Verhelst D, Rossert J, Casadevall N, et al. Treatment of erythropoietin-induced pure red cell aplasia: a retrospective study. Lancet 2004;363:1768–71.

53. Sturgeon P, Smith LE, Chun HM, et al. Autoimmune hemolytic anemia associated exclusively with IgA of Rh specificity. Transfusion 1979;19:324–8.

54. Salama A, Mueller-Eckhardt C. Autoimmune haemolytic anaemia in childhood associated with non-complement binding IgM autoantibodies. Br J Haematol 1987;65: 67–71.

55. Gupta N, Kavuru S, Patel D, et al. Rituximab-based chemotherapy for steroid-refractory autoimmune hemolytic anemia of chronic lymphocytic leukemia. Leukemia 2002; 16:2092–5.

56. Robak T, Bonski JZ, Kasznicki M, et al. Re-treatment with cladribine-based regimens in relapsed patients with B-cell chronic lymphocytic leukemia. Efficacy and toxicity in comparison with previous treatment. Eur J Haematol 2002;69:27–36.

57. Diehl LF, Ketchum LH. Autoimmune disease and chronic lymphocytic leukemia: autoimmune hemolytic anemia, pure red cell aplasia, and autoimmune thrombocytopenia. Semin Oncol 1998;25:80–97.

58. Petz LD. A physician's guide to transfusion in autoimmune haemolytic anaemia. Br J Haematol 2004;124:712–6.

59. Trape G, Fianchi L, Lai M, et al. Rituximab chimeric anti-CD20 monoclonal antibody treatment for refractory hemolytic anemia in patients with lymphoproliferative disorders. Haematologica 2003;88:223–5.

60. Engelhardt M, Jakob A, Ruter B, et al. Severe cold hemagglutinin disease (CHD) successfully treated with rituximab. Blood 2002;100:1922–3.

61. Moyo VM, Smith D, Brodsky I, et al. High-dose cyclophosphamide for refractory autoimmune hemolytic anemia. Blood 2002;100:704–6.

62. Schiffer CA, Miller K, Larson RA, et al. A double-blind, placebo-controlled trial of pegylated recombinant human megakaryocyte growth and development factor as an adjunct to induction and consolidation therapy for patients with acute myeloid leukemia. Blood 2000;95: 2530–5.

63. Archimbaud E, Ottmann OG, Yin JA, et al. A randomized, double-blind, placebo-controlled study with pegylated recombinant human megakaryocyte growth and development factor (PEG-rHuMGDF) as an adjunct to chemotherapy for adults with de novo acute myeloid leukemia. Blood 1999;94:3694–701.

64. Geissler K, Yin JA, Ganser A, et al. Prior and concurrent administration of recombinant human megakaryocyte growth and development factor in patients receiving consolidation chemotherapy for de novo acute myeloid leukemia—a randomized, placebo-controlled, double-blind safety and efficacy study. Ann Hematol 2003;82: 677–83.

65. Gaydos LA, Freireich EJ, Mantel N. The quantitative relation between platelet count and hemorrhage in patients with acute leukemia. N Engl J Med 1962;266:905–9.

66. Norol F, Kuentz M, Cordonnier C, et al. Influence of clinical status on the efficiency of stored platelet transfusion. Br J Haematol 1994;86:125–9.

67. Harkness DR, Byrnes JJ, Lian EC, et al. Hazard of platelet transfusion in thrombotic thrombocytopenic purpura. JAMA 1981;246:1931–3.

68. Gordon LI, Kwaan HC, Rossi EC. Deleterious effects of platelet transfusions and recovery thrombocytosis in patients with thrombotic microangiopathy. Semin Hematol 1987;24:194–201.

69. Babcock RB, Dumper CW, Scharfman WB. Heparin-induced immune thrombocytopenia. N Engl J Med 1976;295: 237–41.

70. Cimo PL, Moake JL, Weinger RS, et al. Heparin-induced thrombocytopenia: association with a platelet aggregating factor and arterial thromboses. Am J Hematol 1979;6: 125–33.

71. Stanworth S, Hyde C, Heddle N, et al. Prophylactic platelet transfusion for haemorrhage after chemotherapy and stem cell transplantation. Cochrane Database Syst Rev 2004;(4):CD004269.

72. Gmur J, Burger J, Schanz U, et al. Safety of stringent prophylactic platelet transfusion policy for patients with acute leukaemia. Lancet 1991;338:1223–6.

73. Schiffer CA, Anderson KC, Bennett CL, et al. Platelet transfusion for patients with cancer: clinical practice guidelines of the American Society of Clinical Oncology. J Clin Oncol 2001;19:1519–38.

74. Guidelines for the use of platelet transfusions. Br J Haematol 2003;122:10–23.

75. Practice guidelines for blood component therapy: a report by the American Society of Anesthesiologists Task Force on Blood Component Therapy. Anesthesiology 1996;84: 732–47.

76. Practice parameter for the use of fresh-frozen plasma, cryoprecipitate, and platelets. Fresh-Frozen Plasma, Cryoprecipitate, and Platelets Administration Practice Guidelines Development Task Force of the College of American Pathologists. JAMA 1994;271:777–81.

77. Blajchman MA. Substitutes and alternatives to platelet transfusions in thrombocytopenic patients. J Thromb Haemost 2003;1:1637–41.

78. Tranholm M, Rojkjaer R, Pyke C, et al. Recombinant factor VIIa reduces bleeding in severely thrombocytopenic rabbits. Thromb Res 2003;109:217–23.

79. Ho CH. The hemostatic effect of packed red cell transfusion in patients with anemia. Transfusion 1998;38:1011–4.

80. Bodey GP, Buckley M, Sathe YS, Freireich EJ. Quantitative relationships between circulating leukocytes and infection in patients with acute leukemia. Ann Intern Med 1966;64:328–40.

81. Crawford J, Dale DC, Lyman GH. Chemotherapy-induced neutropenia: risks, consequences, and new directions for its management. Cancer 2004;100:228–37.

82. Lyman GH, Morrison VA, Dale DC, et al. Risk of febrile neutropenia among patients with intermediate-grade non-Hodgkin's lymphoma receiving CHOP chemotherapy. Leuk Lymphoma 2003;44:2069–76.

83. Bohlius J, Reiser M, Schwarzer G, Engert A. Granulopoiesis-stimulating factors to prevent adverse effects in the treatment of malignant lymphoma. Cochrane Database Syst Rev 2004;(3):CD003189.

84. Ozer H, Armitage JO, Bennett CL, et al. 2000 update of recommendations for the use of hematopoietic colony-stimulating factors: evidence-based, clinical practice guidelines. American Society of Clinical Oncology Growth Factors Expert Panel. J Clin Oncol 2000;18:3558–85.

85. Lyman GH, Kuderer NM, Djulbegovic B. Prophylactic granulocyte colony-stimulating factor in patients receiving dose-intensive cancer chemotherapy: a meta-analysis. Am J Med 2002;112:406–11.

86. Rusthoven J, Bramwell V, Stephenson B. Use of granulocyte colony-stimulating factor (G-CSF) in patients receiving myelosuppressive chemotherapy for the treatment of cancer. Provincial Systemic Treatment Disease Site Group. Cancer Prev Control 1998;2:179–90.

87. Lyman GH, Lyman CG, Sanderson RA, Balducci L. Decision analysis of hematopoietic growth factor use in patients receiving cancer chemotherapy. J Natl Cancer Inst 1993;85:488–93.

88. Uyl-de Groot CA, Vellenga E, Rutten FF. An economic model to assess the savings from a clinical application of haematopoietic growth factors. Eur J Cancer 1996;32A:57–62.

89. Rickles FR, Levine MN, Dvorak HF. Abnormalities of hemostasis in malignancy. In: Colman RW, Hirsh J, Marder VJ, et al, editors. Hemostsis and thrombosis. Philadelphia: Lippincott Williams & Wilkins; 2001. p. 1132–52.

90. Sack GH Jr, Levin J, Bell WR. Trousseau's syndrome and other manifestations of chronic disseminated coagulopathy in patients with neoplasms: clinical, pathophysiologic, and therapeutic features. Medicine (Baltimore) 1977;56:1–37.

91. Gouin-Thibault I, Samama MM. Laboratory diagnosis of the thrombophilic state in cancer patients. Semin Thromb Hemost 1999;25:167–72.

92. Levi M, de Jonge E, Meijers J. The diagnosis of disseminated intravascular coagulation. Blood Rev 2002;16:217–23.

93. Levi M. Current understanding of disseminated intravascular coagulation. Br J Haematol 2004;124:567–76.

94. Abraham E, Reinhart K, Opal S, et al. Efficacy and safety of tifacogin (recombinant tissue factor pathway inhibitor) in severe sepsis: a randomized controlled trial. JAMA 2003;290:238–47.

95. Warren BL, Eid A, Singer P, et al. Caring for the critically ill patient. High-dose antithrombin III in severe sepsis: a randomized controlled trial. JAMA 2001;286:1869–78.

96. Bernard GR, Vincent JL, Laterre PF, et al. Efficacy and safety of recombinant human activated protein C for severe sepsis. N Engl J Med 2001;344:699–709.

97. Sallah S, Wan JY. Inhibitors against factor VIII in patients with cancer. Analysis of 41 patients. Cancer 2001;91:1067–74.

98. Delgado J, Jimenez-Yuste V, Hernandez-Navarro F, Villar A. Acquired haemophilia: review and meta-analysis focused on therapy and prognostic factors. Br J Haematol 2003;121:21–35.

99. Sallah S. Treatment of acquired haemophilia with factor eight inhibitor bypassing activity. Haemophilia 2004;10:169–73.

100. Sallah S, Nguyen NP, Abdallah JM, Hanrahan LR. Acquired hemophilia in patients with hematologic malignancies. Arch Pathol Lab Med 2000;124:730–4.

101. Heit JA, Silverstein MD, Mohr DN, et al. Risk factors for deep vein thrombosis and pulmonary embolism: a population-based case-control study. Arch Intern Med 2000;160:809–15.

102. Heit JA, Silverstein MD, Mohr DN, et al. Predictors of survival after deep vein thrombosis and pulmonary embolism: a population-based, cohort study. Arch Intern Med 1999;159:445–53.

103. Sorensen HT, Mellemkjaer L, Olsen JH, Baron JA. Prognosis of cancers associated with venous thromboembolism. N Engl J Med 2000;343:1846–50.

104. Lee AY, Levine MN. Venous thromboembolism and cancer: risks and outcomes. Circulation 2003;107(23 Suppl 1):I17–21.

105. Piccioli A, Lensing AW, Prins MH, et al. Extensive screening for occult malignant disease in idiopathic venous thromboembolism: a prospective randomized clinical trial. J Thromb Haemost 2004;2:884–9.

106. Thodiyil PA, Kakkar AK. Variation in relative risk of venous thromboembolism in different cancers. Thromb Haemost 2002;87:1076–7.

107. Geerts WH, Pineo GF, Heit JA, et al. Prevention of venous thromboembolism: the Seventh ACCP Conference on Antithrombotic and Thrombolytic Therapy. Chest 2004;126(3 Suppl):338S–400S.

108. Efficacy and safety of enoxaparin versus unfractionated heparin for prevention of deep vein thrombosis in elective cancer surgery: a double-blind randomized multicentre trial with venographic assessment. ENOXACAN Study Group. Br J Surg 1997;84:1099–103.

109. Mismetti P, Laporte S, Darmon JY, et al. Meta-analysis of low molecular weight heparin in the prevention of venous thromboembolism in general surgery. Br J Surg 2001;88:913–30.

110. Agnelli G, Bergqvist D, Cohen AT, Gallus AS, Gent M. Randomized clinical trial of postoperative fondaparinux versus perioperative dalteparin for prevention of venous thromboembolism in high-risk abdominal surgery. Br J Surg 2005;92(10):1212–20.

111. Bergqvist D, Agnelli G, Cohen AT, et al. Duration of prophylaxis against venous thromboembolism with enoxaparin after surgery for cancer. N Engl J Med 2002;346:975–80.

112. Rasmussen MS, Wille-Jorgensen P, Jorgensen LN, et al. Prolonged thromboprophylaxis with low molecular weight heparin (dalteparin) following major abdominal surgery for malignancy [abstract]. Blood 2004;102:56a.

113. Levine M, Hirsh J, Gent M, et al. Double-blind randomised trial of a very-low-dose warfarin for prevention of thromboembolism in stage IV breast cancer. Lancet 1994;343:886–9.

114. Kakkar AK, Levine MN, Kadziola Z, et al. Low molecular weight heparin therapy with dalteparin and survival in advanced cancer: the Fragmin Advanced Malignancy Outcome Study (FAMOUS). J Clin Oncol 2004;22:1944–8.

115. Samama MM, Cohen AT, Darmon JY, et al. A comparison of enoxaparin with placebo for the prevention of venous thromboembolism in acutely ill medical patients. Prophylaxis in Medical Patients with Enoxaparin Study Group. N Engl J Med 1999;341:793–800.

116. Leizorovicz A, Cohen AT, Turpie AG, et al. Randomized, placebo-controlled trial of dalteparin for the prevention of venous thromboembolism in acutely ill medical patients. Circulation 2004;110:874–9.

117. Alikhan R, Cohen AT, Combe S, et al. Prevention of venous thromboembolism in medical patients with enoxaparin: a subgroup analysis of the MEDENOX study. Blood Coagul Fibrinolysis 2003;14:341–6.

118. van den Belt AG, Prins MH, Lensing AW, et al. Fixed dose subcutaneous low molecular weight heparins versus adjusted dose unfractionated heparin for venous thromboembolism. Cochrane Database Syst Rev 2000;(2):CD001100.

119. Gould MK, Dembitzer AD, Doyle RL, et al. Low-molecular-weight heparins compared with unfractionated heparin for treatment of acute deep venous thrombosis. A meta-analysis of randomized, controlled trials. Ann Intern Med 1999;130:800–9.

120. Dolovich LR, Ginsberg JS, Douketis JD, et al. A meta-analysis comparing low-molecular-weight heparins with unfractionated heparin in the treatment of venous thromboembolism: examining some unanswered questions regarding location of treatment, product type, and dosing frequency. Arch Intern Med 2000;160:181–8.

121. van Dongen CJ, van den Belt AG, Prins MH, Lensing AW. Fixed dose subcutaneous low molecular weight heparins versus adjusted dose unfractionated heparin for venous thromboembolism. Cochrane Database Syst Rev 2004, (4), CD001100.

122. Levine M, Gent M, Hirsh J, et al. A comparison of low-molecular-weight heparin administered primarily at home with unfractionated heparin administered in the hospital for proximal deep-vein thrombosis. N Engl J Med 1996;334:677–81.

123. Harrison L, McGinnis J, Crowther M, et al. Assessment of outpatient treatment of deep-vein thrombosis with low-molecular-weight heparin. Arch Intern Med 1998;158:2001–3.

124. Prandoni P, Lensing AW, Piccioli A, et al. Recurrent venous thromboembolism and bleeding complications during anticoagulant treatment in patients with cancer and venous thrombosis. Blood 2002;100:3484–8.

125. Hutten BA, Prins MH, Gent M, et al. Incidence of recurrent thromboembolic and bleeding complications among patients with venous thromboembolism in relation to both malignancy and achieved international normalized ratio: a retrospective analysis. J Clin Oncol 2000;18:3078–83.

126. Warkentin TE. Venous limb gangrene during warfarin treatment of cancer-associated deep venous thrombosis. Ann Intern Med 2001;135(8 Pt 1):589–93.

127. Klein L, Galvez A, Klein O, Chediak J. Warfarin-induced limb gangrene in the setting of lung adenocarcinoma. Am J Hematol 2004;76:176–9.

128. Lee AY, Levine MN, Baker RI, et al. Low-molecular-weight heparin versus a coumarin for the prevention of recurrent venous thromboembolism in patients with cancer. N Engl J Med 2003;349:146–53.

129. Meyer G, Marjanovic Z, Valcke J, et al. Comparison of low-molecular-weight heparin and warfarin for the secondary prevention of venous thromboembolism in patients with cancer: a randomized controlled study. Arch Intern Med 2002;162:1729–35.

130. Hull RD, Pineo GF, Brant RF, et al. Long-term low-molecular-weight heparin versus usual care in proximal-vein thrombosis patients with cancer. Am J Med 2006;119(12):1062–72.

131. Lee AY, Rickles FR, Julian JA, Gent M, Baker RI, Bowden C, et al. Randomized comparison of low molecular weight heparin and coumarin derivatives on the survival of patients with cancer and venous thromboembolism. J Clin Oncol 2005;23(10):2123–9.

132. Klerk CP, Smorenburg SM, Otten HM, et al. The effect of low molecular weight heparin on survival in patients with advanced malignancy. J Clin Oncol 2005;23(10):2130–5.

133. Karthaus M, Kretzschmar A, Kroning H, et al. Dalteparin for prevention of catheter-related complications in cancer patients with central venous catheters: final results of a double-blind, placebo-controlled phase III trial. Ann Oncol 2006;17(2):289–96.

134. Couban S, Goodyear M, Burnell M, et al. Randomized placebo-controlled study of low-dose warfarin for the prevention of central venous catheter-associated thrombosis in patients with cancer. J Clin Oncol 2005;23(18):4063–9.

135. Walshe LJ, Malak SF, Eagan J, Sepkowitz KA. Complication rates among cancer patients with peripherally inserted central catheters. J Clin Oncol 2002;20:3276–81.

136. Masci G, Magagnoli M, Zucali PA, et al. Minidose warfarin prophylaxis for catheter-associated thrombosis in cancer patients: can it be safely associated with fluorouracil-based chemotherapy? J Clin Oncol 2003;21:736–9.

137. Yeh PS, Lin HJ. Cerebrovascular complications in patients with malignancy: report of three cases and review of the literature. Acta Neurol Taiwan 2004;13:34–8.

138. Gallerini S, Fanucchi S, Sonnoli C, et al. Stroke in the young as the clinical onset of non-Hodgkin's lymphoma with paraneoplastic endocarditis. Eur J Neurol 2004;11:421–2.

139. Schattner A, Klepfish A, Huszar M, Shani A. Two patients with arterial thromboembolism among 311 patients with adenocarcinoma of the pancreas. Am J Med Sci 2002;324:335–8.

140. Rogers LR. Cerebrovascular complications in cancer patients. Neurol Clin 2003;21:167–92.

141. Hallahan DE, Chen AY, Teng M, Cmelak AJ. Drug-radiation interactions in tumor blood vessels. Oncology (Huntingt) 1999;13(10 Suppl 5):71–7.

142. Donati MB, Falanga A. Pathogenetic mechanisms of thrombosis in malignancy. Acta Haematol 2001;106:18–24.

143. Falanga A. Mechanisms of hypercoagulation in malignancy and during chemotherapy. Haemostasis 1998;28 Suppl 3:50–60.

144. Saphner T, Tormey DC, Gray R. Venous and arterial thrombosis in patients who received adjuvant therapy for breast cancer. J Clin Oncol 1991;9:286–94.
145. Wall JG, Weiss RB, Norton L, et al. Arterial thrombosis associated with adjuvant chemotherapy for breast carcinoma: a Cancer and Leukemia Group B study. Am J Med 1989; 87:501–4.
146. Kelton JG, Smith JW, Warkentin TE, et al. Immunoglobulin G from patients with heparin-induced thrombocytopenia binds to a complex of heparin and platelet factor 4. Blood 1994;83:3232–9.
147. Warkentin TE. Heparin-induced thrombocytopenia: pathogenesis and management. Br J Haematol 2003;121: 535–55.
148. Chong BH, Eisbacher M. Pathophysiology and laboratory testing of heparin-induced thrombocytopenia. Semin Hematol 1998;35(4 Suppl 5):3–8.
149. Chong BH. Heparin-induced thrombocytopenia. J Thromb Haemost 2003;1:1471–8.
150. Opatrny L, Warner MN. Risk of thrombosis in patients with malignancy and heparin-induced thrombocytopenia. Am J Hematol 2004;76:240–4.
151. Alving BM. How I treat heparin-induced thrombocytopenia and thrombosis. Blood 2003;101:31–7.
152. Greinacher A, Janssens U, Berg G, et al. Lepirudin (recombinant hirudin) for parenteral anticoagulation in patients with heparin-induced thrombocytopenia. Heparin-Associated Thrombocytopenia Study (HAT) investigators. Circulation 1999;100:587–93.
153. Lewis BE, Wallis DE, Berkowitz SD, et al. Argatroban anticoagulant therapy in patients with heparin-induced thrombocytopenia. Circulation 2001;103:1838–43.
154. Ortel TL, Chong BH. New treatment options for heparin-induced thrombocytopenia. Semin Hematol 1998;35 (4 Suppl 5):26–34.
155. Warkentin TE, Kelton JG. A 14-year study of heparin-induced thrombocytopenia. Am J Med 1996;101: 502–7.
156. Rock GA, Shumak KH, Buskard NA, et al. Comparison of plasma exchange with plasma infusion in the treatment of thrombotic thrombocytopenic purpura. Canadian Apheresis Study Group. N Engl J Med 1991;325:393–7.
157. Moake JL, Rudy CK, Troll JH, et al. Unusually large plasma factor VIII:von Willebrand factor multimers in chronic relapsing thrombotic thrombocytopenic purpura. N Engl J Med 1982;307:1432–5.
158. Levy GG, Nichols WC, Lian EC, et al. Mutations in a member of the ADAMTS gene family cause thrombotic thrombocytopenic purpura. Nature 2001;413:488–94.
159. Moore JC, Hayward CP, Warkentin TE, Kelton JG. Decreased von Willebrand factor protease activity associated with thrombocytopenic disorders. Blood 2001;98:1842–6.
160. Mannucci PM, Canciani MT, Forza I, et al. Changes in health and disease of the metalloprotease that cleaves von Willebrand factor. Blood 2001;98:2730–5.
161. Murgo AJ. Thrombotic microangiopathy in the cancer patient including those induced by chemotherapeutic agents. Semin Hematol 1987;24:161–77.
162. Kressel BR, Ryan KP, Duong AT, et al. Microangiopathic hemolytic anemia, thrombocytopenia, and renal failure in patients treated for adenocarcinoma. Cancer 1981;48: 1738–45.
163. Lesesne JB, Rothschild N, Erickson B, et al. Cancer-associated hemolytic-uremic syndrome: analysis of 85 cases from a national registry. J Clin Oncol 1989;7: 781–9.
164. George JN, Li X, McMinn JR, et al. Thrombotic thrombocytopenic purpura-hemolytic uremic syndrome following allogeneic HPC transplantation: a diagnostic dilemma. Transfusion 2004;44:294–304.
165. Roy V, Rizvi MA, Vesely SK, George JN. Thrombotic thrombocytopenic purpura-like syndromes following bone marrow transplantation: an analysis of associated conditions and clinical outcomes. Bone Marrow Transplant 2001;27:641–6.
166. Guinan EC, Tarbell NJ, Niemeyer CM, et al. Intravascular hemolysis and renal insufficiency after bone marrow transplantation. Blood 1988;72:451–5.
167. Holler E, Kolb HJ, Hiller E, et al. Microangiopathy in patients on cyclosporine prophylaxis who developed acute graft-versus-host disease after HLA-identical bone marrow transplantation. Blood 1989;73:2018–24.
168. Schriber JR, Herzig GP. Transplantation-associated thrombotic thrombocytopenic purpura and hemolytic uremic syndrome. Semin Hematol 1997;34:126–33.
169. Atkinson K, Biggs JC, Ting A, et al. Cyclosporin A is associated with faster engraftment and less mucositis than methotrexate after allogeneic bone marrow transplantation. Br J Haematol 1983;53:265–70.
170. Kwaan HC, Gordon LI. Thrombotic microangiopathy in the cancer patient. Acta Haematol 2001;106:52–6.
171. Amorosi EL, Ultmann JE. Thrombotic thrombocytopenic purpura: report of 16 cases and review of the literature. Medicine 1966;45:139–59.
172. George JN, Vesely SK. Thrombotic thrombocytopenic purpura-hemolytic uremic syndrome: diagnosis and treatment. Cleve Clin J Med 2001;68:857–4.
173. Stanworth SJ, Cockburn HA, Boralessa H, Contreras M. Which groups of patients are transfused? A study of red cell usage in London and southeast England. Vox Sang 2002;83:352–7.
174. Wells AW, Mounter PJ, Chapman CE, et al. Where does blood go? Prospective observational study of red cell transfusion in north England. BMJ 2002;325:803.
175. Mathoulin-Pelissier S, Salmi LR, Verret C, Demoures B. Blood transfusion in a random sample of hospitals in France. Transfusion 2000;40:1140–6.
176. Wagner SJ. Pathogen inactivation methods. In: Brecher ME, editor. Bacterial and parasitic contamination of blood components. Bethesda (MD): AABB Press; 2003. p. 201–23.
177. Hart J, Leier B, Nahirniak S. Informed consent for blood transfusion: should the possibility of prion risk be included? Transfus Med Rev 2004;18:177–83.
178. Stramer SL, Glynn SA, Kleinman SH, et al. Detection of HIV-1 and HCV infections among antibody-negative blood donors by nucleic acid-amplification testing. N Engl J Med 2004;351:760–8.
179. Laupacis A, Brown J, Costello B, et al. Prevention of post-transfusion CMV in the era of universal WBC reduction: a consensus statement. Transfusion 2001;41:560–9.
180. Cesaire R, Kerob-Bauchet B, Bourdonne O, et al. Evaluation of HTLV-I removal by filtration of blood cell components in a routine setting. Transfusion 2004;44:42–8.
181. Transfusion-associated transmission of West Nile virus—Arizona, 2004. MMWR Morb Mortal Wkly Rep 2004;53: 842–4.
182. Macedo DO, Beecham BD, Montgomery SP, et al. West Nile virus blood transfusion-related infection despite nucleic acid testing. Transfusion 2004;44:1695–9.
183. Llewelyn CA, Hewitt PE, Knight RS, et al. Possible transmission of variant Creutzfeldt-Jakob disease by blood transfusion. Lancet 2004;363:417–21.
184. Peden AH, Head MW, Ritchie DL, et al. Preclinical vCJD after blood transfusion in a PRNP codon 129 heterozygous patient. Lancet 2004;364:527–9.
185. Murphy EL, David CJ, McEvoy P, et al. Estimating blood donor loss due to the variant CJD travel deferral. Transfusion 2004;44:645–50.
186. Goodnough LT, Shander A, Brecher ME. Transfusion medicine: looking to the future. Lancet 2003;361:161–9.
187. Goldman M, Webert KE, Arnold DM, et al. Proceedings of a consensus conference: towards an understanding of TRALI. Transfus Med Rev 2005;19(1):2–31.
188. Dodd RY. Bacterial contamination and transfusion safety: experience in the United States. Transfus Clin Biol 2003; 10:6–9.
189. Yomtovian R, Lazarus HM, Goodnough LT, et al. A prospective microbiologic surveillance program to detect and prevent the transfusion of bacterially contaminated platelets. Transfusion 1993;33:902–9.
190. Ness P, Braine H, King K, et al. Single-donor platelets reduce the risk of septic platelet transfusion reactions. Transfusion 2001;41:857–61.
191. Goldman M, Blajchman MA. Blood product-associated bacterial sepsis. Transfus Med Rev 1991;5:73–83.
192. Kuehnert MJ, Roth VR, Haley NR, et al. Transfusion-transmitted bacterial infection in the United States, 1998 through 2000. Transfusion 2001;41:1493–9.
193. Sazama K. Bacteria in blood for transfusion. A review. Arch Pathol Lab Med 1994;118:350–65.
194. Fridey. Standards for blood banks and transfusion services. 22[13]. Bethesda (MD): AABB Press; 2003.
195. Webert KE, Blajchman MA. Transfusion-related acute lung injury. Transfus Med Rev 2003;17:252–62.
196. Popovsky MA, Chaplin HC Jr, Moore SB. Transfusion-related acute lung injury: a neglected, serious complication of hemotherapy. Transfusion 1992;32: 589–92.
197. Kopko PM, Paglieroni TG, Popovsky MA, et al. TRALI: correlation of antigen-antibody and monocyte activation in donor-recipient pairs. Transfusion 2003;43:177–84.
198. Popovsky MA, Moore SB. Diagnostic and pathogenetic considerations in transfusion-related acute lung injury. Transfusion 1985;25:573–7.
199. Silliman CC, Boshkov LK, Mehdizadehkashi Z, et al. Transfusion-related acute lung injury: epidemiology and a prospective analysis of etiologic factors. Blood 2003; 101:454–62.
200. Silliman CC, Voelkel NF, Allard JD, et al. Plasma and lipids from stored packed red blood cells cause acute lung injury in an animal model. J Clin Invest 1998;101:1458–67.
201. Lenahan SE, Domen RE, Silliman CC, et al. Transfusion-related acute lung injury secondary to biologically active mediators. Arch Pathol Lab Med 2001;125:523–6.
202. Silliman CC, Paterson AJ, Dickey WO, et al. The association of biologically active lipids with the development of transfusion-related acute lung injury: a retrospective study. Transfusion 1997;37:719–26.
203. Popovsky MA. Transfusion-related acute lung injury (TRALI). In: Popovsky MA, editor. Transfusion reactions. Bethesda (MD): AABB Press; 2001. p. 155–70.
204. Davenport RD. Hemolytic transfusion reactions. In: Popovsky M, editor. Transfusion reactions. Bethesda (MD): AABB Press; 2001. p. 41–4.
205. Inwood MJ, Zuliani B. Anti-A hemolytic transfusion with packed O cells. Ann Intern Med 1978;89:515–6.
206. Chipping PM, Lloyd E, Goldman JM. Haemolysis after granulocyte transfusions. Br Med J 1980;281:1529.
207. Reis MD, Coovadia AS. Transfusion of ABO-incompatible platelets causing severe haemolytic reaction. Clin Lab Haematol 1989;11:237–40.
208. Larsson LG, Welsh VJ, Ladd DJ. Acute intravascular hemolysis secondary to out-of-group platelet transfusion. Transfusion 2000;40:902–6.
209. Sazama K. Reports of 355 transfusion-associated deaths: 1976 through 1985. Transfusion 1990;30:583–90.
210. Davenport RD, Strieter RM, Kunkel SL. Red cell ABO incompatibility and production of tumour necrosis factor-alpha. Br J Haematol 1991;78:540–4.
211. Davenport RD, Strieter RM, Standiford TJ, Kunkel SL. Interleukin-8 production in red blood cell incompatibility. Blood 1990;76:2439–42.
212. Davenport RD, Burdick M, Moore SA, Kunkel SL. Cytokine production in IgG-mediated red cell incompatibility. Transfusion 1993;33:19–24.
213. Davenport RD, Polak TJ, Kunkel SL. White cell-associated procoagulant activity induced by ABO incompatibility. Transfusion 1994;34:943–9.
214. Hess JR, MacDonald VW, Brinkley WW. Systemic and pulmonary hypertension after resuscitation with cell-free hemoglobin. J Appl Physiol 1993;74:1769–78.
215. Capon SM, Goldfinger D. Acute hemolytic transfusion reaction, a paradigm of the systemic inflammatory response: new insights into pathophysiology and treatment. Transfusion 1995;35:513–20.
216. Perrotta PL, Snyder EL. Non-infectious complications of transfusion therapy. Blood Rev 2001;15:69–83.
217. Bigby M, Jick S, Jick H, Arndt K. Drug-induced cutaneous reactions. A report from the Boston Collaborative Drug Surveillance Program on 15,438 consecutive inpatients, 1975 to 1982. JAMA 1986;256:3358–63.
218. Vyas GN, Perkins HA, Fudenberg HH. Anaphylactoid transfusion reactions associated with anti-IgA. Lancet 1968;2:312–5.
219. Sandler SG, Eckrich R, Malamut D, Mallory D. Hemagglutination assays for the diagnosis and prevention of IgA anaphylactic transfusion reactions. Blood 1994;84: 2031–5.
220. Shimada E, Tadokoro K, Watanabe Y, et al. Anaphylactic transfusion reactions in haptoglobin-deficient patients with IgE and IgG haptoglobin antibodies. Transfusion 2002;42:766–73.
221. Vamvakas E, Pineda A. Allergic and anaphylactic reactions. In: Popovsky M, editor. Transfusion reactions. Bethesda (MD): AABB Press; 2001. p. 83–127.
222. Vogelsang G, Kickler TS, Bell WR. Post-transfusion purpura: a report of five patients and a review of the pathogenesis and management. Am J Hematol 1986;21:259–67.
223. McFarland J. Post transfusion purpura. In: Popovsky M, editor. Transfusion reactions. Bethesda (MD): AABB Press; 2001. p. 187–212.
224. Mueller-Eckhardt C. Post-transfusion purpura. Br J Haematol 1986;64:419–24.
225. Shulman NR, Aster RH, Leitner A, Hiller MC. Post-transfusion purpura due to complement fixing antibody against a genetically controlled platelet antigen. A propsed

mechanism for thrombocytopenia and its relevance in autoimmunity. J Clin Invest 1961;40:1597–620.

226. Stricker RB, Lewis BH, Corash L, Shuman MA. Posttransfusion purpura associated with an autoantibody directed against a previously undefined platelet antigen. Blood 1987;69:1458–63.

227. Kickler TS, Ness PM, Herman JH, Bell WR. Studies on the pathophysiology of posttransfusion purpura. Blood 1986; 68:347–50.

228. Valentin N, Vergracht A, Bignon JD, et al. HLA-DRw52a is involved in alloimmunization against PL-A1 antigen. Hum Immunol 1990;27:73–9.

229. Mueller-Eckhardt C, Kuenzlen E, Thilo-Korner D, Pralle H. High-dose intravenous immunoglobulin for post-transfusion purpura. N Engl J Med 1983;308:287.

230. Loren AW, Abrams CS. Efficacy of HPA-1a (PlA1)-negative platelets in a patient with post-transfusion purpura. Am J Hematol 2004;76:258–62.

231. Heddle NM, Klama LN, Griffith L, et al. A prospective study to identify the risk factors associated with acute reactions to platelet and red cell transfusions. Transfusion 1993; 33:794–7.

232. Heddle N, Kelton JG. Febrile nonhemolytic transfusion reactions. In: Popovsky M, editor. Transfusion reactions. Bethesda (MD): AABB Press; 2001. p. 45–82.

233. Dodd RY, Notari EP, Stramer SL. Current prevalence and incidence of infectious disease markers and estimated window-period risk in the American Red Cross blood donor population. Transfusion 2002;42:975–9.

234. Kleinman S, Chan P, Robillard P. Risks associated with transfusion of cellular blood components in Canada. Transfus Med Rev 2003;17:120–62.

235. Chiavetta JA, Escobar M, Newman A, et al. Incidence and estimated rates of residual risk for HIV, hepatitis C, hepatitis B and human T-cell lymphotropic viruses in blood donors in Canada, 1990–2000. CMAJ 2003;169: 767–73.

Rheumatologic Paraneoplastic Syndromes

Megan C. MacNeil, MD
Frank C. Arnett, MD

Neoplastic diseases often present with manifestations in the musculoskeletal system or as mimics of systemic rheumatic diseases. Recognition of these paraneoplastic syndromes and their associated malignancies can lead to earlier cancer diagnosis and treatment. Often treatment of the cancer causes resolution or, at least, stabilization of the rheumatologic disease. At times, however, the paraneoplastic disease can be as morbid as the underlying cancer and require treatment in addition to primary oncologic care. This chapter reviews the most common paraneoplastic rheumatic syndromes and suggestions for their diagnosis and treatment.

Hypertrophic Osteoarthropathy

Hypertrophic osteoarthropathy (HO), also known as Marie-Bamberger syndrome, is characterized by chronic proliferative periostitis of the long bones, clubbing of the fingers and toes, and oligoarticular or polyarticular synovitis.[1] It may be primary or secondary. Primary hypertrophic osteoarthropathy, or pachydermoperiostosis, is usually hereditary, but idiopathic cases have been reported. Secondary causes include malignancy, infectious diseases, especially of the lung, chronic liver disease, inflammatory bowel disease, hyperthyroidism, and cyanotic or congenital heart disease. When HO begins acutely and other causes are not apparent, it almost always indicates an underlying malignancy, usually bronchogenic carcinoma. It also may be seen in a multitude of other malignancies, including carcinoma of the esophagus, colon, liver, and intrathoracic lymphomas.[2–5] More recently, it has been reported in liver rhabdomyosarcoma and nasopharyngeal carcinoma.[6,7]

Clinical Manifestations

Early recognition of HO, especially of rapid onset, should prompt an evaluation for an underlying cancer. HO may precede the symptoms of a malignant diagnosis by as many as 18 months or follow the diagnosis of malignancy by months to years.[1,3]

Clubbing is characterized by[1,8]

1. Softening of the nail bed
2. A loss of the normal 15° angle between the nail and the soft tissue
3. Increased convexity of the nail
4. A shiny appearance of the nail and adjacent skin
5. Local warmth and swelling.

It is usually asymptomatic but may present with dysesthesias and stiffness of the fingers (Figure 1).

Periostitis is inflammation of the fibrous membrane that covers the bones. It may be asymptomatic or may lead to a burning, deep-seated pain, usually located in the distal extremities. The pain is exacerbated when the limb is in a dependent position and is alleviated by elevation.

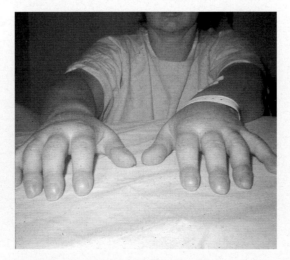

FIGURE 1 Acute clubbing and polyarthritis in a patient subsequently found to have bronchogenic carcinoma (courtesy of the American College of Rheumatology).

Arthritis, with pain, stiffness, and swelling, may involve both the large and small joints; typically, it affects the metacarpophalangeal, wrist, elbow, and knee joints. On physical examination, there may be joint effusions, decreased range of motion, and tenderness of both joints and intervening bony structures. Arthrocentesis typically reveals a noninflammatory fluid, with a synovial white blood cell count usually less than total WBC 1,000 count/min.[9]

Pathophysiology

Clubbing is the result of edema and accumulation of collagen deposition in the nail bed. The etiology of this process is unclear, but it is hypothesized that a growth factor from the tumor enters the systemic circulation and induces endothelial cell activation with vascular and periosteal hyperplasia.[9] Patients with lung cancer have elevated levels of vascular endothelial growth factor, which may play a role in the pathogenesis of HO.[10]

Investigations

There are no definitive laboratory studies of the blood that diagnose HO. Inflammatory parameters such as a sedimentation rate and C-reactive protein may be elevated but more likely reflect the underlying malignancy. Plain radiographs of the involved bones usually reveal the diagnosis. The most consistent finding is periosteal thickening (Figures 2 and 3) and, at times, seeming detachment along the shafts of the long bones.[11] Mild periostosis typically involves only a few bones (usually the tibia and fibula), but severe periostosis may involve all tubular bones. Acro-osteolysis (extensive bone remodeling) may be present in long-standing clubbing. Bone scans also are useful, especially in early disease. Tracer is observed in a pericortical line adjacent to the long bones and occasionally at the digits (referred to as a "string of lights").[12] Once the diagnosis is established, evaluation for age-appropriate malignancy

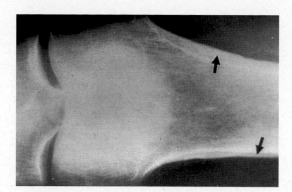

FIGURE 2 Typical periostial thickening and separation along the femur in a patient with HO (courtesy of the American College of Rheumatology).

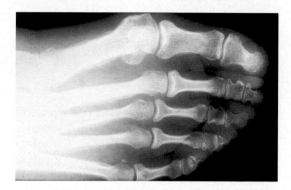

FIGURE 3 Typical periostial thickening and separation along the phalanges and metatarsal bones in a patient with HO.

should begin, with the lung the focus of the initial evaluation, especially in patients who have smoked tobacco or been occupationally exposed to inhaled carcinogens.

Treatment

Treatment of the underlying malignancy usually results in improvement in symptoms of periostosis. If the malignancy is surgically resectable, improvement may occur rapidly over the course of hours to days.[13] Interim treatment involves nonsteroidal anti-inflammatory drugs (NSAIDs) and other analgesics, or, if needed, low-dose corticosteroids may be helpful in controlling pain.[13] For those cases that are refractory to treatment, thoracic vagotomy should be considered.

Carcinoma Polyarthritis

Polyarthritis may be the initial complaint in a patient with an underlying malignancy. Carcinomatous polyarthritis is well described in both solid tumors and hematologic malignancies.[11] However, 80% of cases in women are reported to be associated with breast carcinoma.[14]

Clinical Manifestations

The clinical presentation is most commonly confused with rheumatoid arthritis, although adult-onset Still's disease is a diagnostic consideration when a patient presents with fever.[15] There are clinical features that suggest carcinoma polyarthritis rather than rheumatoid arthritis or Still's disease. These include[16]

1. A close temporal relationship (10 months) between the onset of arthritis and malignancy
2. Late age at onset of inflammatory arthritis
3. Asymmetric joint involvement
4. Explosive onset
5. Lower extremity involvement with sparing of the wrists and small joints of the hands
6. Absence of rheumatoid nodules
7. Absence of rheumatoid factor
8. Absence of family history of rheumatic disease
9. Nonspecific biopsy findings of the synovial lining

Pathophysiology

The pathophysiology of carcinoma polyarthritis is poorly understood. Many theories have been proposed, including antigenic cross-reactivity between the synovium and the tumor, abnormalities in cell-mediated immunity, and circulating immune complex deposition.[11] A study on synovial fluid from a patient with carcinoma polyarthritis failed to reveal any evidence of immune complex deposition, thus calling into question this last theory.[17] Most recently, Schultz and colleagues suggested that tumor-specific T lymphocytes might induce chronic synovitis by cross-reacting with synovial tissue components.[18]

Investigations

Serologic studies in patients with carcinoma polyarthritis are generally unrevealing, although some patients are reported to have positive antinuclear antibodies (ANAs) and rheumatoid factor.[11,19] The sedimentation rate and C-reactive protein also may be elevated. Synovial fluid analyses depict a mildly inflammatory pattern, although studies on synovial fluid are few.[11,20,21] No specific radiographic findings have been reported.

Treatment

The most convincing evidence that carcinoma polyarthritis is a paraneoplastic syndrome is the resolution of symptoms following successful treatment of the malignancy.[11,14] Recurrence of arthritis may indicate a relapse of the primary malignancy.[11,14] Patients also may respond to NSAIDS and intra-articular corticosteroids.[20]

Dermatomyositis and Polymyositis

Clinical Features

Dermatomyositis and polymyositis are inflammatory muscle disorders characterized clinically by progressive, symmetric, proximal muscle weakness. Legs and then arms are most commonly affected, but if the disease is not treated early, pharyngeal muscles may become involved, resulting in dysphagia, aspiration into the lungs, and dysphonia. Eventually, distal, truncal, and extraocular muscles become weak. Dermatomyositis includes cutaneous features such as a heliotrope rash, a violaceous rash that characteristically occurs over the eyelids (Figure 4). Other cutaneous features include erythema over the neck and shoulders (the shawl sign), erythema over the anterior neck and chest (the V sign) (Figure 5), and periungual telangiectasias. Gottron's papules are violaceous or pink plaques located over the interphalangeal joints, elbows, or knees that are diagnostic for dermatomyositis (Figure 6). There may be an associated inflammatory arthritis that typically affects the knees, elbows, wrists, ankles, metacarpophalangeal (MCPs), and proximal interphalangeal (PIP) joints, and, occasionally, symptoms of Raynaud's phenomenon are reported.

A multitude of malignancies have been described in association with dermatomyositis and polymyositis. Most commonly, these are carcinomas, which are age and gender appropriate to the patient. Virtually all types of tumors have

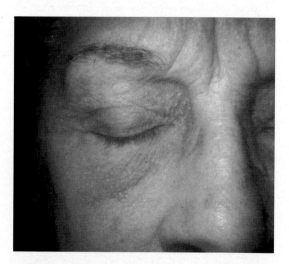

FIGURE 4 Typical heliotrope or lilac discoloration around the eyes of a patient with dermatomyositis.

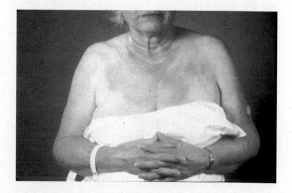

FIGURE 5 Typical "V" sign in a patient with dermatomyositis. Note also lilac discoloration of face, hands and arms.

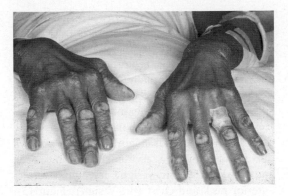

FIGURE 6 Typical Gottron's papules with hypopigmentation over the knuckles and hyperpigmentation around the nailbeds in a patient with dermatomyositis.

been reported. There is much controversy in the literature regarding the incidence of associated malignancy. This stems, at least in part, from the various inclusion and diagnostic criteria applied in previous studies. However, since 1975, most studies have used the Bohan and Peter diagnostic criteria.[11,22] A recent review from Mastaglia and Phillips suggested that the frequency of malignancy varies from 4 to 42%.[23] The association between dermatomyositis and malignancy is stronger than for polymyositis.[23] The incidence of malignancy increases with age [24] and decreases as the duration of the disease course increases.[25] The diagnosis of malignancy may occur prior to, concurrent with, or subsequent to the diagnosis of an inflammatory myopathy.[23]

Pathogenesis

The pathogenesis of malignancy-associated myositis, like that of other inflammatory myopathies, is not entirely understood, but various mechanisms have been proposed. These include environmental triggers, immune complex formation between tumor antigens and muscle and skin antigens, and a tumor myotoxin-inducing inflammation in muscle and skin.[20]

Investigations

An elevated creatinine kinase, adolase, or transaminase level supports the diagnosis of an inflammatory myopathy, but these laboratory results are not elevated in all cases. Muscle biopsies show different and characteristic histopathologic changes for both dermatomyositis and polymyositis, but neither provides clues to the presence of the underlying malignancy. There are no myositis-specific autoantibodies, such as anti-Jo1 or Mi2, that suggest a malignancy-associated myositis. In fact, the presence of any of these autoantibodies makes malignancy less likely. A positive or negative ANA is not at all discriminating. The search for a malignancy should be guided by a thorough history and physical examination.

Baseline laboratory studies should include a complete blood count, chemistries, liver function tests, urinalysis, stool examination for occult blood, and serum protein electrophoresis.[20] Imaging studies should include a chest radiograph and mammograms, but further studies should be pursued based on the findings in the clinical evaluation.[20] The highest risk of malignancy occurs within the first 3 years,[23] but screening for malignancy every 2 to 3 years is recommended by some authors.[20]

Treatment

Myositis associated with malignancy may or may not respond to standard treatment with moderate- to high-dose corticosteroids. Patients who are resistant to standard treatment should raise the clinician's suspicion for malignancy.[11] Treatment of the primary malignancy will occasionally, but not always, improve symptoms.[11,20]

Vasculitis

Vasculitis is characterized by inflammation of blood vessels, which subsequently results in a variety of clinical presentations in many different organ systems. Paraneoplastic vasculitis may involve small- or medium-sized vessels and is chiefly associated with lymphoproliferative disorders, myelodysplastic syndromes, and, occasionally, solid tumors.[11,20,26] It most commonly presents as a leukocytoclastic vasculitis (small vessel) appearing clinically as palpable purpura but may also present as a medium vessel vasculitis mimicking polyarteritis nodosa, which has a well-known association with hairy cell leukemia. Vasculitis may precede the diagnosis of the underlying malignancy, present after the diagnosis, or occur during tumor recurrence or escape from treatment.[26]

Clinical Manifestations

Paraneoplastic vasculitis has various clinical presentations, but it most commonly presents as palpable purpura with or without arthritis.[27] Other cutaneous forms of small vessel vasculitis include urticaria or maculopapular eruptions.[20] Vasculitis of the intestine[26] and nerve and muscles[28] has been reported but is much less frequent.

Hairy cell leukemia deserves special note and has been associated with vasculitis in multiple reports. Hughes and colleagues first noted the association between hairy cell leukemia and polyarteritis nodosa in 1976.[29] There are three general classifications[30]:

1. Leukocytoclastic vasculitis
2. Polyarteritis nodosa–like disease
3. Direct invasion of the vessel wall by hairy cells

Polyarteritis nodosa generally occurs after the diagnosis of hairy cell leukemia and splenectomy and was frequently preceded by infection.[30] Clinical characteristics are variable and may include arthritis, fever, cutaneous vasculitis, digital infarctions, an acute abdomen, mononeuritis multiplex, and/or coronary arteritis.[20]

Pathogenesis

Various mechanisms have been proposed in paraneoplastic vasculitis, including

1. Immune complexes of tumor with associated antigen and antibodies, which may explain most leukocytoclastic vasculitides[26,31]
2. Antibodies directed toward the endothelial cell wall that cross-react with antigens on leukemic cells
3. Leukemic cells that directly affect the vascular wall[26,32,33]

Treatment

Corticosteroids, cyclophosphamide, and treatment of the underlying malignancy may result in improvement in or resolution of the vasculitis. Corticosteroid treatment alone is associated with frequent relapses, and the addition of cyclophosphamide is usually necessary, especially in patients with a polyarteritis-like picture. Prognosis is dependent on the stage and primary malignancy.

Palmar Fasciitis and Polyarthritis Syndrome

Medsger and colleagues first described the palmar fasciitis and polyarthritis syndrome in 1982.[34] The initial case reports included six patients with ovarian cancer. Since that time, a multitude of other malignancies have been reported. The list includes but is not limited to breast,[35] lung, pancreatic,[36] stomach,[37] prostate,[38] uterine,[39] and endometrial[40] cancers. Although palmar fasciitis and polyarthritis syndrome usually indicates an underlying malignancy, the same syndrome may occur in patients on long-term therapy with barbiturates[41] or antituberculous drugs.[42]

Clinical Features

Palmar fasciitis and polyarthritis syndrome is marked by dramatic nodular thickening of the palmar and, at times, plantar fascia (Figure 7). It may extend from the flexor retinaculum to the flexor tendons of the hand, resulting in contractures of fingers owing to palmar fasciitis and "claw hands" (Figure 8).[36] In many ways, it resembles an accelerated and more extensive form of Dupytren's contracture. Paresthesias of the second and third fingers may lead to a diagnosis of carpal tunnel syndrome and may be relieved by carpal tunnel release procedures. The shoulder is commonly affected by an adhesive capsulitis (frozen shoulder), leading to diagnostic confusion with

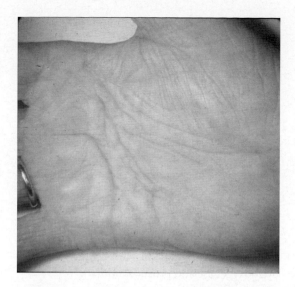

FIGURE 7 Thickening of the palmar fascia with tethering of overlying skin.

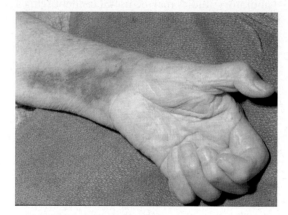

FIGURE 8 Flexure contractures of the fingers resulting in a claw hand.

hand-shoulder syndrome. Hand-shoulder syndrome is a variant of reflex sympathetic dystrophy that is characterized by pain, swelling, and vasomotor changes of the skin over the hand and shoulder. Distinguishing features of palmar fasciitis and polyarthritis syndrome include a more aggressive disease course, bilateral involvement, and a more inflammatory arthritis.[36] In addition, patients commonly complain of morning stiffness and may develop lower extremity involvement and plantar fasciitis. Symptoms may present 1 to 23 months prior to the diagnosis of a malignancy, and, frequently, patients are misdiagnosed as having scleroderma.[34,36]

Investigations

The diagnosis of palmar fasciitis is based on the typical clinical findings; however, biopsies of the fascia will show marked fibrosis with "whorls" of fibroblasts and connective tissue separated by fibrous septae.[36] Immunofluorescence studies have shown immune deposits, suggesting an immunologic pathogenesis.[43–45] Plain hand radiographs may show flexion contractures of the fingers and demineralization but are usually

unremarkable.[36,40] Bone scans have revealed increased uptake of tracer in the involved joints.[40]

Treatment

Treatment of palmar fasciitis is directed toward identification and treatment of the primary malignancy, which may be quite small. In women, attention should be especially directed toward the ovaries. Responses to treatment of the underlying cancer are variable, with some patients improving and others progressing. This may be due to the late stage of presentation in some cases; patients presenting with extensive metastatic disease usually have an overall poor prognosis.[45] Treatment with corticosteroids and anti-inflammatory medications has resulted in variable clinical responses, with appreciable improvement in some patients but not in others.

Panniculitis

Panniculitis is characterized by subcutaneous fat necrosis associated with pancreatitis or pancreatic cancer. Lesions resembling erythema nodosum usually appear over the distal extremities. When they occur in joints or bones, synovitis results from the periarticular fat necrosis.[11] The lesions are generally small and erythematous and range between 1 and 2 cm. Nodules may ulcerate and secrete an oily substance.[46] In addition to the skin and joints, fat necrosis may involve the omentum and peritoneum.[47] A massive release of pancreatic enzymes, including lipase, amylase, and trypsin, results in focal areas of fat necrosis.

Further investigation should be pursued in patients presenting with an unexplained mono- or polyarthritis with subcutaneous nodules. Studies should include a complete blood count; serum levels of lipase, amylase, and trypsin[48]; and a biopsy of the nodule. Eosinophilia is more commonly associated with pancreatic cancer than pancreatitis.[11] If the lipase, amylase, or trypsin level is elevated, the pancreas should be further evaluated with an imaging study. Biopsies of nodules reveal steatonecrosis and "ghost-like cells." These cells have thick cell walls and no nucleus and are pathognomonic for this condition.[11,49] Areas of necrosis are surrounded by inflammatory cells, including neutrophils, lymphocytes, histiocytes, foamy cells, and foreign body giant cells. Basophilic calcium granules are also found in the area of necrosis.

Treatment of panniculitis should be directed at the underlying malignancy.[50] Octreotide has been used with variable results; however, some case reports have shown that the lesions did not progress and new lesions did not develop.[51] Treatment with corticosteroids and anti-inflammatory drugs is generally ineffective.[11] Although subcutaneous fat necrosis tends to occur late in the

disease course of a pancreatic malignancy, its early recognition may prevent long delays in diagnosis and treatment.

Erythema Nodosum

Erythema nodosum is characterized by subcutaneous, firm, red, and tender nodules that may occur anywhere on the body but are most commonly located on the extensor surfaces of the lower extremities (Figure 9). A painful periarthritis and soft tissue swelling that occurs around the ankles and lower legs may be an accompanying feature. Erythema nodosum is often associated with fever, arthralgias, myalgias, abdominal pain, and headaches. Most cases of erythema nodosum usually remit spontaneously after 2 to 3 weeks,[52] but in cases associated with malignancy, the nodules may last longer than 6 months.[43] The female to male ratio is approximately 3 to 6:1.[52] Erythema nodosum has been associated with a number of malignancies but most commonly Hodgkin's and non-Hodgkin's lymphoma and leukemia.[20] Taylor described the first case of erythema nodosum associated with Hodgkin's lymphoma in 1906.[53]

Symptoms may precede the diagnosis of malignancy by up to 24 months or may occur after the diagnosis or with a recurrence.[52] The pathogenesis is not understood but may result from immune complex deposition in the vessels in the dermis and subcutaneous fat.[54] Biopsies of skin lesions show septal panniculitis that is initially characterized by a neutrophilic infiltrate but will eventually progress to lymphocytic and histiocytic infiltration.[55,56] As the lesion matures, a granulomatous lesion develops and there is fibrosis of the septal tissue.[56]

The more common causes of erythema nodosum include infections (streptococcal, mycobacterial, and fungal), medications, and granulomatous diseases, such as sarcoidosis and Crohn's disease. Malignancy should be considered when unexplained lesions last longer than 6 months and respond poorly to conventional treatments.[43,52] Erythema nodosum may respond to NSAIDs or low doses of corticosteroids, but

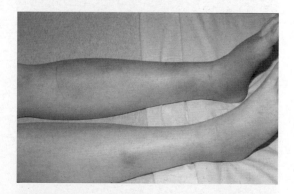

FIGURE 9 Raised tender nodules on the shin, typical of erythema nodosum.

treatment of the underlying malignancy usually leads to resolution of the lesions without recurrence.

Raynaud's Phenomenon and Digital Ischemia

Clinical Manifestations

Raynaud's phenomenon is characterized by intermittent vasospasm, resulting in pallor, cyanosis, and hyperemia of any body part but most commonly the fingers. It is associated with numbness or pain of the fingertips and is precipitated by cold or, less commonly, emotional upsets. It may progress to digital ischemia and ulcers (Figure 10).

The association of digital ischemia and malignancy was first reported in 1884.[57] Reports of malignancy and Raynaud's phenomenon were noted in the early 1900s. It has been reported with solid tumors, including breast, stomach, pancreatic, small bowel, kidney, lung, and ovarian cancer, as well as with lymphoma, leukemia, and myeloma.[20,58–61] It may precede the diagnosis of malignancy by several years.[61] Features that suggest an underlying malignancy include[20,43,58]

1. An older age at onset (over 50 years)
2. An asymmetric presentation (found in 30% of cases)
3. An acute presentation as opposed to a more common insidious one
4. A rapid progression to digital ulcers and gangrene.

Pathogenesis

The pathogenesis is unknown but may be related to circulating immune complexes, paraproteins, cryoglobulins, cryofibrinogens, cold agglutinins, and/or cytokines.[20,58] Inflammatory parameters, such as a sedimentation rate or C-reactive protein, may be elevated but are more likely to be related to the underlying malignancy.

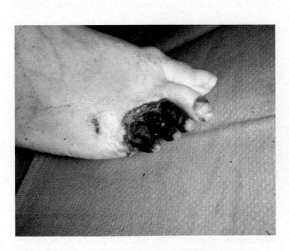

FIGURE 10 Typical findings of dry gangrene.

Prognosis and Treatment

Paraneoplastic Raynaud's syndrome will progress to digital gangrene in 80% of cases. It was previously associated with a dismal prognosis, but treatment of the primary malignancy has led to resolution of symptoms in some cases.[43]

Erythromelalgia

Erythromelalgia is a rare disorder that is characterized by redness, warmth, and pain in the skin of any body part but is most commonly described in the extremities. It was originally described by Mitchell in the 1870s, using the Greek words *erythros* (red), *melos* (extremities), and *algos* (pain).[62] It is generally classified into primary erythromelalgia (an idiopathic form) or secondary erythromelalgia, which is associated with an underlying disease process. In one study, 41% of patients were diagnosed with secondary erythromelalgia and 20% of these patients had a myeloproliferative disorder.[63] The majority of these patients have polycythemia vera (59%) or essential thrombocythemia (38%).[63] Secondary erythromelalgia has also been reported in agnogenic myeloid metaplasia, chronic myelogenous leukemia, and colon cancer.[64,65]

Clinical Manifestations

The median age at onset of myeloproliferation-associated erythromelalgia is 59 years, and it is rarely reported under the age of 30 years.[64] Of note, primary erythromelalgia occurs most commonly in patients younger than 30 years. A 3:2 male to female ratio has been reported in myeloproliferation-associated erythromelalgia; however, this ratio has not been observed in patients with primary forms.[64]

Patients describe a pruritic or prickling sensation that eventually progresses to a burning or throbbing pain. Episodes may last minutes to days. During an episode, there is redness and warmth of the involved area. Limb dependency, exercise, and warm temperatures are common triggers. The patient often describes immersing the hands and feet in ice water to obtain relief. The physical examination is unremarkable when the patient is not having an episode, and this commonly leads to a delay in diagnosis. During an episode, there is erythema and increased temperature of the skin. The patient may have normal or bounding peripheral pulses. Local congestion may develop, leading to acrocyanosis and, rarely, gangrene, requiring amputation. Episodes may result in ischemic ulcers that can become secondarily infected. A few cases of concomitant and alternating episodes of Raynaud's phenomenon have been recorded.

Up to 85% of patients have reported symptoms before the diagnosis of a myeloproliferative disorder was established.[64] The average time

between onset of symptoms and diagnosis of a myeloproliferative disorder is 2.5 years, but symptoms may precede the diagnosis by as many as 16 years.[64,66]

Pathophysiology

The pathophysiology in erythromelalgia associated with myeloproliferative disorders, although not entirely understood, appears to be related to platelet hyperaggregability and arteriolar fibrosis.[66,67] Skin biopsies show arteriolar inflammation, fibromuscular intima proliferation, and thrombotic occlusion.[66] Symptoms often improve with treatment with low-dose aspirin or other NSAIDS, suggesting an important role for cyclooxygenase and prostaglandins.[66]

Investigations

Laboratory studies may be useful in identifying a myeloproliferative disorder. All patients should be evaluated with routine complete blood counts. Elevations in hemoglobin, leukocytes or subsets thereof, and platelets should be further evaluated with bone marrow biopsies.

No specific findings are present on plain radiographs of hands or feet, but bone scans may be useful in excluding other differential diagnoses, such as reflex sympathetic dystrophy. Thermography is rarely necessary but typically shows temperatures between 31°C and 36°C, and differences up to 9°C have been observed.[64]

Skin biopsies will often show arteriolar lesions with swollen endothelial cells, intimal proliferation, and thrombosis, with sparing of the venules, capillaries, and nerves.[66]

Treatment

Local measures, such as elevating or cooling the involved extremity, may be helpful. Aspirin, in a single dose of 650 mg, will often relieve symptoms within hours and last for up to 4 days. Indomethacin and other NSAIDS are also helpful but do not provide long-lasting relief. Sodium-salicylate, dipyridamole, sulfinpyrazone, ticlopidine, and dazoxiben have no significant effect on symptoms.[66]

Treatment of the underlying disease leads to variable responses. Phlebotomy in polycythemia vera and normalization of platelet counts in patients with thrombocytosis have led to improvement in symptoms in many but not all patients.

Lupus-Like Syndrome

A lupus-like syndrome has been associated with a variety of malignancies, including breast carcinoma, hairy cell leukemia, and Hodgkin's and non-Hodgkin's lymphoma.[20,68–70] The syndrome resembles systemic lupus erythematosus and is classically described as a nondeforming polyarthritis, pleuritis, or pnemonitis with a positive ANA.[11,69] The ANA is positive in 70% of cases and anti–double-stranded deoxyribonucleic acid (DNA) positive in 50% of cases.[71] Although a majority of patients will have positive antinuclear antibodies (ANAs), they tend to lack specific antibodies to Smith (Sm), ribonuclear protein (RNP), SS-A (Ro), and SS-B (La).[68] The differential diagnosis includes metastases or radiation-induced injury, but the diagnosis of a lupus-like syndrome should be considered in a patient with these systemic symptoms because they are responsive to treatment with corticosteroids.[11,20]

Multicentric Reticulohistiocytosis

Multicentric reticulohistiocytosis (MRH) is a systemic disease characterized by an insidious onset of papules or nodules in the skin, mucosa, subcutaneous tissue, synovium, periosteum, and bones that may result in a destructive arthritis (Figure 11).[72] The cause of MRH is unknown but is likely related to the proliferation of histiocytes in the nodules. The histiocytes are considered reactive and not malignant cells.[73] Approximately one-third of patients have an underlying malignancy, which is detected after the diagnosis of MRH in 73% of reported cases.[72] It has been associated with a multitude of malignancies; however, there is no association with a predominant type of cancer.[73]

Clinical Manifestations

The mean age at onset of MRH is 50 years, and it is associated with a slight female to male preponderance (1.85:1).[72,74] Eighty-eight percent of cases are reported in Caucasians, which may reflect more reports from developed countries.[74]

The skin lesions are described as reddish brown, pink, or gray papules or nodules that range from a few millimeters to 2 cm in circumference. They typically affect the hands, followed by the face, arms, trunk, legs, ears, mucosa, and

neck.[74] They may be clustered around the nail, forming a "string of coral beads," which is a pathognomonic sign for MRH. Other typical findings may be palpebral xanthelasmas, found in 17% of cases, and vermicular lesions bordering the nostrils in 15% of cases.[74]

The arthritis is typically symmetric and commonly affects the hands and interphalangeal (especially distal) joints (75% cases). However, MRH also may affect the wrists (46%), shoulders (36%), elbows (31%), ankles and hips (9%), feet (6%), and neck and spine (2%).[72,74] It is an erosive arthritis that may progress to arthritis mutilans in as many as 45% of cases.[72] The clinical course is typically relapsing and remitting, and, eventually, most cases will remit spontaneously after 7 to 8 years.[73]

Investigations

Although there is no specific serum laboratory test that is diagnostic for MRH, some patients may have an elevated sedimentation rate or anemia.[72] The skin biopsy contains histiocytic multinucleated giant cells with an eosinophilic, finely granulated, ground-glass cytoplasm.[72] These cells are considered the structural hallmark for MRH. Radiographs of the affected joints reveal periarticular "punched-out" erosions and reabsorption of the juxta-articular zone.[74]

Treatment

There is no therapy that consistently improves MRH. It usually does not follow the same clinical course as the underlying malignancy; however, there have been case reports of regression with successful treatment of the cancer.[75] The patient may be treated symptomatically with NSAIDS and corticosteroids. There have been case reports of successful treatment of MRH with cyclophosphamide[76–79] and methotrexate.[80,81] Treatment regimens with other alkylating agents also have occasionally shown good results,[74,82,83] and, more recently, there have been promising case reports with tumor necrosis factor inhibitors, such as etanercept.[84,85]

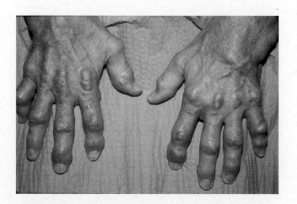

FIGURE 11 Polyarthritis affecting distal and proximal interphalangeal joints and cutaneous nodules over the metacarpal and interphalangeal joints in a patient multicentric reticulohistiocytosis.

REFERENCES

1. Tenebaum J, Altman R. Hypertrophic osteoarthropathy. In: Kelly W, Harris E, Ruddy S, Sledge C, editors. Textbook of rheumatology. Philadelphia: W.B. Saunders; 1981.
2. Morita M, Sakaguchi Y, Kuma S, et al. Hypertrophic osteoarthropathy associated with esophageal cancer. Ann Thorac Surg 2003;76:1744–6.
3. Mendlowitz M. Clubbing and hypertrophic osteoarthropathy. Medicine 1942;21:269.
4. Morgan A, Walker W, Mason M, et al. A new syndrome associated with hepatocellular carcinoma. Gastroenterology 1972;63:340–5.
5. Lofters W, Walker T. Hodgkin's disease and hypertrophic pulmonary osteoarthropathy. Complete clearing following radiotherapy. West Indian Med J 1978;27:227–30.
6. Geary T, Maclennan A, Irwin G. Hypertrophic osteoarthropathy in primary liver rhabdomyosarcoma. Pediatr Radiol 2004;34:250–2.
7. Sohn S, Ryu S, Kwon H, et al. A case of hypertrophic osteoarthropathy associated with nasopharyngeal carcinoma in a child. J Korean Med Sci 2003;18:761–3.
8. Stone O. Clubbing and koilonychia. Dermatol Clin North Am 1986;3:485.
9. Martinez-Lavin M, Pineda C, Valdez T, et al. Primary hypertrophic osteoarthropathy. Semin Arthritis Rheum 1988;17:156–62.
10. Silveira L, Martinez-Lavin M, Pineda C, et al. Vascular endothelial growth factor and hypertrophic osteoarthropathy. Clin Exp Rheumatol 2000;18:57–62.
11. Caldwell DS, McCallum RM. Rheumatic manifestations of cancer. Med Clin North Am 1986;70:385–417.
12. Donnelly B, Johnson P. Detection of hypertrophic pulmonary osteoarthropathy of skeletal imaging with 99mTc-labeled diphosphonate. Radiology 1975;114:389–91.
13. Hammarten J, O'Leary J. The features and significance of hypertrophic osteoarthropathy. Arch Intern Med 1957;99:431–41.
14. Sheon R, Kirsner A, Tangsintanapas P, et al. Malignancy in rheumatic disease: interrelationships. J Am Geriatr Soc 1977;25:20–7.
15. Bennett RM, Ginsberg MH, Thomsen S. Carcinomatous polyarthritis. The presenting symptom of an ovarian tumor and association with a platelet activating factor. Arthritis Rheum 1976;19:953–8.
16. Caldwell DS. Textbook of rheumatology. In: Kelly W, Harris E, Ruddy S, Sledge C, editors. Musculoskeletal syndromes associated with malignancy. Vol II. Philadelphia: W.B. Saunders; 1989. p. 1676–7.
17. Bradley JD, Pinals RS. Carcinoma polyarthritis: role of immune complexes in pathogenesis. J Rheumatol 1983;10:826–8.
18. Schultz H, Krenn V, Tony HP. Oligoarthritis mediated by tumor-specific T lymphocytes in renal-cell carcinoma. N Engl J Med 1999;341:290–1.
19. Mok CC, Kwan YK. Rheumatoid-like polyarthritis as a presenting feature of metastatic carcinoma: a case presentation and review of the literature. Clin Rheumatol 2003;22:353–4.
20. Fam AG. Paraneoplastic rheumatic syndromes. Baillieres Best Pract Res Clin Rheumatol 2000;14:515–33.
21. Simon RD Jr, Ford LE. Rheumatoid-like arthritis associated with a colonic carcinoma. Arch Intern Med 1980;140:698.
22. Bohan A, Peter JB. Polymyositis and dermatomyositis. N Engl J Med 1975;292:344–7, 403–7.
23. Mastaglia FL, Phillips BA. Idiopathic inflammatory myopathies: epidemiology, classification, and diagnostic criteria. Rheum Dis Clin North Am 2002;28:723–41.
24. Buchbinder R, Forbes A, Hall S, et al. Incidence of malignant disease in biopsy-proven inflammatory myopathy: a population based cohort. Ann Intern Med 2001;134:1087–95.
25. Hatron PY MI, Levesque H, Hachulla E, et al. Influence of age on characteristics of polymyositis and dermatomyositis in adults. Medicine 1999;78:139–47.
26. Sanchez-Guerrero J, Gutierrez-Urena S, Vidaller A, et al. Vasculitis as a paraneoplastic syndrome. Report of 11 cases and review of the literature. J Rheumatol 1990;17:1458–62.
27. Longley S, Caldwell DS, Panush RS. Paraneoplastic vasculitis. Unique syndrome of cutaneous angiitis and arthritis associated with myeloproliferative disorders. Am J Med 1986;80:1027–30.
28. Kurzrok R, Cohen PR, Markowitz A. Clinical manifestations of vasculitis in patients with solid tumors. Arch Intern Med 1994;154:334–40.
29. Hughes G, Elkon K, Spiller R, et al. Polyarteritis nodosa and hairy-cell leukemia. Lancet 1979;1:678.
30. Hasler P, Kistler H, Gerber H. Vasculitides in hairy cell leukemia. Semin Arthritis Rheum 1995;25:134–42.
31. Garcias V, Herr H. Henoch-Schonlein purpura associated with cancer of the prostate. Urology 1982;19:155–8.
32. Klima M, Waddell C. Hairy cell leukemia associated with focal vascular damage. Hum Pathol 1984;15:657–9.
33. Posnett D, Marboe C, Knowles D, et al. A membrane antigen (HC1) selectively present on hairy cell leukemia cells, endothelial cells, and epidermal basal cells. J Immunol 1984;132:2700–2.
34. Medsger TA, Dixon JA, Garwood VF. Palmar fasciitis and polyarthritis associated with ovarian carcinoma. Ann Intern Med 1982;96:424–31.
35. Saxman SB, Seitz D. Breast cancer associated with palmar fasciitis and arthritis. J Clin Oncol 1997;15:3515–6.

36. Pfinsgraff J, Buckingham RB, Killian PJ, et al. Palmar fasciitis and arthritis with malignant neoplasms: a paraneoplastic syndrome. Semin Arthritis Rheum 1986;16:118–25.

37. Enomoto M, Takemura H, Suzuki M, et al. Palmar fasciitis and polyarthritis associated with gastric carcinoma: complete resolution after total gastrectomy. Intern Med 2000;39:754–7.

38. Van den Bergh L, Vanneste SB, Knockaert DC. Palmar fasciitis and arthritis associated with cancer of the prostate. Acta Clin Belg 1991;46:106–10.

39. Grados F, Houvenagel E, Cayrolle G, et al. Two new cancer locations accompanied with palmar fasciitis and polyarthritis. Rev Rhum Engl Ed 1998;65:212–4.

40. Docquier C, Majois F, Mitine C. Palmar fasciitis and arthritis: association with endometrial adenocarcinoma. Clin Rheumatol 2002;21:63–5.

41. Mattson RH, Cramer JA, McCutchen CB. Barbiturate-related connective tissue disorders. Arch Intern Med 1989;149:911–4.

42. Seaman JM, Goble M, Madsen L, Steigerwald JC. Fasciitis and polyarthritis during antituberculous therapy. Arthritis Rheum 1985;28:1179–84.

43. Naschitz JE, Rosner I, Rozenbaum M, et al. Rheumatic syndromes: clues to occult neoplasia. Semin Arthritis Rheum 1999;29:43–55.

44. Shiel WCJ, Prete PE, Jason M, Andrews BS. Palmar fasciitis and arthritis with ovarian and non-ovarian carcinomas. New syndrome. Am J Med 1985;79:640–4.

45. Champion D, Saxon JA, Kossard S. The syndrome of palmar fibromatosis (fasciitis) and polyarthritis. J Rheumatol 1987;14:1196–8.

46. Menon P, Kulshreshta R. Pancreatitis with panniculitis and arthritis: a rare association. Pediatr Surg Int 2004;20: 161–2.

47. Potts D, Mass MF, Iseman M. Syndrome of pancreatic disease, subcutaneous fat necrosis and polyserositis. Case report and review of the literature. Am J Med 1975; 58:417–23.

48. Heykarts B, Anseeuw M, Degreef H. Panniculitis caused by acinous pancreatic carcinoma. Dermatology 1999;198: 182–3.

49. Szymanski FJ, Bluefarb SM. Nodular fat necrosis and pancreatic disease. Arch Dermatol 1961;83:224–9.

50. Berkovic D, Hallermann C. Carcinoma of the pancreas with neuroendocrine differentiation and nodular panniculitis. Onkologie 2003;26:473–6.

51. Durden F, Variyam E, Chren M. Fat necrosis with features of erythema nodosum in a patient with metastatic pancreatic carcinoma. Int J Dermatol 1996;35:39–41.

52. Bonci A, Lernia VD, Merli F, Scocco GL. Erythema nodosum and Hodgkin's disease. Clin Exp Dermatol 2001;26: 408–11.

53. Taylor F. The chronic relapsing pyrexia of Hodgkin's disease. Guys Hosp Rep 1906;60:1.

54. Ryan T. Cutaneous vasculitis. Erythema nodosum. In: Rook A, Wilkinson D, Ebling F, editors. Textbook of dermatology. Oxford (UK): Blackwell Scientific Publishers; 1998. p. 2196–202.

55. Lin JT, Chen PM, Huang DF, et al. Erythema nodosum associated with carcinoid tumor. Clin Exp Dermatol 2004;29: 423–36.

56. Bondi EE, Margolis DJ, Lazarus GS. Panniculitis. In: Fitzpatrick TB, Freedberg IM, Eisen AZ, et al, editors. Dermatology in general medicine. New York: McGraw-Hill, Health Professions Division; 1999. p. 1284–8.

57. O'Connor B. Symmetrical gangrene. Br Med J 1884;1:460.

58. Andrasch RH, Bardana EJ Jr, Porter JM, Pirofsky B. Digital ischemia and gangrene preceding renal neoplasm: an association with sarcomatoid adenocarcinoma of the kidney. Arch Intern Med 1976;136:486–8.

59. Bennett TI, Poulton EP. Raynaud's disease associated with cancer of the stomach. Am J Med Sci 1928;176:654–7.

60. Decross AJ, Sahasrabudhe DM. Paraneoplastic Raynaud's phenomenon. Am J Med 1992;92:571–2.

61. Wytock DH, Bartholomew LG, Sheps SG. Digital ischemia asociated with small bowel malignancy. Gastroenterology 1983;84:1025–7.

62. Mitchell SW. On a rare vaso-motor neurosis of the extremities, and on the maladies with which it may be confounded. Am J Med Sci 1878;76:2–36.

63. Babb RR, Alarcon-Segovia D, Fairbairn JF II. Erythermalgia: review of 51 cases. Circulation 1964;29:136–41.

64. Kurzrock R, Cohen PR. Erythromelalgia and myeloproliferative disorders. Arch Intern Med 1989;149:105–9.

65. Mork C, Kalgaard OM, Kvernebo K. Erythromelalgia as a paraneoplastic syndrome in a patient with abdominal cancer. Acta Derm Venereol 1999;79:394.

66. Michiels JJ, Abels J, Steketee J, et al. Erythromelalgia caused by platelet-mediated arteriolar inflammation and thrombosis in thrombocythemia. Ann Intern Med 1985;102: 466–71.

67. Boneu B, Pris J, Guiraud B, et al. [Abnormalities of platelet aggregation during essential thrombocythemia. Effect of aspirin on erythromelalgia]. Nouv Presse Med 1972;1: 2383–8.

68. Strickland RW, Limmani A, Wall JG, Krishnan J. Hairy cell leukemia presenting as a lupus-like illness. Arthritis Rheum 1988;31:566–8.

69. Wallach HW. Lupus-like syndrome associated with carcinoma of the breast. Arch Intern Med 1977;137: 532–5.

70. Houssiau F, Kirkove C, Asherson R, et al. Malignant lymphoma in systemic rheumatic diseases. A report of five cases. Clin Exp Rheumatol 1991;9:515–8.

71. Solans-Laque R, Perez-Bocanegra C, Salud-Salvia A, et al. Clinical significance of antinuclear antibodies in malignant diseases: association with rheumatic and connective tissue paraneoplastic syndromes. Lupus 2004;13:159–64.

72. Barrow M, Holubar K. Multicentric reticulohistiocytosis. A review of 33 patients. Medicine (Baltimore) 1969;48: 287–305.

73. Kurzrock R, Cohen P. Cutaneous paraneoplastic syndromes in solid tumors. Am J Med 1995;99:662–71.

74. Luz F, Gaspar T, Kalil-Gaspar N, Ramos-e-Silva M. Multicentric reticulohistiocytosis. J Eur Acad Dermatol Venereol 2001;15:524–31.

75. Janssen B, Kencian J, Brooks P. Close temporal and anatomic relationship between multicentric reticulohistiocytosis and carcinoma of the breast. J Rheumatol 1992;19: 322–4.

76. Catterall M. Multicentric reticulohistiocytosis: a review of eight cases. Clin Exp Dermatol 1980;5:267–79.

77. Coupe M, Whittaker S, Thatcher N. Multicentric reticulohistiocytosis. Br J Dermatol 1987;116:245–7.

78. Lambert C, Nuki G. Multicentric reticulohistiocytosis with arthritis and cardiac infiltration: regression following treatment for underlying malignancy. Ann Rheum Dis 1992;51:815–7.

79. Doherty M, Martin M, Dieppe P. Multicentric reticulohistiocytosis associated with primary biliary cirrhosis: successful treatment with cytotoxic agents. Arthritis Rheum 1984;27:344–8.

80. Franck N, Amor B, Ayral X, et al. Multicentric reticulohistiocytosis and methotrexate. J Am Acad Dermatol 1995; 33:524–5.

81. Gourmelen O, Le Loet X, Fortier-Beaulieu M, et al. Methotrexate treatment of multicentric reticulohistiocytosis. J Rheumatol 1991;18:627–8.

82. Liang G, Granston A. Complete remission of multicentric reticulohistiocytosis with combination therapy of steroid, cyclophosphamide, and low-dose pulse methotrexate. Case report, review of the literature, and proposal for treatment. Arthritis Rheum 1996;39:171–4.

83. Kenik J, Fok F, Huerter C, et al. Multicentric reticulohistiocytosis in a patient with malignant melanoma: a response to cyclophosphamide and a unique cutaneous feature. Arthritis Rheum 1990;33:1047–51.

84. Kovach B, Calamia K, Walsh J, Ginsburg W. Treatment of multicentric reticulohistiocytosis with etanercept. Arch Dermatol 2004;140:919–21.

85. Matejicka C, Morgan G, Schlegelmilch J. Multicentric reticulohistiocytosis treated successfully with an anti–tumor necrosis factor agent. Arthritis Rheum 2003; 48:864–6.

Rheumatologic Issues in Cancer Patients

Firas Alkassab, MD

Frank C. Arnett, MD

As discussed in the preceding chapter, certain rheumatologic disorders typically or frequently present as paraneoplastic syndromes, thus alerting the physician to a high likelihood of an underlying malignancy. As is presented in this chapter, there are a number of rheumatic and autoimmune diseases that themselves predispose patients to neoplasia, often after many years. Moreover, certain antirheumatic therapeutic agents may augment the risk of these same cancers or predispose patients *de novo* to others. Similarly, a number of oncologic therapies may induce true rheumatic or autoimmune syndromes, or mimics of them. The implications of these interrelationships are highly clinically significant in both diagnosis and management and require recognition by both primary care physicians and specialists alike. Moreover, they even carry over into the care of patients who happen to suffer from both cancer and a rheumatic disease.[1–3]

Rheumatic and Autoimmune Diseases Predisposing Individuals to Cancer

Associations between rheumatic autoimmune diseases and cancer are increasingly being recognized,[4,5] although the pathogenetic mechanisms underling these predispositions are not well understood. It is difficult to demonstrate a causal nature of such relationships owing to the rarity of the co-occurrence of these conditions and the difficulties associated with designing large studies that would answer such questions with certainty.

It has been shown that certain rheumatic or autoimmune conditions carry an increased risk of certain types of malignancies; among these are rheumatoid arthritis (RA), Sjögren's syndrome (SS), dermatomyositis (DM), and systemic sclerosis.[4] Moreover, there is an increased incidence of autoimmune phenomena developing after initiating cancer therapy, as well as an increased malignant potential associated with administration of immunomodulating drugs. This observation makes it even harder to ascertain a causal relationship between rheumatic diseases, cancer and their treatments.

Table 1 displays the suggested associations between the rheumatic diseases and certain malignancies. A brief discussion of the most common diseases and their associations follows.

Rheumatoid Arthritis

The association between (RA) and lymphoproliferative disorders is suggested from epidemiologic data derived primarily from two population-based studies from Sweden[6] and Finland[7] that found an approximately twofold overall increased risk of lymphomas in the RA population. Consistent with these data, in a recent prospective US study, the overall standardized incidence ratio (SIR) for development of lymphoma was reported to be 1.9, which was increased further with the

Table 1 Rheumatic Diseases' Associations with Malignancies

Rheumatic Disease	Associated Neoplasms
Rheumatoid arthritis	Lymphoproliferative diseases (non-Hodgkin's lymphoma, Hodgkin's disease) Paraproteinemia and multiple myeloma[89,90]
Sjögren's syndrome	Lymphoproliferative diseases (non-Hodgkin's lymphoma, Hodgkin's disease) Monoclonal gammopathies,[17,91] angioimmunoblastic lymphadenopathy[92]
Dermatomyositis/polymyositis	Solid tumors (breast, ovarian, lung, pancreatic, gastric, and colorectal cancers)
Systemic sclerosis	Lymphoma at the end after; lung, breast, ovarian, skin, esophageal, and liver cancers; Lymphoma
Systemic lupus erythematosus	? Non-Hodgkin's lymphoma; lung, liver, and vulvar cancers
Giant cell arteritis (temporal arteritis)	? Lymphoid malignancies
Behçet's disease	T-cell lymphoma[93]

use of antirheumatic drugs,[8] as is discussed later. A nested-control study based on the Swedish data found that rheumatoid disease activity is an independent risk factor conferring up to a 25-fold increase in lymphoma risk in severe arthritis with a high inflammatory state.[9,10] Most of the lymphomas appear to be of the non-Hodgkin's disease type, particularly the diffuse large B-cell form.[11]

Sjögren's Syndrome

Many studies have reported an increased incidence of lymphomas ranging from 2 to 9% in patients with primary Sjögren's Syndrome (SS),[12–14] exceeding the frequency of lymphoma in the general population by up to 44-fold.[13] There is, however, a long latency period between the onset of SS, which is often subtle, and the diagnosis of lymphoma ranging from 1.5 to 12 years.[15] There also is an increased incidence of malignant lymphoma with time (2.6% at 5 years compared with 3.9% at 10 years in one study).[16] Similar to RA, most of the lymphomas are of the non-Hodgkin's B-cell type,[12] and some are of the MALT (mucosa-associated lymphoid tissue) type.[17] Hyperstimulation of B cells, an inherent characteristic of SS that has been termed *pseudolymphoma*, appears to be the main pathogenic mechanism that precedes and predisposes patients to the malignant transformation, in conjunction with other suggested mechanisms still under investigation.[18] In patients with primary SS, one in five deaths is attributable to lymphoma.[16]

Dermatomyositis/Polymyositis

The association between Dermatomyositis (DM) and malignancy has long been noted and found to be stronger than polymyositis (PM). An Australian population-based study estimated the SIR for cancer in DM at 6.2 and in PM at 2.0.[19] The incidence was found to be highest within 2 years of the diagnosis of myositis and to fall significantly after that.[19,20] Solid tumors, such as breast, ovarian, lung, pancreatic, gastric, and colorectal cancers, as well as lymphoproliferative malignancies, are overrepresented in the myositis population.[21]

There is no consensus on cancer screening in DM/PM patients, but most authorities advocate routine screening based on the patient's age group, with special attention to those with more risk factors (age 40 years and older, weight loss, previous malignancy, a positive family history of cancer).[22]

Screening should include a thorough history and physical examination along with complete blood counts, serum chemistries that include liver and renal function tests, urinalysis, and a chest radiograph. Thorough pelvic and breast examinations, including PAP smears and mammograms, should be performed in women and digital rectal/prostate examinations in men.[22] Colonoscopy also should be strongly considered.

Myositis may improve with successful treatment of the cancer and return with cancer relapse. Careful follow-up is emphasized. In most cases, however, the myositis requires urgent treatment on its own beginning with high doses of corticosteroids (prednisone 60–80 mg daily) and continuing at those levels (or higher if necessary) until serum levels of creatine kinase (CK) have normalized. Thereafter, corticosteroids should be tapered slowly with close follow-up of the patient's weakness and rash and especially CK levels.[22–25] It should be noted that approximately 5% of myositis patients will never have elevated CK or other muscle enzyme levels despite proximal muscle weakness and positive electromyography and/or muscle biopsy. In such cases, frequent assessment of muscle strength as corticosteroids are tapered is essential.[26,27]

It also is important to note that some DM patients with or without underlying malignancy will have the typical rash but never develop clinically evident myositis (amyopathic DM).[28] Treatment of the rash again usually requires systemic corticosteroids.

Systemic Sclerosis

Associations between Systemic Sclerosis (SSc) and cancer have been studied in two population-based studies from Sweden and South Australia, which reported a 1.5- to 2- fold overall increased risk of malignancy,[29–31] with a high incidence of lung cancer (SIR 5–6) among others. Typically, bronchogenic carcinoma may occur in patients with long-standing pulmonary fibrosis.

Ovarian, liver, breast, and nonmelanoma skin cancers, as well as Lymphoma were overrepresented, and Barrett's esophagus occurs more frequently owing to esophageal dysmotility and gastroesophageal reflux. A subset of patients has been reported in which the onsets of scleroderma and breast cancer occurred contemporaneously.[31]

Systemic Lupus Erythematosus

There are conflicting data regarding the overall risk of cancer in systemic lupus erythematosus (SLE) patients. Non-Hodgkin's lymphoma, in particular, was found to occur four to five times more often in SLE patients than in the general population in two large studies from Denmark and Canada.[32,33] Other malignancies with a suggested increased risk include cancers of the lung, liver, and vagina.

Polymyalgia Rheumatica and Giant Cell Arteritis

Conflicting data exist regarding any association between polymyalgia rheumatica (PMR) or giant cell arteritis (GCA) and malignancy. A prospective study from Norway found no overall increased risk of cancer in patients with PMR or GCA,[34] nor did another Canadian population-based study.[35] There was at least a 2.3-fold increased risk of cancer in patients with biopsy-proven GCA, however, in the Norwegian study, whereas the Canadian study found no such association. Malignancies were reported to be of the lymphoid type in general. Of note, PMR has been reported as a secondary paraneoplastic syndrome associated with renal cell carcinoma.[36] The symptoms of PMR also can be mimicked by multiple myeloma and primary amyloidosis.

Spondyloarthropathies

Spondyloarthropathies per se are not associated with an increased risk of malignancy.[37] Ankylosing spondylitis patients previously treated with spinal irradiation therapy, however, have been found to have an increased risk of developing leukemia and colon cancer.[38]

Cancer and Its Treatment: Implications for Rheumatic Diseases

Acute Monoarthritis

Cancer and its treatment can lead to an acute or chronic monoarthritis, especially in the hospital setting. The possible causes are multiple, and prompt diagnosis is critical to effective treatment (Table 2).

Table 2 Common Causes of Acute and Chronic Monoarthritis in the Causes patient

Acute
   Septic arthritis (bacterial)
   Gout
   Pseudogout
   Hemarthrosis
   Occult trauma/fracture
Chronic
   Septic arthritis (mycobacterial and fungal)
   Avascular necrosis (usually from steroids)
   Metastases

Needle aspiration and laboratory examination of synovial fluid should be performed immediately in patients who develop acute swelling, severe pain, erythema, and warmth in one or more joints or bursae (Table 3).

Bacterial Arthritis

Bacterial arthritis, usually spread hematogenously from another site of infection, is common and life-threatening. Predisposing factors in cancer patients include impaired host defenses by virtue of the malignancy itself or the drugs used to treat it, along with indwelling venous catheters and hospital reservoirs of nosocomial pathogens. It also should be emphasized that patients with preexisting joint diseases, such as RA or osteoarthritis, are more liable to infection in already damaged joints.[39] Patients with prosthetic joints also are at high risk of bacterial seeding during bouts of sepsis, including those occurring during diagnostic and therapeutic manipulations of the oral cavity and respiratory tract, lower gastrointestinal (colonoscopy, surgery) tract, and genitourinary (cystoscopy, catheterization, and surgery) tract.[40]

The most common organism to infect joints is *Staphylococcus aureus*, often methicillin-resistant, originating from cutaneous wounds, cellulitis, decubitus ulcers, or even simple

Table 3 Synovial Fluid Findings in Various Causes of Monoarthritis

Finding	Implication
Appearance	
Clear	Noninflammatory*
Cloudy	Inflammatory
Bloody (does not clot)	Hemarthrosis (bleeding disorder, trauma, tumor)
White blood cell count	
< 2,000/mm³	Noninflammatory
> 2,000/mm³	Inflammatory
Neutrophilic	Bacterial or crystalline
Lymphocytic	Mycobacterial, fungal, tumor
Glucose	
Low (< 25%) of serum level)	Infection
Gram stains and cultures	Diagnostic for bacteria
Mycobacterial and fungal stains and cultures	Diagnostic for mycobacteria and fungi
Wet preparation viewed with polarizing microscope	Diagnostic for MSU and CPPD crystals
	Fat bodies imply bony fractures

CPPD = calcium pyrophosphate dihydrate;
   MSU = monosodium urate.

abrasions, as well as infected venous lines.[41,42] Virtually any bacterial type, gram positive or negative, may cause an infectious arthritis in debilitated and immunocompromised patients. Therefore, bacteriologic identification is imperative from aspirated synovial fluid and/or blood cultures, which should be obtained prior to empiric antibiotic therapy.

Mycobacterial and fungal joint infections tend to be more indolent and chronic. Synovial fluid cultures and stains are less likely to reveal the organisms. Synovial tissue biopsy performed by special needles or arthroscopically with special histopathologic stains and cultures are more likely to yield a correct identification.[42]

Infectious arthritis can rarely be cured with antibiotics alone. Joint drainage is essential in nearly all instances, either arthroscopically or by surgical opening of the joint.[42]

Gouty Arthritis

Gouty arthritis is common in patients with malignancy by virtue of overproduction of uric acid. Proliferating tumor cells, their destruction by chemotherapy or radiation, and cachexia all result in increased cell breakdown and metabolism of purines to uric acid, which may deposit as monosodium urate (MSU) crystals in cartilaginous joint structures, renal interstitium, or both.[43] Renal underexcretion of uric acid may compound hyperuricemia when there is renal insufficiency or medications such as diuretics reduce renal output.[44]

Acute attacks of crystalline arthritis are triggered by sudden changes in serum uric acid levels, either up or down, induced by changes in tumor bulk, drugs and radiocontrast agents, acidosis, or joint trauma. Thus, attacks occurring in the hospital are not unusual. The most commonly affected joints include the first metatarsal phalangeal (podagra), instep and/or dorsal foot, ankle, knee, wrist, or elbow. Gout often mimics cellulitis, thus prompting ineffectual antibiotic coverage. Joint involvement is distinguishable by the exquisite pain elicited by attempts to actively or passively move the adjacent joint. Diagnosis is established by finding the typical intracellular MSU crystals in synovial fluid (see Table 3). It should be noted that even neutropenic patients may have gouty attacks because synoviocyte macrophages can ingest MSU crystals and initiate an inflammatory response.[44]

Treatment of the acute attack must be complete before attempts to lower serum uric acid levels; otherwise, the inflammatory phase may be perpetuated and prolonged. Low-dose colchicine 0.6 mg daily or twice daily may be sufficient in an early or mild episode. Most patients require an additional short-acting nonsteroidal anti-inflammatory drug (NSAID), such as indomethacin 50 mg twice or three times daily,

tolmetin 600 mg three times daily, or naproxen 500 mg twice daily. Patients with any degree of renal impairment or a history of peptic ulcer disease should not receive NSAIDs. Instead, prednisone (or another corticosteroid) 30 to 40 mg daily for 2 to 3 days followed by tapering off over the next week is an effective and far safer option. Another option is injection of a repository corticosteroid into the affected joint.[44]

Once the pain and inflammatory signs are resolved, low-dose colchicine should be continued as prophylaxis against another attack. If there is renal impairment, only a very low dose of colchicine 0.6 mg every 3 to 4 days should be continued so that colchicine-induced neuromyopathy does not occur.[45] The xanthine oxidase inhibitor allopurinol then should be started slowly, beginning at 100 mg daily. The dose should be gradually adjusted upward over the next several weeks, aiming to achieve serum uric acid levels of 6 mg/dL or less. For patients allergic to allopurinol, recombinant uricase therapy may be an option.[46]

Calcium Pyrophosphate Deposition Disease

Calcium pyrophosphate dihydratc (CPPD) deposition disease occurs in approximately 20% of elderly people, as evidenced by the radiographic appearance of stippled calcifications of articular and meniscal cartilage (chondrocalcinosis) in knees, wrists, symphysis pubis, or other joints. The majority of such people remain asymptomatic unless admitted to hospitals for a medical illness or surgery. Similar to uric acid, changes in circulating levels of serum calcium may result in release of CPPD crystals into a joint, causing an acute inflammatory arthritis termed *pseudogout*.

The most commonly affected joints are the knee and wrist. Podagra is exceedingly rare in pseudogout and almost always indicates gout.

CPPD in most patients is likely to be caused by as yet unknown genetic factors. Several metabolic disorders associated with CPPD and acute attacks of pseudogout should be considered and, when found, corrected (Table 4).

Treatment of an acute attack of pseudogout is similar to that described above for gout. Low-dose colchicine may be useful as prophylaxis but is not as effective as in gout.[47]

Table 4 Common Metabolic Causes of Calcium Pyrophosphate Dihydrate and Attacks of Pseudogout
Hypercalcemia (from primary or secondary hyperparathyroidism, metastatic bone disease)
Hypomagnesemia
Hypothyroidism
Hemochromatosis

Acute Polyarthritis

Abrupt onset of acute polyarthritis in a cancer patient should lead to several major considerations. Although usually monoarticular, infections, gout, and pseudogout may present in a polyarticular fashion. The same principles of diagnosis and treatment as discussed above for monoarthritis should apply.

Serum sickness–like reactions (including polyarthritis) owing to drugs, such as sulfonamides, penicillin, and cephalosporins, are not uncommon.

An acute viral infection, especially parvovirus B19, may present in adults in a rheumatoid-like pattern, often with a transient, trunchal, maculopapular rash. Such patients have typically been exposed to young children with erythema infectiosum, or fifth disease. This form of arthritis is typically short-lived (weeks to months) and responds to NSAIDs or low-dose prednisone 5 to 10 mg daily. A more serious aplastic anemia may occur in patients whose bone marrows have been compromised by virtue of malignancy or chemotherapy.[48]

Several cancer chemotherapeutic agents also may cause arthritis and are discussed below.

Finally, a paraneoplastic syndrome, such as hypertrophic osteoarthropathy, palmar fasciitis with polyarthritis syndrome, or carcinomatous polyarthritis, may be emerging (see Chapter 59).

Rheumatic and Autoimmune Diseases Complicating Cancer Therapy

A multitude of rheumatic and autoimmune phenomena have been observed in cancer patients, both before and after initiating certain treatment modalities. Many of these less frequent conditions are based on case reports or small series at best, making the evidence for a true association very weak. Those supported by the most consistent and compelling evidence are summarized in Table 5; a brief discussion of the most relevant associations follows:

Bleomycin, a chemotherapeutic agent used to treat breast cancer, among others, has been linked to pulmonary fibrosis, which resembles that of scleroderma,[49,50] as well as Raynaud's phenomenon and fingertip necrosis. Even local use of bleomycin to treat verrucous skin lesions can induce Raynaud's phenomenon in digits so treated.[51]

Interferon-α, used primarily for the treatment of chronic viral hepatitis but also for malignant lymphoma and carcinoid tumors, has been associated with induction of autoimmune diseases, including RA, PM, SLE, and Hashimoto's thyroiditis.[52,53] Of these, SLE occurred at an incidence of 0.1 to 0.7%. There is increasing evidence that idiopathic SLE and other autoimmune

Table 5 Rheumatic and Autoimmune Syndromes Associated with Cancer Treatments

Cancer Treatment	Associated Rheumatic and Autoimmune Conditions	Comments
Bleomycin	Scleroderma-like pulmonary fibrosis Raynaud's phenomenon	See text
Interferon-α	Rheumatoid arthritis Polymyositis Systemic lupus erythematosus -Hashimoto's thyroiditis	See text
GVHD (after hematopoietic cell transplantation)	Localized and generalized scleroderma (morphea) Cutaneous lupus Sjögren's syndrome Polymyositis	See text
Autologous stem cell transplantation	Spondyloarthropathy Reactive arthritis	See text
BCG immunotherapy	Reactive arthritis Sjögren's syndrome RS3PE syndrome	See text
Radiation therapy	Postradiation morphea	See text
Gemcitabine	Vasculitis (in the form of necrotizing enterocolitis)[94,95]	Used for bladder cancer
Goserelin	Relapsing polychondritis[96]	Used for prostate cancer
Interleukin-2	Rheumatoid-like seronegative polyarthritis[97]	Used to treat melanoma
		Symmetric polyarthritis and seronegative for both RF and ANAs
Uracil-tegafur	Localized and generalized scleroderma (morphea)[98–100]	Cutaneous scleroderma without systemic or vascular manifestations
Melphalan		
Paclitaxel		

ANA = antinuclear antibody; BCG = bacille Calmette-Guérin; GVHD = graft-versus-host disease; RF = rheumatoid factor; RS3PE = remitting seronegative symmetric synovitis with pitting edema.

diseases are driven by interferon-dependent pathways[54]; therefore, this agent should be avoided in such patients because it may exacerbate their autoimmune disease.

Chronic graft-versus-host disease, a known complication after hematopoietic cell transplantation, can cause rheumatic-like syndromes resembling localized and generalized scleroderma (morphea), cutaneous lupus, SS, and PM.[55–57]

Autologous stem cell transplantation, used for lymphoid malignancies, has been linked to the development of spondyloarthropathy in human leukocyte antigen B27–positive patients.[58] Patients who have a history of reactive arthritis (Reiter's syndrome) have been noted to have exacerbations after immunosuppressing chemotherapy, similar to patients with human immunodeficiency virus (HIV) infections[59] (F.C.A., personal observations, 1988).

Bacille Calmette-Guérin immunotherapy, used as an adjunctive treatment for superficial bladder carcinoma, can cause a reactive arthritis (formerly termed Reiter's syndrome), SS, and remitting seronegative symmetric synovitis with pitting edema (RS3PE syndrome).[60–63]

Radiation therapy has been associated with scleroderma skin changes over the irradiated areas (postradiation morphea), especially in patients with preexisting scleroderma.[64–66] In fact, many authorities consider scleroderma a relative contraindication for the use of radiation therapy. A risk-benefit evaluation should be performed in these circumstances.

Rheumatic Disease Treatment: Implications for Cancer Patients

Many agents used to treat rheumatic diseases carry a small but significantly increased risk of the future development of neoplastic diseases.

It has been demonstrated that the increased risk of malignancy associated with certain rheumatic diseases, as discussed above, is independent of drug treatments. This inherent disease association risk, however, is increased even further by the use of these agents.[67] Drugs such as cyclophosphamide, methotrexate, chlorambucil, azathioprine, and possibly tumor necrosis factor (TNF)-α antagonists have been reported to predispose patients to certain types of malignancies.

Little is known about the applications of these antirheumatic drugs in patients with an established diagnosis of cancer. Their concomitant use should be based on expert opinions on a case-by-case basis.

Alkalyting Agents

Cyclophosphamide has been clearly shown to increase the risk of cancer (relative risk 1.5), particularly bladder cancer.[4,67] The duration and dosing of therapy play important roles.[68] Some cases of malignancy, however, have been reported to occur as long as 15 years following drug discontinuance.[67] The incidence was estimated to be approximately 5% in a study of patients with Wegener's granulomatosis, a disease in which cyclophosphamide has proven to be lifesaving.[67,69] The bladder cancer is usually aggressive in nature,[70] justifying a close surveillance program for patients so treated, including periodic examination of the urine for the presence of hematuria and, when indicated, cystoscopy.[69] Finally, monthly intravenous cyclophosphamide pulse therapy rather than daily oral dosing has been found to decrease the malignant potential by reducing the cumulative dose and the total time of exposure to the carcinogenic metabolite acrolein, and it is widely preferred over continuous daily therapy nowadays.[71] Cyclophosphamide also may increase the risk of cutaneous squamous cell carcinomas and lymphoproliferative malignancies, especially B-cell lymphoma, which may present in the brain.[72]

Chlorambucil behaves similarly to cyclophosphamide but has a greater hematotoxic effect and a higher risk of inducing leukemia (1–7%).[73,74]

Antimetabolites

Azathioprine use carries a malignant potential that is smaller in size in patients with RA (1 case of lymphoma per 1,000 patient-years) compared with renal transplant recipients who are receiving the drug,[75] and this risk increases by increasing the cumulative duration of exposure.[68] The most common cancers are squamous cell carcinoma of the skin, B-cell lymphomas, Hodgkin's disease, Kaposi's sarcoma, and carcinoma of the uterine cervix.[76]

Methotrexate increases the risk of lymphoproliferative diseases, generally after long-term use.[77] It has been suggested, albeit still controversially, that Epstein-Barr virus latent infection might play a role in this neoplastic transformation.[78] A French national prospective study found the incidence of Hodgkin's disease to be no higher in RA patients receiving methotrexate than in the general population, a scenario that was not true for non-Hodgkin's lymphoma.[79] These B-cell lymphomas tend to be nonaggressive, and many experts recommend a period of observation off the drug before starting anticancer treatment since spontaneous regression does occur in many cases within a few weeks.[77,80,81] This approach, however, should be coupled with a very careful surveillance program in such patients because recurrence of the lymphoma is a definite possibility.[82] Some of these lymphomas, in complicated cases, can be refractory to conventional chemotherapy but may ultimately respond to newer therapies, such as rituximab.[83]

Anticytokines

Anti-TNF-α agents such as infliximab, adalimumab, and etanercept, used for treatment of moderate to severe RA, psoriasis and psoriatic arthritis, ankylosing spondylitis, and Crohn's disease, have been linked in postmarketing surveillance reports to the development of lymphoproliferative malignancies with SIRs of 2.6 to 3.8.[8,84] The majority of cases have been non-Hodgkin's lymphomas with a median 8-week latency period after starting therapy.[84] Spontaneous regression of the tumor was described in some cases. This association is still controversial, and additional data are needed.

NSAIDs, including aspirin, used to treat many rheumatic diseases, may actually decrease the risk of colon caner (SIR of 0.6–0.7).[6] This finding could be related to the presumed chemoprotective effect that these drugs have against colon neoplasms. Further clinical trials are necessary.

In conclusion, the treatments of both rheumatic and neoplastic diseases in patients who happen to have both interrelate substantially, factoring in all of the associations presented above. Some treatment modalities beneficial for one disease may prove to also be effective,[85–87] or detrimental,[49,66,88] for the other condition. Therapeutic approaches should be decided on an individual basis and after weighing the potential risks and benefits for each intervention.

REFERENCES

1. Benedek TG, Rheumatic diseases and neoplasia. In: Oxford textbook of Rheumatology, 2nd edition, D. Isenberg, P. Maddsion, P. Woo et al, Editors. 1998, Oxford University Press, USA. p. 1665–79.
2. Albert DA, Schumacher HR, Miscellaneous arthropathies, in Rheumatology, 3rd edition, M.C. Hochberg, A.J. Silman, J.S. Smolen et al, Editors. 2003. Mosby. Philadelphia, PA. p. 1753–62.
3. Yazici Y, Kagen LJ, Malignancy and rheumatic disorders, in UpToDate, B.D. Rose, Editor, 2006, Waltham, MA.
4. Benedek, TG, Neoplastic associations of rheumatic diseases and rheumatic manifestations of cancer. Clin Geriatr Med 1988;4(2):333–55.
5. Varoczy L, Gergely L, Zeher M, et al. Malignant lymphoma-associated autoimmune diseases--a descriptive epidemiological study. Rheumatol Int 2002;22(6):233–7.
6. Gridley G, McLaughlin JK, Ekbom A, et al., Incidence of cancer among patients with rheumatoid arthritis. J Natl Cacner Inst 1993;85(4):307–11.
7. Isomaki HA, Hakulinen T, Joutsenlahti U. Excess risk of lymphomas and myeloma in patients with rheumatiod arthritis. Journal of Chronic Diseases 1978;31:691–6.
8. Wolfe F. Lymphoma in rheumatoid arthritis: the effect of methotrexate and anti-tumor necrosis factor therapy in 18,572 patients. Arthritis Rheum 2004;50(6):1740–51.
9. Baecklund E, Ekbom A, Sparen P, et al. Disease activity and risk of lymphoma in patients with rheumatoid arthritis: nested case-control study. BMJ 1998;317:180–1.
10. Baecklund E, Askling J, Rosenquist R, et al. Rheumatoid arthritis and malignant lymphomas. Curr Opin Rheumatol 2004;16(3):254–61.
11. Baecklund E, Sundstorm C, Catrina AI, et al. Lymphoma subtypes in patients with rheumatoid arthritis: increased proportion of diffuse large B cell lymphoma. Arthritis Rheum, 2003;48(6):1543–50.
12. McCurley TL, Collins RD, Ball E. Nodal and extranodal lymphoproliferative disorders in Sjögren's Syndrome; a clinical and immunopathological study. Human Pathology, 1990;21:482–92.
13. Kassan SS, Thomas TL, Moutsopoulos HM, et al. Increased risk of lymphoma in sicca syndrome. Annals of Internal Medicine 1978;89:888–92.
14. Zufferey P, Meyer OC, Grossin M, et al. Primary Sjogren's syndrome (SS) and malignant lymphoma. A retrospective cohort study of 55 patients with SS. Scand J Rheumatol 1995;24(6):342–5.
15. Schmid U, Helborn D, Lennert K. Development of malignant lymphoma in myoepithelial sialadenitis (Sjögren's Syndrome). Archives of Pathological Anatomy 1982; 395(1):11–43.
16. Ioannidis JP, Vassiliou VA, Moutsopoulos HM. Long-term risk of mortality and lymphoproliferative disease and predictive classification of primary Sjögren's Syndrome. Arthritis Rheum 2002;46(3):741–7.
17. Masaki Y, Sugai S. Lymphoproliferative disorders in Sjögren's Syndrome. Autoimmun Rev. 2004;3(3):175–82.
18. Tapinos NI, Moutsopoulos HM. Lymphoma development in Sjogren's syndrome: novel p53 mutations. Arthritis Rheum 1999;42(7):1466–72.
19. Buchbinder R, Forbes A, Hall S, et al., Incidence of malignant disease in biopsy-proven inflammatory myopathy. A population-based cohort study. Ann Intern Med 2001;134(12):1087–95.
20. Sigurgeirsson B, Lindelof B, Edhag O, et al. Risk of cancer in patients with dermatomyositis or polymyositis. A population-based study. N Engl J Med 1992;326(6): 363–7.
21. Hill CL, Zhnag Y, Sigurgeursson B, et al. Frequency of specific cancer types in dermatomyositis and polymyositis: a population-based study. Lancet 2001;357(9250): 96–100.
22. Drake LA, Dinehart SM, Farmer ER, et al. Guidelines of care for dermatomyositis. American Academy of Dermatology. J Am Acad Dermatol 1996;34(5 Pt 1):824–9.
23. Dalakas MC. Current treatment of the inflammatory myopathies. Curr Opin Rheumatol 1994;6(6):595–601.
24. Fafalak RG, Peterson MG, Kagen LJ. Strength in polymyositis and dermatomyositis: best outcome in patients treated early. J Rheumatol 1994;21(4):643–8.
25. Oddis CV, Medsger TAJ. Relationship between serum creatine kinase level and corticosteroid therapy in polymyositis-dermatomyositis. J Rheumatol 1988;15(5): 807–11.
26. Carter JD, Kanik KS, Vasey FB, et al. Dermatomyositis with normal creatine kinase and elevated aldolase levels. J Rheumatol 2001;28(10):2366–7.
27. Kagen LJ, Aram S. Creatine kinase activity inhibitor in sera from patients with muscle disease. Arthritis and Rheumatism 1987;30(2):213–7.
28. Olsen NJ, Park JH, King Jr LE. Amyopathic dermatomyositis. Curr Opin Rheumatol 2001;3(4):346–51.
29. Hill CL, Nguyen AM, Roder D, et al., Risk of cancer in patients with scleroderma: a population based cohort study. Ann Rheum Dis 2003;62(8):728–31.
30. Rosenthal AK, McLaughlin JK, Gridley G, et al. Incidence of cancer among patients with systemic sclerosis. Cancer 1995;76(5):910–4.
31. Roumm AD, Medsger TA Jr. Cancer and systemic sclerosis. An epidemiologic study. Arthritis and Rheumatism 1985; 28(12):1336–40.
32. Mellemkjaer L, Andersen V, Gridley G, et al. Non-Hodgkin's lymphoma and other cancers among a cohort of patients with systemic lupus erythematosus. Arthritis Rheum 1997;40(4):761–8.
33. Abu-Shakra M, Gladman DD, Urowitz MB. Malignancy in systemic lupus erythematosus. Arthritis Rheum, 1996; 39(6):1050–4.
34. Haga HJ, Eide GE, Brun J, et al. Cancer in association with polymyalgia rheumatica and temporal arteritis. J Rheumatol 1993;20(8):1335–9.
35. Myklebust G, Wilsgaard T, Jacobsen BK, et al. No increased frequency of malignant neoplasms in polymyalgia rheumatica and temporal arteritis. A prospective longitudinal study of 398 cases and matched population controls. J Rheumatol 2002;29(10):2143–7.
36. Sidhom OA, Basalaev M, Sigal LH. Renal cell carcinoma presenting as polymyalgia rheumatica. Resolution after nephrectomy. Arch Intern Med 1993;153(17):2043–5.
37. Smith PG, Doll R, Radford EP. Cancer mortality among patients with ankylosing spondylitis not given X-ray therapy. Br J Radiol 1977;50(598):728–34.
38. Darby SC, Smith PG. Long term mortality after a single treatment course with X-rays in patients treated for ankylosing spondylitis. Br J Cancer. 1987;55(2):179–90.
39. Kaandorp CJ, Krijnen P, Moens HJ, et al. The outcome of bacterial arthritis: a prospective community-based study. Arthritis and Rheumatism, 1997;40(5):884–92.
40. Berbari EF, Hanssen AD, Duffy MC, et al. Risk factors for prosthetic joint infection: case-control study. Clin Infect Dis 1998;27(5):1247–54.
41. Byrne PA, Hosein IK, Camilleri J. Methicillin-resistant Staphylococcus aureus septic arthritis: urgent and emergent. Clin Rheumatol 1998;17(5):407–8.
42. Goldenberg DL. Septic arthritis. Lancet, 1998;351(9097): 197–202.
43. Pavithran K, Thomas M. Chronic myeloid leukemia presenting as gout. Clin Rheumatol 2001;20(4):288–9.
44. Terkeltaub RA. Gout. N Engl J Med, 2003;349(17):1647–55.
45. Kuncl RW, Duncan G, Watson D, et al. Colchicine myopathy and neuropathy. N Engl J Med 1987;316(25):1562–8.
46. Bomalaski JS, Clark MA. Serum uric acid-lowering therapies: where are we heading in management of hyperuricemia and the potential role of uricase. Curr Rheum Rep 2004;6(3):240–7.
47. Rosenthal AK. Pathogenesis of calcium pyrophosphate crystal deposition disease. Curr Rheumatol Rep. 2001; 3(1):17–23.
48. Young NS, Brown KE. Parvovirus B19. N Engl J Med 2004; 350(6):586–97.
49. Warner E, keshavjee N, Shupak R, et al. Rheumatic symptoms following adjuvant therapy for breast cancer. Am J Clin Oncol 1997;20(3):322–6.
50. Yamamoto T. Animal model of sclerotic skin induced by bleomycin: a clue to the pathogenesis of and therapy for scleroderma? Clin Immunol. 2002;102(3):209–16.
51. Epstein E. Intralesional bleomycin and Raynaud's phenomenon. J Am Acad Dermatol, 1991;24(5 Pt 1): 785–6.
52. Deutsch M, Dourakis S, Manesis EK, et al. Thyroid abnormalities in chronic viral hepatitis and their relationship to interferon alfa therapy. Hepatology 1997;26(1): 206–10.
53. Ioannou Y, Isenberg DA. Current evidence for the induction of autoimmune rheumatic manifestations by cytokine therapy. Arthritis Rheum 2000;43(7):1431–42.
54. Ivashkiv LB. Type I interferon modulation of cellular responses to cytokines and infectious pathogens: potential role in SLE pathogenesis. Autoimmunity 2003;36(8): 473–9.
55. Sullivan KM, Shulman HM, Storb R, et al. Chronic graft-versus-host disease in 52 patients: adverse natural course and successful treatment with combination immunosuppression. Blood 1981;57(2):267–76.
56. Shulman HM, Sale GE, Lerner KG, et al. Chronic cutaneous graft-versus-host disease in man. Am J Pathol 1978;91(3): 545–70.
57. Parker P, Chao NJ, Niland JC, et al. Polymyositis as a manifestation of chronic graft-versus-host disease. Medicine (Baltimore) 1996;75(5):279–85.
58. Koch B, Kranzhofer N, Pfeundschu M, et al., First manifestations of seronegative spondyloarthropathy following autologous stem cell transplantation in HLA-B27-positive patients. Bone Marrow Transplant, 2000. 26(6):673–5.
59. Dharmasena F, Englert H, Catovsky D, et al. Incomplete Reiter's syndrome following chemotherapy of acute myeloid leukaemia. Postgrad Med J 1986;62(733): 1045–6.
60. Conaghan PG, Brooks PM. Rheumatic manifestations of malignancy. Curr Opin Rheumatol 1994;6(1):105–10.
61. Narvaez J, Castro-Bohorquez FJ, Vilaseca-Momplet J. Sjogren's-like syndrome following intravesical bacillus Calmette-Guerin immunotherapy. Am J Med. 2003; 115(5):418–20.

62. Mouly S, Berenbaum F, Kaplan G. Remitting seronegative symmetrical synovitis with pitting edema following intravesical bacillus Calmette-Guerin instillation. J Rheumatol 2001;28(7):1699–701.

63. Onur O, Celiker R. Polyarthritis as a complication of intravesical bacillus Calmette-Guerin immunotherapy for bladder cancer. Clin Rheumatol 1999;18(1):74–6.

64. Schaffer JV, Carroll C, Dvoretsky I, et al. Postirradiation morphea of the breast presentation of two cases and review of the literature. Dermatology 2000;200(1):61–71.

65. Gollob MH, Dekoven JG, Bell MJ, et al. Postradiation morphea. J Rheumatol 1998;25(11):2267–9.

66. Abu-Shakra M, Lee P. Exaggerated fibrosis in patients with systemic sclerosis (scleroderma) following radiation therapy. J Rheumatol 1993;20(9):1601–3.

67. Radis CD, Kahl LE, Baker GL, et al. Effects of cyclophosphamide on the development of malignancy and on long-term survival of patients with rheumatoid arthritis. A 20-year followup study. Arthritis Rheum 1995;38(8):1120–7.

68. Asten P, Barrett J, Symmons D. Risk of developing certain malignancies is related to duration of immunosuppressive drug exposure in patients with rheumatic diseases. J Rheumatol 1999;26(8):1705–14.

69. Talar-Williams C, Hijazi YM, Walther MM, et al. Cyclophosphamide-induced cystitis and bladder cancer in patients with Wegener granulomatosis. Ann Intern Med 1996;124(5):477–84.

70. Fernandes ET, Manivel JC, Reddy PK, et al. Cyclophosphamide associated bladder cancer--a highly aggressive disease: analysis of 12 cases. J Urol 1996;156(6):1931–3.

71. Boumpas DT, Austin HA 3rd, Vaughn EM, et al. Controlled trial of pulse methylprednisolone versus two regimens of pulse cyclophosphamide in severe lupus nephritis. Lancet 1992;340(8822):741–5.

72. Cras P, Franckx C, Martin JJ. Primary intracerebral lymphoma in systemic lupus erythematosus treated with immunosuppressives. Clin Neuropathol. 1989;8(4):200–5.

73. Kaldor JM, Day NE, Pettersson F, et al. Leukemia following chemotherapy for ovarian cancer. N Engl J Med 1990;322(1):1–6.

74. Cannon GW. Chlorambucil therapy in rheumatoid arthritis: clinical experience in 28 patients and literature review. Semin Arthritis Rheum 1985;15(2):106–118.

75. Silman AJ, Petrie J, Hazleman B, et al. Lymphoproliferative cancer and other malignancy in patients with rheumatoid arthritis treated with azathioprine: a 20 year follow up study. Ann Rheum Dis 1988;47(12):988–92.

76. Penn I. Cancers complicating organ transplantation. N Engl J Med 1990;323:1767.

77. Kamel OW, Weiss LM, van de Rijn M, et al. Hodgkin's disease and lymphoproliferations resembling Hodgkin's disease in patients receiving long-term low-dose methotrexate therapy. Am J Surg Pathol 1996;20(10):1279–87.

78. Feng WH, Cohen JI, Fischer S, et al. Reactivation of Latent Epstein-Barr Virus by Methotrexate: A Potential Contributor to Methotrexate-Associated Lymphomas. J Natl Cancer Inst 2004;96(22):1691–702.

79. Mariette X, Cazals-Hatem D, Warszawki J, et al. Lymphomas in rheumatoid arthritis patients treated with methotrexate: a 3-year prospective study in France. Blood 2002;99(11):3909–15.

80. Fam AG, Perez-Ordonez B, Imrie K. Primary cutaneous B cell lymphoma during methotrexate therapy for rheumatoid arthritis. J Rheumatol 2000;27(6):1546–9.

81. Bachman TR, Sawitzke AD, Perkins SL, et al. Methotrexate-associated lymphoma in patients with rheumatoid arthritis: report of two cases. Arthritis Rheum 1996;39(2):325–9.

82. Moseley AC, Lindsley HB, Skikne BS, et al. Reversible methotrexate associated lymphoproliferative disease evolving into Hodgkin's disease. J Rheumatol 2000;27(3):810–3.

83. Stewart M, Malkovsak V, Krishnan J, et al. Lymphoma in a patient with rheumatoid arthritis receiving methotrexate treatment: successful treatment with rituximab. Ann Rheum Dis 2001;60(9):892–3.

84. Brown SL, Greene MH, Gershon SK, et al. Tumor necrosis factor antagonist therapy and lymphoma development: twenty-six cases reported to the Food and Drug Administration. Arthritis Rheum 2002;46(12):3151–8.

85. Yoo WH, Baek HS. Remission of rheumatoid arthritis with taxol in a patient with breast carcinoma. J Rheumatol 2000;27(6):1572–3.

86. Thomas DA, Kantarjian HM. Current role of thalidomide in cancer treatment. Curr Opin Oncol 2000;12(6):564–73.

87. Enright H, Jacob HS, Vercellotti G, et al. Paraneoplastic autoimmune phenomena in patients with myelodysplastic syndromes: response to immunosuppressive therapy. Br J Haematol 1995;91(2):403–8.

88. Anderlini P, Korbling M, Dale D, et al. Allogeneic blood stem cell transplantation: considerations for donors. Blood 1997;90(3):903–8.

89. Zawadzki ZA, Benedek TG. Rheumatiod arthritis, dysproteinemic arthropathy, and paraproteinemia. Arthritis and Rheumatism 1969;12:555–68.

90. Eriksson M. Rheumatoid arthritis as a risk for mutiple myeloma, a case-control study. Eur J Cancer 1993;29A:259–63.

91. Sugai S, Shimizu S, Hirose Y, et al. Monoclonal gammapathies in Japenese patients with Sjögren's Syndrome. J Clin Immunol. 1985;5(2):90–101.

92. Bignon YJ, Janin-Mercier A, Dubost JJ, et al. Angioimmunoblastic lymphadenopathy with dysproteinaemia (AILD) and sicca syndrome. Ann Rheum Dis 1986;45(6):519–22.

93. Katsura Y, Suzukawa K, Kojima H, et al. Cytotoxic T-cell lymphoma arising in Behcet disease. Int J Hematol 2003;77(3):282–5.

94. Birlik M, Akar S, Tuzel E, et al. Gemcitabine-induced vasculitis in advanced transitional cell carcinoma of the bladder. J Cancer Res Clin Oncol 2004;130(2):122–5.

95. Geisler JP, Schraith DF, Manahan KJ, et al. Gemcitabine associated vasculitis leading to necrotizing enterocolitis and death in women undergoing primary treatment for epithelial ovarian/peritoneal cancer. Gynecol Oncol 2004;92(2):705–7.

96. Labarthe MP, Bayle-Lebey P, Bazex J. Cutaneous manifestations of relapsing polychondritis in a patient receiving goserelin for carcinoma of the prostate. Dermatology 1997;195(4):391–4.

97. Hersh EM, Murray JL, Hong WK, et al. Phase I study of cancer therapy with recombinant interleukin-2 administered by intravenous bolus injection. Biotherapy 1989;1:215–26.

98. Kono T, Ishii M, Negoro N, et al. Scleroderma-like reaction induced by uracil-tegafur (UFT), a second-generation anticancer agent. J Am Acad Dermatol 2000;42(3):519–20.

99. Landau M, Brenner S, Gat A, et al. Reticulate scleroderma after isolated limb perfusion with melphalan. J Am Acad Dermatol. 1998;39(6):1011–2.

100. Kupfer I, Balquerue X, Courville P, et al. Scleroderma-like cutaneous lesions induced by paclitaxel: a case study. J Am Acad Dermatol 2003;48(2):279–81.

Cancer Rehabilitation

Rajesh Yadav, MD
Ki Y. Shin, MD
Ying Guo, MD
Benedict Konzen, MD

Cancer is associated with significant mortality, morbidity, and disability. With improvements in the ability to detect and treat cancer, people are living longer with it.[1] The goal of cancer rehabilitation is to add to quality of life by improving self-reliance and decreasing the burden of care for their caregivers.

Lehman and colleagues first studied this issue of functional deficits in the cancer setting in 1978 with support from the National Cancer Institute.[2] Multiple barriers were also identified, which limited the delivery of cancer rehabilitation care. Many of the remediable cancer rehabilitation problems and barriers remain the same (Table 1).

General Rehabilitation Concepts

One of the differentiating factors in a rehabilitation evaluation is a clear picture of how an illness affects a patient's life and how such an illness precludes what is meaningful to him or her. To describe such changes, the terminology of impairments, disabilities, and handicaps is used but often misunderstood.

Impairment is any loss or abnormality of psychological, physiologic, or anatomic structure or function.[3] Impairment refers to a problem at the organ level. For example, in a postoperative patient with a pathologic fracture of the left hip, impairment would be left lower extremity dysfunction with decreased range of motion about the left hip and decreased weight-bearing status.

Disability is any restriction or lack resulting from an impairment of ability to perform an activity in the manner or within the range considered normal for a human being.[3] Disability refers to a problem at the person level. With the above example, disability would be not being able to perform the activity of getting out of bed on one's own or to ambulate independently.

Handicap is a disadvantage for a given individual resulting from an impairment or a disability that limits or prevents the fulfillment of a role that is normal for that individual. Handicap refers to a problem at the society level. With the above example, if the patient were a postal employee and had to deliver mail, he would be disabled for that job since he is unable to ambulate and fulfill that role. However, if the employment required answering the telephone, then that patient would not be considered handicapped.

A thorough functional history and social support system are also key components of a rehabilitation evaluation.

Types of Cancer Rehabilitation

In the cancer setting, rehabilitation has been described as being preventive, restorative, supportive, and palliative.[4] Preventive interventions are started before or soon after a treatment to prevent functional loss and disability. Restorative interventions include comprehensive restoration of function in a disabled patient with cured or stable disease. Supportive rehabilitation is geared toward patients with progressive disease and disability. Palliative rehabilitation interventions are focused on maintaining comfort and function in terminal phase (Table 2).

Settings for Cancer Rehabilitation

Delivery of rehabilitation can be provided in various settings, including acute inpatient rehabilitation, consultative care, outpatient care (including home care), and even a hospice. Acute inpatient cancer rehabilitation can directly follow cancer treatments such as surgery and/or chemotherapy. After such interventions, patients may be unable to perform basic activities of daily living, such as transfers and ambulation. The goals of acute inpatient rehabilitation include improving mobility and self-care activities to allow for safe discharge. Marciniak and colleagues described functional improvements after acute inpatient rehabilitation in such patients.[5] Some common inpatient rehabilitation diagnoses include

Table 1 Remediable Rehabilitation Problems and Barriers to Delivery of Rehabilitation Care

Remediable Rehabilitation Problems		Barriers to Delivery of Rehabilitation Care
Psychological/psychiatric impairments	Lymphedema management	Lack of identification of patient problems
Generalized weakness	Musculoskeletal difficulties	Lack of appropriate referral by physicians unfamiliar with the concept of rehabilitation
Impairments in activities of daily living	Swallowing dysfunction	Patient too ill to participate
Pain	Impaired communication	Patient denies need
Impaired gait/ambulation	Skin management	Cancer prognosis too limited
Disposition/housing issues	Vocational assessments	Rehabilitation unavailable
Neurologic impairments	Impaired nutrition	No financial resources

Table 2 Benefits of Rehabilitation

Training to maximize functional independence
Facilitation of psychosocial coping and adaptation by patient and family
Improved quality of life through community reintegration: includes resumption of prior home, family, recreational, and vocational activities
Recognition, management, and prevention of comorbid illnesses that limit or impede function

significant asthenia, hemiparesis, severe gait abnormality, dyspnea with exertion, spinal cord injury, and neurogenic bowel and bladder. Significant pain with activity is quite common in patients with musculoskeletal deficits.

Rehabilitation consultation interventions have been linked to functional improvements during acute hospital stay. Outpatient rehabilitation can be prescribed for patients who do not require hospitalization and following acute inpatient rehabilitation to further improve function. Concepts and techniques taught during acute inpatient rehabilitation may also be reinforced during this phase. Common outpatient rehabilitation diagnoses include lymphedema, myofascial pain, rotator cuff dysfunction, peripheral neuropathy, and low back pain.

For terminally ill patients who are declining rapidly, issues of family training, comfort care, and appropriate adaptive equipment(s) may be addressed by the rehabilitation team. These patients may also have limited energy to pursue daily activities. Thus, therapy interventions and exercise may lead to early fatigue and prevent patients from spending quality time toward doing desired activities.

Rehabilitation Team

Rehabilitation is a comprehensive effort and requires an interdisciplinary team of health care professionals, including rehabilitation physicians, rehabilitation nurses, physical therapists, occupational therapists, speech therapists, dietitians, pharmacists, chaplains, social workers, and case managers. Each member of the team is indispensable owing to specific expertise in assisting the patient with a care plan to maximize medical stability, function, financial resources, and caregiver involvement for a meaningful and safe discharge. Medical care is closely coordinated with primary cancer physicians and various consultants. Rehabilitation professionals can give feedback on the patient's functional issues to treating oncologists. Alteration in functional capacity may change the course of medical treatment.

Concept of Safe Discharge

A frequent reason for cancer rehabilitation consultation is to assess the patient's functional status for safe discharge. Important variables here are the patient's physical capacity, cognition, family or caregiver support available, and financial resources. A safe discharge usually requires some combination of these factors. Many of the patients admitted to an acute inpatient rehabilitation unit require some degree of supervision and assistance on discharge owing to physical and cognition dysfunction. Patients usually lose some of their autonomy in exchange for personal safety. More time and financial resources are required

for their care. Often abnormal family dynamics come to the surface at the time of discharge, when the resources of family time and physical and financial assistance are needed. Attention is also directed toward community resources and local support, including church and friends, to fill in the gaps.

Functional Assessment Tools

There are various tools for measuring performance in the cancer setting. The most commonly used scale is the Karnofsky Performance Scale (KPS). In the absence of any medical treatment, the KPS was found to be the best determinant of ultimate patient survival in a national hospice study. With a score of 40, patients lived, on average, less than 50 days; with a score of 20, they lived only 10 to 20 days (Table 3).[6] Another commonly used tool is the Eastern Cooperative Oncology Group (ECOG) scale for performance status (Table 4).

KPS does not address cognitive function or quality of life. Additional limitations of this scale that limit its use as a functional outcomes measure are its inability to objectively quantify the amount of assistance needed and its linkage of physical function with medical status. These criteria fail to accommodate severely disabled but otherwise healthy patients. Its linkage of medical status with work status is often heavily influenced by completely nonmedical factors, such as insurance, family support, and type of work done. These criticisms are also valid for ECOG and similar performance status scales.

Among rehabilitation professions, one of the most commonly used scales has been the Functional Independence Measure (FIM) (Figure 1). This numeric scale is divided into various categories, from self-care to social cognition. In each of these categories, various tasks and patients are assigned a score of 1 through 7 depending on their ability to complete them. Higher scores denote that a lesser amount of assistance is required with a particular task. For example, with a score of 6 with the self-care task of toileting, patients are able to complete the task on their own but require adaptive equipment, such as an elevated commode seat. With the same task, a

Table 4 Eastern Cooperative Oncology Group (ECOG) Scale Performance Status

Grade	Definition
0	Fully active, able to carry on all predisease performance without restriction
1	Restricted in physically strenuous activity; ambulatory; able to perform light or sedentary work
2	Capable of all self-care; ambulatory; unable to perform work activities; up and about more than 50% of waking hours
3	Only capable of limited self-care; confined to bed more than 50% of waking hours
4	Completely disabled; cannot carry out any self-care activity; totally confined to bed or chair

Table 3 Karnofsky Performance Status Scale

Activity Level	Scale (%)	Criteria
Able to carry on normal activity and to work; no special care needed	100	Normal: no complaints; no evidence of disease
	90	Able to carry on normal activity; minor signs or symptoms of disease
	80	Normal activity with effort: some signs or symptoms of disease
Unable to work: able to live at home and care for most personal needs; varying amount of assistance needed	70	Able to care for self; unable to carry on normal activity or to do active work
	60	Requires occasional assistance but is able to care for most of own needs
	50	Requires considerable assistance and frequent medical care
Unable to care for self; requires equivalent of institutional or hospital care; disease may be progressing rapidly	40	Disabled; requires special care and assistance
	30	Severely disabled; hospitalization indicated, although death is not imminent
	20	Very sick; hospitalization is necessary; active supportive treatment is necessary
	10	Moribund; fatal process progressing rapidly
	0	Dead

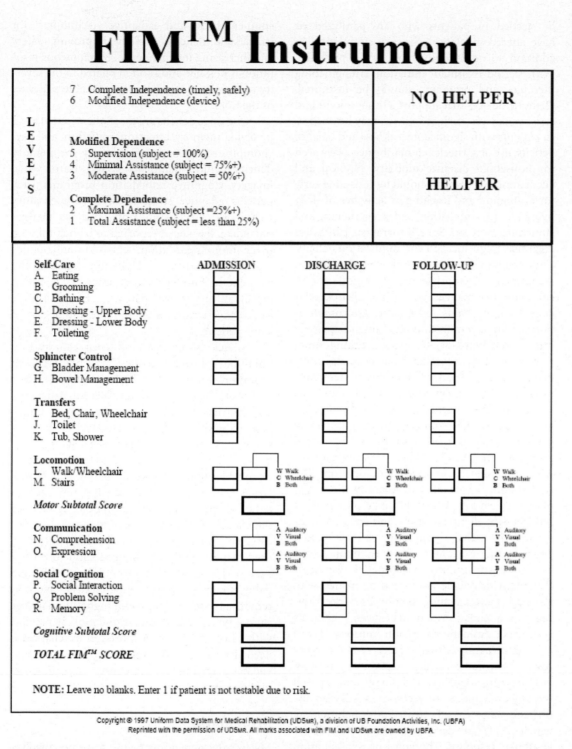

FIM™ Instrument

| LEVELS | 7 Complete Independence (timely, safely)
6 Modified Independence (device) | NO HELPER |
| | **Modified Dependence**
5 Supervision (subject = 100%)
4 Minimal Assistance (subject = 75%+)
3 Moderate Assistance (subject = 50%+)

Complete Dependence
2 Maximal Assistance (subject =25%+)
1 Total Assistance (subject = less than 25%) | HELPER |

	ADMISSION	DISCHARGE	FOLLOW-UP
Self-Care A. Eating B. Grooming C. Bathing D. Dressing - Upper Body E. Dressing - Lower Body F. Toileting			
Sphincter Control G. Bladder Management H. Bowel Management			
Transfers I. Bed, Chair, Wheelchair J. Toilet K. Tub, Shower			
Locomotion L. Walk/Wheelchair M. Stairs	W Walk C Wheelchair B Both	W Walk C Wheelchair B Both	W Walk C Wheelchair B Both
Motor Subtotal Score			
Communication N. Comprehension O. Expression	A Auditory V Visual B Both	A Auditory V Visual B Both	A Auditory V Visual B Both
Social Cognition P. Social Interaction Q. Problem Solving R. Memory			
Cognitive Subtotal Score			
TOTAL FIM™ SCORE			

NOTE: Leave no blanks. Enter 1 if patient is not testable due to risk.

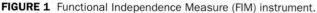

FIGURE 1 Functional Independence Measure (FIM) instrument.

energy, and fewer symptoms. Age has not been demonstrated to be a significant factor.[8,13–15]

Having to motivate and push patients toward functional improvement often brings members of the cancer rehabilitation team closer to the patient. Thus, functional declines owing to advancing disease can be frustrating and disappointing. In a sense, many of the patients may have ever-changing rehabilitation targets. Such a change is not the case in traditional noncancer rehabilitation, in which there is recurrence and relapse. The morbidity and mortality associated with cancer are quite challenging to the cancer rehabilitation process. However, the patient and family's new appreciation and comfort level with everyday activities make the process worthwhile for the patient and team. An important aspect of cancer rehabilitation is alleviation of fear in patients and caregivers, which can decrease the patient's concern about being a burden.[16]

Specific Topics and Rehabilitation

After delineation of basic foundations and principles of cancer rehabilitation, specific topics are presented.

Central Nervous System Tumors

Neurologic tumors can involve the central nervous system (CNS) with either the brain or spinal cord and are either primary or metastatic. Owing to direct injury of neural structures, patients may have motor, sensory, cognitive, and speech deficits. Functional deficits decline further owing to the indirect effects of chemotherapy and radiation treatments. More than 15,000 new cases of primary brain tumor and 4,000 new spinal tumors are diagnosed each year.[17] Metastatic lesions from various sites account for 20 to 40% of brain tumors,[17] occur in approximately 15% of cancer patients,[18] and produce neurologic symptoms in 85,000 patients per year. The lung and breast are the most frequent primary sources of metastatic CNS tumors. Most spinal tumors are extradural and are predominantly metastatic carcinomas, lymphomas, or sarcomas.[19] Spinal cord compression can occur in 5 to 10% of the cancer cases,[20] and resultant functional consequences can include pain, sensory deficits, motor deficits, neurogenic bowel and bladder, and sexual dysfunction (Table 6).

Even a small low-grade malignant tumor in the brain may cause significant functional deficits if present in a critical location, particularly if present close to the brainstem. The location of tumors can determine respectability (Table 7).

Changes in behavior, appetite, memory, and endocrine function may be seen following radiation treatment.[18] Hyponatremia, as seen with syndrome of inappropriate diuretic hormone (SIADH), may lead to mental status changes.[21] Fatigue may be an issue with radiation

score of 4 denotes that minimum assistance is needed. This score implies that patients need somewhere between 1 and 25% assistance and patients are able to perform somewhere between 75 and 99% of the task on their own.

This tool may also be inadequate to assess cancer patients who have fewer persisting motor and communication disorders than patients with neurologic disorders, such as stroke.[7] This scale is also inadequate to assess patients who are clearly able to perform various tasks, but such a performance takes a long amount of time and leaves them fatigued.

Bell and colleagues found that a population of tumor patients admitted to inpatient rehabilitation units had a generally poorer functional prognosis than did noncancer patients.[8]

Quality of Life

General quality of life questionnaires for patients with cancer are listed in Table 5. Quality of life status may be more strongly predictive of survival than performance status.[9–12] Factors associated with a better quality of life include absence of depression, good social involvement, greater

Table 5 General Quality of Life Questionnaires for Patients with Cancer

Name	Acronym
Cancer Rehabilitation Evaluation System Short Form	CARES-SF
European Organization for Research and Treatment of Cancer Core Quality of Life Questionnaire	EORTC QLQ-C-30
Functional Assessment of Cancer Therapy	FACT
Functional Living Index for Cancer	FLIC
Linear Analog Self-Assessment Scale	LASA
Medical Outcomes Study Short Form	MOS SF-36
McGill Quality of Life Questionnaire	MQOL
Quality of Life Index	QLI
Rotterdam Symptom Checklist	RSCL

Table 6 Common Complications of Brain Tumors and Their Treatments

Weakness
Sensory loss
Visuospatial deficits
Hemineglect or bilateral visual deficits
Ataxia
Cognitive deficits: thought processes, memory changes, apraxia, etc.
Speech difficulties
Dysphagia
Bowel and bladder dysfunction
Psychological issues
Behavioral abnormalities
Endocrine issues
Skin issues
Fatigue

treatment. Steroid psychosis may complicate the rehabilitation course also.

With prolonged bed immobility, supportive care is important. Measures should be taken to prevent pressure ulcers and deep venous thrombosis. Range of motion (ROM) of all joints should be done with daily exercises. Passive ROM may be needed in patients who are paralyzed or have altered mentation. Sensory stimulation in addition to socialization should be provided. With steroid treatment initiation, strengthening therapies and programs should be instituted. Orthotic devices that support a limb or joint and assistive devices, such as walkers, may be needed. In patients with significant weakness and balance deficits, use of a wheelchair may be necessary even for household distance mobility. Physical and occupational therapists should be consulted early for evaluation and teaching of activities of daily living (ADL), ambulation, and strengthening and stretching exercises. Speech therapists can assess cognitive, linguistic, and communication deficits. They can also determine swallowing deficits and recommend appropriate dietary modifications, compensatory maneuvers, and therapeutic exercises. Hydrocephalus and seizures are complications of brain tumors and most often negatively impact rehabilitation through declining functional status. Hydrocephalus has been classically described as a triad of subcortical dementia, incontinence, and gait abnormality. It should be suspected when mental status changes occur, when a patient fails to make expected functional gains, or when spasticity, seizures, and emotional problems are present. When training patients with visual deficits, an ophthalmology consultation should be included to quantify the extent of visual field loss. Visual deficits typically affect independent living adversely and must be considered in discharge planning. Patients should be trained to use compensatory techniques such as scanning to improve visuospatial awareness. Patients with double vision can be treated with alternating-eye patching. Before discharge, driving recommendations should be given, with plans for further evaluation as vision improves. Facial and eyelid paralysis may require plastic surgery consultation for corneal protection or cosmesis. For hearing deficits, audiology and speech therapy evaluations are necessary. Vestibular disturbances are typically treated with habituation, which leads to decreased sensitivity of the vestibular response. The goals of rehabilitation are to resolve reversible deficits and to learn compensatory and adaptive techniques for irreversible deficits, thereby improving safety and increasing independence. Spontaneous resolution is possible and is often related to the severity of the initial insult and the possible plasticity of the CNS.

Cognitive deficits are most often seen in areas involving memory, attention, initiation, and psychomotor retardation. Interventions for memory deficits include memory aids and use of visual imagery. Cognitive remediation programs teach patients adaptive strategies and compensatory techniques. Psychostimulants, such as methylphenidate, have been reported to be helpful with psychomotor retardation, depression, and opioid-induced drowsiness.[15,22] Dopamine agonists and stimulating antidepressants improve attention deficits in higher-level patients.[23] Bromocriptine can be effective for motor aphasias and neglect in some patients.[24]

A lack of cortical influence can lead to uninhibited bladder in these patients. Frequent prompting for urination during daytime (every 2 hours) and before sleep is very helpful. Behavioral training may be helpful in patients with unimpaired cognition. This process involves progressively increasing the time between voiding, often by 10 to 15 minutes every 2 to 5 days, until a reasonable interval between voiding is obtained. Drugs to inhibit bladder evacuations, such as anticholinergic and antispasmodic agents for the bladder, should be judiciously used. External catheters can be an option in male patients. A used diaper should be changed soon to protect against skin breakdown. Immobile or sedentary patients may become constipated easily and may require a bowel program with higher fluid intake, stool softeners, and digital stimulation. In patients with stool impaction, a thorough evacuation is needed with an oral laxative, suppositories, and enemas prior to the more conservative measures outlined above.

Myelopathy

Myelopathy may occur owing to tumor involvement, irradiation, and intrathecal chemotherapy. Spinal cord compression eventually occurs in 5% of cancer patients.[25] In addition to myelopathy, radiculopathy is also possible at any level (Table 8).[26,27]

Table 7 Brain Tumor Type and Possible Deficits

Type of Brain Tumor	Possible Deficits
Temporal lobe	Dysnomia, difficulty with comprehension, defective hearing and memory
Parietal lobe	Loss of vision, spatial disorientation, memory loss, dressing apraxia, proprioceptive agnosia
Frontal lobe	Personality changes, libido changes, impulsive behavior, labile emotions, excessive jocularity
Pituitary gland	Headaches, bilateral visual loss, hormonal abnormalities
Acoustic neuromas	Hearing loss, vertigo, facial palsy and numbness, dysphagia, hydrocephalus
Craniopharyngioma (adult)	Visual loss, sexual dysfunction
Craniopharyngioma (children)	Growth failure

Table 8 Symptoms of Myelopathy

Weakness
Sensory deficits
Autonomic disturbance
Pain: spinal or radicular
Incontinence: bowel or bladder
Gait abnormality
Spinal instability

Imaging studies and neurosurgical consultation should be obtained early in patients suspected of having spinal involvement and thus prevent spinal cord damage. In patients with myelopathy, large-dose corticosteroids should be instituted emergently. Spinal stabilization and spinal cord decompression followed by radiation treatment usually provide the best outcome. When spinal surgery is not possible, patients still may be candidates for radiation treatment (Tables 9 and 10).

Radiation-Related Myelopathy

The detrimental effects of radiation are multifactorial and cannot be entirely attributed to dosage, site, or technique. Usually, myelopathy is either transient or delayed. Transient myelopathy is reversible and has a peak onset at 4 to 6 months after radiation.[28] Symmetric paresthesia or shock-like sensation in a nondermatomal pattern is seen from the spine to the extremities.[29] Unfortunately, delayed myelopathy is irreversible and has a latency period of 9 to 18 months. Symptoms typically begin with lower extremity paresthesias and are followed by sphincter incontinence. Central pain can occur in 20% of patients and is characterized by midback pain and dysesthetic pain in the lower extremities. Such pain is treated in a manner similar to that for neuropathic pain.

Rehabilitation

Physical and occupational therapists should be consulted early to address deficits with ADLs and mobility so that appropriate exercises and adaptive equipment may be provided. Spinal immobility may be helpful in patients with pain from forward flexion of the spine. With any new pain or neurologic deficits, additional spinal or spinal cord involvement should be entertained. Adequate pain control is essential and is required for effective rehabilitation outcomes.

Table 9 Findings Associated with a Better Prognosis for Functional Recovery Following Cord Compression
Diagnosis of myeloma, lymphoma, or breast cancer
Slow evolution of symptoms or early neurologic signs
Ambulatory status at time of diagnosis of spinal cord involvement

Table 10 Findings Associated with a Poorer Prognosis for Functional Recovery Following Cord Compression
Sphincter incontinence
Complete paraplegia
Rapid evolution of symptoms (< 72 h)

Patients with myelopathy can develop detrussor-sphincter dyssynergia, a condition in which the bladder contracts but the bladder outlet (sphincters) fails to relax in a timely manner, leading to impaired emptying and increased bladder pressure. Although patients may void on their own, any such attempts should be followed by a postvoid residual volume check on multiple occasions, preferably with a catheter. With residual volumes in excess of 100 to 150 cc, an intermittent catheterization program should be performed every 4 to 6 hours. The goal is to keep urine volumes in the bladder at no more than 350 to 400 cc at any time to prevent overdistention, detrussor muscle injury, and retrograde flow of urine back into the kidneys. More frequent catheterizations may be required with increased fluid intake. Such a program should be taught to patients and their caretakers. In patients who are unwilling to learn such programs, for whom wound care may be an issue, an indwelling Foley catheter should be considered. Patients with injuries at C7 or below should be able to perform such a program on their own. In male patients who have a hyperactive bladder without bladder dyssynergia or those who have normal bladder function but with incontinence owing to impaired cognition or mobility, condom catheters may be used.

Patients with spinal cord injury usually have an upper motoneuron bowel, in which there is difficulty with evacuation. Prior to institution of a regular bowel program, bowel evacuation may be necessary on more than one occasion to rid the patient of hard stool and impaction. Once such cleansing occurs, a program consisting of adequate fluid intake, fiber, stool softeners, and digital stimulation on a daily basis should be started. Warm fluids after meals supplement gastrocolic reflex.

Autonomic Dysreflexia

This medical emergency occurs with a massive sympathetic discharge in response to a noxious stimulus in a spinal cord–injured patient with an injury at T6 or above. The clinical presentation is that of an anxious patient with paroxysmal hypertension, nasal congestion, sweating above the level of the lesion, facial flushing, piloerection, and reflex bradycardia. The most common etiology is a distended bladder, followed by a distended bowel. Other causes include enemas, tight clothing, infection, deep venous thrombosis, and bladder catheterizations. Treatment should focus on finding the underlying cause. Lidocaine jelly should be allowed to sit for some time prior to checking the rectal vault for hard stool or evacuating a distended bladder or bowel. If a cause cannot be found, then treatment with an antihypertensive should be initiated.

Spasticity

In patients with an upper motoneuron lesion (ie, brain or spinal cord injury), spasticity may occur. This motor disorder is characterized by a velocity-dependent increase in resistance to movement across a joint. In addition, there is an increase in tendon reflexes and muscle tone. This tone is the resistance felt by the examiner as passive ROM is tested. Examples of lesions include CNS tumors and myelopathy. Treatment should be initiated with daily ROM exercises, proper positioning, and removal of noxious stimuli. Short-term benefits are obtained with cold modality. In patients in whom spasticity interferes with ADL and mobility, systemic treatment with oral spasmolytic medications should be initiated (ie, baclofen, diazepam, dantrolene, tizanidine). For more severe spasticity, chemical neurolysis, such as phenol block, epidural infusion of medications, and botulinum toxin via an implantable pump should be considered. For patients with deficits with ROM across joints, casting and splinting techniques are helpful.

Peripheral Neuropathy

Peripheral neuropathy symptoms include numbness, paresthesias, weakness, and, occasionally, severe neuropathic pain. Consideration should be given to nonpharmacologic means of pain management, including transcutaneous electrical nerve stimulation and various physical modalities, such as heat and physical therapy. Adaptive strategies such as energy conservation, orthotics, and adaptive equipment can be prescribed. With sensory loss in the lower extremity, preventive measures such as those used for management of diabetic neuropathy and neuropathic ulcers should be considered. Education, nonconstricting footwear, and daily inspection of feet are important.

In patients with lower motoneuron injuries, such as cauda equina syndrome or pudendal nerve injuries, areflexic bowel and a hypotonic external sphincter are present. These patients have difficulty with retaining stool and are more difficult to manage than upper motoneuron bowel patients. Since these patients have bowel accidents, excessive stool softeners, suppositories, and digital stimulation should be avoided. Oral fiber intake with a reduced amount of fluids usually helps.

Leptomeningeal Disease

These patients have a very poor prognosis. Both central and peripheral nervous system involvement may occur, along with cerebrospinal fluid flow obstruction leading to hydrocephalus. Symptoms can include mental status changes, polyradiculopathy with radicular pain, and cauda equina syndrome. Rehabilitation goals are primarily supportive, and management is similar to that outlined earlier depending on the deficits.

Metastatic Bony Disease

Metastatic bony disease is quite common. It is the third most common site of metastases and usually is the most symptomatic. The more commonly involved tumors include breast, lung, kidney, and prostate cancer and multiple myeloma. The axial skeleton is the most common site, with involvement of the spine, ribs, pelvis, skull, proximal femur, and humerus. Osteolytic and osteoblastic activity leads to lytic and sclerotic types of bony lesions, both of which are susceptible to fractures. At the time of diagnosis of an osseous lesion, usually more than one lesion is present. Over two-thirds of the lesions can be painless, and when pain is present with activity, it often heralds fracture. With spinal involvement, the patient may present with new-onset back pain, particularly when recumbent. Consider ruling out a metastatic lesion in a cancer patient with new pain onset.

Treatment consists of primary disease management, radiation, surgical intervention including vertebroplasty, symptom management, and rehabilitation. With mean survival times after fixation of pathologic fractures at roughly 19 months,[30] it is important to maximize quality of life and manage symptoms.

Rehabilitation interventions require comprehensive assessment. Manual muscle testing of the involved limb is contraindicated. Only active movement limited by pain is assessed in the affected limb. Interventions are focused on keeping patients from becoming bedbound, training patients to use residual function or to develop compensatory techniques, use of compensatory techniques, and patient and family education. Prior to chest physical therapy, rib metastases should be ruled out. Resistive exercises are contraindicated.

Although pathologic fractures may occur during rehabilitation, it is uncommon to see them clearly during rehabilitation intervention.[31] Indeed, the fractures may occur even when lying in bed and without any activity in patients with erosive and progressive disease. Alternatives to rehabilitation include bed rest and, if so, then for how long? Complications of bedrest include disuse atrophy, orthostatic hypotension, lower quality of life with more assistance required for ADL, pressure ulcers, and increased risk of deep venous thrombosis.

The majority of nonambulatory patients admitted to a rehabilitation unit after surgical stabilization ambulate with or without assistive device(s).[32] Weight bearing of the affected extremity is usually affected depending on the surgical intervention. With methylmethacrylate cementation, weight bearing as tolerated may be permitted. Such cementation also does not interfere with radiation treatment. With more complicated surgery, touch down or no weight bearing may be allowed. ROM is most often limited during this acute phase. Patients may also have an orthosis in place to limit the joint ROM. Such restrictions may continue for several weeks to months, depending on the surgeon's discretion. A straight-point cane may be used in patients with smaller, painful lesions. With forearm crutches, 40 to 50% weight-bearing reduction may be possible.[33,34] Axillary crutches and walkers allow non–weight bearing in the lower extremities. A rolling walker may be used in patients who are afraid of losing balance while lifting a standard walker.

The hip is a common site of fracture, and patients require partial or total hip arthroplasty. Even nonambulatory patients may be candidates to decrease pain and a low for basic nursing care. Standard hip precautions include hip flexion < 90° and avoidance of adduction and internal rotation for a period of up to 3 months. Early mobilization is crucial. Weight bearing is typically tolerated on postoperative day 1. Patients are generally ambulating independently with assistive devices in a few days at least at a household-level distance (roughly 150 feet). If the trochanters and attached musculature are sacrificed, then an unstable hip is present; thus, a hip abduction brace is required and a more conservative rehabilitation program is instituted. In one study, 28 patients underwent proximal femur surgical resection for metastatic disease and had cementation.[35] Preoperatively, 71% had intractable pain; postoperatively, 81% had no need for analgesics. Over 50% of the patients had good to excellent results with hip ROM and walking ability, and 46% were alive at 12 months.

In patients undergoing pelvis reconstruction for metastatic disease, the mean survival time is of 14.5 months. All of these patients were initially nonambulatory, and with rehabilitation, over 88% were independent with ambulation at 1 month.[36]

Conservative treatment with metastatic lesions to upper extremity consists of bracing and radiation treatment. Surgical treatment options include an intramedullary rod for larger lesions and a compression plate for smaller lesions. Cemented prosthesis may be used with a humeral head and neck metastases. Consideration may be given for prophylactic fixation of a nonfractured upper extremity lesion in patients requiring an assistive device for ambulation. During rehabilitation, active ROM of the affected joint(s) is typically delayed compared with a lower extremity lesion (typically postoperative day 3 or 4). With extensive disease in the upper extremity and lower extremity involvement, a wheelchair may be necessary (Table 11).

Table 11 Effects of Prolonged Immobility
Loss of muscle strength
Joint contractures
Disuse osteoporosis
Cardiac effects: resting tachycardia, orthostatic hypotension, ↓ cardiac output
Venous thrombosis
Pressure ulcers

General Severe Asthenia

Generalized weakness and deconditioning are commonly seen in cancer patients, particularly after various treatments and in advanced disease. Although multifactorial in nature, prolonged bed immobility is a major factor leading to such a state. Rehabilitation interventions are focused on restoring a patient's function through exercises and mitigating decline through compensatory strategies, including environmental modification. Typically, both of these strategies are concurrently applied.

In the muscles of patients with prolonged immobility, declines of 1 to 1.5% of the initial strength have been noted on a daily basis. Such declines correspond to roughly 10 to 20% strength loss per week.[37] Larger muscles are disproportionately affected more severely. A daily stretching program retards muscle atrophy.[38] In addition, isometric exercises on a daily basis can help maintain muscle strength.[37] Generally, it takes two or more times the period of immobilization to recover muscle strength.[39]

Disuse osteoporosis most commonly affects weight-bearing bones with bed immobility. Such a complication is best treated with preventive measures such as active weight-bearing exercises and active muscle contraction. Exercises in bed are not as effective.[40]

Resting heart rate can increase by a half-beat per minute per day for the first 3 to 4 weeks of bed immobilization.[41] Decreased diastolic filling time, myocardial perfusion, stroke volume (with exercise), and cardiac output are all associated with deleterious hemodynamic and orthostatic changes.[40] Such a decline can be reversed by a progressive exercise program and resumption of upright activities. Sudden changes should be avoided with orthostasis. In patients who have been immobilized for a week or more, a tilt table may be needed for an even slower resumption of upright posture. Standing and ambulation may begin when the patient is able to tolerate a 70° angle for 30 minutes.

Although lower-rated (< 20 mm Hg) elastic garments may be effective against deep venous thrombosis, higher ratings (20–30 mm Hg) are helpful with venous insufficiency and orthostasis. Such nonpharmacologic treatments should be supplemented with abdominal binders and medications such as ephedrine and fludrocortisone.

Measures such as frequent turning (preferably every 2 hours) should be taken to prevent pressure ulcers in patients who are totally bed-bound. Irreversible changes can occur with lying in one position for as little as 5 hours. Sitting upright as tolerated should be encouraged.

Breast Cancer and Rehabilitation

The extent of the surgical and usual postoperative radiation treatments typically determines the complications. In lumpectomy, only the tumor and a margin of the breast tissue are removed. With a modified radical mastectomy, all breast tissue with the exception of the pectoralis minor is removed and axillary lymph nodes are sampled (Table 12).

In patients undergoing immediate reconstruction with a transverse rectus abdominis myocutaneous (TRAM) flap, functional gains with ROM are similar to those of non-TRAM patients.[42] Shoulder passive ROM exercise should be started carefully and until tolerance, only earlier. Active movement may be started at the earliest after day 4. More complications are encountered with more aggressive mobilization through range earlier.[43,44] Restrictions with functional activities should be lifted after removal of sutures, typically at 2 weeks.

Lymphedema

The incidence of lymphedema has been variable and reported at up to 37%.[45–47] A median time of 39 months has been noted between treatment and presentation (Table 13).[46]

The patient and involved caretakers should be educated about lymphedema. Skin integrity is crucial. Insect repellents and long-sleeved clothing are typically recommended. Needlesticks

Table 12 Potential Complications after Breast Cancer Treatment(s)

Postoperative wound
Incisional pain
Shoulder range of motion deficits
Lymphedema
Phantom pain
Chest wall pain
Poor cosmesis

Table 13 Lymphedema Management

Education
Elevation of limbs
Exercise
Retrograde massage/manual lymphatic drainage
  techniques
Wrapping
Compression garments
Treatment of infections

and blood pressure measurements should be avoided in the affected extremity. At the earliest sign of skin tenderness and erythema, antibiotics should be considered. Avoidance of heat exposure is helpful.

Exercises should include improvement in ROM for shoulders bilaterally and the neck and improvement in chest wall tightness with stretching of the pectoralis musculature and trapezius. Although a great deal of activity can precipitate lymphedema, no clear data exist in terms of limitation of activity. Heavy lifting should be avoided, typically less than 15 to 20 pounds. Retrograde massage techniques to improve and aid in lymphatic circulation are helpful and should be done daily.

Lymphedema may be acute and chronic in nature. In addition to a difference in limb size and "heaviness," patients note "joint tightness" and decreased ROM in the affected joints. Measurements of the affected limb are typically done with circumferential measurements at various points across the affected limb and with volume displacement techniques.

During an earlier stage, spontaneous resolution of lymphedema may occur. More chronic condition requires a daily long-term regimen and commitment. Exacerbations are treated with early referral to a physical therapist specializing in its management. Compression bandaging with a short stretch bandage for the majority of the day is most useful. At least once a day, this garment should be removed for a short period of time and rewrapped. Once limb volume stabilizes or plateaus with such treatment, a compression garment with a rating of up to 40 mm Hg should be ordered. These garments, when used regularly, should be changed every few months. Consider their use also when traveling via airplane to prevent exacerbation.

Attempts at treatment of chronic lymphedema using benopyrones, which stimulate macrophage-induced protein breakdown, were felt to be promising[48]; however, a recent study did not reveal such benefits.[49]

A rare but serious complication of chronic lymphedema is lymphangiosarcoma. This tumor has a poor prognosis despite aggressive intervention of forequarter amputation in candidates suitable for such surgery.

Head and Neck Cancers

Such cancers and treatments frequently result in deficits with swallowing, communication, nutrition, and musculoskeletal issues. Radical neck dissection is often performed and involves removal of the sternocleidomastoid muscle, spinal accessory nerve (cranial nerve XI), internal and external jugular veins, and submandibular gland. A modified radical neck dissection spares the spinal accessory nerve.

Trapezius impairment leads to shoulder pathology with depression and protraction. Patients have a painful shoulder with decreased ROM, and abduction is typically less than 90°. Rehabilitation focuses on neck ROM, emphasizing flexion and rotation, after suture removal. Active ROM is usually delayed by a few weeks. Transient worsening of dyspnea in patients using the accessory muscle for respiration may be noted. ROM exercises should be continued throughout radiation treatment to combat soft tissue fibrosis and contractures. Scapular stabilizers such as the serratus anterior, rhomboids, and levator scapula should be strengthened.[50] Heavy lifting with the affected side should be avoided.[51] Speech pathology consultation should be obtained early to address communication and swallowing deficits. A dietitian should follow these patients closely also. Use of artificial saliva and good oral care are necessary after radiation treatment for head and neck cancers. ROM with the jaw, tongue, and masticatory muscles and other oral exercises may be needed.

Hematologic Malignancies

Such malignancies include those involving bone marrow and the lymphatics. These malignancies and associated treatments result in fatigue and localized disabling effects. Neurologic deficits, lymphedema owing to local obstruction, pain, and malnutrition may be present.

Walking is very helpful and should be continued to maintain endurance. ROM exercises should be continued and advanced as tolerated. Transfusions are quite common during rehabilitation, especially with bone marrow suppression. Exercise in thrombocytopenic patients is controversial. A major concern in these patients is development of intracranial hemorrhage. In one study, fatal intracranial hemorrhage was found in only 1 of 92 patients receiving chemotherapy.[52] Clinicians should use their judgment when prescribing exercises in this group of patients. However, it may be reasonable to allow nonresistive exercise with platelet counts between 5,000 and 10,000/mm[3] and light resistive exercises with counts above 10,000/mm[3]. Ambulation may be allowed with platelet counts above 5,000/mm[3] with fall precautions.

Conclusions

Successful rehabilitation of patients with cancer requires understanding of the behavior of tumor pathology, flexibility in determining the functional goals and a timeline for achievement of these goals, and awareness of the complications of cancer and its treatments, which negatively impact patient function. The ultimate goals of rehabilitation interventions are to maximize function, promote adaptive and compensatory strategies when full function cannot be restored, and enhance quality of life for cancer patients.

REFERENCES

1. Ries LAG, Eisner MP, Kosary CL, et al. SEER cancer statistics review 1973-1999. Bethesda (MD): National Cancer Institute. Available at: http://seer.cancer.gov/csr/1973 1999/2002.

2. Lehmann JF, DeLisa JA, Warren CG. Cancer rehabilitation: assessment of need, development, and evaluation of a model of care. Arch Phys Med Rehabil 1978;59:410–9.

3. World Health Organization. International classification of impairments, disabilities, and handicaps: a manual of classification relating to the consequences of disease. Geneva: World Health Organization; 1980.

4. Dietz JH. Rehabilitation oncology. New York: John Wiley & Sons; 1981.

5. Marciniak CM, Sliwa JA, Spill G. Functional outcome following rehabilitation of the cancer patient. Arch Phys Med Rehabil 1996;77:54–7.

6. Reuben DB, Mor V, Hiris J. Clinical symptoms and length of survival in patients with terminal cancer. Arch Intern Med 1988;148:1586–91.

7. Meyers CA. Neuropsychological aspects of cancer and cancer treatment. In: Garden FH, Grabois M, editors. Physical medicine and rehabilitation: state of the art reviews. Vol 8. Philadelphia: Hanley & Belfus; 1994. p. 229–41.

8. Bell KR, O'Dell MW, Barr K, et al. Rehabilitation of the patient with brain tumor. Arch Phys Med Rehabil 1998;79: S37–46.

9. Coates A, Gebski V, Signorini D, et al. Prognostic value of quality-of-life scores during chemotherapy for advanced breast cancer. Australian New Zealand Breast Cancer Trials Group. J Clin Oncol 1992;10:1833–8.

10. Kaasa S, Mastekaasa A, Lund E. Prognostic factors for patients with inoperable non-small cell lung cancer, limited disease. The importance of patients' subjective experience of disease and psychosocial well-being. Radiother Oncol 1989;15:235–42.

11. Osoba D, MacDonald N. Disease-modifying management. In: Doyle D, Hanks GWC, MacDonald N, editors. Oxford textbook of palliative medicine. 2nd ed. New York: Oxford University Press; 1999. p. 933–47.

12. Ruckdeschel JC, Piantadosi S. Quality of life assessment. An independent prognostic variable for survival in lung cancer. J Thorac Surg 1991;6:201–5.

13. Giovagnoli AR, Tamburine M, Boiardi A. Quality of life in brain tumor patients. J Neurooncol 1996;30:71–80.

14. Mackworth N, Fobair P, Prados MD. Quality of life self-reports from 200 brain tumor patients: comparisons with Karnofsky performance scores. J Neurooncol 1992;14: 243–53.

15. Weitzner MA, Meyers CA, Byrne K. Psychosocial functioning and quality of life inpatients with primary brain tumors. J Neurosurg 1996;84:29–34.

16. Mackey KC, Sparling JW. Experiences of older women with cancer receiving hospice care: significance for physical therapy. Phys Ther 2000;80:459–68.

17. American Cancer Society. Cancer facts and figures. New York: American Cancer Society; 1990.

18. Black PM. Brain tumors. Part 1 and part 2. N Engl J Med 1991;324:1471–6, 1555–64.

19. Posner JB, Chernik NL. Intracranial metastases from systemic cancer. Adv Neurol 1978;19:579–92.

20. Barron KD, Hirano A, Araki S, et al. Experience with metastatic neoplasm involving the spinal cord. Neurology 1959;9:91–106.

21. Nelson DF, McDonald JV, Lapham LW, et al. Central nervous system tumors. In: Rubin P, McDonald S, Qazi R, editors. Clinical oncology: a multidisciplinary approach for physicians and students. 7th ed. Philadelphia: WB Saunders; 1993. p. 617–44.

22. Bruera E, Brenneis C, Paterson AH, MacDonald RN. Use of methylphenidate as an adjuvant to narcotic analgesics in patients with advanced cancer. J Pain Symptom Manage 1989;4:3–6.

23. Gualtieri T, Chandler M, Coons TB, Brown LT. Amantadine: a new clinical profile for traumatic brain injury. Clin Neuropharmacol 1989;12:258–70.

24. Grujic Z, Mapstone M, Gietelman DR, et al. Dopamine agonists reorient visual exploration away from the neglected hemispace. Neurology 1998;51:1395–8.

25. Casciato Da, Lowitz BB. Manual of bedside oncology. 1st ed. Boston: Little, Brown; 1983. p. 699.

26. Gilbert RW, Kim JH, Posner JB. Epidural spinal cord compression from metastatic tumor: diagnosis and treatment. Ann Neurol 1978;3:40–51.

27. Rodichok LD, Harper GR, Ruckdeschel JC, et al. Early diagnosis of spinal epidural metastases. Am J Med 1981; 70:1181–8.

28. Dropcho EJ. Central nervous system injury by therapeutic irradiation. Neurol Clin 1991;9:969–88.

29. Leibel SA, Guten PH, Davis RL. Tolerance of the brain and spinal cord. In: Guten PH, Leibel SA, Sheline GE, editors. Radiation injury to the nervous system. New York: Raven Press; 1991. p. 239–56.

30. Harrington, KD. The management of acetabular insufficiency secondary to metastatic malignant disease. J Bone Joint Surg Am 1981;63:653–64.

31. Bunting R, Lamont-Havers W, Schweon D, Kilman A. Pathologic fracture risk in rehabilitation of patients with bony metastases. Clin Orthop 1985;192:222–7.

32. Bunting RW, Boublik M, Blevins FT, et al. Functional outcome of pathologic fracture secondary to malignant disease in a rehabilitation hospital. Cancer 1992;69: 98–102.

33. Clark BC, Manini TM, Ordway NR, Ploutz-Snyder LL. Leg muscle activity during walking with assistive devices at varying levels of weight bearing. Arch Phys Med Rehabil 2004;85:1555–60.

34. Joyce BM, Kirby RL. Canes, crutches and walkers. Am Fam Physician 1991;43:535.

35. Haentjens P, DeNeve W, Opdecam P. Prosthetic replacement for pathological fractures of the proximal end of the femur: total prosthesis or bipolar arthroplasty. Rev Chir Orthoped Reparatrice Appar Mot 1994;80:493–502.

36. Vena VE, Hsu JBS, Rosier RN, O'Keefe RJ. Pelvic reconstruciton for severe periacetabular metastatic disease. Clin Orthop 1999;362:171–80.

37. Mueller EA. Influence of training and of inactivity on muscle strength. Arch Phys Med Rehabil 1970;51:449–62.

38. Baker JH, Matsumoto DE. Adaptation of skeletal muscle to immobilization in a shortened position. Muscle Nerve 1988;231–44.

39. Houston ME, Bentzen H, Larsen H. Interrelationships between skeletal muscle adaptations and performance as studied by detraining and retraining. Acta Physiol Scand 1979;105:163–70.

40. Buschbacher RM: Deconditioning, conditioning, and the benefits of exercise. In: Braddom RL, editor. Physical medicine and rehabilitation. Philadelphia: WB Saunders; 1996. p. 687–707.

41. Taylor HL, Henschel A, Brozek J, Keys A. Effects of bed rest on cardiovascular function and work performance. J Appl Physiol 1949;2:223–39.

42. Guo Y, Truong AN. Functional outcome after physical therapy of breast cancer patients status post modified radical mastectomy versus mastectomy and transverse rectus abdominis myocutaneous flap [abstract]. Arch Phys Med Rehabil 1998;79:1157.

43. Jansen RF, van Geel AN, de Groot HG, et al. Immediate versus delayed shoulder exercises after axillary lymph node dissection. Am J Surg 1990;160:481.

44. Dawson I, Stan K, Heslinga JM, et al. Effect of shoulder immobilization on would seroma and shoulder dysfunction following modified radical mastectomy: a randomized prospective clinical trial. Br J Surg 1989;76: 311.

45. Kissin M, Querci della Rovere G, Easton D, Westbury G. Risk of lymphoedema following treatment of breast cancer. Br J Surg 1986;73:580–4.

46. Werner RS, McCormick B, Petrek JA, et al. Arm edema in conservatively managed breast cancer: obesity is a major predictive factor. Radiology 1991;180:177.

47. Ivens D, Hoe A, Podd T, et al. Assessment of arm morbidity from complete axillary dissection. Br J Cancer 1992;66: 1368–73.

48. Casley-Smith JR, Morgan RG, Piller NB. Treatment of lymphedema of the arms and legs with 5,6-benzo-[alpha]-pyrone. N Engl J Med 1993;16:329.

49. Loprinzi CL, Kugler JW, Sloan JA, et al. Lack of effect of Coumarin in women with lymphedema after treatment for breast cancer. N Engl J Med 1999;340:346–50.

50. Saunders WH, Johnson EW. Rehabilitation of the shoulder after radical neck dissection. Ann Otol 1975;84:812–6.

51. Dudgeon BJ, DeLisa JA, Miller RM. Head and neck cancer: rehabilitation approach. Am J Occup Ther 1980;34: 243–51.

52. Gaydos LA Freineich EJ, Mantel N. The quantitative relation between platelet count and hemorrhage in patients with acute leukemia. N Engl J Med 1962;266:905.

Skin Neoplasms Related to Internal Malignancy

Major Michael Murphy, MC, USA, MD
Tri H. Nguyen, MD

The skin is an accessible window through which internal conditions may manifest. Readily seen, touched, and sampled, lesions on the skin may provide valuable clues to internal conditions, especially malignancies. This chapter, therefore, focuses on the myriad of cutaneous clues that may alert one to investigate further for malignant processes. The information in this chapter is organized by an internal body system for ease of use by its intended audience. Some conditions may be associated with multiple malignancies, and these associations are discussed in the order of greatest incidence. Where there is no predominant association, conditions are discussed separately.

When examining the association of the skin to internal malignancy, Curth wrote, "Certain postulates must be fulfilled if the association of benign dermatoses with malignant internal tumors can be considered causal."[1] Those postulates are the following:

1. The dermatosis and malignant internal disease start at the same time or there is only a short interval between the onsets of each.
2. The internal malignant process and the dermatosis run a parallel course.
3. The type of the neoplasm associated with the dermatosis may be uniform or distinctive, i.e., its mechanical, toxic, or biochemical action has specific effects on the skin.
4. The dermatosis is not common.
5. If the association between the dermatosis and malignant disease is based on a genetic relationship, the internal disorder and the dermatosis develop independently of each other and postulates 1 and 2 will not be fulfilled.
6. The incidence of association between dermatosis and malignant disease is statistically important. Such a syndrome will, if one searches further, either fulfill the first four criteria or show a genetic background as postulated in #5.[1]

This chapter delves into many conditions that fulfill Curth's fifth postulate. Many of these conditions are genetic and do not fulfill the definition of a paraneoplastic syndrome as described by McLean, who felt that paraneoplastic manifestations of malignant tumors must fulfill two essential criteria: (1) "The dermatosis must develop after the development of a malignant tumor" and (2) "Both the dermatosis and the malignant tumor must follow a parallel course."[2] This chapter broadens the scope by examining instances that may not fulfill the paraneoplastic definition. Such described neoplasms are markers for syndromes with a higher risk of known internal malignancies. Most importantly, these skin markers of internal malignancy are reliable, recognizable, and relevant.

Skin Neoplasms Related to Malignancies of the Gastrointestinal System

Muir-Torre Syndrome

Skin neoplasm: Sebaceous adenoma, sebaceous epithelioma, and sebaceous carcinoma
Internal malignancy: Colorectal cancer predominantly; less commonly transitional cell cancer of the renal tract, endometrial cancer, ovarian cancer, breast cancer, upper gastrointestinal (GI) tract cancer, laryngeal cancer, and sarcomas
Genetics: Gene: *MSH2* on chromosome 2p and *MLH1* on chromosome 3p
Online Mendelian Inheritance in Man (OMIM): 158320
Inheritance: Autosomal dominant

Muir-Torre syndrome consists of multiple sebaceous neoplasms, keratoacanthomas, and GI, gynecologic, and urologic malignancies in the absence of other predisposing factors. Because of the risk of multiple internal malignancies, early recognition of this syndrome is essential. Twenty-eight percent of skin lesions appear before, 12% appear concurrently with, and 59% occur after the diagnosis of the first internal malignancy.[3]

The skin lesions in Muir-Torre syndrome consist of sebaceous neoplasms and keratoacanthomas. Sebaceous adenomas are slowly growing yellow to skin-colored papules usually found on the head or neck. They are the most sensitive skin marker for Muir-Torre syndrome. Sebaceous epitheliomas are yellowish papules and nodules often resembling a basal cell carcinoma. They are the most specific skin marker for Muir-Torre syndrome.[4] Sebaceous carcinoma can be found at its characteristic location on the eyelid presenting as a painless nodule on the inner eyelid surface or in extraocular locations. Although solitary, sebaceous tumors may occur, multiple lesions are more often the norm. Even though multiple lesions are more typical, the discovery of even one characteristic sebaceous neoplasm should prompt an evaluation for Muir-Torre syndrome. Sebaceous hyperplasia and nevus sebaceous are not associated with Muir-Torre syndrome.

Keratoacanthomas present as rapidly growing crateriform nodules on sun-exposed areas and can be difficult to differentiate from squamous cell carcinoma clinically and histologically. Of 139 patients with Muir-Torre syndrome, 22% had at least one keratoacanthoma.[4] Keratoacanthomas in Muir-Torre syndrome can also be multiple or present with sebaceous differentiation histologically.

Muir-Torre syndrome is associated with multiple internal malignancies. In one study of 139 patients, 282 primary internal malignancies were found. Sixty-one percent of cases have a family history of internal malignancy.[4] Colorectal carcinoma is the most common internal malignancy, accounting for about half of all malignancies in Muir-Torre syndrome. The second most common cancer type is genitourinary, at 24% of primary cancers. Other cancers that have been involved in the syndrome include lymphoma, leukemia, and cancer of the breast, parotid gland, inner ear, tongue, larynx, lung, and cartilage.[4,5] Colorectal carcinoma in Muir-Torre syndrome has some unique features. First, about 58% of all colorectal carcinoma are found proximal to the splenic flexure in this syndrome. It is usually detected about 10 years earlier than the general population. Despite these features, colorectal carcinoma tends to be less aggressive in Muir-Torre syndrome and tends to have a favorable prognosis. One hundred twenty people with Muir-Torre syndrome had a mean survival of 12 years after first diagnosis of malignancy.[5]

Once Muir-Torre syndrome is recognized and diagnosed, preventive screening should be initiated. The initial workup should also include a complete history, a physical examination, laboratory tests (carcinoembryonic antigen, complete blood cell count, erythrocyte sedimentation rate, chemistry, UA, urine cytology), chest radiography, a Pap smear, mammography, endometrial biopsy, and, especially, screening of the colon. Because of the location of colorectal cancer in this syndrome, colonoscopy and barium enema are favored over sigmoidoscopy. Other tests that can be considered include cystoscopy, intravenous pyelography, and computed tomography (CT) of the abdomen and pelvis.[3] All family members should be screened initially and regularly for the skin neoplasms and internal malignancies associated with Muir-Torre syndrome.

Gardner's Syndrome

Skin neoplasm: Epidermal inclusion cysts, desmoid tumors, and fibrous tumors
Internal malignancy: GI carcinoma, thyroid carcinoma
Genetics: Gene: *APC* (adenomatous polyposis coli); Chromosome: 5q21-22
OMIM: 175100
Inheritance: Autosomal dominant

Gardner's syndrome consists of epidermal inclusion cysts, desmoid tumors, fibroid tumors, osteomas, congenital hyperpigmentation of the retinal epithelium, and other less common neoplasms coupled with GI and thyroid malignancies. The diagnostic criteria for Gardner's syndrome are outlined in Table 1.[6] One hundred percent of Gardner's syndrome patients develop GI carcinoma by age 20 to 30 years. Because of this, early recognition and prophylactic treatment are paramount.

Table 1 Diagnostic Criteria for Gardner's Syndrome
1. Presence of all three diagnostic criteria a. colonic polyps b. soft tissue tumors c. osteomas 2. Presence of any one usual finding in an individual, PLUS a family history that individually or collectively has all the criteria outlined in #1.
All based on reference 3.d.5

Epidermal inclusion cysts are the most common skin neoplasms associated with Gardner's syndrome and are found in 35% of patients with Gardner's syndrome. The cysts may even present at birth. Typically, they are firm, mobile, subcutaneous nodules that may aggregate into large masses, usually on the head and neck. Multiple epidermal inclusion cysts should prompt further inquiry for other signs of Gardner's syndrome.[7,8] Desmoid tumors occur in 3 to 17% of cases, with a female predominance (80%). These tumors may occur spontaneously or at sites of surgical incisions. They are nonmetastasizing but may be locally aggressive, causing usual or intestinal obstruction. Desmoid tumors in the retroperitoneum may have a poor prognosis.[8] Fibromas may also be found in the skin, subcutaneous tissue, mesentery, or retroperitoneum.

Osteomas are the most common benign neoplasm found in Gardner's syndrome, being present in 80% of cases. They are most commonly located in the mandible or maxilla as thickenings or masses. Congenital hyperpigmentation of the retinal epithelium (CHRPE) is found in 63% of Gardner's syndrome patients. Dental anomalies, including multiple supernumerary or impacted permanent teeth, are seen in 18% of patients. Other reported neoplasms include lipoma and leiomyomas.[6,8-10]

GI carcinoma is the most common type of malignancy in Gardner's syndrome. Adenomatous polyps develop predominantly in the colon but can also be seen in the small intestine and stomach. Polyps are rarely seen before age 10 years. Early presenting signs of polyposis include bleeding or obstruction. By 20 years of age, 50% of patients with Gardner's syndrome develop polyps. Carcinomatous degeneration occurs in 100% of patients, usually by the second to third decade.[8] The incidence of periampullary cancer increases 100 to 200 times in patients with Gardner's syndrome and also presents a decade earlier (average age of 48 years) than in the general population.[6,8] Treatment consists of early prophylactic total colectomy when polyp formation is detected.

Another malignancy associated with Gardner's syndrome is thyroid carcinoma. It is characterized by an early onset (78% < age 30 years), female predominance (89%), papillary histology (88%), and multicentricity (70%).[9] In 30% of patients, thyroid carcinoma can precede the diagnosis of Gardner's syndrome by as much as 12 years. Because the malignancy is often multicentric, treatment consists of total thyroidectomy.

Caring for patients with Gardner's syndrome should involve gastroenterologists for annual colonoscopy, ophthalmologists (CHRPE), dentists, and regular examinations of the thyroid (neck ultrasonography, physical examination), especially in young women.

Peutz-Jeghers Syndrome

Skin neoplasm: Multiple lentigines
Internal malignancy: GI carcinoma, pancreatic carcinoma, bilateral breast carcinoma, cervical and testicular cancer
Genetics: Gene *STK11* (serine threonine kinase); Chromosome: 19p13.3
OMIM: 175200
Inheritance: Autosomal dominant

Peutz-Jeghers syndrome consists of multiple lentigines predominantly on the face and oral mucosa associated with hamartomatous GI polyps with a small potential for malignant transformation. This syndrome has also been associated with multiple other internal malignancies, many of which can be fatal. The most common GI complaints are abdominal pain, GI bleeding, anemia, vomiting, and rectal prolapse.[8] Clinical signs of the syndrome present at an early age. Early recognition and preventive screenings, therefore, facilitate timely detection and treatment of malignancies.

The skin neoplasms consist of 1 to 5 mm brown/black macules that are predominantly distributed on the central face, lips, and oral mucosa but can be seen on other body areas. These lesions may be present at birth or arise during infancy. Fifty to 60% of patients show clinical manifestations of the syndrome before age 20 years. The lentigines on the mucosa tend to persist throughout life.[8]

The predominant GI manifestations of Peutz-Jeghers syndrome are hamartomatous polyps found throughout the GI tract but most commonly in the ileum and jejunum. A small proportion of these polyps can undergo malignant transformation. The frequency of GI malignancy in Peutz-Jeghers syndrome has been estimated at 2 to 3%.[11] The most common site of malignancy was the large bowel, followed by the duodenum, jejunum, and stomach in a study of 104 patients.[11] The relative risk of death from GI cancer and from all forms of cancer is 13 and 9, respectively. There is a 48% chance of dying of cancer by age 57.[12]

Other malignancies have also been reported in Peutz-Jeghers syndrome. In one study, 36% of patients with Peutz-Jeghers syndrome with a diagnosis of cancer had pancreatic cancer.[13] Several case reports have shown an association between this syndrome and bilateral breast cancer, with a mean age at onset at 42 years.[14] Other reported cancers include ovarian sex cord tumors, adenoma malignum (rare form of cervical cancer), and Sertoli cell testicular tumors in prepubertal boys.[12]

Prophylactic screening in Peutz-Jeghers syndrome should include examination for occult blood, colonoscopy, and upper GI tract endoscopy. Some advocate removal of large or symptomatic colon polyps, whereas others feel that all colon polyps should be removed.[12] Initial screening should be followed by periodic (6–12 months) upper endoscopy and colonoscopy with a small bowel follow-through. Given the risk of bilateral breast cancer, a baseline mammography at age 25 with annual examinations starting at age 40 is recommended. Further, an annual pelvic sonogram and cervical smears are also advisable.[12]

Skin Neoplasms Related to Renal Malignancies

Birt-Hogg-Dubé Syndrome

Skin neoplasm: Fibrofolliculomas, trichodiscomas, acrochordons
Internal malignancy: Renal cancer
Genetics: Gene: Folliculin; Chromosome: 17p11.2
OMIM: 135150
Inheritance: Autosomal dominant

Birt-Hogg Dubé syndrome consists of multiple fibrofolliculomas, trichodiscomas, other skin neoplasms such as lipomas, and collagenomas associated with pulmonary cysts and renal cancer. Pulmonary findings usually precede skin manifestations, which usually occur in the third to fourth decade of life. Renal disease usually presents after skin manifestations.[15]

The skin manifestations of Birt-Hogg-Dubé syndrome include most commonly fibrofolliculomas, trichodiscomas, and acrochordons. Clinically, these lesions can have a similar appearance as 2 to 4 mm smooth, dome-shaped, skin-colored to gray-white papules on the face, neck, and upper trunk that are asymptomatic. There is some contention that, histologically, all of these lesions represent fibrofolliculomas.[16] Other more rarely described skin lesions include deforming lipomas and collagenomas.[15,17,18] Other manifestations of the syndrome include oral papules and pulmonary cysts.

The most common internal neoplasms associated with Birt-Hogg-Dubé syndrome are renal tumors. In one study that included 13 patients with Birt-Hogg-Dubé syndrome, 7 had renal neoplasms.[19] The histologic spectrum of renal tumors in Birt-Hogg-Dubé syndrome is unique (Table 2). The original affected family reported by Birt and colleagues also had hereditary medullary thyroid carcinoma.[15]

Table 2 Histologic Spectrum of Renal Tumors in Birt-Hogg-Dubé (BHD) syndrome

Histologic type	BHD	All renal cancers
chromophobe	34%	5%
oncocytoma	5%	5%
chromophobe/ oncocytic hybrid	50%	NA
clear cell	9%	75%
papillary	2%	15%

Prophylactic screening for patients and family members of patients with Birt-Hogg-Dubé syndrome should include chest radiography, abdominal and chest CT, and renal ultrasonography.[16,20]

Tuberous Sclerosis

Skin neoplasm: Hypomelanotic macules, facial angiofibromas, periungual fibromas, connective tissue nevi
Internal malignancy: Renal cell carcinoma
Genetics: Genes: TSC1 and TSC2; Chromosomes: 9q34 and 16p13
OMIM: 191100
Inheritance: Autosomal dominant with a spontaneous mutation rate as high as 75%

Tuberous sclerosis is a syndrome consisting of several skin findings coupled with tumors of the brain, heart, retinas, kidneys, and lungs, with frequent mental deficiency and epilepsy. The initial skin findings in this syndrome are hypomelanotic macules, which may be present at birth or perinatally. These macules are usually oval- to lance-ovate- (ash leaf) shaped, and their presence is more easily appreciated on Wood's lamp examination. Facial angiofibromas begin to develop next, usually within the first 2 years of life, with full expression by adolescence. These are 1 to 3 mm yellow to pink waxy dome-shaped papules distributed over the nose, cheeks, and forehead. Up to 50% of patients can develop a connective tissue nevus also known as the shagreen patch. These develop in the first decade of life and are usually 1 to 10 cm patches of knobby skin usually found on the lumbrosacral area. At puberty, about 50% of patients develop periungual papules known as Koenen's tumors. These present as firm, digitate, pink, protruding papules that histologically are angiofibromas.

The majority of tumors associated with tuberous sclerosis are benign. The most common renal tumor is an angiomyolipoma. However, renal cell cancer may occasionally develop, with 16 cases having been reported with tuberous sclerosis (bilateral renal cancer in seven patients). The median age at cancer presentation is 28 years, with clear cell carcinoma being the most common histologic subtype.[21] Enlarging renal lesions with intratumoral calcifications that have no fatty tissue as seen by ultrasonography, CT, or MRI are more suspicious. Diagnosis should be confirmed by fine-needle aspiration or surgical exploration. Because renal cancer in tuberous sclerosis is often bilateral, renal-sparing surgery should be performed when possible.[22]

Hereditary Leiomyomatosis and Renal Cell Cancer

Skin neoplasm: Leiomyomas
Internal malignancy: Papillary renal cell carcinoma

Genetics: Gene: HLRCC; Chromosome: 1q42.1
OMIM: 605839
Inheritance: Autosomal dominant

Hereditary leiomyomatosis with renal cell cancer is a familial syndrome with a predisposition to skin leiomyomas, uterine leiomyomas, and papillary renal cell carcinoma. In one study, four unilateral renal cancer cases occurred in females aged 33 to 48 showing papillary histology and all were metastatic at the time of diagnosis.[23] Seven of 11 family members had cutaneous nodules, two of which were confirmed as leiomyomas.

Cutaneous leiomyomas present as erythematous firm nodules that can be painful to the touch. They are rare benign skin tumors thought to arise from the arrector pilorum muscle. Patients and family members with hereditary leiomyomatosis and renal cell cancer should undergo renal ultrasonography. Female patients should also have transvaginal ultrasonography of the uterus because of uterine leiomyosarcomas, which have been reported with this syndrome.

Skin Neoplasms Related to Breast Cancer

Cowden Syndrome

Skin neoplasms: Tricholemmomas, acral keratoses, oral papillomas, sclerotic fibromas, lipomas, angiolipomas, hemangiomas, and multiple acrochordons
Internal malignancy: Breast carcinoma, thyroid carcinoma, rare colon adenocarcinoma
Genetics: Gene: PTEN; Chromosome: 10q22-23
OMIM: 158350
Inheritance: Autosomal dominant with variable expressivity and female predominance

Cowden syndrome consists of multiple skin neoplasms; increased propensity of breast, thyroid, and colon carcinoma; and other features, which can include a high arched palate, bird-like facies, GI polyps, female genital tract neoplasms, an enlarged tongue, and diabetes mellitus.[24] Skin lesions frequently appear before internal manifestations and therefore serve as an important marker for this syndrome.

The mucocutaneous lesions characteristically appear in the second to third decades. Tricholemmomas are a specific cutaneous marker for Cowden syndrome. They usually present as multiple yellow to skin-colored verrucous papules, especially on the face, with a predilection for the ears and periorificial areas. Multiple sclerotic fibromas are another skin marker for the disease. These appear as translucent to skin-colored waxy nodules with a characteristic histology of whorled collagen with significant clefting.[8,25] More than 50% of patients have punctate palmoplantar keratoses. Oral lesions consist of 1 to 3 mm papules that create a cobblestone appearance and can involve the entire oral mucosa and the tongue.

Twenty-five to 36% of female patients with Cowden disease develop breast cancer. Seventy-five percent of female patients have fibrocystic breast disease and fibroadenomas.[26] Breast cancer usually develops around the age of 40 and is a ductal adenocarcinoma that has often metastasized before the diagnosis has been confirmed.[27]

Seven percent of patients with Cowden disease develop thyroid adenocarcinoma. Two-thirds of Cowden disease patients develop some form of thyroid disease, including goiter, adenomas, and thyroglossal duct cysts. Hamartomatous polyps of the GI tract can also develop, and they have a small potential for malignant transformation.[26]

Prophylactic screening for Cowden syndrome should include monthly breast self-examination and periodic mammograms. Some also recommend consideration of bilateral prophylactic mastectomies in women with breast lesions in the third decade of life.[26] Screening should also include a thyroid examination, thyroid function tests, and ultrasonography of the thyroid gland. If nodules are noted on examination, fine-needle aspiration or surgical biopsy is recommended.

Skin Neoplasms Related to Cancer of the Genitourinary System

Extramammary Paget's Disease

Skin neoplasm: Intraepidermal neoplasm consisting of cells with glandular differentiation
Internal malignancy: Bladder, urethra, prostate, endometrial, endocervical, vaginal, colorectal, and breast carcinoma

The current theory is that extramammary Paget's disease arises as a primary intraepidermal neoplasm in most cases. Tumor cells are thought to arise from apocrine gland cells or pluripotent keratinocytes.[28] Approximately 25% of cases are thought to have associated neoplastic disease in adnexal structures or in internal organs with a contiguous epithelial lining. However, an increased incidence of noncontiguous malignancies has also been reported.

Clinically, extramammary Paget's disease presents as an erythematous, edematous, weeping, crusted, and nonhealing plaque with irregular borders. The most common anatomic sites of involvement include the vulva and the perianal area. Patients are usually between 50 and 80 years of age. The normal female to male ratio is 4·1.[29]

Vulvar extramammary Paget's disease usually originates in the epidermis but has been described in association with endometrial,

endocervical, vaginal, vulval, urethral, and bladder neoplasia. Breast cancer is the malignancy that occurs most often in conjunction with vulvar extramammary Paget's disease.[30] Perianal extramammary Paget's disease is rarer and is strongly associated with adenocarcinoma of the colon and rectum. In 70 to 80% of cases, perianal disease arises secondary to invasive malignancy of the anus, rectum, and colon.[28] Disease involving the male genitalia is more commonly associated with internal malignancy (urethra, bladder, and testicles) than vulval disease.

The prognosis for extramammary Paget's disease contained to the epidermis is excellent. When lymphovascular invasion occurs, the prognosis diminishes considerably. The 5-year survival rate with inguinal node metastases is 0%.[28] Treatment for disease in the skin includes wide local excision versus Mohs' micrographic surgery, which provides a higher cure rate with fewer recurrences.

Long-term follow-up is recommended for patients with extramammary Paget's disease to monitor for local skin recurrence and development of an associated cancer. In perianal disease, proctosigmoidoscopy and colonoscopy are recommended at 2- to 3-year intervals.[29] Disease involving the male or female genitalia should prompt examination of the appropriate internal organs looking for associated malignancy.

Skin Neoplasms Related to Cancer of the Endocrine System

Multiple Endocrine Neoplasia Type IIB

Skin neoplasm: Multiple mucosal neuromas
Internal malignancy: Medullary thyroid carcinoma
Genetics: Gene: *RET*; Chromosome: 10q11.2
OMIM: 162300
Inheritance: Autosomal dominant

Multiple endocrine neoplasia type IIB is a syndrome consisting of multiple neuromas, pheochromocytoma, and medullary thyroid carcinoma with a marfanoid body habitus. The skin findings in this syndrome are predominantly neuromas, which present as pedunculated nodules on the eyelid margins, lips, and tongue. Other features include enlarged nerves in the GI tract with megacolon and the eye, leading to corneal nerve thickening.[31–33]

Medullary thyroid cancer occurs in virtually all patients with this syndrome. Surgery is the preferred treatment since this tumor is generally resistant to radiation and chemotherapy. Children as young as 6 months old have been diagnosed with medullary thyroid cancer in this syndrome. Therefore, prophylactic total thyroidectomy within the first 6 months of life is the recommended treatment for patients with

multiple endocrine neoplasia type IIB. Early thyroidectomy is essential for survival. Once medullary thyroid cancer invades the lymph nodes or soft tissue, survival drops to 40% over 7.5 years of follow-up.[31,33,34]

Carney's Syndrome

Skin neoplasm: Myxomas, blue nevi, lentigines, psammomatous melanotic schwannoma
Internal malignancy: Thyroid carcinoma, malignant psammomatous melanotic schwannoma
Genetics: Gene: *PRKAR1A*; Chromosome: 17q23-q24
OMIM: 160980
Inheritance: Autosomal dominant

Carney's syndrome is a complex of myxomas (cardiac, cutaneous, mammary), spotty pigmentation of the skin and mucous membranes, and endocrine gland overactivity (Cushing's syndrome, sexual precocity, and acromegaly) described by Carney in 1985.[35] Patients often have tumors of two or more endocrine glands, including pigmented nodular adrenocortical disease, growth hormone– and prolactin-producing pituitary adenoma, testicular tumors, thyroid adenoma and carcinoma, and ovarian cysts.[36] Detection of this syndrome occurs at a median age of 20 years.

The earliest manifestations of Carney's syndrome are cutaneous. Lesions consist of pigmented brown/black macules and blue/black dome-shaped nodules (lentigines and blue nevi). These lesions are occasionally congenital but usually reach a more characteristic density in the prepubertal years. The typical distribution involves the face, lips, eyelids, ears, trunk, neck, conjunctiva, sclera, vulva, limbs, and back of the hands. Cutaneous myxoma present as sessile papules or subcutaneous nodules, usually less than 10 mm in diameter, some of which are cystic. The most common locations are the eyelid, external ear, and nipple.[35,36]

Malignancy is rare in Carney's syndrome. Up to 75% of patients have thyroid nodules, which usually develop in the first 10 years of life. Five thyroid carcinomas were detected in one series, three of the papillary type and two of the follicular type.[36] Thyroid ultrasonography is an effective method for screening for thyroid involvement in pediatric and young adult patients. Psammomatous melanotic schwannoma is a very rare peripheral nerve sheath tumor found in Carney's syndrome, about 10% of which are malignant and fatal. Screening is difficult because this condition can occur in many anatomic locations, including the esophagus, stomach, and paraspinal sympathetic chain. Fifty-seven percent of deaths in Carney's syndrome are caused by heart-related disease (cardiac myxomas). Cardiac screening should begin at age 5 years in known cases of Carney's syndrome.[36]

Skin Neoplasms Related to the Neural System

Gorlin's Syndrome or Nevoid Basal Cell Carcinoma Syndrome

Skin neoplasm: Multiple basal cell carcinoma, facial milia, epidermoid cysts, palmar/plantar pits

Internal malignancy: Medulloblastomas, fibrosarcoma, ovarian fibromas

Genetics: Gene: *PTCH*; Chromosome: 9q22.3-q31

Inheritance: Autosomal dominant

Gorlin's syndrome consists of multiple basal cell carcinomas that develop at a young age, odontogenic keratocysts, palmar pits, macrocephaly, frontal bossing, calcified falx cerebri, agenesis of the corpus callosum, bifid ribs, spina bifida occulta, calcified diaphragma sellae, and a high arched palate. This syndrome is important to recognize not only for these manifestations but also for the occasional association with medulloblastoma, which occurs at a very young age. The diagnostic criteria for Gorlin's syndrome are outlined in Table 3.

The skin findings in Gorlin's syndrome include basal cell carcinoma, which is found in 76% of affected patients.[37] Basal cell carcinoma has been reported as early as age 2 years, but it more commonly appears in the teenage years and proliferates between puberty and age 35. Basal cell carcinomas number from a few to the hundreds and usually affect the face, back, and

chest. A small proportion of Gorlin's syndrome patients have no basal cell carcinomas.

Other findings include odontogenic keratocysts, which are present in 80% of patients over 20 years old. Palmar pits are found in 60% of patients and present as 2 to 3 mm depressions that develop usually in the second decade of life.[37] Other associated anomalies include macrocephaly, frontal bossing, calcified falx cerebri, rib anomalies, spina bifida occulta, calcified diaphragma sellae, and a high arched palate.

Three to 5% of patients with Gorlin's syndrome develop medulloblastoma. Medulloblastoma in Gorlin's syndrome is unique in that it usually occurs in the first 2 years of life compared with the general population, in which incidence peaks at age 3 to 5 years. Medulloblastoma is a highly invasive embryonal neuroepithelial tumor that arises in the cerebellum and has a tendency to disseminate throughout the central nervous system early in its course. Infants at risk of developing medulloblastoma should be screened by annual MRI until age 8 years.[37] Radiation therapy is contraindicated in patients with Gorlin's syndrome as innumerable basal cell carcinomas later develop within previously irradiated skin. Other rare and possibly coincidental malignancies reported with Gorlin's syndrome include astrocytoma, malignant meningioma, ovarian fibrosarcoma, rhabdomyosarcoma, Hodgkin's lymphoma, leiomyosarcoma, and adenocarcinoma of the rectum.[38–43]

Neurofibromatosis Type 1

Skin neoplasm: Neurofibromas, café au lait macules

Internal malignancy: Malignant peripheral nerve sheath tumors, optic glioma, malignant astrocytoma, ependymoma, meningioma, rhabdomyosarcoma, juvenile chronic myelogenous leukemia, Wilms' tumor, and neuroblastoma[44–57]

Genetics: Gene: *NF1*; Chromosome: 17q11.2

OMIM: 162200

Inheritance: Autosomal dominant

Neurofibromatosis type 1 is an inherited syndrome consisting of cutaneous, ocular, and osseous lesions coupled with malignancies involving the peripheral nerve sheath and central nervous system. The diagnostic criteria for neurofibromatosis are outlined in Table 4. Some of the tumors associated with neurofibromatosis are histologically benign but lethal nonetheless owing to the location.[52] Early detection and management of this syndrome and its associated tumors are essential for the survival of patients with neurofibromatosis.

The cutaneous neoplasms associated with neurofibromatosis include neurofibromas and café au lait macules. Neurofibromas present as pink to tan polypoid or pedunculated rubbery nodules measuring from a few millimeters to

Table 4 Diagnostic Criteria for Neurofibromatosis Type I

Neurofibromatosis Type 1 diagnostic criteria
Must have 2 or more of the following criteria:
1. Six or more café au lait macules. >0.5cm prepuberty; >1.5cm postpuberty
2. Two or more neurofibromas or one plexiform neurofibroma
3. Axillary or inguinal freckling
4. Optic gliomas
5. Osseous lesions – pseudoarthrosis, sphenoid wing dysplasia
6. First degree relative with NF1 by the above criteria

Reference 8.b.13

several centimeters. They invaginate into the skin easily on fingertip pressure, the so-called "buttonhole" sign. Plexiform neurofibromas are firm and tender masses in the subcutaneous tissue that may invade deeper structures. Café au lait macules are tan to brown uniformly pigmented macules with sharp demarcation.

Progression of plexiform neurofibroma to a malignant peripheral nerve sheath tumor occurs in 1 to 5% of patients with neurofibromatosis.[53–56] The relative risk of developing a malignant peripheral nerve sheath tumor in neurofibromatosis versus the general population is 113.[53] The mean age at development of these tumors has been estimated at 26 to 32 years of age.[54,55] Malignant peripheral nerve sheath tumors are often metastatic on presentation or refractory to therapy; therefore, early detection and treatment are paramount. The median survival was 18 months overall. Patients with malignant peripheral nerve sheath tumors on the limbs tend to survive longer (53 months) than those with a nonlimb location (21 months).[55] Pain associated with an enlarging mass is the strongest suggestion that a malignant peripheral nerve sheath tumor has developed. Imaging and biopsy of any painful or enlarging nodular or plexiform neurofibroma should be performed to assess for malignancy.

There is a 30 to 40 times higher than expected rate of association of neurofibromatosis type 1, juvenile chronic myelogenous leukemia, and juvenile xanthogranuloma. The risk of juvenile chronic myelogenous leukemia in children with neurofibromatosis type 1 is 20 to 30 times higher if juvenile xanthogranulomas are present.[56] Juvenile xanthogranulomas present as firm, rubbery, round, pink papules with a yellow tinge found on the head and neck, upper trunk, and upper extremities.

Skin Neoplasms Related to Cancer of the Bone and Cartilage

Maffucci's Syndrome

Skin neoplasm: Subcutaneous hemangiomas
Internal malignancy: Chrondrosarcoma, astrocytoma, ovarian carcinoma, pancreatic carcinoma

Table 3 Diagnostic Criteria for Gorlin's Syndrome

1. 2 major features
2. 1 major feature and an affected 1st degree relative
3. 2 minor features and an affected 1st degree relative
4. Multiple basal cell carcinomas in childhood

MAJOR FEATURES	*MINOR FEATURES*
1. Multiple BCC's or one prior to age 20	1. Congenital skeletal anomaly (bifid ribs vertebral anomaly)
2. Histologically confirmed odontogenic keratocysts	2. Macrocephaly >97th percentile with frontal bossing
3. >3 palmar or plantar pits	3. Cardiac or ovarian fibroma
4. Bilamellar calcification of the falx cerebri	4. Medulloblastoma
	5. Lymphomesenteric cysts
	6. Congential malformations (cleft lip/palate, polydactyly, eye anomalies)

All based on reference 8.a.7

Genetics: Gene: *PTH/PTHRP* type 1 receptor; Chromosome: 3p22-p21.1
OMIM: 166000
Inheritance: Not genetically inherited in a simple mendelian manner

Maffucci's syndrome consists of multiple enchondromas associated with subcutaneous hemangiomas. The symptoms of this syndrome are congenital in 25% of cases but usually begin on average at age 4 to 5 years.[58] The hemangiomas present as soft, compressible, blue-red, and occasionally tender subcutaneous nodules usually located on the hands and feet. Enchondromas occur primarily along the long bones during a time of rapid skeletal growth. Enchondromas represent abnormal cartilage development. Islands of immature cells fail to ossify and later proliferate to form expanding cartilaginous tumors.

Chondrosarcoma develops in 22 to 30% of patients with Maffucci's syndrome.[58] The average age at development of chondrosarcoma is 40 years. They usually present as an enlarging mass that was previously quiescent without a history of preceding trauma. The affected area can be painful and feel heavy. Suspicious lesions should be imaged. Radiologic features that support malignancy include endosteal cortical erosion, cortical destruction with expanding soft tissue mass, or a zone of lucency in a previously mineralized region.[59] Lesions suspicious for malignancy should be biopsied, either by needle aspiration or with open techniques.

A wide variety of noncartilaginous tumors, including astrocytomas, ovarian cancer, and pancreatic cancer, have been reported with Maffucci's syndrome. Periodic assessment and imaging for other tumors involving the brain, abdominal organs, and endocrine glands should be performed.[59]

Skin Neoplasms Associated with Multiple Internal Tumor Types

Multicentric Reticulohistiocytosis

Skin neoplasm: Reticulohistiocytomas
Internal malignancies: Breast, cervix, colon, lung, bronchial, and ovarian carcinoma; lymphoma, leukemia, sarcoma, melanoma[60]

Multicentric reticulohistiocytosis is a noninherited disorder that usually begins around age 40 to 50 years. Eighty-five percent of affected patients are Caucasian.[60] Skin nodules are present in 90% of individuals at the time of diagnosis and present as round, symmetric, pink to brown papules ranging from a few millimeters to 2 cm. They are usually distributed on the face, arms, trunk, mucosa, and neck. In 27% of cases, the "coral bead" sign is present, manifested as papules aligned along the periungual region. Thirty

percent of patients have mucosal involvement, most frequently the buccal mucosa, nasal mucosa, and tongue. Arthritis may precede skin changes by months to years. The arthritis is usually a symmetric polyarthritis involving the hands, knees, wrists, shoulders, elbows, ankles, hips, feet, neck, and spine, in decreasing frequency. Twelve to 45% of patients progress to arthritis mutilans.[61,62] Involvement of the interphalangeal joints can result in "opera glass deformity" owing to telescoping and shortening of the digits.

Malignancy has been reported in association with multicentric reticulohistiocytosis in 20 to 31% of cases.[61,62] No specific type of cancer predominates. In cases associated with malignancy, multicentric reticulohistiocytosis preceded the development of cancer in 73% of cases.[60] Malignancy workup should be guided by a clinician's suspicions after a careful review of systems and physical examination. Various therapeutic regimens have been tried for multicentric reticulohistiocytosis, with variable benefit. These include nonsteroidal anti-inflammatory drugs, methotrexate alone or in combination with other immunosuppressive drugs, hydroxychloroquine, corticosteroids, cyclophosphamide, chlorambucil, and alendronate.[60–66] The disease tends to spontaneously remit after approximately 8 years. Many patients are significantly disabled owing to joint destruction.

REFERENCES

1. Curth HO. Skin manifestations of internal malignant tumors. Md State Med J 1972;17:52–6
2. McLean DI. Cutaneous paraneoplastic syndromes. Arch Dermatol 1986;122:765–7.
3. Cohen PR, Kohn SR, Davis DA, Kurzrock R. Muir-Torre syndrome. Dermatol Clin 1995;13:79–89.
4. Schwartz RA, Torre DP. The Muir-Torre syndrome: a 25-year retrospect. J Am Acad Dermatol 1995;33:90–104.
5. Hall NR, Williams MA, Murday VA, et al. Muir-Torre syndrome: a variant of the cancer family syndrome. J Med Genet 1994;31:627–31.
6. Pauli RM, Pauli ME, Hall JG. Gardner syndrome and periampullary malignancy. Am J Med Genet 1980;6: 205–19.
7. Watne AL. Syndromes of polyposis coli and cancer. Curr Probl Cancer 1982;7:1–31.
8. Mallory SB, Stough DB IV. Genodermatoses with malignant potential. Dermatol Clin 1987;5:221–30.
9. Kelly MD, Hugh TB, Field AS, Fitzsimons R. Carcinoma of the thyroid gland and Gardner's syndrome. Aust N Z J Surg 1993;63:505–9.
10. Herrera-Ornelas L, Elsiah S, Petrelli N, Mittelman A. Causes of death in patients with familial polyposis coli (FPC). Semin Surg Oncol 1987;3:109–17.
11. Flageole H, Raptis S, Trudel JL, Lough JO. Progression toward malignancy of hamartomas in a patient with Peutz-Jeghers syndrome: case report and literature review. Can J Surg 1994;37:231–6.
12. Spigelman AD, Murday V, Phillips RK. Cancer and the Peutz-Jeghers syndrome. Gut 1989;30:1588–90.
13. Hizawa K, Iida M, Matsumoto T, et al. Cancer in Peutz-Jeghers syndrome. Cancer 1993;72:2777–81.
14. Riley E, Swift M. A family with Peutz-Jeghers syndrome and bilateral breast cancer. Cancer 1980;46:851–7.
15. Ubogy-Rainey Z, James WD, Lupton GP, Rodman OG. Fibrofolliculomas, trichodiscomas, and acrochordons: the Birt-Hogg-Dube syndrome. J Am Acad Dermatol 1987;16(2 Pt 2):452–7.
16. Crawford GH, Kim S, James WD. Skin signs of systemic disease: an update. Adv Dermatol 2002;18:1–27.
17. Kovacs G, Akhtar M, Beckwith BJ, et al. The Heidelberg classification of renal cell tumors. J Pathol 1997;183: 131–3.
18. Cohen PR, Kurzrock R. Miscellaneous genodermatoses: Beckwith-Wiedemann syndrome, Birt-Hogg-Dube syndrome, familial atypical multiple mole syndrome, hereditary tylosis, incontinentia pigmenti, and supernumerary nipples. Dermatol Clin 1995;13:211–29.
19. Toro JR, Glenn G, Duray P, et al. Birt-Hogg-Dube syndrome: a novel marker of kidney neoplasia. Arch Dermatol 1999;135:1195–202.
20. Durrani OH, Ng L, Bihrle W III. Chromophobe renal cell carcinoma in a patient with the Birt-Hogg-Dube syndrome. J Urol 2002;168:1484–5.
21. Washecka R, Hanna M. Malignant renal tumors in tuberous sclerosis. Urology 1991;37:340–3.
22. Torres VE, King BF, Holley KE, et al. The kidney in the tuberous sclerosis complex. Adv Nephrol Necker Hosp 1994;23:43–70.
23. Launonen V, Vierimaa O, Kiuru M, et al. Inherited susceptibility to uterine leiomyomas and renal cell cancer. Proc Nat Acad Sci U S A 2001;98:3387–92.
24. Shapiro SD, Lambert WC, Schwartz RA. Cowden's disease. A marker for malignancy. Int J Dermatol 1988;27:232–7.
25. Requena L, Gutierrez J, Sanchez Yus E. Multiple sclerotic fibromas of the skin. A cutaneous marker of Cowden's disease. J Cutan Pathol 1992;19:346–51.
26. Brownstein MH, Wolf, M, Bikowski JB. Cowden's disease. A cutaneous marker of breast cancer. Cancer 1978;41: 2393–8.
27. Starink TM. Cowden's disease: analysis of fourteen new cases. J Am Acad Dermatol 1984;11:1127–41.
28. Lloyd J, Flanagan AM. Mammary and extramammary Paget's disease. J Clin Pathol 2000;53:742–9.
29. Heymann WR. Extramammary Paget's disease. Clin Dermatol 1993;11:83–7.
30. Fever GA, Shevchuk M, Canalog A. Vulvar Paget's disease. The need to exclude an invasive lesion. Gynecol Oncol 1990;38:81–9.
31. Caruso DR, O'Dorisio TM, Mazzaferi EL. Multiple endocrine neoplasia. Curr Opin Oncol 1991;3:103–8.
32. Oberg K, Skogseid B, Eriksson B. Multiple endocrine neoplasia type 1 (MEN-1). Clinical, biochemical and genetical investigations. Acta Oncol 1989;28:383–7.
33. Gardner E, Papi L, Easton DF, et al. Genetic linkage studies map the multiple endocrine neoplasia type 2 loci to a small interval on chromosome 10q11.2. Hum Mol Genet 1993;2:241–6.
34. Leboulleux S, Travagli JP, Caillou B, et al. Medullary thyroid carcinoma as part of a multiple endocrine neoplasia type 2B syndrome: influence of the stage on the clinical course. Cancer 2002;94:44–50.
35. Carney JA. The Carney complex (myxomas, spotty pigmentation, endocrine overactivity, and schwannomas. Dermatol Clin 1995;13:19–26.
36. Stratakis CA, Kirschner LS, Carney JA. Clinical and molecular features of the Carney complex: diagnostic criteria and recommendations for patient evaluation. J Clin Endocrinol Metab 2001;86:4041–6.
37. Gorlin RJ. Nevoid basal cell carcinoma syndrome. Dermatol Clin 1995;13:113–24.
38. Zvulunov A, Strother D, Zirbel G, et al. Nevoid basal cell carcinoma syndrome. Report of a case with associated Hodgkin's disease. J Pediatr Hematol Oncol 1995;17: 66–70.
39. Garcia-Prats MD, Lopez-Carreira M, Mayordoma JI, et al. Leiomyosarcoma of the soft tissues in a patient with nevoid basal-cell carcinoma syndrome. Tumori 1994;80: 401–4.
40. Albrecht S, Goodman JC, Rajagopolan S, et al. Malignant meningioma in Gorlin's syndrome: cytogenetic and p53 gene analysis. Case report. J Neurosurg 1994;81:466–71.
41. Evans DG, Farndon PA, Burnell LD, et al. The incidence of Gorlin syndrome in 173 consecutive cases of medulloblastoma. Br J Cancer 1991;64:959–61.
42. Kraemer BB, Silva EG, Sneige N. Fibrosarcoma of ovary. A new component in the nevoid basal-cell carcinoma syndrome. Am J Surg Pathol 1984;8:231–6.
43. Beddis IR, Mott MG, Bullimore J. Case report: nasopharyngeal rhabdomyosarcoma and Gorlin's naevoid basal cell carcinoma syndrome. Med Pediatr Oncol 1983;11: 178–9.
44. Zollner M, Ermbeck B, Akesson HO, Angervall L. Life expectancy, mortality and prognostic factors in neurofibromatosis type 1. A twelve-year follow-up of an epidemiological study in Goteborg, Sweden. Acta Derm Venereol 1995; 75:136–40.

45. Shearer P, Parham D, Kovnar E, et al. Neurofibromatosis type I and malignancy: review of 32 pediatric cases treated at a single institution. Med Pediatr Oncol 1994;22:78–83.

46. Matsui I, Tanimura M, Kobayashi N, et al. Neurofibromatosis type I and childhood cancer. Cancer 1993;72:27 46–54.

47. Schlumberger M, Gicquel C, Lumbroso J, et al. Malignant pheochromocytoma: clinical, biological, histologic and therapeutic data in a series of patients with distant metastases. J Endocrinol Invest 1992;15:631–42.

48. Hayflick SJ, Hofman KJ, Tunnessen WW Jr, et al. Neurofibromatosis 1: recognition and management of associated neuroblastoma. Pediatr Dermatol 1990;7:293–5.

49. Lederman SM, Martin EC, Laffey KT, Lefkowitch JH. Hepatic neurofibromatosis, malignant schwannoma, and angiosarcoma in von Recklinghausen's disease. Gastroenterology 1987;92:243–9.

50. Warrier RP, Kini KR, Raju U, et al. Neurofibromatosis and malignancy. Clin Pediatr 1985;24:584–5.

51. Ilgren EB, Kinnier-Wilson LM, Stiller CA. Gliomas in neurofibromatosis: a series of 89 cases with evidence for enhanced malignancy in associated cerebellar astrocytomas. Pathol Annu 1985;20 Pt 1:331–58.

52. Hope DG, Mulvihill JJ. Malignancy in neurofibromatosis. Adv Neurol 1981;29:33–56.

53. Evans DGR, Baser ME, McGaurghran J, et al. Malignant peripheral nerve sheath tumours in neurofibromatosis. J Med Genet 2002;29:311–4.

54. King AA, DeBaun MR, Riccardi VM, Gutmann DH. Malignant peripheral nerve sheath tumors in neurofibromatosis I. Am J Med Genet 2000;93:388–92.

55. Leroy K, Dumas V, Martin-Garcia N, et al. Malignant peripheral nerve sheath tumors associated with neurofibromatosis type I: a clinicopathologic and molecular study of 17 patients. Arch Dermatol 2001;137:908–13.

56. Zvulunov A, Barak Y, Metzker A. Juvenile xanthogranuloma, neurofibromatosis, and juvenile chronic myelogenous leukemia. World statistical analysis. Arch Dermatol 1995;131:904–8.

57. Clark RD, Hutter JJ. Familial neurofibromatosis and juvenile chronic myelogenous leukemia. Hum Genet 1982;60:230–2.

58. Kaplan RP, Wang JT, Amron DM, Kaplan L. Maffucci's syndrome: two case reports with a literature review. J Am Acad Dermatol 1994;29(5 Pt 2):894–9.

59. Albregts AE, Rapini RP. Malignancy in Maffucci's syndrome. Dermatol Clin 1995;13:73–8.

60. Rapini RP. Multicentric reticulohistiocytosis. Clin Dermatol 1993;11:107–11.

61. Luz FB, Gaspar TAP, Kalil-Gaspar N, Ramos-e-Silva M. Multicentric reticulohistiocytosis. J Eur Acad Dermatol Venerol 2001;15:524–31.

62. Snow JL, Muller SA. Malignancy-associated multicentric reticulohistiocytosis: a clinical, histological and immunophenotypic study. Br J Dermatol 1995;133:71–6.

63. Goto H, Inaba M, Kobayashi K, et al. Successful treatment of multicentric reticulohistiocytosis with alendronate: evidence for a direct effect of bisphosphonate on histiocytes. Arthritis Rheum 2003;48:3538–41.

64. Bogle MA, Tschen JA, Sairam S, et al. Multicentric reticulohistiocytosis with pulmonary involvement. J Am Acad Dermatol 2003;49:1125–7.

65. Outland JD, Keiran SJ, Schikler KN, Callen JP. Multicentric reticulohistiocytosis in a 14-year-old girl. Pediatr Dermatol 2002;19:527–31.

66. Valencia IC, Colsky A, Berman B. Multicentric reticulohistiocytosis associated with recurrent breast carcinoma. J Am Acad Dermatol 1998;39(5 Pt 2):864–6.

Graft-versus-Host Skin Disease

Sharon R. Hymes, MD

Daniel R. Couriel, MD

Hematopoietic stem cell transplantation (HSCT) using peripheral blood, cord blood, or bone marrow is used to treat a wide variety of genetic and immunologic disorders, as well as advanced malignancies. Since the first bone marrow transplantations, significant advances in technology and immunology have improved the prognosis, rate of engraftment, and quality of life for many stem cell recipients. It is estimated that at least 8,000 HSCTs are performed annually in the United States and more than 15,000 procedures worldwide for a wide variety of indications (Table 1).[1] Graft-versus-host disease (GVHD) is one of the major problems encountered post-transplantation and remains a significant cause of morbidity and mortality. Conversely, in some patients, GVHD is desirable because of a beneficial graft-versus-tumor effect. To take advantage of this, graft manipulation is sometimes employed in an attempt to produce mild GVHD and thereby prevent or treat tumor relapse.[2–4]

Traditionally, two types of cutaneous GVHD are described; the acute form occurs less than 100 days after transplantation, and the chronic form occurs after 100 days. These rigid time-related criteria should serve only as a guide since both acute (aGVHD) and chronic (cGVHD) GVHD are more accurately diagnosed by clinical and, in some cases, histopathologic features. With the advent of new, less intense preparative regimens and the development of other transplantation techniques, such as donor lymphocyte infusions to treat relapsed malignancies following transplantation, the clinical characteristics of GVHD are changing. Now we frequently see delayed or late manifestations of aGVHD or overlapping aGVHD and cGVHD in the same patient.[5,6]

The skin plays a pivotal role in these complex immunologic reactions and manifests changes that are easily accessible for examination and biopsy. Cutaneous GVHD also shares clinical, histopathologic, and immunologic features with other autoimmune disorders, making it a useful model for study. This chapter reviews the pathogenesis, clinical presentation, and diagnostic and treatment dilemmas associated with cutaneous GVHD.

Table 1 Diseases Treatable by Stem Cell Transplantation

Acute leukemias
 Acute lymphoblastic leukemia
 Acute myelogenous leukemia
 Acute biphenotypic leukemia
Chronic leukemias
 Chronic myelogenous leukemia
 Chronic lymphocytic leukemia
 Juvenile chronic myelogenous leukemia
 Juvenile myelomonocytic leukemia
Myelodysplastic syndromes
Stem cell disorders
 Aplastic anemia
 Fanconi's anemia
 Paroxysmal nocturnal hemoglobinuria
 Pure red cell aplasia
Myeloproliferative disorders
 Acute myelofibrosis
 Agnogenic myeloid metaplasia (myelofibrosis)
 Polycythemia vera
 Essential thrombocythemia
Lymphoproliferative disorders
 Non-Hodgkin's lymphoma
 Hodgkin's disease
Phagocyte disorders
Inherited metabolic disorders
Histiocytic disorders
Inherited erythrocyte abnormalities
 β-Thalassemia major
 Sickle cell disease
Inherited immune system disorders
 Ataxia-telangiectasia
 Kostmann's syndrome
 Leukocyte adhesion deficiency
Other inherited disorders
 Lesch-Nyhan syndrome
 Glanzmann's thrombasthenia
Inherited platelet abnormalities
 Amegakaryocytosis/congenital
  thrombocytopenia
Plasma cell disorders
Other malignancies
 Breast cancer, Ewing's sarcoma,
  neuroblastoma
 Renal cell carcinoma

Adapted from National Marrow Donor Program [on-line database www.marrow.org March 2007].

GVHD Risk Factors

Human leukocyte antigen (HLA) disparity is the major factor predisposing individuals to aGVHD.[7] The relative importance of the incompatibility of individual HLA antigens on GVHD is controversial.[8] Thus, it is not yet known whether antigens of class 1 (HLA A, B, and C) or class 2 (HLA-DR and -DQ) play a relatively more important role as triggers of GVHD. Other relevant factors have been identified as predictors of GVHD, and these include sex mismatch (female donor to male recipient),[9] minor histocompatibility antigens in HLA-matched transplants,[10] donor age,[11] source[12] and dose of hematopoietic stem cells (peripheral stem cells more than bone marrow),[13] the intensity of the preparative regimen[5] and GVHD prophylaxis,[13] or other forms of graft manipulation, such as T-cell depletion.[14] aGVHD predominantly affects the skin, the upper and lower gastrointestinal tract, the liver, and, occasionally, the eye and oral mucosa. The staging system is shown in Table 2, and it includes the first three systems but not eye or oral mucosa.[15]

Pathophysiology

Acute GVHD

Both acute and chronic GVHD are forms of immune dysregulation that occur when immunologically competent cells are given to an immunosuppressed or naive host. Donor T cells that recognize recipient alloantigens initiate the process.[16] Rarely, aGVHD may be seen after blood transfusions when viable T cells are given to neonates and fetuses or to patients with iatrogenic or congenital immunodeficiency disorders. To avoid this complication, irradiation of blood products has become the standard of care for immunocompromised recipients. A blood transfusion from a donor who is homozygous for one shared recipient haplotype may cause a similar problem. In this case, the donor lymphocytes recognize the second haplotype in the recipient and may cause an acute graft-versus-host reaction. This is seen most commonly with directed blood donations within family groups or in inbred populations with restricted haplotypes, such as those found in Japan.[17] Transfusion GVHD presents

Stage	Skin	Liver	Gut
	Table 2 Clinical Staging of Acute Graft-versus-Host Disease		
0	No rash owing to GVHD	Bilirubin, <2 mg/dL	None
1	Maculopapular rash <25% of body surface area without associated symptoms	Bilirubin, 2–<3 mg/dL	Diarrhea, >500–1,000 mL/d, nausea and vomiting
2	Maculopapular rash or erythema with pruritus or other associated symptoms covering ≥25 and <50% of body surface area or localized desquamation	Bilirubin, 3–<6 mg/dL	Diarrhea, >1,000–1,500 mL/d, nausea and vomiting
3	Generalized erythroderma or symptomatic macular, papular, or vesicular eruption, with bullous formation or desquamation covering ≥250% of the body	Bilirubin, 6–<15 mg/dL	Diarrhea, >1,500 mL/d, nausea and vomiting
4	Generalized exfoliative dermatitis or ulcerative dermatitis or bullous formation	Bilirubin, ≥15 mg/dL	Severe abdominal pain with or without ileus

Adapted from Przepiorka D et al.[15]

not only with cutaneous, liver, and gastrointestinal problems but may also cause marrow aplasia.[17] GVHD occasionally occurs after transplantation of solid organs that contain lymphoid tissue, such as small bowel transplants.[16,18] However, the most common cause of GVHD remains HSCT, and the most common organ system involved is the skin.[19,20] aGVHD occurs in about 20 to 40% of matched sibling transplants and 60 to 90% of mismatched related or matched unrelated transplants.[20–23]

In 1966, Billingham described the criteria necessary for the development of GVHD.[24] He stated that the graft must contain immunologically competent cells; the host must possess important transplantation alloantigens that are lacking in the donor graft so that the host appears foreign to the graft; the host must be incapable of mounting an effective immunologic reaction against the graft; and the graft must have security of tenure. Current concepts incorporate these criteria with an evolving understanding of the complex immunologic reactions that occur during and after stem cell transplantation.

The major histocompatibility complex (MHC) lies on the short arm of chromosome 6, also called the HLA region. It contains the genes that encode antigens used for tissue typing and the genes that are involved in immune activation. Even in HLA-matched transplants, minor antigens that are expressed on the cell surface as degraded peptides bound to HLA molecules, but not encoded by the genes of the MHC, may be implicated in the development of GHVD.[17,25] The controversy regarding the nature of GVHD after autologous (the donor is also the recipient) or syngeneic (the donor is an identical twin) transplantation complicates the issue even further.

That is, can HLA-identical donor cells produce GVHD without major or minor MHC differences? In these circumstances, what is seen as clinical aGVHD may actually represent the disruption of mechanisms governing self-tolerance, creating an environment conducive to autoreactive T cells.[26,27] The type of conditioning regimen, presence of thymic damage, and type of transplant may be key to this reaction. Removal of T lymphocytes by CD34 (a marker on hematopoietic stem cells) selection may promote this phenomenon of autoaggression and is clinically characterized by a rash, pruritus, eosinophilia, and, less frequently, fever.[28] The skin rash tends to be morbilliform (measles-like) and less severe than that associated with MHC antigen unmatched transplants. Depletion of T cells from the donor infusion may decrease the incidence of GVHD but also may down-regulate the antitumor immune response[27] and is therefore associated with a higher incidence of disease relapse. The introduction or withdrawal of cyclosporine or the addition of interleukin-2 may also potentially induce alloreactivity and GVHD.[29]

aGVHD contributes significantly to morbidity and mortality. Tissue destruction occurs via effector T-cell activation in response to disparate major or minor histocompatibility antigens. The skin reaction is mediated by dendritic cells, T lymphocytes, natural killer (NK) cells, macrophages, and cytokines interacting with cell surface antigens.[20,30–33] Both donor CD4+ and CD8+ cells, as well as NK cells, are found in the dermal infiltrate.[34] Once recruited to the skin, NK cells may mediate significant epidermal damage, despite lacking the ability to be specifically alloreactive.[35] Lymphocytes in apposition to necrotic keratinocytes, or satellite cell necrosis, are a

common histopathologic finding used in diagnosis. However, it is not clear if these cells are directly responsible for the apoptosis.[31,36]

A three-phase model of aGVHD has been proposed, with phase 1 initiated by injury to host tissue induced by the preconditioning regimen.[17,32,37,38] Either total-body irradiation or chemotherapy is necessary to treat residual tumor, as well as to ablate the recipient immune response sufficiently to allow engraftment. However, these modalities are toxic to healthy tissues, and the resultant damage not only releases chemokines and cytokines but also activates host dendritic cells in target tissues. This is confirmed in a skin explant model, where, after conditioning, activated dendritic cells in the dermis are primed for alloreaction at the time of donor T-cell infusion, and the apoptotic machinery in basal keratinocytes is activated.[36] Inflammatory mediators such as tumor necrosis factor (TNF)-α, interleukin (IL)-1,[37,39] and heat shock proteins[30,36] are produced, which then enhance the expression of HLA-DR. In a murine model, dendritic cells from old mice express more TNF-α and IL-12 than young mice, possibly explaining the increased incidence of aGVHD in older recipients.[32]

During the second phase of GVHD, donor T-cell activation and expansion occurs and NK cells, monocytes, and macrophages create an inflammatory milieu composed of activated and recruited immunocytes and soluble mediators. The greater the genetic disparity between host and donor, the greater the T-cell response.[17] If donor T cells are depleted from the infusion, there is a decreased incidence and severity of GVHD.[40] However, engraftment and, as previously mentioned, the desirable graft-versus-tumor effect may also be abrogated. Antigen-presenting cells present transplant recipient antigens to donor lymphocytes. These, in turn, secrete cytokines that damage tissues and further augment the immune response.[17]

Target tissue injury occurs in the third and final phase. Donor T cells respond to the activated host dendritic cells, and inflammatory mediators such as TNF-α perpetuate the apoptosis in basal keratinocytes and other target tissues. The subsequent "cytokine storm" in which IL-1, IL-2, TNF-α, and interferon-γ play an important role continues the process, particularly in the rete ridges. Keratinocytes continue to die by apoptosis and direct satellite cell necrosis.[35,36,41] Fas(CD95)/Fas-Ligand apoptosis plays an important role in cell death, as does a Fas-independent pathway, employing perforin, a protein expressed in functionally active CD8+ and NK cells.[17,42,43] In murine models, the graft-versus-tumor effect may be mediated by the perforin-granzyme pathway.[44] It is hoped that further definition of these processes will lead to unique therapeutic and pharmacologic strategies for regulating epidermal necrosis without losing the antitumor effect.[45]

The skin is furthered targeted for cytotoxic T-cell and NK cell injury by suprabasilar keratinocyte expression of vascular cell adhesion molecule 1 (VCAM-1)[46] and cytokeratin 15.[47] Modified vascular endothelial cells expressing adhesion molecules, including P-selectin, E-selectin, endothelial leukocyte adhesion molecule 1, and VCAM-1,[34,48] as well as up-regulated expression of shear-resistant adhesion molecules within endothelial sites, facilitate the effector cell migration through the vessel wall.[49] Hyaluronic acid expressed on dermal vessels in aGVHD confers this shear-resistant attachment and contributes to cutaneous lymphocytotropism.[50] Polymorphism of platelet endothelial cell adhesion molecule CD31 also increases the risk of GVHD, suggesting that donor lymphocyte recognition of a mismatched endothelial molecule is important.[34,51]

Langerhans' cells are cutaneous dendritic cells that are very important in the pathogenesis of cutaneous GVHD.[52] These cells may renew locally without reconstitution from bone marrow precursors but are replaced by bone marrow–derived precursors after inflammatory injury.[53] Their expression of MHC molecules is sufficient to initiate GVHD even in the absence of MHC expression on host epithelium.[54] Langerhans' cells process antigens and then migrate to the draining lymph nodes to present the information to T lymphocytes.[55] In a murine model, host Langerhans' cells remain for at least 18 months unless donor T cells are administered with the transplant, and these persistent host cells may be crucial targets in perpetuating tissue injury.[38,52] Alloreactive donor T cells may induce Langerhans' cell chimerism through Fas ligand–dependent depletion of host Langerhans' cells and induction of proinflammatory chemokines.[52] During autologous transplantation, dendritic cell activation may be self-limited, producing little or no cutaneous disease.[36]

The prominent role of Langerhans' cells in the initiation and perpetuation of GVHD has created interest into therapeutic modalities that specifically target them. Ultraviolet radiation (UVR) can deplete host Langerhans' cells, leading to their replacement with donor cell–derived cells. An intriguing approach aimed at GVHD prevention uses this modality to replace host Langerhans' cells prior to donor T-cell infusion.[56] A two-step procedure has been suggested, starting with a T cell–depleted stem cell transplant followed by host exposure to UVR. The subsequent depletion of host Langerhans' cells allows donor-derived hematopoietic cells to repopulate the skin. Retransplantation with stem cells plus donor T cells would then, theoretically, decrease the risk of cutaneous GVHD.[52,56]

Chronic GVHD

This profound disorder of immune regulation may evolve from aGVHD or develop de novo in about 20 to 30% of patients. It is characterized by global immune impairment and is seen in 33% of HLA-identical sibling transplants, 49% of HLA-identical related transplants, 64% of matched unrelated transplants, and 80% of 1-antigen HLA-nonidentical unrelated transplants.[57–62]

The exact pathogenesis of cGVHD is largely unknown and ambiguous. In addition to donor-derived alloreactive T cells that are important in aGVHD, post-thymic CD4+ T cells are thought to play an important role in cGVHD. The T-cell precursors may undergo aberrant "thymic education" after HSCT that effectively makes them self-reactive or autoreactive. Additionally, the activation of different helper T-cell subsets (Th1 in acute versus Th2 in cGVHD) may be responsible for distinct manifestations of acute and chronic GVHD. The role of alloreactivity versus autoreactivity in the pathogenesis of cGVHD remains highly controversial. Alloreactivity to minor histocompatibility antigens is believed by some to explain cGVHD as a late phase of aGVHD. On the other hand, the importance of autoreactivity is highlighted by clinical manifestations of cGVHD that frequently mimic those of autoimmune or collagen vascular diseases, the finding of autoantibodies in some patients, and experimental data suggesting the importance of thymic education and damage in the pathogenesis of cGVHD.[63]

Animal studies suggest that transforming growth factor (TGF)-β may be involved in the pathogenesis of cGVHD. Fibrosis in sclerodermatous GVHD may be driven by infiltrating TGF-β$_1$-producing mononuclear cells, and in the murine model, this may be prevented with antibodies to TGF-β given early in the disease. Human latency–associated peptide, a naturally occurring antagonist to TGF-β$_1$, inhibits its up-regulation as well as that of connective tissue growth factor messenger ribonucleic acids and type 1 collagen synthesis in the mouse and may be a potential new therapy in diseases characterized by dermal sclerosis.[64,65]

Clinical Manifestations

Acute Cutaneous GVHD

Depending on the type of transplant and the degree of histocompatibility, the eruption of aGVHD commonly develops 2 to 10 weeks post-transplantation (mean of 10 days) and has suggestive, but not always diagnostic, clinical and pathologic features. Conventionally, GVHD developing before 100 days is called acute.[34,66] Hyperacute forms of cutaneous GVHD, seen almost immediately post-transplantation, are often explosive in onset, as well as complicated by severe systemic involvement, erythroderma, and fever.[67] Cutaneous eruptions resembling aGVHD are sometimes seen after 100 days, especially after donor lymphocyte infusions or infections. They have also been reported with alterations in cyclosporine therapy. These acute-appearing skin changes may be accompanied by cGHVD in other target organs.[68]

Early cutaneous changes may include localized or generalized pruritus, dysesthesias, or pain on the palms, soles, and ears, often accompanied by subtle macular erythema and edema (Figure 1). Affected areas become progressively more edematous and violaceous, mimicking acral erythema or erythema multiforme (Figure 2). A maculopapular morbilliform eruption follows, which often starts on the trunk and becomes confluent (Figure 3) or even folliculocentric.[69] Histologically, follicular GVHD corresponds to involvement of the parafollicular bulge.[70] Erythroderma may result from damage to the epidermal barrier, with associated pruritus and pain. As the disease progresses, patients have difficulty regulating core body temperature and maintaining fluid and electrolyte balance and are at increased risk of infection. Resolution of the erythroderma is characterized by diffuse sunburn-like desquamation. Rarely, aGVHD may present with acquired ichthyosis or "fish scale"–

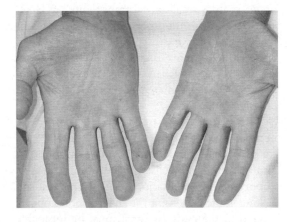

FIGURE 1 Acute graft-versus-host disease (GVHD). Macular erythema on the palm associated with early acute cutaneous GVHD.

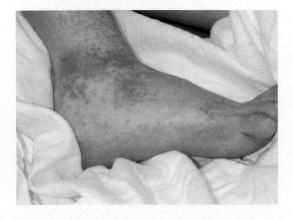

FIGURE 2 Acute graft-versus-host disease (GVHD). Erythema on the sole accompanied by the typical morbilliform eruption of acute cutaneous GVHD.

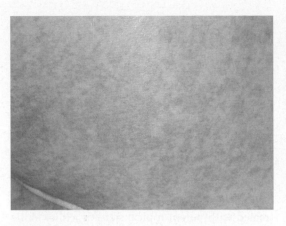

FIGURE 3 Acute graft-versus-host disease (GVHD). Morbilliform (measles-like) eruption of acute cutaneous GVHD.

like changes, which can be distinguished from acquired ichthyosis by biopsy. It is possible that such a condition has been underdiagnosed because acquired ichthyosis-like rashes are often not sampled.[71]

The formation of blisters and the detection of a positive Nikolsky sign (extension of epidermal denudation with pressure) are indicative of even more severe cutaneous disease.[72] Progression produces complete epidermal denudation consistent with toxic epidermal necrolysis (TEN), demonstrated in Figure 4. Loss of epidermal integrity in the setting of profound immunologic impairment places these patients at high risk of infection. The eye may also be severely involved (Figure 5), as well as other epithelial surfaces. Mucous membrane involvement is heralded by erythema, pain, or erosions and is often difficult to distinguish from the mucositis associated with chemotherapy or infection. Grade 3 and 4 GVHD produces bullae and epithelial denudation in the mouth, similar to that seen in TEN.

Localized bullous changes may coexist with a diffuse morbilliform papulosquamous eruption (Figure 6), stressing the importance of a comprehensive skin examination and directed skin biopsy. A clinical grading system as shown

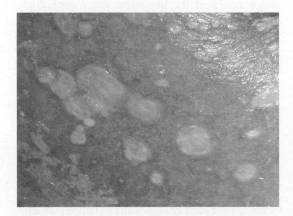

FIGURE 4 Toxic epidermal necrolysis/acute graft-versus-host disease. Islands of necrotic epidermis (white plaques) and exposed dermis.

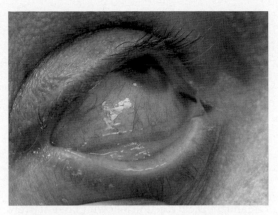

FIGURE 5 Graft-versus-host disease of the eye. Courtesy of Dr. Stella Kim.

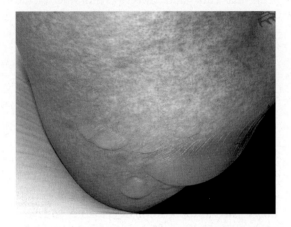

FIGURE 6 Bullous acute graft-versus-host disease (GVHD). Focal bullae associated with the morbilliform eruption of GVHD.

in Table 3[73] is used to define both the extent of involvement and the morphology of the skin changes.

Dyspigmentation of the skin is a postinflammatory change that is distressing to the patient and difficult to treat. Patchy depigmentation or vitiligo, although uncommon, may occur even in the setting of mild cutaneous disease, and the pathophysiology is unclear. Adoptive transfer of donor immunity has been implied when the donor has vitiligo, and the host subsequently develops the problem.[74]

Histopathologic Changes

Skin biopsies are routinely employed to diagnosis acute cutaneous GVHD. However, early changes are not specific and are often difficult to distin-

guish from those induced by chemotherapy, total-body irradiation, or infectious agents. In addition, epidermal changes may be focal and do not always correlate with the clinical presentation.[75,76] Since the importance of therapeutic intervention usually precedes the biopsy results by days, the benefit of serial skin biopsies is questionable.[75,77] However, biopsies are sometimes useful for confirmation of the clinical impression or when entertaining an alternative diagnosis.[78]

Vacuolar change at the basal cell layer is a nonspecific finding but may be the earliest manifestation of disease. As acute cutaneous GVHD progresses, variable intensities of dermal mononuclear cell infiltration, exocytosis (lymphocytes in the epidermis), and spongiosis (inter- and intracellular edema) appear. These changes are also nonspecific and may be found in drug and viral rashes, as well dermatitis. The presence of eosinophils has traditionally been thought to favor a hypersensitivity or drug eruption but also is variably present in GVHD. Therefore, overreliance on the presence of eosinophils to diagnose drug reaction versus GVHD may delay therapy.[77] As aGVHD progresses, dyskeratotic cells become prominent and may be associated with a contiguous or "satellite lymphocyte" (Figure 7).[79,80] Hair follicle and eccrine duct involvement is common, and the presence of necrotic keratinocytes in these locations is quite consistent with the diagnosis. In severe cases, the vacuolar change at the

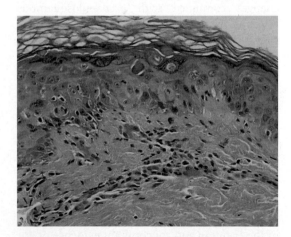

FIGURE 7 Pathology of acute graft-versus-host disease. There is vacuolar change at the dermal-epidermal junction, dyskeratosis, satellite cell necrosis, and an inflammatory infiltrate (grade 2). Courtesy of Dr. Victor Prieto.

Table 3 Overall Clinical Grading of Acute Graft-versus-Host Disease				
Grade	**Stage**			**Functional Impairment**
	Skin	*Liver*	*Gut*	
0 (none)	0	0	0	0
I (mild)	1–2	0	0	0
II (moderate)	1–3	1	1	1
III (severe)	2–3	2–3	2–3	2
IV (life threatening)	2–3	2–3	2–3	2–4

dermal-epidermal junction progress to clefts and then to complete separation of the epidermis from the dermis with epidermal necrosis. Lerner and colleagues standardized these pathologic changes into a useful four-stage grading system as illustrated in Table 4.[81] This grading system is generally reproducible among pathologists, with the most disparity reported in distinguishing grades 1 and 2.[82] It has been suggested that the current system be changed to include dermal lymphoid infiltration as an additional criterion for grade 2 GVHD.[83]

Differential Diagnosis

Early on, the changes of acute cutaneous GVHD are nonspecific. Other eruptions that start on the hands and feet, including acral erythema, must also be considered.[84] The latter is also characterized by pain and erythema of the palms and soles, often occurring after chemotherapy. The morbilliform rash classically associated with aGVHD is also commonly seen in drug and viral eruptions, particularly with human herpesvirus 6.[34] In an attempt to distinguish these entities, drug calendars and meticulous documentation of the onset and progression of the reaction are occasionally helpful. Cutaneous GVHD may be clinically, physiologically, and pathologically identical to erythema multiforme, a hypersensitivity reaction associated with a wide variety of causes. We have found that erythema multiforme–like histologic changes combined with a papulosquamous eruption in the appropriate clinical setting may suggest GVHD over other etiologies but are not diagnostic. Drug-induced erythema multiforme and TEN are often indistinguishable from grade 4 aGVHD. Immunophenotyping of TEN and aGVHD shows a predominance of CD8+ cells and similar serum cytokine profiles, with increased IL-10, TNF-α, and IL-6 in the serum compared with controls.[85,86] This is not surprising since both TEN and aGVHD probably have similar mechanisms of epidermal apoptosis, including the production of TNF-α[87] and dysregulation of Fas expression and/or signaling.[88] The clinical course of the eruption and concomitant evidence of gut or liver GVHD is sometimes necessary to confirm the diagnosis.[89,90]

The cutaneous eruption of lymphocyte recovery can also be mistaken for early cutaneous aGVHD. This maculopapular eruption occurs at the earliest recovery of peripheral lymphocytes, usually starting on the trunk and proximal extremities. It is associated with a sharp transient rise in temperature and nonspecific pathology, demonstrating a superficial perivascular mononuclear cell infiltrate.[91] This transient eruption is less likely to demonstrate necrotic keratinocytes and is self-limiting.

Follicular mucinosis has been reported as a rare and transient reaction following bone marrow transplantation for acute lymphocytic leukemia and is readily identified by biopsy.[92] Both leukemia cutis and Sweet's syndrome (acute febrile neutrophilic dermatosis) may present with erythematous lesions post-transplantation, which are diagnosed by their distinctive pathology.

Treatment of Acute Cutaneous GVHD

The initial management of aGVHD usually consists of corticosteroids. When these alone are ineffective, steroids in combination with cyclosporine[19,93] or, in the case of our center, tacrolimus[94–96] have been considered standard therapy for the initial management of acute GVHD.[19,93,97] Their mechanism of action is unclear but is probably related to suppression of cytokines and lymphocytic activities. Numerous dose schedules have been used in multiple clinical trials, but most centers use methylprednisolone at doses of 2.0 mg/kg. Higher doses are also effective but at the cost of significant side effects and severe catabolic damage, including hyperglycemia, fluid retention, muscular wasting, avascular bone necrosis, and increased rate of infectious complications.[19,93,97–99]

In steroid-refractory cases, antithymocyte globulin has been the most common form of immunosuppression used. Different studies have documented efficacy, but with significant morbidity and mortality, mainly owing to infectious complications.[99,100] Pentostatin, a nucleoside analogue that inhibits adenosine deaminase, is another immunosuppressant that has been increasingly used for the management of aGVHD.[93,101] Objective overall responses in up to

67% have been reported,[93] but the effect on overall survival remains unknown.[102] Other therapies, such as monoclonal antibodies, including daclizumab, visilizumab,[103] and infliximab,[104] as well as denileukin diftitox,[105] have been evaluated in the prevention and treatment of aGVHD, with variable response rates but so far no significant impact on the dismal prognosis of steroid-refractory acute GVHD.

Topical Treatment

Grade 1 and 2 cutaneous GVHD is frequently treated with potent topical steroids, either alone or with occlusion. For symptomatic or extensive disease, "wet wrap" therapy may provide symptomatic relief. Topical steroids are applied to the eruption, followed by warm moist towels, and the patient is then wrapped in a plastic covering followed by blankets to avoid chilling, for approximately 30 minutes. This occlusive dressing increases topical steroid absorption and hydrates the skin. Treatments are repeated several times a day until symptomatic improvement is observed. Over a variable period of time, topical steroid absorption under occlusive dressings may cause enough systemic absorption to cause typical glucocorticoid side effects, as well as striae and skin atrophy. Children are at higher risk than adults for these complications.

Ultraviolet (UV) light initiates inflammation when directed at normal skin but, paradoxically, is useful in treating inflammatory dermatoses.[106] GVHD may occur after UV exposure, prompting the use of sunscreens and photoprotection after HSCT. However, various wavelengths of light, including UVB (290–320 nm), UVA (320–400 nm), and, most recently, narrowband UVB (312 nm), have immunomodulating effects that are useful in the treatment of established disease.[107] UV exposure inhibits contact sensitivity and the proliferative responses of lymphoid cells to mitogens and alloantigens by inactivation of T lymphocytes and antigen-presenting cells. The mechanism of action is not completely known but may reflect the depletion and morphologic alterations of Langerhans' cells and modifications in their capacity to present antigens.[108] Keratinocytes further modify the inflammatory response by producing and releasing immunosuppressive cytokines after exposure to UVB and psoralen plus ultraviolet A (PUVA).[107,109–113]

For many years, psoralens, a photoactivating compound, and UVA light (PUVA) have been successfully employed to treat chronic cutaneous GVHD,[114] but few patients have received PUVA therapy for acute disease. This may change as PUVA has been found to be useful in treating grade 2 to 4 skin changes, thus enabling steroid taper.[115,116] Narrowband UVB therapy has also shown promise in treating acute skin disease in patients who do not respond to systemic

Grade	Histopathologic Features
0	Normal epidermis
1	Focal or diffuse vacuolar alteration of the basal cell layer
2	Grade 1 changes plus dyskeratotic squamous cells in the epidermis and/or hair follicle epithelium
3	Grade 2 changes plus subepidermal vesicle formation
4	Complete separation of the epidermis from the dermis

Table 4 Histopathologic Grading System for Acute Cutaneous Graft-versus-Host Reaction

Adapted from Lerner KG et al.[81]
In grades 1 to 4, there is usually a superficial perivascular lymphocytic infiltrate with exocytosis of these cells into the lower half of the epidermis.

immunosuppression.[112] This approach has the added advantage of avoiding administration of oral psoralens, which may cause nausea and require special protective eyewear to prevent cataracts. There is some evidence that UVB and possibly narrowband UVB therapy carry less risk for cutaneous carcinogenesis than PUVA.[117] However, as all ultraviolet exposure carries with it an increased risk of skin cancer, cumulative doses should be carefully monitored, and patients must have regular skin examinations.[112]

The topical calcineurin inhibitors tacrolimus and pimecrolimus are promising therapeutic agents for diseases characterized by cytokine-induced inflammation. These drugs down-regulate cytokine production by binding to the FK 506 binding protein (tacrolimus) or to macrophilin (pimecrolimus) and blocking calcineurin. This prevents the dephosphorylation necessary for transcription of cytokine genes.[118] Both of these topical medications are marketed as steroid-sparing agents in atopic dermatitis, and they do not cause cutaneous atrophy and striae. In contrast to topical steroids, they do not affect Langerhans' cells, are poorly absorbed, and have a low potential for immunosuppression.[119–121] The long-term side effects of these topical agents in immunosuppressed patients are not known, and large controlled studies have yet to be performed in GVHD.

Topical treatment for grade 3 and 4 GVHD involves supportive care, often in an intensive care setting or burn unit. These patients have severe epidermal necrosis and are subject to all of the complications associated with widespread first-degree body and mucosal burns. The necessity for immunosuppression and the presence of pancytopenia post-transplantation further complicate their treatment. As with TEN in healthy patients, meticulous skin care, antimicrobial agents as indicated, and appropriate dressings are imperative, along with attention to fluid and electrolyte balance.

Chronic Cutaneous GVHD

cGVHD is a multisystem disease with prominent cutaneous manifestations. Similarities to other autoimmune disorders, especially lichen planus, scleroderma, lupus erythematosus, and Sjögren's syndrome, are striking, and autoantibodies are variably present.[122] Skin changes may appear as early as day 31[123] or as late as 2 years after transplantation but most commonly appear at approximately 80 to 100 days. Disease activity may be triggered by infection, UVR, or even trauma. The hematologic system, liver, gastrointestinal tract, eyes, lung, and muscles are often involved, and patients may have problems with wasting. Eosinophilia may herald a flare of the disease in both acute and chronic disease.[77,124]

Classically, cutaneous cGVHD has been described as either lichenoid (lichen planus–like) or sclerodermatous. The lichenoid lesions of cGVHD may demonstrate the classic purple polygonal papules of lichen planus, with variable superficial scale. The distribution can be focal and become confluent (Figure 8), folliculocentric (Figure 9), or even dermatomal.[125] Vesicular lesions occasionally coexist with lichenoid papules and must be distinguished from herpes simplex or varicella-zoster virus superinfection.[126] Disfiguring postinflammatory hyperpigmentation is a common problem with both lichen planus and lichenoid GVHD, especially in darker-skinned individuals, and this may persist despite therapy (Figure 10).[127]

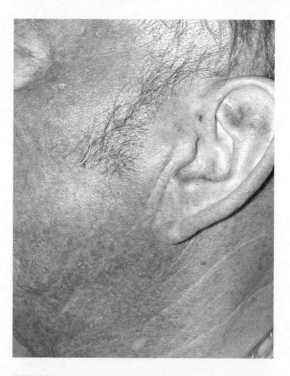

FIGURE 8 Confluent purple papules and plaques of chronic lichenoid graft-versus-host disease.

FIGURE 9 Follicular papules of chronic lichenoid graft-versus-host disease.

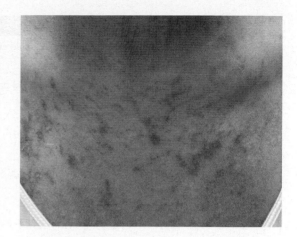

FIGURE 10 Postinflammatory changes of chronic lichenoid graft-versus-host disease.

Although lichenoid GVHD is the most commonly described nonsclerodermatous variant of chronic cutaneous disease, other presentations are possible and not uncommon. Because of the variety of presentations, we prefer to descriptively categorize the lesions of chronic cutaneous GVHD, as shown in Table 5. By specifically describing their morphology, we hope to ascertain which skin lesions are most amenable to a particular therapeutic modality.

Early on, the skin lesions are often subtle and the progression is insidious. Patients complain of photosensitivity, and ambient UV light may flare their disease. There may be marked xerosis (dry skin), or ichthyosis-like changes (Figure 11). As is the case with aGVHD, dyspigmentation may reflect postinflammatory changes or may herald the onset of vitiligo. Extensive loss of pigment after treatment with ganciclovir has been reported in a patient receiving donor T lymphocytes expressing herpes simplex virus thymidine kinase,[128] although adoptive immunity from the donor may also play a role.[74]

Other chronic eruptions that have traditionally been designated "lichenoid" are, in fact, quite polymorphous. Erythematous papules and plaques, some with scale, that are not as well defined as lichen planus are not uncommon. These may be lupus-like in distribution and appearance (Figure 12) or even reminiscent of aGVHD. The morphology and distribution of these plaques are sometimes pityriasiform (annular plaques demonstrating a branny scale) (Figure 13) or folliculocentric (Figure 14). Less common presentations include guttate (small drop-like lesions) (Figure 15) or plaque-like psoriasiform lesions, as well as eczematous plaques (Figure 16). cGVHD of the palms and soles occasionally develops deep-seated vesicles suggestive of hand and foot eczema. Acral keratoses have also been reported.[126,129] After donor lymphocyte infusions, the eruption is often morbilliform and indistinguishable from that seen in acute cutaneous GVHD.

Table 5 Skin Changes in Chronic Graft-versus-Host Disease

Clinical Presentation	Description	Variable Features
Xerosis	Dry skin	Follicular prominence
Lichenoid	Purple, polygonal papules and plaques	Scale
		Vesicles
		Follicular
		Localized or confluent
		Dermatomal
		Dyspigmentation
Papulosquamous	Scaly patches and plaques	Pityriasiform
		Dermatitic
		Localized or confluent
Ichthyosiform	"Fish scales"	Localized or confluent
Depigmention	Vitiligo-like	Localized or confluent
		Dermatomal
Psoriasiform	Well-circumcised lesions with a micaceous scale	Guttate
		Plaque-like
Localized sclerodermatous	Morpheaform plaques	Bullae
		Ulceration
		Follicular plugging
		Joint restrictions
		Poikiloderma
		Dermatomal
Widespread sclerodermatous	Widespread dermal fibrosis	Bullae
		Poikiloderma
		Ulceration
		Vascular tumors
		Joint restriction
		Leopard-like
Fasciitis	Edema, erythema, rippling, peau d'orange changes	Erythema
		Joint restriction
		Coexisting fibrosis
Nail	Various stages of dystrophy	Longitudinal ridging
		Onycholysis
		Pterygium
		Complete destruction
Scalp	Scaling, fibrosis, alopecia	Scarring or nonscarring
		Psoriasiform

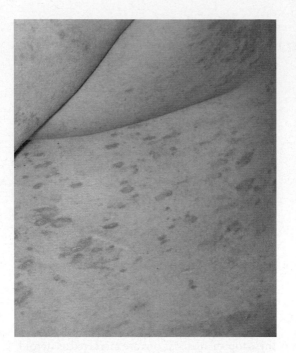

FIGURE 13 Pityriasiform chronic graft-versus-host disease.

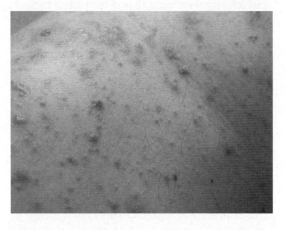

FIGURE 14 Erythematous, folliculocentric chronic graft-versus-host disease.

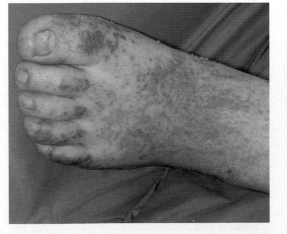

FIGURE 11 Ichthyotic chronic graft-versus-host disease.

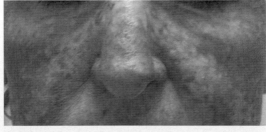

FIGURE 12 Lupus-like, "butterfly" eruption of chronic graft-versus-host disease.

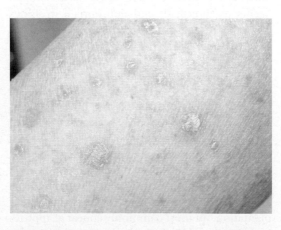

FIGURE 15 Guttate psoriasiform chronic graft-versus-host disease.

Sclerodermatous skin changes may develop concurrently with other lesions or de novo. In some cases, the onset is slow, with localized waxy, bound-down fibrotic plaques of morphea, preceded by variable erythema (Figure 17). The overlying epidermis develops poikilodermatous changes, with prominent atrophy, telangiectasia, and dyspigmentation. Follicular plugging may also be prominent. The skin may appear rippled with linear bands of fibrosis, possibly related to septal panniculitis (Figure 18). Leopard-like changes, with hyperpigmented, scaly macules, may be localized or widespread and precede the sclerotic eruption.[130] When widespread, diffuse sclerodermatous lesions are devastating, and patients are literally "hidebound" with limited mobility, cutaneous erosions, ulcers, and

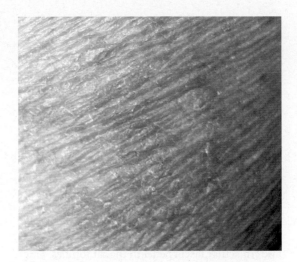

FIGURE 16 Papulosquamous chronic graft-versus-host disease.

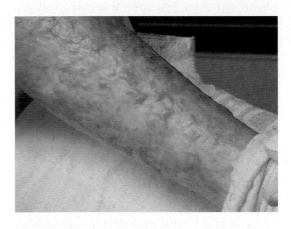

FIGURE 17 Sclerodermoid chronic graft-versus-host disease.

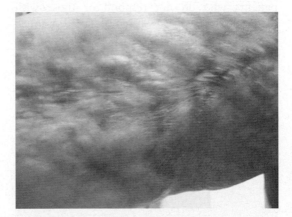

FIGURE 18 Rippled sclerodermoid chronic graft-versus-host disease.

infections. Thalidomide, which is sometimes used to treat this problem, may itself produce ulcers, possibly on the basis of its antiangiogenic properties.[131] Raynaud's phenomenon and acrosclerosis, although common in scleroderma, is infrequently seen in sclerodermatous GVHD.[34] A painful polyneuropathy may be associated with dermal

fibrosis.[132] Extensive sclerodermatous involvement of the thorax may contribute to the restrictive lung problems already associated with chronic pulmonary GVHD.

Alopecia and loss of skin appendages occur as the skin becomes more fibrotic, leading to decreased sweating and hair loss, often with an irreversible scarring alopecia. Rarely, chronic cutaneous GVHD occurs in a dermatomal distribution at the site of antecedent zoster eruption. This striking presentation may reflect changes in keratinocyte antigenicity owing to the virus.[133,134.]

The appearance of bullae heralds a particularly devastating variant of sclerodermatous GVHD and may be localized or widespread.[135] These lesions are not only uncomfortable but also are a nidus for infection, which is slow to heal because of immunosuppression, epidermal atrophy, and dermal fibrosis.

Nails are affected in 50% of patients with chronic cutaneous GVHD, demonstrating variable degrees of dystrophy, thickening, and onycholysis. Pterygium (matrix destruction and damage to the nail plate), similar to that seen in lichen planus, may develop (Figure 19) that affects single or multiple nail units. Longitudinal ridging is the most frequently observed change on both the fingernails and the toenails. Severe nail changes correlate with the duration of the disease and cause considerable morbidity for the patient.[136]

Abrupt and painful skin swelling associated with erythema and subcutaneous edema or a peau d'orange appearance characterizes fasciitis. This is a severe complication, with no specific immunogenetic profile, which resembles the eosinophilia-myalgia syndromes and is resistant to therapy.[137] Patients are functionally disabled,

with widespread skin tightness, joint limitation, and contractures (Figure 20). The face is usually spared, and this may occur independently or concurrently with sclerodermatous changes. Half of the patients also report myalgias, and laboratory evaluation demonstrates an eosinophilia.[137] A full-thickness biopsy through the fascia may be necessary to confirm the diagnosis. It is helpful to objectively document disease progression and treatment response by serial photographs, measurements of joint mobility, and noninvasive 20 MHz sonography.[138]

Mucous membrane are affected in approximately 80% of patients with cGVHD.[61] Oral pain and Sjögren's syndrome–like symptoms are a common and debilitating problem. The salivary glands are a target, resulting in xerostomia and dental caries after damage to major and minor salivary glands.[139] Symptoms of early oral GVHD include burning and erythema, which interferes with nutrition and quality of life. Because of the disturbance in the epidermal barrier, topical or oral antifungal prophylaxis is advisable, as are antiviral agents.

As the oral disease progresses, a lacy, white network called Wickham's striae develops on the buccal mucosa (Figure 21), lips (Figure 22), and palate. Although there may be some differences between oral lichen planus and lichenoid GVHD, both are most probably T cell mediated.[140] These mucosal and gingival lesions may become atrophic, erythematous, or erosive. Atrophy of the tongue is associated with shortened or absent lingual papillae,[34] although elongation of papillae, geographic tongue, and white nondetachable plaques are also seen (Figure 23). Esophageal

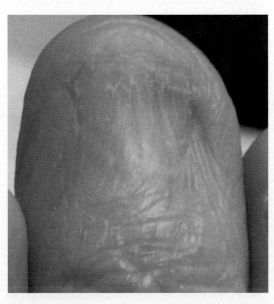

FIGURE 19 Destruction of the nail in chronic graft-versus-host disease.

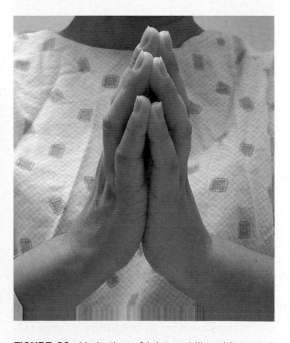

FIGURE 20 Limitation of joint mobility with associated fasciitis—the "prayer" sign.

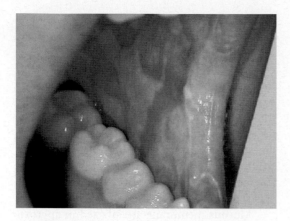

FIGURE 21 Buccal mucosal changes of chronic graft-versus-host disease.

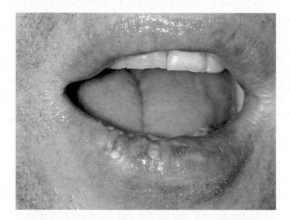

FIGURE 22 Labial lesions of chronic graft-versus-host disease.

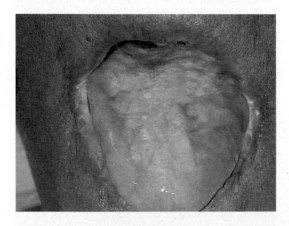

FIGURE 23 Chronic graft-versus-host disease of the tongue.

strictures may develop in conjunction with these mucosal problems. Chronic mucosal lichen planus and lichenoid GVHD may predispose patients to squamous cell carcinoma, and biopsies should be performed if this is suspected.[112,141]

Genital involvement affects sexuality and overall quality of life.[142] After stem cell transplantation, symptoms of inadequate estrogenization can occur secondary to premature ovarian failure, and this should be distinguished from early cGVHD. Vaginal GVHD develops an average of 10 months from transplantation, and symptoms may include dryness, excoriations, ulcerated or thickened mucosa, narrowed or obliterated introitus, frequent vaginal infections, and symptoms of dyspareunia.[143] Similarly, phimosis may occur in men. Topical vaginal treatment includes hormonal therapy, steroids, calcineurin inhibitors, or cyclosporine. Mucosal strictures, such as those of the esophagus, may require dilatation.

Skin Tumors and GVHD

Prolonged immunosuppression and conditioning regimens increase the risk of secondary malignancy of the skin and oral cavity.[144,145] Cutaneous tumors are usually squamous cell carcinoma, but the risk of basal cell carcinoma and melanoma is also increased. This is particularly a problem in individuals with actinic damage or those exposed to therapeutic ionizing irradiation.[146] The pathogenesis of the melanocytic malignancies is unclear as chemotherapy may stimulate nevus growth, but chronic cutaneous GVHD is associated with a decreased number of detectable nevi.[146] The long-term risk of melanoma may be increased when bone marrow transplantation is performed at a young age with a conditioning regimen high in alkylating drugs.[146] Benign vascular tumors have also been described[147] but are uncommon (Figure 24).

As is the case in lichen planus, there is an increased risk of squamous cell carcinoma of the oral mucosa. This may be complicated by coexisting papillomavirus infection. As these tumors may exhibit aggressive behavior, complete and regular skin and dental examinations are recommended.

Pathology of cGVHD

Early disease manifests the vacuolar changes, dyskeratotic cells, and mononuclear cell infiltrate seen in acute GVHD, and this infiltrate may be perifollicular or perineural.[34] Acanthosis, hypergranulosis, and hyperkeratosis are variably present in lichenoid disease, along with a

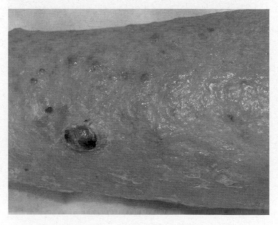

FIGURE 24 Benign vascular tumor associated with chronic graft-versus-host disease.

band-like infiltrate at the dermal-epidermal junction (Figure 25). The rete ridges demonstrate elongation or "sawtooth" changes. As in lichen planus, epidermal atrophy or erosive changes may be evident. Loss of appendages and dermal fat, epidermal atrophy, dermal fibrosis, sclerosis, and minimal infiltrate herald the development of sclerodermatous GVHD.[148] Pan-dermal and deep-dermal sclerosis are characteristic, along with mild vacuolar degeneration and dermal-epidermal junction. Follicular damage and plugging, as well as septal panniculitis, may be prominent.[130]

Patients with early fasciitis showed edema and fibrosis in the septa separating fat lobules and muscular fascia beneath the fat lobules. Later lesions demonstrate a dense lymphocytic infiltrate and thick fibrosis of the fascia.[137] Dermal sclerosis may coexist, as may septal panniculitis.[130] Mucin deposition interspersed between collagen bundles in the papillary and reticular dermis has been reported in association with severe chronic sclerodermoid changes.[149] Both sclerodermatous GVHD and scleroderma are characterized by extracellular matrix deposition of predominantly type 1 collagen. Ultrastructural differences, including absence of beaded filaments and the lack of pericapillary fibrosis, may distinguish the two.[34,150]

Treatment of cGVHD

First-line therapy combines cyclosporine[151,152] or tacrolimus[153] with methylprednisolone. With conventional treatment, the reported response rates have been around 50%, including complete and partial responders. As in the case of aGVHD, patients who do not respond or those with incomplete responses will require an additional, systemic, "steroid-sparing" modality. Some of the most commonly used steroid-sparing immunosuppressants include thalidomide,[154] mycophenolate mofetil,[155,156] sirolimus,[157] and,

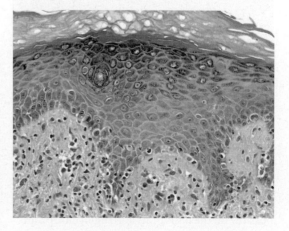

FIGURE 25 Pathology of lichenoid graft-versus-host disease. Note the prominent granular layer, "sawtooth" rete ridges, and dyskeratotic keratinocytes. Courtesy of Dr. Victor Prieto.

more recently, extracorporeal photochemotherapy.[158] All of these modalities have shown activity in small series of patients but were never compared in terms of efficacy. Sirolimus and extracorporeal photochemotherapy have shown promising response rates in the treatment of cutaneous manifestations of cGVHD, particularly sclerodermoid forms. Pain management and psychological support are often necessary for this devastating problem.

Topical Therapy

Topical steroids are routinely used to treat the lichenoid and papulosquamous changes, either alone or under occlusion. Chronic use of topical steroids has the potential to exacerbate the epidermal atrophy or problems with infection. The topical calcineurin inhibitors tacrolimus and pimecrolimus have enjoyed some degree of success in treating the erythema and pruritus of steroid-refractory, chronic cutaneous GVHD in selected patients. These agents are often used in conjunction with systemic therapies, including PUVA and extracorporeal photopheresi.[90,118,119,159] The optimal combination of topical therapeutic modalities is not currently known.

UVR is a useful therapeutic adjunct in certain types of chronic cutaneous GVHD. PUVA,[114,160] PUVA-bath photochemotherapy,[161] and UVA-1 (340–400 nm), alone or combined with other immunosuppressants, may be beneficial.[162] Therapeutic UVB or narrowband UVB has also demonstrated some efficacy.[163] Systemic retinoids have been reported to increase the range of motion, flatten cutaneous lesions, and improve the overall performance status of some patients.[164] Retinoids may act via induction of collagenase activity in fibroblasts or inhibition of fibroblast growth and decreased collagen production in dermal fibroblasts.[165]

Other novel therapies include the use of halofuginone cream. Halofuginone, used to treat coccidiosis in commercial poultry production,[166] is an inhibitor of collagen alpha1(I) gene expression and may inhibit de novo synthesis of collagen on a transcriptional level. The fibroblasts are targeted, and the effect is restricted to dermal fibroblasts. Other proliferating cells, such as keratinocytes, are not affected.[167,168] When applied daily on the left side of the neck and shoulder in one patient with sclerodermatous GVHD, collagen alpha1(I) gene expression, collagen synthesis, and collagen content in skin biopsy specimens were decreased, accompanied by increased neck rotation on the treated side. After cessation of treatment, the sclerosis, skin tightness, and collagen alpha1(I) gene expression returned to baseline levels. No adverse effects were observed, and no plasma levels of the drug were detected.[168]

Oral GVHD

Oral lichenoid cGVHD, like oral lichen planus, is debilitating and difficult to treat. Once an infectious etiology has been excluded, topical steroids, often in the form of dexamethasone mouthwash or rinses, are the mainstay of treatment, along with antifungal and antiviral prophylaxis. As is the case in lichen planus, topical tacrolimus is potentially beneficial in the management of patients with this difficult problem,[169–171] with improvement reported within days to weeks. The major side effect noted by the patients is a burning sensation, and blood levels were very low or undetectable.[171] In some cases, the topical tacrolimus was even more effective for this problem than the systemic drug. Long-term effects, including the risk of intraoral neoplasia, are not yet known. Intraoral PUVA has been tried using a glass fiber extension of a UVA source.[118,172,173] Intraoral UVB irradiation may also be a potential treatment of resistant chronic oral GVHD.[117]

Vaginal GVHD may be treated with topical cyclosporine, which appears to be more efficacious than when used for intraoral disease. Lubricants, dilators, and surgical lysis also may ultimately be needed.[143] Topical calineurin inhibitors may prove useful for recalcitrant cases, but no controlled studies have been performed.

Future Directions

The indications for stem cell transplantation have increased in recent years, as have the number of transplants. To decrease the risk of GVHD, molecular matching of donor and host has replaced the older cellular or serologic techniques. Refinements in conditioning regimens, graft manipulation, and engineering, as well as stem cell sources, have made stem cell transplantation the treatment of choice for many diseases. GVHD, although often an undesirable effect of transplantation, has an antitumor effect that is used to treat relapsed malignancies. The goal is to control the reaction so that remission is maintained without unwanted side effects. Successful identification of the pathogenesis and improved treatment options will have far-reaching repercussions, not only for GVHD but also for other immunologic diseases.

Skin GVHD is common after HSCT and is associated with acute and chronic problems. Severe cutaneous disease produces significant quality of life issues, as well as chronic infections, deformities, and secondary skin tumors. In addition, the cosmetic sequelae of GVHD are often psychologically devastating. A multidisciplinary team approach is often helpful in the diagnosis, treatment, and complications of this disease.

REFERENCES

1. Horrowitz M. Uses and growth of hematopoietic cell transplantation. In: Blume KG, Forman SJ, Appelbaum FR, eds. Thomas'Hematopoietic Cell Transplantation. 3rd ed. Malden, Mass: Blackwell; 2004:9–15

2. Giralt SA, Champlin RE. Leukemia relapse after allogeneic bone marrow transplantation: a review. Blood 1994; 84:3603–12.

3. Slavin S, Morecki S, Weiss L, et al. Immunotherapy of hematologic malignancies and metastatic solid tumors in experimental animals and man. Crit Rev Oncol Hematol 2003;462:139–63.

4. Talmadge JE. Hematopoietic stem cell graft manipulation as a mechanism of immunotherapy. Int Immunopharmacol 2003;38:1121–43.

5. Couriel DR, Saliba RM, Giralt S, et al. Acute and chronic graft-versus-host disease after ablative and nonmyeloablative conditioning for allogeneic hematopoietic transplantation. Biol Blood Marrow Transplant 2004;103: 178–85.

6. Mielcarek M, Martin PJ, Leisenring W, et al. Graft-versus-host disease after nonmyeloablative versus conventional hematopoietic stem cell transplantation. Blood 2003; 102:756–62.

7. Beatty PG, Clift RA, Mickelson EM, et al. Marrow transplantation from related donors other than HLA-identical siblings. N Engl J Med 1985;313:765–71.

8. Nash RA, Pepe MS, Storb R, et al. Acute graft-versus-host disease: analysis of risk factors after allogeneic marrow transplantation and prophylaxis with cyclosporine and methotrexate. Blood 1992;80:1838–45.

9. Weisdorf D, Hakke R, Blazar B, et al. Risk factors for acute graft-versus-host disease in histocompatible donor bone marrow transplantation. Transplantation 1991;51: 1197–203.

10. Goulmy E, Voogt P, van Els C, et al. The role of minor histocompatibility antigens in GVHD and rejection: a mini-review. Bone Marrow Transplant 1991;7 Suppl 1:49–51.

11. Kollman C, Howe CW, Anasetti C, et al. Donor characteristics as risk factors in recipients after transplantation of bone marrow from unrelated donors: the effect of donor age. Blood 2001;98:2043–51.

12. Cutler C, Giri S, Jeyapalan S, et al. Acute and chronic graft-versus-host disease after allogeneic peripheral-blood stem-cell and bone marrow transplantation: a meta-analysis. J Clin Oncol 2001;19:3685–91.

13. Przepiorka D, Smith TL, Folloder J, et al. Risk factors for acute graft-versus-host disease after allogeneic blood stem cell transplantation. Blood 1999;94:1465–70.

14. Goggins TF, Chao N. Depletion of host reactive T cells by photodynamic cell purging and prevention of graft versus host disease. Leuk Lymphoma 2003;44:1871–9.

15. Przepiorka D, Weisdorf D, Martin P, et al. 1994 Consensus conference on acute GVHD grading. Bone Marrow Transplant 1995;15:825–8.

16. Ferrara JL, Deeg HJ. Graft-versus-host disease. N Engl J Med 1991;324:667–74.

17. Vogelsang GB, Lee L, Bensen-Kennedy DM. Pathogenesis and treatment of graft-versus-host disease after bone marrow transplant. Annu Rev Med 2003;54:29–52.

18. Mazariegos GV, Abu-Elmagd K, Jaffe R, et al. Graft versus host disease in intestinal transplantation. Am J Transplant 2004;49:1459–65.

19. Martin PJ, Schoch G, Fisher L, et al. A retrospective analysis of therapy for acute graft-versus-host disease: initial treatment. Blood 1990;76:1464–72.

20. Goker H, Haznedaroglu IC, Chao NJ. Acute graft-vs-host disease: pathobiology and management. Exp Hematol 2001;29:259–77.

21. Gajewski J, Champlin R. Bone marrow transplantation from unrelated donors. Curr Opin Oncol 1996;8:84–8.

22. Basara N, Kiehl MG, Fauser AA. New therapeutic modalities in the treatment of graft-versus-host disease. Crit Rev Oncol Hematol 2001;38:129–38.

23. Chao NJ, Schlegel PG. Prevention and treatment of graft-versus-host disease. Ann N Y Acad Sci 1995;770: 130–40.

24. Billingham RE. The biology of graft-versus-host reactions. Harvey Lect 1966;62:21–78.

25. Goulmy E, Schipper R, Pool J, et al. Mismatches of minor histocompatibility antigens between HLA-identical donors and recipients and the development of graft-versus-host disease after bone marrow transplantation. N Engl J Med 1996;334:281–5.

26. Tokime K, Isoda K, Yamanaka K, et al. A case of acute graft-versus-host disease following autologous peripheral blood stem cell transplantation. J Dermatol 2000;27:446–9.

27. Hess AD. Autologous graft-versus-host disease. J Hematother Stem Cell Res 2000;93:297.

28. Sica S, Chiusolo P, Salutari P, et al. Autologous graft-versus-host disease after CD34+-purified autologous peripheral blood progenitor cell transplantation. J Hematother Stem Cell Res 2000;93:375–9.

29. Fischer AC, Hess AD. Age-related factors in cyclosporine-induced syngeneic graft-versus-host disease: regulatory role of marrow-derived T lymphocytes. J Exp Med 1990;172:85–94.
30. Jarvis M, Marzolini M, Wang XN, et al. Heat shock protein 70: correlation of expression with degree of graft-versus-host response and clinical graft-versus-host disease. Transplantation 2003;76:849–53.
31. Rhoades JL, Cibull ML, Thompson JS, et al. Role of natural killer cells in the pathogenesis of human acute graft-versus-host disease. Transplantation 1993;56:113–20.
32. Gilliam AC. Update on graft versus host disease. J Invest Dermatol 2004;123:251–7.
33. Asagoe K, Takahashi K, Yoshino T, et al. Numerical, morphological and phenotypic changes in Langerhans cells in the course of murine graft-versus-host disease. Br J Dermatol 2001;145:918–27.
34. Aractingi S, Chosidow O. Cutaneous graft-versus-host disease. Arch Dermatol 1998;134:602–12.
35. Horn TD. Effector cells in cutaneous graft-versus-host disease. Who? What? When? Where? How? Br J Dermatol 1999;141:779–80.
36. Hofmeister CC, Quinn A, Cooke KR, et al. Graft-versus-host disease of the skin: life and death on the epidermal edge. Biol Blood Marrow Transplant 2004;106:366–72.
37. Ferrara JL. Pathogenesis of acute graft-versus-host disease: cytokines and cellular effectors. J Hematother Stem Cell Res 2000;93:299–306.
38. Teshima T, Ferrara JL. Understanding the alloresponse: new approaches to graft-versus-host disease prevention. Semin Hematol 2002;39:15–22.
39. Socie G, Stone JV, Wingard JR, et al. Long-term survival and late deaths after allogeneic bone marrow transplantation. Late Effects Working Committee of the International Bone Marrow Transplant Registry. N Engl J Med 1999; 34:14–21.
40. Giralt S, Hester J, Huh Y, et al. CD8-depleted donor lymphocyte infusion as treatment for relapsed chronic myelogenous leukemia after allogeneic bone marrow transplantation. Blood 1995;86:4337–43.
41. Ferrara JL. Cytokine inhibitors and graft-versus-host disease. Ann N Y Acad Sci 1995;770:227–36.
42. Kojima H, Shinohara N, Hanaoka S, et al. Two distinct pathways of specific killing revealed by perforin mutant cytotoxic T lymphocytes. Immunity 1994;15:357–64.
43. Graubert TA, DiPersio JF, Russell JH, et al. Perforin/granzyme-dependent and independent mechanisms are both important for the development of graft-versus-host disease after murine bone marrow transplantation. J Clin Invest 1997;1004:904–11.
44. Tsukada N, Kobata T, Aizawa Y, et al. Graft-versus-leukemia effect and graft-versus-host disease can be differentiated by cytotoxic mechanisms in a murine model of allogeneic bone marrow transplantation. Blood 1999;93:2738–47.
45. Sedghizadeh PP, Allen CM, Anderson KE, et al. Oral graft-versus-host disease and programmed cell death: pathogenetic and clinical correlates. Oral Surg Oral Med Oral Pathol Oral Radiol Endod 2004;97:491–8.
46. Kim JC, Whitaker-Menezes D, Deguchi M, et al. Novel expression of vascular cell adhesion molecule-1 (CD 106) by squamous epithelium in experimental acute graft-versus-host disease. Am J Pathol 2002;161:173.
47. Whitaker-Menezes D, Jones SC, Friedman TM, et al. An epithelial target site in experimental graft-versus-host disease and cytokine-mediated cytotoxicity is defined by cytokeratin 15 expression. Biol Blood Marrow Transplant 2003;99:559–70.
48. Shen N, French P, Guyotat D, et al. Expression of adhesion molecules in endothelial cells during allogeneic bone marrow transplantation. Eur J Haematol 1994;525: 296–301.
49. Sackstein R, Messina JL, Elfenbein GJ. In vitro adherence of lymphocytes to dermal endothelium under shear stress: implications in pathobiology and steroid therapy of acute cutaneous GVHD. Blood 2003;101:771–8.
50. Milinkovic M, Antin JH, Hergrueter CA, et al. CD44-hyaluronic acid interactions mediate shear-resistant binding of lymphocytes to dermal endothelium in acute cutaneous GVHD. Blood 2004;103:740–2.
51. Behar E, Chao NJ, Hiraki DD, et al. Polymorphism of adhesion molecule CD31 and its role in acute graft-versus-host disease. N Engl J Med 1996;334:286–91.
52. Merad M, Hoffmann P, Ranheim E, et al. Depletion of host Langerhans cells before transplantation of donor alloreactive T cells prevents skin graft-versus-host disease. Nat Med 2004;10:510–7.
53. Merad M, Manz MG, Karsunky H, et al. Langerhans cells renew in the skin throughout life under steady-state conditions. Nat Immunol 2002;3:1135–41.
54. Teshima T, Ordemann R, Reddy P, et al. Acute graft-versus-host disease does not require alloantigen expression on host epithelium. Nat Med 2002;8:575–81.
55. Banchereau J, Briere F, Caux C, et al. Immunobiology of dendritic cells. Annu Rev Immunol 2000;18:767–811.
56. Emerson SG. Tanning before transplant: lancing the Langerhans cell. Nat Med 2004;10:451–2.
57. Storek J, Gooley T, Siadak M, et al. Allogeneic peripheral blood stem cell transplantation may be associated with a high risk of chronic graft-versus-host disease. Blood 1997;90:4705–9.
58. Beatty PG, Hansen JA, Longton GM, et al. Marrow transplantation from HLA-matched unrelated donors for treatment of hematologic malignancies. Transplantation 1991;51:443–7.
59. Gaziev D, Polchi P, Galimberti M, et al. Graft-versus-host disease after bone marrow transplantation for thalassemia: an analysis of incidence and risk factors. Transplantation 1997;63:854–60.
60. Urbano-Ispizua A, Garcia-Conde J, Brunet S, et al. High incidence of chronic graft versus host disease after allogeneic peripheral blood progenitor cell transplantation. The Spanish Group of Allo-PBPCT. Haematologica 1997;82:683–9.
61. Sullivan KM, Shulman HM, Storb R, et al. Chronic graft-versus-host disease in 52 patients: adverse natural course and successful treatment with combination immunosuppression. Blood 1981;57:267–76.
62. Martin PJ, Hansen JA, Torok-Storb B, et al. Graft failure in patients receiving T cell-depleted HLA-identical allogeneic marrow transplants. Bone Marrow Transplant 1988;3:445–56.
63. Vogelsang GB. How I treat chronic graft-versus-host disease. Blood 2001;97:1196–201.
64. Zhang Y, McCormick LL, Gilliam AC. Latency-associated peptide prevents skin fibrosis in murine sclerodermatous graft-versus-host disease, a model for human scleroderma. J Invest Dermatol 2003;121:713–9.
65. Zhang Y, McCormick LL, Desai SR, et al. Murine sclerodermatous graft-versus-host disease, a model for human scleroderma: cutaneous cytokines, chemokines, and immune cell activation. J Immunol 2002;168:3088–98.
66. Farmer ER. Human cutaneous graft-versus-host disease. J Invest Dermatol 1985;85 Suppl:124s–8s.
67. Kim DH, Sohn SK, Kim JG, et al. Clinical impact of hyperacute graft-versus-host disease on results of allogeneic stem cell transplantation. Bone Marrow Transplant 2004;33:1025–30.
68. Valks R, Fernandez-Herrera J, Bartolome B, et al. Late appearance of acute graft-vs-host disease after suspending or tapering immunosuppresive drugs. Arch Dermatol 2001;137:61–5.
69. Friedman KJ, LeBoit PE, Farmer ER. Acute follicular graft-vs-host reaction. A distinct clinicopathologic presentation. Arch Dermatol 1988;124:688–91.
70. Sale GE, Beauchamp M. Parafollicular hair bulge in human GVHD: a stem cell-rich primary target. Bone Marrow Transplant 1993;11:223–5.
71. Chao SC, Tsao CJ, Liu CL, et al. Acute cutaneous graft-versus-host disease with ichthyosiform features. Br J Dermatol 1998;139:553–5.
72. Hood AF, Soter NA, Rappeport J, et al. Graft-versus-host reaction. Cutaneous manifestations following bone marrow transplantation. Arch Dermatol 1977;113: 1087–91.
73. Glucksberg H, Storb R, Fefer A, et al. Clinical manifestations of graft-versus-host disease in human recipients of marrow from HL-A-matched sibling donors. Transplantation 1974;18:295–304.
74. Alajlan A, Alfadley A, Pedersen KT. Transfer of vitiligo after allogeneic bone marrow transplantation. J Am Acad Dermatol 2002;46:606–10.
75. Zhou Y, Barnett MJ, Rivers JK. Clinical significance of skin biopsies in the diagnosis and mangement of grraft-vs-host disease in early postallogeneic bone marrow transplantation. Arch Dermatol 2000;136:717–21.
76. Hymes SR, Farmer ER, Lewis PG, et al. Cutaneous graft-versus-host reaction: prognostic features seen by light microscopy. J Am Acad Dermatol 1985;12:468–74.
77. Marra DE, McKee PHN, Ghiem P. Tissue eosinophils and the perils of using skin biopsy specimens to distinguish between drug hypersensitivity and cutaneous graft-versus-host disease. J Am Acad Dermatol 2004;51: 543–6.
78. Farmer E. Why a skin biopsy? Arch Dermatol 2000;136: 779–80.
79. Slavin RE, Santos GW. The graft versus host reaction in man after bone marrow transplantation: pathology, pathogenesis, clinical features, and implication. Clin Immunol Immunopathol 1973;14:472–98.
80. Hymes SR, Farmer ER, Lewis PG, et al. Cutaneous graft-versus-host reaction: prognostic features seen by light microscopy. J Am Acad Dermatol 1985;12:468–74.
81. Lerner KG, Kao GF, Storb R, et al. Histopathology of graft-vs.-host reaction (GvHR) in human recipients of marrow from HL-A-matched sibling donors. Transplant Proc 1974;64:367–71.
82. Massi D, Franchi A, Pimpinelli N, et al. A reappraisal of the histopathologic criteria for the diagnosis of cutaneous allogeneic acute graft-vs-host disease. Am J Clin Pathol 1999;112:791–800.
83. Horn TD, Bauer DJ, Vogelsang GB, et al. Reappraisal of histologic features of the acute cutaneous graft-versus-host reaction based on an allogeneic rodent model. J Invest Dermatol 1994;103:206–10.
84. Ruiz-Genao DP, GF-Villata MJ, Penas PF, et al. Pustular acral erythema in a patient with acute graft-versus-host disease. J Eur Acad Dermatol Venereol 2003;175:550–3.
85. Correia O, Delgado L, Barbosa IL, et al. CD8+ lymphocytes in the blister fluid of severe acute cutaneous graft-versus-host disease: further similarities with toxic epidermal necrolysis. Dermatology 2001;203:212–6.
86. Correia O, Delgado L, Barbosa IL, et al. Increased interleukin 10, tumor necrosis factor alpha, and interleukin 6 levels in blister fluid of toxic epidermal necrolysis. J Am Acad Dermatol 2002;47:58–62.
87. Langley RG, Walsh N, Nevill T, et al. Apoptosis is the mode of keratinocyte death in cutaneous graft-versus-host disease. J Am Acad Dermatol 1996;35 Pt 1:187–90.
88. Wehrli P, Viard I, Bullani R, et al. Death receptors in cutaneous biology and disease. J Invest Dermatol 2000;115: 141–8.
89. Villada G, Roujeau JC, Cordonnier C, et al. Toxic epidermal necrolysis after bone marrow transplantation: study of nine cases. J Am Acad Dermatol 1990;23 Pt 1:870–5.
90. Choi CJ, Nghiem P. Tacrolimus ointment in the treatment of chronic cutaneous graft-vs-host disease: a case series of 18 patients. Arch Dermatol 2001;137:1202–6.
91. Horn TD, Redd JV, Karp JE, et al. Cutaneous eruptions of lymphocyte recovery. Arch Dermatol 1989;125:1512–7.
92. Lee KK, Lee JY, Tsai YM, et al. Follicular mucinosis occurring after bone marrow transplantation in a patient with acute lymphoblastic leukemia. J Formos Med Assoc 2004;103:63–6.
93. Jacobsohn DA, Vogelsang GB. Novel pharmacotherapeutic approaches to prevention and treatment of GVHD. Drugs 2002;62:879–89.
94. Przepiorka D, Devine S, Fay J, et al. Practical considerations in the use of tacrolimus for allogeneic marrow transplantation. Bone Marrow Transplant 1999;24:1053–6.
95. Przepiorka D, Petropoulos D, Mullen CA, et al. Tacrolimus for prevention of graft-versus-host disease after mismatched unrelated donor cord blood transplantation. Bone Marrow Transplant 1999;23:1291–5.
96. Nash RA, Antin JH, Karanes C, et al. Phase 3 study comparing methotrexate and tacrolimus with methotrexate and cyclosporine for prophylaxis of acute graft-versus-host disease after marrow transplantation from unrelated donors. Blood 2000;96:2062–8.
97. Goker H, Haznedaroglu IC, Chao NJ. Acute graft-vs-host disease: pathobiology and management. Exp Hematol 2001;29:259–77.
98. Ruutu T, Hermans J, van Biezen A, et al. How should corticosteroids be used in the treatment of acute GVHD? EBMT Chronic Leukemia Working Party. European Group for Blood and Marrow Transplantation. Bone Marrow Transplant 1998;22:614–5.
99. Ruutu T, Niederwieser D, Gratwohl A, et al. A survey of the prophylaxis and treatment of acute GVHD in Europe: a report of the European Group for Blood and Marrow, Transplantation (EBMT). Chronic Leukaemia Working Party of the EBMT. Bone Marrow Transplant 1997; 19:759–64.
100. Roy J, McGlave PB, Filipovich AH, et al. Acute graft-versus-host disease following unrelated donor marrow transplantation: failure of conventional therapy. Bone Marrow Transplant 1992;10:77–82.
101. Vogelsang GB. Advances in the treatment of graft-versus-host disease. Leukemia 2000;14:509–10.
102. Przepiorka D, Kernan NA, Ippoliti C, et al. Daclizumab, a humanized anti-interleukin-2 receptor alpha chain

antibody, for treatment of acute graft-versus-host disease. Blood 2000;95:83–9.
103. Carpenter PA, Appelbaum FR, Corey L, et al. A humanized non-FcR-binding anti-CD3 antibody, visilizumab, for treatment of steroid-refractory acute graft-versus-host disease. Blood 2002;99:2712–9.
104. Couriel DR, Saliba R, Hicks K, et al. Tumor necrosis factor alpha blockade for the treatment of steroid-refractory acute GVHD. Blood 2004;104:649–54.
105. Ho VT, Zahrieh D, Hochberg E, et al. Safety and efficacy of denileukin diftitox in patients with steroid-refractory acute graft-versus-host disease after allogeneic hematopoietic stem cell transplantation. Blood 2004;104:1224–6.
106. Ozawa M, Ferenczi K, Kikuchi T, et al. 312-nanometer ultraviolet B light (narrow-band UVB) induces apoptosis of T cells within psoriatic lesions. J Exp Med 1999;189:711–8.
107. Kripke ML, Morison WL, Parrish JA. Systemic suppression of contact hypersensitivity in mice by psoralen plus UVA radiation (PUVA). J Invest Dermatol 1983;81:87–92.
108. Ashworth J, Kahan MC, Breathnach SM. PUVA therapy decreases HLA-DR+ CD1a+ Langerhans cells and epidermal cell antigen-presenting capacity in human skin, but flow cytometrically-sorted residual HLA-DR+ CD1a+ Langerhans cells exhibit normal alloantigen-presenting function. Br J Dermatol 1989;120:329–39.
109. Kim TY, Kripke ML, Ullrich SE. Immunosuppression by factors released from UV-irradiated epidermal cells: selective effects on the generation of contact and delayed hypersensitivity after exposure to UVA or UVB radiation. J Invest Dermatol 1990;94:26–32.
110. Kang K, Hammerberg C, Meunier L, et al. CD11b+ macrophages that infiltrate human epidermis after in vivo ultraviolet exposure potently produce IL-10 and represent the major secretory source of epidermal IL-10 protein. J Immunol 1994;153:5256–4.
111. Krueger JG, Wolfe JT, Nabeya RT, et al. Successful ultraviolet B treatment of psoriasis is accompanied by a reversal of keratinocyte pathology and by selective depletion of intraepidermal T cells. J Exp Med 1995;182:2057–68.
112. Grundmann-Kollmann M, Martin H, Ludwig R, et al. Narrowband UV-B phototherapy in the treatment of cutaneous graft versus host disease. Transplantation 2002;74:1631–4.
113. Cooper KD. Cell-mediated immunosuppressive mechanisms induced by UV radiation. Photochem Photobiol 1996; 63:400–6.
114. Hymes SR, Morison WL, Farmer ER, et al. Methoxsalen and ultraviolet A radiation in treatment of chronic cutaneous graft-versus-host reaction. J Am Acad Dermatol 1985; 12 Pt 1:30–7.
115. Wiesmann A, Weller A, Lischka G, et al. Treatment of acute graft-versus-host disease with PUVA (psoralen and ultraviolet irradiation): results of a pilot study. Bone Marrow Transplant 1999;23:151–5.
116. Furlong T, Leisenring W, Storb R, et al. Psoralen and ultraviolet A irradiation (PUVA) as therapy for steroid-resistant cutaneous acute graft-versus-host disease. Biol Blood Marrow Transplant 2002;8:206–12.
117. Elad S, Garfunkel AA, Enk CD, et al. Ultraviolet B irradiation: a new therapeutic concept for the management of oral manifestations of graft-versus-host disease. Oral Surg Oral Med Oral Pathol Oral Radiol Endod 1999; 88:44–50.
118. Elad S, Or R, Resnick I, et al. Topical tacrolimus—a novel treatment alternative for cutaneous chronic graft-versus-host disease. Transpl Int 2003;16:665–70.
119. Ziemer M, Gruhn B, Thiele JJ, et al. Treatment of extensive chronic cutaneous graft-versus-host disease in an infant with topical pimecrolimus. J Am Acad Dermatol 2004; 50:946–8.
120. Stander S, Luger TA. [Antipruritic effects of pimecrolimus and tacrolimus]. Hautarzt 2003;54:413–7.
121. Stuetz A, Grassberger M, Meingassner JG. Pimecrolimus (Elidel, SDZ ASM 981)—preclinical pharmacologic profile and skin selectivity. Semin Cutan Med Surg 2001;20:233–41.
122. Rouquette-Gally AM, Boyeldieu D, Prost AC, et al. Autoimmunity after allogeneic bone marrow transplantation. A study of 53 long-term-surviving patients. Transplantation 1988;46:238–40.
123. Ringden O, Paulin T, Lonnqvist B, Nilsson B. An analysis of factors predisposing to chronic graft-versus-host disease. Exp Hematol 1985;13:1062–7.
124. Nghiem P. The "drug vs graft-vs-host disease" conundrum gets tougher, but there is an answer: the challenge to dermatologists. Arch Dermatol 2001;137:75–6.
125. Beers B, Kalish RS, Kaye VN, et al. Unilateral linear lichenoid eruption after bone marrow transplantation: an unmasking of tolerance to an abnormal keratinocyte clone? J Am Acad Dermatol 1993;28 Pt 2:888–92.
126. Schauder CS, Hymes SR, Rapini RP, et al. Vesicular graft-versus-host disease. Int J Dermatol 1992;31:509–10.
127. Aractingi S, Janin A, Devergie A, et al. Histochemical and ultrastructural study of diffuse melanoderma after bone marrow transplantation. Br J Dermatol 1996;134:325–31.
128. Aubin F, Cahn JY, Ferrand C, et al. Extensive vitiligo after ganciclovir treatment of GvHD in a patient who had received donor T cells expressing herpes simplex virus thymidine kinase. Lancet 2000;355:626–7.
129. Kossard S, Ma DD. Acral keratotic graft versus host disease simulating warts. Australas J Dermatol 1999;40:161–3.
130. Penas PF, Jones-Caballero M, Aragues M, et al. Sclerodermatous graft-vs-host disease: clinical and pathological study of 17 patients. Arch Dermatol 2002;138:924–34.
131. Schlossberg H, Klumpp T, Sabol P, et al. Severe cutaneous ulceration following treatment with thalidomide for GVHD. Bone Marrow Transplant 2001;27:229–30.
132. Aractingi S, Socie G, Devergie A, et al. Localized scleroderma-like lesions on the legs in bone marrow transplant recipients: association with polyneuropathy in the same distribution. Br J Dermatol 1993;129:201–3.
133. Lacour JP, Sirvent N, Monpoux F, et al. Dermatomal chronic cutaneous graft-versus-host disease at the site of prior herpes zoster. Br J Dermatol 1999;141:587–9.
134. Cohen PR, Hymes SR. Linear and dermatomal cutaneous graft-versus-host disease. South Med J 1994;87:758–61.
135. Hymes SR, Farmer ER, Burns WH, et al. Bullous sclerodermalike changes in chronic graft-vs-host disease. Arch Dermatol 1985;121:118–92.
136. Sanli H, Arat M, Oskay T, et al. Evaluation of nail involvement in patients with chronic cutaneous graft versus host disease: a single-center study from Turkey. Int J Dermatol 2004;43:176–80.
137. Janin A, Socie G, Devergie A, et al. Fasciitis in chronic graft-versus-host disease. A clinicopathologic study of 14 cases. Ann Intern Med 1994;120:993–8.
138. Gottlober P, Leiter U, Friedrich W, et al. Chronic cutaneous sclerodermoid graft-versus-host disease: evaluation by 20-MHz sonography. J Eur Acad Dermatol Venereol 2003;17:402–7.
139. Nagler RM, Nagler A. Salivary gland involvement in graft-versus-host disease: the underlying mechanism and implicated treatment. Isr Med Assoc J 2004;6:167–72.
140. Hasseus B, Jontell M, Brune M, et al. Langerhans cells and T cells in oral graft versus host disease and oral lichen planus. Scand J Immunol 2001;54:516–24.
141. Abdelsayed RA, Sumner T, Allen CM, et al. Oral precancerous and malignant lesions associated with graft-versus-host disease: report of 2 cases. Oral Surg Oral Med Oral Pathol Oral Radiol Endod 2002;93:75–80.
142. Spinelli S, Chiodi S, Costantini S, et al. Female genital tract graft-versus-host disease following allogeneic bone marrow transplantation. Haematologica 2003;88:1163–8.
143. Spiryda LB, Laufer MR, Soiffer RJ, et al. Graft-versus-host disease of the vulva and/or vagina: diagnosis and treatment. Biol Blood Marrow Transplant 2003;9:760–5.
144. Kolb HJ, Socie G, Duell T, et al. Malignant neoplasms in long-term survivors of bone marrow transplantation. Late Effects Working Party of the European Cooperative Group for Blood and Marrow Transplantation and the European Late Effects Project Group. Ann Intern Med 1999;131:738–44.
145. Gmeinhart B, Hinterberger W, Greinix HT, et al. Anaplastic squamous cell carcinoma (SCC) in a patient with chronic cutaneous graft-versus-host disease (GVHD). Bone Marrow Transplant 1999;23:1197–9.
146. Andreani V, Richard MA, Blaise D, et al. Naevi in allogeneic bone marrow transplantation recipients: the effect of graft-versus-host disease on naevi. Br J Dermatol 2002; 147:433–41.
147. Garnis S, Billick RC, Srolovitz H. Eruptive vascular tumors associated with chronic graft-versus-host disease. J Am Acad Dermatol 1984;10 Pt 2:918–21.
148. Shulman HM, Sale GE, Lerner KG, et al. Chronic cutaneous graft-versus-host disease in man. Am J Pathol 1978; 91:545–70.
149. Nagler RM, Nagler A. Major salivary gland involvement in graft-versus-host disease: considerations related to pathogenesis, the role of cytokines and therapy. Cytokines Cell Mol Ther 1999;5:227–32.
150. Janin-Mercier A, Saurat JH, Bourges M, et al. The lichen planus like and sclerotic phases of the graft versus host disease in man: an ultrastructural study of six cases. Acta Derm Venereol 1981;61:187–93.
151. Sullivan KM, Witherspoon RP, Storb R, et al. Prednisone and azathioprine compared with prednisone and placebo for treatment of chronic graft-v-host disease: prognostic influence of prolonged thrombocytopenia after allogeneic marrow transplantation. Blood 1988;72:546–54.
152. Sullivan KM, Witherspoon RP, Storb R, et al. Alternating-day cyclosporine and prednisone for treatment of high-risk chronic graft-v-host disease. Blood 1988;72: 555–61.
153. De Jesus J, Ghosh S, Hsu Y, et al. Tacrolimus in combination with steroids for the treatment of chronic GVHD. Biol Blood Marrow Transplant 2004;10:49a.
154. Vogelsang GB, Farmer ER, Hess AD, et al. Thalidomide for the treatment of chronic graft-versus-host disease. N Engl J Med 1992;326:1055–8.
155. Basara N, Blau WI, Romer E, et al. Mycophenolate mofetil for the treatment of acute and chronic GVHD in bone marrow transplant patients. Bone Marrow Transplant 1998;22:61–5.
156. Mookerjee B, Altomonte V, Vogelsang G. Salvage therapy for refractory chronic graft-versus-host disease with mycophenolate mofetil and tacrolimus. Bone Marrow Transplant 1999;24:517–20.
157. Couriel DR. Hicks K, Saliba R, Escalon MP et al. Sirolimus in combination with tacrolimus and corticosteroids for the treatment of resistant chronic graft-versus-host disease. Br J Haematol 2005;130(3):409–17
158. Greinix HT, Volc-Platzer B, Rabitsch W, et al. Successful use of extracorporeal photochemotherapy in the treatment of severe acute and chronic graft-versus-host disease. Blood 1998;92:3098–104.
159. Eckardt A, Starke O, Stadler M, et al. Severe oral chronic graft-versus-host disease following allogeneic bone marrow transplantation: highly effective treatment with topical tacrolimus. Oral Oncol 2004;40:811–4.
160. Vogelsang GB, Wolff D, Altomonte V, et al. Treatment of chronic graft-versus-host disease with ultraviolet irradiation and psoralen (PUVA). Bone Marrow Transplant 1996;17:1061–7.
161. Leiter U, Kaskel P, Krahn G, et al. Psoralen plus ultraviolet-A-bath photochemotherapy as an adjunct treatment modality in cutaneous chronic graft versus host disease. Photodermatol Photoimmunol Photomed 2002;18: 183–90.
162. Grundmann-Kollmann M, Behrens S, Gruss C, et al. Chronic sclerodermic graft-versus-host disease refractory to immunosuppressive treatment responds to UVA1 phototherapy. J Am Acad Dermatol 2000;42 Pt 1:134–6.
163. Enk CD, Elad S, Vexler A, et al. Chronic graft-versus-host disease treated with UVB phototherapy. Bone Marrow Transplant 1998;22:1179–83.
164. Marcellus DC, Altomonte VL, Farmer ER, et al. Etretinate therapy for refractory sclerodermatous chronic graft-versus-host disease. Blood 1999;93:66–70.
165. Gruss C, Reed JA, Altmeyer P, et al. Induction of interstitial collagenase (MMP-1) by UVA-1 phototherapy in morphea fibroblasts. Lancet 1997;350:1295–6.
166. Edgar SA, Flanagan C. Efficacy of Stenorol (halofuginone). III. for the control of coccidiosis in turkeys. Poult Sci 1979;58:1483–9.
167. Pines M, Domb A, Ohana M, et al. Reduction in dermal fibrosis in the tight-skin (Tsk) mouse after local application of halofuginone. Biochem Pharmacol 2001;62: 1221–7.
168. Pines M, Snyder D, Yarkoni S, et al. Halofuginone to treat fibrosis in chronic graft-versus-host disease and scleroderma. Biol Blood Marrow Transplant 2003;9:417–25.
169. Kaliakatsou F, Hodgson TA, Lewsey JD, et al. Management of recalcitrant ulcerative oral lichen planus with topical tacrolimus. J Am Acad Dermatol 2002;46:35–41.
170. Rozycki TW, Rogers RS III, Pittelkow MR, et al. Topical tacrolimus in the treatment of symptomatic oral lichen planus: a series of 13 patients. J Am Acad Dermatol 2002;46:27–34.
171. Morrison L, Kratochvil FJ III, Gorman A. An open trial of topical tacrolimus for erosive oral lichen planus. J Am Acad Dermatol 2002;47:617–20.
172. Tocci MJ, Matkovich DA, Collier KA, et al. The immunosuppressant FK506 selectively inhibits expression of early T cell activation genes. J Immunol 1989;143:718–26.
173. Wolff D, Anders V, Corio R, et al. Oral PUVA and topical steroids for treatment of oral manifestations of chronic graft-vs.-host disease. Photodermatol Photoimmunol Photomed 2004;20:184–90.

Radiation Dermatitis

Sharon R. Hymes, MD
Eric A. Strom, MD

Ionizing radiation is extensively used to treat a wide variety of primary tumors, as well as for the palliation of metastatic disease. Since the discovery of x-rays by Roentgen in 1895 dermatologists, have incorporated radiation into their practices to treat malignant and benign skin tumors, as well as benign skin diseases such as acne, eczema, and dermatophyte infection. In the last 30 years, other modalities have largely supplanted radiation in the treatment of these benign disorders. However, it may still be useful in the treatment of keloids, extraosseous bone formation after prosthesis placement, and post–coronary artery angioplasty.[1,2] Dermatologists today are asked to treat the cutaneous repercussions of radiation therapy (RT), which are a function of technique, target, total dose,[3,4] and individual variations. RT, either as monotherapy or in combination with other treatment modalities, is a powerful tool in tumor control, limited primarily by injury adjacent normal tissue.

Radiation-induced skin changes were recognized soon after the discovery of x-rays and were reported as early as 1902.[5] Even when the skin is not the primary target, it may be injured as an "innocent bystander" and develop profound alterations on a functional, gross, and molecular level. These changes occur not only after therapeutic radiation but also after interventional procedures. Serious radiation-induced skin injuries have been reported after unexpectedly high doses of kilovoltage irradiation exposure during fluoroscopic imaging, including cardiac catheterization.[6,7] Increasingly sophisticated therapeutic regimens and modern equipment have improved the delivery and ameliorated, but not eliminated, these adverse effects. Increased awareness of potential interactions between RT and concomitant chemotherapy has led to new treatment schedules designed to maximize antineoplastic effects while minimizing skin toxicity. However, radiation dermatitis remains a serious side effect, which may limit the duration of treatment and the dose delivered. Multidisciplinary collaboration is useful in identifying the patient at risk of complications and managing acute and chronic treatment problems. As research further defines the mechanisms of radiation-induced cellular damage, new radioprotective agents and techniques have been developed to minimize cutaneous problems. Sophisticated wound care techniques also play an important role in the management of severe cases. This chapter reviews the relevant terminology, pathophysiology, and physical findings associated with radiation-induced skin injury. It also outlines skin care parameters in patients with acute and chronic radiation-induced changes.

Terminology

Ionizing radiation refers to electromagnetic radiation with sufficient energy to eject one or more orbital electrons from an atom or molecule, with the subsequent formation of free radicals. These free radicals alter cellular chemical bonds and the normal structure and function of the cell. Deoxyribonucleic acid (DNA) alterations either are repaired or result in mutations or cell death. The high-energy photons commonly used in RT are known as x-rays when they are created electronically, usually by a linear accelerator (LINAC). This is a megavoltage unit that produces and delivers the desired dose of radiation by accelerating electrons that strike a tungsten target to produce photons. The beam then exits a gantry, which can be rotated around the patient. In general, the higher the photon energy, the more the skin is spared. The LINAC may also be programmed to produce an electron beam. Electron beam therapy, 5 to 20 meV, treats to a depth of 1 to 6 cm with a moderate skin dose that falls off after a few centimeters. These properties make it useful for boost dosing, or localized therapy used to re-treat a defined area of tumor. It is also sometimes used to treat nonmelanoma skin cancer (NMSC), metastatic skin disease, and mycosis fungoides, a form of cutaneous T-cell lymphoma. X-ray contamination of electron beam therapy is carefully monitored to minimize side effects.[8] To control the depth of treatment, correct for missing tissue, or purposely increase the skin dose, a bolus, or gelatin-like tissue equivalent material, is sometimes placed on the patient to bring the surface dose to 100%.

When high-energy photons are produced from the nucleus of radioactive atoms, such as cobalt 60, they are termed gamma rays. Grenz rays, low-energy x-rays in the range of 5 to 15 keV, are produced by orthovoltage units and absorb approximately half of their energy in the first 1 to 2 mm of skin. Although uncommonly used by dermatologists now, grenz rays were frequently employed to treat benign epidermal diseases such as psoriasis, tinea capitis, acne, warts, and dermatitis. In modern dermatologic practices, an arsenal of pharmacologic agents has largely supplanted its use for these benign conditions. Superficial x-ray, 30 to 125 keV, is sometimes used to treat primary or metastatic malignancies involving the skin and nodes and is also produced by an orthovoltage unit. Brachytherapy uses radioactive materials that are implanted directly into the tumor rather than using exogenous sources.

The most common form of measurement of absorbed radiation, the gray, replaces the older term, rad. One gray is the equivalent of 1 J/kg of absorbing material, or 100 rads. Radiation is commonly delivered in a series of smaller fractionated doses, rather than one large dose, to allow time for the recovery of normal tissue and to target the tumor. This technique significantly impacts the development of acute and chronic skin changes as normal stem cells exhibit variable degrees of radiosensitivity.[9] Hyperfractionation uses smaller doses per fraction, often twice daily, impacting both the treatment time and dose. Accelerated fractionation allows the delivery of the standard dose in a shorter period of time to overcome repopulation of rapidly growing tumors.

Depending on the type of tumor and the desired treatment parameters, a special cast, cradle, or mask may be created to immobilize the patient at each radiation session. Pretreatment computed tomography (CT) defines the target and the treatment position (simulation), or simulation may be performed using fluoroscopy. More recently, CT simulators can create a three-dimensional model and digitally reconstructed radiograph. This allows a geometric shaping of the radiation beam that conforms to the shape of the tumor (conformal radiation therapy), allowing directed therapy, with less risk to normal tissue. The radiation physicist, dosimetrist (medical physicist), and oncologist use this information to plan the optimal dose, as well as the placement of physical blocks near the patient, or multileaf collimators mounted in the gantry, to reduce exposure. Wedges, filters using high atomic number material, are used to modify dose distribution. Lines of reference (fiducials) may be painted or tattooed on the patient to ensure proper positioning and localization of the target.

Clinical Manifestations of Radiation Dermatitis

The majority of patients treated with RT develop minor and reversible skin changes. When cutaneous changes do develop, they are commonly graded as acute, consequential late, or chronic and may appear at both the entrance and exit portals.

Acute Radiation-Induced Dermatitis

After RT or accidental exposure, acute changes usually occur within 90 days. The National Cancer Institute common toxicity criteria version 3.0 has become the standard for evaluation (Table 1). Generalized erythema, sometimes undetectable without special instrumentation, may occur hours after radiation exposure and fade within hours to days.[10,11] A second phase consisting of more sustained erythematous changes usually is apparent 10 to 14 days after dosing and is characterized by a blanchable reactive pink color, without other epidermal changes, most likely mediated by cytokines.[12]

Grade 1 changes, usually seen in the fourth or fifth week of therapy, include follicular or generalized erythema and dry desquamation. Other changes include pruritus, epilation, scaling, and dyspigmentation (Figure 1). The

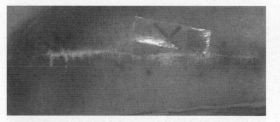

FIGURE 1 Grade 1 radiation dermatitis of the arm with erythema

dryness and hair loss are secondary to injury to sebaceous glands and hair follicles.

Persistent tender or edematous erythema, grade 2 changes, may progress to focal loss of the epidermis, producing moist desquamation in skin folds (Figure 2). This usually occurs after 4 to 5 weeks of therapy, with radiation doses to the skin of 40 Gy or greater.[13] Moist desquamation is characterized by epidermal necrosis, fibrinous exudates, and often considerable pain. Bullae may be present clinically and histologically, and these can rupture or become infected. Histologically, arterioles are obstructed by fibrin thrombi and edema is prominent.[14] At this stage, it is important to identify any superinfection, especially with organisms that may act as superantigens, such as *Staphylococcus aureus*. Superantigens up-regulate cytokine production and inflammation by activating antigen-presenting cells and T cells, resulting in increased skin damage (Figure 3).[15] Depending on the body site, this reaction peaks 1 to 2 weeks after the last treatment and gradually heals, accompanied by increased expression of epidermal growth factor receptors.[16] Epidermal regeneration occurs about the third to fifth week after radiation, with healing within 1 to 3 months.

Confluent moist desquamation in other than skin folds is typical of grade 3 dermatitis (Figure 4), and the formation of ulcers, hemorrhage, and necrosis heralds grade 4 changes

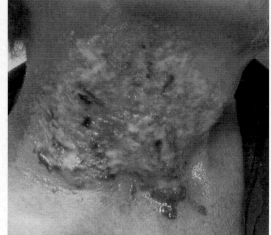

FIGURE 3 Radiation dermatitis of the neck complicated by superinfection

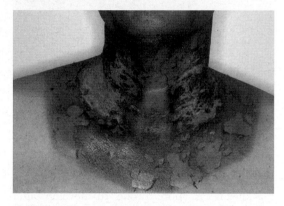

FIGURE 4 Grade 3 radiation dermatitis with confluent moist desquamation of the neck

(Figure 5). These problems may become chronic and lead to consequential late complications (Figure 6). The severity of the acute radiation response may also lead to a late effect in the gut, bladder, and oral mucosa.[17] Disruption of the epithelial basement membrane and breakdown of the barrier function substantially increases the risk of these injuries.[18]

As epidermal function becomes increasing impaired, the permeability of the skin, as measured by transepidermal water loss, increases. Topical treatment may ameliorate radiation dermatitis, as measured by this parameter.[11] A

Grade	Description
0	None
1	Faint erythema or dry desquamation
2	Moderate to brisk erythema or a patchy moist desquamation, mostly confined to skin folds and creases; moderate edema
3	Confluent moist desquamation, ≥ 1.5 cm diameter, not confined to skin folds; pitting edema
4	Skin necrosis or ulceration of full-thickness dermis: may include bleeding not induced by minor trauma or abrasion

Table 1 Radiation Dermatitis: National Cancer Institute Common Terminology Criteria for Adverse Events Version 3

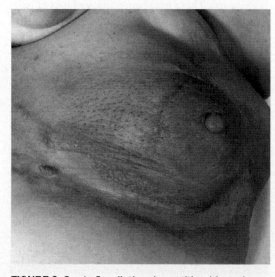

FIGURE 2 Grade 2 radiation dermatitis with erythema of the breast and moist desquamation confined to skin folds

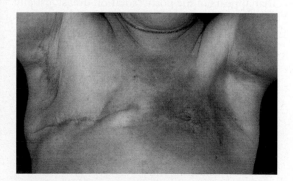

FIGURE 5 Grade 4 radiation dermatitis with skin necrosis of the left chest wall

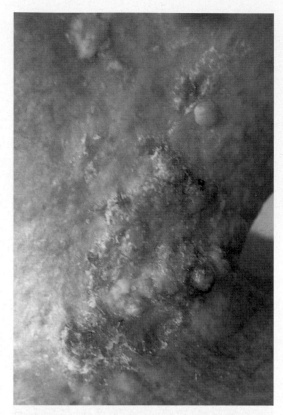

FIGURE 6 Consequential late changes following non-healing acute radiation dermatitis of the neck. There is severe fibrosis complicated by erosions and telangiectasia

"comedo reaction," comprising whiteheads and blackheads, is more prone to develop after head and neck radiation,[19] and pseudorecidives resembling keratoses sometimes appear in the immediate postradiation period. These should be distinguished from tumor recurrences and often spontaneously resolve without treatment.[19,20] Hair loss occurs at skin doses of approximately 30 Gy, and new hair may continue to return for up to a year. Alopecia owing to follicular fibrosis may be permanent at skin doses of 55 Gy or greater.

Chronic Radiation Dermatitis

The skin may appear relatively normal for a varying length of time after RT, and chronic changes may not develop for months to years after exposure. These changes may be transient, such as the edematous peau d'orange appearance that appears in the postirradiation breast, usually resolving in the first year (Figure 7). Postinflammatory hypo- and hyperpigmentation is commonly seen after any disruption of the dermal-epidermal junction and, depending on the severity of the initial reaction and skin type of the patient, may persist or slowly normalize (Figure 8). Certain body sites, such as the scalp, exhibit relatively more tolerance for radiation than the skin of the face, neck, trunk, and extremities.[21] Textural changes, including xerosis (dryness), scale, and hyperkeratosis, are common, and hair follicles and sebaceous glands may be absent. Persistent telangiectasia is more common

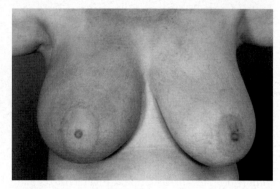

FIGURE 7 Peau d'orange changes in the irradiated breast.

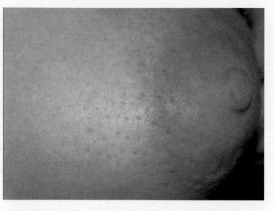

FIGURE 8 Dyspigmentation of the irradiated right breast

after boost dosing, acute grade 3 injury, and moist desquamation, possibly secondary to microvasculature damage (Figure 9).[22,23] However, the development of moist desquamation does not seem to predispose patients to the development of subcutaneous fibrosis,[24] and the boost is not associated with any other late changes.[25]

Poikilodermatous changes, characterized by persistant hyper- and hypopigmentation (dyspigmentation), atrophy, and telangiectasia, are an indication of more severe cutaneous injury (Figure 10). There may be permanent loss of nails and skin appendages, producing alopecia and decreased or absent sweating. The latter is clinically significant when large surface areas are treated, as in the case of electron beam therapy for

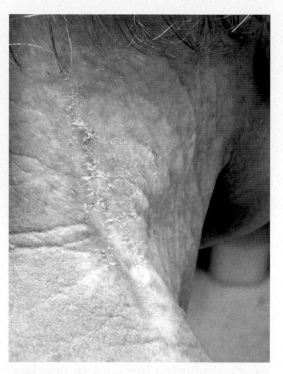

FIGURE 10 Chronic radiation dermatitis of the neck with fibrosis and poikiloderma.

mycosis fungoides. Fibrosis in response to growth factors such as transforming growth factor β (TGF-β)[26] may be focal or widespread, producing tissue retraction, limitation of movement, and pain. Pathologically, the dermis and subcutaneous adipose tissue are replaced by atypical fibroblasts and fibrous tissue (Figure 11). Eccentric myointimal proliferation of the small arteries and arterioles may progress to thrombosis or obstruction, increasing the predisposition for ulcers and skin breakdown.[13] Skin atrophy, related to decreased population of dermal fibroblasts and the reabsorption of collagen,[27] also causes fragility and predisposes patients to erosions and ulcerations, which may be painful, slow to heal, and prone to superinfection (Figure 12). Subungual splinter hemorrhages have been reported on occasion.[28]

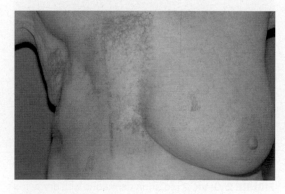

FIGURE 9 Telangiectasia in a rectangular field after boost dosing.

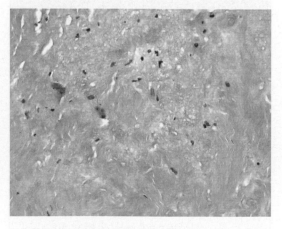

FIGURE 11 Radiation induced fibrosis. Hematoxylin and eosin 50X. Courtesy of Dr. Victor Prieto

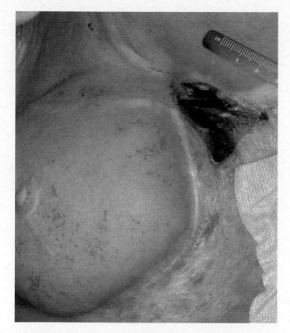

FIGURE 12 Severe radiation fibrosis and a non-healing skin ulcer.

Radiation necrosis is more commonly a consequential late injury associated with high-dose RT, failure to heal acute dermatitis, and dermal ischemia.[29] It is particularly difficult to manage as impaired healing and superinfection are common in tissues rendered relatively avascular. These problems are exacerbated by peripheral vascular disease, diabetes, hypertension, and connective tissue disease.

Pathophysiology

The skin is a continuously renewing organ, and RT not only interferes with normal maturation, reproduction, and repopulation of germinative epidermal and hair matrix cells but also targets fibroblasts and cutaneous vasculature.[30] The radiation-induced injury has been termed a "complex wound," in which structural tissue damage occurs instantaneously, mediated by a burst of free radicals, resulting in DNA damage and alteration of proteins, lipids, and carbohydrates. Each additional exposure or fraction contributes to inflammatory cell recruitment and direct tissue injury.[18] Wound healing is further impaired by inhibition of normal granulation tissue, fibrogenesis, and angiogenesis.[18,31] Acute injury is, therefore, a consequence of reduction in and impairment of functional stem cells, endothelial cell changes, inflammation, and epidermal cell apoptosis and necrosis.

Cutaneous radiation syndrome, occurring after accidental radiation exposure, is also mediated by a combination of inflammatory processes. Alteration of cellular proliferation occurs as a result of a specific pattern of transcriptionally activated proinflammatory cytokines and growth factors.[32] Interaction between epithelial and mesenchymal cells is at least in part initiated by interleukin-1α secreted by the activated epithelial cell during skin injury. This, in turn, may modulate the synthesis of other proinflammatory mediators and proteases in surrounding fibroblasts.[33]

Repetitive radiation exposure delivers a series of tissue insults to skin that has not had time to repair existing damage. During dose fractionation schedules with gaps (extension of the nontreatment period), tissue-specific repopulation is initiated after a lag period. When accelerated repopulation is initiated, there is an increase in the radiosensitivity of the surviving stem cells and a decrease in time for cells to repair sublethal radiation-induced damage.[9] Ionizing radiation also produces epidermal basal cell and endothelial cell damage,[31,34] vascular injury,[14,35] and loss of Langerhans' cells,[36] which are the chief antigen-presenting cells in the skin. Up-regulation of epidermal growth factor receptor[16] may aid in epithelial repair, whereas alterations in epidermal Langerhans' cells may further impair immunologic integrity.[36,37] These events, combined with the intensive inflammation promoted by up-regulation of adhesion molecules such as intercellular adhesion molecule 1 (ICAM-1),[38] contribute to impairment of cutaneous barrier function, bacterial colonization, superinfection, and superantigen production.

Acutely irradiated skin demonstrates a perivascular inflammatory infiltrate around dilated blood vessels with swelling and sloughing of epithelial cells and growth arrest.[39] Lower doses produce clumping of nuclear chromatin, swelling of the nucleus, and apoptosis. Higher doses cause nuclear disfiguration or loss of the nuclear membrane, mitochondrial distortion, and degeneration of the endoplasmic reticulum, as well as direct cellular necrosis. Mitotic activity in the germinal cells of the sebaceous glands, hair follicles, and epidermis is inhibited, and basal layer stem cells are depleted.[13,40] Prostaglandins and thiol compounds are potentially radioprotective agents that have been used to protect normal tissue, with varying degrees of success. In animal models, both have been used to protect hair follicles and other skin structures.[41,42]

TGF-β, a peptide that has a fundamental role in controlling proliferation of many cell types, is intricately involved in the development of chronic radiation dermatitis.[43] This cytokine acts as a "master switch" for tissue fibrosis, activating fibroblasts to secrete extracellular matrix protein.[26,44–46] In the irradiated tissue of pigs, TGF-β₁ also plays an important role in promoting and regulating the late fibrotic process.[47] Its main effect on connective tissues in vivo is to stimulate growth. Endothelial cell proliferation is also stimulated, but epithelial cell growth is inhibited. Mice lacking a downstream mediator of TGF-β, Smad3, demonstrate decreased tissue damage and fibrosis after irradiation, as well as accelerated healing.[48] Up-regulation of TGF-β has been found in fibrotic tissue of irradiated patients but not in the nonirradiated controls,[26] confirming that its induction is a general response of cells to ionizing radiation. It is also chemotactic for mast cells, possibly increasing angiogenesis by inducing macrophages to release factors that lead to neovascularization.[49]

Radiation-induced endothelial cell damage activates components of the coagulation system,[18] which, in turn, promotes inflammation and cytokine overproduction. Thrombin, which is a regulator of cell proliferation, may also modulate the synthesis of TGF-β,[50] vascular endothelial permeability, inflammation, and tissue remodeling.[18,51] Subsequent matrix accumulation, fibrosis, endothelial cell dysfunction, and increased measurable cytokines may ultimately delay reepithelialization.[50]

Long-lasting impairment of the reparative process ultimately affects the integrity of the "healed" radiation-induced wound. Although healed traumatic wounds in nonirradiated skin remodel continuously for years following injury, this capacity is often compromised after RT because of persistent cellular dysfunction or changes in the supporting stroma.[18] Fibroblasts may be permanently altered, causing cutaneous atrophy, contraction, and fibrosis.[52,53] Although total dose is certainly critical in producing cutaneous problems, late effects may be more dependent on the volume, fraction size, and dose/fraction schedules.[14] The underlying pathogenesis of the development of telangiectasia is unknown but may be due in part to inflammatory damage to the microvasculature during the acute injury and the production of platelet-derived growth factor (PDGF) and fibroblast growth factor by damaged endothelial cells or macrophages.[18] Both vascular sclerosis and radiation fibrosis are, in part, related to endothelial cell damage and vascular injury. The identification of genes by microarray analysis may further define the molecular mechanisms of this microvascular insult.[54] Leukocyte infiltration, mediated in part by cell adhesion molecules, is also commonly observed at sites of irradiation and is likely to lead to parenchymal atrophy, fibrosis, and necrosis in normal tissues.[35]

Risk Factors

Dose Fractionation Schedules

The total dose, dose/fractionation, type and quality of the beam, volume, and surface area exposed influence the degree of damage to the epidermis, dermis, adnexal structures, and microvasculature.[9,32,55–57] When photons are absorbed, the energy released produces breakage of chemical bonds and subsequent electron release. These free electrons react with other molecules, particularly water, to form free radicals, which then have the potential to diffuse and damage DNA. In the case of acute radiation dermatitis, the clinical consequences of this reaction are expressed during or immediately after therapy. Usually, these acute changes heal with mild changes. Rarely, the acute dermatitis never completely heals, resulting in consequential late changes, leading to chronic wounds and necrosis. Alternatively, chronic or true late radiation consequences may develop despite minimal acute radiation dermatitis. Unlike acute effects, true late reactions are unlikely to be self-repairing.

Physical Factors

The severity of the skin reaction is both treatment and patient related.[27,58] Physical factors, including smoking,[59] poor nutritional status, problems with skin integrity, actinic damage, body site, obesity,[60] and overlapping skin folds, predispose patients to radiation dermatitis. About 25% of patients receiving parallel-opposed lateral fields will have skin reactions. The intentional use of boost doses to treat malignancies unavoidably produces overlapping fields, and the use of bolus material often results in an increase in the skin dose.[57,61] When the skin is purposefully targeted, as in the case of inflammatory breast cancer, primary skin cancers, or mycosis fungoides, and when dose escalation is used to treat regionally recurrent disease, cutaneous problems should be anticipated. The larger the targeted tumor, the more likely a severe skin reaction is to develop.[59] Tissue expanders, especially in the breast, present a unique dilemma both in delivering the desired dose and maintaining skin integrity (Figure 13). Positioning the patient to reduce apposition of skin folds, skin shields in sensitive areas, and delaying treatment until preexisting skin problems have been addressed may decrease the frequency and severity of radiation-induced skin problems. Deliberate exposure to ultraviolet radiation in treatment areas should be avoided as this may up-regulate cytokine production and serve as a cocarcinogen. Temperature extremes should also be avoided.

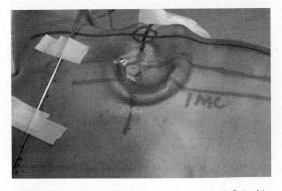

FIGURE 13 Tissue expander of the breast deflated to deliver RT

Genetic Factors

Patients with impaired cellular DNA repair capabilities are at increased risk of radiation-induced problems. Individuals with ataxia-telangiectasia, a rare autosomal recessive disorder resulting from mutations in both copies of the *ATM* gene, are especially prone to develop severe cutaneous complications after RT. It has been suggested that patients who develop serious, unanticipated radiation dermatitis may actually harbor a previously undetected abnormality in ATM or may be heterozygous for this trait. *ATM* heterozygosity occurs in approximately 1% of the general population,[62] and a single mutated copy of the DNA repair gene may predispose patients to cutaneous complications, necessitating dose alterations to reduce cutaneous toxicity.[63] Owing to their increased cellular radiosensitivity, heterozygous *ATM* breast cancer patients may qualify for dose and volume reduction trials.[64]

Other diseases with reduced cellular DNA repair capability call for dose alteration or avoidance of therapeutic radiation entirely. Patients with hereditary nevoid basal cell carcinoma (BCC) syndrome (Gorlin's syndrome) develop multiple BCCs, as well as a variety of phenotypic abnormalities. Abnormalities in the human homologue *Patched* (*PTCH*) gene, the impaired tumor suppressor gene associated with this syndrome, have been identified, and increased cellular proliferation occurs via the hedgehog signaling pathway.[65,66] *Ptc* heterozygous mice exhibit increased radiation-induced teratogenesis, suggesting the role of ptc in the response to ionizing radiation.[67] Nucleoli in fibroblasts of affected individuals are increased after x-radiation, apparently corresponding to increased ribonucleic acid (RNA) synthesis and metabolism.[67,68] Radiation of affected patients may produce devastating results, with the production of widespread cutaneous tumors (Figure 14).

Other chromosomal-breakage syndromes, including Fanconi's anemia, Bloom syndrome, and disorders characterized by defects in DNA repair, such as xeroderma pigmentosum, may experience increased frequency of chromatid breaks and gaps in skin fibroblasts when compared with normal controls after G2 phase x-irradiation. This has also been reported with familial polyposis, Gardner's syndrome, hereditary malignant melanoma, and dysplastic nevus syndrome.[69–71] However, even in patients without known genetic disorders, there may be individual differences in early and late radiation response in the skin. Whether these differences are determined by heterogeneity in intrinsic cell radiosensitivity or by other factors has yet to be elucidated.[72] Attempts have been made in breast cancer patients to predict radiosensitivity and subsequent fibrosis by measuring the number of lethal chromosome aberrations in in vitro irradiated lymphocytes,[73] but there is no clinically standardized method of

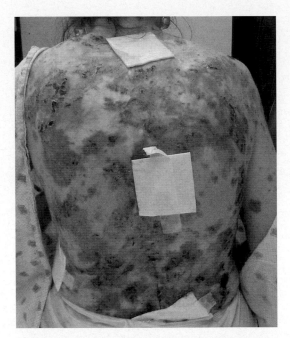

FIGURE 14 A patient with hereditary nevoid basal cell carcinoma who received radiation therapy years earlier. The eroded areas represent basal cell carcinoma, and a bandage covers a biopsy site.

predicting individual variations in response to therapy. Measurements of DNA damage by p53 and p21 protein accumulation have been assayed in the irradiated breast, where no association between the p53 response and degree of erythema was found. Therefore, epidermal p53 response does not reliably predict the degree of radiation-induced epidermal injury.[74] Individual responses to radiation-induced DNA damage vary widely and may be independent of the type of radiation.

Connective Tissue Disease

Preexisting connective tissue or autoimmune disease, including scleroderma, systemic lupus erythematosus (SLE), and perhaps rheumatoid arthritis (RA), unpredictably predispose patients to the development of severe radiation dermatitis.[75–77] Although the mechanism is not known, lymphocytes from patients with RA, SLE, and polymyositis are more radiosensitive than those from healthy volunteers or patients with conditions not associated with autoimmunity. Peripheral blood lymphocytes from patients with SLE, juvenile RA, and systemic sclerosis have significantly greater DNA damage after irradiation than do those from controls.[78,79] Because of this, the presence of connective tissue disease is a relative contraindication to RT.

Infectious Disease

Patients with human immunodeficiency virus (HIV) disease may demonstrate a decreased skin and mucous membrane tolerance to treatment, independent of their risk of infection. They tend to develop cutaneous reactions at a lower dose, as well as more significant systemic problems.[80–82]

Radiosensitizers

An increase in adverse events is well documented after the use of "radiosensitizers" (Figure 15). These are drugs given either immediately prior, during, or less than 7 days postradiation, causing increased cellular damage and impaired repair.[83] It is now known that the timing and dose of any such agents are crucial.[84] For example, when paclitaxel or docetaxel is used in conjunction with radiotherapy in the treatment of breast cancer, it produces synergistic cutaneous toxicity that is both schedule and dose dependent. The concomitant use of tamoxifen with radiation therapy has been implicated in the development of an increased incidence of subcutaneous fibrosis by some investigators.[85]

Differential Diagnosis

Common cutaneous problems, including dermatitis (Figure 16) or infection, may manifest during or after treatment. Even after the acute effects of radiation have subsided, the treated skin may manifest a host of physical and functional changes. Compromised integrity and impaired barrier

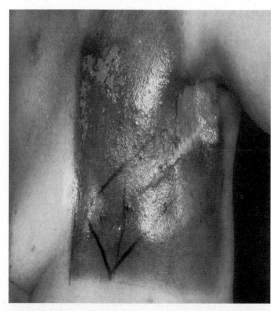

FIGURE 15 Radiation dermatitis in a patient receiving paclitaxel.

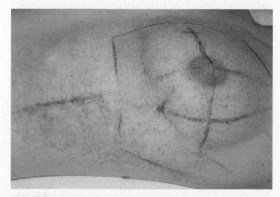

FIGURE 16 Contact dermatitis from the pens used to paint fiducials.

function may produce a *locus minoris resistentiae*, a Latin phrase meaning "a place of less resistance" (Figure 17). It is not unusual to see dermatitis or infection confined to these sites. There have also been case reports of localized Sweet's syndrome in the irradiated skin of the breast,[86] as well as lichen planus confined to a radiation port.[87] Reports of pemphigus, an autoimmune bullous disease, following ionizing radiation exposure are rare. Common to these cases is a prodromal persistent nonspecific dermatitic eruption that is often interpreted as radiation dermatitis and latency of variable duration before the onset of a vesiculobullous eruption that begins at the portal of irradiation.[88]

Cutaneous hypersensitivity syndromes, including erythema multiforme, have been reported to start in irradiated skin and generalize from there.[89] Localized Stevens-Johnson syndrome confined to radiation ports has been reported in conjunction with the administration of oral agents such as phenobarbitol.[90] Other severe complications, including toxic epidermal necrolysis, a skin condition characterized by complete epidermal necrosis, has been reported to occur more frequently when phenytoin and related anticonvulsants are combined with cranial radiation. These reactions also have, on occasion, started in the radiation port,[90–95] prompting some clinicians to avoid phenytoin during RT.[89]

Radiation recall refers to the phenomenon of cutaneous inflammation, limited to the site of radiation, occurring at least 7 days after treatment or after the acute dermatitis has healed (Figure 18).[96] It is graded according to its severity, ranging from erythema to necrosis, ulceration, or hemorrhage (Table 2). Increasingly severe recall dermatitis tends to occur when the offending drugs, usually cytotoxic agents, are introduced shortly after the cessation of RT.[96] It has also been

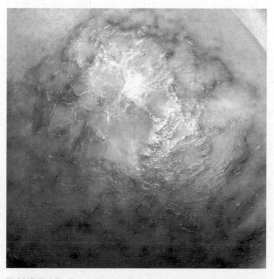

FIGURE 17 Eczema confined to a radiation site, and sparing the non-exposed skin.

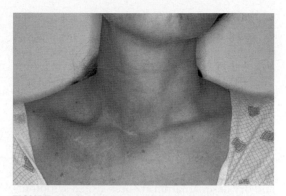

FIGURE 18 Radiation recall of the right neck 2 years after RT.

Table 2 Radiation Recall Reaction: National Cancer Institute Common Terminology Critera Version 3.0

Grade	Description
0	None
1	Faint erythema or dry desquamation
2	Moderate to brisk erythema or a patchy moist desquamation, mostly confined to skin folds and creases; moderate edema
3	Confluent moist desquamation, ≥ 1.5 cm diameter, not confined to skin folds; pitting edema
4	Skin necrosis or ulceration of full-thickness dermis; may include bleeding not induced by minor trauma or abrasion

Reaction following chemotherapy in the absence of additional radiation therapy that occurs in a previous radiation port.

reported after the administration of nonsteroidal antiestrogens, interferon-α2b, simvastatin, and antituberculosis medications.[97] Radiation recall occurs minutes to days after drug exposure and may occur weeks to years after radiation. It unpredictably recurs on reexposure but usually flares after the first exposure to the inciting drug. The longest well-documented hiatus between treatment and recall is 2 years after radiation exposure.[98,99] The etiology of this well-documented phenomenon is uncertain. Impaired cellular repair, gene mutation,[100] vascular damage,[98] epidermal stem cell inadequacy[101] and depletion,[102] drug hypersensitiviy,[96] cumulative direct DNA damage and oxidative stress,[103] koebnerization,[104] nonimmune activation, and up-regulation of cytokines have all been implicated.[97] The latter theory is supported by cases that occur minutes after parenteral infusion, whereas it takes a median 8 days to manifest after oral medications. Although anecdotally beneficial, the role of topical or systemic steroids, mast cell inhibitors, and antihistamines in the prevention and treatment of this problem has not been evaluated in a controlled setting.[96]

Finally, recurrent or secondary tumor should be considered if atypical plaques and nodules develop within the radiation field (Figures 19 and 20). Although irradiated skin may present some difficulty with healing, a biopsy is useful in this clinical situation.

Treatment of Acute Radiation Dermatitis

Early changes (grade 1) characterized by erythema and dry desquamation are best treated symptomatically. The affected area is washed gently with plain water alone or combined with a mild, low-pH cleansing agent that does not exacerbate the existing dermatitis. This has proven to be both physically and psychologically more beneficial than older practices of not washing at all.[105–107] Washing may also reduce the bacterial load and thereby reduce potential superantigen-induced inflammation. Patients should wear well-fitting, nonbinding clothing and avoid unnecessary topical irritants and friction. When required, soft burn nets or other modalities that hold dressings in place without adhesives should replace tape. In the case of breast cancer patients, a sports bra can be used for this purpose. While actively undergoing therapy, aluminum or magnesium salts, such as those found in antiperspirants and talcs, should not be used in the treated area as

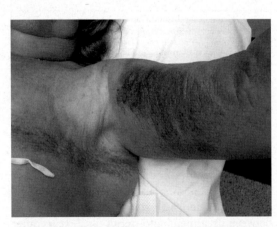

FIGURE 19 Recurrent breast cancer after RT

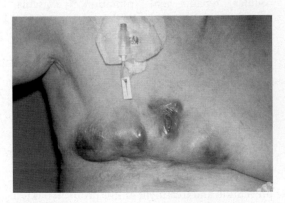

FIGURE 20 Recurrent breast cancer after RT

they can potentially increase the radiation dose to the superficial skin. Ultraviolet exposure should be avoided, and photoprotection in the form of clothing, hats, and sunscreen should be used as tolerated.

Topical Therapy and Wound Care

The goal of treating the erythema and dry desquamation is to avoid a bolus effect, minimize transepidermal water loss, decrease pain, and prevent progression to moist desquamation. Petrolatum-based emollients are commonly used, with or without hydrogel dressings. Radioemulsions containing trolamine were hoped to be "radioprotective" as they are macrophage cell stimulators that remove necrotic tissue, promote fibroblast proliferation, and, ex vivo, reduce vascular alterations, restore CD34 expression, promote epithelial cell proliferation, and decrease interleukin-1 expression and collagen secretion. The oil-in-water formulation also softens nonviable tissues. Although controlled studies show no clinical radioprotective effect over control, many patients express satisfaction with these ointments and find them soothing.[108] Newer non–petroleum-based products combining castor oil, balsam of Peru, and trypsin purportedly stimulate the capillary bed, improve epithelialization, and provide cutaneous protection.[109]

Recommendations for use of other topical skin agents are largely anecdotal, and few randomized studies have been performed. Consequently, a great variety of products have been studied, and many recommendations have emerged. Aloe vera, D-panthenol, hydrophobic and hydrophilic ointments, chamomile, and almond ointment have been tried, with variable results.[110–113] Multiple other creams, including aloe vera, CM-glucan, hydroxyprolisilan C, and Matrixyl (Theta-Cream), have shown no definite benefit in the treatment of radiation dermatitis.[114] The role of antioxidants, including vitamin C, has not been established, and topical ascorbic acid did no better than placebo in preventing skin toxicity after cranial RT.[115] However, when given systemically to mice, higher doses of radiation were required to obtain skin desquamation.[116] Sucralfate (sucrose aluminum), a widely used antiulcer drug, has anti-inflammatory properties and activates cellular proliferation. In a double-blind randomized study comparing the efficacy of sucralfate cream with a base cream in 50 breast cancer patients who received postoperative electron beam therapy to the chest wall, the acute radiation reaction of the skin was statistically decreased and the recovery of the skin was also significantly faster in the sucralfate cream group.[112,113] However, in another study comparing vehicle with vehicle plus 10% sucralfate, there was no significant difference in time to healing or

pain relief.[117] Topical hyaluronic acid has been helpful in some patients undergoing radiation therapy, demonstrating improved healing compared with placebo,[118] as has calendula, an extract from a plant of the marigold family.[119] Barrier films may also prove to be useful when compared with glycerine cream.[120]

The general consensus is that the majority of patients do not need a specific therapy except a moisturizer as tolerated, and there is no agreement on a specific topical agent to manage acute radiation dermatitis.[121] However, as with other forms of dermatitis, creams and ointments are generally better tolerated than lotions in irritated, dry skin. Since approximately 10% of patients have allergic-type reactions with topical agents, this should be considered if exacerbation of the dermatitis occurs.[122]

The use of topical corticosteroids to prevent or treat radiation dermatitis is somewhat controversial. Because these agents have documented anti-inflammatory effects and have been shown to inhibit the up-regulation of interleukin-6 in response to ionizing radiation,[123] they have been used for both treatment and prevention. Comparisons of different topical steroids, instituted either before or during the onset of acute dermatitis, show conflicting results. Some studies show no statistically significant difference between steroid (0.2% hydrocortisone valerate) versus placebo,[124] whereas other groups demonstrate decreased acute radiation dermatitis in the topical steroid group.[125] Comparison of two different steroid creams, 1% hydrocortisone cream and 0.05% clobetasone butyrate, in a double-blind trial was carried out in 54 patients undergoing RT for breast cancer. The cream was administered when patients reached a given dose of 2,000 rad, or earlier, if required. The majority of patients using either cream derived benefit from its soothing effects, but patients using clobetasone butyrate developed more severe skin reactions.[126] Although there is no consensus, at best steroids may ameliorate the dermatitis, but they do not entirely prevent it.[127] It is not known if infection, telangiectasia, or skin atrophy, known side effects of this group of topical agents, is increased. Other anti-inflammatory agents, such as 1% indomethacin cream, were not found to be helpful in preventing radiation-induced erythema.[10,128] The new topical calcineurin inhibitors (topical tacrolimus and pimecrolimus) are potent down-regulators of cytokine production and are currently approved for use in atopic dermatitis. There have been no controlled trials to date documenting their usefulness in radiation dermatitis.

Wound Care for Erosions and Ulcers

Despite the fact that irradiated skin is significantly altered, the care of radiation-induced erosions and ulcers is generally not specific and is adapted from the generic wound care experience (Table 3).[18,52,53,129] From a prognostic standpoint, it may be helpful to distinguish consequential late injury from secondary injury in an irradiated field. Wound dressings are used for multiple

Table 3 Treatment of Radiation Dermatitis*
Acute erythema
Emollients (lotions, creams, or ointments)
Avoid friction, ultraviolet radiation, temperature extremes, and trauma
Symptomatic treatment
Dry desquamation
Emollients (creams or ointments)
Petrolatum based, hydrophilic
Castor oil/balsalm of Peru/trypsin
Trolamine
Miscellaneous (see text)
Gentle cleansing
Topical corticosteroids—controversial
Moist desquamation during RT
As above with the addition of
Hydrogel dressings
Hydrocolloid dressings for minimally exudative wounds (self-adhesive)
Burn pads, alginate or foam dressings for highly exudative wounds
Bacterial culture: treat infected wounds topically or systemically based on culture
Moist desquamation after RT
As above with the addition of
Film dressings for minimally exudative erosions
Infected wounds: ionic silver pads or powder
Topical antibiotics
Cadexomer iodine
Maltodextrin powder
Chronic ulcers
Control secretions, limit bacteria and debris
As above with the addition of
Careful and selective débridement
Mechanical
Enzymatic
Autolytic—moist matrix
Biosurgical
Biologic preparations (GM-CSF, growth factors)
Low-intensity helium laser
Hyperbaric oxygen
Telangiectasia
Vascular lasers (eg, pulsed dye)
Fibrosis
Pentoxifylline with or without vitamin E
Superoxide dismutase
Interferon-γ

GM-CSF = granulocyte-macrophage colony-stimulating factor; RT = radiation therapy; Adapted from Hymes SR, Strom EA, Fife C. Radiation dermatitis: Clinical presentation, pathophysiology, and treatment 2006. J Amer Acad Dermatol 2006; 54:28–46.

reasons, including handling wound secretions and pain control, as well as protecting the skin from outside contamination. In addition, preserving a moist environment enhances reepithelialization, lyses necrotic tissue, and encourages phagocytosis of necrotic debris and bacteria.[13,129,130] To enhance barrier function, hydrophilic and lipophilic creams and ointments are often used alone or with hydrogel dressings. These dressings are soothing but, as they are not self-adherent, must be held in place and removed just prior to treatment. They may be cleaned and reapplied, especially on nonexudative wounds. When refrigerated before use and applied while still cool, patients often find them soothing.

Hydrocolloid dressings provide moderate absorption of secretions and hydrate the wound. Additional benefits include healing of established wounds, simplification of wound care, and pain control.[131] They are self-adherent, which may present a problem when the adhesive is placed on already damaged skin. These dressings are commonly left in place for several days and are, therefore, more useful after completion of RT.

Transparent films allow close observation of the wound, but as they do not absorb exudates, they are more practical in protecting the fragile epidermis or covering early erosions. Heavily exudative wounds are best treated with burn pads or the use of alginate or foam dressings, which are highly absorptive.

Persistent eschars can be removed manually under local anesthesia or treated with enzymatic débridement or autolytic dressings. Biosurgical débridement with sterile live maggots removes necrotic, infected tissue, leaving healthy tissue untouched.[129] Unfortunately, these techniques often leave significant skin and soft tissue defects. Biosynthetic dressings, artificial skin, and bioengineered skin have proved useful in the setting of persistent, nonhealing ulcerations.[132] Novel therapies, including low-intensity helium-neon laser, have benefited some patients with recalcitrant chronic skin ulcers after RT, perhaps by enhancing metabolic pathways, cell proliferation, and motility of fibroblasts and keratinocytes, as well as improving skin circulation and inducing angiogenesis.[13,133,134]

Topical or oral antibacterial agents should be considered in the treatment of wounds that are at high risk or are already infected. Silver-based dressings are antibacterial and have proven to be effective for this purpose. Patients with anal canal or some types of gynecologic tumors undergoing RT and chemotherapy experience close to 100% incidence of dermatitis, often grade 3 or 4. This not only interferes with quality of life but also mandates a hiatus in RT, potentially with a negative impact on patient outcome. In patients in whom the tumor was not close to the skin, silver leaf nylon dressings, removed during

treatments, have been found to be helpful, probably secondary to their antibacterial effects.[135] Cadexemer iodine–based dressings promote autolytic débridement, absorb exudates, control drainage, and are nontoxic to fibroblasts in vitro.[129] Multidextrin powder, a macrophage activator, reduces bioburden by increasing local osmolality and is helpful in odor control.[129]

Targeted Biologic Therapy

Targeted therapy and biologic preparations may be useful in some types of radiation dermatitis. A series of 24 patients with acute radiation-induced vulvar dermatitis found topical granulocyte-macrophage colony-stimulating factor (GM-CSF) plus topical steroid more useful than steroid alone in reducing the severity and duration of the problem.[136] The presumed mechanism of action is the promotion of chemotaxis of monocytes into tissues and the maturation of monocytes into macrophages.

PDGFs are chemotactic for neutrophils, monocytes, macrophages, and fibroblasts. Theoretically, they also stimulate the synthesis of extracellular matrix components, collagen, and additional growth factors. These have shown anecdotal success in producing enough granulation tissue in a chronic radiation wound on the neck to support a skin graft.[137] Chronic radiation ulcers after electron beam therapy were treated successfully with PDGF gel and hydrophilic copolymer membrane.[138] If there is active tumor, there may be some theoretical risk in the use of growth factors, and some topical dressings may partially absorb or inactivate this expensive product.

Treatment of Chronic Fibrosis

Chronic fibrosis is arguably one of the most difficult cutaneous complications to treat. Long thought to be irreversible, supportive measures are often necessary to avoid skin breakdown and infection. Multidisciplinary teams, including specialists in wound care, physical therapy, and pain management, often work together to address important cosmetic and quality of life issues. Physical therapy, deep massage, and active and passive range of motion exercises are important techniques used to maintain mobility and to minimize contractures. Chronic nonhealing ulcers and suspicious lesions may need pathologic examination to exclude the possibility of secondary skin malignancy. Unfortunately, these sites may heal poorly, so biopsies should not be performed early in the evaluation period.

Alternative approaches include the use of pentoxifylline (PTX), a methylxanthine derivative in common use as an inhibitor of platelet aggregation. This drug may also increase phagocytic activity of polymorphonuclear leukocytes and monocytes, as well as antagonizing tumor necrosis factor (TNF)-α and -β. By decreasing the cytokines GM-CSF and interferon-γ, as well as modulating ICAM-1 expression,[139,140] PTX had a significant antifibrotic effect in vivo, reversing gamma ray–induced fibrosis in pigs.[47] The combination of PTX and the antioxidant vitamin E (α-tocopheryl acetate) may further down-regulate TGF-β expression by myofibroblasts and actually reverse the abnormal fibroblast phenotype that perpetuates fibrosis.[44,47,141,142] Other effects include blocking the induction of collagen by TNF-α and GAG synthesis in normal fibroblasts,[143] as well as lowering the levels of type I and III procollagen messenger RNA and of nuclear factor 1, a procollagen gene-activating transcription factor of human dermal fibroblasts.[144]

Studies examining the effect of prophylactic administration of PTX are ongoing. It may reduce late soft tissue pathology but does not affect acute radiation reactions in animals. In patients, late skin changes, fibrosis, and soft tissue necrosis were less severe in the PTX group than controls, possibly by a protective effect against vascular pathology. It also accelerated healing of soft tissue necrosis and reversed some late radiation injuries.[140,145] There were no positive effects on acute skin reactions or pain in some studies,[146] whereas others showed a decrease in pain.[140,145] When PTX was used with vitamin E, arm lymphedema was not prevented following axillary surgery and lymphatic radiotherapy.[147] However, both in patients and in the pig model, some antifibrotic action of this combination was found in established disease.[47,141] In a pig model, there was less subcutaneous fibrotic scar tissue and a decreased immunostaining for TGF-β₁ in the residual fibrotic tissue.[43,47,147] Lipid peroxidation and certain lipid peroxidation products induce genetic overexpression of fibrogenic cytokines, the key molecules in the pathomechanisms of fibrosis, as well as increased transcription and synthesis of collagen.[43,148] Both of these events can be down-regulated, at least in experimental models, by the use of antioxidants. The effect of oxidative stress on cytokine gene expression appears to be an important mechanism by which it promotes connective tissue deposition.[149,150]

Other modalities to treat chronic radiation fibrosis in animals have included intramuscular injections of liposomal CU/ZN superoxide dismutase (SOD) two times a week for 3 weeks. Liposomal SOD may down-regulate TGF-β secretions by myofibroblasts, functioning as an antioxidant and anti-inflammatory agent.[43] Early animal studies show that it may have an immediate radioprotective effect if given prior to radiation, possibly changing genetic programming of cell differentiation and proliferation.[142] It also reverses the radiation-induced fibrotic process in

experimental animals and permits the regeneration of normal tissue in a zone of well-established postirradiation fibrosis.[142]

Another proinflammatory cytokine, interferon-γ, may inhibit collage production in dermal fibroblasts. When used subcutaneously three times a week for 6 months and then once per week for 6 months on five patients with chronic-stage cutaneous radiation syndrome, low-dose interferon-γ was found to be useful for cutaneous fibrosis, as well as the chronic infection in fibrosed skin.[151]

In chronic radiation dermatitis, hyperbaric oxygen can result in reepithelialization of small areas and reduce pain, edema and erythema, or lymphedema,[32] but there is no effect on fibrosis or telangiectasia.[152] Pulsed dye laser treatment has been beneficial in clearing telangiectasia after radiotherapy.[153]

Secondary Cutaneous Malignancy

Ionizing radiation may be used to treat established cutaneous malignancies, but it also increases the frequency of skin cancer and its precursor lesions. The strongest case is made for the increased incidence of BCC, and all available studies show that skin cancer risk is greater from radiation exposure at young ages.[154,155] These tumors arise not only in areas with typical chronic radiation changes but also on normal-appearing irradiated scalp in patients who were treated for tinea capitis.[156] These BCCs may present with aggressive or unusual variants, including keloidal, scarring, or aggressive varieties. Genetic instability may occur in irradiated cells many generations after treatment, possibly accounting for these tumors,[157] and mutations of tumor suppressor genes may play a role in some cases.[156,158]

The growth of other tumors, including radiation keratoses, squamous cell carcinoma, fibrosarcoma, dermatosarcoma, angiosarcoma, and melanoma, has not been as well documented. The observation that fewer skin cancers develop among irradiated African Americans compared with Caucasians despite a comparable dose of ionizing radiation implies that skin susceptibility to ultraviolet exposure may modify the risk from ionizing radiation (Figure 21). Available evidence indicates that the excess risk of skin cancer lasts for 45 years or more following treatment.[154] Most of the studies reporting an increase in NMSC have not distinguished between patients who received radiotherapy versus chemotherapy. Some, but not all, follow-up studies of cancer patients have reported excesses of malignant melanoma as second malignant neoplasms. It is not clear from the studies how much, if any, of the excess melanoma risk is attributable to radiotherapy.[154,155] However, the fact remains that the most common malignancy in the survivors of the bombing of Hiroshima and Nagasaki in

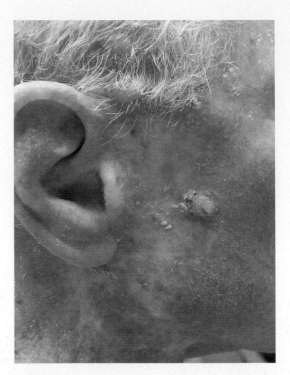

FIGURE 21 Nodular squamous cell carcinoma in the setting of radiation fibrosis and actinic damage.

1945 was NMSC. Squamous cell carcinoma in radiation fields or scars is often ill defined and exhibits aggressive behavior and metastases. Because of this, surgical excision is the preferred modality of treatment. Microscopically monitored surgery with margin control (Mohs' surgery) has a high cure rate, is well tolerated, and is usually performed under local anesthesia in an office setting.

Angiosarcomas are a heterogeneous group of tumors with differing pathogenesis. They may be classified as primary in breast parenchyma, often in younger patients. When found following radical mastectomy with axillary node dissection, Stewart-Treves syndrome, they appear to be associated with chronic edema rather than radiation alone. Angiosarcomas developing in radiation sites should be considered in the clinical setting of late skin thickening, induration, edema, or dyspigmentation.[159]

Because of their premalignant potential, radiation-induced keratoses are often treated. Although there are no studies specifically addressing therapy in irradiated skin, in practice, they are treated like actinically induced premalignancies. Cryotherapy is widely used for localized lesions, but it is of limited usefulness if it does not address large numbers of lesions in the radiation port. Diffuse ill-defined keratoses are candidates for destruction with physical measures such as chemical peels, dermabrasion, or laser. Topical 5-fluorouracil, diclofenac, photodynamic therapy, and imiquimod have also proven beneficial.

Fluorouracil cream is an antineoplastic, antimetabolite drug that interferes with DNA and RNA syntheses, preventing the proliferation of damaged cells.[160] Newer topical modalities, such as diclofenac, are cyclooxygenase 2 (COX-2) inhibitors, inhibiting the enzymes involved in arachidonic acid metabolism. Arachidonic acid metabolites have been shown to play a pivotal role in promoting epithelial tumor growth by stimulating angiogenesis, inhibiting apoptosis, and increasing invasiveness of tumor cells.[161-164] This suggests a possible role for COX-2 inhibitors administered at therapeutically achievable doses in the prevention of radiation-induced malignancy.[165] Diclofenac, a topical COX-2 inhibitor, is typically applied twice a day for 90 days.

Another modality used in the treatment of actinic keratoses and in situ squamous cell carcinoma is topical 5-aminolevulinic acid followed by photodynamic therapy.[166] This uses a photosensitizing compound applied to specific lesions and photoactivated by red-light irradiation. Case reports have found this useful for chronic x-ray dermatitis and particularly helpful in pain relief.[167]

A promising therapeutic option for both keratoses and superficial BCC is topical imiquimod. This immune response modifier affects both the innate and acquired immune responses[168,169] by binding to Toll-like receptor 7 (TLR-7).[170] Subsequent activation of the messenger RNA expression of cytokines, including interferon-α, TNF-α, and interleukin-12, promotes a T helper 1 cell–mediated immune response and reduced Bcl-2 expression, which induces FasR-mediated apoptosis in BCC.[168,171] Currently, imiquimod is approved by the US Food and Drug Administration to treat multiple actinic keratoses[172] and genital warts.

Future Directions

Prevention and treatment of radiation dermatitis are optimally a multidisciplinary mission. Advances in the delivery of radiation include conformal RT, which will target the tumor and minimize exposure to normal tissue. Intensity-modulated RT further shapes the intensity using collimators that focus multiple beams on the target. This results in a smaller high-dose target, but at the cost of increasing the volume of tissue receiving low doses of radiation. CT imaging combined with the LINAC, as well as dedicated operating room suites equipped with a LINAC, provide precision and convenience for the patients and oncologists. The combination of positron emission tomography and CT further defines treatment targets. Newer modalities of therapy, including the use of protons, potentially will avoid the skin and more precisely target the tumor.

Advancements in immunology, including a better understanding of cytokines, inflammation, and their role in producing skin changes, have prompted ongoing investigation of compounds, which may prove to be "cytoprotective." Identification of patients at risk, including those with genetic or autoimmune disorders, and modification of their treatment can help avoid severe complications. Finally, advances in basic wound care management have been invaluable in the treatment of acute and chronic radiation dermatitis. In the future, prospective studies of treatment of radiation dermatitis will provide additional information and guidelines in the treatment of this difficult problem.

REFERENCES

1. Castagna MT, Mintz GS, Waksman R, et al. Comparative efficacy of gamma-irradiation for treatment of in-stent restenosis in saphenous vein graft versus native coronary artery in-stent restenosis: an intravascular ultrasound study. Circulation 2001;104:3020–2.
2. Ahmed JM, Mintz GS, Waksman R, et al. Safety of intracoronary gamma-radiation on uninjured reference segments during the first 6 months after treatment of in-stent restenosis: a serial intravascular ultrasound study. Circulation 2000;101:2227–30.
3. De Conno F, Ventafridda V, Saita L. Skin problems in advanced and terminal cancer patients. J Pain Symptom Manage 1991;6:247–56.
4. King KB, Nail LM, Kreamer K, et al. Patients' descriptions of the experience of receiving radiation therapy. Oncol Nurs Forum 1985;12:55–61.
5. Frieben H. Demonstration eines Cancroid des rechten Handruckens, das sich nach langdauernder Einwirkung von Rontgenstrahlen entwickelt hatte. Fortschr Rontgenstr 1902;6:106–11.
6. Dehen L, Vilmer C, Humiliere C, et al. Chronic radiodermatitis following cardiac catheterisation: a report of two cases and a brief review of the literature. Heart 1999;81:308–12.
7. Huda W, Peters KR. Radiation-induced temporary epilation after a neuroradiologically guided embolization procedure. Radiology 1994;193:642–4.
8. Wilson L, Panizzon RG. Dermatology. In: Bolognia JL, Jorizzo JL, Rapini RP, editors. Radiation therapy. Vol 2. London: Mosby; 2003. p. 2185–95.
9. Hopewell JW, Nyman J, Turesson I. Time factor for acute tissue reactions following fractionated irradiation: a balance between repopulation and enhanced radiosensitivity. Int J Radiat Biol 2003;79:513–24.
10. Simonen P, Hamilton C, Ferguson S, et al. Do inflammatory processes contribute to radiation induced erythema observed in the skin of humans? Radiother Oncol 1998;46:73–82.
11. Schmuth M, Sztankay A, Weinlich G, et al. Permeability barrier function of skin exposed to ionizing radiation. Arch Dermatol 2001;137:1019–23.
12. Kupper TS. The activated keratinocyte: a model for inducible cytokine production by non-bone marrow-derived cells in cutaneous inflammatory and immune responses. J Invest Dermatol 1990;94 Suppl:146S–50S.
13. Mendelsohn FA, Divino CM, Reis ED, et al. Wound care after radiation therapy. Adv Skin Wound Care 2002;15:216–24.
14. Archambeau JO, Pezner R, Wasserman T. Pathophysiology of irradiated skin and breast. Int J Radiat Oncol Biol Phys 1995;31:1171–85.
15. Hill A, Hanson M, Bogle MA, et al. Severe radiation dermatitis is related to *Staphylococcus aureus*. Am J Clin Oncol 2004;27:361–3.
16. Peter RU, Beetz A, Ried C, et al. Increased expression of the epidermal growth factor receptor in human epidermal keratinocytes after exposure to ionizing radiation. Radiat Res 1993;136:65–70.
17. Peters LJ, Ang KK, Thames HD Jr. Accelerated fractionation in the radiation treatment of head and neck cancer. A critical comparison of different strategies. Acta Oncol 1988;27:185–94.
18. Denham JW, Hauer-Jensen M. The radiotherapeutic injury—a complex 'wound.' Radiother Oncol 2002;63:129–45.
19. Goldschmidt H, Breneman JC, Breneman DL. Ionizing radiation therapy in dermatology. J Am Acad Dermatol 1994;30 Pt 1:157–182; quiz 183–6.
20. Goldschmidt H, Sherwin WK. Reactions to ionizing radiation. J Am Acad Dermatol 1980;3:551–79.
21. Dutreix J. Human skin: early and late reactions in relation to dose and its time distribution. Br J Radiol Suppl 1986;19:22–8.
22. Turesson I, Nyman J, Holmberg E, et al. Prognostic factors for acute and late skin reactions in radiotherapy patients. Int J Radiat Oncol Biol Phys 1996;36:1065–75.
23. Bentzen SM, Overgaard J. Patient-to-patient variability in the expression of radiation-induced normal tissue injury. Semin Radiat Oncol 1994;4:68–80.
24. Bentzen SM, Overgaard M. Relationship between early and late normal-tissue injury after postmastectomy radiotherapy. Radiother Oncol 1991;20:159–65.
25. Okumura S, Mitsumori M, Kokubo M, et al. Late skin and subcutaneous soft tissue changes after 10-Gy boost for breast conserving therapy. Breast Cancer 2003;10:129–33.
26. Canney PA, Dean S. Transforming growth factor beta: a promotor of late connective tissue injury following radiotherapy? Br J Radiol 1990;63:620–3.
27. Harper JL, Franklin LE, Jenrette JM, et al. Skin toxicity during breast irradiation: pathophysiology and management. South Med J 2004;97:989–93.
28. Steinert M, Weiss M, Gottlober P, et al. Delayed effects of accidental cutaneous radiation exposure: fifteen years of follow-up after the Chernobyl accident. J Am Acad Dermatol 2003;49:417–23.
29. Hopewell JW. The skin: its structure and response to ionizing radiation. Int J Radiat Biol 1990;57:751–73.
30. Malkinson FD, Hanson WR. Radiobiology of the skin. In: Goldsmith L, editor. Physiology, biochemistry and molecular biology of the skin. Vol II. Oxford: Oxford University Press; 1991. p. 976.
31. Bernstein EF, Harisiadis L, Salomon GD, et al. Healing impairment of open wounds by skin irradiation. J Dermatol Surg Oncol 1994;20:757–60.
32. Gottlober P, Krahn G, Peter RU. [Cutaneous radiation syndrome: clinical features, diagnosis and therapy]. Hautarzt 2000;518:567–74.
33. Boxman I, Lowik C, Aarden L, et al. Modulation of IL-6 production and IL-1 activity by keratinocyte-fibroblast interaction. J Invest Dermatol 1993;101:316–24.
34. Gajdusek C, Onoda K, London S, et al. Early molecular changes in irradiated aortic endothelium. J Cell Physiol 2001;188:8–23.
35. Quarmby S, Kumar P, Kumar S. Radiation-induced normal tissue injury: role of adhesion molecules in leukocyte-endothelial cell interactions. Int J Cancer 1999;82:385–95.
36. Edwards EK Jr, Edwards EK Sr. The effect of superficial x-radiation on epidermal Langerhans cells in human skin. Int J Dermatol 1990;29:731–2.
37. Kawase Y, Naito S, Ito M, et al. The effect of ionizing radiation on epidermal Langerhans cells—a quantitative analysis of autopsy cases with radiation therapy. J Radiat Res (Tokyo) 1990;31:246–55.
38. Behrends U, Peter RU, Hintermeier-Knabe R, et al. Ionizing radiation induces human intercellular adhesion molecule-1 in vitro. J Invest Dermatol 1994;103:726–30.
39. Fajardo LF, Berthrong M. Vascular lesions following radiation. Pathol Annu 1988;23 Pt 1:297–330.
40. Mettler FA Jr, Upton AC Direct effects of radiation in Medical Effects of Ionizing Radiation 2nd Ed. WB Saunders Company, Philadelphia Pa 1995; pg214–221.
41. Geng L, Hanson WR, Malkinson FD. Topical or systemic 16, 16 dm prostaglandin E2 or WR-2721 (WR-1065) protects mice from alopecia after fractionated irradiation. Int J Radiat Biol 1992;61:533–7.
42. Malkinson FD, Geng L, Hanson WR. Prostaglandins protect against murine hair injury produced by ionizing radiation or doxorubicin. J Invest Dermatol 1993;101 Suppl:135S–7S.
43. Martin M, Lefaix J, Delanian S. TGF-beta1 and radiation fibrosis: a master switch and a specific therapeutic target? Int J Radiat Oncol Biol Phys 2000;47:277–90.
44. Vozenin-Brotons MC, Gault N, Sivan V, et al. Histopathological and cellular studies of a case of cutaneous radiation syndrome after accidental chronic exposure to a cesium source. Radiat Res 1999;152:332–7.
45. Schultze-Mosgau S, Wehrhan F, Grabenbauer G, et al. Transforming growth factor beta1 and beta2 (TGFbeta2/TGFbeta2) profile changes in previously irradiated free flap beds. Head Neck 2002;24:33–41.
46. Lorette G, Machet L. [Radiation-induced skin toxicities: prevention, treatment]. Cancer Radiother 2001;5 Suppl 1:116s–20s.

47. Lefaix JL, Delanian S, Vozenin MC, et al. Striking regression of subcutaneous fibrosis induced by high doses of gamma rays using a combination of pentoxifylline and alpha-tocopherol: an experimental study. Int J Radiat Oncol Biol Phys 1999;43:839–47.

48. Flanders KC, Major CD, Arabshahi A, et al. Interference with transforming growth factor-beta/ Smad3 signaling results in accelerated healing of wounds in previously irradiated skin. Am J Pathol 2003;163:2247–57.

49. Gruber BL, Marchese MJ, Kew RR. Transforming growth factor-beta 1 mediates mast cell chemotaxis. J Immunol 1994;1521:5860–7.

50. Yamabe H, Osawa H, Inuma H, et al. Thrombin stimulates production of transforming growth factor-beta by cultured human mesangial cells. Nephrol Dial Transplant 1997;12:438–42.

51. DeMichele MA, Minnear FL. Modulation of vascular endothelial permeability by thrombin. Semin Thromb Hemost 1992;18:287–95.

52. Tibbs MK. Wound healing following radiation therapy: a review. Radiother Oncol 1997;42:99–106.

53. Tokarek R, Bernstein EF, Sullivan F, et al. Effect of therapeutic radiation on wound healing. Clin Dermatol 1994;12:57–70.

54. Kruse JJ, te Poele JA, Russell NS, et al. Microarray analysis to identify molecular mechanisms of radiation-induced microvascular damage in normal tissues. Int J Radiat Oncol Biol Phys 2004;58:420–6.

55. Fernando IN, Ford HT, Powles TJ, et al. Factors affecting acute skin toxicity in patients having breast irradiation after conservative surgery: a prospective study of treatment practice at the Royal Marsden Hospital. Clin Oncol (R Coll Radiol) 1996;8:226–33.

56. Emami B, Lyman J, Brown A, et al. Tolerance of normal tissue to therapeutic irradiation. Int J Radiat Oncol Biol Phys 1991;21:109–22.

57. Lee N, Chuang C, Quivey JM, et al. Skin toxicity due to intensity-modulated radiotherapy for head-and-neck carcinoma. Int J Radiat Oncol Biol Phys 2002;53:630–7.

58. Safwat A, Bentzen SM, Turesson I, et al. Deterministic rather than stochastic factors explain most of the variation in the expression of skin telangiectasia after radiotherapy. Int J Radiat Oncol Biol Phys 2002;52:198–204.

59. Porock D, Kristjanson L, Nikoletti S, et al. Predicting the severity of radiation skin reactions in women with breast cancer. Oncol Nurs Forum 1998;25:1019–29.

60. Twardella D, Popanda O, Helmbold I, et al. Personal characteristics, therapy modalities and individual DNA repair capacity as predictive factors of acute skin toxicity in an unselected cohort of breast cancer patients receiving radiotherapy. Radiother Oncol 2003;69:145–53.

61. Sitton E. Early and late radiation-induced skin alterations. Part I: mechanisms of skin changes. Oncol Nurs Forum 1992;19:801–7.

62. Swift M, Morrell D, Cromartie E, et al. The incidence and gene frequency of ataxia-telangiectasia in the United States. Am J Hum Genet 1986;39:573–83.

63. Iannuzzi CM, Atencio DP, Green S, et al. ATM mutations in female breast cancer patients predict for an increase in radiation-induced late effects. Int J Radiat Oncol Biol Phys 2002;52:606–13.

64. Bremer M, Klopper K, Yamini P, et al. Clinical radiosensitivity in breast cancer patients carrying pathogenic ATM gene mutations: no observation of increased radiation-induced acute or late effects. Radiother Oncol 2003;69:155–60.

65. Hahn H, Wicking C, Zaphiropoulous PG, et al. Mutations of the human homolog of *Drosophila* patched in the nevoid basal cell carcinoma syndrome. Cell 1996;85:841–51.

66. Johnson RL, Rothman AL, Xie J, et al. Human homolog of patched, a candidate gene for the basal cell nevus syndrome. Science 1996;272:1668–71.

67. Hahn H, Wojnowski L, Zimmer AM, et al. Rhabdomyosarcomas and radiation hypersensitivity in a mouse model of Gorlin syndrome. Nat Med 1998;4:619–22.

68. Dezawa M, Fujii K, Kita K, et al. Increase in nucleoli after x-radiation of fibroblasts of patients with Gorlin syndrome. J Lab Clin Med 1999;134:585–91.

69. Sanford KK, Parshad R, Gantt R, et al. Factors affecting and significance of G2 chromatin radiosensitivity in predisposition to cancer. Int J Radiat Biol 1989;55:963–81.

70. Sanford KK, Tarone RE, Parshad R, et al. Hypersensitivity to G2 chromatid radiation damage in familial dysplastic naevus syndrome. Lancet 1987;2:1111–6.

71. Sanford KK, Parshad R, Price FM, et al. Radiation-induced chromatid breaks and DNA repair in blood lymphocytes of patients with dysplastic nevi and/or cutaneous melanoma. J Invest Dermatol 1997;109:546–9.

72. Tucker SL, Turesson I, Thames HD. Evidence for individual differences in the radiosensitivity of human skin. Eur J Cancer 1992;28A:1783–91.

73. Hoeller U, Borgmann K, Bonacker M, et al. Individual radiosensitivity measured with lymphocytes may be used to predict the risk of fibrosis after radiotherapy for breast cancer. Radiother Oncol 2003;69:137–44.

74. Ponten F, Lindman H, Bostrom A, et al. Induction of p53 expression in skin by radiotherapy and UV radiation: a randomized study. J Natl Cancer Inst 2001;93:128–33.

75. Ross JG, Hussey DH, Mayr NA, et al. Acute and late reactions to radiation therapy in patients with collagen vascular diseases. Cancer 1993;71:3744–52.

76. De Naeyer B, De Meerleer G, Braems S, et al. Collagen vascular diseases and radiation therapy: a critical review. Int J Radiat Oncol Biol Phys 1999;44:975–80.

77. Morris MM, Powell SN. Irradiation in the setting of collagen vascular disease: acute and late complications. J Clin Oncol 1997;15:2728–35.

78. McCurdy D, Tai LQ, Frias S, et al. Delayed repair of DNA damage by ionizing radiation in cells from patients with juvenile systemic lupus erythematosus and rheumatoid arthritis. Radiat Res 1997;147:48–54.

79. Harris G, Cramp WA, Edwards JC, et al. Radiosensitivity of peripheral blood lymphocytes in autoimmune disease. Int J Radiat Biol Relat Stud Phys Chem Med 1985;47:689–99.

80. Kao GD, Devine P, Mirza N. Oral cavity and oropharyngeal tumors in human immunodeficiency virus-positive patients: acute response to radiation therapy. Arch Otolaryngol Head Neck Surg 1999;125:873–6.

81. Watkins EB, Findlay P, Gelmann E, et al. Enhanced mucosal reactions in AIDS patients receiving oropharyngeal irradiation. Int J Radiat Oncol Biol Phys 1987;13:1403–8.

82. Smith KJ, Skelton HG, Tuur S, et al. Increased cutaneous toxicity to ionizing radiation in HIV-positive patients. Military Medical Consortium for the Advancement of Retroviral Research (MMCARR). Int J Dermatol 1997;36:779–82.

83. Coleman CN, Turrisi AT. Radiation and chemotherapy sensitizers and protectors. Crit Rev Oncol Hematol 1990;10:225–52.

84. Bentzen SM, Overgaard M, Thames HD, et al. Early and late normal-tissue injury after postmastectomy radiotherapy alone or combined with chemotherapy. Int J Radiat Biol 1989;56:711–5.

85. Azria D, Gourgou S, Sozzi WJ, et al. Concomitant use of tamoxifen with radiotherapy enhances subcutaneous breast fibrosis in hypersensitive patients. Br J Cancer 2004;91:1251–60.

86. Vergara G, Vargas-Machuca I, Pastor MA, et al. Localization of Sweet's syndrome in radiation-induced locus minoris resistentae. J Am Acad Dermatol 2003;49:907–9.

87. Kim JH, Krivda SJ. Lichen planus confined to a radiation therapy site. J Am Acad Dermatol 2002;46:604–5.

88. Low GJ, Keeling JH. Ionizing radiation-induced pemphigus. Case presentations and literature review. Arch Dermatol 1990;126:1319–23.

89. Veness MJ, Dwyer PK. Erythema multiforme-like reaction associated with radiotherapy. Australas Radiol 1996;40:334–7.

90. Duncan KO, Tigelaar RE, Bolognia JL. Stevens-Johnson syndrome limited to multiple sites of radiation therapy in a patient receiving phenobarbital. J Am Acad Dermatol 1999;40:493–6.

91. Aguiar D, Pazo R, Duran I, et al. Toxic epidermal necrolysis in patients receiving anticonvulsants and cranial irradiation: a risk to consider. J Neurooncol 2004;66:345–50.

92. Ahmed I, Reichenberg J, Lucas A, et al. Erythema multiforme associated with phenytoin and cranial radiation therapy: a report of three patients and review of the literature. Int J Dermatol 2004;43:67–73.

93. Eralp Y, Aydiner A, Tas F, et al. Stevens-Johnson syndrome in a patient receiving anticonvulsant therapy during cranial irradiation. Am J Clin Oncol 2001;24:347–50.

94. Khafaga YM, Jamshed A, Allam AA, et al. Stevens-Johnson syndrome in patients on phenytoin and cranial radiotherapy. Acta Oncol 1999;38:111–6.

95. Micali G, Linthicum K, Han N, et al. Increased risk of erythema multiforme major with combination anticonvulsant and radiation therapies. Pharmacotherapy 1999;19:223–7.

96. Camidge R, Price A. Characterizing the phenomenon of radiation recall dermatitis. Radiother Oncol 2001;59:237–45.

97. Ristic B. Radiation recall dermatitis. Int J Dermatol 2004;43:627–31.

98. Bostrom A, Sjolin-Forsberg G, Wilking N, et al. Radiation recall—another call with tamoxifen. Acta Oncol 1999;38:955–9.

99. Parry BR. Radiation recall induced by tamoxifen. Lancet 1992;340:49.

100. Wright EG. Radiation-induced genomic instability in haemopoietic cells. Int J Radiat Biol 1998;74:681–7.

101. Seymour CB, Mothersill C, Alper T. High yields of lethal mutations in somatic mammalian cells that survive ionizing radiation. Int J Radiat Biol Relat Stud Phys Chem Med 1986;50:167–79.

102. Hellman S, Botnick LE. Stem cell depletion: an explanation of the late effects of cytotoxins. Int J Radiat Oncol Biol Phys 1977;2–2:181–4.

103. Smith KJ, Germain M, Skelton H. Histopathologic features seen with radiation recall or enhancement eruptions. J Cutan Med Surg 2002;6:535–40.

104. Camidge R, Price A. Radiation recall dermatitis may represent the Koebner phenomenon. J Clin Oncol 2002;20:4130; author reply 4130.

105. Campbell IR, Illingworth MH. Can patients wash during radiotherapy to the breast or chest wall? A randomized controlled trial. Clin Oncol (R Coll Radiol) 1992;4:78–82.

106. Roy I, Fortin A, Larochelle M. The impact of skin washing with water and soap during breast irradiation: a randomized study. Radiother Oncol 2001;58:333–9.

107. Westbury C, Hines F, Hawkes E, et al. Advice on hair and scalp care during cranial radiotherapy: a prospective randomized trial. Radiother Oncol 2000;54:109–16.

108. Fenig E, Brenner B, Katz A, et al. Topical Biafine and Lipiderm for the prevention of radiation dermatitis: a randomized prospective trial. Oncol Rep 2001;8:305–9.

109. Gray M. Preventing and managing perineal dermatitis: a shared goal for wound and continence care. J Wound Ostomy Continence Nurs 2004;31 Suppl:S2–9; quiz S10–2.

110. Williams MS, Burk M, Loprinzi CL, et al. Phase III double-blind evaluation of an aloe vera gel as a prophylactic agent for radiation-induced skin toxicity. Int J Radiat Oncol Biol Phys 1996;36:345–9.

111. Heggie S, Bryant GP, Tripcony L, et al. A phase III study on the efficacy of topical aloe vera gel on irradiated breast tissue. Cancer Nurs 2002;25:442–51.

112. Maiche AG, Grohn P, Maki-Hokkonen H. Effect of chamomile cream and almond ointment on acute radiation skin reaction. Acta Oncol 1991;30:395–6.

113. Maiche A, Isokangas OP, Grohn P. Skin protection by sucralfate cream during electron beam therapy. Acta Oncol 1994;33:201–3.

114. Roper B, Kaisig D, Auer F, et al. Theta-Cream versus Bepanthol lotion in breast cancer patients under radiotherapy. A new prophylactic agent in skin care? Strahlenther Onkol 2004;180:315–22.

115. Halperin EC, Gaspar L, George S, et al. A double-blind, randomized, prospective trial to evaluate topical vitamin C solution for the prevention of radiation dermatitis. CNS Cancer Consortium. Int J Radiat Oncol Biol Phys 1993;26:413–6.

116. Okunieff P. Interactions between ascorbic acid and the radiation of bone marrow, skin, and tumor. Am J Clin Nutr 1991;54 Suppl:1281S–3S.

117. Delaney G, Fisher R, Hook C, et al. Sucralfate cream in the management of moist desquamation during radiotherapy. Australas Radiol 1997;41:270–5.

118. Liguori V, Guillemin C, Pesce GF, et al. Double-blind, randomized clinical study comparing hyaluronic acid cream to placebo in patients treated with radiotherapy. Radiother Oncol 1997;42:155–61.

119. Pommier P, Gomez F, Sunyach MP, et al. Phase III randomized trial of *Calendula officinalis* compared with trolamine for the prevention of acute dermatitis during irradiation for breast cancer. J Clin Oncol 2004;22:1447–53.

120. Graham P, Browne L, Capp A, et al. Randomized, paired comparison of No-Sting Barrier Film versus sorbolene cream (10% glycerine) skin care during postmastectomy irradiation. Int J Radiat Oncol Biol Phys 2004;58:241–6.

121. Wickline MM. Continuing education: prevention and treatment of acute radiation dermatitis: a literature review. Oncol Nurs Forum 2004;31:237–47.

122. Lokkevik E, Skovlund E, Reitan JB, et al. Skin treatment with bepanthen cream versus no cream during radiotherapy—a randomized controlled trial. Acta Oncol 1996;35: 1021–6.

123. Beetz A, Messer G, Oppel T, et al. Induction of interleukin 6 by ionizing radiation in a human epithelial cell line: control by corticosteroids. Int J Radiat Biol 1997;72: 33–43.

124. Potera ME, Lookingbill DP, Stryker JA. Prophylaxis of radiation dermatitis with a topical cortisone cream. Radiology 1982;143:775–7.

125. Bostrom A, Lindman H, Swartling C, et al. Potent corticosteroid cream (mometasone furoate) significantly reduces acute radiation dermatitis: results from a double-blind, randomized study. Radiother Oncol 2001;59:257–65.

126. Glees JP, Mameghan-Zadeh H, Sparkes CG. Effectiveness of topical steroids in the control of radiation dermatitis: a randomised trial using 1% hydrocortisone cream and 0.05% clobetasone butyrate (Eumovate). Clin Radiol 1979;30:397–403.

127. Schmuth M, Wimmer MA, Hofer S, et al. Topical corticosteroid therapy for acute radiation dermatitis: a prospective, randomized, double-blind study. Br J Dermatol 2002; 146:983–91.

128. Milas L, Nishiguchi I, Hunter N, et al. Radiation protection against early and late effects of ionizing irradiation by the prostaglandin inhibitor indomethacin. Adv Space Res 1992;122:265–71.

129. Smith APS and Fife CE. Advanced therapeutics: the biochemistry and biophysical basis of wound products. In: PJ Sheffield, ED, Wound Care Practice, Best Publishing Company, Flagstaff (AZ) 2004 pp 685–728

130. Varghese MC, Balin AK, Carter DM, et al. Local environment of chronic wounds under synthetic dressings. Arch Dermatol 1986;122:52–7.

131. Margolin SG, Breneman JC, Denman DL, et al. Management of radiation-induced moist desquamation using hydrocolloid dressing. Cancer Nurs 1990;13:71–80.

132. Gonyon DL Jr, Zenn MR. Simple approach to the radiated scalp wound using INTEGRA skin substitute. Ann Plast Surg 2003;50:315–20.

133. Schindl A, Schindl M, Pernerstorfer-Schon H, et al. Low intensity laser irradiation in the treatment of recalcitrant radiation ulcers in patients with breast cancer—long-term results of 3 cases. Photodermatol Photoimmunol Photomed 2000;16:34–7.

134. Schindl A, Schindl M, Schon H, et al. Low-intensity laser irradiation improves skin circulation in patients with diabetic microangiopathy. Diabetes Care 1998;21: 580–4.

135. Vuong T, Franco E, Lehnert S, et al. Silver leaf nylon dressing to prevent radiation dermatitis in patients undergoing chemotherapy and external beam radiotherapy to the perineum. Int J Radiat Oncol Biol Phys 2004;59: 809–14.

136. Kouvaris JR, Kouloulias VE, Plataniotis GA, et al. Topical granulocyte-macrophage colony-stimulating factor for radiation dermatitis of the vulva. Br J Dermatol 2001; 144:646–7.

137. Hom DB, Manivel JC. Promoting healing with recombinant human platelet-derived growth factor-BB in a previously irradiated problem wound. Laryngoscope 2003;113: 1566–71.

138. Wollina U, Liebold K, Konrad H. Treatment of chronic radiation ulcers with recombinant platelet-derived growth factor and a hydrophilic copolymer membrane. J Eur Acad Dermatol Venereol 2001;15:455–7.

139. Samlaska CP, Winfield EA. Pentoxifylline. J Am Acad Dermatol 1994;30:603–21.

140. Dion MW, Hussey DH, Doornbos JF, et al. Preliminary results of a pilot study of pentoxifylline in the treatment of late radiation soft tissue necrosis. Int J Radiat Oncol Biol Phys 1990;19:401–7.

141. Delanian S, Balla-Mekias S, Lefaix JL. Striking regression of chronic radiotherapy damage in a clinical trial of combined pentoxifylline and tocopherol. J Clin Oncol 1999;17:3283–90.

142. Lefaix JL, Delanian S, Leplat JJ, et al. Successful treatment of radiation-induced fibrosis using Cu/Zn-SOD and Mn-SOD: an experimental study. Int J Radiat Oncol Biol Phys 1996;35:305–12.

143. Berman B, Wietzerbin J, Sanceau J, et al. Pentoxifylline inhibits certain constitutive and tumor necrosis factor-alpha-induced activities of human normal dermal fibroblasts. J Invest Dermatol 1992;98:706–12.

144. Duncan MR, Hasan A, Berman B. Pentoxifylline, pentifylline, and interferons decrease type I and III procollagen mRNA levels in dermal fibroblasts: evidence for mediation by nuclear factor 1 down-regulation. J Invest Dermatol 1995;104:282–6.

145. Futran ND, Trotti A, Gwede C. Pentoxifylline in the treatment of radiation-related soft tissue injury: preliminary observations. Laryngoscope 1997;107:391–5.

146. Aygenc E, Celikkanat S, Kaymakci M, et al. Prophylactic effect of pentoxifylline on radiotherapy complications: a clinical study. Otolaryngol Head Neck Surg 2004;130: 351–6.

147. Gothard L, Cornes P, Earl J, et al. Double-blind placebo-controlled randomised trial of vitamin E and pentoxifylline in patients with chronic arm lymphoedema and fibrosis after surgery and radiotherapy for breast cancer. Radiother Oncol 2004;73:133–9.

148. Chiarpotto E, Scavazza A, Leonarduzzi G, et al. Oxidative damage and transforming growth factor beta 1 expression in pretumoral and tumoral lesions of human intestine. Free Radic Biol Med 1997;22:889–94.

149. Poli G, Parola M. Oxidative damage and fibrogenesis. Free Radic Biol Med 1997;22:287–305.

150. Martin M, Vozenin MC, Gault N, et al. Coactivation of AP-1 activity and TGF-beta1 gene expression in the stress response of normal skin cells to ionizing radiation. Oncogene 1997;15:981–9.

151. Gottlober P, Steinert M, Bahren W, et al. Interferon-gamma in 5 patients with cutaneous radiation syndrome after radiation therapy. Int J Radiat Oncol Biol Phys 2001; 50:159–66.

152. Carl UM, Feldmeier JJ, Schmitt G, et al. Hyperbaric oxygen therapy for late sequelae in women receiving radiation after breast-conserving surgery. Int J Radiat Oncol Biol Phys 2001;49:1029–31.

153. Lanigan SW, Joannides T. Pulsed dye laser treatment of telangiectasia after radiotherapy for carcinoma of the breast. Br J Dermatol 2003;148:77–9.

154. Shore RE. Radiation-induced skin cancer in humans. Med Pediatr Oncol 2001;36:549–54.

155. Karagas MR, McDonald JA, Greenberg ER, et al. Risk of basal cell and squamous cell skin cancers after ionizing radiation therapy. For The Skin Cancer Prevention Study Group. J Natl Cancer Inst 1996;88:1848–53.

156. Maalej M, Frikha H, Kochbati L, et al. Radio-induced malignancies of the scalp about 98 patients with 150 lesions and literature review. Cancer Radiother 2004;8:81–7.

157. Tarkkanen M, Wiklund TA, Virolainen MJ, et al. Comparative genomic hybridization of postirradiation sarcomas. Cancer 2001;92:1992–8.

158. Dutrillaux B. [Radiation-induced cancers]. Cancer Radiother 1998;2:541–8.

159. Rao J, Dekoven JG, Beatty JD, et al. Cutaneous angiosarcoma as a delayed complication of radiation therapy for carcinoma of the breast. J Am Acad Dermatol 2003;49: 532–8.

160. Robins P, Gupta AK. The use of topical fluorouracil to treat actinic keratosis. Cutis 2002;70 Suppl:4–7.

161. Marnett LJ. Generation of mutagens during arachidonic acid metabolism. Cancer Metastasis Rev 1994;13:303–8.

162. Masferrer JL, Leahy KM, Koki AT, et al. Antiangiogenic and antitumor activities of cyclooxygenase-2 inhibitors. Cancer Res 2000;60:1306–11.

163. Villa AM, Berman B. Immunomodulators for skin cancer. J Drugs Dermatol 2004;3:533–9.

164. Wolf JE Jr, Taylor JR, Tschen E, et al. Topical 3.0% diclofenac in 2.5% hyaluronan gel in the treatment of actinic keratoses. Int J Dermatol 2001;40:709–13.

165. Bisht KS, Bradbury CM, Zoberi I, et al. Inhibition of cyclooxygenase-2 with NS-398 and the prevention of radiation-induced transformation, micronuclei formation and clonogenic cell death in C3H 10T1/2 cells. Int J Radiat Biol 2003;79:879–88.

166. Guillen C, Sanmartin O, Escudero A, et al. Photodynamic therapy for in situ squamous cell carcinoma on chronic radiation dermatitis after photosensitization with 5-aminolaevulinic acid. J Eur Acad Dermatol Venereol 2000;14:298–300.

167. Escudero A, Nagore E, Sevila A, et al. Chronic x-ray dermatitis treated by topical 5-aminolaevulinic acid-photodynamic therapy. Br J Dermatol 2002;147:394–6.

168. Vidal D, Matias-Guiu X, Alomar A. Open study of the efficacy and mechanism of action of topical imiquimod in basal cell carcinoma. Clin Exp Dermatol 2004;29: 518–25.

169. Stanley MA. Imiquimod and the imidazoquinolones: mechanism of action and therapeutic potential. Clin Exp Dermatol 2002;27:571–7.

170. Stockfleth E, Trefzer U, Garcia-Bartels C, et al. The use of Toll-like receptor-7 agonist in the treatment of basal cell carcinoma: an overview. Br J Dermatol 2003;149 Suppl 66:53–6.

171. Berman B, Sullivan T, De Araujo T, et al. Expression of Fas-receptor on basal cell carcinomas after treatment with imiquimod 5% cream or vehicle. Br J Dermatol 2003;149 Suppl 66:59–61.

172. Lebwohl M, Dinehart S, Whiting D, et al. Imiquimod 5% cream for the treatment of actinic keratosis: results from two phase III, randomized, double-blind, parallel group, vehicle-controlled trials. J Am Acad Dermatol 2004;50: 714–21.

Alopecia

Asra Ali, MD
Sanjay Mehta, MD

Alopecia, or hair loss, is a frequent occurrence in cancer patients. It is typically reported by the patient when approximately 25 to 40% of the person's hair is lost.[1] The precipitating process is often multifactorial and may result from direct or indirect actions on the hair follicles. Hair loss can often occur as a consequence of anticancer therapy, mainly from chemotherapy and radiation therapy.[2,3] A well-recognized but rare presentation of scalp metastasis is alopecia neoplastica,[4] usually owing to metastasis from breast cancer or other primary cancers. Endocrinopathies caused by a direct result of the primary cancer or cancer treatment may be the sole reason for hair loss or may exacerbate an already existing problem.[5] An iatrogenic immunocompromised state predisposes cancer patients to numerous infectious agents that may affect hair growth.[6] Lastly, these patients may suffer from dermatologic conditions that cause alopecia coincidentally with the presentation of their primary malignancy or treatment of their malignancy. Hair loss should be addressed by the physician since it can be a psychologically devastating aspect of cancer therapy. Preparation for such an event and proper interventions after its occurrence will help the patient cope better with this condition.[7]

Hair Functions

Hair has several functions other than its aesthetic importance. It forms a barrier between the skin and environment, therefore helping protect the epidermis from minor abrasions and from ultraviolet light. Hair fiber may also increase the surface area for faster evaporation of sweat from neighboring apocrine glands. Some hair follicles have a highly developed nerve network around them and provide sensory, tactile information about the environment. A key role of hair is to provide protection against heat loss. Although its importance for human survival has diminished, it is still a significant biological entity.[8]

Hair Development

During hair development, epidermal invaginations occur forming columns in the dermis. The central portion of the columns (bulb) along with stem cells, found in the bulge area of the columns, induce hair follicle formation by the overlying epithelium.[9]

Normal Hair Growth

Understanding normal hair growth often aids the physician in correctly interpreting the cause of hair loss. Each day, the scalp hair grows approximately 0.35 mm (6 inches per year); slower growth occurs in elderly people and in patients with a chronic illness. The scalp sheds approximately 100 hairs per day.

Scalp hair grows in an asynchronous pattern. Every hair follicle continually goes through three phases: anagen (growth), catagen (involution, or a brief transition between growth and resting), and telogen (resting) (Figure 2). Since each follicle passes independently through the three stages of growth, the normal process of hair loss usually is unnoticeable. Approximately 80% of hair follicles are in the active growing, or anagen, phase. Follicles remain in anagen for an average of 3 years (range 2–6 years). The hair on the arms, legs, eyelashes, and eyebrows has a very short active growth phase of about 30 to 45 days, explaining why they are so much shorter than scalp hair. The transitional, or catagen, phase, usually affects 2 to 3% of hair follicles from days to a few weeks. Fourteen percent of hair follicles in the resting, or telogen, phase will be shed in a 3 to 5 months period this accounts for normal daily hair shedding. During telogen, hair growth stops and the outer root sheath shrinks and attaches to the root of the hair. This causes the formation of what is known as a club hair. Pulling out a hair in this phase will reveal a solid, hard, dry, white material at the root.

Hair continually cycles through the three phases. Alteration of hair growth cycling can manifest clinically as increased shedding of scalp hair.[10]

Hair Pigment

Hair pigment is formed by melanocytes in hair follicles located in the hair bulb, found at the bottom of hair follicles. Melanocytes are located in other regions of the hair follicle,; however, it is thought that these melanocytes do not significantly contribute to coloring the hair fiber.

Melanocytes produce melanin pigment proteins in their cell cytoplasm. The pigment is accumulated in membrane-bound vesicles in the cell called "melanosomes." The melanocyte cells release their melanosomes to the keratinocytes through dendritic processes. Eumelanin is the pigment of brown or black hair. Pheomelanin is the pigment of blond or red hair. The appearance of white hairs seems to be caused by an interruption of the transmission of pigments from the melanocytes to the keratinocytes, or loss of melanocytes may also be the cause of graying of hair.[8]

Hair Shape

The amount of natural curl a hair has is determined by its cross-sectional shape. The uneven distribution of disulphide bonds is responsible to a variable degree for curling. Hair that is most similar to a circle is straight, and hair that is flattened and elliptical is curly or kinky. In general, people of African origin have rather flat hair viewed in cross-section compared with Caucasian people, whereas people of Asian origin have the most round and even-sized hairs.

The cross-sectional shape also determines the amount of shine the hair has. Straighter hair is shinier because sebum from the sebaceous gland can travel down the hair more easily. The kinkier the hair, the more difficulty sebum has traveling down the hair and therefore the more dry or dull the hair looks.

Evaluation of Hair Loss

The diagnosis of hair disorders is complex, requiring a thorough evaluation of the clinical presentation, history, physical examination, and diagnostic tests.

A careful history often suggests the underlying cause of alopecia. The history should include when the hair loss started; whether the loss was a gradual hair thinning (ie, gradually more scalp appears) or a hair shedding (ie, large quantities of hair falling out); and if any physical, mental, or emotional stressors occurred within the previous 3 to 6 months. Other important components of the history include: The patient's diet, medications, present and past medical conditions (personal or family history of autoimmune conditions, thyroid disease, anemia), associated nail changes, hair care habits (shampooing, bleaching, perming), and family history of alopecia.

The pattern of hair loss can help Establish a possible cause for the hair loss. (Table 1)

The physical examination has three parts. First, the scalp condition is noted. Evidence of erythema, scaling, inflammation, or scarring is noted. Follicular units, on the scalp, are present in nonscarring alopecias but absent in scarring types. Second, the density and distribution of hair are assessed. Third, the hair shaft is examined for caliber, length, shape, and fragility. The nails should also be examined.

Assessment of the amount of alopecia can be done using the World Health Organization criteria for alopecia: grade 0 = no hair loss; grade 1 = minimal hair loss; grade 2 = moderate hair loss; grade 3 = reversible complete hair loss; and grade 4 = irreversible complete hair loss.[11]

Numerous procedures can aid in diagnosing the etiology of the alopecia. One such procedure is the hair-pull test, which gives a rough estimate of how much hair is being lost. It is done by grasping a small portion of hair and gently applying traction while sliding the fingers along the hair shafts. Usually, one to two hairs are removed with this technique. The hairs are then examined under a microscope. A negative test (six or fewer hairs obtained) indicates normal shedding, whereas a positive test (more than six hairs obtained) indicates a process of active hair shedding. Patients should not shampoo their hair 24 hours before the test is performed.

In the hair-pluck test, approximately 50 hairs are grasped with a hemostat and removed with one motion. This test produces a trichogram to assess the telogen to anagen ratio but is rarely needed for clinical diagnosis of hair loss.

Light microscopy examination of hair fibers involves extracting hairs by a slow pull and mounting them between two glass slides. The roots are examined to determine the stage of the hair cycle and the presence of dystrophy. The free ends of the hair are checked to see if they are tapered, cut, fractured, or weathered. Scrapings of scalp scales for bacterial and fungal culture should be performed if indicated. A 20% potassium hydroxide examination under light microscopy will reveal fungal spores and hyphae if present.

Another diagnostic test for alopecia is a scalp biopsy; a 4 mm punch is recommended for patients with a scarring alopecia or for patients with a nonscarring alopecia of unknown origin. Some authorities prefer examination with transverse horizontal sectioning to allow a greater number of follicles to be examined. The biopsy should be taken from an active inflammatory area with hair follicles present.

Laboratory workup, including a complete blood count (CBC), ferritin measurement, and thyroid screening, may also be helpful. Ferritin levels should be higher than 40 µg/L for normal hair growth.[10]

Causes of Alopecia in Cancer Patients

Cancer patients are exposed to many stressors during their treatment regimens. Various etiologies, singly or in combination, may result in alopecia in these patients. The main mechanisms are discussed below. Disorders of alopecia can be divided into those in which the hair follicle is normal but the cycling of hair growth is abnormal (eg, telogen effluvium) and those in which the hair follicle is damaged and may result in a scarring alopecia.

Anagen Effluvium

Anagen effluvium occurs after an insult to the hair follicle impairs its mitotic or metabolic activity. This is a generalized diffuse hair loss from follicles in the anagen growth phase with quite rapid development 1 to 4 weeks after the initial trigger.

Hair follicle growth is affected by many chemotherapeutic agents. Anticancer drugs such as antimetabolites, alkylating agents, and mitotic inhibitors impair metabolic and mitotic processes in actively growing hair follicles, causing an anagen effluvium.[12–15] Table 2 lists the chemotherapeutic agents commonly associated with alopecia. Drugs that are given orally or on a weekly schedule cause significantly less hair loss, even when the total dose of the drug given is greater.[2]

TABLE 2 Anagen Effluvium Caused by Chemotherapies and Other Medications
Most common agents
Nitrosoureas
Cyclophosphamide
Bleomycin
Dactinomycin
Daunorubicin
Fluorouracil
Methotrexate
Less common agents
Levodopa
Bismuth
Cyclosporine
Adapted from Hesketh PJ et al.[17]

The use of multiple agents concurrently increases the risk of alopecia. The inhibition or arrest of cell division in the hair matrix leads to a thin, weakened hair shaft that is susceptible to fracture with minimal trauma; it can also result in complete failure of hair formation. The hair bulb itself may be damaged, and the hairs may separate at the bulb and fall out. Only actively growing anagen follicles are subject to these processes. Since hair bulb cells replicate every 12 to 24 hours, they are highly susceptible to the cytotoxic effects of chemotherapy.[15]

Hair loss usually begins 2 to 4 weeks after the initial chemotherapy dose. The hair loss is clinically most apparent after 1 to 2 months. Pruritus and/or scalp tenderness may be noticeable at the time of shedding. Hair may begin to regrow in about 3 to 6 months (the same time period as telogen).[12,16] The rate of growth can be reduced to 0.004 to 0.1 mm per day as opposed to the normal rate of 0.35 mm per day.[17] When directed at hair-bearing areas such as the scalp, high doses of radiation therapy also cause an anagen arrest. Both chemotherapy and radiation therapy are the main noninflammatory causes of anagen effluvia.[16]

The following list includes other causes of anagen effluvium that may occur concurrently during a patient's chemotherapy treatment regimen. Genetic hereditary diseases, such as Pollitt's syndrome and Marie Unna–type hypotrichosis, can cause anagen effluvium. Defective hormone production can result from hypopituitarism (hypopituitary dwarfism, Simmonds' disease, and Sheehan's syndrome), thyroid gland defects (hypothyroidism, hyperthyroidism), Cushing's syndrome, and, occasionally, juvenile diabetes. Nutritional deficiencies are seen when there is decreased intake of copper, iron, zinc, biotin, essential fatty acids, or vitamin C.

On examination, the hair is thin and tapers to a point (pencil point ends).[16] The slightest external trauma, such as gentle brushing, can cause the distal portion of the shaft to break. Only tapered shafts are shed, not all anagen hairs. Early in the course of an anagen arrest, a gentle hair pull

TABLE 1 Correlation between Common Complaints and Cause of Hair Loss	
Complaint	*Hair Disorder*
Gradual thinning without shedding	Androgenetic alopecia
Diffuse shedding	Telogen effluvium
Hair breakage or hair that does not grow	Structural hair shaft abnormality; tinea capitis
Shedding with circular areas of hair loss	Alopecia areata

test will extract numerous dystrophic hair shafts. As hairs are rapidly shed over a few weeks, fewer and fewer anagen shafts are left in the scalp. Therefore, after most of the hairs have fallen, the remaining hairs should show telogen hairs on a hair-pull test. A trichogram done late in the course of anagen arrest would therefore reveal almost 100% telogen hairs.[16]

On microscopic examination, anagen hairs have long, indented roots covered with intact inner and outer root sheaths and are fully pigmented.

A 4 mm punch biopsy sample of the scalp usually contains 25 to 50 follicles for inspection. Less than 15% of the follicles are normally in the telogen phase. An equal anagen to telogen ratio in a patient with hair loss is characteristic of anagen effluvium. The follicles should show no signs of inflammation, no dystrophic changes of the inner sheath, or traction. These features permit the distinction of anagen effluvium from alopecia areata, androgenetic alopecia, and traction alopecia respectively.[16]

An anagen effluvium is reversible if the underlying disease or treatment is stopped, but occassionally, the process causes irreparable injury. If doses of chemotherapy or radiation therapy are sufficiently high, the stem cells of the follicle may be injured, resulting in a cicatricial alopecia.

Telogen Effluvium

Telogen effluvium is a non-inflammatory diffuse hair loss caused by any condition or situation that shifts the normal distribution of follicles from an anagen to a telogen-predominant distribution.[16] During the telogen phase of hair cycling, the production of hair shafts is temporarily halted. The interval between the inciting event in telogen effluvium and the onset of shedding corresponds to the length of the telogen phase, between 1 and 6 months (the average is 3 months). Acute telogen effluvium is defined as hair shedding lasting less than 6 months, whereas chronic telogen effluvium lasts longer than 6 months. The onset is often insidious, and it can be difficult to identify an inciting event.[18] In the cancer patient, there may be more than one precipitating event, including chemotherapy, radiation therapy, fever, chronic malnutrition, endocrinopathies (hypothyroidism or hyperthyroidism), or surgery. Chronic illness, such as malignancy, particularly lymphoproliferative malignancy; and any chronic debilitating illness, such as systemic lupus erythematosus, end-stage renal disease, or liver disease, can also lead to telogen effluvium.[16] Except for the disruption of hair cycling, hair follicles in telogen effluvium are otherwise normal. Patients with this disorder usually note an increased number of loose hairs on their hairbrush or shower floor. Normal daily loss is

around 100 hairs, whereas in telogen effluvium, the range is from 100 to 300 hairs. If hair loss is at the lower end of the range, it may not be apparent. Axillary and pubic areas often are involved, along with hair of the scalp.

Examination of the scalp may reveal a higher than expected number of short new hairs growing. Because hair grows at a nearly constant rate of approximately 1 cm per month, the duration of the hair shedding can be estimated by measuring the length of the short hairs.

In active telogen effluvium, the gentle hair-pull test will yield at least four hairs with each pull. If the patient's active shedding has ceased, the hair pull will be normal. Telogen hairs are identified by a white bulb, when pulled out, and the lack of a gelatinous hair sheath.

The hair-pluck test, forced extraction of 10 to 20 hairs, usually shows that up to 50% of hairs are in the telogen phase (in contrast to the normal 10 to 15%), although these results can vary.[16] In the typical case of telogen effluvium, the telogen count seldom exceeds 50%. Figures exceeding 80% of telogen hairs are not consistent with a telogen effluvium, and the physician should look for other causes of alopecia.[16]

Laboratory tests that may identify a systemic reason for the hair loss include a thyroid-stimulating hormone test and an antinuclear antibody test if the history suggests the presence of a connective tissue disease. Since iron deficiency is common in premenopausal women, evaluation of CBC, serum iron, iron saturation, and ferritin may be warranted.

Microscopic examination of telogen hairs shows short, club-shaped roots. The hairs lack root sheaths and show depigmentation of the proximal part of the shaft.

Histologic findings in telogen effluvium are subtle and are most easily seen on transverse sections of a punch biopsy. The number and density of hair follicles are normal, but an increased percentage of the hair follicles are in the telogen or catagen phase. If more than 25% of the follicles are in the telogen phase, the diagnosis is confirmed.

Generally, recovery is spontaneous and occurs within 6 months. Any reversible cause of hair shedding, such as poor diet, iron deficiency, hypothyroidism, or medications, should be corrected. No specific treatment for hair loss is required.[16]

Apoptosis of Hair Follicles

Chemotherapeutic drugs may not only cause telogen or anagen effluvium, they may also stimulate premature apoptosis-driven hair follicle regression. Hair loss from apoptosis induced by chemotherapy is mediated by the tp53 and cyclin-dependent kinase 2 molecular signaling pathways. A study by Sharov and colleagues showed that

tp53 is essential for triggering apoptotic cell death in the hair follicle induced by cyclophosphamide (CYP).[19] This was shown through genetic loss of tp53, resulting in complete resistance of murine hair follicles to chemotherapy-induced hair loss.

The tp53 apoptotic pathway uses transcription-dependent and -independent mechanisms[20–23] that are mediated by Fas/APO-1 (CD95), a cell surface receptor and a direct tp53 target. Fas is a gene product that induces apoptosis in multiple cell types.[22] The Fas gene becomes activated when tp53 interacts with the Fas gene's tp53 consensus element in its promoter.[24,25] The Fas receptor requires interaction with the intracellular adaptor molecule Fas-associated death domain, which activates procaspase 8 and recruits it into the death-inducing signaling complex.[23,26] Following proteolytic activation of procaspase 8, caspase 3 is activated along the common final pathway of apoptosis.[26]

CYP up-regulates "death" receptors (Fas/APO-1, p55 kDa tumor necrosis factor receptor) and the mitochondrial proapoptotic protein Bax in the hair follicle. CYP-treated hair follicles display a strong up-regulation of tp53 in the proximal outer and inner root sheaths and in the hair matrix.[19]

The above mechanism raises the possibility of exploring pharmacologic blockade of Fas signaling as part of complex local treatment for inhibiting keratinocyte apoptosis and reducing hair loss induced by chemotherapy of Fas-negative tumors.[19] Another mechanism to inhibit keratinocyte inhibition was studied by Komarove and colleagues in which temporary suppression of tp53 has been suggested as a therapeutic strategy to prevent damage of normal tissues during treatment of tumors.[23] Thus, inhibitors of tp53 may be useful for reducing the side effects of cancer therapy associated with tp53 induction.

Ionizing Radiation

X-rays and gamma rays affect all follicles in an anagen stage of active growth. Anagen effluvium results from the simultaneous inhibition of cell division in hair follicles, leading to a sudden stop in hair fiber production. As noted above, the rapidity with which hair cells grow that makes them sensitive to chemotherapeutic agents also applies to radiation therapy.

The end-organ damage, whether it is the kidney, bowel, or hair, is dependent on both the intrinsic radiosensitivity and the number of target cells comprise an functional subunit (FSU). To illustrate, epilation requires a lower dose of ionizing radiation than desquamation. This is not due to greater radiosensitivity of the hair follicle compared with the basal epithelium but rather to the fact that there are far fewer cells in the FSU that comprises a hair than in a population keratinocytes that can regenerate.[3] Similarly, the depigmentation of hair occurs at lower radiation doses than epidermal depigmentation owing to the relative paucity of melanocytes found in hair follicles compared with the epidermis.[28]

Alopecia Neoplastica

Neoplasia can directly cause permanent hair loss. *Alopecia neoplastica* is the term used for alopecia caused by the direct involvement of the hair follicle and surrounding skin by the neoplastic process. It presents as one or more areas of scarring alopecia and has been reported with both primary and metastatic tumors. The mechanism of alopecia neoplastica is not certain and may result from physical compression from the tumor, reactive fibrosis, release of cytokines, or a combination of factors. The scalp is a site of predilection, possibly because of its abundant blood supply.

The primary tumors associated with alopecia neoplastica are squamous and basal cell carcinomas, lymphoma, melanoma, and angiosarcoma.[29,30] Some other primary skin cancers can also cause alopecia.

Desmoplastic melanoma can cause a scarring alopecia with prominent desmoplasia and infiltration of the hair follicles by tumor cells.[4]

Two variants of mycosis fungoides (cutaneous T-cell lymphoma) can result in permanent alopecia. Alopecia mucinosa (follicular mucinosis) presents as eruptions of follicular papules and/or indurated plaques. The presenting sign of alopecia mucinosa is hair loss. Circulating immune complexes and cell-mediated immunity is associated with the condition.[31] Skin eruptions present as pruritic, pink to yellow-white, follicular papules and plaques. Lesions may be isolated or multiple and are most commonly found on the scalp and face. Usually, the alopecia is reversible unless follicular destruction has occurred owing to excess mucin in the outer root sheath and sebaceous glands. In patients with permanent alopecia, the whole follicle degenerates. On histology, T-cell infiltration and mucinous degeneration of follicular epithelium are seen. Treatments include topical, intralesional, and systemic corticosteroids. In addition, topical and systemic psoralen plus ultraviolet A light therapy, topical nitrogen mustard, and radiation therapy have demonstrated some success. The course of the disease is variable, and there is a likelihood of spontaneous resolution.

Follicular mycosis fungoides is another variant of mycosis fungoides in which the neoplastic cells and reactive inflammation target follicular epithelium.[32] It presents with follicular hyperkeratosis, comedo-like lesions, acquired epidermal cysts, and patchy alopecia. Findings of histopathologic and immunohistochemical studies showed atypical CD4[+] T lymphocytes infiltrating the follicles without follicular mucinosis.

Visceral carcinomas may directly invade underlying skin or metastasize to skin through lymphatics or the bloodstream. Brownstein and Helwig reported that the scalp was the site in 4% of all skin metastases.[33] They found that the source of the primary tumor was usually the lung, colon, stomach, or kidney in men, and metastasis appeared early in the course of the disease. Tumors of the breast and lung were commonest in women, in whom metastasis occurred late in the disease.[34] Other cancers include those of the rectum, ovary, and prostate. Rarely, a scalp metastasis arrives from a pancreas, liver, uterus, or bone primary tumor.

On examination, single or multiple, firm, nontender nodules that rapidly enlarge are the commonest presentation of scalp metastasis. Alopecia neoplastica usually presents as single or multiple areas of cicatricial alopecia. Scleroderma-like plaques may occur, and multiple nodules may simulate turban tumors. Recently, alopecia neoplastica without alopecia has been described. In this case, presented by Mallon and Dawber, there was a unique presentation of scalp metastasis in a patient with breast carcinoma in whom hair loss was clinically inconspicuous.[35]

Lobular breast carcinoma, which accounts for 10% of invasive breast carcinoma, usually elicits a reactive fibrosis that leads to cicatricial alopecia. It is difficult to explain the complete disappearance of the pilosebaceous units, but loss of hair follicles may be the result of fibrosis. Cohen and colleagues considered this to be the major mechanism.[34]

Histopathologic examination of the scalp demonstrates metastatic carcinoma cells in a dense collagenous stroma, which is seen in the deep dermis and the subcutaneous tissue, with loss of pilosebaceous units.

A scarring alopecia that is not readily explained by trauma, infection, or dermatosis should lead to the consideration of an underlying neoplastic process.

Other Common Causes of Alopecia

Nonchemotherapy Medication-Induced Alopecia

Some common medications can also cause either a telogen or anagen effluvium. Androgenic drugs that cause a telogen effluvium include systemic steroids and oral contraceptives.[10] Iatrogenic Cushing's syndrome caused by systemic steroids is also associated with alopecia. The alopecia occurs only after a few months of high-dose treatment with systemic steroids. Alopecia caused by excessive vitamin A is rare but is more commonly observed with vitamin A analogue medications, such as acetretin or isotretinoin. The effects are reversible once treatment stops. Anticoagulation

from warfarin and heparin is responsible for causing alopecia when treatment is long term (eg, 4–6 months) and occurs in more than 10% of patients. Antithyroid drugs cause a reversible alopecia. Several antihypertensive agents are known to cause hair loss, such as β-blockers and captopril. Telogen effluvium occurs in 20 to 30% of patients treated with interferon.[10] There is no relationship between dosage and onset or severity of the hair loss. Agents that block cholesterol synthesis can disrupt keratinization. Cholesterol is a component of cellular lipids, and its synthesis and metabolism are essential for the production of normal epidermal structures. Metal-based treatment, such as gold salt, lithium, and bismuth, may also lead to hair loss. Antiepilepsy medications, such as carbamazepine and sodium valproate–based medications, may also induce alopecia. Colchicine, used to treat gout, can harm the root of the hair after high doses, resulting in an anagen effluvium. Vasopressin can also cause a reversible anagen effluvium.

Androgenetic Alopecia

Androgenetic alopecia is referred to as male pattern hair loss (MPHL) in men and female pattern hair loss (FPHL) in women and is due to the progressive miniaturization of scalp hair. It affects approximately 50% of men and 20 to 53% of women by the age of 50.[36] Dihydrotestosterone (DHT) is a key androgen in the pathogenesis of MPHL and FPHL. The androgen testosterone is converted to DHT by the enzyme 5α-reductase. DHT causes a reduction in protein synthesis by inhibiting adenylyl cyclase in the hair bulb; the result is shorter and finer hair, referred to as miniaturized hair. As the hair growth cycle proceeds, hairs continue to become smaller and finer.[36]

The best treatment option for androgenetic alopecia is minoxidil 5% solution. If it is not effective after 1 year, then antiandrogens can be tried. Hair transplantation can be offered if the occipital donor area is sufficient. Finasteride, a type 2–selective 5α-reductase inhibitor, is also helpful.

Trichotillomania

Trichotillomania is a self-induced primary psychiatric disorder.[10] It results from repetitive hair manipulations by the patient's own hand. On examination, the alopecia patches have unusual shapes and sizes and show broken hairs. A scalp biopsy can be helpful if the diagnosis is difficult clinically. Trichotillomania can be a chronic problem Treatments include: habit reversal training and selective serotonin reuptake inhibitors (SSRIs).

Alopecia Areata

Alopecia areata is an autoimmune disease that targets actively growing (anagen) hair follicles in humans.[10] It is a nonscarring type of hair loss that can affect any hair-bearing area. The process appears to be T cell mediated, but antibodies directed to hair follicle structures also have been found. On examination, there are round to oval, smooth, slightly erythematous, peach colored, or normal-colored patches of nonscarring alopecia. The presence of "exclamation point" hairs, hairs tapered near proximal end, is pathognomonic but is not always found. A positive pull test at the periphery of a plaque usually indicates that the disease is active, and further hair loss can be expected. Nail involvement is found in 6.8 to 49.4% of patients, with the most common finding being pitting.[10] Histologic evaluation shows a characteristic peribulbar lymphocytic infiltrate, which is described as appearing similar to a swarm of bees.

Treatment is not always necessary because the condition is benign, and spontaneous remissions are common. Since alopecia areata is an inflammatory condition, different immunomodulators have been used to treat this condition. These include topical, oral, and intralesional steroids. Topical potent contact allergens that induce an allergic contact dermatitis include squaric acid, dibutyl ester and diphencyprone. These agents are thought to work by inducing the introduction of a second antigen can initiate a new infiltrate containing T-suppressor cells that may modify the preexisting infiltrate and allow regrowth. Cyclosporine has also been used both topically and systemically in the treatment of alopecia areata, with mixed results. Response rates also vary with topical minoxidil 5% treatment. Topical anthralin may work by generating free radicals, which have antiproliferative and immunosuppressive actions.

Tinea Capitis

Tinea capitis is uncommon after puberty.[6] When it occurs in adults, the clinical features may be atypical. Tinea capitis in adults generally occurs in patients who are immunosuppressed. The diagnosis of tinea capitis is suggested by erythema, scaling, and crusting locally on the scalp. When an adult, especially if immunocompromised, presents with a patchy, inflammatory scalp disorder, mycologic samples should be sent for laboratory analysis in all of these patients.

Scarring (Cicatricial) Alopecia

Scarring (cicatricial) alopecia is characterized by follicular destruction and replacement of the interfollicular epidermis by atrophic skin. Hair stem cells are normally localized in the midportion of the follicles, in the mid-dermis. If this area remains undisturbed, the follicles recycle throughout one's life. However, inflammation in this area can destroy the stem cells. In that case, a cicatricial alopecia is established, and no follicle is

able to grow. Some systemic diseases can cause destruction of hair follicles, resulting in a scarring alopecia. Clinically, there is obliteration of the orifices of the follicles. The insult is usually to the bulge zone of the follicle. This process usually occurs as a result of intense inflammation. Some causes of cicatricial alopecia are infectious, (Table 3).[10]

Effects of Chemotherapy on Hair Color

Chemotherapy can cause altered color of regrown hair since melanocytes also represent an unintended target for chemotherapeutic drugs.

An article by Fairlamb noted a graying effect in 40% of individuals, whereas a rejuvenation of color (loss of gray hair) was noted in 20% of patients.[37] Overall, 65% of patients reported some character change in their hair after cytotoxic therapy.

Certain chemotherapies, such as cyclophosphamide (CYP), induce profound changes in tyrosinase and dihydroxyphenylalanine (DOPA) chrome tautomerase activity in murine skin.[38] These are enzymes needed for melanin production. Also, electron microscopy data suggest that after CYP treatment, some melanocytes change their localization and migrate to the bottom of the hair bulb, whereas others undergo apoptosis.[39] Although selected hair bulb melanocytes underwent apoptosis 24 to 48 hours after CYP administration, no cell death was seen in the outer root sheath and bulge melanocytes. Seventy-two hours after CYP administration, the surviving hair bulb melanocytes were proliferative and later migrated up the outer root sheath to the interfollicular epidermis. Five to 7 days after CYP treatment, numerous melanocytes expressing all

TABLE 3 Some Causes of Acquired Scarring Alopecia

Physical injury
Mechanical trauma
Burns
Radiation
Dermatoses
Lichen planus
Lupus erythematosus
Scleroderma
Sarcoidosis
Cicatricial pemphigoid
Follicular mucinosis
Infection
Fungi causing kerion or favus
Lupus vulgaris
Late stages of syphilis
Folliculitis
Herpes zoster and varicella
Leishmaniasis
Neoplasia

three melanogenic proteins had repopulated the epidermis and showed melanogenic activity.

Mitoxantrone, used as adjuvant chemotherapy for breast cancer, has been reported to cause selective loss of white hair.[40]

Hair Loss Prevention

Scalp Tourniquets

This method to prevent hair loss in chemotherapy-induced alopecia (CIA) has been used as far back as 1966, initially by Simister and Hennessey.[12] The idea is to prevent the chemotherapeutic drug from reaching the hair.[41] Drugs with a short half-life and a rapid clearance of active drug and metabolites from the circulation are the most likely to have benefit seen with this procedure.[2] It involves the use of a pneumatic tourniquet placed around the hairline and inflated to a pressure above the systolic arterial pressure. Various studies with differing chemotherapy regimens have been published, making the evaluation of efficacy difficult. The main side effect with this treatment was head discomfort.

Scalp Hypothermia

The end point of scalp hypothermia is to temporarily decrease blood flow to the scalp by vasoconstriction.[42] The use of hypothermia may also result in a decreased metabolic rate of hair follicles, therefore reducing the exposure of hair follicles to the chemotherapeutic agents. Most published studies have evaluated the use of this procedure prior to the administration of doxorubicin since the half-life is short and plasma clearance of the drug and metabolites is rapid.[43] CYP has a longer half-life than doxorubicin, so insufficient hair loss prevention is found with hypothermia when both drugs are used in combination.

The procedure requires that the scalp temperature must be less than 24°C.[44] Different approaches have been used in studies to produce hypothermia. These included ice bags fastened to the patient's head, frozen gel packs that were initially molded around a wig stand,[45–48] and various other investigator-designed devices using circulating cold air or fluid.[2] There has not been a consistent protocol in the various published studies in terms of the amount of time that the cooling process was started before chemotherapy administration and the amount of time that the cooling device was left in place following chemotherapy administration. The chemotherapy regimens and dosages also varied. Therefore, it is difficult to compare the individual studies in regard to efficacy. A recent nonrandomized pilot study by Ridderheim and colleagues used a silicon cap with three temperature monitors.[43] Scalp cooling began 30 minutes prior to administration of chemotherapy, and the temperature was maintained at +5°C throughout the drug administration and for at least 30 minutes after discontinuation. There were 74 treated patients with 13 different chemotherapy regimens used in the cohort study. The results were based on a visual analogue scale (VAS 0–10; 0 = no hair loss, 10 = total hair loss). See Table 4 for chemotherapy protocols and results. This study had a mean follow-up period of 15 months, with no scalp metastases noted among the 74 treated patients. Scalp cooling was well tolerated, with modest patient discomfort. The patients ranked a median value of 1.5 on a scale of 0 = no discomfort to 10 = extreme discomfort. The main complaints involved headache and "being chilled." The time invested by nurses for the procedure was less than 10 minutes per patient. A large clinical trial employing efficient and controlled cooling systems with long-term follow-up is still needed.

The main concern with scalp hypothermia and tourniquet therapy is the potential for scalp metastases. Five cases of scalp metastases among 96 patients treated with hypothermia used for chemotherapy for metastatic breast cancer have been reported. No reports of scalp metastases during adjuvant therapy for breast cancer have been reported.[49,50] The ideal patients for the above two preventive therapies are those receiving single-agent chemotherapy with a palliative intent or for solid tumors that rarely metastasize to the scalp.

Drug Therapies (Established and Experimental)

α-Tocopherol (Vitamin E)

High-dose α-tocopherol has been used at a dose of 1,600 IU orally daily starting 72 hours before chemotherapy to prevent hair loss. A study by Wood reported a 69% success rate using the above regimen prior to an unspecified dose of doxorubicin.[51] However, Martin-Jimenez and colleagues failed to confirm this finding in patients receiving 5-fluorouracil, doxorubicin, and CYP.[52] Another study by Perez and colleagues also did not find

significant benefit for patients receiving doxorubicin alone.[53] Powis and Kooistra revealed that Angora rabbits fed an α-tocopherol-supplemented diet showed evidence of protection against doxorubicin-dependent inhibition of new hair growth.[54] Topical α-tocopherol did not provide any protection from doxorubicin-induced alopecia.

Minoxidil

The effect of induction of hair growth for this medication is thought to result from prolongation of the anagen phase of hair growth. This action has been shown in a mouse model. A few studies have evaluated the use of topical minoxidil to prevent hair loss in patients receiving chemotherapy. A study by Rodriguez and colleagues showed that patients who applied 2% minoxidil to the scalp, beginning 24 hours prior to chemotherapy and continuing throughout therapy with doxorubicin, did not have any improvement of hair loss compared with placebo.[55] A study by Duvic and colleagues revealed that patients who received doxorubicin, CYP, and 5-fluorouracil chemotherapy and applied 2% topical minoxidil solution twice daily throughout chemotherapy and up to 4 months following therapy showed an increased time to maximal hair loss.[56] The time to maximal regrowth from baseline was also improved with minoxidil. It appears that the use of this medication for prevention of hair loss is limited; however, it may decrease the length of time needed for hair regrowth.

AS101: Ammonium Trichloro (dioxoethylente – O, O′) Tellurate

The AS101 compound is an immunomodulator that appears to stimulate lymphocyte secretion of interleukin-1 (IL-1), colony-stimulating factor, and IL-12. It also has been found to have radioprotective effects. Sredni and colleagues evaluated the use of this compound at a dose of 3 mg/m² intravenously three times weekly in patients who

were receiving intravenous carboplatin on day 1 and etoposide on days 3, 5, and 7.[57] AS101 was begun 2 weeks before chemotherapy and was otherwise administered 30 minutes before chemotherapy. The results showed the absence of grade IV alopecia in all patients receiving the active drug versus 9.3% of patients who did not receive AS101. Thirteen percent of patients developed grade 3 alopecia in the AS101 group versus 43.5% of patients who did not receive the active medication. There was no significant difference in chemotherapy response in the two groups. The main side effects of the medication included postinfusional fever and garlic-like halitosis.

Imuvert

Imuvert is an immunomodulator that stimulates IL-1, tumor necrosis factor, and IL-6. IL-1 is a hormone-like polypeptide that mediates a broad spectrum of activities in host defense and in a variety of disease processes.[58–61] Many cell types produce this cytokine, most notably mononuclear phagocytes. Imuvert has been studied in CIA in the newborn rat model. The mechanism of hair protection is based on the fact that IL-1 has been shown to be a potent stimulator for hair follicle keratinocytes.[62] Imuvert may treat alopecia since it is a potent inducer of IL-1.[63,64] Another study by Hussein showed that IL-1 protects against ara-C-induced alopecia in the newborn rats.[65] Imuvert and IL-1 failed to protect against CYP-induced alopecia, suggesting that cell cycle–specific agents (ara-C, doxorubicin) produce alopecia by a different mechanism from that of cell cycle–nonspecific agents, such as CYP.

Calcitriol (1,25-(OH)₂D₃)

Vitamin D_3 analogues directly or indirectly inhibit the apoptosis of normal epithelial cells in vivo, as shown by Schilli and colleagues.[66] The study showed down-regulation of apoptosis in CYP-treated hair follicles by topical calcitriols. The effects are thought to result from genomic interactions of the ligand–vitamin D_3 receptor complex with apoptosis control genes. Certain genes, such as members of the Bcl family, seem to be involved in regulating keratinocyte apoptosis during spontaneous hair follicle regression and possibly during chemotherapy-induced apoptosis.[36] Calcitriol may also induce a change in hair matrix keratinocyte proliferation and/or terminal differentiation, thus rendering follicular keratinocytes less susceptible to the cytotoxic and/or proapoptotic effects of CYP. There may be direct interactions of the selected vitamin D analogues with the vitamin D receptors of follicular keratinocytes, perifollicular macrophages, and mast cells, which subsequently modulate follicular keratinocyte apoptosis. It is still not known if calcitriol may be used therapeutically to protect growing hair follicles without endangering the efficacy of cytostatic drugs.

TABLE 4 Study Results of Scalp Hypothermia			
Chemotherapy Regimen	*Number of Patients*	*VAS Scores, n (range)*	*Wig Necessary (%)*
Anthracycline combinations or single taxane	24	0	0
Combined paclitaxel-carboplatin	30	2.5 (0–6.5)	63
Combined anthracycline and taxanes	6	6 (1.5–8)	
Epirubicin-gemcitabine	18	0 (0–2)	0
ABVD	8	1 (0–7)	0
BEP	2	9 (7.5–10)	100
Topotecan and etoposide	1	0	0
Topotecan	2	2.5 (0–5)	50

Adapted from Ridderheim M et al.[43]
ABVD = Adriamycin (doxorubicin), bleomycin, vinblastine, dacarbazine; ***BEP = bleomycin, etoposide, cisplatin; VAS = visual analogue scale 0–10; 0 = no hair loss, 10 = total hair loss.

Hidalgo and colleagues evaluated topical calcitriol to prevent CIA in patients with breast cancer receiving FAC (5-fluorouracil, Adriamycin [doxorubicin], and cyclophosphamide) chemotherapy.[67] Topitriol cream 0.0025% or 0.005% was administered twice daily; all patients developed grade 2 alopecia between days 20 and 30 postchemotherapy, therefore demonstrating the ineffectiveness of topical topitriol in preventing CIA.

Jimenez and Yunis, however, showed that 0.2 g of topical 1,25-dihydroxyvitamin D_3 protected rats from alopecia induced by etoposide, CYP, and a doxorubicin-CYP combination.[68] It is still not known whether the down-regulation of CYP-induced apoptosis by topical calcitriols reflects direct interactions of the selected vitamin D analogues with the vitamin D receptors of follicular keratinocytes or with those of other resident populations of cells, such as dermal papilla fibroblasts,[69] perifollicular macrophages, or mast cells, which modulate follicular apoptosis.

Cyclosporine

Hussein and colleagues have shown that several agents will protect against CIA in the newborn rat animal model.[70] Such protective agents render the hair follicle keratinocytes resistant to chemotherapy, possibly by the expression of P-glycoprotein (Pgp). Cyclosporine is a potent inhibitor of Pgp. The efficacy of cyclosporine was tested in its effects on CIA in the newborn rat animal model. Cyclosporine, when applied topically, protected rats from local alopecia induced by various agents. The mechanism of protection by cyclosporine and its relationship to Pgp remain uncertain. Paus and colleagues showed that systemic cyclosporine shifts CYP-induced alopecia toward a mild form of dystrophic anagen, thus retarding alopecia and prolonging "primary recovery."[71]

Topical Estrogen

A number of nongenomic 17-β-estradiol (E2)-dependent signaling transductions are involved in various biologic processes. The prototypic estrogen E2 causes a hair follicle response and recovery from chemotherapy to follow a dystrophic catagen pathway.[72] If this pathway is followed, anagen is immediately terminated, followed by a dystrophic catagen and a remarkably shortened telogen phase. Therefore, the hair follicle is able to be reconstructed to a fully functional hair shaft at maximal speed. Hair follicles that follow the dystrophic catagen pathway will exhibit the most severe and fastest alopecia yet also have the fastest regrowth of normally pigmented hair shafts during the recovery phase. Ohnemus and colleagues showed that topical 17β-estradiol significantly altered the cycling response of murine follicles to CYP.[72] The

regrowth of normally pigmented hair shafts after CIA was significantly accelerated. Human studies still need to be explored using topical estrogens as a potential stimulant for hair regrowth after CIA.

Prevention of Radiation-Induced Alopecia

Tempol (4-hydroxy-2,2,6,6,-tetramethylpiperidine-1-oxyl) is a stable nitroxide radical that functions as a superoxide dismutase and can protect mammalian cells from both superoxide hypoxanthine/xanthine oxidase and hydrogen peroxide cytotoxicity. A study by Goffman and colleagues evaluated a topical application of tempol on guinea pigs receiving radiation.[73] There was an increase in the rate of new hair recovery on the skin that had tempol applied to it 15 minutes before radiation exposure compared with unprotected skin. No systemic absorption was noted.

Topical and subcutaneous 16,16-dimethyl prostaglandin E_2 (PGE_2) was studied by Hanson and colleagues in preventing radiation-induced alopecia in mice.[74] Both types of administration of PGE_2 protected the mice to some degree from hair loss.

Parathyroid Hormone–Related Peptide Receptor Agonist

Parathyroid hormone–related peptide (PTHrP) normally causes malignancy-related hypercalcemia but can also regulate keratinocyte proliferation and differentiation.[75] Parathyroid hormone (PTH)/PTHrP-R agonists stimulate insulin-like growth factor 1 production by fibroblasts,[76] which acts as a cell cycle progression factor in keratinocytes. Schilli and colleagues showed increasing evidence that PTH/PTHrP-R mediated signaling is involved in hair growth control, specifically in hair follicle cycling.[77] Holick and colleagues showed that intraperitoneal synthetic PTH/PTHrP-R antagonist PTH (7-34) increased hair growth in hairless mice.[78] PTH (7-34) also accelerated anagen development in infantile C57BL/6 mice with normal hair growth patterns and inhibited spontaneous hair follicle regression (catagen) in adolescent mice. Peters and colleagues demonstrated that PTH/PTHrP-R agonist PTH (1-34) and PTH/PTHrP-R antagonists PTH (7-34) and PTHrP (7-34) can effectively manipulate the hair follicle response to CYP-induced damage as follows: PTH/PTHrP-R antagonists may be given initially during chemotherapy to prevent the acceleration of the hair cycle, thereby decreasing the sensitivity of the hair follicle cells to CYP. After the chemotherapy is completed, a PTH/PTHrP-R agonist may be given, which would accelerate the hair cycle and therefore stimulate regrowth.[75]

Psychological Impact of CIA

CIA is a condition that has significant psychosocial effects, resulting in anxiety, depression, and a negative body image for cancer patients. Alopecia has been cited by 47 to 58% of women with cancer as the most disturbing anticipated aspect of receiving chemotherapy, with 8% of women in one study found to be at risk of avoiding treatment.[79]

Helping patients cope with CIA involves providing accurate information and appropriate support. Support groups and use of a wig can help alleviate some of the anxiety caused by this side effect of cancer therapy. Once alopecia has occurred, self-care strategies to protect the scalp and other areas of hair loss against the sun, cold, or trauma should be encouraged.

Cancer treatment–induced alopecia still remains one of the chief unresolved clinical problems for the oncologist and a substantial source of psychological anguish for the patient. A thorough history, physical examination, and laboratory evaluation should be employed to uncover the etiology of the alopecia in this patient population. Other etiologies, such as systemic disease or nonchemotherapy medications, should not be overlooked. A combination of any of these factors may result in the patient's alopecia. Treatment and prevention will be guided by the etiologic factors. Physicians' recommendations are the most influential factor in cancer treatment choice, but body image concerns are also highly influential factors.[80]

REFERENCES

1. McGarvey EL, Baum LD, Pinkerton RC, et al. Psychological sequelae and alopecia among women with cancer. Cancer Pract 2001;9:283–9.
2. Dorr VJ. A practitioner's guide to cancer-related alopecia. Semin Oncol 1998;25:562–70.
3. Perez C, et al. Biologic basis of radiation therapy. In: McBride W, Withers R, editors. Principles and practice of radiation oncology. 4th ed. Lippincott Williams & Wilkins: Philadelphia; 2004.
4. Crotty K, McCarthy W, Quinn M, et al. Signs, syndromes and diagnoses—alopecia neoplastica caused by desmoplastic melanoma. Australas J Dermatol 2003;44:295–8.
5. Alonso LC, Rosenfield RL. Molecular genetic and endocrine mechanisms of hair growth. Horm Res 2003;60:1–13.
6. Powell J, Stone N, and Dawber RPR. An Atlas of Hair and Scalp Diseases. London, UK: The Parthenon Publishing Group, 2002.
7. Munstedt K, Manthey N, Sachsse S, et al. Changes in self-concept and body image during alopecia induced cancer chemotherapy. Support Care Cancer 1997;5:139–43.
8. Camacho FM, Randall VA, Price VH, et al. (eds). Hair and its Disorders: Biology, Pathology, Management. 2000: Martin Dunitz, London UK
9. Millar SE. Molecular mechanisms regulating hair follicle development. J Invest Dermatol 2002;118:216–25.
10. Shapiro J: Hair Loss. Principles of Diagnosis and Management of Alopecia. London: Martin Dunitz, 2002.
11. Protiere C, Evans K, Camerlo J, et al. Efficacy and tolerance of a scalp-cooling system for prevention of hair loss and the experience of breast cancer patients treated by adjuvant chemotherapy. Support Care Cancer 2002;10:529–37. Epub 2002 Aug 15.
12. Hussein AM. Chemotherapy induced alopecia: new developments. South Med J 1993;86:489–96.
13. Botchkarev VA. Molecular mechanisms of chemotherapy-induced hair loss. J Invest Dermatol Symp Proc 2003;8:72–5.

14. Susser WS, Whitaker-Worth DL, et al. Continuing medical education—mucocutaneous reactions to chemotherapy. J Am Acad Dermatol 1999;40:367–98.

15. Tosi A, Misciali C, Piraccini BM, et al. Drug-induced hair loss and hair growth. Incidence, management and avoidance. Drug Saf 1994;10:310–7.

16. Sperling LC. Hair and systemic disease. Dermatol Clin 2001;19:711–26, ix.

17. Hesketh PJ, Batchelor D, Golant M, et al. Chemotherapy-induced alopecia: psychosocial impact and therapeutic approaches. Support Care Cancer 2004;12:543–9.

18. Headington JT. Telogen effluvium—new concepts and review. Arch Dermatol 1993;129:356–63.

19. Sharov AA, Li GZ, Palkina TN, et al. Fas and c-kit are involved in the control of hair follicle melanocyte apoptosis and migration in chemotherapy-induced hair loss. J Invest Dermatol 2003;120:27–35.

20. Paus R, Cotsarelis G. The biology of hair follicles. N Engl J Med 1999;341:491–8.

21. Paus R, Handjiski B, Eichmuller S, et al. Chemotherapy-induced alopecia in mice. Induction by cyclophosphamide, inhibition by cyclosporine A, and modulation by dexamethasone. Am J Pathol 1994;144:719–34.

22. Paus R, Schilli MB, Handjiski B, et al. Topical calcitriol enhances normal hair regrowth but does not prevent chemotherapy-induced alopecia in mice. Cancer Res 1996;56:4438–43.

23. Komarova EA, Gudkov AV. Could p53 be a target for therapeutic suppression? Semin Cancer Biol 1998;8:389–400.

24. Kastan MB, Onyekwere O, Sidranski D, et al. Participation of p53 protein in the cellular response to DNA damage. Cancer Res 1991;51:6304–11.

25. Friesen C, Herr I, Krammer PH, et al. Involvement of the CD95 (APO-1/FAS) receptor/ligand system in drug-induced apoptosis in leukemia cells. Nat Med 1996;2:574–7.

26. Lindner G, Botchkarev VA, Botchkareva NV, et al. Analysis of apoptosis during hair follicle regression (catagen). Am J Pathol 1997;151:1601–17.

27. Sharov AA, Li GZ, Palkina TN, et al. Fas and c-kit are involved in the control of hair follicle melanocyte apoptosis and migration in chemotherapy-induced hair loss. J invest Dermatol 2003;120:27–35.

28. Vegensa V, Withers HR, Taylor JMB. The effect of depigmentation after multifraction of mouse resting hair follicle. Radiation Res 1987;111:464.

29. Knight TE, Robinson HM, Sina B. Angiosarcoma (angioendothelioma) of the scalp. An unusual case of scarring alopecia. Arch Dermatol 1980;116:683–6.

30. Weedon D. Diseases of cutaneous appendages. In: Skin pathology. 2nd ed. London: Churchill Livingstone; 2002. p. 455–501.

31. Jackow CM, Papadoupoulos E. Follicular mucinosis associated with scarring alopecia, oligoclonal T-cell receptor V beta expansion, and Staphylococcus aureus: when does follicular mucinosis become mycosis fungoides? J Am Acad Dermatol 1997 Nov;37(5 Pt 2):828–31.

32. Lacour JP, Castanet J, Perrin C, et al. Follicular mycosis fungoides. A clinical and histologic variant of cutaneous T-cell lymphoma: report of two cases. J Am Acad Dermatol 1993;29(2 Pt 2):330–4.

33. Brownstein MH, Helwig EB. Patterns of cutaneous metastasis. Arch Dermatol 1972;105:862–8.

34. Cohen I, Levy E, Schreiber H. Alopecia neoplastica due to breast carcinoma. Arch Dermatol 1961;84:490–2.

35. Mallon E, Dawber RP. Alopecia neoplastica without alopecia: a unique presentation of breast carcinoma scalp metastasis. J Am Acad Dermatol 1994;31(2 Pt 2):319–21.

36. Proceedings of the First International Symposium on Androgens–Montpellier. Mol Cell Endocrinol 2002;198:89–95.

37. Fairlamb DJ. Hair changes following cytotoxic drug induced alopecia. Postgrad Med J 1988;64:907.

38. Slominski A, Paus R, Plonka P, et al. Pharmacological disruption of hair follicle pigmentation by cyclophosphamide—a model for studying the melanocyte response to and recovery from cytotoxic drug damage in situ. J Invest Dermatol 1996;106:1203–11.

39. Tobin DJ, Hagen E, Botchkarev VA, et al. Do hair bulb melanocytes undergo apoptosis during hair follicle regression (catagen)? J Invest Dermatol 1998;111:941–7.

40. Arlin ZA, Friedland ML, Atamer MA. Selective alopecia with mitoxantrone. N Engl J Med 1984;310:1464.

41. Hennessey JD. Alopecia and cytotoxic drugs [letter]. Br Med J 1966;2:1138.

42. Peck HJ, Mitchell H, Stewart AL. Evaluating the efficacy of scalp cooling using the Penguin cold cap system to reduce alopecia in patients undergoing chemotherapy for breast cancer. Eur J Oncol Nurs 2000;4:246–8.

43. Ridderheim M, Bjurberg M, Gustavsson A. Scalp hypothermia to prevent chemotherapy-induced alopecia is effective and safe: a pilot study of a new digitized scalp-cooling system used in 74 patients. Support Care Cancer 2003;11:371–7.

44. Anderson JE, Hunt JM, Smith IA. Prevention of doxorubicin-induced alopecia by scalp cooling in patients with advanced breast cancer. Br Med J 1981;282:423–4.

45. Dean JC, Griffith KS, Cetas KS. Scalp hypothermia: a comparison of ice pack and the Kold Kap in the prevention of doxorubicin-induced alopecia. J Clin Oncol 1983;1:33–7.

46. Robinson MH, Jones AC, Durrant KD. Effectiveness of scalp cooling in reducing alopecia caused by epirubicin of advanced breast cancer. Cancer Treat Rep 1987;71:913–4.

47. Middleton J, Franks D, Buchanan RB. Failure of scalp hypothermia to prevent hair loss when cyclophosphamide is added to doxorubicin and vincristine. Cancer Treat Rep 1985;69:373–5.

48. Gregory RP, Cooke T, Middleton J. Prevention of doxorubicin-induced alopecia by scalp hypothermia: relation to degree of cooling. Br Med J 1982;284:1674.

49. Middleton J, Franks D, Buchanan RB. Failure of scalp hypothermia to prevent hair loss when cyclophosphamide is added to doxorubicin and vincristine. Cancer Treat Rep 1985;69:373–5.

50. Vendelbo Johansen L. Scalp hypothermia in the prevention of chemotherapy-induced alopecia. Acta Radiol 1985;24:113–6.

51. Wood LA. Possible prevention of Adriamycin-induced alopecia by tocopherol. N Engl J Med 1985;312:1060.

52. Martin-Jimenez M, Diaz-Rubio E, Gonazalez Larriba JL, et al. Failure of high-dose tocopherol to prevent alopecia induced by doxorubicin [letter]. N Engl J Med 1986;315:894–5.

53. Perez JE, Machiavelli M, Leone BA, et al. High-dose alpha-tocopherol as a preventative of doxorubicin-induced alopecia. Cancer Treat Rep 1986;70:1213–4.

54. Powis G, Kooistra KL. Doxorubicin-induced hair loss in the Angora rabbit: a study of treatments to protect against the hair loss. Cancer Chemother Pharmacol 1987;20:291–6.

55. Rodriguez R, Machiavelli M, Leone B, et al. Minoxidil (Mx) as a prophylaxis of doxorubicin-induced alopecia. Ann Oncol 1994;5:769–70.

56. Duvic M, Lemak NA, Valero V, et al. A randomized trial of minoxidil in chemotherapy-induced alopecia. J Am Acad Dermatol 1996;35:74–8.

57. Sredni B, Albeck M, Tichler T, et al. Bone marrow-sparing and prevention of alopecia by AS101 in non-small-cell lung cancer patients treated with carboplatin and etoposide. J Clin Oncol 1995;13:2342–53.

58. Fibbe WE, Schaafsma R, Falkenburg JHF, et al. The biological activities of interleukin-1. Blut 1989;59:147–56.

59. Platanias LC, Vogelzang NJ. Interleukin-1: biology, pathophysiology, and clinical prospects. Am J Med 1990;89:621–9.

60. Dinarello CA. Interleukin-1 and interleukin-1 antagonism. Blood 1991;77:1627–52.

61. Sauder DN. Interleukin-1. Arch Dermatol 1989;125:679–82.

62. Cairns JI, Cumpstone MB, Kennedy AH, et al. Murine rIL-1-alpha stimulated proliferative and collagenase secretion by cultured hair follicles from neonatal mice [abstract]. J Invest Dermatol 1989;92:410.

63. McCall C, Weimer L, Baldwin S. Stimulation of cytokine production by the bacterially derived biological response modified Imuvert [abstract]. Cytokine 1989;1:113.

64. McCall C, Stable C, Baldwin S. Cytokine secretion stimulated by a biological response modified (BRM) derived from Serratia marcescens [abstract]. Proc Am Assoc Cancer Res 1990;31:302.

65. Hussein AM. Interleukin 1 protects against 1-beta-Darabinofuranosylcytosin induced alopecia in the newborn rat animal model. Cancer Res 1991;51:3329–30.

66. Schilli MB, Paus R, Menrad A.Reduction of intrafollicular apoptosis in chemotherapy-induced alopecia by topical calcitriol-analogs. J Invest Dermatol 1998;111:598–604.

67. Hidalgo M, Rinaldi D, Medina G, et al. A phase I trial of topical topitriol (calcitriol, 1,25-dihydroxyvitamin D3) to prevent chemotherapy-induced alopecia. Anticancer Drugs 1999;10:393–5.

68. Jimenez JJ, Yunis AA. Protection from chemotherapy-induced alopecia by 1,25-dihydroxyvitamin D3. Cancer Res 1992;52:5123–5.

69. Reichrath J, Schilli MB, Kerber A, et al. Hair follicle expression of 1,25-dihydroxyvitamin D3 receptors during the murine hair cycle. Br J Dermatol 1994;131:477–82.

70. Hussein AM, Stuart A, Peters WP. Protection against chemotherapy induced alopecia by cyclosporine A in the newborn rat animal model. Dermatology 1995;190:192–6.

71. Paus R, Handjiski B, Eichmuller S, et al. Chemotherapy induced alopecia in mice: induction by cyclophosphamide, inhibition by cyclosporin A, and modulation by dexamethasone. Am J Pathol 1994;144:719–34.

72. Ohnemus U, Unalan M, Handjiski B, et al. Topical estrogen accelerates hair regrowth in mice after chemotherapy-induced alopecia by favoring the dystrophic catagen response pathway to damage. J Invest Dermatol 2004;122:7–13.

73. Goffman T, Cuscela D, Glass J. et al. Topical application of nitroxide protects radiation-induced alopecia in guinea pigs. Int J Radiat Oncol Biol Phys 1992;22:803–6.

74. Hanson WR, Pelka AE, Nelson AK, et al. Subcutaneous or topical administration of 16,16, dimethyl prostogalndin E2 protects from radiation induced alopecia in mice. Int J Radiat Oncol Biol Phys 1992;23:333–7.

75. Peters EMJ, Foitzik K, Paus R, et al. A new strategy for modulating chemotherapy-induced alopecia, using PTH/PTHrP receptor agonist and antagonist. J Invest Dermatol 2001;117:173–8.

76. Wu TL, Insogna KL, Hough LM, et al. Skin-derived fibroblasts respond to human parathyroid hormone-like adenylate cyclase-stimulating proteins. J Clin Endocrinol Metab 1987;65:105–9.

77. Schilli MB, Ray S, Paus R, et al. Control of hair growth with parathyroid hormone (7-34). J Invest Dermatol 1997;108:928–32.

78. Holick MF, Ray S, Chen TC, et al. A parathyroid hormone antagonist stimulates epidermal proliferation and hair growth in mice. Proc Natl Acad Sci U S A 1994;91:8014–6.

79. Munstedt K, Manthey N, et al. Changes in self-concept and body image during alopecia induced cancer chemotherapy. Support Care Cancer 1997;5:139–43.

80. Margolis GJ, Goodman RL, et al. Psychological factors in the choice of treatment for breast cancer. Psychosomatics 1989;30:192–7.

Paraneoplastic Dermatoses

Jeffrey P. Callen, MD

Bruce H. Thiers, MD

This chapter represents a substantive revision and update of a chapter coauthored by Drs. Thiers, Callen, and Cannick that was written for *Cancer of the Skin*, Rigel DS, Friedman R, Dzubow L, Reintgen DS, Bystryn J-C, Marks R, editors), WB Saunders, Philadelphia, 2005 (with permission of the editors).

Paraneoplastic dermatoses are those disorders in which the skin serves as a marker for an internal malignancy. In its truest sense, the meaning of *paraneoplastic* requires that there be a direct and often parallel course of the dermatosis and the malignancy, or in other words, when the skin manifestation occurs, the malignancy is recognized and if the malignancy is effectively treated, then the dermatosis resolves as well. Most of the conditions that are discussed in this chapter do not have such a course, yet their presence serves as an important marker of a potential malignancy. A wide spectrum of inflammatory, proliferative, metabolic, and neoplastic diseases may affect the skin in association with an underlying malignancy.

Internal cancer may affect the skin both directly and indirectly.[1] Direct involvement may be defined as the actual presence of malignant cells within the skin and includes neoplasms that often first become manifested in the skin but eventually affect internal organs (such as mycosis fungoides), visceral neoplasms metastatic to the skin (such as the Sister Joseph nodule of gastric carcinoma), and tumors arising within or below the skin that ultimately spread to the cutaneous surface (such as Paget's disease of the nipple). In addition, cancer patients offer develop skin changes that are reflective of the therapy directed at the malignancy, such as radiation-induced changes or changes related to chemotherapy. Indirect involvement of the skin in cancer patients implies the absence of tumor cells within the skin. Inherited syndromes associated with skin manifestations and an increased incidence of systemic neoplasia are included in this group, as are cutaneous changes resulting from hormone secretion by tumors and a wide spectrum of proliferative and inflammatory disorders occurring in conjunction with internal malignancy (Table 1).

Table 1 Cutaneous Manifestations of Internal Malignancy

Inherited syndromes (see Table 2)
Hormone-secreting tumors
    Ectopic ACTH syndrome
    Carcinoid syndrome
    Glucagonoma syndrome
Proliferative and inflammatory dermatoses
    Hypertrichosis lanuginosa
    Acanthosis nigricans
    Leser-Trélat sign
    Tripe palms
    Acrokeratosis paraneoplastica (Bazex's syndrome)
    Punctate palmar keratoses
    Bowen's disease
    Primary amyloidosis
    Scleromyxedema
    Kaposi's sarcomoa
    Sweet's syndrome
    Pyoderma gangrenosum
    Blistering diseases: pemphigus, paraneoplastic pemphigus, antiepiligrin cicatricial pemphigoid, dermatitis herpetiformis
    Dermatomyositis
    Digital clubbing
    Vasculitis
    Coagulopathies
    Erythema gyratum repens
    Eczematous and ichthyotic disorders
    Cronkhite-Canada syndrome
    Granuloma annulare
    Extramammary Paget's disease

ACTH = adrenocorticotropic hormone.

History

In *Cancer of the Skin*,[1] Curth outlined a set of criteria that could be used to analyze the relationship between an internal malignancy and a cutaneous disorder.[2] Curth's postulates, consist of five characteristics: (1) a concurrent onset: the malignancy is discovered when the skin disease occurs; (2) a parallel course: if the malignancy is removed or successfully treated, the skin disease remits, and when the malignancy recurs, the cutaneous disease also recurs; (3) a uniform malignancy: there is a specific tumor cell type or site associated with the skin disease; (4) a statistical association: based on sound case-control studies, there is a significantly more frequent occurrence of malignancy in a patient with a cutaneous disease; and/or (5) a genetic association. These criteria are extremely useful in the analysis of the relationship between skin diseases and malignancy. However, not all criteria must be met to believe that there is a relationship. We use these criteria as we analyze the disease entities that are discussed in this chapter.

Inherited Syndromes Associated with Internal Malignancy

Multiple familial cancer syndromes have prominent dermatologic features, and at times, the potential for internal malignancy is first suspected when the skin disease is recognized. In a recent review, Tsao characterized these syndromes into four groups: (1) those with prominent skin cancers with occasional internal malignancies, (2) those with prominent benign cutaneous tumors or rare cutaneous malignancies with internal malignancies, (3) those with prominent non-neoplastic cutaneous features or rare cutaneous tumors with internal neoplasms, and (4) those with minimal well-documented cutaneous features with internal neoplasms (Table 2).[3] In this chapter, we discuss only some of these syndromes.

Cowden's disease, also known as multiple hamartoma syndrome (Mendelian Inheritance in Man [MIM] #158350), is inherited as an autosomal dominant trait but occurs more often in women than in men. This disorder has been linked to mutations in the *PTEN/MMAC1* gene on chromosome 10q22-23. The disorder displays a variety of cutaneous and mucosal manifestations that can occur at any time from childhood to middle age.[4–6] Small (1–4 mm) flesh-colored papules, known as trichilemmomas, are found mainly on the head and neck and may assume a wart-like appearance (Figure 1). Similar papules may coalesce and produce a cobblestone appearance on the tongue and gingiva. Waxy papules or nodules known as sclerotic fibromas are less common but are quite characteristic. Flat wart-like papules may occur on the dorsum of

Table 2 Familial Cancer Syndromes and the Skin

Syndrome	MIM Number	Internal Malignancies
Group 1: prominent skin cancers with occasional internal malignancies		
Nevoid basal cell carcinoma syndrome	109400	Medulloblastomas, meningiomas
Familial multiple atypical mole melanoma pancreatic syndrome	606719	Pancreatic, breast, and, in some families, possibly lung and laryngeal
Xeroderma pigmentosa	194400	10-fold increase in the risk of internal malignancies
Group 2: prominent benign cutaneous tumors or rare cutaneous malignancies with internal malignancies		
Multiple hamartoma syndrome (Cowden's disease)	158350	Breast, thyroid, and colon are the most common, but cancers in many other organs have been reported in individual cases
Gardner's syndrome	175100	Colon and rectal
Muir-Torre syndrome	158320	Colon, rectal, and genitourinary, but also breast, hematologic, and head and neck malignancies have been reported
Multiple endocrine neoplasia type IIA (Sipple's syndrome) and IIB	162300 and 171400	Medullary carcinoma of the thyroid, pheochromocytoma
Neurofibromatosis 1	162200	Neurofibrosarcoma, astrocytoma, pheochromocytoma. Children with juvenile xanthogranuloma and neurofibromatosis 1 have an increased risk of chronic myelomonocytic leukemia
Neurofibromatosis 2	101000	Schwannomas, glioma, astrocytoma, meningioma
Tuberous sclerosis	191100	Cardiac rhabdomyomas, renal malignancies
Group 3: prominent non-neoplastic cutaneous features or rare cutaneous tumors with internal malignancies		
Ataxia-telangiectasia (Louis-Bar's syndrome)	208900	Leukemia
Bloom syndrome	210900	Within the Bloom syndrome registry 71 of 168 patients had an internal malignancy
Peutz-Jeghers syndrome	175200	Gastrointestinal, breast, and ovarian, but a wide variety of cancers have been reported
Rothmund-Thomson syndrome	268400	Osteogenic sarcoma
Werner's syndrome	277700	Increased risk of sarcomas, thyroid cancer, and melanoma

MIM = Mendelian Inheritance in Man.

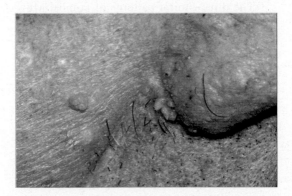

FIGURE 1 Cowden's disease (multiple hamartoma syndrome).

the hands and feet, and keratosis punctata may be present on the soles, sides of the feet, and palms. Lipomas and hemangiomas may also be found.

Internal manifestations are variable. Almost all affected women have fibrocystic disease of the breasts; many of them ultimately develop breast cancer, often bilaterally. Thyroid tumors, both benign and malignant, are frequent (75%). Cancers of the lung and colon have been reported

as well. Hamartomatous polyps of the gastrointestinal tract occur in one-third of patients and are generally benign. The significance of Cowden's disease lies in its value as a marker for the eventual development of breast cancer and, occasionally, thyroid tumors.

Gardner's syndrome (MIM #175100) is another autosomal dominant disorder that is associated with the *APC* (adenomatous polyposis coli) gene on chromosome 5q21. It is characterized by extensive adenomatous polyps of the gastrointestinal tract, especially the colon and rectum.[7] The potential for malignant degeneration of these polyps approaches 100% if not removed; therefore, prophylactic total colectomy should be discussed with the patient and family. The skin lesions that occur in Gardner's syndrome include large, deforming epidermoid cysts, fibromas, lipomas, leiomyomas, trichoepitheliomas, and neurofibromas. Osteomas involving the membranous bones of the face and head occur in about 50% of affected patients.[8] Congenital hypertrophy of the retinal pigment epithelium

has also been associated with Gardner's syndrome.[7]

Peutz-Jeghers syndrome (MIM #175200) is characterized by extensive hamartomatous polyps throughout the gastrointestinal tract. This syndrome is related to mutations in the *STK11/LKB1* gene on chromosome 19p13.3 and is inherited in an autosomal dominant manner. Bleeding and abdominal pain caused by intussusception are the most common gastrointestinal manifestations.[9] The potential for malignant degeneration for these polyps, although possible, is much less than for the adenomatous polyps that occur in Gardner's syndrome.[10] However, certain families appear to have an increased risk of breast and gynecologic cancers.[11–13] The characteristic feature of the condition is freckle-like pigmented macules on the lips, nose, buccal mucosa, and fingertips and in a subungual location.

In Muir-Torre syndrome (also known as Torre syndrome) (MIM #158320), multiple carcinomas, usually of the gastrointestinal tract, are associated with numerous sebaceous gland tumors (benign sebaceous adenomas, malignant sebaceous carcinomas, and others that are hard to classify), primarily on the face and trunk (Figure 2). Other visceral cancers and keratoacanthomas have also been reported.[14] Muir-Torre syndrome appears to be inherited as an autosomal dominant trait and is related to a mutation of the *MSH2* gene located at chromosomes 2p22-p21 and 3p21.3.[15] In contrast, solitary sebaceous gland tumors are not genetically determined, occur most often on the head and neck, and are not associated with visceral malignancy. The diagnosis of gastrointestinal cancer usually precedes the recognition of the cutaneous lesions. The cutaneous tumors can grow quite rapidly but usually do not metastasize. Similarly, the gastrointestinal cancers often behave as low-grade malignancies.

Howel–Evans' syndrome (MIM #148500) represents an association between nonepidermolytic palmoplantar keratoderma (also known as tylosis) and esophageal cancer and was first

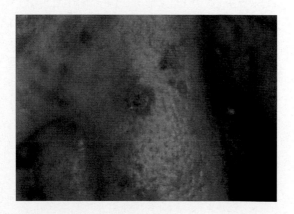

FIGURE 2 Muir-Torre syndrome.

reported in two English families. The keratoderma usually develops during childhood and is accentuated over pressure sites. Onset of the esophageal carcinoma is delayed until middle age. The genetic locus on chromosome 17q25 that appears to be associated with this syndrome is frequently deleted in sporadic esophageal squamous cell carcinoma as well.[16]

Birt-Hogg-Dubé syndrome (MIM #135150) is an autosomal dominant condition characterized by skin tags and benign hair follicle tumors (fibrofolliculomas and trichodiscomas) of the head and neck (Figure 3).[17] This disorder has been mapped to a mutation in the 17p11.2 gene, which encodes folliculin. The incidence of spontaneous pneumothorax, as well as chromophobe and oncocytic types of renal carcinoma, is increased. In some families, a link to colonic polyposis has occurred.[18] Another hereditary syndrome that is associated with renal cell carcinoma is known as hereditary leiomyomatosis and renal cell cancer syndrome (MIM #605839), which is characterized by multiple leiomyomas of the uterus and skin in conjunction with papillary renal cell carcinoma.[19] This disorder is due to a mutation of the gene encoding fumarate hydratase, an enzyme of the tricarboxylic acid cycle. The disorder has been mapped to chromosome 1q42.1.

Melanoma-pancreatic cancer syndrome (also known as familial atypical multiple mole melanoma pancreatic carcinoma syndrome [MIM #606719]) is related to a mutation of the gene encoding cyclin-dependent kinase inhibitor 2A (CDKN2A). In addition to the increased risk of melanoma and pancreatic cancer in these families, there have been reports that link this family cancer syndrome with breast cancer.[20,21]

Patients with the rare autosomal dominant disorder multiple mucosal neuromas syndrome display a constellation of abnormalities, including medullary carcinoma of the thyroid, pheochromocytoma, parathyroid hyperplasia or adenomas, and intestinal ganglioneuromatosis; the latter may give rise to persistent diarrhea.[22] Multiple neuromas appear as whitish nodules mainly on the lips and anterior third of the tongue but also may be noted on the buccal mucosa,

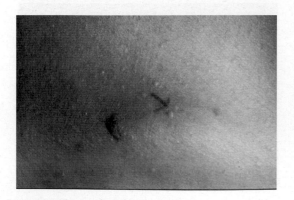

FIGURE 3 Birt-Hogg-Dubé syndrome.

gingiva, palate, pharynx, conjunctivae, and cornea. Affected individuals have characteristic facies, with thick, protuberant, bumpy lips; the eyelids may be thickened and slightly everted. Many patients have a "marfanoid" habitus, with long, slender extremities, poor muscle development, sparse body fat, laxity of joints, pectus excavatum, and dorsal kyphosis. Although multiple mucosal neuromas syndrome is classified as one of the three familial syndromes of multiple endocrine neoplasia (MEN) (see below), many sporadic cases have been reported.

In type 1 neurofibromatosis (von Recklinghausen's disease) (MIM+162200), multiple Schwann cell tumors, malignant degeneration of neurofibromas, and pheochromocytomas (often bilateral) may complicate the clinical course. Gastrointestinal stromal tumors have also been reported.[23] The salient features of this disorder have received extensive review in the recent medical literature.[24] Neurofibromatosis 1, like multiple mucosal neuromas syndrome, may be classified among the apudomas (see below).

Skin Changes Resulting from Hormone-Secreting Tumors

Ectopic hormonal syndromes are best understood in the context of the APUD cell system (ie, cells with a capacity for amino precursor uptake and decarboxylation).[25,26] These cells, which may have a common origin from the neural crest, can secrete a variety of biologically active amines and polypeptide hormones. Neoplastic proliferation of these cells may result in characteristic symptom complexes associated with specific cutaneous changes.

Ectopic adrenocorticotropic hormone (ACTH)-producing tumors cause many of the typical signs and symptoms of Cushing's syndrome. Intense hyperpigmentation, present in only 6 to 10% of patients with Cushing's disease, is especially common in association with ectopic ACTH production and should alert the clinician to the possibility of a hormone-secreting tumor.[27] Although the cause of the hyperpigmentation is unclear, it may be related to tumor production of the peptide β-lipotropin, which contains within its sequence of 91 amino acids the 22–amino acid sequence of beta-MSH (Melanocyte-stimulating hormone). A myasthenia gravis–like syndrome, including profound proximal muscle weakness, may be a striking clinical feature and may reflect either underlying hypokalemia or polymyositis. Oat cell (small cell) carcinoma of the lung is the tumor most often associated with ectopic ACTH production, although other malignancies have been reported.

Carcinoid syndrome is a second example of a hormonal syndrome associated with a nonendocrine tumor.[28] The disorder is probably most

often caused by the release of the enzyme kallikrein from tumor cells, with subsequent conversion of kininogen to vasoactive kinin peptides, including bradykinin; in addition, increased blood levels of histamine may be important in the rare metastatic gastric carcinoid. The most striking cutaneous manifestations are episodes of flushing, initially lasting 10 to 30 minutes and involving only the upper half of the body; as the flush resolves, gyrate and serpiginous patterns may be noted. With successive attacks, more extensive areas may be affected and the redness takes on a cyanotic quality, eventually leading to a more permanent facial cyanotic flush with associated telangiectasia, resembling rosacea. Persistent edema and erythema of the face may result in leonine facies. A pellagra-like picture, noted in some patients, may be due to abnormal tryptophan metabolism. Systemic symptoms associated with the cutaneous flushing include abdominal pain with explosive watery diarrhea, shortness of breath, and hypertension.

Carcinoid tumors are usually found in the appendix or small intestine; extraintestinal carcinoid tumors may arise in the bile ducts, pancreas, stomach, ovaries, or bronchi. The carcinoid syndrome occurs primarily when an intestinal carcinoid tumor metastasizes to the liver or with extraintestinal tumors; flushing attacks can be provoked by palpation of hepatic or abdominal metastases or by alcohol ingestion, enemas, emotional stress, or sudden changes in body temperature. When the syndrome is associated with bronchial adenomas of the carcinoid variety, the flushing is more prolonged and often associated with fever, marked anxiety, disorientation, sweating, salivation, and lacrimation.

The three clinical patterns of familial MEN (types I, IIA, and IIB) are examples of polyglandular endocrine disorders involving the APUD cell system. A carcinoid-like syndrome has been described in MEN IIA (Sipple's syndrome)[29]; otherwise, mucocutaneous lesions occur only in MEN IIB (multiple mucosal neuromas syndrome), which has already been discussed.

Glucagonoma syndrome is associated with an apudoma involving the glucagon-secreting alpha cell of the pancreas.[30] The characteristic cutaneous eruption, necrolytic migratory erythema, usually occurs on the abdomen, perineum, thighs, buttocks, and groin. The perioral region and the distal extremities are often affected. Patches of intense erythema with irregular outlines expand and coalesce, resulting in circinate or polycyclic configurations. Superficial vesicles on the surface rupture quickly to form crusts, but new vesicles may continue to develop along the active margins. An eczema craquelé-like appearance may be noted. Pressure or trauma may initiate or aggravate the eruption, which seems to share features of staphylococcal scalded skin syndrome and acrodermatitis enteropathica. Like the latter disorder, necrolytic migratory erythema sometimes responds to topical application of diiodohydroxyquin; however, zinc levels are normal, and zinc treatment is ineffective. Complete surgical resection is the only curative treatment for the tumor as chemotherapy yields only modest benefit.[31]

Proliferative and Inflammatory Dermatoses Associated with Cancer

Many of the conditions to be discussed in this section are nonspecific and have been reported both in association with and in the absence of underlying malignant disease. Malignancy is most often only one of a number of possible provoking factors.

The association of acquired hypertrichosis lanuginosa (malignant down) with cancer is among the most consistent.[32] The extensive growth of silky, nonpigmented lanugo hair on the face (Figure 4), neck, trunk, and sometimes the extremities usually antedates the discovery of a malignancy. Other causes of hypertrichosis, such as porphyria cutanea tarda and endocrinopathies, should be excluded. The tumors associated with acquired hypertrichosis lanuginosa are often adenocarcinomas and frequently occur in the gastrointestinal tract; however, squamous cell carcinomas have also been reported, and multiple other sites have been associated. A painful glossitis, angular cheilitis, and swollen red fungiform papillae on the anterior half of the tongue may accompany the cutaneous changes.

Acanthosis nigricans is perhaps the best known of the cutaneous markers of internal malignancy.[33] Flexural areas, especially the axillae, groin, and neck, are most often involved; the skin has a hyperpigmented velvety appearance and in severe cases can become quite verrucous (Figure 5). Papillomatous changes may be noted in the oral cavity,[34] and hyperkeratosis in a rugose pattern may develop on the palms and dorsal surfaces of large joints. The cutaneous changes can occur before, coincident with, or after the dis-

covery of an underlying malignancy, which most often is an adenocarcinoma of the stomach. Tumors have also been found in other abdominal organs, with more than 95% being adenocarcinomas. Acanthosis nigricans also occurs in association with insulin resistance and other endocrinopathies, as well as owing to drugs; therefore, a detailed history must be included in the evaluation of all affected patients.[35,36] The possibility of underlying cancer should be strongly considered in any nonobese adult who develops acanthosis nigricans in the absence of a recognizable endocrinopathy. Such an individual should have an extensive gastrointestinal evaluation.

Leser-Trélat sign, the sudden appearance and/or rapid increase in the size of multiple seborrheic keratoses, may be associated with carcinoma of the gastrointestinal tract or female reproductive system.[37] Because most of these patients have coexistent acanthosis nigricans and the malignancy is often an adenocarcinoma of gastrointestinal origin, some clinicians believe that this condition may represent a generalized variant of acanthosis nigricans.

A third related condition is tripe palms. The skin changes manifest as rugose thickening of the palms and, occasionally, the soles (Figure 6). Patients will often have coexistent acanthosis nigricans and sometimes Leser-Trélat sign. Patients with tripe palms and acanthosis nigricans usually have adenocarcinomas of the gastrointestinal tract; however, when tripe palms occur in the absence of acanthosis nigricans, patients tend to have squamous cell carcinoma of the lung.[38]

Patients with Bazex's syndrome (acrokeratosis paraneoplastica) develop an erythematous to violaceous psoriasiform eruption, primarily on acral surfaces (Figure 7).[39,40] The ears, nose, cheeks, hands, feet, and knees are most often affected, but the nails may become dystrophic and the palms and soles may develop a keratoderma in later stages of the disease. The disorder may develop in stages and is associated primarily with carcinomas of the upper respiratory and

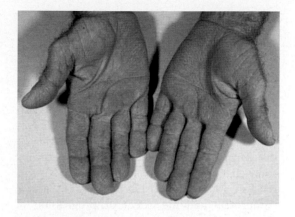

FIGURE 6 Tripe palms. (Courtesy of Dr. Jon Dyer, Columbianm)

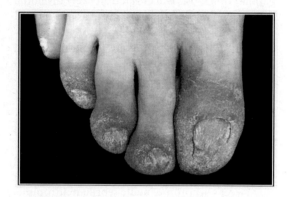

FIGURE 7 Bazex's syndrome.

digestive tracts (larynx, pharynx, trachea, bronchus, and/or upper esophagus), with the malignancy often being detected concurrently. If the tumor is effectively treated, the eruption may resolve but may return with tumor recurrence. There is no known effective treatment for the cutaneous eruption, although corticosteroids and keratolytic agents have been used.

The significance of punctate palmar keratoses as a sign of internal malignancy is controversial,[41] although they have been reported in Cowden's syndrome. Similarly, the purported relationship between Bowen's disease (intraepidermal squamous cell carcinoma) and systemic cancer was recently demonstrated to be nonexistent.[42]

Patients with primary systemic amyloidosis almost always have an underlying plasma cell dyscrasia, usually multiple myeloma.[43] The skin takes on a generalized waxy appearance and bleeds easily when traumatized ("pinch purpura"). Hemorrhagic lesions are especially common around the eyes. Macroglossia is an associated finding. Skin lesions are not seen in secondary amyloidosis.

Scleromyxedema, a cutaneous mucinosis representing the generalized variant of lichen myxedematosus, has been associated with a peculiar serum monoclonal paraprotein.[44,45] The paraprotein is a basic, electrophoretically homogeneous 7S gammaglobulin, usually of the immunoglobu-

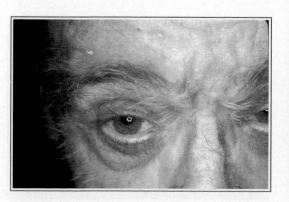

FIGURE 4 Hypertrichosis lanuginosa.

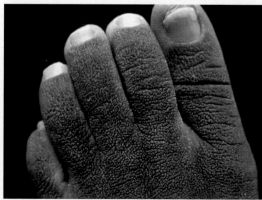

FIGURE 5 Acanthosis nigricans.

lin (Ig)G class, that almost always possesses light chains of the lambda type. Clinically, the disorder appears as a generalized eruption of 2 to 3 mm waxy lichenoid papules, often in a linear arrangement; lesions are most common on the hands, elbows, forearms, upper trunk, face, and neck but may be found anywhere. Induration of the underlying tissue may produce a resemblance to scleroderma; mucin deposition in forehead skin may be disfiguring and lead to longitudinal furrowing somewhat reminiscent of leonine facies. No correlation appears to exist between levels of the paraprotein and the extent or progression of the skin disease. Only a minority of patients with scleromyxedema, lichen myxedematosus, or papular mucinosis will develop an overt myeloma or a detectable plasma cell dyscrasia. Affected patients should have a serum protein electrophoresis, immunofixation electrophoresis, and measurement of Ig levels; these tests should be repeated every 6 months. Therapy of these disorders has been difficult, and although there are reports of chemotherapy and radiotherapy, or stem cell transplants being effective in individual patients, no consistent response has been noted. In a recent report of several patients, the use of thalidomide was promising.[46]

Sweet's syndrome (acute febrile neutrophilic dermatosis) appears to be associated with leukemia or preleukemic conditions in roughly 25% of patients. Sweet's syndrome has been linked to a variety of malignancies, but the vast majority affect myeloid cells.[47,48] The condition is manifest by the acute onset of erythematous, tender, papules, plaques, or nodules on the face, extremities, and upper trunk (Figure 8). The surface appears vesicular and may be studded with pustules. Fever, malaise, and neutrophilia frequently accompany the cutaneous eruption. Biopsy of the skin lesion demonstrates a dense dermal neutrophilic infiltrate, without vasculitis, but recent reports have suggested that some vascular inflammation is possible. The presence of moderate to severe anemia may be helpful in distinguishing Sweet's syndrome associated with a myeloproliferative disease from the idiopathic

variant. Sweet's syndrome will respond to oral corticosteroids, but in a recent report, a patient with recalcitrant Sweet's syndrome and myelofibrosis was successfully treated with oral thalidomide.[49]

Pyoderma gangrenosum is a neutrophilic ulcerative dermatosis. Its superficial form, known as atypical or bullous pyoderma gangrenosum, often occurs on the head and neck and has been associated with hematologic malignancy.[50] Most often the association is with acute myelogenous leukemia, but several cases of chronic myelogenous leukemia, acute lymphoblastic leukemia, and preleukemic states, such as myelofibrosis or agnogenic myeloid metaplasia, have also been reported. The skin and blood disease often present concurrently and run a parallel course.

Classic pyoderma gangrenosum has been associated with a monoclonal gammopathy (and, occasionally, myeloma), with several solid tumors, and with non-Hodgkin's lymphoma. The gammopathy, which has been noted in up to 20% of patients with pyoderma gangrenosum, results from an IgA paraprotein. However, in patients with coexistent pyoderma gangrenosum and IgA paraproteinemia or myeloma, there is no information to suggest a parallel course.[50a]

A variety of blistering diseases have been reported in patients with cancer. Various forms of pemphigus have been associated with thymoma. The occurrence of paraneoplastic pemphigus in patients with cancer, especially lymphoreticular malignancy, is well documented.[51–53] The proposed association of bullous pemphigoid with malignancy probably reflects the tendency of both of these conditions to occur in the elderly rather than any true association. An increased incidence of malignancy has also been reported in the antiepiligrin variant of cicatricial pemphigoid (Figure 9).[54] Individuals with dermatitis herpetiformis may have an increased relative risk of intestinal lymphoma similar to that noted in patients with sprue.[55] Epidermolysis bullosa acquisita has also rarely been reported in patients with lymphoreticular tumors.

Approximately 10 to 30% of adult patients with dermatomyositis have an associated malignancy.[56,57] The neoplasm may occur before, during, or after the diagnosis of dermatomyositis. An awareness of this potential should alert the physician to carefully evaluate all dermatomyositis patients for malignancy. Pathognomonic clinical manifestations include an edematous, violaceous eruption of the upper eyelids (heliotrope rash) and atrophic scaly papules over bony prominences (Gottron's papules) (Figure 10); photosensitivity, malar erythema, poikiloderma, and periungual telangiectasias are important, although less specific, findings. Dermatomyositis is not specific for any particular site or cell type of cancer; however, in Western countries, ovarian and breast carcinoma in women and lung and prostate carcinoma in men are especially frequent. The risk of developing cancer is highest the first 3 years after the diagnosis of dermatomyositis.[56,57] Raynaud's phenomenon or a sclerodermatous change in an adult with dermatomyositis suggests an overlap syndrome; this variant is rarely associated with malignant disease. Childhood dermatomyositis is not associated with malignancy.

A number of musculoskeletal disorders have been reported in patients with cancer. Clubbing is noted in about 10% of individuals with lung cancer and tumors metastatic to the lung.[58] Subperiosteal new bone formation in patients with clubbing (hypertrophic osteoarthropathy) occurs most commonly along the shaft of the phalanges but may affect other bones as well.[59] Joint swelling, synovitis, periarticular swelling, hyperhidrosis, and palmar erythema may be pronounced and create a picture similar to early rheumatoid arthritis. Hypertrophic osteoarthropathy associated with acromegaloid features (pachydermoperiostosis) can occur either in association with lung cancer or as a genetic disease unassociated with malignancy.

A purported association between cutaneous leukocytoclastic vasculitis and cancer has never been proven, although numerous individual case

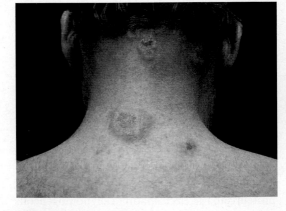

FIGURE 8 Sweet's syndrome.

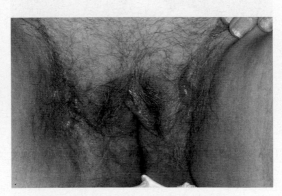

FIGURE 9 Antiepiligrin bullous pemphigoid.

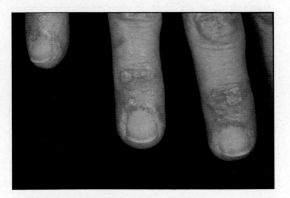

FIGURE 10 Dermatomyositis.

reports have related various vasculitic syndromes to malignancy, including solid tumors and lymphoproliferative disorders.[60,61] Interestingly, both cutaneous leukocytoclastic vasculitis and systemic necrotizing vasculitis have been observed in patients with hairy cell leukemia (leukemic reticuloendotheliosis). Often the patient with coexistent neoplastic disease has the malignancy at the time of diagnosis of the vasculitis. In other cases, release of tumor antigens into the circulation, such as after radiation therapy or chemotherapy, may be the inciting event. A parallel course between the tumor and the vasculitis has not been evident except in a few instances.

Migratory superficial thrombophlebitis and multiple deep venous thromboses have been noted in cancer patients, especially those with tumors arising in the pancreas, lung, stomach, prostate, or hematopoietic system.[62] The neck, chest, abdominal wall, pelvis, and limbs are most frequently affected.

The figurate erythemas may be divided into at least three groups. Erythema chronicum migrans follows a tick bite and may be associated with Lyme disease. Erythema annulare centrifugum may be secondary to a variety of causative factors, including, although rarely, malignancy. Erythema gyratum repens (Figure 11) is almost always associated with cancer,[63] although no one tumor type or site seems to predominate. Multiple wavy urticarial bands with a fine scale migrate over the cutaneous surface, giving it an appearance similar to the grain of wood. The eruption usually occurs within a few months before or after the diagnosis of cancer.

Generalized pruritus, ichthyosis, and exfoliative dermatitis are seen as nonspecific features of lymphoproliferative disorders[64,65]; uncommonly, they may be associated with solid tumors. Pityriasis rotunda may be a variant of acquired ichthyosis; the eruption consists of geometrically perfect, circular patches of scales. The disease was first reported in the Japanese, South African blacks, and West Indian blacks, in whom an associated neoplasm was occasionally described. A familial variant has been recognized in Europe that does not appear to be associated with cancer.[66] Although the exact status of pityriasis rotunda as a paraneoplastic condition remains to be delineated, it seems prudent to rule out concurrent malignancy in affected patients.

Infectious disorders are frequent in cancer patients and may either be directly related to depressed cell-mediated immunity associated with the neoplasm or secondary to pharmacologic immunosuppression. The increased incidence of herpes zoster, either localized or disseminated, in patients with leukemia and lymphoma has been appreciated for years, although such infection usually develops during the course of the illness rather than as a presenting sign.[67] Rarely, herpes zoster may be associated with an underlying carcinoma.

Diffuse cutaneous and, rarely, mucosal hyperpigmentation may also occur in Cronkhite-Canada syndrome; other cutaneous features include onychodystrophy and alopecia.[14] Hamartomatous polyps occur throughout the stomach and intestines, and the incidence of gastrointestinal cancer is approximately 15%.[14] The disease occurs in adults in a sporadic, nongenetic manner. The prognosis is poor.

Granuloma annulare is a common benign skin disease characterized by flesh-colored to erythematous annular dermal plaques. A suggestion of a relationship between granuloma annulare and malignant lymphoma was reported in 13 patients in 1994[68]; however, a subsequent report by Li and colleagues demonstrated no increased risk of malignancy in patients with granuloma annulare.[69]

Extramammary Paget's disease is manifest as an erythematous plaque on locations other than the breast, most often in the inguinal fold, vulva, or scrotum (Figure 12). Malignancy is more common in these patients and is often in a location near the cutaneous lesion but not contiguous with it.[70,71] Therefore, patients with extramammary Paget's disease should be evaluated for possible tumors in the lower gastrointestinal tract (colon and rectum) and in the lower portion of the genitourinary tract (bladder and prostate).

REFERENCES

1. Thiers BH. Dermatologic manifestations of internal cancer. CA Cancer J Clin 1986;36:130–48.
2. Curth HO. Skin lesions and internal carcinoma. In: Andrade R, et al, editors. Cancer of the skin. Philadelphia: WB Saunders; 1976. p. 1308–9.
3. Tsao H. Update on familial cancer syndromes and the skin. J Am Acad Dermatol 2000;42:939–69.
4. Hildenbrand C, Burgdorf WH, Lautenschlager S. Cowden syndrome—diagnostic skin signs. Dermatology 2001; 202:362–6.
5. Waite KA, Eng C. Protean PTEN: form and function. Am J Hum Genet 2002;70:829–44.
6. Zhou XP, Hampel H, Roggenbuck J, et al. A 39-bp deletion polymorphism in PTEN in African American individuals: implications for molecular diagnostic testing. J Mol Diagn 2002;4:114–7.
7. Parks ET, Caldemeyer KS, Mirowski GW. Gardner syndrome. J Am Acad Dermatol 2001;45:940–2.
8. Sayan NB, Ucok C, Karasu HA, Gunhan O. Peripheral osteoma of the oral and maxillofacial region: a study of 35 new cases. J Oral Maxillofac Surg 2002;60:1299–301.
9. Marschall J, Hayes P. Intussusceptions in a man with Peutz-Jeghers syndrome. CMAJ 2003;168:315–6.
10. Boardman LA. Heritable colorectal cancer syndromes: recognition and preventive management. Gastroenterol Clin North Am 2002;31:1107–31.
11. Boardman LA, Pittelkow MR, Couch FJ, et al. Association of Peutz-Jeghers-like mucocutaneous pigmentation with breast and gynecologic carcinomas in women. Medicine (Baltimore) 2000;79:293–8.
12. Boardman LA, Thibodeau SN, Schaid DJ, et al. Increased risk for cancer in patients with the Peutz-Jeghers syndrome. Ann Intern Med 1998;128:896–9.
13. Papageorgiou T, Stratakis CA. Ovarian tumors associated with multiple endocrine neoplasias and related syndromes (Carney complex, Peutz-Jeghers syndrome, von Hippel-Lindau disease, Cowden's disease). Int J Gynecol Cancer 2002;12:337–47.
14. Ward EM, Wolfsen HC. Review article: the non-inherited gastrointestinal polyposis syndromes. Aliment Pharmacol Ther. 2002;16:333–42.
15. Fiorentino DF, Nguyen JC, Egbert BM, Swetter SM. Muir-Torre Syndrome: confirmation of diagnosis by immunohistochemical analysis of cutaneous lesions." J Am Acad Dermatol. 2004; 50:476–8.
16. Risk JM, Evans KE, Jones J, et al. Characterization of a 500 kb region on 17q25 and the exclusion of candidate genes as the familial tylosis oesophageal cancer (TOC) locus. Oncogene 2002;21:6395–402.
17. Vincent A, Farley M, Chan E, James WD. Birt-Hogg-Dube syndrome: a review of the literature and the differential diagnosis of firm facial papules. J Am Acad Dermatol 2003;49:698–705.
18. Zbar B, Alvord WG, Glenn G, et al. Risk of renal and colonic neoplasms and spontaneous pneumothorax in the Birt-Hogg-Dube syndrome. Cancer Epidemiol Biomarkers Prev 2002;11:393–400.
19. Toro JR, Nickerson ML, Wei MH, et al. Mutations in the fumarate hydratase gene cause hereditary leiomyomatosis and renal cell cancer in families in North America. Am J Hum Genet 2003;73:95–106
20. Borg A, Sandberg T, Nilsson K, et al. High frequency of multiple melanomas and breast and pancreas carcinomas in CDKN2A mutation-positive melanoma families. J Natl Cancer Inst 2000;92:1260–6.
21. Lynch HT, Brand RE, Hogg D, et al. Phenotypic variation in eight extended CDKN2A germline mutation familial multiple melanoma-pancreatic carcinoma-prone families. Cancer 2002;94:84–96.
22. Morrison PJ, Nevin NC. Multiple endocrine neoplasia type 2B (mucosal neuroma syndrome, Wagenmann-Froboese syndrome). J Med Genet 1996;33:779–82.
23. Giuly JA, Picand R, Giuly D, et al. Von Recklinghausen disease and gastrointestinal stromal tumors. Am J Surg 2003;185:86–7.
24. Khosrotehrani K, Bastuji-Garin S, Zeller J, et al. Clinical risk factors for mortality in patients with neurofibromatosis 1: a cohort study of 378 patients. Arch Dermatol 2003;139:187–91.
25. DeLellis RA. The neuroendocrine system and its tumors: an overview. Am J Clin Pathol 2001;115:Suppl:S5–16.

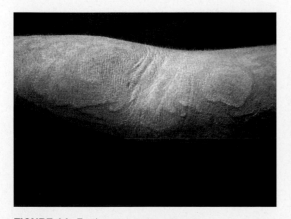

FIGURE 11 Erythema gyratum repens.

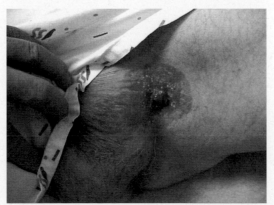

FIGURE 12 Extramammary Paget's disease.

26. Day R, Salzet M. The neuroendocrine phenotype, cellular plasticity, and the search for genetic switches: redefining the diffuse neuroendocrine system. Neuroendocrinol Lett 2002;23:447–51.

27. Torpy DJ, Mullen N, Ilias I, Nieman LK. Association of hypertension and hypokalemia with Cushing's syndrome caused by ectopic ACTH secretion: a series of 58 cases. Ann N Y Acad Sci 2002;970:134–44.

28. McStay MK, Caplin ME. Carcinoid tumour. Minerva Med 2002;93:389–401.

29. Kousseff BG. Multiple endocrine neoplasia 2 (MEN 2)/MEN 2A (Sipple syndrome). Dermatol Clin 1995;13:91–7.

30. Zeng J, Wang B, Ma D, Li F. Glucagonoma syndrome: diagnosis and treatment. J Am Acad Dermatol 2003;48:297–8.

31. Brentjens R, Saltz L. Islet cell tumors of the pancreas: the medical oncologist's perspective. Surg Clin North Am 2001;81:527–42.

32. Kurzrock R, Cohen PR. Cutaneous paraneoplastic syndromes in solid tumors. Am J Med 1995;99:662–71.

33. Anderson SH, Hudson-Peacock M, Muller AF. Malignant acanthosis nigricans: potential role of chemotherapy. Br J Dermatol 1999;141:714–6.

34. Ramirez-Amador V, Esquivel-Pedraza L, Caballero-Mendoza E, et al. Oral manifestations as a hallmark of malignant acanthosis nigricans. Oral Pathol Med 1999;28:278–81.

35. Torley D, Bellus GA, Munro CS. Genes, growth factors and acanthosis nigricans. Br J Dermatol 2002;147:1096–101.

36. Garcia Hidalgo L. Dermatological complications of obesity. Am J Clin Dermatol 2002;3:497–506.

37. Schwartz RA. Sign of Leser-Trelat. J Am Acad Dermatol 1996;35:88–95.

38. Mullans EA, Cohen PR. Tripe palms: a cutaneous paraneoplastic syndrome. South Med J 1996;89:626–7.

39. Bolognia JL, Brewer YP, Cooper DL. Bazex syndrome (acrokeratosis paraneoplastica). An analytic review. Medicine (Baltimore) 1991;70:269–80.

40. Buxtorf K, Hubscher E, Panizzon R. Bazex syndrome. Dermatology 2001;202:350–2.

41. Cuzick J, Babiker A, De Stavola BL, et al. Palmar keratoses in family members of individuals with bladder cancer. J Clin Epidemiol 1990;43:1421–6.

42. Chute CG, Chuang TY, Bergstralh EJ, Su WP. The subsequent risk of internal cancer with Bowen's disease. A population-based study. JAMA 1991;266:816–9.

43. Daoud MS, Lust JA, Kyle RA, Pittelkow MR. Monoclonal gammopathies and associated skin disorders. J Am Acad Dermatol 1999;40:507–35.

44. Pomann JJ, Rudner EJ. Scleromyxedema revisited. Int J Dermatol 2003;42:31–5.

45. Jackson EM, English JC III. Diffuse cutaneous mucinoses. Dermatol Clin 2002;20:493–501.

46. Sansbury JC, Cocuroccia B, Jorizzo JL, et al. Treatment of recalcitrant scleromyxedema with thalidomide in 3 patients. J Am Acad Dermatol 2004;51:126–31.

47. Avivi I, Rosenbaum H, Levy Y, Rowe J. Myelodysplastic syndrome and associated skin lesions: a review of the literature. Leuk Res 1999;23:323–30.

48. Cho KH, Han KH, Kim SW, et al. Neutrophilic dermatoses associated with myeloid malignancy. Clin Exp Dermatol 1997;22:269–73.

49. Browning C, Dixon J, Malone J, Callen JP. Thalidomide effective therapy for myelodysplasia associated Sweet's syndrome with treatment of recalcitrant Sweet's syndrome associated with myelodysplasia. J Am Acad Dermatol. 2005;53:S135–8.

50. Rogalski C, Paasch U, Glander HJ, Haustein UF. Bullous pyoderma gangrenosum complicated by disseminated intravascular coagulation with subsequent myelodysplastic syndrome (chronic myelomonocytic leukemia). J Dermatol 2003;30:59–63.

50a. Jackson JM, Callen JP. Pyoderma gangrenosum and IgA myeloma. J. Cutan Med Surg 1997;2:1–4.

51. Nguyen VT, Ndoye A, Bassler KD, et al. Classification, clinical manifestations, and immunopathological mechanisms of the epithelial variant of paraneoplastic autoimmune multiorgan syndrome: a reappraisal of paraneoplastic pemphigus. Arch Dermatol 2001;137:193–206.

52. Joly P, Richard C, Gilbert D, et al. Sensitivity and specificity of clinical, histologic, and immunologic features in the diagnosis of paraneoplastic pemphigus. J Am Acad Dermatol 2000;43:619–26.

53. Allen CM, Camisa C. Paraneoplastic pemphigus: a review of the literature. Oral Dis 2000;6:208–14.

54. Egan CA, Lazarova Z, Darling TN, et al. Anti-epiligrin cicatricial pemphigoid and relative risk for cancer. Lancet 2001;357:1850–1.

55. Askling J, Linet M, Gridley G, et al. Cancer incidence in a population-based cohort of individuals hospitalized with celiac disease or dermatitis herpetiformis. Gastroenterology 2002;123:1428–35.

56. Hill CL, Zhang Y, Sigurgeirsson B, et al. Frequency of specific cancer types in dermatomyositis and polymyositis: a population-based study. Lancet 2001;357:96–100.

57. Stockton D, Doherty VR, Brewster DH. Risk of cancer in patients with dermatomyositis or polymyositis, and follow-up implications: a Scottish population-based cohort study. Br J Cancer 2001;85:41–5.

58. Myers KA, Farquhar DR. The rational clinical examination. Does this patient have clubbing? JAMA 2001;286:341–7.

59. Kishi K, Nakamura H, Sudo A, et al. Tumor debulking by radiofrequency ablation in hypertrophic pulmonary osteoarthropathy associated with pulmonary carcinoma. Lung Cancer 2002;38:317–20.

60. Spann CR, Callen JP, Yam LT, Apgar JT. Cutaneous leukocytoclastic vasculitis complicating hairy cell leukemia (leukemic reticuloendotheliosis). Arch Dermatol 1982;122:1057–9.

61. Callen JP. Cutaneous leukocytoclastic vasculitis in a patient with an adenocarcinoma of the colon. J Rheumatol 1987;14:386–9.

62. Naschitz JE, Kovaleva J, Shaviv N, et al. Vascular disorders preceding diagnosis of cancer: distinguishing the causal relationship based on Bradford-Hill guidelines. Angiology 2003;54:11–7.

63. Eubanks LE, McBurney E, Reed R. Erythema gyratum repens. Am J Med Sci 2001;321:302–5.

64. Cohen PR. Cutaneous paraneoplastic syndromes. Am Fam Physician 1994;50:1273–82.

65. Callen JP, Bernardi DM, Clark RA, Weber DA. Adult-onset recalcitrant eczema: a marker of noncutaneous lymphoma or leukemia. J Am Acad Dermatol 2000;43: 207–10.

66. Aste N, Pau M, Aste N, Biggio P. Pityriasis rotunda: a survey of 42 cases observed in Sardinia, Italy. Dermatology 1997;194:32–5.

67. Egerer G, Hensel M, Ho AD. Infectious complications in chronic lymphoid malignancy. Curr Treat Options Oncol 2001;2:237–44.

68. Barksdale SK, Perniciaro D, Halling KC, Strickler JG. Granuloma annulare in patients with malignant lymphoma: clinicopathologic study of thirteen new cases. J Am Acad Dermatol 1994;31:42–8.

69. Li A, Hogan DJ, Sanusi ID, Smoller BR. Granuloma annulare and malignant neoplasms. Am J Dermatopathol 2003;25:113–6.

70. Lai YL, Yang WG, Tsay PK, et al. Penoscrotal extramammary Paget's disease: a review of 33 cases in a 20-year experience. Plast Reconstr Surg 2003;112:1017–23.

71. Goldblum JR, Hart WR. Perianal Paget's disease: a histologic and immunohistochemical study of 11 cases with and without associated rectal adenocarcinoma. Am J Surg Pathol 1998;22:170–9.

Cutaneous Reactions to Medications

Steven R. Mays, MD

Joy Kunishige, MD

Cutaneous drug reactions occur both with conventional medications and with chemotherapy agents. The classification of a particular drug rash is primarily based on the morphology and anatomic location of the rash. A drug rash may be maculopapular, for example, or present as acral erythema (erythema of the hands and feet). Sometimes the morphology of a drug rash is highly characteristic and the clinical diagnosis of drug reaction is made without difficulty. Some drug reactions, however, are not so clinically distinct, and the differential diagnosis may easily include other diseases (such as viral exanthems and cutaneous graft-versus-host disease). The first responsibility of the physician in these situations is to decide whether a particular rash does indeed represent a cutaneous reaction to a drug. Once this has been established, the next step is to decide which medication is the culprit. This two-step process requires a familiarity with the common morphologic types of drug reaction and knowledge of the drugs associated with each type. This chapter reviews the relevant data.

Cutaneous reactions to conventional medications are ?? uncommon. One exception is the maculopapular type of drug exanthem that occurs fairly frequently, especially with systemic antibiotics. Some *chemotherapy* reactions (eg, actinic keratosis [AK] recall) are also uncommon. However, some chemotherapy reactions are so common as to be an *expected* result of therapy. Sixty percent of patients receiving capecitabine, for example, develop hand-foot syndrome. A similarly high percentage of patients receiving cetuximab develop an acneiform eruption. In general, in the setting of a cancer hospital, adverse cutaneous reactions to chemotherapy are much more common than those to conventional (non-chemotherapy) medications. This chapter therefore reviews in detail the various types of cutaneous chemotherapy reactions. We review cutaneous reactions to conventional medications as they arise within the differential diagnosis for each particular chemotherapy exanthem.

A single chemotherapy agent may cause different types of reactions in different patients. For example, a particular agent may cause hand-foot syndrome in one patient and cutaneous hyperpigmentation in another.

Most cutaneous chemotherapy reactions are mild to moderate in severity; acneiform eruptions and onycholysis are examples. By contrast, severe cutaneous reactions to chemotherapy (such as a severe episode of hand-foot syndrome may require changes in the scheduled administration of the responsible agent.

Cutaneous reactions to chemotherapy fall into two broad categories. **Specific** cutaneous reactions are those that occur almost exclusively with chemotherapy agents, but not with other medications. **Nonspecific** cutaneous reactions are caused both by conventional medications and by chemotherapy agents. In a patient with a **nonspecific** skin reaction, it may be difficult to determine whether the culprit was a chemotherapy agent or a conventional medication.[1]

Cutaneous Reactions Specific to Chemotherapy

This group of unique reactions occurs only with chemotherapy agents and not with other medications. Examples include hand-foot syndrome and actinic keratosis recall.

Some specific reactions occur with only one or two chemotherapy agents, such as the flagellate cutaneous hyperpigmentation caused by bleomycin. Other specific reactions, such as the hand-foot syndrome, occur with many different chemotherapy agents.

In a patient affected by one of these characteristic reactions, the correct identification of the causative agent is fairly straightforward; this is because one may immediately exclude any nonchemotherapy medications as the cause.

The following sections review the most clinically significant reactions of this type.

Hand-Foot Syndrome

Clinical

Hand Foot Syndrome (HFS) is a localized cutaneous response to certain chemotherapy agents. This reaction is also known as acral erythema, erythrodysesthesia syndrome. Characteristic findings are edema, erythema, and tenderness of the hands and feet. Associated chemotherapy agents are listed in Table 1. The most commonly involved agents are cytarabine, doxorubicin, fluorouracil, and capecitabine.

HFS initially presents with a tingling sensation of the palms or soles, usually within 1 week of drug administration.[2] The patient then develops erythema of the palms and the volar aspect of the fingers; there may also be erythema of the dorsal aspect of the fingers (Figures 1 and 2). The feet may be similarly affected but usually to a lesser extent.[3] There may be edema of the hands, feet, and digits. Tenderness of the palms and soles ranges from mild to severe in intensity. Some patients develop tense blisters of the palms and soles (Figure 3). Occasionally, patients develop a concomitant maculopapular eruption at other sites, such as the wrists, ankles, extremities, or trunk.

HFS usually resolves 1 to 2 weeks after the cessation of chemotherapy. When an episode resolves, there may be impressive desquamation of the palms and soles.

Severe episodes of HFS are a fairly common dose-limiting toxicity for some chemotherapy agents and may necessitate discontinuation of the drug. Severe HFS is defined by the presence of cutaneous ulcerations, bullae, or pain that interferes with the activities of daily living.[4]

The incidence of HFS varies from one chemotherapeutic agent to another. Capecitabine is the agent most likely to cause HFS.[4] Approximately 60% of patients treated with capecitabine develop HFS.[4–6] For other agents, the incidence is much lower. The incidence of **severe** HFS with capecitabine, for example, is 10 to 17%.[4,7–10] Severe HFS is the most common dose-limiting toxicity for capecitabine and for other chemotherapy agents as well.[11,12]

The **first** episode of HFS usually occurs during one of the early cycles of administration of a chemotherapy agent. In a series of 41 patients treated with capecitabine, 93% had their first episode of HFS within the first two cycles.[4] However, the first episode of HFS may occur much later in the treatment phase with some chemotherapy agents.

Table 1 Chemotherapy Agents Associated with Hand-Foot Syndrome

Capecitabine*
Cisplatinum
Clofarabine
Cyclophosphamide
Cytarabine*
Daunorubicin
Docetaxel
Doxorubicin*
Etoposide
Fluorouracil*
Hydroxyurea
Mercaptopurine
Methotrexate
Mitotane
Paclitaxel
Suramin
Tegafur

Adapted from Demircay Z et al[2]; Vakalis D, Ioannides D, Lazaridou E, et al. Acral erythema induced by chemotherapy with cisplatin. Br J Dermatol 1998;139:750-1; Portal I, Cardenal F, Garcia-del-Muro X. Etoposide-related acral erythema. Cancer Chemother Pharmacol 1994;34:181; Bastida J, Diaz-Cascajo C, Borghi S. Chemotherapy-induced acral erythema due to tegafur. Acta Derm Venerol 1997;77:72–3; De Argila D, Dominguez J, Iglesias L. Taxol-induced acral erythema. Dermatology 1996;192:377–8; Lowitt M, Eisenberger M, Sina B. Cutaneous eruptions from suramin: a clinical and histopathological study of 60 patients. Arch Dermatol 1995;131:1147–53.
*Most commonly associated agents.

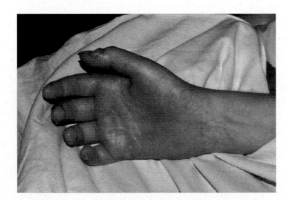

FIGURE 1 Hand-foot syndrome owing to clofarabine.

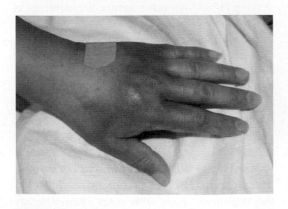

FIGURE 2 Hand-foot syndrome owing to paclitaxel.

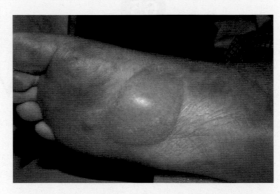

FIGURE 3 Hand-foot syndrome with bullae in a patient receiving clofarabine.

The most **severe** episode of HFS also usually occurs early in the treatment cycle. In the same series of patients treated with capecitabine, 68% had their most severe episode within the first two cycles.[4] However, 14% of the patients in the series had their most severe episode at the fourth cycle or later. By contrast, in a series of 76 patients treated with cytarabine and daunorubicin/ doxorubicin, the recurrences were always milder.[2]

In summary, if a patient has a severe episode of HFS with a particular chemotherapy agent, it can be difficult to predict the severity of HFS with future cycles. Subsequent episodes may be similar in intensity, more severe, or less severe. These are important considerations when oncologists are administering those chemotherapy agents for which HFS is a dose-limiting toxicity.

HFS seems to occur more **commonly** with continuous administration of chemotherapy agents than with bolus infusions.[4] However, bolus infusions seem to be associated with more **severe** episodes of HFS and more rapid time to onset.[3]

Diagnosis

The diagnosis is made clinically in a patient who develops erythema (with or without edema and tenderness) of the palms and soles during the week following administration of a chemotherapy agent associated with HFS.

The differential diagnosis for HFS includes acute cutaneous GVHD. In the post–bone marrow transplantation period, the use of immunosuppressive agents (such as cyclosporine) may limit the expression of acute GVHD to areas of predilection such as the hands and feet; affected patients may present only with erythema and tenderness (sometimes with bullae) of the palms and soles. In this setting, it may be difficult to distinguish between acute cutaneous GVHD and HFS caused by the preceding chemotherapy.[13] Evidence of GVHD at other sites may suggest that hand erythema in a particular patient is an expression of cutaneous GVHD. This evidence may include macular erythema at other sites of predilection (such as the face or ears), the onset of the exanthem at the time of marrow recovery, and/or the presence of signs or symptoms of systemic GVHD

(eg, elevated bilirubin and liver enzymes, diarrhea, abdominal pain). In addition, HFS is likely to resolve by the tenth day post-transplantation, whereas acute cutaneous GVHD is likely to persist well beyond this date.

The histology of HFS is not specific: it may reveal scattered necrotic keratinocytes, vacuolization of the basal layer, and a perivascular lymphocytic infiltrate. This histologic picture is similar to that of cutaneous GVHD.[2] Skin biopsies are not a reliable way of differentiating HFS from acute cutaneous GVHD, especially in the early stages of the two diseases.[3,13]

For those patients who have received only chemotherapy (and no bone marrow transplant), the diagnosis of HFS is usually straightforward. Conventional (nonchemotherapy) medications do not cause HFS. However, when two chemotherapy agents are coadministered, and both may cause HFS, the identification of the actual culprit may be difficult.

Therapy

Treatment of mild to moderate HFS is usually unnecessary. Patients may obtain symptomatic relief with pain medications, cold compresses, and elevation (to reduce edema).[3]

However, patients may be unable to tolerate recurrent episodes of severe HFS owing to intense palmoplantar tenderness, sometimes accompanied by painful blisters, When evaluating patients with an acute, severe episode of HFS, we have not found that potent topical corticosteroids or 4% lidocaine cream give any significant symptomatic relief. It has been our experience that some patients with an acute and severe episode may get relief with systemic steroids; however, this is not a practical therapy for recurrent episodes, nor is it strongly supported by other authors.[14–19]

Treatment of severe HFS is better managed by attempts to prevent future severe recurrences. The most successful approach is probably dose reduction, sometimes accompanied by interruption of therapy.[4]

Severe episodes of HFS caused by 5-fluorouracil may be ameliorated by prophylaxis with pyridoxine 50 mg daily.[12,20] This may also be effective for patients receiving docetaxel.[21]

Onycholysis and Other Nail Disorders

Onycholysis

Chemotherapy agents may cause various disorders of the fingernails and toenails. The particular nail disorder that has the highest associated morbidity is onycholysis.

Onycholysis is the separation of the nail plate from the underlying nail bed. It may affect one or more fingers or toes (Figure 4). In mild onycholysis, there is slight elevation of the distal nail plate from the nail bed; in severe disease, there is complete separation, with resultant loss of the nail plate. Onycholysis is the precursor to the more

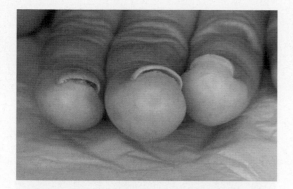

FIGURE 4 Distal onycholysis owing to docetaxel.

unpleasant chemotherapy-associated nail disorders, such as nail plate infections and fingertip cellulitis.

Anthracyclines and taxanes (especially docetaxel) are the chemotherapy agents most likely to cause onycholysis (Table 2). Twenty to 35% of patients treated with docetaxel, for example, develop onycholysis.[22] In one study of weekly paclitaxel, the mean time to onset of onycholysis was 12 weeks.[23] Nonchemotherapy agents, such as tetracycline and captopril, may also cause onycholysis, although rarely.[24]

The onset of onycholysis is probably not related to dose but rather to dose frequency and/or the number of doses. Two separate studies reported patients who did not develop onycholysis with paclitaxel administered every 3 weeks. However, the same patients did develop onycholysis when started on a weekly schedule (even at a lower dose).[23,25,26] Among patients receiving weekly paclitaxel, those who had received more infusions had a higher incidence of onycholysis.[26–28]

Onycholysis and Nail Plate Infections

The space between the nail plate and the nail bed is the subungual zone. When onycholysis occurs,

Table 2 Chemotherapy Agents Associated with Onycholysis
Most common
Paclitaxel
Docetaxel
Daunorubicin
Doxorubicin
Idarubicin
Less common
5-Fluorouracil
Etoposide
Mitoxantrone
Capecitabine

Adapted from Makris A, Mortimer P, Powles TJ. Chemotherapy-induced onycholysis. Eur J Cancer 1996;32A:374–5; Hussain S, Anderson DN, Salvatti ME. Onycholysis as a complication of systemic chemotherapy. Cancer 2000;88:2367–71; Chen GY, Chen YH, Hsu MM, et al. Onychomadesis and onycholysis associated with capecitabine. Br J Dermatol 2001;145:521–2.

this space enlarges, facilitating bacterial colonization or infection. Secondary *Pseudomonas aeruginosa* infections of the subungual area are very common in this patient population and are suggested by green coloration of the nail plate and subungual debris (Figure 5). These infections are often minimally bothersome to patients; the infection may be odoriferous and slightly tender but rarely produces fingertip cellulitis. Daily soaking of the affected digits in 50% acetic acid (white vinegar) is often adequate therapy. Silver sulfadiazine cream also has activity against *Pseudomonas*.[29] Bacterial swab culture of the subungual debris will yield sensitivities should oral antibiotics be necessary. Oral fluoroquinolones are often helpful. Trimming the nail as far back as possible to remove the habitat for bacterial growth under the nail is helpful. In our experience, these infections rarely clear with oral therapy only, and will require topical measures as well.

Some patients with onycholysis develop a low-grade subungual infection with *Staphylococcus aureus* that results in a steady, malodorous, subungual, purulent discharge from beneath one or more nail plates. There may be mixed infections with accompanying *Pseudomonas* or *Candida*. These infections usually respond well to acetic acid soaks and oral antibiotics (as determined by culture sensitivities). Occasionally, this condition may evolve into a more acute, loculated *S. aureus* subungual abscess. In these patients, the nail plate is elevated above a painful purulent subungual mass, often with a cellulitis of the affected fingertip.[22,25,30] Treatment of this condition involves sterile avulsion of the affected nail plate and administration of systemic antibiotics; neutropenic patients should be followed closely.

Patients with chronic onycholysis often develop subungual debris. Although this may clinically resemble a dermatophyte nail infection, potassium hydroxide specimens are usually negative and the patient does not have nail fungus.[25,31] However, we routinely perform potassium hydroxide smears on our affected patients as a small percentage of the specimens do demonstrate fungal hyphae.

Patients with onycholysis may also have subungual hemorrhages, which occur as the nail plate splits off from the nail bed.

Other Nail Disorders

The most common nail disorder caused by chemotherapy is nail pigmentation.[32] This is of cosmetic concern only. The pigmentation may involve the nail plate or the nail bed; there may be patchy pigmentation, longitudinal bands, or transverse bands. The pigment may be blue, gray, brown, black, or white. Many chemotherapy agents cause nail pigmentation.[3,32]

Intense chemotherapy may temporarily arrest nail synthesis and cause a narrow transverse depression of the nail plate (Beau's line) (Figure 6).[25] The number of Beau's lines parallels the number of prior infusions. In extreme cases, there may be resultant loss of the nail plate.

Actinis Keratosis Recall Phenomenon

Clinical

Certain chemotherapy agents will cause inflammation of preexisting subclinical actinic keratosis (AKs). Shortly after the administration of these agents, multiple AKs may spontaneously appear in areas of previous photodamage, such as the forearms. In addition, patients may experience intense inflammation of previously evident AKs.

AK recall occurs most often with 5-fluorouracil but may also occur with other agents (Table 3). In one series of seven patients (who were treated with a variety of chemotherapy agents), the time to onset of AK recall was 2 to 7 days.[33] Typically, there will be an eruption of red scaly papules in a photodistribution. This especially involves the face, exposed scalp, dorsal forearms, dorsal hands, and, to a lesser extent, the chest and upper back (Figure 7). The eruption may be itchy or tender. Occasionally, there may be severe inflammation in and around the keratoses, with large areas of tender erythema of the face, exposed scalp, and dorsal forearms.[33–36]

Diagnosis

This is usually a clinical diagnosis. The differential diagnosis may include lichenoid cutaneous

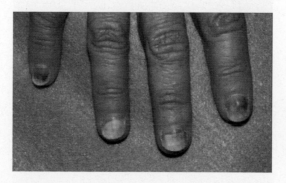

FIGURE 5 Onycholysis owing to paclitaxel, with secondary *Pseudomonas* infection.

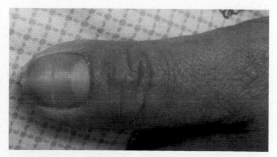

FIGURE 6 Beau's line in a patient receiving paclitaxel.

Table 3 Chemotherapy Agents Associated with Actinic Keratosis Recall

Single agents
    Capecitabine
    Cisplatinum
    Docetaxel
    Doxorubicin
    Fludarabine
    Fluorouracil
    Pentostatin
Combination regimens
    Dactinomycin-vincristine-dacarbazine
    Doxorubicin-cytarabine-6-thioguanine
    Doxorubicin-vincristine

Adapted from Lewis KG et al[34]; Remlinger KA. Cutaneous reactions to chemotherapy drugs: the art of consultation. Arch Dermatol 2003;139:77–81; Susser WS et al[3]; Johnson TM, Rapini RP, Duvic M. Inflammation of actinic keratoses from systemic chemotherapy. J Am Acad Dermatol 1987;17:192–7; Nabai H et al[36]; Revuz J and Valeyrie-Allanore L.[59]

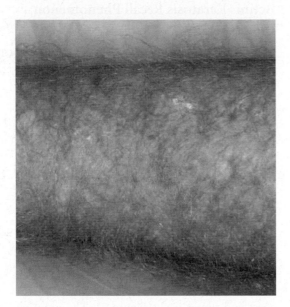

FIGURE 7 Actinic keratosis recall owing to dacarbazine.

GVHD. The morphology of the skin lesions of lichenoid GVHD and AK recall may be similar; however, lichenoid GVHD is not usually confined to photodistributed areas. Skin biopsy will reliably separate the two conditions.

Therapy

Patients with AK recall may have pruritus or tenderness of the affected areas. This generally responds well to topical corticosteroids: low potency (1% hydrocortisone or desonide cream) on the face and medium potency (triamcinolone cream or ointment) at other sites.[3,33] The occurrence of AK recall is not a contraindication to further administration of chemotherapy.[3] Patients with severe, painful AK recall may benefit from dose adjustment of subsequent infusions and from potent topical steroids.[35]

The AKs that occur in the recall phenomenon will generally persist indefinitely, long after the cessation of chemotherapy. Additional infusions of chemotherapy may lead to resolution of some of the AKs.[3] Following the cessation of chemotherapy, residual lesions may be treated with conventional measures, such as cryotherapy and 5-fluorouracil cream.

Acneiform Eruptions

Clinical

Epidermal growth factor receptor (EGFR) inhibitors may cause a striking acneiform eruption; these agents include cetuximab (Erbitux), erlotinib (Tarceva), and gefitinib (Iressa). EGFR inhibitors are chronically administered oral and intravenous agents currently being evaluated for the treatment of various solid tumors, especially non–small cell lung cancer. Occasionally, methotrexate, cisplatinum, and actinomycin D may also cause an acneiform eruption.[37]

Affected patients develop an eruption over the face, back, chest, and shoulders, usually within 5 to 12 days of starting therapy.[38,39] This eruption is clinically identical to inflammatory acne, with pustules and red papules on a background of erythema (Figures 8–10). Usually, there are no acneiform comedones or cysts.[39]

Patients may be distressed by the cosmetic appearance of this eruption. Typically, the acneiform eruption persists throughout the course of EGFR inhibitor therapy. Affected patients may also develop a secondary *S. aureus* impetiginization of the affected areas on the face, with yellow and black crusting superimposed on the pustular eruption (Figure 11). This is partly due to the high rates of nasal colonization in hospital patients.

Of patients treated with EGFR inhibitors, more than 50% develop the acneiform eruption; many develop widespread very dry skin as well.[39–41]

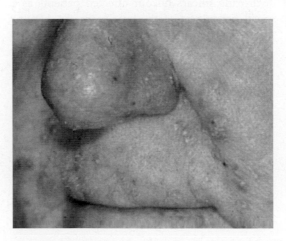

FIGURE 8 Acneiform eruption owing to erlotinib: facial pustules.

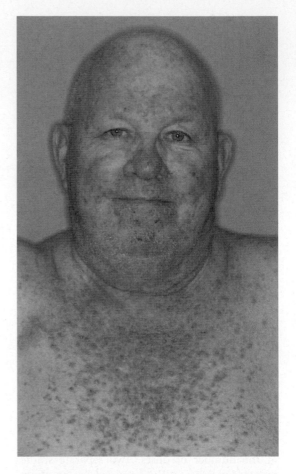

FIGURE 9 Acneiform eruption due to cetuximab: involvement of the scalp, face, and chest.

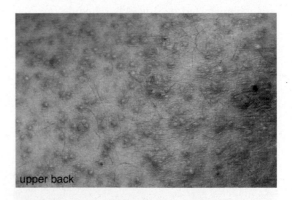

upper back

FIGURE 10 Acneiform eruption owing to cetuximab: pustules on the back.

Diagnosis

The diagnosis is made clinically in a patient who develops a pustular eruption, in the characteristic distribution, 1 to 2 weeks after starting EGFR inhibitor therapy. Skin biopsies are usually not necessary for diagnosis. Histology is not specific and reveals a follicular infiltrate of lymphocytes, neutrophils, and histiocytes. There may be destruction of the follicle in more advanced lesions.[38,42]

At the initial evaluation of the patient, we unroof some of the pustules for bacterial culture and sensitivity to rule out a coexisting *S. aureus* folliculitis or impetigo.

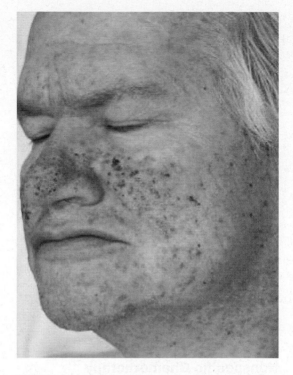

FIGURE 11 Cetuximab-induced acneiform eruption, with secondary *Staphylococcus aureus* infection.

The differential diagnosis includes steroid acne, which also presents with pustules and red papules on the upper trunk; it is less likely to involve the face, however. Bacterial folliculitis may present as perifollicular papules and pustules on a background of erythema as well; however, it is unlikely to have the exact same distribution as the EGFR inhibitor eruption. Miliaria pustulosa is also in the differential diagnosis.

Therapy

Most patients will have at least a fair improvement after 3 to 4 weeks of therapy with oral doxycycline or minocycline (100 mg daily to twice daily), along with the daily application of clindamycin lotion to the face. There have been no controlled studies on the treatment of this problem. Some of us do not use tretinoin cream or clindamycin gel/solution in this setting, as those agents may make the patient's skin wendrier. More impressive results occur with oral isotretinoin (10–40 mg daily), if approved by the referring oncologist.

Patients with superimposed bacterial impetiginization may have thick crusting of their facial skin that is painful for them to remove. In this circumstance, we often do an initial saline soak in clinic, followed by gentle débridement. The patient must then wash the face at least twice daily and apply liberal amounts of mupirocin cream, including to the nares. A course of oral antibiotics may also be necessary as directed by the result of the sensitivities.

Radiation Enhancement

Certain chemotherapy agents enhance the effect of radiation therapy, both on the target tissue and on other exposed areas.[43,44] The increased effect on the tumor is intended and desirable. However, the synergistic effect of radiation therapy and chemotherapy may also involve other tissues in an undesirable manner. The most common side effect of radiation enhancement (RE) is radiation dermatitis; however, RE may also adversely involve the mucosa, lungs, heart, gastrointestinal tract, bladder, brain, and eyes.[3,43]

RE occurs when the chemotherapy and radiation therapy are administered within 1 week of each other.[45,46] Table 4 lists causative agents. An augmented radiation dermatitis develops within the irradiated field and may extend locally.[3] There is tender erythema, edema, vesicles, and erosions of the affected skin. In severe cases, there is cutaneous necrosis and ulceration. The dermatitis usually resolves spontaneously within days or weeks after cessation of the radiation therapy. There may be residual hyperpigmentation, depigmentation, and/or telangiectasias. In severe cases, there may be permanent cutaneous atrophy or fibrosis.[3,43]

The severity of RE is related to the drug dosage, the time sequence of radiation and chemotherapy, and the pharmacologic mechanism of the drug administered.[43] Radiation enhancement may occur with orthovoltage radiation, megavoltage radiation, and electron beam therapy.[37]

Radiation Recall

Radiation recall (RR) is a phenomenon whereby the administration of a chemotherapy agent induces an inflammatory reaction in a previously quiescent radiation field. Radiation recall dermatitis is the most common type.[47] However, RR may also adversely affect the oral mucosa, lungs, esophagus, heart, and intestinal epithelia.[3,43,45]

Table 4 Chemotherapy Agents Associated with Radiation Enhancement Injury to Skin

Single agents
   Bleomycin
   Chlorambucil
   Dactinomycin
   Doxorubicin
   Fluorouracil
   Gemcitabine
   Hydroxyurea
   6-Mercaptopurine
   Methotrexate
Combination regimens
   Cyclophosphamide-dactinomycin-vincristine
   Dactinomycin-amethopterin
   Doxorubicin-cyclophosphamide
   Fluorouracil-cisplatin

Adapted from Susser WS et al.[3]

Usually, patients receive the causative chemotherapy agent a few weeks or months after the radiation therapy and shortly thereafter develop RR dermatitis. Occasionally, the causative agent is administered years later and causes RR at that time.[45] In RR, the minimum period of time between radiation therapy and the administration of the causative agent is 7 days (this distinguishes RR from RE).[45]

RR dermatitis develops in the previously radiated field within hours or days of administration of subsequent chemotherapy.[45] The onset is slower for oral administration than for intravenous administration. Patients develop red macules or plaques that may be painful. The dermatitis is well defined and corresponds exactly to the site of previous irradiation (Figure 12). There may be vesicles, erosions, and, occasionally, ulcerations.[3] Most affected patients had **not** originally experienced acute radiation dermatitis in the involved site at the initial time of radiation therapy.[45]

The differential diagnosis for RR dermatitis includes bacterial cellulitis (especially), early shingles, and cutaneous metastases. The correct diagnosis may initially be difficult for the clinician as some time may have elapsed since the patient received radiation at the involved site.[44]

RR dermatitis resolves spontaneously hours to weeks after the cessation of chemotherapy. It sometimes clears despite continued administration of the agent.[3,45]

The chemotherapy agents most likely to cause RR are doxorubicin, daunorubicin, docetaxel, and paclitaxel. Table 5 lists other associated agents. Rarely, rifampin, isoniazid, and pyrazinamide can cause RR.[48] The recall induced by gemcitabine (unlike other chemotherapy agents) is more likely to involve internal organs rather than the skin.[47]

In the postradiation period, RR usually occurs with the first administration of the causative chemotherapy agent.[45] Drug rechallenge usually causes either mild recurrence of recall or no recurrence.[44]

The severity of RR dermatitis is probably related to (1) the dose of radiation initially

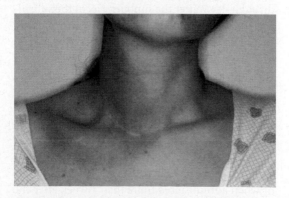

FIGURE 12 Radiation recall dermatitis owing to interferon-α2b.

Table 5 Chemotherapy Agents Associated with Radiation Recall Dermatitis
Bleomycin
Capecitabine
Cyclophosphamide
Cytarabine
Daunorubicin
Docetaxel
Doxorubicin
Epirubicin
Etoposide
Fluorouracil
Gemcitabine
Hydroxyurea
Interferon-α2b
Lomustine
Melphalan
Methotrexate
Paclitaxel
Tamoxifen
Trimetrexate
Vinblastine

Adapted from Susser WS et al[5]; Thomas R, Stea B. Radiation recall dermatitis from high dose interferon alfa-2b. J Clin Oncol 2002;20:355–7; Yeo W, Johnson PJ. Radiation-recall skin disorders associated with the use of antineoplastic drugs. Am J Clin Dermatol 2000;1:113–6; Jeter MD et al[48]; Ortmann E, Hohenberg G. Radiation recall phenomenon after administration of capecitabine. J Clin Oncol 2002;20:3029–34; Kodym E et al.[46]

received and (2) the time period between the radiation and the chemotherapy. Severe RR dermatitis is more likely to occur when that time period is short.[3,45] The radiation dose necessary to induce RR dermatitis when the drug is given weeks after radiation therapy may be inadequate to induce it were the drug to be given months later.

Sunburn Recall

This is an unusual chemotherapy reaction usually caused by methotrexate. Administration of methotrexate to a predisposed patient in the period following sunburn leads to worsening or reactivation of the sunburn. This reaction occurs when methotrexate is administered from day 2 through day 7 after the sunburn (ie, in the subsiding phase of the burn). Patients develop tender erythema and edema (sometimes with vesicles) of the previously sunburned skin.[49,50] Severe reactions may progress to intense blistering and desquamation. The reaction gradually subsides over the following week.[3] Administration of a second dose of methotrexate sometimes leads to further worsening of the recall phenomenon.[50]

Sunburn recall does not occur when methotrexate is administered on the day of the sunburn or when administered more than 1 week after the burn. In general, if an affected patient receives another sunburn, the subsequent administration

of methotrexate should be held for at least 7 days.

Sunburn recall has occurred with methotrexate administered orally, intramuscularly, and intravenously.[49–51] Other occasional causes of sunburn recall are suramin, paclitaxel, and etoposide/cyclophosphamide.[3,52] Rarely, oral antibiotics (such as ciprofloxacin) induce sunburn recall.[52]

Cutaneous Hyperpigmentation

Hyperpigmentation is a common cutaneous side effect of chemotherapy agents and has been reviewed at length.[3,53] Skin, hair, nails, and oral mucosa may all be affected. There are many different reaction patterns of cutaneous hyperpigmentation: photodistributed; pressure accentuated; under occluded areas; widespread (which may resemble Addison's disease); and patches in areas of predilection (such as the palms or soles).[37] An individual chemotherapy agent is often associated with a single type of reaction pattern.

Most chemotherapy agents have the ability to induce some form of hyperpigmentation. The pigmentation may persist long after cessation of the agent. Alkylating agents and antitumor antibiotics are the agents most likely to cause cutaneous hyperpigmentation.[43] Four particularly characteristic patterns are described below.

Bleomycin may induce narrow linear red streaks (flagellate hyperpigmentation) in areas of trauma, especially on the trunk and proximal extremities (Figure 13). This may be quite itchy; it occurs in at least 10% of treated patients.[3,37]

Fluorouracil may induce hyperpigmented serpentine streaks over the arm veins used for intravenous infusion (serpentine supravenous hyperpigmentation). These streaks may extend proximally to the shoulder. This reaction can also occur with vinorelbine, fotemustine, and some multidrug regimens.[3,37]

Thiotepa may cause sharply circumscribed hyperpigmentation under occluded areas, such as bandages, and in intertriginous areas, such as the axillae (Figure 14).[3,54]

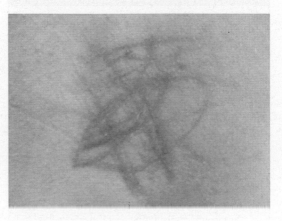

FIGURE 13 Flagellate hyperpigmentation owing to bleomycin.

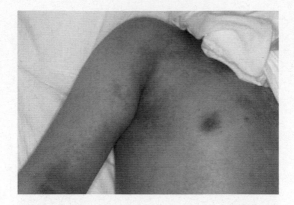

FIGURE 14 Hyperpigmentation of intertriginous areas owing to thiotepa.

Busulfan may cause a diffuse brown or bronze hyperpigmentation (busulfan tan) over the face, neck, chest, abdomen, forearms, and palmar creases. This may clinically resemble Addison's disease.[3,55]

Nonspecific Chemotherapy Reactions

Nonspecific reactions are those that are caused by both conventional medications and chemotherapy agents. Certain chemotherapy agents and conventional medications may, for example, produce clinically indistinguishable maculopapular eruptions. In a patient with a nonspecific skin reaction, it may be difficult to determine whether the culprit was a chemotherapy agent or a conventional medication. The correct identification of the single causative agent will be even more problematic.[1]

Nonspecific reactions include maculopapular eruptions, erythema multiforme, urticaria, anaphylaxis, and Stevens-Johnson syndrome toxic epidermal necrolysis.

The oncology literature often refers to these reactions collectively as hypersensitivity reactions, with a corresponding attempt to classify each as type 1, 2, 3, or 4. However, in many cases, the immunologic mechanism is unknown. In addition, the various types of chemotherapy/drug reactions in this group are clinically quite distinct from each other. We therefore prefer to classify these reactions by their clinical names: urticarial, SJS, maculopapular, etc.

Maculopapular Eruptions

Maculopapular eruptions are usually a clinically trivial side effect of chemotherapy; this is probably why the literature on this subject is slim. In our experience, these eruptions are fairly common and can probably occur with most chemotherapy agents. Associated agents include etoposide, chlorambucil, procarbazine, 5-fluorouracil, melphalan, and hydroxyurea.[1,56–58]

Current knowledge about maculopapular drug exanthems derives mainly from experience with conventional medications. Table 6 lists those conventional medications most likely to cause a maculopapular drug exanthem.

Clinical

Maculopapular drug eruptions usually appear within 1 to 2 weeks of starting a new drug. Reexposure to a previous offender, however, can trigger the reaction in 1 to 2 days. Occasionally, a patient may develop a maculopapular eruption up to 1 week **after** discontinuing a medication.

The skin lesions are clustered pink or red macules or papules or both. Sometimes the skin lesions are edematous and appear to be urticarial. The eruption begins on the trunk and subsequently involves the proximal extremities and neck (Figure 15). It often spares the face and the dorsal aspects of the hands and feet. Occasionally, the eruption progresses to involve the entire cutaneous surface, and the skin lesions may become confluent. The most common complaint is pruritus. Patients often have a low-grade fever. There are no associated mucosal erosions and no cutaneous blisters; the presence of these features should elicit clinical suspicion instead for the Stevens-Johnson Syndrome.

In thrombocytopenic patients, the skin lesions may appear intensely purpuric, especially on the lower legs; this may prompt clinical consideration of a cutaneous small vessel vasculitis (Figure 16). Skin biopsy can reliably differentiate between these two entities.

A maculopapular drug eruption may take up to 2 weeks to resolve following discontinuation of the correct offending agent. In a patient who is receiving multiple medications, this delay in response may make it difficult to correctly identify the causative agent.

Table 6 Conventional Medications Most Likely to Cause a Maculopapular Drug Exanthem
Allopurinol
Amoxicillin
Amphotericin B
Ampicillin
Barbiturates
Captopril
Carbamazepine
Cephalosporins
Chlorpromazine
Enalapril
Gold
Lithium
Naproxen
Oral hypoglycemic agents
Penicillin
Phenytoin
Piroxicam
Quinidine
Sulfonamide antibiotics
Thiazides
Adapted from Nigen S et al.[83]

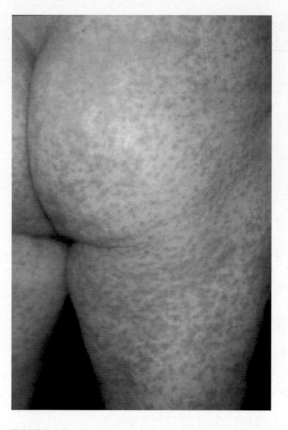

FIGURE 15 Maculopapular drug exanthem due to cephalexin.

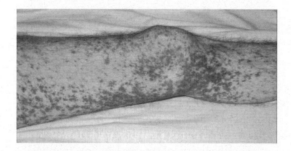

FIGURE 16 Chemotherapy-induced maculopapular eruption with purpura.

If the patient continues to receive the causative agent, the eruption may persist without further change. This may or may not be tolerable to the patient, depending on the severity of the pruritus. In some patients, the eruption will spontaneously resolve despite continued exposure to the medication. On the other hand, a maculopapular drug eruption will occasionally evolve into exfoliative erythroderma, which certainly necessitates discontinuation of the causative agent.[57,59] It is not definitively known whether maculopapular drug reactions may evolve into Stevens-Johnson Syndrome or Toxic Epidermal Necrolysis.[59]

Diagnosis

The approach to the patient with a maculopapular eruption and fever begins with two questions: Does the patient have a drug reaction? If so, which drug is the responsible agent?

In the setting of a cancer hospital, the differential diagnosis may include acute cutaneous GVHD. The cutaneous presentation of maculopapular drug/chemotherapy reactions and cutaneous GVHD may be extremely similar; skin biopsy may not be helpful diagnostically. The diagnosis of acute cutaneous GVHD may be suggested by the presence of signs or symptoms of systemic GVHD (eg, elevated bilirubin and liver enzymes, diarrhea, abdominal pain).

The differential diagnosis also includes viral exanthems. These may be more likely than drug eruptions to start on the head and progress caudally and to display lymphadenopathy and a higher fever.[57] In the absence of suggestive clinical evidence, a drug etiology is favored in adult patients.[59] One rare type of drug reaction may, however, clinically simulate a viral exanthem; DRESS (drug reaction with eosinophilia and systemic signs) is most commonly caused by Dilantin and was previously known in that setting as Dilantin hypersensitivity syndrome.

Early Stevens-Johnson Syndrome (SJS) is also in the differential diagnosis for a maculopapular drug/chemotherapy reaction. The patient almost certainly has only an uncomplicated maculopapular eruption, rather than SJS, if he does not develop mucosal erosions or cutaneous blisters within the first few days of presentation.

Once the diagnosis of drug reaction is reached, an attempt can then be made to identify the probable causative agent. The creation of a drug calendar (Figure 17) is helpful. A patient may receive a new medication or chemotherapy agent for up to 2 weeks before developing a maculopapular eruption; therefore, the time span of the calendar should be at least that long.

Certain drugs (such as acetaminophen and digoxin) almost never cause drug eruptions and can be quickly excluded as candidates.[60] One can then attempt to classify the remaining drugs as a likely or unlikely cause based on the following: (1) time relative to the onset of the rash, (2) information regarding a specific agent from drug databases, (3) experience with other drugs from the same pharmacologic class, and (4) the patient's previous known drug allergies.

Sometimes this process leads to the identification of only one possible causative agent. However, it is often impossible to narrow the field to fewer than two or three highly probable agents. In some cases, it may be impossible to decide whether the eruption was caused by a chemotherapy agent or by a conventional medication.

Therapy

Withdrawal of the causative agent will usually lead to resolution of the eruption within 2 weeks. Discontinuation is not necessarily mandatory if the drug reaction shows no sign of dangerous

DRUG CALENDAR

Patient's name: _____

Rash appears
3/12

DRUG	3/1	3/2	3/3	3/4	3/5	3/6	3/7	3/8	3/9	3/10	3/11	3/12
Enalapril	x	x	x	x	x	x	x	x	x	x	x	x
Bactrim	x	x	x									
Vancomycin									x	x	x	x
Interferon				x	x	x	x	x				
Interleukin-2				x	x	x	x	x				
Dacarbazine				x								
Cisplatinum				x	x	x	x					
Vinblastine				x	x	x	x					
Pepcid				x	x	x	x	x	x	x	x	x
Zofran				x	x	x	x	x	x	x	x	x
Ativan				x	x	x	x	x				
Neulasta										x		
Aranesp										x		

FIGURE 17 Example of a standard drug calendar.

progression and if the patient does not have intolerable pruritus. Obviously, in this scenario, the evolution of the rash should be closely monitored.[59]

Minor pruritus may be alleviated by twice-daily application of triamcinolone 0.1% cream to the affected areas, as well as scheduled dosing of oral hydroxyzine or doxepin (titrated to avoid excessive sedation). In more severe cases, twice-daily topical steroid wet wraps, left in place for 45 minutes, can give considerable relief. Occasionally, systemic steroids are warranted.

Anaphylaxis and Urticaria

Anaphylaxis is a potentially life-threatening reaction that occurs within minutes of exposure to a foreign antigen. Respiratory distress and/or vascular collapse may lead to death. Anaphylaxis is a type 1 hypersensitivity reaction that involves the activation by a foreign antigen of immunoglobulin E bound to mast cells and basophils, with the subsequent release of inflammatory mediators. Responsible agents include drugs, chemotherapy agents, hormones, local anesthetics, and insect venom.[61]

Anaphylactoid reactions are clinically indistinguishable from anaphylaxis. Agents involved in anaphylactoid reactions do not incite type 1 hypersensitivity but probably instead directly cause mast cell degranulation.

The diagnosis of anaphylaxis or anaphylactoid reaction requires the presence of at least one of the following: bronchial obstruction, upper airway obstruction, or acute hypotension. The spectrum of findings may include any of the following: urticaria, angioedema, flushing; laryngeal edema and bronchospasm with dyspnea and wheezing; diarrhea and vomiting; and vascular collapse with hypotension and tachycardia.[61]

Chemotherapy agents associated with these reactions are listed in Table 7. The most commonly Ruana involved agents are asparaginase, docetaxel, paclitaxel, and etoposide.[62]

Because anaphylaxis is a type 1 hypersensitivity reaction, it usually first occurs after repeated infusions of a chemotherapy agent. This is true of asparaginase, for example.[62]

Anaphylactoid reactions may involve direct mast cell degranulation and often occur with the first exposure to the agent; paclitaxel and docetaxel are examples of this process.[62]

Anaphylaxis usually occurs with intravenous administration of chemotherapy but may occasionally occur with oral administration.[1]

Table 7 Chemotherapy Agents Associated with Anaphylaxis

Asparaginase
Carboplatinum
Cisplatinum
Cyclophosphamide
Cytarabine
Daunorubicin
Docetaxel
Doxorubicin
Etoposide
Fluorouracil
Methotrexate
Paclitaxel
Teniposide

Adapted from Weiss RB[1]; Zanotti KM and Markman M[62]; Weiss RB, Donehower RC, Wiernik PH. Hypersensitivity reactions from Taxol. J Clin Oncol 1990;8:1263–8.

Intravesicle administration of cisplatinum may be as likely to cause anaphylaxis as intravenous infusion.[1]

Prophylactic regimens and desensitization protocols may be effective at preventing or minimizing further episodes of anaphylaxis for some chemotherapy agents but not for others.[1,62]

Some chemotherapy agents may cause isolated urticaria in the absence of other clinical findings.[1,63] However, the appearance of isolated urticaria (or other suggestive signs) *during infusion* may herald the onset of anaphylaxis; in that case, the infusion should be discontinued and supportive measures considered.[62]

Stevens-Johnson Syndrome and Toxic Epidermal Necrolysis

TEN is a severe mucocutaneous drug reaction. Affected patients may experience erosive damage to their oral mucosa and lips and slough off large portions of their skin.

SJS can be considered a milder form of TEN, although the exact definition depends on the reference. There is severe mucous membrane involvement and less skin damage.

TEN and SJS likely represent two ends of a spectrum of a severe mucocutaneous drug reaction.[64] We refer to these two entities collectively as SJS-TEN. In some patients, SJS may evolve into TEN.[57]

TEN has an annual incidence of 0.4 to 1.2 per million persons, whereas SJS has an incidence of 1.2 to 6 per million.[64] SJS and TEN are best thought of as drug reactions (with an occasional case reportedly caused by vaccinations or infections).[65] Table 8 lists those drugs that are commonly associated with SJS-TEN. The most common offenders are anticonvulsants, nonsteroidal anti-inflammatory drugs, and antibacterial sulfonamides. Allopurinol and antimalarials follow a close second.[65]

Table 8 Medications Commonly Associated with Stevens-Johnson Syndrome–Toxic Epidermal Necrolysis

Allopurinol
Amathiazone
Amoxicillin
Ampicillin
Carbamazepine
Chlormezanone
Felbamate
Lamotrigine
Penicillin
Phenobarbital
Phenytoin
Piroxicam
Sulfadiazine
Sulfadoxime
Sulfamethoxazole-trimethoprim
Sulfasalazine
Valproic acid

Adapted from Nigen S et al.[83]

Chemotherapy agents also occasionally cause SJS-TEN. Table 9 lists those chemotherapy agents that were identified as the cause in published case reports. For most of these agents, there are only one or two reports of an associated SJS-TEN. The occurrence of SJS-TEN in the setting of chemotherapy is probably highly idiosyncratic. Most of our knowledge about SJS-TEN derives from cases caused by conventional medications.

Clinical

SJS-TEN usually occurs 7 to 21 days after the first exposure to the culprit medication. In a review of

Table 9 Chemotherapy Agents that Have Caused One or More Episodes of Stevens-Johnson Syndrome–Toxic Epidermal Necrolysis

Asparaginase
Bleomycin
Chlorambucil
Cytarabine
Docetaxel
Doxorubicin
Etoposide
Fludarabine
Gemcitabine with radiation therapy
Imatinib mesylate
Interleukin-2
Methotrexate
Mithramycin
Rituximab
Suramin
Thalidomide

Adapted from Solberg LA et al[67]; Cakesen H and Oner AF[68]; Brodsky A et al[69]; Hsiao L-T et al[70]; Ozkan A et al[71]; Stone N et al[72]; Huerta AAS et al[73]; Dourakis SP et al[74]; Sommers KR et al[75]; Hall VC et al[76]; Aydogdu I et al[77]; Houston-Jameson C and Solanki DL[78]; May E and Allolio B[79]; Purpora D et al[80]; Angelopoulou MA et al[81]; Giaccone G et al[82]; Lowndes S, Darby A, Mead G, et al. Stevens-Johnson syndrome after treatment with rituximab. Ann Oncol 2002;13:1948–50.

69 cases of TEN, 78% occurred within 3 weeks of exposure.[66] However, patients may take phenytoin for up to 8 weeks before the onset of SJS-TEN.[57]

Reexposure to an offending medication often results in the onset of SJS-TEN within 48 hours.[64]

In 16 case reports of chemotherapy-associated SJS-TEN, the onset occurred during the first cycle in 56% of cases, during the second cycle in 19% of cases, and during the third cycle in 25% of cases. Of those episodes of SJS-TEN that occurred during the **first** cycle, the majority (7 of 9, or 78%) occurred 2 to 8 days after the first dose of chemotherapy.[67–82]

A febrile prodrome precedes the onset of cutaneous features by 1 to 14 days. Typical features are nausea, vomiting, headache, sore throat, diarrhea, and myalgias.[65,83] Subsequently, there is the abrupt appearance of painful red macules on the trunk and subsequently on the neck, face, and proximal extremities. The skin lesions become dusky or gray, and often coalesce to form large patches. Fragile blisters start to form within the patches; the necrotic blister roofs then slide off, leaving behind large areas of raw and bleeding dermis (Figures 18 and 19).[64]

Measurement of the detached and detachable epidermis allows classification of the patient into one of three groups:

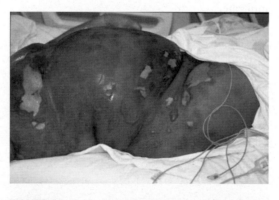

FIGURE 18 Toxic epidermal necrolysis: intact bullae and widespread erosions.

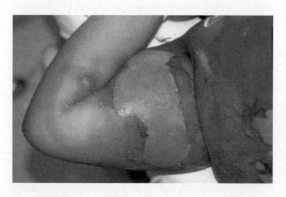

FIGURE 19 Toxic epidermal necrosis: intact bullae and large erosion.

- SJS   <10% of body surface area (BSA)
- TEN   >30% of BSA
- SJS-TEN overlap   10–30% of BSA[64]

Almost all patients with SJS-TEN have oral mucosal disease that may either accompany the onset of skin involvement or precede it by a few days. Patients initially report burning of the buccal mucosa, lips, and sometimes the conjunctiva. Oral mucosal blisters develop and quickly rupture to leave painful erosions on the buccal mucosa; sometimes also on the gingiva, tongue, pharynx, and nasal cavity. Hemorrhagic crusts cover the lips (Figure 20).[65] At this point, most patients are unable to eat or drink.

In the patient with suspected chemotherapy-induced SJS-TEN, it may initially be difficult to differentiate between routine chemotherapy-induced mucositis and the oral mucosal changes of SJS-TEN.

Erosive involvement of the conjunctiva and cornea is fairly common in patients with SJS-TEN. There may also be painful involvement of other mucosal surfaces, such as the genitals, anus, esophagus, nose, and bronchi. Mucous plugs and respiratory obstruction occasionally occur.

Course and Complications

The initial active phase of SJS-TEN includes persistent fever, the formation of mucocutaneous blisters, and the progressive shedding of the oral mucosa and skin. This active phase is complete when the maximum BSA involvement has been reached and no new blisters are appearing. If the offending drug has been discontinued, the active phase lasts for approximately 5 days.[65] Reepithelialization of the denuded skin then occurs over the following 2 to 3 weeks.

During the period in which large cutaneous erosions are present, massive infection of the skin may occur, with subsequent bacteremia or fungemia. *S. aureus* and *Pseudomonas* are the main causative organisms and *Candida albicans* to a lesser extent. Pneumonia and infections of intravenous and urinary tract catheters may occur.[57]

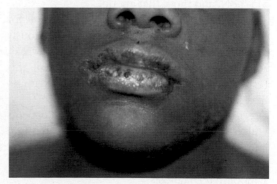

FIGURE 20 Toxic epidermal necrosis: crusting and erosions of the lips.

During this same period, dehydration and electrolyte abnormalities may also occur.

Prognosis

For nonchemotherapy medications, the mortality rate of SJS is 5% and of TEN is 30%; the most common direct cause of death is infection.[64,83] The extent of epidermal detachment is a major prognostic factor.[83] Prompt withdrawal of the offending drug reduces the risk of mortality by 30% per day.[64]

The mortality rate for chemotherapy-induced SJS-TEN is unknown. In 10 case reports of chemotherapy-induced TEN, the cause of death was TEN related in 40%.[67,69,71–74,76,77,79,80] It would seem likely that chemotherapy-induced TEN has a higher mortality rate given that many of the affected patients are neutropenic and are at a greater risk of infection.

Diagnosis

The clinical presentation of an established case of SJS-TEN is characteristic. The patient has fever; painful oral mucositis; hemorrhagic crusts on the lips; painful red macules and patches, especially on the trunk; fragile blisters; and large cutaneous erosions. This presentation often occurs within 7 to 21 days of receiving a drug that is associated with SJS-TEN.

The vigilant physician, however, may suspect the diagnosis of SJS-TEN before the full evolution has occurred. If a patient presents with an early morbilliform eruption and reports **any** tenderness of the oral mucosa or skin, the possibility of SJS-TEN should be considered. Some patients with early disease may present with painful red macules on the palms and soles.

The use of a drug calendar (see Figure 17) may be helpful in correctly identifying the causative medication. In general, most drugs that cause SJS-TEN have been first administered 1 to 3 weeks prior to the onset of the reaction. However, SJS-TEN may occur within 48 hours of reexposure to a previously offending medication.[57] A review of the literature may also point to those drugs that are frequently associated with SJS-TEN, and those that are not.

A medication is unlikely to be responsible for SJS-TEN if it was first given 24 hours previously or if the duration of treatment exceeds 3 weeks. An exception to this is with anticonvulsants (especially phenytoin), which may take up to 8 weeks to cause SJS-TEN.[57]

In general, the medication lists of patients with SJS-TEN should be reduced to a minimum and appropriate substitutions made.[64]

Differential Diagnosis

The most important disease to rule out in the initial evaluation of a patient with possible SJS-TEN is staphylococcal scalded skin syndrome (SSSS); this is because the respective therapies for each of these two diseases are very different. Patients with both disorders may have widespread tender cutaneous erosions. The erosions in SSSS are more superficial, however, "leaving a bed of intact epidermal layers instead of the wet and bright red tissue of TEN."[64] In addition, patients with SSSS do not have oral mucosal involvement. We always perform skin biopsy for frozen section in our cancer patients with possible SJS-TEN; the results are available in a few hours. Frozen section reliably differentiates between SSSS (intraepidermal split) and SJS-TEN (subepidermal split). Some clinicians feel that they can reliably distinguish the two disorders without a biopsy based on the thickness of the sloughing skin and clinical appearance.

Grade IV (severe) acute cutaneous GVHD may strongly resemble SJS-TEN both clinically and histologically. It may be almost impossible to differentiate between these two disorders.[72]

Acute generalized exanthematous pustulosis (AGEP) is a pustular drug eruption. Affected patients have widespread areas of erythema studded with fragile micropustules.[83] Twenty percent of patients have oral mucosal involvement. Skin biopsy of AGEP shows a dense neutrophilic infiltrate with intraepidermal and subcorneal pustules; that of SJS-TEN reveals a necrotic epidermis, a subepidermal split, and a scant inflammatory infiltrate.

Also in the clinical differential diagnosis for SJS-TEN are paraneoplastic pemphigus and drug-induced linear immunoglobulin A disease (particularly associated with vancomycin). These diseases may be suspected when the clinical course of the supposed SJS-TEN seems unusual, for example, a very prolonged course with persistent blistering. Skin biopsy for histology and direct immunofluorescence reliably differentiate between these three diseases.

Phototoxic Reactions

In some patients, the administration of certain drugs causes cutaneous sensitization to ultraviolet (UV) light. Subsequent exposure to UV light causes exaggerated sunburn. There is tender erythema and edema, sometimes with vesicles, in a photodistribution; the typical clinical course of a sunburn follows. Light-protected areas (such as the submental area) and areas covered by clothing are spared.[84]

Phototoxic reactions occur when the patient receives the photosensitizing medication and is exposed to UV light within the following 12 hours. (Sunburn recall is a different phenomenon, in which administration of a medication up to 1 week after UV exposure causes sunburn.)

Offending chemotherapy agents include dacarbazine, fluorouracil, tegafur, and vinblastine.[3,85] Other causative medications include furosemide, thiazide diuretics, phenothiazines, quinolones, sulfonamides, tetracyclines, and tricyclic antidepressants.[84]

Phototoxicity is the result of direct tissue injury caused by the phototoxic agent in conjunction with UV light.[84] (These are not hypersensitivity reactions.) Phototoxic reactions are probably dose dependent.[86] The amount of light necessary to cause a phototoxic reaction may be very low. Theoretically, a phototoxic reaction may occur in any individual exposed to the combination of adequate doses of the agent and the appropriate wavelength of light. UVA light causes most phototoxic reactions.[84]

REFERENCES

1. Weiss RB. Hypersensitivity reactions. Semin Oncol 1992; 19:458–77.
2. Demircay Z, Gurbuz O, Bayik M. Chemotherapy-induced acral erythema in leukemia patients: a report of 15 cases. Int J Dermatol 1997;36:593–8.
3. Susser WS, Whitaker-Worth DL, Grant-Kels JM. Mucocutaneous reactions to chemotherapy. J Am Acad Dermatol 1999;40:367–98.
4. Abushullaih S, Saad ED, Munsell M, Hoff PM. Incidence and severity of hand-foot syndrome in colorectal cancer patients treated with capecitabine: a single institution experience. Cancer Invest 2002;20:3–10.
5. Sakamoto J, Kondo Y, Nishisho I. A phase II Japanese study of a modified capecitabine regimen for advanced or metastatic colorectal cancer. Anticancer Drugs 2004;15: 137–43.
6. Chua DT, Sham JS, Au GK. A phase II study of capecitabine in patients with recurrent and metastatic nasopharyngeal carcinoma pretreated with platinum-based chemotherapy. Oral Oncol 2003;39:361–6.
7. Blum JL, Jones SE, Buzdar AU. Multicenter phase II study of capecitabine in paclitaxel-refractory metastatic breast cancer. J Clin Oncol 1999;17:485–93.
8. Rischin D, Phillips KA, Friedlander M, et al. A phase II trial of capecitabine in heavily pre-treated platinum-resistant ovarian cancer. Gynecol Oncol 2004;93:417–21.
9. Otterson GA, Herndon JE, Watson D, et al. Capecitabine in malignant mesothelioma: a phase II trial by the Cancer and Leukemia Group B. Lung Cancer 2004;44:251–9.
10. Vasey PA, McMahon L, Paul J, et al. A phase II trial of capecitabine (Xeloda) in recurrent ovarian cancer. Br J Cancer 2003;89:1843–8.
11. Gerbrecht BM. Current Canadian experience with capecitabine: partnering with patients to optimize therapy. Cancer Nurs 2003;26:161–7.
12. Fabian CJ, Molina R, Slavik M, et al. Pyridoxine therapy for palmar-plantar erythrodysesthesia associated with continuous 5-fluorouracil infusion. Investig New Drugs 1990;8:57–63.
13. Crider MK, Jansen J, Norins AL, McHale MS. Chemotherapy-induced acral erythema in patients receiving bone marrow transplantation. Arch Dermatol 1986;122: 1023–7.
14. Comandone A, Bretti S, La Grotta G, et al. Palmar-plantar erythrodysesthesia syndrome associated with 5-fluorouracil treatment. Anticancer Res 1993;13:1781–83.
15. Gordon KB, Tajuddin A, Guitart J, et al. Hand-foot syndrome associated with liposome-encapsulated doxorubicin therapy. Cancer 1995;75:2169–73.
16. Hellier I, Bessis D, Sotto A, et al. High-dose methotrexate-induced bullous variant of acral erythema. Arch Dermatol 1996;132:590–1.
17. Kroll SS, Koller CA, Koled S, et al. Chemotherapy-induced acral erythema: desquamating lesions involving the hands and feet. Ann Plast Surg 1989;23:263–5.
18. Walker R, Wilson W, Sauder D, Bengar A, et al. Cytarabine-induced palmar-plantar erythema. Arch Dermatol 1985;121:1240.

19. Brown J, Burck K, Black D, et al. Treatment of cytarabine acral erythema with corticosteroids. J Am Acad Dermatol 1991;24:1023–4.

20. Beveridge RA, Kales AN, Binder RA, et al. Pyrodoxine (BG) and amelioration of hand/foot syndrome. Proc Am Soc Clin Oncol 1990;9:1029.

21. Vukelja SJ, Baker WJ, Burris HA. Pyridoxine therapy for palmar-plantar erythrodysesthesia associated with taxotere. J Natl Cancer Inst 1993;85:1432–3.

22. Nicolopoulos J, Howard A. Docetaxel-induced nail dystrophy. Australas J Dermatol 2002;43:293–6.

23. Flory SM, Solimando DA, Webster GF, et al. Onycholysis associated with weekly administration of paclitaxel. Ann Pharmacother 1999;33:584–6.

24. Brueggemyer CD, Ramirez G. Onycholysis associated with captopril. Lancet 1984;2:1352–3.

25. Correia O, Azeuedo C, Ferreira EP, et al. Nail changes secondary to docetaxel. Dermatology 1999;198:288–90.

26. Spazzopon S, Crivellari D, Lombarali D, et al. Nail toxicity related to weekly taxanes. J Clin Oncol 2002;21:4404–5.

27. Aihara T, Kim Y, Takatsuka Y. Phase II study of weekly docetaxel in patients with metastatatic breast cancer. Ann Oncol 2002;13:286–92.

28. Kuroi K, Bando H, Saji S, et al. Protracted administration of weekly docetaxel in metastatic breast cancer. Oncol Rep 2003;10:1479–84.

29. Stewart LA. Topical antimicrobial agents. In: Bondi EE, Jegasothy BV, Lazarus GS, editors. Dermatology diagnosis and therapy. Norwalk (CT): Appleton and Lange; 1991. p. 336.

30. Van Hooteghem O, Richert B, Vindevoghel A, et al. Subungual abscesses: a new ungual side-effect related to docetaxel therapy. Br J Dermatol 2000;143:462–3.

31. Hussaid S, Anderson DN, Salvatti ME, et al. Onycholysis as a complication of systemic chemotherapy. Cancer 2000;88:2367–71.

32. De Berker DAR, Baran R, Dawber RPR. Handbook of diseases of the nails and their management. Oxford: Blackwell Science; 1995.

33. Johnson TM, Rapini RP, Duvic M. Inflammation of actinic keratoses from systemic chemotherapy. J Am Acad Dermatol 1987;17:192–7.

34. Lewis KG, Lewis MD, Robinson-Bostom L. Inflammation of actinic keratoses during capecitabine therapy. Arch Dermatol 2004;140:367–8.

35. Kirkup ME, Narayan S, Kennedy CTC. Cutaneous recall reactions with systemic fluorouracil. Dermatology 2003;206:175–6.

36. Nabai H, Mohindra R, Mehregan D. Selective inflammatory effect of systemic fluorouracil in actinic keratoses. Cutis 1999;64:43–4.

37. Fitzpatrick JE. Mucocutaneous complications of antineoplastic therapy. In: Freedberg IM, Eisen AZ, Wolff K, et al, editors. Dermatology in general medicine. New York: McGraw-Hill; 2003. p. 1339.

38. Van Doorn R, Scheffer KE, Stoof TJ, et al. Follicular and epidermal alterations in patients treated with Iressa, an inhibitor of the epidermal growth factor receptor. Br J Dermatol 2002;147:598.

39. Lee MW, Seo CW, Kim SW, et al. Cutaneous side effects in non-small cell lung cancer patients treated with Iressa, an inhibitor of epidermal growth factor. Acta Derm Venereol 2004;84:23–6.

40. Interview with Peter Heald, M.D. Skin and Allergy News 2005(Jan).

41. Herbst RS, Lo Russo PM, Purdom M, et al. Dermatologic side effects associated with gefitinib therapy: clinical experience and management. Clin Lung Cancer 2003;4: 366–9.

42. Busam KJ, Capodieci P, Motzer R, et al. Cutaneous side effects in cancer patients treated with the antiepidermal growth factor receptor antibody C225. Br J Dermatol 2001;144:1169–79.

43. Despain JD. Dermatologic toxicity of chemotherapy. Semin Oncol 1992;19:501–7.

44. Ristic B. Radiation recall dermatitis. Int J Dermatol 2004;43:627-31.

45. Camidge R, Price A. Characterizing the phenomenon of radiation recall dermatitis. Radiother Oncol 2001;59: 237–45.

46. Kodym E, Kalinska R, Ehringfeld C. Frequency of radiation recall dermatitis in adult cancer patients. Onkologie 2005;28:18–21.

47. Friedlander PA, Bansal R, Schwartz L. Gemcitabine-related radiation recall preferentially involves internal tissue and organs. Cancer 2004;100:1793–9.

48. Jeter MD, Janne PA, Brooks S, et al. Gemcitabine-induced radiation recall. Int J Radiat Oncol Biol Phys 2002;53: 394–400.

49. Mallory SB, Berry DH. Severe reactivation of sunburn following methotrexate use. Pediatrics 1986;78:514–5.

50. Khan AJ, Marghoob AA, Prestia AE. Methotrexate and the photodermatitis reactivation reaction: a case report and review of the literature. Cutis 2000;66:379–82.

51. Korossy KS, Hood AF. Methotrexate reactivation of sunburn reaction. Arch Dermatol 1981;117:310–1.

52. Ee HL, Yosipovitch G. Photo recall phenomenon: an adverse reaction to taxanes. Dermatology 2003;207:196–8.

53. Pandya AG, Guevara IL. Disorders of hyperpigmentation. Dermatol Clin 2000;18:91–8.

54. Kerker BJ, Hood AF. Chemotherapy-induced cutaneous reactions. Semin Dermatol 1989;8:173–81.

55. Alley E, Green R, Schuchter L. Cutaneous toxicities of cancer therapy. Curr Opin Oncol 2002;14:212–6.

56. Yokel BK, Friedman KJ, Farmer ER, et al. Cutaneous pathology following etoposide therapy. J Cutan Pathol 1987;14:326–30.

57. Breathnach SM, Hintner H. Adverse drug reactions and the skin. Oxford: Blackwell Scientific Publications; 1992.

58. Rapini RP. Cytotoxic drugs in the treatment of skin disease. Int J Dermatol 1991;30:313–22.

59. Revuz J, Valeyrie-Allanore L. Drug reactions. In: Bolognia JL, Jorizzo JL, Rapini RP, editors. Dermatology. Edinburgh: Mosby; 2003. p. 333–53.

60. Arndt KA, Jick H. Rates of cutaneous reactions to drugs. J Am Med Assoc 1976;235:918–23.

61. Austen KF. Allergies, anaphylaxis and systemic mastocytosis. In: Kasper DL, Fauci AS, Longo DL, et al, editors. Harrison's principles of internal medicine. New York: McGraw-Hill; 2005. p. 1947–56.

62. Zanotti KM, Markman M. Prevention and management of antineoplastic-induced hypersensitivity reactions. Drug Saf 2001;24:767–79.

63. Hood AF. Cutaneous side effects of cancer chemotherapy. Med Clin North Am 1986;70:187–209.

64. French LE, Prins C. Toxic epidermal necrolysis. In: Bolognia JL, Jorizzo JL, Rapini RP, editors. Edinburgh: Mosby; 2003. p. 323–31.

65. Fritsch PO, Ruiz-Maldonado R. Erythema multiforme, Stevens-Johnson syndrome, and toxic epidermal necrolysis. In: Freedberg IM, Eisen AZ, Wolff K, et al, editors. Dermatology in general medicine. New York: McGraw-Hill; 2003. p. 543–57.

66. Stern RS, Chan H-L. Usefulness of case report literature in determining drugs responsible for toxic epidermal necrolysis. J Am Acad Dermatol 1989;21:317–22.

67. Solberg LA, Wick MR, Bruckman JE. Doxorubicin-enhanced skin reaction after whole-body electron-beam irradiation for leukemia cutis. Mayo Clin Proc 1980;55:711–5.

68. Cakesen H, Oner AF. Toxic epidermal necrolysis in a girl with leukemia receiving methotrexate. Indian Pediatr 2001;38:426.

69. Brodsky A, Aparici I, Argeri C. Stevens-Johnson syndrome, respiratory distresss and acute renal failure due to synergic bleomycin-cisplatin toxicity. J Clin Pharmacol 1989;29:821–3.

70. Hsiao L-T, Chung H-M, Lin J-T, et al. Stevens-Johnson syndrome after treatment with STI 571: a case report. Br J Hematol 2002;117:620–3.

71. Ozkan A, Apak H, Celkan T, et al. Toxic epidermal necrolysis after the use of high-dose cytosine arabinoside. Pediatr Dermatol 2001;18:38–40.

72. Stone N, Sheerin S, Burge S. Toxic epidermal necrolysis and graft vs host disease: a clinical spectrum but a diagnostic dilemma. Clin Exp Dermatol 1999;24:260–2.

73. Huerta AAS, Tordera P, Cercos AC. Toxic epidermal necrolysis associated with interleukin 2. Ann Pharmacother 2002;36:1171–4.

74. Dourakis SP, Sevastianos VA, Alexopoulou A. Toxic epidermal necrolysis-like reaction associated with docetacel chemotherapy. J Clin Oncol 2002;20:3030–2.

75. Sommers KR, Kong KM, Bui DT, et al. Stevens-Johnson syndrome/toxic epidermal necrolysis in a patient receiving concurrent radiation and gemcitabine. Anticancer Drugs 2003;14:659–62.

76. Hall VC, El-Azhary RA, Bouwhuis S, et al. Dermatologic side effects of thalidomide in patients with multiple myeloma. J Am Acad Dermatol 2003;48:548–52.

77. Aydogdu I, Ozcan C, Harputluoglu M, et al. Severe adverse skin reaction to chlorambucil in a patient with chronic lymphocytic leukemia. Anticancer Drugs 1997;8:468–9.

78. Houston-Jameson C, Solanki DL. Stevens-Johnson syndrome associated with etoposide therapy. Cancer Treat Rep 1983;67:1050–1.

79. May E, Allolio B. Fatal toxic epidermal necrolysis during suramin therapy. Eur J Cancer 1991;27:1338.

80. Purpora D, Ahern MJ, Silverman N. Toxic epidermal necrolysis after mithramycin. N Engl J Med 1978; 299:1412.

81. Angelopoulou MA, Poziopoulos C, Boussiotis VA. Fludarabine monophosphate in refractory B-chronic lymphocytic leukemia: maintenance may be significant to sustain response. Leuk Lymphoma 1996;21:321–4.

82. Giaccone G, Risio M, Bonardi G, et al. Stevens-Johnson syndrome and fatal pulmonary toxicity to combination chemotherapy containing bleomycin: a case report. Tumori 1986;72:331–4.

83. Nigen S, Knowles SR, Shear NH. Drug eruptions: approaching the diagnosis of drug-induced skin diseases. J Drugs Dermatol 2003;2:278–99.

84. Lim HW. Abnormal response to ultraviolet radiation: photosensitivity induced by exogenous agents. In: Freedberg IM, Eisen AZ, Wolff K, et al, editors. Dermatology in general medicine. New York: McGraw-Hill; 2003. p. 1298–307.

85. Treudler R, Georgieva J, Geilen CC, et al. Dacarbazine but not temozolomide induces phototoxic dermatitis in patients with malignant melanoma. J Am Acad Dermatol 2004;50:783–5.

86. Allen JE. Drug-induced photosensitivity. Clin Pharm 1993;12:580–7.

66

Orbital Cellulitis

Dominick I. Golio, MD
Dan S. Gombos, MD, FACS

Orbital cellulitis is a sight- and potentially life-threatening periocular infection. In the cancer patient, early diagnosis and intervention are necessary to avoid secondary complications and negative sequelae. This chapter reviews the clinical features of periocular cellulitis, with an emphasis on rapid diagnosis, workup, and appropriate initiation of antimicrobial therapy.

Presentation

It is useful to distinguish preseptal cellulitis from postseptal disease. In preseptal cellulitis, clinical findings are confined to tissues anterior to the orbital septum. Patients have good central vision, normal ocular motility, and no evidence of pupil or optic nerve abnormalities. Patients with orbital infections (postseptal cellulitis) have more advanced disease, with associated blurry vision, proptosis, and limitation of ocular motility. Abnormalities of the optic nerve or pupillary response can be a harbinger of vision that is potentially threatened.[1,2]

Initial Examination

Patients who develop periocular swelling or injection should have an immediate and thorough ophthalmic assessment. This includes measurement of visual acuity, motility, pupillary response, and color vision and a dilated funduscopic examination. Baseline photographs should be obtained of the periocular structures documenting the extent of the swelling and inflammation (Figure 1). Any proptosis should be measured using an exophthalmometer.

A careful history should be obtained reviewing the onset of symptoms and time course of visual complaints. In the cancer patient, it is important to review the current status of the underlying malignancy and any recent treatment, such as chemo- or radiotherapy. This should include a risk assessment for specific infectious etiologies (eg, neutropenia, recent surgery, central line placement). Once the diagnosis is entertained, a baseline computed tomographic (CT) scan of the orbits and sinuses is obtained, with contrast, thin cuts, and true axial and coronal images. Careful attention must be directed toward the intra- and extraconal space looking for signs of orbital abscesses or associated sinusitis (Figures 2 and 3).[3–5]

Empiric Therapy

In practice, patients with isolated preseptal cellulitis who are in remission of their malignancy with no associated sinusitis can be treated in an outpatient setting with oral antibiotics such as amoxicillin-clavulanate or cefaclor. Close serial observation is necessary to ensure that the periocular findings are responding to treatment.

Patients with concurrent neoplastic disease, neutropenia, recent chemotherapy, and/or a history of bone marrow transplantation are at risk of a broad spectrum of orbital and sinus infections. These patients should be admitted

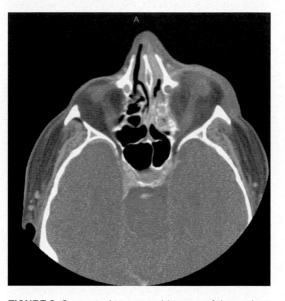

FIGURE 3 Computed tomographic scan of the patient in Figure 1 demonstrating proptosis and adjacent ethmoidal sinusitis.

for empiric intravenous therapy. In the immunocompetent patient, *Staphylococcus aureus*, *Escherichia coli*, and *Streptococcus pneumoniae* are the most common organisms of concern. In the cancer patient, other organisms must also be entertained, including *Pseudomonas*, *Klebsiella*, and methicillin-resistant *S. aureus*. Prompt initiation of broad-spectrum intravenous antibiotics is indicated in most patients. A third- or

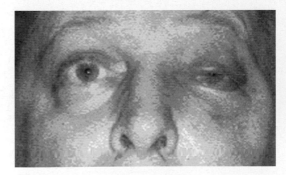

FIGURE 1 Left periorbital cellulitis with associated ptosis, chemosis, and injection.

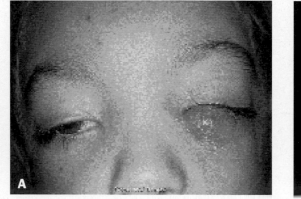
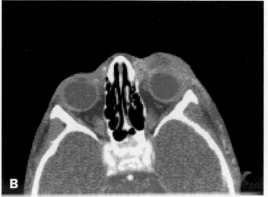

FIGURE 2 A, External photograph of a 4-year-old boy with acute myelogenous leukemia and an anterior orbital abscess. B, Axial computed tomographic scan of the same patient demonstrates the radiographic appearance of the abscess.

fourth-generation cephalosporin (such as ceftri-axone or cefepime) or a carbapenem (such as imipenem) is generally indicated. Vancomycin is also administered to provide appropriate staphylococcus coverage. Individually, each patient should be assessed for the possibility of other rare infections. For example, those patients at risk of anaerobic organisms are also administered metronidazole.[1–4]

Fungal Cellulitis

Cancer patients and those with a history of bone marrow transplantation are at particular risk of disseminated fungal infection. Potential organisms include *Aspergillus* and *Mucor*. These cases can present with fulminant sinusitis and rapid progression of disease in the orbit extending into adjacent structures (including the central nervous system). A biopsy of tissue may be helpful in confirming the diagnosis. In many cases, associated sinusitis can be assessed by the otorhinolaryngologist with débridement and identification of the offending organism.

When suspicion of a fungal cellulitis is made, a multidisciplinary approach works best. Involvement of infectious disease experts is helpful in selecting empiric antifungal coverage, such as liposomal amphotericin B, caspofungin, and/or voriconazole. Traditionally, fungal sinusitis with organisms such as *Mucor* appear in ketoacidotic diabetic patients. One approach is aggressive débridement owing to the fulminant nature of this disease entity. In the cancer setting, particularly among neutropenic and bone marrow transplant patients, a less surgically radical approach is preferred. The otorhinolaryngologist may perform minimal débridement of adjacent paranasal structures. Infectious disease services are consulted regarding the best selection of empiric antifungal agents. This is reviewed in light of the patient's overall systemic situation (ie, renal and hepatic function). Finally, underlying immunosuppression is addressed with granulocyte-stimulating factors.

Follow-Up

Once treatment is initiated, close serial observation is necessary. Generally, frequent ophthalmic examination is recommended to review the patient's visual acuity, motility, and other ocular findings. External photographs can be helpful in documenting a response to therapy (Figure 4).

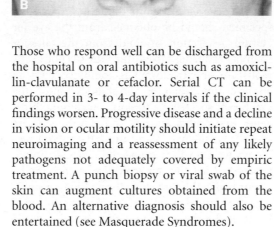

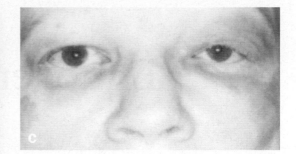

FIGURE 4 Serial external photographs demonstrating resolution of orbital cellulitis in a patient with cutaneous melanoma.

Those who respond well can be discharged from the hospital on oral antibiotics such as amoxicillin-clavulanate or cefaclor. Serial CT can be performed in 3- to 4-day intervals if the clinical findings worsen. Progressive disease and a decline in vision or ocular motility should initiate repeat neuroimaging and a reassessment of any likely pathogens not adequately covered by empiric treatment. A punch biopsy or viral swab of the skin can augment cultures obtained from the blood. An alternative diagnosis should also be entertained (see Masquerade Syndromes).

Surgical Intervention

Identification of an abscess on CT is generally an indication for incision and drainage. Those localized to the lid may be drained with a simple skin incision. More posterior lesions will require orbital surgery. Lesions close to or associated with significant sinusitis can be drained via an ethmoidal or maxillary approach. Tissue that is grossly necrotic should be débrided and sent for fungal stains and culture. Orbital decompression may be necessary in cases in which the optic nerve is compromised secondary to periocular edema. Severe pancytopenia may affect the timing and indications for surgical intervention.

Masquerade Syndromes

In some cases, patients respond poorly to initial therapy and alternative diagnoses must be entertained. Metastatic disease to the orbit can mimic orbital cellulitis. When the diagnosis is in question, an orbital biopsy should be considered. Other entities can also simulate an infection. These include secondary inflammation following radiation therapy, toxic and allergic reactions to medications, orbital inflammatory syndrome, thyroid eye disease, and, rarely, carotid cavernous sinus fistulae.

Conclusion

Orbital cellulitis in the cancer patient can be a serious and life-threatening infection. Patients should be rapidly worked up with neuroimaging and baseline ophthalmic assessment. Treatment should be initiated with empiric broad-spectrum antimicrobials. The complex nature of these cases often lends itself to a multidisciplinary approach with contributions from ophthalmology, infectious disease, and otorhinolaryngology services.

REFERENCES

1. Givner LB. Periorbital versus orbital cellulitis. Pediatr Infect Dis J 2002;21:1157–8.
2. Tovilla-Canales JL, Nava A, Tovilla y Pomar JL. Orbital and periorbital infections. Curr Opin Ophthalmol 2001; 12:335–41.
3. Shuttleworth G, Harrad R. Management of acute eyelid conditions. Practitioner 2000;244:138–43, 145–7.
4. Shovlin JP. Orbital infections and inflammations. Curr Opin Ophthalmol 1998;9:41–8.
5. Eustis HS, Mafee MF, Walton C, Mondonca J. MR imaging and CT of orbital infections and complications in acute rhinosinusitis. Radiol Clin North Am 1998;36:1165–83.

67

Endogenous Endophthalmitis

Dan S. Gombos, MD, FACS

Clinically, endophthalmitis refers to inflammation of the eye associated with an infectious etiology. Broadly speaking, endophthalmitis can be broken down into four different types: postoperative, traumatic, glaucoma associated, and endogenous. This chapter is limited to endogenous endophthalmitis, in which intraocular structures are infected via hematogenous dissemination from other sources.

Risk Factors and Presentation

Patients who are immunocompromised are at particular risk of developing endogenous endophthalmitis. Neutropenia, indwelling catheters (such as central lines and ports), and immunosuppression (from chemo- and radiotherapy) are factors that put the cancer patient at particular risk of this phenomenon. Intravenous drug use further increases this risk.

The presentation of endogenous endophthalmitis can vary. Symptoms may include blurry vision, sensitivity to light, and red eye. There may be varying degrees of pain. Patients who are critically ill may be unable to elicit any symptoms. Restricted motility of the eye, associated inflammation of the lids and periocular structures, or findings of pus in the anterior chamber (hypopyon) are critical signs that necessitate ophthalmic consultation (Figure 1).

Assessment and Workup

Ocular assessment should include measurement of visual acuity and intraocular pressure and a complete dilated fundus examination. If possible, a slit lamp examination is helpful in assessing inflammation in the anterior chamber and vitreous. An eye sonogram may be necessary if there is no view of the posterior segment. Additional workup depends largely on whether a bacterial or fungal etiology is suspected.

If bacterial endophthalmitis is suspected, a specimen should be obtained from the eye for culture. Aspiration of fluid from the anterior chamber (aqueous tap) or the vitreous body (vitreous tap or vitrectomy) is combined with an empiric injection of antibiotics into the eye. Broad-spectrum antibiotics, including third-generation cephalosporins and vancomycin, are injected via the pars plana into the posterior segment with a small-gauge needle.[1] The decision to proceed with a vitreous aspiration (which can be performed in the clinic or at the bedside) or surgical vitrectomy depends on the extent of involvement of the eye at presentation, baseline visual acuity, and the patient's overall general health. In advanced cases, vitrectomy may be indicated from a diagnostic and therapeutic perspective.

In addition, cultures of blood, urine, and any indwelling catheter are obtained on day 1. Systemic and topical antibiotics are administered and directed toward likely pathogens, including *Staphylococcus aureus*, *Bacillus cereus*, streptococci, and *Neisseria meningitides*. Patients are serially monitored with continued topical and intravenous antibiotics.[1,2] In some cases, topical and systemic steroids are administered to address the associated intra- and periocular inflammation.

Fungal endophthalmitis can be distinguished clinically from its bacterial counterpart. It is generally a less fulminant process. Patients may notice redness, decreased vision, floaters, or pain. Examination findings can vary significantly from small yellow-white lesions limited primarily to the retina to (in advanced cases) involvement of the entire posterior segment. The vitreous may become increasingly opacified from cells and debris and obscure visualization of the underlying retina (Figure 2). In some cases, an associated retinal detachment occurs.

Fungal endophthalmitis that primarily infects the retina with no significant vitreal involvement can be treated with systemic intravenous

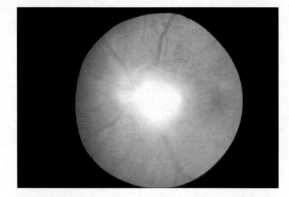

FIGURE 2 Fundus photograph of an eye with a vitreous abscess.

antifungal medications. Amphotericin B, voriconazole, and caspofungin can penetrate the eye and provide adequate treatment.[3,4] When there is more significant ocular involvement associated with inflammation, diagnostic and therapeutic vitrectomy may be necessary. Intraocular administration of antifungal drugs is generally indicated in such cases.[3,4] The most common fungal etiology is disseminated *Candida*, but other species, such as *Aspergillus*, can occur.[5-8]

Patients with both bacterial and fungal endophthalmitis may require prolonged antimicrobial therapy. Patients may need topical cycloplegic agents and monitoring of intraocular pressure, which may become elevated. Management requires a multidisciplinary approach, with the ophthalmologist and infectious disease specialist coordinating care. Ocular prognosis depends greatly on the virulence of the offending organism and the promptness with which treatment is initiated.[9]

Other Infectious Causes

Other potential infectious must be considered when an immunocompromised patient presents with redness of the eye, inflammation, and loss of vision. Viral infections, such as herpes and cytomegalovirus retinitis, can develop indolently. Bloodborne malignancies can also mimic intraocular infection with hypopyon, including leukemia, lymphoma, and retinoblastoma. The appearance of the posterior fundus can distinguish these masquerade syndromes from a true bacterial or fungal endophthalmitis.[10] In

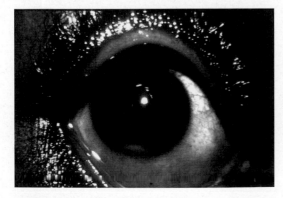

FIGURE 1 Anterior segment photograph of an eye with a hypopyon.

these instances, consultation with an experienced ocular oncologist or retinologist is essential in arriving at the correct diagnosis.

Conclusion

Intraocular inflammation can represent a host of ocular abnormalities in the cancer patient. The most serious is an infectious cause that can lead to rapid and irreversible loss of vision. Cancer patients who present with periocular redness, pain, decline of vision, and floaters should be evaluated by an ophthalmologist. When a bacterial or fungal endophthalmitis is suspected, empiric antimicrobials should be administered

as soon as possible. In advanced cases, therapeutic vitrectomy may be indicated. Prognosis is dependent on early diagnosis and intervention.

REFERENCES

1. Benz MS, Scott IU, Flynn HW Jr, et al. Endophthalmitis isolates and antibiotic sensitivities: a 6-year review of culture-proven cases. Am J Ophthalmol 2004;137:38–42.
2. Jackson TL, Eykyn SJ, Graham EM, Stanford MR. Endogenous bacterial endophthalmitis: a 17-year prospective series and review of 267 reported cases. Surv Ophthalmol 2003;48:403–23.
3. Breit, SM, Hariprasad SM, Mieler WF, et al. Management of endogenous fungal endophthalmitis with voriconazole and caspofungin. Am J Ophthalmol 2005;139:135–40.
4. Sarria JC, Bradley JC, Habash R, et al. *Candida glabrata* endophthalmitis treated successfully with caspofungin. Clin Infect Dis 2005;40:e46–8.
5. Patel AS, Hemady RK, Rodrigues M, et al. Endogenous *Fusarium* endophthalmitis in a patient with acute lymphocytic leukemia. Am J Ophthalmol 1994;117:363–8.
6. Ramsey MS, Willis NR. Endogenous *Candida* endophthalmitis. Can J Ophthalmol 1972;7:126–31.
7. Rao AG, Thool BA, Rao CV. Endogenous endophthalmitis due to *Alternaria* in an immunocompetent host. Retina 2004;24:478–81.
8. Tiribelli M, Zaja F, Fili C, et al. Endogenous endophthalmitis following disseminated fungemia due to *Fusarium solani* in a patient with acute myeloid leukemia. Eur J Haematol 2002;68:314–7.
9. Schiedler V, Scott IU, Flynn HW Jr, et al. Culture-proven endogenous endophthalmitis: clinical features and visual acuity outcomes. Am J Ophthalmol 2004;137:725–31.
10. Rodriguez-Adrian LJ, King RT, Tamayo-Derat LG, et al. Retinal lesions as clues to disseminated bacterial and candidal infections: frequency, natural history, and etiology. Medicine (Baltimore) 2003;82:187–202.

Ocular Side Effects Associated with Chemotherapy

Angela W. Kim, MD

The treatment of cancer frequently includes chemotherapy, radiation therapy (RT), and bone marrow transplantation. In many cases, it is difficult to establish a cause and effect relationship between chemotherapeutic agents and ocular side effects because of overlap of multiple agents, as well as different treatment regimens and modalities used within a short period of time. Chemotherapy can result in direct ophthalmic toxicity. Secondary anemia, thrombocytopenia, and immunosuppression may cause intraocular hemorrhage and infection, which are discussed elsewhere. Drug-induced metabolic changes can also affect vision.

The central nervous system (CNS) is a partially protected environment by way of limited cell division and the blood-brain barrier. Greater CNS toxicity is found in the setting of increased CNS penetration, as occurs through intra-arterial versus intravenous delivery of medication, intrathecal delivery, direct intracranial intratumoral therapy and with osmotic disruption of the blood-brain barrier. Hyperosmotic agents also compromise the blood-retina barrier, which is formed at the tight junctions of the retinal pigment epithelium (RPE) and the retinal blood vessel walls.

The purpose of this chapter is to serve as a very brief summary of known ocular toxicities of different chemotherapeutic agents. For a more comprehensive review of the literature, the reader is referred to Moster's chapter in Walsh and Hoyt's *Clinical Neuro-ophthalmology*.[1]

Antimetabolites

High-dose therapy with methotrexate is associated with reversible periorbital edema, photophobia, ocular pain, and burning associated with keratitis, seborrheic blepharitis, conjunctivitis, and decreased reflex tearing in about 25% of cases.[2,3] Intracarotid artery delivery can cause macular edema with central retinal pigmentary changes.[4,5]

Conjunctivitis and keratitis occur most frequently, with corneal epithelial defects occurring in up to 50% of patients receiving 5-fluorouracil.[2,6] Other complications include blepharitis and other lid changes.[2,7,8] Reversible epiphora occurs in up to 50% of patients and is associated with increased drug concentration in the tears.[6,9] A reversible acute toxic optic neuropathy with optic disc swelling can occur.[10,11]

Cytosine arabinoside (Ara-C) causes a dose-related, reversible keratoconjunctivitis that affects the superficial and deep cornea (Figure 1).[2,12] Symptoms include pain, foreign body sensation, tearing, photophobia, and blurred vision. Bilateral, progressive optic neuropathies have been reported, possibly from potentiation of radiation effects or with intrathecal therapy.[13]

Optic neuropathy is a prominent complication reported with the purine analogue fludarabine (Fludara).[14]

Bromodeoxyuridine is a pyrimidine analogue that, in combination with RT, can cause eyelid erythema, induration, conjunctival chemosis, hyperemia, conjunctivitis, dry-eye syndrome, ectropion, and exposure keratitis.[15]

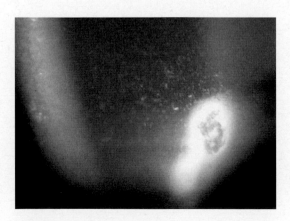

FIGURE 1 Cytosine arabinoside keratopathy manifesting in epithelial opacities seen in the center of the microphotograph. A bright light reflection is seen in the *lower right* aspect of the photograph.

Alkylating Agents

Intracarotid artery infusion of nitrogen mustard may cause a severe ipsilateral necrotizing uveitis.[16]

Delayed posterior subcapsular cataract may occur with busulfan and is related to the dose and duration of treatment.[2]

Nonspecific reversible blurred vision has been reported within 24 hours of high-dose intravenous administration of cyclophosphamide (Cytoxan).[17] Reversible keratoconjunctivitis sicca has been reported in up to 50% of patients.[17] Optic neuropathy has been reported.[18] Transient blurred vision and miosis may be caused by a parasympathomimetic action.[17]

High-dose intravenous therapy with the nitrosoureas causes mild conjunctival hyperemia and nonspecific blurred vision in a small percentage of patients.[2] A delayed, severe, ipsilateral neuroretinal toxicity (probably from ischemia) occurs in up to 70% of patients treated intra-arterially (often with concomitant intracarotid cisplatin), with an approximately 50% incidence of ipsilateral complete blindness.[2] Patients receiving intravenous carmustine (BCNU) and ipsilateral infraophthalmic cisplatin can develop maculopathy.[19] Damage to retinal and choroidal endothelial cells has been suggested as a possible mechanism.[20]

Intracarotid artery infusion of nitrosoureas may cause orbital congestion.[21,22] Ischemia may lead to optic neuropathy and orbital complications.[21,23] Optic neuropathy with and without disc swelling has been reported with intracarotid and supraophthalmic infusion of BCNU.[24–26]

Retinal and CNS toxicities frequently occur after intracarotid or high-dose intravenous delivery of cisplatin.[2,27–29] Cisplatin is associated with RPE changes and maculopathy. When combined with BCNU, patients develop signs of retinal vasculitis and infarction.[20] Toxic, progressive optic neuropathy, including retrobulbar, and papilledema occur in some patients.[30–32]

Antibiotics

Suramin can cause a reversible toxic keratopathy with foreign body sensation and corneal epithelial deposits in approximately 17% of patients; visual blurring may occur from an induced change in the optics of the eyes.[33]

Ocular side effects of doxorubicin (Adriamycin) include excessive tearing, blepharospasm, and periorbital edema with severe keratoconjunctivitis in about 25% of patients during intravenous infusion.[7,34]

Vinca Alkaloids

Optic neuropathy has been described with vincristine but is a diagnosis of exclusion. It may resolve partially or completely off therapy.[2]

Transient ptosis, paresis of extraocular muscles, and brief eye pain have been reported with vinblastine.[35]

Taxoids

Docetaxel (Taxotere) may cause canalicular stenosis with symptomatic epiphora.[36] Transient positive visual phenomena lasting up to a few hours were reported in six patients during paclitaxel (Taxol) infusion at higher than recommended doses.[37]

Hormones

Tamoxifen causes corneal opacities and retinal dysfunction, particularly with high doses.[38] White, refractile opacities, RPE depigmentation, and macular edema may develop. Vision can improve despite the persistence of retinal opacities.[39] Isolated cases of bilateral optic disc swelling with visual loss have been reported.[40,41]

Posterior subcapsular cataracts occur in 10 to 40% of patients who are chronically treated over months with corticosteroids.[2] Corticosteroids can also cause reversible elevation of intraocular pressure, acute myopia with blurry vision, subconjunctival and retinal hemorrhages, scleral discoloration and thinning, exophthalmos, myopathic extraocular muscle paresis, and ptosis.[2,42,43] Immunosuppression secondary to corticosteroids can predispose patients to opportunistic infections. Pseudotumor cerebri (PTC) is a well-documented complication of steroid treatment.[42]

Biologic Response Modifiers

Vaso-occlusive retinopathy can occur in patients treated with interferon-α.[44,45] Preexisting diabetes mellitus is a risk factor. Descriptive cases of oculomotor nerve paralysis, eyelash hypertrichosis, and papilledema have been reported.[46–48]

Reversible dose-dependent effects, such as visual hallucinations, scintillating scotomata,

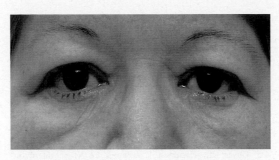

FIGURE 2 Bilateral periorbital edema in a patient treated with STI571. There is soft tissue fullness of both upper eyelids and just below the eyelids, greater on the patient's right side than on the left.

homonymous defects, amaurosis fugax, and diplopia, may occur with interleukin-2.[49–51]

Miscellaneous Drugs

Ocular side effects of retinoids such as retinol and retinoic acid include conjunctivitis and corneal opacities.[52]

Reversible xerophthalmia and nyctalopia have been reported at higher doses of fenretinide (4-HPR).[52,53] Patients with secondary hypervitaminosis A can develop elevated intracranial pressure and a PTC syndrome.

L-Asparaginase is associated with venous thrombosis and can cause dural sinus or cortical vein thrombosis with intracranial hypertension and a PTC syndrome.[54]

Periorbital edema (Figure 2) and epiphora are the most common ocular side effects of STI571 (Gleevec, imatinib mesylate).[55]

Conclusion

Ocular and neuro-ophthalmic toxicity can involve any part of the eye, adnexa, or CNS. Visual abnormalities have numerous potential etiologies, and it is difficult to differentiate the toxic effects of medications from cancer, radiation, infection-related complications, and non–cancer-related diseases. The complexity of this challenge increases with the development of newer agents and protocols and with increased patient survival, often involving multiple therapies.

REFERENCES

1. Moster MM. Complications of cancer therapy. In: Miller NR, Newman NJ, editors. Walsh & Hoyt's clinical neuro-ophthalmology. Vol 2. 5th ed. Baltimore: Williams & Wilkins; 1998. p. 2553–94.
2. Imperia PS, Lazarus HM, Lass JH. Ocular complications of systemic cancer chemotherapy. Surv Ophthalmol 1989; 34:209–30.
3. Doroshow JH, Locker GY, Gaasterland DE, et al. Ocular irritation from high-dose methotrexate therapy: pharmacokinetics of drug in the tear film. Cancer 1981;48: 2158–62.
4. Millay RH, Klein ML, Shults WT, et al. Maculopathy associated with combination chemotherapy and osmotic opening of the blood-brain barrier. Am J Ophthalmol 1986;102:626–32.
5. Neuwelt EA, Howieson J, Frenkel EP, et al. Therapeutic efficacy of multiagent chemotherapy with drug delivery enhancement by blood-brain barrier modification in glioblastoma. Neurosurgery 1986;19:573–82.
6. Christophidis N, Lucas I, Vahda FJE, et al. Lacrimation and 5-fluorouracil. Ann Intern Med 1978;89:574.
7. Vizel M, Oster MW. Ocular side effects of cancer chemotherapy. Cancer 1982;49:1999–2002.
8. Burns LJ. Ocular side effects of chemotherapy. In: Perry MC, Satterfield TS, Pine JW, editors. The chemotherapy source book. Baltimore: Williams & Wilkins; 1992. p. 570–81.
9. Christophidis N, Vajda FJE, Lucas I, et al. Ocular side effects with 5-fluorouracil. Aust N Z J Med 1979;9:143–4.
10. Weiss AJ, Jackson LG, Carabasi R. An evaluation of 5-fluorouracil in malignant disease. Ann Intern Med 1961; 55:731–41.
11. Adams JW, Bofenkamp TM, Kobrin J, et al. Recurrent acute toxic optic neuropathy secondary to 5-FU. Cancer Treat Rep 1984;68:565–6.
12. Hopen G, Mondino BJ, Johnson BL, et al. Corneal toxicity with systemic cytarabine. Am J Ophthalmol 1981;91: 500–4.
13. Margileth DA, Poplack DG, Pizzo PA, et al. Blindness during remission in two patients with acute lymphoblastic leukemia. A possible complication of multimodality therapy. Cancer 1977;39:58–61.
14. Chun HG, Leyland-Jones BR, Caryk SM, et al. Central nervous system toxicity of fludarabine phosphate. Cancer Treat Rep 1986;70:1225–8.
15. Vander JF, Kincaid MC, Hegarty TJ, et al. The ocular effects of intracarotid bromodeoxyuridine and radiation therapy in the treatment of malignant glioma. Ophthalmology 1990;97:352–7.
16. Anderson B, Anderson B Jr. Necrotizing uveitis incident to perfusion of intracranial malignancies with nitrogen mustard or related compounds. Trans Am Ophthalmol Soc 1960;58:95–105.
17. Kende G, Sirin SR, Thomas PRM, et al. Blurring of vision. Cancer 1979;44:69–71.
18. Awidi AS. Blindness and vincristine. Ann Intern Med 1980;93:781.
19. Kupersmith MJ, Seiple WH, Holopigian K, et al. Maculopathy caused by intra-arterially administered cisplatin and intravenously administered carmustine. Am J Ophthalmol 1992;113:435–8.
20. Miller DF, Bay JW, Lederman RJ, et al. Ocular and orbital toxicity following intracarotid injection of BCNU (carmustine) and cisplatin for malignant gliomas. Ophthalmology 1985;92:402–6.
21. Kapp J, Vance R, Parker JL, et al. Limitations of high dose intra-arterial 1,3-bis(2-chloroethyl)-1-nitrosourea (BCNU) chemotherapy for malignant gliomas. Neurosurgery 1982;10:715–9.
22. Gebarski SS, Greenberg HS, Gavrielsen TO, et al. Orbital angiographic changes after intracarotid BCNU chemotherapy. AJNR Am J Neuroradiol 1984;5:55–8.
23. Grimson BS, Mahaley MS Jr, Dubey HD, et al. Ophthalmic and central nervous system complications following intracarotid BCNU (carmustine). J Clin Neuroophthalmol 1981;1:261–4.
24. Shingleton BJ, Bienfang DC, Albert DM, et al. Ocular toxicity associated with high-dose carmustine. Arch Ophthalmol 1982;100:1766–72.
25. Pickrell L, Purvin V. Ischemic optic neuropathy secondary to intracarotid infusion of BCNU. J Clin Neuroophthalmol 1987;7:87–91.
26. Shimamura Y, Chikama M, Taniomoto T, et al. Optic nerve degeneration caused by supraophthalmic carotid artery infusion with cisplatin and ACNU. J Neurosurg 1990; 72:285–8.
27. Wilding G, Caruso R, Lawrence TS, et al. Retinal toxicity after high-dose cisplatin therapy. J Clin Oncol 1985;3: 1683–9.
28. Stewart DJ, Wallace S, Feun LG, et al. A phase I study of intracarotid artery infusion of cis-diamminedichloroplatinum (II) in patients with recurrent malignant intracerebral tumors. Cancer Res 1982;42:2059–62.
29. Feun LG, Wallace S, Stewart DJ, et al. Intracarotid infusion of cis-diamminedichloroplatinum in the treatment of recurrent malignant brain tumors. Cancer 1984;54: 794–9.
30. Ostrow S, Hahn D, Wiernik PH, et al. Ophthalmologic toxicity after cis-dichlorodiammineplatinum (II) therapy. Cancer Treat Rep 1978;62:1591–4.

31. Becher R, Schutt P, Osieka R, et al. Peripheral neuropathy and ophthalmologic toxicity after treatment with cis-dichlorodiaminoplatinum II. J Cancer Res Clin Oncol 1980;96:219–21.

32. Walsh TJ, Clark AW, Parhad IM, et al. Neurotoxic effects of cisplatin therapy. Arch Neurol 1982;39:719–20.

33. Hemady R, Eisenberger M. Ocular complications from suramin therapy for metastatic prostate cancer. Ophthalmology 1994;Suppl:92.

34. Chrousos GA, Oldfield ED, Doppman JL, et al. Prevention of ocular toxicity of carmustine (BCNU) with supraophthalmic intracarotid infusion. Ophthalmology 1986;93:1471–5.

35. Wilson CB. Chemotherapy of brain tumors by continuous arterial infusion. Surgery 1964;55:640–53.

36. Esmaeli B, Burnstine MA, Ahmadi MA, Prieto VG. Docetaxel-induced histologic changes in the lacrimal sac and the nasal mucosa. Ophthalmic Plast Reconstr Surg 2003;19:305–8.

37. Seidman AD, Barrett S. Photopsia during 3-hour paclitaxel administration at doses > 250mg/m2. J Clin Oncol 1994;12:1741–2.

38. Kaiser-Kupfer MI, Lippman ME. Tamoxifen retinopathy. Cancer Treat Rep 1978;62:315–20.

39. Locher D, Tang R, Pardo G, et al. Retinal changes associated with tamoxifen treatment for breast cancer. Invest Ophthalmol Vis Sci 1994;35:1526.

40. Pugesgaard T, Von Eyben FE. Bilateral optic neuritis evolved during tamoxifen treatment. Cancer 1986;58:383–6.

41. Ashford AR, Doney I, Tiwari RP, et al. Reversible ocular toxicity related to tamoxifen therapy. Cancer 1988;61:33–5.

42. Crews SJ. Adverse reactions to corticosteroid therapy in the eye. Proc R Soc Med 1965;88:533–5.

43. David DS, Berkowitz JS. Ocular effects of topical and systemic corticosteroids. Lancet 1969;2:149–51.

44. Guyer DR, Tiedeman J, Yannuzzi LA, et al. Interferon-associated retinopathy. Arch Ophthalmol 1993;111:350–6.

45. Miyamoto N, Takada Y, Miura M. A case of retinopathy associated with interferon therapy for malignant tumor. Folia Ophthalmol Jpn 1997;48:537–40.

46. Bauhertz G, Soeur M, Lustman F. Oculomotor nerve paralysis induced by alpha II-interferon. Acta Neurol Belg 1990;90:111–4.

47. Foon KA, Dougher G. Increased growth of eyelashes in a patient given leukocyte A interferon. N Engl J Med 1984;311:1259.

48. Farkkila M, Iivanainen M, Roine R, et al. Neurotoxic and other side effects of high-dose interferon in amyotrophic lateral sclerosis. Acta Neurol Scand 1984;69:42–6.

49. Parkinson DR. Interleukin-2 in cancer therapy. Semin Oncol 1988;15 Suppl 6:10.

50. Friedman DI, Hu EH, Sadun AA. Neuro-ophthalmic complications of interleukin 2 therapy. Arch Ophthalmol 1991;109:1679–80.

51. Bernard JT, Ameriso S, Kempf RA, et al. Transient focal neurologic deficits complicating interleukin-2 therapy. Neurology 1990;40:154.

52. Costa A, De Palo G, Formelli F, et al. Breast cancer chemoprevention with retinoids. In: Livrea MA, Packer L, editors. Retinoids. Progress in research and clinical applications. New York: Marcel Dekker; 1993. p. 453–5.

53. Chabner BA. Anticancer drugs. In: Devita VT, Hellman S, Rosenberg SA, editors. Principles and practice of oncology. 4th ed. JB Lippincott; 1993. p. 354–6.

54. Cairo MS, Lazarus K, Gilmore RL, et al. Intracranial hemorrhage and focal seizures secondary to use of L-asparaginase during induction therapy of acute lymphocytic leukemia. J Pediatr 1980;97:829–33.

55. Fraunfelder FW, Solomon J, Druker BJ, et al. Ocular side-effects associated with imatinib mesylate (Gleevec). J Ocular Pharm Ther 2003;19:371–5.

Vascular Events, Optic Neuropathies, Paraneoplastic Syndromes, and Visual Loss

Angela W. Kim, MD

Acute and subacute visual loss occurs through many mechanisms and at various locations along the visual pathways. Visual loss can be the result of ocular surface abnormalities, intraocular infection, inflammation, tumor, and hemorrhage, to name a few causes. This chapter discusses retinal hemorrhage from thrombocytopenia and anemia, retinal vascular occlusive disease, optic neuropathies, and paraneoplastic syndromes that affect vision.

Retinal Hemorrhage from Thrombocytopenia and Anemia

Thrombocytopenia and anemia are commonly seen in patients with an underlying hematologic malignancy or as a side effect of chemotherapy. The relatively anticoagulated state with decreased hemostasis may cause vascular leakage.

The diagnosis is based on the ophthalmoscopic presence of retinal hemorrhages in the setting of thrombocytopenia and/or anemia (Figure 1). The presence of multiple comorbid risk factors may make it difficult to pinpoint a single etiology. Therefore, the examination findings must be correlated with the patient's clinical history. With restoration of blood counts, retinal hemorrhages resorb over time. The prognosis is good unless the bleeding is extensive and/or chronic enough to cause permanent photoreceptor damage.

Central Retinal Artery Occlusion

Central retinal artery occlusion (CRAO) is considered a retinal stroke from embolism or thrombosis.[1] It is usually caused by carotid artery disease and has a prevalence of vascular risk factors similar to that of cerebral stroke. The most common emboli are cholesterol, platelet-fibrin, and calcific plaques.[2] Cardiac myxomas can also embolize.

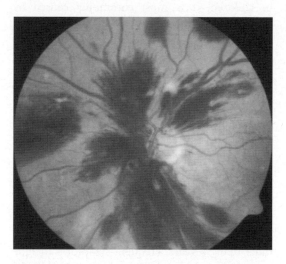

FIGURE 1 A patient with chronic myelogenous leukemia experienced decreased visual acuity. On funduscopic examination, he was found to have prominent, intraretinal hemorrhages and scattered cotton wool spots secondary to thrombocytopenia and anemia.

CRAO usually causes acute unilateral visual loss and may be preceded by amaurosis fugax. The acute ophthalmoscopic findings are diagnostic and include diffuse pale retinal swelling, optic disc pallor, a "cherry-red" spot, attenuated vessels, boxcarring, and, rarely, an embolus. There is no definitive treatment, and the visual prognosis is poor. Patients have often undergone ocular massage, anterior chamber paracentesis, intraocular pressure–lowering medications, and inhalation of carbogen.[3] Early intravascular urokinase or tissue plasminogen activator (t-PA) may be helpful but has associated potential risks.[4,5] Carotid duplex ultrasonography is used to evaluate carotid stenosis, and echocardiography may reveal a cardiac source. In younger patients, cardiac embolism, hypercoagulability, and vasospasm should be sought as the potential etiology and appropriately treated.[6]

Central Retinal Vein Occlusion

CRVO is a common ocular disorder with a strong association with atherosclerotic disease of the central retinal artery as they share a common sheath.[7] Many patients have vascular risk factors[8]; others have associated vasculitis, hyperviscosity, prothrombotic states, or external venous compression. Identification of a specific abnormality may determine a need for anticoagulation or other treatment.

CRVO usually causes acute monocular visual loss. Diagnostic funduscopic findings include dilated, tortuous veins and diffuse, scattered retinal hemorrhages. Severe cases produce the classic "blood and thunder" retinal appearance. The visual prognosis is inversely proportional to the degree of retinal ischemia.[9] There is no standard-specific treatment for the eye, except for potential secondary neovascular complications. Some newer advocated treatments include t-PA, laser-induced chorioretinal anastomosis, radial optic neurotomy, and intravitreal triamcinolone acetonide.[10–13]

Optic Neuropathies

Optic nerve disorders have numerous etiologies. Optic disc edema results from obstruction of axoplasmic transport, which results in swelling of nerve fibers. Mechanical signs of optic disc edema include elevation of the optic nerve head, blurred disc margins, loss of the optic cup, nerve fiber layer edema, and concentric folds around the disc (Figure 2). Vascular signs of disc edema include disc hyperemia, venous dilation and tortuosity, peripapillary hemorrhages, lipid exudates, and nerve fiber layer infarcts (Figure 3). Unilateral or asymmetric involvement may result in a relative afferent pupillary defect (RAPD). Loss of visual acuity, color vision, and visual field may be associated. Permanent damage results in optic disc pallor (Figure 4). Optic neuropathies can be

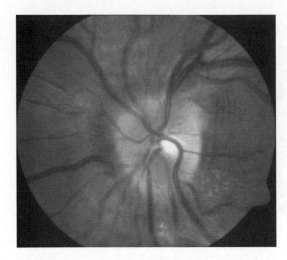

FIGURE 2 This fundus photograph demonstrates optic disc elevation with concentric folds best seen between the 1 o'clock and 2 o'clock positions. Below at the 4 o'clock position, lipid exudates are present.

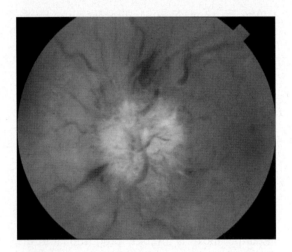

FIGURE 3 This fundus photograph shows a swollen, hyperemic optic disc with venous dilation and tortuosity. There are also nerve fiber layer hemorrhages and white, fluffy cotton wool spots on the disc (nerve fiber layer infarcts).

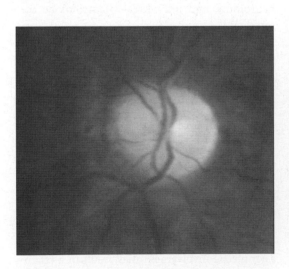

FIGURE 4 Optic disc edema has been replaced with optic disc pallor. Vascular changes, hemorrhages, and infarcts have resolved (same patient as in Figure 3).

divided into many general categories. The following is a very brief discussion of papilledema and ischemic, compressive, and infiltrative optic neuropathies.

Papilledema

Papilledema is optic disc edema caused by elevated intracranial pressure and is diagnosed by lumbar puncture. Acutely, patients typically have normal visual function, with possible blind spot enlargement seen on perimetry. They frequently have headache, nausea, and transient visual obscurations and may have diplopia. Chronic disc swelling can lead to ischemia and any pattern of visual field loss. Papilledema is a neurologic emergency that requires neuroimaging. In adults, the most common causes are primary intracranial tumor, metastasis, and pseudotumor cerebri; in children, it is most commonly caused by posterior fossa tumors.[14]

Anterior Ischemic Optic Neuropathy

Anterior ischemic optic neuropathy (AION) is considered an optic disc stroke and causes sudden, painless infarction of the optic nerve head. It may be arteritic (giant cell arteritis) or nonarteritic (Figure 5). Posterior ischemic optic neuropathy (PION) is usually caused by vasculitis, and, by definition, there is no optic disc swelling. Other ischemic states that can cause disc edema include ischemic CRVO, malignant hypertension, and diabetic papillopathy.

Arteritic AION usually occurs in patients older than 55 years. Frequent symptoms include temporal headache, scalp tenderness, jaw claudication, and constitutional symptoms. Common

laboratory findings include an elevated erythrocyte sedimentation rate and C-reactive protein and anemia of chronic disease. A biopsy proving arteritis is best because of the need for chronic corticosteroid treatment, but highly clinically suspicious cases are also treated.[15] Treatment should begin immediately on suspicion of the possibility of giant cell arteritis.

Nonarteritic AION is the most common cause of acute optic neuropathy in patients over 45 years of age. Visual loss is often noticed on awakening. Often the patient has a crowded disc—the "disc at risk." Most patients have risk factors for atherosclerosis, but some have associated coagulopathies, embolism, acute blood loss, anemia, or hypotension.[16] Greater than 40% of patients can show spontaneous improvement.[17] There is no definitive treatment. Patients may be placed on acetylsalicylic acid for stroke prophylaxis. Infectious, vasculitic, and hypercoagulable etiologies should be sought in patients younger than 50 years without known vascular risk factors.

Radiation Optic Neuropathy

Radiation optic neuropathy (RON) is a rare PION. The pathogenesis is not fully understood, but it is a form of ischemic optic neuropathy. The total dose and daily fractionation size are critical factors and typically should not exceed 55 Gy[18] and 18 Gy,[19] respectively. Most patients experience rapid, painless, and progressive visual loss within 3 years, with a peak incidence at 18 months.[20,21] The diagnosis is clinically suspected and confirmed with T_1-weighted magnetic resonance imaging with contrast, which reveals marked enhancement and enlargement

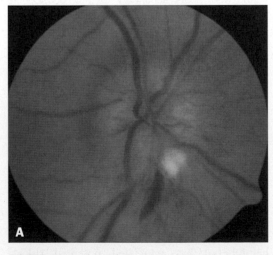

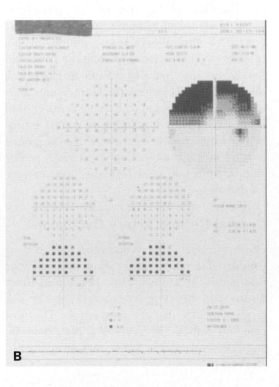

FIGURE 5 A, A patient with nonarteritic ischemic optic neuropathy. The right optic disc is elevated with blurred margins. There is a nerve fiber layer hemorrhage near the inferior pole with an adjacent whitish nerve fiber layer infarct. **B,** Visual field testing demonstrates a superior arcuate defect consistent with infarction in the inferior aspect of the optic disc.

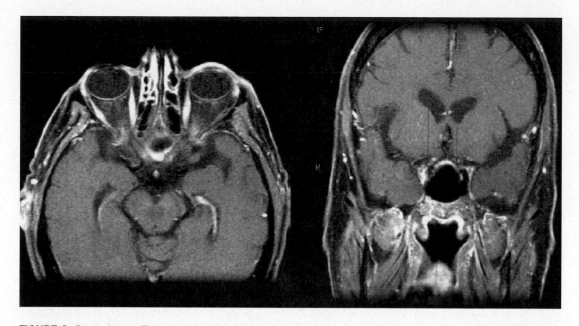

FIGURE 6 Postcontrast T$_1$-weighted magnetic resonance imaging in a patient with radiation optic neuropathy demonstrates bilateral optic nerve enhancement.

of segments of the optic nerve or chiasm (Figure 6).[22,23] Prompt treatment with hyperbaric oxygen is the only treatment associated with any significant visual improvement[24] and should be used alone or in conjunction with other medications (such as high-dose corticosteroids, pentoxyphylline, anticoagulation, or other agents).

Compressive Optic Neuropathy

Compressive optic neuropathy causes progressive visual loss, often a central scotoma, and RAPD. The optic disc can be normal, swollen, or pale. Any unexplained optic disc pallor, progressive visual loss, or corticosteroid-dependent optic neuropathy is considered compressive, until proven otherwise, and the patient must undergo imaging. The differential diagnosis includes primary, secondary, and metastatic tumors; dysthyroid orbitopathy; varix; mucocele; infectious cysts; and others (Figure 7).

Infiltrative Optic Neuropathy

The optic disc may appear grayish-white with hemorrhage or a visible mass owing to infiltrating cancer, inflammatory disease, or infectious processes (Figure 8). Usually, it occurs in patients with leukemia, lymphoma, and other carcinomas that spread to the central nervous system. Lumbar puncture should include high-volume cerebrospinal fluid to look for cytologic evidence of leptomeningeal disease. Infiltrative inflammatory and infectious disorders include sarcoidosis, tuberculosis,[25] and cryptococcosis,[26] to name a few.

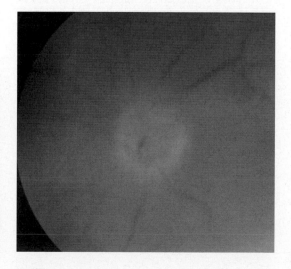

FIGURE 7 A tumor is seen in the lateral aspect of the left orbit on this T$_2$-weighted magnetic resonance image. Pathologic diagnosis was presumed primary orbital melanoma.

FIGURE 8 This fundus photograph shows a grayish-white, fluffy optic disc with central hemorrhage. The patient had an infiltrative optic neuropathy secondary to lymphoma.

Paraneoplastic Retinopathies and Optic Neuropathy

In 1976, Sawyer and colleagues postulated paraneoplastic retinal photoreceptor degeneration in three patients with small cell lung cancer.[27] Since then, several distinct paraneoplastic conditions that affect the eyes have been differentiated by unique clinical characteristics, electrophysiologic abnormalities, and, occasionally, the immunologic profile. The pathogenesis is considered immune mediated. The selected entities that are briefly described are cancer-associated retinopathy (CAR), melanoma-associated retinopathy (MAR), and paraneoplastic optic neuropathy (PON).

Cancer-Associated Retinopathy

CAR is a group of autoimmune conditions that result in photoreceptor degeneration. Recoverin, a 23 kDa protein, was the first and most common retinal antigen linked to CAR.[28] Many other proteins have been identified as potential autoantigens.[29] CAR is the most frequent of the primary visual paraneoplastic disorders and is most commonly related to small cell lung carcinoma, although many other tumor types are also associated.

Most patients experience progressive symptoms of both cone and rod degeneration, including blurry vision, dyschromatopsia, prolonged glare, night blindness, prolonged dark adaptation, and peripheral scotomata, with an initially normal funduscopic appearance. Later, arteriolar narrowing, optic disc pallor, pigmentary changes, and cells may be seen. Electroretinography reveals significantly attenuated or nonrecordable tracings.[30] In the absence of a family history of retinal degeneration, the diagnosis of CAR should be considered. There is no definite effective therapy, and the visual prognosis is very poor. There have been some reports of mild to moderate visual recovery with the use of corticosteroids, plasmapheresis, and/or intravenous immunoglobulin in various combinations.[31–33]

Melanoma-Associated Retinopathy

Berson and Lessell classified MAR as a paraneoplastic disorder that affects rod photoreceptors.[34] Symptoms include shimmering, flickering, pulsating photopsias, difficulty seeing in the dark, and peripheral or paracentral scotomata. Initially, the retinal appearance may be normal. Later, vessel narrowing, pigmentary changes, optic disc pallor, and infrequent vitreous cell or periphlebitis may be seen.[35] MAR produces a characteristic electroretinogram with a negative-appearing waveform.[34,36] Antirod bipolar cell antibodies help make the diagnosis but are not specific for MAR.[37,38] There is no specific therapy for MAR. Keltner and colleagues proposed cytoreductive surgery and radiation, followed by adjuvant immunotherapy.[39] However, there was no difference in survival between those treated and those not treated. A rare patient with MAR and associated uveitis improved after corticosteroid therapy.[40]

Paraneoplastic Optic Neuropathy

PON has been associated with a number of malignancies, especially small cell lung carcinoma.[41–44] Photoreceptor cells, retinal ganglion cells, and nerve fibers exhibit collapsin response mediator protein 5 (CRMP-5, a 62 kDa protein) –specific immunoreactivity.[45]

Clinically, most patients develop subacute, progressive, bilateral, painless visual loss with optic disc edema. This may be accompanied by other neurologic symptoms, including a cerebellar syndrome.[43,44] Vitreous cells, retinal vascular leakage, and retinitis are commonly present.[45] CRMP-5 autoantibodies have been identified in the serum and cerebrospinal fluid of patients with cancer and PON and retinitis.[45] PON should be considered in patients with optic neuropathy and cancer without evidence of central nervous system metastasis. Treatment of the underlying cancer has resulted in significant visual improvement in some patients.[42,44,46] A patient reported by Hoh and colleagues responded to corticosteroids alone.[47]

Conclusion

A number of potential causes of acute and subacute visual loss have been described. However, a vast number of other etiologies of visual loss have not been covered here. All possibilities must be differentiated from one another through careful history taking, examination, ancillary testing, and appropriate ophthalmologic follow-up.

REFERENCES

1. Kollarits CR, Lubow M, Hissong SL. Retinal strokes. I. Incidence of carotid atheromata. JAMA 1972;222:1273–5.
2. Miller NR. Embolic sources of transient monocular visual loss: appearance, source, and assessment. In: Katz B, editor. Ophthalmology clinics of North America. Philadelphia: WB Saunders; 1996. p. 359–80.
3. Atabara NH, Brown GC, Carter J. Efficacy of anterior chamber paracentesis and carbogen in treating acute nonarteritic central retinal artery occlusion. Ophthalmology 1995;102:2029–35.
4. Werner MS, Latchaw R, Baker L, et al. Relapsing and remitting central retinal artery occlusion. Am J Ophthalmol 1994;118:393–4.
5. Mangat HS. Retinal artery occlusion. Surv Ophthalmol 1995;40:145.
6. Greven CM, Slusher MM, Weaver RG. Retinal arterial occlusions in young adults. Am J Ophthalmol 1995;120:776–83.
7. Hayreh SS. Central retinal vein occlusion. In: Mausolf FA, editor. The eye and systemic disease. 2nd ed. St. Louis: CV Mosby; 1980. p. 223–75.
8. Clarkson JG. Central retinal vein occlusion. In: Schachat AP, Murphy RB, editors. Retina. 2nd ed. St. Louis: CV Mosby; 1994. p. 1379–86.
9. Quinlan PM, Elman MJ, Bhatt AK, et al. The natural course of central retinal vein occlusion. Am J Ophthalmol 1990;110:118–23.
10. Weiss JN, Bynoe LA. Injection of tissue plasminogen activator into a branch retinal vein in eyes with central retinal vein occlusion. Ophthalmology 2001;108:2249–57.
11. McAllister IL, Constable IJ. Laser-induced chorioretinal venous anastomosis for treatment of non-ischemic central retinal vein occlusion. Arch Ophthalmol 1995;13:456–62.
12. Opremcak EM, Bruce RA, Lomeo MD, et al. Radial optic neurotomy for central retinal vein occlusion: a retrospective pilot study of 11 consecutive cases. Retina 2001;21:408–15.
13. Greenberg PB, Martidis A, Rogers AH, et al. Intravitreal triamcinolone acetonide for macular oedema due to central retinal vein occlusion. Br J Ophthalmol 2002;86:247–8.
14. Sadun AA, Currie JN, Lessell S. Transient visual obscurations with elevated optic discs. Ann Neurol 1984;16:489–94.
15. Hedges TR III, Gieger GL, Albert DM. The clinical value of negative temporal artery biopsy specimens. Arch Ophthalmol 1983;101:1251–4.
16. Ischemic Optic Neuropathy Decompression Trial Research Group. Characteristics of patients with nonarteritic anterior ischemic optic neuropathy eligible for the Ischemic Optic Neuropathy Decompression Trial. Arch Ophthalmol 1996;114:1366–74.
17. Ischemic Optic Neuropathy Decompression Trial Research Group. Optic nerve decompression surgery for nonarteritic anterior ischemic optic neuropathy (NAION) is not effective and may be harmful. JAMA 1995;273:625–32.
18. Young WC, Thornton AF, Gebarski SS, et al. Radiation-induced optic neuropathy: correlation of MR imaging and radiation dosimetry. Radiology 1992;185:904–7.
19. Goldsmith BJ, Rosenthal SA, Wara WM, et al. Optic neuropathy after irradiation of meningioma. Radiology 1992;185:71–6.
20. Zimmerman CF, Schatz NJ, Glaser JS. Magnetic resonance imaging of radiation optic neuropathy. Am J Ophthalmol 1990;110:389–94.
21. Guy J, Mancuso A, Beck R, et al. Radiation-induced optic neuropathy: a magnetic resonance imaging study. J Neurosurg 1991;74:426–32.
22. Tachibana O, Yamaguchi N, Yamashima T, et al. Radiation necrosis of the optic chiasm, optic tract, hypothalamus, and upper pons after radiotherapy for pituitary edema, detected by gadolinium-enhanced, T1-weighted magnetic resonance imaging: case report. Neurosurgery 1990;27:640–3.
23. McClellan RL, El Gammal T, Kline LB. Early bilateral radiation-induced optic neuropathy with follow-up MRI. Neuroradiology 1995;37:131–3.
24. Borruat F-X, Schatz NJ, Glaser JS, et al. Radiation optic neuropathy: report of cases, role of hyperbaric oxygen therapy, and literature review. Neuroophthalmology 1996;16:255–66.
25. Lana-Peixoto MA, Bambirra EA, Pittella JE. Optic nerve tuberculoma. Arch Neurol 1980;37:186–7.
26. Kupfer C, McCrane E. A possible cause of decreased vision in cryptococcal meningitis. Invest Ophthalmol 1974;13:801–4.
27. Sawyer RA, Selhorst JB, Zimmerman LE, et al. Blindness caused by photoreceptor degeneration as a remote effect of cancer. Am J Ophthalmol 1976;81:606–13.
28. Thirkill CE, Tait RC, Tyler NK, et al. The cancer-associated retinopathy antigen is a recoverin-like protein. Invest Ophthalmol Vis Sci 1992;33:2768–72.
29. Chan JW. Paraneoplastic retinopathies and optic neuropathies. Surv Ophthalmol 2003;48:12–38.
30. Matsui Y, Mehta MC, Katsumi O, et al. Electrophysiological findings in paraneoplastic retinopathy. Graefes Arch Clin Exp Ophthalmol 1992;230:324–8.
31. Klingele TG, Burde RM, Rappazzo JA, et al. Paraneoplastic retinopathy. J Clin Neuroophthalmol 1984;4:239–45.
32. Keltner JL, Thirkill CE, Tyler NK, Roth AM. Management and monitoring of cancer-associated retinopathy. Arch Ophthalmol 1992;110:48–53.
33. Guy J, Aptsiauri N. Treatment of paraneoplastic visual loss with intravenous immunoglobulin: report of 3 cases. Arch Ophthalmol 1999;117:471–7.
34. Berson EL, Lessell S. Paraneoplastic night blindness with malignant melanoma. Am J Ophthalmol 1988;106:307–11.
35. Remulla JFC, Pineda R, Gaudio A, et al. Cutaneous melanoma-associated retinopathy with retinal periphlebitis. Arch Ophthalmol 1995;113:854–5.
36. Kim RY, Retsas S, Fitzke FW, et al. Cutaneous melanoma-associated retinopathy. Ophthalmology 1994;101:1837–43.
37. Milam AH, Saari JC. Autoantibodies against retinal rod bipolar cells in melanoma-associated retinopathy. Invest Ophthalmol Vis Sci 1994;35:2116.
38. Jacobson DM, Adamus G. Retinal anti-bipolar cell antibodies in a patient with paraneoplastic retinopathy and colon carcinoma. Am J Ophthalmol 2001;131:806–8.
39. Keltner JL, Thirkill CE, Yip PT. Clinical and immunologic characteristics of melanoma-associated retinopathy syndrome: eleven new cases and a review of 51 previously published cases. J Neuroophthalmol 2001;21:173–87.
40. Jacobzone C, Cochard-Marianowski C, Kupfer I, et al. Corticosteroid treatment for melanoma-associated retinopathy: effect on visual acuity and electrophysiologic findings. Arch Dermatol 2004;140:1258–61.
41. Grunwald GB, Kornguth SE, Towfighi J, et al. Autoimmune basis for visual paraneoplastic syndrome in patients with small cell lung carcinoma. Retinal immune deposits and ablation of retinal ganglion cells. Cancer 1987;60:780–6.
42. Blumenthal D, Schochet S Jr, Gutmann L, et al. Small-cell carcinoma of the lung presenting with paraneoplastic peripheral nerve microvasculitis and optic neuropathy. Muscle Nerve 1998;21:1358–9.
43. Luiz JE, Lee AG, Keltner JL, et al. Paraneoplastic optic neuropathy and autoantibody production in small-cell carcinoma of the lung. J Neuroophthalmol 1998;18:178–81.
44. de la Sayette V, Bertran F, Honnorat J, et al. Paraneoplastic cerebellar syndrome and optic neuritis with anti-CV2 antibodies: clinical response to excision of the primary tumor. Arch Neurol 1998;55:405–8.
45. Cross SA, Salomao DR, Parisi JE, et al. Paraneoplastic autoimmune optic neuritis with retinitis defined by CRMP-5-IgG. Ann Neurol 2003;54:38–50.
46. Yu Z, Kryzer TJ, Griesmann GE, et al. CRMP-5 neuronal autoantibody: marker of lung cancer and thymoma-related autoimmunity. Ann Neurol 2001;49:146–54.
47. Hoh ST, Teh M, Chew SJ. Paraneoplastic optic neuropathy in nasopharyngeal carcinoma—report of a case. Singapore Med J 1991;32:170–3.

Metastatic Disease to the Eye and Orbit

Dan S. Gombos, MD, FACS
Angela W. Kim, MD

Ocular metastasis to the eye and orbit was first described in the late 1800s by Horner and Perl. At the time, ocular metastasis was felt to be rare; primary uveal melanoma was thought to be the most common malignancy of the eye. In 1967, Albert and Scheie suggested that the incidence of metastatic disease might be higher than previously reported. Since then, numerous studies have confirmed that uveal metastasis from solid tumors is the most common intraocular malignancy.[1-5] Its incidence varies depending on clinical and pathologic surveys ranging between 4 and 12%. Some have suggested rates as high as 30% at the time of death.[1,6] In comparison, the incidence of orbital metastasis is significantly lower than that of intraocular disease. Orbital metastasis accounts for 1.5 to 10% of all orbital tumors. This chapter discusses the clinical presentation, workup, and management of solid tumors that metastasize to the globe (eyeball) and orbit. As these clinical entities differ, they are discussed separately in the sections that follow.

Pathogenesis and Presentation of Intraocular (Uveal) Metastasis

Metastasis to the uvea occurs primarily via hematogenous dissemination through the 20 short posterior ciliary arteries that supply the posterior pole. Patients with intraocular metastasis generally complain of painless loss of vision associated with floaters and flashing lights, but up to 10% may be asymptomatic. The average age of presentation is between 40 and 70 years. Visual acuity can range from 20/20 to no light perception (blindness). Additional clinical findings may include changes in the refractive error (glasses prescription) and dilated injected episcleral vessels (red eye). Examination with an ophthalmoscope demonstrates a flat or dome-shaped subretinal mass with a creamy/yellow to yellow/white appearance (Figures 1 and 2). Larger lesions are often associated with a serous retinal detachment. The most common tumors that present in this fashion are from breast and lung primaries. Up to two-thirds of patients will have a history of cancer. Although less common, metastasis to the iris and ciliary body can also occur. In these cases, the patient may notice a visible mass on the

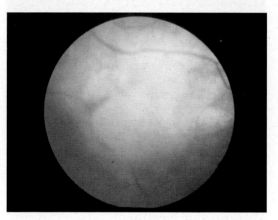

FIGURE 1 Fundus photograph of a metastatic lesion to the uvea from lung cancer. Note the creamy white appearance of this lesion.

eye with pain and increased intraocular pressure (see Figure 2).

Once uveal metastasis is identified, additional workup should be obtained to ensure an accurate diagnosis. The differential diagnosis for an amelanotic intraocular lesion is broad and includes choroidal amelanotic melanoma, hemangioma, choroidal osteoma, posterior scleritis, cytomegalovirus retinitis, choroidal neovascularization with disciform scar, and retinal detachment. Features that assist in conferring the correct diagnosis include the shape, color, and vascular pattern of the lesion. Metastatic lesions have a tendency to grow rapidly; most are located in the posterior segment of the choroid. Additional

testing is often used to confirm the diagnosis. Fluorescein angiography will demonstrate a mottled hyperfluorescence with pinpoint leakage. Ophthalmic ultrasonography demonstrates a mass with medium to high internal reflectivity.[7] These diagnostic tests, in addition to fundus photography and retinal drawings, help serve as a baseline prior to treatment. In most situations, an experienced ophthalmologist can confirm the diagnosis without the need for a biopsy. In selected cases, choroidal biopsy may be necessary via a transvitreal or transcleral approach. Tumors in the iris can be accessed via a paracentesis or anterior chamber tap.

Once the diagnosis is confirmed, systemic workup is indicated. Uveal metastasis has a high association with central nervous system (CNS) involvement. All patients should undergo additional staging, including neuroimaging of the brain and orbits. Malignancies associated with specific tumor markers should have those blood tests reassessed. Management of uveal metastasis varies and depends on the size and intraocular location of the lesion, the presence (or absence) of concurrent CNS disease, and previous therapies administered to the patient.

Observation can be considered for small peripheral asymptomatic lesions that appear to be inactive. Generally, large lesions and those that threaten vision are treated. The most common form of treatment is radiation therapy, which can be administered via external beam or plaque

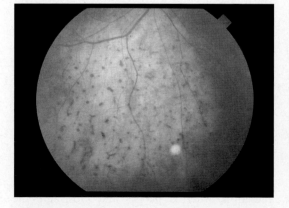

FIGURE 2 Photographs of metastatic lesions to the choroid (A) and iris (B) from breast cancer. Note the injected episcleral blood vessels (B).

brachytherapy. Patients requiring systemic management and those with distant metastasis may be good candidates for chemotherapy.[8,9] All patients need close serial assessment by an ophthalmologist to ensure that their lesions are responding. In advanced cases in which there is no potential for vision and the eye is painful or associated with neovascular glaucoma, enucleation (removal of the eye) can be considered.

Lesions should be monitored closely by an ophthalmologist with serial examinations, photography, and ultrasonography. Over time, tumor foci generally fragment with pigment migration and associated resolution of serous retinal detachment. Even patients with significant visual loss at presentation can regain useful vision following treatment. Recurrences can occur, and patients should be instructed to monitor their vision closely. Those treated with radiation may develop secondary toxicities from treatment such as dry eye and cataract.

Orbital Metastasis

Metastatic disease to the eyelid and orbit is less common than intraocular metastasis. However, with the prolonged survival of patients with cancer, the frequency of orbital metastasis is increasing. Patients may present with droopiness of the lid, a palpable mass, term exophthalmos, enophthalmos, limitation of extraocular motility, double vision, pain, paresthesia, headache, or decreased vision. In some instances, sudden clinical changes may occur owing to hemorrhage or necrosis within the tumor. Rarely, lesions may be pulsatile due to increased vascularity or erosion of adjacent bone with transmission of cerebrospinal pulsations. The lateral orbit is the most common quadrant in which metastasis occurs, followed by the superior, medial, and inferior quadrants. Symptoms precede the diagnosis of a systemic malignancy in up to 42% of patients.[10] Goldberg and colleagues defined five orbital syndromes associated with metastasis.[10] They included: mass effect (causing proptosis); infiltration of orbital tissues; functional (a decrease in cranial nerve function); acute or subacute inflammation; or silent (no orbital symptoms). These patients may be initially misdiagnosed as having alternative diagnoses, such as orbital inflammatory syndrome, cellulitis, or myasthenia gravis.[10]

Two orbital findings are highly associated with specific malignancies. Enophthalmos (an inward displacement of the globe) often occurs in the setting of metastatic breast cancer, but it can also be seen with gastrointestinal, lung, and prostate carcinomas. In this setting, cicatrization with contracture of myofibroblasts causes the retraction of orbital contents (Figure 3). In children, orbital metastasis from neuroblastoma frequently presents with sudden onset of ecchymosis and proptosis with a dramatic

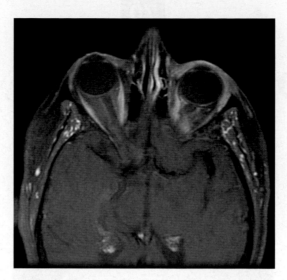

FIGURE 3 Magnetic resonance image demonstrating enophthalmos in a patient with metastatic breast cancer to the left orbit.

clinical progression. Mediastinal involvement may manifest as Horner's syndrome (ptosis, miosis, and anhidrosis); opsoclonus-myoclonus (a paraneoplastic effect) may also be seen.

Workup and Treatment

Once suspected, orbital imaging is indicated. This should include neuroimaging of the brain and adjacent sinus structures. Magnetic resonance imaging (MRI) is helpful in distinguishing metastasis from other simulating lesions, such as optic nerve gliomas, optic nerve sheath meningiomas, and orbital inflammatory syndrome. An MRI should be ordered to include fat-saturated images in both coronal and axial planes, with and without gadolinium. Metastatic lesions are isodense to muscle on T_1-weighted imaging and hyperdense to brain tissue on T_2-weighted imaging. Computed tomography, including axial and coronal views with contrast, is helpful for tumor localization, to aid in identifying small orbital apex lesions, and to confirm or rule out adjacent bone involvement.

In patients with diffuse metastatic disease and involvement of other structures, treatment can proceed empirically. However, in cases for which tissue diagnosis is necessary, biopsy should be performed. This can be done via an open technique or fine-needle aspiration. Orbital metastases are generally treated with palliative radiotherapy or chemotherapy unless considered a solitary isolated metastasis. In the latter case, surgical excision can also be considered. Those tumors that are radiosensitive can respond quickly with dramatic improvement of symptoms. Some studies have suggested that up to 73% of patients show improvement after orbital radiotherapy. Of all symptoms, proptosis is the most responsive to radiation, whereas paresis and ptosis are the least responsive. Alternative modalities are also effective; neuroblastoma and small cell carcinoma

respond well to chemotherapy. Hormonal therapy can be effective in the settings of breast and prostate cancers.

Prognosis

Metastatic lesions to the eye and orbit often respond well to treatment. In many cases, useful vision can be preserved. However, their presence is a grave prognostic indicator for patient survival. Those with orbital metastatic lesions generally live longer than those with metastatic disease to the uvea. The median survival following intraocular metastasis ranges from 9 to 10 months. Median survival following orbital metastasis ranges from 12 to 26 months. Breast, carcinoid, and thyroid tumors are associated with the longest survival, sometimes measured in years. Lung carcinoma, gastrointestinal carcinoma, and cutaneous melanoma usually present in the setting of fulminant dissemination. Accordingly, median survival of less than 6 months is commonly seen in patients with these primary tumors.[1-5]

Conclusion

The diagnosis and management of ocular metastasis require a broad multidisciplinary approach. The primary clinician and oncologist should refer patients to an ophthalmologist whenever patients complain of blurry vision, floaters, pain, and redness. The ophthalmologist must communicate directly with the oncologist to ensure that the appropriate workup is initiated and that the patient is appropriately restaged. Once the extent of metastasis is identified, treatment should be initiated as soon as possible. Although many tumors will respond to therapy with preservation of some vision, the prognosis for patient survival is poor.

REFERENCES

1. Vople NJ, Albert DM. Metastases to the uvea. In: Albert DM, Jakobiec FA, editors. Principles and practice of ophthalmology. Vol 5. 4th ed. Philadelphia: WB Saunders; 1994. p. 3260–70.
2. Shields JA, Shields CL, Gross NE, et al. Survey of 520 eyes with uveal metastases. Ophthalmology 1997;104: 1265–76.
3. Shields JA, Shields CL. Intraocular tumors: a text and atlas. Philadelphia: WB Saunders; 1992.
4. Ferry AP, Font RL. Carcinoma metastatic to the eye and orbit: I. A clinicopathological study of 227 cases. Arch Ophthalmol 1974;92:276–86.
5. Char DH. Clinical ocular oncology. Philadelphia: Lippincott-Raven; 1997.
6. Landis SH, Murray T, Bolden S, et al. Cancer statistics, 1999. CA Cancer J Clin 1999;49:8–32.
7. Coleman DJ, Abramson DH, Jack RL, et al. Ultrasonic diagnosis of tumors of the choroid. Arch Ophthalmol 1974;91:344–54.
8. Letson AD, Davidorf FH, Bruce RA Jr. Chemotherapy for treatment of choroidal metastasis from breast carcinoma. Am J Ophthalmol 1982;93:102–6.
9. Reddy S, Saxena VS, Hendrichson F, et al. Malignant metastatic disease of the eye; management of an uncommon complication. Cancer 1981;47:810–2.
10. Goldberg RA, Rootman J, Cline RA. Tumors metastatic to the orbit: a changing picture. Surv Ophthalmol 1990;35: 1–24.

Obstetric and Gynecologic Issues

Michael Frumovitz, MD, MPH

Brian M. Slomovitz, MD

Diane C. Bodurka, MD

The Pregnant Cancer Patient

The diagnosis of cancer is often overwhelming, especially for the pregnant patient. Medical decision making can become extremely complex as the health of both the mother and the fetus must be considered. Appropriate treatment planning is influenced by the indication for treatment, the safety issues associated with each treatment modality, and the patient's feelings regarding continuation of the pregnancy. The informed consent process disclosing all associated risks and benefits of therapy is crucial.

Maternal cancer complicates approximately 1 in 1,000 to 1 in 5,000 live births in the United States annually,[1] and there are approximately 4,000 cases of concurrent pregnancy and maternal malignancy in the United States each year.[2]

The most frequently diagnosed cancer in pregnancy is cervical cancer, followed by breast cancer, melanoma, ovarian cancer, thyroid cancer, leukemia, lymphoma, and colorectal cancer. Pregnancy does not increase the risk of malignancy, and the incidence of specific malignancies in pregnant women is similar to that in nonpregnant women of the same age range. The incidence of cancer complicating pregnancy may increase as more women delay childbearing until later in life.

Chemotherapy and Pregnancy

All chemotherapeutic regimens are potentially teratogenic and mutagenic. Although controlled studies have been performed on pregnant laboratory animals, one must be cautious when extrapolating animal data to human pregnancies. Since it is not possible to perform prospective studies that evaluate chemotherapy during pregnancy, treatment regimens are frequently based on case reports and small retrospective studies.

Both the mother and the fetus may be affected by chemotherapy. When evaluating the potential effect of a specific antineoplastic agent on the developing fetus, it is important to consider both the maternal physiologic processes that accompany pregnancy and the developmental stage at which the fetus is exposed to the treatment.

Pregnancy may affect the absorption, distribution, and excretion of chemotherapeutic agents.[3] The increase in maternal blood volume affects the distribution of antineoplastic agents, whereas the absorption of oral agents may be influenced by changes in gastrointestinal motility. An increase in the glomerular filtration rate changes the rate of renally excreted agents. Virtually all chemotherapeutic agents cross the placenta.

The developmental stages of the embryo and fetus have been well documented. These stages are divided into the preimplantation period (fertilization to implantation), the embryonic period (gestational weeks 2 through 8), and the fetal period (week 9 to term). Several principles apply to the effects of chemotherapy on the fetus based on these stages.

The first trimester is the most crucial time period and is best characterized by the all-or-none principle in terms of impact on the fetus. Since its circulation has not yet been established, the blastocyst is resistant to teratogens in the preimplantation period. After this time, an exposed blastocyst may be severely damaged and result in a spontaneous abortion. Conversely, the blastocyst may survive without abnormalities.

During the period of organogenesis (gestational weeks 5 through 12), the fetal stem cell population is limited. This is the period of maximal susceptibility to teratogenic insults. Ten to 25% of fetuses exposed to cytotoxic agents during this time period have major malformations.[4] It is generally recommended that chemotherapy administration be delayed until after the first trimester if possible.

Organogenesis is completed by the end of the twelfth gestational week, with the exception of brain and gonadal tissue. Fetal growth restriction owing to chemotherapy surpasses the risk of structural birth defects. However, since the central nervous system continues to develop throughout the fetal period, cortical brain function may be affected by these agents.[3]

Both maternal and fetal physiology during the final weeks of gestation must be taken into consideration when planning and administering chemotherapy. This should also be coordinated with the anticipated time of delivery. In an effort to decrease potential maternal chemotherapy-related complications from delivery, myelosuppressive regimens, which may cause neutropenia or thrombocytopenia, should be avoided approximately 3 weeks prior to the anticipated delivery.

Given that the placenta functions as a route for drug delivery and excretion, the timing of administration of chemotherapy may also affect the neonate. Elevated drug levels may be seen in the newborn if neoplastic agents are administered within close proximity to delivery owing to a lack of elimination. Additionally, a limited ability of the neonatal liver and kidneys to metabolize and excrete specific agents may also elevate the blood levels of these drugs, especially in the preterm infant. Several authors have reported that children born to mothers receiving chemotherapy during pregnancy experienced no physical, neurologic, psychologic, hematologic, or cytogenetic defects.[5,6] However, premature birth and low birth weight for gestational age are likely to be the most common complications associated with maternal chemotherapy administration, and these rates are most likely underreported.[7]

Many chemotherapeutic agents, including cisplatin, cyclophosphamide, doxorubicin, hydroxyurea, and methotrexate, can be found in breast milk. Because of this, breast-feeding is contraindicated in women receiving chemotherapy.[8,9]

Radiation Therapy and the Pregnant Patient

As with chemotherapy, the administration of radiation during pregnancy requires careful consideration of therapeutic and ethical issues. It is difficult to establish accurate estimates of risks owing to a lack of clinical trial data. The majority of available data regarding radiation and pregnancy outcome are extrapolated from animal models or reported in small retrospective series. And as with chemotherapy, the period of fetal development influences the impact of in utero radiation exposure.

The blastocyst is most sensitive to the in utero lethal effects of ionizing radiation during preimplantation and early implantation (the first 10 days after conception). Doses as low as 10 cGy have been shown to increase prenatal death and embryonic resorption in laboratory mice. Virtually all animal experiments, however, reveal that survivors of radiation exposure during this time period develop no congenital anomalies.[10,11]

The greatest incidence of malformations in animals irradiated in utero occurs during organogenesis. This time period is also the time of maximal susceptibility to chemotherapy-induced teratogenicity. Human exposure to radiation during this time period results in intrauterine growth retardation and central nervous system–related anomalies, such as eye abnormalities, severe mental retardation, and microcephaly. Structural abnormalities are not usually seen from radiation therapy. A dose threshold of 5 to 10 cGy has been suggested for the above anomalies, based on data from Japanese survivors of the atomic bomb.[11] This analysis, however, is somewhat compromised by a lack of accurate dosimetry on which to base risk estimates.

Although the fetal stage extends to 12 to 14 weeks' postconception in humans, the central nervous system continues to develop until term. The central nervous system remains sensitive to radiation through approximately 25 weeks after conception. Milder forms of microcephaly and other central nervous system anomalies can occur.[12] Growth retardation may be seen with doses greater than 50 cGy.[11]

The threshold dose below which radiation would not adversely affect a pregnancy is not known. Although several authors suggest that doses less than 10 cGy do not cause adverse effects, any dose of radiation may be capable of inducing genetic mutations, which may not be expressed until future generations.[13] It has been estimated that in utero radiation of 1 cGy may double the risk of childhood malignancies during the first 10 years of life, especially in terms of leukemias.[14] Despite this increase in risk, the absolute risk of future cancers remains low. Table 1 presents the estimated fetal dose of radiation from several common diagnostic procedures.

In utero exposure to 10 cGy is the cutoff point for consideration of therapeutic abortion.[14] Despite this, case reports of 50 cGy administered during the first trimester have not demonstrated a substantial risk of malformation.[11] Radiation therapy directed to the abdomen or pelvis during pregnancy will result in high doses of radiation to the fetus and should be avoided unless pregnancy loss owing to spontaneous abortion or evacuation is expected. Issues regarding radiation exposure of the pregnant patient, including the topic of

Table 1 Estimated Fetal Dose from Common Diagnostic Radiologic Exposure

Type of Examination	Fetal Dose Range in cGy (rad)
Chest radiograph	0.00006
Abdomen flat plate	0.15–0.26
Lumbar spine	0.65
Pelvis	0.2–0.35
Hip	0.13–0.2
Intravenous pyelography	0.47–0.82
Upper GI series	0.17–0.48
Barium enema	0.82–1.14
Mammography	Essentially undetectable
CT of head	0.007
CT of upper abdomen	0.04*
CT of pelvis	2.5
99mTc bone imaging	0.15†

Adapted from Kessel, Rijpkema et al, and Rossouw et al.[23–25]
CT = computed tomography; GI = gastrointestinal.
*For early pregnancy with uterus confined to the pelvis.
†Based on an ovarian dose of 0.015 cGy per mCi of 99mTc, with a typical injected dose of 10 mCi. Bladder drainage should be used owing to a high local dose from urinary excretion of the radiopharmaceutical.

therapeutic abortion, require consideration of all factors affecting the mother and the fetus.

Maternal Hypothyroidism in the First Trimester

Patients treated with radiation therapy, specifically for cancers of the head and neck, are at risk of developing hypothyroidism. Radiation treatment is well recognized as a cause of hypothyroidism. Almost 50% of patients develop hypothyroidism 5 years after radiation therapy, and by 8 years after radiation, almost two-thirds of patients develop hypothyroidism.

For women of childbearing potential, monitoring and correcting thyroid levels are important. Hypothyroidism has been associated with an increased risk of miscarriage, lower infant IQ, placental abruption, and preterm birth.

Prevention of Vaginal Hemorrhage in Cancer Patients of Reproductive Age

Cancer patients of reproductive age are often given treatments that may lead to vaginal bleeding. Once bleeding has started, and if this bleeding is treatment related, the underlying cause, such as thrombocytopenia, should be corrected. Intravenous estrogen (Premarin) may be given at a dose of 25 mg every 4 hours for 24 hours or until bleeding stops. Alternatively, oral contraceptives may be given three times a day for 3 days, then twice a day for 3 days, and then daily.

If there is an increased risk of vaginal bleeding, hormonal agents can be administered, which can function to prevent the incidence of bleeding. Progestins (megestrol, medroxyprogesterone) work by stabilizing the endometrium and

decrease cyclical bleeding if taken continuously. Similarly, oral contraceptive pills can be administered. Depending on the duration of therapy and the nadirs associated with the cytotoxic agents given, oral contraceptive pills can be taken daily for up to 3 months without inducing a menstrual cycle.

Gonadotropin-releasing hormone agonists (eg, leuprolide) have also been used to suppress vaginal bleeding during chemotherapy. In addition, these agents may function to enhance ovarian function and preserve fertility.[15] This is particularly important for adolescent females who are exposed to multiple chemotherapeutic agents.

Vaginal Hemorrhage

The appropriate initial management of the patient who presents with vaginal bleeding requires a stepwise approach to determine the etiology of the bleeding. Vaginal bleeding in postmenopausal women is abnormal. While common causes of vaginal bleeding include endometrial polyps, fibroids, hyperplasia, or atrophic changes (due to lack of estrogen), cancer needs to be considered in the differential diagnosis. In premenopausal women, bleeding may be due to pregnancy-related disease and should be further evaluated with a pregnancy test.

If the pregnancy test is positive, the differential diagnosis includes spontaneous abortion, missed abortion, molar pregnancy, gestational trophoblastic disease, and ectopic pregnancy (discussed later in this chapter). If the patient is bleeding vigorously, large-bore intravenous access should be obtained, fluids should be administered, and blood should be sent to evaluate hematologic and clotting levels. A type and screen should be ordered; a type and crossmatch may be necessary. Careful physical and pelvic examinations should be performed. Any visible lesion in the vagina that may appear bluish in color should not be biopsied as this may precipitate hemorrhage from choriocarcinoma. An obstetrician/gynecologist should be consulted for further evaluation and management.

Women with gestational trophoblastic disease may present with vaginal bleeding and a positive pregnancy test. Although a high index of suspicion is required to diagnose this disease, women may present with a history of multiple emergency room visits for threatened abortion, a uterus larger in size than the reported gestational age, and no fetal movement. They may also experience significant nausea, vomiting, and hypertension. On pelvic examination, the cervical os is usually closed and the uterus is larger than expected for the gestational age. Ultrasonography of the pelvis should be performed; pathognomonic findings include a multiechogenic pattern and absence of fetal parts. A chest radiograph and quantitative serum β-human chorionic gonadotropin (hCG) should be obtained. The patient should be admitted to the hospital. An obstetrician/gynecologist should be consulted for appropriate evaluation, evacuation of the pregnancy, and follow-up.

If the pregnancy test is negative and the bleeding is heavy, a thorough physical examination and pelvic examination should again be performed, with careful attention given to visualization and inspection of the vagina and cervix. If the bleeding is due to an exophytic cervical lesion, a vaginal pack with Monsel's solution should be placed. The patient should be admitted to the hospital for more definitive diagnosis and potential emergent therapy. Treatment options for hemorrhage not controlled by packing include hypogastric artery embolization, transvaginal radiation, and hypogastric artery ligation.

If the cervix is grossly normal in appearance, consideration should be given to an endometrial biopsy if this can be performed. Any vaginal lesion should also be biopsied. If the patient is not bleeding heavily, she may be discharged with immediate referral to a gynecologist or to a gynecologic oncologist if malignancy is suspected.

The vulva and vagina should also be inspected, especially in older women. Packing and hospital admission may be required to establish a definitive diagnosis and begin appropriate treatment.

Ectopic Pregnancy

Ectopic pregnancy is the leading cause of pregnancy-related death during the first trimester. The diagnosis and treatment of tubal pregnancy prior to tubal rupture significantly decrease the risk of maternal death. Early detection of tubal pregnancy increases treatment options, and some patients may be able to receive medical as opposed to surgical intervention.

Since the early 1970s, the incidence of ectopic pregnancy has tripled. In 1992, there were an estimated 109,000 ectopic pregnancies, representing approximately 20 per 1,000 pregnancies and almost 10% of all pregnancy-related deaths.[16] Current Centers for Disease Control and Prevention data do not include ectopic pregnancies diagnosed or treated in physicians' offices, thereby underestimating the true incidence of ectopic pregnancy.

Several factors have been identified as contributing to the increased incidence of ectopic pregnancy. These include the rising incidence of acute and chronic salpingitis, tubal ligation, tubal reconstructive surgery, and conservative management of tubal pregnancy, all of which cause structural damage to the tube; an increase in the use of intrauterine contraceptive devices (IUDs), which assisted reproductive technology/*in vitro* fertilization increase the risk of ectopic pregnancy by a factor of 4; and improved technology, which allows for more definitive diagnosis of

some patients whose condition may have been undetected in the past.

Many retrospective studies have shown that patients with an ectopic pregnancy may be evaluated by a physician on several occasions before the correct diagnosis is made. This delay in diagnosis is usually related to a low index of suspicion on the part of the clinician. An awareness of the risk factors associated with ectopic pregnancy is critical to a prompt diagnosis. Significant risk factors are as follows:

- A history of tubal infection (increases the rate of ectopic pregnancy from 1 in 200 to 1 in 24)
- Previous ectopic pregnancy (15–50% increase in the incidence of ectopic pregnancies in subsequent pregnancies),
- A history of tubal reconstructive surgery
- A history of tubal sterilization within the previous 2 years
- Pregnancy with an IUD in place or a history of IUD use

Although there are no pathognomonic symptoms of ectopic pregnancy, the classic triad consists of history of amenorrhea, new onset vaginal bleeding, and abdominal pain.

Amenorrhea or a history of an abnormal last menstrual period is associated with 75 to 90% of ectopic pregnancies. Vaginal bleeding, which may consist of light spotting or may be as heavy as a menstrual period, results from low hCG production by the ectopic trophoblast; this occurs in 50 to 80% of patients with an ectopic pregnancy. Abdominal pain is present in more than 90% of cases.

Identifying the correct diagnosis in a patient with an acutely ruptured ectopic pregnancy is fairly straightforward. The patient usually presents with symptoms of abdominal pain and distention, as well as hypovolemia (eg, tachycardia, orthostatic blood pressure changes, diaphoresis). Shoulder pain may be present owing to irritation of the phrenic nerve from blood in the peritoneal cavity.

The diagnosis of an unruptured ectopic pregnancy is more difficult to make. Physical examination findings in these patients are extremely variable. Although 90% of patients have abdominal tenderness, only 45% have rebound tenderness. Fifty percent of patients have a palpable adnexal mass. In half of these cases, the mass is contralateral to the ectopic pregnancy and is actually the corpus luteum.[17]

Several critical diagnostic tests should be obtained in patients suspected of having an ectopic pregnancy. These include a urine hCG, transvaginal ultrasonography, and quantitative serum β-hCG. The rapid hCG is obtained to diagnose pregnancy. The β-hCG should be drawn at the time of presentation and then repeated as

necessary. The doubling time of β-hCG in the serum varies from 1.2 days immediately following implantation to 3.5 days 2 months after the last menstrual period. It is important to understand that ectopic gestations may be associated with a normal rise in hCG levels, as well as with plateauing or decreasing titers. If serial quantitative levels of β-hCG do not fall into the normal range, ultrasonography should be performed to attempt to locate the pregnancy. Transvaginal ultrasonography permits the identification of an intrauterine gestational sac at as early as 5 weeks of amenorrhea (2 mm diameter), which virtually rules out an ectopic pregnancy.

The management of an ectopic pregnancy has changed significantly in recent years. Therapeutic options vary from medical therapy to emergent laparotomy. The appropriate treatment depends on the medical status of the patient and the characteristics of the pregnancy. Surgery (either laparotomy or laparoscopy) is indicated in patients with an unstable cardiovascular status, a vaginal sonogram identifies a gestational mass > 3.5 cm, the b-hCG is > 15,000 mIU/dL, or fetal cardiac activity is identified. A patient with stable cardiac status, a gestational mass < 3.5 cm identified on ultrasonography, and b-hCG < 15,000 mIU/dL is an appropriate candidate for medical management with methotrexate. For those patients who are eligible for methotrexate other criteria, such as a willingness to return for follow-up care, must be discussed by the patient and her physician.

The key to successful management of ectopic pregnancy is early diagnosis. Although the number of cases of ectopic pregnancy has steadily increased, the mortality has declined significantly in the past 10 years.[18] A high index of suspicion and vigorous efforts to make an early diagnosis must be made by all physicians evaluating women of reproductive age who present to the emergency room with abdominal pain and a positive pregnancy test.

Rectovaginal Fistulae

A rectovaginal fistula is an epithelium-lined communication between the rectum and the vagina. Although most fistulae are related to obstetric trauma, carcinoma, whether it is primary, recurrent, or metastatic, can lead to a rectovaginal fistula. The most common cancers are rectal, cervical, vaginal, and endometrial. If a patient with a rectovaginal fistula has a history of any of these cancers, a biopsy of the fistula is necessary. Radiation of the pelvis or perineum is another cause of a rectovaginal fistula. The radiation results in tissue damage and decreased vascular supply, which can lead to a proctitis and subsequent ulceration of the rectal wall. The frequency of radiation-induced rectovaginal fistulae is 0.3 to 6%. The incidence increases with higher doses of radiation. These fistulae are usually to the mid- or upper vagina and will occur within 2 years of treatment.

The majority of rectovaginal fistulae are symptomatic, with the patient complaining of the passage of stool or flatus via the vagina. If the fistula cannot be identified on examination, the patient may require additional studies. Contrast studies (eg, barium enema, computed tomography with rectal contrast) are useful.

The treatment of a rectovaginal fistula must be tailored to the individual fistula and the patient's long-term prognosis. A colostomy is often necessary. Depending on medical comorbidities, disease state, and body habitus, a patient can have either a transverse loop colostomy or an end-descending colostomy.

Treatment of Menopausal Symptoms

Menopause, the cessation of ovulation and its accompanying symptoms, marks an important physiologic and social transition in a woman's life. The average age of natural menopause in the United States is 52.6 years.[19] Patients who are postmenopausal at the time of their diagnosis and treatment of cancer are now living longer owing to advances in therapy. Patients who are still having regular menstrual cycles at the time of their cancer diagnosis are often made menopausal by the treatment. For example, the majority of patients with leukemia and lymphoma are under 50 years, and a large proportion of them will be made menopausal with traditional chemotherapy, high-dose chemotherapy, bone marrow transplantation, or radiotherapy.[20] Almost 15% of patients with endometrial cancer will be premenopausal at diagnosis.[21] Standard treatment for these women includes bilateral salpingoophorectomy as part of the surgical staging of the disease. Owing to early detection and improved therapy, women who are iatrogenically made menopausal as a side effect of their cancer treatment may live many decades in a menopausal state.

Vasomotor symptoms are the most commonly reported and often the most distressing symptoms of menopause. Nearly 60% of menopausal women report hot flashes, night sweats, and/or sleep disturbances.[22] Genitourinary symptoms such as vaginal dryness or atrophy and accompanying dyspareunia are also well documented.[22] There is often an accompanying decrease in libido and sexual desire with menopause. The long-term effects of osteoporosis are of particular concern in those cancer patients with an excellent prognosis made menopausal at an early age. For them, the decades without estrogen put them at risk of fractures of the vertebrae, hips, and wrist. In postmenopausal white women, 90% of hip fractures are attributable to

osteoporosis and 20% of them will die within 1 year of sustaining the injury.[23] In addition, long-term deficiency in estrogen has been associated with increasing the risk and mortality of coronary artery disease, as well as the memory loss and cognitive deficits associated with Alzheimer's disease.

In the past, these symptoms and sequelae of the hypoestrogenemic state had been easily managed with hormone replacement therapy. Epidemiologic, observational, and animal studies had repeatedly shown that these medications provided excellent relief of vasomotor and genitourinary symptoms in addition to maintaining bone density. In addition, it was thought that the estrogen component of hormone replacement therapy had an added cardioprotective effect by lowering lipid levels.[24] However, the results from the Women's Health Initiative (WHI), a large randomized control study, showed a significantly higher risk of coronary heart disease in postmenopausal women receiving estrogen and progesterone hormone replacement when compared with controls.[25] Although there were fewer hip fractures in the hormone therapy group, there was a higher rate of breast cancer, stroke, and pulmonary embolism in women receiving estrogen and progesterone. The size and design of the study and the wide media attention to its findings resulted in a sharp decrease in women taking hormone replacement therapy almost immediately on its publication.[26] Over the past years, however, many physicians have reconsidered the initial adverse reaction to the WHI results as women have continued to suffer with vasomotor and genitourinary symptoms in the immediate period after entering menopause. For that reason, many expert panels have recommended the short-term use of hormone replacement therapy (5–7 years) for the control of vasomotor and genitourinary symptoms associated with menopause.[27–29] Women who have not had a hysterectomy should receive combination estrogen and progesterone therapy, whereas women who have had their uterus removed may receive estrogen alone. Continuation of hormone therapy after the initial 5- to 7-year period after entering menopause should be considered carefully and reevaluated on a regular basis.

Hormone replacement therapy for the control of vasomotor and genitourinary symptoms in the immediate postmenopausal period may not be appropriate for all women who have had a cancer diagnosis. Controversy remains as to the effects of hormone replacement therapy in breast cancer survivors. Observational data suggest no increase in the risk of recurrence in patients with breast cancer.[30,31] However, at least one prospective study has demonstrated an increased risk of breast cancer recurrence in women taking hormone replacement therapy when compared

with controls.[32] The hormonal dependence of breast cancer cells and the use of tamoxifen and letrozole (antiestrogenic drugs), coupled with the prospective study findings, make many physicians hesitant to prescribe hormone replacement therapy to women with a history of breast cancer. Likewise, hormonal replacement therapy for women with a history of ovarian and endometrial cancers is felt to be contraindicated by some clinicians owing to the hormonal dependence of the neoplastic cells. Other cancer survivors who should not receive hormone replacement therapy are those women who are at increased risk of thromboembolic events owing to the increase in hypercoagulability events in women taking estrogen with progesterone[25] and estrogen alone.[33] For most women with a diagnosis of cancer, a short course (5–7 years) of hormone replacement therapy for the control of vasomotor symptoms is a reasonable option.

For women with either contraindications to hormone replacement therapy or continued vasomotor symptoms after initial treatment with hormone replacement therapy, other options exist. Behavioral modifications, such as lowering ambient air temperature,[34] exercise,[35] and smoking cessation,[36] may decrease the number and severity of hot flashes. In addition, nonprescription remedies, such as isoflavones, black cohosh, or vitamin E, may be tried for mild hot flashes. These medications may have an effect on vasomotor symptoms. However, there are no conclusive studies demonstrating their efficacy or detailing their absorption. Selective serotonin reuptake inhibitors (SSRIs), such as fluoxetine[37] and venlafaxine,[38] have been shown in randomized, double-blinded, placebo-controlled trials to significantly reduce hot flashes. These medications have an additional benefit of mood elevation in women with depression, a subclinical finding in many postmenopausal patients. The anticonvulsant gabapentin has also been shown to significantly reduce hot flashes.[39] This medication is also well tolerated and might also reduce somatic pain experienced by cancer survivors. Clonidine has been used successfully to treat hot flashes; however, many patients are unable to tolerate the drug-related side effects.[40] There are several treatment options for vasomotor symptoms in addition to hormone replacement therapy. Which regimen to choose will depend on the severity of the symptoms, other comorbidities, and patient and physician preferences. Without treatment, vasomotor symptoms will typically subside spontaneously, although this may take a long period of time.

Menopausal genitourinary symptoms of vaginal dryness, atrophy, and accompanying dyspareunia in addition to dysuria and incontinence can be made worse by cancer treatment. Tamoxifen has been noted to increase these symptoms in women taking this medication for breast cancer.[41] Women who have received pelvic irradiation have significantly increased symptoms of vaginal dryness, atrophy, and dyspareunia.[42] Nonhormonal vaginal lubricants, such as Replens and K-Y jelly, can reduce vaginal dryness and dyspareunia. However, these remedies will not restore the atrophic vaginal and urethral epithelium and therefore will not relieve all of the vaginal or any of the urinary symptoms. Oral hormone replacement therapy has been the most effective in addressing all of these symptoms. Locally administered estrogen in the form of either a vaginal cream or an extended-release vaginal ring or pessary can also alleviate most of the genitourinary symptoms.[43] These routes of estrogen administration are attractive as they do not raise systemic levels of circulating estrogen.[44]

The reduction in libido in postmenopausal women may be partially related to vaginal dryness and dyspareunia. However, a lack of circulating hormones also affects sexual desire. Hormone replacement therapy may alleviate the associated vaginal symptoms that may be physical barriers to sexual intimacy. However, estrogen therapy has little effect on decreased sexual drive.[45] On the contrary, testosterone replacement may be necessary to restore libido.[46] Ongoing studies and drug development continue in an effort to help postmenopausal women regain sexual desire.

As mentioned, osteoporosis and its associated morbidities and mortality are an important consideration for the postmenopausal female. Women with hematologic malignancies such as leukemia, lymphoma, and myeloma are at increased risk of bone loss at baseline. Behavioral modifications such as smoking cessation and weight-bearing exercise help maintain bone strength and structure. Adequate daily intake of both calcium and vitamin D are also important.[47] For patients not taking hormone replacement therapy, other pharmacologic agents may be used to treat osteopenia or osteoporosis. Bisphosphonates have been shown to be equally effective as hormone replacement therapy in preventing postmenopausal bone loss.[48] Side effects such as gastrointestinal distress have made compliance with daily administration of bisphosphonates difficult in the past. However, patients can now take weekly or monthly doses, which greatly reduces the overall side effects and may increase compliance. Selective estrogen receptor modulators (SERMs), such as tamoxifen and raloxifene, also conserve bone mass, thereby reducing the risk fractures. This class of drug also has an additional benefit of reducing the risk of breast cancer and might also decrease the risk of coronary artery disease.[49] Unfortunately, these drugs have no effect on vasomotor or genitourinary symptoms and may actually worsen those symptoms in the acute period just after beginning the medication.

In summary, with more aggressive therapies and improved prognosis, women with cancer are becoming menopausal at a younger age and living longer in this state. Menopause is accompanied by acute vasomotor and genitourinary symptoms. Hormone replacement therapy remains the best treatment for the acute symptoms of menopause and can be safely used for a limited time (5–7 years) in most cancer patients. Patients with breast, ovarian, or endometrial malignancies should discuss this option with their oncologist. Other medications, such as SSRIs and gabapentin, may also alleviate vasomotor symptoms. For women not taking hormonal therapy or other medications, vasomotor symptoms will resolve with time. Despite this, the genitourinary symptoms will persist and worsen with age. For these women, vaginal estrogen may provide good relief of genitourinary symptoms. The decrease in libido, however, will not be affected by this formulation. Research continues as to the role of testosterone to help postmenopausal women maintain their sexual drive.

The long-term effects of menopause include osteoporosis, coronary artery disease, and possible changes in cognitive function. Women with hematologic malignancies are at an increased risk of osteoporosis and should be followed carefully. Exercise, smoking cessation, and dietary intake of calcium and vitamin D are recommended to maintain bone mineral density. Bisphosphonates and SERMs have also been shown to prevent osteopenia and osteoporosis. Newer formulations of the bisphosphonates make administration less frequent and side effects more tolerable. SERMs such as tamoxifen and raloxifene not only have a protective effect on bone, they also reduce the risk of breast cancer and may prevent coronary artery disease in postmenopausal women. They often, however, exacerbate the vasomotor and genitourinary symptoms of hypoestrogenism. To date, there are no recommendations as to how best to manage the heart disease and cognitive loss associated with menopause.

REFERENCES

1. Waalen J. Pregnancy poses tough questions for cancer treatment. J Natl Cancer Inst 1991;83:900–02.
2. Stovall M, Blackwell RC, Cundiff J, et al. Fetal dose from radiotherapy with photon beams: report of AAPM Radiation Therapy Committee Task Committee Task Group No. 36. Med Phys 1995;22:63.
3. Cunningham FG, MacDonald PC, Gant NF, et al. Neoplastic diseases. In: Cunningham FG, MacDonald PC, Gant NF, et al. 19th ed. Norwalk (CT): Appleton & Lange; 1993. p. 1267–9.
4. Caligiuri MA, Mayer RJ. Pregnancy and leukemia. Semin Oncol 1989;16:388–96.
5. Aviles A, Diaz-Magneo JC, Talavera A, et al. Growth and development of children of mothers treated with chemotherapy during pregnancy: current status of 43 children. Am J Hematol 1991;36:243–8.
6. Berry DL, Theriault RL, Holmes FA, et al. Management of breast cancer during pregnancy using a standardized protocol. J Clin Oncol 1999;17:855–61.
7. Garber JE. Long-term follow-up of children exposed in utero to antineoplastic agents. Semin Oncol 1989;16:437–44.
8. Ben-Baruch G, Menczer J, Goshen R, et al. Cisplatin excretion in human milk. J Natl Cancer Inst 1992;84:451–2.
9. Egan PC, Costanza M, Dadion P, et al. Doxorubicin and cisplatin excretion into human breast milk. Cancer Treat Rep 1985;69:1387–9.
10. Hall EJ. Effects of radiation on the embryo and fetus. In: Hall EJ, editor. Radiobiology for the radiologist. 4th ed. Philadelphia: JB Lippincott; 1994. p. 363.
11. Stovall M, Blackwell RC, Cundiff J, et al. Fetal dose from radiotherapy with photon beams: report of AAPM Radiation Therapy Committee Task Group No. 36. Med Phys 1995;22:63–9.
12. Dekabon AS. Abnormalities in children exposed to x-radiation during various stages of gestation: tentative timetable of radiation injury to the human fetus, part I. J Nucl Med 1968;9:471–7.
13. Gaulden ME. Possible effects of diagnostic x-rays on the human embryo and fetus. J Ark Med Soc 1974;70:424–35.
14. Hall EJ. Effects of radiation on the embryo and fetus. In: Hall EJ, editor. Radiobiology for the radiologist. 4th ed. Philadelphia: JB Lippincott; 1994. p. 363.
15. Pereyra Pacheco B, Mendez Ribas JM, Milone G, et al. Use of GnRH analogs for functional protection of the ovary and preservation of fertility during cancer treatment in adolescents: a preliminary report. Gynecol Oncol 2001;81:391–7.
16. Centers for Disease Control and Prevention. Ectopic pregnancy-United States, 1990-1992. MM Weekly Report 1995;44:46–8.
17. Breen JL. A 21 year study of 645 ectopic pregnancies. Am J Obstet Gynecol 1970;106:1004–19.
18. Centers for Disease Control and Prevention. Ectopic pregnancy in the USA. MMWR Morb Mortal Wkly Rep 1989;38:481.
19. Reynolds RF, Obermeyer CM. Age at natural menopause in Spain and the United States: results from the DAMES project. Am J Hum Biol 2005;17:331–40.
20. Piccioni P, Scirpa P, D'Emilio I, et al. Hormonal replacement therapy after stem cell transplantation. Maturitas 2004;49:327–33.
21. Soliman PT, Oh JC, Schmeler KM, et al. Risk factors for young premenopausal women with endometrial cancer. Obstet Gynecol 2005;105:575–80.
22. Obermeyer CM, Reynolds RF, Price K, Abraham A. Therapeutic decisions for menopause: results of the DAMES project in central Massachusetts. Menopause 2004;11:456–65.
23. Kessel B. Hip fracture prevention in postmenopausal women. Obstet Gynecol Surv 2004;59:446–55; quiz 85.
24. Rijpkema AH, van der Sanden AA, Ruijs AH. Effects of postmenopausal oestrogen-progestogen replacement therapy on serum lipids and lipoproteins: a review. Maturitas 1990;12:259–85.
25. Rossouw JE, Anderson GL, Prentice RL, et al. Risks and benefits of estrogen plus progestin in healthy postmenopausal women: principal results from the Women's Health Initiative randomized controlled trial. JAMA 2002;288:321–33.
26. Ettinger B, Grady D, Tosteson AN, et al. Effect of the Women's Health Initiative on women's decisions to discontinue postmenopausal hormone therapy. Obstet Gynecol 2003;102:1225–32.
27. Estrogen and progestogen therapy in postmenopausal women. Fertil Steril 2004;82 Suppl 1:S70–80.
28. Burger H, Archer D, Barlow D, et al. Practical recommendations for hormone replacement therapy in the peri- and postmenopause. Climacteric 2004;7:210–6.
29. Treatment of menopause-associated vasomotor symptoms: position statement of The North American Menopause Society. Menopause 2004;11:11–33.
30. O'Meara ES, Rossing MA, Daling JR, et al. Hormone replacement therapy after a diagnosis of breast cancer in relation to recurrence and mortality. J Natl Cancer Inst 2001;93:754–62.
31. Col NF, Hirota LK, Orr RK, et al. Hormone replacement therapy after breast cancer: a systematic review and quantitative assessment of risk. J Clin Oncol 2001;19:2357–63.
32. Holmberg L, Anderson H. HABITS (hormonal replacement therapy after breast cancer—is it safe?), a randomised comparison: trial stopped. Lancet 2004;363:453–5.
33. Miller J, Chan BK, Nelson HD. Postmenopausal estrogen replacement and risk for venous thromboembolism: a systematic review and meta-analysis for the U.S. Preventive Services Task Force. Ann Intern Med 2002;136:680–90.

34. Molnar GW. Body temperatures during menopausal hot flashes. J Appl Physiol 1975;38:499–503.

35. Ivarsson T, Spetz AC, Hammar M. Physical exercise and vasomotor symptoms in postmenopausal women. Maturitas 1998;29:139–46.

36. Whiteman MK, Staropoli CA, Langenberg PW, et al. Smoking, body mass, and hot flashes in midlife women. Obstet Gynecol 2003;101:264–72.

37. Loprinzi CL, Sloan JA, Perez EA, et al. Phase III evaluation of fluoxetine for treatment of hot flashes. J Clin Oncol 2002;20:1578–83.

38. Evans ML, Pritts E, Vittinghoff E, et al. Management of postmenopausal hot flushes with venlafaxine hydrochloride: a randomized, controlled trial. Obstet Gynecol 2005;105:161–6.

39. Guttuso T Jr, Kurlan R, McDermott MP, Kieburtz K. Gabapentin's effects on hot flashes in postmenopausal women: a randomized controlled trial. Obstet Gynecol 2003;101:337–45.

40. Laufer LR, Erlik Y, Meldrum DR, Judd HL. Effect of clonidine on hot flashes in postmenopausal women. Obstet Gynecol 1982;60:583–6.

41. Day R, Ganz PA, Costantino JP, et al. Health-related quality of life and tamoxifen in breast cancer prevention: a report from the National Surgical Adjuvant Breast and Bowel Project P-1 Study. J Clin Oncol 1999;17:2659–69.

42. Frumovitz M, Sun CC, Schover LR, et al. Quality of life and sexual functioning in cervical cancer survivors. Journal of Clinical Oncology 2005;23:7428–36.

43. Barentsen R, van de Weijer PH, Schram JH. Continuous low dose estradiol released from a vaginal ring versus estriol vaginal cream for urogenital atrophy. Eur J Obstet Gynecol Reprod Biol 1997;71:73–80.

44. Gabrielsson J, Wallenbeck I, Birgerson L. Pharmacokinetic data on estradiol in light of the estring concept. Estradiol and estring pharmacokinetics. Acta Obstet Gynecol Scand Suppl 1996;163:26–31; discussion 32–4.

45. Simon J, Klaiber E, Wiita B, et al. Differential effects of estrogen-androgen and estrogen-only therapy on vasomotor symptoms, gonadotropin secretion, and endogenous androgen bioavailability in postmenopausal women. Menopause 1999;6:138–46.

46. Shifren JL, Braunstein GD, Simon JA, et al. Transdermal testosterone treatment in women with impaired sexual function after oophorectomy. N Engl J Med 2000;343:682–8.

47. Dawson-Hughes B, Harris SS, Krall EA, Dallal GE. Effect of calcium and vitamin D supplementation on bone density in men and women 65 years of age or older. N Engl J Med 1997;337:670–6.

48. Hosking D, Chilvers CE, Christiansen C, et al. Prevention of bone loss with alendronate in postmenopausal women under 60 years of age. Early Postmenopausal Intervention Cohort Study Group. N Engl J Med 1998;338:485–92.

49. Jordan VC, Gapstur S, Morrow M. Selective estrogen receptor modulation and reduction in risk of breast cancer, osteoporosis, and coronary heart disease. J Natl Cancer Inst 2001;93:1449–57.

Sexual Function Issues

Pamela T. Soliman, MD

Kathleen M. Schmeler, MD

Diane C. Bodurka, MD

Normal sexual function depends on multiple factors, including sexual desire, normal response to arousal, and the ability to achieve orgasm. Sexual dysfunction, for various reasons, is a common problem for both patients with cancer and those who survive cancer. Sexual dysfunction may develop early in a patient's disease course, during cancer treatment (related to surgery, radiation, chemotherapy, or hormonal therapy), as a result of symptom management, or after cancer treatment has been completed. Unfortunately, during cancer care, sexual difficulties are rarely addressed, and most patients receive little or no assistance in dealing with the effects of cancer care and treatment on intimacy.[1]

Libido

Libido, or the desire to have sex, is often affected by multiple factors during cancer treatment. Psychological factors, including depression and anxiety, that are often associated with the diagnosis of cancer can have a significant impact on one's desire to be sexually active. Also contributing significantly to loss of sexual desire are the medical interventions that occur during cancer treatment. At the present time, a majority of cancers are treated with a combination of surgery, radiation, and/or chemotherapy. All of these modalities can have some impact on sexual desire.

Surgery

Surgical treatment for cancer often requires hospitalization, anesthesia, exploration of body cavities, and the need to recover from the surgery itself. Postoperative pain and fatigue often affect sexual desire, particularly in the immediate weeks following surgery.[2] Surgeries that have the most impact on sexual desire and function are those involving the pelvis, such as radical prostatectomy, radical cystectomy, abdominoperineal resection for rectal cancer, and radical hysterectomy for gynecologic cancers. This is in part due to changes in body image; however, physiologic effects from the surgery itself also affect sexual function.

Pelvic surgery for both men and women can interfere with the innervation of the pelvic organs and therefore can affect the physiologic response to sexual stimuli. The amount of dysfunction depends on the extent of injury to the sacral plexus. In men, surgery for bladder, rectal, or prostate cancer can affect the ability to have an erection by disruption of the parasympathetic sacral nerve fibers. Although there are procedures designed to spare the sacral nerve fibers, compression or trauma to the nerves can lead to a transient decrease in function, from which it may take a significant amount of time to recover.[3] A list of the most common side effects associated with radical pelvic surgery in men is shown in Table 1.

Table 1 Most Common Physiologic Effects of Pelvic Surgery on Male Sexual Function

Procedure	Common Effects
Radical prostatectomy	Decrease in ability to have an erection May decrease intensity of orgasm Dry orgasm
Radical cystectomy	Decrease in ability to have an erection May decrease intensity of orgasm Dry orgasm Pain with intercourse (rare)
Abdominoperineal resection	Decrease in ability to have an erection May decrease intensity of orgasm Dry orgasm Pain with intercourse (rare)
Total pelvic exenteration	Impaired ability to have an erection May decrease intensity of orgasm Dry orgasm

In women, pelvic surgery can also lead to sexual dysfunction. Jensen and colleagues evaluated sexual function and quality of life in 173 women treated with radical hysterectomy for early-stage cervical cancer.[4] Lack of interest in sex was a common finding among women at 5 weeks (77%) and even up to 2 years after surgery (57%). Dyspareunia, or pain during intercourse, was more common in the immediate time period after surgery; however, a few patients reported dyspareunia 2 years after surgery. Sexual dysfunction associated with pelvic surgery in women is commonly attributed to vaginal shortening and stenosis. In addition, vaginal dryness owing to a lack of estrogen is common in women who undergo oophorectomy at the time of surgery.[5,6] These physiologic changes affect not only affect the ability to function normally but also the desire to engage in sexual activity. The extent of these side effects depends on the type of surgery performed and the organs involved. The most common side effects on sexual function owing to pelvic surgery in women are listed in Table 2.

Radiation

Radiation therapy can result in both immediate and long-term side effects that influence sexual desire and sexual function. During radiation treatment, patients are often fatigued and nauseated and may have skin changes to the radiated areas of the body. All of these symptoms can have a significant effect on the desire to be sexually active, as well as an impact on body image. In a cohort of 118 women who were disease free after treatment with radiation for cervical or vaginal cancer, Jensen and colleagues reported that 91% of patients had low or no sexual interest 1 month after the completion of radiotherapy.[5] Other common symptoms in the immediate period after treatment included a moderate to severe lack of lubrication, vaginal irritation, foul-smelling discharge, and dyspareunia. These symptoms of sexual dysfunction resulted in a high level of distress in this population, and in many of these women, symptoms persisted for at least 2 years after the completion of treatment.

Table 2 Most Common Physiologic Effects of Pelvic Surgery on Female Sexual Function

Procedure	Common Effects
Simple hysterectomy	Vaginal dryness Shortening of the vagina Pain with intercourse (rare)
Radical hysterectomy	Vaginal dryness Shortening of the vagina Pain with intercourse (rare)
Radical cystectomy	Vaginal dryness Pain with intercourse Vaginal dryness
Abdominoperineal resection	Vaginal dryness Pain with intercourse
Total pelvic exenteration and vaginal reconstruction	Loss of erotic zones Need to relearn how to reach orgasm Pain with intercourse (occasional)
Radical vulvectomy	Loss of erotic zones Severe vaginal dryness Need to relearn how to reach orgasm Pain with intercourse

In addition to the short-term side effects of radiation, prolonged external beam radiation can lead to fibrosis of soft tissues, the development of scar tissue, and loss of nerve function. This has a particular effect on patients who have high-dose primary radiotherapy for the treatment of prostate, bladder, cervical, or rectal cancer. External beam radiation to the pelvis also affects the small vessels that help supply the pelvic organs. In men, this can be as damaging as primary surgery to the nerves responsible for erectile function. In contrast to the vascular and nerve damage caused by surgery, the damage related to radiation therapy may not be apparent until months after the completion of therapy.[7] Finally, radiation can cause injury to adjacent normal tissues, including the bladder, rectum, and vagina, which may lead to symptoms that detract from sexual desire, including proctitis, cystitis, and vaginal stenosis.[2]

Improvements in radiation delivery, including the introduction of brachytherapy for the treatment of localized prostate cancer, seem to have had an impact on the side effects associated with pelvic radiation, including those that affect sexual function. Reis and colleagues compared the effects of prostatectomy and primary radiotherapy on sexual function in 158 men with localized prostate cancer.[8] In this cohort, erectile dysfunction was reported in 85% of men who were treated by radical retropubic prostatectomy and in only 23% of men treated with brachytherapy. Other studies have also found that erectile dysfunction may be higher among surgically managed patients; however, there are data to suggest that, over time, the treatment modalities have similar effects on sexual function and desire.[9,10]

Chemotherapy

The effects of chemotherapy on sexual function can also be divided into immediate and long-term effects. During the course of treatment with chemotherapy, many patients experience nausea, vomiting, fatigue, hair loss, and mucositis. Women in particular may experience vaginal or perineal mucositis, causing discomfort during intercourse. These short-term side effects vary depending on the chemotherapy agent used; however, they can all influence a man or woman's feeling of well-being and desire to engage in sexual activity.[2]

In a large cohort of breast cancer patients, Ganz and colleagues found that patients who had received chemotherapy as part of their primary treatment reported more sexual problems at the end of primary treatment than women who did not receive chemotherapy. Lack of interest in sex was reported in 23.4% of all patients in the study, with a greater frequency among women who had received chemotherapy ($p = .002$). They also found that vaginal lubrication problems and pain during intercourse were more severe among women who received chemotherapy. These findings have been reported in previous studies.[11,12] A higher number of women (50%) who received chemotherapy reported that breast cancer had a negative effect on their sex life compared with women who had not received chemotherapy ($p < .001$).[13]

The long-term effects of chemotherapy in women have also been described. These include premature menopause and loss of fertility.[14,15] Up to 50% of premenopausal breast cancer patients report changes in their menstrual periods after the diagnosis of breast cancer. These changes are seen more frequently in women who receive chemotherapy.[13] Goodwin and colleagues found that among patients with early-stage breast cancer, age and systemic chemotherapy were the strongest predictors of early menopause.[16] Physiologic changes associated with menopause, including vaginal dryness, atrophy, and dyspareunia, contribute to discomfort during sexual intercourse and affect a woman's desire to have intercourse and her ability to become aroused. These factors play a major part in a woman's libido and sexual function. There are limited data available on the long-term effects of chemotherapy on libido in the male population.

Hormonal Therapy

In a subset of endocrine-sensitive cancers, hormonal therapy has been used for both prevention and treatment. This type of therapy can also affect sexual desire and sexual function. Tamoxifen, an antiestrogenic compound used in the prevention and treatment of breast cancer, has been shown to increase vaginal discharge and vasomotor symptoms.[11,17,18] Although there are no clear data to suggest that sexual function is statistically different when comparing women on tamoxifen with those taking placebo, some studies have shown that almost 50% of women on tamoxifen complain of pain, burning, or discomfort with intercourse. In addition, a high proportion of these women require the use of vaginal lubricants during intercourse owing to vaginal dryness.[17,19]

Other hormonal therapies used to treat cancer in women include megesterol acetate, gonadotropin-releasing (Gn-RH) analogues, and aromatase inhibitors. Progesterone therapy with megesterol acetate is sometimes used in the treatment of breast or endometrial cancer. Megesterol acetate is also used as an appetite stimulant in cancer and noncancer patients. Consequently, one of the main side effects is weight gain, which can have a negative effect on body image and sexual desire.[20] Gn-RH analogues, which have been used in women with breast or ovarian cancer, are associated with menopausal symptoms, which have also been shown to have a negative impact on sexual desire and sexual function.[21] Aromatase inhibitors are the newest class of hormonal therapy used for postmenopausal breast cancer patients. Although the data are limited, there is some suggestion that use of aromatase inhibitors can result in vaginal dryness, which may result in problems with sexual function.[2]

In men, hormonal therapy is primarily used in the treatment of prostate cancer. Gn-RH analogues are used to eliminate the effects of adrenal androgens. The primary side effect from this therapeutic approach is decreased libido. Although many men can physically achieve an erection and ejaculation despite loss of testosterone, a decrease in libido is commonly reported. In fact, some men who are asymptomatic with a rising prostate-specific antigen choose to delay hormonal therapy for this reason. In men with advanced or progressive disease, other factors have an effect on erectile function and sexual desire, making it difficult to determine the additive effect of the hormonal therapy.[2]

Many patients receive a combination of surgery, radiation, chemotherapy, and hormonal therapy as primary treatment for their cancer. In addition, patients also receive various treatment modalities for recurrent or progressive disease. As such, it is not uncommon for patients to suffer side effects from each of these treatment modalities, which may compound the negative effects on sexual desire and sexual function.

Side Effects of Therapy

In general, single- or multimodality cancer treatment is associated with fatigue, pain, and declining physical function. These factors also have a significant influence on libido and sexual functioning. Fatigue is a common symptom associated with cancer diagnosis and treatment that is associated with decreased libido.[22,23] Chronic fatigue tends to affect most cancer patients but is more prevalent in certain types of cancer, including Hodgkin's lymphoma.[24] This may be related to specific side effects of treatment, such as anemia, but is likely multifactorial and represents the long-term side effects of both chemotherapy and radiation.[2]

Uncontrolled or chronic pain can also contribute to a loss of libido. Pain often manifests itself as psychological distress, poor appetite, and lack of sleep, all of which may have a negative effect on sexual interest. The association between pain and decreased sexual function is intuitive; however, few studies have been conducted to support this relationship. A small study on patients who received high-dose chemotherapy and autologous bone marrow for breast cancer patients found that pain was associated with a decrease in sexual function.[25] There are also some data to support the fact that pain increases psychological distress, which may increase sexual dysfunction.[26]

Medications

In addition to the effects of primary treatment on sexual desire and function, cancer patients are often prescribed multiple medications during their cancer treatment. Many of these medications can affect libido and sexual function. In most cases, the benefits of taking these medications outweigh the side effects; however, it is important to understand what these side effects are to determine if appropriate changes in these medications can be made to alleviate some of the unwanted side effects.

Nausea is a symptom that commonly results from cancer treatment. It is one of the most common short-term side effects associated with both radiation and chemotherapy. In addition, patients who undergo surgery often require antiemetic agents in the postoperative recovery period. Although nausea itself can decrease libido, many of the medications used to treat nausea can also interfere with sexual desire. The primary reason for this effect is that many of these medications also act as sedatives. In addition, certain classes of antiemetics can affect hormone levels that alter sexual desire.[27]

Narcotics are also commonly prescribed at the time of diagnosis or for pain related to cancer treatment. In addition, these medications are often continued in patients who have persistent pain through the course of treatment or for those who have progressive disease. The dose and duration of narcotic use are patient dependent. When narcotics are taken for long periods of time,

tolerance can develop, and patients may require higher doses to achieve the same degree of pain control. When given in large doses, narcotic pain medications can decrease sexual desire.[27]

Difficulty sleeping, anxiety, depression, and chronic pain are often treated with sedatives, anxiolytics, or antidepressants in the cancer patient. In general, sedatives have a negative effect on sexual desire. Similarly, most medications that are used to treat anxiety also decrease sexual desire in men and women. Antidepressant medications, on the other hand, can have a variety of effects on sexual desire. If antidepressant use results in improvement in mood, this may enhance sexual desire. However, the physiologic effects of some of these medicines can have a negative effect on sexual desire. Many of these effects are patient and medication dependent.[27]

Finally, many cancer patients and cancer survivors have other medical comorbidities for which they require medications. Heart disease and hypertension are common medical problems in older men and women. Therefore, medications used to treat these comorbidities are not uncommon in cancer patients. These medications can also complicate the issue of decreased libido and sexual dysfunction.

Sexual desire and sexual function in the cancer patient and cancer survivor are very complicated issues. Multiple factors, including treatment modality, cancer-associated symptoms, medication side effects, and various psychological factors, contribute to a patient's desire or lack of desire for intimacy.

Impotence

Erectile dysfunction is a relatively common problem in the general population. In a large national survey of 18- to 59-year-olds in the United States, 31% of men reported some type of sexual dysfunction. The most common problems reported were premature ejaculation (28.5%), anxiety about performance (17%), lack of interest in sex (15.8%), and inability to maintain an erection (10.4%).[28] As men grow older, the prevalence of erectile dysfunction increases, and by the age of 70, up to 50% of men are impotent.

Erectile dysfunction associated with cancer treatment is primarily due to damage to the sacral nerve plexus, devascularization of the pelvic organs, and changes in hormone levels. These effects can be due to surgery, radiation, chemotherapy, and hormonal therapies. Erectile dysfunction can also result from treatment of other non–cancer-related conditions, such as hypertension and heart disease.

A majority of the studies evaluating erectile dysfunction in cancer patients and survivors have focused on the men who are at the highest risk, those with prostate cancer. Several studies have

suggested that 30 to 50% of men have significant sexual dysfunction at the time of diagnosis with prostate cancer.[29–31] Following treatment with either surgery or definitive radiation therapy, the rates increase to 50 to 80%, and in men who require antiandrogen therapy for advanced prostate cancer, the rates of sexual dysfunction approach 80 to 90%.[32]

Because erectile dysfunction affects such a high proportion of men undergoing therapy for prostate cancer, changes in treatment have been made to help decrease erectile dysfunction. From a surgical standpoint, the nerve-sparing radical prostatectomy has been introduced and has been shown to have some effect on preservation of erectile function. One group reported that up to 86% of men who underwent bilateral nerve-sparing prostatectomy could achieve erections functional for intercourse within 18 months of surgery.[33] Although these data look promising, the patients in this cohort tended to be younger (median age 57 years). Other studies in older populations have reported that approximately 20% of men who undergo bilateral nerve-sparing radical prostatectomy recover to have erections firm enough for vaginal intercourse.[34–37] Although most studies have found that there is some benefit to this approach, further study will be required to determine exactly how effective this procedure is in preserving erectile function.

Modifications in the delivery of radiotherapy, including the use of brachytherapy, three-dimensional conformal therapy, and intensity-modulated therapy, may help preserve erectile function by sparing surrounding tissues.[7,29,35,38–40] Potency after radiation therapy for prostate cancer has been reported to be as high as 30 to 60%.[41] Several studies have suggested that preservation of erectile function is superior after radiotherapy than after surgical therapy; however, there are conflicting reports. Talcott and colleagues did the first prospective study comparing the two treatment modalities, using a validated quality of life questionnaire to evaluate sexual function.[7] They reported that erectile dysfunction was higher initially in the surgery group; however, over time, sexual function declined in the radiotherapy group and improved in the surgically treated group. The longer the follow-up period, the smaller the difference detected between the two treatment groups. This likely relates to the difference in the physiologic damage to the sacral nerve plexus and vasculature of the pelvis that was discussed earlier in the chapter.

Although physicians continue to modify treatments to help prevent erectile dysfunction, impotence continues to affect a large percentage of men treated for prostate cancer. As such, physician and health care workers should also focus on the treatment of erectile dysfunction and sexual rehabilitation.

Psychosocial Issues

Although it is clear that treatment for cancer can affect the physiologic response to sexual stimuli, psychological factors can also have a significant impact on sexual desire and sexual function. Psychological distress is often associated with sexual dysfunction in healthy individuals, and this has also been identified in different cancer populations. Several studies have suggested that the symptoms of depression and anxiety are commonly identified in men and women with cancer. Major depressive disorder has been described in as many as 50% of cancer patients, which is significantly higher than in the general population (8%).[42,43] This is of particular importance because these conditions are often underdiagnosed and therefore undertreated.

Many of the studies evaluating the predictors of psychological distress among cancer patients have been disease specific. In ovarian cancer patients, 30 to 50% of newly diagnosed patients report moderate to severe levels of anxiety.[44,45] This high level of anxiety and psychological distress may be related to the diagnosis of ovarian cancer or related treatments. Completion of therapy and entering the "watching and waiting" period can also be equally distressing. More importantly, many of these women (60%) are not receiving mental health services or psychotropic medications.[46] This suggests that we need to improve detection and treatment of these conditions in cancer patients. Although anxiety and depression can have many implications in the cancer population, these conditions can also affect sexual desire and sexual function.

In a study of newly diagnosed breast cancer patients, Schag and colleagues found that women who were considered at risk of psychological distress based on an evaluation at the time of diagnosis were more likely to report problems with sexual function 1 month and 1 year after diagnosis than women who were categorized as low risk.[47] Reported problems with sexual function included a lack of interest in having sex, difficulty in being sexually aroused, and difficulty reaching orgasm. Similar findings have been described in patients with Hodgkin's disease and acute leukemia.[48]

Cull and colleagues evaluated a group of early-stage cervical cancer patients who were treated successfully with either surgery or radiotherapy.[49] Two years after treatment, approximately 50% of women continued to report persistent tiredness and a lack of energy. There were no differences in outcome or psychological status when comparing the two treatment groups. Overall, the rates of anxiety and depression were higher in patients with early-stage cervical cancer than expected for the general population. Many

patients were found to have high levels of psychological distress, which correlated significantly with both physical complaints and functional outcomes. In the subgroup of women who were sexually active, they felt that their sexual function post-treatment was significantly poorer when compared with pretreatment. Approximately 50% of women reported that they would have liked to receive counseling for their psychological and sexual concerns.

Body Image

In addition to a number of other factors that affect psychological well-being during cancer treatment and diagnosis, body image can have a significant impact on sexual desire and sexual function. The body image changes that are associated with cancer and cancer treatment can be very dramatic. These changes range from surgical defects and deformities (including limb amputation, loss of a breast, and pelvic exenteration) to total body alopecia (loss of scalp hair, eyebrows, pubic and axillary hair). More subtle changes can include weight loss secondary to disease or weight gain from treatment with corticosteroids. All of these factors affect a patient's self-esteem and sexual attractiveness.[2] For some patients, the physical difficulties and the emotional sequelae are so disruptive that they no longer engage in sexual activity.[50]

In a comprehensive evaluation of multiple factors that affect sexual function in ovarian cancer patients, Carmack Taylor and colleagues determined that women who liked the appearance of their body were more likely to be sexually active.[51] Other predictors of sexual activity in these women included being married, being younger than 56 years old, not receiving active treatment at the time of the study, and a longer interval of time between treatment and evaluation of sexual function. This model confirmed that body image, in addition to other factors, was important in the evaluation of sexual function in cancer patients.

In women with breast cancer, breast-conserving procedures have been implemented to help preserve body image. Multiple studies have shown that breast-conserving surgery can have a positive impact on self-image after treatment for breast cancer.[52–54] Women treated with breast-conserving surgery had a more favorable body image, were more satisfied with their surgery, and had better cosmetic results when compared with women treated with mastectomy.[55] Several studies have suggested that issues of body image are more important in a younger population; however, body image has also been shown to be important in the older breast cancer population. Receiving treatment that was consistent with preferences about appearance was important in determining long-term mental health.[56]

A longitudinal study of women with gynecologic cancers treated with pelvic exenteration found that prior to surgery, patients were anxious about or uncomfortable with the body changes that were going to occur as a result of surgery. Many women reported feeling unattractive and uninterested in having sex. After surgery, body image, attractiveness, and self-confidence were all reduced. The extent of surgery and the amount of reconstruction also had a significant impact on body image. Women who had two ostomy sites (to drain bowel and bladder contents) had significantly more problems with physical, sexual, and marital issues when compared with women with one or no ostomy sites. In addition, women who did not have vaginal reconstruction also felt significantly less attractive and self-confident.[57] It is important to recognize that different surgical procedures can have a different impact on quality of life and body image.

It is clear that in the general population, body image and self-esteem have a significant impact on sexual desire and sexual function. Cancer treatment can result in dramatic changes in body image and self-esteem. More conservative organ-preserving surgical approaches and reconstructive surgery, where appropriate, may help alleviate some of the distress associated with these changes in body image.

Sexual Rehabilitation

Assessment

Sexual function is an important aspect of quality of life and should be assessed in all patients diagnosed with cancer. It is important to have a baseline assessment of sexual function to determine if a patient has difficulties with sexual function prior to the initiation of treatment. This may help prevent the patient and the physician from having unrealistic expectations of sexual function during and after completion of treatment.

Evaluating and assessing sexual dysfunction in a cancer patient may require a multidisciplinary approach. Although many oncologists do not have the time or training to address sexual issues, having the primary oncologist perform the initial assessment may have several advantages. It emphasizes to patients that the treating physician sees them as a whole person and not just as someone with a diseased body part. It also indicates to patients that the treating physician understands that sexual function is an important aspect of quality of life. Finally, it gives patients permission and freedom to talk about issues of sexual function during and after cancer treatment.[1]

The initial assessment may be as limited as asking patients if they have any sexual problems or concerns and reassuring them that these issues are common among cancer patients. If a sexual problem is identified or if the oncologist does not feel equipped to address the issue, involvement of a multidisciplinary team may be warranted. This may include mental health professionals trained in sex therapy, gynecologists familiar with concerns regarding hormone replacement or dyspareunia, urologists who specialize in the treatment of erectile dysfunction, and infertility specialists if a patient desires to have children. Once a problem is identified, further questioning may help determine who should be involved in the care of a particular patient. Sample questions to further assess sexual function are shown in Table 3. Topics addressed should include desire, arousal, orgasm, and pain.[2]

The PLISSIT model, which was designed in the 1970s, provides a more structured approach to communicating with patients about sexuality and allows clinicians to gear this communication to their own level of comfort.[58] The acronym PLISSIT was developed from the concepts of permission, limited information, specific suggestions, and intensive therapy. This basic theory starts by giving patients permission to disclose their problem with sexual function and then allowing the clinician to provide information regarding the issues brought forward and make suggestions for future directions. This may include treatment by the primary team or referral to a specialist.

It is important to realize that psychological stressors not related to cancer diagnosis and treatment may also be affecting a patient's sexual desire and sexual function. This may include difficulty with relationships, a history of sexual trauma, unusual guilt about sexuality, other medical problems, and substance abuse.[2],[1] It is also important to consider the influence of aging on sexual function because it is sometimes difficult to distinguish cancer-related changes from the normal slowing of sexual response that is associated with increasing age.

Treatment of Sexual Dysfunction

Once a sexual problem has been identified, the level and type of intervention that are needed must be assessed.[2] In some cases, the sexual problem can be addressed directly by an expert in that field (ie, gynecologist or urologist), although patients who have more complex problems may require referral to a mental health professional trained in sex therapy. The most important step an oncologist can take is to provide information to patients and their partners about sexual functioning, aging, and sexual problems related to cancer treatment. Schover's book, *Sexuality and Fertility after Cancer*, includes a wealth of information and detailed self-help instructions for many of the common sexual problems among cancer patients.[27] This may help ease patients' concerns and facilitate them getting help.

In women, one of the most common symptoms associated with cancer treatment and aging is vaginal dryness. In women who can safely receive estrogen replacement therapy (ERT) after cancer, this is the most effective treatment regimen. Studies suggest that in women who are good candidates for ERT, this should be considered early on in the treatment course to prevent any disruption in normal sexual function. This can be given either in pill form, as a vaginal cream, or as an estradiol-impregnated ring (Estring). Other options include vaginal lubricants and moisturizers such as Vagifem, Astroglide, or K-Y Jelly.

In men, the most common problem is erectile dysfunction. As discussed earlier, erectile dysfunction can be the result of a number of cancer-related issues. It may be related to surgery, radiation, or low testosterone levels after hormonal therapy, or it may be a side effect of a medication. To effectively treat erectile dysfunction, the cause or causes of impotence must be defined. Treatments can then be targeted toward the underlying cause. Some of these issues can be addressed only prior to the initiation of therapy, for example, performing a nerve-sparing prostatectomy or using targeted radiotherapy instead of external beam radiation. After primary therapy, medication changes or correction of abnormal hormone levels may also be effective. If these changes are ineffective, there are oral erectogenic agents and medical devices that can enhance erectile function. It is important that only physicians who have expertise prescribe these modalities as they are not safe for all men.

Summary

Sexual dissatisfaction and/or sexual dysfunction can affect 20 to 90% of adult cancer patients.[59] This may be may related to primary cancer treatment, a result of symptom management, or may occur after cancer treatment has been completed. It is clear that multiple factors affect each cancer patient and his or her desire for sexual activity. The assessment and treatment of these sexual problems can be equally complex.

It is important to have a multidisciplinary approach to effectively diagnose and treat patients with sexual dysfunction.

REFERENCES

1. McKee AL Jr, Schover LR. Sexuality rehabilitation. Cancer 2001;92(4 Suppl):1008–12.
2. Ganz PA LM, Meyerowitz BE. Sexual problems. In: Devita VT, editor. Cancer: principles and practice of oncology. 7th ed. Phililedphia: Lippincott, Williams, and Wilkins; 2005. p. 2662–76.
3. Walsh PC, Donker PJ. Impotence following radical prostatectomy: insight into etiology and prevention. J Urol 1982;128:492–7.
4. Jensen PT, Groenvold M, Klee MC, et al. Early-stage cervical carcinoma, radical hysterectomy, and sexual function. A longitudinal study. Cancer 2004;100:97–106.
5. Jensen PT, Groenvold M, Klee MC, et al. Longitudinal study of sexual function and vaginal changes after radiotherapy for cervical cancer. Int J Radiat Oncol Biol Phys 2003;56:937–49.
6. van Driel MF, Weymar Schultz WC, van de Wiel HB, et al. Female sexual functioning after radical surgical treatment of rectal and bladder cancer. Eur J Surg Oncol 1993;19:183–7.
7. Talcott JA, Rieker P, Clark JA, et al. Patient-reported symptoms after primary therapy for early prostate cancer: results of a prospective cohort study. J Clin Oncol 1998;16:275–83.
8. Reis F, Netto NR Jr, Reinato JA, et al. The impact of prostatectomy and brachytherapy in patients with localized prostate cancer. Int Urol Nephrol 2004;36:187–90.
9. Fulmer BR, Bissonette EA, Petroni GR, Theodorescu D. Prospective assessment of voiding and sexual function after treatment for localized prostate carcinoma: comparison of radical prostatectomy to hormonobrachytherapy with and without external beam radiotherapy. Cancer 2001;91:2046–55.
10. McCammon KA, Kolm P, Main B, Schellhammer PF. Comparative quality-of-life analysis after radical prostatectomy or external beam radiation for localized prostate cancer. Urology 1999;54:509–16.
11. Ganz PA, Rowland JH, Desmond K, et al. Life after breast cancer: understanding women's health-related quality of life and sexual functioning. J Clin Oncol 1998;16:501–14.
12. Berglund G, Nystedt M, Bolund C, et al. Effect of endocrine treatment on sexuality in premenopausal breast cancer patients: a prospective randomized study. J Clin Oncol 2001;19:2788–96.
13. Ganz PA, Kwan L, Stanton AL, et al. Quality of life at the end of primary treatment of breast cancer: first results from the moving beyond cancer randomized trial. J Natl Cancer Inst 2004;96:376–87.
14. Bines J, Oleske DM, Cobleigh MA. Ovarian function in premenopausal women treated with adjuvant chemotherapy for breast cancer. J Clin Oncol 1996;14:1718–29.
15. Knobf MK, Mullen JC, Xistris D, Moritz DA. Weight gain in women with breast cancer receiving adjuvant chemotherapy. Oncol Nurs Forum 1983;10:28–33.
16. Goodwin PJ, Ennis M, Pritchard KI, et al. Adjuvant treatment and onset of menopause predict weight gain after breast cancer diagnosis. J Clin Oncol 1999;17:120–9.
17. Day R, Ganz PA, Costantino JP, et al. Health-related quality of life and tamoxifen in breast cancer prevention: a report from the National Surgical Adjuvant Breast and Bowel Project P-1 Study. J Clin Oncol 1999;17:2659–69.
18. Fallowfield L, Fleissig A, Edwards R, et al. Tamoxifen for the prevention of breast cancer: psychosocial impact on women participating in two randomized controlled trials. J Clin Oncol 2001;19:1885–92.
19. Mortimer JE, Boucher L, Baty J, et al. Effect of tamoxifen on sexual functioning in patients with breast cancer. J Clin Oncol 1999;17:1488–92.
20. Kornblith AB, Hollis DR, Zuckerman E, et al. Effect of megestrol acetate on quality of life in a dose-response trial in women with advanced breast cancer. The Cancer and Leukemia Group B. J Clin Oncol 1993;11:2081–9.
21. Nystedt M, Berglund G, Bolund C, et al. Side effects of adjuvant endocrine treatment in premenopausal breast cancer patients: a prospective randomized study. J Clin Oncol 2003;21:1836–44.

Table 3 Common Questions in the Assessment of Sexual Function

How often do you desire sexual activity?

How difficult is it for you to experience sexual pleasure?

Are you able to achieve and maintain an erection/orgasm?

Do you have adequate vaginal lubrication?

Do you experience any pain during intercourse?

How long have you been experiencing difficulty with sex?

What medications are you currently taking?

22. Andrykowski MA, Curran SL, Lightner R. Off-treatment fatigue in breast cancer survivors: a controlled comparison. J Behav Med 1998;21:1–18.

23. Loge JH, Abrahamsen AF, Ekeberg O, Kaasa S. Hodgkin's disease survivors more fatigued than the general population. J Clin Oncol 1999;17:253–61.

24. Fossa SD, Dahl AA, Loge JH. Fatigue, anxiety, and depression in long-term survivors of testicular cancer. J Clin Oncol 2003;21:1249–54.

25. Winer EP, Lindley C, Hardee M, et al. Quality of life in patients surviving at least 12 months following high dose chemotherapy with autologous bone marrow support. Psychooncology 1999;8:167–76.

26. Passik S. Predictors of psychological distress, sexual dysfunction and physical functioning among women with upper extremity lymphedema related to breast cancer. Psychooncology 1995;4:255.

27. Schover L. Sexuallity and fertility after cancer. New York: John Wiley & Sons; 1997.

28. Laumann EO, Paik A, Rosen RC. Sexual dysfunction in the United States: prevalence and predictors. JAMA 1999;281:537–44.

29. Fossa SD, Woehre H, Kurth KH, et al. Influence of urological morbidity on quality of life in patients with prostate cancer. Eur Urol 1997;31 Suppl 3:3–8.

30. Helgason AR, Adolfsson J, Dickman P, et al. Factors associated with waning sexual function among elderly men and prostate cancer patients. J Urol 1997;158:155–9.

31. Fowler FJ Jr, Barry MJ, Lu-Yao G, et al. Effect of radical prostatectomy for prostate cancer on patient quality of life: results from a Medicare survey. Urology 1995;45:1007–13; discussion 1013–5.

32. Schover LR, Fouladi RT, Warneke CL, et al. Defining sexual outcomes after treatment for localized prostate carcinoma. Cancer 2002;95:1773–85.

33. Walsh PC, Marschke P, Ricker D, Burnett AL. Patient-reported urinary continence and sexual function after anatomic radical prostatectomy. Urology 2000;55:58–61.

34. Bates TS, Wright MP, Gillatt DA. Prevalence and impact of incontinence and impotence following total prostatectomy assessed anonymously by the ICS-male questionnaire. Eur Urol 1998;33:165–9.

35. Fowler FJ Jr, Barry MJ, Lu-Yao G, et al. Outcomes of external-beam radiation therapy for prostate cancer: a study of Medicare beneficiaries in three Surveillance, Epidemiology, and End Results areas. J Clin Oncol 1996;14:2258–65.

36. Gaylis FD, Friedel WE, Armas OA. Radical retropubic prostatectomy outcomes at a community hospital. J Urol 1998;159:167–71.

37. Stanford JL, Feng Z, Hamilton AS, et al. Urinary and sexual function after radical prostatectomy for clinically localized prostate cancer: the Prostate Cancer Outcomes Study. JAMA 2000;283:354–60.

38. Brandeis JM, Litwin MS, Burnison CM, Reiter RE. Quality of life outcomes after brachytherapy for early stage prostate cancer. J Urol 2000;163:851–7.

39. Beard CJ, Propert KJ, Rieker PP, et al. Complications after treatment with external-beam irradiation in early-stage prostate cancer patients: a prospective multiinstitutional outcomes study. J Clin Oncol 1997;15:223–9.

40. Mantz CA, Song P, Farhangi E, et al. Potency probability following conformal megavoltage radiotherapy using conventional doses for localized prostate cancer. Int J Radiat Oncol Biol Phys 1997;37:551–7.

41. Robinson JW, Dufour MS, Fung TS. Erectile functioning of men treated for prostate carcinoma. Cancer 1997;79:538–44.

42. Petty F, Noyes R Jr. Depression secondary to cancer. Biol Psychiatry 1981;16:1203–20.

43. McDaniel JS, Musselman DL, Porter MR, et al. Depression in patients with cancer. Diagnosis, biology, and treatment. Arch Gen Psychiatry 1995;52:89–99.

44. Kornblith AB, Thaler HT, Wong G, et al. Quality of life of women with ovarian cancer. Gynecol Oncol 1995;59:231–42.

45. Portenoy RK, Kornblith AB, Wong G, et al. Pain in ovarian cancer patients. Prevalence, characteristics, and associated symptoms. Cancer 1994;74:907–15.

46. Norton TR, Manne SL, Rubin S, et al. Prevalence and predictors of psychological distress among women with ovarian cancer. J Clin Oncol 2004;22:919–26.

47. Schag CA, Ganz PA, Polinsky ML, et al. Characteristics of women at risk for psychosocial distress in the year after breast cancer. J Clin Oncol 1993;11:783–93.

48. Kornblith AB, Herndon JE II, Zuckerman E, et al. Comparison of psychosocial adaptation of advanced stage Hodgkin's disease and acute leukemia survivors. Cancer and Leukemia Group B. Ann Oncol 1998;9:297–306.

49. Cull A, Cowie VJ, Farquharson DI, et al. Early stage cervical cancer: psychosocial and sexual outcomes of treatment. Br J Cancer 1993;68:1216–20.

50. Andersen BL, van Der Does J. Surviving gynecologic cancer and coping with sexual morbidity: an international problem. Int J Gynecol Cancer 1994;4:225–40.

51. Carmack Taylor CL, Basen-Engquist K, Shinn EH, Bodurka DC. Predictors of sexual functioning in ovarian cancer patients. J Clin Oncol 2004;22:881–9.

52. Kiebert GM, de Haes JC, van de Velde CJ. The impact of breast-conserving treatment and mastectomy on the quality of life of early-stage breast cancer patients: a review. J Clin Oncol 1991;9:1059–70.

53. Moyer A. Psychosocial outcomes of breast-conserving surgery versus mastectomy: a meta-analytic review. Health Psychol 1997;16:284–98.

54. Ganz PA, Schag AC, Lee JJ, et al. Breast conservation versus mastectomy. Is there a difference in psychological adjustment or quality of life in the year after surgery? Cancer 1992;69:1729–38.

55. Hartl K, Janni W, Kastner R, et al. Impact of medical and demographic factors on long-term quality of life and body image of breast cancer patients. Ann Oncol 2003;14:1064–71.

56. Figueiredo MI, Cullen J, Hwang YT, et al. Breast cancer treatment in older women: does getting what you want improve your long-term body image and mental health? J Clin Oncol 2004;22:4002–9.

57. Hawighorst-Knapstein S, Schonefussrs G, Hoffmann SO, Knapstein PG. Pelvic exenteration: effects of surgery on quality of life and body image—a prospective longitudinal study. Gynecol Oncol 1997;66:495–500.

58. Annon J. The PLISSIT model: a proposed conceptual scheme for the behavioral treatment of sexual problems. J Sex Ed Ther 1976;2:1–15.

59. Andersen BL. Sexual functioning morbidity among cancer survivors. Current status and future research directions. Cancer 1985;55:1835–42.

Reproductive Issues

Kathleen M. Schmeler, MD
Pamela T. Soliman, MD
Diane C. Bodurka, MD

The overall survival and cure rates of children and young adults with cancer have improved significantly in recent years (Figure 1).[1,2] This has led to increased emphasis on quality of life issues, including the ability to have children. Many of the chemotherapy and radiation regimens used to treat these young patients are toxic to the gonadal tissues, resulting in infertility and other reproductive problems. These reproductive consequences associated with cancer affect a large number of people. Each year in the United States, over 50,000 men and women of reproductive age and 12,000 children under the age of 15 years are diagnosed with cancer. The most common cancer types diagnosed in children and young adults who develop infertility as a result of the disease or its treatment are shown in Table 1.[1–3]

Effects of Cytotoxic Therapy in Men

Up to 90% of postpubertal young men become azoospermic during cytotoxic chemotherapy.[4–6] The type and dose of agents used for therapy determine the amount of time required for recovery of spermatogenesis. In approximately 50% of men, spermatogenesis is recovered in the 6 months to 5 years following treatment.[7,8] For the remaining patients, severe oligospermia or azoospermia is a permanent effect of treatment.

In men, age at treatment does not appear to be a major factor in recovery from gonadal damage owing to chemotherapy.[9,10]

The effects of radiation on the testes depend on fractionation. Doses given in 3- to 7-week regimens cause more gonadal damage than single doses.[3,11] This is in contrast to all other organ systems, including the female gonads, where fractionation decreases the toxicity of radiation. Azoospermia occurs at doses above 0.6 Gy, with the duration of azoospermia dependent on the total radiation dose received.[12–14]

For male children undergoing cancer treatment, gonadal toxicity is also an important issue as the prepubertal testis is also susceptible to cytotoxic therapy. Similar to adult men, radiation and chemotherapy may produce permanent azoospermia.[3,15] Of note, pubertal development is not usually affected as most of the regimens used do not affect Leydig cell function or testosterone levels.[3,16]

Effects of Cytotoxic Therapy in Women

Unfortunately, the effects of cytotoxic therapy on female gonadal function are almost always irreversible. The effects depend on several factors, including the type of agents used, the cumulative dose, and the patient's ovarian reserve prior to beginning therapy.[17,18] Ovarian reserve refers to the number of primordial follicles within the ovary. A woman is born with all of the primordial follicles she will ever have, and no new oocytes can be generated if all of the primordial follicles are destroyed by cytotoxic therapy. Loss of ovarian reserve owing to chemotherapy will result in early menopause, premature ovarian failure (POF), and infertility.[19] Older women are more susceptible to the sterilizing effects of cytotoxic chemotherapy as they tend to have lower numbers of pretreatment follicles compared with younger patients.[3,19,20]

In women, the degree and persistence of radiation therapy–induced gonadal damage are dependent on patient age, total radiation dose, and the number of treatment fractions.[3] Radiation is more toxic to the ovaries when given in a single dose compared with fractionated doses.[17] Similar to cytotoxic chemotherapy, older women are more susceptible to the sterilizing effects of radiation therapy as they tend to have fewer pretreatment primordial follicles when compared with younger women. The threshold at which POF occurs has been shown to be 3 Gy.[21] If treated with less than 3 Gy, only 11 to 13% of women

Table 1 Most Common Cancer Types Resulting in Infertility

Childhood cancers
  Leukemias
  Lymphomas
  Wilms' tumor
  Neuroblastomas
  Bone and soft tissue sarcomas

Adult cancers
  Breast cancer
  Lymphomas
  Testicular cancer
  Cervical cancer
  Bone and soft tissue sarcomas
  Colorectal cancer

Adapted from Jemal A= and Meistrich ML et al.[1,3]

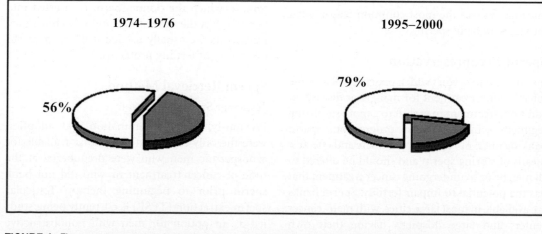

FIGURE 1 Five-year cancer survival rates for children diagnosed under age 15 years.[1]

1974–1976   56%

1995–2000   79%

experience POF. However, treating with 3 Gy or higher results in POF in 60 to 63% of women.[21] It is difficult to say that there is a safe radiation dose as less than 2 Gy of radiation to the ovaries can destroy up to 50% of the oocyte population.[20,22] It is also important to note that even if reproductive function is maintained after treatment, cytotoxic agents will damage some primordial follicles and therefore shorten a patient's reproductive life span. In addition, the sterilizing potentials of radiation and chemotherapy are additive.[20]

Prepubertal girls are less susceptible to the gonadotoxic effects of cytotoxic therapy than young postpubertal women. Most chemotherapy regimens do not cause loss of primordial follicles, and the majority of girls undergo normal pubertal development and menarche. In addition, girls under the age of 12 years who are treated with chemotherapy and in particular with alkylating agents are less likely to experience premature menopause in their twenties or thirties, as is seen in those treated between the ages of 13 and 19 years.[3,23]

Techniques to Protect Gonads

Gonadal Shielding

For patients whose gonads are within or close to the radiation treatment field, special techniques, including field blocking and gonadal shielding, can sometimes be used to reduce gonadal dose. In men being treated with radiation therapy for Hodgkin's disease, testicular shields, also known as clamshells, significantly reduce the radiation dose to the testes.[24] In addition, a special positioning device can be used to retract the remaining testicle out of the radiation field in men being treated with radiation therapy to the hemiscrotum following unilateral orchiectomy for testicular cancer.[25] However, even with these techniques, an appreciable radiation dose may reach the gonads owing to leakage through the accelerator head, radiation scatter from collimators and beam modifiers, and radiation scatter within the patient from the treatment beams.[26,27]

Ovarian Transposition

In women undergoing radiation therapy, surgically transposing the ovaries outside the radiation field can decrease the amount of radiation the ovaries receive and potentially prevent premature ovarian failure and infertility. For patients undergoing radiation treatment for Hodgkin's lymphoma, the ovaries are moved to an area behind the uterus, away from the pelvic lymph node radiation fields. In women with cervical cancer being treated with hysterectomy followed by radiation therapy, the ovaries can be transposed laterally out of the radiation field to potentially prevent premature menopause. This may retain the

possibility of future oocyte retrieval and pregnancy using a surrogate. Transposing the ovaries is estimated to reduce the radiation exposure to approximately 10% of the dose of in situ ovaries.[28,29] However, ovarian failure still occurs in up to 50% of women following ovarian transposition.[30–32] This may be due to not transposing the ovaries far enough out of the radiation field, radiation scatter, vascular compromise, or migration of the ovaries back to their original position.[20]

Pharmacologic Protection

After noting that the prepubertal ovary is less sensitive to cytotoxic drugs,[20,33] investigators attempted to use medications such as gonadotropin-releasing hormone (GnRH) agonists during therapy to help preserve fertility.[34–36] The studies to date have reported conflicting results, and it remains unclear whether administering GnRH agonists during cytotoxic therapy provides any benefit in the prevention of POF. Further prospective study is needed to clarify this issue.

GnRH agonists have also been evaluated in men undergoing chemotherapy and/or radiation for lymphoma and testicular cancer. However, none of the studies have demonstrated a significant protective effect in maintaining spermatogenesis or increasing the rate of spermatogenesis recovery following cancer treatment.[29,34,37,38]

Fertility Preservation for Men

Improved survival rates for many cancers have resulted in an emphasis on quality of life. This is particularly important in men who want to preserve their fertility. A survey of men diagnosed with cancer between the ages of 14 and 40 years was conducted by Schover and colleagues.[39] They found that 51% of men with cancer wanted children in the future, including 77% of men who were childless at the time of their cancer diagnosis. Only 60% of men recalled being informed about infertility as a side effect of cancer treatment, and only 51% had been offered sperm banking. Overall, 24% of men in the study banked sperm, including 37% of childless men. Lack of information was the most common reason cited for failing to bank sperm.

Sperm Cryopreservation

It is difficult to predict which patients will become infertile after treatment for malignant disease. In addition, treatment may shift to a more sterilizing regimen owing to disease progression. Sperm banking or cryopreservation is a safe and effective means of storing sperm and should be offered to all men prior to undergoing cancer treatment that has the potential to impair fertility. Sperm banks are available in most large cities, with many cancer centers and large hospitals having their own sperm banks. If the patient does not live near a

sperm bank, a local laboratory can collect and freeze semen, which can then be shipped to a sperm bank.

The traditional recommendations for sperm cryopreservation are to collect a minimum of three semen samples with at least 48 hours of abstinence between sample collections. This process usually requires 5 to 8 days. However, in many cases, the need to initiate treatment may be urgent, resulting in fewer samples being obtained and shorter time intervals between sample collections. Fortunately, advances in assisted reproductive technology have reduced the number of cryopreserved sperm necessary for the fertilization of eggs. Intracytoplasmic sperm injection (ICSI) can now be performed when undergoing in vitro fertilization (IVF). This involves the injection of a single sperm cell directly into the cytoplasm of each oocyte.[40,41] As a result, even a single ejaculate before starting cancer treatment can provide a reasonable chance of having a biologic child. All semen samples should therefore be accepted for cryopreservation, even if they have only a few motile sperm.

Donor Sperm

Using donated sperm is an option for couples if the male cancer survivor is azoospermic or if the couple is uninterested in pursuing IVF/ICSI. Donated sperm can also prevent transmitting a genetic risk from the male cancer survivor. Major sperm banks in the United States collect sperm from healthy donors who are paid for donating their sperm. The donors undergo detailed screening, including medical history, psychological history, and family history, and in some cases, genetic testing for some diseases is performed. All donors are also screened extensively for sexually transmitted diseases. Information is also provided about the donor's ethnicity, physical traits, education, and profession. Some sperm banks also provide information about the donor's personality and talents.[42–44]

The process of donor insemination is relatively straightforward. The woman who will carry the pregnancy undergoes intrauterine insemination, in which the donor sperm is inserted into her uterus at the time of ovulation. No hormonal treatments are usually needed if the woman has no history of fertility problems.[45]

Sperm Retrieval Methods

Testicular Sperm Extraction

Previously, donor insemination and adoption were the only reproductive options available for azoospermic men who were prepubertal at the time of cancer treatment or who did not bank sperm prior to beginning therapy. Testicular sperm extraction (TESE) is currently being studied as an option for men with nonobstructive azoospermia. Even though these men have no spermatozoa in the ejaculate, they often have small numbers of spermatozoa in the testis tissue.[46] TESE is a procedure involving removal of testicular parenchyma and isolating individual spermatozoa.[47] The spermatozoa are then used for IVF/ICSI.[48–50] Successful sperm retrieval with subsequent live births of healthy children has been reported by a few authors.[47,51–53]

TESE has also been studied as a method to obtain spermatozoa in men who are azoospermic prior to the initiation of cancer therapy. A study by Schrader and colleagues reported successful sperm recovery using TESE in 14 of 31 azoospermic men prior to treatment for testicular cancer or lymphoma.[54] These early findings suggest that TESE may also be an option for fertility preservation in men with pretreatment azoopermia.

Microsurgical Epididymal Sperm Aspiration

Pelvic surgery can result in obstructive azoospermia, where semen is no longer produced, but testicular function is preserved. In these patients, sperm can be retrieved using microsurgical epididymal sperm aspiration. The sperm are then used immediately for IVF/ICSI or cryopreserved for later use. Excellent fertilization rates have been reported using both freshly aspirated or cryopreserved epididymal sperm.[55,56]

Electroejaculation

Some patients with testicular cancer are required to undergo a retroperitoneal lymph node dissection as part of their treatment. Modified nerve-sparing techniques have reduced the extent of dissection necessary to preserve ejaculation; however, up to 50% of patients still experience anejaculation.[57] Medical treatment with sympathomimetics, including pseudoephedrine, ephedrine sulfate, phenylpropanolamine, or imipramine, is sometimes successful in producing emission and ejaculation in these patients. However, if these medications are unsuccessful, electroejaculation can be performed. Following administration of general anesthesia, a rectal probe is inserted and the sympathetic efferent fibers and smooth muscles are electrically stimulated, leading to ejaculation in over 70% of patients.[58,59] Intrauterine insemination can be used following electroejaculation; however, sperm motility tends to be low, so IVF/ICSI may be required to achieve pregnancy.[60]

Future Directions

Testicular stem cell banking is currently under investigation as a method of preserving the fertility of prepubertal boys undergoing potentially sterilizing cancer therapy. The procedure involves the harvesting and cryopreservation of spermatogonial stem cells that are capable of self-renewal, proliferation, and repopulation of the seminiferous tubules. These stem cells could potentially be

transplanted back into the patient's testis after cancer treatment is complete. Encouraging results have been reported in animal studies,[61–63]; however, further research is needed before these advances are applied to the treatment of male infertility.

Fertility Preservation for Women

In general, young female cancer patients, like their male counterparts, are poorly counseled on the effect of cancer treatment on ovarian function and on their options for fertility preservation. Fertility preservation for men is much simpler owing to the availability of sperm banking. The storage of gametes for women is more complex. Fortunately, recent advances in several reproductive technologies may provide the patient with the option of future pregnancy.[18]

Embryo Cryopreservation

Embryo cryopreservation is a widely used method of fertility preservation that has been available to cancer patients for several years. It is a technique that is used regularly by infertility clinics to bank spare embryos for couples undergoing IVF. The woman undergoes treatment with gonadotropins to stimulate her ovaries, followed by a minor surgical procedure to retrieve the oocytes. The oocytes are then fertilized with sperm from a partner or donor. Any resulting embryos are cryopreserved for future use.

Embryo cryopreservation can have several limitations for the woman newly diagnosed with cancer. It requires a male partner or the use of donor sperm. In addition, the woman needs to undergo ovarian stimulation and egg retrieval, possibly resulting in a delay of her cancer treatment. The probability of a successful future pregnancy depends on the number of IVF cycles performed and on the number and quality of embryos obtained. The more cycles performed, the longer the delay in her cancer treatment.[18]

Women with breast cancer make up the largest proportion of women seeking fertility preservation. Many breast tumors are estrogen receptor positive, raising concerns about the high levels of estrogen that result from ovarian stimulation with gonadotropins. Two strategies have been suggested to minimize the exposure to estrogen.[18,20] One is to retrieve oocytes from an unstimulated or natural cycle.[64] This strategy is limited by the possibility that only one or no oocytes may be retrieved, decreasing the probability of a successful future pregnancy. Another strategy is to include a chemopreventive agent such as tamoxifen or letrozole when performing an IVF cycle. These agents have been shown to be efficacious in the prevention of breast cancer recurrence[65,66] and coincidentally have ovulation-inducing properties.[67,68] These agents have been used in

combination with gonadotropins in IVF cycles with good embryo yields and no apparent increase in breast cancer recurrence.[18,67] These preliminary results are very promising; however, further study and long-term follow-up are needed to ensure the safety and effectiveness of using tamoxifen or letrozole in IVF cycles in women with breast cancer.

Oocyte Cryopreservation

Oocyte cryopreservation is an appealing option for women without partners. The patient is treated with gonadotropins to stimulate her ovaries, followed by a minor surgical procedure to retrieve the oocytes. The oocytes are then cryopreserved. Once the patient has completed cancer therapy and is ready to conceive, the oocytes are thawed and fertilized using IVF/ICSI and the embryos are implanted into the patient's uterus. Despite early disappointing results owing to technical challenges associated with cryopreserving oocytes,[18,69] recent studies have reported increased pregnancy rates using IVF/ICSI with thawed oocytes.[70,71]

Donor Eggs

Using another woman's oocytes is an option for women who have lost ovarian function owing to cancer therapy but still have a uterus. The oocytes are retrieved from a donor and are fertilized with sperm from the cancer survivor's partner using IVF. The embryo is then transferred to the cancer survivor's uterus to achieve pregnancy. Although egg donation involves IVF, the cancer survivor does not need to take ovarian-stimulating medications. Because women with ovarian failure no longer produce endogenous estrogen and progesterone, these hormones will have to be taken by the patient to prepare the uterus for implantation and to maintain the early pregnancy until placental function is adequate.[42,72]

Similar to men who donate sperm, women who donate their oocytes go through extensive screening and testing for sexually transmitted diseases. Oocyte donation can be significantly more difficult and expensive than sperm donation. Oocyte donors are required to undergo ovarian stimulation followed by a minor surgical procedure to retrieve the oocytes.[42,44,72]

Future Directions

Ovarian Tissue Cryopreservation and Transplantation

Ovarian tissue cryopreservation and transplantation is an emerging new option for women desiring fertility preservation. The technique involves removing ovarian tissue from the patient prior to undergoing therapy. The tissue is thoroughly examined for any evidence of metastatic disease.

The ovarian cortex is then cut into small strips and cryopreserved. Following completion of cancer therapy, the tissue is thawed and transplanted within the pelvis or in the subcutaneous tissue of the lower abdomen or forearm. The grafts become hormonally active 3 to 4 months after transplantation, at which time oocyte retrieval can be attempted with or without the aid of exogenous gonatropins to stimulate follicular development.[73–77] Oktay and colleagues recently reported on the transplant of cryopreserved ovarian tissue into the subcutaneous abdominal tissue of a breast cancer survivor.[78] Hormonal function was restored, and percutaneous oocyte retrieval was performed following ovarian stimulation. A viable embryo was obtained following fertilization and implanted into the patient's uterus. Unfortunately, no pregnancy occurred.

The potential use of ovarian tissue cryopreservation and transplantation will offer several advantages as a method of preserving fertility. Similar to oocyte cryopreservation, no male partner is needed at the time of the procedure. In addition, pretreatment ovarian stimulation is not required. The ovarian tissue cryopreservation could be performed at ay point in the cycle so that there would be no delay in beginning cancer treatment. In children, ovarian tissue cryopreservation could provide the only available fertility-preserving option as ovarian stimulation and oocyte collection cannot be performed in prepubertal girls. Significant progress is being made with the development of ovarian tissue cryopreservation and transplantation, and it may eventually become a viable option for fertility preservation for girls and women undergoing gonadotoxic cancer treatment.[18]

Adoption

Adoption is also an option for both men and women who are infertile as a result of cancer therapy. Adoption can be domestic, international, public, or private. Most adoption agencies report that they do not exclude cancer survivors as potential parents, especially with documentation from a doctor regarding anticipated life expectancy and quality of life. Some agencies do require patients to be disease free for a certain amount of time, such as 5 years prior to being eligible to adopt.[42,79]

Pregnancy Outcome

One of the major concerns for cancer survivors treated with radiation therapy and/or chemotherapy who retain fertility is whether they will be able to have healthy children. Common areas of concern include pregnancy complications, congenital malformations, and increased risk of cancer in their offspring.

Pregnancy Complications

Several studies have provided information regarding prenatal and perinatal morbidity and mortality in cancer survivors previously treated with radiation and chemotherapy.[80–85] The outcomes vary with cancer diagnosis and with specific therapy. The offspring of female survivors of Wilms' tumor have been shown to have an increase in the risk of intrauterine and peripartum complications. A study by Li and colleagues reported an increased rate of spontaneous abortions, low birth weight babies, and neonatal deaths in women who received 20 to 35 Gy of abdominal radiation with or without chemotherapy for Wilms' tumor.[81] Compared with the general population, their relative risk was 7.9 for perinatal mortality and 4.0 for low birth weight infants (< 2,500 g). These results were confirmed in a study by Byrne and colleagues.[80] The pathogenesis of these radiation-associated adverse pregnancy outcomes remains unclear. It has been hypothesized to be due to damage to the uterine musculature or vascular insufficiency from radiation.[80,86]

For other disease categories, the data are also limited. The available evidence suggests that the offspring of survivors of most other cancers, including acute lymphoblastic leukemia, do not have increased prenatal or perinatal complications.[82,84,85]

Congenital Anomalies

Studies to date have shown no significant increase in congenital malformations over the general population in the offspring of cancer survivors who received radiation or chemotherapy.[80,86,87] In addition, a large case-control study of 45,000 children with congenital anomalies reported no increase in the incidence of parental exposure to alkylating agents or radiation proximal to the gonads in the parents of children with congenital abnormalities compared with the parents of the control group children.[88] A large study of Japanese atomic bomb survivors and their children also showed no significant increase in inherited genetic disease in 30,000 offspring born to radiation-exposed parents.[89]

Currently, a large, ongoing study, the Genetic Consequences of Childhood Cancer Treatment, is evaluating the offspring of childhood cancer survivors treated with chemotherapy and/or radiation.[90] The study population is composed of more than 25,000 childhood cancer survivors in Denmark and the United States who subsequently had nearly 6,500 children of their own. Radiation doses to the gonads are being reconstructed using radiotherapy records. This study will provide important information for cancer survivors who wish to have children.

Cancer in Offspring

Although some cancers have a known genetic component, such as retinoblastoma and familial cancer syndromes including Li-Fraumeni, Lynch syndrome/herediatry nonpolyposis colorectal cancer (HNPCC), and breast cancer, only a small number of cancers affecting children and young adults have any heritable genetic origin.[91,92] Sankila and colleagues studied 5,487 offspring of approximately 14,000 childhood cancer survivors and found that there was less than one excess cancer diagnosis for every 1,000 offspring.[92]

Genetic Counseling

Approximately 5 to 10% of cancers are due to germline mutations in cancer susceptibility genes.[93] Genetic testing has become available for many hereditary cancer syndromes, including breast cancer and Lynch syndrome/HNPCC. Several factors are common in hereditary cancer syndromes and can be used to identify individuals at risk (Table 2).[93] High-risk individuals should be referred for genetic counseling and possible genetic testing. Genetic counseling involves obtaining a detailed family history, performing a risk assessment, providing an explanation of the testing available, and reviewing the options for surveillance and risk reduction.

Genetic counseling and testing can also be of assistance to couples deciding whether to try to conceive a child who may be at risk of cancer. In addition, preimplantation genetic testing may be an option for individuals with hereditary cancer syndromes undergoing IVF. It involves removing one cell from each developing embryo and testing it for the genetic mutation.[94] Only embryos that do not contain the genetic abnormality are then implanted in the woman's uterus. This technology has been used successfully for Tay-Sachs disease, cystic fibrosis, and other genetic disorders. Its use for genetic abnormalities leading to increased cancer risk is currently being evaluated.

Summary

Infertility has become a significant issue for many cancer survivors. Young patients and their families should be informed of the potential effects that their cancer and its treatment can have on reproductive function, including the possibility of sterility. All reproductive-age men undergoing cancer treatment with the potential to impair fertility should be offered sperm cryopreservation. Although fertility preservation in women is more complicated, recent advances in reproductive technologies are providing an increasing number of options for potential future pregnancy.

Further information is available for cancer patients from Fertile Hope (<www.fertilehope. org>), a nonprofit organization dedicated to providing reproductive information, support, and hope to cancer patients whose medical treatments present the risk of infertility.[79]

Table 2 Characteristics of Patients with Hereditary Cancer Syndromes

Cancer onset at an early age (usually ≥ 10 yr earlier than the mean age)
Synchronous or metachronous primary cancers in one individual
Multiple family members with the same cancer or clustering of cancers known to be caused by a single gene
(eg, breast and ovary)
Unusual presentation of cancer, such as breast cancer in a male
Ethnicity (eg, Ashkenazi Jewish ancestry and breast cancer)

Adapted from Matloff ET.[93]

REFERENCES

1. Jemal A, Murray T, Ward E, et al. Cancer statistics, 2005. CA Cancer J Clin 2005;55:10–30.
2. Weir HK, Thun MJ, Hankey BF, et al. Annual report to the nation on the status of cancer, 1975-2000, featuring the uses of surveillance data for cancer prevention and control. J Natl Cancer Inst 2003;95:1276–99.
3. Meistrich ML, Vassilopoulou-Sellin R, Lipshultz LI. Gonadal dysfunction. In: Devita VT, Hellman S, Rosenberg SA, editors. Cancer principles and practice of oncology. 7th ed. Philadelphia: Lippincott Williams & Wilkins; 2005. p. 2560–74.
4. Averette HE, Boike GM, Jarrell MA. Effects of cancer chemotherapy on gonadal function and reproductive capacity. CA Cancer J Clin 1990;40:199–209.
5. Ben Arush MW, Solt I, Lightman A, et al. Male gonadal function in survivors of childhood Hodgkin and non-Hodgkin lymphoma. Pediatr Hematol Oncol 2000;17:239–45.
6. DeSantis M, Albrecht W, Holtl W, et al. Impact of cytotoxic treatment on long-term fertility in patients with germ-cell cancer. Int J Cancer 1999;83:864–5.
7. Heikens J, Behrendt H, Adriaanse R, et al. Irreversible gonadal damage in male survivors of pediatric Hodgkin's disease. Cancer 1996;78:2020–4.
8. Naysmith TE, Blake DA, Harvey VJ, et al. Do men undergoing sterilizing cancer treatments have a fertile future? Hum Reprod 1998;13:3250–5.
9. Pryzant RM, Meistrich ML, Wilson G, et al. Long-term reduction in sperm count after chemotherapy with and without radiation therapy for non-Hodgkin's lymphomas. J Clin Oncol 1993;11:239–47.
10. Meistrich ML, Wilson G, Brown BW, et al. Impact of cyclophosphamide on long-term reduction in sperm count in men treated with combination chemotherapy for Ewing and soft tissue sarcomas. Cancer 1992;70:2703–12.
11. Meistrich ML, van Beek MEAB. Radiation sensitivity of the human testis. In: Lett JR, Altman KI, editors. Advances in radiation biology. New York: Academic Press; 1990. p. 227.
12. Schlappack OK, Kratzik C, Schmidt W, et al. Response of the seminiferous epithelium to scattered radiation in seminoma patients. Cancer 1988;62:1487–91.
13. Hansen PV, Trykker H, Svennekjaer IL, et al. Long-term recovery of spermatogenesis after radiotherapy in patients with testicular cancer. Radiother Oncol 1990;18:117–25.
14. Centola GM, Keller JW, Henzler M, et al. Effect of low-dose testicular irradiation on sperm count and fertility in patients with testicular seminoma. J Androl 1994;15:608–13.
15. Wallace WH, Shalet SM, Crowne EC, et al. Gonadal dysfunction due to cis-platinum. Med Pediatr Oncol 1989;17:409–13.
16. Gerres L, Bramswig JH, Schlegel W, et al. The effects of etoposide on testicular function in boys treated for Hodgkin's disease. Cancer 1998;83:2217–22.
17. Meirow D, Nugent D. The effects of radiotherapy and chemotherapy on female reproduction. Hum Reprod Update 2001;7:535–43.
18. Roberts JE, Oktay K. Fertility preservation: a comprehensive approach to the young woman with cancer. J Natl Cancer Inst Monogr 2005(34):57–9.
19. Speroff L, Glass RH, Kase NG. Regulation of the menstrual cycle. In: Speroff L, Glass RH, Kase NG, editors. Clinical gynecologic endocrinology and infertility. 6th ed. Philadelphia: Lippincott Williams & Wilkins; 1999. p. 201–38.
20. Falcone T, Bedaiwy MA. Fertility preservation and pregnancy outcome after malignancy. Curr Opin Obstet Gynecol 2005;17:21–6.
21. Husseinzadeh N, Nahhas WA, Velkley DE, et al. The preservation of ovarian function in young women undergoing pelvic radiation therapy. Gynecol Oncol 1984;18:373–9.
22. Wallace WH, Thomson AB, Kelsey TW. The radiosensitivity of the human oocyte. Hum Reprod 2003;18:11–21.
23. Byrne J, Fears TR, Gail MH, et al. Early menopause in long-term survivors of cancer during adolescence. Am J Obstet Gynecol 1992;166:788–93.
24. Fraass BA, Kinsella TJ, Harrington FS, et al. Peripheral dose to the testes: the design and clinical use of a practical and effective gonadal shield. Int J Radiat Oncol Biol Phys 1985;11:609–15.
25. Harter DJ, Hussey DH, Delclos L, et al. Device to position and shield the testical during irradiation. Int J Radiat Oncol Biol Phys 1976;1:361–4.
26. Keller B, Mathewson C, Rubin P. Scattered radiation dosage as a function of x-ray energy. Radiology 1974;111:447–9.
27. Kase KR, Svensson GK, Wolbarst AB, et al. Measurements of dose from secondary radiation outside a treatment field. Int J Radiat Oncol Biol Phys 1983;9:1177–83.
28. Haie-Meder C, Mlika-Cabanne N, Michel G, et al. Radiotherapy after ovarian transposition: ovarian function and fertility preservation. Int J Radiat Oncol Biol Phys 1993; 25:419–24.
29. Howell SJ, Shalet SM. Fertility preservation and management of gonadal failure associated with lymphoma therapy. Curr Oncol Rep 2002;4:443–52.
30. Feeney DD, Moore DH, Look KY, et al. The fate of the ovaries after radical hysterectomy and ovarian transposition. Gynecol Oncol 1995;56:3–7.
31. Williams RS, Littell RD, Mendenhall NP. Laparoscopic oophoropexy and ovarian function in the treatment of Hodgkin disease. Cancer 1999;86:2138–42.
32. Yarali H, Demirol A, Bukulmez O, et al. Laparoscopic high lateral transposition of both ovaries before pelvic irradiation. J Am Assoc Gynecol Laparosc 2000;7:237–9.
33. Chiarelli AM, Marrett LD, Darlington G. Early menopause and infertility in females after treatment for childhood cancer diagnosed in 1964-1988 in Ontario, Canada. Am J Epidemiol 1999;150:245–54.
34. Waxman JH, Ahmed R, Smith D, et al. Failure to preserve fertility in patients with Hodgkin's disease. Cancer Chemother Pharmacol 1987;19:159–62.
35. Blumenfeld Z, Avivi I, Linn S, et al. Prevention of irreversible chemotherapy-induced ovarian damage in young women with lymphoma by a gonadotrophin-releasing hormone agonist in parallel to chemotherapy. Hum Reprod 1996; 11:1620–6.
36. Pereyra Pacheco B, Mendez Ribas JM, Milone G, et al. Use of GnRH analogs for functional protection of the ovary and preservation of fertility during cancer treatment in adolescents: a preliminary report. Gynecol Oncol 2001;81:391–7.
37. Kreuser ED, Hetzel WD, Hautmann R, et al. Reproductive toxicity with and without LHRHA administration during adjuvant chemotherapy in patients with germ cell tumors. Horm Metab Res 1990;22:494–8.
38. Brennemann W, Brensing KA, Leipner N, et al. Attempted protection of spermatogenesis from irradiation in patients with seminoma by D-tryptophan-6 luteinizing hormone releasing hormone. Clin Investig 1994;72:838–42.
39. Schover LR, Brey K, Lichtin A, et al. Knowledge and experience regarding cancer, infertility, and sperm banking in younger male survivors. J Clin Oncol 2002;20:1880–9.
40. Kuczynski W, Dhont M, Grygoruk C, et al. The outcome of intracytoplasmic injection of fresh and cryopreserved ejaculated spermatozoa—a prospective randomized study. Hum Reprod 2001;16:2109–13.
41. Opsahl MS, Fugger EF, Sherins RJ, et al. Preservation of reproductive function before therapy for cancer: new options involving sperm and ovary cryopreservation. Cancer J Sci Am 1997;3:189–91.
42. Schover L. Sexuality and fertility after cancer. New York: John Wiley & Sons; 1997.
43. Baker DJ, Paterson MA. Marketed sperm: use and regulation in the United States. Fertil Steril 1995;63:947–52.
44. Garrido N, Zuzuarregui JL, Meseguer M, et al. Sperm and oocyte donor selection and management: experience of a 10 year follow-up of more than 2100 candidates. Hum Reprod 2002;17:3142–8.
45. Speroff L, Glass RH, Kase NG. Male infertility. In: Speroff L, Glass RH, Kase NG, editors. Clinical gynecologic endocrinology and infertility. 6th ed. Philadelphia: Lippincott Williams & Wilkins; 1999. p. 1090–2.
46. Silber SJ, Nagy Z, Devroey P, et al. Distribution of spermatogenesis in the testicles of azoospermic men: the presence or absence of spermatids in the testes of men with germinal failure. Hum Reprod 1997;12:2422–8.
47. Damani MN, Master V, Meng MV, et al. Postchemotherapy ejaculatory azoospermia: fatherhood with sperm from testis tissue with intracytoplasmic sperm injection. J Clin Oncol 2002;20:930–6.
48. Devroey P, Liu J, Nagy Z, et al. Pregnancies after testicular sperm extraction and intracytoplasmic sperm injection in non-obstructive azoospermia. Hum Reprod 1995;10:1457–60.
49. Mercan R, Urman B, Alatas C, et al. Outcome of testicular sperm retrieval procedures in non-obstructive azoospermia: percutaneous aspiration versus open biopsy. Hum Reprod 2000;15:1548–51.
50. Habermann H, Seo R, Cieslak J, et al. In vitro fertilization outcomes after intracytoplasmic sperm injection with fresh or frozen-thawed testicular spermatozoa. Fertil Steril 2000;73:955–60.
51. Chan PT, Palermo GD, Veeck LL, et al. Testicular sperm extraction combined with intracytoplasmic sperm injection in the treatment of men with persistent azoospermia postchemotherapy. Cancer 2001;92:1632–7.
52. Meseguer M, Garrido N, Remohi J, et al. Testicular sperm extraction (TESE) and ICSI in patients with permanent azoospermia after chemotherapy. Hum Reprod 2003; 18:1281–5.
53. Shin D, Lo KC, Lipshultz LI. Treatment options for the infertile male with cancer. J Natl Cancer Inst Monogr 2005(34):48–50.
54. Schrader M, Muller M, Sofikitis N, et al. "Onco-tese": testicular sperm extraction in azoospermic cancer patients before chemotherapy—new guidelines? Urology 2003;61:421–5.
55. Janzen N, Goldstein M, Schlegel PN, et al. Use of electively cryopreserved microsurgically aspirated epididymal sperm and intracytoplasmic sperm injection for obstructive azoospermia. Fertil Steril 2000;74:696–701.
56. Oates RD, Lobel SM, Harris DH, et al. Efficacy of intracytoplasmic sperm injection using intentionally cryopreserved epididymal spermatozoa. Hum Reprod 1996;11:133–8.
57. Sheinfeld J MJ, Bosl G. Campbell's urology. 8th ed. Philadelphia: Saunders; 2002.
58. Ohl DA, Wolf LJ, Menge AC, et al. Electroejaculation and assisted reproductive technologies in the treatment of anejaculatory infertility. Fertil Steril 2001;76:1249–55.
59. Ohl DA, Denil J, Bennett CJ, et al. Electroejaculation following retroperitoneal lymphadenectomy. J Urol 1991;145:980–3.
60. Schatte EC, Orejuela FJ, Lipshultz LI, et al. Treatment of infertility due to anejaculation in the male with electroejaculation and intracytoplasmic sperm injection. J Urol 2000;163:1717–20.
61. Nagano M, Patrizio P, Brinster RL. Long-term survival of human spermatogonial stem cells in mouse testes. Fertil Steril 2002;78:1225–33.
62. Honaramooz A, Behboodi E, Megee SO, et al. Fertility and germline transmission of donor haplotype following germ cell transplantation in immunocompetent goats. Biol Reprod 2003;69:1260–4.
63. Brinster RL, Avarbock MR. Germline transmission of donor haplotype following spermatogonial transplantation. Proc Natl Acad Sci U S A 1994;91:11303–7.
64. Pelinck MJ, Hoek A, Simons AH, et al. Efficacy of natural cycle IVF: a review of the literature. Hum Reprod Update 2002;8:129–39.
65. Fisher B, Costantino J, Redmond C, et al. A randomized clinical trial evaluating tamoxifen in the treatment of patients with node-negative breast cancer who have estrogen-receptor-positive tumors. N Engl J Med 1989; 320:479–84.
66. Goss PE, Ingle JN, Martino S, et al. A randomized trial of letrozole in postmenopausal women after five years of tamoxifen therapy for early-stage breast cancer. N Engl J Med 2003;349:1793–802.

67. Oktay K, Buyuk E, Davis O, et al. Fertility preservation in breast cancer patients: IVF and embryo cryopreservation after ovarian stimulation with tamoxifen. Hum Reprod 2003;18:90–5.

68. Mitwally MF, Casper RF. Aromatase inhibitors for the treatment of infertility. Expert Opin Investig Drugs 2003;12:353–71.

69. Boiso I, Marti M, Santalo J, et al. A confocal microscopy analysis of the spindle and chromosome configurations of human oocytes cryopreserved at the germinal vesicle and metaphase II stage. Hum Reprod 2002;17:1885–91.

70. Porcu E, Fabbri R, Damiano G, et al. Oocyte cryopreservation in oncological patients. Eur J Obstet Gynecol Reprod Biol 2004;113 Suppl 1:S14–6.

71. Yoon TK, Kim TJ, Park SE, et al. Live births after vitrification of oocytes in a stimulated in vitro fertilization-embryo transfer program. Fertil Steril 2003;79:1323–6.

72. Anselmo AP, Cavalieri E, Aragona C, et al. Successful pregnancies following an egg donation program in women with previously treated Hodgkin's disease. Haematologica 2001;86:624–8.

73. Oktay KH, Yih M. Preliminary experience with orthotopic and heterotopic transplantation of ovarian cortical strips. Semin Reprod Med 2002;20:63–74.

74. Oktay K, Buyuk E, Rosenwaks Z, et al. A technique for transplantation of ovarian cortical strips to the forearm. Fertil Steril 2003;80:193–8.

75. Oktay K. Ovarian tissue cryopreservation and transplantation: preliminary findings and implications for cancer patients. Hum Reprod Update 2001;7:526–34.

76. Oktay K, Economos K, Kan M, et al. Endocrine function and oocyte retrieval after autologous transplantation of ovarian cortical strips to the forearm. JAMA 2001;286:1490–3.

77. Oktay K, Kan MT, Rosenwaks Z. Recent progress in oocyte and ovarian tissue cryopreservation and transplantation. Curr Opin Obstet Gynecol 2001;13:263–8.

78. Oktay K, Buyuk E, Veeck L, et al. Embryo development after heterotopic transplantation of cryopreserved ovarian tissue. Lancet 2004;363:837–40.

79. Fertile Hope. Available at: http://www.fertilehope.org.

80. Byrne J, Rasmussen SA, Steinhorn SC, et al. Genetic disease in offspring of long-term survivors of childhood and adolescent cancer. Am J Hum Genet 1998;62:45–52.

81. Li FP, Gimbrere K, Gelber RD, et al. Outcome of pregnancy in survivors of Wilms' tumor. JAMA 1987;257:216–9.

82. Green DM, Hall B, Zevon MA. Pregnancy outcome after treatment for acute lymphoblastic leukemia during childhood or adolescence. Cancer 1989;64:2335–9.

83. Green DM, Whitton JA, Stovall M, et al. Pregnancy outcome of female survivors of childhood cancer: a report from the Childhood Cancer Survivor Study. Am J Obstet Gynecol 2002;187:1070–80.

84. Nygaard R, Clausen N, Siimes MA, et al. Reproduction following treatment for childhood leukemia: a population-based prospective cohort study of fertility and offspring. Med Pediatr Oncol 1991;19:459–66.

85. Pajor A, Zimonyi I, Koos R, et al. Pregnancies and offspring in survivors of acute lymphoid leukemia and lymphoma. Eur J Obstet Gynecol Reprod Biol 1991;40:1–5.

86. Blatt J. Pregnancy outcome in long-term survivors of childhood cancer. Med Pediatr Oncol 1999;33:29–33.

87. Nicholson HS, Byrne J. Fertility and pregnancy after treatment for cancer during childhood or adolescence. Cancer 1993;71(10 Suppl):3392–9.

88. Dodds L, Marrett LD, Tomkins DJ, et al. Case-control study of congenital anomalies in children of cancer patients. BMJ 1993;307:164–8.

89. Neel JV, Schull WJ, Awa AA, et al. The children of parents exposed to atomic bombs: estimates of the genetic doubling dose of radiation for humans. Am J Hum Genet 1990;46:1053–72.

90. Boice JD Jr, Tawn EJ, Winther JF, et al. Genetic effects of radiotherapy for childhood cancer. Health Phys 2003;85:65–80.

91. Olson JE, Shu XO, Ross JA, et al. Medical record validation of maternally reported birth characteristics and pregnancy-related events: a report from the Children's Cancer Group. Am J Epidemiol 1997;145:58–67.

92. Sankila R, Olsen JH, Anderson H, et al. Risk of cancer among offspring of childhood-cancer survivors. Association of the Nordic Cancer Registries and the Nordic Society of Paediatric Haematology and Oncology. N Engl J Med 1998;338:1339–44.

93. Matloff ET. Genetic counseling. In: Devita VT, Hellman S, Rosenberg SA, editors. Cancer principles and practice of oncology. 7th ed. Philadelphia: Lippincott Williams & Wilkins; 2005. p. 2676–83.

94. Grace J, El Toukhy T, Braude P. Pre-implantation genetic testing. Br J Obstet Gynaecol 2004;111:1165–73.

Life after Cancer

Rena Vassilopoulou-Sellin, MD

Pamela N. Schultz, PhD, RN

According to the *SEER Cancer Statistics Review, 1975–2001,* 5-year relative survival rates have increased in recent decades.[1] For example, the survival rate for patients with cancer at all sites in 1954 was 35% but in 2000 had increased to 65.5%. The number of cancer survivors is expected to increase from 1.3 million in 2000 to 2.6 million in 2050.[2] These numbers, in part, will reflect the attainment of a cancer-prone age by the "baby boomers"—hence the increasing annual incidence of cases and the increasing prevalence of cancer survivors.

An important factor complicating the understanding of the impact of cancer treatment on long-term survivors is how one defines "survivor." Survivors' groups have emphasized that one who has been diagnosed with cancer is a "survivor" from the very beginning. How does one differentiate the cancer survivor being treated for active disease from the survivor who has been treated and is now free of disease? Traditionally, cancer-free survival of 5 years or more has been designated as an important milestone; this concept may require revision in the years to come.

Late Effects of Cancer and Cancer Treatment

Several investigators have addressed the presence and complexity of the lasting medical sequelae of cancer throughout the adult lives of the survivors of childhood cancer.[3–5] For example, Stevens and colleagues reported that 58% of survivors had at least one chronic health problem and 32% had two or more, including second primary cancers.[6] In contrast, much less is known about the lasting medical impact of cancer treatment on the survivors of adult-onset cancers. Despite the paucity of information on the physiologic late effects of adult cancers,[7,8] investigators are aware that multiple systems are often affected. For example, pelvic surgery can impair fertility, and splenectomy increases the susceptibility to bacterial infections. Moreover, certain chemotherapy agents and regimens can compromise the health of the cardiovascular, pulmonary, genitourinary, endocrine, and neurologic systems. Radiotherapy may aggravate these complications, impair skeletal development and dental health, and contribute to the risk of second primary cancers. In addition, combining the treatments can increase the number and severity of long-term medical problems.

Recently, attention has been directed toward the impact of cancer treatment on long-term survivors, particularly as it concerns their quality of life. Several investigators have begun to characterize the physiologic health and psychosocial profiles of survivors of childhood cancers. Research regarding the psychosocial profiles of survivors of adult cancers has also increased. However, a stark paucity of data on the physiologic health profile of survivors of adult cancers remains.

Life after Cancer Care Program

The Life After Cancer Care (LACC) program at The University of Texas M. D. Anderson Cancer Center was established to provide follow-up medical care to long-term cancer survivors. Its services include diagnosis and treatment and appropriate referral and consultation for the possible long-term effects of previously treated cancer. The LACC program began a systematic search for living, known cancer survivors who had been treated at the M. D. Anderson Cancer Center. Patients were included if they were diagnosed with a cancer, their cancer was diagnosed at least 5 years before, they were 18 years or older at diagnosis, they had a US address, and they were free of malignant disease at their last contact. Surveys developed to systematically collect health information reported by the survivors themselves were sent out to more than 20,000 individuals who met the above criteria. Simultaneously, the survey was made available through the Internet at <www.mdanderson.org/Departments/LACC>. Our approach has been described in detail.[9]

Data from the more than 10,000 survivors who responded to the survey are presently available for analysis and constitute the focus of this chapter. Complete data are available on 8,739 survivors who are at least 5 years from diagnosis. Sixty-two percent of the sample is female, and 92% of the total sample is white. The mean age ± standard deviation at diagnosis is 47.9 ± 14.2 years. Fifty percent of survivors were diagnosed between the ages of 18 and 48 years, and 25% were diagnosed after the age of 59 years. Approximately 25% of the survivors in our database are more than 20 years from their original diagnosis, and 10% of the survivors are at least 30 years from diagnosis. Figure 1 shows the distribution of survivors by time from diagnosis. Figure 2 illustrates the distribution of survivors by cancer type. The representation of long-term survivors in our database is similar to the incidence of cancer type; for example, thyroid cancer occurs predominantly in women, and head and neck cancer occurs predominantly in men. This is congruent with our database of long-term survivors. In addition, the distribution of cancer survivors by their diagnoses reflects the likelihood of long-term survival with different cancers and perhaps M. D. Anderson referral patterns.

In the survey, the survivors were asked, "Has cancer affected your overall health?" Interestingly, only 37.4% of them replied "yes" to that question, and there were no significant differences between the replies of men and women or among the ethnic groups. Age at diagnosis appeared to be another predictor of how the survivor experienced long-term survival. Survivors who were older when their cancer was diagnosed were less likely to believe that cancer affected their overall health as they aged. On the other hand, survivors who were most likely to report that cancer had affected their overall health tended to be younger at diagnosis (Table 1). Forty-one percent of the survivors who were diagnosed between the ages of 18 and 40 years reported that cancer affected their health in comparison with 36% of those diagnosed between 41 and 65 years of age and 28% of those diagnosed after 65 years of age. Perhaps older individuals expected to develop a number of comorbidities and were less likely to consider them related to their earlier cancer and cancer treatments.

Long-Term Health Problems

We previously reported that the specific health effects reported by long-term cancer survivors

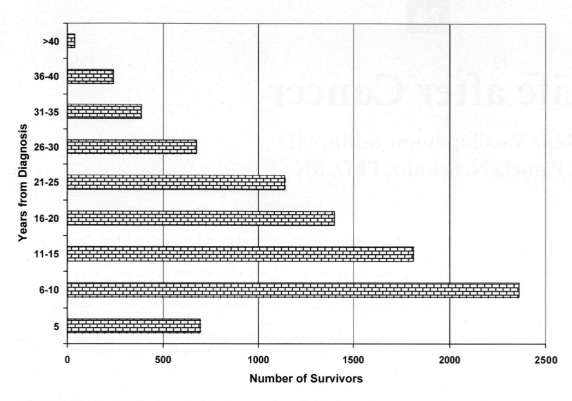

FIGURE 1 Distribution of cancer survivors by years from diagnosis.

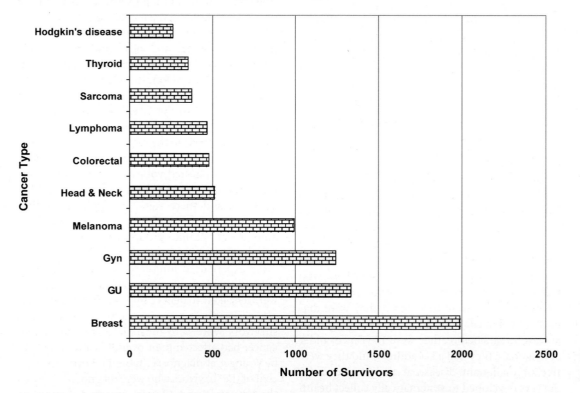

FIGURE 2 Distribution of cancer survivors by the 10 most frequent cancer types within the sample of adult survivors. GU = genitourinary; Gyn = gynecologic.

9.8%) or more hearing loss (14.9% vs 9.9%). These patterns likely reflect a complex interaction of gender-related cancer diagnoses and comorbidities. The pattern of perceived and reported health problems was different among the cancer types. For example, survivors of Hodgkin's disease prominently reported thyroid and lung problems (33.8% of responders with the diagnosis), whereas a previous diagnosis of lymphoma was associated with the frequent mention of memory loss (14.7%).

National Health Interview Survey

A large number of health conditions have been reported by the National Health Interview Survey and categorized by age, ethnicity or race, and gender.[12] Five of these health conditions were comparable to those reported by our cancer-survivor cohort: arthritis symptoms, diabetes, migraine or severe headaches, heart disease, and hearing loss. The frequencies of these conditions in the general population (computed as the number of affected individuals/1,000 population) were compared with those in our cancer-survivor cohort relative to patient age, ethnicity or race, and gender. There were significant differences in the frequencies of these five health conditions between men and women and among ethnic or racial groups. The most common difference in our cancer-survivor cohort for all groups analyzed was a statistically significant loss of hearing.[13] Hispanic American women reported significantly higher rates of diabetes, and African American men reported significantly higher rates of heart disease than the race-adjusted national prevalence rates. Although apparent differences in the frequency of these health conditions may be due to the methodology of the questionnaires, previous cancer or cancer therapy may also play a role in the survivors' health profile. For example, the consistent overreporting of hearing loss may be related to ototoxic chemotherapy. Clearly, further detailed analysis is needed in this area. Further research about comorbidities may also provide information about the health effects from a past cancer diagnosis.

Survivors of Thyroid and Breast Cancers

The importance of the uniqueness of cancer type was made obvious in two studies from our survey cohort of survivors of thyroid and breast cancer. We previously published a report on the thyroid cohort and noted several distinctions.[10] The survivors of thyroid cancer tended to be significantly younger at diagnosis, were significantly closer to their time of diagnosis at contact, were significantly more likely to be women, and reported significantly more specific health effects. We were impressed by the frequent complaints of symptoms that were reminiscent of thyroid

illustrate a complex interplay between age, gender, cancer type, and cancer treatment, as well as ethnicity, race, and social and cultural factors.[9–11] For example, the most frequently reported health problems were arthritis and osteoporosis (1,541 survivors; 26.4%). Men generally reported fewer specific problems; the most frequently mentioned were heart problems (17.2% of responding men), hearing loss (14.9%), and arthritis and

osteoporosis (15.5%). Women generally reported more specific problems; the most frequently mentioned were arthritis and osteoporosis (32.9% of responding women), heart problems (13.9%), and thyroid problems (12.1%). Women were more likely to report thyroid problems (12.1% vs 6.2%) or arthritis and osteoporosis (32.9% vs 15.5%). Men, on the other hand, were more likely to report kidney and bladder problems (14.2% vs

Table 1 Survivors ($N = 3,268$) Who Responded "Yes" to "Has Cancer Affected Your Health?"

Cancer Type	Affected Health (%)	Mean Age at Diagnosis (yr)
Melanoma	16.7	43.4
Colorectal	31.3	50.2
Gynecologic	31.4	44.5
Breast	35.9	46.5
Genitourinary	36.4	55.5
Sarcoma	39.5	40.5
Head and neck	39.8	50.8
Acute leukemia	45.3	39.8
Thyroid	50.3	35.4
Lung	53.3	55.9
Lymphoma	56.9	46.3
Gastrointestinal	57.0	56.0
Chronic leukemia	60.2	49.3
Hodgkin's disease	61.7	30.3

hormone imbalance and described these effects as "thyroid dysregulation." We found that the lifetime supplementation of thyroid hormone was associated with unique problems that compromised the patients' perception of their overall health.

In another study, 291 patients with breast cancer were asked whether they had symptoms commonly associated with menopause, including hot flushes, painful sexual intercourse, inability to concentrate, fatigue, and sleep disturbance.[14] Forty-six percent of these breast cancer survivors indicated that breast cancer had affected their overall health, especially those who had received chemotherapy alone or in combination with radiotherapy. We had a problem differentiating the symptoms of natural menopause from the sequelae of cancer treatment and other physical health problems that affect quality of life. Even though hot flushes and painful sexual intercourse are typically attributed to menopause, in our sample, it was difficult to determine whether they represented normal menopausal symptoms or long-term sequelae of cancer treatment because of the close relationship between these symptoms and the ability to concentrate, fatigue, sleep problems, and general unhappiness.

These findings show that it is sometimes difficult to determine whether specific symptoms should be attributed to cancer treatment or to associated but not causally related conditions. For example, in the case of thyroid and breast cancers, are fatigue and cognitive impairment a result of inappropriate thyroid hormone dosing, a consequence of normal menopause, or a result of cancer treatment? These questions need further clarification.

Ethnic and Racial Influences on Cancer Survivorship

We previously reported that there were significant differences among Caucasian Americans, Hispanic Americans, and African Americans in the types of specific health effects they experienced as long-term survivors of cancer.[11] Moreover, we found significant ethnic or racial differences with respect to age at diagnosis, interval since diagnosis, marital status, educational level, insurability, regular medical care, and the impact on family relationships. These differences among Caucasian Americans, Hispanic Americans, and African Americans probably reflected not only ethnicity or race but also cancer type, gender, type of treatment, and disease stage, to name a few. A complex relationship existed between ethnic or racial group, family and intimate relationships, and treatment types for the survivors of cervical cancer.

Published literature that specifically focuses on the impact of ethnic or racial factors on long-term (> 5 years from diagnosis) cancer survivors is scarce at best. Ethnic or racial differences in the incidence and mortality of various cancers are generally attributed to disparities in the ability of patients to access health care, resulting in their having more advanced disease at the time of diagnosis, the socioeconomic inequities of health care, or both.[1,15–17] In a study examining information from the National Survey of Functional Health, Ren and colleagues reported that race and class discrimination were pervasive and adversely affected the health status of ethnic or racial minorities.[18] Although studies addressing the impact of ethnic or racial differences on health are generally related to diagnosis and treatment-related outcomes, it is plausible that they may also influence other physiologic and psychosocial aspects of health.

When reviewing the information provided by cancer survivors, we found, for the most part, that cancer survivors had a similar view of the impact, or lack thereof, of their cancer experience on their overall physiologic health. There were, however, differences with respect to specific health concerns. For example, African Americans were more likely than Caucasian Americans or Hispanic Americans to report arthritis and osteoporosis, whereas Hispanic Americans were more likely to report abdominal pain and diabetes mellitus. Such differences in health profile and patterns may be partially related to other ethnic or racial propensities; for example, Brooks and colleagues showed that the poor outcomes of African American women who had cervical cancer were associated with preexisting comorbidities.[19]

Grenier and Lipshultz found that African American patients who had been treated with anthracyclines for cancer during childhood might be at a higher risk of cardiotoxicity and suggested that this could also be true for adult cancer survivors.[20] We also found a higher incidence of self-reported heart disease in African American cancer survivors than in Caucasian American or Hispanic American cancer survivors. Although such differences may have a biologic basis, socioeconomic parameters may also play a role.

It is generally thought that marital status is closely related to health.[21] Unmarried people tend to have a higher mortality from all causes, use more health services, and have more psychological distress, and their perceptions of general health are poorer than those of married people. We found differences in health perception among the ethnic or racial groups according to marital status when we did our survey. We did not consistently find a protective effect of marriage; however, our results suggested that there is a positive association between the perception of overall health and the perceived positive impact of the cancer experience on family relationships. It is clear that socioeconomic, psychological, and cultural factors interact with the physiologic factors. Further research on larger, ethnic or racially diverse populations is needed to better understand these interactions.

Work-Related Issues for Cancer Survivors

We analyzed survey information from 4,264 long-term survivors of cancer in which the survivors were asked to respond to questions about their ability to work, job discrimination, and quality of life.[22] Thirty-five percent of the respondents were working at the time of the survey, significantly more men than women and proportionately more Hispanic American than Caucasian American or African American survivors. The younger the survivors were at the time of diagnosis, the more likely they were to be working; age and cancer type were important parameters as well. For most cancer types, the survivors who were working were significantly younger at diagnosis and had a significantly higher quality of life score than those who were not working. Of the survivors working at the time of the survey, 7.3% indicated that they had experienced job discrimination; this was independent of age, gender, or ethnic grouping.

Approximately 10% of survivors indicated that they were unable to work as a result of the effects of cancer, cancer treatment, or both. Significantly more women than men and significantly more African Americans than Caucasian Americans or Hispanic Americans reported being unable to work. Cancer type was also a relevant factor. The role of socioeconomic factors in these findings was not clear. A reassuring finding was that most cancer survivors did not perceive employment-related problems and assimilated back into the workforce. However, for those who did have cancer-related issues, little is known about their experiences because research data for this group were scanty and heterogeneous.

Internet Message Board for Cancer Survivors and Their Families

As a component of the LACC program, a message board was created on the Internet, through which cancer patients and their family members or other loved ones could communicate with and provide support for other patients and families. The message board was accessible to anyone who visited the M. D. Anderson Web page. This message board was monitored, and the findings from the postings were used to further understand the cancer experience and facilitate support for cancer patients.[23] During the initial 16 months since its creation, 972 individuals logged onto the message board ("users") and 284 persons posted 619 messages ("posters"). The messages were read and analyzed for content. The most common cancer types represented by the posted messages were breast, gastrointestinal, lung, gynecologic, head and neck, and colorectal. The most frequent themes were questions about treatment, support, and long-term effects. The message themes differed between those posted by the posters who had cancer and those who were posting a message on behalf of someone who had cancer. For example, friends and relatives who did not have cancer asked most frequently about treatment, whereas most individuals who had cancer posed questions about the long-term effects of cancer. Questions about support and diagnosis appeared to be of similar interest to both groups of posters.

Message board entries reflected yet another aspect of the cancer survivors' experience. In general, literature pertaining to health care and the Internet highlights the significance of this resource. However, little information is available about the types of cancer-related information the Internet users seek. Having such information would allow health care providers and educators to develop materials that are better suited to respond to the needs of consumers and patients.

Concluding Thoughts

Successfully treated cancer patients have much to teach us. Traditionally, cancer research has focused on the diagnosis and treatment of cancer, appropriately so. We have studied those who have not responded to treatment, seeking answers to develop better treatments. We should, in our quest to eradicate cancer, look not only to patients who have succumbed to the disease but also to those who have survived because they provide a living laboratory for the understanding of cancer. We have only scratched the surface in understanding how the cancer survivor has arrived at the place of long-term survivorship. We have accumulated the responses of more than 10,000 cancer survivors to a survey designed to shed some understanding on the cancer survivors' long-term sequelae of cancer treatment. This survivorship project has raised many questions that need further research. For example, this work requires longitudinal and prospective studies of large numbers of survivors. Through programs such as the LACC, the M. D. Anderson Cancer Center is poised to lead the initiative to learn more about cancer survivorship.

REFERENCES

1. Ries LAG, Kosary CL, Hankey BF, et al, editors. SEER cancer statistics review, 1975–2001. Bethesda (MD): National Cancer Institute. Available at: http://seer.cancer.gov/csr/1975_2001/results_merged/topic_survival.pdf.
2. Simmonds MA. Cancer statistics, 2003: further decrease in mortality rate, increase in persons living with cancer. CA Cancer J Clin 2003;53:4.
3. Meadows AT, Hobbie W. The medical consequences of cure. Cancer 1986;15 Suppl 2:524–8.
4. Ried H, Zietz H, Jaffe N. Late effects of cancer treatment in children. Pediatr Dent 1995;17:273–84.
5. Marina N. Long-term survivors of childhood cancer. The medical consequences of cure. Pediatr Clin North Am 1997;44:1021–42.
6. Stevens MC, Mahler H, Parkes S. The health status of adult survivors of cancer in childhood. Eur J Cancer 1998;34:694–8.
7. Loescher LJ, Welch-McCaffrey D, Leigh SA, et al. Surviving adult cancers. Part 1: physiologic effects. Ann Intern Med 1989;111:411–32.
8. Ganz PA. Late effects of cancer and its treatment. Semin Oncol Nurs 2001;17:241–8.
9. Schultz PN, Beck ML, Stava C, Vassilopoulou-Sellin R. Health profiles in 5836 long-term cancer survivors. Int J Cancer 2003;104:488–95.
10. Schultz PN, Stava C, Vassilopoulou-Sellin R. Health profiles and quality of life of 518 survivors of thyroid cancer. Head Neck 2003;25:349–56.
11. Schultz PN, Stava C, Beck ML, Vassilopoulou-Sellin R. Ethnic/racial influences on the physiologic health of cancer survivors. Cancer 2004;100:156–64.
12. Blackwell DL, Collins JG, Coles R. Summary health statistics for U.S. adults: National Health Interview Survey, 1997. National Center for Health Statistics. Vital Health Stat 2002;10.
13. Stava C, Beck ML, Schultz PN, Vassilopoulou-Sellin R. Hearing loss among cancer survivors. Oncol Rep 2006 [In press]
14. Schultz PN, Beck ML, Stava C, Vassilopoulou-Sellin R. Breast cancer: relationship between menopausal symptoms, physiologic health effects of cancer treatment and physical constraints on quality of life on long-term survivors. J Clin Nurs 2006 [In press]
15. President's Cancer Panel. Voices of a broken system: real people, real problems. Bethesda (MD): National Cancer Institute; 2000–2001.
16. Ross H. Lifting the unequal burden of cancer on minorities and the underserved. In: Closing the gap. Washington (DC): Office of Minority Health, Office of Public Health and Science, US Department Health and Human Services; August 2000. p. 1–2.
17. Shavers VL, Brown ML. Racial and ethnic disparities in the receipt of cancer treatment. J Natl Cancer Inst 2002;94:334–57.
18. Ren XS, Amick BC, Williams DR. Racial/ethnic disparities in health: the interplay between discrimination and socioeconomic status. Ethn Dis 1999;9:151–65.
19. Brooks SE, Baquet CR, Gardner JF, et al. Cervical cancer—the impact of clinical presentation, health and race on survival. J Assoc Acad Minor Phys 2000;11:55–9.
20. Grenier MA, Lipshultz SE. Epidemiology of anthracycline cardiotoxicity in children and adults. Semin Oncol 1998;25(4 Suppl 10):72–85.
21. Ren XS. Marital status and quality of relationships: the impact on health perception. Soc Sci Med 1997;44:241–9.
22. Schultz PN, Beck ML, Stava C, Vassiloupoulou-Sellin R. Cancer survivors: work related issues. Am Assoc Occup Health Nurs J 2002;50:220–6.
23. Schultz PN, Stava C, Beck ML, Sellin RV. Internet message board use by patients with cancer and their families. J Clin Oncol Nurs 2003;7:663–7.

Cancer Screening in Cancer Survivors

Sai-Ching Jim Yeung, MD, PhD

Continued advances in cancer treatment have led to improvements in treatment outcomes. The number of cancer survivors aged 18 years and older continues to increase because more childhood cancer patients are surviving to adulthood and adult cancer patients are surviving longer. Currently, more than 70% of pediatric cancer patients will survive long term, and approximately 60% of adult cancer patients will survive for at least 5 years after diagnosis.[1,2] In fact, there are almost 10 million cancer survivors in the United States.

Cancer survivors have a high risk of recurrence of the original cancer and development of second primary malignancies as a result of cancer therapy and other risk factors. In a review of 282 consecutive patients suspected to have a malignancy but no tissue diagnosis, a history of malignancy was a statistically significant predictor of a cancer diagnosis among other predictors, including advanced age, weight loss, thrombocytosis, and monocytosis.[3] Lifelong monitoring and screening for malignancies are thus necessary for cancer survivors. Yet a recent study showed that adult survivors of childhood cancer were not adequately screened for cancer.[4] Often cancer survivors cease to follow up with oncologists because of the lack of active oncologic issues. Furthermore, approximately 70% of cancer patients have comorbid conditions,[5] requiring a comprehensive approach to medical care. Therefore, internists and primary care providers should not only manage active noncancer medical problems but should also ensure continued surveillance for malignancies and provide preventive care.

This chapter summarizes the incidence of and risk factors for second or secondary malignancies and recommendations for cancer screening so that cancer survivors may reap the benefits of early detection. Screening practices for survivors of breast, colorectal, and prostate cancers; childhood acute lymphoblastic leukemia (ALL); and Hodgkin's disease are discussed. These cancers were selected on the basis of their high prevalence or high rates of survival.

Etiologic Factors for Secondary Malignancies

Ionizing Radiation

Many cancer patients have received multimodal therapy, and the separate contributions of chemotherapy and radiotherapy to treatment-related malignancies are not definitively known. Radiation is well known to cause primary cancers. When used as a treatment, radiation is associated with the development of secondary malignancies, including leukemia and brain, bone, thyroid, skin, and breast cancers, which usually develop several years to decades afterward. Typically, these radiation-induced malignancies occur at the margin of or within the irradiated field. Soft tissue sarcomas and osteosarcomas are the most frequent secondary neoplasms after radiotherapy.[6-8]

The risk of developing radiation-induced breast cancer is significantly higher in girls treated with mantle radiation before the age of 21 years than in women treated in their adult years.[6,9] The risk of secondary cancers increases with the total dose of radiation. In one study, a 40-fold increase in the risk of developing bone sarcomas was observed after doses of 60 Gy or more.[7] In another study, a 10-fold increase in the risk of soft tissue sarcoma was seen in retinoblastoma patients receiving ≥ 60 Gy, but even as little as 5 Gy increased the risk 2-fold for this genetically susceptible group.[10] However, high radiation doses do not appear to affect the risk of leukemia and thyroid cancer.

The risk of secondary cancers increases with time since radiation therapy.[11] In the Late Effects Study Group, the median time to develop a secondary neoplasm was 10 years after radiotherapy, but secondary neoplasms might develop as late as > 30 years after radiation exposure.[12] Radiogenic leukemias appear earlier, with a latency of 4 to 8 years, than radiation-induced solid tumors, which are usually diagnosed 10 to 40 years after radiation exposure.[13]

Chemotherapy

Acute myelogenous leukemia (AML) is the most common type of secondary malignancy after chemotherapy, and other types of hematologic malignancies, such as ALL, chronic myelogenous leukemia, and myelodysplastic syndrome, have also been reported.[14] Secondary myeloid leukemias induced by chemotherapy have a low cure rate of 10 to 20% and may be refractory to subsequent chemotherapy, which makes prevention very important.[15] Chemotherapeutic agents that carry a high risk of secondary leukemias are alkylating agents and etoposide, although chemotherapy using multiple drugs, particularly when doxorubicin is included, may increase the risk as well. Alkylating agents, including ifosfamide, cyclophosphamide, melphalan, busulfan, nitrogen mustard, procarbazine, carboplatin, and cisplatin, cause leukemias with deletions on chromosome 5 or 7. Inhibitors of topoisomerase II, such as epipodophyllotoxins, teniposide, and etoposide, cause leukemia with translocation of the *MLL* gene at chromosome band 11q23, and these topoisomerase II inhibitor–induced leukemias have relatively short latency periods of 1 to 3 years. An increase in the risk of secondary leukemia was noted with increasing doses of epipodophyllotoxins; $< 3\%$ of germ cell tumor survivors who received < 2 g/m^2 of etoposide would develop therapy-related acute myeloid leukemia (t-AML), but the incidence of t-AML increased to $> 11\%$ in survivors who received > 2 g/m^2 of etoposide.[13] In survivors of childhood cancers, such as rhabdomyosarcoma, Ewing's sarcoma, and Hodgkin's disease, a dose-response relationship has been demonstrated: alkylating agents increased the risk of a secondary leukemia almost 5-fold, and with the highest doses of alkylating agents, that risk increased to almost 24-fold.[14] Doxorubicin may further increase that risk when used together with high-dose alkylating agents.[14] Alkylating agents may also further increase the risk of radiation-induced secondary bone cancers. In one study[7], the relative risk (RR) of secondary bone sarcomas after radiation therapy was 2.7, but the RR increased to 4.7 when alkylating agents were also used.

Splenectomy

The mechanism by which asplenism aids in the induction of secondary cancers or second primary cancers is unknown, but the spleen may play a significant role in immunosurveillance against malignancies.[16] Standard therapies for Hodgkin's disease and other lymphomas often include splenectomy and splenic irradiation. In a study of 892 Hodgkin's disease survivors, splenectomy increased the risk of treatment-related secondary cancers.[17] In another study of 979 Hodgkin's disease survivors, splenectomy had borderline significance ($p = .09$) in increasing the incidence of secondary malignancies.[18]

Genetic Predisposition

Patients with a genetic predisposition for cancer develop multiple cancers in their lifetime. For instance, patients with Li-Fraumeni syndrome have a 50% probability of developing cancer by age 30 years.[19,20] Genetic predisposition certainly plays a role in the development of secondary cancers. Germline mutations in tumor suppressor genes (eg, the *TP53* tumor suppressor gene mutation in Li-Fraumeni syndrome) and gene mutations for hereditary cancers (eg, hereditary breast cancer genes *BRCA1* and *BRCA2*) may interact with therapeutic exposures, leading to an increased incidence of secondary cancers. Failure to induce apoptotic cell death after deoxyribonucleic acid (DNA) damage, defects in DNA repair, and dysfunction of DNA damage check points are potential mechanisms involved in the development of secondary malignancies after therapeutic exposure to radiation and DNA-damaging chemotherapeutic agents.

Bone Marrow Transplantation

For patients who underwent allogeneic or syngeneic transplantations, the cumulative incidence for secondary solid malignancies was 2.2% at 10 years and 6.7% at 15 years.[21] Patients who have undergone allogeneic transplantation have an increasing risk of new solid malignancies over time.[22,23] The rate of new malignant disease was two- to fourfold higher in these patients than in age-matched control subjects.[21,24] The types of solid malignancies that increased after allogeneic or syngeneic bone marrow transplantations include cancers of the buccal cavity, brain, liver, bone, and connective tissue and melanoma. Higher doses of total-body radiation were associated with a higher risk of solid cancers; and chronic graft-versus-host disease and male sex were closely linked with an increased risk of squamous cell cancers of the buccal cavity and skin.[25] The incidence of secondary solid malignancies after autologous transplantation is estimated to be lower than that after allogeneic transplantation.[22,26] After autologous stem cell transplantation in non-Hodgkin's lymphoma patients, the incidence of second malignancies after 10 years is 21%, with about 10.0% having nonhematologic malignancies.[26] New malignancy after autologous transplantation is the most frequent cause of non–relapse-related death.[27]

Smoking

Continuing to smoke increases the risk of second cancers at the same site or at different sites, regardless of whether the initial cancer is smoking related.[28] When the prognosis is relatively good for the initial malignancy, continued smoking will increase the risk of new primary malignancies for up to 20 years after the initial cancer diagnosis. In survivors of early-stage small cell lung cancer (mostly stages I and II), the risk of a secondary cancer (mostly non–small cell lung cancer) was 3.5- to 4.4-fold higher than that of the general population.[29–31] Continuing to smoke further increases the risk of secondary cancer, particularly in those who had undergone chest irradiation (RR = 21.0) or had received alkylating agents (RR = 19.0).[30] In survivors who ceased to smoke at the time of diagnosis, the risk was the same as in those who had quit smoking at least 6 months before the initial cancer diagnosis. Another study confirmed that patients with small cell lung cancer who survived at least 2 years had a greatly reduced likelihood of a secondary cancer if they quit smoking.[32] In a study of breast cancer survivors who subsequently developed lung cancer, the relationship between lung cancer and thoracic radiation therapy alone was negligible, but the relationship between lung cancer and smoking was substantial and was even stronger for the combination of thoracic radiation therapy and smoking.[33] Similarly, the effect of smoking on the risk of secondary lung cancer has also been observed in Hodgkin's disease survivors.[34,35] In one study, very high risks for subsequent lung cancer were identified for smokers: RR = 20.2 for radiation treatment and smoking and RR = 49.1 for radiation, alkylating agents, and smoking.[34]

Second Primary or Secondary Malignancies in Specific Cancer Survivor Groups

Breast Cancer

The treatment used for breast cancer may affect the subsequent risk of secondary malignancies. For breast cancer patients who were treated with doxorubicin-based regimens, the rates of secondary cancers were 3.8% at 10 years and 7.0% at 15 years.[36] Postmastectomy radiotherapy can increase the risk of secondary lung cancer, particularly in smokers.[37–39] Chemotherapy with alkylating agents increases the risk of acute leukemia, particularly if the patients also receive radiotherapy.[40] Postirradiation sarcomas may also occur.[41] Breast cancer survivors have an increased risk of developing cancer in the breast contralateral to the one where the initial breast cancer has been found. However, radiotherapy does not appear to contribute much to this risk.[42] Antiestrogens and breast cancer screening can reduce the incidence of second breast malignancies and improve survival.[43] Tamoxifen has antiestrogenic effects on breast tissue and significantly decreases the incidence of contralateral breast cancer, but it has proestrogenic effects on the uterus and increases the risk of endometrial cancer.[42] Thus, patients who have undergone long-term adjuvant hormonal therapy should undergo regular gynecologic examination with endometrial screening.

Breast cancer survivors also have increased risk of cancers of the ovaries, endometrium, and colon or rectum.[42,44] These organs share risk factors with breast cancer, that is, diet, obesity, and female hormonal status. Breast cancer genetics has also implicated mutations in *BRCA1* and *BRCA2* as risk factors for breast and ovarian cancers. Screening for ovarian, endometrial, and colorectal cancer should be performed regularly in breast cancer survivors.[45,46]

Prostate Cancer

Radiotherapy for prostate cancer increases the risk of subsequent bladder cancer.[47] Nevertheless, the increase in risk appears to be small and late (some years after radiotherapy).

Testicular Cancer

Testicular cancer is one of the solid tumors with a very favorable outcome, whether it occurs unilaterally or bilaterally.[48] Patients with testicular cancer often receive combination chemotherapy with cisplatin, etoposide, and bleomycin. Although both etoposide and cisplatin can cause secondary leukemia, the risk correlates to the total cumulative dose of etoposide received. Testicular cancer patients treated with a combination of radiotherapy and chemotherapy are at an increased risk of secondary cancers, particularly in the pelvis.[49]

Endometrial and Ovarian Cancer

Survivors of endometrial cancer have increased risk of ovarian, colorectal, and breast cancers.[44,46,48] Therefore, surveillance and screening for these cancers should be performed in survivors of endometrial cancer. Bilateral oophorectomy at the time of hysterectomy for the endometrial cancer may be considered if appropriate because removal of the ovaries will reduce the subsequent risk of ovarian cancer.

Skin Cancer

It is well known that basal cell and squamous cell carcinomas (nonmelanoma skin cancers) tend to develop in the same skin cancer patients. This pattern represents the effect of the shared risk factor: sun exposure. Thus, those who have nonmelanoma skin cancer should avoid sun exposure and should have regular surveillance for new skin malignancies by dermatologists. Patients with dysplastic nevi may develop multiple melanomas. These patients and melanoma survivors should have regular full-body skin examinations by experienced clinicians.[50]

Colorectal Cancer

There are more than 1 million colorectal cancer survivors in the United States now. Colorectal cancer cases are sporadic (approximately 60% of all cases), familial (approximately 30%), or hereditary (approximately 10%, mainly as part of genetic syndromes, such as hereditary nonpolyposis colorectal cancer [HNPCC] and familial adenomatous polyposis [FAP]). FAP has a classic presentation, with the formation of numerous adenomatous polyps in the colon and rectum at a young age. Patients with FAP have almost a 100% probability of developing colorectal cancer by the age of 50 years. Persons with HNPCC have a high risk of colorectal cancers and cancers of the ureter, renal pelvis, and small bowel. Females with HNPCC have a risk of 30 to 60% of developing endometrial cancer in their lifetime. Survivors of colorectal cancer have an elevated risk of second primary malignancies of the colon and rectum, as well as of the breasts, uterus, and ovaries.[46] For colorectal cancer survivors, prompt detection of new primary cancers or recurrent disease can improve subsequent survival. The risk of recurrence is highest during the first 5 years after resection of colorectal cancer; thus, frequent surveillance examination and follow-up care are recommended during this period.

Upper Aerodigestive Tract Cancer

The rate of esophageal cancer that occurs after lung cancer increases after radiotherapy for the initial lung cancer, suggesting a carcinogenic effect of radiation in esophageal cancer's etiology. Even in the absence of radiotherapy, the risk of esophageal carcinoma is still increased after the diagnosis of lung cancer.[51–53] Quitting smoking and discontinuation of tobacco consumption after the diagnosis of the initial primary cancer in the upper aerodigestive tract reduce the risk of other tobacco-related malignancies and thus remain an important strategy to prevent cancer.[54] Particularly in the case of an initial head and neck cancer, it is very important to look carefully for synchronous multiple primary tumors in the upper aerodigestive tract and respiratory system at presentation. For instance, the prognosis is poor if a lung nodule is a recurrence or metastasis from an initial oropharyngeal primary tumor, but cure may still be possible if a lung nodule is a second primary lung cancer that can be surgically removed.

Retinoblastoma

Hereditary retinoblastoma patients are at high risk of developing a secondary malignancy after radiotherapy, and this is primarily due to the genetic predisposition of the retinoblastoma gene (*RB1*) mutation. In the largest study of retinoblastoma survivors, Wong and colleagues reported an RR of 30 for secondary cancers compared with an age-matched control group.[10] The cumulative incidence of secondary cancers for patients with hereditary retinoblastoma was 51% at 50 years compared with 5% at 50 years for patients with the nonhereditary form of retinoblastoma. Two-thirds of the secondary malignancies were soft tissue or osteogenic sarcomas. A radiation dose-response relationship was found for soft tissue sarcomas, with as little as 5 Gy increasing the risk of secondary malignancy 2-fold and >60 Gy increasing the risk 10-fold.

Wilms' Tumor

The National Wilms' Tumor Study Group found an eightfold increase in secondary malignancies in survivors of Wilms' tumor.[49] Most cases of the secondary leukemias were t-AML, which was diagnosed between 1 and 6 years after the original therapy for Wilms' tumor. Secondary lymphomas had similar latency periods. In contrast, much longer latency periods of 3 to 21 years were observed for secondary solid tumors, which were mostly sarcomas and carcinomas (parotid gland, thyroid, breast, hepatocellular, and colon) but also brain tumors. Survivors who received abdominal radiotherapy had twice the risk of secondary cancers compared with those who did not. Doxorubicin may also have potentiated the carcinogenic effect of radiation. In another study, the 20-year cumulative incidence of secondary malignancies after treatment for Wilms' tumor was 3 to 6%.[55]

Hodgkin's Disease

Hodgkin's disease survivors have a RR of 2 to 4 for developing secondary malignancies. The overall cumulative incidences of developing a secondary malignancy, most of which are solid tumors, are 10% at 20 years after treatment for Hodgkin's disease and 26% at 30 years. Young age when treatment began and the use of radiotherapy were important risk factors for secondary cancers in Hodgkin's disease survivors.[56] Compared with the normal population, patients with Hodgkin's disease are more likely to die from secondary cancers and cardiovascular diseases.[57] The RR was 6.6 for death owing to a secondary cancer in a Hodgkin's disease survivor compared with the normal population.

The common secondary solid tumors, in order of incidence, were breast, thyroid, bone, colorectal, lung, and stomach cancers. Breast cancer in the context of Hodgkin's disease is related to mantle radiation therapy and chemotherapy at a young age. Secondary breast cancer differs from sporadic breast cancer because it develops in younger women, is associated with a higher incidence of bilateral disease (both breasts), and is located closer to the midline of the body than sporadic breast cancer.[58]

Hodgkin's disease survivors also have a high risk of acute leukemia[59] and non-Hodgkin's lymphoma[60] after treatment. As many as 25% of the secondary malignancies in Hodgkin's disease survivors are secondary leukemia or lymphoma.[6,61–63] Regimens that contain procarbazine and nitrogen mustard (such as MOPP [nitrogen mustard, Oncovin [vincristine], procarbazine, and prednisone]) convey the highest risk of secondary leukemia compared with regimens that contain cyclophosphamide.[63]

Non-Hodgkin's Lymphoma

Over the past three decades, the combination of cyclophosphamide, doxorubicin, vincristine, and prednisone has cured a significant number of patients with non-Hodgkin's lymphoma. Less than 3% of patients developed secondary cancers after treatment with cyclophosphamide, doxorubicin, vincristine, and prednisone;[64] compared with a control population of patients without non-Hodgkin's lymphoma, this increase was not statistically significant.

Acute Lymphoblastic Leukemia

Current treatment cures more than 80% of children with ALL, but these ALL survivors are at risk of secondary cancers. Radiotherapy appears to be the main contributor to the risk of developing a secondary cancer. Patients with ALL who underwent cranial or craniospinal radiotherapy (about 24 Gy) as central nervous system prophylaxis have an RR of 22 for developing central nervous system tumors. Patients who were less than the age of 5 years at the time of radiotherapy have the highest risk.[65] A high cranial radiation dose is associated with the development of brain tumors; for patients who received >30 Gy, the cumulative incidence of brain tumors is 3.23% at 20 years.[66] Therefore, in recent treatment regimens for ALL, young children (under 10 years old) who have no evidence of central nervous system disease at diagnosis are treated with intensive intrathecal chemotherapy rather than cranial irradiation. The risk of chemotherapy-induced t-AML in ALL survivors varies with the dose and schedule of epipodophyllotoxins, and chemotherapy including epipodophyllotoxins administered weekly or twice weekly resulted in a cumulative secondary AML incidence of 12%.[67]

Screening Recommendations for Secondary Cancer in Cancer Survivors

General Recommendations for All Cancer Survivors

1. Obtain a detailed medical history, including a family medical history. (Discuss the referral

with a clinical genetics service if a significant family history of cancer is identified.)

2. Perform lifelong clinical assessments at yearly intervals that include symptom review, a clinical examination, and screening for secondary malignancies. A careful physical examination with special attention to the radiotherapy field should be performed at long-term follow-up clinic visits; prompt evaluations are needed to address and evaluate new or suspicious signs and symptoms. In the event of unexpected changes in the complete blood count, such as the appearance of macrocytosis, dysplastic changes of any blood cell type, or cytopenia, a bone marrow biopsy and aspiration should be performed.

3. Educate patients regarding the risks of secondary malignancies and the importance of promptly reporting new symptoms or masses.

4. Advise patients on the reduction of risk behaviors, especially smoking and sunbathing.

5. Encourage patients to perform self-examination, such as of the breast, oral cavity, and skin.

Childhood Cancer Survivors

There are more and more survivors of childhood and adolescent cancers in the United States. Late cancer-related complications in these survivors include an increased risk of premature mortality caused by secondary cancers and cardiovascular diseases. The Children's Oncology Group has published guidelines for the long-term follow-up care of survivors of childhood cancers (<http://www.survivorshipguidelines.org>). However, whether surveillance results in measurable reductions in morbidity or mortality has not been proven.

The risk of secondary AML usually manifests within 10 years after treatment; therefore, monitoring should include a complete blood count with differential annually for at least 10 years after therapy (Table 1). Most solid secondary malignancies are related to radiation exposure; therefore, the annual physical examination should pay special attention to the skin and soft tissues in the radiation field together with radiographic (eg, chest radiography if the chest was in the radiation field) or other cancer screening evaluations (eg, dental examination if the mouth was in the radiation field) if indicated.

For female cancer survivors who have undergone radiation therapy with potential effects on the breast (ie, mantle, mediastinal, or lung), a monthly self-breast examination should begin at puberty; clinical breast examination should be performed annually beginning at puberty until 25 years old and then every 6 months; and

Table 1 Cancer Screening for Childhood Cancer Survivors

Cancer	Surveillance	Screening for Second Primary or Secondary Cancers
ALL	Individualized based on chemoradiation treatment regimen*	Brain radiation: central nervous system tumors Acute myelocytic leukemia Cyclophosphamide therapy: bladder cancer
Hodgkin's disease	Individualized*	Breast cancer (in women only) Lung cancer Colorectal cancer Bone cancer Thyroid cancer Nonmelanoma skin cancer

Adapted from guidelines for the long-term follow-up care of survivors of childhood, adolescent, and young adult cancer developed by the Children's Oncology Group. Specific recommendations can be accessed at <http://www.survivorshipguidelines.org>.
ALL = acute lymphoblastic leukemia.
*Frequency based on cumulative anthracycline and chest radiation dose and age at treatment.

mammograms and routine Cleopatra views to screen the inner quadrants should be obtained annually starting 8 years after radiotherapy or at age 25 years. The effectiveness of frequent self- and physician examinations in younger women (<40 years old) with dense breast tissue may be low. However, Hancock and colleagues found that 56% of secondary breast cancers were discovered by physician examination during follow-up and 16% by self-examination.[68] Magnetic resonance imaging (MRI) examinations may be helpful to screen younger females with dense breast tissue and for patients who have undergone mantle field irradiation to treat childhood malignancies.

Although male survivors of childhood cancers are at risk of developing various types of second primary cancers as much as female survivors, they do not appear to have the same risk of breast cancer as do females. A Finnish review of 470,000 registered cancer patients and a Nordic study of 30,880 childhood cancer survivors found no male survivors with secondary breast cancers.[69,70]

Screening for secondary colorectal cancer in cancer survivors at risk (ie, those having received radiation doses of ≥25 Gy to the spine, abdomen, and/or pelvis) involves colonoscopy every 10 years starting at the age of 35 years or 10 years after radiotherapy. Chronic hepatitis, often associated with blood product exposure prior to 1992, increases the risk of hepatocellular carcinoma, which can be screened by measuring serum α-fetoprotein annually; patients who have developed cirrhosis should have annual right upper quadrant ultrasonography.

Breast Cancer Survivors

More than 2.1 million females in the United States are breast cancer survivors. Most breast cancer recurrences occur within the first 5 years after treatment. Nonspecific symptoms (eg, weight loss, persistent cough, or body ache) or physical findings (eg, breast or chest wall changes or

lymphadenopathy) are common in breast cancer recurrence and should be investigated thoroughly during regular follow-up physician visits (Table 2). In addition to monitoring for recurrent disease, cancer screening may benefit breast cancer survivors as they have an increased risk of second primary cancers involving the breasts, colon, rectum, and ovaries.

Current recommendations for surveillance in breast cancer survivors include monthly self-examination of the breasts and chest wall, annual mammography of the remaining breast tissue, and a careful medical history and physical examination every 6 months for 5 years and annually thereafter. Many breast cancer survivors receive treatment with tamoxifen. Although tamoxifen reduces the risk of recurrent breast cancer and maintains bone density, it increases the risk of uterine cancer. To screen for uterine cancer, a pelvic examination and a PAP smear should be performed annually, and vaginal sonography should be performed at 3 and 5 years after the start of tamoxifen therapy to evaluate the endometrium.

Careful compilation of the family history may reveal hereditary breast cancer. Approximately 5 to 10% of breast cancers are caused by germline gene mutations (BRCA1 and BRCA2). Identification of a hereditary component should prompt referral to clinical genetics services for consultation and screening of close relatives.

Mammography may have limited utility in females with dense breast tissue. Other new breast imaging modalities may trivialize the problems encountered in screening women with dense breasts. Ultrasonography may avoid unnecessary biopsies of cysts and may supplement mammography and clinical examination. However, ultrasonography has never been recommended as a routinely used screening tool.[71] Digital mammography and MRI have been introduced for breast cancer screening,[71] and MRI is the most accurate method to determine the size and number of lesions in the breast.[71]

Table 2 Cancer Screening for Survivors of Selected Cancers

Cancer Site	Surveillance for Recurrence	Screening for Second Primary or Secondary Cancers	Genetic Considerations
Breast	Monthly breast self-examinations Medical history and physical examination (including clinical breast examinations) every 6 mo for 5 yr and then annually Annual mammogram	Ipsilateral and contralateral breast Ovarian cancer Colorectal cancer Annual pelvic examination to screen for uterine cancer if patient is taking tamoxifen	Age at diagnosis Family cancer history Consider referral to genetic counseling for BRCA1 or BRCA2 mutations
Colorectal	CEA and clinical examination every 3 mo for 2 yr and then every 6 mo for 3 to 5 yr CT (optimal interval undetermined) Colonoscopy after 1 yr, 3 yr, and then every 5 yr*	Metachronous colorectal cancer Breast cancer Cervical cancer	Family cancer history Genetic counseling and assessment for familial adenomatous polyposis and hereditary nonpolyposis colorectal cancer
Prostate	Clinical evaluation PSA every 6 mo for 5 yr and then annually Digital rectal examination annually	Bladder cancer Colorectal cancer	Age at diagnosis Family cancer history Consider referral for genetic counseling and assessment if strong family history

Adapted from Kattlove H and Winn RJ.[73]
CEA = carcinoembryonic antigen; CT = computed tomography; PSA = prostate-specific antigen.
Surveillance recommendations from the National Comprehensive Cancer Network can be accessed on-line at <http://www.nccn.org>.

Colorectal Cancer Survivors

Survivors of colorectal cancer have a high risk of second malignancies within the lower gastrointestinal tract, as well as in the breasts, uterus, and ovaries.[46] Those with HNPCC have an elevated risk of small bowel and endometrial cancers. The risk of recurrence is highest in the first 5 years after resection. For over 1 million survivors of colorectal cancer in the United States, prompt detection of new or recurrent cancer can improve survival. A meta-analysis has demonstrated a survival benefit of 19% at 5 years among patients undergoing intensive follow-up.

The National Comprehensive Care Network and the American Society of Clinical Oncology guidelines recommend follow-up evaluations to include a medical history, a physical examination, carcinoembryonic antigen (CEA) testing, and colonoscopy. History taking, physical examinations, and measuring CEA are recommended every 3 months for the first 2 years after treatment and then every 6 months for the next 3 years (see Table 2). A CEA blood test should be performed every 3 months for the first 2 years after the initial colon cancer diagnosis and then every 6 months for approximately 5 years after that. CEA measurement, combined with computed tomography (CT) body imaging studies, can improve survival. Colonoscopy should be performed 1 year after the initial colon cancer surgery and then every 3 years.

Patients with elevated CEA levels (which may precede symptoms by as many as 3 to 8 months) should be examined by CT, positron emission tomography, and colonoscopy, as appropriate, to identify the site of recurrent cancer and evaluate whether the recurrent disease can be surgically removed. Surveillance colonoscopy is recommended 12 months after surgery or at 6 months after surgery if a full colonoscopy has not been performed before surgery. If no abnormalities are detected by colonoscopy, then it should be repeated every 3 to 5 years.

Prostate Cancer Survivors

Approximately 98% of prostate cancer patients survive 5 years after diagnosis; thus, the number of prostate cancer survivors is now estimated to exceed 1.7 million in the United States. Disease surveillance of prostate cancer survivors includes a nannual rectal examination and monitoring prostate-specific antigen (PSA) levels every 6 months for 5 years and then annually (see Table 2). Serum PSA declines to undetectable levels after radical prostatectomy; a slower decline occurs after radiotherapy. Elevated serum PSA levels after the initial decline achieved by definitive therapy indicate disease recurrence. Radiotherapy for prostate cancer may be associated with an increased incidence of bladder cancer among prostate cancer survivors;[47] therefore,

signs of hematuria should be thoroughly investigated.

The family history of prostate cancer survivors should be reviewed. Many cases of prostate cancer may have a familial component, and the risk of prostate cancer increases with the number of affected family members. Moreover, men with close relatives affected by breast or ovarian cancer may be at elevated risk of prostate cancer owing to BRCA1 or BRCA2 mutations. If a hereditary or genetic component is suspected, referral to a clinical geneticist for risk assessment and genetic testing may be indicated.

Disclaimer

It is not possible for cancer screening recommendations for cancer survivors to be based on evidence from randomized or controlled trials because secondary cancers are consequences of cancer therapy and cannot be objectives in prospective studies. Therefore, recommendations are based on retrospective studies that have identified secondary cancers in long-term survivors. Under no circumstances should the recommendations be considered as mandatory, and it is common sense that certain recommendations may be inappropriate or contraindicated in individual patients. Furthermore, recommendations must be adapted regularly as our knowledge improves.

REFERENCES

1. Greenlee RT, Murray T, Bolden S, Wingo PA. Cancer statistics, 2000. CA Cancer J Clin 2000;50:7–33.
2. Ries LAG, Smith MA, Gurney JG, et al. Cancer incidence and survival among children and adolescents: United States SEER Program 1975-1995. Bethesda (MD): National Cancer Institute, SEER Program, National Institutes of Health; 1999.
3. Weiser MA, Cabanillas M, Vu K, et al. Diagnostic evaluation of patients with a high suspicion of malignancy: comorbidities and clinical predictors of cancer. Am J Med Sci 2005;330:11–8.
4. Robison LL, Green DM, Hudson M, et al. Long-term outcomes of adult survivors of childhood cancer. Cancer 2005;104:2557–64.
5. Ogle KS, Swanson GM, Woods N, Azzouz F. Cancer and comorbidity: redefining chronic diseases. Cancer 2000;88:653–63.
6. Bhatia S, Robison LL, Oberlin O, et al. Breast cancer and other second neoplasms after childhood Hodgkin's disease. N Engl J Med 1996;334:745–51.
7. Tucker MA, D'Angio GJ, Boice JD Jr, et al. Bone sarcomas linked to radiotherapy and chemotherapy in children. N Engl J Med 1987;317:588–93.
8. Ron E, Lubin JH, Shore RE, et al. Thyroid cancer after exposure to external radiation: a pooled analysis of seven studies. Radiat Res 1995;141:259–77.
9. Ng AK, Bernardo MV, Weller E, et al. Second malignancy after Hodgkin disease treated with radiation therapy with or without chemotherapy: long-term risks and risk factors. Blood 2002;100:1989–96.
10. Wong FL, Boice JD Jr, Abramson DH, et al. Cancer incidence after retinoblastoma. Radiation dose and sarcoma risk. JAMA 1997;278:1262–7.
11. de Vathaire F, Hawkins M, Campbell S, et al. Second malignant neoplasms after a first cancer in childhood: temporal pattern of risk according to type of treatment. Br J Cancer 1999;79:1884–93.
12. Meadows AT, Baum E, Fossati-Bellani F, et al. Second malignant neoplasms in children: an update from the Late Effects Study Group. J Clin Oncol 1985;3:532–8.

13. Hawkins MM, Wilson LM, Stovall MA, et al. Epipodophyllotoxins, alkylating agents, and radiation and risk of secondary leukaemia after childhood cancer. BMJ 1992; 304:951–8.

14. Tucker MA, Meadows AT, Boice JD Jr, et al. Leukemia after therapy with alkylating agents for childhood cancer. J Natl Cancer Inst 1987;78:459–64.

15. Neugut AI, Robinson E, Nieves J, et al. Poor survival of treatment-related acute nonlymphocytic leukemia. JAMA 1990;264:1006–8.

16. Ochsenbein AF. Principles of tumor immunosurveillance and implications for immunotherapy. Cancer Gene Ther 2002;9:1043–55.

17. Dietrich PY, Henry-Amar M, Cosset JM, et al. Second primary cancers in patients continuously disease-free from Hodgkin's disease: a protective role for the spleen? Blood 1994;84:1209–15.

18. Meadows AT, Obringer AC, Marrero O, et al. Second malignant neoplasms following childhood Hodgkin's disease: treatment and splenectomy as risk factors. Med Pediatr Oncol 1989;17:477–84.

19. Malkin D, Jolly KW, Barbier N, et al. Germline mutations of the p53 tumor-suppressor gene in children and young adults with second malignant neoplasms. N Engl J Med 1992;326:1309–15.

20. Russo CL, McIntyre J, Goorin AM, et al. Secondary breast cancer in patients presenting with osteosarcoma: possible involvement of germline p53 mutations. Med Pediatr Oncol 1994;23:354–8.

21. Curtis RE, Rowlings PA, Deeg HJ, et al. Solid cancers after bone marrow transplantation. N Engl J Med 1997;336: 897–904.

22. Baker KS, DeFor TE, Burns LJ, et al. New malignancies after blood or marrow stem-cell transplantation in children and adults: incidence and risk factors. J Clin Oncol 2003;21:1352–8.

23. Bhatia S, Louie AD, Bhatia R, et al. Solid cancers after bone marrow transplantation. J Clin Oncol 2001;19:464–71.

24. Kolb HJ, Socie G, Duell T, et al. Malignant neoplasms in long-term survivors of bone marrow transplantation. Late Effects Working Party of the European Cooperative Group for Blood and Marrow Transplantation and the European Late Effect Project Group. Ann Intern Med 1999;131:738–44.

25. Curtis RE, Metayer C, Rizzo JD, et al. Impact of chronic GVHD therapy on the development of squamous-cell cancers after hematopoietic stem-cell transplantation: an international case-control study. Blood 2005;105: 3802–11.

26. Brown JR, Yeckes H, Friedberg JW, et al. Increasing incidence of late second malignancies after conditioning with cyclophosphamide and total-body irradiation and autologous bone marrow transplantation for non-Hodgkin's lymphoma. J Clin Oncol 2005;23:2208–14.

27. Bhatia S, Robison LL, Francisco L, et al. Late mortality in survivors of autologous hematopoietic-cell transplantation: report from the Bone Marrow Transplant Survivor Study. Blood 2005;105:4215–22.

28. Wynder EL, Mushinski MH, Spivak JC. Tobacco and alcohol consumption in relation to the development of multiple primary cancers. Cancer 1977;40:1872–8.

29. Richardson GE, Tucker MA, Venzon DJ, et al. Smoking cessation after successful treatment of small-cell lung cancer is associated with fewer smoking-related second primary cancers. Ann Intern Med 1993;119:383–90.

30. Tucker MA, Murray N, Shaw EG, et al. Second primary cancers related to smoking and treatment of small-cell lung cancer. Lung Cancer Working Cadre. J Natl Cancer Inst 1997;89:1782–8.

31. Johnson BE. Second lung cancers in patients after treatment for an initial lung cancer. J Natl Cancer Inst 1998;90: 1335–45.

32. Kawahara M, Ushijima S, Kamimori T, et al. Second primary tumours in more than 2-year disease-free survivors of small-cell lung cancer in Japan: the role of smoking cessation. Br J Cancer 1998;78:409–12.

33. Ford MB, Sigurdson AJ, Petrulis ES, et al. Effects of smoking and radiotherapy on lung carcinoma in breast carcinoma survivors. Cancer 2003;98:1457–64.

34. Travis LB, Gospodarowicz M, Curtis RE, et al. Lung cancer following chemotherapy and radiotherapy for Hodgkin's disease. J Natl Cancer Inst 2002;94:182–92.

35. Abrahamsen JF, Andersen A, Hannisdal E, et al. Second malignancies after treatment of Hodgkin's disease: the influence of treatment, follow-up time, and age. J Clin Oncol 1993;11:255–61.

36. Woodward WA, Strom EA, McNeese MD, et al. Cardiovascular death and second non-breast cancer malignancy after postmastectomy radiation and doxorubicin-based chemotherapy. Int J Radiat Oncol Biol Phys 2003;57: 327–35.

37. Neugut AI, Robinson E, Lee WC, et al. Lung cancer after radiation therapy for breast cancer. Cancer 1993;71: 3054–7.

38. Inskip PD, Stovall M, Flannery JT. Lung cancer risk and radiation dose among women treated for breast cancer. J Natl Cancer Inst 1994;86:983–8.

39. Neugut AI, Murray T, Santos J, et al. Increased risk of lung cancer after breast cancer radiation therapy in cigarette smokers. Cancer 1994;73:1615–20.

40. Curtis RE, Boice JD Jr, Stovall M, et al. Risk of leukemia after chemotherapy and radiation treatment for breast cancer. N Engl J Med 1992;326:1745–51.

41. Brady MS, Garfein CF, Petrek JA, Brennan MF. Post-treatment sarcoma in breast cancer patients. Ann Surg Oncol 1994;1:66–72.

42. Boice JD Jr, Harvey EB, Blettner M, et al. Cancer in the contralateral breast after radiotherapy for breast cancer. N Engl J Med 1992;326:781–5.

43. Curtis RE, Boice JD Jr, Shriner DA, et al. Second cancers after adjuvant tamoxifen therapy for breast cancer. J Natl Cancer Inst 1996;88:832–4.

44. Schatzkin A, Baranovsky A, Kessler LG. Diet and cancer. Evidence from associations of multiple primary cancers in the SEER program. Cancer 1988;62:1451–7.

45. Bond JH. Screening guidelines for colorectal cancer. Am J Med 1999;106:7S–10S.

46. Weinberg DS, Newschaffer CJ, Topham A. Risk for colorectal cancer after gynecologic cancer. Ann Intern Med 1999;131:189–93.

47. Neugut AI, Ahsan H, Robinson E, Ennis RD. Bladder carcinoma and other second malignancies after radiotherapy for prostate carcinoma. Cancer 1997;79:1600–4.

48. Travis LB, Curtis RE, Storm H, et al. Risk of second malignant neoplasms among long-term survivors of testicular cancer. J Natl Cancer Inst 1997;89:1429–39.

49. Chaudhary UB, Haldas JR. Long-term complications of chemotherapy for germ cell tumours. Drugs 2003;63: 1565–77.

50. Boland SL, Shaw HM, Milton GW. Multiple primary cancers in patients with malignant melanoma. Med J Aust 1976; 1:517–9.

51. Ahsan H, Neugut AI, Gammon MD. Association of adenocarcinoma and squamous cell carcinoma of the esophagus with tobacco-related and other malignancies. Cancer Epidemiol Biomarkers Prev 1997;6:779–82.

52. Kleinerman RA, Boice JD Jr, Storm HH, et al. Second primary cancer after treatment for cervical cancer. An International Cancer Registries study. Cancer 1995;76: 442–52.

53. Ahsan H, Neugut AI. Radiation therapy for breast cancer and increased risk for esophageal carcinoma. Ann Intern Med 1998;128:114–7.

54. Schottenfeld D, Gantt RC, Wyner EL. The role of alcohol and tobacco in multiple primary cancers of the upper digestive system, larynx and lung: a prospective study. Prev Med 1974;3:277–93.

55. Hawkins MM, Draper GJ, Kingston JE. Incidence of second primary tumours among childhood cancer survivors. Br J Cancer 1987;56:339–47.

56. Bhatia S, Yasui Y, Robison LL, et al. High risk of subsequent neoplasms continues with extended follow-up of childhood Hodgkin's disease: report from the Late Effects Study Group. J Clin Oncol 2003;21:4386–94.

57. Aleman BM, van den Belt-Dusebout AW, Klokman WJ, et al. Long-term cause-specific mortality of patients treated for Hodgkin's disease. J Clin Oncol 2003;21:3431–9.

58. Deniz K, O'Mahony S, Ross G, Purushotham A. Breast cancer in women after treatment for Hodgkin's disease. Lancet Oncol 2003;4:207–14.

59. Josting A, Wiedenmann S, Franklin J, et al. Secondary myeloid leukemia and myelodysplastic syndromes in patients treated for Hodgkin's disease: a report from the German Hodgkin's Lymphoma Study Group. J Clin Oncol 2003;21:3440–6.

60. Rueffer U, Josting A, Franklin J, et al. Non-Hodgkin's lymphoma after primary Hodgkin's disease in the German Hodgkin's Lymphoma Study Group: incidence, treatment, and prognosis. J Clin Oncol 2001;19:2026–32.

61. Kaldor JM, Day NE, Clarke EA, et al. Leukemia following Hodgkin's disease. N Engl J Med 1990;322:7–13.

62. Tucker MA, Coleman CN, Cox RS, et al. Risk of second cancers after treatment for Hodgkin's disease. N Engl J Med 1988;318:76–81.

63. van Leeuwen FE, Chorus AM, van den Belt-Dusebout AW, et al. Leukemia risk following Hodgkin's disease: relation to cumulative dose of alkylating agents, treatment with teniposide combinations, number of episodes of chemotherapy, and bone marrow damage. J Clin Oncol 1994;12:1063–73.

64. Andre M, Mounier N, Leleu X, et al. Second cancers and late toxicities after treatment of aggressive non-Hodgkin lymphoma with the ACVBP regimen: a GELA cohort study on 2837 patients. Blood 2004;103:1222–8.

65. Neglia JP, Meadows AT, Robison LL, et al. Second neoplasms after acute lymphoblastic leukemia in childhood. N Engl J Med 1991;325:1330–6.

66. Walter AW, Hancock ML, Pui CH, et al. Secondary brain tumors in children treated for acute lymphoblastic leukemia at St Jude Children's Research Hospital. J Clin Oncol 1998;16:3761–7.

67. Pui CH, Ribeiro RC, Hancock ML, et al. Acute myeloid leukemia in children treated with epipodophyllotoxins for acute lymphoblastic leukemia. N Engl J Med 1991; 325:1682–7.

68. Hancock SL, Tucker MA, Hoppe RT. Breast cancer after treatment of Hodgkin's disease. J Natl Cancer Inst 1993;85:25–31.

69. Sankila R, Pukkala E, Teppo L. Risk of subsequent malignant neoplasms among 470,000 cancer patients in Finland, 1953-1991. Int J Cancer 1995;60:464–70.

70. Olsen JH, Garwicz S, Hertz H, et al. Second malignant neoplasms after cancer in childhood or adolescence. Nordic Society of Paediatric Haematology and Oncology Association of the Nordic Cancer Registries. BMJ 1993; 307:1030–6.

71. Boetes C, Mus RD, Holland R, et al. Breast tumors: comparative accuracy of MR imaging relative to mammography and US for demonstrating extent. Radiology 1995;197:743–7.

72. Braeuning MP, Pisano ED. New modalities in breast imaging: digital mammography and magnetic resonance imaging. Breast Cancer Res Treat 1995;35:31–8.

73. Kattlove H, Winn RJ. Ongoing care of patients after primary treatment for their cancer. CA Cancer J Clin 2003;53: 172–96.

Disturbances of Growth and Pubertal Development in Childhood Cancer Survivors

Wassim Chemaitilly, MD

Charles Sklar, MD

Cancers occur less frequently during childhood than during adulthood. Around 12,500 individuals under 20 years of age are diagnosed with a new malignancy every year in the United States.[1] Before the age of 15 years, the most frequently observed cancers are leukemia (30.2%, with a majority of patients diagnosed with acute lymphoblastic leukemia [ALL]), central nervous system (CNS) cancers (21.7%), and lymphomas (10.9%, including 6.2% of patients diagnosed with non-Hodgkin's lymphoma [NHL]).[2] The incidence of newly diagnosed malignancies increases during adolescence, with a change in the etiologic distribution due to the rise in the incidence of Hodgkin's disease in that age group. Thus, in adolescence, the most frequently diagnosed cancers are lymphomas (23.6%, including 16.1% of patients diagnosed with Hodgkin's disease) followed by leukemia (10.6%, with a majority of patients diagnosed with ALL) and CNS cancers (10%).[3]

The modest increase in the incidence of childhood and adolescence cancers over the past 20 years comes in sharp contrast to the significant drop in the mortality rates over the same period of time. Cancer incidence rates increased by 1% yearly between 1974 and 1991.[4] In parallel, the five-year survival rates continuously improved and currently exceed 70% in children and adolescents, and reach more than 80% for ALL and 90% for Hodgkin's disease.[2] These improvements are the results of remarkable advances in supportive care and, most importantly, changes in therapy occurring over the past 30 years. Currently, many individuals diagnosed with a malignancy during childhood will receive combined modality therapies, including surgery, aggressive multi-agent chemotherapeutic regimens and radiotherapy.

Approximately two-thirds of pediatric cancer survivors will develop medical complications or disabilities, which can be attributed to their previous cancer treatments.[5] Endocrine disturbances have been documented in 20 to 50% of survivors and frequently occur as late effects of cancer therapy. Survivors of CNS tumors, Hodgkin's disease and those undergoing stem cell transplantation (SCT) are at particular risk of developing endocrine complications as a result of their exposure to radiation therapy and high doses of alkylating agents. These treatments can cause damage to the hypothalamus-pituitary axis, the thyroid gland, and the gonads. The following discusses the common endocrine and growth problems that are observed in survivors of childhood cancer.

Growth Failure

Impaired linear growth with resultant adult short stature occurs frequently in survivors of childhood cancer, particularly in individuals treated at a young age. A variety of factors, including high-dose radiation therapy (particularly to the brain and spine), early pubertal development, hypothyroidism, and growth hormone deficiency (GHD), contribute to the short stature in adult survivors. Both endocrine and non-endocrine factors can contribute to growth retardation.

Non-endocrine Factors

The non-endocrine factors affecting growth are primarily related to intensive chemotherapy and irradiation of skeletal structures.

Chemotherapy

The administration of chemotherapy is often associated with mild to moderate reduced growth. In many instances, the observed growth deceleration is only temporary; however, the adverse effects on growth can persist more long term.[6-8] In a report on a large series of childhood brain tumor survivors, Gleeson and colleagues found that chemotherapy was a significant cause of standing height loss.[7] This is in contrast to a report by Gurney and colleagues on a cohort from the Childhood Cancer Survivor Study of 921 survivors of a childhood brain tumor in which the investigators showed that adjuvant chemotherapy was not an independent risk factor for adult short stature.[8] The negative effects on growth are dependent on the number and dosage of the drugs and the duration of treatment, all of which reflect the intensity of the regimen. Glucocorticoids, mercaptopurine and methotrexate are specific drugs implicated in the inhibition of normal growth. While the mechanisms of chemotherapy-induced growth failure remain uncertain, the data suggest that chemotherapy may act both directly on bone growth by suppressing osteoblast and osteoclast activity and through alterations of the growth hormone–insulin-like growth factor 1 (GH-IGF-1) system.[9,10]

Radiotherapy

Direct external beam radiation to the spine and, to a lesser degree, to the long bones can produce profound losses in growth potential in children. The ultimate impact on final height depends on the dose of radiation therapy, the volume irradiated, and the age of the subject at the time of treatment. Several authors have reported on the skeletal dysplasia that follows total body irradiation (TBI), especially when administered in a single dose, and caused by exposure of the growth plate to radiation.[11-14] In this context, the sitting height is more affected than the standing height, indicating that the irradiation of the vertebrae contributes more to the observed growth impairment.[11-15] Younger patients are more likely to incur a greater loss in final height, and are at risk of having altered body proportions when they reach adulthood.[15] The height reduction that occurs following contemporary radiation regimens for the treatment of diseases such as Hodgkin's disease and Wilms' tumor, where the dose of radiation to the spine and other bones is given at lower doses and in a more conformal fashion, is generally quite modest and usually not clinically important.[16,17]

Endocrine Factors

The most important endocrine factors that disrupt the normal pattern of growth in survivors include GHD and central precocious puberty (CPP). Both of these neuroendocrine disturbances usually are the consequence of hypothalamic-pituitary irradiation. Primary hypothyroidism also may contribute to poor linear growth in these children and will be discussed in the section on thyroid abnormalities.

Growth Hormone Deficiency

Causes (1) Direct insult by tumoral expansion or ablative surgery: Tumors, such as craniopharyngiomas, germinomas, and optic nerve gliomas, which arise near the region of the hypothalamus and pituitary, produce GHD as a direct result of the tumor or of the surgery required to remove it.

(2) Radiotherapy: Cranial irradiation can cause damage to the hypothalamus and, less often, to the pituitary. Growth hormone deficiency is indeed the most common and frequently the only anterior pituitary deficit to develop after cranial irradiation.[18] The site of the damage caused by irradiation is more frequently the hypothalamus, which is more sensitive to radiation than the pituitary.[19] There are two major hypothalamic regulators of GH secretion: growth hormone releasing hormone (GHRH) and somatostatin. The secretion and release of GH by the pituitary is stimulated by GHRH and inhibited by somatostatin. Low doses of radiation (ie,18 gray [Gy] of conventional fractionated radiotherapy) to the hypothalamus/pituitary region are sufficient to cause the loss of the GHRH tone without influencing somatostatin, thus causing GHD.[20] The pituitary gland is damaged at higher doses of irradiation.[19] Risk factors for GHD following radiotherapy can relate to patient characteristics and to the dose of radiation administered to the hypothalamus and pituitary.

(a) Patient characteristics: Younger patients are at an increased risk of developing GHD after radiation of the hypothalamus/pituitary region.[21,22] In a series of 27 patients receiving 24 Gy of cranial prophylactic irradiation for ALL or lymphosarcoma, Brauner and colleagues demonstrated that the GH peak response in stimulation tests strongly correlated with patient age at irradiation, despite similar time

intervals since the completion of treatment, confirming previous reports with similar results from Shalet and colleagues.[21,22]

(b) Dose delivered and time since completion of treatment: Radiation therapy is followed by GHD in both a time- and dose-dependent relationship (Figure 1).[23] External beam radiation doses >30 Gy typically produce GHD within 5 years of treatment; after lower doses, such as 18 to 24 Gy, GHD may not become evident for 10 or more years.[24] In survivors of pediatric SCT, GHD has been shown to develop after TBI, often several years after the completion of cancer treatments.[6,25,26] Once established, radiation-induced GHD is usually permanent.[27] Several authors have reported on a possible improvement in GH secretion in a minority of patients; their findings suggest that retesting patients diagnosed during childhood with irradiation-induced GHD when they reach their final height is warranted before this treatment is continued through adulthood.[28–30]

(3) Chemotherapy: The effects of chemotherapy on the GH-IGF-1 axis are unclear. Slow growth and GHD following chemotherapy have been reported by some authors. Bakker and colleagues recently reported a high incidence of abnormal growth patterns in children receiving a combination of high doses of cyclophosphamide and busulfan for SCT conditioning, with laboratory results suggesting GHD in 4 out of 10 tested patients.[31] Nevertheless, the changes on which the authors based their conclusions were not statistically significant. Rose and colleagues also suggested that some patients may develop

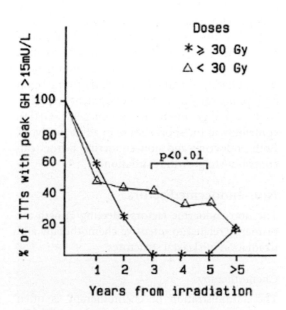

FIGURE 1 Percentage of normal insulin-tolerance tests (ITTs) compared to time from irradiation in patients receiving <30 Gy or ≥30 Gy to the hypothalamic-pituitary axis. Reprinted with permission from Clayton PE, et al.[23]

hypothalamic dysfunction, including GHD, following chemotherapy.[32] Out of 800 cases reviewed by the authors, 31 patients had slow growth patterns and had been exclusively treated with chemotherapy. Out of these 31 patients, 15 were diagnosed with GHD based upon results of stimulation tests alone[32].

Diagnosis Establishing a diagnosis of GHD can be problematic in childhood cancer survivors. There is no "gold standard" diagnostic tool for GHD in general, and some of the available tests are known to be unreliable in cases of hypothalamic or pituitary injury following radiation. The diagnosis is based on the convergence of clinical features and laboratory results.

(1) Clinical features: GHD should be suspected in patients with decreased growth velocity (ie, growth rate below the fifth percentile for age) observed over at least six monthly visits.[33] It is also important to monitor the sitting height in patients who received irradiation to the spine in order to look for the skeletal dysplasia associated with this treatment.[15] Special attention should be paid to the patients' pubertal status because the clinical signs of GHD may be masked by seemingly normal growth rates owing to the inappropriate secretion of sex steroids in patients with precocious puberty, another endocrine complication that can be encountered in this context.[34] As in any pediatric evaluation, the nutritional status (reflected by body weight and body mass index [BMI]), is a key clinical element that can influence linear growth and needs to be taken into account.

(2) Laboratory results: There are three main laboratory diagnostic tools for GHD.

(a) GH provocative tests: The GH peak value is measured after administration of a pharmacologic agent known to stimulate the secretion and release of GH. Several agents are used, but the insulin tolerance test is believed to be the most reliable, despite exposing the patient to the risk of hypoglycemia.[35,36] Although widely used, these tests are non-physiologic and often yield non-reproducible results. The normal peak value has been arbitrarily defined at 10 ng/mL although several authors have lowered the threshold to 7 ng/mL. Despite these caveats, failure to achieve a peak response >10 ng/mL following two pharmacologic stimulation tests is considered part of the standard criteria for a diagnosis of GHD. Nevertheless, failing one stimulation test was considered enough for diagnosing GH deficiency in patients who received irradiation to the hypothalamus and/or pituitary by the GH research society in its consensus guidelines.[27]

(b) GH frequent sampling studies: Spontaneous GH secretion is assessed by obtaining blood samples every 20 minutes over a 12 to 24 hour period. More frequently, the samples are drawn only at night, during sleep ("overnight sampling"), a time when the bulk of GH is produced. GHD is unlikely if a GH peak above 10 ng/mL is observed or if a mean plasma concentration of 3ng/mL or above is derived from the GH levels measured in the collected samples. The overnight sampling appears to be more reliable than the provocative tests, with fewer false negative and false positive results, but it is labor-intensive and continues to be available only in a few academic centers.[37,38]

(c) Measurements of surrogate markers of GH: Growth hormone induces skeletal growth indirectly by stimulating the secretion by the liver of insulin-like growth factor-1 (IGF-1). The effect of IGF-1 on skeletal growth is regulated by its association with IGF binding protein-3 (IGFBP-3). Unlike GH, plasma IGF-1 and IGFBP-3 levels are stable and their measurement does not require performing dynamic tests. They are routinely used as a screening test for the GH status of individuals with short stature.[38] However, IGF-1 and IGFBP-3 are not reliable indicators of the GH status following cranial irradiation, or in cases of a CNS lesion.[39,40] In patients with documented hypothalamic/pituitary injury due to irradiation or tumoral expansion, IGF-1 and IGFBP-3 levels can be in the normal range, despite the presence of GHD.

Central Precocious Puberty

CPP is defined as the onset of puberty before the age of 8 years in girls and 9 years in boys due to the premature activation of the hypothalamic-pituitary-gonadal axis.[41] Over several years, it became evident that cranial irradiation at both lower doses (18 to 35 Gy) and higher doses (35 to 50 Gy) is associated with the development of CPP.[42-44] The presumed mechanism of this activation is the disruption of the cortical inhibitory influence by radiation. Roth and colleagues showed, using animal models, that low-dose hypothalamic irradiation leading to sexual precocity is associated with lower release rates of γ-amino butyric acid (GABA). These findings suggest that irradiation disrupts the inhibitory influence of the GABA-ergic tone, causing the observed activation of the gonadotropin-releasing hormone (GnRH)-gonadotropin-gonadal axis.[45] The age-inappropriate sex steroid secretion can cause rapid bone age progression and further decrease the growth potential of children, the vast majority of whom also suffer from GHD.

Risk Factors   Girls seem more likely than boys to enter puberty at an early age following hypothalamic irradiation.[46] Age at the onset of puberty is directly correlated with age at treatment and inversely correlated with the BMI.[43]

While earlier studies suggested that the tempo of puberty is also accelerated in these patients, recent data have been unable to confirm this.[46] Irradiation doses to the hypothalamus in the range of 35 to 50 Gy can result in CPP, while doses >50 Gy are generally associated with hypogonadotropic hypogonadism within the context of combined hormonal pituitary deficiencies.[47,48]

Diagnosis   (1) Clinical features: Precocious puberty is a clinical diagnosis. In the general pediatric population, it is best characterized by the onset of sustained breast development before the age of 8 years in girls, and by testicular enlargement (testicular volume >4 cc) before the age of 9 years in boys.[41] In childhood cancer survivors, testicular volume may not be a reliable indicator of pubertal growth in boys, and clinicians should be alerted by the early onset of other secondary sexual characters (eg, pubic hair) as well. One of the first signs of pubertal development is an increase in the growth rate, due to the action of the sex steroids. In children who also are likely to have GHD, this may result in falsely reassuring normal growth velocity, as mentioned previously. Therefore, pubertal staging using the Tanner classification is an important part of the regular clinical follow-up of these patients, and any concerns regarding the possibility of early onset of puberty should lead to a referral to an experienced pediatric endocrinologist.[49]

(2) Radiologic findings: The bone age is estimated by performing the standard x-ray examination of the left wrist.[50] Advancement of the bone age more than 2 standard deviations (SD) for chronological age is a consistent finding in children with precocious puberty and is helpful in corroborating the clinical impression of inappropriate sexual development. In girls with CPP, symmetrical uterine growth is evidence of estrogen impregnation, and is an earlier finding than bilaterally enlarged ovaries. It is not, however, a necessary procedure when clinical features and laboratory findings are consistent with the diagnosis.

(3) Laboratory results: In CPP, pubertal development results from the premature activation of the hypothalamic pituitary axis. Therefore, luteinizing hormone (LH) and follicle stimulating hormone (FSH) levels tend to be detectable at baseline and to rise after stimulation by GnRH. An LH/FSH peak ratio above 0.6 unit per liter (U/L) in girls and above 1 U/L in boys indicates a pubertal response.[51] In patients who received gonadotoxic treatments, the LH/FSH response to GnRH will be altered; the FSH response will be augmented, making the results harder to interpret. The plasma estradiol levels in girls and testosterone levels in boys are also important markers of pubertal development.

Management

The final height is most affected in individuals who are diagnosed with cancer at a young age, particularly if they are treated with high doses of radiotherapy (>30 Gy) to the hypothalamus or the hypothalamus and spine.[8] In this context, both GHD and CPP can reduce the growth potential and result in a very impaired final height. While both GHD and CPP are amenable to therapy, growth arrest due to radiation-induced boney dysplasia is not.

Growth hormone replacement therapy improves the growth rate of children who develop GHD following cancer therapy, at least in the short term. Data accumulated several years ago suggested that most patients, however, achieved a final height significantly below their target height.[45,52] The poor response to GH therapy has been attributed both to patient factors, such as spinal irradiation, early pubertal onset, and variables in treatment, such as suboptimal dosing schedules, as well as to the older age of most children started on GH. Recent data suggest that improvements in growth and final height can be achieved with contemporary dosing regimens.[7,53,54] Thus, Gleeson and colleagues reported a significant improvement in the final heights of survivors of childhood brain tumors treated after 1988, compared to patients treated in an earlier era.[7] In a more heterogeneous patient cohort, Adan and colleagues had previously reported a similar trend with a significant improvement of the adult heights in patients treated with contemporary GH replacement regimens.[53] In both studies, the improvement was even more striking in patients with combined GHD and CPP and who received a gonadotropin-releasing hormone agonist to suppress puberty in addition to GH replacement.[7,53] In a more recent report from the Childhood Cancer Survivor Study, supported by final height data on 183 childhood cancer survivors treated with GH, Brownstein and colleagues showed that younger bone age at the beginning of GH replacement and higher doses of GH-positively correlated with a better final height outcome.[55] GH-releasing hormone (GHRH) therapy also may improve growth in subjects with radiation-induced GHD, but the data are quite limited.[20]

Concerns over the safety of GH therapy relate to the fact that GH and IGF-1 are potent growth-promoting agents with anti-apoptotic, mitogenic, and proliferating properties. However, large-scale studies assessing the risk of tumor recurrence in brain tumor survivors treated with GH have now been reported. All have consistently reported no increased risk associated with GH replacement therapy.[56-58] In a report from the Childhood Cancer Survivor Study on 361 GH-treated individuals, including 122 survivors of acute leukemia and 43 survivors of soft tissue sarcomas, Sklar and colleagues did not find evidence for an increased risk of disease recurrence or death following GH-replacement therapy.[58] However, the data suggested that treatment with GH may slightly increase the risk of a secondary solid tumor, especially in survivors of acute leukemia. In view of the small number of second tumors and the wide confidence intervals, the clinical importance of that finding remains uncertain.[58] The risk of developing slipped epiphyses may be increased in cancer survivors (particularly survivors of leukemia) who were treated with GH, compared with children treated with GH for idiopathic GHD.[59]

Young adult survivors with either childhood- or adult-onset GHD, such as that following low-dose cranial irradiation at a young age, also may benefit from GH therapy, especially if they manifest any of the metabolic derangements, such as increased body fat, raised plasma lipids, and decreased bone density and/or quality-of-life issues that have come to be recognized as adult GHD. Murray and colleagues reported on the effects of GH replacement in adulthood in a series of 27 GH-deficient survivors of childhood cancer.[60] After 12 months of replacement, small but significant improvements occurred in the body composition in males and in the cholesterol and triglyceride levels in females. Mild improvement of the bone mineral density occurred after 18 months of treatment. However, the patients reported a significant improvement in their overall quality of life 3 months after beginning the treatment, and this improvement was maintained at 12 months.[60]

Disorders of the Thyroid

Thyroid dysfunction is among the most common endocrine complications of childhood cancer treatments. Thyroid hormones are important for growth and development in childhood, and early recognition of thyroid dysfunction in childhood cancer survivors should be among the objectives of their long-term follow-up.

Hypothyroidism

Apart from its well known neurocognitive and metabolic signs observed in adults, childhood hypothyroidism causes growth deceleration often associated with excessive weight gain. Central hypothyroidism is secondary to hypothalamic and/or pituitary insults and is seen relatively infrequently in this population. In contrast, primary hypothyroidism, due to direct damage to the thyroid following exposure to radiation, is by far the most frequently observed thyroid dysfunction in childhood cancer survivors.

Central Hypothyroidism

Central hypothyroidism is reportedly the second most frequent endocrine disturbance following radiation of the hypothalamus/pituitary region.[61] Its association with chemotherapy, however, remains controversial.

Radiotherapy While early puberty and GHD are the most common neuroendocrine disturbances secondary to irradiation of the hypothalamus/pituitary region, clinically evident alterations of the other hypothalamic-pituitary axes, including thyrotropin thyroid stimulating hormone (TSH) secretion, occur less often and generally only following doses in the range of 30 to 40 Gy.[18,62] Interpretation of the literature about these deficits is complicated by the fact that different investigators employ different hormonal tests and use varying criteria for what constitutes abnormal. For example, Rose and colleagues reported a very high incidence of "hidden" central hypothyroidism secondary to TSH-deficiency following cranial irradiation.[63] According to the authors, the establishment of a diagnosis of TSH-deficiency often requires performing both a thyrotropin-releasing hormone (TRH) test and an assessment of the nocturnal TSH surge. These tests require obtaining multiple blood samples during the day and night. At present, it is unclear whether this subtle form of TSH dysfunction correlates with any clinical findings, and, thus, whether one can justify on clinical grounds the time and expense involved in this diagnostic protocol.

Chemotherapy There are few reports in the literature on the contribution of chemotherapy to the development of central hypothyroidism in childhood cancer survivors. In one report, Rose and colleagues suggested that subtle TSH deficiency was found in as many as 53% of patients exclusively treated with chemotherapy for extracranial malignancies and who were assessed for abnormal growth.[32] The clinical significance of these findings is, again, debatable. Those patients had normal free thyroxine (FT4) levels, and the diagnosis of central hypothyroidism was based upon the absence of a nocturnal surge in TSH secretion. In a previous study including 205 patients, Van Santen and colleagues did not find any damaging effects of chemotherapy on the hypothalamic-pituitary-thyroid axis in young adult survivors of childhood cancer.[64] Schmiegelow and colleagues also reported that chemotherapy did not have a significant influence on the hypothalamic-pituitary-thyroid axis in their 71-patient cohort of childhood brain tumor survivors.[62]

Primary Hypothyroidism

Primary hypothyroidism is the most common thyroid disturbance that occurs in patients whose thyroid gland has been irradiated. It is often detected in survivors who have been treated with neck/mantle irradiation for Hodgkin's disease, craniospinal irradiation for brain tumors, or TBI for cytoreduction before SCT.[25,61,65] Primary hypothyroidism has also been described in individuals treated with a radio-labeled monoclonal antibody such as Iodine-131-meta-iodobenzyl-guanidine (I[131]-MIBG) for neuroblastoma. Chemotherapy alone does not seem to be associated with primary hypothyroidism.[66]

As in other dysfunctions following radiation therapy, the prevalence is determined primarily by the total dose to the thyroid and by the duration of follow-up. In a recent study of 1,791 young adult survivors of Hodgkin's disease, a cumulative incidence of hypothyroidism of 28% was observed.[65] Moreover, the actuarial risk of developing an underactive thyroid 20 years after treatment was 50% for survivors who had received thyroid irradiation with doses ≥ 45 Gy (Figure 2). Additional risk factors for developing hypothyroidism included female gender and/or being older than 15 years of age at the time of diagnosis. Of great clinical importance, new cases have been observed more than 25 years following diagnosis and treatment of Hodgkin's disease. Consequently, all patients previously treated with radiation therapy to the region of the thyroid require lifelong surveillance.

Hyperthyroidism

While far less prevalent than hypothyroidism, hyperthyroidism does develop at an increased rate in certain subsets of childhood cancer survivors. A common setting is following external beam radiation to the neck for Hodgkin's disease, where the chances of becoming hyperthyroid are eight times greater than those observed in the

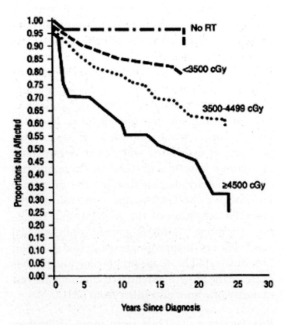

FIGURE 2 Probability of developing an underactive thyroid after diagnosis of Hodgkin's disease. Patients are grouped according to dose of thyroid irradiation. RT = radiation therapy. Reprinted with permission from Sklar, et al.[65]

general population.[65] The major risk factor for development of hyperthyroidism is irradiation of the thyroid involving doses >35 Gy. A second but less common cause of hyperthyroidism is the appearance of autoimmune thyroid disease following allogeneic SCT. The published data are most consistent with the hypothesis that the thyroid disorder is due to adoptive transfer of abnormal clones of T or B cells from donor to recipient.[25] Various types of autoimmune disease have been demonstrated to occur at increased frequency following SCT.

Thyroid Neoplasms

Thyroid neoplasms, both benign and malignant, do occur following irradiation of the thyroid gland as the result of both direct exposure to radiation and scatter irradiation (for example, after prophylactic CNS irradiation in patients treated for ALL). Children at greatest risk are those <10 years of age at the time of treatment and those treated with doses of radiation in the 20 to 29 Gy range. The risk is linear at lower doses of irradiation (0.1 to 1 Gy), but this association seems to become more complex at doses above 30 Gy, showing a downwards curvature in radiation-dose response for thyroid cancer.[67] Nonetheless, the risk of developing a thyroid neoplasm remains elevated following even relatively high-dose radiation therapy. Thyroid nodules are particularly common in females and often occur after a long latency period (>10 years). Sklar and colleagues reported that the risk of thyroid cancer was increased 18-fold in a large cohort of young adult survivors of Hodgkin's disease.[65] The median dose of radiation to the thyroid was 35 Gy, with a range of 25 to 35 Gy. Fortunately, the vast majority of cancers noted after radiation therapy are well differentiated and have excellent prognosis. In a more recent study, Acharya and colleagues studied the characteristics of all patients at our center who developed a thyroid neoplasm after therapeutic radiotherapy during childhood or adolescence.[68] The median dose of radiation to the gland was 24 Gy, with a median interval of 13 years between radiation exposure and clinical recognition of the thyroid neoplasm. Malignant neoplasms represented a high proportion of the observed lesions (39%). Patients who developed malignant lesions differed from those who developed benign lesions only in that the median dose to the thyroid was lower compared to those with benign lesions (20 Gy vs. 29.5 Gy). All of the thyroid malignancies observed after therapeutic radiation were differentiated carcinomas, with papillary carcinoma being most common. In general, the post-irradiation thyroid cancers did not behave in an aggressive fashion.[68] The pathogenesis of irradiation-induced thyroid

neoplasms remains unclear. They may be related to rearrangements of the RET proto-oncogene induced by the exposure to radiation, although the data are conflicting.[69,70] Thyroid neoplasms following radiotherapy may not become evident for many years after irradiation, therefore all individuals at risk require lifelong follow up.[65,68]

Management of Thyroid Disorders

Clinical Assessment

A careful clinical assessment, which includes careful palpation of the neck, should be performed at least annually by an experienced physician to look for a thyroid neoplasm in all childhood cancer survivors who have been treated with neck/mantle irradiation, craniospinal irradiation, or TBI. Linear growth and weight gain, monitored during childhood by plotting on growth curves the heights and weights recorded at visits, can also give some evidence of thyroid dysfunction. Children with hypothyroidism tend to have a deceleration in growth associated with excessive weight gain. Hyperthyroid children tend to have an accelerated growth rate, often associated with weight loss.

Laboratory Assessment

Annual thyroid function tests, including plasma TSH and FT4, should be systematically performed in order to ensure early diagnosis and treatment in patients who received neck/mantle irradiation, craniospinal irradiation, or TBI.

Imaging and Pathology

The role of ultrasonography in screening for thyroid neoplasms in patients treated with radiotherapy remains controversial due to the high prevalence of benign and clinically undetectable thyroid nodules in the general population.[68] Even when the subclinical neoplasms discovered by ultrasonographic screening turn out to be malignant, their clinical importance remains to be proven because their rate of progression into significant lesions may be very low.[71] The diagnostic procedure of choice in evaluating a thyroid nodule in cancer survivors with a history of thyroid exposure to radiation is the fine needle aspiration biopsy.[68]

Treatment

Thyroxine replacement is warranted in patients diagnosed with compensated (normal T4 levels with high TSH) and decompensated (low T4 and high TSH levels) hypothyroidism. The benefit of treating "subtle" forms of hypothyroidism diagnosed by more complex laboratory procedures remains unclear.[32,63] There are no specific guidelines regarding the management of hyperthyroidism and second thyroid neoplasms in

childhood cancer survivors, in whom the same treatments are applied as for the general population.

Disorders of Pubertal Development

Impairments of the Hypothalamic-Pituitary-Gonadal Axis

Central Precocious Puberty

Along with GHD, CPP is one of the most frequent disorders observed after the radiation of the hypothalamus/pituitary region. It was discussed previously, under the growth section of this text.

Hypogonadotropic Hypogonadism

In childhood cancer survivors, insufficient LH and FSH secretions have been reported in the context of hypothalamic and/or pituitary injury following tumor invasion/expansion or the treatments, surgery, and radiation therapy directed against such tumors. Deficits of LH and FSH secretion following irradiation of the hypothalamus/pituitary region, occur less often than GHD, and generally only following doses to the sellar region in the range of >30 to 40 Gy.[18,62,72,73] In female ALL survivors, Bath and colleagues reported lower LH secretion in the 12 adolescents and young adults enrolled in their study, based upon the measurement of the amplitude of the urinary LH surge.[74] The authors attributed this disorder to cranial irradiation, and suggested that doses of 18 to 24 Gy can be sufficient to cause such "subtle" deficits.[74] Byrne and colleagues, in a study of the fertility of women treated with cranial radiotherapy for childhood ALL, found that irradiation of the hypothalamus and/or pituitary with doses in the 18 to 24 Gy range around the time of menarche may affect fertility and suggested that this may be secondary to the impairment gonadotropin secretion.[73] Additional long-term follow-up and data on the fertility of these patients will provide a better sense of the ultimate effect of these lower doses of cranial irradiation.

Little is known on the effects of chemotherapy on LH and FSH secretion. In their recent report on hypothalamic dysfunction after chemotherapy, Rose and colleagues found that three patients out of 27 patients old enough to be assessed for pubertal development, had pubertal delay due to insufficient gonadotropin secretion.[32] Given the lack of clinical information on these patients, and the multiplicity of factors (eg, nutritional, psychological, social) influencing the timing of puberty in a child recovering from cancer, caution is warranted in interpreting these results.

Hyperprolactinemia

Hyperprolactinemia can be observed following high-dose irradiation, particularly when the hypothalamus is exposed to more than 50 Gy. Constine and colleagues reported on a series of 32 patients who received high-dose cranial radiotherapy (39.6 to 70.2 Gy, with a mean 53.6 Gy) as treatment for brain tumors, and showed that 75% of the adult patients and 30% of pediatric patients had elevated baseline prolactin levels.[75] Hyperprolactinemia was symptomatic, however, only in three adult patients, who reported decreased libido.

Primary Gonadal Dysfunction

Males

The human testis is the site of both sex steroid and sperm production. Testosterone, the major male sex steroid, is responsible for normal male secondary sexual characteristics and is also a necessary cofactor in the production of sperm. Although these two functions are interconnected to a certain degree, they are under separate controls, which include a multitude of endocrine, paracrine, and autocrine factors.[76] The testis is composed primarily of three types of cells: germ cells that ultimately form sperm; Sertoli cells that support and nurture developing germ cells and are also the site of production of inhibin; and interstitial Leydig cells responsible for the biosynthesis of testosterone. These three cell types are organized into two functional compartments: germ cells and Sertoli cells form the seminiferous tubules where spermatogenesis takes place, and the network of Leydig cells is responsible for the production of testosterone. Leydig cells lie in close proximity to the basal compartment of the seminiferous tubules, where they can deliver high concentrations of testosterone, which are necessary for normal spermatogenesis.[77] Despite their interconnection, these two functional compartments are affected in different ways by the treatments (eg, chemotherapy, radiation) given to individuals with cancer.

Leydig Cell Dysfunction   Treatment-induced Leydig cell failure and/or dysfunction results from damage or loss of the machinery required for testosterone synthesis and release. Leydig cell failure and androgen insufficiency are relatively uncommon compared to the damage to germ cells and infertility following cancer therapy.

Diagnosis   If it occurs prior to or during normal puberty, individuals with Leydig cell failure will experience delayed/arrested pubertal maturation and lack of secondary sexual characteristics. If the insult is sustained following the completion of normal pubertal development, one can observe lack of libido, erectile dysfunction, decreased bone density, decreased muscle mass and other metabolic disturbances.[78] Raised plasma concentrations of LH combined with low

levels of testosterone are the hormonal hallmarks of Leydig cell dysfunction. It is important to note, however, that these changes may not become apparent until the individual has reached mid-adolescence.[79,80] Thus, it can be very difficult to assess or predict Leydig cell function in the preadolescent male.

Chemotherapy-Induced Leydig Cell Failure   In general, Leydig cells, with their slow rate of turnover, are much less vulnerable to damage from cancer therapy than are germ cells. Chemotherapy-induced Leydig cell failure resulting in androgen insufficiency and requiring testosterone replacement therapy is quite rare.[78,81,82] Nonetheless, prior studies suggest that Leydig cell dysfunction may be observed following treatment with alkylating agent regimens.[78,83-85] These reports indicate that from 10 to 57% of male subjects can develop elevated serum concentrations of LH following treatment.[72,83,86-89] Insofar as the majority of males undergo a normal puberty, and most produce adult levels of testosterone, it appears that Leydig cell dysfunction is generally subclinical when it occurs. For instance, in a report by Kenney and colleagues on 17 male survivors of childhood sarcoma treated with high-dose cyclophosphamide, while baseline LH was elevated in 40% of the patients, testosterone secretion was normal in 93.8% of the cases.[86] Young boys and adolescent males who receive standard-dose cyclophosphamide alone (200 mg/kg) as conditioning regimen before SCT for aplastic anemia appear to retain normal Leydig cell function; the vast majority are reported to have normal plasma concentrations of LH and testosterone and to normally enter and progress through puberty.[90] In patients whose SCT conditioning regimen combined high doses of busulfan and cyclophosphamide, Leydig cell function also appears to be preserved in most adult males despite damage to the germinal epithelium.[31,91]

Radiation-Induced Leydig Cell Failure
External irradiation is more likely than chemotherapy to cause Leydig cell damage. The doses required are much higher than the doses needed to cause germ cell failure. The interpretation of the impact of radiation on Leydig cell function is confounded by the concurrent use of chemotherapy in most subjects as well as the potential effects of the malignancy itself (eg, testicular relapse in ALL). Nonetheless, the data obtained from individuals treated with radiation therapy for a variety of malignancies show that the likelihood of sustaining radiation-induced Leydig cell failure is directly related to the dose delivered and inversely related to age at treatment.[92-95] Normal amounts of testosterone are produced by the majority of males who receive

≤20 Gy fractionated radiation to the testes.[78] Shalet and colleagues noted that Leydig cell function was preserved in a group of adult males who, as children, were exposed to doses up to 9.8 Gy of testicular irradiation.[96] Both, Sklar and colleagues and Castillo and colleagues described age-appropriate levels of testosterone and normal pubertal maturation in males who were treated prophylactically with 12 Gy of testicular irradiation for ALL.[82,97] Because raised plasma concentrations of LH, both at baseline and following GnRH stimulation, are found in many of these young men, one must assume that subclinical injury to the Leydig cell is common at this dose range. A dose of > 24 Gy of fractionated irradiation as therapy for young males with testicular relapse of ALL is associated with a very high risk for Leydig cell dysfunction. One should anticipate that the majority of boys who are prepubertal at the time they receive 24 Gy testicular irradiation will develop frank Leydig cell failure and require androgen replacement.[80,94,95] Most, but not all, boys who are older and/or in early puberty at the time they are treated with 24 Gy will also ultimately need therapy with testosterone.[95] It has been estimated that testicular doses in excess of 33 Gy are needed to induce Leydig cell failure in 50% of adolescent and young adult men.[98] Of note, Sklar reported normal adult testosterone levels in two young men who received in excess of 40 Gy testicular irradiation during late adolescence.[78]

Germ Cell Dysfunction   Treatment-induced germ cell failure in males occurs frequently, in contrast to what occurs in Leydig cells, which are resistant to most chemotherapeutic agents and lower doses of radiation.

Diagnosis   Infertility resulting from radiation therapy or chemotherapy is often associated with reduced testicular volume, increased FSH concentrations, and reduced plasma concentrations of inhibin B. While there are good correlations overall between these markers and sperm counts in large groups of survivors, considerable overlap occurs between normal and abnormal individuals; many male survivors with documented azoospermia fail to manifest either a reduced testicular volume or an elevated level of FSH.[86] Thus, currently, there is no substitute for sperm analysis to determine a male's current fertility status.[99]

Chemotherapy-Induced Germ Cell Failure
The chemotherapeutic agents most commonly associated with impaired male fertility include the alkylating agents listed in Table 1. Importantly, the concept derived from studies suggesting that the germ cells of younger individuals were less vulnerable to the toxic effects of chemotherapy compared with older boys and young adults has been called into question by more recent studies.[86]

TABLE 1 Chemotherapeutic Agents
Associated with Germ Cell Damage

Alkylating Agents
Cyclophosphamide
   Ifosfamide
   Procarbazine
   Busulfan
   Melphalan
   Thiotepa

Nitrosoureas
   BCNU (carmustine)
   CCNU (lomustine)

Etoposide

Cisplatin

Impaired fertility occurs in 40 to 60% of young adult survivors of childhood cancer. A high probability of oligospermia, azoospermia and infertility exists in those exposed to >20 g/m^2 of cyclophosphamide. In contrast, many individuals treated with a cumulative dose of 7.5 to 10 g/m^2 or less retain normal sperm production.[72,86] Procarbazine, another alkylating agent commonly used in the treatment of Hodgkin's disease has also been shown to induce gonadal dysfunction in a dose-dependent fashion. In a study by van den Berg and colleagues, patients with Hodgkin's disease who received three mechlorethamine, vincristine, procarbazine, and prednisone (MOPP) cycles alternating with three cycles of doxorubicin hydrochloride, bleomycin, vinblastine, and dacarbazine seemed to suffer less testicular damage than patients who received 6 MOPP cycles.[100] The sperm counts available in this study were too few to enable any definite conclusions, but these findings are consistent with an earlier report from Mackie and colleagues.[89] Most of the young men treated with the combination of busulfan and cyclophosphamide in preparation for SCT do appear to sustain damage to their germinal epithelium. Anserini and colleagues, in a small sample of post-SCT patients, demonstrated that recovery of some spermatogenetic activity occurred in 50% of cases after such conditioning regimens, but semen quality was impaired.[101] Grigg and colleagues had previously suggested that recovery of spermatogenetic activity occurred more frequently in patients receiving lower doses of cyclophosphamide (120 mg/kg) and busulfan (16 mg/kg) than in patients who receive the usual higher doses.[102] Overall, the ultimate effect of this combination on male fertility remains unclear.

Radiotherapy-Induced Germ Cell Failure

Testicular irradiation in doses as low as 0.15 Gy has produced impaired sperm production. If the dose is under 1 to 2 Gy, recovery is generally common. At doses >2 to 3 Gy, recovery of sperm production is rare.[103] Germ cell dysfunction is present in essentially all males treated with TBI.[104] The vast majority of subjects will have increased plasma levels of FSH as well as reduced testicular volume, indices that correlate with impaired spermatogenesis. Azoospermia is the rule for patients studied in the first few years after treatment with TBI. Recovery of germ cell function has occurred rarely and primarily following single-dose irradiation.[105] A few men have been reported to father a child following TBI.[104]

Females

Ovarian failure results in disruption of and damage to both ovarian germ cells and the hormone-producing cells. This results from the structural and functional interdependence within the follicle between sex–hormone-producing cells and oocytes.[78] This contrasts with testicular pathology where, despite the loss of the germ cells following cytotoxic therapy, production of sex hormones is often preserved. As the ovarian follicular reserve decreases naturally with age, older patients are more at risk of ovarian failure following childhood cancer and its treatments.[78]

Diagnosis Ovarian failure that occurs prior to the onset of puberty will result in delayed puberty and primary amenorrhea. If ovarian function is lost during or after pubertal maturation, one generally observes arrested puberty, secondary amenorrhea, and menopausal symptoms (ie, hot flashes, vaginal dryness). Women who experience premature loss of estrogen production are also predisposed to developing osteoporosis and coronary artery disease.[106] Increased plasma concentrations of gonadotropins, especially FSH, and reduced levels of estradiol are typically found in the adolescent and young adult with ovarian failure. As in the male, plasma levels of LH/FSH may remain normal in the prepubertal child, despite coexisting ovarian failure.[107] Thus, it may not be possible to establish the status of ovarian function in young girls until they reach 10 to 12 years of age.

Chemotherapy-Induced Ovarian Failure The ovaries of prepubertal females, with their greater complement of follicles, are relatively resistant to chemotherapy-induced damage compared with the ovaries of adults.[102,107] Nonetheless, certain chemotherapeutic agents (see Table 1) when given at high doses are toxic, even to young ovaries, especially alkylating agents, including cyclophosphamide, ifosfamide, busulfan, cisplatin, carmustine (BCNU), and lomustine (CCNU).[108–110] Fortunately, the majority of prepubertal girls and adolescent females receiving standard combination chemotherapy will retain or recover ovarian function during the immediate post-treatment period.[78,111–113] However, histologic examination of ovarian tissue in prepubertal and postpubertal girls treated for solid tumors or leukemia has revealed a decreased number of ovarian follicles and inhibition of follicular growth compared to age-matched controls.[114,115] In a recent study combining data from strictly timed ovarian ultrasonography and hormonal assessment, Larsen and colleagues reported on the ovarian function of 100 childhood cancer survivors.[116] Interestingly, the authors found that survivors with spontaneous menses at the time of the study (70 patients) had similar LH and FSH concentrations but smaller ovarian volumes, lower numbers of antral follicles per ovary, and lower inhibin B levels when compared to age-matched controls, suggesting a reduced ovarian reserve in the survivors' group.

Increased plasma concentrations of FSH, a sensitive index of ovarian damage and reproductive aging, have been noted in young women treated with alkylating agents for acute leukemia, brain tumors, and Hodgkin's disease.[89,113,117–122] Fortunately, many of these women demonstrate normalization of their FSH levels over time, and only a minority seem to experience irreversible ovarian failure requiring long-term hormone-replacement therapy. Of note, however, recovery may not occur for many years following the completion of therapy.[78,123] However, some of these young women may experience a premature menopause when they reach their 20s and 30s.[124] Females who receive high-dose myeloablative therapy with alkylating agents such as busulfan, melphalan, and thiotepa in the context of SCT are at high risk of developing ovarian failure.[31,91,125] This has been observed in patients treated before and after pubertal development, is characterized by menopausal levels of LH and FSH, delayed or arrested puberty, and amenorrhea. Recovery of function has been recorded only rarely, but the follow-up time has been relatively brief for most of the patients.[104,126] When female childhood cancer survivors treated with chemotherapy do get pregnant, no adverse pregnancy outcomes were identified in a large study conducted by Green and colleagues within the framework of the Childhood Cancer Survivor Study.[127]

Radiotherapy-Induced Ovarian Failure

Females receiving abdominal, pelvic, or spinal irradiation are at increased risk of ovarian failure, especially if both ovaries were within the treatment field.[26,128–130] The data suggest that the ovary of a younger individual is more resistant to damage from irradiation than is the ovary of an older (adult) individual.[111,131–133] Thus, while radiation doses of 6 Gy may be sufficient to produce irreversible ovarian damage in women >40 years of age, doses in the range of 10 to 20 Gy are needed to induce permanent ovarian failure in the majority of females treated during childhood.[128,129,131,133] Moreover, it is important to keep in mind that, if irradiation is being given in association with alkylating agent chemotherapy, ovarian dysfunction may occur despite the use of lower doses of radiation.

Administration of spinal radiation for the treatment of ALL and brain tumors appears to result in clinically significant ovarian damage in some young women.[44,118,120,121] The incidence of raised plasma concentrations of FSH was 19% and 67% in young women treated for ALL with 18 and 24 Gy spinal irradiation, respectively. Long-term follow-up data, however, indicate that the majority of these young women go on to experience normal puberty and menarche, albeit at an older age.[44] Several groups report raised plasma concentrations of FSH in the majority (64 to 86%) of female subjects treated with chemotherapy and craniospinal irradiation.[120,121] Normalization of FSH levels occurs over time in the majority of these young women.[120] In our experience, essentially all female brain tumor survivors treated with craniospinal irradiation and standard doses of chemotherapy have entered puberty at a normal or early age and few has required hormone-replacement therapy.[43]

Girls treated with whole abdominal and/or pelvic irradiation for Hodgkin disease or Wilms' tumor or other solid tumors (eg, rhabdomyosarcoma, neuroblastoma) are at high risk of ovarian failure.[122,128,134] In the study by Wallace and colleagues, 27 of 38 females treated with whole abdominal radiation therapy (total dose 22 to 30 Gy) during early childhood for a variety of solid tumors failed to undergo or complete pubertal development.[128] A further 10 experienced an early menopause at a median of 23.5 years of age, including three who had conceived at an earlier time. When ovarian transposition is performed prior to radiotherapy, however, ovarian function is retained in the majority of young girls and adolescent females.[78,133] In a report from the Childhood Cancer Survivor Study including data on 1,915 female survivors and 4,029 pregnancies, Green and colleagues reported, however, a significant risk of low birth weight in the offspring of female survivors treated with pelvic irradiation.[127]

The outcome of ovarian function following TBI appears to be determined to a large extent by the age of the patient at the time of irradiation.[135] Our data, as well as the data of others, indicate that approximately 50% of prepubertal girls given fractionated TBI will enter puberty spontaneously and achieve menarche at a normal age.[82,92,136] While plasma gonadotropins have been elevated in up to two-thirds of these patients early after transplant, normalization of the plasma concentrations of LH and FSH can occur over time.[92] Ovarian failure is seen in essentially all patients who are greater than age 10 years at the time they are treated with TBI.[92,135–137] Patients require

hormonal support in order to achieve normal sexual development and to maintain normal menstruation. Recovery of ovarian function has been documented in a small number of women who have received TBI.[104] These women had increased risks of miscarriage and premature delivery of low birth weight infants.[104] This can be due to the uterine consequences of TBI. Holm and colleagues, Bath and colleagues, and Larsen and colleagues demonstrated that the uterine volume of patients treated with TBI is smaller than in normal controls and cancer survivors exclusively treated with chemotherapy.[138–140] The blood supply of the uterus was significantly decreased after TBI, suggesting a vascular mechanism for the observed abnormalities, with increased risks in younger patients.[138–140] Overall, the full impact of SCT on reproduction and on the health of future offspring will remain in question until we have data from large numbers of survivors followed long-term.

Hormone-Replacement Therapy

Males

Testosterone-replacement therapy is indicated in Leydig cell failure resulting from both primary hypogonadism and hypogonadotropic hypogonadism. In boys with pubertal delay, defined as the lack of signs of puberty and/or prepubertal levels of testosterone after 14 years of age, testosterone replacement therapy induces the development of secondary sexual characters and the pubertal growth spurt; it also contributes to the restoration of normal body composition and normal bone mineral density (BMD).[141] Low doses of long-acting testosterone esters (eg, testosterone enanthate starting at doses of 50 mg administered intramuscularly every month) are used to induce puberty, the dose being gradually increased thereafter to full replacement doses at adulthood.[142,143] The transdermal forms of testosterone, available for adult patients, deliver high doses of treatment and are not suitable for pediatric use. Oxandrolone, a non-aromatizable androgen is sometimes used to stimulate the growth velocity and induce the pubertal growth spurt without advancing the bone age.[142] Its benefits in comparison to the low doses of testosterone used to induce puberty are uncertain, and it lacks the virilizing effect of testosterone.[143]

Young men with mild testosterone deficiency (borderline low plasma testosterone levels and raised LH levels) may have a low BMD and some impairment of their sexual function.[144] However, in a randomized, placebo-controlled study of patients from that population, Howell and colleagues showed that testosterone replacement therapy did not result in significant changes in BMD, body composition, and quality of life. The authors concluded that androgen replacement

in this population cannot be recommended as a routine practice.[145]

In patients with hypogonadotropic hypogonadism retaining the potential for spermatogenesis, treatment with chronic GnRH or human chorionic gonadotropin will stimulate testicular growth and germ cell production. This treatment is generally restricted to adult men at the time they desire paternity.

Females

Despite recent reports on the possible association between cardiovascular disease, breast cancer and estrogen replacement without progesterone in post-menopausal women estrogen-replacement therapy is still indicated in young girls with ovarian failure in order to induce secondary sexual characters and optimal bone density[146,147]. Treatment can be initiated with a low dose of estrogen (eg ethinyl estradiol, 2 to 10 micrograms, conjugated equine estrogen 0.15–0.3 mg according to age at which replacement therapy is started). The dose can be slowly escalated over an 18–24 month period of time, followed by cyclic estrogen-progesterone therapy (eg low estrogen birth control pill). If breakthrough bleeding occurs on estrogen monotherapy, cyclic estrogen-progesterone should be initiated earlier[142].

Alterations in Body Composition

Overweight

The most widely accepted measurement to define childhood adiposity uses the BMI, calculated as the ratio between the weight (in kilograms) divided by the height^2 (in m^2) and expressed in percentiles with regards to both gender and chronological age. Overweight is defined in children whose BMI is above the 95th percentile for gender and chronological age. Patients whose BMI is between the 85th and 95th percentile are described as "at risk" for being overweight.[148] Obesity and being overweight are well-established sequelae of cancer therapy and are often observed in survivors of acute leukemia and various brain tumors.

Sklar and colleagues examined BMI in a group of 126 survivors of ALL, and a high incidence of being overweight was observed but was confined to those survivors who received cranial irradiation (Figure 3).[149] Additional risk factors for obesity other than cranial irradiation include female gender and exposure to dexamethasone. van der Sluis and colleagues compared the body composition parameters (BMI, lean body mass, and percentage of body fat measured with dual X-ray absorptiometry [DEXA]) of childhood ALL survivors exposed to high-dose dexamethasone and cranial irradiation to those of patients only treated with dexamethasone.[150] Their findings suggest that the deleterious effects of dexamethasone on body composition may be

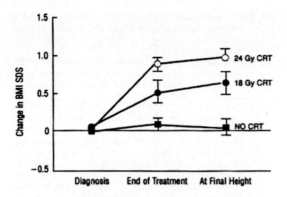

FIGURE 3 Change in body mass index (BMI) — standard deviation score (SDS) [mean ± Standard Error of Mean (SEM)] in survivors of acute lymphoblastic leukemia according to type of central nervous system prophylaxis. CRT = cranial irradiation. Reprinted with permission from Sklar, et al.[149]

temporary. Oeffinger and colleagues, in a report from the Childhood Cancer Survivor Study using data from 1,765 adult survivors of childhood ALL, found that cranial radiotherapy ≥ 20 Gy, especially in females treated at a young age (< 4 years) was significantly associated with obesity (ie, BMI ≥ 30).[151] The mechanisms underlying these propensities remain unsolved. One possible explanation is that radiation damages centers within the brain that normally control eating behaviors and/or regulate body composition. For instance, Brennan and colleagues found higher leptin levels in ALL survivors treated with cranial radiotherapy (18 to 25 Gy), when compared to BMI-matched controls, suggesting that cranial irradiation may induce a state of relative leptin resistance.[152] Growth hormone deficiency in adulthood has been associated with obesity and may contribute to the observed changes in body composition in ALL survivors who received high-dose cranial radiotherapy.[153] Childhood ALL survivors have also been shown to have reduced physical activity, even a long time after remission, but the contribution of this behavioral factor has yet to be proven.[154] Premature adiposity rebound, believed to be a predictor of adult obesity, was also described in childhood ALL survivors in a study by Reilly and colleagues, and may partly explain the increased risk for obesity in patients treated at a very young age (< 5 years).[155]

Brain tumors developing near the sellar region and their treatments can also disrupt hypothalamic and pituitary functions and induce severe states of morbid obesity.[156] In a large retrospective study, Lustig and colleagues analyzed data compiled over 30 years on 148 patients surviving childhood brain tumors.[157] Their findings showed that the development of obesity in those patients was associated with the degree of hypothalamic damage (tumoral proximity to the hypothalamus, hypothalamic exposure to radiation, especially to doses above 51 Gy, and extent of the surgical resection) and with the histology of

the tumor (craniopharyngioma, pilocytic astrocytoma and medulloblastoma). In a report on 921 patients from the Childhood Cancer Survivor Study, Gurney and colleagues also showed that hypothalamic/pituitary irradiation was associated with a greater risk of obesity in female patients, and that this association was dose dependent.[8] However, the authors did not find an overall significant difference in BMI in their population of childhood brain cancer survivors compared to the general population and related that observation to the exclusion of patients with craniopharyngioma from their study.[8] While the hypothalamic insult is believed to alter satiety centers and cause hyperphagia, another mechanism involving an increased parasympathetic tone leading to hyperinsulinemia (the latter promoting fat storage) has been suggested as a contributing factor to obesity in these patients.[158] It is with regards to that latter mechanism that treatment with octreotide has been tried in a small number of patients with hypothalamic obesity and has yielded some encouraging results.[157] Otherwise, there are no specific strategies for the prevention and treatment of obesity in childhood cancer survivors.

Osteoporosis

Young adult survivors of childhood cancer have reduced BMD, and many of them are at an increased risk for osteoporosis and fractures.[106] Osteopenia and osteoporosis can occur in childhood cancer survivors for several reasons. Firstly, the disease itself and its progression can affect bone structure and metabolism. For instance, in a prospective study, Crofton and colleagues had findings consistent with a low bone turnover in children who had just been diagnosed with ALL and before starting any treatments.[9] Secondly, chemotherapy and exposure to glucocorticoids can also adversely affect the bone mineral density. Methotrexate, in particular, a cytotoxic drug frequently used in treating ALL, has been shown to alter bone metabolism and to be associated with an increased risk for fractures.[159,160] Finally, the hormonal deficiencies associated with cancer and its treatments (and described earlier in the text), GHD, and sex-hormone deficiencies, are additional factors for osteoporosis.[106,161]

Subjects deemed at high risk for the development of osteoporosis should undergo periodic bone density studies. While the DEXA remains the most widely used tool for measuring bone mineral density, its results should be interpreted according to age, pubertal stage and height in the pediatric population using the z-score values. Failure to take these elements into account may result in over-diagnosing osteoporosis.[162] Preventive measures (for example, supplementation with calcium and vitamin D, smoking cessation, weight-bearing exercise) should be encouraged

in all individuals with low or borderline bone mineral density. Therapeutic interventions (for example, sex hormone therapy, GH replacement, bisphosphonates) may prove beneficial for those with abnormally reduced bone density, but long-term follow-up data are currently not available.

Conclusion

Endocrine sequelae occur frequently following childhood cancer and its treatments. Our understanding of the consequences on growth and pubertal development of cancer therapy, as well as the alterations it induces on body composition, has increased substantially over the past few years. Radiation therapy and chemotherapy are capable of causing damage to the endocrine systems, which control these functions. These endocrine abnormalities may remain subclinical for many years. Physicians who follow children or adolescents who have been treated with chemotherapy and/or radiation therapy for cancer must encourage the patients to continue lifelong surveillance for potential endocrine disease. The prevention, early recognition and treatment of these complications will help reduce long-term morbidity and improve the quality of life of childhood cancer survivors.

REFERENCES

1. Ries LAG, Smith MA, Gurney JG, et al. Cancer incidence and survival among children and adolescents. United States SEER program 1975–1995. NCI SEER program. Bethesda (MD): NIH publication No. 99-4649;1999.
2. Linet M, Ries LAG, Smith MA, et al. Cancer surveillance series: recent trends in childhood cancer incidence and mortality in the United States. J Natl Cancer Inst 1999;91: 1051–8.
3. Stiller C. Epidemiology of cancer in adolescents. Med Pediatr Oncol 2002;39:149–55.
4. Gurney JG, Davis S, Severson RK, et al. Trends in cancer incidence among children in the US. Cancer 1996;78: 532–41.
5. Sklar CA. Overview of the effect of cancer therapies: the nature, scale and breadth of the problem. Acta Pediatr Scand 1999;433 (Suppl):1–4.
6. Sklar CA. Growth and neuroendocrine dysfunction following therapy for childhood cancer. Pediatr Clin North Am 1997;44:489–503.
7. Gleeson HK, Stoeter R, Ogilvy-Stuart AL, et al. Improvements in final height over 25 years in growth hormone (GH)-deficient childhood survivors of brain tumours receiving GH replacement. J Clin Endocrinol Metab 2003; 88:3682–9.
8. Gurney JG, Ness KK, Stovall M, et al. Final height and body mass index among adult survivors of childhood brain cancer: Childhood Cancer Survivor Study. J Clin Endocrinol Metab 2003;88:4731–9.
9. Crofton PM, Ahmed SF, Wade JC, et al. Effects of intensive chemotherapy on bone and collagen turnover and the growth hormone axis in children with acute lymphoblastic leukemia. J Clin Endocrinol Metab 1998;83:3121–9.
10. Argüelles B, Barrios V, Pozo J, et al. Modifications of growth velocity and the insulin-like growth factor system in children with acute lymphoblastic leukemia: a longitudinal study. J Clin Endocrinol Metab 2000;85:4087–92.
11. Probert JC, Parker BR, Kaplan HS. Growth retardation in children after megavoltage irradiation of the spine. Cancer 1973;32:634–9.
12. Shalet SM, Gibson B, Swindell R, Pearson D. Effects of spinal irradiation on growth. Arch Dis Child 1987;62:461–4.
13. Brauner R, Fontoura M, Zucker JM, et al. Growth and growth hormone secretion after bone marrow transplantation. Arch Dis Child 1993;64:458–63.

14. Thomas BC, Stanhope R, Plowman PN, Leiper AD. Growth following single fraction and fractionated total body irradiation for bone marrow transplantation. Eur J Pediatr 1993;152:888–92.
15. Clayton PE, Shalet SM. The evolution of spinal growth after irradiation. Clin Oncol 1991;3:220–2.
16. Papadakis V, Tan C, Heller G, Sklar C. Growth and final height after treatment for childhood Hodgkin's disease. J Pediatr Hematol Oncol 1996;18:272–6.
17. Hogeboom CJ, Glosser SC, Guthrie KA, et al. Stature loss following treatment for Wilm's tumor. Med Pediatr Oncol 2001;36:295–304.
18. Sklar CA, Constine LS. Chronic neuro-endocrinological sequelae of radiation therapy. Int J Radiat Oncol Biol Phys 1995;31:1113–21.
19. Costin G. Effects of low-dose cranial radiation on growth hormone secretory dynamics and hypothalamic pituitary function. Am J Dis Child 1988;142:847–52.
20. Oglivy-Stuart AL, Wallace WH, Shalet SM. Radiation and neuroregulatory control of growth hormone secretion. Clin Endocrinol 1994;41:163–8.
21. Brauner R, Czernichow P, Rappaport R. Greater susceptibility to hypothalamopituitary irradiation in younger children with acute lymphoblastic leukemia. J Pediatr 1986;108:332.
22. Shalet SM, Beardwell CG, Pearson D, Morris Jones PH. The effect of varying doses of cerebral irradiation on growth hormone production in children. Clin Endocrinol 1976; 5:287–290.
23. Clayton PE, Shalet SM. Dose dependency of time of onset of radiation-induced growth hormone deficiency. J Pediatr 1991;118:226–8.
24. Brennan BM, Rahim A, Mackie EM, et al. Growth hormone status in adults treated for acute lymphoblastic leukaemia in childhood. Clin Endocrinol 1998;48:777–83.
25. Boulad F, Sands S, Sklar C. Late complications after bone marrow transplantation in children and adolescents. Curr Probl Pediatr 1998;28:277–97.
26. Goddard AG, Harris SJ, Plowman PN, et al. Growth hormone deficiency following radiotherapy for orbital and parameningeal sarcomas. Pediatr Hematol Oncol 1999;16:23–33.
27. Growth Hormone Research Society. Consensus guidelines for the diagnosis and treatment of growth hormone (GH) deficiency in childhood and adolescence: summary statement of the GH Research Society. J Clin Endocrinol Metab 2000;85:3990–3.
28. Gleeson HK, Gattamaneni HR, Smethurst C, et al. Reassessment of growth hormone status is required at final height in children treated with growth hormone replacement after radiation therapy. J Clin Endocrinol Metab 2004;89: 662–6.
29. Couto-Silva AC, Trivin C, Esperou H, et al. Changes in height, weight and plasma leptin after bone marrow transplantation. Bone Marrow Transplant 2000;26:1205–10.
30. Holm K, Nysom K, Rasmussen MH, et al. Growth, growth hormone and final height after bone marrow transplantation: possible recovery of irradiation-induced growth hormone insufficiency. Bone Marrow Transplant 1996;18: 163–70.
31. Bakker B, Oostdijk W, Bresters D, et al. Disturbances of growth and endocrine function after busulfan-based conditioning for haematopoeitic stem cell transplantation during infancy and childhood. Bone Marrow Transplant 2004;33:1049–56.
32. Rose SR, Schreiber RE, Kearney NS, et al. Hypothalamic dysfunction after chemotherapy. J Pediatr Endocrinol Metab 2004;17:55–66.
33. Reiter EO, Rosenfeld RG. Normal and abnormal growth. In: Larsen PR, Kronenberg HM, Melmed S, editors. Williams textbook of endocrinology. Philadelphia: WB Saunders; 2003. p. 1003–14.
34. Sklar C. Endocrine complications of the successful treatment of neoplastic diseases in childhood. Growth Genet Horm 2001;17:37–42.
35. Lissett CA, Saleem S, Rahim A, et al. The impact of irradiation on GH responsiveness to provocative agents is stimulus dependent: results in 161 individuals with radiation damage to the somatotropic axis. J Clin Endocrinol Metab 2001;86:663–8.
36. Darzy KH, Aimaretti G, Wieringa G, et al. The usefulness of the combined growth hormone (GH) releasing hormone and arginine stimulation test in the diagnosis of radiation-induced GH deficiency is dependent on the post irradiation interval. J Clin Endocrinol Metab 2003;88: 95–102.
37. Albertsson-Wikland K, Lannering B, Marky I, et al. A longitudinal study on growth and growth hormone (GH) secretion in children with irradiated brain tumors. Acta Pediatr Scand 1987:966–973.
38. Chemaitilly W, Trivin C, Souberbielle JC, Brauner R. Assessing short statured children for growth hormone deficiency. Horm Res 2003;60:34–42.
39. Weinzimer SA, Homan SA, Ferry RJ, Moshang T. Serum IGF-1 and IGFBP-3 concentrations do not accurately predict growth hormone deficiency in children with brain tumours. Clin Endocrinol 1999;51:339–45.
40. Sklar C, Sarafoglou K, Whittam E. Efficacy of insulin-like growth factor binding protein-3 (IGFBP-3) in predicting the growth hormone response to provocative testing in children treated with cranial irradiation. Acta Endocrinol 1993;129:511–5.
41. Sigurjonssdottir T, Hayes A. Precocious puberty: a report of 96 cases. Am J Dis Child 1968;1115:309–21.
42. Brauner R, Czernichow P, Rappaport R. Precocious puberty after hypothalamic and pituitary irradiation in young children. N Engl J Med 1984;311:920.
43. Oberfield SE, Soranno D, Nirenberg A, et al. Age at the onset of puberty following high-dose central nervous system radiation therapy. Arch Pediatr Adolesc Med 1996;150: 589–92.
44. Mills JL, Fears TR, Robison LL, et al. Menarche in a cohort of 188 long-term survivors of acute lymphoblastic leukemia. J Pediatr 1997;131:589–602.
45. Roth C, Schmidberger H, Lakomek M, et al. Reduction of gamma-aminobutyric acid-ergic neurotransmission as a putative mechanism of radiation induced activation of the gonadotropin releasing-hormone-pulse generator leading to precocious puberty in female rats. Neurosci Lett 2001;297:45–8.
46. Ogilvy-Stuart AL, Shalet SM. Growth and puberty after growth hormone treatment after irradiation for brain tumours. Arch Dis Child 1995;73:141–6.
47. Constine LS, Woolf PD, Cann D, et al. Hypothalamic-pituitary dysfunction after radiation for brain tumors. N Engl J Med 1993;328:87–94.
48. Lam KSL, Tse VKC, Wang C, et al. Effects of irradiation on hypothalamic pituitary function: a 5-year longitudinal study in patients with nasopharyngeal carcinoma. Q J Med 1991;78:165–76.
49. Tanner JM. Growth at adolescence. Oxford: Blackwell; 1978. p. 28–39.
50. Greulich W, Pyle S. Radiographic atlas of skeletal development of the hand and wrist. 2nd ed. Stanford: University Press; Stanford CA 1959.
51. Oerter KE, Uriarte MM, Rose SR, et al. Gonadotropin secretory dynamics during puberty in normal girls and boys. J Clin Endocrinol Metab 1990;71:1251–8.
52. Sulmont V, Brauner R, Fontoura M, Rappaport R. Response to growth hormone treatment and final height after cranial or craniospinal irradiation. Acta Paediatr Scand 1990;79:542–9.
53. Adan L, Sainte-Rose C, Souberbielle JC, et al. Adult height after growth hormone (GH) treatment for GH deficiency due to cranial irradiation. Med Pediatr Oncol 2000;34: 14–9.
54. Leung W, Rose SR, Zhou YM, et al. Outcomes of growth hormone replacement therapy in survivors of childhood acute lymphoblastic leukemia. J Clin Oncol 2002;20: 2959–64.
55. Brownstein CM, Mertens AC, Mitsby PA, et al. Factors that affect final height and change in height standard deviation scores in survivors of childhood cancer treated with growth hormone: a report from the Childhood Cancer Survivor Study. J Clin Endocrinol Metab 2004;89: 4422–7.
56. Swerdlow AJ, Reddingius RE, Higgins CD, et al. Growth hormone treatment of children with brain tumours and risk of tumour recurrence. J Clin Endocrinol Metab 2000; 85:4444–9.
57. Packer RJ, Boyett JM, Janns AJ, et al. Growth hormone replacement therapy in children with medulloblastoma: use and effect on tumor control. J Clin Oncol 2001;19: 480–7.
58. Sklar CA, Mertens AC, Mitsby P, et al. Risk of disease recurrence and second neoplasm in survivors of childhood cancer treated with growth hormone: a report from the Childhood Cancer Survivor Study 2002;87:3136–41.
59. Blethen SL, Rundle AC. Slipped capital femoral epiphyses in children treated with growth hormone. A summary of the natural cooperative growth experience. Horm Res 1996; 46:113–6.
60. Murray RD, Darzy KH, Gleeson HK, Shalet SM. GH-deficient survivors of childhood cancer: GH replacement during adult life. J Clin Endocrinol Metab 2002;87: 129–35.
61. Chin D, Sklar C, Donahue B, et al. Thyroid dysfunction as a late effect in survivors of pediatric medulloblastoma/primitive neurectodermal tumors: a comparison of hyperfractionated versus conventional radiotherapy. Cancer 1997;80:798–804.
62. Schmiegelow M, Feldt-Rasmussen U, Rasmussen AK, et al. A population-based study of thyroid function after radiotherapy and chemotherapy for a childhood brain tumor. J Clin Endocrinol Metab 2003;88:136–40.
63. Rose SR, Lustig RH, Pitukcheewanont P, et al. Diagnosis of hidden central hypothyroidism in survivors of childhood cancer. J Clin Endocrinol Metab 1999;84:4472–9.
64. Van Santen HM, Vulsma T, Dijkgraaf MG, et al. No damaging effect of chemotherapy in addition to radiotherapy on the thyroid axis in young adult survivors of childhood cancer. J Clin Endocrinol Metab 2003;88:3657–63.
65. Sklar C, Whitton J, Mertens, et al. Abnormalities of the thyroid in survivors of Hodgkin's disease: data from the Childhood Cancer Survivor Study. J Clin Endocrinol Metab 2000;85:3227–32.
66. Bethge W, Guggenberger D, Bamberg M, et al. Thyroid toxicity of treatment for Hodgkin's disease. Ann Haematol 2000;79:114–8.
67. Sigurdson AJ, Ronckers CM, Mertens AC, et al. Primary thyroid cancer after a first tumour in childhood (the Childhood Cancer Survivor Study): a nested case-control study. Lancet. 2005;365:2014–23.
68. Acharya S, Sarafoglou K, LaQuaglia M, et al. Thyroid neoplasms after therapeutic radiation of malignancies during childhood or adolescence. Cancer 2003;97:2397–403.
69. Bounacer A, Wicker R, Caillou B, et al. High prevalence of activating ret proto-oncogene rearrangements, in thyroid tumors from patients who had received external radiation. Oncogene 1997;15:1263–76.
70. Elisei R, Romei C, Vorontsova T, et al. RET/PTC rearrangements in thyroid nodules: studies in irradiated and non irradiated malignant and benign thyroid lesions in children and adults. J Clin Endocrinol Metab 2001;86: 3211–6.
71. Liel Y. Screening without efficacy, thyroid ultrasonography is another example. BMJ 2004; 328:521.
72. Relander T, Gavallin-Stahl E, Garwicz S, et al. Gonadal and sexual function in men treated for childhood cancer. Med Pediatr Oncol 2000;35:52–63.
73. Byrne J, Fears TR, Mills JL, et al. Fertility of long-term male survivors of acute lymphoblastic leukemia diagnosed during childhood. Pediatr Blood Cancer 2004;42:364–72.
74. Bath LE, Anderson RA, Critchley HOD, et al. Hypothalamic-pituitary-ovarian dysfunction after prepubertal chemotherapy and cranial irradiation for acute leukaemia. Hum Reprod 2001;16:1838–44.
75. Constine LS, Woolf PD, Cann D, et al. Hypothalamic-pituitary dysfunction after radiation for brain tumors. N Engl J Med 1993;328:87–94.
76. Griffin JE, Wilson JD. Disorders of the testes and the male reproductive tract. In: Wilson JD, Foster DW, editors. Williams textbook of endocrinology, Vol. 8. Philadelphia: W.B. Saunders; 1992. p. 799–852.
77. Morris ID. The testis: endocrine function. In: Hiller SG, Kitchener HC, Neilson JP, editors. Scientific essentials of reproductive medicine. London, U.K.; W.B. Saunders; 1996. p. 160–71.
78. Sklar C. Reproductive physiology and treatment-related loss of sex-hormone production. Med Pediatr Oncol 1999; 33:2–8.
79. Lustig RH, Conte FA, Kogan BA, Grumbach MM. Ontogeny of gonadotropin secretion in congenital anarchism: sexual dimorphism versus syndrome of gonadal dysgenesis and diagnostic considerations. J Urol 1987;138:587–91.
80. Shalet SM, Horner A, Ahmed SR, Morris-Jones PH. Leydig cell damage after testicular irradiation for lymphoblastic leukemia. Med Pediatr Oncol 1985;13:65–8.
81. Blatt J, Poplack DG, Sherins RJ. Testicular function in boys after chemotherapy for acute lymphoblastic leukemia. N Engl J Med 1981;304:1121–4.

82. Sklar CA, Kim TH, Ramsay NKC. Testicular function following bone marrow transplantation performed during or after puberty. Cancer 1984;53:1498–501.
83. Papadakis V, Vlachopapadopoulou E, Van Syckle K, et al. Gonadal function in young patients successfully treated for Hodgkin's disease. Med Pediatr Oncol 1999;32: 366–72.
84. Tsatsoulis A, Whitehead E, St John J, et al. The pituitary-Leydig cell axis in men with severe damage to the germinal epithelium. Clin Endocrinol 1987;27:683–9.
85. Siimes MA, Rautonen J, Makipernaa A, Sipila I. Testicular function in adult males surviving childhood malignancy. Pediatr Hematol Oncol 1995;12:231–41.
86. Kenney LB, Laufer MR, Grant FD, et al. High risk of infertility and long term gonadal damage in males treated with high dose cyclophosphamide for sarcoma during childhood. Cancer 2001;91:613–21.
87. Bramswig JH, Heimes U, Heiermann E, et al. The effect of different cumulative doses of chemotherapy on testicular function. Cancer 1990;65:1298–302.
88. Heikens J, Behrendt H, Adriaanse R, Berghout A. Irreversible gonadal damage in male survivors of pediatric Hodgkin's disease. Cancer 1996;78:2020–4.
89. Mackie EJ, Radford M, Shalet SM. Gonadal function following chemotherapy for childhood Hodgkin's disease. Med Pediatr Oncol 1996;27:74–8.
90. Sanders JE. Endocrine complications of high-dose therapy with stem cell transplantation. Pediatr Transplant 2004; 8 (Suppl 5):39–50.
91. Afify A, Shaw PJ, Clavano-Harding A, Cowell CT. Growth and endocrine function in children with acute myeloid leukemia after bone marrow transplantation using busulfan/cyclophosphamide. Bone Marrow Transplant 2000; 25:1087–1092.
92. Sarafoglou K, Boulad F, Gillio A, Sklar C. Gonadal function after bone marrow transplantation for acute leukemia during childhood. J Pediatr 1997;130:210–6.
93. Shalet SM, Tsatsoulis A, Whitehead E, Read G. Vulnerability of the human Leydig cell to radiation damage is dependent upon age. J Endocrinol 1989;120:161–5.
94. Leiper AD, Grant DB, Chessels JM. Gonadal function after testicular radiation for acute lymphoblastic leukemia. Arch Dis Child 1986;61:53–6.
95. Brauner R, Caltabiano P, Rappaport R, et al. Leydig cell insufficiency after testicular irradiation for acute lymphoblastic leukemia. Horm Res 1988;30:111–4.
96. Shalet SM, Beardwell CG, Jacobs HS, Pearson D. Testicular function following irradiation of the human prepubertal testis. Clin Endocrinol 1978;9:483–90.
97. Castillo LA, Craft AW, Kernahan J, et al. Gonadal function after 12-Gy testicular irradiation in childhood acute lymphoblastic leukemia. Med Pediatr Oncol 1990;18: 185–9.
98. Izard MA. Leydig cell function and radiation: a review of the literature. Radiother Oncol 1995;34:1–8.
99. Andreu JAL, Fernandez PJ, i Tortajada JF, et al. Persistent altered spermatogenesis in long-term childhood cancer survivors. Pediatr Hematol Oncol 2000;17:21–30.
100. van den Berg H, Furstner F, van den Bos C, Begrendt H. Decreasing the number of MOPP courses reduces gonadal damage in childhood Hodgkin's disease. Pediatr Blood Cancer 2004;42:210–5.
101. Anserini P, Chiodi S, Costa M, et al. Semen analysis following allogeneic bone marrow transplantation. Additional data for evidence-based counselling. Bone Marrow Transplant 2002;30:447–51.
102. Grigg AP, McLachlan R, Zajac J, Szer J. Reproductive status in long-term bone marrow transplant survivors receiving busulfan-cyclophosphamide (120 mg/kg). Bone Marrow Transplant 2000;26:1089–95.
103. Meistrich ML, Vassillopoulou-Sellin R, Lipshultz LI. Gonadal dysfunction. In: DeVita VT Jr, Hellman S, Rosenberg SA, editors. Cancer: principles and practice of oncology. Vol 5. Philadelphia: Lippincott-Raven; 1997. p. 2758–73.
104. Sanders JE, Hawley J, Levy W, et al. Pregnancies following high-dose cyclophosphamide with or without high-dose busulfan or total-body irradiation and bone marrow transplantation. Blood 1996;87:3045–52.
105. Sklar CA, Kim TH, Ramsay NKC. Testicular function following bone marrow transplantation performed during or after puberty. Cancer 1984;53:1498–501.
106. Aisenberg J, Hsieh K, Kalaitzoglou G, et al. Bone mineral density (BMD) in long-term survivors of childhood cancer. J Pediatr Hematol Oncol 1998;20:241–5.
107. Carr BR. Disorders of the ovary and the reproductive tract. In: Wilson JD, Foster DW, editors. Williams textbook of endocrinology. Vol 8. Philadelphia: W.B. Saunders; 1992. p. 733–98.
108. Rivkees SA, Crawford JD. The relationship of gonadal activity and chemotherapy-induced gonadal damage. JAMA 1988;259:2123–2125.
109. Wallace WH, Shalet SM, Crowne EC, et al. Gonadal dysfunction due to cis-platinum. Med Pediatr Oncol 1989;17: 409–13.
110. Schilsky R, Lewis B, Sherins R, Young RC. Gonadal dysfunction in patients receiving chemotherapy for cancer. Ann Intern Med 1980;93:109–14.
111. Horning SJ, Hoppe RT, Kaplan HS, Rosenberg SA. Female reproductive potential after treatment for Hodgkin's disease. N Eng J Med 1981;304:1377–82.
112. Siris ES, Leventhal BG, Vaitukaitis JL. Effects of childhood leukemia and chemotherapy on puberty and reproductive function in girls. N Eng J Med 1976;294:1143–6.
113. Hudson MM, Greenwald C, Thompson E, et al. Efficacy and toxicity of multiagent chemotherapy and low-dose involved field radiotherapy in children and adolescents with Hodgkin's disease. J Clin Oncol 1993;11:100–8.
114. Himelstein-Braw R, Peters H, Faber M. Morphological studies of the ovaries of leukaemic children. Br J Cancer 1978;38:82–7.
115. Nicosia SV, Matus-Ridley M, Meadows AT. Gonadal effects of cancer therapy in girls. Cancer 1985;55:2364–72.
116. Larsen E, Muller J, Schmiegelow K, et al. Reduced ovarian function in long-term survivors of radiation and chemotherapy-treated childhood cancer. J Clin Endocrinol Metab 2003;88:5307–14.
117. Wallace WHB, Shalet SM, Tetlow LJ, Morris–Jones PH. Ovarian function following the treatment of childhood acute lymphoblastic leukaemia. Med Pediatr Oncol 1993;21:333–9.
118. Hamre MR, Robison LL, Nesbit ME, et al. Effects of radiation on ovarian function in long term survivors of childhood acute lymphoblastic leukemia: a report from the Children Cancer Study Group. J Clin Oncol 1987;5: 1759–65.
119. Ahmed SR, Shalet SM, Campbell RHA, Deakin DP. Primary gonadal damage following treatment of brain tumours in childhood. J Pediatr 1983;103:562–5.
120. Clayton PE, Shalet SM, Price DA, Jones PH. Ovarian function following chemotherapy for childhood brain tumours. Med Pediatr Oncol 1989;17:92–6.
121. Livesey EA, Brook CGD. Gonadal dysfunction after treatment of intracranial tumours. Arch Dis Child 1988; 63:495–500.
122. Sy Ortin TT, Shostak CA, Donaldson SS. Gonadal status and reproductive function following treatment for Hodgkin's disease in childhood. The Stanford experience. Int J Radiat Oncol Biol Phys 1990;19:873–80.
123. Nasir J, Walton C, Lindow SW, Masson EA. Spontaneous recovery of chemotherapy-induced primary ovarian failure: implication for management. Clin Endocrinol 1997;46:217–9.
124. Byrne J, Fears TR, Gail MH, et al. Early menopause in long-term survivors of cancer during adolescence. Am J Obstet Gynecol 1992;166:788–93.
125. Michel G, Socie G, Gebhard F, et al. Late effects of allogeneic bone marrow transplantation for children with acute myeloblastic leukemia in first complete remission: the impact of conditioning regimen without total-body irradiation—a report from the Société Française de Greffe de Moelle. J Clin Oncol 1997;15:2238–46.
126. Thibaud E, Rodriguez-Macias K, Trivin C, et al. Ovarian function after bone marrow transplantation during childhood. Bone Marrow Transplant 1998;21:287–90.
127. Green DM, Whitton JA, Stovall M, et al. Pregnancy outcome of female survivors of childhood cancer: a report from the Childhood Cancer Survivor Study. Am J Obstet Gynecol 2002;187:1070–80.
128. Wallace WHB, Shalet SM, Hendry JH, et al. Ovarian failure following abdominal irradiation in childhood: the radiosensitivity of the human oocyte. Br J Radiol 1989; 62:995–8.
129. Wallace WHB, Shalet SM, Crown EC, et al. Ovarian failure following abdominal irradiation in childhood: natural history and prognosis. Clin Oncol 1989;1:75–9.
130. Stillman RJ, Schinfeld JS, Schiff I, et al. Ovarian failure in long term survivors of childhood malignancy. Am J Obstet Gynecol 1981;139:62–6.
131. Lushbaugh CC, Casarett GW. The effect of gonadal irradiation in clinical radiation therapy: a review. Cancer 1976; 37:1111–20.
132. Damewood MD, Grochow LB. Prospects for fertility after chemotherapy or radiation for neoplastic disease. Fertil Steril 1986;45:443–59.
133. Thibaud E, Ramirez M, Brauner R, et al. Preservation of ovarian function by ovarian transposition performed before pelvic irradiation in childhood. J Pediatr 1992;12: 880–4.
134. Green DM, Brecher ML, Lindsay AN, et al. Gonadal function in pediatric patients following treatment for Hodgkin's disease. Med Pediatr Oncol 1981;9:235–44.
135. Mertens AC, Ramsay NKC, Kouris S, et al. Patterns of gonadal dysfunction following bone marrow transplantation. Bone Marrow Transplant 1998;22:345–50.
136. Matsumoto M, Shinohara O, Ishiguro H, et al. Ovarian function after bone marrow transplantation performed before menarche. Arch Dis Child 1999;80:452–4.
137. Sanders JE, Buckner CD, Amos D, et al. Ovarian function following marrow transplantation for aplastic anemia or leukemia. J Clin Oncol 1988;6:813–8.
138. Holm K, Nysom K, Brocks V, et al. Ultrasound B-mode changes in the uterus and ovaries and Doppler changes in the uterus after total body irradiation and allogeneic bone marrow transplantation in childhood. Bone Marrow Transplant 1999;23:259–63.
139. Bath LE, Critchley HOD, Chambers SE, et al. Ovarian and uterine characteristics after total body irradiation in childhood and adolescence: response to sex steroid replacement. Br J Obstet Gyneacol 1999;106:1265–72.
140. Larsen EC, Schmiegelow K, Rechnitzer C, et al. Radiotherapy at a young age reduces uterine volume of childhood cancer survivors. Acta Obstet Gynecol Scand 2004;83:96–102.
141. Mulder JE. Benefits and risks of hormone replacement therapy in young adult cancer survivors with gonadal failure. Med Pediatr Oncol 1999;33:46–52.
142. Brook CGD. Treatment of late puberty. Horm Res 1995; 51 (Suppl 3):101–3.
143. De Luca F, Argente J, Cavallo L, et al. Management of puberty in constitutional delay of growth and puberty. J Pediatr Endocrinol Metab 2001;14:953–7.
144. Howell SJ, Radford JA, Adams JE, Shalet SM. The impact of mild Leydig cell dysfunction following cytotoxic chemotherapy on bone mineral density (BMD) and body composition. Clin Endocrinol 2000;52:609–16.
145. Howell SJ, Radfordt JA, Adams JE, et al. Randomized placebo-controlled trial of testosterone replacement in men with mild Leydig cell insufficiency following cytotoxic chemotherapy. Clin Endocrinol 2001;55: 315–24.
146. Writing group for the Women's Health Initiative Investigators. Risks and benefits of estrogen plus progestin in healthy postmenopausal women: principal results from the Women's Health Initiative randomized controlled trial. JAMA 2002;288:321–33.
147. Mulder JE. Benefits and risks of hormone replacement therapy in young adult cancer survivors with gonadal failure. Med Pediatr Oncol 1999;33:46–52.
148. Barlow SE, Dietz WH. Obesity evaluation and treatment: Expert Committee recommendations. The Maternal and Child Health Bureau, Health Resources and Services Administration and the Department of Health and Human Services. Pediatrics 1998;102(3):E29.
149. Sklar CA, Mertens AC, Walter A, et al. Changes in body mass index and prevalence of overweight in survivors of childhood acute lymphoblastic leukemia: role of cranial irradiation. Med Pediatr Oncol 2000;35:91–5.
150. van der Sluis IM, van den Heuvel-Eibrink MM, Hahlen K, et al. Altered bone mineral density and body composition, and increased fracture risk in childhood acute lymphoblastic leukemia. J Pediatr 2002;141:204–10.
151. Oeffinger KC, Mertens AC, Sklar CA, et al. Obesity in adult survivors of childhood acute lymphoblastic leukemia: a report from the childhood cancer survivor study. J Clin Oncol 2003:21;1359–65.
152. Brennan BM, Rahim A, Blum WF, et al. Hyperleptinemia in young adults following cranial irradiation in childhood: growth hormone deficiency or leptin insensitivity? Clin Endocrinol 1999;50:163–9.
153. Talvensaari KK, Lanning M, Tapanainen P, Knip M. Long term survivors of childhood cancer survivors have an

increased risk of manifesting the metabolic syndrome. J Clin Endocrinol Metab 1996;81:3051–5.

154. Reilly JJ, Vetham JC, Ralston JM, et al. Reduced energy expenditure in pre-obese children treated for acute lymphoblastic leukemia. Pediatr Res 1998;44:557–62.

155. Reilly JJ, Kelly A, Ness P, et al. ALSPAC Study Team. Premature adiposity rebound in children treated for acute lymphoblastic leukaemia. J Clin Endocrinol Metab 2001;86:3742–5.

156. Lustig RH, Post SR, Srivannaboon K, et al. Risk factors for the development of obesity in children surviving brain tumors. J Clin Endocrinol Metab 2003;88:611–6.

157. Lustig RH, Hinds PS, Ringwald-Smith K, et al. Octreotide therapy of pediatric hypothalamic obesity: a double-blind, placebo-controlled trial. J Clin Endocrinol Metab 2003;88:2586–92.

158. Brennan BMD, Rahim A, Adams JA, et al. Reduced bone mineral density in young adults following cure of acute lymphoblastic leukaemia in childhood. Br J Cancer 1999; 79:1859–63.

159. Stanislavejic S, Babcock AL. Fractures in children treated with methotrexate for leukemia. Clin Orthpaed Related Res 1997;125:139–144.

160. De Boer H, Blok GJ, Van Lingen A, et al. Consequences of childhood onset growth hormone deficiency for adult bone mass. J Bone Mineral Res 1994;9:1319–26.

161. Nysom K, Holm K, Michaelsen KF, et al. Bone mass after allogeneic bone marrow transplantation for childhood leukaemia or lymphoma. Bone Marrow Transplant 2000; 25:191–6.

Preoperative Considerations in the Cancer Patient Undergoing Surgery

Sean Malone, MD, FACP

Harrison G. Weed, MD, MS, FACP

General internists and family practice physicians frequently act as primary care physicians or consultants in the perioperative assessment and management of patients with cancer. Approximately 75% of patients with solid tumors undergo surgical resection for cure, and about 90% undergo surgery for cure or palliation. Perhaps the primary consideration is the patient's cancer diagnosis, including the extent of the disease and cancer-related treatments that are planned or have already been performed. The natural history of the cancer, including prognosis, and the possible side effects of any previous chemotherapy or radiation therapy should also be considered. For example, some chemotherapies can cause permanent adverse effects on pulmonary or cardiac function that should be considered prior to surgery.

In the preoperative evaluation of a cancer patient, as with any preoperative evaluation, the physician should have a basic understanding of the surgical procedure and should know whether the surgery is intended for cure or palliation. The physician must also obtain a thorough medical history and physical examination to adequately assess comorbid conditions, such as hypertension, diabetes, cardiac, pulmonary, or renal disease. The preoperative medical evaluation should include an assessment of the patient's functional status, nutritional status and pain. Patients with cancer vary widely in their performance status. Some patients are ambulatory and fully functional in activities of daily living, whereas others are severely debilitated. A patient's performance status depends on many factors, including the type of cancer, extent of disease, side effects of cancer-related treatments, and presence of comorbid medical conditions. The Karnofsky performance status scale is a general and robust prognostic indicator for both cancer and surgical outcome and mortality. However, to assess risks for specific perioperative complications, such as cardiac complications or deep vein thrombosis, it is important to use more specific measures of risk as are described in the following sections. In addition, a careful assessment of nutritional status can help identify patients who might benefit from delaying surgery for a week of intensive nutritional supplementation.

In general, organ dysfunction is managed with standard treatments, regardless of the patient's cancer. Physicians should pay particular attention to pain management, which is too frequently overlooked by clinicians despite the high priority patients place on this aspect of their care. Finally, because most patients with cancer who are undergoing surgery have many caregivers, including surgeons, oncologists, and radiation oncologists, one common role of the primary care physician is to coordinate the patient's overall care. Frequently, the physician knows the patient well enough to have a frank conversation with the patient and the patient's family about their expectations. This conversation can provide an opportunity to ascertain the patient's wishes regarding resuscitation. In summary, primary care physicians frequently play an important and complex role in the perioperative care of patients with cancer. Indeed, the complexity of this role has led to proposals that hospitals should implement coordination mechanisms to improve delivery of multidisciplinary care to patients with cancer.[1]

REFERENCE

1. Bickell NA, Young, GJ. Coordination of care for early-stage breast cancer patients. J Gen Intern Med, 2001;16: 737–42.

Perioperative Nutritional Issues

Sean Malone, MD, FACP
Harrison G. Weed, MD, MS, FACP

Malnutrition has been recognized as a risk factor for poor surgical outcome for at least 70 years.[1,2] It is associated with infection, poor wound healing, prolonged postoperative recovery, and sepsis with multiorgan failure. Clinical trials, many of them exclusively or predominantly in cancer patients, have demonstrated the benefits of vigorous perioperative nutritional support for severely malnourished patients.[3] The nutritional state of all cancer patients should be evaluated prior to surgery, and, in general, patients with a recent, sustained loss of more than 15% of body weight or with a severely cachectic appearance and with a serum albumin below 2.5 gm/dL should be considered for at least a week of vigorous nutritional support prior to surgery.[3,4] Whenever feasible, enteral feeding is preferred, because it provides more benefit with less risk than does parenteral feeding.[5,6]

Causes and Effects of Malnutrition on Surgical Outcome

From 40 to 80% of patients anticipating major cancer surgery are malnourished.[7] There are many causes of malnutrition in cancer patients, including pain-induced and medication-induced anorexia, mechanical obstruction of the oropharynx or gastrointestinal tract, the side effects of chemotherapy and radiation therapy (including anorexia, nausea, and stomatitis), the use of restrictive alternative diets or dietary supplements, and a fear of "feeding" the cancer. In addition, an inflammatory response to the cancer can lead to the release of tumor necrosis factor-α (formerly called cachectin), interleukin 6 (IL-6) and other inflammatory mediators causing both anorexia and a general catabolic state. The catabolic state is manifested by insulin resistance, depletion of fat stores, and increased protein turnover.[8] Malnutrition can be exacerbated by the metabolic demands of the cancer and by surgery-related fasting and stress. Immune suppression as a direct consequence of the cancer, or as a side effect of treatments makes patients more susceptible to infection, and infection causes additional inflammation that can further exacerbate cachexia. Whatever the causes of preoperative malnutrition, it is associated with worse surgical outcomes, including poor surgical site healing, more frequent infection, and increased 30-day mortality.[9]

Preoperative Nutritional Assessment and Treatment

Most single measures of nutrition are relatively poor predictors of postoperative outcome because people can be sustained on a wide variety of diets, because there is a broad range of normal for body habitus, and because most measures are affected by factors other than nutritional status. Anthropometrics (measures and formulae of weight, height, limb circumferences and skinfold thicknesses) do not predict surgical outcome. Although serum albumin concentration is a simple and robust measure of nutrition, it has a relatively long half-life (up to 20 days) and is affected by factors other than nutrition, including the patient's hydration status. Nonetheless, an observational trial of more than 54,000 patients undergoing major noncardiac surgery at Veterans Administration hospitals found that, in a multivariable model, serum albumin concentration was the single best predictor of 61 variables for 30-day operative morbidity and mortality.[9] As serum albumin concentration dropped from 4–6 gm/dL to below 2.1 gm/dL, mortality increased from 1% to 29%, and morbidity increased from 10% to 60%. Combining serum albumin with gross measures of nutrition, including recent weight loss, body mass index, and patient appearance, yields a subjective nutritional index that is perhaps the most robust indicator of nutritional status: the Subjective Global Assessment.[10]

One purpose of assessing risk is to help decide which patients might benefit from perioperative nutritional support. There have been a number of studies that showed apparent benefit of total parenteral nutrition (TPN); however, they were poorly controlled and meta-analysis showed a high complication rate that negated the benefits.[5] Complications that are more frequent in patients receiving TPN include pneumothorax, sepsis, and abdominal abscesses.[11] A Veterans Affairs Medical Center (VAMC) trial of almost 400 malnourished patients undergoing major abdominal or thoracic surgery, who were randomized to receive perioperative TPN or usual care, showed no benefit overall but a trend toward benefit in severely malnourished patients (as measured by the Subjective Global Assessment) or by just considering those who had lost more than 15% of their baseline weight.[12] Over 60% of these patients had cancer. Therefore, general surgery should not be delayed for intensive preoperative nutritional support except for patients who are severely malnourished as assessed by a greater than 15% loss of body weight, a cachectic appearance with a low body mass index, and a serum albumin below 2.5 gm/dL. Furthermore (when feasible), enteral nutrition, either oral or via feeding tube, is preferred over TPN because enteral nutrition yields a lower complication rate, including a lower rate of infections.

Postoperative Nutritional Support

Although the benefits of preoperative nutritional support are often diminished by the continued presence of the factors that led to malnutrition and must be weighed against the risks of postponing surgery, postoperative nutritional support is more uniformly effective and beneficial. Many patients are unable to maintain adequate nutritional intake after cancer surgery. This can be due to postoperative compromise in the gastrointestinal tract (for example, postoperative ileus) or to medication side effects such as anorexia and slowed bowel transit from narcotic analgesics or chemotherapy. It can also be due to mechanical compromise of chewing and swallowing. Over 93% of patients who undergo resection of oropharyngeal cancers required at least some postoperative nutritional support. The National Institutes of Health, the American Society for Parenteral and Enteral Nutrition, and the American Society for Clinical Nutrition jointly reviewed prospective, controlled trials of perioperative nutritional support involving over 2,500 surgical patients, most of whom had cancer. They reached three main conclusions: (1) TPN given to severely malnourished patients with gastrointestinal cancer for 7 to 10 days before surgery decreases postoperative complications by approximately 10%; (2) routine use of early postoperative TPN in malnourished general surgical patients who did not receive preoperative TPN increases postoperative complications by approximately 10%; and (3) postoperative nutritional support is necessary to prevent starvation of patients unable to eat for more than a week after surgery. In sum, most patients will benefit from postoperative nutritional support if they are malnourished and/or will be unable to eat for more than a week after surgery; however, TPN should be reserved for patients without enteral access who are severely malnourished.

REFERENCE

1. Studley HO. Percentage of weight loss: basic indicator of surgical risk in patients with chronic peptic ulcers. JAMA 1936;106:458–60.
2. Studley HO. Percentage of weight loss: a basic indicator of surgical risk in patients with chronic peptic ulcer. Nutr Hosp 2001;16:141–3.
3. Salvino RM, Dechicco RS, Seidner DL. Perioperative nutrition support: who and how. Cleve Clin J Med 2004;71:345–51.
4. Baker JP, Detsky AS, Wesson DE, et al. Nutritional assessment: a comparison of clinical judgement and objective measurements. N Engl J Med 1982;306:969–72.
5. Detsky AS, Baker JP, O'Rourke K, Goel V. Perioperative parenteral nutrition: a meta-analysis. Ann Intern Med 1987;107:195–203.
6. McGeer AJ, Detsky AS, O'Rourke K. Parenteral nutrition in cancer patients undergoing chemotherapy: a meta-analysis. Nutrition 1990;6:233–40.
7. Ollenschlager G, Viell B, Thomas W, et al. Tumor anorexia: causes, assessment, treatment. Recent Results Cancer Res 1991;121:249–59.
8. Kern KA, Norton JA. Cancer cachexia. J Parenter Enteral Nutr 1988;12:286–98.
9. Gibbs J, Cull W, Henderso W, et al. Preoperative serum albumin level as a predictor of operative mortality and morbidity: results from the National VA Surgical Risk Study. Arch Surg 1999;134:36–42.
10. Detsky AS, Smalley PS, Chang J. The rational clinical examination. Is this patient malnourished? JAMA 1994;271:54–8.
11. Brennan MF, Pinkers PW, Posner M, et al. A prospective randomized trial of total parenteral nutrition after major pancreatic resection for malignancy. Ann Surg 1994;220:436–41.
12. The Veterans Affairs Total Parenteral Nutrition Cooperative Study Group. Perioperative total parenteral nutrition in surgical patients. N Engl J Med 1991;325:525–32.

79

Perioperative Neurologic Issues

Herbert B. Newton, MD

Harrison G. Weed, MD, MS, FACP

Neurological complications are common in patients with cancer. Delirium is perhaps most common, but seizures, stroke, focal weakness, back pain, and gait disturbances also occur.[1,2] These complications can be due to medication toxicity, infection, metabolic abnormalities, and both direct and indirect effects of cancer on the nervous system. It is important to detect and address neurologic complications before surgery, to continue appropriate treatments through the perioperative period, and to anticipate special risks and needs that may arise after surgery.

Brain metastases can present with headache, confusion or new focal neurologic deficits, such as hemiparesis. Papilledema is unreliable as a diagnostic sign of brain metastases because it occurs in less than one-fourth of patients. Leptomeningeal metastases should be suspected in patients who develop multifocal neurologic deficits, especially the combination of cranial neuropathies with spinal nerve root deficits. Lung and breast cancers, melanomas, and lymphomas are common causes of leptomeningeal metastases. Spinal cord compression presents with severe acute back pain and myelopathy. Myelopathy can include the physical findings of leg weakness and spasticity, lower extremity hyperreflexia, abnormal Babinski's reflex, and urinary incontinence. Emergent treatment of spinal cord compression with high-dose corticosteroids, radiation therapy, or surgical decompression is necessary to preserve neurologic function.

Delirum

Delirium, including confusion and encephalopathy is common in cancer patients and has many potential causes, including medication side effects, metabolic disturbances, metastatic intracranial tumors, strokes, seizures, and side effects of cancer treatments (Table 1). Patients undergoing chemotherapy often have both baseline and chemotherapy-induced cognitive dysfunction in areas such as attention, learning, and processing speed. Chemotherapy-induced effects resolve in some, but not all patients.[3] Delirium is often due to medications, especially narcotics, sedatives, and antiemetics exacerbating underlying age or

Table 1 Disorders Associated with Postoperative Mental Status Changes in Cancer Patients

Structural
Hydrocephalus/elevated intracranial pressure
Primary or metastatic brain tumor, including leptomeningeal metastases
Stroke: thrombotic or hemorrhagic, including tumor hemorrhage
Radiation therapy to the head

Medications
Anticonvulsants
Antidepressants
Antiemetics
Anxiolytics
Chemotherapy
Narcotics
Neuroleptics
Sedatives
Steroids

Metabolic Abnormalities
Endocrine disorders
Fluid/electrolyte imbalances
Hepatic failure
Hypoxemia
Nutritional deficiencies: Wernicke's encephalopathy
Renal failure

Infections
Meningitis
Pneumonia
Urinary tract infection
Sepsis
Surgical site infection

disease-related deficits; however, infections (eg, sepsis, pneumonia, meningitis, encephalitis) must be kept in mind as possible causes. Delirium can be the only manifestation of infection in patients who are immunosuppressed from the cancer and/ or chemotherapy.

Stroke

Stroke can be caused by a variety of tumor-related conditions, including direct tumor invasion, side effects of chemotherapy, cancer-related coagulopathy, and thrombotic (marantic) endocarditis.[1] Certain types of operations can also place patients at risk for stroke due to arterial embolus from manipulation of the heart and great vessels or the cerebral vasculature. In addition, perioperative hypotension can cause ischemia distal to a narrowed vessel that was adequately perfused at the patient's usual blood pressure.

Seizures

Prior to surgery, it is important to thoroughly assess any new or chronic seizures. New onset seizures can be caused by cancer metastatic to the brain, brain hemorrhage or infarction, infection, or metabolic disturbances. The preoperative report should include a basic description of the patient's usual seizure pattern, including seizure frequency, when the most recent seizure occurred, and the current anticonvulsant regimen. The patient's baseline anticonvulsant serum concentrations should be determined. Often, this information is available from the physician who usually prescribes the patient's anticonvulsant medication, but it can be obtained as a preoperative blood test. For patients whose seizures are well controlled, a baseline anticonvulsant level can help to determine whether any postoperative seizure might be due to insufficient medication or if another explanation must be sought. If feasible, before surgery a neurologist should evaluate and adjust the medications of any patient whose seizures are not fully controlled. In general, on the day of surgery, anticonvulsant medications should be taken with a sip of water. During the time a patient is unable to take enteral medications, there are several alternative intravenous anticonvulsants that can be considered, including phenytoin (Dilantin), fosphenytoin (Cerebyx) and valproate sodium (Depacon). A substitute intravenous anticonvulsant should be selected and ordered prior to surgery to minimize the patient's risk for breakthrough seizure activity in the perioperative period.

Neuromuscular Disorders

Paraneoplastic syndromes that affect neuromuscular function are rare but are of particular concern in the perioperative period because treatment with anesthetic agents can exacerbate muscular weakness leading to delayed recovery of mechanical lung function or even respiratory failure. Symptoms and signs of Eaton-Lambert syndrome include proximal muscle weakness, diminished or absent deep tendon reflexes, and autonomic neuropathy with varied manifestations, including gastroparesis and orthostatic hypotension. Some medications, such as calcium channel antagonists, can exacerbate symptoms, and treatment of the cancer can occasionally improve them.[4]

Pain Management

Pain is also common in patients with cancer who are anticipating surgery and almost universal immediately after surgery. Cancer-related pain can be due to tumor compression or invasion of nerves, to healing of the surgical site, to side effects of treatments, and to other causes.[5] At the time of the preoperative evaluation every patient should be asked specifically about pain. The cause of any new pain should be adequately investigated, and the patient's need for pain medication should be addressed. New or worsening pain in the spine should suggest epidural spinal cord compression and warrants an immediate evaluation, probably including spinal MRI. Treatment of pain should not wait for a determination of cause, but should be initiated simultaneously with any indicated evaluation.

In general, pain medications should be taken as usual on the day of surgery with a sip of water. Because nonsteroidal anti-inflammatory analgesics can increase perioperative blood loss, it is important to establish the surgeon's wishes for use of these medications around the time of surgery. In general, aspirin is discontinued one to two weeks before surgery, and other nonsteroidal anti-inflammatory drugs are discontinued at least two days before surgery. Acetaminophen and opiates can be taken up to the time of surgery.

Because cancer patients are sometimes taking substantial doses of opiate pain medication, an accurate record of a patient's opiate use prior to surgery is helpful in estimating approximate doses of medication needed for pain control after surgery. Ensure that all caregivers are aware if the patient is receiving a transdermal analgesic, such as fentanyl, because it can be overlooked and the patient inadvertently under- or overdosed.

Preoperative Evaluation

In the preoperative period, it is important to obtain a complete neurologic history. In particular, it is helpful to obtain any prior history of stroke, TIA, or seizure disorder.

It is equally important to seek a few specific neurologic physical findings in the preoperative evaluation of cancer patients. A standard screening neurologic evaluation should include assessment of alertness, orientation, gross cranial nerve function, gross motor function, major deep tendon reflexes, gross sensation to light touch, speech, and gait. Any suggestion of somnolence, forgetfulness, confusion, or agitation should be further characterized with a Mini-Mental Status examination. Depression should be in the differential diagnosis of causes. Any asymmetry of strength or reflexes, or any evidence of speech or gait dysfunction should be investigated by a more thorough neurologic examination. Patients at risk for neuropathy from chemotherapy should also be tested for fine touch, vibration, and proprioception in their distal extremities.

Postoperative Evaluation

In the postoperative period, a neurologic assessment is an important part of the patient evaluation. Postoperative delirium is usually due to medication and the stress of surgery exacerbating underlying age or disease-related deficits; however, metabolic disturbances, stroke, seizure, and infection must be kept in mind as possible causes (see Table 1). Some types of chemotherapy are more commonly associated with seizures, including cisplatin, ifosfamide, interferon, L-asparaginase, and methotrexate.

Hospital Discharge

Medications, pain control, follow-up and communication are four fundamentals to ensure a patient is adequately prepared for hospital discharge. Ensure that the patient is on the appropriate medications and that medications have not been accidentally duplicated or dropped when therapeutically equivalent medications were substituted to conform to the hospital formulary. Prior to discharge, ensure that every patient has adequate access to pain control, including both medication and non-medication methods. Ensure that the patient has all necessary follow-up appointments, including follow-up with a neurologist for any new neurologic developments. Finally, ensure that all of the patient's many physicians and other health care providers receive reports of the hospitalization.

REFERENCES

1. Newton HB Shah SM. Neurological syndromes and emergencies in the cancer patient: differential diagnosis, assessment protocols, and targeted clinical interventions. Emerg Med Reports 1997;18:149–58.
2. Newton H. Neurologic complications of systemic cancer. Am Fam Physician 1999;63:2211–8.
3. Wefel JS, et al. The cognitive sequelae of standard-dose adjuvant chemotherapy in women with breast carcinoma: results of a prospective, randomized, longitudinal trial. Cancer 2004;100:2292–9.
4. McEvoy KM, et al. 3, 4-diaminopyridine in the treatment of lambert-eaton myasthenic syndrome. N Engl J Med 1989;321:1567.
5. Grossman SA, Staats PS. Current management of pain in patients with cancer. Oncology 1994;8:93–107.

80

Hematologic Issues

Spero R. Cataland, MD

Anemia

Causes

Anemia in patients who have been, or are actively being, treated with chemotherapy or radiation therapy may require special attention during the perioperative period because of the patients' inability to respond adequately to acute blood loss. This compromise of marrow function can have several causes, including recent marrow-suppressive chemotherapy, reactive anemia of cancer, replacement of the bone marrow by infiltrating malignant cells, and, rarely, a myelodysplastic syndrome secondary to chemotherapy or radiation therapy. In the perioperative period, patients undergoing chemotherapy may require transfusion with packed red cells more frequently than comparable patients who are not actively receiving chemotherapy. However, as with any patient, red blood cell transfusion should not be based on an arbitrary hemoglobin level, but upon need demonstrated by the patient's clinical condition.[1,2] The risk for chemotherapy-related anemia does not completely disappear after patients have been cured of the cancer and have recovered from adverse treatment effects. Within five years, about 1% of patients who receive adjuvant chemotherapy for breast cancer may develop a chemotherapy-induced myelodysplastic syndrome or acute myeloid leukemia. Higher rates are seen with more intense chemotherapy regimens.[3]

Treatment

The acute perioperative treatment of anemia in patients actively receiving cancer therapy is not different from that for non-cancer patients; packed red cell transfusion is the mainstay of therapy. Patients being actively treated for a malignancy may require transfusion support sooner and may require more transfusions in the perioperative period than comparable patients not undergoing chemotherapy or radiation therapy. If the surgery is not urgent, then delaying surgery until the patient's marrow function recovers can help to minimize transfusion requirements; however, this usually requires several months. For some patients, it might be appropriate to stimulate bone marrow function with erythropoietic medications. One month of treatment with epoetin alpha (Epogen, Procrit) or darbepoetin alpha (Aranesp) can usually stimulate erythropoiesis sufficiently to significantly increase hemoglobin levels.[4]

Neutropenia, Lymphopenia, Lymphocytosis

Causes

The most common clinically significant effect of cancer chemotherapy is neutropenia. Although the administration of granulocyte colony stimulating factors can reduce the severity and the duration of neutropenia, patients can still have a period of neutropenia that is associated with a significantly increased risk of postoperative infection and other complications. In one series of 56 neutropenic cancer patients requiring urgent abdominal surgery, half had a major postoperative complication, and 30-day postoperative mortality was 32%.[5] Hematologic malignancies can also cause neutropenia directly. Patients with acute myeloid and lymphoid leukemias, as well as patients with advanced chronic myelogenous leukemia, may have a clinically significant neutropenia, not because of chemotherapy, but because of replacement of normal bone marrow by cancer cells. Finally, patients with chronic lymphoblastic leukemia (CLL) are likely to be at higher risk for postoperative infectious complications because of both neutropenia and hypogammaglobulinemia from CLL and from chemotherapy.

Treatment

Patients with neutropenia are at increased risk for perioperative complications, including death. The administration of granulocyte colony stimulating factors can shorten the duration of neutropenia after chemotherapy, but is unlikely to have a significant effect on neutropenia that is caused directly by an underlying hematologic malignancy. If feasible, postpone elective and semi-elective surgeries until the patient's granulocyte count rises above 1,000/mm[3].

Thrombocytopenia and Thrombocytosis

Thrombocytopenia

Causes

Transient thrombocytopenia is a frequent finding in patients undergoing chemotherapy. Similar to neutropenia, the severity and duration of thrombocytopenia depends on agent-specific factors as well as patient-specific factors that include age and previous response to myelosuppressive therapy.[6] Although studies rarely report rates of myelosuppression and complications, almost all chemotherapeutic agents will produce some degree of myelosuppression, with most agents producing a nadir 7 to 14 days after treatment, and recovery requiring 21 to 28 days.[7] Patients with a lymphoproliferative disorder can also develop immune-mediated thrombocytopenia (ITP). In addition, thrombocytopenia can be caused by infiltration of the bone marrow by the cancer, independently of the myelosuppressive effects of chemotherapy. Finally, up to 1% of patients previously treated with chemotherapy or radiation therapy develop a recalcitrant chronic thrombocytopenia due to a therapy-related myelodysplastic syndrome.

Treatment

Thrombocytopenia can pose a significant danger in the perioperative period. If the thrombocytopenia is likely to be transient (for example, if it is caused by recent chemotherapy) and the surgery can be safely postponed, then the procedure should be postponed until the thrombocytopenia resolves. If the surgery cannot be safely postponed, then platelet transfusions can usually achieve a platelet count sufficient to provide hemostasis. In contrast to chemotherapy-induced thrombocytopenia, thrombocytopenia due to ITP in patients with an underlying lymphoproliferative disorder is less likely to respond to platelet transfusion, and hemostasis is unlikely to be adequate for surgery. Direct treatment of the ITP with corticosteroids and intravenous immunoglobulins is a reasonable approach, but is also often ineffective. However, successful treatment of the underlying lymphoproliferative disorder usually leads to resolution of the ITP. Therefore, if feasible, the surgery should be postponed to allow time for treatment of the underlying lymphoproliferative disorder.

Thrombocytosis

Causes and Treatment

Because platelets are an acute phase reactant, patients can develop a reactive thrombocytosis as part of the inflammatory reaction to a cancer or to cancer treatments. Reactive thrombocytosis can reach platelet counts of 106/mm³; however, regardless of the platelet count, reactive thrombocytosis does not increase the risk of thrombosis.[8] Therefore, cytoreductive therapy is unnecessary and anticoagulant treatment beyond that indicated for the patient's clinical situation is unnecessary. As the inflammatory reaction resolves, the patient's platelet count will also gradually return to baseline. In contrast to a reactive thrombocytosis, a thrombocytosis caused by an underlying myeloproliferative disorder (eg, myelofibrosis, essential thrombocytosis, or polycythemia vera) is characterized by qualitative abnormalities in platelet function. Patients with this type of thrombocytosis are at increased risk, both for thrombotic and for hemorrhagic perioperative complications. Cytoreductive therapy or acute removal of platelets via apheresis can improve surgical hemostasis and may be appropriate.

REFERENCES

1. Carson J, et al. Perioperative blood transfusion and postoperative mortality. JAMA 1998;279:199–205.
2. Leal-Noval S, et al. Transfusion of blood components and postoperative infection in patients undergoing cardiac surgery. Chest 2001;119:1461–8.
3. Smith R, et al. Acute myeloid leukemia and myelodysplastic syndrome after doxorubicin-cyclophosphamide adjuvant therapy for operable breast cancer: the National Surgical Adjuvant Breast and Bowel Project Experience. J Clin Oncol 2003;21:1195–204.
4. Macdougall IC, et al. Correction of anaemia with darbepoetin alfa in patients with chronic kidney disease receiving dialysis. Nephrol Dial Transplant 2003;18: 576–81.
5. Glenn J, Funkhouser WK, Schneider PS. Acute illnesses necessitating urgent abdominal surgery in neutropenic cancer patients: description of 14 cases and review of the literature. Surgery 1989;105:778–89.
6. Crawford A, Dale DC, Lyman GH. Chemotherapy-induced neutropenia. Cancer 2004;100:228–37.
7. Ciark HH and Dennis AC. Heuatologic Complications of Cancer Chemotherapy. Boltimure 1996;559–69.
8. Schafer AI. Current concepts: thrombocytosis. N Engl J Med 2004;350:1211–9.

Prevention of Postoperative Venous Thromboembolism and Perioperative Management of Anticoagulation in the Cancer Patient

Amir K. Jaffer, MD
Daniel J. Brotman, MD

Venous thromboembolism (VTE) is one of the most common complications of cancer. Patients with cancer have an approximate sixfold increased risk of VTE compared to those without cancer.[1] Active cancer accounts for ≈ 20% of all new VTE events occurring in the community.[1] The estimated annual incidence of VTE in cancer patients is about 1 in 200.[2] The number may be higher in patients undergoing chemotherapy and in those with indwelling central venous catheters. There may also be a relationship between VTE and the stage of disease, type of malignancy and type of ongoing cancer therapy.[3] Cancer is also a well-recognized major risk factor for the development of postoperative VTE. The incidence of fatal pulmonary embolism (PE) after major abdominal and pelvic cancer surgery may be as high as 5% in the absence of VTE prophylaxis.[4] Therefore, when a patient with cancer is planning to undergo surgery, close attention to prevention of this potentially fatal illness is essential.

Cancer and Thrombosis

All three components of Virchow's triad, namely hypercoagulability, endothelial damage and stasis, are responsible for the increased risk of VTE in surgical patients with cancer. In cancer, macrophages and monocytes interact with malignant cells to release tumor necrosis factor (TNF), interleukin-1 (IL-1), and interleukin-6 (IL-6), causing endothelial injury. Chemotherapy also leads to the release of these factors.[5] Interactions between cancer cells and macrophages also activate platelets, factor X, and factor XII, which lead to thrombin generation. Tissue factor and other procoagulants released by cancer cells can

activate factor VII and factor X directly.[5] Additional prothrombotic insults affecting cancer patients may include cytotoxic chemotherapies, hormonal therapy such as tamoxifen, and growth factors such as granulocyte colony stimulating factor (GCSF) and erythropoietin.[5]

The increased risk of VTE in breast cancer patients treated with tamoxifen plus chemotherapy is clear. In two large clinical trials of women with node negative breast cancer, the 5-year incidence of VTE was 4.2% in those who received chemotherapy and tamoxifen, 0.9% in those receiving tamoxifen alone, and 0.2% in the placebo group.[6,7] In general, cancer patients receiving chemotherapy or immunosuppressive therapy have about a 6.5-fold increased risk of VTE compared to non-cancer patients.[8]

Pharmacologic Prophylaxis

Commonly used antithrombotic pharmacologic options include unfractionated heparin (UFH), low-molecular-weight heparins (LMWHs), and vitamin K antagonists (eg, warfarin). Newer agents such as subcutaneous fondaparinux (a synthetic pentasaccharide that inhibits factor Xa) and direct thrombin inhibitors (DTIs) show promise in clinical trials. UFH has been evaluated in clinical trials for the prevention of VTE after cancer surgery. UFH is a heterogenous mixture of repeating polysaccharide chains of varying sizes, averaging about 15,000 daltons. It binds antithrombin (AT-III) and facilitates AT-III-mediated inactivation of factors IIa, Xa, IXa and XIIa. Of these, IIa and Xa are most responsive to inhibition. Due to its large size, UFH is not well absorbed from subcutaneous tissue, and it has a

variable anticoagulant response due to interactions with plasma proteins, macrophages, and endothelial cells.[9] It also binds to platelets and platelet factor-4 (PF4), and may precipitate heparin-induced thrombocytopenia (HIT). LMWHs have also been evaluated in clinical trials for the prevention of VTE after cancer surgery. LMWHs are derived from UFH through a chemical depolymerization or de-fractionation process. They are about one-third the size of UFH, with a molecular weight of approximately 5,000 daltons. These smaller molecules are readily absorbed from the subcutaneous tissue, eliciting a more predictable anticoagulant response than UFH. Unlike UFH, LMWHs have only minimal nonspecific binding to plasma proteins, endothelial cells, and monocytes,[9] resulting in a predictable dose response, which obviates the need for lab monitoring. The longer plasma half-life of LMWH compared to UFH allows these drugs to be dosed subcutaneously once or twice daily. LMWHs do not bind platelets as readily as UFH and may carry a lower risk of heparin-induced thrombocytopenia than UFH. Because of their smaller size, LMWHs tend to preferentially inhibit factor Xa, whereas UFH tends to inhibit both factor Xa and IIa equally.[9]

Fondaparinux is a synthetic analogue of the unique pentasaccharide sequence that mediates the interaction of heparin with antithrombin. It inhibits both free and platelet-bound factor Xa. It binds antithrombin with high affinity, has close to 100% bioavailability, and has a plasma half-life of 17 hours that permits once-daily administration. The drug is excreted unchanged in the urine and is contraindicated in patients with severe renal impairment (ie, CrCl < 30 mL/min). It does not bind PF4 and therefore should not cause HIT. At this time, there is no antidote for fondaparinux; however, if uncontrolled bleeding does occur, a procoagulant such as recombinant factor VII might be effective.[9] Fondaparinux effectively prevents thrombosis following major abdominal cancer surgery, and can also be used in the acute treatment of VTE.

Warfarin is a coumarin derivative that exerts its anticoagulant effects by limiting hepatic production of the biologically active vitamin K-dependent clotting factors (factors II, VII, IX, X). Additionally, warfarin interferes with the production of the anticoagulant proteins C and S and can potentially exert a transient procoagulant effect following initiation of treatment. In addition, it takes approximately 96 hours to decrease the levels of factor IIa enough to provide a clinical anticoagulant effect, even though depletion of the short-lived factors VII and IX can increase the international normalized ratio (INR) in less than 24 hours. Although warfarin monotherapy has been shown to be effective in preventing VTE after orthopedic surgery in several trials, a recent meta-analysis[10] and a case-control study suggest that it is inferior to LMWH. Therefore, it is our own preference to avoid warfarin monotherapy as VTE prophylaxis after major surgery, especially since the patient is unprotected from thrombosis during the first few days of treatment.

Ximelagatran is an oral direct thrombin inhibitor. It is a prodrug that is rapidly hydrolyzed to form melagatran, the active drug that binds thrombin. It has a plasma half-life of 4 to 5 hours and is given twice daily in fixed doses. It does not have drug and food interactions like warfarin. It is renally cleared. The drug has been shown in phase III trials to be effective for VTE prevention after major orthopedic surgery, for stroke prevention in atrial fibrillation, for acute treatment of VTE, and for secondary prevention of VTE after an acute episode.[11] The drug, however, has not been evaluated for VTE prevention in cancer patients undergoing surgery. Although ximelagatran was approved for use in several European countries for VTE prevention after major orthopedic surgery, it was later withdrawn. The United States Food and Drug Administration (FDA) recently declined to approve its use in the United States based on its potential hepatotoxicity as shown in clinical trials.

The details of selected trials evaluating UFH, LMWH, and fondaparinux in cancer surgery patients are outlined in Table 1. There is evidence that UFH effectively reduces the risk of VTE after cancer surgery; however, the dose of the UFH may be important. In an early gynecologic cancer surgery trial, UFH 5,000 units (U) subcutaneously (SC) twice daily (bid) was not significantly superior to placebo with rates of VTE 14.8% and 12.4%, respectively.[12] Other clinical trials outlined in Table 1 suggest that UFH 5,000 U SC every 8 hours (q8h) or three times

a day (tid) is as effective as LMWH (eg. enoxaparin sodium 40 mg SC four times a day [qd] or Dalteparin 5,000 U SC qd) with similar bleeding rates in most studies.[13] Although some studies have reported fewer wound hematomas with LMWH than with UFH, other studies have suggested the opposite. It is our recommendation, therefore, for cancer surgery patients to receive either UFH 5,000 U SC q8h or tid or a LMWH for most types of cancer-related surgeries.

The results of the 2,927-patient, randomized, double-blind, dalteparin-controlled, Pentasaccharide in General Surgery Study) trial show that fondaparinux is at least as safe and efficacious as a low molecular weight heparin (dalteparin) for the prevention of VTE following major abdominal surgery. The rate of VTE in the fondaparinux and dalteparin groups were 4.6% and 6.1%, respectively ($p = .14$). For those patients who underwent abdominal cancer surgery (approximately 70% of the overall sample), VTE incidence was significantly reduced for fondaparinux recipients compared to dalteparin recipients (4.7% to 7.7%, $p = .02$). Fondaparinux's adverse effect profile was reassuring in patients with and without malignancy.

The duration of prophylaxis has also been evaluated in at least two clinical trials.[14,15] The evidence suggests that cancer patients undergoing major orthopedic surgery, pelvic surgery, or abdominal surgery should receive extended prophylaxis with an LMWH for up to 28 days postoperatively; extended prophylaxis may reduce the risk of postoperative thrombosis by 60% compared to standard prophylaxis that is stopped after 6 to 10 days of treatment.[14]

Mechanical Prophylaxis

The options for mechanical prophylaxis include graduated compression stockings (GCSs) and intermittent pneumatic compression (IPC) devices. They are attractive options in those patients who are actively bleeding or at high risk for bleeding. Studies in gynecologic surgery patients suggest that the patients most likely to fail IPCs are those with underlying cancer.[16] In another study, the rate of VTE was 4% with IPCs and 6.9% with UFH 5,000 U SC bid, these results were not statistically different, and UFH 5,000 U bid is probably inferior to tid dosing, as suggested in Table 82-1. Therefore, the potential role of IPCs for preventing postoperative thrombosis in cancer patients remains ill-defined. Some practical problems with IPCs include that they need to be on for at least 15 hours a day to achieve maximal benefit; ambulation is restricted if patients wear the IPCs all day, and sleep may be adversely affected.

Three meta-analyses demonstrated that GCSs are superior to placebo.[17-19] In the Cochrane

review, the rate of DVT with placebo was 27% and, while with GCSs, about 13% (an NNT of 7).[18] However, this was in all general surgery patients and not just cancer surgery patients. GCSs in combination with UFH may provide added efficacy, increasing the protective effect of UFH by as much as 75%.[18] Therefore, combining this modality with either LMWH or UFH in cancer surgery patients may be helpful, although this dual modality has never systematically studied specifically in cancer surgery patients. Some practical problems with GCSs include difficulty with fitting and poor compliance by patients and health care providers.[13]

Our recommendations for VTE prophylaxis in surgical patients with cancer are evidence-based and adapted from recent guidelines of the American College of Chest Physicians.[13] These recommendations are outlined in Table 82-2.

Non-Surgery Cancer Patients

Primary prevention of VTE in non-surgical cancer patients has only been studied to a limited extent; limited data do support using warfarin, but this has not been embraced in clinical practice. The data with LMWH for primary prevention of VTE in the cancer patient not undergoing surgery do not show any benefit. In a trial of 311 women with metastatic breast cancer, warfarin at an INR of 1.3 to 1.9 was found to be both clinically effective (rate of VTE = 0.6% vs. 4.4% in the placebo group; $p = .031$) and cost-effective, with no increased risk of bleeding compared to placebo.[20,21] In a recently published trial termed the fragmin advanced malignancy outcome study,[22] 382 patients with advanced cancer were randomized to receive either a once-daily subcutaneous injection of dalteparin (5,000 IU) or placebo for 1 year. The survival rates in the dalteparin group were 46%, 27%, and 21%, at 1, 2, and 3 years, respectively, compared with 41%, 18%, and 12%, respectively, for patients receiving placebo ($p = .19$). The rates of symptomatic venous thromboembolism were no different at 2.4% and 3.3% for dalteparin and placebo, respectively, and with bleeding rates of 4.7% and 2.7%, respectively.

Cancer Patients with Central Venous Catheters

Central venous catheters (CVCs) predispose to upper extremity DVT in the general population.[8] Cancer patients with indwelling catheters are probably at even higher risk for developing upper extremity DVT, but the overall incidence of clinically apparent CVC-associated DVT is still low at ≈ 3.4% (1.14 per 1,000 catheter days) amongst those with peripherally inserted central catheters.[13] There is one study that supports the use of a 1 mg daily dose of warfarin for DVT

Table 1 Selected Randomized Control Trials of LMWH, UFH, and IPC Trials in Cancer Surgery

Study	Type of Surgery	No. of Patients	Prophylaxis	Rate of VTE	Diagnostic Modality
Enoxacan I[53]	Abdominal or pelvic surgery for cancer	1115	UFH 5,000 U SC tid vs Enoxaparin 40 mg SC qd	18.2% (UFH) 14.7% (enoxaparin) (*p* = NS)	Venography Venography or ultrasonography
Mcleod et al[54]	Colorectal surgery (1/3 of patients with cancer)	936	UFH 5,000 U SC tid vs enoxaparin 40 mg SC qd	9.4% (UFH) 9.4% (enoxaparin) (*p* = NS)	
Clarke-Pearson et al[55]	Gynecologic cancer surgery	208	UFH 5,000 U bid vs IPC*	6.9% (UFH) 4.0% (IPC) (*p* = NS)	I-125 fibrinogen
Clarke-Pearson et al[12]	Gynecologic cancer surgery	185	UFH 5,000 U bid vs placebo	14.8% (UFH) 12.4% (placebo) (*p* = NS)	I-125 fibrinogen + IPG†
Clarke-Pearson et al[56]	Gynecologic cancer surgery	304	UFH 5,000 U SC q8h vs placebo	8.0% (UFH) 18.4% (placebo) ($p < 0.05$)	I-125 fibrinogen
Bergqvist et al[14]	Abdominal or pelvic surgery for cancer	332	Enoxaparin 40 mg SC qd vs placebo (for 3 weeks after all patients recd. 6 to 10 d of LMWH)	4.8% (enoxaparin) 12.0% (placebo) (*p* = 0.02)	Venography
Agnelli et al[57]	High-risk abdominal surgery	2927	Fondaprinux 2.5 mg SC qd vs. dalteparin 5,000 IU SC qd	4.6% (fondaprinux) 6.1% (dalteparin) *p* = 0.14 In the subroup with Cancer: 4.7% (fondaprinux) 7.7% (dalteparin) *p* = 0.02	Ultrasonography

bid = twice daily; d = dalton; LMWH = low-molecular-weight heparin; IPC = intermittent pneumatic compression; IU = international units; NS = not significant; qd = four times a day; SC = subcutaneous; tid = three times a day; U = units; UFH = unfractionated heparin.
* intermittent pneumatic compression
† impedence plethysmography

Table 2 Patients with underlying cancer undergoing surgery for a non-cancer related condition

Type of Surgery	Type of Prophylaxis	Duration
Moderate risk general surgery	UFH 5,000 U SC tid or LMWH*	Until ambulation or discharge
High risk general surgery	UFH 5,000 U SC tid or LMWH plus IPC or GCSs	Up to 28 days
Vascular surgery	UFH 5,000 U SC tid or LMWH	Until ambulation or discharge
Laparoscopic gynecologic surgery > 30 min.	UFH 5,000 U SC tid or LMWH plus IPC or GCSs	Until ambulation or discharge
Major gynecologic surgery	UFH 5,000 U SC tid or LMWH plus M IPC or GCSs	Until ambulation or discharge
Urologic surgery other than low-risk	UFH 5,000 U SC tid or LMWH plus IPC or GCSs	Until ambulation or discharge
Major orthopedic surgery	LMWH or VKA or Fondaparinux†	28 to 35 days
	Neurosurgery	
	Extracranial	
	Intracranial	
	LMWH plus IPC ± GCSs	
	LMWH plus IPC ± GCSs	
	Until ambulation or discharge	

Adapted from Geerts et al.[13]
GCSs = graded compression stockings; IPC = intermittent pneumatic compression; IU = international units; LMWH = low-molecular-weight heparin; qd = four times a day; SC = subcutaneously; tid = three times a day; U = units; VKA=Vitamin K antagonists (warfarin).
*LMWH dosing = enoxaparin 40 mg SC qd, dalteparin 5,000 IU SC qd or tinzaparin 75 IU/kg qd
†2.5 mg SC qd

prevention. In this trial, the rate of upper extremity DVT by mandatory venography at day 90 was 37.5% with placebo and 9.5% with warfarin ($p < .001$).[23] However, two subsequent trials failed to show any benefit from 1 mg daily dosing compared to placebo in preventing clinically apparent DVT.[13] In addition, the safety of 1 mg of daily warfarin without monitoring in cancer patients may be of concern because these patients may be more susceptible to small doses of warfarin due to their nutritional status and their vitamin K stores.

LMWH has also been evaluated for prevention of CVC-associated thrombosis. In one small study, dalteparin 2,500 U SC once daily was superior to no therapy for the prevention of venographically detectable thrombosis.[24] In a larger trial of 425 cancer patients receiving chemotherapy, dalteparin 5,000 IU SC once daily did not show superiority over placebo. The rate of clinically relevant VTE was ≈3.5% in both groups.[25] Therefore, based on this evidence, we and the ACCP do not endorse routine prophylaxis for cancer patients with CVCs.

Postoperative VTE in Cancer Patients

Patients with cancer are at higher risk for postoperative VTE than patients without cancer undergoing similar surgeries,[26] and clinicians should have a high index of suspicion for postoperative VTE in these patients. Objective radiographic tests, such as lower extremity duplex ultrasonography or helical computed tomography, should be used for diagnosis in postoperative cancer patients. Given the ongoing hemostatic activation in postoperative hospitalized patients,[27] there is no role for D-dimer testing.[28]

Table 3 Recommendations for VTE prophylaxis for Cancer Surgery

UFH 5,000 U SC q8h or tid at least until ambulation or discharge with a preoperative dose of 5,000 U SC given 2 hours prior to surgery

OR

LMWH (enoxaparin 40 mg SC qd or dalteparin 5000 U SC qd) or Fondaparinux 2.5mg SC qd

Extended prophylaxis for 28 days with LMWH for major abdominal, pelvic or orthopedic surgery in cancer patients.

LMWH = low-molecular-weight heparin; q8h = every 8 hours; qd = four times a day; SC = subcutaneously; tid = three times a day; U = units; VTE= venous thromboembolism.

When postoperative VTE is diagnosed in a patient with cancer, the treatment options are similar to the options in patients without cancer. However, the optimal management strategy may be different. Cancer patients who undergo successful curative surgery are probably no different from patients without cancer and can be viewed as having situational thromboses. In such cases, 3 months of anticoagulation is reasonable. However, many cancer patients are not cured of their disease and have ongoing chronic activation of the clotting cascade, particularly those with adenocarcinomas of the viscera, brain tumors, or certain hematologic malignancies. In these patients, although the precipitating event (surgery) may be situational, ongoing hypercoagulability places them at higher risk for recurrent thrombosis following discontinuation of therapy. Indefinite anticoagulation may be considered in patients who suffer VTE following surgery who have uncured malignancies known to be associated with hypercoagulable states (such as visceral adenocarcinomas or brain tumors), but this strategy may expose patients to a high risk of bleeding[29] and should be considered only on a case-by-case basis.

Given the high rates of warfarin-resistant thrombosis and warfarin-associated bleeding in patients with cancer,[29] consideration of long-term LMWH treatment is justified when a cancer patient develops a thrombosis. The CLOT investigators[30] recently examined the safety and efficacy of dalteparin (200 IU/kg/d for the first month, followed by 150 IU/kg/d for 5 months) compared to oral anticoagulation for the treatment of VTE in cancer patients. Of 336 patients, 27 (8.0%) in the LMWH group suffered recurrence, compared to 53 of 336 (15.8%) in the oral anticoagulation group (hazard ratio 0.48; *p* = .002). Most recurrences occurred while on anticoagulation. The frequencies of major and minor bleeding were similar. Although this trial did not specifically enroll patients with postoperative

VTE, the relatively high recurrence rates illustrate that cancer patients with VTE are at high risk for recurrence even in the face of ongoing warfarin treatment. A smaller study using enoxaparin 1.5 mg/kg/d demonstrated a similar risk reduction that failed to reach statistical significance.[29] However, any increased efficacy of LMWH in the treatment of cancer-associated VTE compared to oral anticoagulation must be weighted against the cost of the drug[31] and the willingness of the patient or family members to administer daily injections.

Inferior Vena Cava Filters

Inferior vena cava (IVC) filter placement has increased during the last two decades in patients with PE, patients with DVT alone, and patients at risk for VTE who have not yet had an event.[32] Some authors have argued against placement of IVC filters in patients with advanced cancer because the filters may have little overall clinical benefit in terminally ill patients, and may not be cost-effective. In a case series of 308 patients with cancer-associated VTE who received IVC filters,[33] the filters appeared to be safe and effective in preventing PE-related deaths. Although overall mortality was high in these patients (median survival < 1 year), less than 5% of patients suffered PE-related death. It is our opinion, however, that IVC filters be reserved for cancer patients with contraindication to anticoagulation, recurrent thromboembolic disease despite LMWH therapy, or a significant complication from anticoagulation therapy. The FDA recently approved three different types of retrievable filters. Although long-term safety data for these devices was not available as of this writing, they may be attractive options for cancer surgery patients who have a very high risk of developing perioperative VTE and transient contraindication to anticoagulation (such as intracranial surgery). In our opinion, prophylactic filter placement is not generally warranted and should be tested in prospective trials before we can recommend this strategy for our patients.

Perioperative/Periprocedural Management of Warfarin in Cancer Patients

Although some patients with cancer may suffer recurrent VTE despite warfarin treatment, warfarin is effective for treatment and secondary prevention of VTE for most cancer patients.[30] Other cancer patients may be on warfarin for other indications, such as atrial fibrillation or valvular heart disease. When a cancer patient on warfarin is scheduled to undergo surgery, there are a few key questions that must be addressed. First, does the nature of the procedure warrant discontinuation

of therapeutic anticoagulation? Second, if anticoagulation must be reversed, is the patient at high enough risk for short-term thrombosis to justify "bridging" anticoagulation with short-acting anticoagulants prior to the procedure? If so, which agent should be used? Finally, which anticoagulation regimen should be employed following the procedure? Although these questions need to be addressed prior to surgery for all patients on warfarin—regardless of whether or not they have cancer—the second and third questions require special thought for cancer patients who are often at particularly high risk for VTE and VTE recurrence.

Some minor procedures, such as dental, cutaneous, and ophthalmologic surgeries and gastrointestinal endoscopy without biopsy, can be performed safely in patients who are fully anticoagulated.[35–39] Cancer patients requiring such procedures can continue their warfarin without interruption. If this approach is considered, the surgeon must agree that the procedure can safely be performed while the patient is anticoagulated, and care should be taken to ensure that the patient does not have a supra-therapeutic INR on the morning of the procedure. Other procedures such as prostate biopsy, endoscopic biopsy, and even herniorrhaphy may be performed with a reduced dose (but not full reversal) of oral anticoagulation, targeting an INR of 1.5 to 2.0 on the morning of surgery.[40] If anticoagulation must be discontinued, then approximately 5 to 6 days are required for anticoagulant effects of warfarin to wear off in most non-cancer patients.[41] Provided that hepatic synthetic function is normal or near-normal, there is no reason to suspect that a longer duration of cessation is needed in patients with cancer.

During the few days prior to surgery, while the oral anticoagulation is wearing off, the patient is relatively unprotected from VTE. The risk of recurrence during a brief period of warfarin cessation depends upon the timing of the most recent thrombotic event, the duration of anticoagulant cessation, and the intensity of the underlying proclivity to develop thrombosis. In general, for patients with a thrombosis in the preceding month, the average daily recurrence rate is approximately 0.3% to 1.3%.[42–45] This high rate may stem from the likelihood that residual, unstabilized thrombus is still present. Over the next two months, the daily recurrence rate is approximately four- to tenfold lower.[42–44] However, these figures apply to all patients on warfarin for acute VTE, and there is reason to suspect that patients with underlying hypercoagulable states (such as malignancy) may be at higher risk for thrombosis than these figures suggest. Therefore, we recommend that all cancer patients with a thrombotic episode in the preceding three months receive short-acting anticoagulants prior to surgery starting 2 days after the warfarin is discontinued. If the most recent event occurred in the preceding month, consideration should be given to delaying the procedure or placing an inferior vena cava filter. In patients with more distant thrombosis (> 3 months prior) without evidence of underlying active cancer, it may be reasonable to simply let the warfarin wash out without any preoperative bridging therapy. However, this latter approach should be exercised cautiously in patients with a history of life-threatening, recurrent thromboses and active cancer. Patients with cancer without history of VTE, but who are on warfarin for other conditions (such as atrial fibrillation), may also need bridging therapy. The need for bridging therapy in these cancer patients is summarized in Table 4. As a general rule, patients at very high risk (ie, > 10% annual risk for arterial embolism or > 10% monthly risk for venous thromboembolism) should receive bridging anticoagulation. For patients at low-risk (ie, < 5% annual risk for arterial embolism, or < 5% monthly risk for venous thromboembolism), however, bridging therapy prior to surgery may involve unnecessary risk. The need for bridging in intermediate-risk patients may need to be decided on a case-by-case basis.

If a decision is made that bridging therapy with short-acting anticoagulants is warranted, LMWHs allow for effective outpatient treatment. Unless the thrombosis was very recent (in the preceding 3 months), we believe that prophylactic doses of LMWH are appropriate. It is important to recognize that the doses of LMWH used in the initial treatment of VTE ("full-intensity" treatment) may, in fact, be higher intensity then necessary, with potential risk of bleeding.[45] Although full-intensity treatment with heparin products is clearly indicated for the initial treatment of VTE, lower doses may be reasonable following the first few weeks of therapy. For example, in the CLOT study, which compared dalteparin to oral anticoagulation following cancer-associated VTE,[30] the dose of dalteparin was decreased from full-intensity (200 IU/kg/d) to 75% of the full-intensity (150 IU/kg/d) after the first month of therapy to reduce the risk of bleeding. Despite this dose reduction, there was a > 50% reduction in VTE recurrence in those assigned to dalteparin (compared to oral anticoagulation) and comparable bleeding rates in both groups. This supports the concept that full-dose treatment with LMWH may be excessive and unnecessary beyond the first month of VTE treatment. Observational bridging studies of LMWH in patients who require temporary interruption of warfarin therapy have utilized full doses of LMWH (ie, dalteparin 200 IU/kg SC qd, enoxaparin 1 mg/kg SC q12h or enxoaprin 1.5 mg/kg SC qd).[46] However, the ideal dosing regimen remains to be determined in a randomized

---

Table 4 Risk for Thromboembolism

High risk: Annual risk of arterial thromboembolism > 10% or monthly risk of venous thromboembolism > 10% without anticoagulation] (bridging advised)

Known hypercoagulable state as documented by a thromboembolic event and one of the following: protein C deficiency, protein S deficiency, antithrombin III deficiency, homozygous factor V Leiden mutation or antiphospholipid antibody syndrome

Hypercoagulable state suggested by recurrent (two or more) arterial or idiopathic venous thromboembolic events (not including primary atherosclerotic events, such as stroke or myocardial infarction due to intrinsic cerebrovascular or coronary disease)

Venous or arterial thromboembolism within the preceding 3 months

Rheumatic atrial fibrillation

Acute intracardiac thrombus visualized by echocardiogram

Atrial fibrillation plus mechanical heart valve in any position

Older mechanical valve model (single disk or ball-in-cage) in mitral position

Recently placed mechanical valve (< 3 months)

Atrial fibrillation with history of cardioembolism

Intermediate risk [annual risk of arterial thromboembolism 5 to 10% or monthly risk of venous thromboembolism 5 to 10% without anticoagulation] (Bridging decision to be made on a case-by-case basis)

Cerebrovascular disease with multiple (two or more) strokes or TIAs without risk factors for cardiac embolism

Newer mechanical valve model (eg, St. Jude) in mitral position

Older mechanical valve model in aortic position

Atrial fibrillation without a history of cardiac embolism but with multiple risks for cardiac embolism (eg, low ejection fraction (< 40%), diabetes, hypertension, non-rheumatic valvular heart disease, recent (within preceding month) transmural myocardial infarction)

VTE > 3 to 6 months ago

Low risk [annual risk of arterial thromboembolism < 5% or monthly risk of venous thromboembolism < 5% without anticoagulation] (bridging not advised)

One remote VTE (> 6 months ago)

Intrinsic cerebrovascular disease (such as carotid atherosclerosis) without recurrent strokes or TIAs

Atrial fibrillation without multiple risks for cardiac embolism

Newer model prosthetic valve in aortic position

---

clinical trial. In the absence of prospective randomized clinical trials, we believe that established prophylactic doses (eg, 40 mg daily or 30 mg twice daily of enoxaparin, or dalteparin 5,000 IU) are probably appropriate for "bridging" therapy in most patients with a history of cancer-associated

---

VTE, and that 75% of full-dose treatment can be considered (eg, 1.125 mg/kg daily or 0.75 mg/kg twice daily of enoxaparin, or 150 IU/kg/d of dalteparin) if the thrombosis was recent (1 to 6 months prior). The last dose of LMWH should be approximately 24 hours before surgery if full-dose or 75% of full-dose LMWH is used and at least 12 hours prior to surgery if prophylactic doses of LMWH are used. This is important to prevent unnecessary surgical bleeding and complications related to spinal or epidural anesthesia. In patients with renal insufficiency, subcutaneous UFH or dose-reduced enoxaparin may be appropriate options,[40,47,48] but we discourage the use of intravenous heparin except in patients at extremely high risk (eg, those with thrombosis in the preceding month) since it necessitates hospitalization, and prophylactic dosing regimens are not established for intravenous heparin. In patients with a history of heparin-induced thrombocytopenia, LMWH and UFH should be avoided. Consideration can be given to the off-label use 2.5 mg daily of fondaparinux (a pentasaccharide with no in-vitro cross-reactivity to antibodies against platelet-factor 4).[49,50] In patients with a history of HIT who are at very high risk for recurrence (eg, thrombosis in the preceding month), admission to the hospital for administration of perioperative intravenous direct thrombin inhibitors (such as lepirudin or argatroban) is appropriate.

Following surgery, the daily risk for recurrent VTE is much higher than prior to surgery, since surgery itself is a major risk factor for VTE. However, there is also an increased risk for anticoagulant-mediated bleeding, especially from the surgical site.[50] Major postoperative bleeding is a problem in its own right but also necessitates cessation of anticoagulation, placing patients at high risk for thrombosis. For this reason, it is appropriate to use prophylactic doses of agents with demonstrated efficacy in VTE prevention following major surgery (eg, enoxaparin 40 mg daily or 30 mg twice daily, dalteparin 5,000 IU SC qd or fondaparinux 2.5 mg daily),[50–52] rather than full-intensity anticoagulation. Since the antithrombotic effects of warfarin are delayed, warfarin can be restarted the day of surgery or on the following day. Once the INR approaches therapeutic intensity, the parenteral antithrombotic drugs can be discontinued. Figure 1 outlines a protocol bridging them copy.

Conclusion

VTE is a common complication in cancer patients especially those undergoing surgery, and patients who develop this complication have a higher rate of dying compared to non-cancer patients with VTE. It is clear that cancer patients undergoing major surgery need both aggressive and extended

Pre-op Protocol:
- If pre-op INR 2-3, stop warfarin 5 days before surgery (4 doses).
- If pre-op INR 3-4.5, stop warfarin 6 days before surgery (5 doses).
- Start LMWH* about 2 days after last warfarin dose.
- Last dose of LMWH* approximately 24 hours prior to procedure.
- Patient educated in self injection and provided with written instructions
- Discuss plan with Surgeon and Anesthesiologist.
- Check stat INR in am of surgery to ensure <1.5 and in some cases <1.2

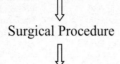

Surgical Procedure

Post-op Protocol:
- Restart LMWH* approximately 24 hours post procedure; consider thromboprophylaxis dose of LMWH on post-op if patient is at high risk for bleeding.
- Discuss above with Surgeon.
- Start warfarin at patient's pre-op dose on day of surgery or post-op day 1.
- Daily PT/INR until patient is discharged and periodically thereafter until INR therapeutic.
- Make arrangements for frequent patient contact following hospital discharge to ensure adherence to therapy and no anticoagulant related bleeding
- CBC with platelets at day 3 and day 7 post-op to screen for HIT
- Discontinue LMWH when INR is 2-3 for two consecutive days.

*Enoxaparin 1mg/kg SC q12h or 1.5mg/kg SC 24hr
or Dalteparin 120U/kg q12h or Dalteparin 200U/kg SC q24h. and adjsuted dose LMWH for patients with CrCl<30ml/min*

INCLUSION CRITERIA:
- Treating physician thinks patient needs bridge therapy.
- Medically and hemodynamically stable.
- Scheduled for elective procedure or surgery.

EXCLUSION CRITERIA
- Allergy to UFH or LMWH.
- Morbid obesity (eg. BMI > 40 kg/m^2, or weight > 150 kg in a patient of average height)
- Pregnant woman with a mechanical valve .
- History of bleeding disorder or intracranial hemorrhage.
- GI bleeding within the last ten days.
- Major trauma or stroke within the past two weeks.
- History of HIT or severe thrombocytopenia (< 30-50K).
- Language barriers that may interfere with successful drug administation.
- Potential for medication noncompliance.
- Unsuitable home environment to support therapy.
- Severe Liver Disease.

FIGURE 1 Outlines a brigding protocol for caucer patients on warfarin in head of a surgery requiring short acting parenteral antithrombotic. BMI = body mass index; CBC = complete blood count; CrCl = ; GI = gastrointestinal; HIT = heparin-induced thrombocytopenia; INR = international normalized ratio; K = ; kg = kilograms; LMWH = low-molecular-weight heparin; PT = ; q12h = every 12 hours; q24h = every 24 hours; SC = subcutaneously.
*Enoxaparin 1mg/kg SC q12h or 1.5mg/kg SC 24 hours or dalteparin 100 U/kg q12h or dalteparin 200 U/kg SC q24h and adjusted dose Enoxaparin for patients with CrCl < 30 mL/min.

pharmacologic prophylaxis for up to 28 days postoperatively. At this time, we believe that LMWHs are the agents of choice; however, encouraging data are emerging for newer agents such as fondaparinux. Patients on long-term warfarin with recent VTE, high-risk atrial fibrillation or mechanical valves may need parenteral bridging therapy with short acting anticoagulants such as LMWHs in preparation for their surgery to decrease the risk of thromboembolism.

REFERENCES

1. Heit JA, O'Fallon WM, Petterson TM, et al. Relative impact of risk factors for deep vein thrombosis and pulmonary embolism: a population-based study. Arch Intern Med 2002;162:1245–8.
2. Lee AY, Levine MN. Venous thromboembolism and cancer: risks and outcomes. Circulation 2003;107(23 Suppl 1):17–21.
3. Kakkar AK. Thrombosis and cancer. Hematol J 2004;5 Suppl 3:20–3.
4. Kakkar AK, Williamson RC. Prevention of venous thromboembolism in cancer patients. Semin Thromb Hemost 1999;25:239–43.
5. Bick RL. Cancer-associated thrombosis. N Engl J Med 2003;349:109–11.
6. Fisher B, Costantino J, Redmond C, et al. A randomized clinical trial evaluating tamoxifen in the treatment of patients with node-negative breast cancer who have estrogen-receptor-positive tumors. N Engl J Med 1989;320:479–84.
7. Fisher B, Dignam J, Wolmark N, et al. Tamoxifen and chemotherapy for lymph node-negative, estrogen receptor-positive breast cancer. J Natl Cancer Inst 1997;89:1673–82.
8. Heit JA, Silverstein MD, Mohr DN, et al. Risk factors for deep vein thrombosis and pulmonary embolism: a population-based case-control study. Arch Intern Med 2000;160:809–15.
9. Hirsh J, Raschke R. Heparin and low-molecular-weight heparin: the Seventh ACCP Conference on Antithrombotic and Thrombolytic Therapy. Chest 2004;126(3 Suppl):188–203.
10. Mismetti P, Laporte S, Zufferey P, et al. Prevention of venous thromboembolism in orthopedic surgery with vitamin K antagonists: a meta-analysis. J Thromb Haemost 2004;2:1058–70.
11. Weitz JI, Hirsh J, Samama MM. New anticoagulant drugs: the Seventh ACCP Conference on Antithrombotic and Thrombolytic Therapy. Chest 2004;126(3 Suppl):265–86.
12. Clarke-Pearson DL, Coleman RE, Synan IS, et al. Venous thromboembolism prophylaxis in gynecologic oncology: a prospective, controlled trial of low-dose heparin. Am J Obstet Gynecol 1983;145:606–13.
13. Geerts WH, Pineo GF, Heit JA, et al. Prevention of venous thromboembolism: the Seventh ACCP Conference on Antithrombotic and Thrombolytic Therapy. Chest 2004;126(3 Suppl):338–400.
14. Bergqvist D, Agnelli G, Cohen AT, et al. Duration of prophylaxis against venous thromboembolism with enoxaparin after surgery for cancer. N Engl J Med 2002;346:975–80.
15. Rasmussen MS. Preventing thromboembolic complications in cancer patients after surgery: a role for prolonged thromboprophylaxis. Cancer Treat Rev 2002;28:141–4.
16. Clarke-Pearson DL, Dodge RK, Synan I, et al. Venous thromboembolism prophylaxis: patients at high risk to fail intermittent pneumatic compression. Obstet Gynecol 2003;101:157–63.
17. Agu O, Hamilton G, Baker D. Graduated compression stockings in the prevention of venous thromboembolism. Br J Surg 1999;86:992–1004.
18. Amarigiri SV, Lees TA. Elastic compression stockings for prevention of deep vein thrombosis. Cochrane Database Syst Rev 2000:CD001484.
19. Wells PS, Lensing AW, Hirsh J. Graduated compression stockings in the prevention of postoperative venous thromboembolism. A meta-analysis. Arch Intern Med 1994;154:67–72.
20. Levine M, Hirsh J, Gent M, et al. Double-blind randomised trial of a very-low-dose warfarin for prevention of thromboembolism in stage IV breast cancer. Lancet 1994;343(8902):886–9.
21. Rajan R, Gafni A, Levine M, et al. Very low-dose warfarin prophylaxis to prevent thromboembolism in women with metastatic breast cancer receiving chemotherapy: an economic evaluation. J Clin Oncol 1995;13:42–6.
22. Kakkar AK, Levine MN, Kadziola Z, et al. Low molecular weight heparin, therapy with dalteparin, and survival in advanced cancer: the fragmin advanced malignancy outcome study (FAMOUS). J Clin Oncol 2004;22:1944–8.
23. Bern MM, Lokich JJ, Wallach SR, et al. Very low doses of warfarin can prevent thrombosis in central venous catheters. A randomized prospective trial. Ann Intern Med 1990;112:423–8.

24. Monreal M, Alastrue A, Rull M, et al. Upper extremity deep venous thrombosis in cancer patients with venous access devices—prophylaxis with a low molecular weight heparin (fragmin). Thromb Haemost 1996;75:251–3.

25. Reichardt P, Kretzschmar, A, Biakhov, M et al. A phase III double blind , placebo controlled study evaluating the efficacy and safety of dalteparin in preventing catheter-related complications in cancer patients with central venous catheters [abstract]. Clin Oncol 2002;21:Abstract 1474.

26. Prandoni P, Sabbion P, Tanduo C, et al. Prevention of venous thromboembolism in high-risk surgical and medical patients. Semin Vasc Med 2001;1:61–70.

27. Iversen LH, Okholm M, Thorlacius-Ussing O. Pre- and postoperative state of coagulation and fibrinolysis in plasma of patients with benign and malignant colorectal disease—a preliminary study. Thromb Haemost 1996; 76:523–8.

28. Brotman DJ, Segal JB, Jani JT, et al. Limitations of D-dimer testing in unselected inpatients with suspected venous thromboembolism. Am J Med 2003;114:276–82.

29. Meyer G, Marjanovic Z, Valcke J, et al. Comparison of low-molecular-weight heparin and warfarin for the secondary prevention of venous thromboembolism in patients with cancer: a randomized controlled study. Arch Intern Med 2002;162:1729–35.

30. Lee AY, Levine MN, Baker RI, et al. Low-molecular-weight heparin versus a coumarin for the prevention of recurrent venous thromboembolism in patients with cancer. N Engl J Med 2003;349:146–53.

31. Hull RD, Raskob GE, Pineo GF, et al. Subcutaneous low-molecular-weight heparin vs warfarin for prophylaxis of deep vein thrombosis after hip or knee implantation. An economic perspective. Arch Intern Med 1997;157:298–303.

32. Stein PD, Kayali F, Olson RE. Twenty-one-year trends in the use of inferior vena cava filters. Arch Intern Med 2004;164:1541–5.

33. Wallace MJ, Jean JL, Gupta S, et al. Use of inferior vena caval filters and survival in patients with malignancy. Cancer 2004;101:1902–7.

34. Kinney TB. Update on inferior vena cava filters. J Vasc Interv Radiol 2003;14:425–40.

35. Konstantatos A. Anticoagulation and cataract surgery: a review of the current literature. Anaesth Intensive Care 2001;29:11–8.

36. Kadakia SC, Angueira CE, Ward JA, Moore M. Gastrointestinal endoscopy in patients taking antiplatelet agents and anticoagulants: survey of ASGE members. American Society for Gastrointestinal Endoscopy. Gastrointest Endosc 1996;44:309–16.

37. Eisen GM, Baron TH, Dominitz JA, et al. Guideline on the management of anticoagulation and antiplatelet therapy for endoscopic procedures. Gastrointest Endosc 2002;55:775–9.

38. Wahl MJ. Dental surgery in anticoagulated patients. Arch Intern Med 1998;158:1610–6.

39. Thumboo J, O'Duffy JD. A prospective study of the safety of joint and soft tissue aspirations and injections in patients taking warfarin sodium. Arthritis Rheum 1998;41:736–9.

40. Marietta M, Bertesi M, Simoni L, et al. A simple and safe nomogram for the management of oral anticoagulation prior to minor surgery. Clin Lab Haematol 2003;25:127–30.

41. White RH, McKittrick T, Hutchinson R, Twitchell J. Temporary discontinuation of warfarin therapy: changes in the international normalized ratio. Ann Intern Med 1995;122:40–2.

42. Kearon C, Hirsh J. Management of anticoagulation before and after elective surgery. N Engl J Med 1997;336:1506–11.

43. Hull R, Delmore T, Genton E, et al. Warfarin sodium versus low-dose heparin in the long-term treatment of venous thrombosis. N Engl J Med 1979;301:855–8.

44. Coon WW, Willis PW 3rd. Recurrence of venous thromboembolism. Surgery 1973;73:823–7.

45. Brotman DJ, Kaatz S. Should patients on warfarin for 3 months for idiopathic proximal deep venous thrombosis receive bridging therapy precolonoscopy (with expected biopsy)? Med Clin North Am 2003;87:1205–14.

46. Jaffer AK, Brotman DJ, Chukwumerije N. When patients on warfarin need surgery. Cleve Clin J Med 2003;70:973–84.

47. Chow SL, Zammit K, West K, et al. Correlation of antifactor Xa concentrations with renal function in patients on enoxaparin. J Clin Pharmacol 2003;43:586–90.

48. Nagge J, Crowther M, Hirsh J. Is impaired renal function a contraindication to the use of low-molecular-weight heparin? Arch Intern Med 2002;162:2605–9.

49. Weitz JI. New anticoagulants for treatment of venous thromboembolism. Circulation 2004;110(9 Suppl 1):19–26.

50. Turpie AG, Eriksson BI, Lassen MR, Bauer KA. A meta-analysis of fondaparinux versus enoxaparin in the prevention of venous thromboembolism after major orthopaedic surgery. J South Orthop Assoc 2002;11:182–8.

51. Bergqvist D. Low molecular weight heparin for the prevention of venous thromboembolism after abdominal surgery. Br J Surg 2004;91:965–74.

52. Leclerc JR, Geerts WH, Desjardins L, et al. Prevention of venous thromboembolism after knee arthroplasty. A randomized, double-blind trial comparing enoxaparin with warfarin. Ann Intern Med 1996;124:619–26.

53. Efficacy and safety of enoxaparin versus unfractionated heparin for prevention of deep vein thrombosis in elective cancer surgery: a double-blind randomized multicentre trial with venographic assessment. ENOXACAN Study Group. Br J Surg 1997;84:1099–103.

54. McLeod RS, Geerts WH, Sniderman KW, et al. Subcutaneous heparin versus low-molecular-weight heparin as thromboprophylaxis in patients undergoing colorectal surgery: results of the Canadian colorectal DVT prophylaxis trial: a randomized, double-blind trial. Ann Surg 2001;233:438–44.

55. Clarke-Pearson DL, Synan IS, Dodge R, et al. A randomized trial of low-dose heparin and intermittent pneumatic calf compression for the prevention of deep venous thrombosis after gynecologic oncology surgery. Am J Obstet Gynecol 1993;168:1146–54.

56. Clark-Pearson DL, DeLong E, Synan IS, et al. A controlled trial of two low-dose heparin regimens for the prevention of postoperative deep vein thrombosis. Obstet Gynecol 1990;75:684–9.

57. Agnelli G BD, Cohen et al. A randomized double-blind study to compare the efficacy and safety of fondaparinux with dalteparin in the prevention of venous thromboembolism after high-risk abdominal surgery: the Pegasus study [abstract]. J Thromb Haemost 2003;July 2003:Abstract OC006.

Surgery in the Patient with Endocrine Disease

Gail A. Welsh, MD

Karen F. Mauck, MD, MSc

Endocrine disorders are common in cancer patients who undergo surgery. Patients may have a chronic endocrine disease, such as diabetes mellitus, in addition to their malignancy. They may have primary or metastatic disease of an endocrine organ, such as the thyroid or adrenal gland. Finally, treatment of their malignancy, whether by surgery, radiation or chemotherapy, may affect endocrine function. This chapter discusses perioperative evaluation and management of cancer patients with diabetes mellitus, thyroid disorders, adrenal dysfunction due to exogenous steroids, and electrolyte abnormalities.

The Patient with Diabetes Mellitus

Introduction

Diabetes mellitus is a common medical condition with a prevalence of about 8% in the United States population.[1] Complications from diabetes such as hyperglycemia, ischemic heart disease, peripheral vascular disease and renal insufficiency can contribute to adverse perioperative outcomes that include postoperative infection, myocardial infarction, and acute renal failure.[2] The cancer patient with diabetes may have additional risk factors for complications that must be identified in the perioperative period. Chemotherapy with corticosteroids can worsen insulin resistance and precipitate or maintain hyperglycemia. Immunosuppression from both malignancy and its therapies can add to an increased risk of infection from both hyperglycemia and poor wound perfusion secondary to vascular disease. Anorexia and cachexia from cancer may affect the patient's need for diabetic medications and lead to hypoglycemia. Careful preoperative evaluation and meticulous perioperative management of diabetic cancer patients undergoing surgery can modify risk factors and prevent both medical and surgical complications.

Preoperative Assessment

Patients with known diabetes should be identified preoperatively, but up to a third of patients with diabetes may be undiagnosed.[3] Those with risk factors for diabetes, including family history, advanced age, obesity, inactivity, dyslipidemia, polycystic kidney disease or a history of gestational diabetes, and those with symptoms of diabetes, such as polyuria, polydipsia, weight loss or weight gain, should be tested for it before surgery.[1] Nonurgent surgery may need to be postponed in the newly diagnosed diabetic if blood sugars are very high or ketosis is present.

Duration of disease, episodes of diabetic ketosis, complications from previous surgeries, and medications should be documented. An A1C may be helpful in determining how well controlled the patient has been and how effective his or her current medication regimen is. All diabetics should be tested preoperatively for renal disease with electrolytes and a creatinine.

One of the greatest risks for the diabetic undergoing surgery is perioperative ischemia and infarction. Diabetic patients without previous myocardial infarction have the same risk for myocardial infarction as nondiabetic patients with a previous myocardial infarction.[4] The Relative Cardiac Risk Index (RCRI) includes insulin-requiring diabetes mellitus as one of six well-validated independent predictors of major perioperative cardiac complications.[5] Therefore, all diabetics should be screened for heart disease with a pertinent history, cardiac exam and EKG. Early studies suggested that treatment of patients at risk for cardiac complications with beta-blockade could prevent perioperative morbidity and death,[6] but subsequent randomized trials have not demonstrated similar efficacy. Based on the most recent guidelines from the American College of Cardiology (ACC), beta-blockade should be continued in diabetics going to surgery who are already on them for cardiac disease. There is also probable benefit in initiating perioperative beta-blockade in diabetics going for vascular or intermediate surgery who have a history of or newly diagnosed coronary heart disease, or who have a history of heart failure, a history of

cerebrovascular disease or a serum creatinine greater than 2.0 mg/dL.[5] If possible, beta-blockade should be initiated days to weeks prior to the procedure, and the target heart rate should be 70 or less. The ACC guideline is also useful in determining which patients should undergo additional cardiac studies prior to surgery, but invasive studies and interventions may not be warranted in the cancer patient with a poor prognosis who is undergoing palliative rather than curative surgery. Medical treatment for presumptive disease can be used to modify cardiac risk after discussion and agreement with the patient and surgical team.

Perioperative Management

Type 1 diabetics have an absolute deficiency of insulin due to pancreatic islet cell failure, and always require insulin. Type 2 diabetics have a relative insulin deficiency with peripheral insulin resistance and increased hepatic gluconeogenesis.[1] Management options in them include diet and exercise, oral medications, or insulin, but a patient's usual regimen may need to be modified in the perioperative period. Surgery is a stress that releases counterregulatory hormones such as cortisol, glucagon, catecholamines, and growth hormone that oppose insulin, increase insulin resistance, and exacerbate hyperglycemia.

There is an increasing body of evidence that suggests that hyperglycemia contributes not only to a higher incidence of wound and other postoperative infections, but may predict higher morbidity and mortality in hospitalized patients as well. Additional studies have suggested that closer management of hyperglycemia, usually with insulin infusions, can decrease the risk of postoperative infection, affect long-term outcomes of myocardial infarction, and reduce mortality in intensive care unit (ICU) patients.

In a study that prospectively monitored glucose control in 100 diabetic patients undergoing major surgery at a tertiary care center, a glucose level >220 on postoperative day 1 increased the relative risk of a serious postoperative infection to 5.7 compared to patients with blood sugars less than 220.[7] In another study, the mean of six blood sugars was used to evaluate perioperative glycemic control in the first 36 hours after coronary artery surgery in 411 diabetic patients. Postoperative hyperglycemia greater than 200 was an independent predictor of short term postoperative infectious complications.[8] In a prospective study of 2,467 diabetic patients who underwent open heart surgeries over a period of 10 years, those who were treated with a continuous intravenous insulin infusion to maintain blood sugars less than 200 had a clinically significant decrease in sternal wound infections compared to those who were treated with intermittent subcutaneous insulin injections based on a sliding scale.[9]

Several studies in stroke and myocardial infarction patients have shown that higher blood sugars at admission correlate with poorer outcomes, even in patients without diabetes.[10,11] The hyperglycemia may be an indicator of insulin resistance due to the stress of the illness or a marker for the extent of injury. A retrospective study of 1,826 patients admitted to a single ICU for a wide range of medical and surgical diagnoses showed that hospital mortality increased as glucose levels increased and that the lowest mortality occurred among patients with mean glucose values between 80 and 99 mg/dL.[12] Records of 2,030 consecutive adult patients with and without diabetes admitted to the general wards of a single hospital were reviewed for hyperglycemia. Of the study patients, 38% had either a fasting glucose of 126 or greater or two or more random glucose levels of 200 or more. Newly diagnosed hyperglycemia was associated with a higher in-hospital mortality rate (16%) compared to those patients with known diabetes (3% mortality) and patients with normoglycemia (1.7% mortality).[13]

Some authors argue that close monitoring and modification of hyperglycemia with intravenous insulin infusions can decrease hospital mortality. The Diabetes and Insulin-Glucose Infusion in Acute Myocardial Infarction study showed that long-term mortality was decreased in diabetic patients whose blood sugars were tightly controlled after an acute myocardial infarction.[14] A prospective controlled study randomized 1,548 patients admitted to a surgical ICU on mechanical ventilation either to intensive insulin therapy to maintain blood glucose between 80 and 110 mg/dL or conventional treatment with maintenance of blood glucose between 180 to 200 mg/dL. Intensive insulin therapy reduced mortality during intensive care from 8% with conventional treatment to 4.6% ($p < .04$) with the benefit attributable to its effect on mortality in patients who remained in ICU for more than 5 days. Intensive insulin therapy also reduced overall hospital mortality by 34%, bloodstream

infection by 46%, acute renal failure requiring dialysis by 41%, the median number of red-cell transfusions by 50%, and critical-illness polyneuropathy by 44%.[15] In another study, 800 consecutive patients admitted to a single ICU were placed on a protocol to monitor and maintain blood glucose levels lower than 140 mg/dL. A continuous insulin infusion was begun if a patient had a glucose reading of 200 on two separate occasions. The patients were matched to 800 patients previously admitted prior to initiation of the protocol. The protocol resulted in significantly improved glycemic control and was associated with decreased mortality (29.3% reduction, $p = .002$) and decreased length of ICU stay (10.8% reduction, $p = .01$).[16]

These studies, which assessed the correlation between hyperglycemia and hospital mortality, looked at patients with and without diabetes admitted mainly to ICUs and did not specifically address postoperative diabetic patients. However, a study of 3,554 diabetics undergoing coronary artery bypass grafting compared aggressive treatment of hyperglycemia with subcutaneous insulin (1987 to 1991) versus a continuous insulin infusion (1992 to 2001). Glucose control was significantly better with a continuous infusion (177 ± 30 mg/dL vs. 213 ± 40 mg/dL). Observed mortality was significantly lower in patients on a continuous insulin infusion (2.5%) compared to those patients on subcutaneous insulin (5.3%, $p < .0001$). Multivariable analysis revealed that continuous insulin infusion added an independently protective effect against death.[17] A smaller study of 141 diabetics undergoing coronary artery bypass grafting prospectively randomized patients to tight glycemic control (serum glucose of 125 to 200 mg/dL) with an intravenous glucose, insulin, and potassium solution versus standard treatment with intermittent subcutaneous insulin and a serum glucose target of less than 250 mg/dL. Patients with tight glycemic control had improved perioperative outcomes, enhanced survival and decreased incidence of both ischemic events and wound complications.[18]

Continuous insulin infusions are labor-intensive, and, so far, there is insufficient evidence to justify a continuous insulin infusion in all diabetics undergoing surgery. However, critically ill surgical patients and those undergoing major surgeries should be considered for this therapy. Perioperative blood sugars less than 200 mg/dL should be a target in all diabetic patients to decrease risk of infections. Postoperative ICU patients should be more tightly controlled with blood sugars between 80 to 110 mg/dL.[15] More studies need to be done to see if tighter glucose control in diabetic patients undergoing noncardiac surgery reduces postoperative ischemia, infarction, and mortality.

The timing, type and duration of surgery will determine perioperative management of oral

hypoglycemics as well as insulin dosing in the diabetic. Oral hypoglycemics should be held the morning of surgery. Insulin may be needed in the patient who is only on oral medication if the patient's diabetes is poorly controlled. Table 1 details preoperative dosing of insulin based on a patient's type and scheduled regimen of insulin as well as the time and duration of surgery. Patients on basal insulin regimens such as glargine or continuous infusion pumps should receive their basal medication during surgery without boluses. Insulin-treated patients undergoing major surgery should be treated with a continuous insulin infusion.[19]

The patient who receives insulin prior to surgery should be given D5 in the intravenous fluids at 100 to 150 cc/hr to prevent hypoglycemia while taking nothing by mouth. All diabetics should have their blood glucose checked preoperatively and then frequently throughout the surgery and in the postoperative period. Postoperative blood sugars can be managed with a continuous insulin infusion or sliding scale subcutaneous insulin with reintroduction of the patient's preoperative regimen when he or she resumes a full diet. An exception is a patient on metformin hydrochloride who receives intravenous contrast during a procedure. The medication should be held for 72 hours after the procedure, and a creatinine should be checked before it is restarted.[19] Metformin should not be resumed in a patient who develops postoperative heart failure, hypotension, renal insufficiency or hepatic dysfunction.[20] Metabolic and hormonal changes can continue up to 4 days after major surgery, but are most pronounced through the first postoperative day.[21] Persistence of hyperglycemia may reflect a perioperative complication such as infection. Providers must be alert throughout the perioperative period for neuropsychiatric symptoms in a diabetic that may be due to hypoglycemia or ketosis.

The Patient with Hypothyroidism

Introduction

Hypothyroidism is a common disease with a prevalence of 1 to 2% in the general population, though it is ten times more common in women than men.[22] Genetics, environmental factors, such as dietary iodine deficiency, and autoimmune disease play a role in its development. Medications such as lithium or amiodarone, surgery for benign or malignant thyroid disease, and radiation to the head and neck or to the mediastinum in lymphoma, head and neck, or breast cancer can cause hypothyroidism.[23,24]

Thyroid function affects the physiology of many of the body's organs, and its dysfunction can influence perioperative outcome through myocardial contractility and heart rate, lowered

Table 1 Perioperative Management of Diabetes Mellitus Insulin Regimens

Duration and Type of Surgery	Anticipated Meals	Usual Insulin Regimen	Perioperative Management
Short Early am	Breakfast will be eaten	Single or multiple doses	Delay and give after procedure with breakfast
		Peakless (glargine)	Usual am dose
		Insulin pump	Basal rate, bolus with breakfast if needed
Short Late am	Breakfast will be missed	Single am dose	2/3 TDD as IAI
	Lunch will be eaten	2 or 3 daily doses MDI	1/2 TMD as IAI
			1/3 am dose of SAI
		Peakless (glargine)	Usual am dose
		Insulin pump	Basal rate only
Short Afternoon	Breakfast will be missed	Single am dose	½ TDD as IAI
	Lunch will be missed	2 or 3 daily doses MDI	1/3 TMD as IAI
			1/3 am, 1/3 lunch doses of SAI
or	or	Peakless (glargine)	Usual am dose
Uncertain	Uncertain	Insulin pump	Basal rate only
Complex	NPO	Any	Continuous IV insulin
Prolonged			

Adapted from Jacober SJ and Sowers JR.[19]
IAI = intermediate-acting insulin; MDI = multiple doses of short-acting insulin; SAI = short-acting insulin; TDD = total daily dose (short plus intermediate-acting insulin); TMD = total morning dose (short plus intermediate-acting insulin).

metabolic rate, hemostasis, gastrointestinal motility, and free water balance.[25] There are case reports of intraoperative hypotension, cardiovascular collapse, and myxedema coma in undiagnosed hypothyroid patients undergoing anesthesia and surgery.[26,27] Yet there are no randomized, prospective studies that compare surgical outcomes in untreated hypothyroid patients versus controls.

However, two studies from the 1980s did evaluate the hypothyroid patient undergoing surgery with retrospective case-matched controls. In one study, anesthetic and surgical outcomes were compared in 59 hypothyroid and 59 paired euthyroid patients. There was no difference in surgical outcome, hospital length of stay, or perioperative complications that included pulmonary or myocardial infarction, sepsis, arrhythmias, need for postoperative ventilatory assistance, fluid and electrolyte imbalances, or bleeding complications. In addition, no differences in outcome were found based on level of thyroxine, although only a few patients in the sample were severely hypothyroid.[28] A second retrospective study looked at perioperative complications in 40 hypothyroid patients matched to 80 euthyroid controls. Hypothyroid patients had more intraoperative hypotension in noncardiac surgery, more heart failure in cardiac surgery, more postoperative gastrointestinal and neuropsychiatric complications and were less likely to mount a fever with infection. However, there were no differences between the two groups in duration of hospitalization, perioperative arrhythmias, delayed anesthetic recovery or death.[29]

Preoperative Assessment

Despite its prevalence, preoperative screening for thyroid disease is not justified in the general population. Furthermore, assessment of thyroid function is complicated in the hospitalized patient by the euthyroid sick syndrome, which significantly reduces the specificity of the serum thyroid-stimulating hormone.[30] Nevertheless, cancer patients who have undergone radiation to the thorax or head and neck or who have undergone prior thyroidectomy or head and neck surgery should be assessed for hypothyroidism.[31] Increased risks for hypothyroidism were found in post-laryngectomy patients who were female, received preoperative radiation therapy, had invasion of the thyroid gland by tumor, had cervical metastasis, and had postoperative fistula.[32] Studies have shown a higher prevalence of hypothyroidism in patients with cutaneous melanoma,[33] as well as those with autoimmune diseases such as autoimmune pancreatitis, Sjögren's syndrome, polymyalgia rheumatica and giant cell arteritis.[34–36] Hypothyroidism should be considered in any of these patients. In addition, thyroid function should be assessed in all patients with known hypothyroidism prior to surgery.

Perioperative Management

Clinical and laboratory euthyroidism is the optimal management goal for hypothyroid patients undergoing elective surgery, but patients with mild to moderate hypothyroidism may undergo urgent or emergent surgery without delay. Postoperative complications in subtherapeutic patients such as ileus, delirium, or infection without fever, should be anticipated and managed. Patients with severe hypothyroidism manifested by heart failure, pericardial effusion, mental status changes, or very low levels of thyroxine should be treated with perioperative intravenous triiodothyronine (T_3) or thyroxine (T_4) along with glucocorticoids if they undergo urgent or emergent surgery.

Thyroid replacement therapy can be initiated in the newly diagnosed patient with mild to moderate disease who undergoes noncardiac surgery at the same dose and schedule that would have been initiated in the outpatient setting. Patients already on therapy can take their usual dose of medication the morning of surgery. Levothyroxine (synthetic T_4) has a half-life of 5 to 9 days and so oral doses can be missed for several days after surgery in a patient who is not eating. Liothyronine (synthetic T_3) has a shorter half-life of 1.5 days. About 80% of levothyroxine is absorbed enterally in the duodenum and proximal jejunum, and, therefore, patients who are fed with a percutaneous jejunostomy tube may not adequately absorb levothyroxine over a prolonged period of time.[37] In those cases, infusion intravenously or through a nasogastric tube may be warranted. Intravenous levothyroxine should be reduced to 80% of the oral dose.

There is controversy regarding the initiation of thyroid hormone replacement in those patients who undergo cardiac surgery. A common concern is that treatment may provoke or exacerbate ischemia, though a large early study showed that less than 1% of newly diagnosed hypothyroid patients developed angina in the first 6 months of therapy.[38] A small retrospective study showed no difference in outcome in coronary artery bypass graft (CABG) between hypothyroid patients with mild to moderate hypothyroidism compared to those who were euthyroid on replacement.[39] A prospective study showed no difference in outcome from CABG between patients with mild to moderate hypothyroidism and those without the disease.[40] A more recent prospective study evaluated 58 consecutive patients on thyroid replacement in a sample of 3,631 patients who underwent CABG over a 7-year period. Women with hypothyroidism on hormone replacement had an excess 30-day mortality compared to men with hypothyroidism on replacement. Levothyroxine dose and serum thyroxine level were inversely associated with mortality. However, the study was limited in several ways. The number of hypothyroid patients was small, and the prevalence of hypothyroidism in the study sample was likely underestimated because thyroid hormone levels were not checked preoperatively in all patients.[41] Given the conflicting studies, the need for thyroid replacement in newly diagnosed or undertreated hypothyroid patients undergoing cardiac surgery needs to be assessed on an individual basis.

In a case series of 136 post-laryngectomy head and neck cancer patients, wound complications were twice as frequent in those who were hypothyroid.[32] Case reports documented rapid healing of fistulas refractory to conservative therapy in head and neck cancer patients if occult hypothyroidism was treated.[42] Hypothyroidism should be suspected in any postoperative patient who develops unexplained heart failure, prolonged ileus or neuropsychiatric complications. Myxedema coma is rare, but surgery can precipitate it.[43-44] It should be considered in any hypothyroid patient who develops seizures, shock or coma and should be treated in an ICU with intravenous T_3 and T_4 as well as glucocorticoids.[45]

The Patient with Hyperthyroidism

Introduction

Thyrotoxicosis carries risk for the perioperative patient. Thyroid hormone exerts direct inotropic and chronotropic effects on cardiac muscle, and it influences the sympathetic nervous system and vasculature. Manifestations of thyrotoxicosis include systolic hypertension with a widened pulse pressure, tachycardia, decreased systemic vascular resistance, and increased cardiac output, all of which can lead to angina, congestive heart failure and arrhythmias.[46-48] Thyroid storm is a rare but life-threatening complication of thyrotoxicosis. It can present with fever, tachycardia, and confusion, and can quickly progress to cardiovascular collapse and death.[49] The stress of surgery can provoke perioperative complications in the undiagnosed or undertreated hyperthyroid patient.

Preoperative Assessment

Like hypothyroidism, the prevalence of hyperthyroidism is higher in women and increases with age.[50-52] It may also be higher in patients with thyroid cancer. Two European studies showed a prevalence of hyperthyroidism of 9.1% in 217 patients[53] and 14% in 110 patients who underwent thyroidectomies for differentiated cancer.[54] Struma ovarii is a teratoma of the ovaries that contains thyroid tissue. Tumors may be benign or malignant, but in either case, a small percentage of patients can develop ectopic hyperthyroidism from them.[55] Patients with previous radiation therapy for Hodgkin's disease have an elevated risk, not just for hypothyroidism but for Graves' disease.[23] Patients who have undergone past treatment for hyperthyroidism may develop recurrent disease.[56] While screening for hyperthyroidism is not warranted in the general surgical population, patients with previous thyroid surgery or treatment, patients with clinical symptoms suggestive of hyperthyroidism and patients with cancers associated with it should be tested for thyroid function.

Perioperative Management

Elective surgery in a patient with hyperthyroidism should be postponed until the patient is clinically and biochemically euthyroid. Preoperative treatment should include a combination of therapies directed against the thyroid gland, against peripheral effects of thyroid hormone, and against systemic decompensation (Table 2).[57] The thionamides, propylthiouracil (PTU) and methimazole, block thyroid hormone synthesis but not its release. Though it may take 3 to 8 weeks for the patient to become euthyroid while on them, they are preferred therapy. Methimazole has a longer duration of action and once-daily dosing, while PTU has the advantage of blocking peripheral T_4 to T_3 conversion. Both can cause agranulocytosis in less than 1% of patients.

Iodine can be beneficial in patients who need rapid preparation or combination therapy for severe thyrotoxicosis. It decreases the synthesis

---

Table 2 Management of Thyrotoxicosis

Treatment directed against the thyroid gland
Inhibition of new hormone synthesis
　Thionamide drugs (PTU, MMI)
Inhibition of thyroid hormone release
　Iodine
　Potassium iodide, Lugol's solution,
　　iopanoic acid
　Lithium carbonate

Treatment Directed against Peripheral Effects of Thyroid Hormone
Inhibition of T_4 to T_3 conversion
　PTU
　Corticosteroids
　Iopanoic acid, amiodarone
　Propranolol
　Anti-adrenergic agents
　Reserpine
　Guanethidine
Removal of excess circulating thyroid hormone
　Plasmapheresis
　Charcoal plasmaperfusion

Treatment Directed against Systemic Decompensation
Treatment of hyperthermia
　Acetaminophen
　Cooling
　Correction of dehydration and nutritional
　　deficit
　Fluids and electrolytes
　Glucose
　Vitamins
Supportive therapy
　Corticosteroids
　Vasopressors
　Treatment of congestive heart failure
　Treatment of arrhythmia

Treatment Directed at a Precipitating Event in Thyroid Storm
Etiology-dependent therapy

Adapted from Langley RW and Burch HB.[57]

---

of new hormone,[58] but in hyperthyroid patients it may paradoxically worsen thyrotoxicosis by temporarily providing substrate for more thyroid production.[59] Thus a thionamide should be given at least an hour before its administration. Iodine can be given orally through, Lugol's solution, or iopanoic acid, a radiographic contrast agent. It can also be given intravenously or rectally.

All thyrotoxic patients should be treated with beta-blockade unless there are contraindications to its use. At high doses propranolol blocks peripheral conversion of T_4 to T_3, but other β-blockers have no effect on hormone production. Rather, they treat tachycardia and help prevent cardiac complications such as arrhythmia. Higher and more frequent doses of β-blockers than usual may be necessary because of increased metabolism in the hyperthyroid patient.[60] Heart rate and blood pressure should be used as a guide for dosing. Longer acting β-blockers such as atenolol given the morning of surgery provide longer perioperative blockade.[61] Intravenous propranolol, metoprolol or esmolol can be used for the patient who cannot take oral medication.

Some patients may need rapid preparation for urgent or emergent surgery, and reports have shown this can be done safely in an average of seven days.[62,63] A regimen for this preparation is detailed in Table 3.

All patients should be monitored closely for intraoperative and postoperative cardiac complications, including ischemia, heart failure, and arrhythmia. Thionamides should be continued in the postoperative patient who has not undergone thyroidectomy. These can be given rectally for the patient who cannot take them orally.[64,65] Adrenal reserve may be low in the thyrotoxic patient, and corticosteroid replacement should be considered in the decompensating or critically ill postoperative patient. Corticosteroids treat adrenal insufficiency and may block peripheral conversion of T_4 to T_3. Thyroid carcinoma, an elevated free thyroxine level and substernal thyroid disease are risk factors for post-thyroidectomy hypocalcemia, and postoperative calcium should be checked in those cases.[66]

Although thyroid storm is now rare, it should be considered in patients with high fever, gastrointestinal symptoms (such as nausea, vomiting, diarrhea or abdominal pain), and cardiac or neuropsychiatric decompensation.[49] Therapy is similar to the patient with severe thyrotoxicosis but is given at higher doses and includes beta-blockade, thionamides, iodinated contrast agents, iodine and corticosteroids. Supportive care in the ICU is essential and should include hydration, nutrition with glucose and vitamins, antipyretics, cooling blankets, and treatment of cardiac decompensation. Acetaminophen should be given for fever because aspirin may increase thyroid hormone concentrations by

Table 3 Rapid Preparation of Thyrotoxic Patients for Emergent Surgery

Drug Class	Recommended Drug	Dosage	Mechanism of Action	Continue Postoperatively?
Beta-adrenergic blockade	Propranolol	40 to 80 mg PO tid-qid	Beta-adrenergic blockade; decreased T_4 to T_3 conversion (high dose)	Yes
	or Esmolol	50 to 100 µg/kg/min	Beta-adrenergic blockade	Change to oral propranolol
Thionamide	Propylthiouracil	200 mg PO q4h	Inhibition of new thyroid hormone synthesis; decreased T_4 to T_3 conversion	Stop after near total thyroidectomy Continue after nonthyroid surgery
	or Methimazole	20 mg PO q4h	Inhibition of new thyroid hormone synthesis	Stop after near total thyroidectomy Continue after nonthyroid surgery
Oral cholecysto-graphic agent	Iopanoic acid	500 mg PO bid	Decreased release of thyroid hormone, decreased T_4 to T_3 conversion	Stop immediately after surgery
Cortico-steroids	Hydrocortisone	100 mg PO or IV q8h	Vasomotor stability; decreased T_4 to T_3 conversion	Taper over 72 hours
	or Dexamethasone	2 mg PO or IV q6	Vasomotor stability; decreased T_4 to T_3 conversion	Taper over 72 hours
	or Betamethasone	.5 mg PO IM or IV q6h	Vasomotor stability; decreased T_4 to T_3 conversion	Taper over 72 hours

Adapted from Langley RW and Burch HB.[57]

bid = twice a day; IM = intramuscularly; IV = intravenously; PO = by mouth; qid = four times a day; q4h = every 4 hours; q6h = every 6 hours; q8h = every 8 hours; T_3 = triiodothyronine; T_4 = thyroxine; tid = three times a day.

interfering with protein binding of T_3 and T_4 (see Table 2).

The Patient on Exogenous Corticosteroids

Introduction

Millions of prescriptions for oral corticosteroids are written yearly in the United States for autoimmune and inflammatory diseases such as asthma or rheumatoid arthritis.[67] Corticosteroids are also frequently used in cancer patients in chemotherapy regimens and as treatment for complications of malignancy and chemotherapy, such as nausea or increased intracranial pressure and swelling from primary and metastatic brain tumors.

Adrenal gland production of cortisol is an essential endocrine response to stress and is caused by activation of the hypothalamic-pituitary-adrenal (HPA) axis and increased serum corticotropin (also called ACTH). Cortisol maintains vascular tone, endothelial integrity, and vascular permeability, and also potentiates the vasoconstrictor actions of catecholamines.[68] Destruction of the adrenal glands through infection, infarction, hemorrhage, or autoimmune disease leads to primary adrenal insufficiency. Secondary adrenal insufficiency can be caused by

exogenous corticosteroids that can suppress the normal feedback loop of the HPA axis. Chronic suppression may prevent sufficient innate cortisol production by otherwise normal adrenals during stress. Recovery of adequate adrenal function may be delayed after cessation of exogenous corticosteroids.

The stress of surgery can precipitate adrenal crisis in the cancer patient with underlying adrenal insufficiency and lead to fever, hypotension, shock, and death. Early case reports in the 1950s suggested that acute adrenal insufficiency occurred when patients' chronic corticosteroids were withheld in the perioperative period. In response to those reports, "stress dose" supplemental steroid regimens were devised to give to patients currently or previously on corticosteroids who underwent surgery to ensure adequate cortisol coverage and to prevent adrenal crisis. Patients often received large doses of corticosteroids for several days in the perioperative period. More recent authors have questioned the need for, or the amount of, supplemental perioperative corticosteroids.[69] Some have argued that patients only need to continue on their usual dose of corticosteroids in the surgical period.[70] Although other recent studies have shown that perioperative corticosteroids may carry additional benefits, such as prevention of postoperative nausea and

modulation of inflammatory mediators that may improve surgical outcomes, they can also increase the risk of infection and mask a febrile response to it.[71–73] Corticosteroids can provoke or increase hyperglycemia, affect wound healing, and contribute to gastrointestinal hemorrhage and perforation.[74–77] Management of patients on chronic corticosteroids must balance the risk of adrenal crisis from insufficient corticosteroid supplementation against the risk of complications from excessive corticosteroid supplementation.

The dose and duration of exogenous corticosteroids that cause suppression of the HPA axis are highly variable among individuals. It seems clear that doses equivalent to less than 5 mg of morning prednisone or prednisone given on an every-other-day regimen do not cause HPA axis suppression no matter how long they are given.[78,79] Long-acting corticosteroids such as dexamethasone, which are frequently given to cancer patients, may cause HPA suppression sooner than those with shorter half-lives. A number of small studies showed that patients recover HPA function quickly (within one to two weeks) after given high doses of corticosteroids for 5 to 30 days, but a few patients may remain suppressed for much longer.[80,81] There are studies that show biochemical evidence of HPA axis suppression in patients on chronic, high-dose, inhaled or potent topical steroids, and case reports of adrenal insufficiency with stress in patients, especially children, on those medications.[82,83] There are only a few older, poorly designed studies that look at how long it takes for the HPA axis to recover after a course of prolonged corticosteroids.

Some have argued that the corticotropin stimulation test should be used to assess patients preoperatively for HPA axis suppression so that only those who need supplemental corticosteroids receive them. Though it is a very sensitive test for primary adrenal insufficiency, its sensitivity is less for secondary adrenal insufficiency.[84] Furthermore, there may not be time for the patient to undergo the test prior to surgery. In addition, a few small studies showed that even those patients who have documented HPA axis suppression from exogenous corticosteroids do not develop adrenal insufficiency—even when they go to surgery without corticosteroid coverage.[70,85,86] Laboratory evidence of HPA axis suppression does not always correlate with clinical adrenal insufficiency.

Without a sufficient number of well-designed studies to provide reliable evidence for decisions on which patients on chronic corticosteroids need perioperative supplementation, the consultant must rely on consensus. The likelihood of adrenal crisis in a surgical patient on chronic corticosteroids is low, but the morbidity and mortality from untreated adrenal crisis is high, and, therefore, it must be prevented. A conservative approach is to consider any patient who has been on greater than 5 mg of prednisone for more than a week as possibly suppressed. Though there is still disagreement among experts on what dose and duration to use as a cut-off for presumed HPA axis suppression, there is more agreement on what amount of corticosteroid needs to be given for specific types of procedures.

Cortisol levels peak postoperatively in the early recovery period, probably in response to pain, but usually return to normal 24 hours after surgery.[87,88] The average corticosteroid requirement for minor surgery is 25 mg/d of hydrocortisone; for moderate stress surgery, it is 50 to 75 mg/d; and for major surgery, 100 to 150 mg/d.[69] Though the response to severe stress or critical illness can be 200 to 500 mg of cortisol per day, responses of more than 200 mg/d in the first 24 hours after surgery are rare. Therefore, many patients on corticosteroids will only need to take their usual dose for minor or moderate stress surgery to meet the hydrocortisone needs of the procedure. For example, patients on 7.5 mg daily of prednisone who undergo a minor procedure, such as an inguinal hernia repair, are already on the equivalent of more than 25 mg of hydrocortisone. They should take the usual dose the morning of surgery and do not need supplementation with additional corticosteroids (Table 4).

Preoperative Assessment

A patient's type and dose of corticosteroid and duration of use should be documented. Use in the 6 months to a year before surgery should be investigated, especially in patients with underlying diseases that are treated with corticosteroids. Previous complications from corticosteroids, such as osteoporosis or infections. should be noted. The decision to continue with the usual corticosteroid dose or to add a supplemental dose needs to be communicated to the patient and the anesthesiologist. The consultant must be familiar with corticosteroid equivalencies in order to choose dosing compatible with the patient's corticosteroid regimen and the stress of the anticipated surgery (Table 5).

Table 5 Supplemental Corticosteroid Regimen

Type of surgical procedure	Corticosteroid supplementation
Minor	If currently taking corticosteroids take usual dose in am, no supplementation needed
	If not currently on corticosteroids, take the equivalent of 25 mg of hydrocortisone
Moderate	50 to 75mg hydrocortisone equivalent over the day of surgery
	Resume usual dose POD 1
Major	100 to 150 mg of hydrocortisone equivalent over day of surgery
	Taper by 1/2 to usual dose over 24-48 hours
Critical Illness	50 to 100 mg hydrocortisone IV q6 to 8 or .18 mg/kg/h continuous infusion plus 50ug fludrocortisone until shock resolved.

Reproduced with permission from.

Perioperative Management

Usual and supplemental oral corticosteroids can be given the morning of surgery if it is minor or of short duration. Supplemental corticosteroids given in addition to the patient's usual oral dose should be given intravenously prior to intubation for prolonged or complex procedures. Additional doses may need to be given intraoperatively or in recovery depending on the length and stress of surgery and half-life of the corticosteroid used. Corticosteroids with longer half-lives such as dexamethasone may be preferred over ones with shorter half-lives, such as hydrocortisone, to achieve longer lasting coverage and less fluctuation in cortisol levels in the surgical period. Supplemental corticosteroids do not need to be given to patients on high-dose inhaled or topical

corticosteroids unless they have documented HPA axis suppression. However, if they develop perioperative hypotension or other signs of adrenal insufficiency, they should be assessed and treated promptly.

In the absence of complications such as bleeding, ischemia, or infection, the patient can resume his or her usual corticosteroid dose the day after minor or moderate stress surgery. Patients who undergo major surgery should probably be tapered over 24 to 48 hours to their usual dose.

Adrenal insufficiency should be suspected in any patient who develops fever, hypotension, or shock, postoperatively. Confusion, hyperkalemia, and hyponatremia may also be indications of adrenal insufficiency. Though acute primary adrenal insufficiency is uncommon in the surgical period, it can occur in response to prolonged hypotension or overwhelming infection or hemorrhage involving both adrenals.

The surgical patient in the ICU may need special evaluation of adrenal function. In critical illness, and in particular septic shock, inflammatory mediators may suppress the HPA axis. Tissues and receptors may become resistant to corticosteroids, and, despite normal or even high levels of cortisol, a relative adrenal insufficiency may develop. Some studies have shown that, in these patients, supplemental corticosteroids may decrease mortality.[89,90] Therefore, surgical patients with septic shock resistant to vasopressors should have a random cortisol level checked. If it is less than 20, they should be treated with corticosteroids. If the level is 20 to 34, an ACTH stimulation test should be done. If the rise in cortisol in response to the test is less than 9, corticosteroids should be given (see Table 5).

The Patient with Electrolyte Abnormalities

Hypercalcemia

General Overview

Malignancy associated hypercalcemia is a life-threatening disorder with high morbidity and mortality. Approximately one-third of all outpatients who present with hypercalcemia and half of all hospitalized patients with hypercalcemia have a malignancy-related etiology.[91] It is the most common life-threatening metabolic disorder associated with cancer.[92] Hypercalcemia is estimated to occur in 10% to 20% of cancer patients during the course of their disease, but the symptoms are often overlooked because they are nonspecific and are dismissed as being due to the underlying malignant process or its therapy.[93,94]

Various types of malignancies have been associated with hypercalcemia. However, over half of the patients with malignancy-associated hypercalcemia have a lung or breast carcinoma.

Table 4 Corticosteroid Equivalents

Corticosteroid	Relative Potency	Equivalent Dose (mg)	Biological Half-life (hr)
Hydrocortisone (cortisol)	1	20	8 to 12
Cortisone	.8	25	8 to 12
Prednisone	4	5	18 to 36
Prednisolone	4	5	18 to 36
Methylprednisolone	5	4	18 to 36
Triamcinolone	5	4	18 to 36
Dexamethasone	25 to 50	.5	35 to 54

Adapted from Krasner AS. Glucocorticoid-induced adrenal insufficiency. JAMA 1999;282:671–6.

Other malignancies frequently associated with hypercalcemia include multiple myeloma, squamous carcinomas of the head and neck, and carcinomas of the kidney and ovary.[95] The relative frequency of the type of malignancies associated with hypercalcemia is outlined in Table 6.

Malignancy-associated hypercalcemia is predominantly due to increased mobilization of calcium from bone, and to a minor degree from increased renal tubular calcium reabsorption. There are three major mechanisms by which this occurs: tumor cell release of parathyroid–hormone-related peptide, induction of local osteolysis by tumor cell mediators, and increased production of calcitriol (1, 25 hydroxy-vitamin D$_3$) by tumor cells.[96]

Preoperative Assessment

Free intracellular calcium initiates or regulates muscle contraction, neurotransmitter release, hormone secretion, enzyme action, and energy metabolism. Thus, symptoms of hypercalcemia are due to the various end-organ abnormalities associated with these functions.[97] The degree of symptomatology is linked more to the rate of increase in serum calcium than to that of the absolute serum calcium level.[98] Mild to moderate hypercalcemia is often asymptomatic, but symptoms could include anorexia, nausea, vomiting, constipation, polydipsia and polyuria, muscle weakness, and fatigue. When the hypercalcemia is more severe (corrected serum calcium of more than 14.0 mg/dL), the patient will often develop mental status changes such as lethargy, headache, confusion or obtundation. Cardiac abnormalities are also common and include shortened QT intervals, bradycardia, ST-T wave abnormalities and arrhythmias. Peptic ulcer disease is more prevalent in hypercalcemic patients because the production of gastrin and gastric acid is increased. Approximately one-third of all hypercalcemic patients are hypertensive; the hypertension usually resolves with successful treatment of the primary disease.

Table 6 Malignancies Associated with Hypercalcemia

	No. of Patients	Percent of Total
Breast	40	36
Lung	26	23
Myeloma	15	14
Head and Neck	9	8
Kidney	9	8
Gastrointestinal	6	5
Bladder	3	3
Undifferentiated	3	3
Total	111	100

Reproduced with permission from Adami S and Rossini M.[95]

It is important to check calcium levels in the perioperative assessment of patients with malignancy—regardless of symptomatology. In this population, ionized calcium levels are a better alternative than total serum calcium levels. Because half of the total extracellular calcium is protein-bound (mainly albumin) or complexed with anions, decreased serum albumin levels can markedly affect the result of the measured total serum calcium. In a patient with abnormal albumin levels, the total serum calcium needs to be corrected; every change in total serum albumin of 1 g/dL is associated with a 0.8 mg/dL change in total serum calcium. This is important to keep in mind because of the high prevalence of low serum albumin in this population. Alternatively, plasma concentrations of ionized calcium represent the hormone-regulated and biologically active form of calcium and do not need to be corrected for albumin. Ionized calcium levels are therefore a better alternative for calcium measurement in the cancer patient.

The acute treatment of hypercalcemia is hydration with normal saline. The benefit of hydration is twofold. Hydration lowers serum calcium concentrations by dilution and sodium acts to inhibit renal tubular absorption of calcium. Once the patient is volume-expanded, furosemide-induced diuresis will facilitate renal elimination of calcium. Complications of these interventions include hypomagnesemia and hypokalemia, and, thus, magnesium and potassium need to be followed closely and replaced as necessary. Phosphate levels should be monitored and replaced because hypophosphatemia decreases calcium uptake into bone, increases calcium, and stimulates breakdown of bone. Hydration and diuresis, accompanied by phosphate repletion, suffice for the acute management of most hypercalcemic patients.

Intraoperative Management (Communication with Anesthesia)

Patients with mild or moderate hypercalcemia (12 to 14 mg/dL) who have normal renal and cardiovascular function present no special preoperative problems. Because severe hypercalcemia (>14 mg/dL) can result in hypovolemia, normal intravascular volume and electrolyte status should be restored before anesthesia and surgery are begun. However, asymptomatic hypercalcemia is associated with minimal risk in the euvolemic patient if the corrected calcium concentration is less than 12 mg/dL. The anesthetic management of a patient with hypercalcemia should involve maintenance of hydration and urine output with sodium-containing fluids.[97]

Intraoperative monitoring of the electrocardiogram is useful to detect cardiac conduction defects with prolonged PR or QT intervals and/or widening of the QRS complex. Hypercalcemic patients who have skeletal muscle weakness may have decreased requirements for muscle relaxants, whereas hypercalcemia might also antagonize the effects of nondepolarizing muscle relaxants. In view of this unpredictable response to muscle relaxants, many anesthesiologists will decrease the initial dose of these drugs and monitor the patient's response with a peripheral nerve stimulator.[99]

Postoperative Management

Postoperative management of hypercalcemia in this population should include more definitive treatment of the hypercalcemia. The most effective way to control the hypercalcemia of malignant disease is by expedited therapy (chemotherapy, radiation therapy or surgical therapy) aimed at eradicating or reducing the tumor burden.[94] To control the serum calcium level in the interim, an antihypercalcemic drug can be used.

There have been several antihypercalcemic therapies used in the past, but bisphosphonates have become the drug of choice because they inhibit osteoclast function—which is the final common pathway for bone resorption in both humoral and local osteolytic hypercalcemia (bone resorption is increased in the majority of patients with malignancy-induced hypercalcemia).[100] An infusion of either intravenous zoledronic acid or pamidronate is most commonly used. In the presence of more severe or symptomatic hypercalcemia, intramuscular calcitonin can be used in conjunction with the bisphosphonate.[94] The serum calcium will usually reach a nadir at 5 to 7 days. The duration of normocalcemia is variable, depending on the tumor type, tumor burden, and patient differences. Calcium concentrations should be monitored on a weekly basis and repeat treatment with zoledronic acid or pamidronate at 2- to 3-week intervals is recommended until the patient has definitive treatment of the malignancy and the hypercalcemia has resolved. Unfortunately, the malignant process is often quite advanced when hypercalcemia occurs and the patient usually dies within a few weeks.

Hyponatremia

General Overview

Hyponatremia is defined as a decrease in serum sodium concentration below 136 milliequivalents per liter (mEq/L).[101] It is one of the most common electrolyte disorders in the general population, occurring in 1 to 20% of all hospitalizations.[102–107] Similarly, hyponatremia has been reported in about 4% of cancer patient hospitalizations.[108]

Many malignancies have been associated with hyponatremia. However, more than 50%

of patients with malignancy-associated hyponatremia have lung (both non-squamous cell and squamous cell), breast and head/neck carcinomas. Other malignancies that are occasionally associated with hyponatremia are gastrointestinal neoplasms, acute leukemias, non-Hodgkin lymphomas and other hematological malignancies.[108]

Hyponatremia in the setting of malignancy has several potential etiologies. The most common causes are syndrome of inappropriate antidiuretic hormone (SIADH) secretion and depletional (gastrointestinal, renal losses or poor oral [PO] intake) states, occurring in 35% and 33%, respectively, of hospitalized cancer patients.[108] Of course, hyponatremia in this population can also be secondary to certain antineoplastic drugs, by iatrogenic causes, and by other comorbid conditions. Table 7 outlines the common causes of hyponatremia in cancer patients categorized into one of three categories: 1) related to tumor or metastasis, 2) related to therapy, or 3) related to secondary complications.[109]

Preoperative Assessment

The symptoms of hyponatremia are primarily neurologic, and the severity is dependent on the rapidity of onset and absolute decrease in plasma sodium. Early on, patients may be asymptomatic or may complain of nausea and malaise. As the plasma sodium falls, the symptoms progress to include headache, lethargy, confusion, and obtundation. Stupor, seizures, and coma do not usually occur unless the plasma sodium falls acutely below 120 mEq/L.[110] Cardiac symptoms (ventricular tachycardia and fibrillation) usually occur late, at levels of 110 mEq/L or lower.[97] However, electrocardiogram (ECG) changes (widened QRS and elevated ST segment) are noted at levels of 115 mEq/L.[99] In chronic hyponatremia, adaptive mechanisms designed to preserve cell volume occur and tend to minimize the increase in intracellular fluid volume, and, thus, patients are less symptomatic at lower sodium levels.[110] Since serum sodium concentrations of less than 130 mEq/L have been associated with a 60-fold increase in mortality, early recognition and appropriate therapy are important.[109]

A careful history and physical examination is important to help identify the etiology of the hyponatremia. An assessment of fluid intake and output should include oral and parenteral intake, as well as extracellular volume losses from gastrointestinal sources, from skin and from urine. The physical exam should focus on volume status. Postural hypotension, dry mucous membranes, and poor skin turgor suggest decreased extracellular fluid volume. Peripheral edema and jugular venous distention suggest increased extracellular fluid volume. However, commonly, the patient is euvolemic, and none of these findings are present.

Laboratory evaluation should include plasma osmolality, electrolytes, blood urea nitrogen and creatinine, glucose, urine sodium and urine osmolality. The results of the history, physical examination findings, and the laboratory evaluation should help to narrow down the etiology of the hyponatremia, which is crucial to implementing an appropriate treatment plan aimed at normalizing the serum sodium levels.

Acute treatment of hyponatremia and the urgency of sodium correction depend on the presence and severity of the symptoms and the rapidity in which the hyponatremia has developed. The treatment of hyponatremia is directed by the presumed etiology and by the extracellular fluid volume status. For patients with hypovolemic hyponatremia, treatment should involve replacing the extracellular fluid volume with isotonic saline, which will restore normal intrarenal hemodynamics and suppress vasopressin release. For patients with hypervolemic hyponatremia, the mainstay of treatment consists of sodium and water restriction, often with the use of loop diuretics to facilitate free water excretion. Those patients with euvolemic hyponatremia are the most common and, perhaps, the most difficult to treat in that patients usually have to adhere to strict water restriction.

In any patient with severe, symptomatic hyponatremia, a concentrated solution of saline can be used cautiously to replace the serum sodium up to 125 mEq/L, and then less aggressive measures can be instituted. If hypertonic saline is necessary, the patient should be closely monitored in an intensive care setting where sodium levels and urine output can be monitored on an hourly basis. The rate of correction of the serum sodium concentration has been the subject of debate. A good rule of thumb is to correct the serum sodium at the rate in which the hyponatremia developed. If the patient developed hyponatremia and symptoms within 48 hours, a more rapid correction is safe. If the timeline of onset is unknown or greater than 48 hours, it is best to replace the serum sodium more slowly (10 to 12 mEq/L per day) to prevent delayed neurologic complications.[109]

Intraoperative Management

Asymptomatic hyponatremia is not associated with increased perioperative risk, provided that normal extracellular fluid volume is normalized.[111] Patients with symptomatic hyponatremia, however, need to be treated urgently and should not undergo any surgical procedure until the symptoms resolve.

Due to the decreased excitability of cells as a result of the hyponatremia, patients may have poor myocardial contractility and increased sensitivity to nondepolarizing muscle relaxants. Patients with hyponatremia may also develop unexpected hypotension in response to cardiac depressant anesthetic drugs due to the hyponatremic effect on myocardial function.[99]

Preventive measures, such as preference for the use of isotonic saline for intraoperative fluid replacement in patients who are "at risk" for hyponatremia are also important. Those felt to be "at risk" are patients with malignancies known to be associated with SIADH, patients with CNS lesions, patients on positive pressure ventilation, and patients who are currently on chemotherapy. For these patients, it is important to monitor sodium levels closely and to avoid the use of hypotonic fluid replacement if at all possible.

Postoperative Management

The sodium levels need to be monitored closely in the postoperative period, as well, because pain, stress, and opiate use can also stimulate ADH secretion. In addition, postoperative oral intake is usually reduced, and fluid replacement can often be excessive. All these factors can worsen hyponatremia.

The postoperative management of patients with malignancy-associated hyponatremia should be directed at treating the underlying neoplasm or correcting the underlying disorder felt to be contributing to the hyponatremia. The cornerstone of hyponatremia treatment is fluid management. However, for patients who are unresponsive or noncompliant with water restriction, there are pharmacologic agents that interfere with

Table 7 Major Causes of Hyponatremia in Cancer Patients

Related to Tumor or Metastasis
Syndrome of inappropriate antidiuretic hormone (SIADH) secretion
Adrenal insufficiency
Cirrhosis with ascites
Reset osmostat

Related to Therapy
Vincristine
Cyclophosphamide
Cisplatin
Hydration with hypotonic fluids
Overhydration

Related to Secondary Complications
Vomiting
Diarrhea
Lung disease (eg, pneumonia, TB or metastasis)
Central nervous system involvement
Acute renal failure
Salt-losing nephropathy

Reproduced with permission from McDonald GA, Dubose TD.[109]

vasopressin action—the most common of which is demeclocycline. Demeclocycline interferes with the effect of antidiuretic hormone at the level of the collecting tubule and is most effective for patients with hyponatremia due to SIADH, but can also be used for patients with other causes of hyponatremia in whom loop diuretics are either contraindicated or ineffective.[112]

REFERENCES

1. Weinstock RS. Treating type 2 diabetes mellitus: a growing epidemic. Mayo Clin Proc 2003;78:411–3.
2. Keighley MR, Razay G, Fitzgerald MG. Influence of diabetes on mortality and morbidity following operations for obstructive jaundice. Ann R Coll Surg Engl 1984;66: 49–51.
3. Coursin DB, Connery LE, Ketzler JT. Perioperative diabetic and hyperglycemic management issues. Crit Care Med 2004;32(4):S116–125.
4. Haffner SM, Lehto S, Ronnemaa T, et al. Mortality from coronary heart disease in subjects with type 2 diabetes and in nondiabetic subjects with and without prior myocardial infarction. N Engl J Med 1998;339:229–34.
5. Fleisher LA, Beckman JA, Brown KA, et al. ACC/AHA guidelines on perioperative cardiovascular evaluation for noncardiac surgery. Circulation 2007;116:1971–96.
6. Lindenauer PK, et al. Perioperative beta-blocker therapy and mortality after major noncardiac surgery. N Engl J Med. 2005;353:349–61.
7. Pomposelli JJ, et al. Early postoperative glucose control predicts nosocomial infection rate in diabetic patients. J Parent & Enter Nutr 1998;22:77–81.
8. Golden SH, et al. Perioperative glycemic control and the risk of infectious complications in a cohort of adults with diabetes. Diab Care 1999;22:1408–14.
9. Furnary AP, et al. Continuous intravenous insulin infusion reduces the incidence of deep sternal wound infection in diabetic patients after cardiac surgical procedures. Ann Thor Surg 1999;67:352–60.
10. Capes SE, et al. Stress hyperglycemia and increased risk of death after myocardial infarction in patients with and without diabetes: a systematic overview. Lancet 2000;355:773–78.
11. Capes SE, et al. Stress hyperglycemia and prognosis in nondiabetic and diabetic patients: a systematic overview. Stroke 2001;32:2426–32.
12. Krinsley JS. Association between hyperglycemia and increased hospital mortality in a heterogeneous population of critically ill patients. Mayo Clin Proc 2003;78: 1471–8.
13. Umpierrez GE, et al. Hyperglycemia: an independent marker of in-hospital mortality in patients with undiagnosed diabetes. J Clin Endocrinol Metab 2002;87:978–82.
14. Malmberg K, et al. Glycometabolic state at admission: important risk marker of mortality in conventionally treated patients with diabetes mellitus and acute myocardial infarction-long term results from the Diabetes and Insulin-Glucose Infusion in Acute Myocardial Infarction (DIGAMI) study. Circulation 1999;99:2626–32.
15. Van den Berghe G, et al. Intensive insulin therapy in critically ill patients. N Engl J Med 2001;345:1359–67.
16. Krinsley JS. Effect of an intensive glucose management protocol on the mortality of critically ill adult patients. Mayo Clin Proc 2004;79:992–1000.
17. Furnary AP, et al. Continuous insulin infusion reduces mortality in patients with diabetes undergoing coronary artery bypass grafting. J Thor Cardiovasc Surg 2003; 125:1007–21.
18. Lazar HL et al. Tight glycemic control in diabetic coronary artery bypass graft patients improves perioperative outcomes and decreases recurrent ischemic events. Circulation 2004;109:1497–502.
19. Jacober SJ, Sowers JR. An update on perioperative management of diabetes. Arch Intern Med 1999;159:2405–11.
20. Bailey CJ, Turner RC. Drug therapy: metformin. N Engl J Med 1996;334:574–9.
21. Schiff RL, Welsh GA. Perioperative evaluation and management of the patient with endocrine dysfunction. Med Clin N Am 2003;87:175–92.
22. Vanderpump MP, Tunbridge WM. Epidemiology and prevention of clinical and subclinical hypothyroidism. Thyroid 2002;12:839–47.

23. Hancock SL, Cox RS, McDougall IR. Thyroid diseases after treatment of Hodgkin's disease. N Engl J Med 1991;325:500–605.
24. Joensuu H, Viikari J. Thyroid function after postoperative radiation therapy in patients with breast cancer. Acta Radiologica-Oncology 1986;25:167–70.
25. Lee HT, Levine M. Acute respiratory alkalosis associated with low minute ventilation in a patient with severe hypothyroidism. Canadian J Anaesth 1999;46:185–9.
26. Abbott TR. Anaesthesia in untreated myxoedema. Br J Anaesth 1967;39:510–4.
27. Kim JM, Hackman L. Anesthesia for untreated hypothyroidism: report of three cases. Anesth Analg 1977;56: 299–302.
28. Weinberg AD, Brennan MD, Gorman CA. Outcome of anesthesia and surgery in hypothyroid patients. Arch Intern Med 1983;143:893–7.
29. Ladenson PW, et al. Complications of surgery in hypothyroid patients. Am J Med 1984;77:261–6.
30. Attia J, Margetts P, Guyatt G. Diagnosis of thyroid disease in hospitalized patients. Arch Intern Med 1999;159:658–65.
31. Shafer RB, et al. Thyroid function after radiation and surgery for head and neck cancer. Arch Intern Med 1975;135: 843–6.
32. Gal RL, et al. Risk factors associated with hypothyroidism after laryngectomy. Otolaryngology 2000;123:211–7.
33. Ellerhorst JA, et al. High prevalence of hypothyroidism among patients with cutaneous melanoma. Oncology Reports 2003;10:1317–20.
34. Komatsu K, et al. High prevalence of hypothyroidism in patients with autoimmune pancreatitis. Dig Dis Sci 2005;50:1052–7.
35. Perez B, et al. Autoimmune thyroid disease in primary Sjögren's syndrome. Am J Med 1995;99:480–4.
36. Bowness P, et al. Prevalence of hypothyroidism in patients with polymyalgia rheumatica and giant cell arteritis. Br J Rheumatol 1992;31:349–51.
37. Smyrniotis V, et al. Severe hypothyroidism in patients dependent on prolonged thyroxine infusion through a jejunostomy. Clin Nutrition 2000;19:65–7.
38. Keating FR, Parkin TW, Shelby JB. Treatment of heart disease associated with myxedema. Prog Cardiovasc Dis 1960;3:364–81.
39. Myerowitz PD, et al. Diagnosis and management of the hypothyroid patient with chest pain. J Thorac Cardiovasc Surg 1983;86:57–60.
40. Drucker DJ, Burrow GN. Cardiovascular surgery in the hypothyroid patient. Arch Intern Med 1985;145:1585–7.
41. Zindrou D, Taylor KM, Bagger JP. Excess coronary artery bypass graft mortality among women with hypothyroidism. Ann Thor Surg 2002;74:2121–5.
42. Talmi YP, Finkelstein Y, Zohar Y. Pharyngeal fistulas in postoperative hypothyroid patients. Ann Otol Rhinol Laryngol 1989;98(4 Pt 1):267–8.
43. Appoo JJ, Morin JF. Severe cerebral and cardiac dysfunction associated with thyroid decompensation after cardiac operations. J Thor Card Surg 1997;114:496.
44. Catz B, Russell S. Myxedema, shock and coma. Arch Intern Med 1961;108:407–17.
45. Holvey DN, et al. Treatment of myxedema coma with intravenous thyroxine. Arch Intern Med 1964;113: 89–95.
46. Klein I, Ojamaa K. Mechanisms of disease: thyroid hormone and the cardiovascular system. N Engl J Med 2001;344: 501–9.
47. Woeber KA. Thyrotoxicosis and the heart. N Engl J Med 1992;327:94–7.
48. Frost K, Vestergaard P, Mosekilde L. Hyperthyroidism and risk of atrial fibrillation or flutter: a population-based study. Arch Int Med 2004;164:1675–8.
49. Burch HB, Wartofsky L. Life-threatening thyrotoxicosis. Thyroid storm. Endocrinol Metab Clin North Am 1993;22:263–77.
50. Flynn RW, et al. The thyroid epidemiology, audit and research study: thyroid dysfunction in the general population. J Clin Endocrinol Metab 2004;89:3879–84.
51. Bjoro T, et al. [Prevalence of hypothyroidism and hyperthyroidism in Nord-Trondelag].[Norwegian] Tidsskr Nor Laegeforen 2002;122:1022–8.
52. Wang C, Crapo LM. The epidemiology of thyroid disease and implications for screening. Endocrinol Metab Clin North Am 1997;26:189–218.
53. Bolko P, et al. [Is hyperthyroidism often present in patients with thyroid differentiated carcinoma]. [Polish] Pol Arch Med Wewn 2002;107:555–9.

54. Calo PG, et al. [Differentiated thyroid carcinoma and hyperthyroidism: a frequent association?] [Italian] Chirurgia Italiana 2005;57:193–7.
55. Devaney K, Snyder R, Norris HJ. Proliferative and histologically malignant struma ovarii: a clinicopathologic study of 54 cases. Int J Gynecol Pathol 1993;12:333–43.
56. Sivanandan R, et al. Postoperative endocrine function in patients with surgically treated thyrotoxicosis. Head & Neck 2004;26:331–7.
57. Langley RW, Burch HB. Perioperative management of the thyrotoxic patient. Endocrinol Metab Clin North Am 2003;32:519–34.
58. Wartofsky L, Ransil BJ, Ingbar SH. Inhibition by iodine of the release of thyroxine from the thyroid glands of patients with thyrotoxicosis. J Clin Invest 1970;49:78–86.
59. Vagenakis AF, Braverman LE. Adverse effects of iodides on thyroid function. Med Clin N Am 1975;59:1075–88.
60. Feely J, Sevenson IH, Crooks J. Increased clearance of propranolol in thyrotoxicosis. Ann Intern Med 1981:94: 472–4.
61. Gerst PH, et al. Long-acting beta-adrenergic antagonists as preparation for surgery in thyrotoxicosis. Arch Surg 1986;121:838–40.
62. Panzer C, Beazley R, Braverman L. Rapid preoperative preparation for severe hyperthyroid Graves' disease. J Clin Endocrinol Metab 2004;89:2142–4.
63. Baeza A, Aguayo J, Barria M, Pineda G. Rapid preoperative preparation in hyperthyroidism. Clin Endocrinol 1991;32:439.
64. Nabil N, Miner DJ, Amatruda JM. Methimazole: an alternative route of administration. J Clin Endocrinol Metab 1982;54:180–1.
65. Walter RM, Bartle WR. Rectal administration of propylthiouracil in the treatment of Graves' disease. Am J Med 1990;88:69–70.
66. McHenry CR, et al. Risk factors for postthyroidectomy hypocalcemia. Surgery 1994;116:641–7.
67. Axelrod L. Perioperative management of patients treated with glucocorticoids. Endocrinol Metab Clin North Am 2003;32:367–83.
68. Lamberts SWJ, Bruining HA, deJong FH. Corticosteroid therapy in severe illness. N Engl J Med 1997;337: 1285–92.
69. Salem M, et al. Perioperative glucocorticoid coverage. A reassessment 42 years after emergence of a problem. Ann Surg 1994;219:416–25.
70. Bromberg JS, et al. Adrenal suppression and steroid supplementation in renal transplant recipients. Transplantation 1991;51:385–90.
71. Bisgaard T, et al. Preoperative dexamethasone improves surgical outcome after laparoscopic cholecystectomy: a randomized double-blind placebo-controlled trial. Ann Surg 2003;238:651–60.
72. Shimada H, et al. Clinical benefits of steroid therapy on surgical stress in patients with esophageal cancer. Surgery 2000;128:791–8.
73. Stuck AE, Minder CE, Frey FJ. Risk of infectious complications in patients taking glucocorticoids. Rev Infect Dis 1989;11:954–63.
74. London MJ, et al. Association of fast-track cardiac management and low-dose to moderate-dose glucocorticoid administration with perioperative hyperglycemia. J Cardiothorac Vasc Anesth 2000;14:627–30.
75. Anstead GM. Steroids, retinoids and wound healing. Adv Wound Care 1998;11:277–85.
76. Cetindag IB, et al. Postoperative gastrointestinal complications after lung volume reduction operations. Ann Thorac Surg 1999;68:1029–33.
77. Weiner HL, Rezai AR, Cooper PR. Sigmoid diverticular perforation in neurosurgical patients receiving high-dose corticosteroids. Neurosurgery 1993;33:40–43.
78. LaRochelle GE, et al. Recovery of the hypothalamic-pituitary-adrenal axis in patients with rheumatic diseases receiving low-dose prednisone. Am J Med 1993;95: 258–64.
79. Ackerman GL, Nolsn CM. Adrenocortical responsiveness after alternate-day corticosteroid therapy. N Engl J Med 1968;278:405–9.
80. Carella MJ, et al. Hypothalamic-pituitary-adrenal function one week after a short burst of steroid therapy. J Clin Endocrinol Metab 1993;76:1188–91.
81. Henzen C, et al. Suppression and recovery of adrenal response after short-term, high-dose glucocorticoid treatment. Lancet 2000:355:542–5.
82. Lipworth BJ. Systemic adverse effects of inhaled corticosteroid therapy: a systematic review and meta-analysis. Arch Intern Med 1999:159:941–55.

83. Walsh P, et al. Hypothalamus-pituitary-adrenal axis suppression by superpotent topical steroids. J Am Acad Dermatol 1993;29:501–3.

84. Dorin RI, Qualls CR, Crapo LM. Diagnosis of adrenal insufficiency. Ann Intern Med 2003;139:194–204.

85. Glowniak JV, Loriaux DL. A double-blind study of perioperative steroid requirements in secondary adrenal insufficiency. Surgery 1997;121:123–9.

86. Kehlet H, Binder C. Adrenocortical function and clinical course during and after surgery in unsupplemented glucocorticoid-treated patients. Br J Anaesth 1973;45: 1043–8.

87. Udelsman R, et al. Responses of the hypothalamic-pituitary-adrenal and renin-angiotensin axes and the sympathetic system during controlled surgical and anesthetic stress. J Clin Endocrinol Metab 1987;64:986–94.

88. Chernow B, et al. Hormonal responses to graded surgical stress. Arch Intern Med 1987;147:1273–8.

89. Rivers EP, et al. Adrenal insufficiency in high-risk surgical ICU patients. Chest 2001;119:889–96.

90. Annane D, et al. Effect of treatment with low doses of hydrocortisone and fludrocortisone on mortality in patients with septic shock. JAMA 2002:288:862–71.

91. Dent DM, et al. The incidence and causes of hypercalcemia. Postgrad Med 1987;63:745–50.

92. Raue F. Epidemiological aspects of hypercalcemia and malignancy. Recent Results Cancer Res 1994;137:99–106.

93. Burt ME, et al. Incidence of hypercalcemia and malignant neoplasm. Arch Surg 1980;115:704–7.

94. Morton AR, Lipton A. Hypercalcemia In: Clinical oncology. 3rd ed. Abeloff, editor. 2004; Elsevier. p. 957–72.

95. Adami S, Rossini M. Hypercalcemia of malignancy: pathophysiology and treatment. Bone 1992;13:S51–55.

96. Flombaum C. Metabolic emergencies in the cancer patient. Sem in Oncol 2000;27:322–34.

97. Miller R, editor. Anesthesia. 5th ed. 2000; Philadelphia: Churchill Livingstone, Inc. p. 930–1.

98. Body J. Hypercalcemia of malignancy. Sem in Nephrol 2004;24:48–54.

99. Stoelting RK, Dierdorf S, editors. Anesthesia and co-existing disease. 4th ed. 2002; Philadelphia: Churchill Livingstone, Inc.

100. Hurtado J, Dsbrit P. Treatment of malignant hypercalcemia. Expert Opin Pharmacother 2002;3:521–7.

101. Adrogue HJ. Hyponatremia. N Engl J Med 2000;342: 1581–9.

102. Flear CT, Gill GV, Hyponatremia: mechanisms and management. Lancet 1981;2:16–31.

103. Hochman I, Cabili S. Hyponatremia in internal medicine ward patients: causes, treatment and prognosis. Isr J Med Sci 1989;25:73–6.

104. Jamieson M. Hyponatremia. Br Med J 1985;290:1723–8.

105. Kennedy PG, Mitchell DM. Severe hyponatremia in hospital inpatients. Br Med J 1978;2:1251–3.

106. Natkunam A, Shek CC. Hyponatremia at hospital admission. J Med 1991;22:83–96.

107. Tierney WM, et al. The prognosis of hyponatremia at hospital admission. J Gen Intern Med 1986;1:380–5.

108. Berghmans T, Paesmans M, Body J. A prospective study on hyponatremia in medical cancer patients: epidemiology, etiology and differential diagnosis. Support Care Cancer 1999;8:192–7.

109. McDonald GA, Dubose TD. Hyponatremia in the cancer patient. Oncol 1993;7:55–64.

110. Green GB, et al, eds. The Washington manual of medical therapeutics. 2004; Lippincott, Williams, & Wilkins.

111. Sendak M. Monitoring and management of perioperative fluid and electrolye therapy in principals and practice of anesthesiology. T.J. Rogers MC, Covino BG, editors. 1992; St. Louis:Mosby. p. 863.

112. Heideman RL. Hyponatremia. In: Clinical oncology. 3rd ed. Abeloff, editor. 2004; Elsevier. p. 973–86.

Perioperative Cardiopulmonary Complications and Consideration in the Cancer Patient

Valerie Seabaugh, MD

Cancer patients are prone to many cardiothoracic complications, even if their primary tumor site is distant from the chest. Complications, such as pleural effusions, pulmonary embolism (PE), and cardiac compromise (from a variety of mechanisms), are commonly encountered in the oncology patient. These cardiothoracic complications can be particularly devastating—if not lethal—to this already physiologically compromised patient population. In fact, oncology patients admitted to the intensive care unit (ICU) with a complication requiring mechanical ventilation have a 65 to 75% mortality rate.[1,2] Needless to say, in patients at increased risk for cardiothoracic complications, it is not surprising that there are unique considerations for cancer patients in the perioperative phase of their treatment. This chapter will focus on these special considerations, as well as the frequent and infrequent complications encountered in thoracic surgery for cancer patients.

Pre-Operative Considerations

Lung cancer consistently remains one of the leading causes of cancer death in the United States.[3] The 5-year mortality of nonoperative treatment for stage one lung cancer is almost 83%.[4] In contrast, mortality from lung resection surgery is about 3 to 4 %.[5] Because resection remains the only hope for cure, every patient presenting with a lung tumor deserves careful consideration for surgery.

In evaluating patients preoperatively for pulmonary resection, a balance must be struck between the patient's mortality risk of nonoperative treatment versus the mortality risk of surgical lung resection. Because many of the patients presenting for lung resection have a smoking history, the concurrence of chronic obstructive pulmonary disease (COPD) with lung cancer is quite high. The challenge becomes predicting which patient with already compromised pulmonary function will tolerate loss of lung tissue (Figure 1).

Forced expiratory volume in one second (FEV1) is a commonly used spirometry study that has been shown to be a predictor of postoperative complications.[6] Although this test is effort-dependent, it does help quantify the extent of disease in COPD patients. In the patient being considered for pneumonectomy, an FEV1 greater than 2 L indicates the patient is in a lower risk category and can proceed to surgery. Alternatively, in the case of smaller adults, an FEV1 greater than 80% of predicted suggests the patient will tolerate pneumonectomy. If the FEV1 is greater than 1.5 L the patient is a suitable candidate for lobectomy. Additionally, each patient must be assessed for radiographic evidence of interstitial disease and queried about level of dyspnea during exercise. If there is interstitial disease or a history of undue dyspnea on exertion, the diffusing capacity of carbon monoxide (DLCO) should also be measured. A predicted postoperative DLCO (ppoDLCO) of greater than 80% has been shown to have a very low postoperative mortality. A ppoDLCO value less than 40% of predicted is very sensitive as an indicator of a high postoperative mortality risk, and a ppoDLCO less than 80% is indicative of a threefold increased risk of pulmonary complications.[7] Therefore, patients with a ppoDLCO greater than 80% may proceed to surgery without further testing. For patients with ppoDLCO less than 40%, the product of the ppoDLCO and ppoFEV1 has been shown to be a sensitive predictor of surgical outcome. If the ppoDLCO × ppoFEV1 is less than 1,650, there is a high risk of mortality, and other options should be considered.[8] For patients where the ppoFEV1 is 30 to 80% and the ppoDLCO is 40 to 80%, additional exercise testing is recommended.

The maximal oxygen consumption (VO$_2$ max) is calculated from measuring exhaled gases during exercise. During exercise, oxygen uptake increases incrementally up to a maximum amount. Beyond this level of activity, there is no increase in oxygen entering the circulation from the lungs. This peak uptake is the VO$_2$ max and is thought to be a reflection of a patient's pulmonary reserve. A VO$_2$ max less than 10 mL/kg/min portends an unacceptably high risk for postoperative complications and death. If the VO$_2$ max is greater than 20 mL/kg/min, the risk is acceptable for surgery. If the VO$_2$ is less than 15 mL/kg/min and the ppoFEV1 and DLCO are both less than 40%, the danger of death is too high for surgical treatment.[8] For patients testing between 10 to 20 mL/kg/min, decision-making should be based on overall clinical picture and additional testing. Additional exercise testing to consider is the patient's ability to climb a flight of stairs or to walk at a progressively faster pace. Stair climbing is a rather simple form of exercise testing that was used to evaluate lung resection candidates prior to the availability of pulmonary function testing. A patient unable to climb one flight of stairs has been shown in several studies to be in danger of serious postoperative complications.[9–12] Shuttle walking is a test that estimates pulmonary reserve based on walking between two points that are 10 m apart. Each trip between the markers is timed by an audio signal that is shorter for each repetition, forcing the patient to walk at an escalating pace. The number of completed trips between the markers before the patient must stop due to dyspnea is their shuttle-walking score. Inability to complete at least 25 shuttles during two tests correlates with a high mortality risk and approximates a VO$_2$ less than 10 mL/kg/min.[9–12]

For patients with conflicting test results or on the borderline of acceptability for surgical treatment, a broader approach must be used to consider their surgical candidacy. Age should not be used as a selection criteria since there is suggestion that elderly patients with adequate

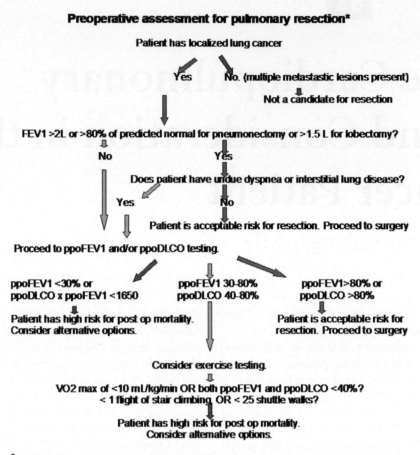

FIGURE 1 Preoperative assessment for pulmonary resection.

pulmonary reserve can tolerate resection.[13] Rather, patients need to be presented with the options and known risks based on their cardiopulmonary function profile and allowed to weigh the risks versus the potential benefits for themselves.

Pulmonary Complications

Pleural Effusions

Pleural effusions are a common and troublesome complication in oncology patients in both the acute inpatient and the chronic office-based setting. Because of their frequent presence in patients with all types of neoplasms, a discussion of the physiology of the pleura and the mechanism of fluid accumulation is necessary to understand their treatment.

Physiology of the Pleura

The pleura is a membranous surface covering the lungs, mediastinum, diaphragm, and intrathoracic chest wall. This surface comprises the parietal and visceral pleura. The visceral pleura covers the lung parenchyma, including the intralobar fissures. The parietal pleura provides coverage to the thoracic wall. The parietal pleura is made of loose, irregular connective tissue over which lies a single layer of mesothelial cells. Vessels and initial lymphatics are within this irregular connective tissue matrix. The connective tissue within the visceral pleura contains collagenous fibers (woven in a pleated fashion) which have two discrete functions in lung physiology. This woven layer helps create the elastic recoil of the lung allowing for passing exhalation.

Additionally it provides the lung with resistance to overinflation.[14]

Physiology of Pleural Fluid Accumulation

There are two main pathophysiologic perturbations which lead to the formation of pleural fluid accumulation. Either the rate of pleural fluid accumulation has exceeded the rate of maximal fluid absorption, or the pleural space's ability to absorb the fluid has decreased. Of course, a combination of these two variables can also lead to fluid accumulation.

Ordinarily, there is a balance between the oncotic and hydrostatic pressure gradients, so that the net accumulation of fluid in the pleural space is zero. Under normal conditions, the hydrostatic fluid tension favoring movement from the capillaries to the pleural space is about 35 cm H_2O. This number reflects about 5 cm H_2O of negative pleural pressure pulling across the capillary, as well as 30 cm of H_2O in capillary hydrostatic pressure within the vessel wall. Opposing this force out of the capillaries is the oncotic pressure exerted by protein and solute within the plasma of the capillary, which totals about 34 cm H_2O. However, there is an oncotic pressure from the normal pleural fluid protein found within the space. This small amount of fluid contains some protein, even at baseline conditions. This protein opposes the capillary oncotic pressure by about 5 cm H_2O. Therefore, the net oncotic pressure working against the hydrostatic pressure totals 29 cm H_2O.[14]

As demonstrated in Figure 2, there is a 6 cm H_2O pressure gradient favoring movement of fluid from the capillaries to the pleural space (35 cm H_2O − 29 cm H_2O = 6 cm H_2O). In animal models, the rate of pleural fluid formation is 0.01 mL/kg/h.[15] The mechanism to clear this constantly forming pleural fluid is the lymphatic system. When challenged with increasing pleural fluid formation, the lymphatic system has the ability to absorb between 0.22 to 0.40 mL/kg/h.[16,17] Therefore, a 70-kg human can clear over 670 mL of pleural fluid in a 24-hour period (or 28 mL per hour).

With the physiologic and respiratory changes that accompany surgery, formation of pleural effusions is unfortunately common. In the setting of surgery (in the cancer patient, in particular), there are additional causative factors for the formation of pleural effusions.

In the setting of a gastrointestinal/abdominal tumor, cancer patients are at increased risk of malnutrition and, consequently, hypoproteinemia. Hypoproteinemia can decrease plasma oncotic pressure and, therefore, contribute to net movement of fluid out of the pleural capillary. Up to 8% of effusions may be associated with

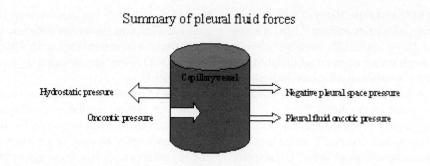

FIGURE 2 Summary of pleural fluid forces.

hypoproteinemia/hypoalbuminemia.[18] Hypoalbuminemia as the sole cause of pleural effusion, however, is controversial. In studies of four patient groups (divided into four discrete groups with serum proteins above 3.5 g/dL, from 2.1 to 3.5 g/dL, from 1.0 to 2.0 g/dL, and less than 1.0 g/dL), the incidence of an effusion was comparable among all the groups. In each patient in the group with serum albumin less than 1.0 g/dL, there was an additional causative factor for the effusion.[19] Hypoproteinemia may be a contributing factor more than a causative factor in the formation of pleural effusion.

Patients with abdominal neoplasms also frequently develop paradoxical pleural effusions. The mechanism for this fluid accumulation may be due to anatomic defects in the diaphragm. Porous openings in the diaphragm, as well as defects around the esophageal junction, which allow ascitic fluid to freely flow into the thoracic cavity, have been described.[20]

Obviously, cancer patients with metastatic disease many times have obstructed lymphatic channels, as well as plugged porous endopenings, and may not have the ability to accommodate even the normal rate of pleural fluid formation leading to fluid collection. Local tumor growth may also block the thoracic duct and create an effusion comprised of chyle (chylothorax). Cancer (specifically lymphoma) is responsible for about 75% of non-traumatic chylothoraces.[14]

Any perturbation that increases the rate of formation has the potential to create a large effusion. Compounding the inability to reabsorb normal pleural fluid, is the additional risk factor for congestive heart failure from prior cancer treatments. Chest radiation and chemotherapy can both contribute to the development of heart failure as well as edematous tissues with leaky capillary beds. In these patients, as pulmonary capillary pressure increases, fluid begins to leak out of the vessel wall and into the interstitium. This edema in the interstitium elevates the interstitial pressure and drives fluid across the visceral pleura into the pleural space.[21,22]

In the critically ill patient, the systemic inflammatory response (SIR) and sepsis (which can both be seen frequently in the postoperative oncology patient) also cause capillary leak. Both the sepsis and SIR syndromes similarly result in effusion formation. Both syndromes are associated with the release of mediators that affect capillary permeability and create leaky vessels.

Indications for Drainage of Effusions

Simply stated, there are three indications for drainage of pleural fluid. If the patient has a parapneumonic effusion or empyema, drainage of the infected fluid is indicated to clear the infection. Secondly, if the fluid is of unknown origin, drainage for diagnostic purposes is a reasonable approach. Thirdly, effusions can be drained for symptomatic relief in patients who have chronic or acute accumulations of a known origin.

Whether the effusion is of lung, pleural, or paramalignant origin the approach to management is similar. When constructing therapy plans for cancer patients with pleural effusions, symptomatology must first be assessed. Complaints of dyspnea and fatigue are not only associated with pleural effusions, but also concurrent cardiopulmonary disease, respiratory complications (such as PE & infection), and complications of chemotherapy or radiation therapy. If a symptomatic patient with a pleural effusion reports relief of dyspnea with thoracentesis and the post-procedure chest x-ray shows lung re-expansion, there are several options for long-term management. In patients deemed to have only a few months expected survival, periodic therapeutic thoracentesis is a reasonable approach to palliate symptoms. In patients with longer expected survival, chemical pleurodesis by chest tube or thorascopic technique can be considered. Pleuroperitoneal shunting, permanent pleural drainage catheters, pleurectomy/pleural abrasion and systemic therapy are additional options. In patients with non–small cell lung cancer, recurrent effusion, and improvement with thoracentesis, pleurodesis is recommended.[23] In patients with small cell lung cancer, systemic chemotherapy is recommended. There is also data to suggest that effusions from other types of cancer, such as breast, lymphoma, prostate, ovarian, thyroid, and germ cell neoplasms, may respond to systemic chemotherapy.[24]

Preoperative Pleural Fluid Drainage

In a symptomatic patient being considered for surgery or a general anesthetic, drainage of a large effusion may be indicated for the potential benefit of increasing lung expansion and facilitating ventilation.[25] However, in the surgical candidate without symptoms of dyspnea, preoperative drainage is not necessary given the continued ability to effectively ventilate and oxygenate the patient.[26]

Postoperative Pleural Fluid Drainage

In the immediate postoperative setting, pleural effusion drainage may be indicated if there is difficulty in ventilator weaning or if a pleural effusion is felt to be the source of dyspnea threatening a patient to be reintubated. If there is any suspicion of an effusion becoming contaminated and developing into an empyema, then surgical intervention is absolutely necessary for drainage and decortication of the infected material.

Perioperative Pulmonary Embolism

The association between pulmonary thromboembolism and malignancy has been known since 1865. Malignancy along with stroke, immobilization, recent surgery, and a history of previous thromboembolism are the five most common risk factors for developing pulmonary embolism.[27] In one study, 17% of patients initially presenting with pulmonary embolism or deep venous thrombosis (DVT) had a known cancer diagnosis.[28] Another 5% of these patients went on to have a malignancy diagnosed either at presentation or within one-year follow up. Patients receiving certain chemotherapy regimens, such as asparaginase for acute lymphoblastic leukemia (ALL), tamoxifen combined with chemotherapy for breast cancer, and docetaxel with thalidomide for prostate cancer, have all been reported to have increased rates of thromboembolism.[29–31] It is well established that oncology patients are at increased risk for thromboembolism, but the additional risk factor of surgery can double their likelihood for pulmonary embolism.[32]

Most pulmonary embolisms arise from the venous system of the lower extremities. Having a high index of suspicion for DVT and pulmonary embolism is necessary due to the vague and unreliable symptomatology associated with both PE and DVT. Patients with symptomatic DVT have been shown to have asymptomatic pulmonary embolisms, and patients with pulmonary embolisms do not necessarily have any preexisting symptomatology of a DVT.[33–37] The most frequent symptoms of PE are dyspnea, pleuritic pain, cough, and hemoptysis. The most common signs of acute PE are tachypnea, rales, tachycardia, a fourth heart sound, and an accentuated pulmonic component of the second heart sound.[34] Fever is associated with PE in 14% of patients.[38]

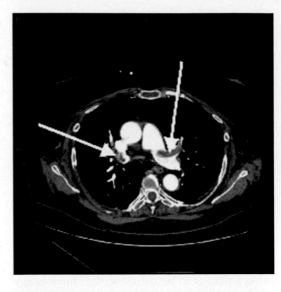

FIGURE 3 Chest computed tomography scan demonstrating bilateral pulmonary artery filling defects consistent with massive pulmonary embolism.

Diagnostic Modalities for PE

Diagnosing acute PE can be challenging, and a variety of diagnostic studies are available to the clinician. Simple studies such as EKG, chest radiography, and arterial blood gas can be completed rapidly at the bedside, but are nonspecific for diagnosing pulmonary embolism. Generally, these studies are useful to rule out other conditions that may be mimicking a suspected PE.

Pulmonary venography is the gold standard for diagnosing PE. It is performed by injecting contrast (usually by a transfemoral approach) into a pulmonary artery branch under fluoroscopy. The drawback to pulmonary angiography is that it is an invasive study that requires a skilled clinician, who may not always be available to perform the study.[39]

Pooled data suggests that contrast-enhanced spiral CT has a 70% sensitivity and an 88% specificity with a 76% positive predictive value and an 84% negative predictive value.[40] It has the advantage of being fairly expeditious to perform and readily available. Another advantage is the benefit of imaging the chest to rule out other possible intrathoracic pathology. Advances in computed tomography (CT) have now made it possible to scan with 1 mm resolution in a single 10-second breathhold for the patient. Although some studies have shown a sensitivity of only 70% for standard CT angiography,[41] with multidetector row CT, the improved resolution appears to have the ability to detect PE in sixth-order branches of the pulmonary vasculature and is recommended as a first-line imaging modality by Schoepf and Costello.[42]

Magnetic resonance imaging (MRI) is an evolving area in the diagnosis of PE. It has a sensitivity of 88% and a specificity of 90% in diagnosing central pulmonary emboli.[43] MRI has the advantage of being minimally invasive without the need for nephrotoxic contrast administration. However, many patients have contraindications to MRI and it does not appear to be as sensitive for segmental pulmonary emboli.[40]

Transesophageal echocardiography can be utilized in diagnosing a central PE with a specificity of 100% but a sensitivity of 76%.[44] It has severe limitations in diagnosing segmental pulmonary emboli and can be poorly tolerated in nonintubated patients already experiencing respiratory compromise from a suspected PE.

D-dimer blood assays quantify the cross-linked fibrin degradation products in the circulation. They are not only elevated in the setting of PE, but trauma, surgery, disseminated intravascular coagulation, inflammatory states, and malignancy have been known to elevate D-dimer levels as well. The D-dimer assay has a high negative predictive value and is useful in excluding the diagnosis of PE together with the clinical presentation.[45,46]

Lung scintigraphy or a ventilation/perfusion scan will study the consequence of a PE occluding flow within the pulmonary artery(s). Comparison of blood flow to air flow is used to predict the presence of a PE. This comparison of the ventilation to perfusion (V/Q scan) has the ability to predict the presence of a PE when the scan is interpreted as high probability. In high probability scans, the prevalence of PE is about 85% (however, this does leave 15% of patients receiving anticoagulation unnecessarily). In low probability to intermediate probability studies, the prevalence of PE is 25%. However, in the setting of a patient with a low probability scan but high clinical likelihood, the prevalence of PE can

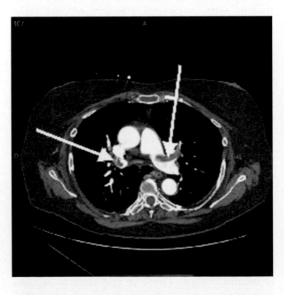

FIGURE 4 Chest computed tomography scan demonstrating large anterior and posterior pericardial effusion. Image courtesy of Mylen Truong, MD, The University of Texas M. D. Anderson Cancer Center.

be as high as 40%.[27] The disadvantage of the V/Q scan for clinicians lies in the difficulty of formulating the best treatment course for a patient when 73% of V/Q scans are reported as intermediate probability.[27]

Lower extremity venous ultrasonography is another option available to diagnose DVT. Lower extremity ultrasonography has limitations in the availability of staff to perform the study; and the presence of casts, dressings, or other lower extremity fixation devices can prevent the performance of complete studies. Most importantly, a normal venous sonogram does not exclude the possibility of a pulmonary embolism already occurring. In patients with objective evidence of a PE, lower extremity ultrasonography is only able to diagnose a DVT in 50% of cases.[47] This may be due to the possibility that the entire thrombus has already embolized out of the lower extremity venous system or that the PE originated from another source, such as the pelvis. Therefore ultrasonography is probably most useful to the clinician in surveillance of DVT formation and prevention of the occurrence of PE.[47]

Treatment of PE and DVT

Recent treatment guidelines were developed by the American College of Chest Physicians concerning the treatment of both DVT and PE.[48] The following discussion provides a summary specific to cancer patients.

When there is objective evidence of DVT, anticoagulation with unfractionated heparin or low-molecular-weight heparin (LMWH) is recommended. If unfractionated heparin is used intravenously (IV), the initial loading dose can be

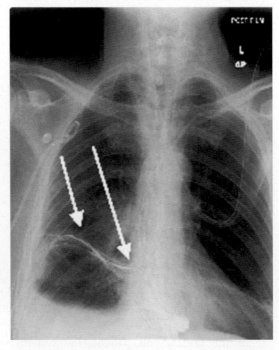

FIGURE 5 Chest radiograph demonstrating contrast leaking from esophageal anastomosis.

either 5,000 units or weight-adjusted to 80 units per kilogram of body weight. This dose is followed by 30,000 units over the first 24 hours or 18 units/kg/h by continuous infusion. Although activated partial thromboplastin time (aPTT) is most commonly used to titrate the heparin infusion, it is important to realize that the PTT study is a global coagulation test that does not always correlate to the antithrombotic activity of heparin or its concentration in the plasma. Laboratories should therefore standardize the aPTT assay to correspond with plasma heparin levels between 0.3 to 0.7 IU/mL anti-Xa activity by the amidolytic assay.[49] Subcutaneous administration is as effective and safe as IV administration.[50] If the subcutaneous route is utilized, 5,000 units should be given IV followed by 17,500 units subcutaneously twice on the first day. The dose is then adjusted to achieve 1.5 to 2.5 prolongation based on an aPTT drawn 6 hours after the morning administration.

LMWH is another treatment option for DVT. Recent meta-analysis failed to show any benefit in bleeding risk or recurrence of embolus with LMWH compared to unfractionated heparin.[51] However, other studies have shown the benefit of decreased hospital time with home use of LMWH in the treatment of DVT and that it can be administered in once- or twice-daily dosing.[52,53]

If the patient has reversible risk factors for DVT (such as surgery within the last 3 months) it is recommended that treatment be initiated with several days of LMWH or unfractionated heparin followed by 3 months of vitamin K antagonist therapy. However, in a patient with nonreversible risk factors such as cancer, treatment with LMWH for a minimum of 6 months is recommended (dalteparin 200 IU/kg body weight subcutaneously daily for one month followed by 150 IU/kg, or tinzaparin sodium 175 IU/kg body weight subcutaneously daily). Discontinuation after 6 months can be considered if the cancer is felt to be resolved. In the case of patients with ongoing presence of malignancy, indefinite anticoagulant therapy is appropriate.

Since PE and DVT are different manifestations of the same disease process, recommendations for the treatment of pulmonary embolism are similar to the treatment of DVT. The exception is that anticoagulant therapy should be initiated prior to definitive diagnostic testing in the setting where there is a high clinical suspicion of PE. Again, unfractionated heparin and low-molecular-weight heparin are both options. LMWH allows for earlier discharge in some cases. In the cancer patient, LMWH is preferable to unfractionated heparin. Duration of therapy for PE is identical to the recommendations for DVT treatment. Several days of unfractionated heparin or LMWH should be followed by long-term

anticoagulation. For patients with malignancy still present, LMWH is superior to vitamin K antagonists unless the cancer is felt to be resolved. In the case where anticoagulation is contraindicated or there is recurrent DVT or PE despite adequate therapy, a vena caval filter is indicated.

Cardiac Complications

Pericardial Effusion

The pericardium and heart can be a common site for metastatic disease as opposed to primary neoplasia. Up to one in five post mortem exams of cancer patients showed evidence of metastatic disease to the heart or pericardium.[54] Adenocarcinoma of the esophagus, breast, and lung are the most common malignancies known to metastasize to this area, but it is possible for nearly any cancer type.[55,56] It is therefore not surprising to be faced with the issue of pericardial effusion in the perioperative period either from neoplastic origin or as a secondary sequelae of the patient's systemic disease state (chemotherapy, chest radiation, myocardial infarction, uremia, hypothyroidism, trauma to pericardium such as cardiac surgery, tuberculosis, viral/bacterial/fungal pericarditis). Although low voltage changes and tachycardia are nonspecific electrocardiogram findings, pericardial effusion is best evaluated by echocardiography.[57]

Treatment decisions are best made on an individual basis, taking into consideration the patient's symptoms, the effusion etiology, if the patient is being evaluated preoperatively, and the patient's prognosis. If an effusion within the pericardial sac is creating pressure that impairs cardiac function, then by definition a cardiac tamponade exists. Tamponade can be either acute or chronic. Accumulation of a very small amount of fluid in a short amount of time can lead to serious tamponade symptomatology. Conversely, if given time to expand, the pericardium can hold a surprising amount of fluid while a patient remains asymptomatic. In the acute situation, as pressure begins to equalize in the chambers of the heart due to the extrinsic pericardial pressure, filling of the heart is severely compromised. As the right-sided pressure approaches 20, emergent evacuation of the fluid is indicated by the most expeditious method. Usually, this is accomplished with percutaneous drainage through a subxiphoid approach. If the etiology of the accumulation is known, a catheter may be left in place for future sclerosis.

Other treatment options include creation of a pericardial window or pericardioperitoneal shunt.[58] Large effusions or those with any evidence of hemodynamic compromise should be drained.[59] Because of the hemodynamic lability associated with general anesthesia and even the regional anesthetic techniques (spinal/epidural)

preoperative drainage of significant pericardial effusions should be strongly considered.

Perioperative Thoracic Mechanical Complications

Lobar Lung Collapse and Torsion

Lobar torsion is a recognized but rare complication of pulmonary resection. However, undiagnosed lobar torsion can have serious sequelae. The incidence of lobar torsion is between 0.3 to 0.089%.[60,61] The presentation of lobar torsion is nonspecific and includes fever, tachycardia, loss of breath sounds over the affected field, and sudden cessation of air leak. On chest radiography, there may be rapid opacification of the affected lobe. A high index of suspicion is required to make the diagnosis. In the clinical setting of lobar opacification on chest radiography, it is prudent to proceed with a bronchoscopic evaluation. On bronchoscopy, complete or partial airway occlusion can usually be seen. If the diagnosis is not clear, follow-up CT can be a useful adjunct. Treatment for torsion is thoracotomy to detorse the lobe and resect any infarcted tissue.[61]

Lobar collapse is a much more common complication in postsurgical patients, particularly post-thoracotomy patients. The incidence of lobar collapse in a surgical ICU setting has been stated to be as high as 8.5 %.[62] Lobar collapse can result from mucous plugging a bronchus. Inflammation of bronchial mucosa can also create an elliptically shaped channel that decreases air flow and mucous clearing, resulting in collapse.[63] In the setting of an upper lobectomy, the pulmonary anatomy is altered such that the remaining lung is shifted upward in the chest creating a partial torsion or narrowing of the bronchi to the lower lobes (23).[64] Treatment includes bronchoscopy (to rule out torsion as well as to clear retained secretions) and supportive pulmonary physiotherapy.

Post-pneumonectomy Syndrome

Pneumonectomy creates an empty pleural cavity, which can be associated with anatomic changes creating the post-pneumonectomy syndrome. As the remaining lung overinflates, the entire mediastinum can shift into the empty thorax, creating a torsion-type compression of the trachea and bronchus. The shifting of the mediastinum can be evident on a plain chest film, but is also diagnosed on chest CT and bronchoscopy. This complication can occur anywhere from 6 months to many years postoperatively. Patients who develop this syndrome present with cough, recurrent pneumonia, and stridor.[65] Treatment is a surgical procedure to reposition the mediastinum and fill the empty cavity with a nonabsorbable material such as saline breast implants, thereby shifting the mediastinum back to the original anatomic position.[66]

Bronchopleural Fistula

Bronchopleural fistulas can develop as a complication of pneumonectomy and carry anywhere from a 30 to 80% mortality rate. Patients with a large (> 25 mm) bronchial stump are at risk.[67] Other risk factors include right-sided surgery and age above 60 years. Unresolved tumor which requires chemotherapy or radiation also places patients at additional risk.

The possible sequela of a postoperative bronchopleural fistula is the development of an empyema. Early development of an air leak in the chest tube of the operative side may herald fistula formation. In the first postoperative week, empyema is not as large of a concern as it is in the 2 to 3 weeks following surgery.

Treatment includes draining the empyema and systemic antibiotics. When the acute infection is resolved, surgical repair of the fistula is required.

Chylothorax

Chylothorax usually develops within the first 1 to 3 postoperative days after thoracotomy and has an incidence of 1 to 2% in post-thoracotomy patients.[68] It presents as rapid filling of the empty thoracic cavity after pneumonectomy and/or chylous drainage from chest tubes. Although it more commonly occurs after procedures involving lymph node resection and dissection near the thoracic duct in the mediastinum, it can occur with any cardiovascular or pulmonary surgery.[69] Diagnosis is confirmed by the presence of triglycerides (> 110 mg/dL) as well as chylomicrons in the drainage fluid.[70] Conservative treatment has a 70 to 80% success rate and consists of a nothing-by-mouth (NPO) diet with total parenteral nutrition support.[68,71] Reoperation with thoracic duct ligation should be considered if chest tube drainage does not decrease to less than 1,500 mL/day for 5 days, if drainage does not considerably decrease over 2 weeks of treatment, or if the patient's nutrition status is impaired by treatment.[72]

Cardiac Herniation

Although cardiac herniation is a rare complication following pneumonectomy in cancer patients, it merits discussion because missing this diagnosis can be lethal to the patient. With either right or left pneumonectomy, the heart can herniate through a defect in the pericardium and into the empty pleural space. It is most common within 3 days of surgery, although it has been reported as far as 6 months postoperatively.[73] The presentation can mimic many other acute catastrophic cardiopulmonary events such as pulmonary

embolism, massive myocardial infarction, and great-vessel rupture. Patients have a sudden onset of hypotension, chest pain, cyanosis, elevated central venous pressure, and shock, which can quickly progress to cardiovascular collapse. Chest radiography can be useful in diagnosis by showing a shift of the heart shadow out of the thoracic cavity with the remaining lung and into the empty pleural space. Treatment is emergent thoracotomy to reposition the heart and repair the defect.[74]

Esophageal Leak

In experienced centers, postoperative mortality from esophagectomy is 5%, with about a 35% five-year survival.[75] Although there is no uniformity in the definition of anastomotic leak, some authors report a post-esophagectomy leak rate as high as 53%.[76] Lerut and colleagues suggest dividing anastomotic leaks into four categories.[77] Small leaks lacking major symptomatology, but visualized with a radiographic contrast study, may be managed conservatively with a nothing-by-mouth regimen for several days. In leaks of a cervical anastomosis with wound inflammation and containment on contrast study, wound drainage, antibiotics, and NPO are recommended. Somatostatin (to decrease gastric secretion) and proton pump inhibitors (to neutralize gastric secretion) can also be of additional benefit in these cases. In clinically major leaks, with patients showing signs of sepsis and severe anastomotic disruption on endoscopy, CT-guided drainage is indicated for well-contained fluid collections. Reoperation for débridement and temporary esophagostomy and feeding jejunostomy are recommended in the case of a poorly contained thoracic leak with a large anastomotic defect on endoscopy. Otherwise, conservative treatment is favored. At the fourth level of anastomotic leak, there is evidence of tissue necrosis on endoscopy. These cases also require reoperation with débridement, esophagostomy, and feeding jejunostomy.

Tumor Embolization

Dyspnea in a cancer patient can have a variety of etiologies and presents a challenge to clinicians. There are a host of reasons for oncology patients to complain of shortness of breath. Infection, thromboembolism, cardiopulmonary disease (induced by prior chemotherapy or radiation therapy), baseline cardiopulmonary disease (from COPD and coronary artery disease), metastases, and effusions are all common occurrences in patients with cancer. However, embolization of solid tumor cells is probably underdiagnosed. Autopsy series estimate the incidence of tumor embolization in patients with solid tumors to be anywhere from 3 to 26 %.[78-80] Tumor embolization is not necessarily the same entity as

tumor metastasis to the lung. Tumor emboli can occur in large proximal vessels (similar to thromboembolism), in the microvasculature, in the lymphatic system, or a combination of these.[78] Although tumor cells have broken away from the primary site and traveled through the venous system to lung vasculature, the cells ability to grow in a distant site depends on interactions with local inflammatory mediators and signaling pathways.

Tumor emboli are more tenacious compared to thromboemboli owing to the inability of tumor cells to be reorganized. If a patient survives a thromboembolic event, symptomatology will eventually improve due to the reorganization of the clot and recannulation of the vessel. In contrast, tumor emboli lack this reorganizational capability and their presence represents a continued problem for the patient.

The most common presenting complaint is dyspnea, but patients may also experience cough, chest pain, and abdominal pain.[12] Patients can develop cor pulmonale symptomatology over weeks to months. Presenting examination findings include peripheral edema, ascites, jugular venous distention, and an augmented second heart sound. Patients may be hypoxic with a respiratory alkalosis on arterial blood gas sampling. Echocardiogram can show a dilated right heart. Definitive diagnosis is difficult with conventional imaging modalities. Chest radiography may only show prominent pulmonary vasculature or an enlarged cardiac silhouette. Because the emboli are most commonly found in the microvasculature, CT angiography is usually normal. Pulmonary angiography is considered the definitive diagnostic modality for thromboembolism, but it is insensitive to tumor emboli.[81] Ventilation perfusion scanning may be the only abnormal radiologic exam in the tumor embolism patient. Small, peripheral, subsegmental perfusion defects may appear concomitantly with a normal ventilation scan.[82,83]

Pulmonary artery wedge aspiration cytology is possibly the most definitive test for diagnosis of tumor embolus (although negative cytology does not rule out the diagnosis). After a pulmonary artery catheter is inserted, the catheter is wedged with the balloon inflated as if to measure a wedge pressure. The first 10 to 15 mL of aspirated blood is discarded. The next 10 mL are sent in a heparinized tube for cytologic analysis. In order to avoid misinterpretation of normal megakaryocytes as tumor cells, an experienced pathologist should review the cytology.[84]

Treatment of tumor emboli is directed toward treatment of the underlying tumor. If the patient has a larger central embolus, it may be worthwhile to consider a vena caval filter, or even embolectomy. However, most emboli will not be amenable to this type of therapy, and the best response will probably be gained from eradication of the presenting mass with conventional methods.

Summary

Cancer patients frequently experience cardiopulmonary complications. Patients with primary pulmonary tumors require careful testing to evaluate their suitability for lung resection. Pleural effusions are a troublesome and common occurrence in patients in the perioperative setting. An understanding of the physiology of the pleura as well as the patients expected disease course is paramount in the consideration of the treatment of pleural effusion. Cancer patients are well known to be at increased risk for thromboembolism. Thromboembolism may require an indefinite therapeutic time period as long as tumor is still present. Pericardial effusion and tamponade can occur secondary to tumor metastasis to the pericardium and must be ruled out in any oncology patient. Although rare, lobar torsion and cardiac herniation can be deadly post-lobectomy and post-pneumonectomy complications. Elderly, right-sided pneumonectomy patients with larger bronchial stumps are at greatest risk of developing bronchopleural fistula. Bronchopleural fistula is associated with empyema. A rapidly developing effusion after thoracotomy may represent chylothorax and must be investigated. Esophageal leaks after esophagectomy may develop relatively well-contained cavities with mild symptomatology or cause life-threatening septic shock, depending on their location and size. Tumor embolus is probably underdiagnosed and can cause symptoms of cor pulmonale.

REFERENCES

1. Hauser M, Tabak J, Baier H. Survival of patients with cancer in a medical critical care unit. Arch Intern Med 1982; 142:527–9.
2. Staudinger T, Stoiser B, Mullner M, et al. Outcome and prognostic factors in critically ill cancer patients admitted to the intensive care unit. Crit Care Med 2000;28: 1322–8.
3. Jemal A, Tiwari RC, Murray T, et al. Cancer statistics, 2004;CA Cancer J Clin 2004;54:8–29.
4. Motohiro A, Ueda H, Komatsu H, et al. Prognosis of non-surgically treated, clinical stage I lung cancer patients in Japan. Lung Cancer 2002;36:65–9.
5. Damhuis RA, Schutte PR. Resection rates and postoperative mortality 7,899 patients with lung cancer. Eur Respir J 1996;9:7–10.
6. Datta D, Lahiri B. Preoperative evaluation in patients undergoing lung resection surgery. Chest 2003;123: 2096–103.
7. Ferguson MK, Little L, Rizzo L, et al. Diffusing capacity predicts morbidity and mortality after pulmonary resection. Thorac Cardiovasc Surg 1988;96:894–900.
8. Beckles MA, Spiro SG, Colice GL, et al. The physiologic evaluation of patients with lung cancer being considered for resectional surgery. Chest 2003;123:1050114.
9. Van Nostrand D, Kjelsberg MD, Humphrey EW. Preresectional evaluation of risk from pneumonectomy. Surg Gynecol Obstet 1968;127:306–12.
10. Olsen FN, Bolton JWR, Weiman DS, et al. Stari climbing as an exercise test to predict the post-operative complications of lung resection Chest 1991;99:587–90.
11. Holden DA, Rice TW, Stelmach K. Exercise testing, 6 minute walk and stair climbing in the evaluation of patients

12. Firish M, Trayner E, Dammann O, et al. Symptom-limited stair climbing as a predictor of postoperative cardiopulmonary complications after high-risk surgery. Chest 2001;120:1147–51.
13. BTS guidelines: guidelines of the selection of patients with lung cancer for surgery. Thorax 2001;56:89–108.
14. Light R. Pleural diseases. Philadelphia: Lippincott, Williams, and Wilkins; 2001.
15. Broaddus VC, Araya M, Carlton DP, et al. Developmental changes in pleural liquid protein concentration in sheep. Am Rev Respir Dis 1991;143:38–41.
16. Stewart PB. The rate of formation and lymphatic removal of fluid in pleural effusions. J Clin Invest 1963;42:258–62.
17. Leckie WJH, Tothill P. Albumin turnover in pleural effusions. Clin Sci 1965;29:339–52.
18. Mattison LE, Coppage L, Alderman DF, et al. Pleural effusion in the medical ICU. Prevalence, causes and clinical implications. Chest 1997;111:1018–23.
19. Eid AA, KeddissiJI, Kinasewitz GT. Hypoalbuminemia as a cause of pleural effusions. Chest 1999;115:1066–9.
20. Lieberman FL, Hidemura R, Peters RL, et al. Pathogenesis and treatment of hydrothorax complicating cirrhosis with ascites. Ann Inter Med 1966;64:341–51.
21. Wiener-Kronish JP, Broaddus VC. Interrelationship of pleural and pulmonary interstitial liquid. Annu Rev Physiol 1993;55:209–26.
22. Bhattacharya J, Gropper MA, Staub NC. Interstitial fluid pressure gradient measured by micropuncture in excised dog lung. J Appl Physiol 1990;68:384–90.
23. Kvale P, Simoff M, Prakash U, et al. Lung cancer. Palliative care. Chest 2003;123:284S–311S.
24. Antony VB, Loddenkemper R, Astoul P, et al. Management of malignant pleural effusions. Eur Respir J 2001;18: 402–19.
25. Grant IS. Anaesthesia and respiratory disease. In: Nimmo WS, Smith G, editors. Anaesthesia. Oxford: Blackwell Scientific Publications; 1989. p. 860–861.
26. Lee BB, Critchley LAH. Pleural effusions and Aneaesthesia 1994;49:178–9.
27. Value of the ventilation/perfusion scan in acute pulmonary embolism. Results of the prospective investigation of pulmonary embolism diagnosis (PIOPED). The PIOPED Investigators. JAMA 1990;263:2753–9.
28. Monreal M, Lensing AWA, Prins MH, et al. Screening for occult cancer in patients with acute deep vein thrombosis or pulmonary embolism. J Thromb Haemost 2004;2: 876–81.
29. Priest JR, Ramsay NKC, Steinherz PG, et al. A syndrome of thrombosis and hemorrhage complicating L-asparaginase therapy for childhood acute lymphoblastic leukemia. J Pediatr 1982;100:984.
30. Clahsen PC, Van de Velde CJ, Julien JP, et al. Thromboembolic complications after perioperative chemotherapy in women with early breast cancer: a European Organization for Research and Treatment of Breast Cancer Cooperative Group study. J Clin Oncol 1994;12:1266.
31. Horne MK III, Figg WD, Arlen P, et al. Increased frequency of venous thromboembolism with the combination of docetaxel and thalidomide in patients with metastic androgen-independent prostate cancer. Pharmacotherapy 2003;23:315–8.
32. Kakkar AK, Williamson RC. Prevention of venous thromboembolism in cancer patients. Semin Thromb Hemost 1999;25:239–43.
33. Stein PD, Terrin ML, Hales CA, et al. Clinical, laboratory, roentgenographic and electrocardiographic findings in patients with acute pulmonary embolism and no pre-existing cardiac or pulmonary disease. Chest 1991; 100:598–603.
34. Stein PD, Saltzman HA, Weg JG. Clinical characteristics of patients with acute pulmonary embolism. Am J Cardiol 1991;68:1723–4.
35. Moser KM. Venous thromboembolism. Am Rev Respir Dis 1990;141:235–49.
36. Moser KM, LeMoine JR. Is embolic risk conditioned by location or deep venous thrombosis? Ann Intern Med 1981;94:439–44.
37. Girard P, Decousus M, Laporte S, Buchmuller A. Diagnosis of pulmonary embolism in patients with proximal deep vein thrombosis: specificity of symptoms and perfusion defects at baseline and during anticoagulant therapy. Am J Respir Crit Care Med 2001;164:1033–7.
38. Stein PD, Afzal A, Henry JW, Willareal CG. Fever in acute pulmonary embolism. Chest 2000;117:39–42.

39. VanBeek EJ, Brouwerst EM, Song B, et al. Clinical validity of a normal pulmonary angiogram in patients with suspected pulmonary embolism—a critical review. Clin Radiol 2001;56:838–42.
40. Stein PD, Hull RD, Pineo GF. The role of newer diagnostic techniques in the diagnosis of pulmonary embolism. Curr Opin Pulm Med 1999;5:212–5.
41. Perrier A, Howarth N, Didier D, et al. Performance on helical computed tomography in unselected patients width suspected pulmonary embolism. Ann Intern Med 2001; 135:88–97.
42. Schoepf UJ, Costello P. CT angiography for the diagnosis of pulmonary embolism: state of the art. Radiology 2004;230: 329–37.
43. Erdman WA, Clarke GD. Magnetic resonance imaging of pulmonary embolism. Semin Ultrasound CT MR 1997;18: 338–48.
44. Pruszczyk P, Tobicki A, Kuch-Wocial A, et al. Transesophageal echocardiography for definitive diagnosis of hemodynamically significant pulmonary embolism. Eur Heart J 1995;16:534–8.
45. Riedel M. Diagnosing pulmonary embolism. Postgrad Med J 2004;80:309–19.
46. Perrier A, Desmarais S, Miron MJ, et al. Non-invasive diagnosis of venous thromboembolism in outpatients. Lancet 1999;353:190–5.
47. Kearon C. Diagnosis of pulmonary embolism. CMAJ 2003; 168:183–94.
48. Buller H, Agnelli G, Hull R, et al. Antithrombotic therapy for venous thromboembolic disease: The seventh ACCP conference on antithrombotic and thrombolytic therapy. Chest 2004;126 (S):401S–428S.
49. Hirsh J, Raschke R. Heparin and low molecular weight heparin. The seventh ACCP conference on antithrombotic and thrombolytic therapy. Chest 2004;126: 188S–203S.
50. Hommes DW, Bura A, Mazzolai L, et al. Subcutaneous heparin compared with continuous intravenous heparin administration in the initial treatment of deep vein thrombosis: a meta-analysis. Arch Intern Med 1995;155: 601–7.
51. Dolovich LR, Ginsberg JS, Douketis JD, et al. A meta-analysis comparing low-molecular-weight heparins with unfractionated heparin in the treatment of venous thromboembolism: examining some unanswered questions regarding location of treatment, product type, and dosing frequency. Arch Intern Med 2000;160:181–8.
52. Wells PS. Outpatient treatment of patients with deep-vein thrombosis or pulmonary embolism. Curr Opin Pulm Med 2001;7:360–4.
53. Harrison L, McGinnis J, Crowther M, et al. Assessment of outpatient treatment of deep-vein thrombosis with low molecular weight heparin. Arch Intern Med 1998;158: 2001–3.
54. Lam KY, Dickens P, Chan ACL. Tumors of the heart. A 20-year experience with a review of 12485 consecutive autopsies. Arch Pathol Lab Med 1993;117:1027–31.
55. Zayas R, Anguita M, Torres F, et al. Incidence of specific etiology and role of methods for specific etiologic diagnosis of primary acute pericarditis. Am J Cardiol 1995;75: 378–82.
56. Wilkes JD, Fidias P, Vaickus L, et al. Malignancy-related pericardial effusion. 127 cases from the Roswell Parek Cancer Institute. Cancer 1995;76:1377–87.
57. Cheitlin MD, Armstrong WF, Aurigemma GP, et al. ACC/AHA/ASE 2003 guideline update for the clinical application of echocardiography: summary article: a report of the American College of Cardiology/American Heart Association Task Force on Practice Guidelines (ACC/AHA/ASE Committee to Update the 1997 Guidelines for the Clinical Application of Echocardiography). Circulation 2003;108: 1146–62.
58. Lefor A. Perioperative management of the patient with cancer. Chest 1999;115:165S–171S.
59. Keefe D. Cardiovascular emergencies in the cancer patient. Semin Oncol 2000;27:244–55.
60. Keagy BA, Lores ME, Starek PJK. Elective pulmonary lobectomy: factors associated with morbidity and operative mortality. Ann Thorac Surg 1985;40:349–52.
61. Cable DG, Deschamps C, Allen MS, et al. Lobar torsion after pulmonary resection: presentation and outcome. J Thorac Cardiovasc Surg 2001;122:1091–3.
62. Shevland J, Hirleman M, Hoang K, Kealey G. Lobar collapse in the surgical intensive care unit. Br J Radiol 1983;56: 531–4.
63. Uzieblo M, Welsh R, Pursel SE, Chmielewski GW. Incidence and significance of lobar atelectasis in thoracic surgical patients. Am Surg 2000;May 66:476–80.

64. Massard G, Wihlm J. Postoperative atelectasis. Chest Surg Clin North Am 1998;8:503–28.

65. Mehran RJ, Deslauriers J. Late complications. Postpneumonectomy syndrome. Chest Surg Clin N Am 1999;9: 655–73.

66. Valji AM, Maziak DE, Shamji FM, et al. Postpneumonectomy syndrome: recognition and management. Chest 1998;114:1766–9.

67. Hollaus PH, Setinek U, Lax F, et al. Risk factors for bronchopleural fistula after pneumonectomy: stump size does matter. Thorac Cardiovasc Surg 2003;51:162–6.

68. Shimizu K, Yoshida J, Nishimura M, et al. Treatment strategy for chylothorax after pulmonary resection and lymph node dissection for lung cancer. J Thorac Cardiovasc Surg 2002;124:499–502.

69. Cevese PG, Vecchioni R, D'Amico DF, et al. Postoperative chylothorax. Six cases in 2500 operations, with a survey of the world literature. J Thorac Cardiovasc Surg 1975;69: 966–71.

70. Staats BA, Ellefson RD, Budahn LL, et al. The lipoprotein profile of chylous and non-chylous pleural effusions. Mayo Clin Proc 1980;55:700–4.

71. Kutlu CA, Sayar A, Olgac G, et al. Chylothorax: a complication following lung resection in patients with NSCLC. Thorac Cardiov Surg 2003;51:342–5.

72. Selle JG, Snyder WH III, Schreiber JT. Chylothorax: indications for surgery. Ann Surg 1973;177:245–9.

73. Zandberg F, Verbeke SJME, Snijder R, et al. Sudden cardiac herniation 6 months after right pneumonectomy. Ann Thorac Surg 78:1095–7.

74. Fouroulis C, Kotoulas C, Konstantinou M, et al. The use of pedicled pleural flaps for the repair of pericardial defects, resulting after intrapericardial pneumonectomy. Eur J Cardiothorac Surg 2002;21:92–3.

75. Lerut T, Coosemans W, DeLeya P, et al. Optimizing treatment of carcinoma of the esophagus and gastroesophageal junction. Surg Oncol Clin of N Am 2001;10: 863–84.

76. Bardina R, Bonavina L, Asolati M, et al. Single-layered cervical esophageal anastomoses: a prospective study of two suturing techniques. Ann Thorac Surg 1994;58:1087–90.

77. Lerut T, Coosemans W, Decker G, et al. Anastomotic complications after esophagectomy. Dig Surg 2002;19: 92–8.

78. Kane RD, Hawkins HK, Miller JA, et al. Microscopic pulmonary tumor emboli associated with dyspnea. Cancer 1975; 36:1473–82.

79. Bast RC, Kufe DW, Pollack RE, et al. Cancer Medicine. 5th ed. Hamilton (ON): BC Decker Inc; 2000.

80. Shields DJ, Edwards WD. Pulmonary hypertension attributable to neoplastic emboli: an autopsy study of 20 cases and a review of the literature. Cardiovasc Pathol 1992; 1:279–87.

81. Schriner RW, Ryu JH, Edwards WD. Microscopic pulmonary tumor embolism causing subacute cor pulmonale: a difficult antemortem diagnosis. Mayo Clin Proc 1991;66: 143–8.

82. Crane R, Rudd TG, Dail D. Tumor microembolism: pulmonary perfusion pattern. J Nucl Med 1984;25: 877–80.

83. Boudreau RJ, Lisbona R, Sheldon H. Ventilation-perfusion mismatch in tumor embolism. Clin Nucl Med 1982;7: 320–2.

84. Lukl P. Pulmonary microvascular cytology in the dyspneic cancer patient. Merits and caution. Arch Pathol Lab Med 1992;116:129–30.

Psychosocial Issues

Kathleen Young Bellamy, MSW, LISW
Harrison G. Weed, MD, MS, FACP

The Importance of Social Support

Treatment plans can be undermined by a lack of consideration of the patient's social context, including the patient's financial and emotional needs, the patient's family concerns and the patient's belief systems (Table 1). Addressing a patient's psychosocial needs is an essential aspect of good perioperative patient care; however, doing so can be difficult and time-consuming.[1,2] Furthermore, patients are sometimes embarrassed to bring social issues, such as finances, to a physician's attention. Other professionals can help to address these issues, including social workers, psychologists, psychiatrists and chaplains (Table 2). Two critical tasks for the physician are, (1) to recognize the importance of social issues in successfully implementing a treatment plan, and (2) to communicate early and often with the other professionals who can help to address the social issues. Before surgery, it is important to establish the kinds of support that the patient will need after the procedure. As we have reduced the length of the perioperative hospital stay, we have placed more responsibility

Table 1 Psychosocial Issues for Cancer Patients in the Perioperative Period

Financial Needs
Paying for treatment
Communication with insurers
Time off from work
Obtaining needed medical equipment

Emotional Needs
Impact—response to diagnosis of cancer
Depression: diagnosis and treatment including counseling

Family Concerns
Care for a child, spouse, pet or other family member
Keeping family members informed

Belief System
Treatment proscriptions (eg prohibition of blood transfusion)
Disposition of removed body parts
Rituals, including those in case of death

Table 2 Professionals Who Provide Psychosocial Support

Social Worker
Financial
   Communicating with Insurers, eg reimbursement
   Communicating with Employer, eg time off of work
   Obtaining resources, eg tube feeds, medical equipment
   Helping to navigate disability application process
Completing forms for physician/patient
Counseling of patient/family, less-intimidating source of information
Discharge planning and arrangements
Placement—Aftercare Needs

Psychologist and Psychiatrist
Counseling of patient and family
Recommendations on approach to patient and family

Psychiatrist
Prescription of treatment for psychiatric illness

Chaplain
Counseling of patient and family
Advice on ritual needs and religious proscriptions

Hospice
Palliative therapies

outside of the hospital on patients and families to prepare for, and to recover from, surgery. Having the appropriate support available at home can sometimes enable a patient to recover from surgery at home instead of at an extended care facility (nursing home). Furthermore, patients with adequate social support are less likely to have complications than clinically similar patients without social support.[3,4] Note that the patient's family might also require psychosocial support. For example, the patient might be the primary care provider for a family member, such as a child, spouse or parent, and alternate sources of care will be needed to enable the patient to have surgery and recover. Usually, the sooner these needs are discovered, the easier it is to address them. Therefore, a thorough preoperative evaluation should include an assessment of the patient's

psychosocial needs and referral to appropriate professional help.

Procedure-Specific Issues

Different surgical procedures may bring up different psychosocial issues. For example, although sexuality can be an issue with any serious illness, it is even more likely to be an issue for patients with breast and genital cancers. Therefore, providing these patients with information, and, if needed, referral to a counselor can be important to postoperative recovery. Perioperative patient education and supplies must be tailored to the surgery and to the patient. For example, patients with cancers involving the airway are likely to require information (and even training) about keeping the airway patent, and are likely to need suction equipment if they will go home with a tracheotomy. Failure to plan for these considerations can not only delay hospital discharge, but can be fatal. As another example, patients with oropharyngeal and gastrointestinal cancers, and their families often have questions about foods and diets. Patients with oropharyngeal cancers usually have difficulty chewing and swallowing, and may even have difficulty speaking, before and/or after surgery. Patients, and the families of patients with cancers of the face, neck, and breast are often concerned about how they will appear after surgery and what cosmetic and prosthetic options are available. If these issues are not adequately addressed prior to surgery, then the patients and their families can suffer unnecessary shock and consternation, and have a negative perception of a surgery that was technically successful.

Write a List of Psychosocial Issues

In the same way that physicians keep a medical "problems list," it is useful to write out a psychosocial problems list for patients with cancer who are anticipating surgery. This list should include tests and treatments that might be unusual or experimental, and therefore not reimbursed. A social worker can often help to generate this list, and to garner the necessary resources. The list should also include special needs during hospitalization, such as diet or visitation, and the patient's anticipated needs for postoperative rehabilitation or placement. There are many government and private programs to help patients with cancer. The two keys to obtaining assistance from these programs are (1) learning about them, and (2) applying for them early in the clinical course. Therefore, the earlier a social worker or other qualified person is engaged in this task, the more likely the patient is to obtain needed resources. The patient will not receive the care, no matter how medically necessary, if it is not both feasible and paid for. Therefore, sometimes the care plan must be modified to accommodate social realities, including transportation, religious proscriptions, and reimbursement limitations.

Resources for the Primary Care Physician

A primary care physician whose patient is undergoing cancer surgery may not have the resources to address the patient's many psychosocial issues. Hospitals often have professional social work staff that can be a useful resource for the primary care physician. Clerical staff and nurses in oncologists' and surgeons' offices are another useful resource because they usually have experience working with similar patients and addressing cancer-specific psychosocial issues. They can often refer the patient to additional financial and counseling services. Written, faxed, or phoned communication with the oncologist's or the surgeon's office as soon as an issue is identified can often speed resolution of the problem.

Psychosocial Issues for Children of Parents undergoing Cancer Surgery

The young children of a cancer patient can present additional psychosocial issues. These issues include relatively straightforward problems, such as obtaining childcare, to more subtle problems, such as a child's magical thinking (blaming himor herself for the parent's illness). Additional issues can include helping young children cope with separation from a hospitalized parent (for example, by arranging for hospital visits). Teenage children are often dealing with issues of separation and independence that can be complicated by the parent's cancer and hospitalizations. The American Cancer Society has information, pamphlets, and videotapes in a "Kids Can Cope with Cancer" program that can be accessed via their Web site (www.cancer.org) or through the local society.

Working with the Patient's Belief System

The patient's religious/spiritual belief system can determine which treatments are acceptable.[5] The classic perioperative example is the proscription against blood transfusions by some religions. Another consideration is the disposition of any removed body parts. This information must be ascertained and communicated to the surgeon prior to surgery. Although the surgeon is ultimately responsible, the internist and the primary case physician are often in a good position to know such information and to work closely with the patient and family. Information on the patient's religious beliefs is usually collected on nursing intake forms, but must be explicitly reviewed and addressed to avoid inconvenience and religious transgression. When faced with the diagnosis of cancer, and with the need for surgery, many patients are overwhelmed with issues of mortality.[6] This can complicate their care and can lead to avoidance and even refusal of therapeutically indicated procedures. Unless these issues are addressed, they can continue to plague the patient and interfere with care. A physician can make significant progress in addressing these issues simply by acknowledging them.[5] In the inpatient setting, the hospital chaplain can also often provide substantial comfort and reassurance to patients and families.

Complementary and Alternative Therapies in the Perioperative Period

Most studies find that complementary and alternative therapies are used by about half of cancer patients, and find that, about half the time, the patient's doctors' are unaware of them.[7] Some alternative therapies are being actively investigated for their potential benefits; however, they can also directly interfere with surgery. The Society for Integrative Oncology (http//:www.inegativeon.org) is a useful source of current knowledge. In the perioperative period, some relatively noninvasive treatments, such as massage, can help to relieve anxiety and discomfort without adverse effects.[8, 9] Other complementary treatments (such as herbal medicines) can have adverse effects. For example, ginseng, garlic, and ginkgo biloba can increase perioperative bleeding. It is generally recommended that all herbal medications be discontinued two weeks prior to surgery.[10] The physician must recognize that alternative therapies are often an important part of the patient's belief system, and that the patient's belief in the alternative therapy can be stronger than the patient's belief in conventional medicine. Compassionate and open communication is critical to developing a care plan that is agreeable to the patient and concordant with our best current understanding of pathophysiology and therapeutics.

Additional Psychosocial Issues for an Inpatient

One key to effective inpatient management is keeping the hospital social worker or discharge planner updated on the treatment plan. It is a useful practice to include an estimate of the discharge date and a summary list of the patient's discharge needs (including any placement issues) in the patient's daily progress note. This note is usually written by a social worker or discharge planner, but must be reviewed and updated by the physician to ensure good communication.

Billing for Psychosocial Care

Payment for psychosocial support is often considered to be "bundled" with the perioperative care; but specific interventions, such as counseling, can be appropriately billed and are covered by some health plans. To be reimbursed, both the medical diagnosis and the time spent counseling must be documented in the patient's medical record.

REFERENCES

1. Trijsburg RW, van Knippenberg FCE, Rijpma SE. Effects of psychological treatment on cancer patients: a critical review. Psychosomatic Med 1992;54:489–517.
2. Meyer TJ, Mark MM. Effects of psychosocial intervention with adult cancer patients: a meta-analysis of randomized experiments. Health Psychology 1995;14:101–8.
3. Cwikel JG, Behar LC, Zabora JR. Psychosocial factors that affect the survival of adult cancer patients: a review of research. J Psychosocial Oncology 1997;15:1–34.
4. Houts P, et al. Unmet psychological, social, and economic needs of persons with cancer in Pennsylvania. Cancer 1986;58:2355–61.
5. King DE, Bushwick B. Beliefs and attitudes of hospital inpatients about faith healing and prayer. J Fam Pract 1994;39:349–52.
6. Gallup H. Spiritual beliefs and the dying process. A report on a national survey. The George H. Gallup International Institute, 1997.
7. Cassileth BR, Deng G. Complementary and alternative therapies for cancer. Oncologist 2004;9:80–9.
8. Fellowes D, Barnes K, Wilkinson S. Aromatherapy and massage for symptom relief in patients with cancer. Cochrane Database Syst Rev 2004. CD002287(2).
9. Deng G, Cassileth BR, Yeung KS. Complementary therapies for cancer-related symptoms. J Support Oncol 2004;2:419–26.
10. Hodges PJ, Kam PC. The peri-operative implications of herbal medicines. Anaesthesia 2002;57:889–99.

Emergency Care: Special Considerations in Cancer Patients

Margaret B. Row, MD, MBA

Sai-Ching Jim Yeung, MD, PhD

The emergency care of patients with cancer presents many challenges. To formulate an appropriate treatment plan, clinicians providing emergency care for cancer patients (newly diagnosed patients, patients currently receiving cancer treatments, patients with stable disease, patients in remission, and patients dying from cancer) must not only be guided by the standard emergency protocols but also by the prognosis, the quality of life, and the patient's and family's wishes.

There are few emergency centers that provide care to large numbers of cancer patients. Each year at The University of Texas M. D. Anderson Cancer Center, approximately 18,000 patients with acute care issues are evaluated in the emergency center. About 40% of those patients require hospitalization, and about one quarter of these require critical care. Patients with cancer present to emergency centers with medical complaints related to the malignancy, related to treatments for the malignancy, or completely unrelated to the malignancy. The emergency physician must determine quickly and methodically whether the patient's presenting complaint is a true oncologic emergency or just an unscheduled consultation for a non-emergency condition. The key to accurate diagnosis is being able to identify common complaints associated with various cancer types at different stages of the natural history or treatment. Medical problems unrelated to the malignancy must always be considered in the differential diagnosis of the presenting complaint.

The goal of this chapter is to share our experience and discuss selected issues in the emergency care of cancer patients. Rather than discussing a laundry list of topics traditionally considered oncologic emergencies—such a discussion could fill volumes[1,2]—we shall address the major presenting complaints seen among patients at our emergency center. The major topics we will cover are cardiopulmonary emergencies, thromboembolic disease, hemostatic disorders, central nervous system emergencies, tumor lysis syndrome, and infection.

Cardiopulmonary Emergencies

Sudden Cardiopulmonary Arrest

When a cancer patient is brought to an emergency center in full or impending cardiopulmonary arrest, the emergency care provider may never have met the patient before, which makes assessing prognosis difficult. The success rate of cardiopulmonary resuscitation and the hospital discharge rate of resuscitated patients are similar for cancer patients and non-cancer patients.[3] If a cancer patient has good performance status and is not expected to die soon, the patient should be resuscitated with the same vigorous effort as non-cancer patients. However, when cardiopulmonary arrest comes as the last events in the disintegration of bodily functions caused by cancer, resuscitation will generally be futile.

The emergency care provider faces the major decision on whether to initiate or continue resuscitative efforts or stop because of futility. The decision is based on the patient's physical status, the events leading to the cardiopulmonary arrest, duration of arrest, initial cardiac rhythm; presence of rigor mortis or algor mortis, the stage and prognosis of cancer, prospects for cancer treatment success, directives of the patient or family, comorbid conditions, performance status, nutritional status, advanced age, and potential quality of life if the patient survives.

Resuscitation generally follows the algorithms outlined in the advanced cardiac life support protocols.[4] However, if the specific causes of cardiopulmonary arrest are identified, the clinician may be able to tailor resuscitative efforts accordingly. For example, prior knowledge of the presence of pericardial effusion would help the physician tailor the resuscitative effort. Emergent pericardiocentesis will relieve the pressure on the cardiac chambers and rapidly restore cardiac output in pulseless electrical activity due to cardiac tamponade. Acute carcinoid syndrome is another example of a treatable cause of cardiopulmonary arrest in cancer patients. Anesthesia, chemotherapy, adrenergic drugs (eg, dopamine and epinephrine), biopsy, or surgery may precipitate a carcinoid crisis in carcinoid tumor patients. Hypotension, arrhythmias, and bronchospasm due to massive release of serotonin and other vasoactive humors from the tumor can be treated effectively with a somatostatin analogue (octreotide acetate 150 to 500 μg intravenously).[5]

Arrhythmia

Arrhythmia is a common presenting problem of cancer patients in emergency centers. Arrhythmia may be related to cancer, cancer treatment, or unrelated medical problems. Signs and symptoms of arrhythmia can be subtle and intermittent, and may include isolated or recurrent syncope, lightheadedness, dizziness, dyspnea (Table 1), hypotension (Table 2), palpitation, chest pain, transient or persistent neurologic deficits of acute onset, and peripheral vascular embolization.

Sustained arrhythmia can be diagnosed easily by electrocardiography. However, transient or intermittent arrhythmia, which is common, may present a diagnostic challenge. Normal findings on a brief period of continuous monitoring do not exclude the presence of an intermittent or latent, but potentially life-threatening, rhythm disturbance. If the symptoms suggest arrhythmia, Holter monitoring for 24 to 48 hours is warranted. Cardiac rhythm analysis can be challenging in cancer patients because exaggerated respiratory variations of the electrical axis and changes in mean QRS voltage due to pleural or pericardial effusions, pulmonary surgery or radiation-induced lung damage may be confused with heart rhythm irregularity.

Primary arrhythmia is caused by focal or diffuse abnormalities in cardiac and pericardial structures. Common causes of primary

Table 1 Differential Diagnosis of Dyspnea in a Cancer Patient
Cardiac
Congestive heart failure (comorbid heart diseases, chemotherapy-induced cardiomyopathy, amyloidosis, … etc.)
Cardiac arrhythmia (comorbid heart diseases, cancer treatment-induced arrhythmia, arrhythmia secondary to electrolyte abnormalities, … etc.)
Valvular heart disease (carcinoid cardiac disease, comorbid valvular diseases)
Pericardial tamponade
SVC syndrome
Pulmonary
Pneumothorax
Infectious pneumonia (bacterial, fungal, mycobacterial, viral, and protozoal (PCP))
Radiation pneumonitis
Bronchiolitis obliterans
Drug-induced toxicity (infiltrates, fibrosis)
Alveolar hemorrhage
Pleural effusion
Lymphangitic carcinomatosis
Leukostasis
Extensive pulmonary metastasis
Pulmonary embolism
Restrictive lung disease (including massive ascites)
Air way
Tracheal or bronchial obstruction
Pharyngeal or laryngeal obstruction
Angioedema
Asthma
Chronic obstructive pulmonary diseases
Psychogenic
Anxiety
Systemic
Transfusion reaction
Anaphylaxis or anaphylactoid reaction
Metabolic acidosis
Anemia

Table 2 Differential Diagnosis of Hypotension in a Cancer Patient
Autonomic dysfunction
Toxins (medications, illicit drugs, alcohol)
Amyloidosis
Hypovolemia
Dehydration
Hemorrhage
Dialysis
Cardiac
Cardiomyopathy
Myocardial infarction
Cardiac arrhythmia
Valvular dysfunction
Infection
Sepsis
Endocarditis

arrhythmia in cancer patients include increased intracardiac pressure and wall stress; ischemic heart disease; hypertrophic, congestive and infiltrative cardiomyopathy; and fibrosis related to aging. The major cancer-related causes of primary arrhythmia are intracardiac tumors (primary or metastatic),[6] amyloid infiltration,[7] myocarditis,[8] pericarditis,[9] and chemotherapy-induced cardiomyopathy (especially anthracyclines).[10]

Secondary arrhythmia arises from abnormal electrolyte concentrations, toxic reactions to drugs, thyroid disorders, vasoactive mediator release (by pheochromocytomas and carcinoid tumors), and radiation-induced heart damage. Arrhythmogenic cancer drugs include anthracyclines,[11] arsenic trioxide,[12] 5-fluorouracil,[13] irinotecan,[14] gemcitabine,[15] and interferon.[16]

Treatment of Arrhythmia

The urgency and etiology of arrhythmia guide the therapy. Specific treatment aimed at reversing the causative factor is preferred.

Treatment of stable secondary arrhythmia usually involves restoring metabolic homeostasis (particularly glucose, potassium, calcium, and magnesium) and removal of offending drugs or substances. When antiarrhythmic treatment is necessary, standard guidelines for arrhythmia management may be followed.[4] Except for beta-adrenergic blockers, many antiarrhythmic agents are potentially proarrhythmic,[17] and the cardiac rhythm should be monitored during the initiation of therapy.

Supraventricular tachycardia is the most common arrhythmia in cancer patients. Paroxysmal supraventricular tachycardia can be aborted by vagus-stimulating maneuvers such as carotid sinus massage. Adenosine administered as one or two rapid intravenous boluses is frequently effective in restoring normal sinus rhythm. When the mechanism of supraventricular tachycardia is unclear on electrocardiographic monitor strips, adenosine is sometimes used to help determine the mechanism. However, adenosine for diagnostic purpose is usually unnecessary with careful analysis of standard electrocardiograms. In cancer patients, sustained supraventricular tachycardia often cannot be terminated by drug therapy. While drugs are used to regulate the excessive pulse rate, elective synchronized cardioversion should be considered and planned soon after diagnosis. Anticoagulation therapy may be avoided if supraventricular tachycardia can be terminated within 48 hours of the onset. In the absence of a reliable time of arrhythmia onset, anticoagulation therapy is needed, and transesophageal echocardiography may be

performed to exclude the presence of intracardiac thrombi prior to elective cardioversion.

Arrhythmias due to structural cardiac abnormalities are likely to persist and progress to life-threatening arrhythmias. In the emergency setting, the treatment goals are stabilization of blood pressure and oxygenation, diagnosis of correctable causes, and symptom control. Emergent consultation with cardiologists, cardiothoracic surgeons may be required to arrange for emergent diagnostic or interventional procedures to address the root cause of arrhythmias.

In the absence of do-not-resuscitate (DNR) orders, cancer patients with unstable arrhythmia should be treated with pharmacologic or electrical interventions according to the current standard of care, such as the guidelines recommended by the American Heart Association.[18] These interventions include administration of a vasopressor, (vasopressin or epinephrine), administration of antiarrhythmic drugs (amiodarone, lidocaine, or procainamide), electrical cardioversion or defibrillation, intravenous infusion of crystalloid fluid, airway management and ventilation with oxygen, and chest compression. Torsades de pointes may be treated by intravenous magnesium, electrical overdrive pacing or pharmacologic overdrive with isoproterenol, and antiarrhythmic agents such as phenytoin or lidocaine. As for emergent synchronized cardioversion, the initial energy level for atrial fibrillation may be 200 joules,[19] although higher energy levels for cardioversion are appropriate when cancer patients are significantly overweight or have concomitant effusions. Lower initial energy levels (ie, 50 to 100 joules) should be used to for atrial flutter.

Pericardial Tamponade

Pericardial tamponade occurs when hemodynamics is impaired by accumulation of fluid in the pericardial cavity. Not including hemopericardium, the etiology of pericardial tamponade is usually either malignant or infectious. Infectious causes of pericardial tamponade include pericardial abscess[20] and *Candida* pericarditis.[21] Excess pericardial fluid accumulation due to malignancy can be caused by (1) obstruction of lymphatic drainage and (2) tumor nodules on pericardial surfaces secreting excess fluid. Pericardial fluid cytologic tests have a 70 to 80% diagnostic yield for malignant pericardial effusion.

Pericardial tamponade can be caused by a number of cancers. The most common malignancy that actually arises from the pericardium is mesothelioma. Cancers in the chest, such as carcinoma of the lung and malignant thymoma, may extend directly into the pericardium. Yet the most frequent routes of spread to the pericardium by cancer are by retrograde lymphangitic spread or hematogenous dissemination, which occur frequently in cancers arising in the chest (eg, breast and lung carcinomas). Malignant melanoma is the most likely cancer to metastasize to the heart. Leukemias and lymphomas (both Hodgkin's and non-Hodgkin's) may cause pericardial effusions as well[22].

Usually pericardial effusion is a late complication in patients with known metastatic disease although it may occasionally be the first clinical manifestation of malignancy. Less than one third of patients with malignant pericardial effusion are symptomatic. The most common complaints are shortness of breath, dyspnea on exertion, orthopnea, pleuritic chest pain and general weakness. Physical findings may range from normal to hemodynamic collapse. Signs of compromised cardiac output include tachypnea, hypotension, tachycardia, jugular venous distention and peripheral edema. The severity of hemodynamic impairment is determined by both the amount of pericardial fluid and the rate of fluid accumulation. Exaggerated decrease in systolic blood pressure with inspiration (pulsus paradoxus) is a classic finding of cardiac tamponade, but it is nonspecific because it can also be present in patients with significant lung disease, or cor pulmonale.

In the course of investigating the signs and symptoms of cancer patients with pericardial tamponade, electrical alternans in electrocardiographs or widening of the cardiac silhouette on plain chest radiographs are very helpful findings when present. (Figure 1.) Computed tomography (CT) or magnetic resonance imaging (MRI) studies provide information on the size, location, and presence of loculation of pericardial effusions but do not provide adequate assessment of the hemodynamic significance of the effusions. In contrast, two-dimensional echocardiography can not only diagnose pericardial effusion but can also evaluate its hemodynamic significance (ie, determine whether there is cardiac tamponade). Compression of the right atrium, diastolic collapse of the right ventricle, and a side-to-side or front-to-back movement of the heart (cardiac rocking) are common echocardiographic signs of pericardial tamponade. Doppler study of respiration-induced alterations in the blood flow across the mitral valve is also helpful in evaluating the hemodynamic significance of pericardial effusions.

Initial management of a malignant pericardial effusion depends on its hemodynamic significance. In patients with severe symptoms and compromise in cardiac output, echocardiography-guided pericardiocentesis may be performed in the emergency center or intensive care unit. Placement of a drainage catheter into the pericardial space may be required to prevent rapid recurrence of tamponade. The catheter

can remain in place until the pericardial fluid drainage is <50 mL over 24 hours.

Long-term management aims at preventing reaccumulation of pericardial fluid, which occurs in >50% of patients with malignant effusions. In patients with rapidly reaccumulating effusion with significant hemodynamic compromise, creating a pleuropericardial window using one of a variety of approaches can help the patient to avoid repeated pericardiocentesis. The pleuropericardial window procedure is usually performed in an operating room, but can also

be performed at the intensive care unit using local anesthesia (eg, the use of a percutaneous intrapericardial balloon catheter to create a pleuropericardial window).[23] Creating a pericardioperitoneal shunt through a laparoscopic transdiaphragmatic approach is another treatment option.[24] In hemodynamically stable patients, pericardial radioactive colloid, systemic chemotherapy or external-beam irradiation may be used for tumors that are sensitive to these treatments. Instillation of chemotherapeutic agents or sclerosing agents into the pericardial cavity can

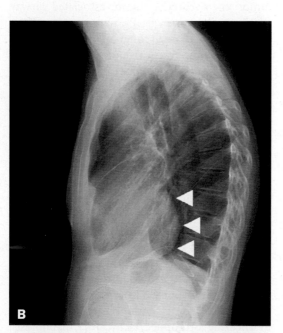
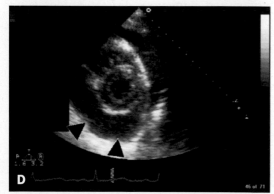
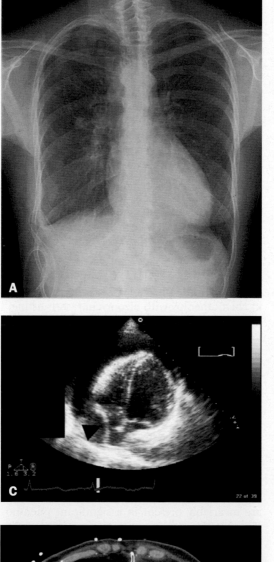
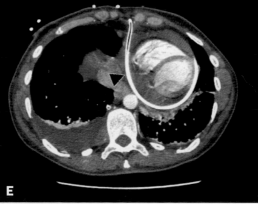

FIGURE 1 Cardiac tamponade by malignant pericardial effusion. A 48 year-old female with non–small cell lung cancer and malignant right pleural effusion presented with dyspnea and mild hypotension to our emergency center. *A*, Chest radiography showed a small residual right pleural effusion and the presence of an indwelling Denver pleural catheter. *B*, Mild posterior fullness of the cardiac silhouette was apparent in the lateral view (white arrow heads). *C*, Two-dimensional echocardiography demonstrated right atrial collapse (black arrow head) and *D*, a large circumferential pericardial effusion. A pericardial catheter was inserted emergently to drain the pericardial effusion. *E*, The pericardial catheter was shown on the CT scan image (black arrow head).

also prevent reaccumulation of pericardial fluid in many patients.[25]

Acute Airway Obstruction

Acute airway obstruction usually involves the upper airway. Nonmalignant causes of upper airway obstruction in cancer patients include foreign body or food aspiration, severe tracheomalacia, tracheal stenosis, airway edema, and fungal, viral, or bacterial infections. Upper airway obstruction due to angioedema can occur in 2 to 3% of patients receiving paclitaxel.[26] Causes of airway obstruction related to cancer include tumor encroachment, tumor-associated airway edema, or hemorrhage. Primary tumors of the head and neck (base of tongue, larynx, hypopharynx, thyroid, or trachea) and lung can directly extend to the upper airway and cause obstruction. Metastatic spread of cancers to the neck or mediastinum can also cause obstruction of the upper airway.

For the lower airway, the most common cause of obstruction is primary bronchogenic carcinoma. Other, less common causes are metastases from cancers of the colon, breast, thyroid, or kidney; melanoma; lymphoma; or sarcoma. Severe bronchospasm due to release of hormone mediators is a major component of the acute carcinoid syndrome.

Dyspnea is the primary symptom of airway obstruction. As the airway diameter narrows, dyspnea on exertion will progress to dyspnea at rest. Further progression of obstruction will lead to wheezing, orthopnea, tachycardia, diaphoresis, stridor, and respiratory distress. Stridor is an ominous sign that can rapidly be followed by bradycardia, obtundation, and death.

The oral cavity should be quickly inspected to exclude the presence of foreign body or food. Clinical diagnosis of upper airway obstruction is often confirmed by direct visualization with either a laryngoscope or bronchoscope. Endotracheal intubation may be difficult, and laryngoscopy or bronchoscopy may be necessary to guide the endotracheal tube. Severe upper airway obstruction that is immediately reversible may require tracheotomy. Other supportive therapies include corticosteroids, bronchodilators, and helium-oxygen mixtures.

For patients with lower airway obstruction, chest radiographs identify the obstruction in 75% of cases. In other cases, CT scan of the chest can usually reveal the diagnosis. (Figure 2.) Interventional pulmonary treatments using rigid or flexible bronchoscopes and may involve balloon bronchoplasty,[27] placement of stents,[28,29] laser bronchoplasty,[29,30] cryosurgery,[31] and brachytherapy.[37] Other surgical interventions may be considered as appropriate for the patient's cancer prognosis, functional performance status, and comorbid conditions.

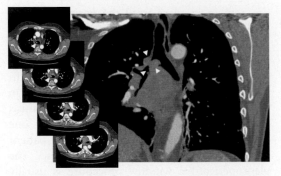

FIGURE 2 Carinal mass obstructing right main stem bronchus. A 65 year-old man with adenocarcinoma of the lower esophagus presented with subacute onset of dyspnea on exertion. Computed tomography of the chest revealed a subcarinal mass encasing the right main stem bronchus with endobronchial extension (white arrow heads) that caused obstruction of right main stem bronchus.

Pneumothorax

In cancer patients, procedures often associated with iatrogenic pneumothorax include percutaneous lung biopsy, transbronchial biopsy, and insertion of central venous lines. Even nasogastric tube placement may occasionally result in pneumothorax. Secondary Spontaneous pneumothorax is most often due to chronic obstructive pulmonary diseases, and may be common among smokers with lung cancers and head-and-neck cancers. Primary and metastatic pulmonary neoplasms may also lead to spontaneous pneumothorax. Pneumothorax has been reported in chemotherapy with bleomycin,[33] carmustine,[34] and lomustine. Rupture of mycetoma (aspergillosis, coccidioidomycosis, cryptococcosis, and mucormycosis) into the pleural space may result in pneumothorax. Other infectious agents associated with pneumothorax include *Klebsiella, Staphylococcus,* and *Pseudomonas* species, jiroveci (formerly Pneumocystis carinii), and *Mycobacterium* species.

Patients with underlying lung disease often cannot tolerate decreases in vital capacity and have a higher risk for respiratory failure when pneumothorax occurs. Dyspnea and chest pain are invariably present in a significant pneumothorax. Other symptoms, such as cough, hemoptysis, or orthopnea, are less common. Small pneumothoraces (<20% of lung volume) are undetectable on physical examination. In a large pneumothorax, examination usually reveals absent or decreased breath sounds on auscultation, absent tactile fremitus, and hyperresonance of the affected side of the chest. Deviation of the trachea to the side contralateral to the affected lung and decreased movement of the affected hemithorax may also be present. In a tension pneumothorax, increased central venous and intrapleural pressures may manifest as jugular venous distension. When venous return and cardiac output are impeded by the tension pneumothorax, hypotension, severe hypoxemia, and respiratory acidosis will occur.

Chest radiographs are the most valuable diagnostic tools for pneumothorax. Pneumothorax is diagnosed when a chest radiograph reveals a visceral pleural line beyond which there are no lung markings. About one-third of pneumothoraces are undetected on semi-erect and supine chest radiographs.[35] In a small pneumothorax, the pleural line may be difficult to see. Therefore, a good-quality upright chest radiograph and a bright light for viewing are needed, and in some cases, expiratory films may be helpful. Recently, digital processing of digitized chest radiographs to enhance edges are becoming popular to help to detect visceral pleural lines.

For small pneumothoraces without significant symptoms, close observation will suffice. Serial chest radiographs should be obtained several hours after the initial radiograph to rule out further expansion of the pneumothorax. If the small pneumothorax is stable in size, the patient may be discharged with appropriate instructions and follow-up arrangement, and scheduled for repeat chest radiographs in 12 to 48 hours.[36]

Intrapleural catheter aspiration may be performed for symptomatic pneumothoraces, rapidly expanding pneumothoraces, and pneumothoraces of more than 15% of the ipsilateral pleural space (Figure 3). A pneumothorax

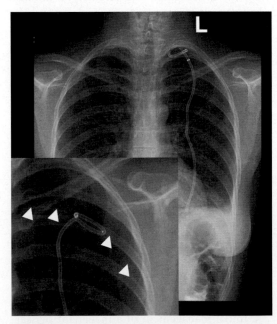

FIGURE 3 Pneumothorax. A 38 year-old female suffered pneumothorax during attempts for central venous catheter insertion. A small residual pneumothorax persisted despite placement of a pig-tail catheter into the pleural cavity connected to a Heimlich valve (enlarged inset: the pleural line indicated by the arrow heads). The left lung became fully expanded after repositioning of the pig-tail catheter (full chest radiograph).

that fails to reexpand or recurs after catheter aspiration requires tube thoracostomy. Heimlich valves are often used. Initial treatment with tube thoracostomy is indicated for a traumatic pneumothorax and hemothorax, a pneumothorax occupying more than 15% of the ipsilateral pleural space with retained secretions or lung infections on the affected side, or a pneumothorax that developed while on mechanical ventilation. Thoracotomy or thoracoscopic surgical repair may be considered for patients with only partial lung expansion 5 to 7 days after a tube thoracostomy and for patients with a persistent air leak due to bronchopleural fistula. Thoracoscopic pleurodesis with talc or other drugs, thoracoscopic pleurectomy, thoracoscopic pleural abrasion, or chest tube pleurodesis may be considered to prevent recurrence.[37]

Thromboembolic Diseases

Venous Thromboembolism

The association between malignancy and venous thromboembolism (VTE) is well established; numerous studies have demonstrated that almost all types of cancer may be associated with an increased risk for thromboembolic disease. VTE is the second leading cause of death in patients with cancer. VTE comprises two related conditions: deep venous thrombosis (DVT) and pulmonary embolism (PE). DVT is often a precursor of PE. Unfortunately, even one and a half centuries after Armand Trousseau reported the association between VTE and malignancy in 1865, the pathophysiology of VTE remains poorly understood.

Compared with non-cancer patients, cancer patients have higher rates of initial thrombosis, recurrence of thrombosis, and fatal PE.[38] Patients with malignancy and no underlying comorbid condition have a 15 to 20% risk of developing thromboembolic disease. Compared with patients without cancer undergoing similar procedures, cancer patients undergoing surgery have two to three times the risk of developing postoperative VTE.[39] The most common cancers associated with VTE include prostate, colon, lung, and brain cancer (in men), and breast, lung, and ovarian cancer (in women).[40,41] In one retrospective analysis, pancreatic cancer was also associated with a high incidence of VTE and a 12.1% per-hospitalization risk of VTE.[42] In another study, genitourinary and gynecologic malignancies were commonly associated with VTE.[43] The incidence of DVT after surgery for brain tumors has been reported to be 1.6 to 4%. PE occurs in as many as 5% of patients after neurosurgery, and the associated mortality rate is 9 to 50%.[44,45]

Extrinsic factors play an important role in cancer patients' predisposition to VTE. These include cytotoxic chemotherapeutic agents which increase the risk 6.5-fold[54] hormonal treatments (estrogens and anti-estrogens), radiotherapy, and central venous catheters. Radiotherapy causes endothelial damage, making a nidus for the formation of platelet clumping.

The presence of a central venous catheter, commonly used in cancer patients to facilitate chemotherapy administration and blood draws, is an independent risk factor for VTE and carries the same weight as other risk factors, such as malignancy, chemotherapy, and oral contraceptive therapy.[46] Approximately 13 to 35% of patients with subclavian venous catheters develop axillary-subclavian vein thrombosis, with catheterization estimated to account for 39% of all subclavian vein thromboses.[47] The question of whether cancer patients with central venous catheters should receive prophylaxis with warfarin is controversial, and a need for more randomized studies is recognized.[48]

Patients with a prior episode of VTE are at increased risk for recurrence, especially if other risk factors are present. In a case-control study, patients with prior VTE had eight times the risk of a subsequent episode compared to patients without prior VTE.[49]

Diagnostic Strategies in the Emergency Setting

In the emergency room, the diagnostic evaluation of patients with suspected VTE should include history and complete physical examination, radiologic imaging, and, as more recent evidence suggests, laboratory studies. The clinician needs to be astute to elicit additional risk factors that would predispose the cancer patient to VTE, as discussed previously.

In the case of DVT, the patient may be asymptomatic or have complaints such as pain or swelling in the involved extremity. It is difficult to diagnose PE in cancer patients because the signs and symptoms are vague and difficult to differentiate from those related to the malignancy process or side effects of cancer treatments. The most common presenting symptoms of PE are dyspnea, tachypnea, and pleuritic chest pain.[50,51] Sometimes, fever and a pleural rub may be detected. When massive PE occurs, increase in pulmonary vascular resistance and right ventricular afterload causes right ventricular failure. The patient may have angina due to right ventricle ischemia. Cardiovascular collapse and death may ultimately occur following development of ischemia, right ventricular dysfunction, tricuspid regurgitation, and forward flow failure. Hemoptysis is rare and is associated with pulmonary infarction, a complication happening 12 to 36 hours after PE.

Although DVT in the lower extremities occurs in fewer than half of all patients with PE,[52] the lower extremities should be examined for evidence of thrombosis. Assessment of oxygen saturation by pulse oximetry or arterial blood gas measurements and calculation of alveolar-arterial oxygen gradient can be helpful. A chest radiograph is needed to exclude causes of pulmonary symptoms other than PE. An electrocardiogram commonly shows sinus tachycardia, inverted T waves, or nonspecific ST-T wave abnormalities, but the S_1-Q_3-T_3 pattern classical for PE is uncommon. Other electrocardiographic changes associated with right ventricular abnormalities such as right axis deviation, atrial arrhythmia, P-pulmonale, and right bundle branch block may occur. Electrocardiography, chest radiography, and measurement of arterial blood gases, although routinely performed in patients with clinically suspected PE, may not be of value in confirming the diagnosis.[53]

D-dimer, a marker of endogenous fibrinolysis, has been studied in a variety of settings to determine whether it can be used alone or in combination with radiologic studies to exclude the diagnosis of VTE. Elevated D-dimer levels usually occur in patients with VTE but may also be elevated in other conditions, including infection, trauma, and malignancy. Several studies in the 1990s showed that the D-dimer has a high negative predictive value and is a sensitive but nonspecific marker of VTE. In a meta-analysis of studies from 1983 to 2003 comparing results of different D-dimer assays with findings on objective tests for VTE (compression ultrasonography, venography, and lung scanning) in patients with suspected DVT or PE, Stein and colleagues concluded that the D-dimer enzyme-linked immunosorbent assay (ELISA) had 95% sensitivity and negative likelihood ratios (about 0.1) for excluding DVT and PE.[54]

The usefulness of a D-dimer test coupled with clinical suspicion of DVT was tested in a study of 1,096 outpatients.[55] The patients were divided into two groups by using the "Clinical Model for Predicting the Pretest Probability of Deep-Vein Thrombosis".[56] Completely normal findings on D-dimer testing may exclude the possibility of VTE in a low-risk population. Recent data suggest that D-dimer testing may be also be used to determine if a patient has a recurrent DVT. Plasma D-dimer measurement seems to provide a simple method for excluding acute recurrent DVT in symptomatic patients.[57]

Venous compression ultrasonography is the radiologic diagnostic test of choice for suspected DVT.[58] Normally, the veins are compressible. In the presence of a DVT, the vein is non-compressible.[59] Contrast venography remains the reference standard for diagnosis of DVT, but is rarely used because it is invasive, expensive, and not readily available.[53]

The degree of clinical suspicion should guide the clinician in the diagnostic work-up of VTE, especially PE. A patient with a high clinical suspicion of PE should undergo imaging testing immediately. D-dimer is not the diagnostic test of choice when there is a high clinical suspicion of PE but may be useful if the clinical probability is low.[60,61]

The radionuclide ventilation-perfusion (V/Q) scan is a common initial test for diagnosing PE. When V/Q scans are interpreted as having an "intermediate probability" of PE, other tests such as spiral CT, MRI, and pulmonary angiography may be indicated to further investigate the diagnosis of PE. Spiral CT and MRI are relatively new diagnostic modalities with sensitivities and specificities of about 80% and 90%, respectively.[62,63] Despite those rates, PE in the distal pulmonary vasculature is not reliably detected with these modalities[64]; the negative predictive value of spiral CT angiography for PE is 98% (Figure 4).[65] Spiral CT is increasingly becoming the diagnostic method of choice for acute PE at many institutions. Moores and colleagues performed a meta-analysis of the literature from 1966 through 2004, assessing the safety of withholding anticoagulation in patients with suspected PE and negative results on spiral CT, and concluded that it was safe to withhold anticoagulation after negative spiral CT results since the rate of subsequent VTE was the same as that seen after negative results on conventional pulmonary angiography.[66] Nevertheless, the gold standard for the diagnosis of PE is pulmonary angiography, which should be considered in patients with strong clinical suspicion of PE and negative initial diagnostic tests.[67]

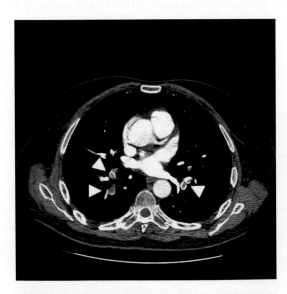

FIGURE 1 Bilateral pulmonary embolism. A CT chest angiogram demonstrated multiple filling defects in the lumen of pulmonary vasculature on both sides (arrow heads) in a pancreatic cancer patient with chest pain and dyspnea.

Treatment Options in the Emergency Setting

In cases of massive PE, hemodynamic instability and hypoxia must be treated emergently with intravenous crystalloid fluids, inotropic agents, and oxygen administration by mask or endotracheal tube. For patients in whom PE is strongly suspected, heparin or low-molecular-weight heparin (LMWH) should be administered unless clinically contraindicated. Unfractionated heparin is administered in a bolus injection of 80 U/kg, and then a continuous intravenous infusion of 18 U/kg/h is used, adjusted to maintain the activated partial thromboplastin time at 1.5 to 2.0 times the baseline control value.[68] LMWHs are alternatives for unfractionated heparin[69] with the same or lower risk of bleeding complications as unfractionated heparin,[70] and have the advantage of not requiring intravenous access and partial thromboplastin time monitoring. Thrombolysis is generally considered in patients with massive PE and hemodynamic instability.[71] Criteria for thrombolytic therapy are emboli occlusion of more than 40% of the pulmonary vasculature,[72] echocardiographic evidence of right ventricular dysfunction, and severe hypoxemia.[73] Compared to anticoagulation alone, thrombolytic therapy doubles the rate of major complications, including intracranial hemorrhage.[74] Although thrombolysis accelerates fibrinolysis and clot dissolution and improves cardiopulmonary function, a definite beneficial effect on mortality remains to be demonstrated by large-scale studies.[75] Surgical and catheter embolectomy is reserved for patients in whom the usual treatment approaches fail.

In hemodynamically stable patients with VTE, treatment should begin with administration of unfractionated heparin or LMWHs to prevent thromboembolic recurrence. The therapy should begin immediately after the diagnosis is established. Studies comparing the LMWHs and unfractionated heparin have found that they are equally effective, but LMWHs have the advantage of potential outpatient administration and no need for coagulation laboratory monitoring.[40,76,77] For cancer patients, anticoagulation therapy should be continued until the malignancy is no longer active,[78] and LMWHs may be superior to warfarin in the prevention of recurrent VTE.[79] The high drug cost of LMWHs may be offset by the cost of coagulation laboratory monitoring required for wafarin therapy.

Outpatient treatment of DVT with LMWHs and close monitoring has become standard practice. Patients treated on an outpatient basis need to have follow-up with their primary physicians within 3 to 5 days for monitoring of the platelet count and coagulation parameters and decide whether or not to transition to oral anticoagulation.[80] Outpatient treatment of PE has been investigated in a limited number of studies of the general patient population. Patients with low

risk according to a quantitative risk score were treated successfully in the outpatient setting with LMWH.[81] Another prospective cohort study showed that outpatient LMWH treatment was feasible and safe for patients with non-massive PE.[82] Outpatient treatment of PE needs to be investigated further in cancer patients. Exclusion criteria for the outpatient treatment of VTE with LMWH should include the need for hospitalization (because of the severity of the disease and comorbidities), active bleeding, and severe coagulopathy.

Patients with VTE who are severely thrombocytopenic, who are at risk of serious bleeding, who are actively bleeding, or who are allergic to heparin products present a therapeutic challenge to the emergency center physician. The accepted indications for the placement of an inferior vena caval filter include active bleeding, risk of serious bleeding that precludes the use of anticoagulant therapy, and failure of anticoagulant therapy. However, the use of inferior vena caval filters is associated with an increased long-term risk of recurrent DVT despite concurrent oral anticoagulant therapy.[83]

Hemostatic Disorders and Acute Hemorrhage

After organ failure due to tumor invasion and infection, bleeding is the third most common cause of death in patients with metastatic cancer and the second most common cause of death in patients with hematologic malignancies.[84,85] Causes of hemorrhage in cancer patients include coagulopathies due to the malignancy or its treatment, tumor invasion of vascular structures, and bleeding from the tumor itself.

In the hemorrhaging cancer patient, no matter where the bleeding site is, the immediate treatment goal is to achieve hemostasis, establish hemodynamic stability, determine the cause, and correct any coagulopathy. Prompt action on the part of the emergency physician will limit morbidity and mortality.

In the emergency setting, direct compression of the bleeding vessel or site should be applied whenever feasible while the cardiopulmonary status is rapidly assessed. Intravenous fluid resuscitation is vital to maintain intravascular volume, cardiac output, and adequate vital organ perfusion. Isotonic crystalloid fluids (lactated Ringer's solution, normal saline, etc.) are the appropriate first-line agents because colloids (eg, hetastarch) have not been proven to improve survival compared with crystalloids.[86] Coagulopathy and thrombocytopenia should be corrected by transfusion of blood products as quickly as possible. Whether to transfuse red blood cells depends on hemodynamic stability, estimated blood loss, persistence of hemorrhage, and comorbid conditions (eg, ischemic heart disease and cerebrovascular disease). Typed and cross-matched red blood cells are preferred, but in the case of massive life-threatening hemorrhage, non-cross-matched type-specific blood or type-O blood may have to be administered during emergent resuscitation. Specific procedures to control bleeding, such as balloon tamponade, embolization, or surgical ligation of bleeding vessels, should be performed rapidly.

Massive Hemoptysis

Massive hemoptysis can be defined as expectoration of 100 mL of blood in a single episode or more than 600 mL of blood over a 24-hour period.[87,88] Mortality increases with increased bleeding. Nearly a third of patients with massive hemoptysis have a fatal hemorrhage.[89] Death results from asphyxiation rather than exsanguination.

Patients at greatest risk for massive hemoptysis are those with tumors involving the airway (eg, endobronchial tumor or tumor invading the pulmonary or bronchial vessels). Other causes of massive hemoptysis include infection (eg, necrotizing pneumonia or lung abscess due to various organisms, including mycobacteria and fungi), PE with infarction, and bronchiectasis. Hemostatic abnormalities, such as severe thrombocytopenia and coagulopathy, may result from malignancy or its treatment, and impaired hemostasis will worsen pulmonary hemorrhage. Hemoptysis may be the presenting symptom of malignancy, especially in patients with lung cancer. Metastatic disease from breast cancer, melanoma, laryngeal cancer, sarcoma, or lymphoma may also lead to massive hemoptysis.[90]

The airway should be protected. Intubation is recommended for patients with rapid bleeding, hemodynamic instability, severe dyspnea, ventilatory impairment, or hypoxia.[87] Patients with hemodynamic instability also require volume resuscitation, administration of supplemental oxygen, correction of underlying coagulopathies, and cough suppressants. Attempts should be made to localize the site of bleeding, and the patient should be positioned bleeding side down to prevent aspiration of blood into the unaffected lung. Maintenance of the airway is important, and the patient should be intubated in preparation for bronchoscopy. If the bleeding can be localized, unilateral intubation should be done to protect the non-bleeding lung.[91] A balloon occlusion (Fogarty) catheter may be used temporarily to tamponade the bleeding. Emergency thoracic surgery and pulmonary medicine consultations should be arranged.[92] Nonsurgical options include arterial embolization of bronchial arteries,[93] bronchoscopic laser photocoagulation and electrocautery,[29,94–96] or radiation treatment.[93,97,98]

Carotid Artery Rupture

Rupture of the carotid artery (or "carotid blowout") is one of the most devastating complications of head and neck cancer and its treatment and is now considered a syndrome. Carotid blowout syndrome (CBS) is defined as the rupture of the extracranial carotid arteries or their major branches. It is most commonly seen in squamous cell carcinoma of the head and neck. Additional risk factors include previous neck dissection, irradiation, previous CBS with stent placement, and wound infection.[99–102]

Carotid artery rupture often occurs as a sudden and massive arterial spurting. Occasionally, ominous minor and transient sentinel bleeding episodes herald the massive carotid blowout. In some cases, bleeding through a fistula into the esophagus, trachea, hypopharynx or pharynx may masquerade as massive hematemesis or hemoptysis. Even with prompt management, many such patients will rapidly deteriorate with hypotension, hypovolemic shock, and loss of consciousness, ending in death.

Prompt control of the bleeding site is key in reducing mortality. Firm, constant pressure with a gauze bandage at the site of bleeding is mandatory until the patient arrives in the operating room or interventional radiology suite. Initial management should also include airway management and aggressive fluid resuscitation. Large-bore intravenous access with crystalloid infusion should be immediate. Transfusion of packed red blood cells should be started promptly. Vasopressor agents may be necessary for hemodynamic support until the bleeding can be stopped. The bleeding very rarely stops spontaneously. With emergent operative ligation of the common carotid artery or internal carotid artery, a mortality rate of 40% and a neurologic morbidity rate of 60% have been reported.[103–105] More recently, management of carotid blowout syndrome with intraluminal balloon occlusion and endovascular stenting has shown promising results: reported morbidity and mortality rates are less than 10%.[106–108]

Splenic Rupture

Acute leukemia, chronic myelogenous leukemia and non-Hodgkin's lymphoma are malignancies commonly associated with spontaneous splenic rupture. Other associated malignancies include hairy cell leukemia, Hodgkin's lymphoma, gastric cancer, prostate cancer, and lung cancer. The mechanism of spontaneous splenic rupture is not clear but may involve minor trauma to the spleen, infiltration of the splenic capsule by malignant cells, severe splenomegaly, splenic infarction, thrombocytopenia, and coagulopathy.

Pain in the left shoulder or abdomen (left upper quadrant), tachycardia, and hypotension are typical signs and symptoms of splenic rupture, the severity of which depends on the extent of bleeding. Diagnostic peritoneal lavage is rarely used in non-trauma cases. Imaging studies often can provide a definitive diagnosis of splenic rupture. The diagnostic study of choice is CT, which is noninvasive and can provide detailed information about the severity of retroperitoneal or intraperitoneal hemorrhage. Splenic rupture can also be diagnosed by ultrasonography,[109] the portability of which allows bedside evaluation for hemodynamically unstable patients.

Prompt splenectomy is indicated for patients with hematologic malignancies having splenic rupture because the mortality rate is high without surgery. In selected patients with contraindications to surgery, selective arterial embolization or external-beam irradiation of the ruptured site may control bleeding.[110] Patients who are not surgical candidates should be supported with intravenous crystalloid fluid, supplemental oxygen, pain medications, and blood products.

Gastrointestinal Hemorrhage

Upper gastrointestinal bleeding is a common problem, both in the general patient population and in cancer patients. Fewer than 20% of cases of upper gastrointestinal bleeding can be attributed to cancer[111–113]; most cases of upper gastrointestinal bleeding are due to non-cancer causes, such as hemorrhagic gastritis and peptic ulcer disease, esophagitis, esophageal varices, and Mallory-Weiss tears. When cancer is the cause, the malignancies most commonly implicated include adenocarcinoma, lymphoma or sarcoma of the gastrointestinal tract, and metastatic tumors.

Treatment of upper gastrointestinal bleeding in cancer patients should address the cause. Fluid resuscitation and blood transfusions are warranted to maintain hemodynamic stability. Correction of coagulopathy is necessary, and, if the patient is actively bleeding, platelet transfusions should be given to maintain the platelet count above 50,000 per microliter. H_2-antagonists or proton-pump inhibitors are routinely given to reduce or neutralize gastric acid, but this has not been shown to stop active bleeding or prevent rebleeding.[114] Endoscopic therapies such as epinephrine injections, bicap electrocoagulation, heater probe, and the argon plasma laser coagulator may be used to achieve hemostasis.

Retroperitoneal Hemorrhage

Any damage to retroperitoneal organs (eg, the kidneys, adrenal glands, pancreas, duodenum, major blood vessels) may cause retroperitoneal hemorrhage. Retroperitoneal or intraperitoneal invasive procedures (including radiofrequency coagulation for treatment of liver tumors[115]) and placement of a central venous catheter through a femoral vessel can also cause severe retroperitoneal hemorrhage. Malignancies rarely cause spontaneous retroperitoneal hemorrhage; cases involving renal cell carcinoma (primary or metastatic),[116] angiolipoma,[117] or adrenal-gland tumors[118] have been reported. Hemostatic abnormalities are predisposing factors for spontaneous retroperitoneal hemorrhage.

Retroperitoneal hemorrhage causes nonspecific signs and symptoms that may vary according to the rate of, and the site of, bleeding. Patients may present with abdominal pain, a tender mass in the flank, tachycardia, and hypotension. Some may have hematuria or hematochezia if the blood somehow finds its way into the ureter or gastrointestinal tract. Diagnosis of retroperitoneal hemorrhage is difficult on the basis of clinical findings, and a high level of clinical suspicion and early imaging studies are keys to successful diagnosis and treatment. CT of the abdomen and pelvis is the noninvasive study most commonly used to diagnose retroperitoneal bleeding. (Figure 5.) Ultrasonography can be performed at the bedside for rapid diagnosis of unstable patients.

In the emergency center, stabilizing treatments for acute retroperitoneal hemorrhage—such as intravenous crystalloid fluid, blood transfusion, and correction of coagulopathy and thrombocytopenia—should be started immediately. The patient should be monitored closely for hemodynamic stability. In life-threatening cases of acute retroperitoneal hemorrhage, most patients require emergent laparotomy and surgical removal of the bleeding tumor or organ. Selective arterial embolization may control the bleeding of a renal lesion since renal cell carcinomas are often hypervascular. Preoperative embolization may also help minimize intraoperative blood loss. In hemodynamically stable patients with subacute bleeding, external-beam irradiation of the bleeding tumor may be performed.[119]

Epistaxis

Epistaxis is common in patients with malignancies, especially in those who are thrombocytopenic or coagulopathic. Epistaxis is the most frequent otolaryngologic complication in patients undergoing leukemia treatment or bone marrow transplantation.[120] Most minor episodes of epistaxis result from drying of the nasal mucosa and local trauma to the anterior nasal vessels.[121] Epistaxis in cancer patients is usually not life-threatening. The physician's approach should be to maintain an adequate airway while reassuring the patient. If blood is aspirated and then expectorated or swallowed and then vomited, epistaxis may mimic hemoptysis or hematemesis, respectively. Maneuvers to control the bleeding may include pinching the nose, applying an ice pack to the face and nose, and applying pressure to the gingival buccal junction above the maxillary incisors to compress the anterior nasal artery. In cases of more severe bleeding, topical vasoconstrictors/decongestants [eg, phenylephrine hydrochloride, oxymetazoline] can be used to constrict the mucosal vessels to stop the bleeding. Electrocautery may also be used if the bleeding site can be identified. Nasal packing may be used for anterior bleeds. Posterior artery bleeding necessitates posterior packing and endoscopic evaluation. Correction of thrombocytopenia and coagulopathy by transfusion of blood products is essential to control the bleeding.

Urinary Tract Hemorrhage

Hematuria is common in patients with cancer, and it may be massive and life-threatening, requiring aggressive management. Causes include tumor involving the bladder, chemotherapy, radiation-induced or viral hemorrhagic cystitis,

and severe coagulopathy. Bladder and prostate carcinomas are the tumors that most often cause massive hematuria. Cervical and rectal carcinomas may also cause bleeding if they invade the bladder.[122] The oxazaphosphorine drugs (cyclophosphamide, ifosfamide, and busulfan) are the chemotherapy agents most commonly associated with hemorrhagic cystitis.[123,124] Prophylactic measures aimed at minimizing the formation of the offending metabolite and its contact with the bladder epithelium include aggressive hydration to encourage frequent urination, continuous bladder irrigation, and administration of the uroprotective agent 2-mercaptoethane sulfonate.[122] Patients who have undergone bone marrow transplantation may develop severe hemorrhagic cystitis associated with adenovirus and parvovirus infections.[125,126] Pelvic irradiation may result in bladder complications, including massive hematuria; the tumors most commonly associated with this finding include bladder, rectal, cervical, and prostate carcinoma.

Massive hematuria may lead to intravesicular clot formation and urinary retention. In such cases, after a urology consultation, the bladder should be lavaged to evacuate clots via a three-way Foley catheter, and continuous bladder irrigation with normal saline should be continued until bleeding subsides. Aggressive volume resuscitation with crystalloid intravenous fluid and packed red blood cell transfusion may be necessary. Any coagulation abnormalities must be promptly addressed. If hemorrhage persists, formalin, alum, prostaglandins, phenol, iced saline, or silver nitrate may be instilled in the bladder in an attempt to stop the bleeding. Should conservative measures fail, surgical measures may be required to control bleeding.[127]

Central Nervous System Emergencies

Altered Mental Status

"Altered mental status" is a general phrase describing reduced levels of mentation, including impaired cognition, diminished attention, altered level of consciousness, and/or reduced awareness, and may range from intermittent mild disturbance to coma. Altered mental status is a common chief complaint in emergency departments, accounting for 4 to 10% of emergency visits in the general population, and may be a confounding complaint with other clinical presentations (Table 3). Elderly patients are more likely (up to 30%) to present with altered mental status for emergency care than are younger patients.[128]

The evaluation of altered mental status in an emergency setting requires complete evaluation of the patient. A reliable history is often not attainable from the patient, and family members and/or bystanders offer important components

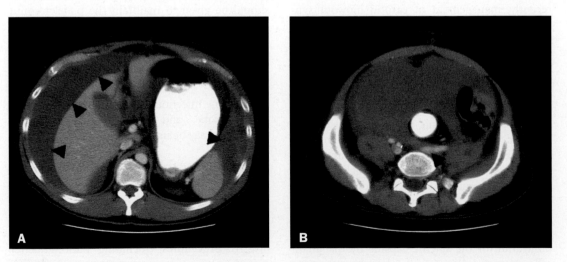

FIGURE 5 Retroperitoneal bleeding from left iliac artery with hemoperitoneum. A 44 year-old male with retroperitoneal malignant fibrous histiocytoma had surgical resection of the cancer 6 weeks prior to presentation at the emergency center with mild abdominal pain and hypotension. CT scan of the abdomen demonstrated hemoperitoneum (left panel: arrow heads) and extravasation of intravenous contrast from the left iliac artery (right panel: arrow head).

Table 3 Differential Diagnosis of Altered Mental Status in a Cancer Patient
Hypoxia
Hypoglycemia or hyperglycemia
Thiamine deficiency
Hypothermia or hyperthermia
Seizures
Toxins (medications, illicit drugs, alcohol)
Electrolyte abnormalities
Infectious causes (meningitis, encephalitis, abscess)
Stroke
Subarachnoid hemorrhage
Intracerebral hemorrhage
Tumors
Metabolic encepholapathyencephalopathy (hepatic, uremic, sepsis, etc.)
Hypercapnia
Vasculitis

of the history. Underlying medical conditions—including diabetes mellitus, hypertension, coronary artery disease, chronic obstructive pulmonary disease, and alcohol abuse—may point to a possible cause (Table 3).[129]

Patients with altered mental status should be examined to ensure that their vital signs are sufficient to support brain function. The "ABCs"—airway, breathing, and circulation—are of utmost importance. Blood pressure, respiration rate, and oxygen saturation must be checked, and testing must be done to ensure that the patient is not hypoglycemic. Once these basic functions are examined, a complete physical examination, including a complete neurologic examination, should be completed. Essential laboratory studies should be ordered, including a complete blood cell count, prothrombin time, partial thromboplastin time, chemistry panel, toxicologic screen, and blood cultures.[130] Arrhythmias and acute myocardial infarction should be ruled out by obtaining an electrocardiogram and measuring appropriate cardiac enzymes. Arterial blood gas values should be obtained if hypoxemia, hypercapnia, drug intoxications, or metabolic encephalopathies are being considered. A head CT scan or a lumbar puncture should be emergently obtained if intracranial pressure or meningitis is considered in the differential diagnosis.

In all patients with coma, a 100 mg intravenous dose of thiamine, an important cofactor for several enzymes, should be replaced since its depletion can lead to Wernicke's encephalopathy. If opiate overdose is a possible cause, intravenous naloxone, 0.4 to 2.0 mg, should be given. Flumazenil, a specific benzodiazepine receptor blocker, can reverse benzodiazepine-induced coma. However, the benefits of reversing coma induced

by benzodiazepine must be weighed against the risk of flumazenil-induced seizures or cardiac arrhythmias.[131]

Spinal Cord Compression

About 1 to 5% of cancer patients may develop spinal cord compression, and they should be treated emergently because delays may result in permanent neurologic deficits.[132] Spinal cord compression due to cancer most commonly involves the thoracic spine: 70% of cases involve the thoracic spine; 20%, the lumbosacral spine; and 10%, the cervical spine. Spinal cord compression may be the initial presentation of lung cancer, breast cancer, prostate cancer, multiple myeloma, lymphoma, renal cell cancer, or sarcoma.

Either direct compression or interruption of the vascular supply causes injury to the spinal cord by the tumor. Pain is the most prevailing presenting symptom—present in over 90% of patients. Unlike the pain in degenerative intervertebral disc disease, the pain in spinal cord compression tends to worsen when the patient is supine, moving the back, coughing, or sneezing. Pain (radicular or local, constant or intermittent) may be present for days or months before the emergence of other neurologic deficits. Associated neurologic symptoms may include motor and sensory deficits in the spinal cord levels below the highest point of compression, and autonomic dysfunction (bowel or bladder dysfunction). Physical examination may reveal bone tenderness over the involved area, sensory loss, ataxic gait, or muscle paralysis. Paraplegia with difficulty in ambulation is present at diagnosis in almost three-quarters of patients with spinal cord compression.[133] Dense paralysis and urinary retention before treatment are predictors of a poor neurologic outcome.

The differential diagnosis includes intramedullary metastasis, disc herniation, vertebral body fracture with retropulsion of bone fragment, epidural abscesses, and hematoma. Plain radiographs of the spine may demonstrate bony abnormalities but offer no information on soft tissue lesions. The diagnostic test of choice is MRI of the spine with gadolinium enhancement (Figure 6).[134]

Prompt adequate analgesic therapy will facilitate patient cooperation for physical examination and diagnostic imaging studies. High-dose corticosteroids should be started when the spinal cord compression by tumor is clinically suspected. There is no clear clinical study data to support the superiority of one particular corticosteroid dosing regimen over others. The initial dose of dexamethasone varies from 10 to 100 mg in common clinical practice, and this is usually followed by 4 to 10 mg every 4 to 6 hours.[135] An emergent neurosurgical consultation should be sought to

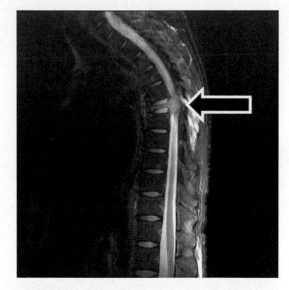

FIGURE 6 Thoracic spinal cord compression. A 43 year-old male with adenocystic cancer of the left lacrimal gland presented with severe back pain between his scapulae plus bilateral chest pain. Magnetic resonance imaging of the spine demonstrated tumor replacement of T6 thoracic vertebral body with complete collapse of the vertebral body and epidural extension of the tumor compressing the spinal cord. The patient was treated by emergent T6 diskectomy, corpectomy and stabilization, and postoperative radiotherapy.

determine if surgery is indicated. If surgical intervention is not warranted, radiotherapy at the level of the compression should be initiated, although prior radiotherapy to the involved anatomic region must also be taken into consideration.

Increased Intracranial Pressure with Brain Herniation

Increased intracranial pressure may be caused by primary brain tumors, brain metastases, intracranial hemorrhage, infection, or trauma. Cancers that most frequently metastasize to the brain include lung cancer, breast cancer, and melanoma. Depending on the underlying process, the presentation may be acute or subacute. Processes that develop gradually usually allow early diagnosis and treatment in the clinic setting before herniation develops. Acute processes (eg, hemorrhage) may cause rapid deterioration of neurologic function and require emergency intervention. Patients with hematologic malignancies are likely to have prolonged thrombocytopenia, which increases the risk of intracranial hemorrhage.

The patient with elevated intracranial pressure and brain herniation is often unconscious on arrival at the emergency department. The examination must focus on signs of brain herniation, including level of consciousness, presence of papilledema, papillary size and light responses, whether the patient is exhibiting decerebrate or decorticate posturing, and the presence of nuchal rigidity or opisthotonos. Uncal herniation, and central transtentorial herniation produce characteristic clinical syndromes, but foraminal or tonsillar cerebellar herniation and transfalcial (cingulated) herniation are difficult to recognize due to the lack of specific features. Cushing reflex (systemic hypertension and bradycardia) is a late finding in elevated intracranial pressure.[136]

If clinical findings suggest increased intracranial pressure or brain herniation and the patient is neurologically unstable, treatment to decrease intracranial pressure should be instituted immediately, even before brain imaging studies. Emergent treatments for brain herniation are hyperventilation, mannitol, and corticosteroids. Hyperventilation is the fastest way to decrease intracranial pressure, but the effects generally last only a few hours. After endotracheal intubation, the ventilator is set to hyperventilate, targeting a PCO_2 of 25 to 30 mm Hg. Hypocapnia causes cerebral vasoconstriction, decreases cerebral blood volume, and, consequently, decreases intracranial pressure. Mannitol, a hyperosmotic agent, also has fast onset but short-lived effects. Solutions of 20 to 25% mannitol are infused intravenously (IV) at 0.5 to 2 g/kg over 20 to 30 minutes. Additional doses may be given if the patient's clinical condition continues to deteriorate. Corticosteroids may be helpful, especially when vasogenic edema is present. Dexamethasone is most often used, and is usually administered IV as an initial bolus of 40 to 100 mg, followed by 40 to 100 mg IV per day in divided doses. Immediate neurosurgical consultation should be sought in the emergency department to determine whether surgical intervention is indicated. Once the patient is stabilized, treatment should be directed at the underlying cause.

Status Epilepticus

Seizures in cancer patients may be due to metabolic, infectious, structural, and cancer–treatment-related causes, but the majority of cancer patients presenting to an emergency center with seizures are due to brain lesions.[137] Status epilepticus is defined as continuous seizure activity or successive seizures without full recovery between seizures for more than 30 minutes. It can lead to devastating neurologic damage from neuronal injury and cell death, as well as serious systemic complications (eg, neurogenic pulmonary edema and rhabdomyolysis with renal failure).

After seizure activity, physical examination may show bruises, bitten tongue, and signs of urinary or fecal incontinence. Patients may have focal neurologic deficits and altered mental status (confused or unresponsive) in a postictal phase, which may last for up to 24 hours. Laboratory findings may reveal increases in lactic acid and muscle enzyme levels. The status of the malignancy, cancer treatment history, seizure history, and current medications should also be reviewed.

When a cancer patient presents with status epilepticus, airway, breathing, and circulation should be quickly assessed, and then anticonvulsant therapy with a benzodiazepine (lorazepam or diazepam) should be administered parenterally. Phenytoin (or given as the prodrug fosphenytoin sodium) and phenobarbital are second-line and third-line agents, respectively. After a seizure, the unconscious patient should be placed lying on his or her side in the recovery position to prevent aspiration. Supplemental oxygen and airway suctioning may be needed. For patients with continuing seizure activity refractory to anticonvulsants, combination anticonvulsant therapy with complete sedation or anesthesia is required in the intensive care unit with endotracheal intubation, mechanical ventilation, and monitoring with electroencephalography.

The precipitating factor in provoked seizures needs to be identified by measurement of electrolytes, serum glucose, calcium and magnesium, and hepatic and renal function testing. A complete blood cell count, blood cultures, arterial blood gases, drug screens and electrocardiography may be appropriate. Lumbar puncture may also be needed, depending on the suspected precipitating factor, the patient's condition, and findings on brain imaging by CT or MRI.[138]

Tumor Lysis Syndrome

Tumor lysis syndrome (TLS) is caused by the death of a large number of cancer cells,[139] and is characterized by hyperuricemia, hyperkalemia, azotemia, hyperphosphatemia, hypocalcemia, and metabolic acidosis out of proportion to the degree of renal insufficiency. TLS usually occurs after chemotherapy (including corticosteroid alone in sensitive lymphomas),[140] immunotherapy,[141] or radiotherapy,[142] but can also occur spontaneously. Historically, TLS has usually occurred less than 72 hours after chemotherapy in patients with leukemia and lymphoma. New effective treatments have caused TLS in patients with chronic lymphocytic leukemia, which is an indolent and chronic disease.[141] TLS also has been reported in patients with solid tumors, including small-cell carcinomas,[143] breast cancer,[144] non–small-cell lung cancer,[145] and ovarian cancer.[146] The dreaded consequences of TLS are life-threatening arrhythmia secondary to the severe electrolyte abnormalities (especially hyperkalemia) and renal failure. Early recognition of metabolic abnormalities in TLS and prompt treatment can minimize morbidity and avoid mortality.

Common symptoms of TLS include nausea, vomiting, weakness, fatigue, cloudy urine, muscle cramps, and arthralgia. Physical signs include neuromuscular irritability, seizures, muscle weakness, and arrhythmias. Hyperphosphatemia, hyperkalemia, and hypocalcemia may lead to cardiac arrhythmia or tetany. Arrhythmia in TLS may cause sudden death.[147] Precipitation of uric acid or calcium phosphate in the renal tubules may lead to acute renal failure.

Factors associated with high risk of TLS include the type of malignancy (eg, the risk is high in patients with Burkitt's lymphoma), responsiveness of the malignancy to treatment, rapid cell cycle turnover, and large tumor burden. Other risk factors are acute renal failure developing shortly after chemotherapy, preexisting renal insufficiency, and poor response to hydration. Pretreatment lactate dehydrogenase levels, which correlate with tumor bulk in patients with stage C or D lymphoma, can predict the development of azotemia after chemotherapy, but pretreatment uric acid levels are not predictive. Preventive measures in patients at risk for TLS include aggressive hydration with intravenous crystalloid fluid up to 3 L/m²/d to maintain a urine output of >100 mL/h with or without loop or osmotic diuretics, and the xanthine oxidase inhibitor allopurinol (100 to 300 mg orally per day).

There are few or no signs or symptoms in early TLS, and the diagnosis requires a high level of suspicion. In cancer patients with risk factors for TLS, routine uric acid and electrolyte screening (including calcium and phosphorus levels) is indicated. Once diagnosed, patients with severe TLS should have intravenous fluid hydration coupled with diuresis by loop diuretics (eg, furosemide 20 to 200 mg IV every 4 to 6 hours), acetazolamide (250 to 500 mg IV daily) and mannitol. If aciduria is present, sodium bicarbonate or sodium acetate infusion may be used to alkalinize the urine between pH 7.1 and 7.5. To treat hyperuricemia, allopurinol may be increased up to 900 mg/d. Recombinant urate oxidase (uricozyme or rasburicase, an enzyme that oxidizes uric acid to allantoin) (200 μg/kg IV daily) may be used to prevent or treat urate nephropathy.[148] The high potassium level can be lowered rapidly by shifting potassium into cells with IV administration of insulin plus dextrose, IV sodium bicarbonate, and beta-adrenergic stimulation. To remove potassium from the body, loop diuretics, oral potassium ion-exchange resins (sodium polystyrene sulfonate), and dialysis may be used. Intravenous calcium infusion can stabilize excitable membranes and decrease the risk of arrhythmia and tetany in hyperkalemia. In hyperphosphatemic patients with hypocalcemia, oral calcium-based phosphate-binding compounds (eg, calcium acetate or calcium carbonate) will reduce phosphate absorption and increase calcium absorption. Intravenous calcium administration can potentially cause precipitation of calcium phosphate in severe hyperphosphatemia, and should be used cautiously.

Indications for dialysis in patients with TLS include: (1) symptomatic hypocalcemia and a serum phosphorus level greater than 3.3 mmol/L ($>$ 10.2 mg/dL), (2) severe azotemia and renal failure (creatinine $>$ 10 mg/dL), (3) persistent hyperkalemia ($>$ 6 mEq/L), (4) severe hyperuricemia ($>$ 10 mg/dL), (5) oliguria or anuria despite diuretic use, (6) refractory acidemia, and (7) volume overload. Hemodialysis is commonly performed intermittently; continuous venovenous hemofiltration and continuous arteriovenous hemodialysis with a high dialysate flow rate are also effective.

Infection

Febrile Neutropenia

The most common reason for a visit to the emergency center at M. D. Anderson Cancer Center is fever. Infection remains the leading cause of morbidity and mortality in cancer patients with neutropenia.[149] A clinically evident source of infection will guide antibiotic therapy. In addition, a variety of factors in cancer patients will influence antibiotic therapy: immune compromise, the presence of vascular access devices, breach of host-defense barriers, and the probability of exposure to multi-drug-resistant microbes. Neutropenic fever is a true medical emergency, in which the timely administration of antibiotics may prevent sepsis or death. Neutropenia is defined as an absolute neutrophil count $<$ 500/μl or $<$ 1000/μl, depending on the reference cited.[150,151] A patient who is neutropenic for weeks is at greater risk for developing life-threatening infections than one who is neutropenic for less than one week.[150,151]

In a general emergency department review of the treatment of patients with neutropenia and fever, less than 50% of these patients had an identifiable source of infection.[152] The type of infection with prolonged or profound neutropenia can also be different that that seen in an immunocompetent host. Invasive fungal infections (*Candida*, *Aspergillus*), viral infections (cytomegalovirus), and life-threatening bacteremia (gram-negative rods) are seen with greater frequency in patients with prolonged neutropenia. In addition, patients who have been hospitalized are at risk for nosocomial infection with multi-drug–resistant organisms such as *Escherichia coli* with extended-spectrum β-lactamase and vancomycin-resistant enterococcus. Patients receiving prophylactic antibiotics may also have infection with organisms resistant to these antibiotics.[153]

During neutropenia, the mucosa of the alimentary tract may be altered, and mucositis and stomatitis may give bacteria an entryway into the bloodstream, resulting in both gram-positive and gram-negative bacteremia. Perirectal and perineal infections may also occur and must be considered.

Guidelines have been published for the treatment of cancer patients with febrile neutropenia.[154] Low-risk patients with solid tumors (ie, patients with no evidence of infection, able to tolerate oral antibiotics, and able to return for close follow-up) may be treated with oral antibiotics on an outpatient basis.[155,156] These patients can be treated with a combination of oral amoxicillin/clavulanate 500 mg three times a day and ciprofloxacin 500 mg three times a day for a total of 7 days. Patients with solid tumors who have evidence of sepsis, soft tissue infection, or pneumonia, and who are unable to return for close follow-up in the case of a change in status, should be admitted to the hospital and receive intravenous antibiotics.

Most cancer patients with neutropenic fever require hospitalization and intravenous antibiotics—especially leukemia patients and bone marrow transplant recipients. Patients with no obvious infectious source can be treated with monotherapy. Other patients should receive combination therapy with a glycopeptide if there is a suspected gram-positive source of infection and/or receive combination therapy with an aminoglycoside if a gram-negative etiology is possible. Agents that have been studied for monotherapy include the broad-spectrum antibiotics, such as cefepime, carbapenems, and piperacillin/tazobactam.[154,157–163]

Other causes of fever in neutropenic cancer patients are medications used to treat the malignancy, such as monoclonal antibodies, other chemotherapeutic agents (eg, cytarabine), and granulocytic growth factors. Patients may also develop fever while receiving blood transfusions. Drug-induced fever from antibiotics has also been reported; the agents most commonly involved include ciprofloxacin, rifampin, and trimethoprim/sulfamethoxazole.[164–166]

Prophylactic antibiotics should be considered for neutropenic patients who are undergoing emergency invasive procedures because the invasive procedure may lead to bacteremia. Examples include rectal introduction of contrast material for a CT scan in a patient with potential neutropenic colitis and emergent endoscopy in a neutropenic patient.

In formulating an antibiotic regimen, the emergency physician must follow the hospital's antibiogram and be aware of the presence of antibiotic-resistant organisms in the institution and community. In addition, the patient's past culture results and sensitivities must be taken into account. Recent cultures revealing vancomycin-resistance enterococcus should alert the clinician to the risk of failure of empiric therapy using vancomycin to cover gram-positive organisms. Linezolid or daptomycin should be considered as alternative therapy.[167] The current local *Pseudomonas* resistance patterns should alert the clinicians to the need for double empiric antibiotic coverage for *Pseudomonas*.

Sepsis

The goal of treatment in patients with sepsis or septic shock is to decrease mortality by rapidly instituting appropriate therapy. With in-hospital mortality approaching 50% in some studies, prompt identification of the septic patient and initiation of therapy are key factors in improving clinical outcomes.[168] In 2003, experts in critical care and infectious diseases from 11 international organizations developed guidelines for managing severe sepsis and septic shock. The Surviving Sepsis Campaign, a worldwide effort, has increased awareness and improved clinical outcomes in sepsis.[169] Many hospitals have instituted "severe sepsis bundles" (a "bundle" being defined as a group of synergistic interventions) to facilitate organized, evidence-based health care in the critical care setting, and emergency departments have started to adopt the Surviving Sepsis Campaign guidelines. A major recommendation by the Surviving Sepsis Campaign is early goal-directed therapy, which is reported to reduce absolute mortality by 16%.[170] In the emergency center, therapy for sepsis must start early and continue throughout the hospital course.

Once a patient with signs and symptoms suggestive of sepsis is identified, the components of the "severe sepsis bundle" should be implemented within 6 hours. Diagnostic studies aimed to identify the infectious process and organisms should include blood cultures from two separate sites, appropriate cultures of body fluid and sites, and radiologic studies. Undisputedly, early appropriate empiric antibiotic therapy is the cornerstone of treating sepsis. Broad-spectrum antibiotics should be administered as soon as possible, preferably within 1 hour of diagnosis. Empiric antibiotic therapy should be chosen on the basis of the current bacterial susceptibility patterns in the hospital and community. Crystalloid and colloid volume resuscitation should begin immediately. Urine output, mental status, and changes in blood pressure should guide treatment. A septic patient may require as much as 6 L of intravenous fluid during the first 24 hours of treatment. Vasopressor support may include norepinephrine and dopamine (pressor doses of $>$ 5 μg/kg/min) as first-line choices. Glucocorticoid supplementation in adrenal insufficiency produced a 10% benefit.[170,171] Stress dose steroids (eg, hydrocortisone 200 to 300 mg/d) may be necessary if adrenal insufficiency is suspected. Packed red blood cells should be replaced as necessary to maintain a hemoglobin level of 7 to

9 g/dL.[172] Other therapies such as recombinant activated protein C, tight glucose control, and low-tidal-volume ventilation strategies have also led to improved survival.[170]

REFERENCES

1. Yeung SC, Escalante CP, editors. Oncologic emergencies. Hamilton (ON), Canada: BC Decker, Inc; 2002.

2. Johnston PG, Spence RAJ, editors. Oncologic emergencies. Oxford, UK: Oxford University Press; 2002.

3. Hendrick JM, Pijls NH, van der Werf T, Crul JF. Cardiopulmonary resuscitation on the general ward: no category of patients should be excluded in advance. Resuscitation 1990;20:163–71.

4. Cummins RO (Editor). ACLS Provider Manual. Dallas, TX: American Heart Association, 2004.

5. Kvols LK. Therapy of the malignant carcinoid syndrome. Endocrinol Metab Clin North Am 1989;18:557–68.

6. Lopez FF, Mangi A, Mylonakis E, et al. Atrial fibrillation and tumor emboli as manifestations of metastatic leiomyosarcoma to the heart and lung. Heart Lung 2000;29:47–9.

7. Mathew V, Olson LJ, Gertz MA, Hayes DL. Symptomatic conduction system disease in cardiac amyloidosis. Am J Cardiol 1997;80:1491–2.

8. Pentz WH. Advanced heart block as a manifestation of a paraneoplastic syndrome from malignant thymoma. Chest 1999;116:1135–6.

9. Donnelly MS, Weinberg DS, Skarin AT, Levine HD. Sick sinus syndrome with seroconstrictive pericarditis in malignant lymphoma involving the heart: a case report. Med Pediatr Oncol 1981;9:273–7.

10. Bristow MR, Billingham ME, Mason JW, Daniels JR. Clinical spectrum of anthracycline antibiotic cardiotoxicity. Cancer Treat Rep 1978;62:873–9.

11. Friess GG, Boyd JF, Geer MR, Garcia JC. Effects of first-dose doxorubicin on cardiac rhythm as evaluated by continuous 24-hour monitoring. Cancer 1985;56:2762–4.

12. Unnikrishnan D, Dutcher JP, Varshneya N, et al. Torsades de pointes in 3 patients with leukemia treated with arsenic trioxide. Blood 2001;97:1514–6.

13. Aziz SA, Tramboo NA, Mohi-ud-Din K, et al. Supraventricular arrhythmia: a complication of 5-fluorouracil therapy. Clin Oncol (R Coll Radiol) 1998;10:377–8.

14. Miya T, Fujikawa R, Fukushima J, et al. Bradycardia induced by irinotecan: a case report. Jpn J Clin Oncol 1998;28:709–11.

15. Santini D, Tonini G, Abbate A, et al. Gemcitabine-induced atrial fibrillation: a hitherto unreported manifestation of drug toxicity. Ann Oncol 2000;11:479–81.

16. Sonnenblick M, Rosin A. Cardiotoxicity of interferon. A review of 44 cases. Chest 1991;99:557–61.

17. Frumin H, Kerin NZ, Rubenfire M. Classification of antiarrhythmic drugs. J Clin Pharmacol 1989;29:387–94.

18. Kern KB, Halperin HR, Field J. New guidelines for cardiopulmonary resuscitation and emergency cardiac care: changes in the management of cardiac arrest. JAMA 2001;285:1267–9.

19. Gallagher MM, Guo XH, Poloniecki JD, et al. Initial energy setting, outcome and efficiency in direct current cardioversion of atrial fibrillation and flutter. J Am Coll Cardiol 2001;38:1498–504.

20. Muto M, Ohtsu A, Boku N, et al. *Streptococcus milleri* infection and pericardial abscess associated with esophageal carcinoma: report of two cases. Hepatogastroenterology 1999;46:1782–4.

21. Rabinovici R, Szewczyk D, Ovadia P, et al. Candida pericarditis: clinical profile and treatment. Ann Thorac Surg 1997;63:1200–4.

22. McKenna RJ Jr, Ali MK, Ewer MS, Frazier OH. Pleural and pericardial effusions in cancer patients. Curr Probl Cancer 1985;9:1–44.

23. Galli M, Politi A, Pedretti F, et al. Percutaneous balloon pericardiotomy for malignant pericardial tamponade. Chest 1995;108:1499–501.

24. Pataki N, Szelig L, Horvath OP, et al. Pericardial drainage using the transdiaphragmatic route: refinement of the laparoscopic technique. Surg Endosc 2002;16:1105.

25. Maher EA, Shepherd FA, Todd TJ. Pericardial sclerosis as the primary management of malignant pericardial effusion and cardiac tamponade. J Thorac Cardiovasc Surg 1996;112:637–43.

26. Price KS, Castells MC. Taxol reactions. Allergy Asthma Proc 2002;23:205–8.

27. Sheski FD, Mathur PN. Long-term results of fiberoptic bronchoscopic balloon dilation in the management of benign tracheobronchial stenosis. Chest 1998;114:796–800.

28. Colt HG, Dumon JF. Airway stents. Present and future. Clin Chest Med 1995;16:465–78.

29. Lee P, Kupeli E, Mehta AC. Therapeutic bronchoscopy in lung cancer. Laser therapy, electrocautery, brachytherapy, stents, and photodynamic therapy. Clin Chest Med 2002;23:241–56.

30. Morice RC, Ece T, Ece F, Keus L. Endobronchial argon plasma coagulation for treatment of hemoptysis and neoplastic airway obstruction. Chest 2001;119:781–7.

31. Walsh DA, Maiwand MO, Nath AR, et al. Bronchoscopic cryotherapy for advanced bronchial carcinoma. Thorax 1990;45:509–13.

32. Chella A, Ambrogi MC, Ribechini A, et al. Combined Nd-YAG laser/HDR brachytherapy versus Nd-YAG laser only in malignant central airway involvement: a prospective randomized study. Lung Cancer 2000;27:169–75.

33. Leeser JE, Carr D. Fatal pneumothorax following bleomycin and other cytotoxic drugs. Cancer Treat Rep 1985;69:344–5.

34. Wilson KS, Brigden ML, Alexander S, Worth A. Fatal pneumothorax in "BCNU lung". Med Pediatr Oncol 1982;10:195–9.

35. Tocino IM, Miller MH, Fairfax WR. Distribution of pneumothorax in the supine and semirecumbent critically ill adult. AJR Am J Roentgenol 1985;144:901–5.

36. Baumann MH, Strange C, Heffner JE, et al. Management of spontaneous pneumothorax: an American College of Chest Physicians Delphi consensus statement. Chest 2001;119:590–602.

37. Baumann MH. Treatment of spontaneous pneumothorax. Curr Opin Pulm Med 2000;6:275–80.

38. Levitan N, Dowlati A, Remick SC, et al. Rates of initial and recurrent thromboembolic disease among patients with malignancy versus those without malignancy. Risk analysis using Medicare claims data. Medicine (Baltimore) 1999;78:285–91.

39. Hirsh JD, Hull RD. Pathogenesis of venous thromboembolism and clinical risk factors. In: Venous thromboembolism: natural history, diagnosis and management. Boca Raton (FL): CRC Press; 1987. p. 5–16.

40. Levine M, Gent M, Hirsh J, et al. A comparison of low-molecular-weight heparin administered primarily at home with unfractionated heparin administered in the hospital for proximal deep-vein thrombosis. New Engl J Med 1996;334:677–81.

41. Rickles FR, Edwards RL. Activation of blood coagulation in cancer: Trousseau's syndrome revisited. Blood 1983;62:14–31.

42. Khorana AA, Fine RL. Pancreatic cancer and thromboembolic disease. Lancet Oncol 2004;5:655–63.

43. Escalante CP, Kurtin D, Rivera E, Elting LS. Severity of illness, outcomes, and resource use in elderly cancer patients with deep venous thrombosis. Clin Appl Thromb Hemost 2000;6:175–8.

44. Walsh DC, Kakkar AK. Thromboembolism in brain tumors. Curr Opin Pulm Med 2001;7:326–31.

45. Levi AD, Wallace MC, Bernstein M, Walters BC. Venous thromboembolism after brain tumor surgery: a retrospective review. Neurosurgery 1991;28:859–63.

46. Anderson FA Jr, Spencer FA. Risk factors for venous thromboembolism. Circulation 2003;107:(Suppl 1)9–16.

47. Kerr TM, Lutter KS, Moeller DM, et al. Upper extremity venous thrombosis diagnosed by duplex scanning. Am J Surg 1990;160:202–6.

48. Schafer AI, Levine MN, Konkle BA, Kearon C. Thrombotic disorders: diagnosis and treatment. Hematology, Am Soc Hematol Educ Program Book 2003;520–39.

49. Samama MM. An epidemiologic study of risk factors for deep vein thrombosis in medical outpatients: the Sirius study. Arch Intern Med 2000;160:3415–20.

50. The PIOPED Investigators. Value of the ventilation/perfusion scan in acute pulmonary embolism. Results of the prospective investigation of pulmonary embolism diagnosis (PIOPED). JAMA 1990;263:2753–9.

51. Stein PD, Saltzman HA, Weg JG. Clinical characteristics of patients with acute pulmonary embolism. Am J Cardiol 1991;68:1723–4.

52. Davidson BL, Elliott CG, Lensing AW. Low accuracy of color Doppler ultrasound in the detection of proximal leg vein thrombosis in asymptomatic high-risk patients. The RD Heparin Arthroplasty Group. Ann Intern Med 1992;117:735–8.

53. Gao S, Escalante C. Venous thromboembolism and malignancy. Expert Rev Anticancer Ther 2004;4:303–20.

54. Stein PD, Hull RD, Patel KC, et al. D-dimer for the exclusion of acute venous thrombosis and pulmonary embolism: a systematic review. Ann Intern Med 2004;140:589–602.

55. Wells PS, Anderson DR, Rodger M, et al. Evaluation of D-dimer in the diagnosis of suspected deep-vein thrombosis. New Engl J Med 2003;349:1227–35.

56. Wells PS, Anderson DR, Bormanis J, et al. Value of assessment of pretest probability of deep-vein thrombosis in clinical management. Lancet 1997;350:1795–8.

57. Rathbun SW, Whitsett TL, Raskob GE. Negative D-dimer result to exclude recurrent deep venous thrombosis: a management trial. Ann Intern Med 2004;141:839–45.

58. Lensing AW, Prandoni P, Brandjes D, et al. Detection of deep-vein thrombosis by real-time B-mode ultrasonography. New Engl J Med 1989;320:342–5.

59. Kearon C, Julian JA, Newman TE, Ginsberg JS. Noninvasive diagnosis of deep venous thrombosis. McMaster Diagnostic Imaging Practice Guidelines Initiative. Ann Intern Med 1998;128:663–77.

60. Righini M, Aujesky D, Roy PM, et al. Clinical usefulness of D-dimer depending on clinical probability and cutoff value in outpatients with suspected pulmonary embolism. Arch Intern Med 2004;164:2483–7.

61. Siragusa S, Anastasio R, Porta C, et al. Deferment of objective assessment of deep vein thrombosis and pulmonary embolism without increased risk of thrombosis: a practical approach based on the pretest clinical model, D-dimer testing, and the use of low-molecular-weight heparins. Arch Intern Med 2004;164:2477–82.

62. Oudkerk M, van Beek EJ, Wielopolski P, et al. Comparison of contrast-enhanced magnetic resonance angiography and conventional pulmonary angiography for the diagnosis of pulmonary embolism: a prospective study. Lancet 2002;359:1643–7.

63. Herold CJ. Spiral computed tomography of pulmonary embolism. Eur Respir J Suppl 2002;35:13s–21s.

64. Sostman HD, Layish DT, Tapson VF, et al. Prospective comparison of helical CT and MR imaging in clinically suspected acute pulmonary embolism. J Magn Reson Imaging 1996;6:275–81.

65. Tillie-Leblond I, Mastora I, Radenne F, et al. Risk of pulmonary embolism after a negative spiral CT angiogram in patients with pulmonary disease: 1-year clinical follow-up study. Radiology 2002;223:461–7.

66. Moores LK, Jackson WL Jr, Shorr AF, Jackson JL. Meta-analysis: outcomes in patients with suspected pulmonary embolism managed with computed tomographic pulmonary angiography. Ann Intern Med 2004;141:866–74.

67. van Beek EJ, Brouwerst EM, Song B, et al. Clinical validity of a normal pulmonary angiogram in patients with suspected pulmonary embolism—a critical review. Clin Radiol 2001;56:838–42.

68. Hirsh J. Heparin. N Engl J Med 1991;324:1565–74.

69. The Columbus Investigators. Low-molecular-weight heparin in the treatment of patients with venous thromboembolism. N Engl J Med 1997;337:657–62.

70. Simonneau G, Sors H, Charbonnier B, et al. A comparison of low-molecular-weight heparin with unfractionated heparin for acute pulmonary embolism. The THESEE Study Group. Tinzaparine ou Heparine Standard: Evaluations dans l'Embolie Pulmonaire. N Engl J Med 1997;337:663–9.

71. Dalen JE, Alpert JS, Hirsch J. Thrombolytic therapy for pulmonary embolism: is it effective? Is it safe? When is it indicated? Arch Intern Med 1997;157:2550–6.

72. Thrombolytic therapy in treatment: summary of an NIH Consensus Conference. Br Med J 1980;280:1585–7.

73. Goldhaber SZ, Haire WD, Feldstein ML, et al. Alteplase versus heparin in acute pulmonary embolism: randomised trial assessing right-ventricular function and pulmonary perfusion. Lancet 1993;341:507–11.

74. Marder VJ. Thrombolytic therapy: overview of results in major vascular occlusions. Thromb Haemost 1995;74:101–5.

75. Kucher N, Rossi E, De Rosa M, Goldhaber SZ. Thrombolysis Massive pulmonary embolism. J Thromb Haemost 2001;86:444–51. Circulation. 2006; 113:577–82.

76. Gould MK, Dembitzer AD, Doyle RL, et al. Low-molecular-weight heparins compared with unfractionated heparin for treatment of acute deep venous thrombosis. A meta-analysis of randomized, controlled trials. Ann Intern Med 1999;130:800–9.

77. Koopman MM, Prandoni P, Piovella F, et al. Treatment of venous thrombosis with intravenous unfractionated

heparin administered in the hospital as compared with subcutaneous low-molecular-weight heparin administered at home. The Tasman Study Group. New Engl J Med 1996;334:682–7.

78. Schulman S, Granqvist S, Holmstrom M, et al. The duration of oral anticoagulant therapy after a second episode of venous thromboembolism. The Duration of Anticoagulation Trial Study Group. N Engl J Med 1997;336:393–8.

79. Lee AY, Levine MN, Baker RI, et al. Low-molecular-weight heparin versus a coumarin for the prevention of recurrent venous thromboembolism in patients with cancer. N Engl J Med 2003;349:146–53.

80. Bates SM, Ginsberg JS. Clinical practice. Treatment of deep-vein thrombosis. New Engl J Med 2004;351:268–77.

81. Wicki J, Perrier A, Perneger TV, et al. Predicting adverse outcome in patients with acute pulmonary embolism: a risk score. Thromb Haemost 2000;84:548–52.

82. Kovacs MJ, Anderson D, Morrow B, et al. Outpatient treatment of pulmonary embolism with dalteparin. Thromb Haemost 2000;83:209–11.

83. Decousus H, Leizorovicz A, Parent F, et al. A clinical trial of vena caval filters in the prevention of pulmonary embolism in patients with proximal deep-vein thrombosis. Prevention du Risque d'Embolie Pulmonaire par Interruption Cave Study Group. New Engl J Med 1998;338:409–15.

84. Klastersky J, Daneau D, Verhest A. Causes of death in patients with cancer. Eur J Cancer 1972;8:149–54.

85. Hersh EM, Bodey GP, Nies BA, Freireich EJ. Causes of death in acute leukemia: a ten-year study of 414 patients from 1954-1963. JAMA 1965;193:105–9.

86. Bellomo R. Fluid resuscitation: colloids vs. crystalloids. Blood Purif 2002;20:239–42.

87. Cahill BC, Ingbar DH. Massive hemoptysis. Assessment and management. Clin Chest Med 1994;15:147–67.

88. Hirshberg B, Biran I, Glazer M, Kramer MR. Hemoptysis: etiology, evaluation, and outcome in a tertiary referral hospital. Chest 1997;112:440–4.

89. Panos RJ, Barr LF, Walsh TJ, Silverman HJ. Factors associated with fatal hemoptysis in cancer patients. Chest 1988;94:1008–13.

90. Shannon N. Noninfectious pulmonary emergencies. In: Yeung SC, Escalante CP, editors. Oncologic emergencies. Hamilton (ON), Canada: BC Decker Inc; 2002. p. 191–248.

91. Lordan JL, Gascoigne A, Corris PA. The pulmonary physician in critical care — Illustrative case 7: Assessment and management of massive haemoptysis. Thorax 2003; 58:814–9.

92. Sehhat S, Oreizie M, Moinedine K. Massive pulmonary hemorrhage: surgical approach as choice of treatment. Ann Thorac Surg 1978;25:12–5.

93. Marshall TJ, Jackson JE. Vascular intervention in the thorax: bronchial artery embolization for haemoptysis. Eur Radiol 1997;7:1221–7.

94. Tsukamoto T, Sasaki H, Nakamura H. Treatment of hemoptysis patients by thrombin and fibrinogen-thrombin infusion therapy using a fiberoptic bronchoscope. Chest 1989;96:473–6.

95. Freitag L. Development of a new balloon catheter for management of hemoptysis with bronchofiberscopes. Chest 1993;103:593.

96. Colt HG. Laser bronchoscopy. Chest Surg Clin N Am 1996;6:277–91.

97. Bhattacharyya P, Dutta A, Samanta AN, Chowdhury SR. New procedure: bronchoscopic endobronchial sealing; a new mode of managing hemoptysis. Chest 2002; 121:2066–9.

98. Shneerson JM, Emerson PA, Phillips RH. Radiotherapy for massive haemoptysis from an aspergilloma. Thorax 1980;35:953–4.

99. Ketcham AS, Hoye RC. Spontaneous carotid artery hemorrhage after head and neck surgery. Am J Surg 1965; 110:649–55.

100. Heller KS, Strong EW. Carotid arterial hemorrhage after radical head and neck surgery. Am J Surg. 1979;138: 607–10.

101. Chaloupka JC, Roth TC, Putman CM, et al. Recurrent carotid blowout syndrome: diagnostic and therapeutic challenges in a newly recognized subgroup of patients. AJNR Am J Neuroradiol 1999;20:1069–77.

102. Maran AG, Amin M, Wilson JA. Radical neck dissection: a 19-year experience. J Laryngol Otol 1989;103:760–4.

103. Marchetta FC, Sako K, Maxwell W. Complications after radical head and neck surgery performed through previously irradiated tissues. Am J Surg 1967;114:835–8.

104. Coleman JJ 3rd. Treatment of the ruptured or exposed carotid artery: a rational approach. South Med J 1985; 78:262–7.

105. Citardi MJ, Chaloupka JC, Son YH, et al. Management of carotid artery rupture by monitored endovascular therapeutic occlusion (1988–1994). Laryngoscope 1995; 105:1086–92.

106. Cohen J, Rad I. Contemporary management of carotid blowout. Curr Opin Otolaryngol Head Neck Surg 2004; 12:110–5.

107. Lesley WS, Chaloupka JC, Weigele JB, et al. Preliminary experience with endovascular reconstruction for the management of carotid blowout syndrome. AJNR Am J Neuroradiol 2003;24:975–81.

108. Morrissey DD, Andersen PE, Nesbit GM, et al. Endovascular management of hemorrhage in patients with head and neck cancer. Arch Otolaryngol Head Neck Surg 1997; 123:15–9.

109. Siniluoto TM, Paivansalo MJ, Lanning FP, et al. Ultrasonography in traumatic splenic rupture. Clin Radiol 1992; 46:391–6.

110. Athale UH, Kaste SC, Bodner SM, Ribeiro RC. Splenic rupture in children with hematologic malignancies. Cancer 2000;88:480–90.

111. Wilcox CM, Spenney JG. Stress ulcer prophylaxis in medical patients: who, what, and how much? Am J Gastroenterol 1988;83:1199–211.

112. Klein MS, Ennis F, Sherlock P, Winawer SJ. Stress erosions. A major cause of gastrointestinal hemorrhage in patients with malignant disease. Am J Dig Dis 1973;18:167–71.

113. Lightdale CJ, Kurtz RC, Boyle CC, et al. Cancer and upper gastrointestinal tract hemorrhage. Benign causes of bleeding demonstrated by endoscopy. JAMA 1973; 226:139–41.

114. Schnoll-Sussman F, Kurtz RC. Gastrointestinal emergencies in the critically ill cancer patient. Semin Oncol 2000;27:270–83.

115. Mulier S, Mulier P, Ni Y, et al. Complications of radiofrequency coagulation of liver tumours. Br J Surg 2002; 89:1206–22.

116. Heyman J, Leiter E. Spontaneous retroperitoneal hemorrhage: unusual presentation of renal cancer. Urology 1987;30:259–61.

117. Pode D, Caine M. Spontaneous retroperitoneal hemorrhage. J Urol 1992;147:311–8.

118. Yamada AH, Sherrod AE, Boswell W, Skinner DG. Massive retroperitoneal hemorrhage from adrenal gland metastasis. Urology 1992;40:59–62.

119. Berney CR, Roth AD, Allal A, Rohner A. Spontaneous retroperitoneal hemorrhage due to adrenal metastasis for non-small cell lung cancer treated by radiation therapy. Acta Oncol 1997;36:91–3.

120. DiNardo LJ, Hendrix RA. The infectious and hematologic otolaryngic complications of myelosuppressive cancer chemotherapy. Otolaryngol Head Neck Surg 1991; 105:101–6.

121. Kirchner JA. Current concepts in otolaryngology. N Engl J Med 1982;307:1126–8.

122. deVries CR, Freiha FS. Hemorrhagic cystitis: a review. J Urol 1990;143:1–9.

123. Stillwell TJ, Benson RC Jr. Cyclophosphamide-induced hemorrhagic cystitis. A review of 100 patients. Cancer 1988;61:451–7.

124. Millard RJ. Busulfan-induced hemorrhagic cystitis. Urology 1981;18:143–4.

125. Mufson MA, Belshe RB. A review of adenoviruses in the etiology of acute hemorrhagic cystitis. J Urol 1976;115: 191–4.

126. Kohno A, Takeyama K, Narabayashi M, et al. Hemorrhagic cystitis associated with allogeneic and autologous bone marrow transplantation for malignant neoplasms in adults. Jpn J Clin Oncol 1993;23:46–52.

127. EK, Klotz AD, Vaze AA, Grasso V. Nephrologic and urologic emergencies. In: Yeung S-CJ, Escalante CP, editors. Oncologic emergencies. Hamilton (ON), Canada: BC Decker Inc; 2002. pp. 280–303.

128. Wofford JL, Loehr LR, Schwartz E. Acute cognitive impairment in elderly ED patients: etiologies and outcomes. Am J Emerg Med 1996;14:649–53.

129. American College of Emergency Physicians: Clinical policy for the initial approach to patients presenting with penetrating extremity trauma. Ann Emerg Med 1999;33: 612–36.

130. Kanich W, Brady WJ, Huff JS, Perron AD, Holstege C, Lindbeck G, Carter CT. Altered mental status: evaluation and etiology in the ED. Am J Emerg Med. 2002; 20: 613–7

131. Weinbroum AA, Flaishon R, Sorkine P, et al. A risk-benefit assessment of flumazenil in the management of benzodiazepine overdose. Drug Saf 1997;17:181–96.

132. Byrne TN. Metastatic epidural cord compression. Curr Neurol Neurosci Rep 2004;4:191–5.

133. Helweg-Larsen S, Sorensen PS. Symptoms and signs in metastatic spinal cord compression: a study of progression from first symptom until diagnosis in 153 patients. Eur J Cancer 1994;30A:396–8.

134. Loughrey GJ, Collins CD, Todd SM, et al. Magnetic resonance imaging in the management of suspected spinal canal disease in patients with known malignancy. Clin Radiol 2000;55:849–55.

135. Sorensen S, Helweg-Larsen S, Mouridsen H, Hansen HH. Effect of high-dose dexamethasone in carcinomatous metastatic spinal cord compression treated with radiotherapy: a randomised trial. Eur J Cancer 1994; 30A:22–7.

136. Grady PA, Blaumanis OR. Physiologic parameters of the Cushing reflex. Surgical Neurology 1988;29:454–61.

137. Singh G, Rees JH, Sander JW. Seizures and epilepsy in oncological practice: causes, course, mechanisms and treatment. J Neurol Neurosurg Psychiatry 2007; 78: 342–49.

138. Roth HL, Drislane FW. Seizures. Neurol Clin 1998;16: 257–84.

139. Flombaum CD. Metabolic emergencies in the cancer patient. Semin Oncol 2000;27:322–34.

140. Loosveld OJ, Schouten HC, Gaillard CA, Blijham GH. Acute tumour lysis syndrome in a patient with acute lymphoblastic leukemia after a single dose of prednisone. Br J Haematol 1991;77:122–3.

141. Yang H, Rosove MH, Figlin RA. Tumor lysis syndrome occurring after the administration of rituximab in lymphoproliferative disorders: high-grade non-Hodgkin's lymphoma and chronic lymphocytic leukemia. Am J Hematol 1999;62:247–50.

142. Schifter T, Cohen A, Lewinski UH. Severe tumor lysis syndrome following splenic irradiation. Am J Hematol 1999;60:75–6.

143. Kalemkerian GP, Darwish B, Varterasian ML. Tumor lysis syndrome in small cell carcinoma and other solid tumors. Am J Med 1997;103:363–7.

144. Drakos P, Bar-Ziv J, Catane R. Tumor lysis syndrome in nonhematologic malignancies. Report of a case and review of the literature. Am J Clin Oncol 1994;17:502–5.

145. Persons DA, Garst J, Vollmer R, Crawford J. Tumor lysis syndrome and acute renal failure after treatment of non-small-cell lung carcinoma with combination irinotecan and cisplatin. Am J Clin Oncol 1998;21:426–9.

146. Bilgrami SF, Fallon BG. Tumor lysis syndrome after combination chemotherapy for ovarian cancer. Med Pediatr Oncol 1993;21:521–4.

147. Van Der Klooster JM, Van Der Wiel HE, Van Saase JL, Grootendorst AF. Asystole during combination chemotherapy for non-Hodgkin's lymphoma: the acute tumor lysis syndrome. Neth J Med 2000;56:147–52.

148. Mahmoud HH, Leverger G, Patte C, et al. Advances in the management of malignancy-associated hyperuricaemia. Br J Cancer 1998;77:18–20.

149. Husni R, Raad I. Emergent and serious infections in cancer patients. In: Yeung S-CJ, Escalante CP, editors. Oncologic emergencies. Hamilton (ON), Canada: BC Decker Inc; 2002. p. 145–61.

150. Bodey GP, Buckley M, Sathe YS, Freireich EJ. Quantitative relationships between circulating leukocytes and infection in patients with acute leukemia. Ann Intern Med 1966;64:328–40.

151. Dale DC, Guerry DT, Wewerka JR, et al. Chronic neutropenia. Medicine 1979;58:128–44.

152. Perrone J, Hollander JE, Datner EM. Emergency department evaluation of patients with fever and chemotherapy-induced neutropenia. J Emerg Med 2004;27:115–9.

153. Picazo JJ. Management of the febrile neutropenic patient: a consensus conference. Clin Infect Dis 2004;39 Suppl 1:1–6.

154. Hughes WT, Armstrong D, Bodey GP, et al. 2002 guidelines for the use of antimicrobial agents in neutropenic patients with cancer. Clin Infect Dis 2002;34:730–51.

155. Rubenstein EB, Rolston K, Benjamin RS, et al. Outpatient treatment of febrile episodes in low-risk neutropenic patients with cancer. Cancer 1993;71:3640–6.

156. Rolston KV. New trends in patient management: risk-based therapy for febrile patients with neutropenia. Clin Infect Dis 1999;29:515–21.

157. Raad, II, Escalante C, Hachem RY, et al. Treatment of febrile neutropenic patients with cancer who require hospitalization: a prospective randomized study comparing imipenem and cefepime. Cancer 2003;98:1039–47.

158. Bohme A, Shah PM, Stille W, Hoelzer D. Piperacillin/tazobactam versus cefepime as initial empirical antimicrobial therapy in febrile neutropenic patients: a prospective randomized pilot study. Eur J Med Res 1998; 3:324–30.

159. Jandula BM, Martino R, Gurgi M, et al. Treatment of febrile neutropenia with cefepime monotherapy. Chemotherapy 2001;47:226–31.

160. Cordonnier C, Herbrecht R, Pico JL, et al. Cefepime/amikacin versus ceftazidime/amikacin as empirical therapy for febrile episodes in neutropenic patients: a comparative study. The French Cefepime Study Group. Clin Infect Dis 1997;24:41–51.

161. Gorschluter M, Hahn C, Fixson A, et al. Piperacillin-tazobactam is more effective than ceftriaxone plus gentamicin in febrile neutropenic patients with hematological malignancies: a randomized comparison. Support Care Cancer 2003;11:362–70.

162. Hess U, Bohme C, Rey K, Senn HJ. Monotherapy with piperacillin/tazobactam versus combination therapy with ceftazidime plus amikacin as an empiric therapy for fever in neutropenic cancer patients. Support Care Cancer 1998;6:402–9.

163. Del Favero A, Menichetti F, Martino P, et al. A multicenter, double-blind, placebo-controlled trial comparing piperacillin-tazobactam with and without amikacin as empiric therapy for febrile neutropenia. Clin Infect Dis 2001; 33:1295–301.

164. Deamer RL, Prichard JG, Loman GJ. Hypersensitivity and anaphylactoid reactions to ciprofloxacin. Ann Pharmacother 1992;26:1081–4.

165. Martinez E, Collazos J, Mayo J. Hypersensitivity reactions to rifampin. Pathogenetic mechanisms, clinical manifestations, management strategies, and review of the anaphylactic-like reactions. Medicine 1999;78:361–9.

166. Gluckstein D, Ruskin J. Rapid oral desensitization to trimethoprim-sulfamethoxazole (TMP-SMZ): use in prophylaxis for *Pneumocystis carinii* pneumonia in patients with AIDS who were previously intolerant to TMP-SMZ. Clin Infect Dis 1995;20:849–53.

167. Smith PF, Birmingham MC, Noskin GA, et al. Safety, efficacy and pharmacokinetics of linezolid for treatment of resistant gram-positive infections in cancer patients with neutropenia. Ann Oncol 2003;14:795–801.

168. Rivers E, Nguyen B, Havstad S, et al. Early goal-directed therapy in the treatment of severe sepsis and septic shock. New Engl J Med 2001;345:1368–77.

169. Dellinger RP, Carlet JM, Masur H, et al. Surviving Sepsis Campaign guidelines for management of severe sepsis and septic shock. Crit Care Med 2004;32:858–73.

170. Shapiro NI, Howell M, Talmor D. A blueprint for a sepsis protocol. Acad Emerg Med 2005;12:352–9.

171. Minneci PC, Deans KJ, Banks SM, et al. Meta-analysis: the effect of steroids on survival and shock during sepsis depends on the dose. Ann Intern Med 2004;141:47–56.

172. Zimmerman JL. Use of blood products in sepsis: an evidence-based review. Crit Care Med 2004;32:S542–7.

Geriatric Considerations in the Care of Cancer Patients

Claudia Beghe, MD
Lodovico Balducci, MD

A reduction of cancer-related morbidity and mortality in older individuals is essential for cancer control for at least two reasons. First, cancer already affects more persons aged 65 and older than those younger, and this difference is going to widen with the aging of the population (Figure 1).[1] Second, cancer-related mortality has decreased for people younger than 65 but has increased for those older, during the past 50 years.[2] The management of cancer in the older aged person involves an answer to new questions germane to the aging of the population:

1. Why do incidence and prevalence of cancer increase with age?
2. Is cancer equally lethal and morbid in both younger and older individuals?
3. Which older persons may benefit from cancer prevention and cancer treatment (that is, which ones have a life expectancy long enough to die of cancer or to suffer the complications of cancer)? Which ones are able to tolerate cancer treatment?
4. What type of clinical trials are necessary to assess benefits and risks of cancer prevention and cancer treatment in older persons? How can we increase the participation of older individuals in clinical trials?
5. What is the role of the primary care physician in cancer control?

These questions will be addressed after reviewing the extent of the problem (that is, the epidemiology of cancer and aging).

Epidemiology of Cancer and Aging

At the beginning of the past century, the age-weighted profile of the population appeared as a pyramid, with a wide base of individuals younger than 20 and a small tip representing those over 85. Today the pyramid has become closer to a square (what epidemiologists like to call the squaring of the pyramid), due to a prolongation of the average life expectancy and a reduction in fatality

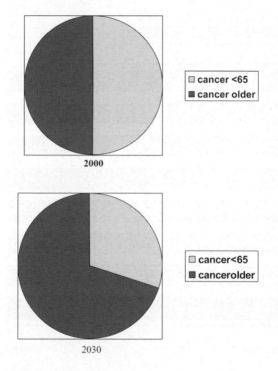

FIGURE 1 Cancer burden of people aged 65+ in 2000 and 2030.

rate.[3] Of interest, the segment of the population undergoing the most rapid expansion in the United States and in the developed world is that aged 85 and over!

The aging of the population has been associated with an increased incidence and prevalence of chronic disease, among which cancer is prominent (Figure 2) since the incidence of most common cancers increases with age. While the mortality rate of cardiovascular disease is decreasing, that of cancer is increasing,[4] and, in a nondistant future, cancer may become the number one cause of mortality for older individuals.

Six epidemiologic observations are highlighted, as they may have clinical implications.

First, Figure 2 indicates that the incidence of most cancers increases until age 65 and levels

off, or even declines, thereafter. Autopsy studies indicate that the incidence of cancer—even occult cancers—declines after age 95, and cancer is only a minor cause of mortality after this age.[5,6] So, when discussing cancer in the elderly, one refers to cancers occurring in the age window of 65 to 95.

Second, some neoplasms (including breast and colorectal cancer) tend to present at a more advanced stage in older rather than younger patients.[7] This suggests a number of remediable causes, including the fact that older individuals may not be utilizing optimal cancer screening[8] and may not be as attentive as the younger ones to early symptoms of cancer. Cognitive decline, increased threshold for visceral pain,[9] symptoms of previous conditions that may mask the symptoms of cancer, and the prejudice that pain is a natural result of aging, may lessen one's alertness to cancer presentation.[10]

Third, in the past two decades the incidence of two neoplasms, non-Hodgkin's lymphomas and malignant brain tumors, has increased unexpectedly among the elderly.[1,2] This phenomenon may be accounted for by the fact that older tissues are more susceptible to environmental carcinogens than younger tissues. In other words, older individuals may represent a natural monitor system for new environmental carcinogens, because an epidemic of cancer in older individuals may predict the same epidemics, to come years later, among the younger ones. Another important clinical implication is that the epidemiology of neoplastic diseases is evolving, and the clinician should be alerted to the possibility that previously rare diseases are becoming more common among the elderly.

Fourth, in the past two decades, there has been an age-related shift in mortality for some cancers, most notably lung cancer. Whereas the mortality has declined for individuals under 60, it has increased for those over 75.[2] In the meantime, a large portion of lung cancers, if not

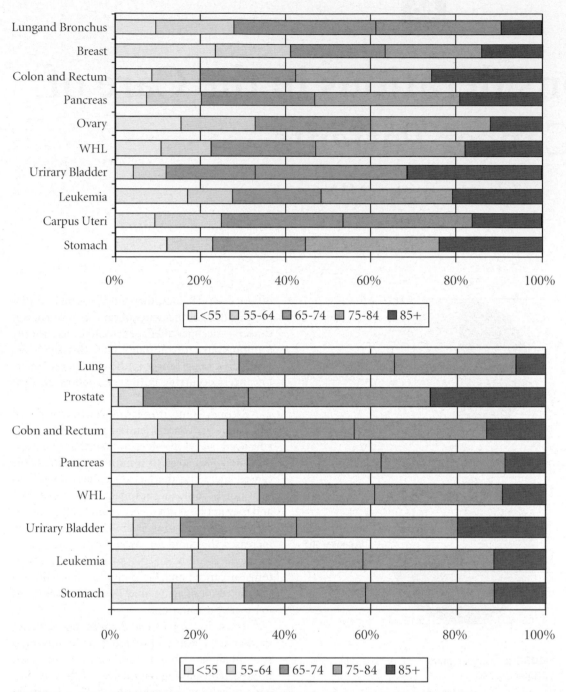

FIGURE 2 Incidence of different cancer and age. Reproduced with permission from Berlin NI.[4]

aggressive tumors that may shorten a patient's survival.

Sixth, cancer affects preferentially older individuals in good general conditions. Repetto and colleagues and Ferrucci and colleagues established in Italy that older individuals with cancer had a lower prevalence of comorbidity and of functional dependence than individuals of the same age without cancer.[14,15] In an analysis of the Surveillance, Epidemiology and End-Result (SEER) data, Diab and colleagues found that women who developed breast cancer at age 80 and older had a more prolonged life expectancy than women of the same age without breast cancer.[16] These findings support aggressive investigation and treatment of cancer in older individuals since, in the majority of cases, cancer is the cause of death.

Biologic Interactions of Cancer and Age

Aging involves a progressive reduction of the functional reserve of multiple organs and systems, increased prevalence of diseases, appearance of a number of pathologic conditions that are called geriatric syndromes and restriction in personal and social resources. The final result is a progressive reduction in life expectancy and tolerance of stress, and increased prevalence and degree of functional dependence. An elegant way to summarize the different dimensions of aging is loss of entropy,[17] which is a loss of energy available, a decline in the amount of energy that can be wasted, and the need to economize energy.

A number of molecular cellular and physiologic changes underlie aging and have been partly identified. At the molecular level, aging cells in vitro accumulate genomic abnormalities that make them more susceptible to environmental toxins, including environmental carcinogens.[18] In addition, aging cells may lose the self-replicative ability (proliferative senescence).[19] At a physiologic level, aging is seen as a chronic and progressive inflammation that leads to accumulation of catabolic cytokines in the circulation.[20,21] These substances may be responsible to some extent for many age-related changes, including sarcopenia, fatigue, osteoporosis, cognitive decline, immune senescence, and reduced hemopoiesis.[22,23] Other important physiologic aspects of aging include endocrine senescence, with reduced production of sexual hormones and growth hormone.

Age and Carcinogenesis

At least three mechanisms may account for the association of aging and cancer. The first is duration of carcinogenesis. As carcinogenesis is a multistep process that may take several years, it is reasonable to expect a linear increase in the incidence of cancer with age.[18] The second involves

the majority, develop in ex-smokers, are better differentiated, and have a much more indolent clinical course.[11,12] This finding is a direct result of smoking cessation that has resulted in prolongation of survival, decreased incidence of coronary death and chronic obstructive lung disease, and in more indolent forms of lung cancer.

Fifth, the incidence and prevalence of multiple cancers increases with age.[13] In part, this may be due to "field carcinogenesis" and, in part, to the fact that aging is a risk factor for multiple, different cancers. Field carcinogenesis implies that all cells of susceptible tissues have been exposed to the same dose of the same carcinogens during a lifetime, and persons with history of cancer are at increased risk for a second cancer in the same

organ and system (breast cancer, colorectal cancer, etc.). As smoking is a carcinogen for different tissues, it is not unusual to see in the same smoker a primary cancer of the lung, the upper airways, the esophagus, the bladder, or the pancreas. The suspicion for two simultaneous cancers should be high, when older patients present with lesions in different organs. While metastatic cancer is rarely curable, two primary cancers may both be curable. In addition, older individuals may harbor indolent metastatic neoplasms, with a median survival of several years. These include prostate cancer, breast cancer metastatic to the bones and soft tissues, and low-grade lymphomas. The presence of such neoplasms should not preclude the investigation and treatment of more increased susceptibility of aging cells to environmental carcinogens. Both experimental and epidemiologic findings support this possibility. In rodents, cutaneous, hepatic, lymphatic, and nervous tissues are more likely to develop cancer after exposure to carcinogens if they are obtained from older animals.[18] In humans, the incidence of some neoplasms, including non-melanomatous skin and prostate cancer, increases logarithmically with age, suggesting that carcinogenesis is enhanced.[24] Increased susceptibility to environmental carcinogens may also explain the increased incidence of non-Hodgkin's lymphomas, anaplastic astrocytomas and glioblastoma multiforme in older individuals during the past 30 years.

Age-related increased susceptibility to environmental carcinogens suggests that cancer prevention strategies may be effective in older individuals. These include elimination of the carcinogen, or blockage and reversal of carcinogenesis via chemoprevention.

Third, proliferative senescence, paradoxically, may enhance the risk of cancer. Senescent cells lose the ability to undergo apoptosis, may become immortal, and give origin to slowly growing tumors, such as follicular lymphoma.[19]

Aging and Tumor Growth

Aging may influence tumor growth by two mechanisms. First, the tumor cell may have different biologic characteristics in the younger and in the older person. Second, the older tumor host may modulate the tumor growth in a different way.

It is reasonable to expect a concentration of more indolent tumors among older individuals (Figure 3) by a process of natural selection. This is certainly the case with breast cancer, as the prevalence of well-differentiated, hormone–receptor-rich tumors increases with age.[25,26] The influence of the tumor host on cancer growth was

demonstrated in a now classical experiment by Ershler and colleagues, who demonstrated the same load of Lewis lung carcinoma and B16 melanoma were associated with shorter survival and higher incidence of metastasis in younger animals.[27] In successive studies, these authors demonstrated that the tumor growth rate seemed to decrease for poorly immunogenic—and increase for highly immunogenic—tumors, highlighting the influence of immune senescence on tumor growth. In humans, Kurtz, and colleagues, demonstrated a reduction in the growth rate of primary breast cancer among older women directly related to the degree of mononuclear cell reactions.[28] This observation suggested that immune senescence may mitigate tumor growth in poorly immunogenic tumors. In addition to immune senescence, endocrine and proliferative senescence may play a role in modulating tumor growth. Clearly, decline in sexual hormone production may affect the growth of hormone-dependent tumors, such as breast, prostate, and endometrial cancer. In addition, a decline in growth hormone may deprive tumor cells of insulin-like growth factor 1, one of the most powerful tumor growth factors. Proliferative senescence of stromal cells is associated with increased production of heregulin, a powerful tumor growth factor, and of metalloproteinases, enzymes that facilitate tumor metastasis with the dissolution of collagen.[19]

Age-related changes in tumor behavior have clinical relevance (Table 1). Table 1 contains two important messages. The first is that both the biology of the tumor cells and the influence of the tumor host may change with the age of the patient. The second is that tumors may become more aggressive and more lethal (as well as more indolent) with the age of the patient. This information is contrary to common wisdom holding that age is always associated with less aggressive and less lethal neoplasms.

At this point, one should emphasize that age by itself cannot be considered prognostic. While 80% of breast cancers in women aged 70 and older are rich in hormone receptor, 20% of these cancers are poor in hormone receptor and may need cytotoxic chemotherapy. While 67% of patients aged 60 and over with acute myeloid leukemia express Multidrug resistance 1 gene, 33% do not and have a disease responsive to chemotherapy.

Irrespective of age, each case should be treated on its own merits based on an estimate of risks and benefits.

Biology of Age and Decisions Related to Cancer Prevention and Cancer Treatment

Age may lessen the benefits and increase the risk of cancer prevention and cancer treatment, owing to a reduction in both life expectancy and tolerance of therapy. Prior to involving an older individual in a preventative or therapeutic program, it is important to assess risk and benefit based on individual life expectancy and functional reserve, as well as on the aggressiveness of the tumor. Since aging is highly individualized, chronologic age is not a good predictor of the risk-to-benefit ratio in individual situations. To provide this judgment, the patient's primary care physician and the oncologist need to work together, to share information and to participate in the treatment plan.

Clinical Evaluation of the Older Patient

A comprehensive geriatric assessment (CGA) reflecting the multidimensional nature of aging is the backbone of any geriatric practice (Table 2). In addition to the medical condition and the function of the patient, the CGA examines the personal and social resources that may compensate for the loss in functional reserve.

In general geriatrics, the CGA has achieved important goals, including reduced rate of functional dependence and of admission to hospital and adult living facilities.[29–32] According to some studies, the CGA has also improved the life expectancy of older individuals.

In geriatric oncology the CGA has succeeded in the following:

- Discovering conditions that may compromise cancer treatment, including unsuspected comorbidity, early cognitive decline, subclinical depression, functional limitations, malnutrition, polypharmacy, and adequacy of the caregiver.[14,33–35] In a pilot study involving 15 women aged 70 and older with early breast cancer, the performance of the CGA resulted in additional 17.2 interventions per patient.[35]

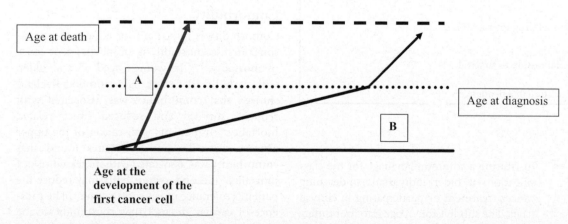

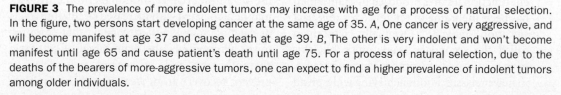

FIGURE 3 The prevalence of more indolent tumors may increase with age for a process of natural selection. In the figure, two persons start developing cancer at the same age of 35. *A*, One cancer is very aggressive, and will become manifest at age 37 and cause death at age 39. *B*, The other is very indolent and won't become manifest until age 65 and cause patient's death until age 75. For a process of natural selection, due to the deaths of the bearers of more-aggressive tumors, one can expect to find a higher prevalence of indolent tumors among older individuals.

Table 1 Age and Changes in Cancer Prognosis

Neoplasm	Age-Related Changes in Prognosis	Mechanism(s)
Acute myelogenous leukemia[111]	Worse: Increased resistance to chemotherapy Increased mortality during induction	Increased prevalence of MDR1 expressing cells; Increased prevalence of stem-cell leukemia
Non-Hodgkin's lymphoma[112–114]	Worse: Decreased duration of complete remission	Increased circulating concentration of interleukin 6
Breast cancer[26-28]	More indolent disease	Increased prevalence of hormone receptor-rich well-differentiated tumors Decreased production of sexual hormones Immune senescence
Coelomic ovarian cancer[115]	Worse: Decreased remission duration Decreased survival	Unknown
Non–small cell lung cancer[7]	Better prognosis Presentation at an earlier stage	Unknown

MDR1 = ;

Table 2 Comprehensive Geriatric Assessment and Clinical Implication

Functional Status Activities of Daily (ADL) and Instrumental Activities of Daily Living (IADL)	Relation to life expectancy, functional dependence and tolerance of stress
Comorbidity Number of comorbid conditions and comorbidity indices	Relation to life expectancy and tolerance of stress
Mental Status Folstein mini mental status	Relation to life expectancy and dependence
Emotional Conditions Geriatric Depression Scale (GDS)	Relation to life expectancy; may indicate motivation to receive treatment
Nutritional Status Mini-nutritional assessment (MNA)	Reversible condition; possible relationship to survival
Polypharmacy	Risk of drug interactions
Geriatric Syndromes Delirium, dementia, depression, falls, incontinence, spontaneous bone fractures, Neglect and abuse, failure to thrive, vertigo.	Relationship to survival Functional dependence

- Providing an estimate of life expectancy and tolerance of treatment. Life-expectancy declines with the degree of functional dependence and with the seriousness of both comorbidity and geriatric syndromes.[36–38] Two recent studies demonstrated that the risk of chemotherapy-induced myelosuppression increased for patients who were dependent in some instrumental activities of daily living (IADLs).[39]

- Instituting a common language for the classification of older individuals undergoing cancer treatment or participating in clinical trials. The subdivision of age into four different functional states proposed by Hamerman has been the frame of reference for this classification (Table 3).[40] Originally, Hamerman called the secondary state frailty, but this term may give rise to some confusion because, in newer classifications achieving widespread

acceptance, frailty is more germane to the intermediate state and is intended as a condition of increased vulnerability to environmental stress, rather than a condition of functional reserve exhaustion.

In the following discussion, the aspects of the geriatric assessment[41] with special interest for the oncologist are highlighted.

Function

Function is assessed by examining performance status (PS), activities of daily living (ADLs) and instrumental activities of daily living (IADLs). ADLs include transferring, bathing, dressing, eating, toileting, and continence; dependence in one or more of these activities, with the exception of incontinence, assigns an individual to the secondary state defined by Hamerman, and is associated with a two-year mortality rate of 27%. ADL dependence may prompt admission to an assisted living facility.[36,42,43] IADLs are activities necessary to maintain an independent life; they include use of transportation, shopping, the ability to take medications independently, to provide to one's own meals, to use the telephone, and to manage finances. Dependence in one or more IADLs is associated with a 16% two-year mortality rate, a 50% risk of dementia,[36,42–44] and increased risk of neutropenia from cytotoxic chemotherapy.[39] Two studies found a poor correlation between functional dependence and PS, and recommended that both be evaluated.[34,35] Although they are not part of the CGA, advanced activities of daily living (AADLs) are generating increasing interest. AADLs are those that make life pleasurable and include leisure activity as well as professional and other working activities.[41] Assessing AADLs may be considered an indirect measurement of quality of life as well as of psychological health and motivation to undergo treatment.

Comorbidity

Comorbidity is important for at least three reasons. First, comorbidity is an independent cause of mortality.[45–46] In women aged 65 and older, with early breast cancer, Satariano and Regland showed that comorbidity was associated with reduced survival and reduced cancer-related mortality.[45] In patients with cancer of the upper airways, Piccirillo and colleagues found that comorbidity was associated with increased risk of mortality.[46] Second, comorbidity may reduce the patient's tolerance of cancer treatment. The presence of cardiac diseases may contraindicate the use of anthracyclines; multiple chronic diseases may be associated with increased circulating levels of catabolic cytokines, sarcopenia that compromises hemopoiesis, the main target of cytotoxic chemotherapy, and, in general, may delay or prevent recovery from treatment. (The multiple

Table 3 Taxonomy of Age

Group	Characteristics	Treatment Implications
Primary	No functional dependence Negligible comorbidity	Standard treatment
Intermediate (Functional reserve substantially reduced; some degree of reversibility)	Dependence in one or more IADLs Stable comorbidity (for example, stable angina, chronic renal insufficiency, etc.)	Attempt to rehabilitation and correction of reversible conditions Special precautions such as provision of caregiver and reduction of initial chemotherapy dose

Secondary or frailty (negligible functional reserve, no reversibility; rehabilitation directed only to prevent further deterioration)	One of the following criteria:
	• Dependence in one or more ADLs
	• Three or more comorbid conditions or one poorly controlled comorbid conditions
	• One or more geriatric syndrome
	Alternative definition: at least three of the following:
	  • Involuntary weight loss ($\geq 10\%$ original weight over one year)
	  • Steady fatigue
	  • Difficulty in initiating movements
	  • Slow movements
	  • Reduced grip strength
		Symptom management, that may include chemotherapy at low doses, is the main goal of treatment

Near death (irreversible decline toward death)		Terminal care

Adapted from Hamerman D.[40]
ADLs = activities of daily living; IADLs = instrumental activities of daily living;

drugs associated with comorbidity may also suppress hemopoiesis).[22,23,47,48] Third, comorbidity may alter the prognosis of cancer. Meyerhardt and colleagues reported that patients with colonic cancer and diabetes experienced higher cancer recurrence rate than those without diabetes.[48] Polypharmacy resulting from comorbidity may alter the metabolism of antineoplastic agents. This possibility has been well established in children with acute lymphatic leukemia, in whom the use of antiepileptic drugs was associated with decreased time to progression and overall survival.[49] Polypharmacy may also have some beneficial effect on cancer. Recent studies showed that chronic use of nonsteroidal anti-inflammatory drugs was associated with lower risk of death from cancer of the large bowel,[50–52] and use of statins was associated with decreased risk of both colorectal and breast cancer.[53] The assessment of comorbidity is controversial.[54] Satariano and Ragland identified seven conditions associated with reduced life expectancy and demonstrated that the risk of mortality increased with the number of comorbid conditions. Other authors devised comorbidity scales, accounting for the degree of severity of each condition. Of these, the Cumulative Index of Related Symptoms-Geriatrics (CIRS-G) proved in some studies as the most sensitive.[54] Another advantage of the CIRS-G is that its final score may be translated into the score of another scale of common use in epidemiologic studies: Charlson's scale, which is also commonly used.

Among the comorbid conditions, anemia should be highlighted because its incidence and prevalence increase with age[23] and it has a pervasive effect on cancer treatment.[55] Anemia is an independent risk factor for death, and chemotherapy-related toxicity[56]; it is the main cause of fatigue and functional dependence[23] and may be associated with congestive heart failure, coronary deaths, and cognitive decline.[56] Controversy lingers on the definition of anemia. The common definition of the World Health Organization (WHO), defines anemia as hemoglobin levels below 12 g/dL for women and 13 g/dL for men.[55] This definition was recently challenged by a number of studies. The Women's Health and Aging Study (WHAS) showed that hemoglobin levels lower than 13.4 g/dL were an independent risk factor for death among 1,003 home-dwelling women aged 65 and over, followed prospectively for a period of 8 years.[57] The same study demonstrated that the risk of functional dependence increased inversely with hemoglobin levels lower than 13 g/dL.[58] Other studies showed that the risk of functional dependence and mobility impairment increased inversely for levels of hemoglobin lower than 14 g/dL both in men and women.[59,60] Clearly, the values proposed by the WHO should be reexamined in light of these results.

More than 50% of the causes of anemia in older individuals are reversible and include iron deficiency and B_{12} deficiency, for which prevalence increases with age.[23] Particular mention is deserved for anemia related to renal insufficiency and chronic infection that can be reversed by erythropoietin.[59] In these conditions, one observes a form of "relative erythropoietin insufficiency" in that older individuals may be unable to produce an adequate amount of erythropoietin to reverse anemia.

Geriatric Syndromes

These conditions are typical, if not specific, of aging and include dementia, depression, delirium, incontinence, vertigo, falls, spontaneous bone fractures, failure to thrive, and neglect and abuse. Geriatric syndromes are associated with reduced life expectancy, and may be considered a hallmark of the secondary state in the Hamerman classification (see Table 2).[40] To be considered as geriatric syndromes, these conditions must interfere with a person's daily life: dementia must be moderate to severe, delirium must occur as a result of medications or organic diseases that do not commonly affect the central nervous system (eg urinary or upper respiratory infections); incontinence must be complete and irreversible, falls must occur at least three times a month or the fear of falling must prevent regular activities such as walking. Depression is associated with a decreased life expectancy, even when it is subclinical,[60–62] that is diagnosed only by screening tests. Depression interferes with treatment compliance and may be fully reversible by medication. A simple 15-item questionnaire, the Geriatric Depression Scale 15 (GDS 15) speedily and reliably detects individuals with subclinical depression and is part of the CGA.[62]

Social Resources

The home caregiver is the fulcrum of social resources. Ideally, the caregiver should be able to recognize and manage emergencies, to support the patient physically and emotionally, to mediate conflicts among family members, and to act as spokesperson of the family with the health care provider.[63] By assuring compliance with treatment plans and positive interactions among health care professionals, family, and patients, the caregiver is an important resource for the practitioner managing older individuals. The practitioner should then assume responsibility for the selection, training, and support of the caregiver.

In the majority of cases, the only available caregiver is an older spouse with health problems of his or her own, or a married daughter who needs to balance her care-giving duties with family and work responsibilities.

Nutrition

The prevalence of protein/calorie malnutrition increases with age. Isolation, depression, economic restriction, and reduced appreciation of hunger, may all contribute to insufficient food intake, while chronic diseases and inflammatory cytokines may impede the synthesis of new proteins.[22] The Mini Nutritional Assessment is a simple nutritional screening test of worldwide use that identifies patients who are malnourished and those at risk of becoming malnourished and allows the prevention and early reversal of malnutrition.[64]

Polypharmacy

The prevalence of polypharmacy increases with age, and, among cancer patients aged 70 and older, was found to be as high as 41%.[33,34] Polypharmacy includes redundant prescriptions as well as the consumption of drugs with dangerous interactions; it highlights a common problem of older individuals in developed countries: the absence of a primary care provider.[65] According to one study, more than 50% of individuals aged 70 and older in the United States, Canada, and Israel, while attending multiple specialty clinics, lacked a primary care physician.

Other Forms of Geriatric Assessment

While the CGA represents the standard form of geriatric assessment, it may be complemented by laboratory data and by so-called tests of physical performances.

Laboratory Markers of Aging

The circulating levels of inflammatory markers increase with age and so does the prevalence of disability and geriatric syndromes. Not surprisingly, functional dependence and geriatric syndromes are associateed with increased levels of inflammatory cytokines in the circulation.[21] As chronic inflammation may activate coagulation, markers of intravascular coagulation, such as D-dimer, may also have prognostic value.[20,21] In home-dwelling individuals aged 70 and over, Cohen and colleagues demonstrated that increased concentrations of interleukin 6 (IL-6) or D-dimer were associated each with a 50% increased risk of functional dependence and death.[20] When the concentration of both substances was elevated, however, the risk increased more than threefold. These encouraging results suggest that in a non-distant future, laboratory markers of aging may become available

Tests of Physical Performance

The difficulty in performing some activities is considered a predictor of functional dependence and disability. Of particular interest, one study showed that the risk of mortality and functional dependence can be predicted by the "get up and go test."[66] This consists of asking an older individual to get up from an armchair and walk 10 feet forward and back. Inability to get up without using the chair arms, and requiring more than 10 seconds to walk the distance are both highly predictive of functional decline.

The Geriatric Assessment in Clinical Practice

Very little doubt exists on the benefits of geriatric assessment, but practical application is not well defined, especially in a time of shrinking health care resources. Three practical questions concern the subjects, the executors, and the extent of the CGA.

Who should undergo a CGA? The National Cancer Center Network (NCCN) recommended that all patients aged 70 and over undergo some form of geriatric assessment.[67] The basis of this recommendation is three prospective studies demonstrating that CGA discovered a number of relevant clinical conditions that otherwise would have been missed in patients of this age group.[17,33,34]

Who should perform the CGA? In our opinion, the primary care physician is best positioned to perform the CGA in older patients at regular intervals, and to communicate the findings to the oncologist and other specialists. At the meantime, all specialists caring for older individuals should at least be able to interpret the CGA and, ideally, should be able to perform it when needed.

What extent of geriatric assessment should all older patients undergo? Though most of the CGA may be based on patients' self-report,[34] the CGA may still be time-consuming, especially for patients who are unable to fill out a questionnaire on their own. A cost-effective approach to the CGA is to screen all patients with a simple, user-friendly test and to perform an in-depth assessment only in those patients who screen positive. For this purpose, the "get-up and go" test is commonly used because of simplicity.[66] The test we recommend is the one proposed by the Cardiovascular Health Study (CHS) and which involves five simple parameters (Table 4). The CHS investigators followed more than 8,500 individuals aged 65 and over for more than 8 years and found that, on the basis of these parameters, they could describe three groups of patients of different life expectancy and risk of functional dependence(Figure 4).[68] These were "the fit," who had no abnormalities, the "pre-frail," who presented one or two abnormalities, and the "frail," with three or more abnormalities. We propose that both the pre-frail and the frail undergo a more in-depth assessment. The advantage of this classification is threefold: first, it has been well validated; second, it may become the standard classification of older individuals, according to one consensus conference; and third, it is very simple to execute.

Geriatric Assessment and Life Expectancy

Life-expectancy is crucial for determining the benefits and risks of cancer prevention and cancer treatment in older individuals. The CGA may be utilized to estimate life expectancy with the caveat that this determination is always associated with some degree of uncertainty. Walter and colleagues proposed two methods to estimate both short-term (Table 5)[69] and long-term life expectancy (Figure 5).[70] In patients who had been discharged from the hospital these investigators validated a scoring system for a number of conditions (see Table 5). The one-year mortality rate was less that 10% for scores 0 to 1 and more than 60% for scores ≥ 6. The main limitation of this system is that it was developed in a Veterans Administration Hospital, and metastatic cancer probably involved lung and colorectal cancer and androgen refractory prostate cancer metastatic to the bones, all of which have a median survival longer than 1 year. If patients with breast cancer and hormone sensitive prostate cancer had been included, the score for metastatic cancer would probably have turned out much lower. Also, thanks to new forms of treatment, the median survival of even these more malignant cancers has improved: in the case of colorectal cancer, it is now close to 2 years; in the case of hormone refractory prostate cancer, it is close to 3 years. For long-term life expectancy, the authors proposed the use of life tables: they proposed dividing the life expectancy of each age cohort into quartiles and deciding (on the basis of the CGA) to which quartile each individual belonged (Figure 6). Another method utilizes a program available free online (www.adjuvantonline.com).[71] Originally designed to calculate the benefit of adjuvant chemotherapy for breast and colon cancer for patients of different age and comorbidity, it may be utilized to estimate individual life expectancies, based on the results of the CGA.

Cancer Prevention in Older Individuals

As the incidence of cancer increases with age, older individuals appear more likely than the younger ones to benefit from cancer prevention, but other conditions, such as reduced life expectancy and decreased tolerance of treatment, may lessen these benefits. Given these opposite influences of age, it is legitimate to ask what is a meaningful end point for cancer prevention in the elderly. Traditionally , reduction in cancer-related mortality has been considered a proof of the effectiveness of cancer prevention. Clinical trials in older individuals should consider alternative end points, such as preservation of function and of quality of life.[72]

Table 4 Cardiovascular Health Study Functional Assessment

Evaluation of Frailty

1. Weight loss. Unintentional weight loss of {140} 10 pounds on prior year, by direct measurement of weight.
2. Grip strength < 20% below standard for BMI measured with Jamar Hydraulic Dynamometer (see below).
3. Walk time below a cut-off point for sex and height (see below).
4. Exhaustion. Measured as two staments from the CES-D depression scale.
5. Physical activity, measured on the short version of the Minnesota Leisure Time activity (see below). Men, kilocalories per week < 383; women, < 270.

Grip Strength by Body Mass Index*

Man

Body Mass Index	Cut-off Grip Strength (kg)
≤ 24	≤ 29
24.1–26	≤ 30
26.1–28	≤ 30
28	≤ 32

Woman

≤ 23	≤ 17
23.1–26	≤ 17.3
26.1–29	≤ 18
> 29	≤ 21

Walk time

Man

Height (cm)	Cut-off Point (sec)
≤ 173	≥ 7
> 173	≥ 6

Woman

≤ 159	≥ 7
> 159	≥ 6

Exhaustion: score 2 or 3 on two questions of the CES-D
a. I felt everything I did was an effort
b. I could not get going
Sores: 0 = never 1 = 1–2 days a week; 2 = 3–4 days a week; 3 = most of the time

Physical Activity
Patients will be asked whether they engaged in any of the following activities in the past two weeks.
High-Intensity Activities
- Swimming
- Hiking
- Anaerobics
- Tennis
- Jogging
- Racquetball
- Walked for exercise for at least 1 hour {140} 4 miles per hour

Moderate or Light-Intensity Activities
- Gardening
- Mowing
- Raking
- Golfing
- Bowling
- Biking
- Dancing
- Calisthenics
- Exercise Cycle
- Walked for exercise for at least 1 hour at a strolling pace

Patients who did not engage in any of these activities over the past 2 weeks will be considered at low physical activity.

*Derived from height and body surface

Chemoprevention

Preventative interventions of common use include chemoprevention and early detection of cancer.

At least three groups of substances (hormonal agents, retinoids, and the non-steroidal anti-inflammatory drug [NSAID]) have demonstrated ability to prevent cancer in randomized clinical trials.[51,73–75] The selective estrogen receptor modulator (SERM) tamoxifen causes a number of complications, including endometrial cancer, deep venous thrombosis, strokes, and vasomotor and genitourinary manifestations of menopause, whose incidence increases with age.[73] In a decision analysis, Gail and colleagues calculated that tamoxifen may be beneficial for women aged 70 if their risk of developing breast cancer over five years is as high as 7% and if they don't present other contraindications to the drug.[76] The 5α-reductase inhibitor finasteride prevents prostate cancer, but those individuals who develop prostate cancer on treatment present a more aggressive form of disease.[74]

Retinoids delay occurrence of a second head and neck cancer in smokers, but their use is complicated by substantial side effects.[75] A number of cohort and retrospective studies have suggested that aspirin may prevent death from cancer of the large bowel,[51,52] while the COX-2 inhibitor celecoxib has reduced the number and the size of colonic polyps in patients with familial polyposis,[50] which are predisposed to colon cancer. There is no agreement on the safest and most effective agent, on the doses and duration of treatment, and on the potential therapeutic complications. While chemoprevention of cancer appears promising, it is not yet ready for clinical use.

Screening and Early Detection

As the prevalence of common cancers increases with age, the positive predictive value of screening tests also increases.[72] Improved accuracy is counterbalanced by the fact that older individuals might have undergone previous cancer screening, and that previous screening examination might have eliminated most prevalencet cases of cancer.

Breast Cancer

Serial mammograms reduce by 20 to 30% the cancer-related mortality among women aged 50 to 70.[77] The benefits of mammography after age 70 have been suggested by three reports. A cohort, historically controlled study, the Nijmegen study, showed a reduction in cancer-related mortality up to age 75[78]; two retrospective studies of the Survey Epidemiology and End Results (SEER) data showed that there was a more than twofold decrement of breast cancer related mortality for women 70 to 79 who had undergone at least two

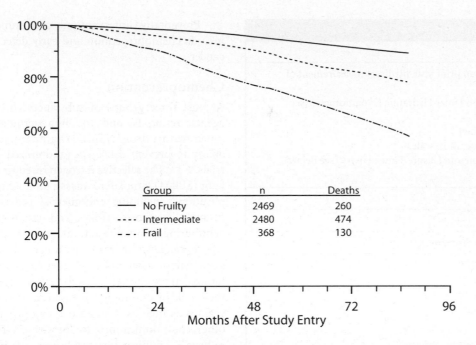

FIGURE 4 Survival of fit, pre-frail, and frail individuals in the CHS. Reproduced with permission from Fried et al.[67]

Table 5 Determination of One-Year Life Expectancy after Hospital Discharge

A: Scoring System

Risk Factors	Odds Ratio	p Value	Score
Male	1.4 (1.1–1.8)	.01	1
ADLs: 1–4	2.1 (1.6–1.6)	< .0001	2
All	5.7 (4.2–7.7)	< .0001	5
Comorbidity			
Congestive heart failure	2.0 (1.5–2.5)	< .001	2
Solitary cancer	2.6 (.17–3.9)	< .001	3
Metastatic cancer	13.4 (6.2–39)	< .001	8
Creatinine > 3.0	1.7 (1.2–2.5)	.01	2
Albumin 3.0–3.4 < 3	1.7 (1.2–2.3)	.001	1
	2.1 (1.4–3.0)	< .001	2

B: Score and One-Year Mortality

Score	1 Year Mortality
0–1	< 10%
2–3	18%
4–6	32%
> 6	64%

Adapted from Walter LC, et al.[69]
ADLs = activities of daily living.

mammograms after age 70[79] and that the benefit was largely independent from comorbidity.[80] Based on these reports, it is reasonable to recommend that older women undergo some form of breast cancer screening, if their life expectancy is 5 years or longer. A number of issues still need to be addressed.

The first issue is the role of new screening techniques, such as digital mammography or breast magnetic resonance imaging (MRI), that appear more sensitive than conventional mammography. The second is the role of clinical examination of the breast (CBE), which is cheaper and more practical than mammography. In the Canadian study, CBE was as effective as screening mammography in women aged 50 to 60,[81] and in the Breast Cancer Detection Demonstration Project, it was as sensitive as mammography for invasive cancer.[82] The third issue is whether only women at high risk of cancer should undergo serial mammograms. As the risk of breast cancer increases with the degree of bone density, Kerlikowske and colleagues calculated that 90% of early breast cancer would still be detected in women aged 70 to 79 if only those with bone density underwent regular mammography. With this approach, both cost and inconvenience of screening would be reduced.[83] The cost would be reduced by half. Clearly, new studies should focus on the most cost-effective screening strategy for older women.

Colorectal Cancer

Early detection of cancer of the large bowel reduces the cancer-related mortality for persons aged 50 to 80. Though the only screening strategy tested in randomized controlled studies involves serial examination of the stools for occult blood, a recent decision analysis suggests that the most cost-effective approach may involve full colonoscopy every 10 years.[84] In selected case, virtual colonoscopy may be utilized because it is less invasive.

Prostate Cancer

With exception for individuals at high risk (African Americans and those with a family history of prostate cancer) the value of screening asymptomatic men for prostate cancer with serial prostate-specific antigen (PSA) determinations is controversial. Also controversial is the level of PSA that should be considered abnormal[85] and the time interval at which the test should be performed.[86] According to a recent study, approximately 30% of invasive prostate cancers occur in patients with PSA < 4.0 ng/mL and 15% in those with PSA levels < 2.6 ng/dL.[85] If screening is instituted, it should be continued up to age 75, as a recent Swedish study demonstrated that radical prostatectomy reduces the prostate cancer-related mortality up to age 75.[87]

Other Cancers

No benefits of screening women over age 60 for cervical cancer have been recognized, if these women have undergone regular Papanicolau smear (Pap smear) examinations of the cervix earlier in life.[72]

In recent years, there has been a lot of interest in early detection of lung cancer. This interest stems from different reasons. First, lung cancer occurs more frequently in ex-smokers, and, in these subjects, it is a more indolent disease, amenable to cure with surgery.[21,22] Second, a new imaging technique, helical CT, is more sensitive to small lesions than chest. The Prostate, Colon Lung and Ovary (PCLO) study examining the value of early detection of cancer in these sites may solve some of the controversial issues.

Cancer Treatment

Surgery

According to Medicare data, age 70 and over is associated with increased incidence of surgical

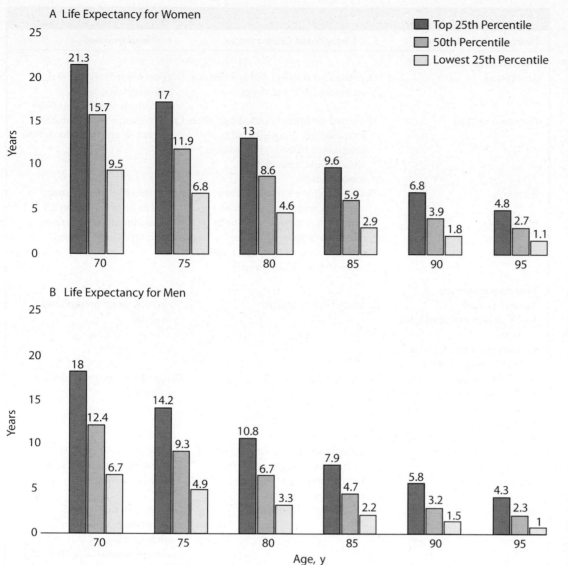

FIGURE 5 Median life expectancy for patients of different age cohort, according to the life-tables. Reproduced with permission from Walter LC, Covinsky KE.[70]

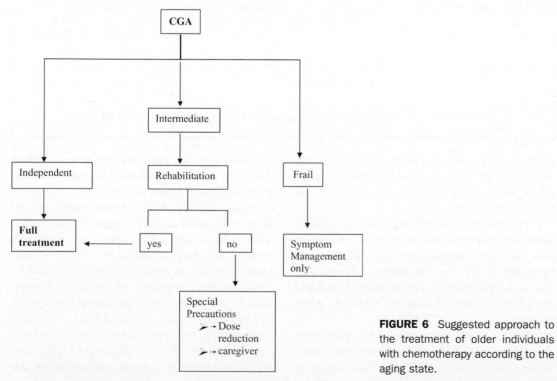

FIGURE 6 Suggested approach to the treatment of older individuals with chemotherapy according to the aging state.

complications and of surgical mortality, and with more prolonged postoperative hospitalization.[88] The difference in outcome is mainly due to emergency surgery for obstructing cancer of the large bowel and the resulting gram-negative sepsis. With the possible exception of pneumonectomy,[89] elective surgery is well tolerated by independent older individuals in the absence of comorbidity. Age should never be a reason to avoid life-saving surgery . More timely and consistent screening for cancer of the large bowel may prevent most of the emergency surgery and consequent mortality.

Recent advances in anesthesia have minimized the risk of cardiovascular complications and respiratory suppression.[90] Thanks to the evolution of surgical techniques, surgery has become less radical and lengthy and allows the use of local anesthesia in a number of procecures, such as partial and total mastectomy, local resection of rectal tumors, and many forms of laparoscopic surgery.

Radiation Therapy

External beam irradiation is well tolerated, even in individuals over age 80, according to a number of studies.[91] As the risk of mucositis increases with age, ensure adequate nutritional support for patients receiving radiation of the upper airways, the esophagus, and the pelvis. Conformational radiation therapy has greatly improved the therapeutic index of the treatment by minimizing toxicity. Another radiation technique of special interest in the elderly is brachytherapy, which has substantially reduced the duration and the toxicity of the treatment for prostate cancer and appears very promising in the postoperative management of breast cancer.

Hormonal Therapy

The main considerations related to the use of hormonal therapy in older individuals include the following.

- The risk of deep venous thrombosis and cerebrovascular ischemia from SERMs increases with age. Age also appears to be a risk factor for endometrial cancer from tamoxifen and toremifene citrate.[73] It appears prudent to avoid such compounds in women at risk for the following complications: uterus present, previous venous or arterial thrombosis, or cerebrovascular disease (especially when long-term treatment is planned, as in the adjuvant or preventative setting).

- Aromatase inhibitors are now the preferred front-line hormonal treatment for metastatic breast cancer, and are preferred by many practitioners, even in the adjuvant setting. The main risk of aromatase inhibitors over the long term is osteoporosis and long bone fractures.[92] It is customary to obtain a bone density measurement prior to institution of treatment and to manage with bisphosphonates women with osteoporosis or osteopenia. Though this strategy is reasonable, its effectiveness is unproven.

- Luteinizing hormone-releasing hormone (LH-RH) analogs are today the preferred form of androgen deprivation in prostate cancer. It has been a common trend during the last few years to treat patients with PSA relapse. These individuals have an expected survival in excess of 10 years and, consequently, are at risk to experience long-term complications of androgen deprivation, including osteoporosis, sarcopenia, and anemia. Intermittent androgen deprivation may minimize these complications and is compared to continuous deprivation in a randomized controlled study.[93] Prior to LH-RH, estrogen in low dose was the preferred form of androgen deprivation. This treatment, which prevented osteoporosis and sarcopenia, has become obsolete owing to concerns for cardiovascular and thrombotic complications. Other advantages of estrogen therapy include low cost, low incidence of hot flashes and preservation of libido.

Cytotoxic Chemotherapy

Though the risk of chemotherapy complications increases with age, it should be emphasized that older individuals may benefit from chemotherapy to the same extent as younger individuals. Pfreundschuh and colleagues demonstrated that patients aged 60 to 75 with large cell lymphoma had better survival when they received dose-intense rather than standard treatment.[94] Sargent and colleagues showed that adjuvant chemotherapy for cancer of the large bowel was as effective in individuals over 70 as it was in younger ones.[95] Langer demonstrated similar response rate and survival for patients aged 70 and older with metastatic non–small cell lung cancer as for those younger.[96] Furthermore, chemotherapy may provide the best form of palliation in patients with most metastatic cancer. Proper patient selection and supportive care are the mainstay of safe and effective chemotherapy in the elderly.

Age is associated with a number of pharmacologic changes that may influence effectiveness and toxicity of chemotherapy (Table 6).[97]

Oral antineoplastic drugs appear very convenient for older individuals, due to dose flexibility and home administration. There is concern, however, that the bioavailability of these agents may decrease with age, especially after age 80, due to decreased absorption. Phase II studies of these agents in older individuals are desirable.

The initial dose of antineoplastic agents should be adjusted to glomerular filtration rate (GFR) in individuals over 65, as renal excretion declines with age. To avoid undertreatment, subsequent doses should be escalated as tolerated.[67]

The volume of distribution of hydrosoluble agents is determined by the body water content and by the concentration of albumin and hemoglobin in the circulation. Predictably, anemia is a risk factor for chemotherapy-induced myelotoxicity and should be reversed, when feasible.[58]

Myelosuppression, mucositis, peripheral neuropathy, and cardiomyopathy are the complications of chemotherapy that become more common with age. The risk of neutropenic infections, as well as the duration and complications of hospitalization from neutropenic infections increases after age 65.[98,99] Myelopoietic growth factors filgrastim and PEG-filgrastim (filgrastim with polyethylene glycol [PEG] attached) are effective in older individuals and should be used prophylactically in individuals aged 65 and older with treatment regimens of moderate toxicity such as the combination of cyclophosphamide, hydroxydaunomycin (doxorubicin), Oncovin (vincristine), and prednisone (CHOP) for large cell lymphoma.[100] PEG-filgrastim (pegylated filgrastim) requires a single administration per

Table 6 Pharmacological Changes of Age

Pharmacologic changes	Changes and Consequences	Considerations
Pharmacokinetics		
Absorption	Decreased for nutrient. No information on bioavailability of drugs	Support phase II trial of oral anti-neoplastic agents in individuals aged 70 and older
Distribution (Vd)	Decreased for hydrosoluble drugs, with increased risk of toxicity. Vd is determined by body composition, albumin and hemoglobin concentration	Correct anemia; when possible prevent or reverse malnutrition
Excretion	Decreased renal excretion; biliary excretion probably maintained	Adjust doses of chemotherapy to GFR in individuals over 65
Metabolism	Decreased liver metabolism due to decreased hepatocytic mass, splanchnic circulation and activity of Cy-P-450 related enzymes	No clear clinical consequences. Issue needs to be studied
Pharmacodynamics		
Normal Tissues • Decreased ability of DNA repair • Decreased intracellular metabolism of drugs	Increased risk of toxicity	No known direct prevention of overturn
Neoplastic tissue • Increased expression MDR1 • Decreased cell proliferation • Tumor anoxia • Increased stromal attachment	Multidrug resistance	Drugs that over-turn multidrug resistance
Increased susceptibility of normal tissues Hemopoietic tissue	Increased risk of neutropenia and neutropenic infections, increased risk of anemia and thrombocytopenia	Prophylactic treatment with myelopoietic growth factors after chemotherapy
Mucosas	Increased risk of mucositis	Substitute IV fluorinated pyrimidines with capecitabine, when feasible Timely hospital admission and fluid resuscitation Consider AES-14 and keratinocyte growth factor
Peripheral and central nervous tissue	Increased risk of peripheral neuritis, and increased risk of chemo-brain	Avoid combination of two neurotoxic agents; avoid combination of chemotherapy and radiation to the brain
Myocardium	Increased risk of anthracycline-related cardiomyopathy	Consider use of pegylated liposomal doxorubicin "in lieu" of doxorubicin

AES-14 = ; Cy-P-450 = ; DNA = deoxyribonucleic acid; GFR = glomerular filtration rate; IV = intravenously; MDR1 = ; Vd = distribution.

cycle of chemotherapy and has become the agent of choice. Anemia is also a common manifestation of myelosuppression. In addition to enhancing the risk of chemotherapy-related toxicity, anemia causes fatigue and functional dependence.[58,100] Epoetin or darbepoetin ameliorate anemia in 60 to 70% of patients.

Mucositis may lead to volume depletion from lack of fluid intake and diarrhea.[97] The management of mucositis may include substitution of intravenous fluorinated pyrimidines (fluorouracil and floxuridine) with oral capecitabine. Capecitabine is a prodrug activated in the neoplastic tissue that minimizes the exposure of normal tissues to the active agent. Other provisions include timely fluid resuscitation, and use of AES-14, a oral preparation of glutamine.[101] A recombinant keratinocyte growth factor proved effective in preventing the mucositis from high-dose chemotherapy and may be beneficial to older patients.

No antidotes to neurotoxicity are available. Precautions include avoidance of combination of neurotoxic drugs (eg, cisplatin and paclitaxel), and discontinuance of a neurotoxic drug in the presence of weakness.

Age is a risk factor for anthracycline-induced cardiomyopathy.[102,103] The incidence of this complication increases for total doses of doxorubicin higher than 300 mg/m^2. Pegylated liposomal doxorubicin has a favorable toxicity profile with respect to doxorubicin and may be preferred in older individuals for the indications for which it was proven effective (myeloma, lymphoma, metastatic breast and ovarian cancer).[104] Other ways to prevent cardiomyopathy include continuous intravenous infusion of doxorubicin, which is cumbersome, and concomitant administration of dexrazoxane, which may increase the risk of myelodepression and mucositis.[97]

The selection of patients who can tolerate treatment is essential to safe and effective management of older individuals. On the basis of the Hamerman classification of older individuals[40] we recommend using the algorithm in Figure 6.

Targeted Therapy

Targeted therapies promise to minimize the toxicity and enhance the effectiveness of treatment and, for this reason, appear almost ideal for older individuals. Limited data suggest that these agents are indeed safer. Appropriate caveats for the elderly include:

- Myelosuppression from radioisotope-tagged (tositumomab [Bexaar] and ibritumomab tiuxetan, [Zevalin]) and cytotoxic-tagged (gemtuzumab ozogamicin, Mylotarg) antibodies may increase with age . Mylotarg has also been associated with deep venous thrombosis.

- The CD-33 targeted monoclonal antibodies alemtuzumab (Campath) may cause prolonged and irreversible myelosuppression, especially if used at doses higher than recommended. Campath may also cause severe suppression of T-cell immunity and lead to infection with intracellular organisms

- Angiogenesis inhibitors (thalidomide, bevacizumab) are associated with increased risk of deep venous thrombosis in older individuals. Bevacizumab has also been associated with bleeding and hypertension.

Supportive Care of the Older Cancer Patient

In addition to the management of treatment complications, supportive care of the older person involves management of symptoms and of conditions that may interfere with cancer treatment.

The NCCN has issued a series of guidelines to ameliorate treatment complications (Table 7). The basis of these guidelines has already been discussed.

The most common symptoms of cancer include fatigue and pain. Fatigue is common in older individuals, and may lead to prolonged functional dependence.[105] Management of anemia is the first step in relieving fatigue. This includes evaluation and management of the causes of anemia. Even in the absence of chronic bleeding, iron deficiency becomes more common with age, and is due at least in part to hepcidin, a

---

Table 7 Guidelines for the Management of the Older Person with Cancer

1. All patients aged 70 and older should undergo some form of geriatric assessment prior to institution of treatment.
2. The dose of compounds that are excreted through the kidneys or that give origin to active and toxic metabolites excreted through the kidneys, should be adjusted to individual GFRs in persons aged 65 and older. The doses should be escalated if no toxicity is encountered.
3. Patients aged 70 and older treated with moderately toxic chemotherapy (of dose intensity comparable to CHOP, should receive prophylactic growth factors (G-CSF or pegylated G-CSF).
4. Hemoglobin levels should be maintained at ≥ 12 g/dL with epoetin.

Patients aged 65 and older experiencing grade 3 to 4 mucositis should be admitted to the hospital and receive aggressive fluid resuscitation.

Adapted from the National Cancer Center Network
GFR = glomerular filtration rate; CHOP = cyclophosphamide, hydroxydaunomycin (doxorubicin), Oncovin (vincristine), and prednisone; G-CSF = Granulocyte stimulating factor

---

liver-synthesized protein that prevents the absorption of iron from the intestinal tract as well as from the red blood cell precursors.[23] Oral iron has limited activity in this situation, and parenteral iron repletion may be the treatment of choice. Vitamin B_{12} deficiency, due to decreased digestion of food, is present in at least 5% of individuals aged 60 and older. In addition to anemia, B_{12} deficiency may be associated with cognitive decline. Probably the most common cause of anemia in the older cancer patient is anemia of chronic disease or of chronic inflammation. This form of anemia responds well to erythropoietin. One study showed that the addition of parenteral iron enhances the response to erythropoietin.[106] Other causes of fatigue include increased concentration of catabolic cytokines in the circulation and sarcopenia.[105] When fatigue persists, despite the correction of anemia, the use of neuroanaleptic drugs or antidepressants is recommended . In addition, anecdotal reports suggest that daily exercise may prevent or limit fatigue.

Though the threshold for perception of pain increases with age, pain is a common problem in older cancer patients.[107] The majority of older patients, even when cognitively impaired, may report pain and its severity. In general, a vertical pain scale is preferred in older individuals owing to the possible loss of vision later. The so-called pain thermometer is probably the instrument of most common use to assess pain in the elderly . In the rare case where a patient cannot communicate, the observation of the so-called pain behavior is useful to guide pain management. Pharmacologic treatment of pain should take into account some basic principles:

- Acetaminophen is the preferred non-opioid drug, but it does not have anti-inflammatory activity and, consequently, is not very helpful with bone metastases
- The COX-2 inhibitors should be used "in lieu" of the COX-1 inhibitors in patients at high risk of bleeding (anticoagulant therapy, bleeding disorders, peptic ulcer or *Helicobacter pylori* gastritis)
- Of the COX-1 inhibitors, one should avoid indomethacin and piroxicam, due to high risk of bleeding complications
- Mild opioids (codeine, tramadol) have little place in the management of older individuals, because they need to be activated by the Cy-P450 enzymatic complex. The activity of this system declines with age and might be altered by a large number of drugs
- Age is associated with increased sensitivity to the effects of morphine and hydromorphone. These drugs are metabolized into 3- and 6-glucuronides, that are excreted from the kidneys. The 3-glucuronide is mainly responsible for the toxicity, and the 6-glucuronide for the activity, of the drugs. In older individuals, it

is recommended that the therapy be started with short-acting agents at escalating doses and that sustained-release compounds be used only when the total dose need has been determined.

- Oxycodone, hydrocodone, and fentanyl may be easier to handle, but in the presence of liver insufficiency, the half-life of these drugs may be increased
- Intrathecal administration of opioid is probably the safest, and should be considered in all patients with severe chronic pain and a life expectancy of three months or longer.

Any practitioner dealing with older individuals should be familiar with delirium, an alteration of mental status, whose peculiar characteristic is continuous variation in attention. Delirium may be a common manifestation of multiple causes, including new drugs, infections, electrolyte abnormalities, neoplastic involvement of the central nervous system. Less common causes of delirium include new pain, angina, or myocardial infarction. The management includes the treatment of the primary cause and the use of phenothiazines or haloperidol.

The importance of nutrition, home safety, and the caregiver have already been described in the section related to the geriatric assessment.

Clinical Trials in the Older Patient

Individuals aged 65 and older have been underrepresented in clinical trials of cancer treatment, despite the increased incidence and prevalence of cancer with age.[108,109] Most of the recommendations we presented are inferred from clinical trials in younger individuals. In this section we examine age-related questions that should be addressed in clinical trials, the barrier to the enrollment of older individuals in clinical trials, and strategies to overcome these barriers.

Age-Related Questions

These include the pharmacology of antineoplastic agents, patient selection, patient classification end points, and long-term outcome.

In view of the pharmacologic changes of aging, it appears necessary to conduct phase II trials of novel agents reserved to older individuals. The goals of these trials may include effectiveness and toxicity, as well as pharmacologic parameters, such as Area Under the Curve, half-life and disposal of the drug. These trials appear particularly necessary for oral agents because intestinal absorption declines with age. While somebody advocates phase I trials reserved to older individuals, we don't concur with this recommendation since these trials may unnecessarily delay the development of life-saving drugs due to excess of complications in older individuals. Of course, age should not be a criterion of exclusion from phase I trials.

Patient selections should be based on the nature of the trial. In trials of adjuvant treatment, only patients with a significant risk of cancer recurrence and cancer death should be enrolled in the trial. This can be estimated from individual life expectancy and the tumor stage. The Web site Adjuvant! Online <www.adjuvantonline.com> and its accompanying computer program provide a standardized means to assess this risk for cancers of the breast and of the large bowel.[71]

In clinical trials, patients are generally stratified according to performance status. In older individuals, performance status may not be sufficient to explain the variations in outcome.[33] Hopefully, a common language to classify older individuals may be adopted. The CHS classification of older individuals in fit, pre-frail, and frail appears as a reasonable complement of performance status.[68] At the very least, the patient's dependence in IADLs should be accounted for since this appears to be an independent predictor of chemotherapy-related toxicity.

While overall survival should still be the main end point of clinical trials with life-prolonging treatment, functional preservation and quality of life appear more important in older individuals whose life expectancy is limited.

Barriers to Clinical Trial Enrollment

One study in patients with breast cancer and showed that women aged 65 and older were as willing as younger women to enter clinical trials, but physicians were less likely to offer the clinical trials to older women.[110] Hopefully, better understanding of aging will make clinicians more comfortable in offering clinical trials to older individuals. In the meantime, it is important to recognize that simply designed clinical trials with minimal diagnostic investigations may catalyze the enrollment of older patients. The Geriatric Oncology Consortium (GOC), which involves approximately 150 practices around the United States, was organized for this purpose and completed a study of 750 older individuals with solid tumors in a record time of less than two years. Hopefully, this achievement heralds the abatement of the last barriers to the participation of older individuals in clinical trials.

Conclusions

Cancer in the older patient is becoming increasingly common. Older individuals with adequate life expectancy and treatment tolerance benefit from cancer prevention and treatment to an extent comparable with that of younger individuals.

Early detection of breast and colorectal cancer is beneficial for individuals with a life expectancy of at least five years. Ongoing studies may establish the benefits of screening asymptomatic older persons for cancer of the lung, of the prostate, and of the ovaries.

Older individuals are more vulnerable to the complications of cancer chemotherapy, including myelosuppression, mucositis, peripheral and central neurotoxicity, and cardiotoxicity. Proper dose adjustments, prophylactic treatment of older individuals with filgrastim or PEG-filgrastim, management of anemia, and drug selection may ameliorate the risk of chemotherapy in the majority of older patients.

The primary care physician has a central role in the management of older individuals with cancer. It behooves this practitioner to estimate the patient's life expectancy and functional research, and to manage concomitant conditions that may interfere with cancer treatment, including the adequacy of social resources. The oncology specialist and the primary care physician should work together to manage incoming problems and treatment complications and should present a common front to the patients and their families.

REFERENCES

1. Yancik R, Ries L. Cancer in the older person: an international issue in an aging world. Semin Oncol 2004;31:128–36.
2. Wingo PA, Cardinez CJ, Landis SH, et al. Long term trends in cancer mortality in the United States, 1930–1998. Cancer 2003;97, S21:56–66.
3. Yancik RM, Ries L. Cancer and age: magnitude of the problem. In: Balducci L, Lyman GH, Ershler WB, Extermann M, editors. Comprehensive geriatric oncology. 2nd ed. London, UK: Taylor and Francis; 2004. p. 38–46.
4. Berlin NI. The conquest of cancer. Cancer Invest 1995;11:540–50.
5. Stanta G, Campagner L, Cavallieri F, et al. Cancer of the oldest old: what we have learned from autopsy studies. Clin Ger Med 1997;13:55–68.
6. Caranasos GJ. Prevalence of cancer in older persons living at home and in institutions. Clin Ger Med 1997;13:15–32.
7. Goodwin JS. Presentation of cancer in older patients. In: Balducci L, Lyman GH, Ershler WB, Extermann M, editors. Comprehensive geriatric oncology. 2nd ed. London, UK: Taylor and Francis; 2004.
8. Randolph WM, Mahnken JD, Goodwin JS, et al. Using Medicare data to estimate the prevalence of breast cancer screening in older women: comparison of different methods to identify screening mammograms. Health Serv Res 2002;37:1643–57.
9. Balducci L. Management of cancer pain in the older patient. J Supp Oncol 2003;1:175–91.
10. Balducci L. Perspectives on quality of life of older patients with cancer. Drugs Aging 1994;4:313–24.
11. Tony L, Spitz MR, Feuger JJ, et al. Lung cancer in former smokers. Cancer 1996;78:1004–10.
12. Ebbert JO, Yang P, Vachon CM, et al. Lung cancer risk reduction after smoking cessation: observation of a prospective cohort of women. J Clin Oncol 2003;21:921–6.
13. Luciani A, Balducci L. Multiple primary malignancies. Semin Oncol 2004;31:264–73.
14. Repetto L, Fratino L, Audisio RA, et al. Comprehensive geriatric assessment adds information to the Eastern Cooperative Group Performance Status in Elderly cancer patients. An Italian group for geriatric oncology study. J Clin Oncol 2002;20:494–502.
15. Ferrucci L, Cavazzini C, Corsi A, et al. Biomarkers of frailty in older persons. J Endocrinol Invest 2002;25 (Suppl 10):10–5.
16. Diab SG, Elledge RM, Clark GM. Tumor characteristics and clinical outcome of elderly women with breast cancer. J Natl Cancer Inst 2000;92:550–6.
17. Lipsitz LA. Physiologic complexity, aging and the path to frailty. Sci Aging Knowledge Environ 2004;21:16.

18. Anisimov VN. Age as a risk factor in multistage carcinogenesis. In: Balducci L, Lyman GH, Ershler WB, Extermann M, editors. Comprehensive geriatric oncology. 2nd ed. London, UK: Taylor and Francis; 2004, 75–101.
19. Hornsby PJ. Replicative senescence and cancer. In: Balducci L, Extermann M. Biologic basis of geriatric oncology; Kluwer; 2005. Springer, NY, 53–74
20. Cohen HJ, Harris F, Pieper CF. Coagulation and activation of inflammatory pathways in the development of functional decline and mortality in the elderly. Am J Med 2003;114:180–7.
21. McDermott MM, Guralnick JM, Greenland P, et al. Inflammatory and thrombotic blood mark and walking-related disability in men and women with and without peripheral vascular disease. J Am Ger Soc 2004;52:1888–94.
22. Hamerman D, Berman JV, Albers W, et al. Emerging evidence of inflammation in conditions frequently affecting older adults: reports of a symposium. J Am Ger Soc 1999;47:1016–102.
23. Guralnik JM, Eisenstadt RS, Ferrucci L, et al. Prevalence of anemia in persons 65 years and older in the USA: evidence for a high rate of unexplained anemia. Blood 2004;104:2262–8.
24. Balducci L, Aapro M. Epidemiology of cancer and aging. In: Balducci L, Extermann M, editors. Biologic basis of geriatric oncology. Kluwer; 2005. Springer NY, 1–16.
25. Martoni A, Cucinotta D, Balducci L. Meeting report: breast cancer in the older woman. Tumori 2004;90:437–45.
26. Balducci L, Silliman RA, Diaz N. Breast cancer in the older woman: an oncologic perspective. In: Balducci L, Lyman GH, Ershler WB, Extermann M. Comprehensive geriatric oncology. 2nd ed. London, UK: Taylor and Francis; 2004, 662–703.
27. Ershler WB. Influence of tumor host on the tumor growth in older patients. In: Balducci L, Lyman GH, Ershler WB, Extermann M, editors. Comprehensive geriatric oncology. 2nd ed. London, UK: Taylor and Francis; 2004.
28. Kurtz JM, Jacquemier J, Amalric R, et al. Why are local recurrences after breast-conserving therapy more frequent in younger patients. J Clin Oncol 1990;10:141–52.
29. Cohen HJ, Feussner JR, Weinberger M, et al. A controlled trial of inpatient and outpatient geriatric assessment. N Engl J Med 2002;346:147–157.
30. Reuben DB, Franck J, Hirsch S, et al. A randomized clinical trial of outpatient geriatric assessment (CGA), coupled with an intervention, to increase adherence to recommendations. J Am Ger Soc 1999;47:269–76.
31. Bula CJ, Berod AC, Stuck AE, et al. Effectiveness of preventive in-home geriatric assessment in well functioning, community dwelling older people: secondary analysis of a randomized trial. J Am Ger Soc 1999;47:389–95.
32. Caplan GA, Williams AJ, Daly B, et al. A randomized controlled trial of comprehensive geriatric assessment and multidisciplinary intervention after discharge of elderly from the emergency department: the DEED II study. J Am Ger Soc 2004;52:1417–23.
33. Extermann M, Overcash J, Lyman GH, et al. Comorbidity and functional status are independent in older cancer patients J Clin Oncol 1998;16:1582–7.
34. Ingram SS, Seo PH, Martell RE, et al. Comprehensive assessment of the elderly cancer patient: the feasibility of self-report methodology. J Clin Oncol 2002;20:770–5.
35. Extermann M, Meyer J, McGinnis M, et al. A comprehensive geriatric intervention detects multiple problems in older breast cancer patients. Crit Rev Oncol Hematol 2004;49:69–75.
36. Inouye SK, Peduzzi PN, Robison JT, et al. Importance of functional measures in predicting mortality among older hospitalized patients. JAMA 1998;279:1187–1193.
37. Stump TE, Callahan CM, Hendrie HC. Cognitive impairment and mortality in older primary care patients. J Am Ger Soc 2001;49:934–40.
38. Extermann M, Chen A, Cantor AB, et al. Predictors of toxicity from chemotherapy in older patients. Eur J Cancer 2002;38:1466–73.
39. Zagonel V, Fratino L, Piselli P, et al. The comprehensive geriatric assessment predicts mortality among elderly cancer patients [abstract]. Proc Am Soc Clin Oncol 2002; 21:365.
40. Hamerman D. Toward an understanding of frailty. Ann Intern Med 1999;130:945–50.
41. Burns R, Nichols LO, Martindale-Adams J, et al. Interdisciplinary geriatric primary care evaluation and management. Two year outcomes. J Am Ger Soc 2000; 48:8–13.
42. Ramos LR, Simoes EJ, Albert MS. Dependence in activities of daily living and cognitive impairment strongly predicted mortality in older urban residents in Brazil. J Am Ger Soc 2001;49:1168–75.
43. Barbeger-Gateau P, Fabrigoule C, Helmer C, et al. Functional impairment in instrumental activities of daily living: an early clinical sign of dementia? J Am Ger Soc 1999;47:456–62.
44. Katz P. Function, disability, and psychological well being. Adv Psychosom Med 2004;25:41–62.
45. Satariano WA, Ragland DR. The effect of comorbidity on 3-year survival of women with primary breast cancer. Ann Int Med 1994;120:104–10.
46. Piccirillo JF, Tierney RM, Costa I, et al. Prognostic importance of comorbidity in a hospital-based cancer registry. JAMA 2004;291:2441–7.
47 Astani A, Smith RC, Allen BJ. The predictive value of body proteins for chemotherapy induced toxicity. Cancer 2000;88:796–903.
48. Meyerhardt JA, Catalano PJ, Haller DG, et al. Impact of diabetes mellitus on outcome of patients with colon cancer. J Clin Oncol 2003;21:433–40.
49. Relling MV, Pui CH, Sandlund JT, et al. Adverse effect of anticonvulsivant on efficacy of chemotherapy for adult lymphoblastic leukemia. Lancet 2000;356:285–90.
50. Steinbach G, Phillips RKS, Lynch PM. The effect of celecoxib, a cyclooxygenase 2 inhibitor in familial adenomatous polyposis. N Engl J Med 2000;342: 1946–52.
51. Terry MB, Gammon MD, Zhang FF, et al. Association of frequency and duration of aspirin use and hormone receptor status with breast cancer risk. JAMA 2004;291:2433–40.
52. Poynter JN, Rennert G, Bonner JD, et al. HMG CoA reductase inhibitors and risk of colorectal cancer. ASCO Proc 2004;23:1.
53. Extermann M. Measuring comorbidity in older cancer patients. Eur J Cancer 2000;36:453–71.
54. Schijvers D, Highley M, DeBruyn E, et al. Role of red blood cell in pharmakinetics of chemotherapeutic agents. Anticancer Drugs 1999;10:147–53.
55. Knight K, Wade S, Balducci L. Prevalence and outcome of anemia in cancer: a systematic review of the literature. Am J Med 2004;116 Suppl 7a:11–26.
56. Chaves PH, Xue QL, Guralnik JM, et al. What constitutes normal hemoglobin concentration in community-dwelling disabled older women? J Am Ger Soc 2004;52: 1811–6.
57. Chaves PH, Ashar B, Guralnik JM, et al. Looking at the relationship between hemoglobin concentration and prevalent mobility difficulty in older women. Should the criteria currently used to define anemia in older people be reevaluated? J Am Ger Soc 2002;50:1527–64.
58. Balducci L, Hardy CL, Lyman GH. Hemopoiesis and aging. In: Balducci L, Extermann M. Biological basis of geriatric oncology. Kluwer; 2004. Springer, NY, 171–184.
59. Salive ME, Cornoni-Huntley J, Guralnik JM, et al. Anemia and hemoglobin levels in older persons: relationship with age, gender and health status. J Am Ger Soc 1992;40: 489–96.
60. Blazer DG, Hybels CF, Pieper CF. The association of depression and mortality in elderly persons: a case for multiple independent pathways. J Gerontol Med Sci 2001;56A; M505–9.
61. Covinsky KE, Kahana E, Chin MH, et al. Depressive symptoms and three year mortality in older hospitalized medical patients. Ann Int Med 1999;130:563–9.
62. Lyness JM, Ling DA, Cox C, et al. The importance of subsyndromal depression in older primary care patients. Prevalence and associated functional disability. J Am Ger Soc 1999;47:647–52.
63. Weitzner MA, Haley WE, Chen H. The family caregiver of the older cancer patient. Hematol Oncol Clin 2000;14; 269–82.
64. Guigoz Y, Vellas B, Garry PJ. Mininutritional assessment: a practical assessment tool for grading the nutritional state of elderly patients. In: Vellas B, Facts, research, interventions in geriatrics. New York: Serdi Publishing Company; 1997. p. 15–60.
65. Clarfield AM, Bergman H, Kane R. Fragmentation of care for frail older people-an international problem. Experience from three countries: Israel, Canada, and the United States. J Am Ger Soc 2001;49:1714–21.
66. Gill TM, Baker DI, Gottschalk M, et al. A program to prevent functional decline in physically frail elderly persons who live at home. N Engl J Med 2002;347:1068–74.
67. Balducci L. Guidelines for the management of the older person with cancer. J Natl Compr Canc Netw 2005. [In press]
68. Fried LP, Tangen CM, Walston J, et al. Frailty in older adults: evidence for a phenotype. J Gerontol Med Sci 2001;56A: M146–M156.
69. Walter LC, Linquist K, Covinsky KE, et al. Relationship between health status and use of screening mammography and papanicolau smears among women older than 70 years of age. Ann Intern Med 2004;140:681–8.
70. Walter LC, Covinsky KE. Cancer screening in elderly patients: a framework for individual decision-making. JAMA 2001;285:2750–6.
71. Ravdin PM, Siminoff LA, Davis GJ, et al. Computer program to assist in making decisions about adjuvant therapy for women with early breast cancer. J Clin Oncol 2001;19: 980–91.
72. Balducci L, Beghe C. Cancer prevention in the older person. Clin Ger Med 2002;18;505–528.
73. Fisher B, Costantino JP, Wickerham DL, et al. Tamoxifen for prevention of breast cancer: report from the national adjuvant breast and bowel project. J Natl Cancer Inst 1998;90:1371–88.
74. Thompson IM, Goodman DJ, Tanger CM, et al. The influence of finasteride on the development of prostate cancer. N Engl J Med 2003;349:215–24.
75. Hong WK, Spitz MR, Lippman SM. Chemoprevention in the 21st century: genetics, risk modeling, and molecular targets. J Clin Oncol 2000;18 Suppl:9–18.
76. Gail MH, Costantino JP, Bryant J, et al. Weighing the risks and benefits of tamoxifen treatment for preventing breast cancer. J Natl Cancer Inst 1999;91:1829–46.
77. Kerlikowske K, Grady D, Rubin SM, et al. Efficacy of screening mammography. A meta-analysis. JAMA 1995;273: 149–54.
78. Van Dijck JAAM, Holland R, Verbeeck ALM, et al. Efficacy of mammographic screening in the elderly: a case-referent study in the Nijmegen program in the Netherland. J Natl Cancer Inst 1994;86:934–8.
79. McCarthy EP, Burns RB, Freund KM, et al. Mammography use, breast cancer stage at diagnosis, and survival among older women. J Am Ger Soc 2000;48:1226–33.
80. McPherson CP, Swenson KK, Lee MW. The effects of mammographic detection and comorbidity on the survival of older women with breast cancer. J Am Ger Soc 2002;50:1061–8.
81. Miller AB, Baines CJ, To T, et al. Canadian national breast screening study 2: breast cancer detection and death rates among women aged 50-59 years. Can Med Assoc J 1992;147:1477–88.
82. Mitra I. Breast screening: the case for physical examination without mammography. Lancet 1994;343:342–4.
83. Kerlikowske K, Salzman P, Phillips KA, et al. Continuing screening mammography in women aged 70 to 79 years. JAMA 1999;282:2156–63.
84. Frazier AL, Colditz GA, Fuchs CS. Cost-effectiveness of screening for colorectal cancer in the general population. JAMA 2000;284:1954–61.
85. Thompson IM, Pauler DK, Goodman PJ, et al. Prevalence of prostate cancer among men with a prostate specific antigen level < 4.0 ng/milliliter. N Engl J Med 2004; 350;2239–46.
86. Punglia R, D'Amico AV, Catalona WJ, et al. Effect of verification bias on screening for prostate cancer by measurement of prostate specific antigen. N Engl J Med 2003;349:335–42.
87. Holmberg L, Bill-Axelson A, Hegelsen F, et al. A randomized trial comparing radical prostatectomy with watchful waiting in early prostațe cancer. N Engl J Med 2002; 347:781–9.
88. Kemeny MM, Bush-Devereaux E, Merriam LT, et al. Cancer surgery in the elderly. Hematol Oncol Clin North Am 2000;14:169–92.
89. Dexter EU, Jahangir N, Kohman LJ. Resection for lung cancer in the elderly patients. Thor Surg Clin 2004;14: 1163–71.
90. Miguel R, Vila H. Perioperative considerations in the geriatric oncology patient. In: Balducci L, Lyman GH, Ershler WB, Extermann M, editors. Comprehensive geriatric oncology. 2nd ed. London, UK: Taylor and Francis; 2004. p. 415–26.
91. Zachariah B, Balducci L. Radiation therapy of the older patient. Hematol Oncol Clin N Am 2000;14:131–67.
92. Goss P. Anti-aromatase agents in treatment and prevention of breast cancer. Cancer Control 2002;9 (Suppl 2):2–8.

93. Diamond TH, Bucci J, Kersley JH, et al. Osteoporosis and spinal fractures in men with prostate cancer. Risk factors and effects of androgen deprivation therapy. J Urol 2004;172:529–32.

94. Pfreundschuh M, Trumper L, Kloess M, et al. Two weekly or three-weekly CHOP chemotherapy with or without etoposide for the treatment of elderly patients with aggressive lymphoma. Results of the NHL-B trial of the DSHNHL. Blood 2004;104:634–41.

95. Sargent DJ, Goldberg RM, Jacobson SD, et al. A pooled analysis of adjuvant chemotherapy for resected colon cancer in elderly patients. N Engl J Med 2001;345:1091–7.

96. Langer CJ. Elderly patients with lung cancer: biases and evidence. Curr Treat Opt Oncol 2002;3:85–102.

97. Cova D, Balducci L. Cancer chemotherapy in the older patient. In: Balducci L, Lyman GH, Ershler WB, Extermann M, editors. Comprehensive geriatric oncology. 2nd ed. London, UK: Taylor and Francis; 2004. p. 463–488.

98. Morrison VA, Picozzi V, Scotti S, et al. The impact of age on delivered dose-intensity and hospitalizations for febrile neutropenia in patients with intermediate –grade non-Hodgkin's Lymphoma receiving initial CHOP chemotherapy: a risk factor analysis. Clin Lymphoma 2001;2:47–56.

99. Chrischilles E, Delgado DI, Stolshek BS, et al. Impact of age and colony stimulating factor use in hospital length of stay for febrile neutropenia in CHOP treated non-Hodgkin's lymphoma patients. Cancer Control 2002;9:203–11.

100. Balducci L, Hardy CL, Lyman GH. Hematopoietic growth factors in the older cancer patient. Curr Opin Hematol 2001;8:170–87.

101. Sonis ST. A biological approach to mucositis. J Supp Oncol 2004;2:21–36.

102. Swain SM, Whaley FS, Ewer MS. Congestive heart failure in patients treated with doxorubicin. Cancer 2003;97:2869–79.

103. Hequet O, Le QH, Moullet I, et al. Sub-clinical late cardiomyopathy after doxorubicin therapy for lymphoma in adults. J Clin Oncol 2004;22:1864–71.

104. O'Brien ME, Wigler N, Inbar M, et al. Reduced cardiotoxicity and comparable efficacy in a phase III trial of pegylated liposomal doxorubicin versus conventional doxorubicin for first line treatment of metastatic breast cancer. Ann Oncol 2004;15:440–9.

105. Tralongo P, Respini D, Ferrau F. Fatigue and aging. Crit Rev Oncol Hematol 2003;48 Suppl:57–64.

106. Auerbach M, Ballard H, Trout JR, et al. Intravenous iron optimizes the response to recombinant human erythropoietin in cancer patients with chemotherapy–related anemia: a multicenter open-label randomized trial. J Clin Oncol 2004;22:1301–7.

107. Balducci L. Management of cancer pain the geriatric patient. J Supp Oncol 2003;1:175–191.

108. Talarico L, Chen G, Pazdur R. Enrollment of elderly patients in clinical trials for cancer drug registration: a 7 year experience by the US Food and Drug Administration. J Clin Oncol 2004;22:4626–31.

109. Unger JM, Hutchins LF, Albain KS. Under-representation of elderly patients in cancer clinical trials: causes and remedial strategies. In: Balducci L, Lyman GH, Ershler WB, Extermann M, editors. Comprehensive geriatric oncology. 2nd ed. London, UK: Taylor and Francis; 2004. p. 259–274.

110. Kemeny MM, Peterson BL, Kornblith AB, et al. Barriers to clinical trial participation by older women with breast cancer. J Clin Oncol 2003;21:2268–75.

111. Lancet JE, Willman CL, Bennett JM. Acute myelogenous leukemia and aging: clinical interactions. Hematol Oncol Clin North Am 2000;16:251–268.

112. The International Non-Hodgkin's Lymphoma Prognostic Factors Project: a predictive model for aggressive non-Hodgkin's Lymphoma. N Engl J Med 1993;329:987–94.

113. Solal-Celigny P, Roy P, Colombat P, et al. Follicular lymphoma international prognostic index. Blood 2004;104:202–8.

114. Preti HA, Cabanillas F, Talpaz M, et al. Prognostic value of serum interleukin 6 in diffuse large-cell lymphoma. Ann Intern Med 1997;127:186–94.

115. Thigpen JT. Gynecological cancer in the older woman. In: Balducci L, Lyman GH, Ershler WB, Extermann M. Comprehensive geriatric oncology. 2nd ed. London, UK: Taylor and Francis; 2004, 771–83.

Integrative Medicine: Complementary and Alternative Therapies

Gary E. Deng, MD, PhD

Barrie R. Cassileth, PhD, MS

Definition

Many practices previously termed unorthodox or unconventional are increasingly recognized for their therapeutic value, evolving over time to become complementary and alternative medicine (CAM). That language shift was exemplified by the creation over a decade ago of the National Institutes of Health Office of Alternative Medicine, which in 1999 was renamed the "National Center for Complementary and Alternative Medicine" (NCCAM). NCCAM defines CAM as "a group of diverse medical and health care systems, practices, and products that are not presently considered to be part of conventional medicine."

A necessary distinction between "complementary" and "alternative" therapies is required. Complementary therapies, used as adjuncts to mainstream care, are supportive measures that help control symptoms, enhance well-being, and contribute to overall patient care (Table 1).[1,2] Alternative therapies, conversely, are unproved or disproved, often promoted for use instead of mainstream treatment or offered as viable therapeutic options. This is especially problematic in oncology, when delayed treatment can diminish the possibility of remission and cure.[3] Over time, some complementary therapies are proven safe and effective. These become integrated into mainstream care, producing integrative medicine, a combination of the best of mainstream cancer care and rational, data-based, adjunctive complementary therapies.[4]

Current Status

The most comprehensive and reliable findings on Americans' use of CAM in general come from the National Center for Health Statistics (NCHS) 2002 National Health Interview Survey (NHIS). NCHS is an agency of the Centers for Disease Control and Prevention.[5] Of 31,044 adults surveyed, 75% used some form of CAM. When prayer specifically for health reasons are excluded, the number was still at 50%. The survey shows most common use among women, better-educated people, those hospitalized in the previous year, and former smokers, indicating a more health conscious segment of the population. Common reasons given for use of CAM are shown in Figure 1.

By various accounts, 10% to over 60% of cancer patients have used CAM, depending primarily on the definitions applied.[2,6-9] The Datamonitor 2002 Survey indicated that 80% of cancer patients used an alternative or complementary modality.[10] There is some indication of a growth in CAM use by cancer patients in recent years.[11] In our clinical experience, cancer patients most commonly use CAM to help get through chemotherapy, radiation, or surgery; to confront a poor prognosis and explore all treatment options; and to prevent cancer recurrence.

In 1997, consumer expenditures related to CAM were estimated at $36 billion to $47 billion, including $12 billion to $20 billion paid out-of-pocket to CAM practitioners.[8] Sale of vitamins and minerals in the United States approximated $2.1 billion in 1999, including $6.6 billion for vitamins and $4.2 billion for herbs.[12]

The advent of the Internet facilitates dissemination of information and misinformation. The keywords "alternative cancer medicine" on Google.com revealed close to 3 million results at the end of 2004 and about 28 million at the beginning of 2007. It is difficult, if not impossible, for the public to distinguish between evidence-based information and scientific-sounding infomercials promoting services and products. (Reputable sources of information are listed in Table 2.)

Many mainstream medical professionals are reluctant to accept complementary therapies, often because supporting scientific evidence, until recently, was rarely available. That many CAM practices are based on ancient philosophical and health care paradigms also reduces their credibility, as does the language used to describe underlining theories and mechanisms that may appear strange or ridiculous to those trained in the contemporary biomedical sciences. Fortunately, recent rigorous research has produced data on the safety, efficacy, and biologic mechanisms of some complementary therapies, and presents data in scientific language.

The definition of complementary therapies is evolving. As more is learned, those shown to be safe and effective are adopted into mainstream health care. This is reflected in the establishment of integrative or complementary medicine programs in major academic medical centers, including major National Cancer Institute-designated cancer centers such as Memorial Sloan-Kettering, M. D. Anderson, Dana-Faber, and others.[13] Similar programs have been initiated in Canada, Australia, and Europe.

In this chapter, we introduce first the principles of Eastern medical systems, on which many current CAM therapies are based. We then introduce and review research data on complementary modalities that have been studied in cancer patients. These modalities include mind-body therapies, manual therapies and bodywork, dietary measures and supplements for cancer prevention, herbal medicine, and acupuncture. Those without a substantial body of research evidence are not discussed in detail here.

Eastern Therapeutic Models

Complete therapeutic systems of theory and practice were developed by ancient cultures.

Table 1 Categories and Examples of Useful Complementary Therapies

Biologically based practices	Dietary supplements (vitamins, some herbal remedies)
Mind-body practices	Meditation, guided imagery, hypnosis, relaxation techniques
Manipulative and body-based practices	Massage, reflexology
Practices from ancient medical systems	Acupuncture, Yoga

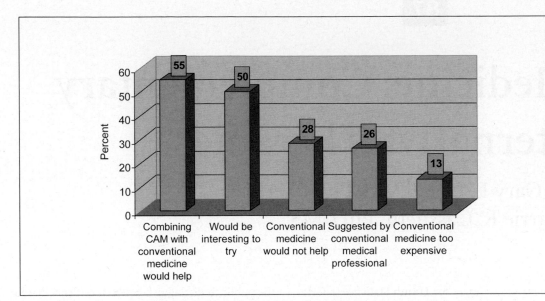

FIGURE 1 Common reasons people use CAM. Adapted from Barnes PM et al.[5]

Table 2 Reputable Sources of Online Information on Complementary and Alternative Medicine

National Center for Complementary and Alternative Medicine (NCCAM): http://nccam.nih.gov
National Cancer Institute: http://www.cancer.gov/cam/index.html
American Cancer Society: http://www.cancer.org/docroot/ETO/ETO_5.asp?sitearea=ETO
USDA Food and Nutrition Information Center: http://www.nal.usda.gov/fnic
NIH Office of Dietary Supplements: http://dietary-supplements.info.nih.gov
U.S. Pharmacopeia: http://www.usp.org/dietarySupplements
Memorial Sloan-Kettering Cancer Center: http://www.mskcc.org/aboutherbs
M. D. Anderson Cancer Center: http://www.mdanderson.org/departments/CIMER
Institute of Medicine: http://www.iom.edu/board.asp?id=3788

Although the beliefs on which they are based may be outmoded, some of their practices, such as herbal remedies and acupuncture, have value today. The two most prominent Eastern systems are traditional Chinese medicine (TCM) and India's ayurvedic medicine.[14] These paradigms embody a holistic approach to health maintenance, emphasizing interactions among internal "life forces" and harmony between individuals and their environments. These systems hold the belief that health requires a strong and balanced body and mind. If the balance is disturbed, disease occurs. Therapeutic interventions aim to restore the balance.

Traditional Chinese Medicine

The earliest TCM text, Huang Di Nei Jing (Yellow Emperor's Canon of Internal Medicine) dates from 500 to 300 BCE. Its theory centers on the balance between Yin and Yang. Anything with cold, dark, weak, and hollow qualities are Yin; those that are hot, bright, strong, and solid are Yang. "Qi" (pronounced chee), the vital energy or life force, and "Xue," the blood, circulate around the body to regulate the balance of Yin and Yang in the major organ systems (heart, lung, spleen, liver, kidney) of the body. These organ systems are functional entities, responsible for modern medicine's cardiovascular, respiratory, digestive, emotional and genitourinary activities, respectively.[15]

Traditional TCM diagnostic techniques include observation, listening, inquiry and palpation, which includes pulse taking. Findings that fit specific patterns lead to a diagnosis. TCM practitioners then prescribe herbal and/or acupuncture treatment. Herbal remedies are usually a formulation of multiple ingredients (mainly botanicals) but also, occasionally, minerals and animal products. The herbal remedies are most commonly prepared by brewing the ingredients in hot water. The ingredients are said to work in combination to achieve a synergistic effect and to balance out side effects.[15]

Acupuncture remains an important TCM practice. Inserting and manipulating needles at specific body points, originally to regulate the flow of Qi and restore harmony, is a viable treatment for many symptoms, and modern research shed light on its mechanisms. Many acupuncture points are rich in nerves, and contemporary investigation suggests that acupuncture may regulate nervous system activities.[16,17] Acupuncture is discussed in greater detail later in this chapter.

Ayurvedic Medicine

The term "ayurveda" is a combination of Sanskrit words "ayur" (life) and "veda" (knowledge). Ayurvedic ("knowledge of life") medicine can be traced back to 1500 BCE. It was originally described in the Hindu scriptures called the Vedas and the texts known as the Samhitas. Its root is deeply embedded in Indian civilization and Hindu philosophy. Ayurveda remains intertwined with India's moral, spiritual, and cultural values to this day.[18]

There is much similarity between ayurveda medicine and TCM. Both view the balance of mind, body, and spirit, as well as balanced adaptation to external forces, as essential to optimal health. Three basic forces (doshas), believed to exist in all beings, include vata (motion), pitta (metabolism), and kapha (structure). "Prana" (similar to the Chinese "Qi") flows through the body and concentrates in "Chakras" (body points alone the midline thought to be the focal points of interaction among the internal organs and external elements). Imbalance results in diseases.

Ayurvedic diagnostic techniques include observation, questioning the patient, and palpation, with special attention paid to pulse, tongue, eyes, and nails. Diagnoses are described as discordance of doshas in relationship to specific organ systems. Therapies are directed to balance the doshas based on the individual's body type. Main methods of treatment are cleansing and detoxifying (shodan), palliation (shaman), rejuvenation (rasayana) and spiritual healing (satvajaya).[18] Ayurvedic medicine has a strong mind-body component. Spiritual healing is aimed at relieving stress and negative thoughts, and achieving enlightenment. Sound therapy, imagery, exercise, and meditation are common techniques to keep consciousness in balance. Therapies used in ayurvedic medicine that have relevance to cancer care, such as yoga and meditation, are discussed in the following sections.

Mind-Body Therapies

Current-day mind-body therapies are based on the reciprocal relationship between mind and body. Chronic stress and depression are associated with cardiovascular risk and impaired immune function.[19,20] Physical problems are exacerbated by social and emotional stress. Cancer is not amenable to treatment only through attention to patients' psychological needs, but relief from mood disturbance, anxiety and other mental distress greatly improves the patient's quality of life. In addition to conventional psychiatric care, several mind-body techniques are helpful.[21]

Mind-body modalities, including meditation, hypnosis, relaxation techniques, cognitive-behavioral therapy, biofeedback, and guided imagery have become part of mainstream care over the years. A survey found that 19% of American adults used at least one mind-body therapy in a one-year period.[22] A meta-analysis of 116 studies found that mind-body therapies could reduce anxiety, depression, and mood disturbance in cancer patients, and assist their coping skills.[23] Mind-body techniques can also help reduce chronic low-back pain, joint pain, headache, and procedural pain.[24]

Meditation

Meditation can be grouped into two categories. Concentrative mediation focuses attention on increasing mental awareness and clarity of mind. Here, attention is focused on an image, a sound, or on one's breathing. Mindfulness meditation, instead, opens attention to whatever goes through the mind and to the flow of sensations experienced from moment to moment, without attempts to discover their meaning. The emphasis on the present helps release the mind from negative past memories and from worries about the future. A common goal of many mind-body therapies is to achieve "inner peace."

Changes in brain electrical activity and immune functions have been reported in individuals who underwent a training program in mindfulness meditation. In a randomized, wait-list controlled study, significant increases in left-sided anterior activation, a pattern previously associated with positive affect, were found in the meditators. When the subjects were immunized with influenza vaccine, significant increases in specific antibody titers were observed. There was no correlation between the magnitude of increase in left-sided activation and that of the rise in antibody titer.[25]

In a randomized wait-list control study of 109 cancer patients, participation in a seven-week mindfulness-based stress reduction program was associated with significant improvement in mood disturbance and symptoms of stress.[26] A single arm study of breast and prostate cancer patients showed significant improvement in overall quality of life, stress, and sleep quality, but symptom improvement was not significantly correlated with program attendance or minutes of home practice.[27]

Yoga, which combines physical movement, breath control, and meditation, improved sleep quality in a trial of 39 lymphoma patients. Practicing a form of yoga that incorporates controlled breathing and visualization significantly decreased sleep disturbance when compared to wait-list controls.[28] Mindfulness-based stress reduction techniques must be practiced to produce beneficial effects.[29]

Hypnosis

Hypnosis is an artificially induced state of consciousness in which a person is highly receptive to suggestion. A hypnotherapist or one's own self (self-hypnosis) can induce the trancelike state (similar to deep daydreaming) by first inducing relaxation and then directing attention to specific thoughts or objects. The World Health Organization (WHO) estimates that 90% of the general population can be hypnotized, with 20 to 30% able to enter the deeper somnambulistic state. For best results, the patient and the therapist must have a good rapport with a certain level of trust; the environment must be comfortable and free from distractions; the patient must be willing to undergo the process and must desire to be hypnotized. Hypnosis was endorsed by the British Medical Society in 1955 and the American Medical Association in 1958. Research shows that hypnosis is beneficial in reducing pain, anxiety, phobias, nausea, and vomiting.

In one study, 20 excisional breast biopsy patients were randomly assigned to a hypnosis or control group (standard care). Post-surgery pain and distress were reduced in the hypnosis group.[30] In another study, children undergoing multiple painful procedures such as bone marrow aspiration or lumbar puncture were randomized to receive hypnosis, a package of cognitive behavioral coping skills, or no intervention. Those who received either hypnosis or cognitive behavioral therapy experienced more pain relief than control patients. The effects were similar between hypnosis and cognitive behavioral therapy. Both therapies also reduce anxiety and distress, with hypnosis showing greater effectiveness.[31] Hypnosis was studied in a randomized controlled trial of 60 patients undergoing elective plastic surgery. Peri- and postoperative anxiety and pain were significantly reduced in the hypnosis group when compared to the control group, who received only stress reduction training. Reduction in anxiety and pain was achieved along with significant reduction in intraoperative requirements for sedatives and analgesics.[32]

In a study of 67 bone marrow transplant patients, subjects were randomized to one of the four intervention groups: hypnosis training, cognitive behavioral coping skills training, therapist contact control, or usual care. Oral pain from mucositis was reduced in the hypnosis group.[33] A National Institutes of Health (NIH) Technology Assessment Panel found strong evidence for hypnosis in alleviating cancer-related pain.[34] Hypnosis effectively treats anticipatory nausea in pediatric[35] and adult cancer patients[36] and reduces postoperative nausea and vomiting.[32]

Selection of proper patients and the qualifications of the hypnotherapist contribute to safe hypnotherapy. The WHO cautions that hypnosis should not be performed on those with psychosis or certain personality disorders. A small percentage of patients may experience dizziness, nausea, or headache. These symptoms usually result from patients brought out of trance by inexperienced hypnotherapists.

Relaxation Techniques

Randomized, controlled trials demonstrate that relaxation training and guided imagery significantly ameliorate anxiety and distress. A randomized study of relaxation therapy versus alprazolam showed that both approaches significantly decreased anxiety and depression, although the effect of alprazolam was slightly quicker for anxiety and stronger for depressive symptoms.[37] Relaxation achieves the effect without side effects and at a lower cost. A randomized trial of 82 radiation therapy patients found significant reductions in tension, depression, anger, and fatigue for those who received relaxation training or imagery.[38]

A meta-analysis of 59 studies showed improved sleep induction and maintenance with psychological interventions.[39] Although pharmaceuticals may produce a rapid response, some studies suggest that behavioral therapies help to maintain longer-term improvement in sleep quality. The NIH consensus panel concluded that behavioral techniques, particularly relaxation and biofeedback, produce improvements in some aspects of sleep, but the magnitude of improvement in sleep onset and time may not achieve clinical significance.[34]

Manual Therapies and Bodywork

The many types of bodywork have in common the manipulation or movement of parts of the body to achieve health benefits. Osteopathy and chiropractic teach complete systems of diagnosis and treatment. Massage therapy has variations, such as Swedish massage and shiatsu. Other bodywork techniques, such as the Alexander Technique and Pilates, address posture and movement, while yoga, tai chi, Reiki, and polarity therapy incorporate strong mind-body components.[14]

Osteopathic and Chiropractic Manipulation

Osteopathy was developed in late 19th century by Andrew Taylor Still, a trained engineer and physician who believed that "structure governs function." Osteopathy is taught as a complete system of medical care. In the United States, training blends conventional medical, surgical, and obstetrical practices with osteopathic manipulative treatments (OMT), involving manipulation of the bones, muscles, and tendons to promote blood flow and enhance the body's healing powers. Doctors of Osteopathy (DOs) are licensed to perform surgery and prescribe medicine in the United States after completion of licensure examinations and graduate medical education.

Some DOs focus on the conventional medical approach and provide general medical care, while others focus more on manipulative treatment. In Europe, osteopaths rely more on the latter.[40]

Chiropractic was also originated in the late 19th century in the United States. The founder, Daniel David Palmer, believed that the proper alignment of the spinal column is essential to optimal health. Palmer believed that subluxations impede normal function of the nervous system and lead to illness, and that spinal manipulation (adjustment) was required to correct the problem. Chiropractic is widely accepted by the regulatory authority and third-party payers, if not by mainstream medicine. In 1987, the US Supreme Court upheld a lower-court finding charging the American Medical Association of antitrust violations in its attempt to eliminate the chiropractic profession. Chiropractic services are included in Medicare, in over half of health maintenance organizations, and in 75% of private health insurance plans.[41,42]

Although manipulative techniques in osteopathic and chiropractic care are offered to treat many medical conditions, most controlled clinical trials of these techniques were conducted in patients with lower back pain.[43] Systematic reviews and meta-analysis supported its benefits in acute[44] and chronic[45] back pain. A randomized controlled trial compared standard medical therapies to osteopathic manipulation in the treatment of chronic lower back pain. No statistically significant difference was found for pain and range of motion, although those receiving osteopathy required significantly less medication and used less physical therapy.[46] A recent systemic review of spinal manipulation concluded that there is moderate evidence of its short-term efficacy in treating acute and chronic lower back pain, but insufficient data to draw conclusions regarding its efficacy for lumbar radiculopathy.[47]

Massage Therapy

Massage therapists apply pressure to muscle and connective tissue to reduce tension and pain, improve circulation, and encourage relaxation. Swedish massage, the most common type in the US, is gentle and comprises five basic strokes (stroking, kneading, friction, percussion, and vibration). The movement is rhythmic and free-flowing. The practice of massage therapy requires state certification or licensure.

Massage therapy helps relieve symptoms commonly experienced by cancer patients. It reduces anxiety and pain[48–51] as well as fatigue, distress, nausea, and anxiety.[48] Anxiety and pain were evaluated in a crossover study of 23 inpatients with breast or lung cancer receiving reflexology (foot massage) or usual care. Patients experienced significant decreases in anxiety,

and in one of three pain measures, breast cancer patients experienced significant decreases in pain as well.[49] In another study, 87 hospitalized cancer patients were randomized to receive foot massage or control. Pain and anxiety scores fell with massage, with differences between groups achieving statistical and clinical significance.[50] The use of aromatic oil seemed to enhance the effect of massage in early studies,[51,52] but significant enhancement was not seen in more recent randomized controlled trials.[53–55] For non-cancer subacute and chronic back pain, massage therapy was found effective in a systematic review of randomized controlled trials, and preliminary data suggest it may help reduce the costs of care.[56]

Manual lymphatic drainage (MLD), which provides a gentle pumping action through specific hand movements, helps breast–cancer-related lymphedema. A randomized, controlled, crossover study compared the effects of MLD with those of simple lymphatic drainage (a less-robust massage regimen), in 31 women with breast–cancer-related lymphedema. MLD significantly reduced excess limb volume and dermal thickness and significantly improved quality-of-life end points.[57,58]

Safety

Osteopaths and chiropractors are educated and should be well aware of contraindications for manipulation, such as acute fractions, underlying aneurysm, bone metastasis, etc. There are no data on the frequency of adverse effects from OMT, as the total number of OMT performed per year is unknown. A review of 128 articles published between 1925 and 1993 revealed 185 cases of major complications. The majority was cerebrovascular accidents (66%), the rest, disk herniations, pathologic fractures or dislocations, and an increase in pain.[59] There have been reports of rare, serious complications from chiropractic spinal manipulation. A Danish retrospective cohort study examined the incidence of cerebrovascular accidents after manipulation. The frequency is between 1 in every 120,000 to 900,000 cervical manipulations.[60,61] Complications from lumbar manipulations are rarer.[42] Many oncologists warn cancer patients against the use of chiropractic manipulation.

Massage therapy is safe when practiced by credentialed practitioners. Serious adverse events are rare and associated with exotic types of massage or untrained practitioners.[62] In work with cancer patients, the application of deep or intense pressure should be avoided, especially near lesions or anatomic distortions such as postoperative changes. Patients with bleeding tendencies should receive only gentle, light-touch massage.

Dietary Measures and Supplements for Cancer Prevention

Epidemiologic studies show that some cancers are more or less prevalent in specific populations. This phenomenon cannot be explained entirely by genetics since, for example, Asian-American women born in the West are at greater risk for breast cancer than Asian-American women born in the East. Attempts have been made to identify "active ingredients" in diets and to see whether oral supplementation with such ingredients may reduce cancer risk.

Diet

In general, diets high in saturated fat and caloric intake are associated with higher cancer risk. Conversely, epidemiologic as well as animal studies show that fruit and vegetable intake assists cancer prevention. Large, prospective studies are under way to determine whether dietary supplementation can reduce cancer risk. Given other health benefits, such as reduced risk of cardiovascular disease, a diet high in fruits and vegetables and low in saturated fat is advisable.

Diet plays an important role in the prevention of gastrointestinal (GI) cancers. Obesity increases the risk of esophageal and colon cancers, and high alcohol intake elevates the risk of esophageal and liver cancers. Ingestion of aflatoxin-contaminated peanuts or grains increases the risk of liver cancer. Salt-preserved foods and high salt intake are linked to stomach cancer. Dietary fiber significantly lowers the risk of colon cancer.[63]

Although most animal studies show that dietary fat increases the development of breast tumors, data from case-control or cohort human studies are less strong.[64] Type of fat is important because there is an inverse relationship between consumption of olive oil (monounsaturated fat) or fish oil (polyunsaturated fat) and breast cancer risk. Excess body weight is a significant risk factor for recurrence and for shorter survival in breast cancer patients, especially in Stage I and II patients.[65] Several clinical trials (the Women's Health Initiative, the Women's Intervention Nutrition Study, and the Women's Healthy Eating and Lifestyle Study) are ongoing to address the relationship between dietary fat, other components of diet, and the risk of breast cancer and other diseases.

Epidemiologic studies suggest a role for low-fat diets in prostate cancer prevention. Data from case-control and prospective studies are mixed. In animal studies, low-fat diets decrease tumor growth.[66] Some demonstrate a direct association between increased saturated and monounsaturated fat and increased risk of prostate cancer,[67,68] while others find no relationship.[69,70] In a cohort study of more than 58,000 men, prostate cancer risk was not associated with the intake of total fat, total saturated fatty acids, or total trans-unsaturated fatty acids, in general, although lower risk was weakly associated with increased intake of linolenic acid.[71]

Dietary Supplements

Antioxidants are the best studied supplements for cancer prevention, based on their assumed protective effect against oxidative stress to the genome, proteins, and lipids. Compounds that can induce differentiation of immature cells constitute another major class of chemopreventive agents.

The largest chemoprevention study to date is the α-Tocopherol, β-Carotene Cancer Prevention Study, a randomized controlled trial of 29,000 male smokers in Finland. Dietary supplementation with α-tocopherol, a form of Vitamin E, or β-carotene, a precursor of Vitamin A, did not reduce the incidence of lung cancer among male smokers. On the contrary, β-carotene was associated with increased risk of lung cancer in current smokers and recent quitters.[72] Although supplementation of α-tocopherol did not reduce overall incidence of lung cancer, higher serum α-tocopherol status was associated with lower lung cancer risk, particularly among younger persons and those with less cumulative smoke exposure. This suggests that high levels of α-tocopherol, if present during the early critical stages of tumorigenesis, may inhibit lung cancer development. Both the beneficial and the adverse effects of supplemental α-tocopherol and β-carotene disappeared during post-intervention follow-up.[73]

In the β-Carotene and Retinol Efficacy Trial, another large chemoprevention trial of 18,000 smokers, former smokers, and workers exposed to asbestos, β-carotene and vitamin A supplementation again was associated with a higher risk of lung cancer.[74] Interestingly, subanalyses revealed that fruit and vegetable consumption reduced lung cancer risk only in the placebo arm. The association was strongest with Rosaceae fruit or Cruciferae vegetables.[75] This illustrates that plant foods have a role in preventing lung cancer in high-risk populations, and that purified β-carotene supplements do not provide the protective effects associated with foods.

Selenium is a trace element required for the activity of the antioxidant enzyme glutathione peroxidase, which protects cell membranes from damage caused by the peroxidation of lipids.[76] Dietary selenium and serum selenium levels correlate inversely with the risk of several types of cancer.[77] Plants that grow in selenium-rich soil or animals that eat such plants are good sources of dietary selenium, and Brazil nuts are a particularly rich source of selenium.

In a multi-center, randomized, placebo-controlled study of 1,312 patients with history of non-melanoma skin cancer (the Nutritional Prevention of Skin Cancer Trial), daily intake of 200 μg of selenium lowered the incidence of prostate cancer by two-thirds.[78] The incidence of lung and colorectal cancers also was reduced. There was no significant effect on other cancers. In the Health Professionals Follow-Up Study, higher selenium levels were associated with reduced risk of advanced prostate cancer.[79] The association became stronger with additional controls for family history of prostate cancer, body mass index, calcium intake, lycopene, and saturated fat intake, vasectomy, and geographical region.

A randomized, placebo-controlled, double-blind, phase III prostate cancer prevention trial of 32,400 men (the Selenium and Vitamin E Cancer Prevention Trial) is under way to test the preventive efficacy of selenium and vitamin E.[80,81] Final results are anticipated in 2013. This study will also generate strong data regarding the safety of vitamin E; one meta-analysis of mostly cardiovascular chemopreventive trials found slightly higher mortality associated with high-dose (> 400 IU/d) vitamin E supplementation.[82]

Lycopene is a natural pigment found in tomato, watermelon, guava, rose hips, and pink grapefruit. It is classified as a non-provitamin A carotenoid. Epidemiologic studies suggest an inverse relationship between lycopene consumption and lung, prostate, and stomach cancers.[83] A prospective study of male health professionals, the Health Professionals Follow-up Study, found an association between frequent tomato or lycopene intake and reduced risk of prostate cancer. Intake of tomato sauce, in which lycopene is more bioavailable, was associated with an even greater reduction in prostate cancer risk, especially for extraprostatic cancers. The associations persisted even when fruit, vegetable, and olive oil consumption were controlled.[84]

Calcium may lower the risk of colorectal adenomas by suppressing cell proliferation. Increasing the daily intake of calcium via low-fat dairy food reduces the proliferative activity of colonic epithelial cells and restores markers of normal cell differentiation in patients with a history of polypectomy for colonic adenomatous polyps. Recurrence of adenoma and the average number of adenomas were both significantly reduced by calcium intake in a large placebo-controlled, double-blind trial. In another large randomized study, calcium supplementation was associated with a modest, but not significant, reduction in risk of adenoma recurrence.

Anti-inflammatory drugs such as nonsteroidals or COX-2 inhibitors also show promise in colon cancer prevention, and good evidence indicates that sulindac, aspirin, and celecoxib help prevent colonic adenomas. Unfortunately, increased risk of heart attack and stoke is found in patients taking COX-2 inhibitors.[85] How this finding affects the future of this class of drugs remains to be seen.[86]

Soy contains isoflavones, including phytoestrogens, genistein, and daidzein. Genistein and daidzein are selective estrogen-receptor modulators (SERMs). Dietary intake of soy and high serum phytoestrogen levels are associated with lower risk of prostate cancer. In vitro studies indicate that genistein inhibits the growth of prostate cancer cells, apparently independent of genistein's estrogenic effects.[87,88] Prospective intervention trials have not yet been conducted to evaluate the role of soy in preventing prostate cancer. Most prospective trials included men following a diagnosis of prostate cancer.[89,90]

Some research suggests that soy products may decrease breast cancer risk, but the effect appears dependent on when in the woman's lifetime soy products were consumed. In animal studies, rats fed soy-enriched diets through puberty had a decreased incidence of mammary tumors later in life, but this effect was not seen when the soy-enriched diet started after puberty. Epidemiologic studies in general fail to show a protective effect for soy products, except in women who consume them during adolescence or in large amounts.[91] The phytoestrogen activity in soy products raises concerns about their use by breast cancer patients or survivors with estrogen–receptor-positive cancer. In theory, these products may increase the risk of breast cancer recurrence or progression. It is possible these phytoestrogens produce paradoxical effects, as both estrogenic and antiestrogenic effects are observed in vitro. The effect may depend on the concentration or other co-factors in the cells, not unlike other selective estrogen receptor modulators.

Based on existing data, the consumption of soy products in moderation is neither encouraged nor discouraged for the prevention of breast cancer. Women with estrogen–receptor-positive breast cancer should not consume large amounts of phytoestrogen-rich foods such as concentrated soy products.

Herbal Medicine

Botanicals have been the major source of medicinal materials for millennia prior to the 20th century. Even today, a large percentage of people in developing countries rely on herbal medicines for their health care. About one-quarter of prescription drugs contain active ingredients derived from plants, including several chemotherapeutic agents (paclitaxel, docetaxel), camptothecins (irinotecan hydrochloride, topotecan hydrochloride), and vinca alkaloids (vincristine, vinorelbine tartrate).

Botanicals are a valuable source for the development of therapeutic agents, where they are carefully studied for safety and efficacy. Sold as dietary supplements, however, they are rarely produced to the same high standards. Many therapeutic claims remain unproven, and some herbs cause significant side effects. Detrimental herb-drug interactions may occur. Finally, product inconsistency and contamination have been reported.[92]

Problems and Potential of Herbal Supplements

Most claims made by producers of herbal supplements are based on historical experience, unconfirmed by clinical trials. Many herbs show direct antitumor activity from in vitro or animal experiments,[93,94] but translating preclinical to clinical use often fails because the active constituents, often unknown, are insufficiently potent or metabolized before reaching their target. The composition of herbs is complex, typically containing hundreds of constituents. Moreover, some herbal remedies function through the synergistic effects of their multiple constituents, hindering identification of active components.

Herbs and other botanical products that enhance immune function are especially popular among cancer patients and may prove useful in cancer treatment or prevention. Some show immunomodulatory effects in preclinical studies, assisting tumor rejection or resistance to pathogens.[95-97] However, the most popular immune-boosting herb in the United States used commonly to treat colds—Echinacea—shows disappointing results in randomized controlled trials.[98-100]

The popular use of herbal supplements has important public health implications (see "Herb-Drug Interactions" and "Quality Control Issues"). In order to evaluate the effectiveness and safety of herbal supplements and guide their use by the consumers, rigorous clinical trials are under way. The United States Food and Drug Administration (FDA) issued "Guidance for Industry—Botanical Drug Products" in 2004 to aid the drug development process.[101]

Side Effects

Because botanicals contain biologically active constituents, they carry health risks if not used properly. The botanical kava kava, for example, proved more effective than placebo in treating anxiety, stress, and insomnia,[102,103] and it was considered a viable alternative to benzodiazepines because of its benefits and absence of dependency and addiction. However, later reports associate this herbal remedy with severe hepatotoxicity resulting in death.[104]

Red clover and black cohosh are promoted and used as "natural hormone replacement therapy" to treat postmenopausal symptoms. Red clover preparations, however, failed to significantly reduce the numbers of hot flashes, although one preparation reduced hot flashes more rapidly than another. This may be an example of the inconsistent standardization that characterizes supplement development.[105] Products containing red clover should not be used by patients with estrogen–receptor-positive breast cancer as they contain phytoestrogens. Black cohosh reduced menopausal symptoms without systemic estrogenic effect in an open-label study,[106] but another trial of women with breast cancer showed no overall benefit.[107] Whether black cohosh has estrogenic activity remains under debate. Recent laboratory research showed no direct interaction of black cohosh extract with estrogen receptors.[108]

Herbal medicine was practiced historically by those with at least some knowledge of side effects of the herbs. Today, however, many herbal and other botanical products are readily available to US consumers under the Dietary Supplement Health and Education Act of 1994, which regulates them only as food supplements and requires no prior studies of safety and efficacy. A few herbal products have been removed from the market by the FDA due to adverse events. A recent example is agents that contain ephedrine, as its sympathomimetic activity has been associated with cardiovascular complication, including death.

Herb-Drug Interactions

Herbs may attenuate or lessen the effect of a drug either by direct action on its target or by altering its pharmacokinetics.[109,110] Herbs such as fever-few, garlic, ginger, and ginkgo have anticoagulant effects and should be avoided by patients on warfarin, heparin, aspirin, and related agents. Red clover, Dong quai, and licorice, because of their phytoestrogen components, should not be used by patients on tamoxifen or aromatase inhibitors. St. John's wort was a popular product for depression, at least equivalent in efficacy to tricyclics and selective serotonin reuptake inhibitors (SSRIs) in mild to moderate depression and with a side-effect profile superior to both.[111,112] It was found, however, that St. John's wort induces cytochrome P450 CYP3A4. Reduced plasma levels of SN38, an active metabolite of irinotecan, have been reported following simultaneous use.[113] Such metabolic interactions preclude St. John's wort for patients on medications metabolized by CYP3A4.[114]

Although not an herb, grapefruit juice was found to significantly change the plasma level of many prescription drugs. Further study found that furanocoumarin derivatives inhibit intestinal CYP3A4, which consequently increases the bio-availability of drugs that are substrate to first pass metabolism by this enzyme.[115,116] Interestingly, the interaction was initially discovered by accident in an ethanol-calcium channel blocker interaction study in which grapefruit juice was used as the vehicle for the alcohol.[117] Details of herb-drug interaction can be found at several sources.[92,118]

Quality Control Issues

The story of PC-SPES illustrates the quality control problems in herbal medicine. This 8-herb formulation was in popular use to treat prostate cancer. Although its exact mechanism of action is unclear, the constituents had been shown in preclinical studies to stimulate natural killer cells, inhibit growth of cancer cell lines, and bind to estrogen receptors where they inhibit 5α-reductase. Four small clinical studies demonstrated that patients with androgen-dependent or -independent prostate cancer had lower prostate-specific antigen (PSA) levels following use of PC-SPES.[119,120] Patients whose disease progressed after chemotherapy or ketoconazole treatment (a difficult-to-treat population) still responded to PC-SPES.[119,120] Toxicities in those trials were similar to those expected from estrogen treatment, including gynecomastia (common), loss of libido, and venous thrombosis (uncommon).[119,120]

Unfortunately, despite promising clinical activity against prostate cancer, PC-SP was found to be contaminated with undeclared synthetic drugs, including indomethacin, warfarin, alprazolam and diethylstilbestrol (DES).[121] In 2002, the FDA warned consumers to stop using PC-SPES, and the manufacturer (BotanicLab, Brea, CA) recalled the product and went out of business. One report compared PC-SPES with DES head-to-head in 90 androgen-insensitive prostate cancer patients. In this prospective, multicenter, randomized phase II trial, decline of PSA, median response duration, and median time to progression were all superior in the PC-SPES group. DES was detected in several lots of PC-SPES, the amount ranging from 0.01% to 3.1% of the dose in the DES arm.[122] Apparently PC-SPES clinical activity is not attributable entirely to DES contamination. The studies of PC-SPES serve as a good illustration of the promise, the problems, the complexity, and the importance of rigorous scientific research of herbal products.

Acupuncture

Acupuncture is the stimulation of certain points on the body with needles. Recent scientific research suggests that the effects of acupuncture are likely mediated by the nervous system. Release of neurotransmitters and change of brain-functional magnetic resonance imaging (MRI) signals are observed during acupuncture.[16,123] Traditionally, it is used for almost every ailment, but most indications are not confirmed by rigorous clinical study. However, evidence supports the use of acupuncture in treating some common symptoms experienced by cancer patients and others.

Pain

Pain is the most common and the best studied indication for acupuncture. Acupuncture relieves both acute (eg, postoperative dental pain) and chronic (eg, headache) pain.[124,125] Whether it helps musculoskeletal pain remains controversial.[126,127] An NIH consensus statement in 1997 supported acupuncture for adult postoperative pain, chemotherapy-related nausea and vomiting, and postoperative dental pain.[124] Insufficient evidence was available to support other claims of efficacy at that time, but in the ensuing years, many publications have documented the utility of acupuncture as an adjunct treatment for pain, emesis, and other symptoms.

A randomized controlled trial of 570 patients with osteoarthritis of the knee found that a 26-week course of acupuncture significantly improved pain and dysfunction when compared to sham-acupuncture control. In this study, all patients received other usual care for osteoarthritis. At week 8, improvement in function (but not in pain) was observed, indicating that long-term treatment may be required to achieve full effect.[128] A companion paper reported the results of a randomized controlled trial of acupuncture for chronic neck pain.

Acupuncture appears effective against cancer-related pain. A randomized placebo-controlled trial tested auricular acupuncture for patients with pain despite stable medication. A total of 90 patients were randomized to have needles placed at correct acupuncture points (treatment group), versus acupuncture or pressure at non-acupuncture points. Pain intensity decreased by 36% at 2 months from baseline in the treatment group, a statistically significant difference compared with the two control groups, for whom little pain reduction was seen.[129] Skin penetration per se showed no significant analgesic effect. The authors selected acupuncture points by measuring electrodermal signals. These results are especially important because most of the patients had neuropathic pain, which is often refractory to conventional treatment.

Brain imaging technology is now being used to examine the specific nervous pathways involved in acupuncture. In functional MRI studies, true acupuncture induces brain activation in the hypothalamus and nucleus accumbens, and deactivates areas of the anterior cingulate cortex, amygdala, and hippocampus. Such changes are not observed in control stimulations, which affect only sensory cortex change. Deactivation of the amygdala and hippocampus has also been observed with electroacupuncture. These data

suggest that acupuncture modulates the affective-cognitive aspect of pain perception.[123] Correlations between signal intensities and analgesic effects have also been reported.[130]

Nausea and Vomiting

Acupuncture helps lessen chemotherapy-induced nausea and vomiting.[131] In one study, 104 breast cancer patients receiving highly emetic chemotherapy were randomized to receive electroacupuncture at the PC6 acupuncture point, minimal needling at non-acupuncture points, or pharmacotherapy alone. Electroacupuncture significantly reduced the number of episodes of total emesis (from a median of 15, down to 5) when compared with pharmacotherapy only. Most patients did not know the group to which they had been assigned.[132] The effects of acupuncture do not appear entirely due to attention, clinician-patient interaction, or placebo.

Acupressure wrist bands that render continuous stimulation of the PC6 point have also been tested for chemotherapy-related nausea and vomiting. In a randomized, controlled trial of 739 patients, nausea on the day of chemotherapy was reduced significantly in patients wearing wrist bands compared with no-band controls. No significant differences were found for delayed nausea or vomiting.[133] Acupuncture also suppresses nausea and vomiting caused by pregnancy,[134] surgery,[135] and motion sickness.[136,137]

The combination of acupuncture and serotonin receptor antagonists, the newest generation of antiemetics, showed mixed results. In a trial of patients with rheumatic disease, the combination decreased the severity of nausea and the number of vomiting episodes more than ondansetron alone in patients receiving methotrexate (an agent also used in chemotherapy).[138] However, a study of cancer patients receiving high-dose chemotherapy and autologous stem cell transplantation reported no significant benefit for ondansetron plus acupuncture versus ondansetron plus placebo acupuncture.[139]

Other Symptoms

Acupuncture has been reported to reduce xerostomia (severe dry mouth). Radiotherapy for head and neck cancer causes acute and chronic xerostomia, which may persist despite the use of pilocarpine (Salagen) and amifostine (Ethyol). Acupuncture improved xerostomia inventory scores in 18 patients with head and neck cancer and pilocarpine-resistant xerostomia. However, a controlled trial of acupuncture versus superficial needling found increased salivary flow in patients with both conditions (68% and 50%, respectively). Although real acupuncture produced greater improvement and a longer latency phase, the difference was not significant.[140] Randomized

trials with proper controls and adequate power are needed before conclusions can be drawn.

Patients with breast or prostate cancer may experience vasomotor symptoms (hot flashes) during estrogen or androgen ablation therapy. A few uncontrolled studies investigated acupuncture to treat these symptoms. Self-stimulation of implanted miniature acupuncture needles attenuated tamoxifen-related hot flashes in 8 of 12 patients with breast cancer,[141] and similar results were found in a case series of patients with breast[142,143] and prostate cancer.[144] Controlled trials are under way at several centers.

Fatigue following chemotherapy or irradiation, another major and common problem, has few reliable treatments in patients without a correctable cause such as anemia.[145] In an uncontrolled trial of fatigue after chemotherapy, acupuncture reduced fatigue 31% after 6 weeks of treatment. Among those with severe fatigue at baseline, 79% had non-severe fatigue scores at follow-up,[146] whereas fatigue was reduced only in 24% of patients receiving usual care in another center.[147]

Adverse Effects

Acupuncture needles are regulated as a medical device in the United States. They are filiform, sterile, single-use, and very thin (28 to 40 gauge) (Figure 2). Insertion of acupuncture needles causes minimal or no pain and less tissue injury than phlebotomy or parenteral injection. Acupuncture performed by experienced, well-trained practitioners is safe. Only 6 cases of potentially serious adverse events were reported in a recent study of 97,733 patients receiving acupuncture in

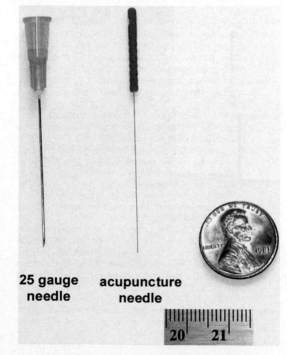

25 gauge needle   **acupuncture needle**

20   **21**

FIGURE 2 Acupuncture needle.

Germany. They included exacerbation of depression, hypertensive crisis, vasovagal reaction, asthma attack, and pneumothorax. The most common minor adverse events included local bleeding and needling pain, both in fewer than .05% of patients.[148] It is prudent to avoid acupuncture at the site of tumor or metastasis, limbs with lymphedema, areas with considerable anatomic distortion due to surgery, and in patients with thrombocytopenia, coagulopathy or neutropenia. Cancer patients require certified practitioners who are experienced in treating patients with malignant diseases.

Summary

The use of complementary and alternative therapies is prevalent among cancer patients and survivors. They seek these therapies because some of their health care needs are not adequately addressed by mainstream medicine. Whereas alternative therapies can be harmful to patients, complementary therapies play an important role in the overall care of cancer patients. Increased research on the safety and efficacy of complementary therapies enables evidence-based guidance for physicians and patients. Health care professionals should ask patients about their use of CAM, recognize and explore the underlying needs, discuss the pros and cons in a receptive, evidence-based manner, advise the patient after considering the balance of benefits and risks, and know where to find reliable additional information.

REFERENCES

1. Deng G, Cassileth BR, Yeung KS. Complementary therapies for cancer-related symptoms. J Support Oncol 2004;2: 419–26.
2. Weiger WA, Smith M, Boon H, et al. Advising patients who seek complementary and alternative medical therapies for cancer. Ann Intern Med 2002;137:889–903.
3. Cassileth BR, Deng G. Complementary and alternative therapies for cancer. Oncologist 2004;9:80–9.
4. Cassileth B, Deng G, Vickers A, Yeung KS. PDQ integrative oncology. Hamilton (ON), Canada: BC Decker Inc; 2005.
5. Barnes PM, Powell-Griner E, McFann K, Nahin RL. Complementary and alternative medicine use among adults: United States, 2002. Adv Data 2004;343:1–19.
6. Adams J, Sibbritt DW, Easthope G, Young AF. The profile of women who consult alternative health practitioners in Australia. Med J Aust 2003;179:297–300.
7. Chrystal K, Allan S, Forgeson G, Isaacs R. The use of complementary/alternative medicine by cancer patients in a New Zealand regional cancer treatment centre. N Z Med J 2003;116:PMID 15728227.
8. Eisenberg DM, Davis RB, Ettner SL, et al. Trends in alternative medicine use in the United States, 1990–1997: results of a follow-up national survey. JAMA 1998;280:1569–75.
9. Lee MM, Chang JS, Jacobs B, Wrensch MR. Complementary and alternative medicine use among men with prostate cancer in 4 ethnic populations. Am J Public Health 2002; 92:1606–9.
10. Exploring complementary and alternative medicine. Paper presented at: The Richard and Hinda Rosenthal Lectures 2001, 2003; Wshington (DC).
11. Ernst E, Cassileth BR. The prevalence of complementary/ alternative medicine in cancer: a systematic review. Cancer 1998;83:777–82.
12. National Nutritional Foods Association. Available at: http:// www.nnfa.org/facts/#Supplements (accessed December 27, 2004).
13. Cassileth BR. The Integrative Medicine Service at Memorial Sloan-Kettering Cancer Center. Semin Oncol 2002;29: 585–8.
14. Cassileth BR. The Alternative medicine handbook: the complete reference guide to alternative and complementary therapies. New York: W.W. Norton & Company, Inc.; 1998.
15. Wisemann N, Ellis A. Fundamentals of Chinese medicine: Zhong Yi Xue Ji Chu. Brookline (MA): Paradigm Publications; 1996.
16. Han JS. Acupuncture: neuropeptide release produced by electrical stimulation of different frequencies. Trends Neurosci 2003;26:17–22.
17. Shen J. Research on the neurophysiological mechanisms of acupuncture: review of selected studies and methodological issues. J Altern Complement Med 2001;7 Suppl 1: 121–7.
18. Lad V. Textbook of Ayurveda: Ayurvedic Pr; 2000.
19. Rozanski A, Blumenthal JA, Kaplan J. Impact of psychological factors on the pathogenesis of cardiovascular disease and implications for therapy. Circulation 1999;99: 2192–217.
20. Reiche EM, Nunes SO, Morimoto HK. Stress, depression, the immune system, and cancer. Lancet Oncol 2004;5: 617–25.
21. Astin JA, Shapiro SL, Eisenberg DM, Forys KL. Mind-body medicine: state of the science, implications for practice. J Am Board Fam Pract 2003;16:131–47.
22. Wolsko PM, Eisenberg DM, Davis RB, Phillips RS. Use of mind-body medical therapies. J Gen Intern Med 2004; 19:43–50.
23. Devine EC, Westlake SK. The effects of psychoeducational care provided to adults with cancer: meta-analysis of 116 studies. Oncol Nurs Forum 1995;22:1369–81.
24. Astin JA. Mind-body therapies for the management of pain. Clin J Pain 2004;20:27–32.
25. Davidson RJ, Kabat-Zinn J, Schumacher J, et al. Alterations in brain and immune function produced by mindfulness meditation. Psychosom Med 2003;65:564–70.
26. Speca M, Carlson LE, Goodey E, Angen M. A randomized, wait-list controlled clinical trial: the effect of a mindfulness meditation-based stress reduction program on mood and symptoms of stress in cancer outpatients. Psychosom Med 2000;62:613–22.
27. Carlson LE, Speca M, Patel KD, Goodey E. Mindfulness-based stress reduction in relation to quality of life, mood, symptoms of stress and levels of cortisol, dehydroepiandrosterone sulfate (DHEAS) and melatonin in breast and prostate cancer outpatients. Psychoneuroendocrinology 2004;29:448–74.
28. Cohen L, Warneke C, Fouladi RT, et al. Psychological adjustment and sleep quality in a randomized trial of the effects of a Tibetan yoga intervention in patients with lymphoma. Cancer 2004;100:2253–60.
29. Shapiro SL, Bootzin RR, Figueredo AJ, et al. The efficacy of mindfulness-based stress reduction in the treatment of sleep disturbance in women with breast cancer: an exploratory study. J Psychosom Res 2003;54:85–91.
30. Montgomery GH, Weltz CR, Seltz M, Bovbjerg DH. Brief presurgery hypnosis reduces distress and pain in excisional breast biopsy patients. Int J Clin Exp Hypn 2002; 50:17–32.
31. Liossi C, Hatira P. Clinical hypnosis versus cognitive behavioral training for pain management with pediatric cancer patients undergoing bone marrow aspirations. Int J Clin Exp Hypn 1999;47:104–16.
32. Faymonville ME, Mambourg PH, Joris J, et al. Psychological approaches during conscious sedation. Hypnosis versus stress reducing strategies: a prospective randomized study. Pain 1997;73:361–7.
33. Syrjala KL, Cummings C, Donaldson GW. Hypnosis or cognitive behavioral training for the reduction of pain and nausea during cancer treatment: a controlled clinical trial. Pain 1992;48:137–46.
34. Integration of behavioral and relaxation approaches into the treatment of chronic pain and insomnia. NIH Technology Assessment Panel on Integration of Behavioral and Relaxation Approaches into the Treatment of Chronic Pain and Insomnia. JAMA 1996;276:313–8.
35. Zeltzer LK, Dolgin MJ, LeBaron S, LeBaron C. A randomized, controlled study of behavioral intervention for chemotherapy distress in children with cancer. Pediatrics 1991;88:34–42.
36. Morrow GR, Morrell C. Behavioral treatment for the anticipatory nausea and vomiting induced by cancer chemotherapy. N Engl J Med 1982;307:1476–80.
37. Holland JC, Morrow GR, Schmale A, et al. A randomized clinical trial of alprazolam versus progressive muscle relaxation in cancer patients with anxiety and depressive symptoms. J Clin Oncol 1991;9:1004–11.
38. Decker TW, Cline-Elsen J, Gallagher M. Relaxation therapy as an adjunct in radiation oncology. J Clin Psychol 1992; 48:388–93.
39. Morin CM, Culbert JP, Schwartz SM. Nonpharmacological interventions for insomnia: a meta-analysis of treatment efficacy. Am J Psychiatry 1994;151:1172–80.
40. Howell JD. The paradox of osteopathy. N Engl J Med 1999;341:1465–8.
41. Jensen G, Mootz R, Shekelle P, et al. Insurance coverage of chiropractic services. In: Cherkin D, Mootz R, editors. Chiropractic in the United States: training, practice, and research. Rockville (MD): Agency for Health Care Policy and Research; 1997. p. 39–47.
42. Meeker WC, Haldeman S. Chiropractic: a profession at the crossroads of mainstream and alternative medicine. Ann Intern Med 2002;136:216–27.
43. Lesho EP. An overview of osteopathic medicine. Arch Fam Med 1999;8:477–84.
44. Shekelle PG, Adams AH, Chassin MR, et al. Spinal manipulation for low-back pain. Ann Intern Med 1992;117: 590–8.
45. van Tulder MW, Koes BW, Bouter LM. Conservative treatment of acute and chronic nonspecific low back pain. A systematic review of randomized controlled trials of the most common interventions. Spine 1997;22:2128–56.
46. Andersson GB, Lucente T, Davis AM, et al. A comparison of osteopathic spinal manipulation with standard care for patients with low back pain. N Engl J Med 1999;341: 1426–31.
47. Bronfort G. Spinal manipulation: current state of research and its indications. Neurol Clin 1999;17:91–111.
48. Ahles TA, Tope DM, Pinkson B, et al. Massage therapy for patients undergoing autologous bone marrow transplantation. J Pain Symptom Manage 1999;18:157–63.
49. Stephenson NL, Weinrich SP, Tavakoli AS. The effects of foot reflexology on anxiety and pain in patients with breast and lung cancer. Oncol Nurs Forum 2000;27: 67–72.
50. Grealish L, Lomasney A, Whiteman B. Foot massage. A nursing intervention to modify the distressing symptoms of pain and nausea in patients hospitalized with cancer. Cancer Nurs 2000;23:237–43.
51. Wilkinson S, Aldridge J, Salmon I, et al. An evaluation of aromatherapy massage in palliative care. Palliat Med 1999;13:409–17.
52. Ballard CG, O'Brien JT, Reichelt K, Perry EK. Aromatherapy as a safe and effective treatment for the management of agitation in severe dementia: the results of a double-blind, placebo-controlled trial with Melissa. J Clin Psychiatry 2002;63:553–8.
53. Graham PH, Browne L, Cox H, Graham J. Inhalation aromatherapy during radiotherapy: results of a placebo-controlled double-blind randomized trial. J Clin Oncol 2003;21:2372–6.
54. Soden K, Vincent K, Craske S, et al. A randomized controlled trial of aromatherapy massage in a hospice setting. Palliat Med Mar 2004;18:87–92.
55. Gedney JJ, Glover TL, Fillingim RB. Sensory and affective pain discrimination after inhalation of essential oils. Psychosom Med 2004;66:599–606.
56. Cherkin DC, Sherman KJ, Deyo RA, Shekelle PG. A review of the evidence for the effectiveness, safety, and cost of acupuncture, massage therapy, and spinal manipulation for back pain. Ann Intern Med 2003;138:898–906.
57. Williams AF, Vadgama A, Franks PJ, Mortimer PS. A randomized controlled crossover study of manual lymphatic drainage therapy in women with breast cancer-related lymphoedema. Eur J Cancer Care (Engl) 2002;11: 254–61.
58. Badger C, Preston N, Seers K, Mortimer P. Physical therapies for reducing and controlling lymphoedema of the limbs. Cochrane Database Syst Rev 2004:CD003141.
59. Vick DA, McKay C, Zengerle CR. The safety of manipulative treatment: review of the literature from 1925 to 1993. J Am Osteopath Assoc 1996;96:113–5.
60. Klougart N, Leboeuf-Yde C, Rasmussen LR. Safety in chiropractic practice, Part I; the occurrence of cerebrovascular accidents after manipulation to the neck in Denmark from 1978–1988. J Manipulative Physiol Ther 1996;19: 371–7.

61. Klougart N, Leboeuf-Yde C, Rasmussen LR. Safety in chiropractic practice. Part II: treatment to the upper neck and the rate of cerebrovascular incidents. J Manipulative Physiol Ther 1996;19:563–9.

62. Ernst E. The safety of massage therapy. Rheumatology (Oxford) 2003;42:1101–6.

63. Diet, nutrition and the prevention of chronic diseases: WHO; 2003.

64. Carroll KK. The role of dietary fat in breast cancer. Curr Opin Lipidol 1997;8:53–6.

65. Tretli S, Haldorsen T, Ottestad L. The effect of pre-morbid height and weight on the survival of breast cancer patients. Br J Cancer 1990;62:299–303.

66. Connolly JM, Coleman M, Rose DP. Effects of dietary fatty acids on DU145 human prostate cancer cell growth in athymic nude mice. Nutr Cancer 1997;29:114–9.

67. Whittemore AS, Kolonel LN, Wu AH, et al. Prostate cancer in relation to diet, physical activity, and body size in blacks, whites, and Asians in the United States and Canada. J Natl Cancer Inst 1995;87:652–61.

68. Bairati I, Meyer F, Fradet Y, Moore L. Dietary fat and advanced prostate cancer. J Urol 1998;159:1271–5.

69. Mills PK, Beeson WL, Phillips RL, Fraser GE. Cohort study of diet, lifestyle, and prostate cancer in Adventist men. Cancer 1989;64:598–604.

70. Severson RK, Nomura AM, Grove JS, Stemmermann GN. A prospective study of demographics, diet, and prostate cancer among men of Japanese ancestry in Hawaii. Cancer Res 1989;49:1857–60.

71. Schuurman AG, van den Brandt PA, Dorant E, et al. Association of energy and fat intake with prostate carcinoma risk: results from The Netherlands Cohort Study. Cancer 1999;86:1019–27.

72. The effect of vitamin E and beta carotene on the incidence of lung cancer and other cancers in male smokers. The Alpha-Tocopherol, Beta Carotene Cancer Prevention Study Group. N Engl J Med 1994;330:1029–35.

73. Virtamo J, Pietinen P, Huttunen JK, et al. Incidence of cancer and mortality following alpha-tocopherol and beta-carotene supplementation: a postintervention follow-up. JAMA 2003;290:476–85.

74. Omenn GS, Goodman GE, Thornquist MD, et al. Effects of a combination of beta carotene and vitamin A on lung cancer and cardiovascular disease. N Engl J Med 1996;334:1150–5.

75. Neuhouser ML, Patterson RE, Thornquist MD, et al. Fruits and vegetables are associated with lower lung cancer risk only in the placebo arm of the beta-carotene and retinol efficacy trial (CARET). Cancer Epidemiol Biomarkers Prev 2003;12:350–8.

76. Gronberg H. Prostate cancer epidemiology. Lancet 2003; 361(9360):859–64.

77. Willett WC, Polk BF, Morris JS, et al. Prediagnostic serum selenium and risk of cancer. Lancet 1983;2(8342):130–4.

78. Clark LC, Combs GF Jr, Turnbull BW, et al. Effects of selenium supplementation for cancer prevention in patients with carcinoma of the skin. A randomized controlled trial. Nutritional Prevention of Cancer Study Group. JAMA 1996;276:1957–63.

79. Yoshizawa K, Willett WC, Morris SJ, et al. Study of prediagnostic selenium level in toenails and the risk of advanced prostate cancer. J Natl Cancer Inst 1998;90:1219–24.

80. Hoque A, Albanes D, Lippman SM, et al. Molecular epidemiologic studies within the Selenium and Vitamin E Cancer Prevention Trial (SELECT). Cancer Causes Control 2001;12:627–33.

81. Klein EA, Thompson IM, Lippman SM, et al. SELECT: the next prostate cancer prevention trial. Selenum and Vitamin E Cancer Prevention Trial. J Urol 2001;166: 1311–5.

82. Miller ER 3rd, Pastor-Barriuso R, Dalal D, et al. Meta-analysis: high-dosage vitamin e supplementation may increase all-cause mortality. Ann Intern Med. 2005 Jan 4;42(1):37–46.

83. Giovannucci E. A review of epidemiologic studies of tomatoes, lycopene, and prostate cancer. Exp Biol Med (Maywood) 2002;227:852–9.

84. Giovannucci E, Rimm EB, Liu Y, et al. A prospective study of tomato products, lycopene, and prostate cancer risk. J Natl Cancer Inst 2002;94:391–8.

85. Fitzgerald GA. Coxibs and cardiovascular disease. N Engl J Med 2004;351:1709–11.

86. Couzin J. Clinical trials: halt of Celebrex study threatens drug's future, other trials. Science 2004;306(5705):2170a.

87. Hempstock J, Kavanagh JP, George NJ. Growth inhibition of prostate cell lines in vitro by phyto-oestrogens. Br J Urol 1998;82:560–3.

88. Peterson G, Barnes S. Genistein and biochanin A inhibit the growth of human prostate cancer cells but not epidermal growth factor receptor tyrosine autophosphorylation. Prostate 1993;22:335–45.

89. Kumar NB, Cantor A, Allen K, et al. The specific role of isoflavones in reducing prostate cancer risk. Prostate 2004;59:141–7.

90. deVere White RW, Hackman RM, Soares SE, et al. Effects of a genistein-rich extract on PSA levels in men with a history of prostate cancer. Urology 2004;63:259–63.

91. Peeters PH, Keinan-Boker L, van der Schouw YT, Grobbee DE. Phytoestrogens and breast cancer risk. Review of the epidemiological evidence. Breast Cancer Res Treat 2003; 77:171–83.

92. Cassileth B, Lucarelli C. Herb-drug interactions in oncology: Hamilton (ON), Canada: BC Decker Inc; 2003.

93. Cohen I, Tagliaferri M, Tripathy D. Traditional Chinese medicine in the treatment of breast cancer. Semin Oncol 2002;29:563–74.

94. Vickers A. Botanical medicines for the treatment of cancer: rationale, overview of current data, and methodological considerations for phase I and II trials. Cancer Invest 2002;20:1069–79.

95. Kodama N, Harada N, Nanba H. A polysaccharide, extract from Grifola frondosa, induces Th-1 dominant responses in carcinoma-bearing BALB/c mice. Jpn J Pharmacol 2002;90:357–60.

96. Ooi VE, Liu F. Immunomodulation and anti-cancer activity of polysaccharide-protein complexes. Curr Med Chem 2000;7:715–29.

97. Wasser SP, Weis AL. Therapeutic effects of substances occurring in higher Basidiomycetes mushrooms: a modern perspective. Crit Rev Immunol 1999;19:65–96.

98. Taylor JA, Weber W, Standish L, et al. Efficacy and safety of echinacea in treating upper respiratory tract infections in children: a randomized controlled trial. JAMA 2003;290: 2824–30.

99. Yale SH, Liu K. Echinacea purpurea therapy for the treatment of the common cold: a randomized, double-blind, placebo-controlled clinical trial. Arch Intern Med 2004; 164:1237–41.

100. Barrett BP, Brown RL, Locken K, et al. Treatment of the common cold with unrefined echinacea. A randomized, double-blind, placebo-controlled trial. Ann Intern Med 2002;137:939–46.

101. U.S. Food and Drug Administration. Guidance for Industry Botanical Drug Products. 2004; [80 screens]. Available at: http://www.fda.gov/cder/guidance/4592fnl.htm (accessed December 30, 2004).

102. Geier FP, Konstantinowicz T. Kava treatment in patients with anxiety. Phytother Res 2004;18:297–300.

103. Lehrl S. Clinical efficacy of kava extract WS 1490 in sleep disturbances associated with anxiety disorders. Results of a multicenter, randomized, placebo-controlled, double-blind clinical trial. J Affect Disord 2004;78: 101–110.

104. From the Centers for Disease Control and Prevention. Hepatic toxicity possibly associated with kava-containing products—United States, Germany, and Switzerland, 1999–2002. JAMA 2003;289:36–7.

105. Tice JA, Ettinger B, Ensrud K, et al. Phytoestrogen supplements for the treatment of hot flashes: the Isoflavone Clover Extract (ICE) Study: a randomized controlled trial. JAMA 2003;290:207–14.

106. Liske E, Hanggi W, Henneicke-von Zepelin HH, et al. Physiological investigation of a unique extract of black cohosh (Cimicifugae racemosae rhizoma): a 6-month clinical study demonstrates no systemic estrogenic effect. J Womens Health Gend Based Med 2002;11:163–74.

107. Jacobson JS, Troxel AB, Evans J, et al. Randomized trial of black cohosh for the treatment of hot flashes among women with a history of breast cancer. J Clin Oncol 2001;19:2739–45.

108. Mahady GB. Is black cohosh estrogenic? Nutr Rev 2003; 61(5 Pt 1):183–6.

109. Gurley BJ, Gardner SF, Hubbard MA, et al. In vivo assessment of botanical supplementation on human cytochrome P450 phenotypes: Citrus aurantium, Echinacea purpurea, milk thistle, and saw palmetto. Clin Pharmacol Ther 2004;76:428–40.

110. Sparreboom A, Cox MC, Acharya MR, Figg WD. Herbal remedies in the United States: potential adverse interactions with anticancer agents. J Clin Oncol 2004;22: 2489–503.

111. Linde K, Mulrow CD. St John's wort for depression. Cochrane Database Syst Rev 2000:CD000448.

112. Schrader E. Equivalence of St John's wort extract (Ze 117) and fluoxetine: a randomized, controlled study in mild-moderate depression. Int Clin Psychopharmacol 2000;15: 61–8.

113. Mathijssen RH, Verweij J, de Bruijn P, et al. Effects of St. John's wort on irinotecan metabolism. J Natl Cancer Inst 2002;94:1247–9.

114. Markowitz JS, Donovan JL, DeVane CL, et al. Effect of St John's wort on drug metabolism by induction of cytochrome P450 3A4 enzyme. JAMA 2003;290:1500–4.

115. Kane GC, Lipsky JJ. Drug-grapefruit juice interactions. Mayo Clin Proc 2000;75:933–42.

116. Bailey DG, Dresser GK. Interactions between grapefruit juice and cardiovascular drugs. Am J Cardiovasc Drugs 2004;4: 281–97.

117. Bailey DG, Spence JD, Edgar B, et al. Ethanol enhances the hemodynamic effects of felodipine. Clin Invest Med 1989;12:357–62.

118. Memorial Sloan-Kettering Cancer Center. About Herbs, Botanicals & Other Products; [1 screen]. Available at: http://www.mskcc.org/aboutherbs (accessed March 28, 2007).

119. Small EJ, Frohlich MW, Bok R, et al. Prospective trial of the herbal supplement PC-SPES in patients with progressive prostate cancer. J Clin Oncol 2000;18:3595–603.

120. Oh WK, George DJ, Hackmann K, et al. Activity of the herbal combination, PC-SPES, in the treatment of patients with androgen-independent prostate cancer. Urology 2001;57: 122–6.

121. Sovak M, Seligson AL, Konas M, et al. Herbal composition PC-SPES for management of prostate cancer: identification of active principles. J Natl Cancer Inst 2002;94: 1275–81.

122. Oh WK, Kantoff PW, Weinberg V, et al. Prospective, multicenter, randomized phase ii trial of the herbal supplement, PC-SPES, and diethylstilbestrol in patients with androgen-independent prostate cancer. J Clin Oncol. 2004 Sep 15;22(18):3705–12.

123. Wu MT, Hsieh JC, Xiong J, et al. Central nervous pathway for acupuncture stimulation: localization of processing with functional MR imaging of the brain—preliminary experience. Radiology 1999;212:133–41.

124. NIH Consensus Conference. Acupuncture. JAMA 1998;280: 1518–24.

125. Melchart D, Linde K, Fischer P, et al. Acupuncture for recurrent headaches: a systematic review of randomized controlled trials. Cephalalgia 1999;19:779–86.

126. Ernst E, White AR. Acupuncture for back pain: a meta-analysis of randomized controlled trials. Arch Intern Med 1998;158:2235–41.

127. Tulder MV, Cherkin DC, Berman B, et al. Acupuncture for low back pain. Cochrane Database Syst Rev 2000: CD001351.

128. Berman BM, Lao L, Langenberg P, et al. Effectiveness of acupuncture as adjunctive therapy in osteoarthritis of the knee: a randomized, controlled trial. Ann Intern Med 2004;141:901–10.

129. Alimi D, Rubino C, Pichard-Leandri E, et al. Analgesic effect of auricular acupuncture for cancer pain: a randomized, blinded, controlled trial. J Clin Oncol 2003;21:4120–6.

130. Zhang WT, Jin Z, Cui GH, et al. Relations between brain network activation and analgesic effect induced by low vs. high frequency electrical acupoint stimulation in different subjects: a functional magnetic resonance imaging study. Brain Res 2003;982:168–78.

131. Lee A, Done ML. Stimulation of the wrist acupuncture point P6 for preventing postoperative nausea and vomiting. Cochrane Database Syst Rev 2004:CD003281.

132. Shen J, Wenger N, Glaspy J, et al. Electroacupuncture for control of myeloablative chemotherapy-induced emesis: a randomized controlled trial. JAMA 2000;284: 2755–2761.

133. Roscoe JA, Morrow GR, Hickok JT, et al. The efficacy of acupressure and acustimulation wrist bands for the relief of chemotherapy-induced nausea and vomiting. A University of Rochester Cancer Center Community Clinical Oncology Program multicenter study. J Pain Symptom Manage 2003;26:731–42.

134. Rosen T, de Veciana M, Miller HS, et al. A randomized controlled trial of nerve stimulation for relief of nausea and vomiting in pregnancy. Obstet Gynecol 2003;102: 129–35.

135. Streitberger K, Diefenbacher M, Bauer A, et al. Acupuncture compared to placebo-acupuncture for postoperative

nausea and vomiting prophylaxis: a randomised placebo-controlled patient and observer blind trial. Anaesthesia 2004;59:142–9.

136. Bertolucci LE, DiDario B. Efficacy of a portable acustimulation device in controlling seasickness. Aviat Space Environ Med 1995;66:1155–8.

137. Ming JL, Kuo BI, Lin JG, Lin LC. The efficacy of acupressure to prevent nausea and vomiting in post-operative patients. J Adv Nurs 2002;39:343–51.

138. Josefson A, Kreuter M. Acupuncture to reduce nausea during chemotherapy treatment of rheumatic diseases. Rheumatology (Oxford) 2003;42:1149–54.

139. Streitberger K, Friedrich-Rust M, Bardenheuer H, et al. Effect of acupuncture compared with placebo-acupuncture at P6 as additional antiemetic prophylaxis in high-dose chemotherapy and autologous peripheral blood stem cell transplantation: a randomized controlled single-blind trial. Clin Cancer Res 2003;9:2538–44.

140. Blom M, Dawidson I, Fernberg JO, et al. Acupuncture treatment of patients with radiation-induced xerostomia. Eur J Cancer B Oral Oncol 1996;32B(3):182–90.

141. Towlerton G, Filshie J, O'Brien M, Duncan A. Acupuncture in the control of vasomotor symptoms caused by tamoxifen. Palliat Med 1999;13:445.

142. Tukmachi E. Treatment of hot flushes in breast cancer patients with acupuncture. Acupunct Med 2000;18:22–7.

143. Porzio G, Trapasso T, Martelli S, et al. Acupuncture in the treatment of menopause-related symptoms in women taking tamoxifen. Tumori 2002;88:128–30.

144. Hammar M, Frisk J, Grimas O, et al. Acupuncture treatment of vasomotor symptoms in men with prostatic carcinoma: a pilot study. J Urol 1999;161:853–6.

145. Mock V, Atkinson A, Barsevick A, et al. NCCN practice guidelines for cancer-related fatigue. Oncology (Huntingt) 2000;14(11A):151–61.

146. Vickers AJ, Straus DJ, Fearon B, Cassileth BR. Acupuncture for postchemotherapy fatigue: a phase II study. J Clin Oncol 2004;22:1731–5.

147. Escalante CP, Grover T, Johnson BA, et al. A fatigue clinic in a comprehensive cancer center: design and experiences. Cancer 2001;92(6 Suppl):1708–13.

148. Melchart D, Weidenhammer W, Streng A, et al. Prospective investigation of adverse effects of acupuncture in 97 733 patients. Arch Intern Med 2004;164:104–5.

Survivorship—A Reversal of Fortune

Sai-Ching Jim Yeung, MD, PhD

Carmen Escalante, MD

Robert F. Gagel, MD

A fundamental characteristic of the human condition is the desire to survive. Parents will often sacrifice their own lives to ensure the survival of their offspring, and individuals confronted with overwhelming danger will struggle heroically. This tenacious behavior in a cancer patient, combined with the oncologic advances of the past several decades, has created a dramatic reversal of fortune for patients with cancer. For the average cancer patient, there is now a greater than 50% probability of survival; even for those with cancer who will ultimately die, survival periods have steadily lengthened in recent years.

A challenge faced by those of us who have not experienced cancer is the question of what normality is for a cancer patient who has survived a near-death experience. One answer could be that normality probably does not exist for this group. In the same way that prisoners of military conflicts, battle-hardened veterans of bloody wars, or concentration camp survivors move on with their lives, but never completely rid themselves of the terrible memories, cancer survivors move forward but are left with permanent reminders of their journey. Like the war veteran, these scars not only affect the psyche, but also other organ systems. As we cross a threshold, one where more patients survive than die, it is important to ask whether the experience during—and the unhealthful sequelae of—therapy can be improved. Although there is the sincere hope that targeted therapies currently being developed will substantially lower toxicity, a more realistic expectation is that these newer therapies will also target normal tissues where these signal transduction pathways are important.

Several trends in cancer survivorship are emerging. Perhaps the most significant is that the number of cancer survivors is growing, and they are now recognizing shared experiences with other survivors. This has led to the development of embryonic survivorship groups who are in the initial stages of organization to demand solutions to the variety of residual ailments that have resulted from their journey through cancer treatment. The initial stages had the feeling of other nascent movements: calls for action without a clear idea of what would make things better. In recent years, this has been replaced by more clearly focused efforts that, in turn, have forced the oncology community to broaden its definition of the cancer experience to include survivorship. Not only do these survivors want to live, they not unexpectedly want to live with some semblance of the quality of life they experienced before the illness.

The major dilemma faced by this field is the difficulty of delivering a lethal blow to a cancer without causing toxicity to other organ or tissue sites. In this text, we have provided an up-to-date compilation of current knowledge and approaches, but implicit in these discussions is the recognition that we are only at the beginning of understanding mechanisms of long-term effects. Furthermore, and with good reason, there has been little effort expended to study basic mechanisms of disease in survivors beyond descriptive studies. The focus has been on creating survivorship; now that we have moved past the midpoint, it is time to reexamine priorities and include these issues as an important component of the research agenda.

In truth, the landscape is uneven. Great strides have been made in reducing death in breast cancer, Hodgkin's disease, and testicular cancer, whereas there has been little or no improvement in overall survival in lung cancer, malignant brain tumors, or pancreatic cancer. In these latter areas, the focus (by necessity) will remain on control of the malignancy.

At least two strategies can be envisioned for addressing long-term sequelae in patients with malignancies. The first is to develop therapies that are effective but less toxic. For malignancies where substantial progress has been made on improving outcomes, there are active efforts to maintain or improve efficacy while reducing long-term effects. Specific examples include the use of aromatase inhibitors in breast cancer,[1] the use of monoclonal antibodies for treatment of a variety of malignancies,[2–4] and small organic molecules that target specific molecular targets in certain cancers.[5] As outcomes improve for other malignancies, it seems likely the pace of this process will increase.

A second strategy is to study the molecular mechanisms of toxicity and use this information to develop preventive therapies. This approach has proven challenging in the past because therapies effective in the treatment of cancer have a broad spectrum of activities, making it difficult to dissect the mechanisms causing a particular effect. Nonetheless there has been some success. Recognizing that anthracycline effects on cardiac muscle (free radical formation in cardiac cells)[6] differed from its effects in the transformed cell (inhibition of ribonucleic acid [RNA] and deoxyribonucleic acid [DNA] synthesis), investigators in this field have developed several pharmacologic agents (dexrazoxane and its analogues) that inhibit free radical formation in cardiac muscle, thereby blunting the damaging effects of anthracyclines on cardiac muscle.[7] Although the protection is imperfect and used predominantly in patients treated with high-dose anthracycline therapy, it highlights an example where elucidation of a difference between a mechanism of cancer therapy and organ toxicity has proven useful.

A question that will be asked is whether it makes sense, in this fast moving field of molecular targeting of cancer, to initiate studies of mechanisms of toxicity for first- and second-generation therapies with higher toxicity, those most likely to be replaced as cancer therapy moves forward. A more robust and forward-looking strategy is to focus energy on the large number of new therapeutic agents under development. This seems a more practical approach for several reasons. First, it is already clear that molecular targeting of specific biochemical pathways, singly or in combination, will be an effective therapeutic approach for treatment of cancer. As many of the same pathways have broad importance in normal tissues, it will be important to develop strategies for preventing unwanted effects in normal tissue. One example that comes immediately to mind is the effect of a broad spectrum of tyrosine kinase inhibitors that target the vascular endothelial growth factor and epidermal growth factor receptors to cause hypertension and a broad spectrum of dermatologic disorders.[8,9] These findings have already spawned some research into mechanisms,[10,11] although there is at present no clear understanding of why inhibition of these receptor tyrosine kinases cause these effects. Although there is the temptation to treat the hypertension and dermatologic manifestations with currently available therapies as best as can be done, omitting any research into the underlying mechanisms, it is important to study the mechanisms because it is likely these agents (or others that target the same pathways) will become the mainstays of cancer therapy for the foreseeable future. Indeed, such investigation may yield insight that will not only be helpful in the treatment of these manifestations in the cancer patient, but also in the greater population, because these same signal transduction pathways are likely to be of importance in the genesis of the same medical problems during normal aging. None of this will occur quickly, but it will be important to move forward on this agenda, linked arm in arm, with the development of new treatments for cancer.

It will also be important to develop social and psychological support systems for cancer survivors. Just as survivors of war-time experiences struggle throughout their lives, cancer survivors are misunderstood by the general medical community. There is incomplete understanding outside of major cancer centers of the profound physical and psychological effects that cancer and its treatments cause. One of the areas highlighted by one Institute of Medicine report on cancer survivorship was the importance of developing a care plan for survivorship.[12] This report specifically suggested that patients being discharged from active cancer treatment/surveillance be provided with a "comprehensive care summary and follow-up plan that is clearly and effectively explained." The suggested components of this care plan are shown in Table 1.

We believe that at least one additional step is needed: the development of a body of expertise to address the unique needs of cancer survivors. The

---

Table 1 Components of Care Plan

Summary of Cancer Type and Treatment
Specific recommendations regarding follow up
Recommendations regarding specific preventive and healthy living practices
Information on legal protections regarding employment and access to health insurance
Information on the availability of psychosocial services in the community

---

fast pace of cancer therapy today has left the general physician woefully unprepared to participate actively in the care of the cancer survivor. New therapies sprout up on a regular basis; the only exposure the general physician has is with the one or two patients undergoing a newly developed therapy. He/she generally has no experience with anticipated long-term problems. Indeed, even the oncologic community may not understand the long-term sequelae of a treatment approved in the last year or two, an inevitable outgrowth of the fast-track approval of oncologic therapies today. Thus the growing number of these patients and the explosion of new therapeutic approaches argue persuasively for the development of a subspecialty of medicine dedicated to these issues. This issue was also highlighted in the Institute of Medicine's report, although there was no mention in the report of the development of a group of physicians who see their role as different and separable from the role played by the oncologist. Although it is conceivable that oncologists could fulfill this need, they have been more appropriately focused on cancer treatment; and general physicians, uniquely suited for this role by their situation in the community, do not have enough exposure to a the myriad therapeutic agents used to treat cancer, nor a large enough patient population to gain this experience.

As the discipline of geriatrics was spawned by the increasing longevity of the population, so to will the growth in numbers of long-term survivors lead to development of a unique and separable subspecialty of internal medicine. There has been a proliferation of medical and scientific groups focused on supportive care for cancer patients and internal medicine in the cancer patient that will, over time, consolidate and define this discipline of medical practice. As is the case with the geriatrician, the total number of these individuals will be small, but as they move through the medical community to educate, inform, and perform research on these topics, their presence will be noted. We anticipate that the next 50 years will be exciting years as survivorship becomes commonplace.

REFERENCES

1. Morandi P, Rouzier R, Altundag K, et al. The role of aromatase inhibitors in the adjuvant treatment of breast carcinoma: the M. D. Anderson Cancer Center evidence-based approach. Cancer 2004;101:1482–9.
2. Hagemeister FB. Rituximab and chemotherapy for aggressive lymphomas: a significant advance in therapy. Clin Adv Hematol Oncol 2003;1:120–5.
3. O'Brien S, Albitar M, Giles FJ. Monoclonal antibodies in the treatment of leukemia. Curr Mol Med 2005;5:663–75.
4. Ross JS, Gray KE, Webb IJ, et al. Antibody-based therapeutics: focus on prostate cancer. Cancer Metastasis Rev 2005;24:521–37.
5. Benjamin RS, Blanke CD, Blay JY, et al. Management of gastrointestinal stromal tumors in the imatinib era: selected case studies. Oncologist 2006;11:9–20.
6. Myers CE, McGuire WP, Liss RH, et al. Adriamycin: the role of lipid peroxidation in cardiac toxicity and tumor response. Science 1977;197(4299):165–7.
7. Swain SM, Whaley FS, Gerber MC, et al. Delayed administration of dexrazoxane provides cardioprotection for patients with advanced breast cancer treated with doxorubicin-containing therapy. J Clin Oncol 1997;15:1333–40.
8. Faivre S, Delbaldo C, Vera K, et al. Safety, pharmacokinetic, and antitumor activity of SU11248, a novel oral multitarget tyrosine kinase inhibitor, in patients with cancer. J Clin Oncol 2006;24:25–35.
9. Holden SN, Eckhardt SG, Basser R, et al. Clinical evaluation of ZD6474, an orally active inhibitor of VEGF and EGF receptor signaling, in patients with solid, malignant tumors. Ann Oncol 2005;16:1391–7.
10. Carter RW, Kanagy NL. Tyrosine kinases regulate intracellular calcium during alpha(2)-adrenergic contraction in rat aorta. Am J Physiol Heart Circ Physiol 2002;283:H1673–80.
11. Endemann D, Touyz RM, Yao G, Schiffrin EL. Tyrosine kinase inhibition attenuates vasopressin-induced contraction of mesenteric resistance arteries: alterations in spontaneously hypertensive rats. J Cardiovasc Pharmacol 2002;40:123–32.
12. Life CoCS-ICaQo, Board NCP. From cancer patient to cancer survivor: lost in transition. Washington (DC): The National Acadamies Press; 2006.

Index